P9-DDX-898

HANDBOOK OF OBESITY

HANDBOOK OF OBESITY

Etiology and Pathophysiology

Second Edition

edited by

GEORGE A. BRAY
CLAUDE BOUCHARD
Pennington Biomedical Research Center
Louisiana State University
Baton Rouge, Louisiana, U.S.A.

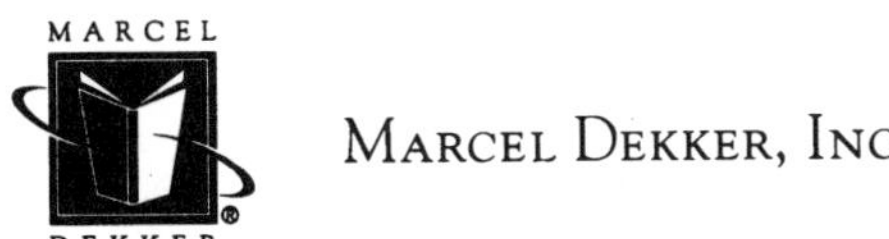

Marcel Dekker, Inc.   New York • Basel

The first edition of this book (and its companion volume, *Handbook of Obesity: Clinical Applications, Second Edition*) was published as *Handbook of Obesity* edited by George A. Bray, Claude Bouchard, and W. P. T. James (Marcel Dekker, Inc., 1998).

Although great care has been taken to provide accurate and current information, neither the author(s) nor the publisher, nor anyone else associated with this publication, shall be liable for any loss, damage, or liability directly or indirectly caused or alleged to be caused by this book. The material contained herein is not intended to provide specific advice or recommendations for any specific situation.

Trademark notice: Product or corporate names may be trademarks or registered trademarks and are used only for identification and explanation without intent to infringe.

Library of Congress Cataloging-in-Publication Data
A catalog record for this book is available from the Library of Congress.

ISBN: 0-8247-0969-1

This book is printed on acid-free paper.

Headquarters
Marcel Dekker, Inc.
270 Madison Avenue, New York, NY 10016, U.S.A.
tel: 212-696-9000; fax: 212-685-4540

Distribution and Customer Service
Marcel Dekker, Inc.
Cimarron Road, Monticello, New York 12701, U.S.A.
tel: 800-228-1160; fax: 845-796-1772

Eastern Hemisphere Distribution
Marcel Dekker AG
Hutgasse 4, Postfach 812, CH-4001 Basel, Switzerland
tel: 41-61-260-6300; fax: 41-61-260-6333

World Wide Web
http://www.dekker.com

The publisher offers discounts on this book when ordered in bulk quantities. For more information, write to Special Sales/Professional Marketing at the headquarters address above.

Copyright © 2004 by Marcel Dekker, Inc. All Rights Reserved.

Neither this book nor any part may be reproduced or transmitted in any form or by any means, electronic or mechanical, including photocopying, microfilming, and recording, or by any information storage and retrieval system, without permission in writing from the publisher.

Current printing (last digit):

10 9 8 7 6 5 4 3 2 1

PRINTED IN THE UNITED STATES OF AMERICA

Preface to the Second Edition

The publication of the first edition of the *Handbook of Obesity* occurred just as the Food and Drug Administration requested the recall of fenfluramine and dexfenfluramine. Each drug alone and in combination with phentermine had been associated with a rash of valvular heart disease. These cases were similar to some seen with the carcinoid syndrome that secretes serotonin. There was an accumulation of material on the aortic valves in the heart that made them leaky. The good news is that many of these valvular lesions have been reversible when the drugs were discontinued, and there are no cases known to us of progression after the drugs were stopped.

Thus, at the time the first edition of the *Handbook of Obesity* was published, the chapters dealing with fenfluramine and combination therapy were already out of place. In addition, there were few drug treatments on the horizon.

In spite of this negative impact, the scientific advances preceding the publication of the first edition had been substantial. As we began to plan the second edition, we reviewed each of the 49 chapters in the first edition. The major changes were in the therapeutic area where many new drugs were under evaluation and where new strategies for prevention of obesity were being evaluated.

Based on these advances in the therapeutic area, we added 12 new chapters, which made a substantially longer volume with 61 chapters. We thus decided to divide the handbook into two separate volumes. The first deals with the prevalence, etiology, and consequences of obesity. In the second volume we have included the chapters dealing with evaluation, prevention, and treatment.

In this volume we cover the history, definition, prevalence, etiology, and pathophysiology of obesity. The prevalence of obesity continues to increase rapidly (Chaps. 4, 6, and 7). At present more than 60% of adult Americans are overweight and more than 30% are obese. Important ethnic differences led to the addition of a chapter dealing with this important subject (Chaps. 2 and 3). We also have a new chapter on the fetal origins of obesity and the impact that the intra-uterine environment has on future risks for developing obesity. The costs of obesity have become more important for individual nations, and the chapter on this subject has been expanded (Chap. 8).

Genetic and molecular biology are important areas for research and are promising the pharmaceutical industry new approaches to the problem (Chaps. 9 and 10). The importance of animal models has resulted in the addition of a second chapter on this area (Chap. 12). The regulation of food intake in animals and humans provides important new insights into the ways they choose and regulate their energy intake (Chaps. 13–16). The epidemic of AIDS has added a new variety of fat accumulation associated with treatment with proteases and we have added a chapter to cover this area (Chap. 19). The importance of visceral and total body fat continues to expand. One of the key new developments of the 1990s was the recognition that the fat cell is one of the most important endocrine cells in the body. We have recognized this with several chapters on adipose tissue (Chaps. 17, 18, 20, 21, and 22). We have also recognized the importance of obesity in the function of the classical endocrine glands such as the adrenal, thyroid, pituitary and gonads (Chaps. 25, 26, and 27). The other side of the energy balance from food intake is energy expenditure. This subject too receives substantial discussion in several chapters (Chaps. 23, 24, and 28). Muscle metabolism and nutrient partitioning are the final two chapters in this section.

Obesity has a myriad of effects on the health of human beings. Obesity increases the risk of death, as discussed in Chapter 31. The metabolic syndrome, as a collection of findings that predict health risks, has become considerably more important in the past decade and has been discussed by one of the scientists who originated this concept (Chap. 32). We have also invited chapters dealing with the cardiovascular system, blood pressure, lipoproteins, diabetes, gall bladder disease, pulmonary function, arthritis, and pregnancy. To end this volume we have included a discussion of the role of physical activity in health and the effect of obesity on the quality of life (Chaps. 42 and 43).

We are indebted to a number of people for this volume. Ms. Nina Laidlaw and Ms. Heather Miller at the Pennington Biomedical Research Center have provided able assistance to the editors. At Marcel Dekker, Inc., Ms. Moraima Suarez has taken the principal role. We are both indebted to each of these three people. Without the excellent writing from each of the authors and their collaborators, we would not have the superb chapters that make up this volume. We thank all of them.

George A. Bray
Claude Bouchard

Preface to the First Edition

This volume has been designed to provide up-to-date coverage of the range of subjects that make up the field of obesity research. The chapters have been written by many of the leading scientists and clinicians in the field.

We have divided the book into four sections. Part one deals with the history, definitions, and prevalence of obesity. The first of these nine chapters outlines the history of obesity using a series of timelines to put the important events in the development of obesity research into the historical context. This is followed by a chapter written by the three editors on definitions that can be used to frame the subject matter of obesity. A chapter on the measurement of body composition follows. The global prevalence of obesity in children and in the elderly is then presented in three separate chapters. This section ends with a discussion of the behavioral and psychological correlates of obesity, and the cultural context in which obesity is viewed by different ethnic groups.

The second section focuses on the etiological factors involved in the development of this problem. The first chapter is a detailed presentation of the genetics of human obesity. A genetic approach has proved particularly important since the discovery of leptin and the rapid mapping of genetic loci that are associated with the development of obesity. A great deal has been learned about obesity from the study of animals models, a variety of which are presented by two of the experts in the field. The third chapter deals with the rise of genetic approaches to obesity, which has been aided by advances in molecular biology. There follow three chapters on the intake of food. One of these deals with this problem in humans, the second with the problem in animals, and the third with the neural basis for the intake of food in both humans and animals. Together these chapters provide a vivid view of the current standing of the field of nutrient intake.

Our understanding of the importance of adipose tissue has steadily increased, from regarding it as a simple storage organ to recognizing it as a secretory organ as well. The important differences between white and brown adipose tissue have also been elucidated, and their role in the development and maintenance of human obesity defined. These concepts are developed in the next four chapters. The final group of chapters in the second section deals with energy expenditure. There is a chapter on energy expenditure and thermogenesis during rest and one on physical activity and its relation to obesity and food intake. Finally, the roles of the endocrine system, the autonomic nervous system, and substrate handling are discussed. From this second section the reader should obtain a detailed understanding of the genetic basis of obesity; the role and control of food intake in the development of obesity; the way fat cells function as a storage, thermogenic, secretory organ; and, finally, the way in which energy expenditure is controlled and involved in the development of obesity.

The third section deals with the pathophysiology of obesity, that is, the mechanisms by which obesity produces damaging effects on health. The first two chapters in this section deal with the role of central fat and the metabolic syndrome. This is followed by a detailed discussion of the effects of obesity on a variety of individual organ systems. Three chapters are devoted to problems of the cardiovascular system and lipoprotein abnormalities, which are important consequences of obesity. Diabetes is one of the most frequent problems associated with obesity, as explained in one chapter. The ways in which obesity enhances the risk of gall bladder disease are developed in another chapter. This is followed by a clear discussion of the pulmonary problems arising from obesity, one of which (the Pickwickian syndrome, or sleep apnea) is named after the famous fat boy, Joe, in Dicken's *Pickwick Papers*. Obesity has important effects on the risk for gout and arthritis and this is discussed in a separate chapter. Two chapters in this section deal with the effects of obesity on endocrine function and pregnancy. Finally, the problem of weight cycling and the risk of intentional and unintensional weight loss are discussed in two chapters that have picked up important themes of obesity research and put them into a valuable perspective.

The final section deals with prevention and treatment. Since an ounce of prevention is worth a pound of cure, the section begins with a chapter on prevention. This is followed by a clinically useful set of guidances for the evaluation of the overweight patient. The cornerstones for treatment of obesity—behavior therapy, diet, and exercise—are presented in three separate chapters. These are followed by three important chapters on the management of diabetes, hypertension, and hyperlipidemia in the obese individual. Finally, there is a chapter on the current status of pharmacological treatment of obesity and a chapter on the surgical approaches that can be used for an individual for whom other approaches to treatment have failed.

The preparation of this volume has required the work of many people. First, we want to thank the authors and their secretarial assistants for submitting the chapters so promptly. This will make the entire volume timely. Several individuals in the editors' office have also played key roles in moving this forward. We want to thank especially Ms. Millie Cutrer and Terry Hodges in Baton Rouge, Ms. Karen Horth and Ms. Diane Drolet in Quebec City, and Ms. Jean James in Aberdeen. The guiding hand at Marcel Dekker, Inc., who has been so valuable in nudging and cajoling us along when we needed, is Ms. Lia Pelosi. We thank you all and hope that the readers appreciate the important role each of you, and others we have not mentioned, including especially our long-suffering families, has made to the success of this volume.

George A. Bray
Claude Bouchard

Contents

Preface to the Second Edition *iii*
Preface to the First Edition *v*
Contributors *xi*

PART I HISTORY, DEFINITIONS, AND PREVALENCE

1. Historical Framework for the Development of Ideas About Obesity 1
George A. Bray

2. Evaluation of Total and Regional Adiposity 33
Steven B. Heymsfield, Richard N. Baumgartner, David B. Allison, Wei Shen, ZiMian Wang, and Robert Ross

3. Ethnic and Geographic Influences on Body Composition 81
Paul Deurenberg and Mabel Deurenberg-Yap

4. Prevalence of Obesity in Adults: The Global Epidemic 93
Jacob C. Seidell and Aila M. Rissanen

5. Fetal Origins of Obesity 109
David J. P. Barker

6. Pediatric Overweight: An Overview 117
Bettylou Sherry and William H. Dietz

7. Obesity in the Elderly: Prevalence, Consequences, and Treatment 135
Robert S. Schwartz

8. Economic Costs of Obesity 149
Ian D. Caterson, Janet Franklin, and Graham A. Colditz

PART II ETIOLOGY

9. Genetics of Human Obesity 157
Claude Bouchard, Louis Pérusse, Treva Rice, and D. C. Rao

10. Molecular Genetics of Rodent and Human Single Gene Mutations Affecting Body Composition 201
Streamson Chua, Jr., Kathleen Graham Lomax, and Rudolph L. Leibel

11. Rodent Models of Obesity 255
David A. York

12. Primates in the Study of Aging-Associated Obesity 283
Barbara C. Hansen

13. Behavioral Neuroscience and Obesity 301
Sarah F. Leibowitz and Bartley G. Hoebel

14. Experimental Studies on the Control of Food Intake 373
Henry S. Koopmans

15. Diet Composition and the Control of Food Intake in Humans 427
John E. Blundell and James Stubbs

16. Central Integration of Peripheral Signals in the Regulation of Food Intake and Energy Balance: Role of Leptin and Insulin 461
L. Arthur Campfield, Françoise J. Smith, and Bernard Jeanrenaud

17. Development of White Adipose Tissue 481
Gérard Ailhaud and Hans Hauner

18. Lipolysis and Lipid Mobilization in Human Adipose Tissue 515
Dominique Langin and Max Lafontan

19. Lipodystrophy and Lipoatrophy 533
Steven R. Smith

20. Uncoupling Proteins 539
Daniel Ricquier and Leslie P. Kozak

21. Peroxisome Proliferator–Activated Receptor γ and the Transcriptional Control of Adipogenesis and Metabolism 559
Lluis Fajas and Johan Auwerx

22. Biology of Visceral Adipose Tissue 589
Susan K. Fried and Robert R. Ross

23. Resting Energy Expenditure, Thermic Effect of Food, and Total Energy Expenditure 615
Yves Schutz and Eric Jéquier

24. Energy Expenditure in Physical Activity 631
James O. Hill, W. H. M. Saris, and James A. Levine

25. Endocrine Determinants of Obesity 655
Jonathan H. Pinkney and Peter G. Kopelman

26. Endocrine Determinants of Fat Distribution 671
Renato Pasquali, Valentina Vicennati, and Uberto Pagotto

27. Sympathoadrenal System and Metabolism 693
Eric Ravussin and Ian Andrew Macdonald

28. Energy Expenditure and Substrate Oxidation 705
Jean-Pierre Flatt and Angelo Tremblay

29. Skeletal Muscle and Obesity 733
David E. Kelley and Len Storlien

30. Nutrient Partitioning 753
Samyah Shadid and Michael D. Jensen

PART III PATHOPHYSIOLOGY

31. Obesity and Mortality Rates 767
Kevin R. Fontaine and David B. Allison

32. Etiology of the Metabolic Syndrome 787
Per Björntorp

33. Obesity as a Risk Factor for Major Health Outcomes 813
JoAnn E. Manson, Patrick J. Skerrett, and Walter C. Willett

34. Effects of Obesity on the Cardiovascular System 825
Edward Saltzman and Peter N. Benotti

35. Obesity and Lipoprotein Metabolism 845
Jean-Pierre Després and Ronald M. Krauss

36. Obesity and Blood Pressure Regulation 873
Albert P. Rocchini

37. Obesity and Diabetes 899
Jeanine Albu and F. Xavier Pi-Sunyer

38. Obesity and Gallbladder Disease 919
Cynthia W. Ko and Sum P. Lee

39. Obesity and Pulmonary Function 935
Shyam Subramanian and Kingman P. Strohl

40. Obesity, Arthritis, and Gout 953
Anita Wluka, Tim D. Spector, and Flavia M. Cicuttini

41. Obesity, Pregnancy, and Infertility 967
Stephan Rössner

42. Physical Activity, Obesity, and Health Outcomes 983
William J. Wilkinson and Steven N. Blair

43. Obesity and Quality of Life 1005
Donald A. Williamson and Patrick M. O'Neil

Index *1023*

Contributors

Gérard Ailhaud, Ph.D. Professor, Department of Biochemistry, Unité Mixte de Recherche 6543, Centre National de la Recherche Scientifique, Nice, France

Jeanine Albu, M.D. Division of Endocrinology, Diabetes, and Nutrition, Department of Medicine, Columbia University College of Physicians and Surgeons, and St. Luke's-Roosevelt Hospital Center, New York, New York, U.S.A.

David B. Allison, Ph.D. Professor and Head, Division of Statistical Genetics, Department of Biostatistics, The University of Alabama at Birmingham, Birmingham, Alabama, U.S.A.

Johan Auwerx, M.D., Ph.D. Professor of Medicine, Institut de Génétique et de Biologie Moléculaire et Cellulaire, Illkirch, and Université Louis Pasteur, Strasbourg, France

David J. P. Barker, M.D., Ph.D., F.R.S. Director, Medical Research Council Environmental Epidemiology Unit, University of Southampton, Southampton, England

Richard N. Baumgartner, Ph.D. Professor, Department of Internal Medicine, University of New Mexico School of Medicine, Albuquerque, New Mexico, U.S.A.

Peter N. Benotti, M.D. Department of Surgery, Valley Hospital, Ridgewood, New Jersey, U.S.A.

Per Björntorp, M.D., Ph.D., F.R.C.P.(Edin) Professor, Department of Heart and Lung Diseases, University of Göteborg, Göteborg, Sweden

Steven N. Blair, P.E.D. President and CEO, The Cooper Institute, Dallas, Texas, U.S.A.

John E. Blundell, Ph.D., F.B.P.s.S. Chair of Psychobiology, Department of Psychology, University of Leeds, Leeds, England

Claude Bouchard, Ph.D. Executive Director, Pennington Biomedical Research Center, Louisiana State University, Baton Rouge, Louisiana, U.S.A.

George A. Bray, M.D. Boyd Professor, Chronic Disease Prevention, Pennington Biomedical Research Center, Louisiana State University, Baton Rouge, Louisiana, U.S.A.

L. Arthur Campfield, Ph.D. Professor, Department of Food Science and Human Nutrition, Colorado State University, Fort Collins, Colorado, U.S.A.

Ian D. Caterson, M.B.B.S., B.Sc.(Med), Ph.D., F.R.A.C.P. Boden Professor of Human Nutrition, Human Nutrition Unit, University of Sydney, Sydney, New South Wales, Australia

Streamson Chua, Jr., M.D., Ph.D. Associate Professor, Division of Molecular Genetics, Department of Pediatrics, Columbia University College of Physicians and Surgeons, New York, New York, U.S.A.

Flavia M. Cicuttini, M.B.B.S., F.R.A.C.P., Ph.D. Associate Professor, Department of Epidemiology and Preventive Medicine, Monash University, Melbourne, Victoria, Australia

Graham A. Colditz, M.D., Dr.PH. Professor, Departments of Medicine and Epidemiology, Harvard School of Public Health, Harvard Medical School, and Brigham & Women's Hospital, Boston, Massachusetts, U.S.A.

Jean-Pierre Després, Ph.D. Chair Professor of Human Nutrition, Quebec Heart Institute, Laval Hospital Research Center, Laval University, Sainte-Foy, Quebec, Canada

Paul Deurenberg, Ph.D. Consultant, Research and Information Management, Health Promotion Board, Singapore, Republic of Singapore

Mabel Deurenberg-Yap, M.D., Ph.D. Director, Research and Information Management, Health Promotion Board, Singapore, Republic of Singapore

William H. Dietz, M.D., Ph.D. Director, Division of Nutrition and Physical Activity, National Center for Chronic Disease Prevention and Health Promotion, Centers for Disease Control and Prevention, Atlanta, Georgia, U.S.A.

Lluis Fajas, Ph.D. Institut de Génétique et de Biologie Moléculaire et Cellulaire, Illkirch, and Université Louis Pasteur, Strasbourg, France

Jean-Pierre Flatt, Ph.D. Department of Biochemistry and Molecular Pharmacology, University of Massachusetts Medical School, Worcester, Massachusetts, U.S.A.

Kevin R. Fontaine, Ph.D. Assistant Professor, Division of Rheumatology, Johns Hopkins University, Baltimore, Maryland, U.S.A.

Janet Franklin, B.Med.Sci.(Hons), M.Nutr/Diet A.P.D. Metabolism and Obesity Services, Department of Endocrinology, Royal Prince Alfred Hospital, Sydney, New South Wales, Australia

Susan K. Fried, Ph.D. Professor, Division of Gerontology, Department of Medicine, University of Maryland, and Baltimore Veterans Administration Medical Center, Baltimore, Maryland, U.S.A.

Barbara C. Hansen, Ph.D. Professor, Department of Physiology, and Director, Obesity and Diabetes Research Center, University of Maryland, Baltimore, Maryland, U.S.A.

Hans Hauner, M.D. Professor, Clinical Department, German Diabetes Research Institute, Dusseldorf, Germany

Steven B. Heymsfield, M.D. Professor, Department of Medicine, Columbia University College of Physicians and Surgeons, and New York Obesity Research Center, St. Luke's-Roosevelt Hospital, New York, New York, U.S.A.

James O. Hill, Ph.D. Director, Center for Human Nutrition, University of Colorado Health Sciences Center, Denver, Colorado, U.S.A.

Bartley G. Hoebel, M.D. Professor, Department of Psychology, Princeton University, Princeton, New Jersey, U.S.A.

Bernard Jeanrenaud, M.D. Professor Emeritus, Geneva Faculty School of Medicine, University of Geneva, Geneva, Switzerland

Michael D. Jensen, M.D. Professor, Department of Internal Medicine, Mayo Clinic, Rochester, Minnesota, U.S.A.

Eric Jéquier, M.D. Professor Emeritus, Institute of Physiology, University of Lausanne, Lausanne, Switzerland

David E. Kelley, M.D. Professor, Department of Medicine, University of Pittsburgh, Pittsburgh, Pennsylvania, U.S.A.

Cynthia W. Ko, M.D. Assistant Professor, Division of Gastroenterology, Department of Medicine, University of Washington, Seattle, Washington, U.S.A.

Henry S. Koopmans, Ph.D. Department of Physiology and Biophysics, University of Calgary, Calgary, Alberta, Canada

Peter G. Kopelman, M.D., F.R.C.P. Professor of Clinical Medicine, Department of Metabolic Medicine, Barts and the London Queen Mary's School of Medicine and Dentistry, University of London, London, England

Leslie P. Kozak, Ph.D. Professor, Experimental Obesity, Pennington Biomedical Research Center, Louisiana State University, Baton Rouge, Louisiana, U.S.A.

Ronald M. Krauss, M.D. Director, Atherosclerosis Research, Children's Hospital Oakland Research Institute, Oakland; Senior Scientist, Department of Genome Science, Lawrence Berkeley National Laboratory; and Adjunct Professor, Department of Nutritional Sciences, University of California, Berkeley, Berkeley, California, U.S.A.

Max Lafontan, Ph.D., D.Sc. Director of Research, Obesity Research Unit, INSERM U586, Louis Bugnard Institute, Université Paul Sabatier-Centre Hospitalier Universitaire de Rangueil, Toulouse, France

Dominique Langin, D.V.M., Ph.D. Director of Research, Obesity Research Unit, INSERM U586, Louis Bugnard Institute, Université Paul Sabatier-Centre Hospitalier Universitaire de Rangueil, Toulouse, France

Sum P. Lee, M.D., Ph.D. Professor and Head, Division of Gastroenterology, Department of Medicine, University of Washington, Seattle, Washington, U.S.A.

Rudolph L. Leibel, M.D. Professor and Head, Division of Molecular Genetics, Department of Pediatrics, and Naomi Berrie Diabetes Center, Columbia University College of Physicians and Surgeons, New York, New York, U.S.A.

Sarah F. Leibowitz, Ph.D. Associate Professor of Behavioral Neurobiology, The Rockefeller University, New York, New York, U.S.A.

James A. Levine, M.D., Ph.D. Professor, Division of Endocrinology, Department of Internal Medicine, Mayo Clinic, Rochester, Minnesota, U.S.A.

Kathleen Graham Lomax, M.D. Postdoctoral Fellow, Institute of Human Nutrition, Department of Pediatrics, Columbia University College of Physicians and Surgeons, New York, New York, U.S.A.

Ian Andrew Macdonald, Ph.D. Professor, School of Biomedical Sciences, University of Nottingham Medical School, Nottingham, England

JoAnn E. Manson, M.D., Ph.D., F.A.C.P. Professor, Department of Medicine, Harvard Medical School, and Chief, Division of Preventive Medicine, Brigham & Women's Hospital, Boston, Massachusetts, U.S.A.

Patrick M. O'Neil, Ph.D. Professor, Department of Psychiatry and Behavioral Sciences, and Director, Weight Management Center, Medical University of South Carolina, Charleston, South Carolina, U.S.A.

Uberto Pagotto, M.D., Ph.D. Assistant Professor, Departments of Internal Medicine and Gastroenterology, University of Bologna, and Endocrine Unit, S. Orsola-Malpighi General Hospital, Bologna, Italy

Renato Pasquali, M.D. Director, Endocrinology Unit, Departments of Internal Medicine and Gastroenterology, University of Bologna, and S. Orsola-Malpighi General Hospital, Bologna, Italy

Louis Pérusse, Ph.D. Professor, Department of Social and Preventive Medicine, Faculty of Medicine, Laval University, Sainte-Foy, Quebec, Canada

Jonathan H. Pinkney, M.D. Senior Lecturer, Department of Medicine, University of Liverpool, Liverpool, England

F. Xavier Pi-Sunyer, M.D. Professor and Director, Division of Endocrinology, Diabetes, and Nutrition, Columbia University College of Physicians and Surgeons, and St. Luke's-Roosevelt Hospital Center, New York, New York, U.S.A.

D. C. Rao, Ph.D. Professor and Director, Division of Biostatistics, Washington University School of Medicine, St. Louis, Missouri, U.S.A.

Eric Ravussin, Ph.D. Professor, Health and Performance Enhancement, Pennington Biomedical Research Center, Louisiana State University, Baton, Rouge, Louisiana, U.S.A.

Treva Rice, Ph.D. Division of Biostatistics, Washington University School of Medicine, St. Louis, Missouri, U.S.A.

Daniel Ricquier, Ph.D. Professor, Unité Mixte de Recherche, UPR 9078, Centre National de la Recherche Scientifique, Faculty of Medicine, Necker-Sick Children, Paris, France

Aila M. Rissanen, M.D., Ph.D. Professor, Obesity Research Unit, Helsinki University Hospital, Helsinki, Finland

Albert P. Rocchini, M.D. Professor and Director of Pediatric Cardiology, Department of Pediatrics, University of Michigan, Ann Arbor, Michigan, U.S.A.

Robert R. Ross, Ph.D. Associate Professor, Division of Endocrinology and Metabolism, Department of Medicine, School of Physical and Health Education, Queen's University, Kingston, Ontario, Canada

Stephan Rössner, M.D., Ph.D. Obesity Unit, Huddinge University Hospital, Huddinge, Sweden

Edward Saltzman, M.D. Jean Mayer USDA Human Nutrition Research Center on Aging at Tufts University, and Director, Obesity Consultation Center, Tufts–

New England Medical Center Boston, Massachusetts, U.S.A.

W. H. M. Saris, M.D., Ph.D. Scientific Director, Nutrition and Toxicology Research Institute, University of Maastricht, Maastricht, The Netherlands

Yves Schutz, Ph.D. Lecturer, Institute of Physiology, University of Lausanne, Lausanne, Switzerland

Robert S. Schwartz, M.D. Goodstein Professor of Medicine/Geriatrics, Department of Medicine, University of Colorado Health Sciences Center, Denver, Colorado, U.S.A.

Jacob C. Seidell, Ph.D. Professor, Department of Nutrition and Health, Faculty of Earth and Life Sciences, Free University of Amsterdam and Free University Medical Center, Amsterdam, The Netherlands

Samyah Shadid, M.D. Department of Internal Medicine, Mayo Clinic, Rochester, Minnesota, U.S.A.

Wei Shen, M.D. Research Scientist, Obesity Research Center, St. Luke's-Roosevelt Hospital, and Institute of Human Nutrition, Columbia University College of Physicians and Surgeons, New York, New York, U.S.A.

Bettylou Sherry, Ph.D., R.D. Epidemiologist, Maternal and Child Nutrition Branch, Division of Nutrition and Physical Activity, National Center for Chronic Disease Prevention and Health Promotion, Centers for Disease Control and Prevention, Atlanta, Georgia, U.S.A.

Patrick J. Skerrett, M.S. Senior Editor, Division of Preventive Medicine, Department of Medicine, Brigham & Women's Hospital, and Editor, Harvard Health Publications, Harvard Medical School, Boston, Massachusetts, U.S.A.

Françoise J. Smith, M.S. Senior Research Scientist, Department of Food Science and Human Nutrition, Colorado State University, Fort Collins, Colorado, U.S.A.

Steven R. Smith, M.D. Associate Professor, Endocrinology Laboratory, Pennington Biomedical Research Center, Louisiana State University, Baton Rouge, Louisiana, U.S.A.

Tim D. Spector, M.D., F.R.C.P., M.Sc. Consultant Rheumatologist and Professor, Department of Genetic Epidemiology, Guy's and St. Thomas' Hospital NHS Trust, London, England

Len Storlien, Ph.D. Professor, Faculty of Health and Behavioural Sciences, University of Wollongong, Wollongong, New South Wales, Australia, and AstraZeneca, Mölndal, Sweden

Kingman P. Strohl, M.D. Professor, Department of Medicine, Case Western Reserve University School of Medicine, Cleveland, Ohio, U.S.A.

James Stubbs, Ph.D. Department of Appetite and Energy Balance, Rowett Research Institute, Aberdeen, Scotland

Shyam Subramanian, M.D. Fellow, Division of Pulmonary, Critical Care and Sleep Medicine, Department of Medicine, Case Western Reserve University School of Medicine, Cleveland, Ohio, U.S.A.

Angelo Tremblay, Ph.D. Professor, Department of Social and Preventive Medicine, Faculty of Medicine, Laval University, Sainte-Foy, Quebec, Canada

Valentina Vicennati, M.D. Endocrinology Unit, Department of Internal Medicine and Gastroenterology, University of Bologna, and S. Orsola-Malpighi General Hospital, Bologna, Italy

ZiMian Wang, Ph.D. Research Associate, Columbia University College of Physicians and Surgeons, and Obesity Research Center, St. Luke's-Roosevelt Hospital, New York, New York, U.S.A.

William J. Wilkinson, M.D., M.S. Director, Weight Management Research Center, Centers for Integrated Health Research, The Cooper Institute, Dallas, Texas, U.S.A.

Walter C. Willett, M.D., D.Ph. Professor and Chair, Department of Nutrition, Harvard School of Public Health, Boston, Massachusetts, U.S.A.

Donald A. Williamson, Ph.D. Professor and Chief, Health Psychology, Pennington Biomedical Research Center, Louisiana State University, Baton Rouge, Louisiana, U.S.A.

Anita Wluka, M.B.B.S., F.R.A.C.P. Department of Epidemiology and Preventive Medicine, Monash University, Melbourne, Victoria, Australia

David A. York, Ph.D. Boyd Professor, Experimental Obesity, Pennington Biomedical Research Center, Louisiana State University, Baton Rouge, Louisiana, U.S.A.

HANDBOOK OF OBESITY

1

Historical Framework for the Development of Ideas About Obesity

George A. Bray

Pennington Biomedical Research Center, Louisiana State University, Baton Rouge, Louisiana, U.S.A.

I INTRODUCTION

Religions dissipate like fog, kingdoms vanish, but the works of scientists remain for eternity.

Ulug Beg, 15th century (cited in Uzbekistan: Macleod and Maghew, p 17.)

We do not live in our own time alone; we carry our history within us.

Gaarder (1:152)

The goal of historical scholarship is said to be to reconstruct the past, but the only past available for reconstruction is that which we can see from the present. The nature of science as an analytical discipline, involved at one and the same time in the uncertainties of discovery and in the accumulation of a body of objective knowledge, raises some special problems of historical reconstruction.

Crombie (2:4)

This last quote applies admirably to this chapter on the history of obesity "as an analytical discipline. . . and the accumulation of a body of objective knowledge." In this chapter I will explore the historical framework in which this accumulation of a body of objective knowledge about obesity has occurred. I am not a historian and thus lack the perspective of someone trained in that field. I am rather a practicing scientist who has tried to understand the processes of experimental science to apply them to improving my own science. In an earlier review (3) I covered a number of concepts in the history of obesity. Other historical milestones for obesity have been examined in the selections I wrote for the Classics in Obesity section of the journal *Obesity Research* (4–33). This book will build on these earlier papers and attempt to place these contributions to the field of obesity into a broader historical context (34,35).

This part of the chapter is divided into sections. The first will review the limited data on obesity in prehistoric times. The second section will consider obesity from the beginning of recorded history (ca 3600 BC) to the onset of the scientific era (ca AD 1500). The third section will cover the development of concepts about obesity in the scientific era from AD 1500 to 1900, and the fourth section will deal briefly with the 20th century. Although these divisions are arbitrary, they provide the framework that will be used in this chapter.

To facilitate placing the scientific events discussed in this chapter into a broader historical context, I have prepared a series of timelines beginning in AD 1500. Each one covers one century, and places historical developments in the fields of science and other social and political events in relation to milestones in obesity. Although the discussion will range into fields prior to the beginning of the period called the "scientific era" (AD 1500 to the present), the timeline begins with the period which I have called the scientific era (ca AD 1500) and continues to the present. The prescientific era is defined for the purpose of this paper as prior to the development of the printing press by Gutenberg in 1456, but for convenience, it will be dated at AD 1500.

Clearly, there were many important scientific and mathematical advances before 1500 (36,37). However, the advent of printing with movable type and the appearance of the scientific method led to an accelerating rate of scientific advance after AD 1500. The timeline consists of 11 separate lines, showing developments in science and technology, anatomy and histology, physiology, chemistry/biochemistry, genetics, pharmacology, neuroscience, and clinical medicine. Observations in clinical medicine related to obesity antedate 1500, but the impact of many discoveries on scientific medicine was delayed until the beginning of the 19th century. If one wanted a demarcation line for the beginning of modern medicine, it might well be the French Revolution (1789–1800) (38,39).

II PREHISTORIC MEDICINE (~3000 BC)

A Paleomedicine

The study of medicine prior to written history can be done from artistic representations, from skeletal finds and related artifacts. Among the earliest evidence of man's therapeutic efforts were those aimed at the relief of fevers and burns, attempts to relieve pain and to stop bleeding. Trepanning, or drilling holes in the skulls to let out "evil spirits," to treat "epilepsy," or to relieve skull fractures, was practiced in many parts of the world up to the 19th century. The medicine man and the relation of magic and religion to healing and disease are prominent features of prehistoric medicine are present and in some rural cultures, even today. That obesity was known in this early period is evident from Stone Age artifacts.

B Stone Age Obesity

1 Paleolithic Artifact

Table 1 is a list of several artifacts from the paleolithic stone age that depict obesity. These artifacts were found across Europe from southwestern France to Russia north of the Black Sea. The location in which they were found and their appearance is shown in Figure 1. They were produced during a fairly narrow time frame in the early Upper Paleolithic period (Upper Perigordian or Gravettian) some 23,000–25,000 years ago (40). They

Table 1 Paleolithic Venus Figurines with Prominent Obesity

Place found	Number found	Height	Composition
Willendorf, Austria	One	11 cm	Limestone
Dolni Vestonice, Czeckoslovakia	Many	11.4 cm	Terracotta
Savignano, Italy	One	24 cm	Serpentine
Lespugue, France	One	14.7 cm	Ivory
Grimaldi, France	Many		Terracotta
Laussel, France	Many	40 cm	Terracotta
Kostenki, Russia	Many	47 cm	Ivory
Gagarino, Russia	Many		Ivory

are distributed over > 2000 km from west to east. Their composition is ivory, limestone, or terracotta (baked clay). The most famous of these is the Venus of Willendorf, a small statuette measuring 12 cm in height with evidence of abdominal obesity and pendulous breasts (41). The similarity in design of these artifacts as shown in Figure 2 suggests that there may have been communication across Europe during this period of glaciation.

This and the other paleolithic female figurines are frequently viewed as primordial female deities, reflecting the bounty of the earth (42). In a review of historical ideas published as a thesis in 1939, Hautin (43) concludes that these figures prove the existence of obesity in the paleolithic era and that they also symbolize the expression and possible esthetic ideals of the period. "The women immortalized in stone age sculpture were fat; there is no other word for it. . . [O]besity was already a fact of life for paleolithic man—or at least for paleolithic woman" (42).

2 Neolithic Artifacts

The Neolithic period spans the time from 8000 BC to ca 5500 BC. This period saw the introduction of agriculture and establishment of human settlements. The Neolithic age and the Chalcolithic or Copper age, which continued to 3000 BC, were notable for numerous Mother Goddess artifacts found primarily in Anatolia (currently Turkey). The richest finds are from the excavations at Catalhoyuk and Hacilar and are from the period between 5000 and 6000 BC. Most of these figurines are made of terracotta, but a few are of limestone or alabaster. Their corpulence is abundantly evident in the pendulous breasts and large abdominogluteal areas. They range in height from 2.5 to 24 cm, but most are between 5 and 12 cm. They are seated,

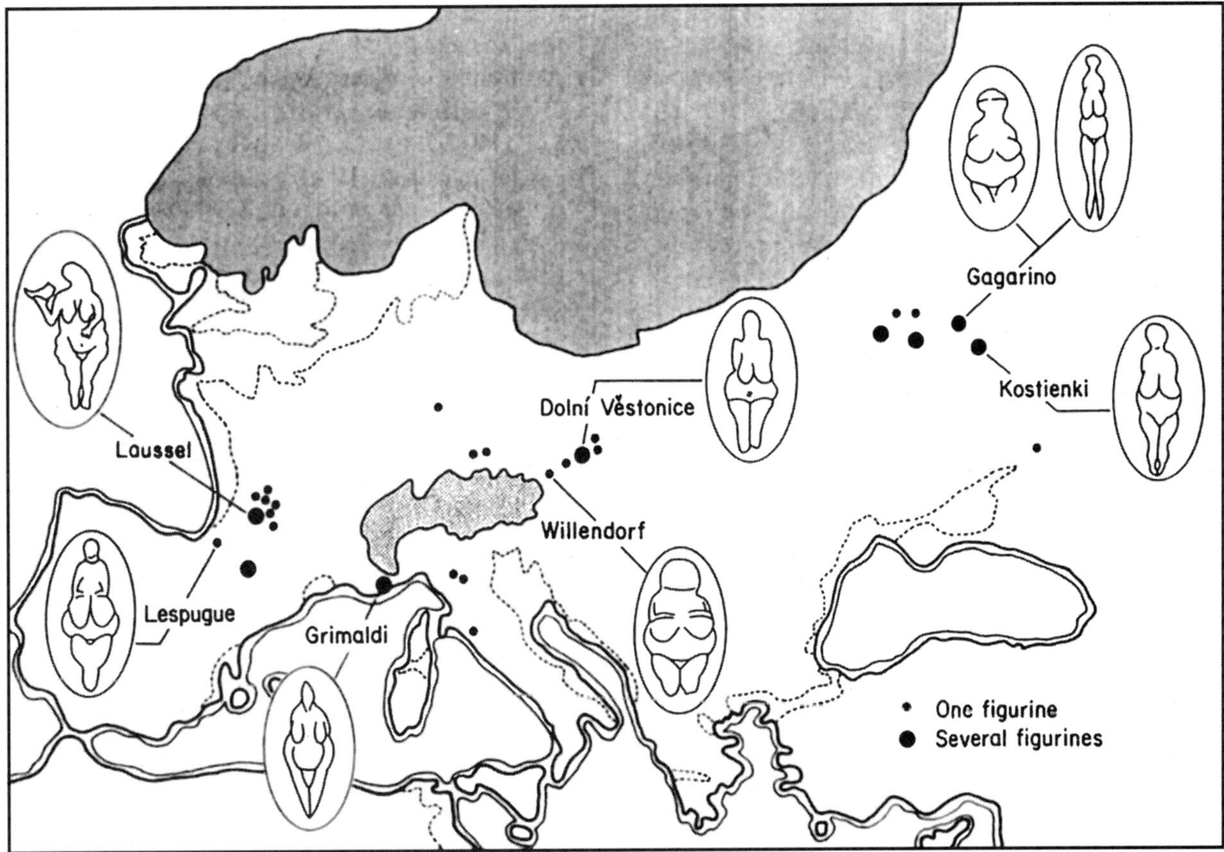

Figure 1 Map showing location of the paleolithic "Venus" figurines. Note that obese figurines have been found throughout Europe and in the Middle East.

standing, or lying. One of the most famous from Catalhoyuk is 20 cm tall. She sits on a throne with two lions serving as her arm rests. The figurines from this period show exaggeration of the hips, belly, and breasts, with genital areas indicated by triangular decoration, symbolizing motherhood and womankind, attributes which are shared by later Mother Goddess figurines from Kybele to Artemis. It is important to note that no deity or mythological figure has ever borne as many different names as the Mother Goddess. On the Kultepe tablets (1800 BC) she is known as Kubaba; the Lydians called her Kybebe; the Phrygians, Kybele; and the Hittites, Hepat. In ancient Pontic Comana (near Tokat) and Cappadocian Comana (Kayseri), she was known by the ancient Anatolian name of Ma. She was Marienna and Lat to the Sumerians, Arinna to the people of the Late Hittite period, Isis to the Egyptians, Rhea to the Greeks, Artemis to the Ephesians, and Venus to the Romans. The name Kybele has even survived into modern times as the Anglo-Saxon Sybil and its variants, and Turkish Sibel. At Catalhoyuk she is depicted as giving birth to a child; at Hacilar she is holding a child. This child is represented in later mythology by gods such as Attis, Adonis, and Tammuz (44).

III MEDICINE AND OBESITY FROM RECORDED HISTORY TO AD 1500 (PRESCIENTIFIC MEDICINE)

Medical traditions have developed in all cultures. Several of these are described below, along with evidence that obesity was present. Evidence for obesity has been identified in all of these medical traditions and geographic regions, suggesting that independent of diet, the potential to store nutrients as fat was selected for by evolution at an early period in human development.

Medical traditions are an integral part of all societies. Many factors influence the cultural sophistica-

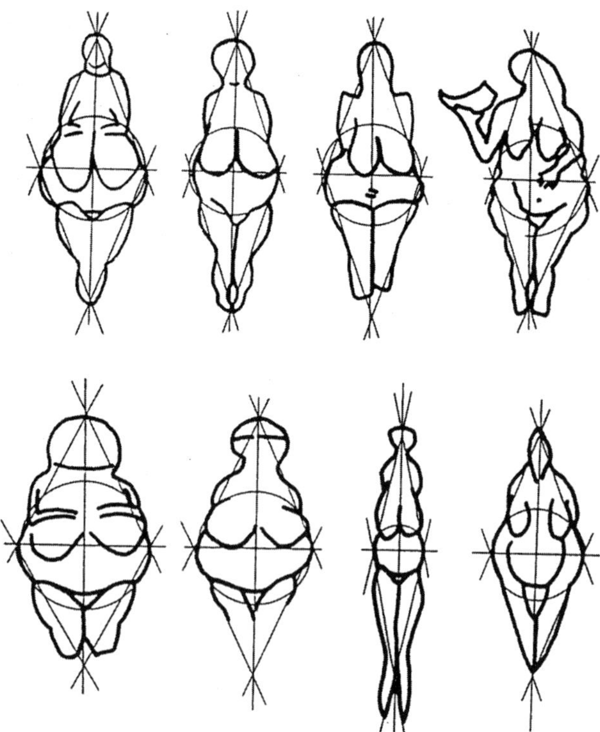

Figure 2 Similarity in design of the "Venus" figurines. All of the figures identified have similar structural features, although they were composed of several different materials. This similarity suggests that there may have been communication or migration among these sites during the Upper Paleolithic period.

tion achieved by these societies, including agricultural practices, development of writing and metallurgy, and the political climate. Several of the most sophisticated cultures have developed between two great river systems, and this has given rise to the two-rivers hypothesis of cultural development. These rivers are the Yellow River and the Yangtse River in China; the Ganges and Indus Rivers in India; the Amu Darya and Syr Darya Rivers in Central Asia; and the Tigris and Euphrates Rivers in the fertile crescent of the Middle East. In all of these societies, whether in two rivers or otherwise, there have been many examples of "obesity."

A Mesopotamian Medicine

The Tigris and Euphrates River basin was the land of healers and astrologers. Cuneiform writing, libraries, sanitation, and medical knowledge are evident by 3600 BC. Of the 30,000 clay tablets with cuneiform writing that were recovered in the library at Ninevah from ca 2000 BC, 800 are related to medical matters. The medical armamentarium of Sumerian physicians consisted of more than 120 minerals and 250 herbs including cannabis, mustard, mandragora, belladonna, and henbane (45). A terracotta statuette showing enormously fat thighs and arms was found at Susa in the middle Elamite period in the 12th century BC (46,47), indicates the continuing representation of obesity in artifacts of the female body.

B Egyptian Medicine

Paralleling the Mesopotamian medical tradition was the tradition of medicine in Egypt where the relationship between priests and physicians was very close. Imhotep, who became the god of healing, began as a Viser to King Zoser (2900 BC). Imhotep was a man of great accomplishment who in addition to being a physician was an architect, a poet, and a statesman. Two major archeological finds, the Edwin Smith papyrus (48), written between 2500 and 2000 BC, and the Ebers papyrus, written ca 1550 BC, provide major knowledge about medicine in Egypt. Obesity was known to the Egyptians. A study of royal mummies showed that both stout women (Queens Henut-Tawy and Inhapy) and stout men were not uncommon in Egypt, at least not among the higher classes, although "obesity was regarded as objectionable" (49). Several examples of obesity are also seen in the stone reliefs which were the principal artistic medium. A doorkeeper in the temple of Amon-Ra Khor-en-Khonsu; a cook in Ankh-ma-Hor's tomb (6th dynasty) (50); a fat man enjoying food presented to him by his lean servants in Mereruka's tomb; the local yeoman, the famed Sheikh et Balad (49); and the grossly obese harpist playing before the prince Aki (Middle Kingdom) (51). Studies of the skinfolds of mummies such as Amenophis III and Ramses III show that they were fat (51). One of the most interesting figures is that of the Queen of Punt from the temple of Queen Hatshepsut, Deir el-Bahri (18th dynasty). She has marked steatopygia and appears to have shortening of the lower extremities, suggesting dyschondroplasia or dislocated hips (49–52).

C Chinese and Tibetan Medicine

The early Chinese believed that disease was sent by the gods or by demons. Bone inscriptions indicate the presence of leprosy, typhoid fever, cholera, and plague. Anatomic dissection was not permitted because of ancestor worship. The Yellow Emperor (Huang Di) and the Divine Farmer (Shen Nong Bencaojing) are the legendary founders of Chinese Medicine (53). The Chinese pharmacopeia contains 365 herbal medicines. The Hung Tu Hei Ching (Yellow Emperor's Inner Canon) dates from 200 BC and is a dialogue on bodily functions and disease. In China, Zhang Zhongjing was considered the Father of Medicine, the equivalent of Hippocrates in Greece. Zhang described symptoms and treatment for many diseases. Hua Toh (3rd century AD) is the only known surgeon from ancient China. Acupuncture, the art of treatment by inserting sharp needles into the body, was developed and reached its zenith in China. This technique of placing sharp objects in the pinna of the ear to reduce "appetite" has been used to treat obesity.

The Tibetan offspring of the Chinese Tradition is beautifully illustrated in the 17th-century treatise *The Blue Beryl*, composed by Sangye Gyamtso, the scholar and regent of Tibet. It is an erudite yet practical commentary on the ancient text entitled *The Four Tantras* (54). In this text obesity is described as a condition requiring catabolic treatment. It also notes that "overeating... causes illness and shortens life span. It is a contraindication to the use of compresses or mild enemas." For treatment of obesity two suggestions are made: "The vigorous massage of the body with pea flour counteracts phlegm diseases and obesity.... The gullet, hair compress and flesh of a wolf remedy goiters, dropsy and obesity" (54).

D Indian Medicine

The fourth great medical tradition is that of Indian medicine (53). In the sacred medical texts of Ayurvedic medicine, sin was viewed as the cause of disease, and medical knowledge was closely interwoven with religion and magic. The Caraka Samhita was the first document on Indian medicine, and the Susruta Samhita was the second great medical Sanskrit text. The Caraka Samhita described 20 sharp and 101 blunt instruments as well as an operating table. At least 500 drugs are listed along with 700 medicinal herbs including, among others, cinnamon, borax, castor oil, ginger, and sodium carbonate. The Ayurveda recommended the administration of testicular tissue (organotherapy) as a cure for impotence as well as for obesity (55).

E Meso-American medicine

Prior to the "discovery" of the New World by Columbus in 1492, there were three high cultures in the Meso-American world. The Incas occupied the highlands along the west coast of what is now Peru. The Mayan culture occupied the Yucatan Peninsula and surrounding areas of Central America, and the Aztecs controlled the central plateaus of Central America. When Columbus, Cortez, and their compatriots arrived in the new world, the Meso-American cultures were exposed to several devastating diseases, including measles, smallpox, and chickenpox, which were more lethal than the military armaments the invaders brought. The Pre-Columbian Americans still lived in a Stone Age culture, but were highly sophisticated in their knowledge of mathematics, astronomy, and language. Among the most useful drugs discovered in the New World was the Cinchona bark (quinine), which was used to treat fevers, including malaria. Diseases were believed to be caused by supernatural, magical, and natural causes. Treatment was related to the cause (56). One of the sources of information about disease in Pre-Columbian societies is their sculptured artifacts. These figurines represent malnutrition, deformity, and physical illness (57). Some of the individuals represent people suffering from various diseases including spinal defects, endemic goiter, obesity, eye diseases, and skin ailments (57).

F Greco-Roman Medicine

From the vantage point of Western civilization, Greco-Roman medicine has been the major source of our medical tradition. The health hazards associated with obesity were clearly noted in the medical writings of Hippocrates, where he states, "Sudden death is more common in those who are naturally fat than in the lean" (58). These traditions also note that obesity was a cause of infertility in women and that the frequency of menses was reduced in the obese.

Galen was the leading physician of Roman times. His influence on medicine and medical teaching lasted more than 1000 years. He identified two types of obesity, one he called "moderate" and the other "immoderate." The former is regarded as natural and the other as morbid.

Descriptions of sleep apnea associated with obesity also date from Roman times. Dionysius, the tyrant of Heracleia of Pontius, who reigned ca 360 BC, is one of the first historical figures afflicted with obesity and somnolence. This enormously fat man frequently fell asleep. His servants used long needles inserted through his skin and fat to awaken him when he fell asleep. Kryger cites a second case of Magas, King of Cyrene, who died in 258 BC. He was a man "weighted down with monstrous masses of flesh in his last days; in fact he choked himself to death" (59,60).

G Arabic Medicine

With a decline of Roman influence after AD 400, scholarly activity shifted from Rome to Byzantium and then to the broader Arabic world following the rise of Islam in the 7th century. One of the leading figures of this medical tradition was Abu Ali Ibn Sina, or Avicenna in its Westernized form. Like Galen, he was an influential author who published more than 40 medical works and 145 works on philosophy, logic, theology, and other subjects. Obesity was well known to this Arabic physician. His approach to treating obesity is described later.

With increasing trade and travel, the European culture gradually reestablished contact with Arabian medicine and the Roman traditions it absorbed. Both the Crusades and the invasions by the Arabs of the Peloponessus and southern Spain brought an infusion of classical knowledge from which came the Renaissance and the beginning of the "scientific era" (2,61).

IV SCIENTIFIC MEDICINE (1500 TO PRESENT)

The remainder of this chapter will focus on science and medicine since 1500. Medieval science (1150–1450) was constrained by the earlier Greek paradigm of Aristotelian science and the Arabic renderings of these teachings by Avicenna. With the introduction of instruments such as the mechanical watch, the magnetic compass, and the magnifying glass, it became possible to quantify and critically examine some features of human experience and the underlying philosophical tradition. Out of this interaction grew the experimental method of verification and falsification which provides the basis of the Scientific Era (62).

In the following sections, I will review each of the major areas that affect the development of the "science of obesity." To put this in the broader context, the reader is referred to the timeline in Figures 3–7.

A Anatomy

The date 1543 is pivotal in the story of anatomy and for scientific thought in general. That was the year that Vesalius published his treatise on human anatomy (63), the first truly modern anatomy based on his own dissections. Andreas Vesalius was only 28 years old when he published his masterpiece. In 1543, Copernicus (64) also published his book on the solar system, arguing that planets revolved around the sun. In his accurate and careful dissections, Vesalius showed that the human body could be directly explored by appropriate experimental methods. In so doing, he applied the concept of direct verification and experimental manipulation and identified a number of inaccuracies in the anatomy of Galen, which appears to have been based on animal dissections and treatment of wounded gladiators.

A key element in communicating these discoveries, including those of Vesalius and Copernicus, was the process of movable type and printing invented by Gutenberg. This technical development was followed by the steady distribution of printing presses throughout Europe over the next 50 years. The printing press made classical literature widely available and made it possible to communicate original observations to an ever-growing audience in a relatively short time, as contrasted to handwritten books. The revolution in communication had begun, and the age of anatomy, ushered in at the beginning of the 16th century, expanded rapidly. This was also the peak of the Renaissance. Up to the 16th century, Galen and his writings from Roman times and the Canons of Avicenna from Arabic medicine had been the main source of information about anatomy, physiology, and clinical medicine. Although there is no clear evidence that either Galen or Avicenna ever dissected a human cadaver, their influence was only broken by the application of direct observation and verification after hundreds of years.

The first anatomical dissections of obese individuals are attributed to Bonetus (65). Other descriptions appear in the publications by Morgagni (66), by Haller (67,68), and most particularly by Wadd (69). Of the 12 cases presented in Wadd's book, *Comments on Corpulency, Lineaments of Leanness*, two had been examined at postmortem and had been found to have enormous accumulations of fat. This was the first instance of a monograph devoted to obesity that contained anatomical dissections.

B Microscopic Anatomy (Histology)

The invention of the microscope in the 17th century moved anatomy to the next level. By the middle decades of the 17th century, early microscopists had begun to publish the results of their histologic investigation using simple microscopes. The important initial observations by Malpighi (70), Hooke (71), and Leeuwenhoek (72)

TIMELINE 1500 - 1600

Science and Technology	1543 - Copernicus - Heliocentric theory of the solar system 1589 - Galileo's law of falling bodies
Anatomy and Histology	1543 - Vesalius - *Human Anatomy* published 1549 - Anatomic Theater built in Padua
Physiology	1540 - Servetus describes pulmonary circulation
Chemistry / Biochemistry	
Genetics	
Pharmacology	1526 - Paracelsus founds "chemotherapy"
Neuroscience	
Clinical Medicine	1505 - Royal College of Surgeons, Edinburgh 1518 - Royal College of Physicians, London 1524 - First hospital in Mexico City 1530 - Frascatorius Poem on Syphilis 1544 - St. Bartholomew's Hospital, London *1595- First thesis on obesity*
	1500 1510 1520 1530 1540 1550 1560 1570 1580 1590
Presidents of the United States	
Events	1492 - Columbus discovers America 1517-1521 - Luther reformation 1519-1522 - Magellan circumnavigates the globe 1545-1563 - Council of Trent 1558 - 1603 - Reign of Queen Elizabeth I 1564-1616 - Shakespeare 1588-Spanish armada destroyed 1589-Reign of Henry IV of France 1598- Edict of Nantes

Figure 3 Timeline for developments in science, obesity, and contemporary events in the 16th century.

TIMELINE 1600 - 1700

Science and Technology	1620 - Bacon's *Organum Novum*; 1662-Descartes *De Homine Figuris*; 1662-Newton and Leibniz develop calculus; 1665 - Newton's law of gravity; 1687-Newton's *Principia*
Anatomy and Histology	1610-Galileo devises microscope; 1658 - Swammerdam describes red corpuscles; 1661-Malpighi publishes *Pulmonary Circulation*; 1665-Hooke's *Micrographia* published; 1672-DeGraaf, ovarian follicle; 1675-Leeuwenhoek, protozoa
Physiology	1614-Santorio, father of metabolic obesity, describes metabolic scale, pulse counting, thermometer; 1628 Harvey publishes *Circulation of Blood*; 1665-Lower transfuses blood in dogs
Chemistry / Biochemistry	1661 Boyle defines chemical element; 1674 - Mayow, animal heat in muscles
Genetics	
Pharmacology	
Neuroscience	
Clinical Medicine	1639 - First hospital in Canada; 1642 - Jacob Bontius describes beri beri; 1650 - Glisson describes rickets; 1656 - Wharton publishes *Adenographia*; 1659 -Willis describes puerperal fever; 1670 - Willis describes "sweet" urine in diabetes; 1683- Sydenham treatise on gout
	1600 · 1610 · 1620 · 1630 · 1640 · 1650 · 1660 · 1670 · 1680 · 1690
President of the United States	
Events	1607-Jamestown, VA, settled; 1618-1648 -The 30 Years War; 1620-Plymouth, MA, settled; 1636-Harvard College founded; 1640-1688- Reign of Frederick the Great Elector; 1642-1661-English civil war and Cromwell rule; 1654-1715-Reign of Louis XIV; 1660-1689-Reign of Charles II of England; 1666-London fire; 1682-1725-Reign of Peter the Great of Russia; 1690-Locke publishes *On Human Under-standing*; 1692-Salem witch hunt

Figure 4 Timeline for developments in science, obesity, and contemporary events in the 17th century.

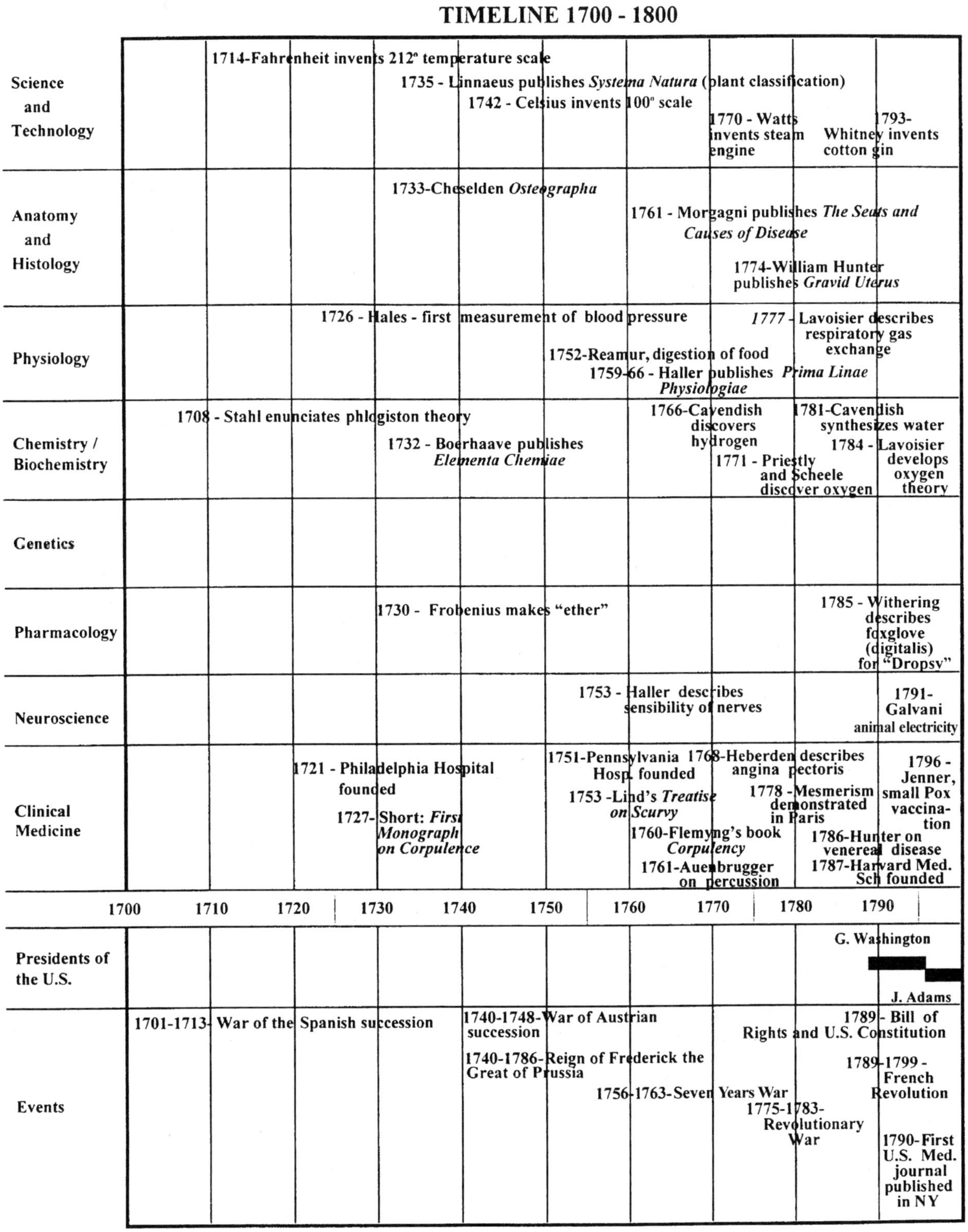

TIMELINE 1700 - 1800

Science and Technology	1714-Fahrenheit invents 212° temperature scale; 1735 - Linnaeus publishes *Systema Natura* (plant classification); 1742 - Celsius invents 100° scale; 1770 - Watts invents steam engine; 1793- Whitney invents cotton gin
Anatomy and Histology	1733-Cheselden *Osteographa*; 1761 - Morgagni publishes *The Seats and Causes of Disease*; 1774-William Hunter publishes *Gravid Uterus*
Physiology	1726 - Hales - first measurement of blood pressure; 1752-Reamur, digestion of food; 1759-66 - Haller publishes *Prima Linae Physiologiae*; *1777* - Lavoisier describes respiratory gas exchange
Chemistry / Biochemistry	1708 - Stahl enunciates phlogiston theory; 1732 - Boerhaave publishes *Elementa Chemiae*; 1766-Cavendish discovers hydrogen; 1771 - Priestly and Scheele discover oxygen; 1781-Cavendish synthesizes water; 1784 - Lavoisier develops oxygen theory
Genetics	
Pharmacology	1730 - Frobenius makes "ether"; 1785 - Withering describes foxglove (digitalis) for "Dropsy"
Neuroscience	1753 - Haller describes sensibility of nerves; 1791- Galvani animal electricity
Clinical Medicine	1721 - Philadelphia Hospital founded; 1727- Short: *First Monograph on Corpulence*; 1751-Pennsylvania Hosp. founded; 1753 -Lind's *Treatise on Scurvy*; 1760-Flemyng's book *Corpulency*; 1761-Auenbrugger on percussion; 1768-Heberden describes angina pectoris; 1778 - Mesmerism demonstrated in Paris; 1786-Hunter on venereal disease; 1787-Harvard Med. Sch founded; 1796 - Jenner, small Pox vaccination
	1700 · 1710 · 1720 · 1730 · 1740 · 1750 · 1760 · 1770 · 1780 · 1790
Presidents of the U.S.	G. Washington; J. Adams
Events	1701-1713- War of the Spanish succession; 1740-1748-War of Austrian succession; 1740-1786-Reign of Frederick the Great of Prussia; 1756-1763-Seven Years War; 1775-1783- Revolutionary War; 1789- Bill of Rights and U.S. Constitution; 1789-1799 - French Revolution; 1790-First U.S. Med. journal published in NY

Figure 5 Timeline for developments in science, obesity, and contemporary events in the 18th century.

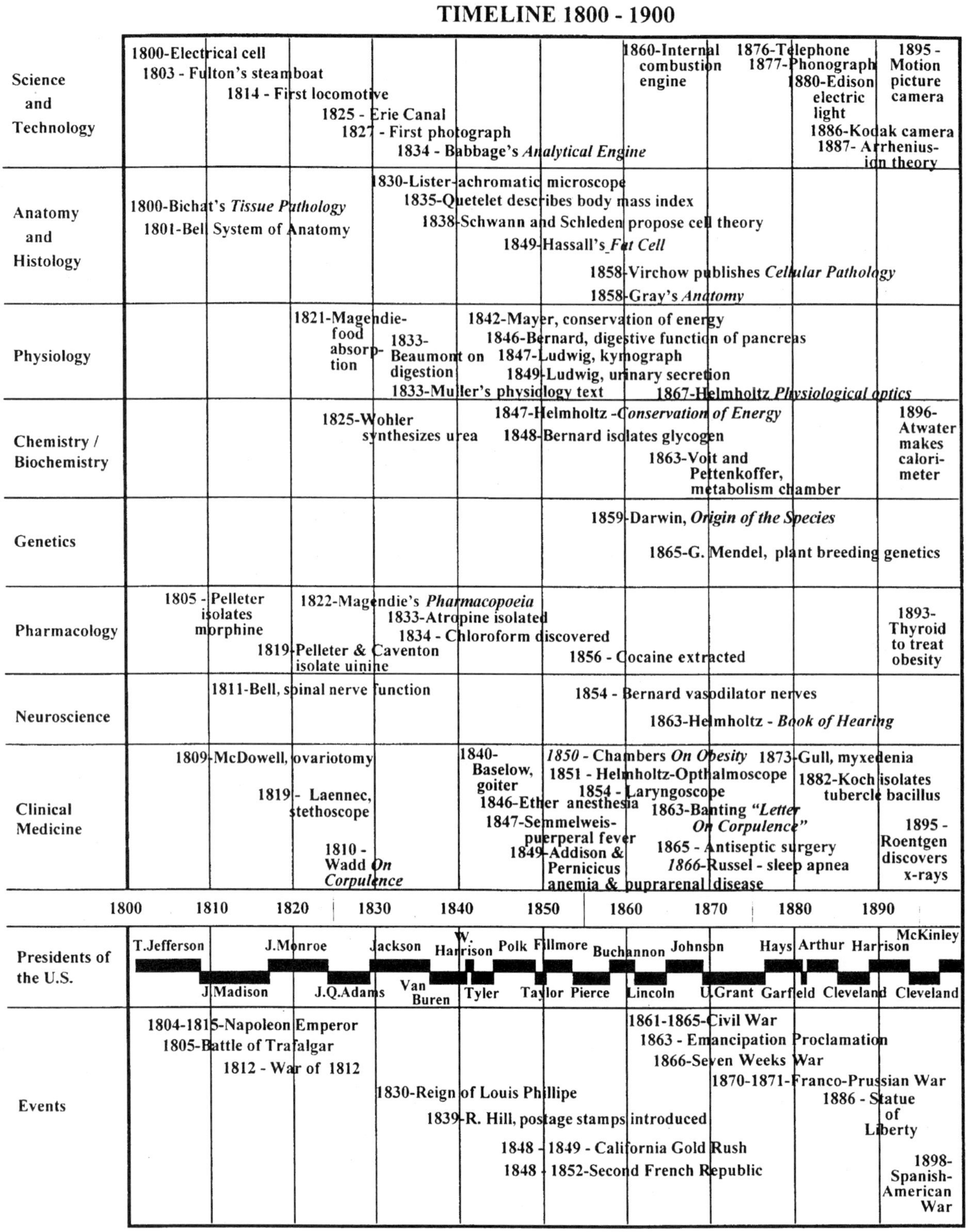

TIMELINE 1800 - 1900

Science and Technology	1800-Electrical cell; 1803 - Fulton's steamboat; 1814 - First locomotive; 1825 - Erie Canal; 1827 - First photograph; 1834 - Babbage's *Analytical Engine*; 1860-Internal combustion engine; 1876-Telephone; 1877-Phonograph; 1880-Edison electric light; 1886-Kodak camera; 1887- Arrhenius-ion theory; 1895 - Motion picture camera
Anatomy and Histology	1800-Bichat's *Tissue Pathology*; 1801-Bell System of Anatomy; 1830-Lister-achromatic microscope; 1835-Quetelet describes body mass index; 1838-Schwann and Schleden propose cell theory; 1849-Hassall's *Fat Cell*; 1858-Virchow publishes *Cellular Pathology*; 1858-Gray's *Anatomy*
Physiology	1821-Magendie- food absorption; 1833- Beaumont on digestion; 1833-Muller's physiology text; 1842-Mayer, conservation of energy; 1846-Bernard, digestive function of pancreas; 1847-Ludwig, kymograph; 1849-Ludwig, urinary secretion; 1867-Helmholtz *Physiological optics*
Chemistry / Biochemistry	1825-Wohler synthesizes urea; 1847-Helmholtz -*Conservation of Energy*; 1848-Bernard isolates glycogen; 1863-Voit and Pettenkoffer, metabolism chamber; 1896- Atwater makes calori- meter
Genetics	1859-Darwin, *Origin of the Species*; 1865-G. Mendel, plant breeding genetics
Pharmacology	1805 - Pelleter isolates morphine; 1819-Pelleter & Caventon isolate uinine; 1822-Magendie's *Pharmacopoeia*; 1833-Atropine isolated; 1834 - Chloroform discovered; 1856 - Cocaine extracted; 1893- Thyroid to treat obesity
Neuroscience	1811-Bell, spinal nerve function; 1854 - Bernard vasodilator nerves; 1863-Helmholtz - *Book of Hearing*
Clinical Medicine	1809-McDowell, ovariotomy; 1819 - Laennec, stethoscope; 1810 - Wadd *On Corpulence*; 1840- Baselow, goiter; 1846-Ether anesthesia; 1847-Semmelweis- puerperal fever; 1849-Addison & Pernicicus anemia & suprarenal disease; *1850* - Chambers *On Obesity*; 1851 - Helmholtz-Opthalmoscope; 1854 - Laryngoscope; 1863-Banting *"Letter On Corpulence"*; 1865 - Antiseptic surgery; *1866*-Russel - sleep apnea; 1873-Gull, myxedenia; 1882-Koch isolates tubercle bacillus; 1895 - Roentgen discovers x-rays
	1800 1810 1820 1830 1840 1850 1860 1870 1880 1890
Presidents of the U.S.	T.Jefferson; J.Madison; J.Monroe; J.Q.Adams; Jackson; Van Buren; W. Harrison; Tyler; Polk; Taylor; Fillmore; Pierce; Buchannon; Lincoln; Johnson; U.Grant; Hays; Garfield; Arthur; Cleveland; Harrison; Cleveland; McKinley
Events	1804-1815-Napoleon Emperor; 1805-Battle of Trafalgar; 1812 - War of 1812; 1830-Reign of Louis Phillipe; 1839-R. Hill, postage stamps introduced; 1848 - 1849 - California Gold Rush; 1848 - 1852-Second French Republic; 1861-1865-Civil War; 1863 - Emancipation Proclamation; 1866-Seven Weeks War; 1870-1871-Franco-Prussian War; 1886 - Statue of Liberty; 1898- Spanish-American War

Figure 6 Timeline for developments in science, obesity, and contemporary events in the 19th century.

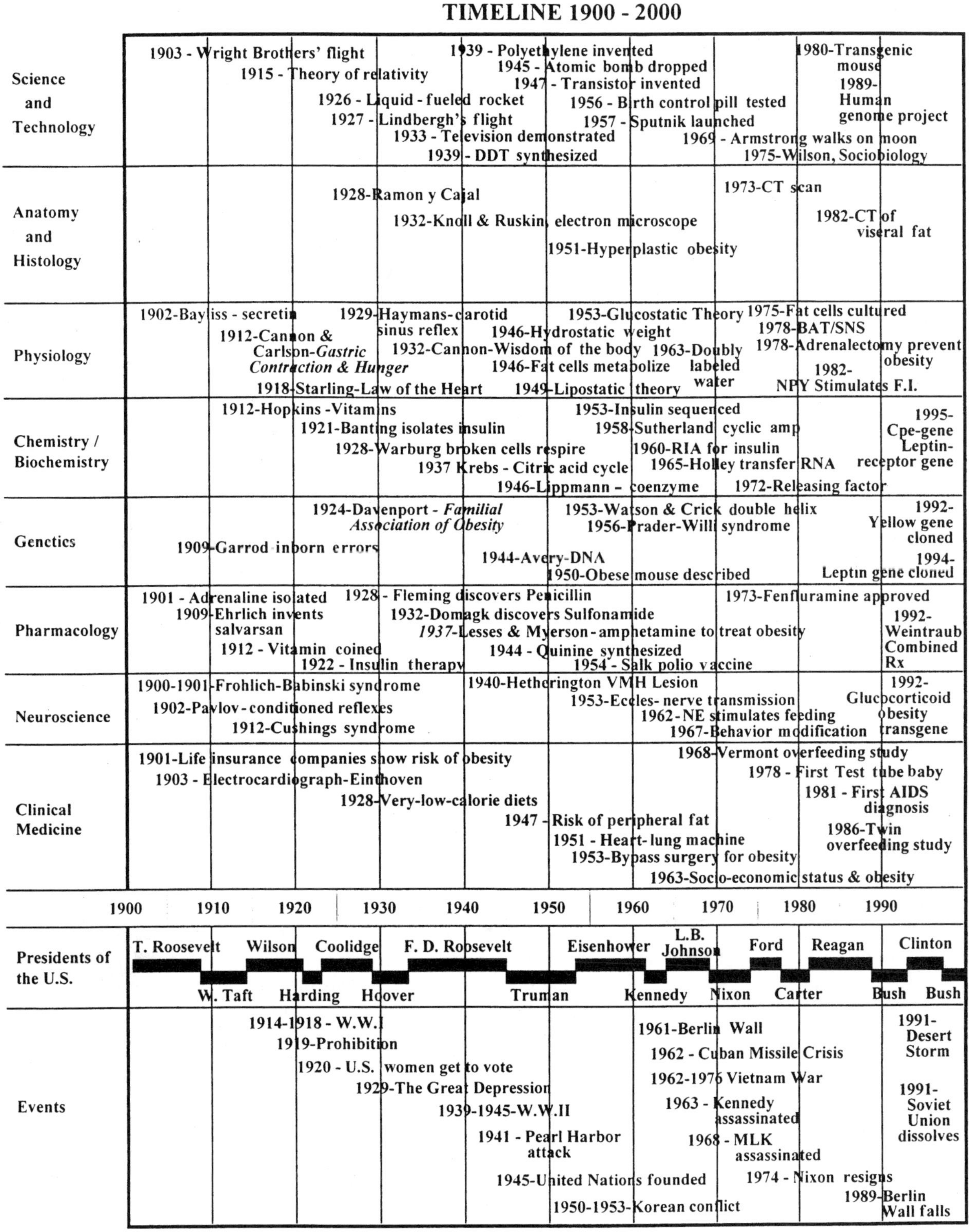

TIMELINE 1900 - 2000

Science and Technology	1903 - Wright Brothers' flight; 1915 - Theory of relativity; 1926 - Liquid - fueled rocket; 1927 - Lindbergh's flight; 1933 - Television demonstrated; 1939 - DDT synthesized; 1939 - Polyethylene invented; 1945 - Atomic bomb dropped; 1947 - Transistor invented; 1956 - Birth control pill tested; 1957 - Sputnik launched; 1969 - Armstrong walks on moon; 1975-Wilson, Sociobiology; 1980-Transgenic mouse; 1989- Human genome project
Anatomy and Histology	1928-Ramon y Cajal; 1932-Knoll & Ruskin, electron microscope; 1951-Hyperplastic obesity; 1973-CT scan; 1982-CT of visceral fat
Physiology	1902-Bayliss - secretin; 1912-Cannon & Carlson-*Gastric Contraction & Hunger*; 1918-Starling-Law of the Heart; 1929-Haymans-carotid sinus reflex; 1932-Cannon-Wisdom of the body; 1946-Hydrostatic weight; 1946-Fat cells metabolize; 1949-Lipostatic theory; 1953-Glucostatic Theory; 1963-Doubly labeled water; 1975-Fat cells cultured; 1978-BAT/SNS; 1978-Adrenalectomy prevent obesity; 1982-NPY Stimulates F.I.
Chemistry / Biochemistry	1912-Hopkins -Vitamins; 1921-Banting isolates insulin; 1928-Warburg broken cells respire; 1937 Krebs - Citric acid cycle; 1946-Lippmann – coenzyme; 1953-Insulin sequenced; 1958-Sutherland cyclic amp; 1960-RIA for insulin; 1965-Holley transfer RNA; 1972-Releasing factor; 1995- Cpe-gene Leptin-receptor gene
Gencties	1909-Garrod inborn errors; 1924-Davenport - *Familial Association of Obesity*; 1944-Avery-DNA; 1950-Obese mouse described; 1953-Watson & Crick double helix; 1956-Prader-Willi syndrome; 1992- Yellow gene cloned; 1994- Leptin gene cloned
Pharmacology	1901 - Adrenaline isolated; 1909-Ehrlich invents salvarsan; 1912 - Vitamin coined; 1922 - Insulin therapy; 1928 - Fleming discovers Penicillin; 1932-Domagk discovers Sulfonamide; *1937*-Lesses & Myerson - amphetamine to treat obesity; 1944 - Quinine synthesized; 1954 - Salk polio vaccine; 1973-Fenfluramine approved; 1992- Weintraub Combined Rx
Neuroscience	1900-1901-Frohlich-Babinski syndrome; 1902-Pavlov-conditioned reflexes; 1912-Cushings syndrome; 1940-Hetherington VMH Lesion; 1953-Eccles- nerve transmission; 1962-NE stimulates feeding; 1967-Behavior modification; 1992- Glucocorticoid obesity transgene
Clinical Medicine	1901-Life insurance companies show risk of obesity; 1903 - Electrocardiograph-Einthoven; 1928-Very-low-calorie diets; 1947 - Risk of peripheral fat; 1951 - Heart- lung machine; 1953-Bypass surgery for obesity; 1963-Socio-economic status & obesity; 1968-Vermont overfeeding study; 1978 - First Test tube baby; 1981 - First AIDS diagnosis; 1986-Twin overfeeding study
	1900 1910 1920 1930 1940 1950 1960 1970 1980 1990
Presidents of the U.S.	T. Roosevelt; W. Taft; Wilson; Harding; Coolidge; Hoover; F. D. Roosevelt; Truman; Eisenhower; Kennedy; L.B. Johnson; Nixon; Ford; Carter; Reagan; Bush; Clinton; Bush
Events	1914-1918 - W.W.I; 1919-Prohibition; 1920 - U.S. women get to vote; 1929-The Great Depression; 1939-1945-W.W.II; 1941 - Pearl Harbor attack; 1945-United Nations founded; 1950-1953-Korean conflict; 1961-Berlin Wall; 1962 - Cuban Missile Crisis; 1962-1975 Vietnam War; 1963 - Kennedy assassinated; 1968 - MLK assassinated; 1974 - Nixon resigns; 1989-Berlin Wall falls; 1991- Desert Storm; 1991- Soviet Union dissolves

Figure 7 Timeline for developments in science, obesity, and contemporary events in the 20th century.

identified the pulmonary circulation, the fine structure of small animals and red blood cells, among others.

Gradually, the sophistication of the microscope improved, first with the introduction of the compound microscope and then with achromatic lenses. These developments made microscopes sufficiently powerful to define intracellular structures. This led to the concept of the "cell" as the basic unit of life by the middle of the 19th century. It was the combination of the compound achromatic microscope, which allowed sufficient resolution to distinguish the multiple intracellular components of cells, coupled with the intellectual genius of Schwann (73) and of Schleiden (74) that recognized the unifying principles of the cell wall, nucleus, and an area of structures surrounding this nucleus as the basic elements of cell biology. Shortly afterward, the first substantial textbooks of microscopic anatomy were published (75,76), and shortly after that, the recognition of the fat cell as a member of this group. A description of the growth and development of fat cells was published in 1879 by Hoggan and Hogan (77). In his early observations on the development of the fat vesicle, Hassall (78) suggested that certain types of obesity might result from an increased number of fat cells. It was more than a century later that the work of Bjurlf (79), of Hirsch (80), and of Bjorntorp (81) elaborated this important concept as the "hyperplastic" form of obesity. Within 20 years following the promulgation of the cellular theory of biology (73,74), Virchow (82) provided a cellular interpretation of pathology. The next advance in microscopic anatomy was the introduction of the electron microscope by Knoll and Ruska in 1932 (83), which has provided a detailed look at all elements of the fat cell (84).

C Physiology

The application of experimental methods is nowhere better illustrated than in the discovery of the circulation of the blood by William Harvey in 1616, which he published in 1628 (85). His theory is monumental in the way that experimental observations and human reasoning were brought together. His theory of the circulation of the blood was published before the capillaries that connect the arterial and venous circulations had been described (70). While in medical school in Padua, Harvey had seen his professor, Fabrizio of Aquapendente, demonstrate the presence of valves in the veins that only allowed blood to flow one way. At some point between his graduation from Padua in 1596 and his anatomic dissections at the Royal College of Physicians in London in 1616, he realized the importance of the valves in the veins (86). He presented his "discovery" to the Royal College of Physicians in 1616 to a ho-hum reception. Gradually, the importance of the discovery and of the method by which he argued its cogency became apparent. He demonstrated experimentally that the valves in the veins allowed blood to travel in only one direction. From the limited quantity of blood in the body, he argued that the blood must circulate and be reused. It was, however, not for another 50 years that the capillary circulation was demonstrated by Malpighi (70).

The early physiological studies by Harvey on the circulation of the blood set the stage for further work in physiology. Two of these themes are particularly relevant to obesity. The first is metabolism and the second digestion. In 1614, Santorio (87,88) described his metabolic balance, a pulse watch for measuring the pulse and a way of measuring temperature. He was following the dictum of his contemporary, Gallileo, who said: "Measure what can be measured, and make measurable what cannot be measured" (1). The balance that Santorio constructed consisted of a platform on which he could sit, counterbalanced by a beam to which weight could be added or subtracted to record changes in his weight related to bodily functions. With this system, he could measure his food intake and his excretory losses. In more recent times, Newburgh and his colleagues (89) used a similar method to record the loss of water with respiration and showed that it accounted for ~24% of the heat produced by the body. The seminal contributions to metabolic work qualify Santorio Santorio for the title of Father of Metabolic Obesity.

The second group of physiological studies that relate to obesity were those on the gastrointestinal tract and digestion. In 1752, Reamur (90) succeeded in isolating the gastric juice from his pet kite and showed that it digested food. Later in the 18th century, Spallanzani (91,92) showed that gastric juice would digest food and prevent putrefaction outside the body. The American William Beaumont (93) published data from his direct observation of digestion made possible by studies of a patient, Alexis St. Martin, who suffered a bullet wound in his abdomen that healed with a fistula allowing direct observation of the stomach and its contents (93). Understanding of the way food was digested and absorbed was advanced by Magendie and his distinguished pupil Claude Bernard, one of the leaders of the French physiological school. It was Bernard who demonstrated the digestive function of the pancreas (94).

These 18th- and 19th-century observations on digestion were followed in the early 20th-century by the seminal and long-lasting theory that hunger resulted from gastric contractions. This theory was based on direct measurements of the association of gastric contraction with hunger by Washburn and Cannon (95) and independently by Carlson (96).

D Chemistry and Biochemistry

Modern chemistry might be traced to the 17th century work of Robert Boyle, who established the concept of chemical elements (97,98). By the late 17th century, Boyle (98) recognized that when a lighted candle went out, a mouse living in the same environment rapidly died. It was clear that some important element was present in the air that was essential for life and for the candle to burn. At the beginning of the 18th century, Georg Stahl (99) postulated that this substance was phlogiston. It was not until the work of Priestley (100), of Scheele (who simultaneously discovered what we now call oxygen) (101), and particularly of Lavoisier (102), that the Phlogiston Theory was replaced by the Oxygen Theory of Combustion.

The Oxygen Theory culminated from the research of Lavoisier in the last three decades of the 18th century. Lavoisier recognized that oxidation meant combining with oxygen. His experimental work showed that metabolism was similar to combustion (102). Lavoisier's death at the hands of Revolutionary French government in 1794 deprived humanity of one of its great intellects.

The legacy of Lavoisier from the 18th century served as the basis for the laws of the conservation of mass and energy (103) and formed the basis for the work of Rubner (104,105), who formulated the Law of Surface Area based on the observation of a linear relationship between metabolic expenditure of animals of many sizes and their surface area [body weight]$^{0.7}$. This Law of Surface Area and the work of Voit and Pettenkofer (106) in Germany were the framework on which Atwater and Rossa constructed the first functional human calorimeter at Wesleyan College in Middletown, CT, in 1896 (107). The instrument served as a tool for extensive studies on metabolic requirements during food intake and on the effects of starvation by Atwater (108) and by Benedict (109,110).

Following the work of Atwater and Benedict in the early 20th century, studies using metabolic chambers languished until after World War II. The earliest of these post–World War II chambers was built in Paris, France, and at the National Institutes of Health in Bethesda, MD. However, it was the chamber built in Lausanne, Switzerland, by Jequier (111) that provided the most extensive and continuing series of studies on energy expenditure in human subjects in the post–World War II period. This chamber and similar units built in Phoenix, AZ, are patterned after the one in Lausanne and the one in London built by Garrow (112), have shown that for human beings, fat-free mass provides a slightly better relationship for energy expenditure than surface area. Utilizing this information, several predictors of obesity have been developed including a low metabolic rate, a high rate of carbohydrate oxidation as indicated by a high RQ, and insulin sensitivity (113).

The study of energy expenditure in human beings and animals has advanced rapidly in the past two decades following the introduction of doubly labeled water as a technique for measuring total energy expenditure in free-living subjects (114). Doubly labeled water measures energy expenditure by following the path of deuterium and oxygen through the metabolic pathways in the body. Deuterium can only be excreted as water, while ^{18}O can be excreted as water or as carbon dioxide following respiratory combustion of carbon containing compounds. Thus, the ratio of deuterium to ^{18}O gradually diverges following the administration of these isotopes as water, and this rate of diversion can be used to calculate energy expenditure if the respiratory quotient is known. Application of this technique to human beings shows that overweight people underestimate their dietary intake more than do normal-weight people (111,115). This tool has provided a new paradigm in which to assess energy needs and questions the validity of data obtained from dietary records.

The chemistry of biological systems was the natural outgrowth of chemistry. The term "biology," as the study of living things with the "cell" as its basal unit, was a 19th-century concept. Biological chemistry or biochemistry is also a 19th-century concept that may be dated from the demonstration by Wohler (116) in 1828 that urea, an organic molecule, could be synthesized from inorganic materials.

The study of body composition was also an important 19th-century contribution to the biochemistry of obesity. Chemical analysis of human cadavers was conducted, and the fat stores in adipose tissue were demonstrated to be primarily triglyceride (116).

Biological chemistry in the mid-19th century was dominated by Claude Bernard (117) and his teacher Magendie (118) France and by Liebig and his studies of food chemistry in Germany (119). Magendie was a leader in the application of the experimental method to the study of living animals. His pupil, Claude Bernard, discovered liver glycogen as the source of blood glucose (117). He also showed that damage (piqure) to the hypothalamus could produce glycosuria. His scientific philosophy was one of "gradualism." Scientific theory would naturally lead to step-by-step progress, a concept that was a dominant element in the 19th-century philosophy of science. This concept of gradualism is in sharp contrast to the concept of paradigm shifts (120) and scientific revolutions (121) (see Sec. V).

Claude Bernard's contemporary in Germany was Liebig. His concept that the carbohydrates, proteins, and fat were all that were needed for human nutrition served as the basis for nutritional science during much of the 19th century. Overthrow of this theory by the discovery of vitamins at the turn of the 20th century gave birth to a new and broader field of nutrition (122). The development of nutrition through the first half of the 20th century is epitomized by the discovery of vitamins and their function. This era largely closed in 1948 with the elucidation of the structure of vitamin B_{12}. With the closing of this era, the impact of macronutrients again took center stage through the recognition of the role of dietary fats and obesity as "causes" of chronic disease (123,124).

The 20th century saw an explosion in the application of chemical and biochemical techniques to the study of obesity. Sophistication in the measurement of body components has greatly expanded. The work by Benke, Feen, and Wellman applied the techniques of density for quantitating the fat and nonfat compartments of the body (125). This methodology has been supplemented since World War II by the application of radioactive isotopes (126) to the study of body composition by many workers (127). New techniques have continued to provide ever better ways of characterizing the human body. Radioactive isotopes have largely been replaced by stable isotopes. The introduction of ultrasound for measuring fat thickness, of computed axial tomographic (CT) scans, and magnetic resonance imaging (MRI) scans to measure regional fat distribution, the use of dual-energy x-ray absorptiometry to measure body fat, lean body compartments, and bone mineral, and the use of whole body neutron activation have provided sophisticated techniques for accurate and detailed determination of body composition in vivo (128).

E Genetics and Molecular Biology

The setting for the biological revolution of the last quarter of the 20th century had its roots in the mid-19th century with the publication by Darwin of the *Origin of the Species* (129) and by Mendel of the unitized inheritable traits subsequently called genes (130). In the early 20th century, Garrod suggested the concept of "metabolic" disorders in a classic monograph (131). Genetic work was greatly aided by the use of the fruitfly, *Drosophila*, with their giant chromosomes, and of mice, whose breeding cycle was relatively short. Gradually, genetic material was traced to the nucleus and to deoxyribonucleic acid (DNA). A new field of molecular biology was born from the seminal work of Watson and Crick published in 1953 (132), who proposed the double-helix model for the structure of this DNA leading to the "cracking" of the genetic code and the development of the tools of molecular biology. With these techniques it became possible to identify and isolate the genes underlying the rare forms of inherited obesity in animals and human beings (133–135). The Human Genome Project has now completed the sequencing of all of the genes in *Drosophila melanogaster* (136) and the human genome.

The first genetic breakthrough in the study of obesity came in 1992 with the identification of the genetic defect in a mouse called the Yellow Obese mouse. The agouti gene that produces this defect provides the information to make a 133–amino acid peptide (133). In the Yellow Obese mouse, the agouti gene is expressed in many tissues where it is not normally expressed. The resulting agouti protein serves as a competitor for melanocortin receptors and through this mechanism can account for the yellow coat color, hyperphagia, and obesity present in these animals.

Shortly after the discovery of the agouti gene, the genetic defect in the ob/ob mouse was identified (134). The ob gene is altered with a stop message (codon) at amino acid 105. This truncates the normal 167–amino acid protein called leptin. Leptin in the normal animal appears to signal the brain about the state of peripheral fat stores and their adequacy for reproduction. Leptin is also involved in modulating a number of other steroid messages. In the obese (ob/ob) mouse, leptin will reverse the obesity and correct the other defects.

The third obesity gene to be cloned was the gene for the recessively inherited FAT mouse (135). The nature of this gene defect was suspected from the high levels of pro-insulin in these animals. Cleavage of insulin to proinsulin requires the enzyme carboxypeptidase-E. It was subsequently determined that this gene was defective, resulting in defective synthesis of hormones and neuromediators, from prohormones and pro-neuromediators.

Genetic susceptibility for human obesity has also benefited from the advances in genetics and molecular biology (136). Beginning with the work of Davenport

(137) on the inheritance of body mass index in families and the work of Verscheuer on identical twins (138), a growing body of data argues that important components of total body fat mass and fat distribution are inherited (139,140). From this basis in epidemiological data, a search has begun for the genes involved in human (141) and animal forms of obesity. From the studies of responsiveness to dietary fat in animals, at least 12 different genes have been identified as playing a role (142,143). In human beings, a large and growing number of candidate genes have been explored for their possible relationship with the development of obesity and several have been shown to contribute in small ways to this syndrome (141).

F Pharmacology

The field of pharmacology, the study of drugs and their biological effects, grew from a base in chemistry (144) and the early findings in biology. Its early successes included the isolation of morphine, strychnine, emetine, and quinine, and the publication of the first Pharmacopeia by Magendie in 1822 (145). One of the major advances in this field in the 19th century was the introduction of anesthesia, which was discovered almost simultaneously by three Americans—Crawford Long, W.T.G. Morton, and Horace Wells—between 1842 and 1846 (146–148). The first effective public demonstration was given in the Ether Dome of the Massachusetts General Hospital in Boston in October 1846. This was followed by the introduction of carbolic acid to reduce infection in the operating room by Sir Joseph Lister in 1865 (149,150).

The 19th century also saw a number of efforts at "pharmacologic" treatment of obesity. Among these were the use of hydrotherapy and various laxatives and purgatives. Thyroid extract was also initially used to treat obesity in the late 19th century, beginning in 1893 (151).

A key element in the entire field of pharmacology was the discovery of aniline in the 19th century (152). Developed by the dye industry, aniline served as the base for synthesizing numerous drugs in the 20th century and for the "magic bullet" concept of Ehrlich (153). Dinitrophenol was one of those aniline products. It was introduced for treatment of obesity, when weight loss was noted in workers in the chemical industry who handled dinitrophenol. This drug was subsequently abandoned after it produced cataracts and neuropathy. This tragedy of treatment shows the need for careful clinical evaluation of drugs before they are made available for general clinical use (154).

Amphetamine was a second product of the synthetic organic chemical industry that was used for treatment of obesity. In the 1930s, dextroamphetamine, which was synthesized in 1887 (155), was shown to produce weight loss in individuals being treated for narcolepsy (156). Because amphetamine is addictive, it fell into disrepute and led to a negative view of all drugs with a similar chemical structure. However, the similarity of chemical structure on paper proved misleading pharmacologically. The β-phenethylamine chemical structure is the backbone of amphetamine (α-methyl-β-phenethylamine). Amphetamine affects two neurotransmitters, dopamine and norepinephrine. Modifying the β-phenethylamine structure can completely change the effect on neurotransmitters. Phentermine is a β-phenethylamine cousin of amphetamine that affects primarily norepinephrine. Fenfluramine, another β-phenethylamine cousin, is pharmacologically unrelated to amphetamine since it only affects serotonin.

G Neuroscience

A neural basis for some kinds of obesity became evident at the beginning of the 20th century. The case reports by Babinski (157) and by Frohlich (158) were preceded by a case reported by Mohr (159). Each report described single individuals who developed obesity in association with a tumor at the base of the brain. This important clinical finding opened a new field of research and heralded the development of techniques to produce obesity by injection of toxic material such as chromic oxide at the base of the brain (160) or, more specifically, by localized electrolytic or thermal damage to specific hypothalamic nuclei (161). Such a specific anatomic localization of hypothalamic centers where damage would produce either increased food intake (damage to ventromedial hypothalamus) or decreased food intake (damage to lateral hypothalamus) (162) led, in 1954, to the dual center hypotheses of Stellar (163), which served as the basis for thinking about hunger and satiety for the next 20 years.

It soon became clear that hyperphagia was not essential for the development of obesity after a hypothalamic lesion (164) or in genetically obese mice (165). One explanation for the development of obesity without hyperphagia was provided by the autonomic hypothesis (166) based on the observations of increased activity of the parasympathetic nervous system (vagus nerve) (167) and reduced activity of the sympathetic nervous system (168). This insight, coupled with the role of brown adipose tissue and the thermogenic component of the sympathetic nervous system in heat generation in small animals and in inhibiting food intake, has been central to the development of β-adrenergic drugs as potential agents for treating obesity (169).

The discovery of a number of peptides that are present in both the brain and the gastrointestinal tract has brought together the areas of neuroscience and physiology in the control of body fat and obesity. Secretin was the first GI hormone found (170). Subsequently, cholecystokinin was found to stimulate contraction of the gallbladder and then to reduce food intake (171). Of the many peptides now known, neuropeptide-Y is among the more interesting because it will stimulate food intake and produce obesity when given continuously (172).

H Clinical Medicine and Obesity

Well before the Scientific Era, which I have dated as beginning in AD 1500, individuals with massive obesity have been noteworthy. Table 2 lists some of the largest individuals on record. Cases of monstrous obesity have been noted since antiquity (59,60,173,174). In the 19th century, Dubourg (175) discussed 25 cases, Schindler (176) identified 17 such cases, and Maccary 11 (177). Individual cases have also been reported by many other authors (178–187). These individuals were frequently noted for their "odd" or "monstrous" appearance. The outlook for this group was particularly bleak from both a clinical and a social perspective.

These case reports beg a very important question that has only recently begun to be answered: Are all cases of obesity the same? Classification of obesity can be viewed as one component of the more general efforts to classify diseases that began when Galen labeled them moderate or immoderate. Although many classifications of disease exist, one of the most interesting was the effort to classify disease based on the classification of plants and animals introduced by Linnaeus (188). His system involved giving each individual a genus and species name and categorizing the genera into classes, orders, and phyla. Although Sydenham began such a systematic classification of disease, the two best-known efforts to classify diseases in this way were published by Sauvages (189) and Cullen (190). In both of them obesity was called "polysarcie." In the English translation of Cullen's work, Obesity is in Class III, The Cachexieas: It is listed under the second order called Intumescentiae with a genus name of *Polysarcia* (*Corrporis pinguedinosa intumescentiamolesta*). Obesity, as a word to describe increased fatness, gradually replaced polysarcie, embonpoint, and corpulence during the 19th century. A more detailed discussion of the classifications of obesity beginning with the division into endogenous and exogenous by Von Noorden can be found in elsewhere (155).

Table 2 Cases of Extraordinary Obesity

Name	Gender	Age at death	Maximum weight (kg)	Ref.
Lambert	M	39	335	(1)
Bright	M		280	(182)
Darden	M	59	462	(3)
Campbell	M	22	332	(174)
Valenzuela	M	39	385	(3)
Titman	—	36	318	(2)
Zadina	M	29	332	(2)
Raggio	M	27	381	(2)
	F		385	(174)
Maguire	M	31	367	(2)
Karns	F	28	338	(2)
Nunez	F	23	343	(2)
Hall	M	37	318	(2)
Pontico	F	35	350	(2)
Hughes	M	32	485	(3)
Craig	M	38	411	(3)
Knorr	M	46	408	(3)
King	F	35	381	(3)

Sporadic cases of obesity have been noted since antiquity. Gould and Pyle (174) describe a large number of cases of massive obesity in children and adults. They cite the writings of Athenaeus who described Denys, the tyrant of Heraclea, as so enormous that he was in constant danger of suffocation, which was treated by putting needles in the back of his chair. Several other very fat people identified by Gould and Pyle are William the Conqueror; Charles le Gros; Louis le Gros; Humbert II, Count of Maurienne; Henry I, King of Navarre; Henry III, Count of Champagne; Conan III, Duke of Brittany; Sancho I, King of Leon; Alphonse II, King of Portugal; the Italian poet Bruni who died in 1635; Vivonne, a general under Louis XIV; Frederick I, King of Wurtemberg, and Louis XVII.

The small monograph written by William Wadd in 1829, entitled *Comments on Corpulency, Lineaments of Leanness* (69), presents a series of clinical cases of morbidly obese individuals presented both descriptively and in several cases graphically. Most of the cases were from his medical correspondence, a characteristic way of evaluating patients by "consulting physicians" since the physical examination was not a part of the usual clinical visit in the early 1800s. Of the 12 cases in his book, all but one was in men. Weights were noted in five cases and ranged from 106 kg (16 st; 10 lb; or 234 pounds) to 146 kg (23 st; 21b; or 324 pounds). Two of the cases examined at postmortem had enormous accumulations of fat. Although autopsy observations of obese individuals had been made previously, this was the first instance in which they were included in a monograph devoted to obesity and leanness.

Wadd notes that sudden death is not uncommon in the corpulent, thus revalidating Hippocrates. His statement, "A sudden palpitation excited in the heart of a fat man has often proved as fatal as a bullet through the thorax" is consistent with the association of obesity and sudden death noted in the ongoing Framingham Study. In several of the cases, corpulent patients were seeking specific pills to treat their obesity. Wadd makes a distinction between the therapeutic activists and those favoring less aggressive therapy with the homeopathists being at the far extreme with minimal dosage of medication. "Truly it has been said—some Doctors let the patient die, for fear they should kill him; while others kill the patient, for fear he should die."

One important lesson from the study of massively obese individuals was the association of obesity with sleep apnea, a disease often referred to as the Pickwickian syndrome (191,192). Patients with alveolar hypoventilation, which produces this syndrome, date back to Greco-Roman times (59,60). The earliest published medical report of hypoventilation and its consequences was that by Russell in 1866 (193), although he did not know its cause.

Other clinical subtypes of obesity, in addition to the massively obese, have been gradually defined. Cases of hypothalamic injury with obesity have been identified since 1840 (159), and received particular attention following the reports by Babinski (157) and by Frohlich (158). In the early 20th century, Cushing recognized (194) that obesity was associated with basophilic adenomas of the pituitary gland (195). Cushing's syndrome can also be caused by medication with adrenal steroids. A number of nonsteroidal drugs, including phenothiazines, some antidepressants (amitriptyline), some anticonvulsants (valproate), antiserotonin drugs (cyproheptadine), and antidiabetic drugs can also cause weight gain. Other endocrine diseases such as hypogonadism and isolated growth hormone deficiency are also associated with increased fat deposits. Several rare genetic disorders have obesity as finding (141). Finally, a sedentary life-style and a high-fat diet, particularly in animals, have been reported to produce obesity.

Besides the lessons from individual patients, which have been provided by these case reports, there are the lessons that come from evaluation of collective data. Quetelet (196) was one of the leaders in developing "mathematical" methods to evaluate populations. He developed the concept of the "average man" and used the ratio of weight divided by the square of stature or height (kg/m^2) as a measure of an individual's fatness. This unit, the body mass index, might be termed the Quetelet Index (QI) in honor of the man who developed what has become a widely used way of evaluating weight status.

The life insurance industry has extended the population-based view of obesity (124). As early as 1901, data began to appear showing that both excess amounts of weight and central distribution of this weight were associated with shortened life expectancy. Because of the financial need to relate risk to the cost of life insurance, the insurance industry has continued to provide data showing these relationships. These data were responsible for stimulating evaluation of the association of weight status with mortality risks in several population-based studies (197–201). In all of these studies, a curvilinear increase in risk of mortality is associated with rising weight or body mass or QI index.

Although the relationship of central fat to increased mortality could be discerned in these early insurance studies, it remained for Vague (202) to bring this concept to the attention of health professionals. Although Vague's data are clear, the adipomuscular ratio that he used to measure fat distribution was a complex one and it remained for the simpler measurement of waist circumference divided by hip circumference (WHR) and the subscapular skinfold measurement to provide the wide recognition for the risk that centrally located fat poses. With better methods of measuring fat distribution with CT and MRI scans, it is now clear that increased visceral fat is an important component in the health risks associated with obesity.

I Treatment of Obesity

1 Treatment with Diet and Exercise

> *In America there are fewer cures for obesity undertaken than abroad ... because ... there are fewer obese people here.*
>
> Carter et al. (203)

This statement was made in 1917, but time and the tides have now produced an epidemic of obesity in America (204).

The clinical approach to treatment of obesity long antedates the Scientific Era. From the time of Hippocrates (205) and Galen (206) in the prescientific era, diet and exercise were an integral part of the therapeutic regimen for obese patients. Hippocrates, the "Father of Medicine," suggested in the 5th century BC:

> Obese people and those desiring to lose weight should perform hard work before food. Meals

should be taken after exertion and while still panting from fatique and with no other refreshment before meals except only wine, diluted and slightly cold. their meals should be prepared with a sesame or seasoning and other similar substances and be of a fatty nature as people get thus, satiated with little food. They should, moreover, eat only once a day and take no baths and sleep on a hard bed and walk naked as long as possible (205).

Galen, nearly 2000 years ago, outlined his approach to treatment of the obese as follows:

> I have made any sufficiently stout patient moderately thin in a short time, by compelling him to do rapid running, then wiping off his perspiration with very soft or very rough muslin and then massaging him maximally with diaphoretic unctions, which the younger doctors customarily call restoratives, and after such massage leading him to the bath after which I give him nourishment immediately but bade him rest for a while or do nothing to which he was accustomed, then lead him to a second bath and then gave him abundant food of little nourishment so as to fill him up but distribute little of it to the entire body (206)

From this Greco-Roman beginning dietary treatment can be traced to the Arabic tradition in medicine. In the first book of his Cannon, Avicenna describes how to reduce the overweight individual:

> The regimen which will reduce obesity. (1) Produce a rapid descent of the food from the stomach and intestines, in order to prevent completion of absorption by the mesentery. (2) Take food which is bulky but feebly nutritious. (3) Take the bath before food often. (4) Hard exercise... (207)

When the Western medical tradition moved to Europe in the 11th to 13th centuries, so did the concepts of hygiene, diet, and exercise. These were embodied in the "institutes of medicine," a major component of medical education for centuries. One of the most widely used guides was the Regimen Sanitatis (208) developed in the school at Salerno, Italy, in the 12th century, which did not specifically provide advice for obesity. Chaucer, the 14th-century poet, did reiterate the advice flowing from Hippocrates when he said; "Agonys glotonye, the remedie is abstinence." (Against gluttony the remedy is abstinence.)

Dietary treatment in the 18th century was summarized by Tweedie:

> In attempting its cure, when the habit is threatened with any morbid effects, from the plethora existing either in the head or lungs, this must be removed by a bleeding or two; and as corpulent people do not bear blood-letting well, purging is most to be depended upon for the removal of the plethora (209).

He also says, "The diet should be sparing. They should abstain from spirits, wines and malt liquors, drinking in their stead, either spring water, toast and water or else water agreeably acidulated by any pure vegetable acids." Finally he increases exercise gradually.

The 18th-century Italian layman Cornaro (210) became a champion of dietary moderation after he successfully conquered his own obesity. At the beginning of his book he says: "O wretched, miserable Italy! Does not though plain see, that gluttony deprives [us] of more soul years, than either war, or the plague itself could have done?" Cornaro's doctor's advice was to eat or drink nothing that was not wholesome and that only in small quantities.

Comments on obesity have occasionally come from the field of gastronomy, the classic work by Brillat-Savarin in 1826 being the best known. This masterpiece has been published in many attractive and beautifully illustrated editions (211). He attributes obesity to several causes:

1. The first is the natural temperament of the individual.
2. The second principal cause of obesity lies in the starches and flours which man uses as the base for his daily nourishment.
3. A double cause of obesity results from too much sleep combined with too little exercise.
4. The final cause of obesity is excess, whether in eating or drinking.

From this, Brillat-Savarin moves to treatment. He says: "Any cure of obesity must begin with the three following and absolute precepts: discretion in eating, moderation in sleeping, and exercise on foot or on horseback." Having said this much he goes on to say: "Such are the first commandments which science makes to us: nevertheless I place little faith in them. . ." He then goes on to recommend a diet low in grains and starches.

In spite of the long history of dietary recommendations for treatment of obesity, it wasn't until 1863 that the first "popular" diet book appeared. This was a small, 21-page pamphlet published privately by William Banting entitled "A Letter on Corpulence Addressed to the Public" (212). The demand was so great that a second, hardcover edition was published within a year. In this pamphlet, he recounted his successful weight loss experience using a diet prescribed by his ear surgeon, William Harvey (213). The immediate success of this pamphlet led to reprinting worldwide and a popularization of the term "Bantingism" as a reference to dieting.

Banting's Cure (very severe)

Breakfast, 8 AM: 150–180 g (5–6 oz) meat or broiled fish (not a fat variety of either); a small biscuit or 30 g (1 oz) dry toast; a large cup of tea or coffee without cream, milk, or sugar.

Dinner, 1 PM: Meat or fish as at breakfast, or any kind of game or poultry, same amount; any vegetable except those that grow underground, such as potatoes, parsnips, carrots, or beets; dry toast, 30 g (1 oz); cooked fruit without sugar; good claret, 300 cc (10 oz). Madeira or sherry.

Tea, 5 PM: Cooked fruit, 60–90 g (2–3 oz); one or two pieces of zwieback; tea, 270 cc (9 oz) without milk, cream, or sugar.

Supper, 8 PM: Meat or fish, as at dinner, 90–120 cc (3–4 oz); claret or sherry, water, 210 cc (7 oz).

Fluids restricted to 1050 cc (35 oz) per day.

From these humble beginnings, diet books by professionals, self-styled professionals, and lay people have continued to appear, particularly as the concerns about obesity as a health and cosmetic problem have increased (35).

I have summarized two diets from the early 20th century to show the approaches that were used at that time (203).

Von Noorden's Diet

Von Noorden, one of the leading scholars of obesity at the beginning of the 20th century, based his dietary approach on an estimate of an individual's caloric requirement. Basal calorie needs were estimated from ideal weight. For this he assumed that a 70-kg individual would require 37 kcal/kg, or 2590 calories. If the individual weighed an extra 30 kg, they would need 1110 extra calories to feed this extra 30 kg. Von Noorden's first-degree reduction diet reduced energy to 80% of the basal needs, or for the 70-kg individual to 2000 kcal/day. His second-degree reduction diet reduced intake to 60% or 1500 kcal/day for the individual requiring 2500 kcal/day. His third-degree reduction, which was only infrequently used, lowered calories to 40% or 1000 kcal/day. His dietary approach also reduced fat to 30 g/day. His protein allowance was 120–180g/day with carbohydrate in the neighborhood of 100 g/day. His menu plan, adapted from Carter et al. (203), is summarized below:

	Minimal	Maximal
Protein	120 g (4 oz)	180 g (6 oz)
	492 cal	738 cal
Fat	30 g (1 oz)	30 g (1 oz)
	280 cal	280 cal
Carbohydrate	100 g (3 1/3 oz)	120 g (4 oz)
	410 cal	*492* cal
	1182 cal	1510 cal

A sample of the Von Noorden Diet is shown below:

Breakfast: Lean meat, 80 g (2 2/3 oz); bread, 25 g (1 oz); tea, 1 cup with milk, no sugar

Midforenoon: One egg

Luncheon: Soup, 1 small portion; lean meat, 160 g (5 1/3 oz); potatoes, 100 g (3 1/3 oz); fruit, 100 g (3 1/3 oz);

Afternoon: 3 PM: Cup of black coffee,
4 PM: Fruit, 200 g (6 2/3 oz)
6 PM: Milk, 250 cc (8 oz)

Dinner: Meat, 125 g (3 1/6 oz); bread (graham), 30 g (1 oz); fruit, small portion as sauce without sugar; salad, vegetable or fruit, radishes, pickles

Ebstein's Diet

At the other extreme is the high-fat diet illustrated by Ebstein. Ebstein modified existing diets by allowing a considerable amount of fat and restricting the carbohydrates by forbidding all sugar, sweets, and potatoes, but allowing 180–210 g (6–7 oz) of bread. Vegetables that grow aboveground are allowed, and all sorts of meat, especially fat meat, is permitted. Fats are allowed, 120–180 g (4–6 oz) per day. He used a three-meal plan with the largest meal at midday.

Breakfast: One large cup of black tea, without cream or milk, or sugar; white or brown bread, 60 g (2 oz) with plenty of butter

Dinner: 2 PM. Clear soup, meat 120–180 g (4–6 oz) with gravy, and fat meat is especially recommended; vegetables in abundance (as noted above); small amount of fresh or stewed fruit (without sugar) or salad; two or three glasses of light white wine. Shortly after dinner a cup of tea is allowed with sugar or milk.

Supper: 7:30 PM. Large cup of tea, without sugar or milk; one egg with or without a small portion of meat, preferably fat. Occasionally a little cheese or fresh fruit.

Total values: Protein, 100 g (3 1/3 oz); fat, 85 g (3 oz); carbohydrate, 50 g (2 2/3 oz)

These two themes, the low-fat/high-protein/high-carbohydrate diet and the high-fat/low-carbohydrate diet were repeating themes through the 20th century, but their origins were in the late 19th century. Had either of these approaches "cured" obesity, as their proponents often suggested, there would have been no need for the continual supply of new diets which we saw throughout the 20th century (35).

As a prelude to its clinical application the metabolic features of starvation were explored by Benedict using metabolic chambers (109,110) and the suggestion that calories could be dissipated by *luxuskonsumption*, or burning off of unneeded calories, was promulgated by Gulick (214) and Neumann (215) but challenged by the critical studies of Wiley and Newburgh (216).

A practical application of the work on starvation was published by Evans et al. (217), who showed the potential benefits of a very low calorie diet. Although Evans continued to publish on this approach to diet until the beginning of World War II (217), this idea was lost sight of until "fasting" was reintroduced as a treatment for obesity by Bloom in 1959 (218). Following his enthusiastic report, the use of liquid formula diets that were initially popularized from the Rockefeller University metabolic ward increased gradually and then rapidly increased until a major crisis followed with the report of 17 deaths in patients using a formula diet compounded from gelatin (219). Although the Gelatin Commission in France in the 19th century (220) had concluded that gelatin was an inadequate protein, this lesson was relearned painfully in the 1970s (122,221). New diets subsequently appeared using high-quality protein, and sales reached another peak in the late 1980s. When the U.S. Government raised concerns about these diets and other "commercial weight control" programs (222), there was a rapid and sudden decrease in public interest and a loss of commercial profitability.

2 Behavior Modification

One of the central developments in the treatment of obesity in the 20th century was in the behavioral field. Following the introduction of psychoanalytic techniques by Freud and his colleagues (223), several theories were proposed suggesting that obesity might result from "personality" disorders. These were carefully tested and found to be wanting (224). That obesity had important social components, however, became clear from its relation to socioeconomic status (225). The prevalence of obesity was found to be much higher in the lower social and economic groups than in the higher social and economic groups in the seminal Manhattan study.

Although psychoanalytic approaches were unproductive as a basis for treatment, other avenues of behavioral research were productive. One of these flows from the work on conditioned reflexes by Pavlov and his followers (226), and another from the work on operant behavior by Skinner (227,228). It was an adaptation of these latter techniques that was used by Stuart (229) in his classic study in 1967. Stuart treated 11 patients, 8 of whom were available for follow-up at the end of the year. In this group, weight losses using techniques of monitoring food intake and manipulating the environment in which it was eaten were indeed striking. Subsequent to this seminal work, the principles of behavior modification have been widely applied, and some would consider them to have been central to the treatment of obesity in the late 20th century.

3 Pharmacotherapy

As the understanding of pharmacology has increased, so too has its application to treatment of obesity become more focused. Although one might call Withering the Father of Pharmacology because he published his findings on digitalis (230) in 1785, the first chemical work was in the early 19th century and during the important period of French hegemony in medicine (38). A summary of 19th century treatments is provided by Sajous (231):

> Besides the familiar dietetic treatment, thyroid gland is used to enhance catabolism, but not in the large doses usually prescribed, which provide hypercatabolism and greatly weaken the patient. From 2 to 3 grains (132 to 196 mg) t.i.d. are enough to increase gradually the lipolytic power of the blood. Potassium iodide in increasing doses can be used instead, when thyroid extract cannot be obtained. Hyoscine hydrobromate 1/100 grain t.i.d. assists the reducing process by increasing the propulsive activity of the arterioles and causing them to drive an excess of blood into the fat-laden areas. Carlsbad, Homburg, and Marienbad waters owe their virtues mainly to the alkaline

and purgative salts they contain, especially sodium sulphate. As a beverage alkaline Vichy water is advantageous to enhance the osmotic properties of the blood and facilitate the elimination of wastes.

Shortly after their discovery in the 19th century, endocrine organ extracts were used for the treatment of obesity as early as the 1890s (231):

> The fact that thyroid preparations in sufficient doses promote the rapid combustion of fats has caused them to be used extensively in this disorder. In large doses (thyroid gland) . . . imposes hyperoxidation upon all cells . . . we behold gradual emaciation beginning with the adipose tissues, which are the first to succumb. Hence the use of thyroid preparations in obesity. Sajous goes on to say that small doses (66 mg or 1 grain) are indicated in all cases to begin with: "Briefly, in all cases of obesity in which thyroid gland is rationally indicated, the feature to determine is whether directly or indirectly hypothyroidia underlies the adiposis" (231).

Sajous also describes the use of testicular extracts: "Testicular preparations, including spermine, have been recommended in a host of disorders, particularly . . .obesity . . . but others again have failed to obtain any favorable results" (231).

The first serendipitous observation on the use of aniline-derived drugs was the publication by Lesses and Myerson (156) of the hypothesis that amphetamines might be useful in the treatment of obesity. This molecule underwent many chemical medications including the synthesis of fenfluramine, a drug that was shown to act on serotonergic mechanisms. Realizing that both serotonergic and noradrenergic receptors were involved in modulating food intake, Weintraub et al. in 1992 published a 4-year study showing that combination therapy might be better than monotherapy (232). This classic series of papers has opened a whole new pharmacologic approach to obesity. As has often happened in obesity, this strategy came to an abrupt end in 1997 when valvular insufficiency was reported (233), leading to withdrawal of fenfluramine and dexfenfluramine from the market.

4 Surgery

Surgical intervention for excess fat can be dated from Talmudic days. According to Preuss (234), Rabbi Eleazar was given a sleeping potion and taken into a marble chamber where his abdomen was opened and many basketfuls of fat were removed. "Plinius also describes a very similar 'heroic cure for obesity': the son of the Consul L. Apronius had fat removed and thus his body was relieved of a disgraceful burden." More recently, in AD 1190, a surgeon cut open the abdomen of Count Dedo II of Groig in order to remove the excessive fat from him (p 215). Following the advent of anesthesia in 1846, this procedure has been revived.

The historical view of gastrointestinal function in relation to obesity may be perceived to have reached its zenith (or nadir, depending on one's perspective) with the introduction of gastrointestinal operations for obesity. Three operative approaches have been developed to treat obesity.

The first procedure reported by Kremen (235) was a jejunoileal bypass on a single patient. Believing that if weight were lost, patients would be able to maintain the weight loss, Payne and DeWind performed a series of 11 jejunocolic anatamoses that produced significant diarrhea and weight loss (236). When the patients were reanastamosed, they regained weight. Against this background, these authors and many others carried out jejunoileal bypass operations that were associated with numerous metabolic and infectious complications and were largely discontinued as a surgical approach to obesity in the 1970s.

An alternative approach to altering gastrointestinal function to treat obesity was developed by Mason and Ito (237) who performed the first gastric reduction operation. These procedures have now become the dominant operative procedures for the treatment of obesity and are the subject of a major clinical trial in Sweden (238).

V TOWARD A SCIENCE OF OBESITY

Toward the end of the Middle Ages, two historical and philosophic traditions, one of Indo-European origin with Greco-Roman philosophy as its base, and the other of Semitic origin with the Hebrew and Christian traditions as its base, reached a form of resolution synthesis in the Hegelian sense (239) from which the Renaissance and Modern Science both took their roots (1,240).

The modern scientific tradition is the tradition of "experimental" science. That is, progress was made by designing "experiments" to test hypotheses and apply mathematical analysis to the results. The fruitfulness of this tradition is everywhere around us. Its application to obesity has come, as it has come to all other areas, but progress has been slow. From the beginning of the Scientific Era (AD 1500) to the beginning of Modern Medicine (AD 1800), only a few scholarly theses with obesity as the subject matter had been published (241–246). In general, these theses reflected the traditions of Hippocrates, Galen, or Avicenna, as interpreted in the more contemporary traditions provided by the iatrochemical and iatromechanical views of the words originating in the mechanical and chemical explanations of life. As interest in obesity increased, a much larger number of theses with obesity as the subject were published in the 18th century (247–280), which also saw publication of the first monographs on the subject (281,282). Table 3 is a list of most English, French, and German monographs up to 1950 (281–321).

There were two works published in English before 1800. The first of these was by Thomas Short (281). He begins by saying, "I believe no age did ever afford more instances of corpulency than our own." From Short's perspective, treatment of obesity required restoring the natural balance and removal of the secondary causes. One should, if possible, pick a place to live where the air is not too moist or too soggy, and one should not reside in flat, wet countries or in the city or the woodlands. He thought that exercise was important and that the diet should be "moderate spare and of the more detergent kind."

Table 3 Monographs on Obesity

English	French	German
18th century		
Short (281)		
Flemyng (282)		
19th century		
Wadd (69,296)	Maccary (177)	Kisch (302)
Chambers (297)	Dancel (300)	Ebstein (303)
Harvey J (298)	Worthington (301)	
Harvey W (299)		
20th century		
Williams (304)	Leven (313)	Von Noorden (318)
Christie (305)	Haeckel (314)	Pfaundler (319)
Rony (306)	Le Noir (315)	Gries et al. (320)
Rynearson and Gastineau (307)	Boivin (316)	Bray (321)
Craddock (308)	Cref and Herschberg (317)	
Bruch (309)		
Mayer (310)		
Garrow (311)		
Stunkard (312)		

A second monograph by Flemyng (282) listed four causes of corpulency. The first cause is "the taking in of too large a quantity of food, especially of the rich and oily kind." He went on to note that not all obese people were big eaters. The second cause of obesity is "too lax a texture of the cellular or fatty membrane. . .whereby its cells or vesicles are liable to be too easily distended." The third cause was an abnormal state of the blood that facilitated the storage of fat in the vesicles.

Finally, defective evacuation was also an important cause. Since Flemyng believed that sweat, urine, and feces all contained "oil," he believed that the treatment for obesity was to increase the loss of "oil" by each of these three routes. Thus, laxatives and diuretics could be used for treatment.

From the beginning of the 19th century, the base of medical literature relating to obesity increased rapidly. *Corpulency* and *polysarcy* were the terms most in use at the beginning of the 19th century, but by the end of the century, *obesity* had replaced both of them. Additional monographs on obesity appeared in English, French, and German. The cell theory was proposed and fat cells were identified. The laws of thermodynamics were developed and tested in animals and human beings by the first part of the 20th century.

I have picked the year 1850 as a dividing line for the beginning of a modern science of obesity (283). This was the time when the French Clinical School which began at the French Revolution went into its long decline and the German Laboratory School began its rapid ascent. This was after the fat cell had been described, the Quetelet (BMI) Index had been published, and the conservation of energy had been proposed (284). From 1850 to the beginning of World War II, the hegemony of German Laboratory Science in the field of obesity and elsewhere was evident (283).

With the advent of the 20th century, concerns about the relation of obesity to health risks gradually replaced concerns about being underweight (35). As the 20th century progressed, four themes coalesced to form the basis of a modern science of obesity. These include the behavioral or psychological aspects of obesity, the physiological approach to a controlled system of food intake, the cellular basis for obesity centered in the growing diversity of cellular functions for the fat cell, and the genetic and molecular biological approaches to understanding the problem.

From the beginning of World War II and the monograph by Rony (306), a period of American hegemony began. In the post–World War II period, the growth of the National Institutes of Health has served as a major stimulus for research in obesity

(285). Several important events occurred which brought the scientific threads of obesity together. The first was the formation of many associations for the study of obesity. The first of them was formed in the United Kingdom and held its first meeting in 1968 (286). This was followed in 1972 by the first Fogarty Center Conference on Obesity (287), and 1 year later by the First International Congress on Obesity (288). Following that congress, it was clear that a journal devoted to obesity was needed, and the *International Journal of Obesity* began publication in 1976 under the editorship of Dr. Alan Howard and Dr. George Bray. The first meeting of the North American Association for the Study of Obesity was held at Vassar College in Poughkeepsie, NY, in 1982. Subsequent International Congresses were held in 1977 in Washington, DC (289); in 1980 in Rome (290); in 1983 in New York City (291); in 1986 in Jerusalem (292) in 1990 in Kobe, Japan (293); in 1994 in Toronto (294); in 1998 in Paris (295); and in 2002 in Sao Paulo. In 1986 the International Association for the Study of Obesity was formed under the leadership of Dr. Barbara Caleen Hansen. As growth continued, a second journal appeared in 1980 under the title *Obesity and Weight Regulation*. This journal, like so many others, succumbed in part because it was not part of one of the national associations. *Obesity Surgery* was the third journal to be founded and was followed in 1993 by *Obesity Research*, published by the North American Association for the Study of Obesity. This rapid growth of scientific institutions surrounding a scientific discipline is characteristic of developments which have sprung up throughout the scientific sphere to provide a way of focusing the activities of scientists in a *manageable way*.

REFERENCES

1. Gaarder J. Sophie's World. (Translated by P. Moller.) London: Phoenix House, 1995.
2. Crombie AC, ed. Scientific Changes. Historical Studies in the Intellectual, Social and Technical Conditions for Scientific Discovery and Technical Investigation, from Antiquity to the Present. New York: Basic Books, 1963.
3. Bray GA. Obesity: historical development of scientific and cultural ideas. Int J Obes 1990;14:909–926.
4. Bray GA. Temperature, food intake, and the internal milieu. Obes Res 1997;5(6):638–640.
5. Bray GA. Anorexia nervosa and socio-economic status. Obes Res 1997;5(5):489–491.
6. Bray GA. Amino acids, protein, and body weight. Obes Res 1997;5(4):373–376.
7. Bray GA. Growth of a molecular base for feeding: the mind body dualism. Obes Res 1997;5(3):271–274.
8. Bray GA. Archeology of mind—obesity and psychoanalysis. Obes Res 1997;5(2):153–156.
9. Bray GA. Energy expenditure using doubly labeled water: the unveiling of objective truth. Obes Res 1997; 5(1):71–77.
10. Bray GA. Methods and obesity research: the radioimmunoassay of insulin. Obes Res 1996;4(6):579–582.
11. Bray GA. Static theories in a dynamic world: a glucodynamic theory of food intake. Obes Res 1996;4(5): 489–492.
12. Bray GA. Eat slowly—from laboratory to clinic; behavioral control of eating. Obes Res 1996;4(4):397–400.
13. Bray GA. Obesity and surgery for a chronic disease. Obes Res 1996;4(3):301–303.
14. Bray GA. Body fat distribution and the distribution of scientific knowledge. Obes Res 1996;4(2):189–192.
15. Bray GA. Hereditary adiposity in mice: human lessons from the yellow and obese (OB/OB) mice. Obes Res 1996;4(1):91–95.
16. Bray GA. The tide shifts again: the ebb and flow of history. Obes Res 1995;3(6):605–608.
17. Bray GA. Luxuskonsumption—myth or reality? Obes Res 1995;3(5):491–495.
18. Bray GA. Laurence, Moon, Bardet, and Biedl: reflections on a syndrome. Obes Res 1995;3(4):383–386.
19. Bray GA. The indexing waltz. Obes Res 1995;3(4): 357–359.
20. Bray GA. Measurement of body composition: an improving art. Obes Res 1995;3(3):291–293.
21. Bray GA. From very-low-energy diets to fasting and back. Obes Res 1995;3(2):207–209.
22. Bray GA. Life insurance and overweight. Obes Res 1995;3:97–99.
23. Bray GA. Obesity research and medical journalism. Obes Res 1995;3:65–71.
24. Bray GA. The inheritance of corpulence. Obes Res 1994;2:601–605.
25. Bray GA. Harvey Cushing and the neuroendocrinology of obesity. Obes Res 1994;2:482–485.
26. Bray GA. What's in a name? Mr. Dickens' "Pickwickian" fat boy syndrome. Obes Res 1994;2:380–383.
27. Bray GA. Lavoisier and scientific revolution: the oxygen theory displaces air, fire, earth and water. Obes Res 1994;2:183–188.
28. Bray GA. Commentary on classics in obesity. 6. Science and politics of hunger. Obes Res 1993;1(6): 489–493.
29. Bray GA. Commentary on Classics in Obesity 5. Fat cell theory and units of knowledge. Obes Res 1993; 1(5):403–407.
30. Bray GA. Commentary on Classics of Obesity 4. Hypothalamic obesity. Obes Res 1993;1(4):325–328.

31. Bray GA. Commentary on Atwater classic. Obes Res 1993;1(3):223–227.
32. Bray GA. Letter on corpulence. Obes Res 1993;1:153–163.
33. Bray GA. Commentary on Banting letter. Obes Res 1993;1(2):148–152.
34. Martinie J. Notes sur l'Histoire de l'Obesité. Thesis de Paris 1934. Paris: Les Presses Universitaires de France, 1934.
35. Schwartz H. Never Satisfied. A Cultural History of Diets, Fantasies and Fat. New York: Doubleday, 1986.
36. Needham J. Science and Civilization in China. Cambridge: Cambridge University Press, 1988, 6 vols.
37. Singer C, Homyard EJ, Hall AR, Williams TI. A History of Technology. New York: Oxford University Press, 1954–1958, 5 vols.
38. Ackerknecht EH. Medicine at the Paris Hospital. Baltimore: Johns Hopkins University Press, 1967.
39. Foucault M. The Birth of the Clinic. An Archaeology of Medical Perception. New York: Vintage Books, 1973.
40. Gamble C. The Palaeolithic Settlement of Europe. Cambridge: Cambridge University Press, 1986.
41. Stephen-Chauvet. La Médicine chez les Peuples Primitifs. Paris: Librairie Maloine, 1936.
42. Beller AS. Fat & Thin. A Natural History of Obesity. New York: Farrar, Straus and Giroux, 1977.
43. Hautin RJR. Obesity. Conceptions actuelles Thèse pour le Doctorat en Médicine. Bordeaux: Imprimerie Bier, 1939.
44. Kulacoglu, B. Gods and Goddesses. (Translated by J. Ozturk.) Anhura: Museum of Anatolian Civilizations, 1992.
45. Garrison F. An Introduction to the History of Medicine. Philadelphia: W.B. Saunders, 1914.
46. Contenau G. La médicine en Assyrie et en Babylonie. Paris: Librairie Maloine, 1938.
47. Spycket A. Kassite and middle Elamite sculpture. In: Later Mesopotamia and Iran. Tribes and Empires 1600–538 BC. London: British Museum Press, 1995, p 30 plate 18.
48. Smith E. The Edwin Smith Surgical Papyrus. (Published in facsimile and hieroglyphic transliteration with translation and commentary in two volumes by James Henry Breasted.) Chicago: University of Chicago Press, 1930. Classics of Medicine, Special Edition, 1984.
49. Darby WJ, Ghalioungui P, Grevetti L. Food: The Gift of Osiris. London: Academic Press, 1977, p 60.
50. Nunn JF. Ancient Egyptian Medicine. London: British Museum Press, 1996.
51. Reeves C. Egyptian Medicine. London: Shire Publications, 1992.
52. Eiler I. Egyptian Bookshelf Disease. London: British Museum Press, 1995.
53. Alphen JV, Aris A. Oriental Medicine: An Illustrated Guide to the Asian Arts of Healing. Boston: Shambhala, 1996.
54. Tibetan Medical Paintings. Illustrations to the Blue Beryl Treatise of Sangye Gyamtso. (1635–1705). New York: Henry N. Abrams, 1992.
55. Iason AH. The Thyroid Gland in Medical History. New York: Frobin Press, 1946.
56. Ortiz de Montellano BR. Aztec Medicine, Health and Nutrition. New Brunswick: Rutgers University Press, 1990.
57. Vogel VJ. American Indian Medicine. Norman: University of Oklahoma Press, 1970.
58. Hippocrates. Oeuvres Complètes d'Hippocrate. (Traduction nouvelle avec le texte grec en regard. . .par E. Littre.) Paris: J.B. Ballière, 1839.
59. Kryger MH. Sleep apnea. From the needles of Dionysius to continuous positive airway pressure. Arch Intern Med 1983;143:2301–2303.
60. Kryger MH. Fat, sleep, and Charles Dickens: literary and medical contributions to the understanding of sleep apnea. Clin Chest Med 1985;6:555–562.
61. Campbell D. Arabian medicine and its influence on the Middle Ages. London: Kegan Paul, Trench, Trubner & Co, 1926, 2 vols.
62. Beaujouan G. Motives and opportunities for science in the medieval universities. In: Scientific Change. Historical Studies in the Intellectual, Social and Technical Conditions for Scientific Discovery and Technical Invention, from Antiquity to the Present. Crombie AC, ed. New York: Basic Books, 1963, pp 232–234.
63. Vesalius A. De humani corporis fabrica. Basileae: ex off. Joannis Oporini, 1543.
64. Copernicus N. De revolutionibusorbium colestium. Libri VI. Norimberg: Apud Ioh. Petrium, 1543.
65. Bonetus T. Sepulchretum, sive anatomia practica, ex cadaveribus morbo denatis, proponens historias omnium humani corporis affectum. Genevae: Sumptibus Cramer & Perachon, 1700.
66. Morgagni GB. De sedibus, et causis morborum per anatomen indagatis libriquinque. Venetiis: typog. Remordiniana, 1761.
67. Haller A. Corpulence ill cured; large cryptae of the stomach (etc). Path Observ 1756;44–49.
68. Haller A. Elementa physiologiae corporis humani. Lausanne: Marci–Michael Boursquet & Sociorum, 1757.
69. Wadd W. Comments on corpulency lineaments of leanness mems on diet and dietetics. London: John Ebers & Co., 1829.
70. Malpighi M. Opera Omnia. Londini: R. Scott, 1686.
71. Hooke R. Micrographia or some physiological descriptions of minute bodies made by magnifying glasses; with observations and inquiries thereupon. London: J. Martyn & J. Allestry, 1665–1667.

72. Van Leeuwenhoek A. The Select Works of Antony van Leeuwenhoek, Containing His Microscopical Discoveries in Many of the Works of Nature. (Translated from the Dutch and Latin editions by Samual Hoole.) London: G. Sidney, 1800.
73. Schwann T. Mikroscopische Untersuchungen uber di Ubereinstimmung in der Struktur un dem Wachstum der Thiere und Pflanzen. Berlin: Sander, 1839.
74. Schleiden MJ. Beitrage zur Phytogenesis. Arch Anat Physiol Wiss Med 1839;137–176.
75. Henle FGJ. Allgemeine Anatomie. Leipzig: L. Voss, 1841.
76. Hassall A. The microscopic anatomy of the human body, in health and disease. London: Samuel Highley, 1849.
77. Hoggan G, Hogan FE. On the development and retrogression of the fat cell. J R Microsc Soc 1879;2:353.
78. Hassall A. Observations on the development of the fat vesicle. Lancet 1849;i:63–64.
79. Bjurlf P. Atherosclerosis and body build with special reference to size and number of subcutaneous fat cells. Acta Med Scand 1959;166 (suppl 349):99.
80. Hirsch J, Kittle JL. Cellularity of obese and nonobese human adipose tissue. Fed Proc 1970;29:1516–1521.
81. Bjorntorp P, Sjostrom L. Number and size of adipose tissue fat cells in relation to metabolism in human obesity. Metabolism 1971;20:703–713.
82. Virchow R. Die Cellularpathologiein inrer Begrundung auf physiologische and pathologische Gewebelehre. Berlin: August Hirschwald, 1858.
83. Knoll M, Ruska E. Beitrag zur geometrischen Electronenoptik. Ann Physik 1932;12:607–661.
84. Renold AE, Cahill GF, eds. Handbook of Physiology. Section 5. Adipose Tissue. Bethesda, MD: American Physiological Society, 1965.
85. Harvey W. The Anatomical Exercises of Dr. William Harvey. De Motu Cordis 1628: De Circulatione Sanguinis 1649. (The first English text of 1653 edited by Geoffrey Keynes.) London: Nonesuch Press, 1928.
86. Osler W. The Evolution of Modern Medicine. New Haven: Yale University Press, 1921.
87. Santorio S. A new art of Physick. Contained in eight sections of aphorisms, concerning insensible perspiration; being a vapor of breathing from the body. Plainly shewing that health and sickness is best discerned by weighing the body. (Translated by Abdiah Cole.) London: Peter Cole, 1663.
88. Santorio, Santorio. Medicina Statica: Being the aphorisms of Sanctorius, translated into English with large explanations. The second edition. To which is added Dr. Keil's Medicina statica Britannica, with comparative remarks and explanations. As also medic-physical essays. . .by John Quincy. London: W. and J. Newton, A. Bell, W. Taylor and J. Osborne, 1720.
89. Newburgh LH, Johnston MW. The exchange of energy between man and the environment. Springfield, IL: Charles C. Thomas, 1930.
90. Reamur RAF. Sur la digestion des oiseaux. His Acad R Sci 1756;266–307, 461–495.
91. Spallanzani L. Opusculi di fisica animale e vegetabile. Moedena: Soc: tipografica, 1776, 2 vols.
92. Spallanzani L. Dissertationsrelative to the natural history of animals and vegetables. London: J. Murray and S. Highley, 1796. 2 vols.
93. Beaumont. Experiments and Observations on the Gastric Juices and the physiology of digestion. Plattsburgh: FP Allen, 1833.
94. Bernard C. De l'origine du sucre dans l'économie animale. Arch Gen Med 1848;18(4th ser):303–319.
95. Cannon WB, Washburn AL. An explanation of hunger. Am J Physiol 1912;29:441–454.
96. Carlson AJ. The control of hunger in health and disease. Chicago: University of Chicago Press, 1916.
97. Partington JR. A Short History of Chemistry, 2d ed. London: Macmillan, 1951.
98. Boyle R. The Works of the Honourable Robert Boyle. London: A. Millar, 1764.
99. Stahl GE. Theoria medica vera. Physiologiam & pathologiam. Halae, Literis Ophanotrophei, 1708.
100. Priestley J. Experiments and Observation on Different Kinds of Air. London: J. Johnson 1775.
101. Scheele CW. The Discovery of Oxygen, Part 2. Edinburgh: William F. Clay, 1894.
102. Lavoisier AL. Traité Elédmentiare de Chemie, Présenté dans un Order Nouveau et d'Après les Couvertes Modernes. Paris: Chez Cuchet, 1789.
103. Helmholtz HLF. Uber die Erhaltung der Kraft, eine physikalische Abhandlung. Berlin: G. Reimer, 1847.
104. Rubner M. Die gesetze des Energieverbrauchs bei der Ernahrung. Leipzig: Franz Deuticke, 1902.
105. Rubner M. The Laws of Energy Consumption in Nutrition. New York: Academic Press, 1982.
106. Pettenkofer MJ, Voit C. Untersuchuingenuber die Respiration. Ann Chem Pharm (Heidelberg) 1862–63 (suppl 2):52–70.
107. Atwater WO, Rosa EB. Description of a new respiration calorimeter and experiments on the conservation of energy in the human body. US Department of Agriculture Office of Experimental Station 1899; 63.
108. Atwater WO, Benedict FG. Experiments on the Metabolism of Matter and Energy in the Human Body, 1900–1902. Washington: Government Printing Office, 1903.
109. Benedict FG. A study of prolonged fasting. Washington: Carnegie Institution, Report No. 203, 1915.
110. Benedict FG, Miles WR, Roth P, Smith HM. Human Vitality and Efficiency Under Prolonged Restricted Diet. Washington: Carnegie Institute, 1919, pub. No. 280.
111. Jequier E, Schutz Y. Long-term measurements of

energy expenditure in humans using a respiration chamber. Am J Clin Nutr 1983;989–998.
112. Garrow J. Energy Balance and Obesity in Man, 2d ed. Amsterdam: Elsevier/North Holland, 1978.
113. Ravussin E, Swinburn BA. Pathophysiology of obesity. Lancet 1992;340:404–408.
114. Schoeller DA, Van Santen E, Peterson DW, Dietz W, Jaspan J, Klein PD. Total body water measurement in humans with O and H labeled water. Am J Clin Nutr 1980;33:2686–2693.
115. Lichtman SW, Pisarska K, Berman ER, et al. Discrepancy between self-reported and actual caloric intake and exercise in obese subjects. N Engl J Med 1992;327:1893–1898.
116. Wohler F. Ueber kunstliche Bildung des Harnstoffs. Ann Phys Chem (Leipzig) 1828;12:253–256.
117. Bernard C. Sur le méchanisme de la formation du sucre dans le foie. C R Acad Sci 1855;41:461–469.
118. Magendie F. Précis ÉlÉmentaire de Physiologie. Paris: Mequignon-Marvis, 1816.
119. Liebeg JV. Chemistry and its application to agriculture and physiology. (Translated by Lyon Playfair.) London: Taylor and Walton, 1842.
120. Bernard C. Memoire sur le pancréas et sur le role du suc pancréatique dans les phénomènes digestif. Suppl C R Acad Sci (Paris)1856;1:379–563.
121. Kuhn TS. The Structure of Scientific Revolutions. Chicago: University of Chicago Press, 1962.
122. McCollum EV. A history of nutrition. The sequence of ideas in nutrition investigations. Boston: Houghton Mifflin, 1957.
123. Select Committee on Nutrition and Human Needs (hearing) of the United States Senate 95th Congress. Diet Related to Killer Diseases. Washington: Government Printing Office, 1977. Vols VI, VII (2VI, 2VII).
124. Society of Actuaries. Build Study of 1979. City Recording and Statistical Corp, 1980.
125. Behnke AR Jr, Feen BG, Welham WC. The specific gravity of healthy men. Body weight divided by volume as an index of obesity. JAMA 1942;118:495–498.
126. Hevesy G. Radioactive Indicators. Their Application in Biochemistry, Animal Physiology, and Pathology. New York: Interscience Publishers, 1948.
127. Moore FD, Olesen KH, McMurrey JD, Parker HV, Ball MR, Boyden CM. The Body Cell Mass and Its Supporting Environment. Philadelphia: W.B. Saunders, 1963.
128. Wang Z, Pierson RN, Heymsfield SB. The five-level model: a new approach to organizing body composition. Am J Clin Nutr 1992;56(1):19–28.
129. Darwin C. On the Origin of Species by Means of Natural Selection or the Preservation of Favoured Races in the Struggle for Life. London: John Murray, 1859.
130. Bateson W. Mendel's Principles of Heredity: A Defence. London: Cambridge University Press, 1902.
131. Garrod AE. Inborn Errors of Metabolism. The Coonian Lectures Delivered Before the Royal College of Physicians of London, in June, 1908. London: Henry Frowde, Hodder & Stoughton, Oxford University Press, 1909.
132. Watson JD, Crick FH. Molecular structure of nucleic acids: a structure for deoxyribose nucleic acid. Nature 1953;171(4356):737–738.
133. Bultman SJ, Michaud EJ, Woychik RP. Molecular characterization of the mouse agouti locus. Cell 1992;71:1195–1204.
134. Zhang YY, Proenca R, Maffei M, Barone M, Leopold L, Friedman JM. Positional cloning of the mouse obese gene and its human homolog. Nature 1994;372: 425–432.
135. Naggert JK, Fricker LD, Varlamov O, et al. Hyperproinsulinaemiain obese fat/fat mice associated with a carboxypeptidase-e mutation which reduces enzyme-activity. Nat Genet 1995;10:135–142.
136. Rankinen T, Perusse L, Weisnagel SJ, Snyder E, Chagnon Y, Bouchard C. The human obesity gene map: the 2001 update. Obes Res 10:196–243.
137. Davenport CB. Body Build and Its Inheritance. Washington: Carnegie Institution, 1923;329:37.
138. Verschuer OV. Die VerebungsbiologischeZwillingsforschung.Ihre Biologischen Grundlagen. Mit 18 Abbildungen. Ergebnisse der Inneren Medizin und Kinderheilkunde, 31st ed. Berlin: Verlag Von Julius Springer, 1927.
139. Vogler GP, Sorensen TI, Stunkard AJ, Srinivassen MR, Rao DC. Influences of genes and shared family environment on adult body mass index assessed in an adoption study by a comprehensive path model. Int J Obes 1995;19:40–45.
140. Bouchard C, Despres J, Mauriege P. Genetic and nongenetic determinants of regional fat distribution. Endocrin Rev 1993;14(l):72–93.
141. Bouchard C, Perusse L. Current status of the human obesity gene map. Obes Res 1996;4:81–90.
142. Warden CH, Fisler JS, Shoemaker SM, et al. Identification of 4 chromosomal loci determining obesity in a multifactorial mouse model. J Clin Invest 1995;95: 1545–1552.
143. West DB, Goudey-Lefevre J, York B, Truett GE. Dietary obesity linked to genetic-loci on chromosome-9 and chromosome-15 in a polygenic mouse model. J Clin Invest 1994;94:1410–1416.
144. Paracelsus. Wunder artzney, vonn allerley leibs gebrochen, unnd zu fallende Krankheiten, ohn sondere Beschwerung, Unlust unnd Verdrusz, kurtzlich zu heilen, unnd die Gesundheit widerumb mit geringem Kosten zun Wegen zubringen.... Basel: Sebastian Henricpetri, 1573. Sm 8vo modern calf. History of Medicine, not in Osler, Wellcome or Waller.
145. Magendie F. Formulary for the preparation and employment of several new remedies, namely, resin

of nux vomica, strychnine, morphine, hydrocyanic acid, preparations of cinchona.... (Translated from the Formulaire of M. Magendie, published in Paris, October 1827.) London: T. and G. Underwood, 1828.
146. Wells H. A History of the Discovery of the Application of Nitrous Oxide Gas, Ether, and Other Vapors to Surgical Operations. Hartford: J. Gaylord Wells, 1847.
147. Warren E. Some Account of the Letheon: Or, Who Is the Discoverer of Anesthesia. Boston: Dutton and Wentworth, 1847.
148. Bowditch NL. The Ether Controversy. Vindication of the Hospital Report of 1848. Boston: John Wilson, 1848.
149. Lister J. On the effects of the antiseptic system of treatment upon the salubrity of a surgical hospital. Lancet 1870;1:4–6, 40–42.
150. Lister JB. The Collected Papers of Joseph, Baron Lister. Member of the Order of Merit, Fellow and Sometime President of the Royal Society, Knight Grand Cross of the Danish Order of the Danebrog Knight of the Prussian Order pour le Mérite Associé Etranger de l'Institut de France. Oxford: Clarendon Press, 1909.
151. Bray GA. Use and abuse of appetite-suppressant drugs in the treatment of obesity. Ann Intern Med 1993;119(7 pt 2):707–713.
152. Canguilhem G. Ideology and Rationality in the History of the Life Sciences. (Translated by A. Goldhammer.) Cambridge, MA: MIT Press, 1988.
153. Ehrlich P, Hata S. Die experimentelle Chemotherapie der Spirillosen. Berlin: Julius Springer, 1910.
154. Tainter ML, Stockton AB, Cutting WC. Use of dinitrophenol in obesity and related conditions. JAMA 1933;101:1472–1475.
155. Bray GA. The Obese Patient, 9th ed. Philadelphia: W.B. Saunders, 1976.
156. Lesses MF, Myerson A. Human autonomic pharmacology XVI: benzedrine sulfate as an aid in the treatment of obesity. N Engl J Med 1938;218:119–124.
157. Babinski MJ. Tumeur du corps pituitaire sans acromégalie et avec le développement des organes génitaux. Rev Neurol 1900;8:531–533.
158. Frohlich A. Ein fall von tumor der hypophysis cerebri ohne akromegalie. Wiener Klin Rdsch 1901;15:883–886.
159. Mohr B. Hypertrophie der Hypophysis cerebri und dadurch bedingter Druck auf die Hirngrundflache, insebesondere auf die Sehnerven, das Chiasma derselben und den linkseitigen Hirnschenkel. Wschr Ges Heilk 1840;6:565–571.
160. Smith PE. The disabilities caused by hypophysectomy and their repair. The tuberal (hypothalamic) syndrome in the rat. JAMA 1927;88:159–161.
161. Hetherington AW, Ranson SW. Hypothalamic lesions and adiposity in the rat. Anat Rec 1940;78:149–172.
162. Anand BK, Brobeck JR. Hypothalamic control of food intake in rats and cats. Yale J Biol Med 1951;24: 123–146.
163. Stellar E. The physiology of motivation. Psychol Rev 1954;5:22
164. Han PW. Hypothalamic obesity in rats without hyperphagia. Ann NY Acad Sci 1967;30:229–242.
165. Coleman DL. Obese and diabetes: two mutant genes causing diabetes-obesity syndromes in mice (review). Diabetologia 1978;14:141–148.
166. Bray GA, York DA. Hypothalamic and genetic obesity in experimental animals: an autonomic and endocrine hypothesis. Physiol Rev 1979;59:719–809.
167. Powley TL, Opsahl CA. Ventromedial hypothalamic obesity abolished by subdiaphragmatic vagotomy. Am J Physiol 1974;226:25–33.
168. Nishizawa Y, Bray GA. Ventromedial hypothalamic lesions and the mobilization of fatty acids. J Chem Invest 1978;61(3):714–721.
169. Rothwell NJ, Stock MJ. A role for brown adipose tissue in diet-induced thermogenesis. Nature 1979;281: 31–35.
170. Bayliss WM. Principles of General Physiology. London: Longmans, Green, 1918, 2d ed rev.
171. Gibbs J, Young RC, Smith GP. Cholecystokinin elicits satiety in rats with open gastric fistulas. Nature 245(5424):323–325,1973.
172. Stanley BG, Kyrkouli SE, Lampert S, Leibowitz SF. Neuropeptide Y chronically injected into the hypothalamus: a powerful neurochemical inducer of hyperphagia and obesity. Peptides 1986;7:1189–1192.
173. Celsus AAC. De Medicina with an English Translation by W.G. Spencer. London: Heinemann, 1935–1938, 3 vols.
174. Gould GM, Pyle WL. Anomalies and Curiosities of Medicine. New York: Julian Press, 1956.
175. Dubourg L. Recherches sur les causes de la polysarcie. Paris: A. Parent, 1864;54.
176. Schindler CS. Monstrose Fettsucht. Wiener Med Presse 1871;12:410–412, 436–439.
177. Maccary A. Traite sur la Polysarcie. Paris: Gabon, 1811.
178. Glais J. De la Grossesse Adipeuse. Paris: A. Parent, 1875;1–36.
179. Dupytren. Observation sur un cas d'obesité, suivie de maladie du coeur et de la mort. J Med Chir Pharm 1806;12:262–273.
180. Anonymous. The Life of That Wonderful and Extraordinarily Heavy Man, Daniel Lambert, from His Birth to the Moment of His Dissolution; with an Account of Men Noted for Their Corpulency, and Other Interesting Matter. New York: Samuel Wood & Sons, 1818.
181. Barkhausen. Merkwurdige allgemeine Fettablagerung bei einem Knaben von 5 1/4 Jahren. Hannov Ann f ges Heilk. 1843; 8:200–203.

182. Coe T. A letter from Dr. T. Coe, Physician at Chelmsford in Essex, to Dr. Cromwell Mortimer, Secretary R. S. concerning Mr. Bright, the fat man at Malden in Essex. Phil Trans 1751–1752;47:188–193.
183. Don WG. Remarkable case of obesity in a Hindoo boy aged twelve years. Lancet 1859;1:363.
184. Eschenmeyer. Beschreibung eines monstrosen fett Madchen, das in einem Alter von 10 jahren starb, nach dem es eine hohe van 5 fuss 3 zoll und ein Gewicht von 219 pfund erreicht hatte. Tubing Bl Naturw Arznk 1815;1:261–285.
185. Gordon S. Art. XV.—Reports of rare cases. IV. Case of extensive fatty degeneration in a boy 14 years of age. Death from obstructed arterial circulation. Dublin Q J Med Sci 1862; 33:340–349.
186. McNaughton J. Cases of Polysarcia Adiposa in Childhood. New York: C.S. Francis, 1829: 317–322.
187. Wood T. A sequel to the case of Mr. Thomas Wood, of Billericay, in the Country of Essex, by the same. Med Trans 1785;3:309–318.
188. Linnaeus Cv. Species *Plantarum*, Stockholm: Salvius, 1753.
189. Sauvages FB. Nosologia methodica sistens morborum classes juxta Sydenhami menen and botanicorum ordinem. Amstelodami: Fratrum de Tournes, 1768, 2 vols.
190. Cullen W. First Lines of the Practice of Physic, by William Cullen, M.D., Late Professor of the Practice of Physic in the University of Edinburgh, and Including the Definitions of the Nosology; with Supplementary Notes Chiefly Selected from Recent Authors, Who Have Contributed to the Improvement of Medicine by Peter Reid, M.D. Edinburgh: Abernethy and Walker, 1810, 2 vols.
191. Burwell CS, Robin ED, Whaley RD, Bickelman AG. Extreme obesity associated with alveolar hypoventilation: a Pickwickan syndrome. Am J Med 1956; 21:811–818.
192. Robin ED, ed. Claude Bernard and the Internal Environment. A Memorial Symposium. New York; Marcel Dekker, 1979.
193. Russell J. A case of polysarka, in which death resulted from deficient arterialisation of the blood. Br Med J 1866; i:220–221.
194. Cushing H. The Pituitary Body and Its Disorders. Clinical States Produced by Disorders of the Hypophysis Cerebri. Philadelphia: J.B. Lippincott, 1912.
195. Cushing H. The basophil adenomas of the pituitary body and their clinical manifestations. Pituitary basophilism. Bull Johns Hopkins Hosp 1932; L:137–195.
196. Quetelet A. Sur l'Homme et le Développement de ses Facultés, ou Essai de Physique Sociale. Paris: Bachelier, 1835.
197. Dawber TR. The Framingham Study: The Epidemiology of Atherosclerotic Disease. Cambridge: Harvard University Press, 1980.
198. Keys A, Aravanis C, Blackburn HW, et al. Epidemiological studies related to coronary heart disease: Characteristics of men aged 40–59 in seven countries. Acta Med Scand Suppl 1966;460:1–392.
199. Lew EA, Garfinkel L. Variations in mortality by weight among 750,000 men and women. J Chronic Dis 1979; 32:563–576.
200. Waaler HT. Height, weight and mortality: the Norwegian experience. Acta Med Scand 1984; 679:1–56.
201. Manson JE, Willett WC, Stampfer MJ, et al. Body weight and mortality among women. N Engl J Med 1995;333:677–685.
202. Vague J. La differenciation sexuelle. Facteur déterminant des furmes de l'obesité. Presse Med 1947;55:339–340.
203. Carter HS, Howe PE, Mason HH. Nutrition and Clinical Dietetics. Philadelphia: Lea and Febiger, 1917.
204. Flegal KM, Carroll MD, Kuczmarski RJ, Johnson CL. Overweight and obesity in the United States: prevalence and trends, 1960–1994. Int J Obes Relat Metab Disord 1998; 22(1):39–47.
205. Precope J. Hippocrates on Diet and Hygiene. London: Zeno, 952.
206. Green RM. A Translation of Galen's Hygiene (De Sanitate Tuenda). Springfield, IL: Charles C. Thomas, 1951.
207. Gruner OC. A Treatise on the Canon of Medicine of Avicenna Incorporating a Translation of the First Book. London: Luzac, 1930.
208. Harington J. The School of Salernum Regimen Sanitatis Salernitanum. New York: Paul Hoeber, 1920.
209. Tweedie J. Hints on Temperence and Exercise, Shewing Their Advantage in the Cure of Dyspepsia, Rheumatism, Polysarcia, and Certain States of Palsy. London: T. Rickaby, 1799.
210. Cornaro L. Sure and Certain Methods of Attaining a Long and Healthful Life: With Means of Correcting a Bad Constitution. London: D. Midwinter, 1737, 5th English ed, p 11.
211. Brillat-Savarin JA. The Physiology of Taste or, Meditations on Transcendental Gastronomy. (Translated from the French by M.F.K. Fisher.) San Francisco: Arion Press, 1994.
212. Banting W. A Letter on Corpulence Addressed to the Public. London: Harrison and Sons, 1863.
213. Harvey W. On Corpulence in Relation to Disease: With Some Remarks on Diet. London: Henry Renshaw, 1872.
214. Gulick A. A study of weight regulation in the adult human body during over-nutrition. Am J Physiol 1922;60:371–395.
215. Neumann RO. Experimentel Beitrage zur Lehre von dem taglichen Nahrungsbedarfdes Menschen unter besonderer Berucksichtigung der notwendigen Eiweifsmenge. Arch Hyg 1902;45:1–87.
216. Wiley FH, Newburgh LH. The doubtful nature of

"Luxuskonsumption." J Clin Invest 1931;10:733–744.
217. Evans FA. A radical cure of simple obesity by dietary measures alone. Atlantic Med J 1926;30:140–141.
218. Bloom WL. Fasting as an introduction to the treatment of obesity. Metabolism 1959;8:214–220.
219. Sours HE, Frattali VP, Brand CD, Feldman RA, Forbes AL, Swanson RC, Paris AL. Sudden death associated with very low calorie weight reduction regimens. Am J Clin Nutr 34:453–461, 1981.
220. Magendie F. Rapport fait à l'Academie des Sciences au nom de la Commission dite "de la gelatine." C R Acad Sci (Paris) 1841:237–283.
221. Carpenter KF. Protein and Energy: A Study of Changing Ideas in Nutrition. Cambridge: Cambridge University Press, 1994.
222. U.S. House of Representatives. Hearing before the Subcommittee on Regulation, Business Opportunities, and Energy of the Committee on Small Business. Deception and Fraud in the Diet Industry, Part I. Washington: Government Printing Office, 1990.
223. Freud S. The Interpretation of Dreams. (Authorized translation of third edition with introduction by A.A. Brill, PhD, MD.) New York: Macmillan, 1913.
224. Stunkard AJ, Mendelson M. Obesity and the body image. I. Characteristics of disturbances in the body image of some obese persons. Am J Psychiatry 123: 1296–1300,1967.
225. Moore ME, Stunkard AJ, Srole L. Obesity, social class, and mental illness. JAMA 1962;181:962–966.
226. Pavlov IP. Conditioned Reflexes: An Investigation of the Physiological Activity of the Cerebral Cortex. (Transl by G.V. Anrep.) London: Oxford University Press, 1928.
227. Skinner BF. Science and Human Behavior. New York: Macmillan, 1953.
228. Ferster CB, Nurenberger JI, Levitt EB. The control of eating. J Math 1962;1:87–109.
229. Stuart RB. Behavioral control of overeating. Behav Res Ther 1967;5:357–365.
230. Withering W. An Account of the Foxglove and Some of Its Medical Uses: With Practical Remarks on Dropsy and Other Diseases. Birmingham: M. Swinney, 1785.
231. De Sajous CE. The Internal Secretion and the Principles of Medicine. Philadelphia: F.A. Davis Company, 1916. 7th ed, pp 710, 724, 782.
232. Weintraub M, Sundaresan PR, Schuster B, et al. Long term weight control: the National Heart, Lung and Blood Institute funded multimodal intervention study. I–VII. Clin Pharmacol Ther 1992;51:581–646.
233. Connolly HM, Crary JL, McGoon MD, Hensrud DD, Edwards BS, Edwards WD, Schaff HV. Valvular heart disease associated with fenfluramine-phentermine. N Engl J Med 1997;337(9):581–588.
234. Preuss J. Biblical and Talmudic Medicine. (Translated and edited by F. Rosner, MD.) New York: Hebrew Publishing Company, 1978.
235. Kremen AJ, Linner JH, Nelson CH. Experimental evaluation of nutritional importance of proximal and distal small intestine. Ann Surg 140:439–448, 1954.
236. Payne JH, DeWind LT, Commons RR. Metabolic observations in patients with jejunocolic shunts. Am J Surg 1963;106:273–289.
237. Mason EE, Ito C. Gastric bypass. Ann Surg 1970; 170:329–339.
238. Sjostrom CD, Lissner L, Wedel H, Sjostrom L. Reduction in incidence of diabetes, hypertension and lipid disturbances after intentional weight loss induced by bariatric surgery: the SOS Intervention Study. Obes Res 1999;7(5):477–484.
239. Sarton G. The History of Science and the New Humanism. New York: Henry Holt, 1931.
240. Sarton G. A History of Science. Ancient Science Throughout the Golden Age of Greece. Cambridge, MA: Harvard University Press, 1952.
241. Schenkio MM. De pinguedinis in animalibut generatione et concretione. In: Erastus Th. Philosophi et Medici Celeberrimi Disputationum et Episolarum Medicalium, Volumen Doctissimum. Tiguri: Johan Wolphium, 1595.
242. Ettmueller M. Pratique de Médicine Speciale ... sur les Maladies Propres des Hommes, des Femmes & des Petits Enfants, avec des Dissertations ... sur l'Épilepsie, l'Yvresse, le Mal Hypochondriaque, la Douleur Hypochondriaque, la Corpulence, & la Morsure de la Vipère (trad. nouv.) Lyon: Thomas Amaulry, 1691.
243. Gosky AU. Disputatio solennis de marasmo, sive marcore: macilentia item & gracilitate sanorum; macilentia & gracilitate aegrotatium; crassitie & corpulentia sanorum naturali; crassitie & magnitudine corporis morbosa aegrorum. Argentinae: Typis Eberhardii Welperi, 1658.
244. Held JF. Disputationem medica de corpulentia nimia. Publicae. . .censurae. . .submittit. Jenae: Nisianis, 1670.
245. Leisner KC. Dissertatio medica de obesitate exsuperante. Jenae: Typ Gollnerianis, 1683.
246. Widemann GM. Disputatio medica de corpulaentia nimia. Lipsiae: typ Krugerianus, 168l.
247. Vaulpre JM. De obesitate, comodis et noxis. Montepellier: Joannem-Franciscum Picot, 1782.
248. Fecht EH. Disputatio medica inauguralis de obesitate nimia. Rostochi: J. Wepplingii, 1701.
249. Triller DW. De pinguedine seu succo nutritio superfluo. Halae: Type C. Henklii, 1718.
250. Bass G. Dissertationem inauguralem medicam de obesitate nimia. Erfordiae: Preolo Heringii, 1740.
251. Bertram JW. Dissertatio inauguralis medica de pinguedine. Halae Magdeb: J.C. Hilligéri, 1739.
252. Bon J. Dissertatio medica inauguralis. De mutatione pinguedinis. Harderovici: Apud Johannem Moojen, 1742.

253. Bougourd O. An obesis somnus brevis salubrior? Paris: 1733 [thesis].
254. Dissertatio inauguralis medica de obesitate: Viennae: Typis Joan Thomae Nobil. de Trattnern, 1776.
255. Ebart FCW. Dissertatio inauguralis medica de obesitate nimia et morbis inde orindus. Small quarto ed. Gottingen: Lit J.H. Schulzii, 1780.
256. Hoelder FB. Obesitatis corporis humani nosologia. Tubingae: Lit Schrammianis, 1775.
257. Homeroch CF. De pinguedine ejusque sede tam secundum quam preaeter naturam constitutis. Lipsiae: Ex Offician Langenhemiana, 1996.
258. Hulsebusch JF. Dissertatio inauguralis medica sistens pinguedinis corporis humani, sive panniculi adiposi veterum, hodie membranae cullulosae dictae fabricam, ejusque, & contenti olei historiam, usum, morbos. Lugduni Batavorum: Joh Arnold Langerak, 1728.
259. Jansen WX. Pinguedinis animalis consideratio physiologica et pathologica. Lugduni Batavorum: J. Hazebroek, A. van Houte et Ardream Koster, 1784.
260. Kroedler JS. Theses inauguralis medicae de eo quod citius moriantur obesi, quam graciles secundum Hippocratis aphorismum XLIV. Sect II. Erfordiae: Typis Groschianis, 1724.
261. La Sone JMF. An in macilentis liberior quam in obesis circulatio. Paris: Quillau, 1740.
262. Locke SCJ. De celeri corporum incremento causa debilitatis in morbis. Lipsiae: ex officina Langenhemia, 1760.
263. Lohe AW. Exhibens de morbis adipis humani principia generalia. Duisburg, 1772.
264. Muller PA. Dissertatio physiologica de pinguedine corporis. Hafniae: Typis Andreae Hartvigi Godiche, 1766.
265. Oswald JH. Obesitatis corporis humani therapia. Tubingae: Litteris Schrammianis, 1775.
266. Person C. An parcior obesis, quam macilentis sanguinis missio. Paris: Quillau, 1748.
267. Pohl JC. Dissertationem inauguralem de obesis et voracibus eorumque vitae incommodis ac morbis. Lipsiae: J.C. Langenhemii, 1734.
268. Polonus SI. Dissertatio medica inauguralis de pinguedine. Harderovici: Typis Everardi Tyhoff, 1797.
269. Quabeck KJ. Dissertatio inauguralis medica de insolito corporis augmento frequenti morborum futurorum signo. Halae Magdeb: J.C. Hendelii, 1752.
270. Redhead J. Dissertatio physiologica-medica, inauguralis, de adipe, quam annuente summo numine. Edinburgh: Balfour et Smellie, 1789.
271. Riegels ND. De usu glandularum superrenalium in animalibus nec non de origine adipis. Hafniae, 1790.
272. Reussing HCT. Dissertatio inauguralis medica de pinguedine sana et morbosa. Jenae: Ex Officina Fiedleriana, 1791.
273. Riemer JA. De obesitatis causis praecipuis. Halae and Salem: Stanno Hendeliano, 1778.
274. Schroeder PG. Dissertatio inauguralis medica de obesitate vitanda. Rintelii. J.G. Enax, 1756.
275. Schulz C. Disputatio medica inauguralis de obesitate quam, annuente summo numine. Lugduni Batavorum: Conradum Wishoff, 1752.
276. Seifert PDB. Dissertatio phyiologico-pathologico de pinguedine. Gryphiswaldiae: I.H. Eckhardt, 1794.
277. Steube JS. Dissertatio medica de corpulentia nimia. Jenae: Litteris Mullerianus, 1716.
278. Tralles BL. Dissertatio de obesorum ad morbos mortemque declivitte. Halae Magdeb: Litteris Hilligerianis, 1730.
279. Trouillart G. Dissertatiio physiologico-practica inauguralis de pinguedine, et morbis ex nimia ejus quantitate. Harderovici: Apud Joannem Moojen, 1767.
280. Verdries JM. Dissertatio medica inauguralis de pinguedinis usibus et nocumentis in corpore humano, 8th ed. Giessae Hassorum: J.R. Vulpius, 1702.
281. Short T. A Discourse Concerning the Causes and Effects of Corpulency Together with the Method for Its Prevention and Cure. London: J. Robert, 1727.
282. Flemyng M. A Discourse on the Nature, Causes and Cure of Corpulency. London: L. Davis and C. Reymers, 1760.
283. Bray GA. Commentary on paper by Chambers. Obes Res 1:85–86, 1993.
284. Bray GA. Quetelet: quantitative medicine. Obes Res 2:68–71, 1994.
285. Harden VA. Inventing the NIH. Federal Biomedical Research Policy, 1887–1937. Baltimore: Johns Hopkins University Press, 1986.
286. McLean BI, Howard AN. A double-blind trial of mazindol using a very low calorie formula diet. Int J Obes 1977;1:271–278.
287. Bray GA. Obesity in Perspective. Fogarty International Center Series on Preventive Med. Washington: Govt Printing Office, 1976. DHEW publication No. 75–708. Parts 1 and 2.
288. Howard AN. Recent advances in obesity research. In: Proceedings of the 1st International Congress on Obesity. London: Newman Publishing, 1975.
289. Bray GA. Recent Advances in Obesity Research. II. Proceedings of the 2nd International Congress on Obesity 23–26 October 1977, Washington D.C. London: Newman Publishing, 1978.
290. Bjorntorp P, Cairella M, Howard A.N. eds. Recent Advances in Obesity Research: III. Proceedings of the 3rd International Congress on Obesity. London: John Libbey, 1981:374–387.
291. Hirsch J, Van Itallie TB, eds. Recent advances in obesity research: IV. Proceedings of the 4th International Congress on Obesity 5–8 October, 1983. New York; USA. London John Libbey, 1985.
292. Berry EM, Blondheim SH, Eliahou E, Shafrir E, eds. Recent Advances in obesity: V. Proceedings of the 5th

International Congress on Obesity. London: John Libbey, 1987:290–292.
293. Oomura Y, Tarui S, Inoue S, Shimazu T, eds. Progress in Obesity Research, 1990. London: John Libbey, 1991.
294. Angel A, Anderson H, Bouchard C, Lau D, Leiter L, Meldelson R, eds. Progress in Obesity Research: 7. London: John Libbey, 1996.
295. Guy-Grand B, Ailhaud G, eds. Progress in Obesity Research: 8. London: John Libbey, 1999.
296. Wadd W. Cursory remarks on corpulence; or obesity considered as a disease: with a critical examination of ancient and modern opinions, relative to its causes and cure. London: J. Callow, 1816.
297. Chambers TK. Corpulence; Or, Excess of Fat in the Human Body; Its Relation to Chemistry and Physiology, Its Bearings on Other Diseases and the Value of Human Life and Its Indications of Treatment. London: Longman, Brown, Green and Longmans, 1850.
298. Harvey J. Corpulence, Its Diminution and Cure Without Injury to Health. London: Smith, 1864.
299. Harvey W. On Corpulence in Relation to Disease: With Some Remarks on Diet. London: Henry Renshaw, 1872.
300. Dancel JF. Traite Théorique et Pratique de l'Obésité (Trop Grand Embonpoint). Aveo Plusieurs Observations de Guérison de Maladies Occasionées ou Entretienues par Cet État Anormal. Paris: J.B. Baillière et Fils, 1863, pp 1–357.
301. Worthington LS. De l'obésité Etiologie, therapeutiqueet hygiène. Paris: E. Martinet, 1875, p 188.
302. Kisch EH. Die fettleibigkeit (lipomatosis universalis). Auf gurndlage Zahlreicher beobachtungen klinisch Dargestellt. Stuttgart: Ferdinand Enke, 1988.
303. Ebstein W. Die Fettleibigkeit (Korpulenz) un ihre Behandulung nach physiologicschen Grundsatzen. Weisbaden: Bergmann, 1882.
304. Williams LLB. Obesity. London: Milford, 1926.
305. Christie WF. Obesity: A Practical Handbook for Physicians. London: William Heinemann, 1937.
306. Rony HR. Obesity and Leanness. Philadelphia: Lea and Febiger, 1940.
307. Rynearson EH, Gastineau CF. Obesity. Springfield, IL: Charles C. Thomas, 1949.
308. Craddock D. Obesity and Its Management. Edinburgh and London: E. and S. Livingstone, 1969.
309. Bruch H. The Importance of Overweight. New York: W.W. Norton, 1957.
310. Mayer J. Overweight: Causes, Cost and Control. Englewood Cliffs, NJ: Prentice-Hall, 1968.
311. Garrow JS. Treat Obesity Seriously. A Clinical Manual. Edinburgh and London: Churchill Livingstone, 1981.
312. Stunkard AJ. The Pain of Obesity. Palo Alto, CA: Bull Publishing, 1976.
313. Leven G. Du Obésité. Paris: G. Steinheil, 1901.
314. Haeckel F. Grandes et Petites Obésité. Cure Radicale. Paris: Masson, 1911.
315. LeNoir P. L'Obésité et Son Traitement. Paris: J.B. Baillière and Fils, 1907.
316. Boivin F. La cure physiologique de l'obésité. Paris: Jules Rousset, 1911: 1–191.
317. Cref AF, Herschberg AD. Abrège d'Obésité Paris: Masson,1979.
318. Von Noorden K. Die fettsucht. Vienna: Holder, 1910.
319. Pfaundler M. Korpermass-studien an Kindern. Berlin: Springer, 1916.
320. Gries FA, Berchtold P, Berger M. Adipositas, pathophysiologie,klinik und therapie. Berlin: Springer-Verlag, 1976.
321. Bray GA. The obese patient. In: Smith LH Jr, ed. Major Problems in Internal Medicine, Vol IX. Philadelphia: W.B. Saunders, 1976.

2

Evaluation of Total and Regional Adiposity

Steven B. Heymsfield, Wei Shen, and ZiMian Wang

Columbia University College of Physicians and Surgeons and St. Luke's-Roosevelt Hospital, New York, New York, U.S.A.

Richard N. Baumgartner

University of New Mexico School of Medicine, Albuquerque, New Mexico, U.S.A.

David B. Allison

The University of Alabama at Birmingham, Birmingham, Alabama, U.S.A.

Robert Ross

Queen's University, Kingston, Ontario, Canada

I INTRODUCTION

Quantifying the amount and distribution of adipose tissue and its related components is integral to the study and treatment of human obesity. Body composition research is a field devoted specifically to the development and extension of methods for in vivo quantification of adipose tissue and other biochemical and anatomical components of the body. This review focuses on methods of estimating body composition components in the context of evaluating human obesity and its associated risks.

The chapter first describes the organization of human body composition with an emphasis on body adiposity. The human body can be organized into five levels of increasing complexity—atomic, molecular, cellular, tissue system, and whole body. Obesity-related components are recognized at each of the five body composition levels.

A general review is next provided on approaches to measuring body composition components, especially fat mass, adipose tissue, and related components. Two main groups of methods are reviewed: those that are useful mainly in research laboratories as reference methods, including whole-body ^{40}K counting, neutron activation analysis, hydrometry, underwater weighing/air plethysmography, dual-energy x-ray absorptiometry, multicomponent models, and imaging methods such as computerized axial tomography and magnetic resonance imaging; and those that are applicable in field settings including anthropometry and bioimpedance analysis. An overview of method errors is included in the next section.

Body composition methods for quantifying regional and whole-body obesity-related components are now available for the quantitative in vivo study of human obesity.

II BODY COMPOSITION AND ENERGY EXCHANGE

An individual's body mass reflects total lifetime nutrient and energy balance. Energy balance, or stores, the difference between energy ingested as food and organic compounds oxidized as fuel, can be physiologically allocated into three main molecular components—the small storage carbohydrate glycogen pool, the larger structural and functional protein pool, and the variable lipid or fat storage pool (Fig. 1) (1). Taken together with associated water and minerals, the collective energy compartment is reflected by and changes parallel with body mass. It is within this dynamic model of energy exchange and storage that the study of human body composition and obesity resides.

While the molecular level is ideally suited for thermodynamic analysis, energy stores can be envisaged as comprising the six classic levels of biology, atomic, molecular, cellular, tissue-organ, whole-body, and population. The first four of these levels are depicted in Figure 2 (2). In this review we examine each of the major compartments at these four levels and explore means by which they can be quantified in laboratory and field settings. Our focus is on measurement of adiposity-related components in the overall context of this book. Other reviews and monographs examine body composition in general with specific areas of focus including elements, molecular components, body cell mass, tissues including bone and skeletal muscle, and visceral organs (see Appendix).

III ADIPOSITY COMPONENTS

Adiposity generally reflects energy stores, and excess stored energy and body weight are the hallmark of human obesity. Each body composition level of the individual has a representation of adiposity (3). We now review the main features of the five body composition levels with a focus on adiposity-related components.

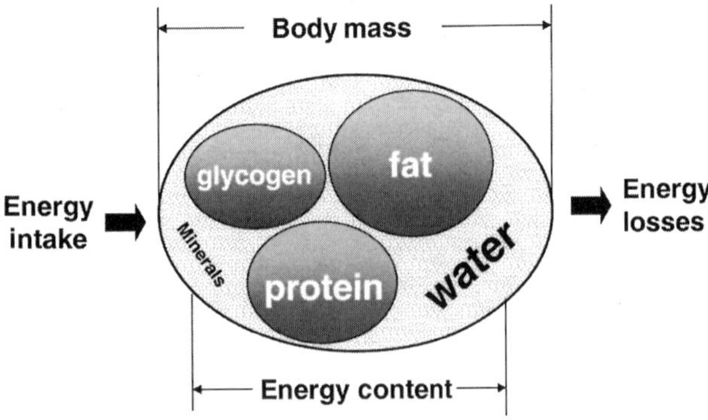

Figure 1 Interrelations between energy intake, output, and stores. (From Ref. 1.)

Atomic	Molecular	Cellular	Tissue-Organ
N, Ca, P, K, Na, Cl	**Lipid**	**Adipocytes**	**Adipose tissue**
H	Water	Cells	Skeletal muscle
C	Proteins	ECF	Visceral organs and residual
O	Glycogen	ECS	Skeleton
	Minerals		

Figure 2 First four of the five levels of human body composition. Components related to "fatness" are identified by bold enclosure. ECS and ECF are extracellular and intracellular solids, respectively. (From Ref. 2.)

A Atomic Level

The human body is composed of 11 elements that account for > 99.5% of body weight (Fig. 3) (1). Three of these elements, carbon, hydrogen, and oxygen, are found in storage triglycerides or "fat" (Table 1). The average proportions of triglyceride as carbon, hydrogen, and oxygen are considered stable at ~76.7%, 12.0%, and 11.3%, respectively. These stable elemental proportions allow the development of methods for deducing total body fat from total body carbon and other elements.

Carbon is the characteristic component of adiposity at the atomic level. Reference Man, for example, contains 16 kg carbon, and 60% or 9.6 kg of carbon exits in adipose tissue (4).

B Molecular Level

The main atomic level elements, including trace elements that occur in low but essential concentrations, combine to form various chemical compounds that may be grouped into the broad classes that define the molecular level of body composition. The main components of the molecular level are shown in Figure 4 and include water, lipids, proteins, minerals, and glycogen (3). Each of the nonaqueous components represents many differ-

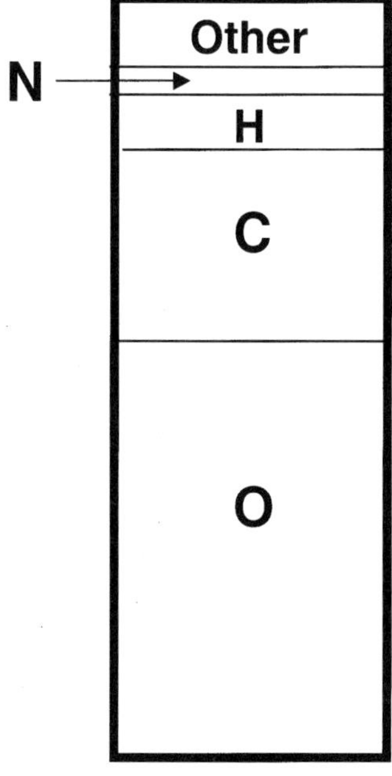

Figure 3 Atomic level of body composition. (From Ref. 3.)

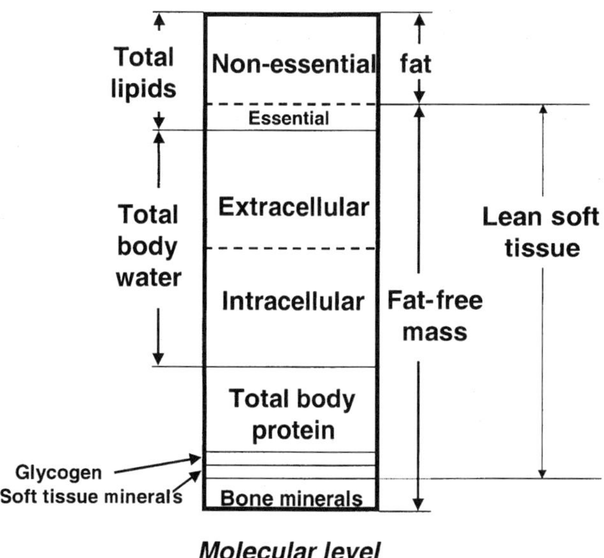

Figure 4 Main components of the molecular level of body composition. (From Ref. 3.)

ent but closely related chemical compounds. For example, the "protein" component consists of several hundred different specific proteins.

Lipid is the main molecular-level component of interest in the study of human obesity. The term lipid refers to all chemical compounds that are insoluble or weakly soluble in water, but are soluble in organic solvents such as chloroform and diethyl ether (5). Lipids isolated from human tissues include triglycerides, sphyngomyelin, phospholipids, steroids, fatty acids, and terpenes. Triglycerides, commonly referred to as "fats," are the primary storage lipids in humans, and comprise the largest fraction of the total lipid component. At present there is limited information on the exact proportion of total lipids as triglycerides, or the amount of within and between-person variability. Comizio et al. (6) examined the proportion of total body lipid as triglyceride in the adult rat under usual dietary conditions and with dietary energy restriction without and with swimming exercise. The authors observed that with negative energy balance and weight loss there were parallel losses of total body triglyceride and lipid. The fraction (mean $\pm$ SD) of total lipids as triglyceride was 0.83 $\pm$ 0.08 in the control rats with lowering at 2 and 9 weeks of energy restriction to 0.82 $\pm$ 0.04 (P = NS vs. control) and 0.70 $\pm$ 0.15 (P = .05) and at 9 weeks for energy restriction plus exercise to 0.67 $\pm$ 0.09 (P = .003). The Reference Man reportedly has 13.5 kg of total lipid, of which 12.0 kg, or 89%, is "fat" (4).

A summary of molecular-level component characteristics is presented in Table 2. These characteristics are used in developing body composition methods, and their application will be presented in later sections. An important feature of the molecular level is the "stable" relationships that exist between the various components. These stable relations form the basis of many widely used body composition methods. The three most important of these are the hydration of fat free mass (i.e., TBW/FFM), potassium content of fat free mass

Table 1 Chemical Formulae and Elemental Stoichiometry of Representative Triglycerides

	Elemental content (%)		
Formulae	Carbon	Hydrogen	Oxygen
$C_{57}H_{104}O_6$	77.4	11.8	10.9
$C_{51}H_{98}O_6$	75.9	12.2	11.9
$C_{55}H_{102}O_6$	76.9	11.9	11.2
$C_{55}H_{104}O_6$	76.7	12.1	11.2
"Average" triglyceride	76.7	12.0	11.3

Source: Ref. 4.

Table 2 Characteristics of Molecular-Level Components

Component	Density (g/cm^3)	Elemental stoichiometry
Water	0.99371 at 36°C 0.9934 at 37°C	0.111 H; 0.889 O
Protein	1.34 at 37°C	0.532 C; 0.070 H; 0.161 N; 0.227 O; 0.01 S
Glycogen	1.52 at 37°C	0.444 C; 0.062 H; 0.494 O
Minerals	3.042	
Bone[a]	2.982 at 36-36.7°C	0.398 Ca; 0.002 H; 0.185 P; 0.414 O
Nonbone	3.317	
Lipid		
Adipose tissue extracts	0.9007 at 36°C	0.767 C; 0.120 H; 0.113 O

[a] Calculated from the largest component of bone mineral, calcium hydroxyapatite $[Ca_3(PO_4)_2]_3Ca(OH)_2$. Other small elemental contributions to bone, such as Na, are recognized.
Sources: Refs. 4–6.

(i.e., TBK/FFM), and densities (D) of fat and FFM. These assumed stable or relatively stable relations allow development of two component molecular level models consisting of fat and FFM.

The hydration of FFM is among the most important stable relations applied in body composition research (7–9). A strong correlation with an intercept not significantly different from zero was observed between total body water (TBW) and FFM across mammals ranging in body mass from mouse to gray seal (10). The mean ratio of TBW/FFM for the mammals was ~0.73 and this ratio is among the best-known stable body composition associations. This constancy provides a means of estimating total body fat in vivo: body fat = body mass − FFM = body mass − TBW/0.73.

The total body potassium (TBK) to FFM ratio was historically important as it formed the basis of many classic body composition studies that explored fat and FFM relations. A mean TBK/FFM ratio of 68.1 ± 3.1 mmol/kg was derived by Forbes et al. (11) based on the whole-body chemical analysis of four human cadavers. This ratio was then introduced and applied as an in vivo method for estimating total body fat mass in vivo: body fat = body mass − FFM; = body mass − TBK/68.1. However, this ratio actually varies considerably across sex and age (12). The total body potassium to FFM ratio is thus not widely used today as improved methods of evaluating total body fat in vivo are available.

The relatively stable densities of fat (0.9007 g/cm^3) and FFM (1.100 g/cm^3) are the basis of many body composition models and were first suggested six decades ago by Behnke et al. (13). The simplest model consists of two components and is derived from two simultaneous equations:

$$\text{body mass} = \text{fat} + \text{FFM} \tag{1}$$

$$\text{body mass}/D_b = \text{fat}/0.9007 + \text{FFM}/1.100 \tag{2}$$

Solving the two simultaneous equations,

$$\text{body fat mass} = (4.95/D_b - 4.50) \times \text{body mass} \tag{3}$$

where D_b is body density measured by the underwater weighing technique. However, the assumption of a constant FFM density of 1.100 g/cm^3 causes some model error as FFM density actually varies, although within a relatively narrow range (14). To avoid this model error, three-, four-, and/or five-component models were developed for measuring total body fat with improved accuracy (15).

C Cellular Level

The cellular level includes three main components, cell mass, extracellular fluid, and extracellular solids (Fig. 5). Cells can be divided into specific types such as connective, epithelial, nervous, and muscular. Adipocytes or fat cells serve as the primary storage site for triglycerides. All mass can be separated into two components, one metabolically active "body cell mass," and the other triglycerides, or "fat." The concept of body cell mass was originated by Moore and refers to the compartment actively involved in energy consumption and heat production (7). Extracellular solids consist mainly of bone minerals and collagen, reticular, and elastic fibers.

The following are some of the important assumed stable cellular level relationships applied in body composition models: K/intracellular water = 159 mmol/kg H_2O = 6.22 g/kg H_2O; K/body cell mass = 4.69 g/kg; Ca/extracellular solids = 0.177 kg/kg; and extracellular water/ extracellular fluid = 0.92.

D Tissue Organ Level

The main components at this level are adipose tissue, skeletal muscle, bone, and visceral organs (e.g., liver, kidneys, heart, etc.) (Fig. 6). The adipose tissue component includes adipocytes with collagenous and elastic fibers, fibroblasts, capillaries, and extracellular fluid.

Human adipose tissue is often assumed to have an average composition consisting of 80% lipid, 14%

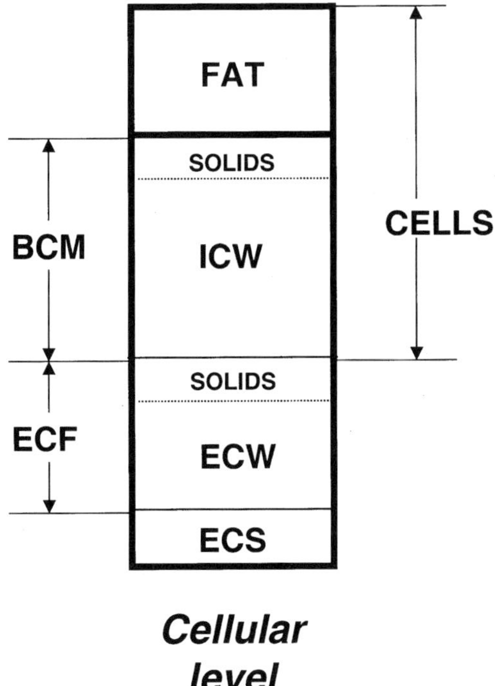

Figure 5 Cellular level of body composition. BCM, body cell mass; ECF, extracellular fluid; ICW, intracellular water; ECS, extracellular solids; and ECW, extracellular water. (From Ref. 3.)

water, 5% protein, and < 1% mineral, and a density of 0.92 g/cm^3 at body temperature (4). However, this average belies the large variation observed in adipose tissue composition. Level of adiposity, age, gender, and heredity all play an important role in determining adipose tissue composition, notably fat content. Martin and colleagues suggest that for every 10% increase in relative adiposity there is a corresponding rise in adipose tissue lipid fraction of 0.124 (16). A notable feature of adipose tissue is the large extracellular fluid compartment relative to cell mass. Of the 14% of average adipose tissue samples as water, 11% is extracellular water.

An important aspect of obesity research is examination of regional adipose tissue biology. Adipose tissue can be classified as two main types, subcutaneous and internal (Table 3) (4,17). Adipose tissue occurs in abundance in subcutaneous sites and is known to gross anatomists as superficial fascia, defined as the adipose tissue between the skin and the muscles. Subcutaneous adipose tissue also occurs in and around female breasts. Subcutaneous adipose tissue has also been partitioned by Kelly et al. into the plane superficial to the fascia within subcutaneous adipose tissue and that below this fascia, so-called deep subcutaneous adipose tissue (18).

Internal adipose tissue is found in the visceral compartment and in nonvisceral sites. The most important internal adipose tissue component in the obesity field is found in the visceral compartment. The word *viscera* is Latin for "organs in the cavities of the body," usually applied to the heart and lungs as thoracic viscera and the stomach and intestines as abdominal viscera. Since there are three main body cavities—thoracic, abdominal, and pelvic—there are three corresponding visceral adipose tissue (VAT) components (Table 3). However, the medical literature varies widely in defining VAT based on imaging methods. This topic is reviewed in the section on imaging methods. Very few human studies in the obesity field examine intrathoracic VAT, including pericardial, epicardial, and periaortic adipose tissue.

Of the nonvisceral internal adipose tissue, interstitial adipose tissue is interspersed within the cells of a tissue (e.g., skeletal muscle) so tightly that it may be included with the tissue/organ at dissection. Adipose tissue is almost absent in some anatomic sites such as the penis,

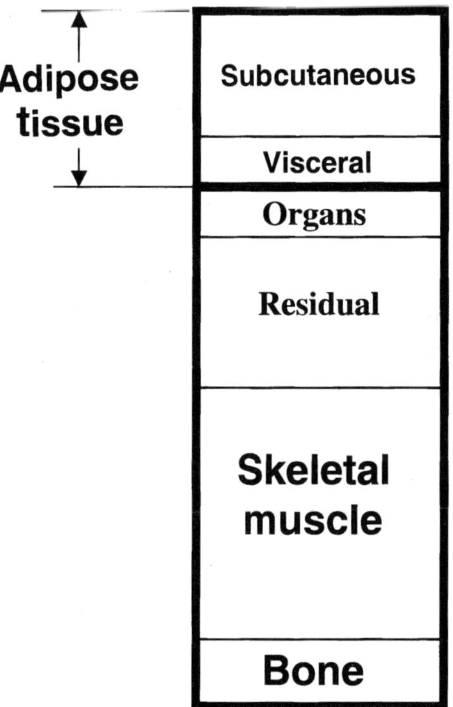

Figure 6 Tissue-organ level of body composition. (From Ref. 3.)

Table 3 Anatomic Distribution of Adipose Tissue

Subcutaneous adipose tissue
  including adipose tissue of female breast
    Retromammary adipose tissue
    Intramammary adipose tissue
Internal adipose tissue
  Visceral adipose tissue
    Intrathoracic
      Cardiac adipose tissue
        Pericardial adipose tissue
        Epicardial adipose tissue
        Periaortic adipose tissue
      Retrosternal adipose tissue
      Adipose tissue of superior mediastinal areas
    Intra-abdominal adipose tissue
      Intraperitoneal adipose tissue
        Omental adipose tissue
        Mesenteric adipose tissue
      Retroperitoneal adipose tissue
        Perirenal adipose tissue
        Pararenal adipose tissue
        Periaortic adipose tissue
        Peripancreatic adipose tissue
    Intrapelvic
      Intraperitoneal adipose tissue
        Mesenteric adipose tissue
      Retroperitoneal adipose tissue
      Postabdominal wall adipose tissue
  Nonvisceral internal adipose tissue
      Adipose tissue in bone marrow
      Interstitial adipose tissue
      Paravertebral adipose tissue
      Retro-orbital adipose tissue
      Localized pads in the synovial membrane of many joints

scrotum, labia minora, nipple, nose, ear, eyelids, and brain. Some triglyceride exists within skeletal muscle, liver, and other nonadipose tissue cells, although this component is classified as intracellular lipid. Each anatomic adipose tissue component has specific metabolic and functional characteristics.

Illustrations of the subcutaneous, visceral (i.e., peri- and pararenal, mesenteric, omental), interstitial, and marrow adipose tissue compartments of the Visible Man are shown in Figures 7 and 8 for the midabdominal region and leg, respectively (17).

E Whole-Body Level

Skinfolds, circumferences, and linear dimensions are all measurements at the whole-body level. These measurements are often used with prediction equations to estimate components at the other four body composition levels.

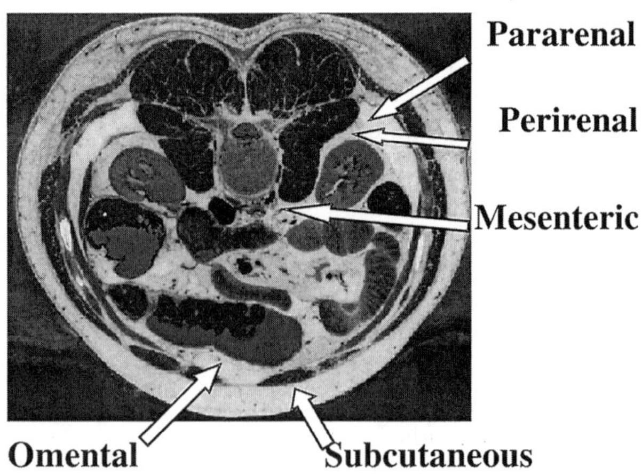

Figure 7 Cross-sectional photograph of National Library of Medicine's Visible Man at the midabdominal region with identified adipose tissue components. (From Ref. 17.)

IV MEASUREMENT METHODS

A Body Weight and Stature

Standardized methods have been described for measuring weight and stature, as well as other anthropometric variables (19). For most clinical research purposes, it is desirable to measure body weight to the nearest $\pm$ 0.1 kg using a high-quality calibrated beam-balance or electronic scale. Subjects should be measured either nude or wearing standardized light clothing of known weight.

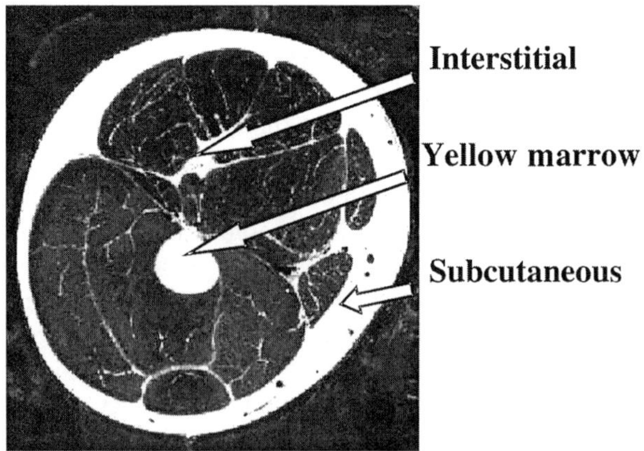

Figure 8 Cross-sectional photograph of National Library of Medicine's Visible Man at the mid–upper arm region with identified adipose tissue components. (From Ref. 17.)

If heavier clothing is worn, it is necessary to estimate and record the additional weight of this clothing. The presence of edema, a common problem in severely obese subjects, should be noted. A variety of practical problems may be encountered when measuring the weight of obese subjects. Severely obese patients may have difficulty standing on standard scales, which may be too narrow or too high above the floor for an individual with balance problems. Specially designed chairs or sling-scales may be used.

The preferred method of measuring stature is to the nearest $\pm$ 1 cm using a wall-mounted stadiometer. Inexpensive, plastic stadiometers are available for clinical use that have acceptable accuracy. Close attention should be paid to standardized positioning of the subject when making the measurement (19). As for weight, a variety of practical problems may be encountered when measuring the stature of obese subjects. For example, the standard method requires the subject to stand erect with head, shoulders, and buttocks against the stadiometer board. This positioning may be difficult to achieve for obese individuals with large, protruding buttocks.

It is sometimes considered difficult and expensive to measure weight and stature in very large epidemiological surveys, and it is usually not possible to obtain measurements of past weight or stature for retrospective studies. In these settings many investigators have relied on self-reported weight and stature. This requires the assumption that the subjects know and can report their weight and stature both accurately and reliably. It is possible to verify this assumption in a subsample of participants with measured values in a cross-sectional survey, but this is difficult in retrospective studies where recalled weight or stature may be many years in the past.

Among adults, self-reported weight and height are generally highly correlated with measured weight and height. Correlations for reported stature range from 0.53 (20) to 0.99 (21); and those for weight range from 0.89 to 0.99 (21). The magnitudes of the correlations vary somewhat across studies and in relation to age and sex. In any event, high correlations do not necessarily reflect accuracy, since systematic differences (i.e., constant and relative biases) between self-reported and measured values may exist regardless of the strength of the correlations. Biases in the self-reporting of weight and height have been documented. Obese people tend to underreport their weight more than nonobese people. Women consistently underreport their weight and men tend to underreport it when they are overweight and over-report it when they are underweight.

Recall of weight and height at earlier ages, reports by surrogates (e.g., parents, spouses, children, siblings), and records from driver's licenses (22) can also be used in place of measured variables. These can be expected generally to have less reliability and accuracy than self-reported current weight, and correlations with measured weight are considerably less. There is little evidence that self-measurements are any more accurate or reliable than simple self-reported estimates.

Body weight and stature can be used to estimate "relative weight." The more common approach now used worldwide is to calculate body mass index (BMI) (weight/stature^2). The objective of weight-stature indices such as body mass index is to obtain a measure of body weight (W) that is independent of stature (S). An example of such an index is given in Eqs. (4) and (5), which are based on the assumed relationship

$$W/S^b = a \tag{4}$$

and

$$W = aS^b \tag{5}$$

In Eq. (4) and (5), a and b are constants. These equations indicate that for any increment in S^b, body weight changes in a proportional manner so as to keep the W/S^b ratio constant. The great statistician and anthropometrist Lambert-Adolphe-Jacques Quetelet first observed that among adults weight in kilograms seemed to increase in proportion to the square of stature in meters (23). Quetelet's Index, W/S^2, was further established to be a useful index for grading adiposity in population studies by Keys, who appears to have been responsible for renaming it the "body mass index" (24). It is now conventional to refer to W/S^2 as the BMI, but the reader should be aware that an infinite number of weight-stature indices can be constructed using different powers of stature, as well as weight (25). Historically, various investigators have presented arguments for the merits of different values of b in W/S^b, based on the influence of age, gender, race, and even disease risk on the association between weight and stature (26–30). Benn even suggested that the power coefficient, b, should be established empirically within a population rather than applying a common coefficient across all populations (31).

It is important to keep in mind that the underlying assumption in the use of body mass indices is that they reflect variation among people in body adiposity (32). Garn et al. (33) cogently reminded us of three limitations to this assumption: (1) the correlation of BMIs with stature may be influenced by age; (2) BMIs may be influenced by body proportions, specifically leg length relative to trunk size; and (3) BMIs may be correlated with lean as well as fat mass. Quetelet's Index, or BMI, is not perfectly correlated with body fatness: r's with percent body fat range widely from about .40 to .90 across various studies. Moreover, the association of BMI with percent body fat may be nonlinear, especially at higher levels of adiposity (34). This suggests that the index can vary in sensitivity for grading body fatness among populations. Abdel-Malek and associates (25) presented a method for empirically determining powers for both weight and stature that would maximize the association between total body fat or percent body fat and weight-stature indices in a group or subsample of a population. As for the approach of Benn (31), this method has not been widely applied.

A potentially more troublesome problem is the fact that body mass indices are also associated with FFM. This is because weight includes FFM and stature is not correlated perfectly with FFM. As a result, body mass indices tend to retain significant correlations with FFM even when powers of b are found that minimize the correlation between weight and stature. The net result is that there may be a considerable range of body fatness (or leanness) among individuals with the same body mass index (35,36). The magnitudes of the associations of body mass indices with fat and fat free components are also influenced by age, gender, and racial differences in body composition, and by variation in body proportions. Substantial misclassification bias can result when people are classified as "overweight" or "obese" using cutoff values that do not take these factors into consideration (36,37).

Body weight and stature, or indices such as BMI, can also be used in equations to estimate body composition. As an example, percent body fat can be calculated using the following equation:

$$\begin{aligned}\%\text{fat} = {} & 64.5 - 848 \times (1/\text{BMI}) + 0.079 \times \text{age} \\ & -16.4 \times \text{sex} + 0.05 \times \text{sex} \times \text{age} + 39.0 \\ & \times \text{sex} \times (1/\text{BMI}) \qquad (6)\end{aligned}$$

with sex = 1 for male and 0 for female (38). Body fat in this investigation was evaluated using a four-component model as the reference method. The percent fat prediction formula is applicable in Caucasians and African Americans and a separate equation is available for use in Asian subjects.

B Component Reference Methods

Body composition methods vary in several characteristics including cost, safety, technical complexity, portability, accuracy, reproducibility, and requirement for subject participation. In the section that follows we organize methods for convenience into two main groups, "reference" methods that are often applied in small-scale studies requiring high accuracy and reproducibility, and "field" methods that require reference method calibration and that are appropriate for use in epidemiological studies.

1 ^{40}K Counting

Whole-body ^{40}K counting is a classic and widely used technique for evaluating adiposity (11). The natural abundance of ^{40}K in the human body is constant at 0.0118% of total body potassium. ^{40}K is radioactive and emits a characteristic 1.46 MeV γ-ray that can be counted by detection systems with appropriate shielding from natural background radioactivity.

The procedure is to first measure ^{40}K in a whole-body counter and then calculate total body potassium from ^{40}K. Once total body potassium is known, FFM can be estimated by assuming a constant relationship between total body potassium and FFM,

$$\text{FFM} = \text{TBK}/\text{ratio} \qquad (7)$$

where "ratio" is the assumed constant proportion of FFM as potassium. The estimated ratio for Reference Man is 63.3 mmol/kg and reflects the summed potassium proportions of all organs and tissues, notably skeletal muscle mass (Table 4) (4,39). Relative organ proportions vary among individuals and, accordingly, several suggested sex- and age-specific TBK/FFM ratios are recognized and applied in estimating FFM (12). Total body fat is calculated as the difference between body weight and FFM.

The total body potassium method of estimating FFM and fat mass is of great historical significance. Many early obesity studies were carried out with total body potassium measured by whole-body counting as the reference method for fat and FFM. Whole-body and regional counters are costly, and there are important technical issues that require attention to achieve accurate results. Today there are methods of equivalent, if not greater, accuracy for quantifying fat and FFM that are more available to research laboratories and are of equal or lower cost.

Total body potassium can also be measured using dilution of the radioactive isotope ^{42}K (7). This method is useful in specialized whole-body counter calibration studies, but has no practical application in the study of human obesity. The 12.4-hr half-life of ^{42}K and the radiation exposure involved preclude the routine use of

Table 4 Reference Man's TBK/FFM Ratio Calculated from 14 Tissues/Organs

Tissue/organ	Fat-free mass (kg)	fFFM$_i$	(K/FFM)$_i$	(K/FFM)$_i$× fFFM$_i$
Skin	2.34	0.041	24.0	0.98
GI tract	1.13	0.020	33.9	0.68
Adipose tissue	3.00	0.053	40.9	2.17
Blood	5.46	0.096	41.2	3.96
Skeleton	8.10	0.143	47.4	6.77
Lung	0.99	0.018	49.1	0.88
Kidney	0.29	0.005	52.0	0.26
Urinary bladder	0.095	0.002	53.8	0.11
Heart	0.30	0.005	61.4	0.31
Pancreas	0.09	0.002	65.4	0.13
Liver	1.68	0.030	68.5	2.06
Skeletal muscle	27.38	0.483	78.5	37.90
Spleen	0.18	0.003	79.6	0.24
Brain	1.25	0.022	85.9	1.89
Total	52.29	0.922		58.34

Abbreviations: fFFM$_i$, fraction of whole-body fat free mass (56.7 kg) as individual tissue/organ fat free mass; (K/FFM)$_i$, ratio of potassium to fat free mass of individual tissue/organ. Whole-body TBK/FFM can be calculated as $\text{TBK/FFM} = \Sigma\,[(\text{K/FFM})_i \times f\text{FFM}_i]/\Sigma\,(f\text{FFM}_i) = 58.34/0.922 = 63.3$ mmol/kg.
Source: Ref. 39.

this isotope. Exchangeable potassium (K_e), which accounts for most of total body potassium, can also be measured using a combination of exchangeable sodium and total-body water measurements and this might be a useful approach at centers in which whole-body counters are unavailable.

Although the application of total body potassium as a measure of adiposity in human obesity research in limited, total body and exchangeable potassium provide useful measures of body cell mass. The body cell mass compartment is often considered a measure of metabolically active tissue. The measurement and interpretation of body cell mass is discussed in detail by Moore and colleagues (7). Recent studies also support the use of total body potassium in skeletal muscle mass measurement.

2 In Vivo Neutron Activation Analysis

A group of methods referred to as whole-body counting/in vivo neutron activation analysis can be used to estimate adiposity-related components. The methods share in common the ability to quantify all main elements at the atomic body composition level in vivo including H, C, N, O, P, Ca, Cl, K, and Na (3). Once these elements are known, it is possible to calculate, using simultaneous equations, the main molecular level components such as fat, protein, water, and minerals. Components at other levels, such as body cell mass, extracellular fluid, intracellular fluid, and skeletal muscle can also be calculated using models based on measured elements.

Only a few centers throughout the world are capable of measuring all of the major elements, while several additional centers are capable of measuring one or two elements. Whole-body counting alone can measure naturally occurring ^{40}K. When subjects are activated with a neutron source first and then placed back in a whole-body counter, additional elements such as Na, Cl, Ca, and P can be quantified by "delayed-gamma" neutron activation. Two other methods, prompt-gamma neutron activation and inelastic neutron scattering methods are used to measure elements such as N, H, C, and O. Each neutron activation system is unique and many alternative methods have been advanced over the years.

In this section we provide a selective review of one representative adiposity measurement method, the multicomponent total body carbon method of estimating total body fat mass. This method provides the main concepts related to all in vivo neutron activation methods.

The total-body carbon method represents an evolution of neutron activation methods at the Brookhaven National Laboratory in Upton, NY. The total body carbon method provides fat estimates that are independent of the two-component total body potassium, water, and underwater weighing methods. This method can be used as a reference method for evaluating other body composition methods.

The initial model for estimating fat mass developed by Cohn and colleagues at Brookhaven was relatively simple (40). There were two measured elements, N and Ca, which were used to calculate total body protein and bone mineral, respectively. Tritium dilution volume was used to estimate total body water, and fat mass was then calculated as the difference between body weight and the sum of total body protein, water, and minerals. Additional improvements in the model were made by Heymsfield et al. as new information became available (41). The most recent advance occurred when Kehayias and colleagues introduced inelastic neutron scattering for measuring total body carbon (42,43).

The total body carbon method is based on the observation that almost all body carbon is incorporated into four components at the molecular level of body composition, fat, protein, glycogen, and bone mineral. Kyere and colleagues (44) first proposed a model in which fat could be calculated from total body carbon. This model was later improved by Kehayias et al., who proposed four simultaneous equations (42,43),

$$\text{TBC} = 0.77 \times \text{fat} + 0.532 \times \text{protein} + 0.444 \times \text{glycogen} + \text{carbon in bone mineral} \quad (8)$$

$$\text{TBN} = 0.16 \times \text{protein} \quad (9)$$

$$\text{Glycogen} = 0.044 \times \text{protein} \quad (10)$$

$$\text{Carbon in bone mineral} = 0.05 \times \text{TBCa} \quad (11)$$

where all units are in kg, and TBC, TBN, and TBCa represent total body carbon, nitrogen, and calcium, respectively. Solving the simultaneous equations for fat mass,

$$\text{total body fat} = 1.30 \times \text{TBC} - 4.45 \times \text{TBN} - 0.06 \times \text{TBCa} \quad (12)$$

This last equation indicates that the total body carbon method measures total body fat as a function of three elements, C, N, and Ca.

There are two important issues to consider with respect to Eq. (12) are the coefficients constant, and can total-body carbon, nitrogen, and calcium be measured accurately? Equation (8) includes the proportions of total body carbon as fat, protein, glycogen, and bone mineral. Equations (9), (10), and (11) include the ratios between protein and nitrogen, glycogen and protein, and carbon and calcium in bone mineral. All of the ratios in Eqs. (9)–(11) are assumed constant, and it is useful to consider this assumption in some detail.

Although triglycerides extracted from human tissues vary in fatty acid composition, their carbon/triglyceride ratios (C/TG) are very close to 0.77 (Tables 1 and 2). The various stoichiometries indicate that the C/TG ratio varies within a narrow range (0.759–0.774). It is therefore reasonable to assume a constant C/TG ratio of 0.77 in Eq. (8), (13).

Total-body protein can be calculated from total body nitrogen, and nitrogen can be measured by prompt-γ neutron activation analysis. This calculation is based on the assumption that a constant ratio (0.16) exists between nitrogen and protein [Eq. (9)]. Protein includes almost all compounds containing nitrogen, varying from simple amino acids to complex nucleoproteins (45). The current suggested chemical formula for protein is $C_{100}H_{159}N_{26}O_{32}N_{0.7}$. The C/protein and N/protein ratios in this widely accepted formula are 0.532 and 0.16, respectively. Chemical analysis confirmed the ratios' validity for most proteins analyzed, although a few specific proteins have N contents that are different from 0.16 (e.g., 0.137 and 0.172 for albumin and collagen, respectively). The chemical analysis of two cadavers, however, yielded whole body N/protein ratios of 0.156 and 0.158, close to the assumed value of 0.16 (46).

Glycogen is not included in most body composition models owing to its small amount. In the total body carbon method for estimating fat, glycogen content was included because of the high C/glycogen ratio of 0.444. In the model of Kehayias et al. the glycogen/protein ratio was assumed constant at 0.044 (42). This consideration must be approximate because the concentrations of glycogen in liver, skeletal muscle, and heart vary significantly with fasting and feeding. Total body glycogen content is ~ 0.3–0.5 kg and thus the total amount of carbon in glycogen is only ~0.2 kg. The model error from the assumed constant glycogen/protein ratio therefore has only a small effect on the accuracy of total body fat estimates.

The main compound of bone mineral, calcium hydroxyapatite $[Ca_3(PO_4)_2]_3\,Ca(OH)_2$, does not contain carbon. Biltz and Pellegrino found that the ratio of carbon to bone calcium is 0.05 g/g (47). It is known that almost all body calcium is incorporated into bone mineral. The total body carbon method estimates carbon in bone mineral, presumably incorporated as carbon in bicarbonate, from total body calcium [Eq. (6)]. Although the carbon/calcium ratio is an approximation, errors in this proportion have only a small effect on fat estimates as with glycogen.

The total body carbon method does not consider the carbon in soft tissue minerals as HCO_3^-. This is because the very small amount of carbon in soft tissue minerals has almost no impact on fat estimates.

From the above discussion it is clear that many assumptions are needed in developing the total body carbon method for measuring total body fat. The main assumptions, however, appear to be highly stable, and position the total body carbon-fat estimation method as a means of analyzing human chemical composition in vivo. Returning to the second aspect of the total body carbon method, measurement of C, N, and Ca, all three elements are quantified by neutron activation analysis.

Total body carbon is measured by inelastic scattering which is based on the reaction (42,43)

$$^{12}C + n \longrightarrow {}^{12}C^* \overset{\nearrow n'}{\longrightarrow} {}^{12}C + \gamma(4.44\ \text{MeV}) \quad (13)$$

Fast incoming neutrons that interact with matter by inelastic collisions result in prompt nuclear de-excitation with γ-ray release $(n,n'\gamma)$. Total-body nitrogen is measured using prompt-γ neutron activation analysis, and its reaction is (48):

$$^{14}N + n \longrightarrow {}^{15}N^* \xrightarrow{\sim 10^{-15}s} {}^{15}N\ (\text{stable}) + \gamma\ (10.83\ \text{MeV}) \tag{14}$$

Delayed-γ neutron activation is used to measure total body calcium based on the reaction (49):

$$^{48}Ca + n \longrightarrow {}^{49}Ca \longrightarrow {}^{49}Sc^* \xrightarrow{+\beta^-} {}^{49}Sc + \gamma\ (3.084\ \text{MeV}) \tag{15}$$

The notation for this reaction is given as [$^{48}Ca(n,\gamma)^{49}Sc$] for [target nucleus (incident particle, emitted particle) residual nucleus]. All three of the neutron activation analysis methods involve radiation exposure, and this is the main disadvantage of the total body carbon method. The average exposure is 80, 575, and 50 mrem for prompt-γ, delayed-γ, and inelastic scattering neutron activation analysis, respectively.

The between-measurement coefficients of variation for total body carbon, nitrogen, and calcium are 3.0%, 2.7%, and 0.8%, respectively. The propagated error in the total body carbon method of measuring total body fat is 3.4–4.0% (42).

The total body carbon method is not widely used in the study of body composition since only a few laboratories in the world have the necessary three neutron activation systems. However, the total body carbon method is important because it is based on highly stable models that are not affected to an appreciable degree by age, sex, ethnicity, or disease. In some respects, at least conceptually, the total body carbon method approaches the potential accuracy in estimating total body fat afforded by lipid extraction of human cadavers.

3 Hydrometry

Dilution methods, including those for total body water, or "hydrometry," include a group of body composition methods designed to quantify fluid compartments and the components that exist entirely within body fluid compartments such as exchangeable potassium, sodium, and chlorine. All dilution methods are based on the use of a labeled tracer with three properties: (1) it has the same or similar distribution space as the component analyzed; (2) it has a distinct property (e.g., radioactivity or color) that can be quantitatively measured; and (3) it is nontoxic in the amounts used. A dose of tracer (T) is administered to the subject, and after an equilibration interval, a portion of the tracer exchanges with other molecules or is excreted; any excreted tracer can be measured in urine. The tracer that remains in the body (T') then homogeneously distributes within the unknown component (C) volume. The following model then applies (50),

$$P^* = R \times (C + T') \tag{16}$$

where T' represents the known amount of tracer in the body at equilibrium, P* is the known measured distinct tracer property, and R is the ratio of P* to the sum of C and T'. Because T' is much smaller than C, the model can be simplified to

$$P^* = R \times C \tag{17}$$

One can analyze a sample of the unknown component such as blood or a piece of tissue. Because the tracer is homogeneously distributed in the unknown component,

$$\Delta P^* = R \times \Delta C \tag{18}$$

where ΔC and ΔP* are the measured unknown component mass and tracer property, respectively. Combining this formula with the above equation, a dilution model is derived,

$$C = [P^* \times \Delta C]/AP^* \tag{19}$$

In the model, P* is known and ΔC and ΔP* can be measured in samples. The unknown component (C) volume can thus be calculated.

Although dilution methods are widely used in the measurement of extracellular fluid, plasma volume, and exchangeable electrolytes (K_e, Na_e, and Cl_e) (50), the most important use in the obesity field is measurement of total body water. This is because water is the largest component at the molecular body composition level in normal adults and also because water occupies a relatively constant fraction of FFM, usually assumed as 0.73 based upon classic in vitro experiments. The stable hydration fraction of ˜0.73 is recognized from human cadaver studies (Table 5) and, within a reasonable range, is also observed across all adult mammals (Fig. 9)(8–10).

Water labeled with either of two isotopes of hydrogen (deuterium, ^2H_2O; tritium, ^3H_2O) or oxygen ($H_2{}^{18}O$) has been used to quantitate total body water by the dilution method in healthy and diseased individuals (51). The use of deuterium and ^{18}O-labeled water-stable isotopes is safe and preferred for children and pregnant women. The assays for these two isotopes in biological fluids rely on labor intensive techniques such as mass spectrometry. Tritium is radioactive and should not be used in children or in pregnant women. On the

Table 5 Fat-Free Body Mass Hydration (TBW/FFM) Evaluated in Nine Adult Human Cadavers

Gender	Age (yr)	BM (kg)	TBW (kg)	FFM (kg)	TBW/FFM	Cause of death
M	46	53.8	29.7	43.3	0.686	Skull fracture
M	60	73.5	37.2	53.0	0.702	Heart attack
M	25	71.8	44.4	61.1	0.726	Uremia
M	63	58.6	35.0	48.0	0.729	Esophageal cancer
F	59	25.9	13.3	18.2	0.731	Extreme cachexia
F	42	45.1	25.3	34.5	0.733	Drowning
M	48	62.0	43.9	59.3	0.740	Infective endocarditis
M	35	70.6	47.9	61.7	0.776	Mitral insufficiency
F	67	43.4	32.0	39.6	0.808	Advanced malignancy
Mean	49	50.1	34.3	46.6	0.737	
SD	14	15.8	10.8	14.5	0.036	

BM, body mass; F, female; FFM, fat-free body mass; M, male; TBW, total body water; TBW/FFM, ratio of total body water to fat-free body mass.
Source: Ref. 10.

other hand, it is somewhat easier to measure with widely available scintillation counters (51).

Once the dilution volume is known, total body water volume and mass can be calculated from isotope exchange fraction and water density. Each of the three isotopes measures a specific dilution volume that is somewhat larger than the actual volume. For the two hydrogen isotopes, tritium and deuterium, the dilution volume is larger than actual total body water because the H atoms in the tracer exchange with H atoms bound to carboxyl, hydroxyl, and amino groups (52). Similarly, the ^{18}O tracer exchanges with oxygen atoms in carboxyl and phosphate groups (53). Exchange of labeled atoms

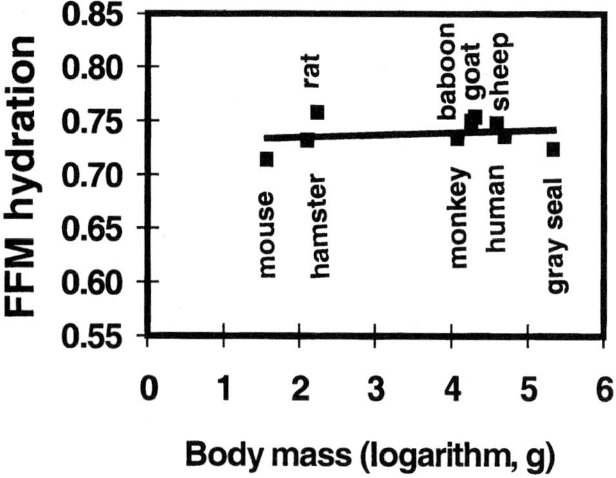

Figure 9 Total body water versus fat-free body mass, both expressed in logarithms, for humans and eight mammalian species. (From Ref. 10.)

with unlabeled atoms from molecular components may vary owing a number of factors, but most investigators assume a stable exchange of ~4% for tritium and deuterium and ~1% for ^{18}O(53). Thus, total body water is calculated as the product of isotope dilution volume and a correction factor that accounts for isotope exchange (e.g., ^3H_2O and ^2H_2O dilution volumes × 0.96; $H_2{}^{18}O$ dilution volume × 0.99). At present, there does not appear to be a universally accepted, fully valid method of estimating isotope exchange. Total-body water volume is converted to mass using the density of water at body temperature (0.9937 g/cc at 36°C or 0.9934 g/cc at 37°C). Total body water, once known, can then be used to estimate total body fat and FFM as: FFM = 1.37 × TBW, and fat = body weight − FFM.

The total body water method is widely used, and the specific isotope selected depends on available funds, analytical facilities, and subject characteristics. An important feature of the total body water method is the availability of stable isotopes, thus eliminating radioactivity from the analysis for use in children or pregnant women. The subject evaluation portion of the total body water method can be carried out in field settings, and some investigators use this approach in phenotyping subjects in remote settings. The total body water method can also be used as the reference for total body fat in remote settings when developing ethnic-specific calibration equations for calibrating bioimpedance and anthropometric methods. The total body water method is also a reasonable approach for estimating adiposity in morbidly obese patients for whom other methods may not be suitable. The validity of the assumed stable FFM hydration (0.73) in morbidly obese subjects is unknown.

An important concern is bias error due to systematic variation in the TBW/FFM ratio with age, gender, race, obesity, disease, or other factors. As an example, TBW/FFM is known to be higher in infants and young children than in adults (54). Some have speculated that the TBW/FFM ratio is decreased in obesity and elevated in elderly people (55,56). Certain diseases (e.g., renal disease, congestive heart failure) clearly result in alterations in the TBW/FFM ratio. Lastly, the early phase of weight loss (i.e., the first 1–2 weeks) with obesity treatment may be associated with relatively greater water loss than of other FFM components and thus the assumed TBW/FFM ratio may not be constant during the phase of dynamic weight change (57).

4 Hydrodensitometry/Air Displacement Plethysmography

a. *Hydrodensitometry*

Hydrodensitometry, often referred to as underwater weighing, is one of the oldest in vivo methods of analyzing human body composition as a two-component (i.e., fat and FFM) model (58).

Hydrodensitometry is based on the Archimedean principle that a solid object submerged in water is subject to a buoyant force that is equal to the weight of the water displaced by the object, or the loss in weight of the object when it is weighed while submerged in the water. Thus, the specific gravity or "density" of the object can be determined from the weight of the object divided by the loss in weight when submerged in water. The human body generally has a density close to that of water (i.e., 1.0 g/cm^3). Individual deviations from this value are mainly due to the amount of fat in the body. Because fat is less dense than water, the lower the body density, the greater the amount of body fat. Behnke was the first to show that this method could be used to deduce the percentage of weight that is fat from body density using a simple two-component model that assumes specific densities for fat and fat-free fractions of body weight (13,59).

Lipid extracts of human adipose tissue, which are mostly triglycerides, have a mean density of 0.9007 g/cm^3 at body temperature (60) (Table 2). The density of FFM has been estimated to be 1.100 g/cm^3 based on data from cadaver studies (61). Fat-free body mass is assumed to be composed of constant proportions of water (73.2%), minerals (6.8%), and protein (19.5%) with residual amounts (< 1%) of other chemical components (e.g., glycogen). The densities of these individual chemical components are also considered to be constants at body temperature (Table 2). Human body densities generally vary between 1.08 g/cm^3 (very lean) and 1.03 g/cm^3 (moderately obese). Obese subjects will have body densities < 1.03 g/cm^3, and severely obese people may have densities < 1.00 g/cm^3.

The most commonly used two-component model for estimating body composition from body density measured by underwater weighing was derived originally by Siri [Eq. (1)](62). A revised model proposed by Brozek et al. (61) gives slightly lower estimates in obese subjects due to somewhat different underlying assumptions regarding the densities of fat (0.8888 g/cc) and fat-free (1.1033 g/cc) components. Additional revised models have been proposed that adjust the coefficients in two-component equations for systematic differences in the composition of FFM associated with age, sex, ethnicity, and level of fatness (14,54,56). These adjusted equations should not be applied without, verifying in a random subsample of a study population that the assumed deviations in fat-free composition actually occur. None of these equations consider human individual variability in the composition of FFM that may occur independent of age, sex, ethnicity, or obesity. As the composition of FFM may change with short-term weight loss, two-component models based on body density alone may provide inaccurate estimates of the amount of fat lost during the early phase of obesity treatment (63).

A limitation of the underwater weighing method is that accurate measurements require active participation and effort by the subject being measured. In the conventional approach, the subject must submerge their body completely while exhaling maximally, and then hold their breath and body position for several seconds until a weight measurement is obtained. Some individuals cannot perform adequately, and underwater weighing is not feasible in very young children, frail elderly, or those with serious cardiovascular or pulmonary diseases. In those who can perform the procedure, errors may occur owing to body movement and the buoyant effects of air in the gastrointestinal tract and lungs. Errors due to movement during submersion may be reduced by the use of electronic load cells and stable chair systems, rather than spring scales and body slings. It is not feasible to measure the amount of air and gas in the stomach and intestinal tract, and a fixed value is usually assumed (~ 100 mL).

The larger air volume in the lungs is adjusted for by measuring residual lung volume when the subject is out of the water using a spirometer with He dilution or N washout, or during weighing with systems designed for this purpose. The simultaneous measurement of residual lung volume and underwater weight may be preferred because it controls for the effects of the increased pressure of water on the thorax during immersion. Some studies suggest, however, that these effects are small and result in only a slight reduction in residual volume in normal subjects (64). Maximum effort and compliance by the subject during spirometry, whether in or out of the water, and repeated measurements of residual lung volume may be more important. Inaccurate measurements of air in the lungs can be a major source of error when estimating body density from underwater weighing.

Although feasible, underwater weighing of obese subjects may present special problems. Obesity is often association with respiratory problems and reduced lung function, which may make it more difficult to obtain accurate measurements of residual lung volume. As obese subjects have a strong tendency to float owing to their low body density, it may be necessary to use a weight belt, or other tare weight system, to completely submerge the body. The tare weights must be measured and recorded carefully to obtain an accurate underwater weight. Despite these limitations, high levels of precision can be achieved in most obese subjects with underwater weighing. Moreover, underwater weighing may be the only practical method of measuring body fat in very obese subjects who cannot be evaluated by other methods. The minimum possible technical and biological errors from all sources for percent body fat by underwater weighing has been estimated to be about ± 2.5% (65). This represents an ideal, however, that can be achieved only if careful attention is given to optimizing the performance of subjects and the quality of the equipment, and if all model assumptions are valid.

Assuming subjects are comfortable with water submersion, the hydrodensitometry method is very safe. Underwater weighing systems range in price and at the low end can be built quickly at low cost. Once built, the systems are usually not transportable.

b. *Air Displacement Plethysmography*

Air displacement plethysmography (ADP) is a technique designed to replace hydrodensitometry in the approximation of body composition (66). The governing principle is essentially that of hydro-densitometry—that the density of a human body can be used to approximate two-compartment body composition, fat and FFM. In ADP, however, body volume is evaluated by measuring air displaced by a body's introduction to a controlled environment.

Attempts in a number of forms have been made throughout the years to replace hydrodensitometric measurement with ADP. However, these approaches were unsatisfactory for a number of reasons, but owing particularly to complications arising from the introduction into the measurement chamber of the human body itself (e.g., changes in temperature, air composition, etc.). Such problems have largely been addressed with the commercial ADP system now available (BOD POD Body Composition System, Life Measurement Instruments, Concord, CA) (66).

The BOD POD measurement system is comprised of an electronic scale and the BOD POD unit itself, both routed through a computer operated by a technician (66). The measuring process is relatively simple. First, the subject, wearing a form-fitting bathing suit and swim cap, is weighed on the scale. The subject is then seated in the front chamber of the calibrated BOD POD unit. An egg-shaped capsule, the unit has a large window that allows the subject to see outside, making for a more comfortable environment. A moving diaphragm mounted between the front and rear chambers, 450 and 300 L, respectively, oscillates during the measurement process to create in the two chambers volume perturbations of exactly equal magnitude. Air between the two chambers is constantly mixed during measurement, and the subject breathes through a filtered tube as thoracic volume change due to breathing is recorded. Thus are addressed the effects of changes in isothermal conditions and air composition.

Once measurement is complete, the software provided with the system records the subject's volume and density and, using the Siri equation [Eq. (1)], calculates and records the subject's body composition. Studies have indicated that the reproducibility of percent adiposity measurement using the BOD POD is high, with between-trial SD reported at 0.4% and CV 1.7% ± 1.1%, both marginally lower than for hydrostatic weighing (67). Some investigators have found a trend in the BOD POD toward underestimation of body density as compared to hydrodensitometry, creating a small but statistically significant difference in percent fat (68). There are now many studies reporting good agreement between BOD POD percent fat estimates and those provided by other reference methods such as DXA. Systems are reportedly in development that are suited for young children for whom the present BOD POD is not ideally designed.

Benefits of this ADP system include the ease of use relative to hydrodensitometry, minimal requirement for subject participation, and high level of reproducibility. Subjects and technicians also require a minimal amount of instruction, the process takes only a few minutes for each subject, and the chamber is relatively accessible for the elderly, disabled, and obese. A limitation of the ADP system is that the chamber, while mobile for field use, weighs > 135 kg, and transporting the entire system might prove difficult. Nevertheless, BOD POD systems are in use at settings involved in phenotyping remote populations. Clothing restrictions can be of some concern for individual patients; for example, the manufacturer's instructions advise that subjects should wear a swim cap and tight-fitting swimsuit to ensure accuracy. Furthermore, the size of the chamber may be restrictive for very large people. Finally, the cost of the BOD POD may be prohibitive for some who would wish to use the system.

5 Dual-Energy X-Ray Absorptiometry

Anthropologists and health care workers in the field of metabolic bone disease have long required a means for quantifying bone mass. In the past, the preferred approach was to expose one side of the subject's wrist to a photon-emitting radioactive source while a scintillation counter was positioned on the other side of the wrist (69). The number of counts detected served to indicate the amount of attenuating calcium or bone present. The wrist was typically the site of choice for measurement because at that part bone is the main attenuating tissue, unlike conditions at the hip or spine where soft tissue is also present. Later, investigators explored means of evaluating hip and spine, as those are two bone areas of clinical concern for the study of osteoporosis. The single-photon system evolved to a dual-photon system, and is now based on a filtered x-ray source and is commonly called dual-energy x-ray absorptiometry (DXA) (69). In order to quantify bone mineral within a soft-tissue containing pixel, DXA systems required information about soft tissue composition. The capacity for quantifying the fat and lean soft tissue content of a pixel evolved into DXA's central role in modern body composition analysis.

All DXA systems in general operate on similar principals, although important technical details prevail (70) (Fig. 10). An x-ray source provides a broad photon beam that is usually filtered, thus yielding two main energy peaks. Some systems use a pulsating voltage source to produce the two energy peaks. The emitted photons traverse the subject's tissues; the extent of the attenuation that follows depends on the tissue's elemental makeup. Elements of low atomic weight, such as hydrogen, minimally attenuate photons whereas elements such as calcium are highly attenuating. The difference in attenuation between the two energy peaks is particular to each element, and thus to each tissue. The characteristic attenuation signature for fat, lean, and bone mineral allows one to develop pixel-by-pixel composition estimates using a series of

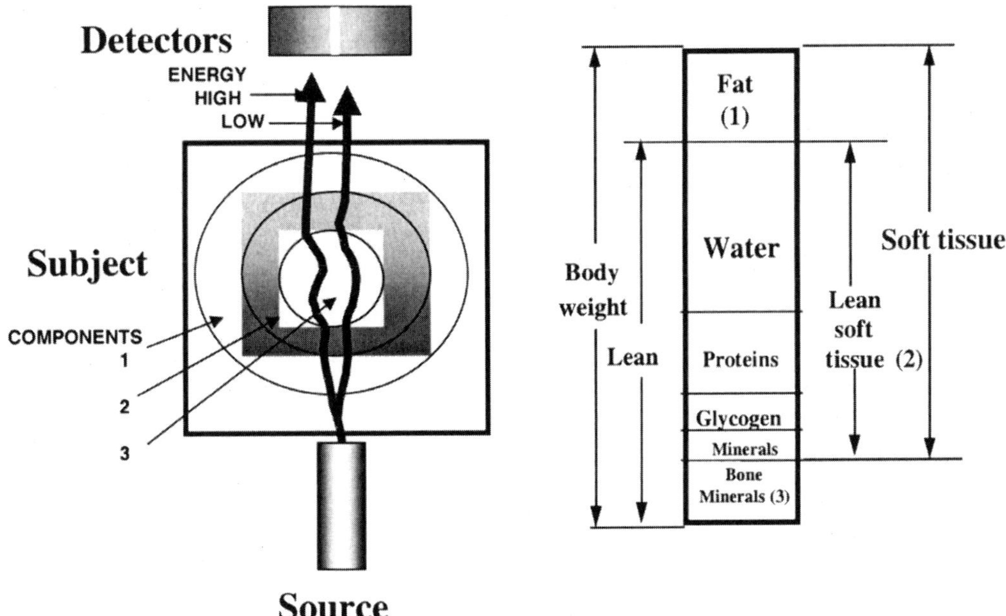

Figure 10 Schematic representation of DXA system (left) and three-component model consisting of bone mineral, lean soft tissue, and fat. (From Ref. 17.)

assumptions and reconstruction algorithms (70). Some systems use a simple "pencil beam" configuration as the patient is scanned, while others are based on a "fan beam" configuration of x-ray source and detector. Fan beam systems tend to be faster, requiring just several minutes for each scan; pencil beam models have a longer scan time. Accuracy varies between system designs and software. The manufacturer performs calibrations that allow resolution of the three molecular level components, bone mineral, fat, and lean soft tissue (Fig. 4). Once systems are operational, system calibration and functional evaluations are also carried out on a regular basis. DXA x-ray exposure is minimal (< 1 mrem), allowing for safe longitudinal studies in children and adults.

DXA estimates the three molecular level components for the whole body and separately for the arms, legs, and trunk. The body segment estimates are somewhat less precise and accurate than those for the whole body (69). The accuracy of DXA systems is influenced by the thickness of the energy-absorbing tissues in the path of the x-ray beam, and accuracy decreases with increasing thickness due to beam hardening. Manufacturers of DXA systems include correction algorithms in their operating software for the effects of body thickness, although different versions of software may provide somewhat different body composition estimates (71).

Several studies have compared DXA with physicochemical analyses of pig carcasses, and generally show better results for larger animals, and application in infants and small children is now well accepted (72–74). New, specially designed DXA systems are proving useful in phenotyping fatness in small animals such as the mouse. DXA has also been evaluated using experimental models composed of measured amounts of biological tissues or non-biological tissue-equivalent materials (75,76).In vivo studies of DXA accuracy can be separated into experimental versus observational groups. In experimental studies, packets of lard have been placed on lean subjects to simulate increased amounts of adipose tissues (74,77). These studies have produced mixed results that seem to depend on where the additional lard was placed on the body (trunk vs. legs), the type of scanner, and the version of software used. Other experiments have tested the effects of changes in hydration of the FFM using either patients undergoing hemodialysis or volunteers ingesting large amounts of water. Generally, DXA has been shown to measure changes in body fluids accurately and to correctly attribute these changes to the lean soft tissue mass (78). A recent study with phantoms supported by theoretical calculations suggests that percent fat estimates by DXA are minimally influenced by changes in hydration within the physiological range (79). Observational studies have compared DXA, with favorable outcomes, to estimates from hydrodensitometry, total body water, and multicomponent models in subject groups over wide ranges of body fatness (80,81). It is important to note that few studies were specifically designed to test the accuracy of DXA in moderately or severely obese subjects.

Most studies show that DXA estimates of body composition are highly reproducible. This has been evaluated in a variety of experiments. Reported technical errors for estimates of percent fat ranged from 0.3% to 1.4%; errors for FFM range from 0.3 to 0.9 kg (69,80). Reported coefficients of variation range from 0.5% to 4% for percent body fat, 1% to 1.7% for fat mass, and 0.7%, to 1.0% for FFM (78,82). Although there is substantial evidence that DXA estimates lose accuracy with increasing body thickness, reports are conflicting as to whether thickness results in a systematic bias toward either over- or underestimation of body fatness (76). These conflicting results might be attributable to the use of different scanners and versions of software incorporating different calibration standards and thickness corrections. In any event, it is reasonable to expect that DXA estimates will lose both accuracy and precision in thicker obese subjects.

The DXA approach is rapidly becoming the most available and established of the reference body composition methods as systems are well designed and provide accurate and reproducible results, studies in children are possible, and there exists the possibility of transporting systems in a mobile van. The disadvantages of DXA are that it cannot be used in pregnant women, the cost of purchasing and operating the system is relatively high, and very large or obese subjects cannot be easily accommodated on most available systems. An ongoing and unresolved debate centers on the superiority of fan beam versus pencil beam systems, and on other system characteristics that differ among manufacturers.

The application of DXA to the body composition analysis of obese patients is subject to additional practical limitations. Many obese individuals will simply be too wide for the scan field (~ 190 × 60 cm) as the soft tissue falling outside of the scan field will not be included in the body composition analysis, resulting in biased estimates. As a result, DXA manufacturers generally do not recommend scanning individuals > 100 kg body weight. This represents a serious limitation to the application of DXA body composition analysis, and it also may limit the accuracy of regional body composition data. For example, it may not be possible to abduct the arms sufficiently from the trunk, or to separate the legs sufficiently at the thighs, in obese subjects to obtain accurate estimates of separate arm and leg soft-tissue masses. Tataranni and Ravussin (82) described an approach that combines information from two DXA scans taken for each side of the body in obese subjects. This approach appears to provide reasonably accurate estimates, compared to those from hydrodensitometry, but requires careful attention to subject positioning in the scan field and also adds significantly to total scan and data analysis time. As an alternative, the authors suggest multiplying body weight by percent fat estimates from a half-body scan in order to derive total body estimates. This method is likely to be accurate, albeit only in subjects with little anatomical asymmetry between the right and left halves of the body.

6 Multicomponent Models

A supplementary approach to the two-compartment hydrodensitometry or ADP methods is to use multicomponent methods that include measures of total body water, bone mineral mass, and soft tissue mineral mass in addition to body density, assuming fixed densities for each component (Table 2) (83–85). Multicomponent models are designed to provide estimates of three or more components. Adding more measured components reduces the number of applied model assumptions and multicomponent methods are often applied as the criterion against with other methods are compared (86).

Selected examples are provided in Table 6 of three-, four-, and five-component methods of estimating fat mass along with the measurable quantities and simultaneous equations upon which they are based (83–90). The equations in Table 6 are based on component densities at body temperature, which ranges between 36°C and 37°C (Table 2). In certain groups, such as children, elderly, African-American, or sick patients, these methods may provide more accurate estimates of body fatness than the simpler, two-component models. Precise measures of total body water, bone mineral mass, and soft tissue mineral mass are required, however, to avoid swamping the gain in accuracy with increased propagated errors of the additional measurements (91). In addition, the benefit in terms of improved accuracy should always be evaluated in relation to the increased cost associated with obtaining the additional measurements of total body water, total body bone mineral, and soft tissue mineral (86). These costs may be justified when the goal is to estimate changes in body fat over time, as in clinical weight loss studies, and in evaluating the accuracy of other potential reference methods.

7 Imaging Methods

Imaging methods, such as CT and MRI, are considered the most accurate means available for in vivo quantification of body composition on the tissue system level. Although access and expenses remain obstacles to routine use, these imaging approaches are now used extensively in body composition research. CT and MRI are the methods of choice for calibration of field methods designed to measure adipose tissue and skeletal muscle in vivo, and are the only methods available for measurement of internal tissues and organs. More recently both methods have been employed to measure the quality of various tissues, in particular, skeletal muscle tissue.

a. Computed Tomography

The basic CT system consists of an x-ray tube and receiver that rotate in a perpendicular plane to the subject. CT measures are 0.1–0.2 Å, 60–120 kVp x-rays that are attenuated as they pass through tissues (92). Attenuation is expressed as the linear attenuation coefficient or CT number. The CT number is a measure of attenuation relative to air and water. The CT numbers of air and water are defined as −1000 and 0 Hounsfield number (HU), respectively. The x-ray beam attenuation is related to three factors: coherent scattering, photoelectric absorption, and Compton interactions (92). Physical density is the main determinant of attenuation and, therefore, CT number. There is a linear correlation between CT number and tissue density (93,94). Each of the image pixels or voxels has a CT number which gives contrast to the image. Image reconstruction is usually done with mathematical techniques based on either two-dimensional Fourier analysis, filtered back-projection, or a combination of these methods.

CT body composition methods are designed to quantify components at the tissue system level of body composition. The main components are adipose tissue, skeletal muscle, bone, visceral organs, and brain. Cross-sectional images are composed of picture elements or pixels, usually 1 × 1 mm squares. Slice thicknesses vary, and when considered in three dimensions, the image consists of volume elements or voxels. Each pixel/voxel is assigned a value on a gray scale that reflects the composition of the tissue.

Table 6 Representative Multicomponent Methods for Measuring Total Body Fat

Reference	Required measurements		Simultaneous equations	Fat mass equation
	Properties	Components		
Siri(62)	BW, BV	Water	BW = FM + water + protein + mineral BV = FM/0.900 + water/0.994 + protein/1.34 + mineral/3.04 protein = 2.40 × mineral	FM = 2.057 × BV − 0.786 × water − 1.286 × BW
Lohman (54)	BW, BV	Mineral	BW = FM + water + protein + mineral BV = FM/0.9007 + water/0.994 + protein/1.34 + mineral/3.04 water = 4.00 × protein	FM = 6.386 × BV + 3.961 × mineral − 6.09 × BW
Baumgartner et al. (88)	BW, BV	Water, TBBM	BW = FM + water + protein + TBBM + Ms BV = FM/0.9007 + water/0.994 + protein/1.34 + TBBM/2.982 + Ms/3.317 Ms = 0.235 × TBBM	FM = 2.75 × BV − 0.714 × water + 1.148 × mineral − 2.05 × BW
Selinger (89)	BW, BV	Water, TBBM	BW = FM + water + protein + TBBM + Ms BV = FM/0.9007 + water/0.994 + protein/1.34 + TBBM/2.982 + Ms/3.317 Ms = 0.0105BW	FM = 2.75 × BV − 0.714 × water + 1.129 × TBBM − 2.037 × BW
Heymsfield (90)	BW, BV	Water, TBBM	BW = FM + water + TBBM + residual BV = FM/0.9907 + water/0.99371 + TBBM/2.982 + residual/1.404	FM = 2.513 × BV − 0.739 × water + 0.947 × TBBM − 1.79 × BW
Wang (86)	BW, BV	Water, Mo, MS	BW = FM + water + protein + Mo + Ms BV = FM/0.9007 + water/0.99371 + Protein/1.34 + Mo/2.982 + Ms/3.317	FM = 2.748 × BV − 0.715 × water + 1.129 × Mo + 1.222 × Ms − 2.051 × BW

Abbreviations: BV, body volume (liter); BW, body weight (kg); FM, fat mass (kg); Mo, osseous mineral; Ms, soft tissue mineral (kg); TBBM (kg) = ashed bone from DXA × 1.0436.
Source: Ref. 15.

Quantifying tissue volume by CT requires two steps. First, the tissue area (cm^2) on each cross-sectional CT image is determined using one of two methods (95,96). In one technique, the investigator traces the perimeter of the target tissue with a light pen or track ball controlled cursor. The area of the circumscribed tissue is then calculated, usually with software installed on the CT scanner console. The second approach employs a computerized edge detection procedure that identifies the area of the target tissue by selecting pixels within a given HU range, for example −190 to − 30 HU for adipose tissue (96). Automated procedures are now becoming available. Once the tissue areas (cm^2) are quantified for a series of images, the total volume can be calculated by integrating data from multiple contiguous slices. The tissue mass can be then calculated if a value for the density of the tissue is assumed.

CT tissue area and volume measurements have been shown to be highly reproducible. Kvist et al. (96) reported an average error of ± 0.6% for whole body adipose tissue volume for duplicate measures in four subjects. Chowdhury et al. (95) reported intraobserver errors for a large number of CT-measured body composition components. Some examples are for skin = 2.4%, total adipose tissue = 0.4%, and heart = 3.4%. An earlier report by Brummer et al. (97) indicated interobserver errors of 0.7%, 0.4%, and 2.1% for total adipose tissue, skeletal muscle, and visceral organs, respectively.

Several studies have established the accuracy of area and volume measurements from CT. Heymsfield et al. (98) reported that organ masses estimated using CT were highly reproducible and agreed with actual mass to within 5–6%. Rossner and colleagues (99) found good agreement between CT and cadaver adipose tissue areas and ratios (r's ranged from .77 to .94). Chowdhury and colleagues (95) reported that the average difference between body weight and mass determined from CT measured tissue volumes was 0.024 ± 0.65 kg and the coefficient of variation was 0.85%. Wang and colleagues (100) reported that body volume calculated from 22 CT slices was highly correlated with body volume from underwater weighing in seventeen men ($r = .99$, $P = .0001$, SEE = 1.9 L, n = 17), although there was a statistically significant difference between the mean values (CT = 74.8 ± 13.9 L vs. UWW = 73.6 ± 13.7 L, $P < .02$). This difference between mean volumes may be due to difficulty in accurately estimating residual lung volumes and in quantifying lung parenchymal volume by CT.

Heymsfield and colleagues were among the first to explore the use of CT in body composition research. They initially used CT to quantify the cross-sectional area of arm muscle in 1979 (101); subsequent reports described methods of estimating visceral organ volumes (98) and VAT (102). Borkan and colleagues were the first to systematically evaluate VAT in 1982 (103). Sjöström and colleagues introduced whole-body imaging and multicomponent analysis to quantify total body and regional adipose tissue, skeletal muscle, bone, and other organ/tissue volumes (104).

In recent years CT has been employed to measure the quality of various tissues—in particular, skeletal muscle tissue. The focus has been to establish the lipid content as altered fat deposition in skeletal muscle is linked to reduced insulin-stimulated glucose uptake. An increased muscle lipid content has also been noted in older persons and is associated with muscle wasting diseases (105,106). As noted above, CT is capable of distinguishing different tissue types on the basis of their attenuation characteristics, which in turn are a function of tissue density and chemical composition. Skeletal muscle attenuation is determined by measuring the mean attenuation value from all pixels within the range of 0–100 HU. The lower the mean attenuation value, the greater the infiltration of lipid within the muscle. As an additional means of characterizing muscle composition, the distribution of attenuation values is described as representing two components on the basis of muscle density. One-component, normal-density muscle is defined as muscle pixels with attenuation values within 2 SD of the mean attenuation value observed in lean, normal muscle (31–100 HU). The second component, low density muscle, is defined as muscle with below normal attenuation values (0–30 HU).

The reliability and validity of in vivo measurement of skeletal muscle attenuation was recently studied by Goodpaster et al. (107). Single-slice CT scans performed on phantoms of varying lipid concentrations revealed good agreement between attenuation and lipid concentration ($r^2 = .995$). The test-retest coefficient of variation for mean attenuation values obtained from two CT scans performed on six volunteers was 0.51% for the midthigh and 0.85% for the midcalf. Although additional validation studies would be useful, preliminary findings suggest that the variability of muscle composition values by CT is low and that the method provides accurate estimates of lipid content, albeit by comparison to phantoms.

Early studies that employed CT to measure muscle composition found associations between reduced skeletal muscle attenuation and aging (108), Duchenne muscular dystrophy, and other myopathies (109). More recently, Goodpaster et al. have observed that the mean muscle attenuation within skeletal muscle is reduced in obesity and type 2 diabetes mellitus (110), and that weight loss increases the mean attenuation value of muscle (111). These unique applications of CT represent a major advance in the study of altered muscle composition in vivo with numerous applications in both applied and clinical medicine. An example of this approach is given in Figure 11.

In a manner similar to that used to determine skeletal muscle density, CT has also been employed to determine the density of liver tissue (112). As with muscle, the lower the Hounsfield units, the lower the liver density and the greater the fat content of the liver. Therefore liver density is inversely related to liver fat and thus is a surrogate for it (113). Several investigators have employed CT to measure liver composition in various cohorts. A focus of this research has been to determine possible links between fatty liver and insulin resistance (114). Determination of liver fat "fatty liver" may provide novel insight into the relationship between abdominal obesity, in particular visceral fat, and increased metabolic risk. Björntorp hypothesized that the metabolic importance of visceral fat may be due to the delivery of free fatty acids into the portal system exerting potent and direct effects on the liver. Indeed, it is now well established that the plasma free fatty acid

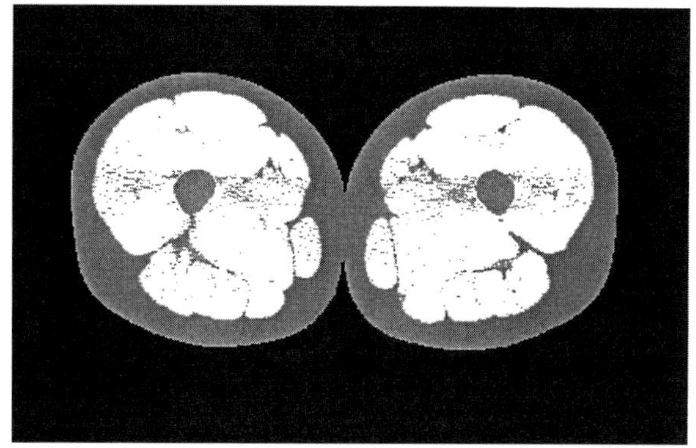

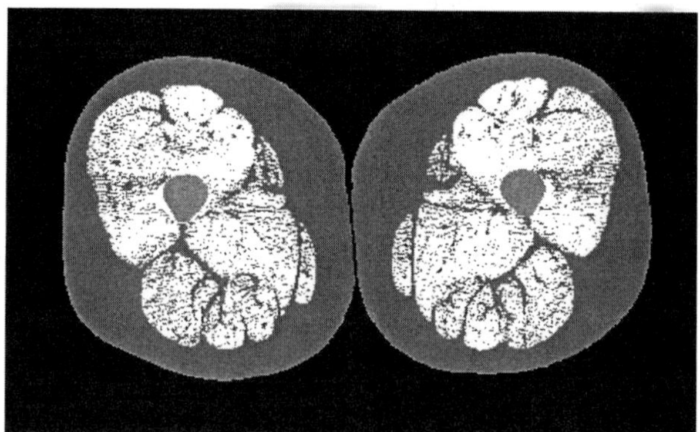

Figure 11 CT images of the proximal thigh for a lean (left) and obese (right) subject. The darker-appearing pixels within the skeletal muscle tissue of both subjects have attenuation values (Hounsfield Units) between 0 and 100. Skeletal muscle attenuation is determined by measuring the mean attenuation value from all pixels within the range of 0 to 100 HU. The lower the mean attenuation value, the greater the infiltration of lipid within the muscle. The mean attenuation value of the skeletal muscle of the obese subject is lower (i.e., darker pixels) by comparison to the lean subject.

concentration is a primary modulator of hepatic insulin resistance (115). This is consistent with the knowledge that in men and women omental and mesenteric adipocytes are metabolically more active by comparison to abdominal subcutaneous adipocytes. Thus sustained differences in portal concentration of free fatty acids may at least partially explain the hepatic and peripheral insulin resistance that characterize viscerally obese older persons. Although it is not possible to readily access the portal circulation in vivo, it is reasonable to expect that sustained delivery of free fatty acids to the liver would cause an increase in the infiltration of lipid within the liver—hepatic steatosis or "fatty liver." Consistent with this position, evidence suggests that visceral fat is a positive correlate of liver fat in men (112), but not women (116).

b. Magnetic Resonance Imaging

The estimation of body composition components on the tissue system level using MRI is essentially the same as for CT. The two methods differ mainly in the manner in which the images are acquired, which has subsequent bearing on practical considerations of cost and applicability, as well as technical aspects of image analysis, relative accuracy, and reliability.

MRI does not use ionizing radiation. Instead, it is based on the interaction between hydrogen nuclei (i.e., protons), which are abundant in all biological tissues, and the magnetic fields generated and controlled by the MRI system's instrumentation. Hydrogen protons have a nonzero magnetic moment which cause them to behave like tiny magnets. When a subject is placed inside the magnet of a magnetic resonance imager, where the field strength is typically 10,000 times stronger than the earth's, the magnetic moments of the protons align themselves with the magnetic field. Having aligned the H protons in a known direction, a pulsed radiofrequency field (RF) is applied to the body tissues causing a number of hydrogen protons to absorb energy. When the RF is turned off, the protons gradually return to their original positions, releasing in the process the energy that they absorbed in the form of an RF signal. It is this signal that is used to generate the magnetic resonance images by computer.

Foster et al. (117) were among the first to illustrate the applicability of MRI to body composition analysis. Hayes et al. (118) first demonstrated the quantification of subcutaneous adipose tissue distribution in human subjects using MRI. A variety of studies have subsequently used MRI to quantify adipose tissue and/or lean tissue areas or volumes in children (119), normal males and females (120–122), obese males and females (123,124), diabetics (124), and elderly people (125). To date several groups have employed MRI to evaluate whole body adipose tissue and lean tissue distribution in human subjects (120–122c).

Historically, an important problem with the application of MRI to body composition analysis has been the substantial time needed to obtain images of sufficient quality and resolution for reliable measurements. For example, depending on the pulse sequence used, the acquisition of a set of MRI images for the abdomen could require between 8 (120) and 16 min (126). Recent advances in MRI technology have reduced the time needed to obtain the same quality images of the abdomen to ~25 sec, and a series of images for whole body analysis can be acquired in <30 min (127). These advances should make MRI a much more accessible instrument for body composition studies in the future.

A multislice MRI protocol for whole body analysis is illustrated in Figure 5 (127). The pulse sequence used to obtain images of the abdomen in this protocol requires 26 sec. During this time the subject must hold his/her breath to reduce the effects of respiratory motion on image quality.

A factor that has impeded the use of MRI in body composition analysis has been the availability of appropriate image analysis software. In contrast to CT, this software is not generally included on most MRI control consoles. As a result, MRI image data usually must be translated and downloaded to a separate workstation with image analysis software. Once this is accomplished, the approach to the analysis of MRI images is similar to that used for CT images. The perimeter of the tissue of interest can be traced using a light pen or mouse-controlled pointer, and the area within the perimeter can be calculated by multiplying the number of pixels in the highlighted region by their known area (128,129). Alternatively, image segmentation algorithms can be used that highlight all pixels within a selected range of intensities believed to be representative of a specific tissue. The latter approach, however, is considered more problematic when applied to MRI than to CT images for three reasons: (1) the distributions of pixel intensity (gray scale) values for different tissues overlap more for MRI than for CT images; (2) noise due to respiratory motion blurs the borders between tissues in the abdomen to a greater extent in MRI than in CT; and (3) inhomogeneity in the magnetic field can produce "shading" at the peripheries of MRI images.

Once tissue areas have been quantified from MRI images, volumes (cm^3) and masses may be calculated in a manner similar to that described above for CT. Ross (120), however, has defined a somewhat different mathematical formula for deriving tissue volumes from measurements of a series of axial MRI images. This formula recognizes that each image has a slice thickness and that the pixels identified for a tissue are actually volume elements, or voxels. Thus, the formula is based on volumes of truncated cones defined by pairs of consecutive images as follows:

$$V = d \times \sum_{i=1}^{n} \left\{ h/3 \times \left[(A_i + A_{i+1}) + (A_i + A_{i+1})^{0.5} \right] \right\} \tag{20}$$

where V is total tissue volume, A and A_{i+1} are the two consecutive images, and h is the distance between slices.

Several studies support the accuracy of MRI estimates of human adipose tissue and skeletal muscle and some examples are presented in Table 7. Using a rat model, Ross et al. (130) reported that whole carcass chemically extracted lipid was highly correlated with MRI adipose tissue mass ($r = .99$, $P < .01$) and that the standard error of estimate was 8.7%. Fowler et al. (128) compared MRI adipose tissue measurements to those obtained by dissection in a group of lean and obese pigs. The authors observed that the distribution of MRI adipose tissue correlated strongly with adipose tissue distribution by dissection ($r = .98$), and that the mean square error was 2.1%. Engstrom et al. (131) compared the cross-sectional area measurements of skeletal muscle determined from the proximal thigh in cadavers to the corresponding MRI-measured cross-sectional areas and reported that the correlation coefficient between the two approached unity ($r = .99$). Abate et al. (129) compared MRI measures of abdominal subcutaneous and visceral adipose tissue to that obtained by direct weighing of the same adipose tissue compartments after dissection in three human cadavers. In this study the authors subdivided VAT into intraperitoneal and retroperitoneal depots. For the various compartments the mean difference between the two methods was 0.076 kg or 6%.

Overall, the reported reliability of body composition estimates from MRI is somewhat less than that for CT as shown by the examples in Table 8. Seidell et al. (134) reported CV%'s for repeated measurements of total, visceral, and subcutaneous adipose tissue areas for the abdomen of 5.4, 10.6 and 10.1%, respectively. Baumgartner et al. (135,136) reported CV%'s of <5% for total and subcutaneous adipose tissue and 16% for VAT, which were calculated from two repeated measurements by two independent observers on 25 sets of images. For skeletal muscle, Mitsiopoulos et al. (133) report that the intraobserver correlation for duplicate MRI measurements obtained at the midthigh level in vivo is 0.99 with a standard error of 8.7 cm^2 or <3%.

It is important with MRI to distinguish error associated with repeated analyses of the same image from that associated with repeated acquisition of the image. There are at least three studies that report reliability

Table 7 MRI Validation Studies

Reference	Subjects (N)	IV	Correlation (SEE, %)			
			SCAT	Visceral AT	Total AT	SM
Comparison with CT						
Seidell et al. (126)	Human (7)	Midabdomen	0.79 (4.9)	0.79 (12.8)	0.99 (4.4)	—
Sobel et al. (132)	Human (11)	Umbilicus	0.98 (8)	0.93 (20)	—	—
Ross et al. (130)	Rats (21)	Whole body	0.98 (12)	0.98 (13.6)	0.99 (8.7)	—
Comparison with cadavers						
Engstrom et al. (131)	Human (3)	Thigh muscle CSA	—	—	—	0.99
Mitsiopoulos et al. (133)	Human	Arm and leg muscle CSA	0.99 (7.6)	—	—	0.97 (10)

AT, adipose tissue; IV, independent variable; SC, subcutaneous; SEE, standard error of estimate; SM, skeletal muscle; SCAT, subcutaneous adipose tissue; %, percent; CSA, cross-sectional area.
Source: Ref. 129a.

data for repeated image acquisitions (128,129,160,188). The CVs for measurements of subcutaneous abdominal adipose tissue areas measured for two images taken at the same level range from 1% to 10%. The reported CVs for VAT are somewhat higher, ranging from 6% to 11% (Table 8) Overall, these reported CVs for MRI are about two to three times greater than those for studies using CT.

Ross et al. (120) described special, interactive image analysis software that allows the analyst to correct misclassified pixels. Although training and experience are needed to use this software, reliability equivalent to those for CT can be achieved. Decreased scan times and other improvements in imaging techniques should further increase the reliability of future MRI body composition analyses. A more detailed review of the procedures used to determine body composition using MRI can be found elsewhere (138,140).

To date the principal application of MRI in human body composition research has been to characterize the quantity and distribution of adipose tissue and skeletal muscle. MRI has been employed to measure adipose tissue and lean tissue in fetuses (142), children (119), normal-weight males and females (120–122), obese males and females (123,124), and diabetic (124) and (125) elderly populations. While the aforementioned studies base their observations in large measure on a single MR image, it is also possible to acquire whole body MRI data in ~30 min (Fig. 12). The acquisition of whole-body MRI offers distinct advantages in assessing the influence of weight loss on body composition. For example, weight reduction scenarios may induce re-

Table 8 Reliability Studies[a]

Reference	Subject (N)	T	MRI Sequence	Anatomical position	Coefficient of variation (%)			
					SCAT	Visceral AT	Total AT	LT
Staten et al.	Human (6)	0.5	SE	Midabdomen	5.0	10.0	3.0	—
Seidell et al. (134)	Human (7)	1.5	IR	Umbilicus	10.1	10.6	5.4	—
Garard et al. (138)	Human (4)	1.5	SE	6 Abd. images	3.0	9.0	—	—
Ross et al. (130)	Rats (11)	1.5	SE	Whole body	—	—	4.3	—
Ross et al. 1993 (139)	Human (3)	1.5	SE	L4-L5	1.1	5.5	—	—
				Whole body	—	—	2.5	—
Sohlström et al. (121)	Human (3)	0.02	SR	Whole body	1.7	5.3*	1.5	—
Ross et al. (140)	Human (11)	1.5	SE	Proximal thigh	—	—	—	1.2
Abate et al. (129)	Cadavers (3)	0.35	SE	Abdomen	2.2	6.0	—	—
Ross et al. (141)	Human (19)	1.5	SE	L4-L5	—	—	—	1.0
Mitsiopoulos et al. (133)	Cadavers (6)	1.5	SE	Arm and leg slices	2.5	—	—	2.6

[a] Reported as nonsubcutaneous adipose tissue (SCAT).
AT, adipose tissue; IR, inverse recovery; SC, subcutaneous; LT, lean tissue; SE, spin-echo; SR, saturation recovery; T, strength of magnet in Tesla.

gional changes in adipose tissue or muscle. Thus, if an increase in skeletal muscle in one anatomical region is masked by a loss of skeletal muscle in another, only MRI studies could discover it. Indeed, whole-body MRI protocols have been employed to make important observations with respect to the effects of various perturbations on total and regional adipose tissue (143,144) and skeletal muscle distribution (145). Whole-body MRI has also been used to describe age-related muscle loss "sarcopenia" (146). Using fewer images, several investigations have employed MRI to assess the influence of weight loss (145), inactivity (146,147), and resistance training (148) on region-specific changes in skeletal muscle.

Similar to CT, recent evidence suggests that MRI may also be employed to measure the quality of in vivo skeletal muscle (149). Because proton MR imaging integrates, rather than separates, the signals from distinct protons within the image voxel, conventional MRI is not useful for determining, for example, the concentration of lipid or water in skeletal muscle. To obtain basic information within the tissue volume of interest requires application of "chemical shift" imaging techniques. Several chemical shift methods have been developed which separate the water and fat signals from the region of interest, creating the potential to determine water and fat contents of skeletal muscle. Tsubahara et al. (150) demonstrated a ^{1}H chemical shift imaging technique (Dixon method) to measure the fat and water content of skeletal muscle in men and women varying widely in age. Ross et al. reported preliminary findings using a spiral MR imaging scheme for direct quantification of the lipid MRI signal in skeletal muscle (149). In this approach, the signal from the water protons is selectively spoiled prior to excitation and spatial encoding of the signal from the lipid protons. The acquisition scheme is combined with the use of a three-point Dixon technique, short echo times, and mapping of radiofrequency inhomogeneities in order to minimize known biases in the MRI signal.

Figure 13 illustrates a representative comparison between conventional and lipid images obtained from

Protocol (Abdomen)

T1-weighted, spin-echo pulse sequence
Each image = 10 mm thickness, 40 mm spaces
TR = 210 ms; TE = 17 ms; 1/2 NEX
FOV = 48 cm X 36 cm (rectangular)
Matrix = 256 X 256
Each acquisition = 7 images
Time = 26 seconds (breath hold)

Protocol (Appendicular)

T1-weighted, spin-echo pulse sequence
Each image = 10 mm thickness, 40 mm spaces
TR = 210 ms; TE = 17 ms; 1 NEX
FOV = 48 cm X 36 cm (rectangular)
Matrix = 256 X 256
Each acquisition = 7 images
Time = 43 seconds

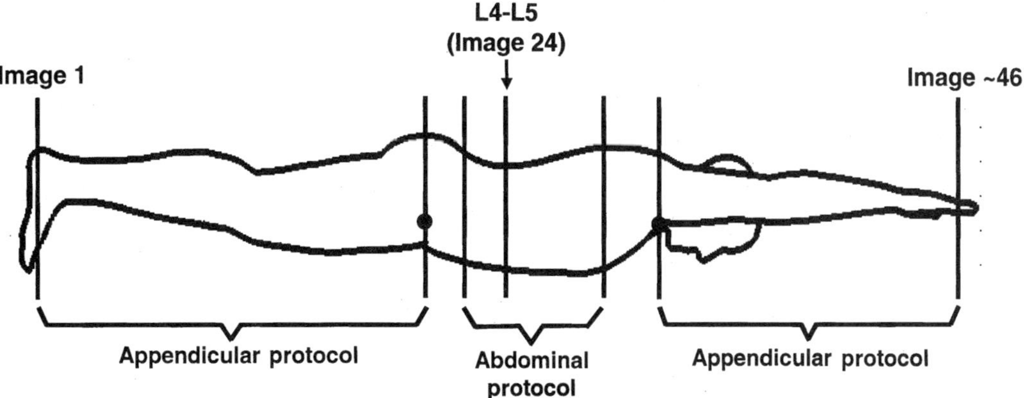

Figure 12 Illustration of the MRI protocol used to acquire axial images throughout the whole body. Both sequences employ a T1-weighted spin-echo scheme. The principal difference is that the abdomen sequence uses a one-half Fourier transformation pulse sequence (1/2 NEX). Using these parameters reduces the time required to obtain the data set to 26 sec during which the subject is asked to hold his/her breath. Although the signal-to-noise ratio is decreased using this scheme, the limitation is offset by the reduction in respiratory motion artifact normally associated with the acquisition of MR images in the abdomen region.

a single subject. Absolute lipid concentration is achieved by aligning cylindrical lipid phantoms of known concentration within the field of view during image acquisition. The signal intensity for each phantom is determined and subsequently used to derive a regression equation (i.e., signal intensity vs. concentration). The signal intensity from various regions of interest (ROIs) within skeletal muscle are then obtained and applied within the regression formula to determine absolute lipid concentration for the given ROI. Although preliminary evidence suggests that this method may be employed to characterise and distinguish the lipid concentration in lean and obese muscle (149), it is noted that with this MRI method it is not possible to separate the lipid measurement into intra- and extramyocellular compartments. Partitioning the lipid signal into separate compartments is accomplished using ^{1}H MRS (magnetic resonance spectroscopy), details of which are reported elsewhere (151).

In addition to quantification of muscle lipid using ^{1}H MRI, Constandinides et al. (152) have recently demonstrated the feasibility of using sodium (^{23}Na) MRI to quantify sodium concentration in human muscle and, using a 3D Twisted Projection Imaging scheme with a 1.5-T scanner, provide evidence that ^{23}Na MRI can accurately and reliability measure variations in sodium content that are characteristic of normal and diseased muscle. In this study it was also shown that ^{23}Na MRI may be used to characterize the selective recruitment of muscle during exercise, knee cartilage degeneration in osteoarthritis, and atrophy in myotonic dystrophy. The potential application of ^{23}Na MRI for the diagnosis of muscle dystrophy in aging muscle is particularly promising. Although ^{1}H MRI facilitates diagnosis of muscle atrophy in advanced states, elevations in sodium concentration within skeletal muscle, characteristic of the imbalance in sodium homeostasis in muscle dystrophy, by ^{23}Na MRI may foreshadow the onset of muscle dystrophy and/or muscle wasting commonly observed in the elderly.

Although these initial observations for both ^{1}H and ^{23}Na MRI are restricted to skeletal muscle of the lower limb, they represent unique applications of MRI that can be utilized to obtain novel insight into the composition of skeletal muscle and its metabolic capacities, insights which are highly relevant to the adverse health consequences of, for example, obesity, diabetes and aging.

c. *Imaging Abdominal Adipose Tissues*

One of the more common applications of CT and MRI imaging methods in obesity-related body com-

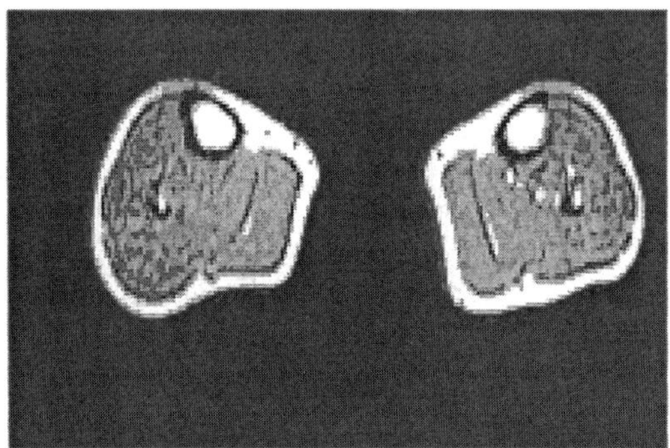

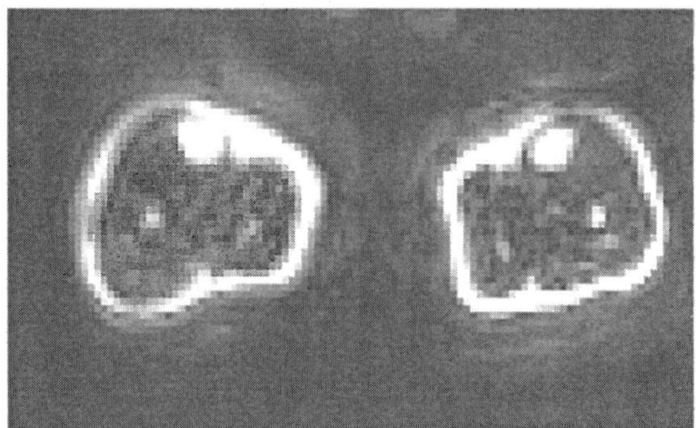

Figure 13 Illustration of conventional T1-weighted image (left) with corresponding water suppressed lipid images (right) obtained from a normal weight subject. The lipid image is obtained using a spiral MR imaging scheme for direct quantification of the lipid MRI signal in skeletal muscle.

position is the measurement of abdominal adipose tissue distribution. CT and MRI are uniquely capable of distinguishing between the subcutaneous and visceral adipose tissue depots that comprise abdominal obesity. Clearly, the ability to measure abdominal subcutaneous and visceral adipose tissue using these methods represents a major advance in our understanding of the relationships between obesity phenotype and health risk. Numerous studies have now clearly identified that division of abdominal adipose tissue into visceral and subcutaneous depots provides novel insight into the relationship between abdominal obesity and related comorbid conditions; however, the independent contribution of these adipose tissue depots to metabolic risk remains a topic of debate (153,154).

Abdominal subcutaneous and intraabdominal adipose tissue depots can be further subdivided according to differences in anatomical and metabolic characteristics. This topic was introduced in an earlier section and an anatomic classification of adipose tissue is presented in Table 3. Abdominal subcutaneous adipose tissue measured by CT can also be subdivided into superficial and deep compartments using the fascia superficialis (Fig. 14). The rationale for such a division comes from animal studies indicating that adipocytes within the deep compartment are more metabolically active than superficial adipocytes (155). If the same heterogeneity exists in humans, segmentation of the subcutaneous depots may clarify which subcutaneous abdominal adipose tissue depot is the stronger correlate of insulin resistance. Indeed, Kelley et al. (18) report that among men and women combined, glucose uptake is strongly correlated with both visceral and deep subcutaneous adipose tissue.

As the fascia superficialis is not visible with MRI, it is not possible to determine deep and superficial adipose tissue depots in a manner similar to CT. However, because the majority of deep subcutaneous adipose tissue is located in the posterior half of the abdomen, a line can be drawn dissecting the abdomen into posterior and anterior depots (Fig. 14). In this way it is assumed that posterior subcutaneous AT measured by MRI is analogous to deep subcutaneous AT measured by CT. This is reasonable given that approximately three-fourths of the "deep" subcutaneous AT is located in the posterior abdomen (18,156). Using this method Misra et al. (157) report that the posterior compartment (analogous to deep subcutaneous AT), when compared

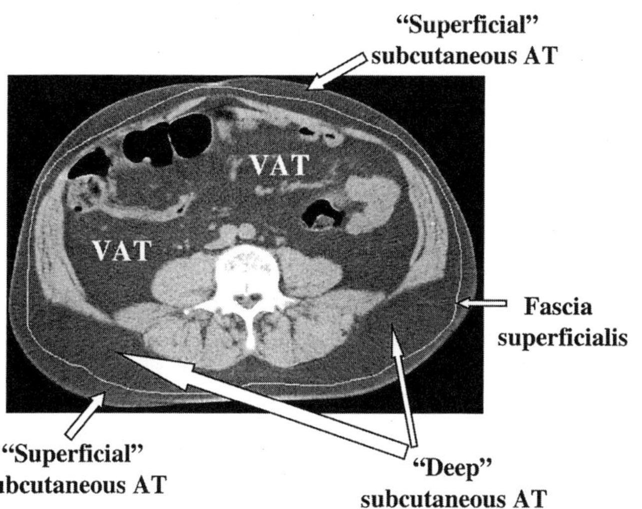

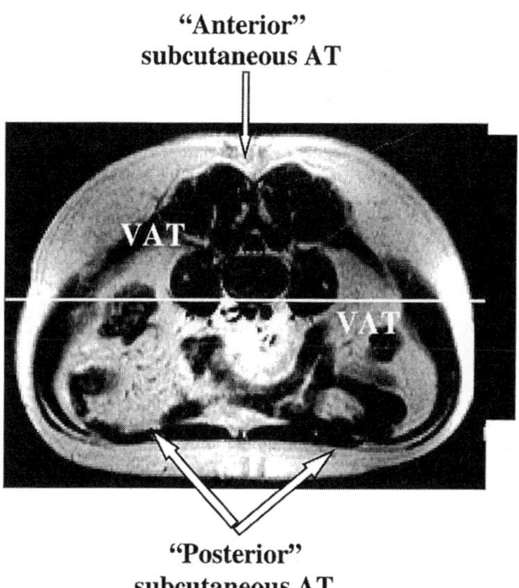

Figure 14 (Left) CT image of the abdomen illustrating the subdivision of abdominal subcutaneous adipose tissue (AT) into "deep" and "superficial" depots using the fascia superficialis (highlighted for clarity). The "deep" layer surrounds the abdomen but the majority of deep subcutaneous AT is located posteriorly. (Right) MRI image of the abdomen at the L4-L5 level. The fascia superficialis on MR images is often difficult to observe using standard acquisition sequences thus, an arbitrary line is drawn horizontally using the vertebral disk as an anatomical landmark to divide abdominal subcutaneous AT into "anterior" and "posterior" depots. In men "posterior" AT is analogous to "deep" subcutaneous AT because a majority the deep AT is located in the posterior region. This assumption is likely untrue for women.

to anterior compartment mass, displayed a stronger relationship with insulin-mediated glucose disposal.

The subdivision of abdominal subcutaneous adipose tissue based on metabolic characteristics is analogous to the partitioning of intra-abdominal adipose tissue into intraperitoneal and retroperitoneal depots on the premise that nonesterified fatty acids from intraperitoneal adipose tissue alone (i.e., omental and mesenteric adipocytes) are delivered directly to the liver, the so-called portal theory (115). Subdivision of visceral AT into intraperitoneal and retro-peritoneal depots on MRI or CT images is not straightforward because the peritoneum is not visible using either method (Fig. 14). Thus intra-abdominal adipose tissue is subdivided into intraperitoneal and extraperitoneal adipose tissue areas (cm^2) at the L4-L5 level using the mouse pointer to draw a straight line across the anterior border of the L4-L5 disk and the psoas muscles continuing on a tangent toward the inferior borders of the ascending and descending colons and extending to the abdominal wall. For images in which the kidneys appear, an oblique line is drawn from the anterior border of the aorta and inferior vena cava to the anterior border of the kidney extending to the abdominal wall. On all images extraperitoneal adipose tissue is defined as the adipose tissue located posterior to the lines drawn (Fig. 14). Whether subdivision of visceral adipose tissue into intraperitoneal and retroperitoneal depots provides additional insight into the relationships between visceral adipose tissue and metabolic risk per se remains unclear. Whereas some report that intraperitoneal adipose tissue is a srong correlate of insulin resistance (158), others report that subdivision of visceral adipose tissue into intraperitoneal and retroperitoneal depots provides no additional insight (159).

Apart from the segmentation of abdominal adipose tissue depots, there is considerable variation among studies using multiple image protocols for both the number and location of the CT or MRI images used to determine either abdominal subcutaneous or intra-abdominal adipose tissue volume (121,160). This may also partly explain large differences among studies for estimated intraabdominal adipose tissue volumes in apparently similar populations. To be consistent with the definition of intra-abdominal adipose tissue as adipose tissues that are portally drained, it is suggested that the L9-L10 and S2-S3 intervertebral spaces be used to define the upper and lower intra-abdominal adipose tissue landmarks. The L9-L10 space corresponds to an anatomical position marginally above the hilar region of the spleen, whereas the S2-S3 space corresponds anatomically to the rectosigmoid junction. These two landmarks define a region within which the majority of intra-abdominal adipose tissue is portally drained.

It is not yet firmly established whether single or multiple images are needed to accurately estimate intra-abdominal adipose tissue. The area of intra-abdominal adipose tissue from a single L4/L5 image correlates highly with intraabdominal adipose tissue volume (96,120). In addition, intra-abdominal adipose tissue area determined from a single slice appears to correlate as strongly with metabolic variables as do volumes from multiple images (122). On the other hand, it may be preferable to quantify intra-abdominal adipose tissue volumes in studies designed to develop anthropometric prediction equations. Sjöström et al. (104) presented data suggesting that the error associated with total adipose tissue prediction by anthropometry can be reduced if intra-abdominal adipose tissue volume is measured using multiple images.

d. Imaging Summary

Several factors should be considered when choosing a study imaging method. Both CT and MRI produce high-resolution scans of all major tissue system level body composition components. Both methods are very expensive and require high technical skill for application. In general, CT has been shown to provide more reliable data than MRI, although this is changing rapidly with the introduction of new imaging techniques and image analysis software. A major advantage of MRI is the lack of ionizing radiation. There are no known health risks associated with MRI at the current magnet field strengths of about 1.5 T. Newer scanning protocols are rapid and cost is usually reduced. The small-bore magnets create a problem for claustrophobic patient, and very obese patients cannot usually fit within the magnet core. An important advantage of CT is that instruments are widely available. A second advantage of CT is the high resolution of images and the consistency of tissue attenuation values from scan to scan. Within reasonable limits, water, skeletal muscle, adipose tissue, and other components have similar Hounsfield unit distributions within and between scans. The consistency of attenuation data allows development of standardized protocols for reading scans and separating various tissues from each other.

The cost of CT scanning is variable and access during peak patient hours may be limited. The major disadvantage of CT is the associated radiation exposure. This limits the study of children and of women in childbearing years. Regional studies with appropriate scanner settings substantially lower radiation dose compared to whole-body studies. Radiation exposure is still a concern in long-term longitudinal studies with repeated measurements over time. Lastly, some very obese patients may be too large to fit within the scanner and our experience is that CT study is limited to patients below about BMI 35 kg/m^2.

C Component Field Methods

1 Anthropometry

Anthropometry is the least expensive, most widely used method of assessing human body composition. Anthropometric measurements are used in clinical and epidemiological studies to grade the degree of adiposity in individuals and groups and to estimate the prevalence of overweight and obesity in populations. The measurements are also used to describe the anatomical distribution of adipose tissue and to classify individuals and groups with regard to the "type" of obesity—"centralized" or "peripheral." The various measures, and the ratios or indices derived from them, are important for evaluating the health risks associated with excess body fatness or obesity and any changes that occur during treatment of obese patients (36,161).

The anthropometric measurements considered as most useful in assessing obesity include weight, stature, skinfold thicknesses, circumferences of the trunk and limbs, and sagittal trunk thickness. Ultrasound is considered in this section as a "quasi-anthropometric" method that is being applied increasingly in clinical studies to quantify adipose tissue distribution. It is placed here, instead of in the section on imaging, because of the limited nature of the regional body composition information provided.

Anthropometric variables do not correspond directly to body composition components but are superficial, somatic measures that are influenced by, and consequently correlated with, variation in the underlying components. Anthropometric variables can therefore be used either as "proxy variables" for the underlying components or in body composition prediction equations. The following sections will consider the merits and limitations of these two different approaches to using weight, stature, skinfold thicknesses, circumferences, and sagittal trunk thickness to grade or predict body adiposity, classify individuals or groups as "obese," and describe adipose tissue distribution.

a. *Skinfolds*

These are measurements of a double thickness or "fold" of skin, underlying fascia, and subcutaneous adipose tissue that are taken using calipers at standardized locations on the body. The essential technique is to pinch and elevate a skinfold at specific anatomical sites using the thumb and fingers and to measure the thickness of the fold with specially designed calipers. These measurements are correlated with, but are not directly representative of, the actual thickness of subcutaneous adipose tissue. This has been illustrated by comparisons of skinfold thickness measurements with radiographic and ultrasound measurements of subcutaneous adipose tissue thickness at different anatomical sites (51,162,163). Because ~70–90% of total adipose tissue is subcutaneous, skinfold thicknesses can be used to grade or predict total body fat (164). In addition, since the thickness of subcutaneous adipose tissue varies among anatomical locations, skinfold thicknesses are useful for describing subcutaneous adipose tissue distribution or "fat patterning." They are not useful, however, for predicting amounts of intra-abdominal adipose tissues.

Carefully standardized methods of measuring skinfold thicknesses have been developed and it is important to adhere strictly to these to ensure reliable measurements that are comparable with published tables of reference data, and that can be used in appropriate equations for predicting body fat (165). A variety of skinfold calipers are available and measurements may differ systematically among brands depending on quality and the control of pressure between the jaws of the calipers. Jaw pressure is important because skinfolds vary within and between individuals in compression when measured (162,165). Variability in compression is a major factor affecting the reliability of skinfold thickness measurements. Calipers with different jaw pressures will produce systematically different readings, and those with manually controlled jaw pressures will be less reliable than those with built-in spring mechanisms. As a result, the use of different brands of skinfold calipers within a study is not recommended unless their systematic differences are known. Research-quality calipers (e.g., Holtain, Lange, Harpenden) exert a constant pressure of 10 g/cm^3 between the jaws and have a finer scale of measurement (i.e., 0.1-mm intervals) than the inexpensive, plastic calipers marketed for clinical use (165).

In theory, skinfold thicknesses can be measured anywhere on the body that a double fold of skin and subcutaneous adipose tissue can be pinched and elevated. In practice, only a few standard sites are commonly measured based on their accessibility, ease of measurement, and high correlation with measures of total body fat. The triceps and subscapular sites meet these criteria best in most sex, ethnic, and age groupings, and are used widely for grading adiposity (19,165).

Skinfold thicknesses are also used in equations that predict body density, total body fat mass, or percent body fat. The most widely used equations are those of Jackson and Pollock (163) and Dumin and Womersely (164). When applied with close attention to proper measurement technique, these equations can predict percent body fat with errors of 3.5–5% and a 95% confidence interval between ±7–10% (65). An advantage to the use of skinfold thickness prediction equations is that they estimate rather than grade the underlying variables of interest (e.g., body density, total body fat, percent body fat). Subsequent analyses can then deal directly with associations between the estimates and the various outcomes of interest, rather than with indirect associations with imperfect proxy variables or indices. This can greatly facilitate interpretation of some associations as long as the predicted values can be considered accurate. A disadvantage is that body composition prediction equations based on skinfold thicknesses are "population specific." As a result, they must always be cross-validated in at least a subsample of a study population before general application. This clearly adds to the expense and difficulty of using these equations. Lohman (65) and Roche and Gue (165) have developed explicit criteria for the evaluation of the accuracy of prediction equations in cross-validation studies.

An important problem is the simple feasibility of obtaining reliable data for very obese subjects. Skinfold calipers can accurately measure skinfolds only up to 40 mm (Holtain) or 60 mm (Lange) in thickness. This may limit the ability to measure skinfolds at some sites and in obese subjects. In addition, the reliability of the measurements may decrease with increasing thickness (162). As a result of these limitations, some may prefer the use of circumference measurements for grading or predicting body fatness or quantifying adipose tissue distribution in obese subjects.

b. *Ultrasound*

Ultrasonic measurements of subcutaneous adipose tissue thickness have been explored as an alternative to skinfolds (166). The benefits to ultrasound are: (1) the measurements theoretically have greater validity in relation to actual subcutaneous adipose tissue thickness; (2) they are not affected by variation within and between persons for tissue compressibility; (3) greater thicknesses can be measured than with currently available skinfold calipers; and (4) sites can be measured that are inaccessible to calipers, for example, paraspinal adipose tissue in the lumbar region. There are also two major drawbacks: (1) the measurements are obtained at considerably increased cost; and (2) reliable meaurements can only be made using B-mode imaging ultrasound by highly trained technicians (167). B-mode imaging ultrasound provides a real-time two-dimensional image of skin and subcutaneous adipose tissue and underlying interface with muscle. The image can be frozen and printed, providing a permanent record, and the subcutaneous adipose tissue thickness can be measured using a ruler or digitizer. Considerable skill may be needed in obtaining the images, depending on the ultrasound equipment used, and in identifying correctly the adipose tissue–muscle interface on the image. At some sites, this interface may be easily confused with other fibrous tissue interfaces and bone reflections.

Ultrasound has also been explored as a method of quantifying the amount of intra-abdominal adipose tissues (166,167). This approach appears promising and merits further development since the alternatives are either very expensive (e.g., CT or MRI) or inaccurate (e.g., circumference ratios or prediction equations).

c. *Circumferences*

Body circumferences are useful in that, unlike skinfold thicknesses, they can always be measured, even in extremely obese subjects. Circumferences reflect internal as well as subcutaneous adipose tissue, but are also influenced by variation in muscle and bone. As a result, the interpretation of circumference measurements, and especially circumference ratios, is often not straightforward. As for all anthropometric variables, body circumferences should be measured with close attention to standardized procedures (19). Flexible, inelastic cloth or steel tapes are recommended.

The most useful circumferences for grading or predicting body fat and for describing adipose tissue distribution are upper arm, chest, waist or abdomen, hip or buttocks, proximal or midthigh, and calf (19,165). Waist or abdomen circumferences are usually very highly correlated with total fat mass and percent body fat in men ($r > .85$); in women, hip or thigh circumferences may have slightly higher correlations. Correlations of upper arm, thigh, and calf circumferences with measures of body fat are somewhat lower, and these circumferences tend to be more strongly influenced by variation in appendicular skeletal muscle.

d. *Adipose Tissue Distributions*

Numerous epidemiological and clinical studies have established that centralized obesity, in which fat is stored preferentially in adipocytes on and within the trunk rather than the extremities, represents the obesity phenotype that conveys the largest risk for morbidity and mortality from the major chronic diseases: heart disease, cancer, and diabetes (36,168). A variety of anthropometric approaches have been developed to grade or classify centralized adipose tissue distribution. Recent efforts have been focused on developing equations for predicting the amount of VAT, which is believed to be the main aspect of centralized obesity associated with risk. The following section reviews the merits and limitations of these anthropometric approaches.

Skinfold thicknesses have been used to describe primarily the distribution of subcutaneous adipose tissues. This aspect of the adipose tissue distribution has been called "fat patterning," to distinguish it from the more general form that includes the amounts and distribution of internal adipose tissues (169,170). Historically, three main approaches have been used to describe fat patterning: pattern profile, ratio, and principal-components methods. The pattern profile method was first applied by Garn (169) and compares two or more groups graphically for mean values of skinfold thicknesses across several anatomical sites. It provides a useful, visual comparison of differences or similarities between groups for anatomical variation in subcutaneous adipose tissue thickness. Cluster analysis provides a more sophisticated, statistical approach to defining pattern profiles (171).

A variety of skinfold thickness ratios have been used to index fat patterning. The ratio of the subscapular to triceps skinfolds is one of simplest and most widely used. Some consider it to be important to include a skinfold on the leg, such as the lateral calf or medial thigh skinfold (172). The advantages of the ratio approach are that it requires few variables and simple computation, and provides a single continuous variable for grading subjects. Three problems can be identified, however, with ratio indices of fat patterning: (1) they tend to be correlated with total fat mass or percent body fat; (2) they may have poor sensitivity and validity with regard to the latent variable, subcutaneous adipose tissue distribution; and (3) it may be difficult to determine whether a correlation with another variable (e.g., serum HDL cholesterol) is due to variation in the numerator or denominator of the ratio. The use of a greater number of skinfolds and the sum of all skinfolds in the denominator may partly alleviate these problems. Principal components analysis is a more sophisticated statistical approach to constructing fat pattern indices. This approach summarizes the information in several skinfold variables in a smaller number of new, statistically independent indices (173). When this method is applied to data for several skinfold variables, it provides the best "reference" measures for judging the validity and sensitivity of simpler ratio indices.

The main criticism of skinfold thickness methods in the study of obesity is that they do not capture variation in the amounts of internal adipose tissues, especially those surrounding the viscera. Visceral adipose tissue has been recognized as the main aspect of adipose tissue distribution that is associated with increased risk for chronic disease (168). As a result, many prefer indices based on circumferences that are believed to include variation in VATs. The most popular circumference index is the "waist/hip ratio" (WHR), followed by the "waist/thigh ratio" (WTR). The waist/hip ratio was the first used to assess the associations between adipose tissue distribution and chronic disease morbidity and mortality (173–177). Numerous studies have now shown that WHR is an independent predictor of metabolic disturbances including insulin resistance, dyslipidemia, hypertension, and atherosclerosis (178–180). Similar associations have been also been reported for WTR, as well as for skinfold thickness indices and some other circumference indices such as the "conicity index" (180,181). In general, the association of risk factors, as well as morbidity and mortality, with circumference indices tends to be somewhat stronger than with skinfold thickness indices of adipose tissue distribution. This is generally thought to be due to either the increased measurement error in skinfold thicknesses, or the influence of VAT volume on waist circumference. As for BMI or skinfolds, cutoff values for WHR have been recommended for defining "upper-body obesity" (179). The recommended values generally used are >0.95 in men and >0.80 in women. It is important to recognize that these values were selected based on the increase in risks with increasing WHR and not on the association with adipose tissue distribution.

There are several problems in the use of circumference ratios as indices of adipose tissue distribution. First, standard definitions of the circumferences are not always followed, making it difficult to compare results across studies (182). For example, the "waist" circumference has been defined variously as at the level of: the smallest circumference on the torso below the sternum, the umbilicus, the lower margin of the ribs, and the iliac crests. The "hip" circumference has been defined as at the level of: the iliac crests, the anterior iliac spines, the greater trochanters, or maximum posterior protrusion of the buttocks. There may be considerable differences among circumferences measured at these locations. Some may vary between subjects in relation to bone landmarks (e.g., smallest circumference on torso below the sternum), or may be difficult to identify in obese subjects. There is scarcely any difference between a "waist" circumference measured at the level of the umbilicus and a "hip" circumference measured at the level of the iliac crests in most subjects. Obviously, "waist" circumference in one study may be the same as "hip" circumference in another when both are defined as at the level of the iliac crests.

In obese subjects, the identification of the "waist" may be extremely subjective, if not impossible, and the measurement is more correctly defined as an abdominal circumference. The location of the abdominal circumference in relation to a soft tissue landmark, such as the umbilicus, is not recommended because many obese subjects will have an extremely pendulous abdominal adipose panniculus. The umbilicus may be directed downward and located well below the horizontal, transverse plane of the midabdomen. This may lead to considerable variation among subjects in the definition of this measurement. In addition, a pendulous panniculus may result in overlapping of abdominal and hip circumferences or interfere with the standard measurement of hip circumference.

A second problem is that circumferences are influenced by variation in muscle and bone as well as adipose tissues, as noted previously. These influences may be particularly difficult to sort out when ratio indices are used. It has been assumed conventionally that increased WHRs mainly reflect increased VAT, based on studies that report significant correlations between WHR and VAT area, as measured using imaging methods. Some studies, however, have reported significant correlations with measures of cross-sectional muscle area also, in particular those for the pelvis or hips (135). Thus, variation in WHR may reflect the effects of increased VAT on waist circumference (i.e., numerator) as well as decreased gluteofemoral muscle on hip circumference (i.e., denominator). This influence of muscle has been recognized increasingly and may be important in understanding the relationship of WHR to chronic disease risk. Larsson et al. (175) reported that the risk of heart disease was greatest in those with lower BMIs and high WHRs. Filipovsky et al. (181) reported that all-cause and cancer mortality over 20 years of follow-up in the Paris Prospective Study was greatest in those with low BMIs but high WTRs. The low BMIs in this study might reflect low muscle mass, rather than low fat; subsequently, the high WHRs or WTRs might reflect a combination of increased VAT and muscle loss (36). It should be remembered that the phenotype originally described by Vague (183), who first drew attention to the association of body composition and metabolic disease, consisted of an expanded abdominal fat mass in conjunction with thin legs. The latter might reflect muscle atrophy associated with disease as much as lack of subcutaneous adipose tissue on the extremities. This potentially important association between visceral adiposity and skeletal muscle was reemphasized by Björntorp (168).

A third problem is the strong correlation of circumferences and circumference ratios with total adiposity. This makes it difficult statistically to separate the effects of centralized adipose tissue distribution from obesity. This confounding is further exacerbated by the moderate positive correlations of body fatness and centralized adipose tissue distribution with age. Many early studies that reported significant correlations between WHR and VAT did not control for the confounding influences of age and BMI. Seidell et al. (134) reported that WHR did not correlate significantly with the ratio of visceral to subcutaneous adipose tissue, as measured using CT, after adjustment for age and BMI. Similarly, Ross et al. (120) reported that, after controlling for both age and adiposity, WHR explained only 12% of the variation in absolute levels of VAT in men. Furthermore, the observed relationship between WHR and relative VAT was nonexistent. Thus, while WHR is an independent predictor of numerous metabolic aberrations, its association with risk may not be attributed simply to its association with the amounts of either absolute or relative VAT.

Several investigators have argued that simple waist circumference is a better index of variation in VAT than WHR (184,185a–185c); it is important to note, however, that waist circumference is very highly correlated with total adiposity ($r > 90$) in most populations. Also, the error of prediction of VAT from waist circumference, alone or in combination with other variables, is large (120,134). Ross et al. (120) reported that the sensitivity and specificity of waist circumference for predicting absolute values of VAT was poor. These observations are explained in large measure by the intraindividual variation in the visceral to subcutaneous adipose tissue ratio. It is important to establish whether reductions in VAT are related to concurrent reductions WHR or waist circumference. Some have reported that WHR changes with weight loss, while others do (120,186,187). Ross et al. (188) reported that diet and exercise induced reductions in VAT that were significantly associated with reduced waist circumferences in obese male ($r = .69$) and female ($r = .47$) subjects. For the two groups combined, a 1-cm reduction in waist circumference was associated with a 4% reduction in VAT ($P < .01$). The standard deviation associated with the 4% reduction in VAT per centimeter reduction in waist circumference, however, was also 4%. This suggests that the ability to quantify small changes in VAT volume from waist circumference is limited by interindividual variations in the reduction of abdominal subcutaneous and lean tissue. Thus, whereas changes in visceral obesity are clearly associated with changes in waist circumference, it is not possible to accurately predict small changes in VAT.

A final proviso is that hip circumference may have predictive value for outcome in a direction opposite to that of waist circumference. In a recent study, Seidell et al. (185c) observed the traditional association between a large waist circumference, dyslipidemia, insulin levels, and glucose concentrations in Quebec City residents. Narrow hips were also independently associated with an adverse metabolic profile. Accordingly, a narrow waist and large hips may be protective against cardiovascular disease and the authors suggest that the specific effects of each circumference measurement are not well captured in the WHR.

Efforts to develop equations for predicting VAT have not generally been successful. The errors associated with these equations tend to be large: 25–40% (120,134,184–187). This level of accuracy is clearly insufficient for estimating changes in individuals and may be inadequate for comparing groups. Few of these equations have been cross-validated in independent samples. Future efforts to develop this approach have value, however, given the inadequacies described above for skinfold and circumference indices. At present, it would appear that new or different anthropometric measurements will be needed to increase the accuracy of prediction equations to acceptable levels. One measure that has been suggested is the sagittal thickness of the trunk or abdomen.

Several studies have suggested that sagittal trunk thickness correlates more highly than other anthropometric variables with the volume of VAT quantified by imaging methods (185,189). As a result, it may be useful both as a simple index, like waist circumference, or as an independent variable in equations for predicting VAT. There is present no standardized technique for measuring sagittal trunk thickness, and, to date, its at use has been limited mostly to clinical studies.

Sagittal trunk thickness may be defined as the maximum diameter of the abdomen in the sagittal plane. As for circumferences, this measurement may be obtained technically in all subjects regardless of obesity level. Bony landmarks for the standard location of this measurement have not been identified: alternative possibilities include the xiphoid process of the sternum, the fourth lumbar vertebrae, or the iliac crests. It is important to note that the choice between these landmarks will result in measurements at very different levels on the trunk or abdomen. Sliding calipers with long, parallel blades are necessary for this measurement.

Although sagittal trunk thickness may be taken with the participant standing, measurement in the supine recumbent position may be preferred to maximize the association with the latent variable, intra-abdominal adipose tissue volume. Theoretically, when a person with an enlarged intra-abdominal adipose tissue mass lies supine, the mass shifts cranially, causing anterior projection of the abdomen, which is measured as increased sagittal thickness (189). When a person is standing, gravity pulls the intra-abdominal adipose tissue mass downward, and the maximum sagittal thickness may be located somewhat lower. It is important to keep in mind that the level of the maximum measurable diameter, either supine or standing, will likely vary among some subjects. The extent to which these measurements are influenced by the amount of subcutaneous abdominal adipose tissue, and shifts in its distribution between supine and standing measurements, is not well established.

Results for the use of sagittal thickness to grade or predict VAT volume in several Swedish studies have been summarized by Sjöström (189). VAT volume was estimated using seven cross-sectional CT scans of the abdomen. Sagittal thickness was measured on the CT image at the level of L4-L5. VAT volume was regressed on sagittal thickness (ST) in 17 men producing an equation, VAT (L) $= 0.731 \times$ ST (cm)-11.5, ($R^2 = 0.81$). This equation was later cross-validated in two independent samples of 7 and 13 men, respectively, with virtually indistinguishable results. A similar regression equation was developed using data for 10 women and cross-validated in nine independently selected women: VAT (L) $- 0.370 \times$ ST(cm) $- 4.85$, ($R^2 = .80$). Sjöström and associates also showed that changes in VAT volume were accurately tracked by changes in sagittal thickness in six patients with Cushing's disease during treatment.

Pouliot et al. (185) analyzed associations of sagittal thickness with VAT area on CT images at L4-L5 in 81 men and 70 women, 30–42 years of age. Sagittal thickness correlated better with VAT area than waist/hip ratio in both sexes; however, it was also correlated strongly with subcutaneous abdominal adipose tissue area. Taken together, the results of the studies by Sjöström et al. (189) and Pouliot et al. (185) indicate that sagittal thickness is somewhat more sensitive than conventional indices such as waist/hip ratio for grading or predicting the amounts of VAT.

The measurements of sagittal thickness in these studies were taken from the CT scans, rather than anthropometrically. Sjöström and associates, however, reported that the squared difference between sagittal thicknesses measured anthropometrically and on the CT images in their studies was only 1.7%. In an independent study, Van der Kooy et al. (190) reported a high correlation ($r = .94$) between sagittal thickness measured with the subject standing and from MRI images at the same level. It may be important to consider that the errors of estimation for VAT averaged ~20% in these studies, which could allow for considerable misclassification when subjects are grouped by sagittal thickness. Lastly, the strong correlation with abdominal subcutaneous adipose tissue areas reported by Pouliot et al. (185) is bothersome since it suggests that sagittal thickness may not accurately discriminate visceral from subcutaneous abdominal adipose tissue.

Whereas establishment of the association of sagittal diameter with the latent variable of interest, VAT, is important, it is also important to examine the sensitivity of this measure in relation to risk factors associated with visceral obesity. Richelsen and Pedersen (191) recently analyzed associations of sagittal thickness and other indices of VAT with serum total cholesterol, triglyceride, LDL and HDL, fasting insulin, and glucose concentrations in 58 middle-aged men. They concluded that sagittal thickness was slightly better correlated with an adverse lipid, insulin, and glucose risk profile than waist/hip ratio. Similar findings were also reported in the study by Pouliot et al. (185). Taken together, these studies suggest that sagittal diameter may be preferred to other indices of VAT as a risk factor in epidemiologic studies of obesity-associated chronic diseases. In this regard, Seidell et al. (192) reported that abdominal sagittal thickness was a strong predictor of mortality in younger adult men enrolled in the Baltimore Longitudinal Study. Further studies are needed to establish the usefulness of sagittal thickness for grading or predicting VAT and as a risk factor in different age, sex, and ethnic groups.

2 Bioimpedance Analysis

Bioimpedance analysis (BIA) is a technique for predicting body composition based on the electrical conductive properties of the human body. The ability of the body to conduct an electric current is due to the presence of free ions, or electrolytes, in the body water. The amount of electricity that can be conducted is determined mainly by the total volume of electrolyte-rich fluid in the body. Measures of bioelectric conductivity are therefore proportional to TBW and to body composition components with high water concentrations such as the fat-free and skeletal muscle masses. As a result, these methods predict FFM, and fat must be derived secondarily as the difference between body weight and predicted FFM (193).

Many factors other than the amount and electrolyte concentration of body water, however, influence measurements of electrical conductivity. These include body temperature, distribution of fluids between intra- and extracellular spaces, body proportions or "geometry," the amounts and structures of different conductive, as well as nonconductive, tissues, and technical issues such as correct calibration and application of the equipment. The net result is that exact functional relationships between measurements of bioelectric conductivity and TBW or other fat-free components cannot be derived from either physicochemical models or experimentally. Thus, relationships between conductivity measurements and body composition components must be established indirectly by statistical calibration against criterion measures (e.g., estimates of TBW from deuterium dilution analysis or DXA) in a sample of subjects.

Because it is portable, BIA is suitable for field use and is being applied increasingly as a phenotyping method in field settings. The most commonly used BIA method injects a high-frequency, low-amplitude alternating electric current (50 kHz at 500–800 mÅ) into the body using distally placed electrodes and measures the voltage drop due to resistance with proximal electrodes. Conventionally, surface gel electrodes are used with standardized placements on the right ankle and hand, although other electrode arrangements have been described that allow estimation of segmental (e.g., arm or leg) electrical properties (194). Stainless-steel contact electrodes are also now used in some systems in place of the conventional gel electrodes. The amount of resistance measured (R) is inversely proportional to the volume of electrolytic fluid in the body. It is also dependent on the proportions or "geometry" of this volume (i.e., ratio of length [L] to cross-sectional area [A], or $R \alpha L/A$). These relationships have led to the use of the simple formula $V = \rho L^2/R$ as the theoretical basis of most BIA applications, where V is conductive volume (e.g., TBW), L is a measure of body length (usually stature), R is measured resistance, and ρ is an estimate of the "specific resistivity" of the conductive material (195).

There are a number of limitations to the validity of this simple formula. The formula is accurate only for a cylindrical conductor with uniform cross-sectional area and homogeneous composition (e.g., a wire). The human body could be described as a series of roughly cylindrical conductors with variable cross-sectional area and heterogeneous, highly structured composition. The value of ρ is influenced by all of these factors and consequently cannot be deduced directly. As a result, equations for predicting body composition must be developed based on independent measurements of resistance, stature, and other anthropometric variables, and TBW or FFM in a sample of subjects. Least-squares regression techniques are applied to the data to derive an equation of the basic form:

$$V(\text{i.e., TBW or FFM}) = a + bS^2/R + e \quad (21)$$

where a is intercept, b is slope, and e is residual error or unexplained variation in V due to random measurement errors and/or misspecification of the parameters (a and b) in the equation. It is not possible to interpret the parameter b in this equation as an estimate of ρ in the formula $V = \rho L^2/R$, unless the intercept (a) and residual error (e) approach zero. These conditions are rarely, if ever, met for the reasons given above. The equation may also contain body circumferences and skinfold thickness, although the inclusion of these additional variables reduces the main benefit of BIA relative to anthropometric prediction equations. The reason BIA is becoming increasingly popular is that only a few simple, highly reproducible measurements are needed. Multiple frequency systems are available, but only a small advantage over the conventional 50-kHz systems are noted for estimation of TBW and FFM.

As for most prediction methods, BIA equations tend to lose accuracy when applied to subjects who do not resemble those included in the sample from which the equations were developed. Thus, their generalizability may be limited and all BIA equations should be cross-validated in independent samples to verify their applicability. Few, if any, equations have been developed that can be demonstrated to be applicable to all individuals without regard to age, gender, ethnicity, or obesity. Our experience is that the performance of a particular equation can be unpredictable, even when applied with close attention to measurement techniques and equipment to a sample with characteristics closely similar to those of the source-sample. As a result, it is recommended that any externally-developed BIA equation be cross-validated in a random subsample against estimates from an accepted reference method before general extension to an entire study population.

The relatively low cost, portability, ability to track long-term body composition changes, operation simplicity, and lack of radiation exposure make appropriately developed BIA methods a good choice for field applications.

V ERRORS OF ESTIMATION

All in vivo body composition methods attempt to estimate or predict the size, volume, or mass of an unknown component from measurements of associated properties or other components using various equations or models. An important area of body composition methodology is quantitative analysis of the magnitudes and directions of the different types of errors that may occur. A variety of previous efforts have been made to address this complicated area (65,196–198), and it would not be appropriate to provide a detailed review in this chapter. The following provides a general overview of basic concepts.

Measurement error can be caused by instrument error and observer error. Instrument error can be minimized by appropriately and rigorously calibrating all measuring devices on a regular basis. Training, periodic evaluations, and a quality control program will help to reduce observer error.

Accuracy is the level of agreement between the measured value and the "true" dimension. Accuracy of a component measurement is usually established by comparison to an accepted reference method or "gold standard." For example, subcutaneous adipose tissue thickness estimated using a skinfold caliper can be compared to corresponding reference estimates by CT or MRI. Of course any such analysis also includes instrument, observer, and model errors. In clinical situations measurements by an anthropometrist are usually compared to those of a designated "expert" as the reference.

Some body composition measurements are used directly, as for example triceps skinfold thickness as a measure of fatness. Mathematically transforming a skinfold measurement to a component estimate, such as body fat, involves error sources. Methods based upon statistically derived prediction formulas are population specific, and error may arise when applying the prediction formula to a new subject group or outside of the original subject range for age, weight, and stature. Methods based on biological models, such as fat-free mass density (i.e., 1/100 g/cc), include "model" errors. For example, calculation of fat-free mass from the assumed hydration of 0.73 is based on average population values. Actual subject hydration may deviate from the assumed model, and this introduces error into the component (i.e., fat-free mass) estimate.

Precision, as distinct from accuracy, defines the quality of a measurement in terms of being sharply defined or exact. In this sense precision refers to the scale of measurement, as for example a skinfold measured to the nearest 1 mm is more precise than one measured to the nearest 0.5 cm. A highly precise measurement (e.g., body weight measured to the nearest gram) is not necessarily accurate if the weight scale used is improperly calibrated. The definition of precision overlaps to some extent with that of "reliability." Reliability is the degree to which a measurement is replicable using the same instrument by the same or a different observer. The linkage to precision comes in that it is difficult for a measurement to be precise or exact if it is unreliable.

The precision of a body composition estimate can be quantified as the variability among repeated measurements over a short time period in the same subject. One approach for expressing precision is the technical error of measurement, which is the standard deviation (SD) of repeated measurements on the same subject by the same or different observers. The technical error of measurement, which is expressed in the same units as the measured quantity, can also be expressed in percent as a coefficient of variation (i.e., SD/mean × 100).

Reliability is also referred to as "reproducibility" or "repeatability." Reliability, as distinct from precision, is more commonly expressed in terms of the intraclass correlation among repeated measurements (197), sometimes called the "reliability coefficient." Measures of reliability often include both measurement error and physiological variation.

The total variation of a component's mass monitored over time includes measurement variation and biological variation (199). Biological variation occurs even in the healthy individual as weight and fluid balance fluctuate over time. This aspect of measurement variability is the difference between total component mass variation over time and that due to measurement error. Some measures, such as height, are extremely stable in adults while others, such as fluid status, are moderately variable over time. In practice, this biological component of variability is often included in component reliability estimates.

It is important to minimize biological variation for some measurements, as for example impedance with BIA. Impedance varies normally with posture, fluid status, time of day, and menstrual status. Controlling these factors, to the extent possible, will keep the biological component of measurement variability to a minimum.

VI REFERENCE VALUES

Once collected, body composition data are usually compared to corresponding data from a reference population. Some reference data for the United States noninstitutionalized population are available from the National Health and Nutrition Examinations Surveys (NHANES) (200). Body weight, height, and BMI values by age, sex, and race from NHANES III are presented in Tables 9–11 (unpublished data).

Extensive reference data are available for skinfold thicknesses at the triceps and subscapular sites that are stratified by sex, ethnicity, and age (200). Additional skinfolds that may be useful for grading adiposity or describing adipose tissue distribution include suprailiac and paraumbilical for abdominal adipose tissue, and medial thigh and medial or lateral calf or leg adipose tissue. Fewer reference data, however, are available for these sites, which limits their usefulness in some contexts.

The commonest way to use skinfold thickness data is to compare individual values or group means to tabulated reference values for appropriate sex, ethnic, and age groupings (200). An implicit assumption is that the reference data are "representative," in the sense of being collected from a randomly selected sample of a well-defined population as in the NHANES studies.

Skinfold thicknesses can also be used as continuous variables grading adiposity or adipose tissue distribution within a study population. This approach works well if the study population is relatively homogeneous. It works less well if the study population is heterogeneous and the association of the selected skinfold thickness with total fat mass or percent body fat varies by sex, ethnicity, age, or other characteristics. As a result, stratification on sex, ethnicity, and age is generally recommended when skinfold thicknesses are used as continuous measures grading levels of body adiposity in analyses of relative risks or correlations with risk factors. Nationally representative reference data are available for abdominal, hip, and midthigh circumferences from the NHANES III on CD-ROM (National Center for Health Statistics, Hyattsville, MD).

Absolute compartment estimates are often adjusted for body mass and expressed as a percentage or as a height-normalized index (e.g., FFM/Ht^2) (201). There are as yet no appropriately derived and reported "healthy" body composition ranges, and investigators have suggested two interim measures. The first involves population means and ranges based on the NHANES III bioimpedance analysis database (e.g., mean % fat values vs. age by ethnic group; Tables 9–11) (unpublished data). This information allows comparison of the study subject or group to the sex-, age-, and race-specific value observed in the U.S. population. Other large subject databases with group averages for specific populations are reported. The second approach provides predicted percent fat estimates for sex, age, race, and

Table 9 Selected Anthropometric and Impedance Measures According to Age and Sex for Non-Hispanic Whites: NHANES III (unpublished data)

		Non-Hispanic white males				Non-Hispanic white females			
Age (years)	Anthropometric measure	N	Mean	Standard deviation	Standard error	N	Mean	Standard deviation	Standard error
12–13.9	Weight (kg)	88	51.7	12.3	1.5	101	52.1	13.3	1.6
	Stature (cm)		159.6	8.4	0.9		157.8	8.2	1.0
	BMI (kg/m^2)		20.1	3.5	0.4		20.9	4.7	0.6
	TBW (L)		31.3	6.3	0.8		28.5	4.2	0.6
	%fat		18.4	7.3	1.0		24.8	9.7	1.2
14–15.9	Weight (kg)	82	68.3	20.5	2.5	120	57.8	10.5	1.2
	Stature (cm)		172.2	7.6	0.8		162.6	6.0	0.7
	BMI (kg/m^2)		23.0	6.3	0.8		21.9	3.8	0.4
	TBW (L)		40.6	7.0	0.9		29.9	3.7	0.5
	%fat		18.4	8.3	1.2		29.1	6.5	0.8
16–17.9	Weight (kg)	96	70.9	13.8	1.6	104	61.1	14.5	1.7
	Stature (cm)		177.0	7.9	0.8		164.5	6.6	0.8
	BMI (kg/m^2)		22.6	4.0	0.5		22.5	4.9	0.6
	TBW (L)		43.1	6.2	0.8		30.7	4.0	0.5
	%fat		17.7	6.8	0.9		30.7	6.9	0.9
18–19.9	Weight (kg)	76	73.1	15.0	1.9	90	63.7	15.0	1.9
	Stature (cm)		176.9	6.7	0.8		164.9	5.8	0.7
	BMI (kg/m^2)		23.3	4.2	0.6		23.4	5.5	0.7
	TBW (L)		43.2	5.8	0.8		31.9	4.2	0.6
	%fat		19.6	6.9	1.0		30.8	7.9	1.0
20–29.9	Weight (kg)	384	79.2	16.6	0.9	426	63.2	14.3	0.8
	Stature (cm)		177.5	6.7	0.3		163.6	6.7	0.4
	BMI (kg/m^2)		25.1	4.9	0.3		23.6	5.1	0.3
	TBW (L)		45.5	6.9	0.4		31.8	4.5	0.3
	%fat		21.8	6.2	0.4		31.0	7.5	0.5
30–39.9	Weight (kg)	436	84.0	17.1	0.9	543	69.1	18.0	0.9
	Stature (cm)		177.8	6.8	0.3		164.6	6.3	0.3
	BMI (kg/m^2)		26.5	4.6	0.3		25.5	6.5	0.3
	TBW (L)		47.2	7.6	0.4		33.5	5.1	0.3
	%fat		23.6	5.8	0.4		33.0	8.5	0.5
40–49.9	Weight (kg)	410	86.0	17.0	0.9	454	70.7	16.8	1.0
	Stature (cm)		177.3	6.7	0.3		163.4	6.1	0.3
	BMI (kg/m^2)		27.3	4.9	0.3		26.6	6.5	0.4
	TBW (L)		48.0	7.8	0.5		33.3	5.2	0.3
	%fat		24.2	5.7	0.4		35.4	6.9	0.4
50–59.9	Weight (kg)	396	86.9	15.0	0.8	454	73.9	17.4	1.0
	Stature (cm)		176.7	6.2	0.3		162.4	6.0	0.3
	BMI (kg/m^2)		27.8	4.6	0.3		28.0	6.4	0.4
	TBW (L)		47.9	6.5	0.4		33.8	5.1	0.3
	%fat		25.1	6.0	0.4		37.3	7.1	0.4
60–69.9	Weight (kg)	465	84.9	14.7	0.8	447	70.3	15.1	0.9
	Stature (cm)		175.3	6.3	0.3		160.8	6.1	0.4
	BMI (kg/m^2)		27.6	4.2	0.2		27.2	5.6	0.3
	TBW (L)		46.2	6.6	0.4		32.5	4.8	0.3
	%fat		26.2	5.5	0.3		36.9	6.9	0.4
70–79.9	Weight (kg)	447	79.3	13.3	0.7	538	67.1	14.5	0.8
	Stature (cm)		172.4	6.7	0.3		158.3	6.8	0.4
	BMI (kg/m^2)		26.7	4.0	0.2		26.7	5.3	0.3
	TBW (L)		44.0	6.4	0.4		31.6	4.9	0.3
	%fat		25.1	5.5	0.3		35.9	6.9	0.4

Table 10 Selected Anthropometric and Impedance Measures According to Age and Sex for Non-Hispanic Blacks: NHANES III (unpublished data)

		Non-Hispanic black males				Non-Hispanic black females			
Age (years)	Anthropometric measure	N	Mean	Standard deviation	Standard error	N	Mean	Standard deviation	Standard error
12–13.9	Weight (kg)	124	52.1	16.7	1.5	156	55.1	13.3	1.2
	Stature (cm)		157.9	10.1	1.0		159.6	7.3	0.7
	BMI (kg/m^2)		20.7	5.2	0.5		21.5	4.4	0.4
	TBW (L)		30.7	7.0	0.7		29.3	4.1	0.4
	%fat		19.5	8.9	1.1		26.9	8.8	0.8
14–15.9	Weight (kg)	131	64.4 171.5	15.4	1.4	102	62.0	16.3	1.8
	Stature (cm)		21.8	7.7	0.8		163.1	7.1	0.8
	BMI (kg/m^2)		38.9	4.7	0.4		23.2	5.3	0.6
	TBW (L)		17.8	6.7	0.7		30.9	5.3	0.7
	%fat			7.5	9.0		30.9	8.0	0.9
16–17.9	Weight (kg)	126	68.7	14.5	1.3	126	64.0	15.8	1.6
	Stature (cm)		173.8	7.2	0.7		163.9	7.0	0.7
	BMI (kg/m^2)		22.7	4.1	0.4		23.8	5.7	0.6
	TBW (L)		41.2	6.6	0.7		31.0	4.2	0.5
	%fat		18.6	6.4	0.8		32.6	8.5	0.9
18–19.9	Weight (kg)	118	74.7	16.4	1.5	110	65.8	18.6	2.0
	Stature (cm)		176.6	7.2	0.7		163.6	6.3	0.7
	BMI (kg/m^2)		23.8	4.4	0.4		24.6	6.7	0.8
	TBW (L)		44.1	7.5	0.8		31.4	5.5	0.7
	%fat		19.9	6.0	0.8		33.3	8.7	1.0
20–29.9	Weight (kg)	462	82.9	20.5	1.0	510	70.4	16.7	0.8
	Stature (cm)		177.1	7.4	0.4		163.7	6.1	0.3
	BMI (kg/m^2)		26.3	5.8	0.3		26.2	6.0	0.3
	TBW (L)		46.1	8.0	0.4		32.8	4.9	0.3
	%fat		23.7	7.0	0.4		35.5	7.5	0.4
30–39.9	Weight (kg)	454	82.9	17.9	0.9	569	76.7	20.2	1.0
	Stature (cm)		177.2	6.6	0.3		163.7	6.7	0.3
	BMI (kg/m^2)		26.4	5.4	0.3		28.6	7.4	0.4
	TBW (L)		46.5	7.7	0.4		34.4	5.8	0.3
	%fat		23.6	6.7	0.4		38.0	7.7	0.4
40–49.9	Weight (kg)	339	83.6	17.2	1.0	395	81.5	21.1	1.2
	Stature (cm)		176.5	7.3	0.4		164.2	6.1	0.4
	BMI (kg/m^2)		26.8	4.8	0.3		30.2	7.4	0.4
	TBW (L)		46.1	7.5	0.5		35.8	6.0	0.4
	%fat		24.9	6.1	0.5		39.4	7.0	0.4
50–59.9	Weight (kg)	191	83.7	19.4	1.4	231	80.7	19.4	1.5
	Stature (cm)		175.2	6.6	0.5		162.5	5.8	0.5
	BMI (kg/m^2)		27.2	5.7	0.4		30.6	7.1	0.6
	TBW (L)		45.9	8.5	0.7		35.2	5.8	0.5
	%fat		25.1	6.7	0.7		40.0	7.5	0.6
60–69.9	Weight (kg)	258	80.9	16.2	1.0	258	77.6	18.3	1.3
	Stature (cm)		173.6	6.6	0.5		161.1	6.3	0.5
	BMI (kg/m^2)		26.8	4.9	0.3		29.9	7.0	0.5
	TBW (L)		44.7	7.7	0.5		34.0	5.6	0.4
	%fat		24.9	6.6	0.6		39.8	6.9	0.5
70–79.9	Weight (kg)	145	77.0	15.5	1.3	149	74.0	16.5	1.5
	Stature (cm)		171.6	7.1	0.7		159.4	5.7	0.6
	BMI (kg/m^2)		26.2	4.8	0.4		29.1	6.3	0.6
	TBW (L)		43.2	7.4	0.7		33.4	5.3	0.6
	%fat		24.3	6.3	0.7		38.5	6.7	0.6

Table 11 Selected Anthropometric and Impedance Measures According to Age and Sex for Mexican-Americans: NHANES III (unpublished data)

		Mexican-American males				Mexican-American females			
Age (years)	Anthropometric measure	N	Mean	Standard deviation	Standard error	N	Mean	Standard deviation	Standard error
12–13.9	Weight (kg)	132	52.7	14.1	1.5	139	53.3	12.3	1.2
	Stature (cm)		156.0	9.2	0.9		155.4	6.5	0.7
	BMI (kg/m^2)		21.4	4.6	0.5		21.9	4.5	0.5
	TBW (L)		30.2	6.2	0.7		27.9	4.2	0.5
	%fat		22.0	8.2	1.0		28.6	7.6	0.8
14–15.9	Weight (kg)	108	62.5	16.6	1.9	113	56.2	10.7	1.2
	Stature (cm)		167.2	8.5	0.9		157.7	6.0	0.7
	BMI (kg/m^2)		22.2	5.1	0.6		22.5	3.7	0.4
	TBW (L)		37.2	6.9	0.9		28.1	3.7	0.4
	%fat		18.8	7.7	1.1		31.8	6.3	0.7
16–17.9	Weight (kg)	126	67.9	12.2	1.3	112	62.2	15.5	1.7.
	Stature (cm)		170.5	6.7	0.7		159.3	5.8	0.7
	BMI (kg/m^2)		23.3	3.7	0.4		24.5	5.7	0.7
	TBW (L)		39.6	5.5	0.6		30.2	4.5	0.6
	%fat		21.3	5.4	0.7		33.3	7.1	0.8
18–19.9	Weight (kg)	109	72.8	13.9	1.6	90	59.6	13.1	1.6
	Stature (cm)		171.9	6.3	0.7		157.7	5.7	0.7
	BMI (kg/m^2)		24.6	4.4	0.5		23.9	4.9	0.6
	TBW (L)		41.5	5.9	0.7		28.9	3.7	0.5
	%fat		22.7	5.7	0.8		33.5	6.8	0.9
20–29.9	Weight (kg)	631	73.9	13.9	0.7	509	64.8	14.5	0.8
	Stature (cm)		170.0	6.4	0.3		157.6	6.2	0.3
	BMI (kg/m^2)		25.6	4.2	0.2		26.1	5.5	0.3
	TBW (L)		41.6	6.1	0.3		30.5	4.3	0.2
	%fat		24.1	6.0	0.4		35.8	7.0	0.4
30–39.9	Weight (kg)	443	78.4	14.2	0.8	451	70.6	17.1	1.0
	Stature (cm)		170.6	7.0	0.4		156.9	6.3	0.4
	BMI (kg/m^2)		26.9	4.3	0.2		28.6	6.4	0.4
	TBW (L)		43.4	6.5	0.4		32.2	4.8	0.3
	%fat		25.4	5.4	0.4		38.0	7.1	0.4
40–49.9	Weight (kg)	361	82.0	14.5	0.9	334	73.4	13.9	0.9
	Stature (cm)		169.7	6.3	0.4		157.2	5.4	0.4
	BMI (kg/m^2)		28.4	4.4	0.3		29.7	5.6	0.4
	TBW (L)		44.7	6.6	0.5		32.6	4.3	0.3
	%fat		26.6	5.3	0.4		39.9	5.5	0.4
50–59.9	Weight (kg)	165	82.6	15.1	1.4	171	71.3	13.7	1.2
	Stature (cm)		169.3	6.0	0.5		155.7	5.4	0.5
	BMI (kg/m^2)		28.7	4.5	0.4		29.5	5.5	0.5
	TBW (L)		45.0	7.1	0.7		32.1	4.4	0.4
	%fat		26.7	5.3	0.6		39.4	5.7	0.5
60–69.9	Weight (kg)	301	78.2	12.7	0.9	278	70.0	14.1	1.0
	Stature (cm)		168.3	6.0	0.4		154.3	5.9	0.4
	BMI (kg/m^2)		27.6	4.0	0.3		29.5	5.9	0.4
	TBW (L)		42.6	5.9	0.4		31.6	4.6	0.4
	%fat		26.7	5.2	0.4		39.4	5.7	0.4
70–79.9	Weight (kg)	118	72.3	12.5	1.4	101	65.0	13.0	1.5
	Stature (cm)		165.5	5.7	0.6		153.0	5.9	0.7
	BMI (kg/m^2)		26.3	4.0	0.4		27.8	5.5	0.7
	TBW (L)		39.9	6.3	0.7		30.1	4.4	0.6
	%fat		26.1	5.2	0.7		37.8	6.8	0.8

BMI (38). A BMI-based prediction equation [Eq. (21)] was presented in an earlier section for white and black subjects. The prediction lines for this model are provided in Figure 15 for males and females in three age groups (30, 50, and 70 years).This information allows linkage of percent fat ranges with corresponding BMI ranges for normal weight $>17.5<25$ kg/m^2), overweight ($\geq 25<30$ kg/m^2), and obesity ≥ 30 kg/m^2.

At present there are inadequate data for appropriately derived population or other range categories of subcutaneous, visceral, or other adipose tissue depots.

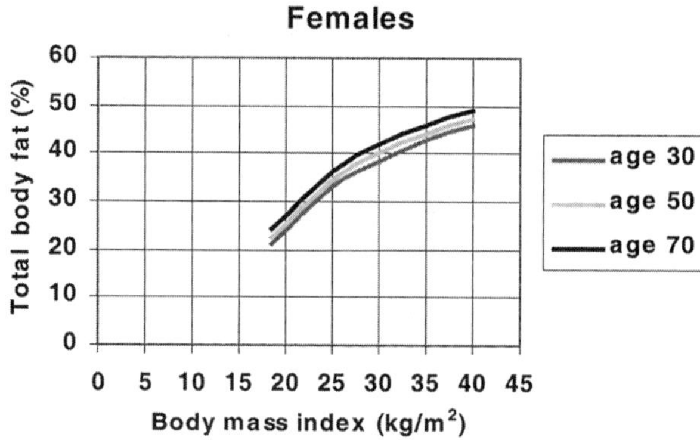

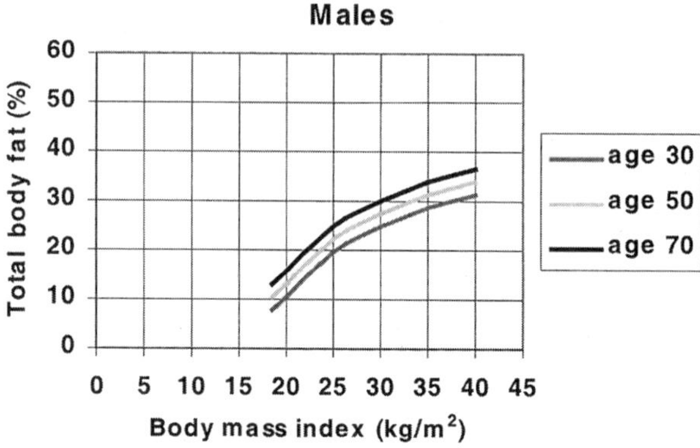

Figure 15 Total body fat, expressed as a percentage of body weight, versus body mass index in females (upper panel) and males (lower panel). The regression lines were developed based upon the formula of Gallagher et al. (38).

VII SUMMARY AND CONCLUSIONS

The remarkable technological advances over the past decade provide investigators with the tools needed to evaluate components at all five body composition levels. The applications for body composition analysis abound and dictate the selected method requirements. While our method organization was separated into two categories, laboratory and field, each method has an array of definable characteristics that ultimately determine research and clinical utility. Most methods are capable of providing estimates of more than one adiposity-related component so that the investigator can choose among them depending on instrument availability and specific method features. Some of the qualitative characteristics of the methods reviewed in this chapter are summarized in Table 12. These "gradings" are subjective but should give the reader some idea of how to select a method among those available with consideration for the evaluated subject population. The present overview should be supplemented by the interested reader with in-depth body composition reviews and the available texts published since 1985 are presented in the Appendix.

Body composition analysis is an indispensable research and clinical component that provides important insights into the pathogenesis and treatment of obese animals and humans.

APPENDIX

Monographs on Body Composition Research Published Since 1985

Norgan NG, ed. Human Body Composition and Fat Distribution. EUR-NUT Report 8, 1985.

Roche AF, ed. Body-Composition Assessments in Youth and Adults. Columbus, OH: Ross Laboratory, 1985.

Forbes GB. Human Body Composition: Growth, Aging, Nutrition and Activity. New York: Springer-Verlag, 1987.

Ellis KJ, Yasumura S, Morgan WD, eds. In Vivo Body Composition Studies. Institute of Physical Sciences in Medicine, 1987.

Lohman TG, Roche AF, Martorell R, eds. Anthropometric Standardization Reference Manual. Champaign, IL: Human Kinetics, 1988.

Yasumura S, Harrison JE, McNeill KG, Woodhead AD, Dilmanian FA eds. In Vivo Body Composition Studies: Recent Advances. New York: Plenum, 1990.

Gibson RS. Principles of Nutritional Assessment. Oxford: Oxford University Press, 1990.

Fidanza EF. Nutritional Status Assessment. London: Chapman and Hall, 1991.

Himes JH, ed. Anthropometric Assessment of Nutrition Assessment of Nutritional Status. Wiley-Liss, 1991.

Roche AF. Growth, Maturation and Body Composition: The Fels Longitudinal Study 1929-1991. Cambridge: Cambridge University Press, 1992.

Table 12 Main Qualitative Features of Available Body Composition Methods Used to Evaluate Adiposity-Related Components

	^{40}K	IVNA	TBW[a]	UWW	ADP	DXA	MCM	MRI[b]	CT[c]	ANTH	BIA
Accurate?	•••	••••	•••	•••	•••	•••	••••	••••	••••	•	••
Reproducible?	••	••	••	••	••	••••	•••	•••	•••	•	••••
Cost to purchase?	••••	••••	•	••	•••	•••	•••	••••	••••	•	•
Cost to operate?	•••	•••	••	••	••	••	••	•••	•••	•	•
Technician training?	••	••	••	••	••	••	••	•••	•••	••	•
Radiation exposure?	•	••••	•	•	•	••	••	•	••••	•	•
Requires subject participation	•	•	•	•••	••	•	•••	•	•	•	•
Transportable?	•	•	••••	•	••	••	•	•	•	••••	••••
Regional estimates?	Y √	Y √	NX	NX	NX	Y √	NX	Y √	Y √	Y √	Y √
Appropriate for:											
Very obese adults?	N √	N √	Y √	Y √	NX	NX	YX	NX	NX	YX	Y √
Children?	Y √	NX	Y √	Y √	Y √	Y √	Y √	Y √	NX	Y √	Y √
Elderly?	Y √	Y √	Y √	Y √	Y √	Y √	Y √	Y √	N √	Y √	Y √

Abbreviations: ANTH, anthropometry; ADP, air displacement plethysmography; BIA, bioimpedance analysis; CT, computerized axial tomography; DXA, dual-energy x-ray absorptiometry; IVNA, in vivo neutron activation analysis; K, potassium; MCM, multicomponent models; MRI, magnetic resonance imaging; N, no; TBW, total body water; UWW, underwater weighing; Y, yes.

Scale: • (least or none)–•••• (most).

[a] Assumes stable isotope.

[b] Assumes four or more components and stable isotope for TBW.

Marriott BM, Grumstrup-Scott J, eds. Body Composition and Physical Performance: Applications for the Military Services. Washington: National Academy Press, 1992.

Lohman TG. Advances in Body Composition Assessment. Champaign, IL: Human Kinetics, 1993.

Ellis KJ, Eastman JD, eds. Human Body Composition: In Vivo Methods, Models, and Assessment. New York: Plenum, 1993.

Kral JG, VanItallie TB, eds. Recent Development in Body Composition Analysis: Methods and Applications. London: Smith-Gordon, 1993.

Kreitzman SN, Howard AN, eds. The Swansea Trial: Body Composition and Metabolic Studies with a Very-Low-Calorie Diet (VLCD). London: Smith-Gordon, 1993.

WHO Expert Committee. Physical Status: The Use and Interpretation of Anthropometry. Geneva: WHO Technical Report Series 854, 1995.

Davies PSW, Cole TJ, eds. Body Composition Techniques in Health and Disease. Cambridge: Cambridge University Press, 1995.

Heyward VH, Stolarczyk L. Applied Body Composition Assessment. Champaign, IL: Human Kinetics, 1996.

Roche AF, Heymsfield SB, Lohman TG, eds. Human Body Composition: Methods and Findings. Champaign, IL: Human Kinetics, 1996.

Grimnes S, Martinsen ØG. Bioimpedance and Bioelectricity Basics. San Diego: Academic Press, 2000.

Yasamura S, Wang J, Pierson RN Jr, eds. In Vivo Body Composition Studies. New York: New York Academy of Sciences, 2000.

Pierson RN Jr, ed. Quality of the Body Cell Mass: Body Composition in the Third Millenium. New York: Springer-Verlag, 2000.

REFERENCES

1. Heymsfield SB, Hoffman DJ, Testolin C, Wang ZM. Evaluation of human adiposity. In: Björntorp P, ed. International Textbook of Obesity. Chichester: John Wiley & Son, 2001:85–97.
2. Heymsfield SB, Baumgartner RN, Ross R, Allison DB, Wang ZM. Evaluation of total and regional body composition. In: Bray GA, Bouchard C, James WPT, eds. Handbook of Obesity. New York: Marcel Decker, 1998;41–77.
3. Wang ZM, Pierson RN Jr, Heymsfield SB. The five level model: a new approach to organizing body composition research. Am J Clin Nutr 1992; 56:19–28.
4. Snyder WS, Cook MJ, Nasset ES, Karhausen LR, Howells GP, Tipton IH. Report of the Task Group on Reference Man. Oxford: Pergamon Press, 1975.
5. Gurr MI, Harwood JL, Lipid Biochemistry. 4th ed. London: Chapman and Hall, 1991.
6. Comizio R, Pietrobelli A, Tan YX, Wang ZM,

Withers R, Heymsfield SB, Boozer CN. Total body lipid and triglyceride response to energy deficit: relevance to molecular level body composition model. Am J Physiol 1998; 274:E860–E866.

7. Moore FD, Olsen KH, McMurray JD, Parker HV, Ball MR, Boyden CM. The Body Cell Mass and Its Supporting Environment: Body Composition in Health and Disease. Philadelphia: W.B. Saunders, 1963.
8. Pace N, Rathbun EN. Studies on body composition. III. The body water and chemically combined nitrogen content in relation to fat content. J Biol Chem 1945; 158:685–691.
9. Sheng HP, Huggins RA. A review of body composition studies with emphasis on total body water and fat. Am J Clin Nutr 1979; 32:630–647.
10. Wang ZM, Deurenberg P, Wang W, Pietrobelli A, Baumgartner RN, Heymsfield SB. Hydration of fat-free body mass: review and critique of a classic body composition constant. Am J Clin Nutr 1999; 69:833–841.
11. Forbes GB, Hursh J, Gallup J. Estimation of total body fat from potassium-40 constant. Science 1961; 133:101–102.
12. Ellis KJ. Whole-body counting and neutron activation analysis. In: Roche AF, Heymsfield SB, Lohman TG, eds. Human Body Composition. Champaign, IL: Human Kinetics, 1996, 45–62.
13. Behnke AR, Feen BG, Welham WC. The specific gravity of healthy men. JAMA 1942; 118:495-498.
14. Visser M, Gallagher D, Deurenberg P, Wang J, Pierson RN Jr, Heymsfield SB. Density of fat-free body mass relationship with race, age, and level of body fatness. Am J Physiol 1997; 272:E781–787.
15. Heymsfield SB, Wang ZM, Withers R. Multicomponent molecular-level models of body composition analysis. In: Roche A, Heymsfield SB, Lohman T, eds. Human Body Composition. Champaign, IL: Human Kinetics, 1996:129–147.
16. Martin AD, Daniel MZ, Drinkwater DT, Clarys JP. Adipose tissue density, estimated adipose lipid fraction and whole body adiposity in male cadavers. Int J Obes 1994; 18:79–83.
17. Hoffman DJ, Huber RK, Allison DB, Wang Z, Shen W, Heymsfield SB. Human Body Composition. Philadelphia: Saunders. In press.
18. Kelley DE, Thaete EL, Troost F, Huwe T, Goodpaster BH. Subdivisions of subcutaneous abdominal adipose tissue and insulin resistance. Am J Physiol 2000; 278:E941–E948.
19. Lohman TG, Roche AF, Martorell R. Anthropometric Standardization Reference Manual. Champaign, IL: Human Kinetics, 1988.
20. Kuskowska-Wolk A, Karlsson P, Stolt M, Rossner S. The predictive validity of body mass index based on self reported weight and height. Int J Obes 1989; 13:441–453.
21. Lass NJ, Mitchell KK, Pellegrino JE, Shumate KS. Correlational analysis of speakers' heights, weights, and temporal speech features. Percept Mot Skills 1979; 48(1):297–298.
22. Le Marchand L, Yoshizawa CN, Nomura AMY. Validation of body size information on driver's licenses. Am J Epidemiol 1988; 128:874–877.
23. Quetelet LAJ. Anthropométrie ou measure des differents facultés de l'homme. Brussels; C. Marquardt, 871:479
24. Keys A, Aravanis C, Blackburn H, Van Buchem FSP, Buzina R, Djordjevic BS, Fidanza F, Karvonen MJ, Menotti A, Puddu V, Taylor HL. Coronary heart disease: overweight and obesity as risk factors. Ann Intern Med 1972; 77:15–27.
25. Abdel-Malek AK, Mukherjee D, Roche AF. A method of constructing an index of obesity. Hum Biol 1985; 57:415–430.
26. Billewicz WZ, Kemsley WFF, Thomson AM. Indices of adiposity. Br J Prev Soc Med 1962; 16:183–188.
27. Khosla T, Lowe CR. Indices of obesity derived from body weight and height. Br J Prev Soc Med 1967; 21:122–128.
28. Florey C du V. The use and interpretation of ponderal index and other weight-height ratios in epidemiological studies. J Chron Dis 1970; 23:93–103.
29. Lee J, Kolonel LN, Hinds MW. The use of an inappropriate weight-height derived index of obesity can produce misleading results. Int J Obes 1982; 6:233–239.
30. Lee J, Kolonel LN. Are body mass indices interchangeable in measuring obesity-disease associations? Am J Public Health 1984; 74:376–377.
31. Benn RT. Some mathematical properties of weight-far-height indices used as measures of adiposity. Br J Prev Soc Med 1971; 25:42–50.
32. Roche AF, Siervogel RM, Chumlea WC, Webb P. Grading body fatness from limited anthropometric data. Am J Clin Nutr 1981; 34:2831–2838.
33. Garn SM, Leonard WR, Hawthorne VM. Three limitations of the body mass index. Am J Clin Nutr 1986; 44:996–997.
34. Garrow JS, Webster J. Quetelet's index (W/H2) as a measure of fatness. Int J Obes 1985; 9:147–153.
35. Bouchard C. Genetics of human obesities: introductory notes. In: Bouchard C, ed. The Genetics of Obesity. Boca Raton: CRC Press, 1994:1–16.
36. Baumgartner RN, Heymsfield SB, Roche AF. Human body composition and the epidemiology of chronic disease. Obes Res 1995; 3:73–95.
37. Gallagher D, Visser M, Sepulveda D, Pierson RN Jr, Harris T, Heymsfield SB. How useful is body mass index for comparison of body fatness across age, sex, and ethnic groups? Am J Epid 1996; 143:228–239.
38. Gallagher D, Heymsfield SB, Heo M, Jebb SA, Murgatroyd PR, Sakamoto Y. Healthy percent body fat ranges: an approach for developing guidelines

based upon body mass index. Am J Clin Nutr 2000; 72:694–701.

39. Wang ZM, Pi-Sunyer FX, Kotler DP, Wang J, Pierson RN Jr, Heymsfield SB. Magnitude and variation of ratio of total body potassium to fat-free mass: a cellular level modeling study. Am J Physiol 2001; 281:E1–E7.
40. Cohn SH, Vaswani AN, Yasumura S. Improved model for determination of body fat by in vivo neutron activation. Am J Clin Nutr 1984; 40:255–259.
41. Heymsfield SB, Waki M, Kehayias J, Lichtman S, Dilmanian FA, Kamen Y, Wang J, Pierson RN Jr. Chemical and elemental analysis of humans in vivo using improved body composition models. Am J Physiol (Endocrin Metab) 1991; 261:E190–E198.
42. Kehayias JJ, Heymsfield SB, LoMonte AF, Wang J, Pierson RN Jr. In vivo determination of body fat by measuring total body carbon. Am J Clin Nutr 1991; 53:1339–1344.
43. Kehayias JJ, Heymsfield SB, Dilmanian FA, Wang J, Gunther DM, Pierson RN Jr. Measurement of body fat by neutron inelastic scattering: comments on installation, operation and error analysis. In: Yasumura S, Harrison JE, McNeill KG, Woodhead AD, Dilmanian FA, eds. Advances in In Vivo Body Composition Studies. New York: Plenum Press, 1990:339–346.
44. Kyere K, Oldroyd B, Oxby CB, Burkinshaw L, Ellis RE, Hill GL. The feasibility of measuring total body carbon by counting neutron inelastic scatter gamma rays. Phys Med Biol 1982; 27:805–817.
45. Cunningham JJ. N×6.25: Recognizing a bivariate expression for protein balance in hospitalized patients. Nutrition 1994; 10:124–127.
46. Knight GS, Beddoe AH, Streat SJ, Hill GL. Body composition of two human cadavers by neutron activation and chemical analysis. Am J Physiol 1986; 250:E179–E185.
47. Biltz RM, Pellegrino ED. The chemical anatomy of bone. J Bone Joint Surg Am 1969; 51A:456–466.
48. Kehayias JJ, Ellis KJ, Cohn SH, Weinlein JH. Use of a pulsed neutron generator for in vivo measurement of body carbon. In: Ellis KJ, Yasumura S, Morgan WD, eds. In Vivo Body Composition Studies. London: Institute of Physical Sciences in Medicine, 1987: 427–435.
49. Dilmanian FA, Weber DA, Yasumura S, Kamen Y, Lidofsky L, Heymsfield SB, Pierson RN Jr, Wang J, Kehayias JJ, Ellis KJ. The performance of the BNL delayed-gamma neutron activation systems. In: Yasumura S, Harrison JE, McNeill KG, et al., eds. Advances in In Vivo Body Composition Studies: Recent Advances. New York: Plenum Press, 1990: 309–315
50. Shizgal HM, Spanier AH, Humes J, Wood CD. Indirect measurement of total exchangeable potassium. Am J Physiol 1977; 233:F253–F259.
51. Pierson RN Jr, Wang J, Colt E, Neumann P. Body composition measurements in normal men: the potassium, sodium, sulfate, and tritium space in 58 adults. J Chron Dis 1982; 35:419–428.
52. Culebras JM, Moore FD. Total body water and the exchangeable hydrogen. 1. Theoretical calculation of nonaqueous exchangeable hydrogen in man. Am J Physiol 1997; 232:R54–R59.
53. Wong WW, Cochran WJ, Klish WJ, Smith EO, Lee LS, Klein PD. In vivo isotope-fractionation factors and the measurement of deuterium, and oxygen-18 dilution spaces from plasma, urine, saliva, respiratory water vapor, and carbon dioxide. Am J Clin Nutr 1988; 47:1–6.
54. Lohman TG. Applicability of body composition techniques and constants for children and youths. Exerc Sport Sci Rev 1986; 14:325–357.
55. Waki M, Kral JG, Mazariegos M, Wang J, Pierson RN Jr, Heymsfield SB. Relative expansion of extracellular fluid in obese vs. nonobese women. Am J Physiol 1991; 261:E199–E203.
56. Deurenberg P, Leenen R, Van der Kooy K, Hautvast JGAJ. In obese subjects the body fat percentage calculated with Siri's formula is an overestimate. Eur J Clin Nutr 1989; 43:569–575.
57. Kooy KVD, Leenen R, Deurenberg P, Seidell JC, Westerterp KR, Hautvast JGAJ. Changes in fat-free mass in obese subjects after weight loss: a comparison of body composition measures. Int J Obes 1992; 16:675–683.
58. Wang ZM, Heshka S, Pierson RN Jr, Heymsfield SB. Systematic organization of body composition methodology: overview with emphasis on component-based methods. Am J Clin Nutr 1995; 61:457–465.
59. Behnke AR, Wilmore JH. Evaluation and Regulation of Body Build and Composition. Englewood Cliffs, NJ: Prentice-Hall, 1974.
60. Fidanza F, Keys A, Anderson JT. Density of body fat in man and other mammals. J Appl Physiol 1953; 6:252–256.
61. Brozek J, Grande F, Anderson T, Keys A. Densitometric analysis of body composition: a revision of some assumptions. Ann NY Acad Sci 1963; 110:113–140.
62. Siri WE. Body composition from fluid spaces and density. In: Brozek J, Henschel A, eds. Techniques in the Measurement of Body Composition. Washington: National Academy of Sciences, 1961:223–244.
63. Murgtroyd PR, Coward WA. An improved method for estimating changes in whole-body fat and protein mass in man. Br J Nutr 1989; 62:311–314.
64. Sawka MN, Weber H, Knowlton RG. The effect of total body submersion on residual lung volume and body density measurements in man. Ergonomics 1978; 21:89–94.
65. Lohman TG. Advances in Body Composition Assessment. Champaign, IL: Human Kinetics, 1992.
66. McCrory MA, Gomez TD, Bernauer EM, Molé PA. Evaluation of a new air displacement plethysmograph

for measuring human body composition. Med Sci Sports Exerc 1995; 27(12):1686–1691.

67. Collins MA, Millard-Stafford ML, Sparling PB, Snow TK, Rosskopf LB, Webb SA, Omer J. Evaluation of the BOD POD for assessing body fat in collegiate football players. Med Sci Sports Exerc 1999; 31(9): 1350–1356.
68. Wells JCK, Fuller NJ. Precision of measurement and body size in whole-body air-displacement plethysmography. Int J Obes Relat Metab Disord 2001; 25:1161–1167.
69. Mazess RB, Barden HS, Bisek JP, Hanson J. Dual-energy x-ray absorptiometry for total-body and regional bone-mineral and soft-tissue composition. Am J Clin Nutr 1990; 51:1106–1112.
70. Pietrobelli A, Formica C, Wang ZM, Heymsfield SB. Dual-energy x-ray absorptiometry body composition model: review of physical concepts. Am J Physiol 1996; 271: E941–E951.
71. Van Loan MD, Keim NL, Berg K, Mayclin PL. Evaluation of body composition by dual energy x-ray absorptiometry and two different software packages. Med Sci Sport Exerc 1995; 27:587–591.
72. Brunton JA, Bayley HS, Atkinson SA. Validation and application of dual-energy x-ray absorptiometry to measure bone mass and body composition in small infants. Am J Clin Nutr 1993; 58:839–845.
73. Ellis KJ, Shypailo RJ, Pratt JA, Pond WG. Accuracy of dual energy x-ray absorptiometry for body-composition measurements in children. Am J Clin Nutr 1994; 60:660–665.
74. Svendsen OL, Haarbo J, Hassager C, Christiansen C. Accuracy of measurements of body composition by dual-energy x-ray absorptiometry in vivo. Am J Clin Nutr 1993; 57:605–608.
75. Heymsfield SB, Wang J, Heshka S, Kehayias JJ, Pierson RN. Dual-photon absorptiometry: comparison of bone mineral and soft tissue mass measurements in vivo with established methods. Am J Clin Nutr 1989; 49:1283–1289.
76. Laskey MA, Lyttle KD, Flaxman ME, Barber RW. The influence of tissue depth and composition on the performance of the Lunar dual-energy x-ray absorptiometer whole-body scanning mode. Eur J Clin Nutr 1992; 46:39–45.
77. Snead DB, Birge SJ, Kohrt WM. Age-related differences in body composition by hydrodensitometry and dual-energy x-ray absorptiometry. J Appl Physiol 1993; 74:770–775.
78. Going SB, Massett MP, Hall MC, Bare LA, Root PA, Williams DP, Lohman TG. Detection of small changes in body composition by dual-energy x-ray absorptiometry. Am J Clin Nutr 1993; 57:845–850.
79. Testolin CG, Gore R, Rivkin T, Horlick M, Arbo J, Wang ZM, Chiumello G, Heymsfield SB. Dual-energy x-ray absorptiometry: analysis of pediatric fat estimate errors due to tissue hydration effects. J Appl Physiol 2000; 89:2365–2372.
80. Clark RR, Kuta JM, Sullivan JC. Prediction of percent body fat in adult males using dual energy x-ray absorptiometry, skinfolds, and hydrostatic weighing. Med Sci Sport Exerc 1993; 528–535.
81. Pritchard JE, Nowson CA, Strauss BJ, Carlson JS, Kaymakci B, Wark JD. Evaluation of dual energy x-ray absorptiometry as a method of measurement of body fat. Eur J Clin Nutr 1993; 47:216–228.
82. Tatarrani PA, Ravussin E. Use of dual-energy x-ray absorptiometry in obese individuals. Am J Clin Nutr 1995; 62:730–734.
83. Friedl KE, DeLuca JP, Marchitelli LJ, Vogel JA. Reliability of body-fat estimations from a four-component model by using density, body water, and bone mineral measurements. Am J Clin Nutr 1992; 55:764–770.
84. Fuller NJ, Jebb SA, Laskey MA, Coward WA. Four compartment model for the assessment of body composition in humans: comparison with alternative methods, and evaluation of the density and hydration of the fat-free mass. Clin Sci 1992; 82:687–693.
85. Heymsfield SB, Waki M. Body composition in humans: advances in the development of multicompartment chemical models. Nutr Rev 1991; 49:97–108.
86. Wang ZM, Pi-Sunyer FX, Kotler DP, Wielopolski L, Withers RT, Pierson RN Jr, Heymsfield SB. Multicomponent methods: evaluation of new and traditional soft-tissue mineral models by in vivo neutron activation analysis. Am J Clin Nutr. In press.
87. Siri WE. The gross composition of the body. In: Larence JH, Tobias CS, eds. Biological and Medical Physics. New York: Academic Press, 1956:239–280.
88. Baumgartner RN, Heymsfield SB, Lichtman S, Wang J, Pierson RN Jr. Body composition in elderly people: effect of criterion estimates on predictive equations. Am J Clin Nutr 1991; 53:1345–1353.
89. Selinger A. The body as a three component system. Unpublished doctoral dissertation, University of Illinois, Urbana, 1977.
90. Heymsfield SB, Lichtman S, Baumgartner RN, Wang J, Kamen Y, Aliprantis A, Pierson RN Jr. Body composition of humans: comparison of two improved four compartment models that differ in expense, technical complexity, and radiation exposure. Am J Clin Nutr 1990; 52:52–58.
91. Lohman TG, Going SB. Multicomponent models in body composition research: opportunities and pitfalls. In: KJ Ellis, JD Eastman, eds. Human Body Composition, New York: Plenum Press, 1993:53–58.
92. Sprawls P. The Physical Principles of Diagnostic Radiology. Baltimore: University Park Press, 1977: 101–117.
93. Wang ZM, Heshka S, Heymsfield SB. Application of computerized axial tomography in the study of body

composition: evaluation of lipid, water, protein, and mineral in healthy men. In: Ellis KJ, Eastman JD, eds. Human Body Composition: In Vivo Methods, Models, and Assessment. New York: Plenum Press, 1993: 3–4.

94. Heymsfied SB, Noel R, Lynn M, Kutner M. Accuracy of soft tissue density predicted by CT. J Comput Assist Tomogr 1979; 3:859–860.
95. Chowdhury B, Sjöström L, Alpsten M, Kostanty J, Kvist H, Löfgren R. Multi-compartment body composition technique based on computerized tomography. Int J Obes 1994; 18:219–234.
96. Kvist H, Sjöström L, Tylen U. Adipose tissue volume determinations in women by computed tomography: technical considerations. Int J Obes 1986; 10:53–67.
97. Brummer RJM, Lonn L, Grangard UI, Bengtsson BA, Kvist H, Sjöström L. Adipose tissue and muscle volume determinations by computed tomography in acromegaly, before and one year after adenectomy. Eur J Clin Invest 1993; 23:199–205.
98. Heymsfield SB, Fulenwider T, Nordlinger B, Balow R, Sones P, Kutner M. Accurate measurement of liver, kidney, and spleen volume and mass by computerized axial tomography Ann Intern Med 1979; 90:185–187.
99. Rossner S, Bo WJ, Hiltbrandt E, Hinson W, Karstaedt N, Santago P, Sobol WT, Crouse JR. Adipose tissue determinations in cadavers—comparison between cross-sectional planimetry and computed tomography. Int J Obes 1990; 14:893–902.
100. Wang ZM, Visser M, Ma R, Baumgartner RN, Kotler D, Gallagher D, Heymsfield SB. Skeletal muscle mass: evaluation of neutron activation and dual-energy x-ray absorptiometry methods. J Appl Physiol 1996; 80(3):824–831.
101. Heymsfield SB, Olafson RP, Kutner NM, Nixon DW. A radiographic method of quantifying protein–calorie undernutrition. Am J Clin Nutr 1979; 32:693–702.
102. Heymsfield SB, Noel R. Radiographic analysis of body composition by computerized axial tomography. In: Ellison N, Newell G, eds. Nutrition and Cancer. 1981; 17:161–172.
103. Borkan GA, Gerzof SG, Robbins AH, Hults DE, Silbert CK, Silbert JE. Assessment of abdominal fat content by computerized tomography. Am J Clin Nutr 1982; 36:172–177.
104. Sjöström L. A computer-tomography based multicomponent body composition technique and anthropometric predictions of lean body mass, total and subcutaneous adipose tissue. Int J Obes 1991; 15:19–30.
105. Ryan AS, Nicklas BJ. Age-related changes in fat deposition in midthigh muscle in obese women: relationships with metabolic cardiovascular disease risk factors. Int J Obes 1999; 23:126–132.
106. Liu M, Chino N, Ishihara T. Muscle damage progression in Duchenne muscular dystrophy evaluated by a quantitative computed tomography method. Arch Phys Med Rehabil 1993; 74:507–514.
107. Goodpaster BH, Kelley DE, Thaete FL, Jing HE, Ross R. Skeletal muscle attenuation determined by computed tomography is associated with skeletal muscle lipid content. J Appl Physiol 2000; 90:104–110.
108. Overand TJ, Cunningham DA, Patterson DH, Lefcoe MS. Thigh composition in young and elderly men determined by computed tomography. Clin Physiol 1992; 12:629–640.
109. Nordal HJ, Dietrichson P, Eldevik P, Gronseth K. Fat infiltration, atrophy and hypertrophy of skeletal muscles demonstrated by x-ray computed tomography in neurological patients. Acta Neurol Scand 1988; 77: 115–122.
110. Goodpaster BH, Thaete FL, Simoneau JA, Kelley DE. Subcutaneous abdominal fat and thigh muscle composition predict insulin sensitivity independent of visceral fat. Diabetes 1997; 46:1579–1585.
111. Goodpaster BH, Kelley DE, Wing RR, Meier A, Thaete FL. Effects of weight loss on regional distribution and insulin sensitivity in obesity. Diabetes 1999; 48:839–847.
112. Banerji MA, Buckley MC, Chaiken RL, Gordon D, Lebovitz HE, Kral JG. Liver fat, serum triglycerides and visceral adipose tissue in insulin-sensitive and insulin-resistant black men with NIDDM. Int J Obes 1995; 19:846–850.
113. Ricci C, Longo R, Gioulis E, Bosco M, Pollesello P, Masutti F, Croce LS, Paoletti S, De Bernard B, Tiribelli C, Dalla Palma L. Noninvasive in vivo quantitative assessment of fat content in human liver. J Hepatol 1997; 27:108–113.
114. Goto T, Onuma T, Takebe K, Kral JG. The influence of fatty liver on insulin clearance and insulin resistance in non-diabetic Japanese subjects. Int J Obes 1995; 19:841–845.
115. Björntorp P. "Portal" adipose tissue as a generator of risk factors for cardiovascular disease and diabetes. Arteriosclerosis 1990; 10:493–496.
116. Mahmood S, Taketa K, Imai K, Kajihara Y, Imai S, Yokobayashi T, Yamamoto S, Sato M, Omori H, Manabe K. Association of fatty liver with increased ratio of visceral to subcutaneous adipose tissue in obese men. Acta Med Okayama 1998; 52:225–231.
117. Foster MA, Hutchison JMS, Mallard JR, Fuller M Nuclear magnetic resonance pulse sequence and discrimination of high- and low-fat tissues. Mag Res Imaging 1984; 2:187–192.
118. Hayes PA, Sowood PJ, Belyavin A, Cohen JB, Smith FW. Subcutaneous fat thickness measured by magnetic resonance imaging, ultrasound, and calipers. Med Sci Sports Exerc 1988; 20(3):303–309.
119. De Ridder CM, De Boer RW, Seidell JC, Nieuwenhoff CM, Jeneson JAL, Bakker CJG, Zonderland ML, Erich WBM. Body fat distribution in pubertal girls quantified by magnetic resonance imaging. Int J Obes 1992; 16:443–449.

120. Ross R, Léger L, Morris DV, De Guise J, Guardo R. Quantification of adipose tissue by, MRI: relationship wit anthropometric variables. J Appl Physiol 1992; 72(2):787–795.
121. Sohlström A, Wahlund LO, Forsum E. Adipose tissue distribution and total body fat by magnetic resonance imaging, underwater weighing, and body-water dilution in healthy women. Am J Clin Nutr 1993; 58:830–838.
122. Thomas EL, Saeed N, Hajnal JV, Brynes A, Goldstone AP, Frost G, Bell JD. Magnetic resonance imaging of total body fat. J Appl Physiol 1998; 85(5):1778–1785.
122a. Busetto L, Tregnaghi A, Bussolotto M, Sergi G, Beninca P, Ceccon A, Giantin V, Fiore D, Enzi G. Visceral fat loss evaluated by total body magnetic resonance imaging in obese women operated with laparascopic adjustable silicone gastric banding. Int J Obes 2000; 24(1):60–69.
122b. LeBlanc A, Lin C, Shackelford L, Sinitsyn V, Evans H, Belichenko O, Schenkman B, Kozlovskaya I, Oganov V, Bakulin A, Hedrick T, Feeback D. Muscle volume, MRI relaxation times (T2), and body composition after spaceflight. J Appl Physiol 2000; 89(6):2158–2164.
122c. Heymsfield SB, Gallagher D, Kotler DP, Wang Z, Allison DB, Heshka S. Body-size dependence of resting energy expenditure can be attributed to non-energetic homogeneity of fat-free mass. Am J Physiol Endocrinol Metab 2002: 282(1):E132–E138.
123. Ross R, Shaw KD, Rissanen J, Martel Y, De Guise J, Avruch L. Sex differences in lean and adipose tissue distribution by magnetic resonance imaging: anthropometric relationships. Am J Clin Nutr 1994; 59:1277–1285.
124. Gray D, Fujioka K, Colletti PM, Kim H, Devine W, Cuyegkeng T, Pappas T. Magnetic-resonance imaging used for determining fat distribution in obesity and diabetes. Am J Clin Nutr 1991; 54:623–627.
125. Baumgartner RN, RL Rhyne C, Troup S, Wayne, Garry PJ. Appendicular skeletal muscle areas assessed by magnetic resonance imaging in older persons. J Gerontol 1992; 47:M67–M72.
126. Seidell JC, Bakker CJC, Van der Kooy K. Imaging techniques for measuring adipose-tissue distribution—a comparison between computed tomography and 1.5-T magnetic resonance. Am J Clin Nutr 1990; 51:953–957.
127. Ross R, Pedwell H, Rissanen J. Effects of energy restriction and exercise on skeletal muscle and adipose tissue in women as measured by magnetic resonance imaging. Am J Clin Nutr 1995; 61:1179–1185.
128. Fowler PA, Fuller MF, Glasbey CA, Cameron GG, Foster MA. Validation of the in-vivo measurement of adipose tissue by magnetic resonance imaging of lean and obese pigs. Am J Clin Nutr 1992; 56:7–13.
129. Abate N, Burns D, Peshock RM, Garg A, Grundy SM. Estimation of adipose tissue mass by magnetic resonance imaging: validation against dissection in human cadavers. J Lipid Res 1994; 35:1490–1496.
129a. Heymsfield SB, Ross R, Wang ZM, Frager D. Imaging techniques of body composition: advantages of measurement and new uses. In: Carlson-Newberry SJ, Costello RB, eds. Emerging Technologies for Nutrition Research: Potential for Assessing Military Performance Capability. Washington: National Academy Press, 1997:127–150.
130. Ross R, Léger L, Guardo R, De Guise J, Pike BG. Adipose tissue volume measured by magnetic resonance imaging and computerized tomography in rats. J Appl Physiol 1991; 70(5):2164–2172.
131. Engstrom CM, Loeb GE, Reid JR, Forrest WJ, Avruch L. Morphometry of the human thigh muscles. A comparison between anatomical sections and computer tomographic and magnetic resonance images. J Anat 1991; 176:139–156.
132. Sobel W, Rossner S, Hinson B, Hiltbrandt E, Karstaedt N, Santago P, Wolfman N, Hagaman A, Crouse JR III. Evaluation of a new magnetic resonance imaging method for quantitating adipose tissue areas. Int J Obes 1991; 15:589–599.
133. Mitsiopoulos N, Baumgartner RN, Heymsfield SB, Lyons W, Gallagher D, Ross R. Cadaver validation of magnetic resonance imaging and computerized tomography measurement of human skeletal muscle. J Appl Physiol 1998; 85:115–122.
134. Seidell JC, Oosterlee A, Thijssen M, Burema J, Deurenberg P, Hautvast J, Josephus J. Assessment of intra-abdominal and subcutaneous abdominal fat: relation between anthropometry and computed tomography. Am J Clin Nutr 1987; 45:7–13.
135. Baumgartner RN, Rhyne RL, Troup C, Wayne S, Garry PJ. Appendicular skeletal muscle areas assessed by magnetic resonance imaging in older persons. J Gerantol 1992; 47(3):M67–M72.
136. Baumgartner RN, Rhyne RL, Garry PJ. Body composition in the elderly from MRI: associations with cardiovascular disease risk factors. In: Ellis K, Eastman J, eds. Human Body Composition: In Vivo Methods, Models, and Assessment. New York: Plenum Press, 1993:35–38.
137. Staten MA., Totty WG, Kohrt WM. Measurement of fat distribution by magnetic resonance imaging. Invest Radiol 1989; 24:345–349.
138. Garard EL, Snow RC, Kennedy DN, Frisch RE, Guimaraes AR, Barbieri RL, Sorensen AG, Egglin TK, Rosen BR. Overall body fat and regional fat distribution in young women: quantification with MR imaging. Am J Radiol 1991; 157:99–104.
139. Ross R, Shaw KD, Martel Y, de Guise J, Avruch L. Adipose tissue distribution measured by magnetic resonance imaging in obese women. Am J Clin Nutr 1933; 57:470–475.
140. Ross R, Shaw KD, Rissanen J, Martel Y, De Guise J,

Avruch L. Sex differences in lean and adipose tissue distribution by magnetic resonance imaging: anthropometric relationships. Am J Clin Nutr 1994; 59:1277–1285.
141. Ross R, Pedwell H, Rissanen J. Effects of energy restriction and exercise on skeletal muscle and adipose tissue in women as measured by magnetic resonance imaging. Am J Clin Nutr 1995; 61:1179–1185.
142. Deans HE, Smith FW, Lloyd DJ, Law AN, Sutherland HW. Fetal fat measurement by magnetic resonance imaging. Br J Radiol 1989; 62:603–607.
143. De Ridder CM, De Boer RW, Seidell JC, Nieuwenhoff CM, Jeneson JAL, Bakker CJG, Zonderland ML, Erich WBM. Body fat distribution in pubertal girls quantified by magnetic resonance imaging. Int J Obes 1992; 16:443–449.
144. Sohlström A, Forsum E. Changes in adipose tissue volume and distribution during reproduction in Swedish women as assessed by magnetic resonance imaging. Am J Clin Nutr 1995; 61:287–295.
145. Janssen I, Ross R. Effects of sex on the change in visceral, subcutaneous and skeletal muscle in response to weight loss. Int J Obes 1999; 23:1035–1046.
146. Janssen I, Heymsfield SB, Wang Z, Ross R. Skeletal muscle mass and distribution in 468 men and women aged 18–88 years. J Appl Physiol 2000; 89(1): 81–88.
147. Ferrando AA, Stuart CA, Brunder DG, Hillman GR. Magnetic resonance imaging quantitation of changes in muscle volume during 7 days of strict bed rest. Aviat Space Environ Med 1995; 66:976–981.
148. Treuth MS, Ryan AS, Pratley RE, Rubin MA, Millar JP, Nicklas BJ, Sorkin J, Harman SM, Goldberg AP, Hurley BF. Effects of strength training on total and regional body composition in older men. J Appl Physiol 1994; 77(2):614–620.
149. Ross R, Goodpaster B, Kelley D, Boada F. Magnetic resonance imaging in human body composition research: from quantitative to qualitative tissue measurement. Ann NY Acad Sci 2000; 904:12–18.
150. Tsubahara A, Chino N, Akaboshi K, Okajima Y, Takahashi H. Age-related changes of water and fat content in muscles estimated by magnetic resonance (MR) imaging. Disabil Rehabil 1995; 17(6):298–304.
151. Boesch C, Slotboom J, Hoppeler H, Kreis R. In vivo determination of intra-myocellular lipids in human muscle by means of localized ^{1}H-MR-spectroscopy. Magn Reson Med 1997; 37:484–493.
152. Constantinides CD, Gillen JS, Boada FE, Pomper MG, Bottomly PA. Sodium MRI and quantification in human muscle: potential applications in exercise and disease. Radiology 2000; 216(2):559–568.
153. Seidall JC, Bouchard C. Visceral fat in relation to health: is it a major culprit of simply an innocent bystander. Int J Obes 1997; 21:626–631.
154. Frayn KN. Visceral fat and insulin resistance—causative or correlative? Br J Nutr 2000; 83:S71–S77.
155. Hood R, Allen C. Lipogenic enzyme activity in adipose tissue during the growth of swine with different propensities to fatten. J Nutr 1973; 103: 353–362.
156. Goodpaster BH, Kelley DE, Wing RR, Meier A, Thaete FL. Effects of weight loss on regional fat distribution and insulin sensitivity in obesity. Diabetes 1999; 48:839–847.
157. Misra A, Garg A, Abate N, Peshock R, Stray-Gundersen J, Grundy S. Relationship of anterior and posterior subcutaneous abdominal fat to insulin sensitivity in nondiabetic men. Obes Res 1997; 5:93–99.
158. Abate N, Garg A, Peshock R, Stray-Gundersen J, Adama-Huet B, Grundy S. Relationship of generalized and regional adiposity to insulin sensitivity in men with NIDDM. Diabetes 1996; 45:1684–1693.
159. Rissanen J, Hudson R, Ross R. Visceral adiposity, androgens and plasma lipids in obese men. Metabolism 1994; 43(10):1318–1323.
160. Fowler PA, Fuller MF, Glasby CA, Foster MA, Cameron GG, McNiel G, Maughan RJ. Total and subcutaneous adipose tissue distribution in women: the measurement of distribution and accurate prediction of quantity by using magnetic resonance imaging. Am J Clin Nutr 1991; 54:18–25.
161. Roche AF, Baumgartner RN, Guo S. Anthropometry: classical and modem approaches. In: Whitehead RG, Prentice A, eds. New Techniques in Nutritional Research. New York: Academic Press, 1991:241–260.
162. Himes JH, Roche AF, Siervogel RM. Compressibility of skinfolds and the measurement of subcutaneous fatness. Am J Clin Nutr 1979; 32:1734–1740.
163. Jackson AS, Pollock ML. Generalized equations for predicting body density of women. Med Sci Sports Exerc 1980; 12:175–182.
164. Durnin JVGA, Womersely J. Body fat assessment from total body density and its estimation from skinfold thickness: measurements on 481 men and women aged 16 to 72 years. Br J Nutr 1974; 32:77–97.
165. Roche AF, Guo S. Development, testing and use of predictive equations for body composition measures. In: Kral JG, VanItallie TB, eds. Recent Developments in Body Composition Analysis: Methods and Applications. London: Smith-Gordon, 1993:1–16.
166. Armellini F, Zamboni M, Rigo L, Tedesco T, Bergamo-Andreis IA, Procacci C, Bosello O. The contribution of sonography to the measurement of intra-abdominal fat. J Clin Ultrasound 1990; 18:563–567.
167. Bellisari A, Roche AF, Siervogel RM. Reliability of B-mode ultrasonic measurements of subcutaneous adipose tissue and intra-abdominal depth: comparisons with skinfold thicknesses. Int J Obes 1993; 17:475–480.
168. Björntorp P. Visceral obesity: a "civilization syndrome." Obes Res 1993; 1:206–222.
169. Garn SM. Relative fat patterning: an individual characteristics. Hum Biol 1955; 27:75–89.
170. Bouchard C. Introductory notes on the topic of fat

distribution. In: Bouchard C, Johnston F, eds. Fat Distribution During Growth and Later Health Outcomes. New York: Alan R. Liss, 1988:1–8.

171. Bailey SM, Garn SM, Katch VL, Guire KE. Taxonomic identification of human fat patterns. Am J Phys Anthrop 1982; 59:361–366.
172. Mueller WH, Stallones L. Anatomical distribution of subcutaneous fat: skinfold site choice and construction of indices. Hum Biol 1981; 53:321–335.
173. Baumgartner RN, Roche AF, Guo S, Lohman TG, Boileau RA, Slaughter M. Adipose tissue distribution: the stability of principal components by sex, ethnicity and maturation stage. Hum Biol 1986; 58:719–735.
174. Lapidus L, Bengtsson C, Larsson B, Pennart K, Rybo E, Sjöström L. Distribution of adipose tissue and risk of cardiovascular disease and death: a 12 year follow up of participants in the population study of women in Gothenburg, Sweden. Br Med J 1984; 289:1257–1261,
175. Larsson BK, Svardsudd L, Welin L, Wilhelmsen, Bjorntorp P, Tibblin G. Abdominal adipose tissue distribution, obesity and risk of cardiovascular disease and death: 13 year follow up of participants in the study of men born in 1913. Br Med J 1984; 288:1401–1404.
176. Ohlson LO, Larsson B, Svardsudd K, Welin L, Eriksson H, Wilhelmsen L, Bjorntorp P, Tibblin G. The influence of body fat distribution on the incidence of diabetes mellitus, 13.5 years of follow-up of the participants of the study of men born in 1913. Diabetes 1985; 34:1055–1058.
177. Seidell JC, Deurenberg P, Hautvast JGAJ. Obesity and fat distribution in relation to health—current insights and recommendations. World Rev Nutr Diet 1987; 50:57–91.
178. Kissebah AH. Insulin resistance in visceral obesity. Int J Obes 1991; 15:109–115.
179. Després JP. Lipoprotein metabolism in visceral obesity. Int J Obes 1991; 15:45–52.
180. Bray GA. Pathophysiology of obesity. Am J Clin Nutr 1992; 55:488S–494S.
181. Filipovsky J, Ducimetiere P, Darne B, Richard JI. Abdominal body mass distribution and elevated blood pressure are associated with increased risk of death from cardiovascular diseases and cancer in middle-aged men. The results of a 15-20-year follow-up in the Paris prospective study I. Int J Obes 1993; 17:197–203.
182. Houmard JA, Wheeler WS, McCammon MR, Wells JM, Truitt N, Hamad SF, Holbert D, Israel RG, Barakat HA. An evaluation of waist to hip ratio measurement methods in relation to lipid and carbohydrate metabolism in men. Int J Obes 1991; 15:181–188.
183. Vague J. The degree of masculine differentiation of obesities: a factor determining predisposition to diabetes, atherosclerosis, gout and uric calculous diseases. Am J Clin Nutr 1956; 4:20–34.
184. Kekes-Szabo T, Hunter GR, Nyikos I, Nicholson C, Snyder S, Lincoln B. Development and validation of computed tomography derived anthropometric regression equations for estimating abdominal adipose tissue distribution. Obes Res 1994; 2:450–457.
185. Pouliot MC, Després JP, Lemieux S, Moorjani S, Bouchard C, Tremblay A, Nadeau A, Lupien PJ. Waist circumference and abdominal sagittal diameter: best simple anthropometric indexes of abdominal visceral adipose tissue accumulation and related cardiovascular risk in men and women. Am J Cardiol 1994; 73:460–468.
185a. Janssen I, Heymsfield SB, Allison DB, Kotler DP, Ross R. The combination of body mass index and waist circumference identifies a unique obesity phenotype. Am J Clin Nutr 2002. In press.
185b. Rankinen T, Kim SY, Pérusse L, Després JP, Bouchard C. The prediction of abdominal visceral fat level from body composition and anthropometry: ROC analysis. Int J Obes 1999; 23:801–809.
185c. Seidell JC, Pérusse L, Després JP, Bouchard C. Waist and hip circumferences have independent and opposite effects on cardiovascular disease risk factors: the Quebec Family Study. Am J Clin Nutr 2001; 74:315–321.
186. Zamboni M, Armellini F, Turcato E, Todesto T, Bissoli L, Bergamo-Andreis IA, Bosselo O. Effect of weight loss on regional body fat distribution in premenopausal women. Am J Clin Nutr 1993; 58:29–34.
187. Ross R, Rissanen J, Hudson R. Sensitivity associated with the identification of visceral adipose tissue levels using waist circumference in men and women: effects of weight loss. Int J Obes 1996; 20:533–538.
188. Ross R, Pedwell H, Rissanen J. Effects of energy restriction and exercise on skeletal muscle and adipose tissue in women as measured by magnetic resonance imaging. Am J Clin Nutr 1995; 61:1179–1185.
189. Sjöstrom L. Body composition studies with CT and with CT-calibrated anthropometric techniques. In: Kral JG, Vanltallie TB, eds. Recent Developments in Body Composition Analysis: Methods and Applications. London: Smith-Gordon, 1993:17–34.
190. Van der Kooy K, Leenen R, Seidell JC, Deurenberg P, Visser M. Abdominal diameters as indicators of visceral fat: comparison between magnetic resonance imaging and anthropometry. Br J Nutr 1993; 70:47–58.
191. Richelsen B, Pedersen SB. Associations between different anthropometric measurements of fatness and metabolic risk parameters in non-obese, healthy, middle-aged men. Int J Obes 1995; 19:169–174.
192. Seidell JC, Andres R, Sorkin JD, Muller DC. The sagittal waist diameter and mortality in men: the Baltimore Longitudinal Study on Aging. Int J Obesity 1994; 18:61–67.
193. Baumgartner RN, Chumlea WC, Roche AF. Bioelectric impedance for body composition. Exerc Sport Sci Rev 1990; 18:193–224.
194. Baumgartner RN, Chumlea WC, Roche AF. Estima-

tion of body composition from segmental impedance. Am J Clin Nutr 1989; 50:221–225.
195. Baumgartner RN. Electrical Impedance and TOBEC. In: Roche AF, Lohman TG, Heymsfield SB, eds. Human Body Composition: Methods and Findings. Champaign, IL: Human Kinetics, 1996.
196. Mueller SH, Martorell R. Reliability and accuracy of measurement. In: Lohman TB, Roche AF, Martorell R, eds. Anthropometric Standardization Reference Manual. Champaign, IL: Human Kinetics 1988:83–87.
197. Dunn G. Design and Analysis of Reliability Studies: The Statistical Evaluation of Measurement Errors. London: Edward Arnold, 1989.
198. Bland JM, Altman DG. Statistical methods for assessing agreement between two methods of clinical measurement. Lancet 1986; 307–310.
199. Habicht JP, Yarbrough C, Martorell R. Anthropometric field methods: criteria for selection. In: Jelliffe DB, Jelliffe EFP, eds. Nutrition and Growth. New York: Plenum Press, 1979:365–387.
200. Frisancho AR. Anthropometric Standards for the Assessment of Growth and Nutritional Status. Ann Arbor, MI: University of Michigan Press, 1993.
201. VanItallie TB, Yang MU, Heymsfield SB, Funk RC, Boileau RA. Height-normalized indices of the body's fat-free mass and fat mass: potentially useful indicators of nutritional status. Am J Clin Nutr 1990; 52: 953–959.

3

Ethnic and Geographic Influences on Body Composition

Paul Deurenberg and Mabel Deurenberg-Yap

Health Promotion Board, Singapore, Republic of Singapore

I INTRODUCTION

Body composition information on humans can be collected at various levels, such as atomic, molecular, cellular, tissue, or whole-body level (1). In the case of obesity, the main component of interest is body fat, at the tissue [adipose tissue obtained by computer tomography (CT) or magnetic resonance imaging (MRI) scanning] or molecular level [body fat mass or body fat percent as assessed by densitometry or dual-energy x-ray absorptiometry (DXA) scans]. In addition, the distribution of fat over the body is important. The latter can be evaluated by CT or MRI scans or by anthropometry.

There are many methods to measure or assess body composition, especially for body fat and body fat distribution. Apart from direct methods (chemical carcass analyses or in vivo neutron activation analyses, *IVNAA*), these methods can be described as indirect and doubly indirect (2). Indirect methods are validated against experimentally found or calculated quantitative relationships between body parameters and components of body composition as obtained from carcass analyses or *IVNAA*. Doubly indirect methods assess body composition based on statistical relationships between easy measurable body parameters and an indirect method. The resulting formulas are usually population specific and have an estimation error of 4–5% compared to the method of reference. Table 1 lists methods for the determination of body composition with special reference to body fat. Generally the error of indirect methods is $<3\%$. For doubly indirect methods, the estimation error is larger and is usually $\sim 5\%$.

Chemical carcass analyses revealed that the chemical composition of the body varies widely among subjects. This is especially true for the amount of body fat. It was found that the variation in body composition among subjects is greatly reduced if the various components are expressed in relation to the fat free body (3,4), and with this the concept of the two-compartment model of body composition was born (5). This concept divides the body into a fat mass, which contains all ether-soluble fat, and a fat-free mass, which is the difference between body weight and the fat mass (FM). Chemically the fat-free mass (FFM) consists of water, minerals, protein, and a small amount of carbohydrate (mainly glycogen and glucose). The carbohydrate component is small and is normally neglected. Carcass analyses revealed that the mean composition of the fat free mass is $\sim 73\%$ water, 20% protein, and 7% minerals (5). This chemical composition of the fat-free mass is confirmed in many modern studies in young adults using in vivo techniques (6), although there are slight variations among population groups (7–10). These figures are the basis for a number of indirect

Table 1 Methods to Determine Body Fat

Direct	Indirect	Doubly indirect
Chemical carcass analyses	Densitometry	Weight/height indices, e.g., BMI
In vivo neutron activation analyses (IVNAA)	Dilution techniques, e.g., deuterium oxide dilution	Skinfold thickness measurements
	Dual-energy x-ray absorptiometry (DXA)	Bioelectrical impedance
	More compartment models	Body circumferences
	CT/MRI scanning	

CT, computed tomography; MRI, magnetic resonance imaging; BMI, body mass index.

measures of body fat, i.e., for densitometry and for dilution methods.

Assuming a constant composition of the fat-free mass (as above) and given the densities for water (0.993 kg/L), protein (1.340 kg/L) and minerals (3.038 kg/L) at body temperature, the density of the fat-free mass can be calculated as 1.100 kg/L. As the density of the fat mass is 0.900 kg/L, it is obvious that the density of the body will vary between 0.9 kg/L and 1.1 kg/L depending on the amount of body fat. This forms the basis for the densitometric method for the determination of body fat. The volume of the body is measured by either water displacement, air displacement, or underwater weighing (11), and body density is then calculated as weight/volume. Using Siri's (5) formula ($BF\% = 495/\text{density}_{\text{body}} = 450$) or other similar equations, body fat percent can be calculated. Principles and description of different densitometric techniques are given elsewhere (11,12).

The amount of water in the human body can be determined by dilution techniques (13). With these techniques, the subject is given a tracer (usually deuterium oxide, tritium oxide or ^{18}O-labeled water), and after a suitable dilution time the concentration of the tracer is determined in the body fluids (saliva, blood, or urine). The amount of body water can be calculated from the given dose and the tracer concentration in the body fluid, and, assuming a constant water fraction of the fat-free mass (i.e. 73%), fat-free mass and consequently fat mass can be calculated (14).

II ACCURACY AND VALIDITY OF REFERENCE BODY COMPOSITION METHODS

How accurate are these techniques? The technical error of these methodologies is small and is in experienced hands with adequate instrumentation not beyond one percentage point of body fat percent (15). Siri (5) calculated that owing to variations in the assumed constant composition of the fat-free mass, the densitometric method has a methodological error of maximally 2–3%. This was confirmed, for example, in a study by Heymsfield et al. (6) Deuterium dilution results in about the same level of error. For example, if an obese, edematous subject is weighed underwater, the normal calculation formula to convert body density into body fat could overestimate body fat percent by two or three percentage points (due to a larger amount of body water in the fat free mass its density is < 1.100 kg/L). In the same subject deuterium oxide dilution would, however, underestimate body fat percent by some two or three percentage points.

With the development of new body composition techniques such as *IVNAA* and dual-energy x-ray absorptiometry (DXA), and their combined use with densitometry and deuterium oxide dilution, it has become possible to measure body composition using chemically defined multicompartment models (11). The most popular models are a three-compartment model (fat mass, water, and dry fat-free mass) in which variation of the water fraction in the fat-free mass is accounted for, and a four-compartment model (fat mass, water, minerals, and protein). In the latter model, the variation of both the water and the mineral fraction in fat-free mass is accounted for. Although the technical error of these multicompartment models is not lower compared to two-compartment models (15), they do have a smaller methodological error, as the variation in the composition of the fat-free mass is accounted for. This makes the three- and especially the four-compartment model suitable as a reference when it comes to comparing groups in which the composition of the fat-free mass might differ. Such differences are known to exist between age groups (children vs. adults vs. elderly), males and females, and also ethnic groups.

Table 2 provides examples for females from various ethnic groups for body fat percent measured by densitometry alone, (assuming a density of the fat-free mass of 1.1 kg/L) and a four-compartment model. As can be seen, body fat calculated from the Siri formula is gen-

Table 2 Body Fat Percent in Females of Different Ethnic Groups Measured by Two Body Composition Methods[a]

Race	Ref.	BF2c	BF4c	Difference
Blacks	17	21.2	21.8	+0.6
Blacks	18	26.5	28.1	+1.6
Blacks	8	35.1	35.3	+0.2
Chinese	10	26.7	29.7	+3.0
Chinese	9	30.3	33.5	+3.2
Indian	9	35.5	38.2	+2.7
Malays	9	35.9	37.8	+1.9
Whites	17	24.2	23.6	−0.6
Whites	18	30.2	29.3	−0.9
Whites	8	30.2	30.5	+0.3
Whites	10	27.7	28.9	+1.2

[a] BF2c: body fat from two-compartment model; BF4c: body fat from four-compartment model.

erally lower in blacks and in Asians than body fat from the four-compartment model. In Caucasian groups, the differences between two- and four-compartment models are not so obvious.

There are numerous studies (in vitro as well as in vivo) showing that blacks (most studies refer to African-Americans) compared to Caucasians have higher bone density and bone mineral content as well as higher muscle mass (16). The amount of water in the fat-free mass, however, is not different. As minerals and proteins are the densest components in the fat-free mass, it can be calculated that the density of the fat-free mass blacks is higher than in Caucasians (17,18), although this was not found in all studies (8).

The same holds for the comparison between Asians (Chinese) and Caucasians (10), although less information is available on Asians. Recently it was shown that there are also small differences in the composition of the fat-free mass (in terms of water, mineral, and protein fraction) among (Singaporean) Chinese, Malays, and Indians (9).

Generally, studies among ethnic groups suggest that the use of the classical densitometric method and the use of the Siri (5) formula is likely to lead to biased measurements of body fat percent. Thus for comparative studies among ethnic groups this method is not suitable, unless formulas based on measured rather than assumed densities of the fat-free mass are used (11). For comparative studies, the use of multicompartment models is recommended to avoid any systematic bias. Multicompartment methods are, however, expensive, and the instrumentation is not available to many researchers. As the water content in the fat-free mass is (in most studies) not found to be different from the assumed value of 73%, dilution methods may be a good alternative for comparative studies among ethnic groups (9,14). The method has the advantage that it is "portable," and even researchers who do not have the necessary instrumentation could use the methodology as samples can be sent to specialized laboratories for analyses.

III ACCURACY AND VALIDITY OF PREDICTIVE BODY COMPOSITION METHODS

Doubly indirect methods rely on a statistical relationship between easily measurable body parameters and body composition as measured by a direct or an indirect method. There are many examples of such methods, and the most often used for the prediction or assessment of body fat are skinfold thickness measurements, bioelectrical impedance measurements, and weight/height indices. All these methods have in common that the standard error of estimate (SEE) of the equation is ~4–5 percentage body fat points and that the prediction equations are not "general" but are population specific. It has to be kept in mind that a SEE of 5% means, that, even if the mean bias is zero in 34% of the population, the differences between measured and predicted body fat percent will exceed −5 or +5 percentage body fat points. In 5% of the population, the error will be higher than −10 or +10 percentage points. Thus, for individual assessments, these methods are not very reliable. Unfortunately, many prediction formulas also have a systematic bias if applied to other populations than the one in which they were developed.

Table 3 gives for three methods an example of systematic bias. In this table, the predictive values from a BMI-based prediction formula (19), an impedance-based formula (20) and a skinfold based formula (21) are compared in Indonesian and Caucasian males and females of comparable age. It is obvious that in Caucasians the differences between measured and predicted values are much lower than in Indonesians. This is not surprising, as the formulas used to predict were all developed in Caucasians. These data show that the interpretation of predicted values from formulas developed in other populations has to be approached with caution.

The reasons for those systematic biases are easy to understand from the principles of the predictive

Table 3 Measured and Predicted Body Fat Percent in Dutch and Indonesian Adult Males and Females

	Females				Males			
	Indonesian (51)		Dutch (42)		Indonesian (59)		Dutch (64)	
	Mean	SD	Mean	SD	Mean	SD	Mean	SD
Age (years)	35	9	34	8	41	7	40	8
BMI (kg/M^2)	22.7	4.7	24.4	4.9	24.3	3.3	26.2	3.6
BF deuterium %	36.0	6.4	33.2	9.2	28.3	6.2	26.5	7.6
BF BMI (%)	29.8	7.1	31.7	7.0	22.3	4.9	24.4	5.7
BF imp (%)	27.4	8.9	33.1	6.9	22.3	4.9	26.4	7.3
BF skfd (%)	32.6	6.4	33.9	5.2	27.3	6.6	25.8	6.1

BMI: body mass index; BF deuterium, body fat from deuterium oxide dilution; BF BMI: body fat predicted from body mass index using a sex- and age-specific Caucasian prediction formula (19); BF imp: body fat predicted from bioelectrical impedance (20); BF skfd: body fat predicted from skinfolds (21).

methods. The skinfold methodology assumes that the thickness of the subcutaneous fat layer, as it can be measured using skinfold calipers, is representative of the total-body fatness. Skinfold thicknesses at exactly defined sites are then used in a formula that regresses the skinfold thicknesses against a measure of body fat, generally body density. Differences between sexes and age groups are accounted for in most formulas, but less is known about the relationship between subcutaneous fat layer and total fat among ethnic groups. Little is also known about the representativeness of different body sites for the total subcutaneous fat layer in various ethnic groups. What is known, however, suggests that ethnic groups differ in subcutaneous fat pattern. For example, blacks tend to have less subcutaneous fat in the extremities and more subcutaneous fat on the back of the trunk, resulting in a higher trunk-to-extremity skinfold ratio compared to Caucasians. The amount of intra-abdominal or visceral fat is, however, for the same amount of total body fat, lower in blacks. There are indications that the skinfold patterns of other ethnic groups differ also from that of Caucasians (23,24). It is therefore not surprising that the application of skinfold formula often results is biased mean estimates of body fat percent (24). Differences in subcutaneous fat pattern also may explain why formulas using different combinations of skinfolds [as for example the Dumin and Womersley equations (21)] can give different results in the same population. Apart from the problem of different fat patterning, there is the additional problem that the method of reference used to develop the prediction equation may give biased values of body fat in various ethnic populations. Also, different types of skinfold calipers measure different skinfold thicknesses (25). Generally, the skinfold methodology is less valid in very thin subjects and in the very obese, and the methodology needs trained observers to obtain valid and reproducible results. More research in various ethnic groups has to be done in the area of subcutaneous fat pattern and its relationship with body fat percent based on valid reference methods.

Total body bioelectrical impedance is related to the water content of the body, but it is affected by many other parameters, some of which can be controlled for. The formulas for the prediction of body fat percent using bioelectrical impedance analyses generally have an estimation error of about five percentage body fat points (11). As for skinfolds, also impedance formulas are population specific, and thus predictive values are often strongly biased (see Table 3). The reason for those biases are, in most situations, differences in body build. Also technical error due to lack of standardisation or the use of different instruments can contribute to systematic biases.

In total-body bioelectrical impedance analysis a small alternating current is applied to the body and the resistance or impedance of the body to that current is measured. It is assumed that the human body is a homogeneous conductor. However, the conductivity of the total body is for a large part (> 80%) determined by the extremities, whereas most of the body water is in the trunk. This leads to the observation that subjects with relatively long legs and/or long arms will have relatively (too) high impedance values for their total body water. As a consequence, total body water and fat-free mass will be underestimated by the usual formulas and hence body fat will be overestimated. Relative leg length was discussed as one of the reasons that in Indonesians and Chinese bioelectrical impedance underestimates BF%, as Asians have relatively short legs compared to Caucasians (23,26,27). As relative leg length and relative arm length differ remarkably among ethnic groups (see also Fig. 1), this is something to keep in mind if impedance is used for body composition analyses.

In addition to the "classical" total-body impedance analyzers, which measure the conductivity of the subject from foot to hand while lying supine, there are now various commercially available impedance analyzers that measure impedance from hand to hand (standing) or from foot to foot while standing on a weighing scale. Weight, height, age, and gender are included in the formulas that are incorporated in these instruments. Although these instruments are more convenient to use than the classical impedance analyzers where the subjects had to lie supine, they do not provide better information, and the population specificity of formulas may be even a greater problem. This is understandable, as the "assessed" water content of the extremities (arms or legs) is assumed to be representative for the whole body. It is obvious that this is not true across populations where there are obvious differences in relative leg and/or arm length, but also not in ethnically homogeneous populations. For example, in a subject with relatively highly developed leg muscles, the foot-to-foot impedance analyzer is likely to underestimate body fat percent.

Apart from biases caused by body build differences, the impedance methodology has many other pitfalls, despite its easy and convenient application. Standardization is very important, not only regarding body position but also regarding environmental temperature. In addition different machines give different readings, and the correct type of electrodes is important as well. However, when compared to skinfold measurements, less experience is needed to perform an accurate measurement. A report of a consensus meeting on the use of bioelectrical impedance in body composition studies has been published (28).

Both the impedance methodology and skinfold thickness measurements are "portable" methods, which can be used in large population studies. Skinfold measurements have the disadvantage that the subject has to be partly undressed and that there is physical contact between the researcher and the subject, which may limit its practical application in certain populations. As increasing fatness results in increasing weight, weight corrected for height methods can also be used as indicators for body fatness.

An appropriate weight/height index has to have a high correlation with body fat, but also a low correlation with body height, as otherwise body fat percent would be systematically over- or underestimated in short people. The most popular of all indices is the body mass index (BMI) or Quetelet Index. The WHO (29,30) recommends the BMI as an indicator of overweight and obesity. The correlation between BMI and body fat percent body fat percent (BF%) is high (depending on the age group ranging from 0.6 to 0.8), and the correlation found with body height is generally low and not significant.

The BMI can also be used as a predictor for BF%. Several studies have demonstrated a good relationship between the BMI and the amount of body fat if age and sex are accounted for (19,31–33). When using such age- and sex-specific equations percent body fat can be predicted with an error of 3–5%, an error comparable with the prediction error of skinfold thickness or impedance measurements.

In some subjects or groups of subjects, BMI cannot be used to predict body fat, as for example in pregnancy and in body builders. It has to be kept in mind, however, that the BMI also correlates with the fat-free mass. The BMI is in fact not more than a weight index, and as a measure of body fatness it assumes that a fixed part of the index consists of fat-free mass, whereas all exceeding mass is body fat. The situation is not so simple, however, as with increasing body fatness the amount of fat-free mass also tends to increase (more muscle needed to "carry" excess body fat and more bone mass to support the heavier weight).

Biodata	Dutch	Asian
Age (yrs)	21	22
Height (cm)	175.6	158.0
Weight (kg)	77.2	43.9
Relative leg length	0.47	0.45
Wrist (cm)	5.6	4.4
Knee (cm)	9.1	8.4
Armspan (cm)	177.0	157.5
Waist (cm)	82.0	62.2
Hip (cm)	104.0	87.0
BMI (kg/m^2)	25.0	17.6
BF4c (%)	31.1	29.6

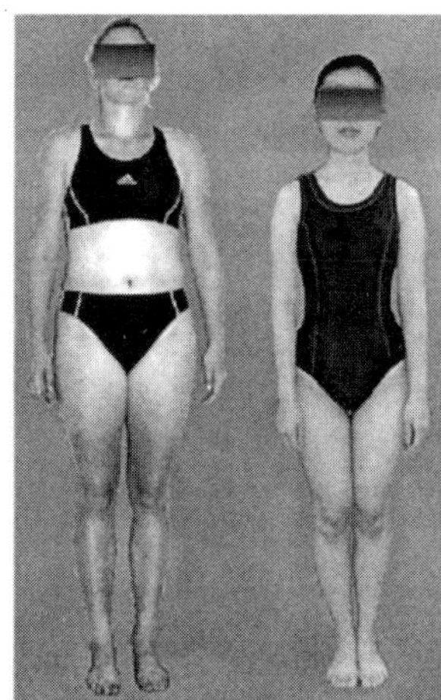

Figure 1 Body build and composition data from a Caucasian (Dutch) subject and a Chinese (Singaporean) subject. BMI, body mass index; BF4c, body fat from four-compartment model. (From Ref. 1.)

Moreover, the index assumes that the weight distribution over the body length is homogeneous. However, weight per unit length is higher in the trunk than in the legs. This means that subjects with relatively longer legs will generally have a lower BMI, and thus in those subjects body fat tends to be underestimated with a BMI-based formula. It has been discussed in the literature (34) that the long-leggedness in the Australian Aboriginal accounts for about 2 kg/m^2 of their low BMI. There are considerable differences in relative leg lengths among ethnic groups (27), with blacks generally having longer legs than Caucasians and some Asians groups having shorter legs than Caucasians. It is clear that this has an impact on the validity of the BMI as predictor of BF%. However, it has to be kept in mind that differences in relative leg length also exist among various African groups (e.g., Ethiopians vs. West African groups) and Asian groups (e.g., Chinese vs. Indians). Also, there is generally a wide variation in relative leg length within a given (homogeneous) ethnic group.

In addition, body build has been shown to have an impact on the BMI/BF% relationship. Although the effect of body build is often not found to be strong in homogeneous populations (35,36), comparisons between different (ethnic) population groups have shown that body build is a contributing factor (37–39).

Figure 2 demonstrates how body build and leg length affect relationship between BMI and body fatness, and Figure 3 shows the impact of relative leg

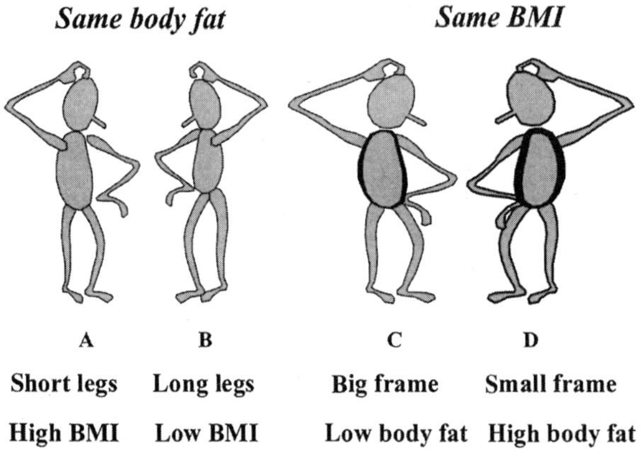

Figure 2 Subject A has the same BF% as subject B, but because he has shorter legs his BMI will be higher (more mass per cm length in the trunk. Subject C has the same BMI as subject D, but as his frame is bigger (stockier), he will have more skeletal mass, more muscle mass, and more connective tissue. Therefore for the same BMI he will have less BF%.

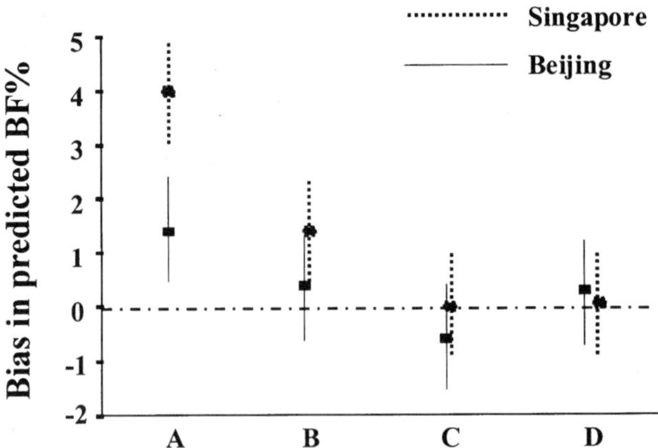

Figure 3 BF%: body fat percent. Bias: measured BF% minus predicted BF% (19). A: without correction; B: corrected for relative leg lengths; C: corrected for frame size; D: corrected for relative leg lengths and frame size. (From Ref. 38.)

length and body build on the BMI/BF% relationship in a group of sex- and age-matched Beijing Chinese, Singapore Chinese, and Dutch Caucasians. As can be seen the relationship between BMI and BF% is different among the three groups, but after correction for relative leg length and/or body build, the differences completely disappear (38). The effect of body build on the BMI/BF% relationship was confirmed in two other studies among ethnic groups (37,39). To visualize how different Caucasians are in relation to Singapore Chinese, two typical subjects from recent studies are shown in Figure 1.

Several studies in different ethnic groups confirm a fairly good relationship between BMI and BF% as long as age and sex are taken into account. In addition ethnicity can have a clear impact on the relationship. From this it may be concluded that if BMI is used to classify people in categories of body fatness, the cutoff points for those categories should ideally be ethnic specific (40).

IV DEFINITION OF OBESITY AND BMI CUT-OFF POINTS

The WHO (30) defines obesity as a condition with excess body fat to the extent that health and well-being are adversely affected. The body mass index is used for the purpose of classification. The suggested cutoff points for overweight (BMI $\geq$25 kg/m^2) and obesity (BMI $\geq$30 kg/m^2) are based on observational studies on the relationship between morbidity and mortality and BMI primarily in Caucasians from Europe and the United States. In Caucasians, a BMI of 30 kg/m^2 corresponds to a BF% of ~25% in young adult males and ~35% in young adult females (29), although there are variations around those estimates.

In cross-country or cross-ethnic group comparisons on obesity, two factors should be kept in mind: the body composition part, i.e., the level of body fatness; and the health risks related to overweight/obesity. Because of the differences in the BMI/BF% relationship among ethnic groups, it is clear that a general BMI cutoff point can be questioned. More specifically, a comparison between groups should be based on comparable levels of body fatness, which could be at different levels of BMI. Figure 4 shows calculated BMI cutoff points for obesity in different ethnic groups having the same body fat percent (40). According to this, the cutoff points for obesity might be considerably lower in many ethnic groups than the advocated level of 30 kg/m^2 in Caucasians. The main limitation of the data in Figure 4 is that BF% in the different populations was determined using different techniques, of which the validity in the population under study is not sure. For a comparative study on the relationship between BF% and BMI among (ethnic) groups, a prerequisite is that the reference method to determine body fat percent is valid. As discussed earlier in this chapter, such a method should ideally be a multicompartment model or, alternatively, deuterium oxide dilution.

A recent study in Singapore using a four-compartment model clearly showed differences in BMI/BF% relationship among Chinese, Malays, Indians, also in comparison to Caucasians (39). The cutoff point that was calculated based on this study was 27 kg/m^2, which is similar to that suggested by Guricci et al. (22) and currently used in Indonesia. This BMI cutoff point is slightly higher than the one suggested by Ko et al. (41) for Hong Kong Chinese, which is 26 kg/m^2. Unfortunately, in the study of Ko et al. (41) BF% was assessed by impedance. Although the methodology was validated against DXA, no correction was made for the slight overestimation of impedance against DXA. Moreover, DXA cannot be regarded as a reference technique, and there are numerous studies showing either an under- or overestimation (9,42,43) of BF% from DXA, in some studies also ethnic dependent (9,44). Studies on the relationship between BMI and BF% from impedance were published earlier (45,46). The validity of those studies remains obscure, BIA is too much affected by body build factors (that may differ among groups) to be a reliable reference method. A study showing that the relationship between weight and impedance among some different ethnic groups has similar slopes has been published (47), but this study does not allow any conclusion as the different groups may have differed in body composition. More information on the relationship between BMI and BF% in different (ethnic) groups is needed and ideally multicentre studies have to be carried out with strict standardisation of methodologies. Those studies should include parameters of body build to enable explanations of possible differences and perhaps to enable corrections of BMI for differences in body build. Implementation of these lower BMI cut-off points for obesity in the population will result in a much

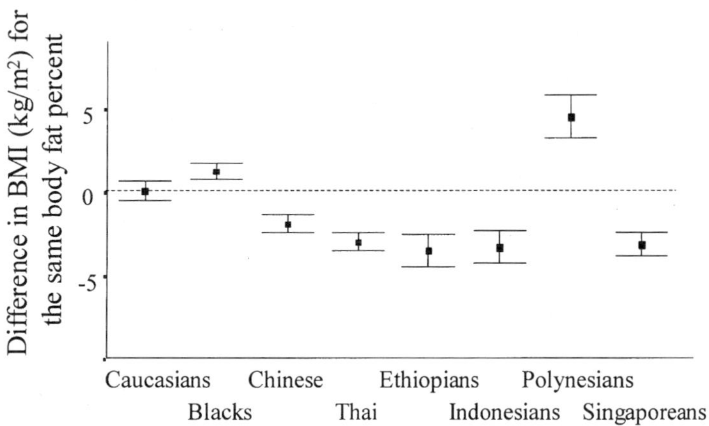

Figure 4 Adjustments to be made in BMI to reflect equal levels of body fat percent compared to Caucasians of the same age and sex. (From Refs. 39, 40.)

higher prevalence of obesity in many countries/ethnic groups, whereas in other groups the prevalence might become lower.

However, a lowering of cutoff point is not appropriate if there would be no elevated health risk at those lower levels of body mass index. This second aspect should also be carefully studied among different ethnic groups. It is known that in several Asian populations, cardiovascular morbidity and mortality are high and that the risk factors for CVD are high already at very low levels of BMI. For example, Ko et al. (48) showed that Hong Kong Chinese have at a very low BMI a high odds ratio for diabetes, hypertension, dyslipidemia, and albuminuria. Similarly, Figure 5 shows that in Singapore, the odds ratio of having at least one CVD risk factor is high at very low levels of BMI (49,50). Currently the International Obesity Task Force (IOTF) (51) is discussing a revision of BMI-based cutoff points for obesity in the Asian region, suggesting a BMI cutoff as low as 23 kg/m^2 for overweight and a BMI of 25 kg/m^2 for obesity. It seems necessary that redefining cutoff points should be extended to other ethnic groups as well. In the earlier-mentioned meta-analyses (40), it was shown not only that there are differences among clearly different ethnic groups (as Caucasians and Asians), but also that within the "same" ethnic group there might be differences in the BMI/BF% relationship. For example, American Caucasians apparently have a lower body fat percent at the same BMI than do Caucasians in Europe (33,40). As both the American and the European data came from various laboratories, most of them using densitometry, it is unlikely that this difference is due to differences in methodology. The black populations groups studied by Luke et al. (46) differed as well, which is confirmed by a study of Long et al. (52). Also, Northern and Southern Chinese differ (38,40), a difference that could be ascribed to body build differences. Wagner et al. (16), in a recent review also stress the need for in-depth studies in blacks to avoid biased estimations of obesity prevalence.

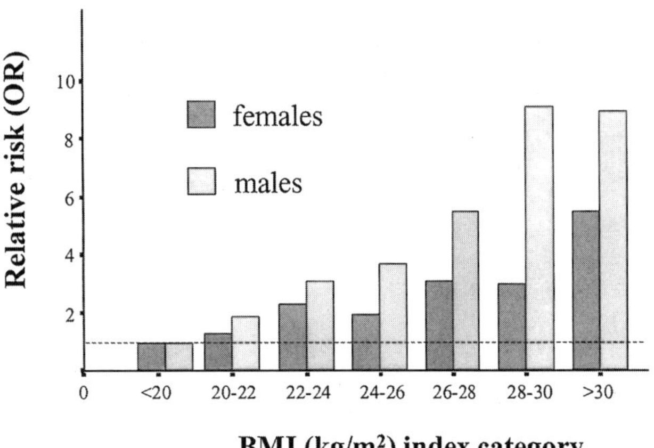

Figure 5 Risk factors: elevated serum cholesterol (≥6.2 mmol/L), elevated total cholesterol/HDL cholesterol ratio (>4.4), elevated triglyceride (≥1.8 mmol/L), elevated blood pressure (≥140/90mmHg), diabetes mellitus (OGGT ≥11.1 mmol/L). Data are corrected for age, ethnicity, educational level, occupation, physical activity, smoking, and waist/hip ratio. (From Ref. 20.)

With regard to the relationship between BMI and body composition in different ethnic groups, there are two other interesting points to consider. There is first the definition of underweight. Many Asian populations have a large number of people with a BMI lower than 20 kg/m^2 or even lower than 18.5 kg/M^2, the BMI value that is suggested by the WHO as cutoff for underweight (30). Those low BMI values are hardly prevalent in adult Western (Caucasian) populations. In the recent (1998) National Health Survey in Singapore, as many 11% of the females and 7% of the males had a BMI below 18.5 kg/m^2. The proportion of Singaporeans with a BMI <20 kg/km^2 were 25% and 15% for females and males, respectively (50). There is no reason at all to assume that undernutrition is epidemic among Singaporeans. This suggests that "healthy" BMI values in those populations could be shifted to the left, causing on the one hand higher obesity prevalences, and on the other hand lower undernutrition prevalences.

A second point is that if some ethnic groups have higher body fat percent at a given BMI, their fat-free mass will be lower, resulting in lower metabolic rates for a given weight and height (age and sex). This may shed new light on some reported low values of resting metabolic rate and total daily energy expenditure in certain population groups (53).

V BODY FAT DISTRIBUTION

Since the early work of Vague (54), confirmed by many other studies [e.g., by Larson et al. (55)], it is clear that body fat distribution, specifically the amount of intra-abdominal (visceral) fat, is a more important risk factor for metabolic disorders than total body fat. The amount of visceral and subcutaneous abdominal adipose tissue can be assessed by computer tomography (CT) or magnetic resonance imaging (see Sec. 3).

Various anthropometric techniques have been used to predict body fat distribution, for example trunk to total skinfold thickness ratio, sagittal diameter, waist-thigh circumference ratio, waist-hip circumference ratio (WHR), or waist circumference (WC) alone (56). Many epidemiological studies have shown that there is a clearly increased risk for metabolic disorders such as hypertension, glucose intolerance, and hyperlipidemia with increased WHR or WC, and the WHO (30) defines cutoff points for abdominal obesity at a waist circumference level of 80 cm and 95 cm for females and males, respectively, and a WHR of 0.85 and 1.00 for females and males, respectively. Like BMI, these cutoff values are based on observational studies mainly among Caucasians (30). Although all studies in various ethnic groups show a positive relationship between parameters of body fat distribution and morbidity, recent studies suggest that the relationship between anthropometric parameters and the actual amount of visceral fat might differ among ethnic groups. Data from the MONICA study (57) suggest that optimal screening cut-off points (action levels) for WC may be population (ethnic) specific.

However, there is not yet sufficient evidence on the relationship between these indices and visceral fat to justify ethnic specific cutoff points for body fat distribution (58–61), and there is not yet enough information about the relation with these indices with morbidity. Generally African-Americans (children as well as adults) have less visceral adipose tissue as found by CT or MRI than their white counterparts (59,60,62,63). On the other hand, a comparative study among Pima Indians showed that there were no differences in visceral and subcutaneous abdominal fat areas (MRI) with age-, sex-, and BMI-matched Caucasians (64). The main limitation of most studies is the relatively small number of subjects, due to the nature (cost and radiation exposure) of the measurements. Data from NHANES III (65) show that for the same level of apparent body fatness (BMI) the corresponding WC values are higher in Caucasians than in Hispanics and African-Americans. This seems contradictive to the fact that African-Americans have a relatively higher truncal (subcutaneous) fat distribution (16). This shows that anthropometric indicators for body fat distribution have to be interpreted with caution, as the correlation with visceral fat is relatively low (0.4–0.7), which can easily result in misclassification.

Several comparative studies concluded that American blacks and whites differ in their metabolic relationships with body fat and body fat distribution (66,67). On the contrary, Despres et al. (68) showed that ethnicity per se contributed only little to the variation in lipid profile between blacks and whites after controlling for differences in other variables (among them body mass index and body fat distribution).

In a recent study in Singapore we found that the relative risk for having at least one cardiovascular risk factor (e.g., elevated cholesterol, hypertension, diabetes mellitus) is elevated at levels of WC or WHR far below the WHO cutoff points (50). Using WHO cutoff points for classification of abdominal obesity (30) would miss a large part of the population at risk. This elevated risk could be due to a higher amount of visceral fat at low WC or to other factors, e.g., genetic factors. Further studies in Singapore are needed to determine the relationship between anthropometric measurements (WC and WHR) and the amount of visceral fat by CT or MRI.

Generally, more studies among ethnic groups have to be done to establish the relation between anthropometric indices of body fat distribution and visceral fat. These studies should be complementary to epidemiological studies on the relationship between indices of body fat distribution and disease risks. Results of both laboratory studies and epidemiological studies will provide necessary information to accept existing universal WC and WHR cutoff points or to redefine ethnic-specific cutoff points. As in the case of the relation between BMI and BF%, the use of standardized methodology is of utmost importance to avoid biased outcomes of studies. This standardization would include landmarks for waist and hip circumference and measurements of CT/MRI.

VI SUMMARY

There is a need for multicenter multiethnic studies on body composition in which methodologies are highly standardized and in which reference methods like a chemically defined four-compartment model or (as a second choice) deuterium oxide dilution for total body fat and scanning techniques for body fat distribution are used. Ideally, those studies should also investigate the validity of predictive methods and search for possible explaining factors in order to possibly generalize prediction equations. Such studies could help in redefining BMI cutoff values for obesity and underweight when combined with data on risk factors such as cardiovascular disease. Similarly, cutoff points for body fat distribution (i.e. waist or waist-hip ratio, skinfold thickness ratios) should be validated and if needed redefined in different ethnic groups.

REFERENCES

1. Wang ZM, Pierson RN, Heymsfield SB. The five-level model: a new approach to organising body composition research. Am J Clin Nutr 1992;56:19–28.
2. Deurenberg P. The Assessment of Body Composition: Use and Misuse Annual Report. Lausanne; Nestlé Foundation, 1992: 35–72.
3. Pfeiffer L. Uber den Fettgehalt des Körpers und verschiedener Teile desselben bei mageren und fetten Tieren. Zeitschr Biol 1887;23:340–380.
4. Magnus-Levy A. Physiology des Stoffwechsels. In: Van Noorden C, ed. Handbuch der Pathologie des Stoffwechsels. Berlin; Hirschwald, 1906:446.
5. Siri WE. Body composition from fluid spaces and density: analysis of methods. In: Brozek J, Henschel A, eds. Techniques for Measuring Body Composition. Washington: National Academy of Sciences, 1961:223–244.
6. Heymsfield SB, Wang J, Kehayias J, Heshka S, Lichtman S, Pierson RN. Chemical determination of human body density in vivo: relevance to hydrodensitometry. Am J Clin Nutr 1989;50:1282–1289.
7. Baumgartner RN, Heymsfield SB, Lichtman S, Wang J, Pierson RN. Body composition in elderly people: effect of criterion estimates on predictive equations. Am J Clin Nutr 1990;53:1345–1353.
8. Visser M, Gallagher D, Deurenberg P, Wang J, Pierson RN, Heymsfield SB. Density of fat-free body mass: relationship with race, age and level of body fatness. Am J Physiol 1997;272:E781–E789.
9. Deurenberg-Yap M, Schmidt G, Van Staveren WA, Hautvast JGAJ, Deurenberg P. Body fat measurements among Singaporean Chinese, Malays and Indians: a comparative study using a four-compartment model and different two-compartment models. Br J Nutr 2001; 85:491–498.
10. Werkman A, Deurenberg-Yap M, Schmidt G, Deurenberg P. A comparison between the composition and density of the fat-free mass of young adult Singaporean Chinese and Dutch Caucasiains. Ann Nutr Metab 2000; 44:235–242.
11. Roche AF, Heymsfield SB, Lohman TG. Human Body Composition. Champaign, IL: Human Kinetics, 1996.
12. Dempster P, Aitkens S. A new air displacement method for the determination of human body composition. Med Sci Sports Exerc 1995;27:419–425.
13. Forbes GB. Human Body Composition. New York: Springer-Verlag, 1987.
14. Wang ZM, Deurenberg P, Wang W, Pietrobelli A, Baumgartner RM, Heymsfield SB. Hydration of fat-free body mass: review and critique of a classic body composition constant. Am J Clin Nutr 1999;69:833–841.
15. Jebb SA, Elia M. Multi-compartment models for the assessment of body composition in health and disease. In: Davies PSW, Cole TJ, eds. Body Composition Techniques in Health and Disease. Cambridge: Cambridge University Press, 1995: 240–254.
16. Wagner DR, Heyward VH. Measures of body composition in blacks and whites: a comparative review. Am J Clin Nutr 200;71:1392–1402.
17. Deck-Côté K, Adams WC. Effects of bone density on body composition estimates in young black and white women. Med Sci Sports Exerc 1993;25:290–296.
18. Ortiz O, Russell M, Daley TL, Baumgartner RN, Waki M, Lichtman S, Wang J, Pierson RN Jr, Heymsfield SB. Differences in skeletal muscle and bone mineral mass between black and white females and their relevance to estimate body composition. Am J Clin Nutr 1992;55: 8–13.
19. Deurenberg P, Weststrate JA, Seidell JC. Body mass index as a measure of body fatness: age and sex specific prediction formulas. Br J Nutr 1991;65:105–114.
20. Deurenberg P, Tagliabue A, Schouten FJM. Multi-frequency impedance for the prediction of extra-cellular water and total body water. Brit J Nutr 1995;73:349–358.
21. Durnin JVGA, Womersley J. Body fat assessed from total body density and its estimation from skinfold thickness: measurements on 481 men and women aged from 17 to 72 years. Br J Nutr 1974;32:77–97.
22. Guricci S, Hartriyanti Y, Hautvast JGAJ, Deurenberg P. Relationship between body fat and body mass index: differences between Indonesians and Dutch Caucasians. Eur J Clin Nutr 1998;52:779–783.
23. Deurenberg P, Deurenberg-Yap M, Wang JJ, Lin FP, Schmidt G. Prediction of body fat percent from anthropometry and impedance in Singapore and Beijing Chinese. Asia Pacific J Clin Nutr 2000;9:93–98.
24. Norgan NG. The assessment of the body composition of populations. In: Davies PSW, Cole TJ, eds. Body Composition Techniques in Health and Disease. Cambridge: Cambridge University Press, 1995:195–221.
25. Zillikens MC, Conway JM. Anthropometry in blacks: applicability of generalized skinfold equations and differences in fat patterning between blacks and whites. Am J Clin Nutr 1990;52:45–51.
26. Guricci S, Hartriyanti Y, Hautvast JGAJ, Deurenberg P. The prediction of extracellular water and total body water by multi-frequency bio-electrical impedance in a South East Asian population. Asia Pacific J Clin Nutr 1999;8:155–159.
27. Eveleth PB, Tanner JM. World-wide Variation in Human Growth. Cambridge: Cambridge University Press, 1976.
28. Bioelectrical impedance analysis in body composition measurement. NIH Technology Assessment Statement 1994, Dec 12–14, pp 1–35.
29. WHO. Physical Status: The Use and Interpretation of Anthropometry. Technical Report Series 854. Geneva: WHO, 1995.

30. WHO. Obesity: Preventing and Managing the Global Epidemic. Report on a WHO Consultation on Obesity, Geneva, 3–5 June 1997. Geneva: WHO, 1998.
31. Womersley J, Durnin JVGA. A comparison of the skinfold method with extent of overweight and various weight-height relationships in the assessment of obesity. Br J Nutr 1977;38:271–284.
32. Norgan NG, Ferro-Luzzi A. Weight-height indices as estimators of fatness in men. Hum Nutr Clin Nutr 1982;36c:363–372.
33. Gallagher D, Visser M, Sepulveda D, Pierson RN, Harris T, Heymsfield SB. How useful is BMI for comparison of body fatness across age, sex and ethnic groups. Am J Epidemiol 1996;143:228–239.
34. Norgan NG. Interpretation of low body mass indices: Australian Aborigines. Am J Phys Anthropol 1994;94: 229–237.
35. Fehily AM, Butland BK, Yarnell JWG. Body fatness and frame size: the Caerphilly study. Eur J Clin Nutr 1990;44:107–111.
36. Baecke JAH, Burema J, Deurenberg P. Body fatness, relative weight and frame size in young adults. Br J Nutr 1982;48:1–6.
37. Guricci S, Hartriyanti Y, Hautvast JGAJ, Deurenberg P. Differences in the relationship between body fat and body mass index between two different Indonesian ethnic groups: the effect of body build. Eur J Clin Nutr 1999:53:468–472.
38. Deurenberg P, Deurenberg-Yap M, Wang J, Lin Fu Po, Schmidt G. The impact of body build on the relationship between body mass index and body fat percent. Int J Obes 1999;23:537–542.
39. Deurenberg-Yap M, Schmidt G, Staveren WA, Deurenberg P. The paradox of low body mass index and high body fat percent among Chinese, Malays and Indians in Singapore. Int J Obes 2000;24:1011–1017.
40. Deurenberg P, Yap M, Van Staveren WA. Body mass index and percent body fat: a meta-analysis among different ethnic groups. Int J Obes 1998;22: 1164–1171.
41. Ko GTC, Tang J, Chan JCN, Sung R, Wu MMF, Wai HPS, Chen R. Lower BMI cut-off value to define obesity in Hong Kong Chinese: an analysis based on body fat assessment by bioelectrical impedance. Br J Nutr 2001;85:239–242.
42. Roubenoff R, Kehayia JJ, Dawson Hughes B, Heysmfield SB. Use of dual energy X-ray absorptiometry in body composition studies: not yet a golden standard. Am J Clin Nutr 1993;58:589–591.
43. Clarck RR, Kuta JM, Sullivan JC. Prediction of percent body fat in adult males using dual energy x-ray absorptiometry, skinfolds and hydrostatic weighing. Med Sci Sports Exerc 1993;25:528–535.
44. Wang K, Russel M, Mazariegos M, Burastero S, Thornton J, Lichtman S. Heymsfield SB, Pierson RN. Body fat by dual photon absorptiometry: comparison with traditional methods in Asians, blacks and whites. Am J Hum Biol 1992;4:501–510.
45. Swinburn BA, Craig PL, Daniel R, Dent DPD, Strauss BJG. Body composition differences between Polynesians and Caucasians assessed by bioelectrical impedance. Int J Obes 1996;20:889–894.
46. Luke A, Durazo-Arvizzu R, Rotimi C, Prewitt E, Forrester T, Wilks R, Ogunbiyi OL, Schoeller DA, McGee D, Cooper RS. Relation between BMI and body fat in black population samples from Nigeria, Jamaica and the United States. Am J Epidemiol 1997; 145:620–628.
47. Heitmann BL, Swinburn BA, Carmichael H, Rowley K, Plank L, McDermont R, Leonard D, O'Dea K. Are there ethnic differences in the association between body weight and resistance, measured by bioelectrical impedance? Int J Obes 197;21:1085–1092.
48. Ko GTC, Chan JCN, Cockram CS, Woo J. Prediction of hypertension, diabetes, dyslipidemia or albuninuria using simply anthropometric indexes in Hong Kong Chinese. Int J Obes 1999;23:1136–1142.
49. Deurenberg-Yap M, Tan BY, Chew SK, Deurenberg P, Van Staveren W. Manifestation of cardiovascular risk factors at low levels of body mass index and waist-hip-ratio in Singaporean Chinese. Asia Pacific J Clin Nutr 1999;8:177–183.
50. Deurenberg-Yap M, Chew SK, Lin FP, Van Staveren WA, Deurenberg P. Relationships between indices of obesity and its co-morbidities among Chinese, Malays and Indians in Singapore. Int J Obes 2001;25:1554–1562.
51. Steering Committee. The Asia Perspective: Redefining Obesity and Its Treatment. Melbourne: International Diabetes Institute, 2000.
52. Long AE, Prewitt TE, Kaufman JS, Rotimi CN, Cooper RS, McGee DL. Weight-height relationships among eight populations of West African Origin: the case against constant BMI standards. Int J Obes 1998;22:842–846.
53. Henry CJK, Rees DG. New prediction equations for the estimation of basal metabolic rate in tropical people. Eur J Clin Nutr 1991;45:177–185.
54. Vague J. The degree of masculine differentiation of obesities: a factor determining predisposition to diabetes, atherosclerosis, gout and uric calculous disease. Am J Clin Nutr 1956;4:20–34.
55. Larsson B, Svardsudd K, Welin L, Wilhelmsen L, Bjorntorp P, Tibblin G. Abdominal adipose tissue distribution, obesity and risk of cardiovascular disease and death: a 13 year follow up of participants in the study of men born in 1913. Br Med J 1984;288: 1401–1404.
56. Van der Kooy K, Seidell JC. Techniques for the measurement of visceral fat: a practical guide. In J Obes 1883;17:187–196.

57. Molarius A, Seidell JC, Sans S, Tuomilehto J, Kuulasma K. Varying sensitivity of waist action levels to identify subjects with overweight of obesity in 19 populations of the WHO MONICA project. J Clin Epidemiol 1999;52:1213–1224.
58. Lovejoy JC, De la Bretonne JA, Klemperer M, Tulley R. Abdominal fat distribution and metabolic risk factors: effect of race. Metabolism 1996;45:1119–1124.
59. Albu JB, Murphy L, Frager DH, Johnson JA, Pi-Sunyer FX. Visceral fat and race dependent risks in obese nondiabetic premenopausal women. Diabetes 1997;46:456–462.
60. Conway JM, Yanovski Sz, Avila NA, Hubbard VS. Visceral adipiose tissue differences in black and white women. Am J Clin Nutr 1995;61:765–771.
61. Dowling HJ, Pi-Sunyer FX. Race dependent health risk of upper body obesity. Diabetes 1993;42:537–543.
62. Yanovski JA, Yanosvki SZ, Filmer KM, Hubbard VS, Avila N, Lewis B, Reynolds JC, Flood M. Differences in body composition of black and white girls. Am J Clin Nutr 1996;64:833–839.
63. Goran MI, Nagy TR, Treuth MS, Trowbridge C, Dezdenberg C, McGloin A, Gower BA. Visceral fat in white and African American prepubertal children. Am J Clin Nutr 1997;65:1703–1708.
64. Gautier JF, Milner MR, Elam E, Chen K, Ravussin E, Pratley RE. Visceral adipose tissue is not increased in Pima Indians compared with equally obese Caucasians and is not related to insulin action or secretion. Diabetologica 1999;42:28–34.
65. Okusun IS, Tedders SH, Choi S, Dever GEA. Abdominal adiposity associated with established body mass indexes in white, black and Hispanic Americans. A study from the third National Health and Nutrition Examination Survey. Int J Obes 2000;24: 1279–1285.
66. Harris NM, Stevens J, Thomas N, Schreiner P, Folsom AR. Associations of fat distribution and obesity with hypertension in a bi-ethnic population, Atherosclerosis Risk in Communities Study. Obes Res 2000;8: 516–524.
67. Berman DM, Rodrigues LM, Nicklas BJ, Ryan AS, Dennis KE, Goldberg AP. Racial disparities in metabolism, central obesity, and sex hormone-binding globulin in postmenopausal women. J Clin Endocrinol Metab 2001;86:97–103.
68. Despres JP, Couillard C, Cagnon J, Bergeron J, Leon AS, Rao DC, Skinner JS, Wilmore JH, Bouchard C. Race, visceral adipose tissue, plasma lipids, and lipoprotein lipase activity in men and women: the Health, Risk Factors, Exercise Training and Genetics Family Study. Arterioscler Thromb Vasc Biol 2000;20:1932–1938.

4

Prevalence of Obesity in Adults: The Global Epidemic

Jacob C. Seidell

Free University of Amsterdam and Free University Medical Center, Amsterdam, The Netherlands

Aila M. Rissanen

Helsinki University Hospital, Helsinki, Finland

I CLASSIFICATION OF OBESITY AND FAT DISTRIBUTION

The epidemiology of obesity has for many years been difficult to study because many countries had their own specific criteria for the classification of different degrees overweight. Gradually during the 1990s, however, the body mass index (BMI) (weight/height^2) became a universally accepted measure of the degree of overweight and now identical cutoff points are recommended. This most recent classification of overweight in adults by the World Health Organization is the following (1):

Classification	*BMI (kg/m^2)*	*Associated health risks*
Underweight	< 18.5	Low (but risk of other clinical problems increased)
Normal range	18.5–24.9	Average
Overweight	25.0 or higher	
Preobese	25.0–29.9	Increased
Obese class I	30.0–34.9	Moderately increased
Obese class II	35.0–39.9	Severely increased
Obese class III	40 or higher	Very severely increased

In many community studies in affluent societies, this scheme has been simplified and cutoff points of 25 and 30 kg/m^2 are used for descriptive purposes. Both the prevalence of very low BMI (< 18.5 kg/m^2) and very high BMI (40 kg/m^2 or higher) are usually low, in the order of 1–2% or less. Already researchers in Asian countries have criticized these cut points. The absolute health risk (particularly of type 2 diabetes mellitus) seems to be higher at any level of the body mass index in Chinese and South Asian people, which is probably also true for Asians living elsewhere. There are some suggestions to lower the cut points to designate obesity or overweight by several units of body mass index (e.g., 23 kg/m^2 for overweight and 25 kg/m^2 for obesity) in Asian populations. In countries such as China and India, each with over a billion inhabitants, small changes in the criteria for overweight or obesity potentially increase the world estimate of the number of obese people by several hundred million (current estimates are ~ 250 million worldwide).

Much research over the last decade has suggested that, for an accurate classification of overweight and obesity with respect to the health risks, one needs to factor in abdominal fat distribution. Traditionally this has been indicated by a relatively high waist-to-hip circumference ratio. Recently it has been proposed that the waist circumference alone may be a better and simpler measure of the health risks associated with abdominal fatness (2). In 1998 the National Institutes of Health (National Heart, Lung, and Blood Institute) adopted the BMI classification and combined this with waist cutoff points (3). In this classification the combination of overweight (BMI between 25 and 30 kg/m^2) and moderate obesity (BMI between 30 and 35 kg/m^2) with a large waist circumference ($\geq$102 cm in men or $\geq$88 cm in women) is proposed to carry additional risk (3).

In this chapter, we focus on the prevalence of overweight and obesity as indicated by the body mass index. The emphasis is on recent surveys and time-trends, and data have been selected that are based on representative population surveys with measured weight and height.

II PREVALENCE OF OBESITY BY WHO REGION

A Africa

Table 1 shows the levels of overweight and obesity in women living in Sub-Saharan African countries (4). Obesity is relatively uncommon in all countries. This region is increasingly devastated by the AIDS epidemic and by chronic malnutrition due to wars and natural disasters. A closer inspection of the data revealed that obesity is relatively more common in urban than in rural areas and more prevalent in women with high socio-economic status. Data on men are very scarce from this region. There are fragmented data from South Africa which suggest that obesity is relatively common there in both rural and urban areas (5). Table 2 shows the prevalence of obesity in various regions and ethnic groups in South Africa. Mauritius is one of the best-studied parts of Africa with respect to cardiovascular risk factors, but it is also one of the least representative. Over 5000 people were studied in 1987 and 1992. The prevalence of obesity increased from 3.4% to 5.3% in men and from 10.4% to 15.1% in women (6).

B The Americas

Figure 1 shows the time trends of the prevalence of obesity in men and women throughout the 1990s. The prevalence increased by about 1 percent point per year (7). These data are based on self-reported weight and height, and this probably leads to a considerable underestimation of the prevalence of obesity. The most recent (1988–1994) estimates of obesity in adults in the United States, based on measured weight and height, are ~20% in men and ~25% in women (8).

Table 1 Overweight (BMI 25–29.9 kg/m^2) and Obesity (BMI $\geq$ 30 kg/m^2) Levels in Women Aged 15–49 Years in Sub-Saharan Africa

Country	Year of survey	Sample size	% Overweight	% Obese
Benin	1996	2266	6.9	2.1
Burkina Faso	1992/1993	3161	5.9	1.0
Central African Republic	1994/1995	2025	5.5	1.1
Comoros	1996	773	15.9	4.4
Cote d'Ivoire	1994	3108	11.0	3.0
Ghana	1993	1773	9.3	3.4
Kenya	1993	3294	11.4	2.4
Malawi	1992	2323	8.1	1.1
Mali	1996	4327	7.2	1.2
Namibia	1992	2205	13.8	7.1
Niger	1992	3292	6.2	1.2
Senegal	1992/1993	2895	12.0	3.7
Tanzania	1991/1992	4597	9.3	1.9
Tanzania	1996	3721	10.8	2.6
Uganda	1995	3199	7.3	1.2
Zambia	1992	3239	11.8	2.4
Zambia	1996/1997	3838	10.5	2.3
Zimbabwe	1994	1968	17.4	5.7

Source: Ref. 4.

Table 2 Prevalence of Obesity (BMI $\geq$ 30 kg/m^2) in South Africa

Year	Area	Ethnic group	Men %	Women %
1982	Urban Cape Town	"Coloured"	7.2	31.4
1990	Urban Cape Town	African	13.9	48.6
1990	Rural Western Cape	White	17.6	20.4
1990	Rural QwaQwa	African	12.7	40.2
1990	Urban Mangaung	African	12.9	43.9
1990	Urban Durban	Indian	3.5	17.6

Source: Ref. 5.

There are important ethnic differences in the prevalence of obesity, particularly in women (Table 3). The women/men prevalence ratio is highest among non-Hispanic blacks (ratio ~1.8), lower in Mexican-Americans (ratio ~1.5) and lowest in non-Hispanic whites (ratios ~1.1).

The prevalence of obesity in Canada is less than in the United States although the most recent estimates are already a decade old. Canada has experienced also an increase in the prevalence of overweight and obesity, particularly in men (Fig. 2, top). The most recent estimates of the prevalence of obesity are 13.4 percent in men and 15.4 in women (9).

Table 4 summarizes some of the prevalence data found in Latin American countries (10–12). Surveys show that obesity is quite common throughout South America and Mexico, particularly among women. Table 5 shows lower estimates of obesity among young adult women, but with the exception of Haiti, all prevalences are of the order of 10% (4). It is likely that these lower estimates are due to the fact that the studies by Filozof et al. (10) also covered middle-aged men and women among whom obesity is much more common than at younger ages.

Socioeconomic conditions in many developing countries are very different from those in countries

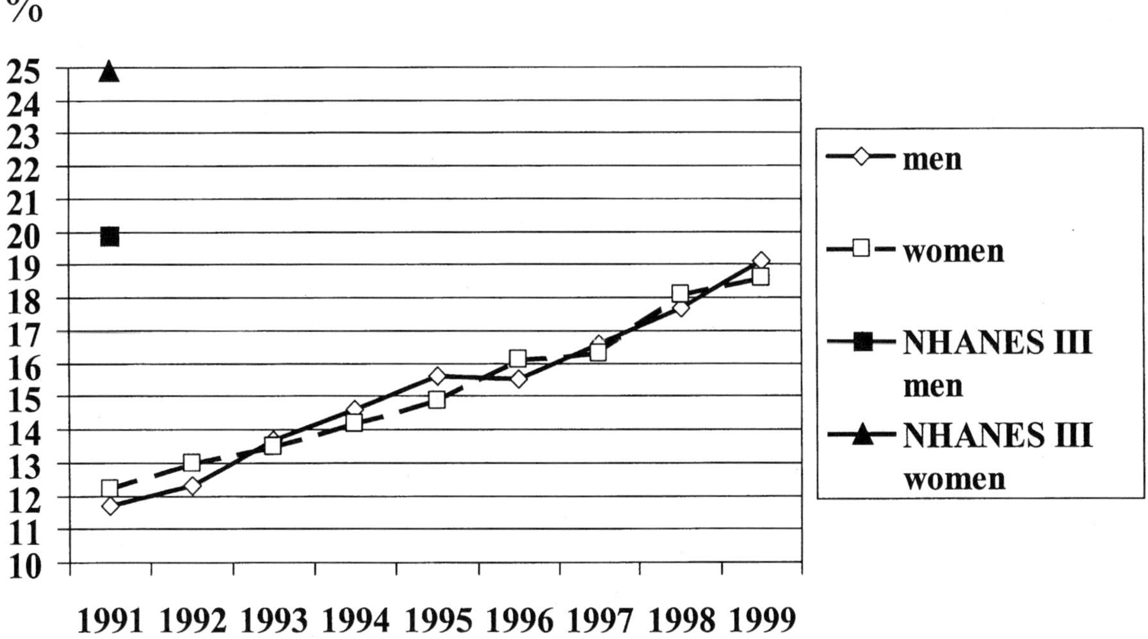

Figure 1 Time trends of the prevalence of obesity (BMI $\geq$ 30 kg/m^2) in the United States based on the behavioral risk factor surveillance system (self-reported height and weight). The NHANES III (National Health and Nutrition Examination Survey III) was conducted between 1998 and 1994 (depicted here as the midpoint of the survey in 1991) in a nationally representative sample based on measured weight and height. (From Refs. 7 and 8.)

Table 3 Sex-Specific Prevalence Data of Obesity (BMI ≥ 30 kg/m^2) and Sex Ratio by Ethnicity in Men and Women Aged 20–74 in the United States, 1988–1994

Race/ethnic group	Men	Women	Sex ratio
Non-Hispanic white	20.0	22.4	1.12
Non-Hispanic black	21.3	37.4	1.76
Mexican-American	23.1	34.2	1.48

Source: Ref. 8.

with established market economies. In such affluent countries, obesity is increasingly limited to those with low socioeconomic status whereas in developing countries obesity is more common in those with relatively high socioeconomic status. In countries undergoing economic transition these socioeconomic relations to obesity may change over time. Opposing trends may be seen within a single country. One interesting illustration of the changing socioeco-

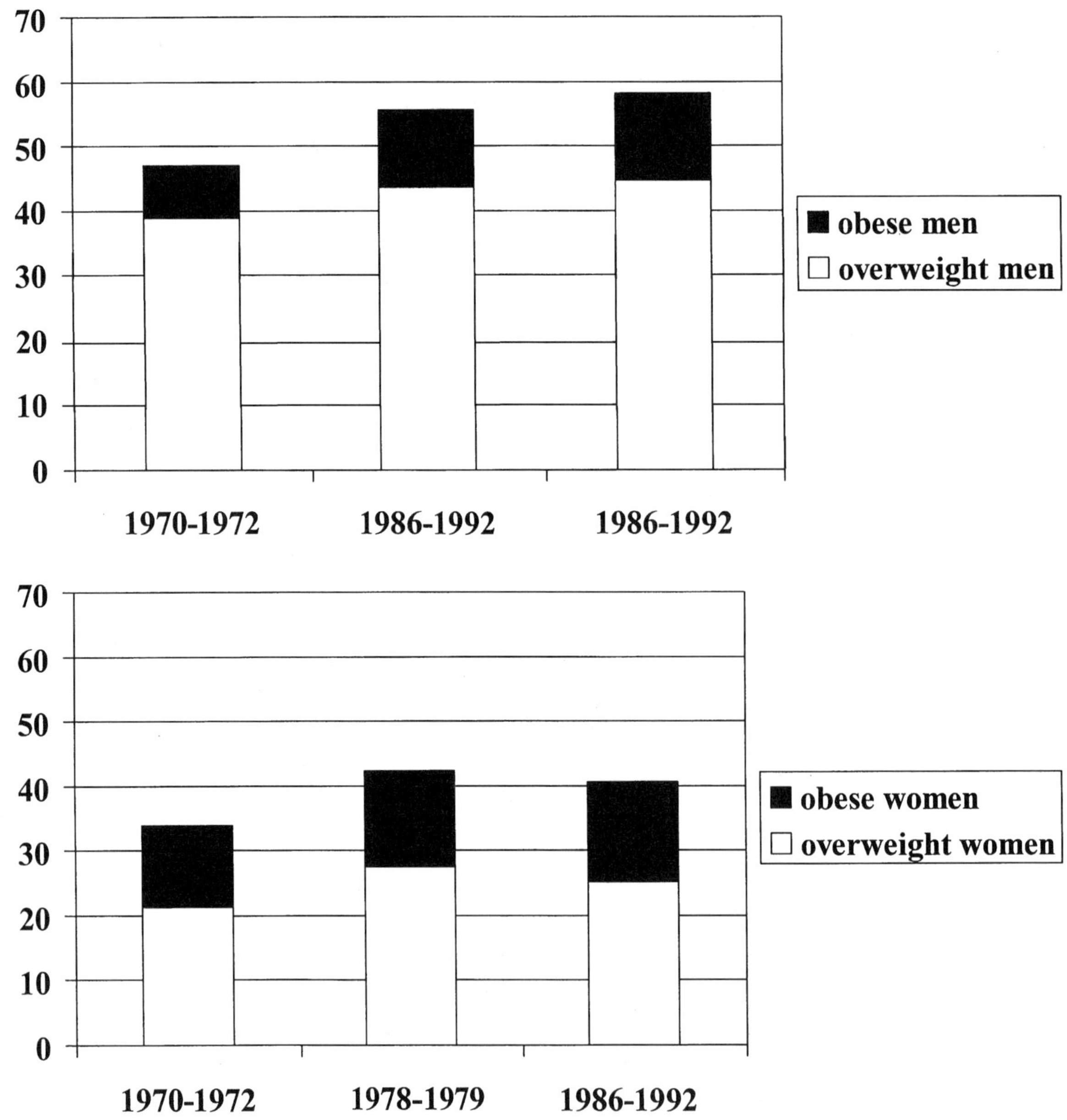

Figure 2 Time trends in the prevalence of overweight (BMI 25–29.9 kg/m^2) and obesity (BMI ≥ 30 kg/m^2) in Canadian men (top) and women (bottom). (From Ref. 9.)

Table 4 Overweight (BMI 25–29.9 kg/m^2 and Obesity (BMI ≥ 30 kg/m^2) in Adults in Latin American Countries

		% Overweight		% Obese	
Country	Year of survey	Men	Women	Men	Women
Argentina	1997	—	—	28.4	25.4
Brazil	1997	—	—	6.9	12.5
Chile	1992	—	—	15.7	23.0
Mexico[a]	1992/1993	41	36	14.9	25.1
Mexico[b]	1995	39	35	11	23
Paraguay	1991/1992	—	—	22.9	35.7
Peru	1996	—	—	7.2	16.4

[a] Arroyo et al. (11).
[b] Sanchez-Castillo et al. (12).
Source: Ref. 10 except where noted.

nomic dimensions can be found in a paper by Monteiro et al. (13), who have looked at time trends in Brazil by income and degree of urbanization (11). Their results show rapid increases in obesity in Brazilian men in all groups (Fig. 3, top), although the levels of obesity in those with low income from rural areas are still only slightly above 1%. This is low compared to the prevalence of ~10% in urban men with high incomes.

In women, the situation is quite different. Obesity rates are generally higher compared to men in all groups. There were rapid continuing increases in women with low income but in those with high income there seems to be a stabilization or even a decline (Fig. 3, bottom). Such data highlight the profound effect of socioeconomic conditions on the prevalence of obesity.

Cuba is one of the few examples of Latin American countries where the prevalence of obesity has decreased (14). The collapse of the Soviet Union in 1990 had dramatic effects on the food supply and transportation, leading to decreased energy intake and increased energy expenditure. The resulting drop in the prevalence of obesity is unique in the world (see Fig. 4).

C Southeast Asia

Overweight and obesity are still relatively uncommon in Asia, but this is rapidly changing (15). Table 6 shows that the prevalence of obesity in most large countries is still in the order of 1–5%.

Despite the relatively low prevalence of obesity in Asian populations, the situation there is of particular concern for two reasons. The first is that the prevalence seems to be increasing rapidly, particularly in urban areas (16). Secondly, Asian populations already seem to be particularly prone to develop type 2

Table 5 Overweight (BMI 25–29.9 kg/m^2) and Obesity (BMI ≥ 30 kg/m^2) Levels in Women Aged 15–49 Years in Latin America

Country	Year of survey	Sample size	% Overweight	% Obese
Bolivia	1994	2347	26.2	7.6
Brazil	1989	10189	25.0	9.2
Brazil	1996	3158	25.0	9.7
Colombia	1995	3319	31.4	9.2
Dominican Republic	1991	2163	18.6	7.3
Dominican Republic	1996	7356	26.0	12.1
Guatamela	1995	4978	26.2	8.0
Haiti	1994/1995	1896	8.9	2.6
Honduras	1996	885	23.8	7.8
Mexico	1987	3681	23.1	10.4
Peru	1992	5200	31.1	8.8
Peru	1996	10747	35.5	9.4

Source: Ref. 4.

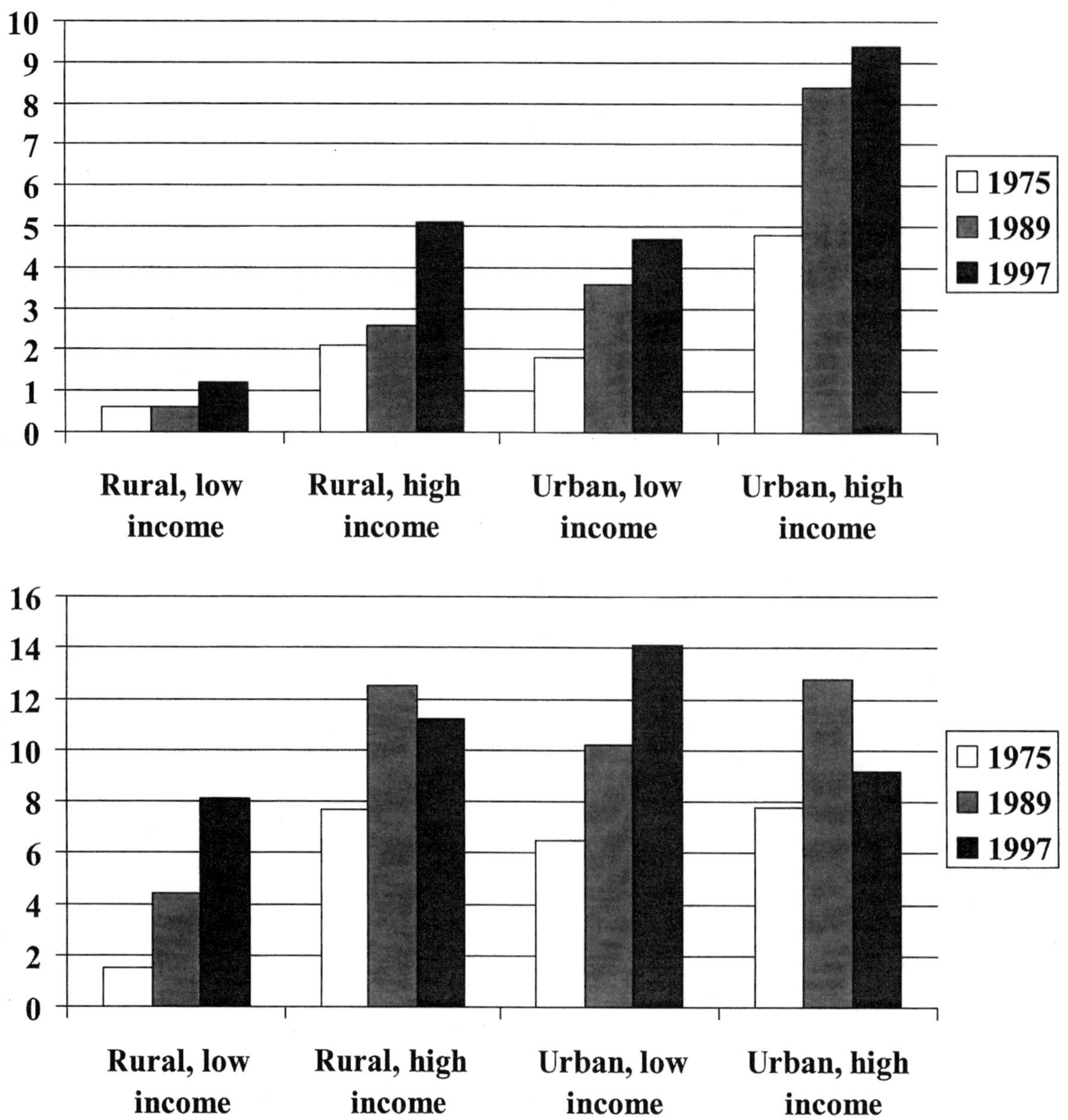

Figure 3 Time trends in the prevalence of obesity (BMI $\geq$ 30 kg/m^2) in Brazil by income (highest and lowest quartile of income) and degree of urbanization, in (top) men and (bottom) women. (From Ref. 11.)

diabetes mellitus at low levels of fatness. Uncontrolled diabetes mellitus is a major cause for nephropathy, neuropathy, retinopathy, and arteriosclerosis. The WHO has projected that the number of diabetics worldwide will increase from ~130 million patients today to ~300 million in 25 years (see Fig. 5). The largest contribution to this increase is expected to come from Asian populations, particularly China and India (17).

D Europe

In many reviews it has been shown that obesity (defined as a body mass index of 30 kg/m^2 or higher) is a prevalent condition in most countries with established market economies (8,16). There is a wide variation in the prevalence of obesity between and within these countries. It is quite easy to find places with at least a twofold difference in the prevalence of obesity within one single

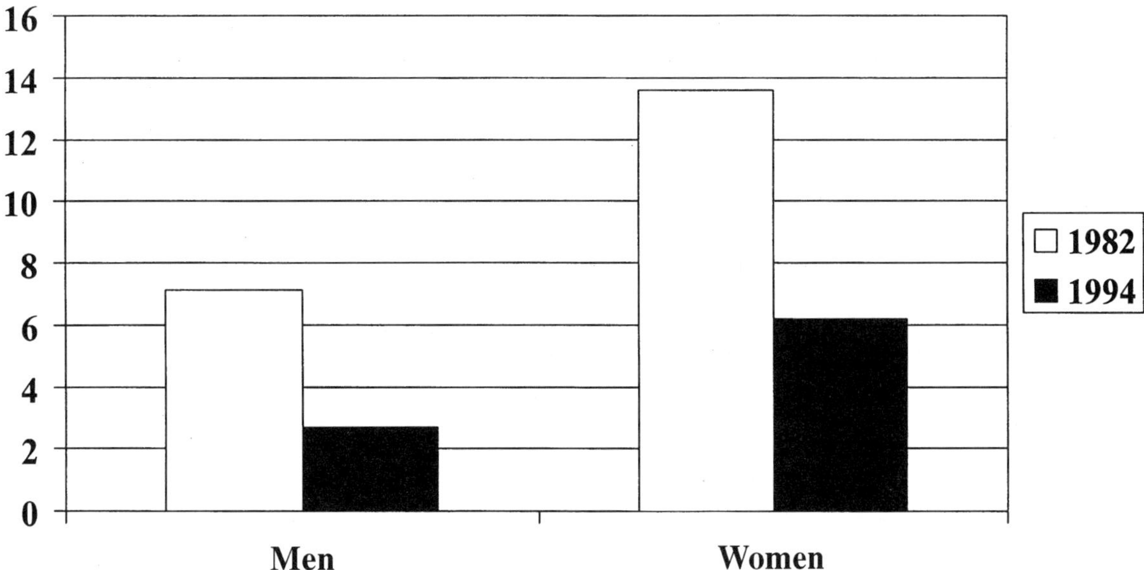

Figure 4 Time trends in the prevalence of obesity (BMI $\geq$ 30 kg/m^2) in Havana, Cuba (before and after the collapse of the Soviet Union). (From Ref. 14.)

country. In countries with established market economies, obesity is usually more frequent among those with relative low socioeconomic status, and the prevalence increases with age until ~60–70 years of age after which the prevalence declines (18). In most of these established market economies it has been shown that the prevalence is increasing over time (8,16). Tables 7 and 8 show the increases in the prevalence of obesity in men and women aged 35–64 years in several centers participating in the WHO MONICA project (19). It is clear that there is a rapid increase in the prevalence of obesity in most centers from countries in the European Union, particularly in men. The prevalence of obesity in men and women in European countries in the EU region (Table 7) is similar with a women/men prevalence ratio of 1.07 (range 0.56–1.29). In central and eastern European countries (Table 8), the prevalence is generally much higher in women than in men (average women/men prevalence ratio 2.03; range: 1.27–2.87).

In central and eastern Europe countries, the prevalence of obesity in women may have stabilized or even slightly decreased but still it still remains among the highest in Europe. A study by Molarius et al. (19) showed that the social class differences in the prevalence of obesity are increasing with time. Obesity is fast becoming a lower-class problem in Europe.

Figure 6 shows the secular time trends of the prevalence of obesity in the United Kingdom and the Netherlands. In the mid-1980s the prevalence of obesity in men was similar in these two countries but in the United Kingdom the increase in the prevalence has been much more dramatic than in the Netherlands.

Figure 7 shows the women/men prevalence ratio in 1997 in the United Kingdom. The prevalence is similar in 25 to 65-year-old men and women but is progressively higher in women aged > 65 years. It is also higher in women than men in the youngest age group (16–24 years). There are several possible explanations for the higher prevalence in women at older ages. It may be the result of a secular trend in which the prevalence of obesity has increased more in men from more recent birth cohorts than in women of the same age. An

Table 6 Sex-Specific Prevalence Data of Obesity (BMI $\geq$ 30 kg/m^2) and Sex Ratio in Selected Studies in Southeast Asia

Country	Study	Age	Men	Women
India	1988–1990	Adults	0.5[a]	
Malaysia	1990	18–64	7.9	6.1
Thailand	National Health Examination Survey 1991, n = 13,300	20+	4.0	5.6

[a] Men and women combined.
Source: Ref. 1.

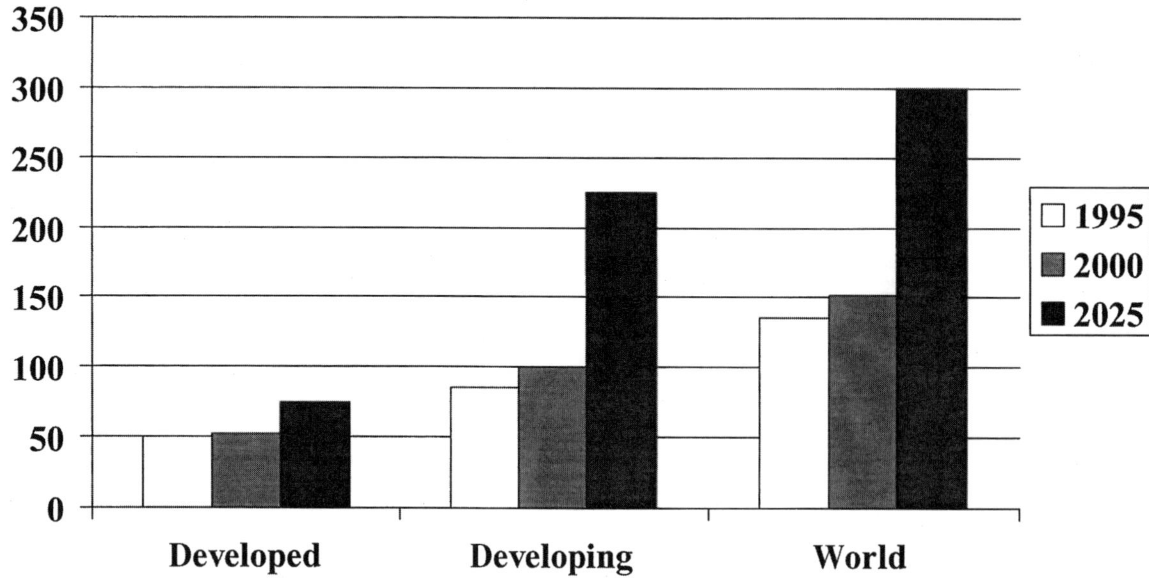

Figure 5 Current and predicted worldwide prevalence of type 2 diabetes mellitus. (From Ref. 17.)

Table 7 Prevalence of Obesity (age-standardized % with BMI $\geq$ 30) of Centers in EU Countries Participating in the First Round of the MONICA Study (May 1979 to February 1989) and the Third Round (June 1989 to November 1996)

	Men		Women		
Country (center)	1st	3rd	1st	3rd	Women/men (sex ratio) 3rd
Belgium (Ghent)	9	10	11	11	1.10
Denmark (Glostrup)	11	13	10	12	0.92
Finland (north Karelia)	17	22	23	24	1.09
Finland (Kuopio)	18	24	20	25	1.04
Finland (Turku/Loimaa)	19	22	17	19	0.86
France (Toulouse)	9	13	11	10	0.77
France (Lille)	13	17	17	22	1.29
Germany (Augsburg, urban)	18	18	15	21	1.17
Germany (Augsburg, rural)	20	24	22	23	0.96
Iceland (Iceland)	12	17	14	18	1.06
Italy (area Brianza)	11	14	15	18	1.29
Italy (Friuli)	15	17	18	19	1.12
Spain (Catalonia)	10	16	23	25	1.56
Sweden (North)	11	14	14	14	1.00
Switzerland (Vaud/Fribourg)	12	16	12	9	0.56
Switzerland (Ticino)	19	13	14	16	1.23
United Kingdom (Belfast)	11	13	14	16	1.23
United Kingdom (Glasgow)	11	23	16	23	1.00
Mean	*13.7*	*17.0*	*16.4*	*18.8*	*1.07*

Source: Ref. 19.

Table 8 Prevalence of Obesity (age-standardized % with BMI $\geq$ 30 kg/m^2) in Centers of Countries in Central and Eastern Europe Participating in the First Round of the MONICA Study (May 1979 to February 1989) and the Third Round (June 1989 to November 1996)

	Men		Women		
Country (center)	1st	3rd	1st	3rd	Women/men (sex ratio) 3rd
Poland (Warsaw	18	22	26	28	1.27
Poland (Tarnobrzeg)	13	15	32	37	2.47
Russia (Moscow)	14	8	33	21	2.63
Russia (Novosibirsk)	13	15	43	43	2.87
Czech Republic (rural CZE)	22	22	32	29	1.32
Yugoslavia (Novi Sad)	18	17	30	27	1.59
Mean	*16.3*	*16.5*	*32.7*	*30.8*	*2.03*

Source: Ref. 19.

alternative plausible explanation is a biological one. After menopause women may experience a greater increase in body fat mass compared to men as a result of the drop in estrogen levels. A third explanation may be that obese men die more often prematurely than obese women do. The age-standardized absolute risk of some obesity-related diseases such as coronary heart disease is higher among men than among women.

Table 9 shows the prevalence of obesity in some less-studied countries including some countries that were previously part of the former Soviet Union. In most of these surveys, the prevalence in women was in the order 15–20%, considerably higher than the prevalences observed in men.

E Eastern Mediterranean

Generally, there is a lack of good representative data (e.g., national surveys) from this region. Table 10 shows the prevalence of overweight and obesity in Northern

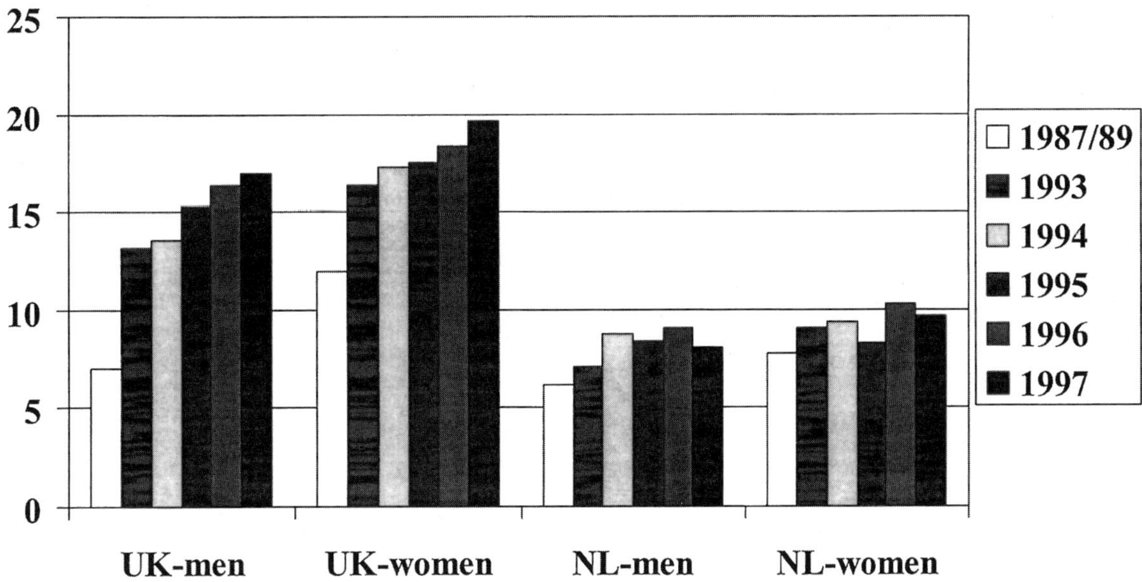

Figure 6 Time trends in the prevalence of obesity (BMI $\geq$ 30 kg/m^2) in the United Kingdom (Health Survey for England) and the Netherlands (data from the National Institute of Public Health in Bilthoven). (From Ref. 17.)

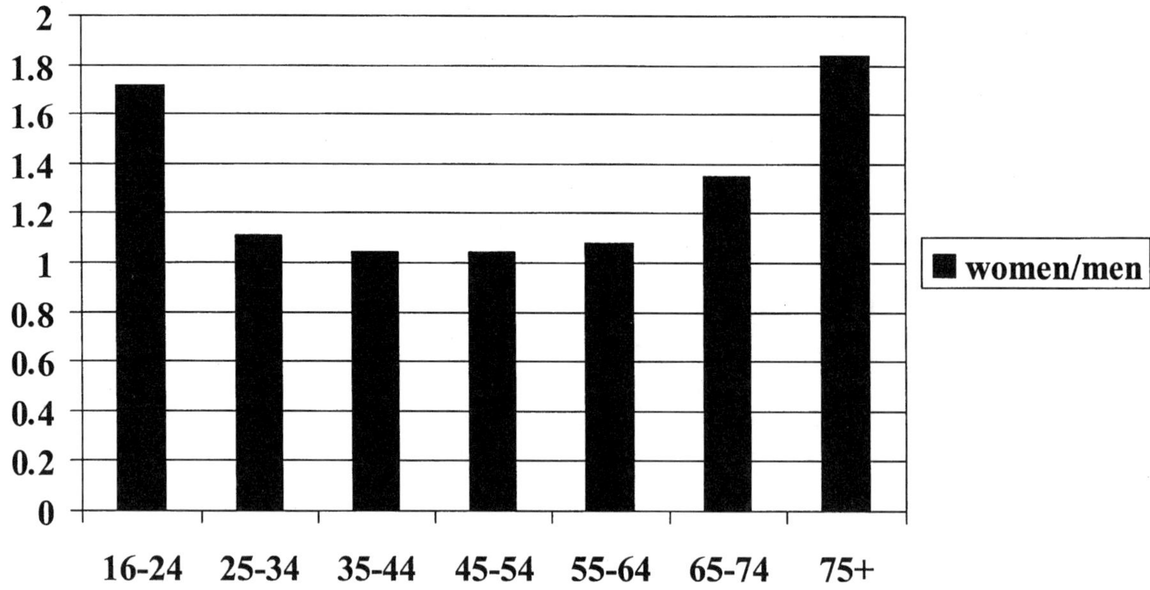

Figure 7 The gender ratio (women/men) of the prevalence of obesity (BMI $\geq$ 30 kg/m^2) by age in the Health Survey for England (ages 16+), 1997. (From Refs. 17 and 18.)

Africa and the Middle East. The results show that the prevalence of obesity is higher in women than in men (particularly in the Middle East and the Gulf states).

F Western Pacific Region

Table 11 shows the prevalence of obesity in selected countries from the western Pacific region (15). Trend data on the prevalence of overweight and obesity are available for Australia, China, Japan, and Samoa. The prevalence of obesity in Australia and New Zealand appears to be in the order of 10–15%, but recent data from the 1990s are not available (1). Aboriginals have, depending on their degree of "Westernization," a much higher or lower prevalence of obesity compared to the general Australian population. In Japan, the prevalence of obesity is of the order of 2–3%. In the 1992 Nationwide Nutritional Survey, the prevalence of obesity in China was ~1.2% in men and ~1.6% in women. Some of the Pacific Island populations have extremely high rates of obesity. The prevalence of obesity in Nauru, for example, was reported in 1987 to be ~65% in men and ~70% in women (1). Similar high rates have been observed in urban areas of Papua

Table 9 Overweight (BMI 25–29.9 kg/m^2) and Obesity (BMI $\geq$ 30 kg/m^2) Levels in the Baltic States

			% Overweight		% Obese	
Country	Year of survey	Sample size	Men	Women	Men	Women
Estonia	1997	1154	32.0	23.9	9.9	6.0
Latvia	1997	2292	41.0	33.0	9.5	17.4
Lithuania	1997	2096	41.9	32.7	11.4	18.3
Lithuania[a]	2000	2195	45.6	31.6	16.9	23.4
Kazakstan[b]	1995	3538	—	21.8	—	16.7
Uzbekistan[b]	1996	4077	—	16.3	—	5.4

[a] Finbalt study based on self-reported height and weight (Janina Petkeviciene, personal communication).
[b] Adapted from Martorell et al. (4).
Source: Ref. 20 except where noted.

Table 10 Overweight (BMI 25–29.9 kg/m^2) and Obesity (BMI ≥ 30 kg/m^2) Levels in Women Aged 15–49 Years in North Africa and the Middle East

			% Overweight		% Obese	
Country	Year of survey	Sample size	Men	Women	Men	Women
Bahrain	1991/1992	290	16.0	31.3	26.3	29.4
Kuwait	1993/1994	3435	35.2	32.3	32.3	40.6
Saudi Arabia	1996	13177	29.0	27.0	16.0	24.0
Jordan	1994/1996	2836	—	—	32.7	59.8
Morocco	1984/1985	41921	18.7[a]		5.2[a]	
Morocco[b]	1992	2850	—	22.3	—	10.5
Morocco[c]	1998/1999	17320	28.0	33.0	5.7	18.3
Tunisia[c]	1997	2760	23.3	28.2	6.7	22.7
Egypt[b]	1995/1996	6769	—	31.7	—	20.1
Turkey[b]	1993	2401	—	31.7	—	18.6

[a] Men and women combined.
[b] Adapted from Martorell et al. (4).
[c] Adapted from Mokhtar et al. (22).
Source: Ref. 21 except where noted.

New Guinea (36% in men and 54% in women), whereas the prevalence in the highlands was not higher than ~5% in men and women. Urban Samoans in 1991 had a prevalence of 58% in men and 77% in women, and the figures were high in rural areas as well (42% in men and 59% in women).

The International Diabetes Institute has proposed that the international classification of obesity should be modified for Asian countries (15). It recommended that overweight be classified as a BMI >23 and obesity as a BMI of 25 or higher. If such a classification is adapted, then the prevalence of obesity in large countries such as China will be high and rapidly increasing (Fig. 8) (21). There is, however, as of yet, no consensus on this issue, and a large and coherent body of data would be needed before such a proposal could be implemented.

III EXPLANATIONS FOR THE GROWING EPIDEMIC OF OBESITY

A Life-Style Changes

On an ecological or population level these time trends are not too difficult to explain, although the exact quantification of the various factors involved is almost impossible. On the one hand there is an increase in the average energy supply per capita. The World Health Report (23) has estimated that the average energy supply per capita in the world was 2300 kcal in 1963, 2440 kcal in 1971, 2720 kcal in 1992, and will be 2900 kcal by 2010. These increases are obviously not evenly distributed across the world's population and, sadly, many remain undernourished although in Asia (particularly China and India) and most of Latin

Table 11 Sex-Specific Prevalence Data of Obesity (BMI ≥ 30 kg/m^2) and Sex Ratio in Selected Studies in the Western Pacific Region

Country	Study	Age (years)	Men	Women	Ratio women/men
China	Chinese National Nutrition Survey, 1992	20–45	1.0 (urban) 0.5 (rural)	1.7 (urban) 0.7 (rural)	1.70 1.40
Japan	National Nutrition Survey, 1990–1994 n = 12,926	35–64	1.9	2.9	1.53
Philippines	Food and Nutrition Research Institute, 1993 n = 9585	20+	1.7	3.4	2.00

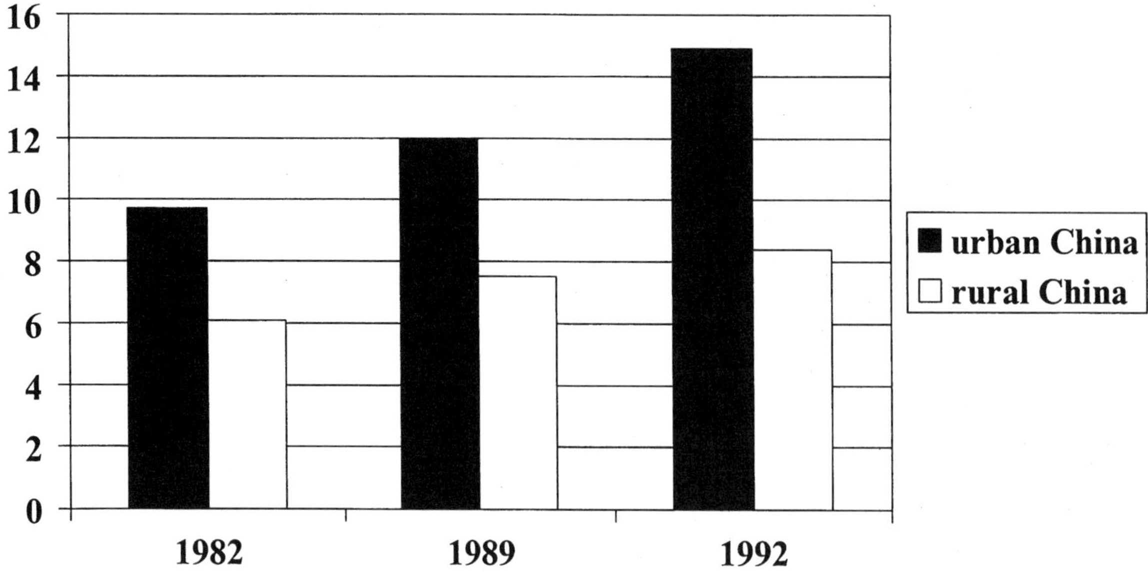

Figure 8 Time trends in the prevalence of overweight (BMI $\geq$ 25 kg/m^2) in China. (From Ref. 21.)

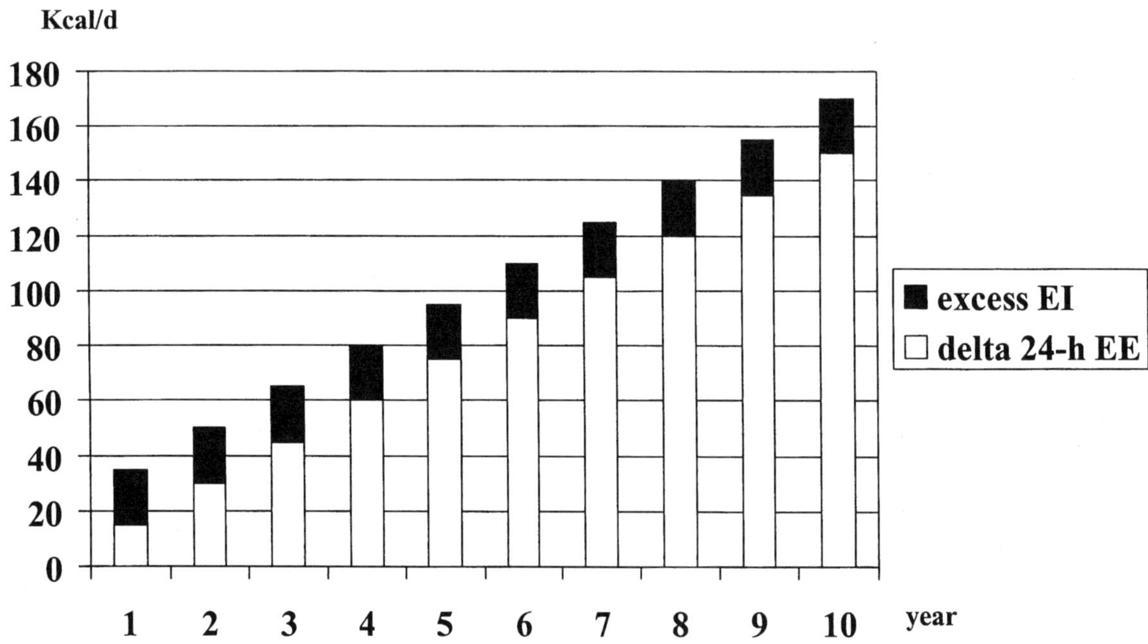

Figure 9 Hypothetical calculations of the magnitude of a positive energy balance to gain 10 kg over 10 years. It is estimated that an excess of 20 kcal/day over a 1-year period leads to a weight gain of about one 1 kg. One kilogram of weight gain is estimated to lead to about a 15 kcal/day increase in 24-hr energy expenditure. (From Ref. 24.)

America, these numbers are declining. The number of people with access to at least 2700 kcal has increased from 0.145 billion in 1969–1971 to 1.8 billion in 1990–1992 and is estimated to grow to 2.7 billion in 2010. Even when corrected for the increase in the world's population, this implies a more than 10-fold increase in the number of people having access to high-calorie diets. The globalization of agricultural production and food processing has affected not only the quantity of energy available per capita, but also the energy density.

At the same time there are continuing changes in the physical demands of work and leisure time. Mechanization of many types of work and changes in transportation are causing ever-increasing numbers of people to be sedentary for most of the time.

Increasing sedentary behavior has been proposed to be one of the principal reasons for a further increase in the prevalence of obesity in countries with established market economies. Sedentary behavior is poorly measured by the number of hours engaged in sports only. Large and important differences can be seen in the number of hours spent at sedentary jobs and in front of television or computer screens during leisure time. Transportation is almost certainly a factor as well. For example, in the Netherlands, 30% of short trips are done by bicycle and 18% by walking. In the United Kingdom these percentages are 8% by cycling and 12% walking, and in the United States 1% by bicycle and 9% by walking. Accumulated over a year, these daily activities can easily explain the small but persistent changes in energy balance needed to greatly increase the prevalence of obesity.

Figure 9 shows the disturbances in energy balance necessary to shift one individual's BMI from 23 to 26 kg/m^2. Energy intake in excess of energy expenditure needs only to be 20 kcal/day to produce weight gain over a year. This is in the order of 5 min less of brisk walking per day or an additional can of beer per week. There are compensating increases in energy expenditure, however, which may range from 15 to 25 kcal/day per kilogram of weight gain in women and men respectively (24), so that the actual increase in energy intake or reduction in energy expenditure to achieve major weight change is much larger.

Given the changes in life-styles over recent decades in many parts of the world, it is not surprising that people gain weight on average. With small changes in average body weight, the prevalence of obesity increases rapidly. For every unit increase in BMI, there is an increase in the prevalence of obesity of about five percentage points (1).

B Social, Economic, and Cultural Determinants of the Prevalence of Obesity

Many factors affect energy balance and determine obesity. The major determinants can be grouped into three groups (25):

1. Biological influences and unalterable factors (e.g., age, sex, hormonal factors, and genetics).
2. Behavioural influences (which are the result of complex psychological factors, including habits, emotions, attitudes, beliefs, and cognitions developed through a background of learning history).
3. Environmental influences (physical, economic, and sociocultural environment).

With respect to the behavioural and sociocultural factors that affect energy balance and obesity, there are many that relate to eating habits and physical activity. Of the many gender-related social determinants of obesity, we briefly discuss the perception of overweight as a desirable or undesirable trait. The attitudes toward obesity vary greatly across social and ethnic groups, and are related to the economic position of individuals and groups. In many affluent countries women experience social pressures to be thin. Katzmarzyk and Davis (26) studied the body weight and shape of Playboy centerfolds in the period 1978 to 1998 as an example of culturally "ideal" women, and noted that 70% of them were underweight by WHO standards (BMI < 18.5 kg/m^2). They speculate that this phenomenon helps to explain the high levels of body dissatisfaction and disordered eating among young women. It has been observed that these social pressures toward thinness are greater among women than among men, and greater in women with high educational level compared to those with a low educational level.

The prevalence of obesity is also sharply inversely associated with educational level. Black women in the United States are more likely to be obese than white women, even when adjusted for socioeconomic status, but they are less likely to perceive themselves as being overweight (27). Such epidemiological data would suggest that the perception overweight as un undesirable characteristic may play a role in the prevention of overweight, particularly in young white women of high socioeconomic background in affluent countries. This is undoubtedly an oversimplification, but if true it does so against the potential cost of an increased risk of body dissatisfaction and perhaps disordered eating.

Perceptions of overweight in black women in South Africa from disadvantaged communities in Cape Town, where food insecurity is a continuous concern, are in sharp contrast (28). From a qualitative in-depth survey of overweight women, it was shown that in these communities the concept of an individual voluntarily regulating food intake when food was available was completely unacceptable. Increased body mass index was regarded as a token of well-being in that marital harmony was perceived to be reflected in increased body weight. Overweight children were regarded as reflecting health as it was associated with sufficient food supply and intake. According to a survey in an urban black population in the Cape Peninsula of South Africa, more than half of the women above the age of 35 years were obese (BMI > 30 kg/m^2) whereas a considerable proportion of the children were undernourished (5). The Cape Peninsula is an example of a population that has undergone rapid economic transition and which has moved from undernutrition to extreme overnutrition.

Doak et al. (29) similarly described the coexistence of overweight and underweight within households in Brazil, China, and Russia. An underweight child coexisting with an overweight nonelderly adult was the predominant pair combination in all three countries. On an international level, Martorell et al. (4) studied the prevalence of obesity in women aged 15–49 years in different regions of developing countries. The prevalence of obesity was estimated to be ~17% in the Middle East and North Africa, >15% in Central Eastern Europe/Commonwealth of Independent States, ~6% in Latin America and the Caribbean, and <3% in Sub-Saharan Africa. There was a clear positive association between the gross national product (GNP) and the percentage of obesity up to a level of $1500 GNP. With higher GNPs, the relationship was no longer present. In these countries, obesity was more prevalent in urban than rural areas and in those with high educational level compared to those with low educational level. The relationships between obesity and these indicators of social class sharply diminished with an increase in the countries' GNP.

Such observations illustrate the complexities of the social determinants of obesity. In affluent countries, the social pressures to thinness seem to be more intense in women than in men, and in developing countries the pressures toward high body mass index seem also to be directed mainly to women. In affluent countries, the preoccupation with diet is more common in those with high socioeconomic status, whereas in developing countries a high body mass index is particularly appreciated in those with low socioeconomic status. These social pressures may reflect many underlying issues among which the food insecurity may be an important and often neglected element (30). In societies where food security is never a problem, obesity is common but not appreciated (particularly in women) whereas in food-insecure societies obesity is uncommon in women but regarded as a desirable trait. In countries undergoing an economic transition and in immigrants from developing to developed countries, their traditional perceptions of ideal body weight in women may be sustained. At the same time, increases in food availability and decreases in energy expenditure promote weight gain. Such a mixture of attitudes and changes of socioeconomic conditions may, in part, explain the exceptionally rapid increase in the prevalence of obesity, particularly in the women in such populations. Why the sociocultural ideals vary more by socioeconomic conditions among women than among men may be explained by the relative importance of energy reserves in women under conditions where the food supply is insecure. The energy reserves required for pregnancy and lactation may provide a biological basis for the cultural perception of an association between obesity and fertility. In situations where food is abundant throughout the year and no strenuous physical activity is required, the cultural ideals about body shape seem to disappear.

IV CONCLUSIONS

The prevalence of obesity is increasing at an alarming rate in many parts of the world. In white populations living in the west and north of Europe, in Australia, and in the United States, the prevalence of obesity is equally high in men and women. In countries with relatively low gross national product, such as those in central and eastern Europe, Asia, Latin America, and Africa, the prevalence is 1.5–2 times higher among women than among men. Within affluent societies, the rates of obesity seem to be higher among women at older ages (65 years) and in groups with relatively low socioeconomic status. Obesity is particularly common among women living in relatively poor conditions.

REFERENCES

1. World Health Organization. Obesity: Preventing and Managing the Global Epidemic. WHO Technical Report Series, No. 894, 2000.
2. Lean MEJ, Han TS, Seidell JC. Impairment of health

and quality of life in men and women with a large waist. Lancet 1998; 351:853–856.
3. NIH. Clinical Guidelines on the Identification, Evaluation, and Treatment of Overweight and Obesity in Adults. The Evidence Report. NIH, NHLBI, June 1998.
4. Martorell R, Kahn LK, Hughes ML, Grummer-Strawn LM. Obesity in women from developing countries. Eur J Clin Nutr 2000; 54:247–252.
5. Steyn K, Bourne L, Jooste P, Fourie JM, Rossouw K, Lombard C. Anthropometric profile of a black population of the Cape Peninsula in South Africa. East Afr Med J 1998; 75:35–40.
6. Hodge AM, Dowse GK, Gareeboo H, Tuomilehto J, Alberti KG, Zimmet PZ. Incidence, increasing prevalence, and predictors of change in obesity and fat distribution over 5 years in the rapidly developing population of Mauritius. Int J Obes Relat Metab Disord 1996;2:137–146.
7. Mokdad AH, Serdula MK, Dietz WH, Bowman BA, Marks JS, Koplan JP. The spread of the obesity epidemic in the United States, 1991–1998. JAMA 1999;282:1519–1522.
8. Seidell JC, Flegal KM. Assessing obesity: classification and epidemiology. Br Med Bull 1997;53; 238–252.
9. Torrance GM, Hooper MD, Reeder BA. Trends in overweight and obesity among adults in Canada (1970–1992): evidence from national surveys using measured height and weight. Int J Obesity 2002; 26:797–804.
10. Filozof C, Gonzalez C, Sereday M, Mazza C, Braguinsky J. Obesity prevalence and trends in Latin-Amencan counties. Obes Rev 2001; 2:99–106.
11. Arroyo P, Loria A, Fernandez V, Flegal KM, Kuri-Morales P, Olaiz G, Tapia-Conyer R. Prevalence of pre-obesity and obesity in urban adult Mexicans in comparison with other large surveys. Obes Res 2000; 8:179–185.
12. Sanchez-Castillo CP, Lara JJ, James WPT. Diet and nutritional trends in Mexico. In: Fitzpatrick DW, Anderson JE, L'Abbe ML, eds. Proceedings of the 16th International Congress on Nutrition. Ottawa: Canadian Federation of Biological Sciences, 1998: 266–267.
13. Monteiro CA, Benicio D'A, Conde WL, Popkin BM. Shifting obesity trends in Brazil. Eur J Clin Nutr 2000; 54:342–346.
14. Porrata C, Rodriguez-Ojea A, Jimenez S. The epidemiologic transition in Cuba. In: Pena M, Bacallao J, eds. Obesity and Poverty—A New Public Health Challenge. Pan American Health Organization, Washington DC: Scientific Publication No. 576, 2000:51–66.
15. International Diabetes Institute. The Asia-Pacific perspective: redefining obesity and its treatment. Health Communications Australia Pty. ISBN # 0-9577082-1-1, 2000.
16. Seidell JC, A Rissanen. World-wide prevalence of obesity and time-trends. In: Bray GA, Bouchard C, James WPT, eds. Handbook of Obesity. New York: Marcel Dekker, 1997:79–91.
17. Seidell JC. Obesity, insulin resistance and diabetes—a world-wide epidemic. Br J Nutr 2000; 83(suppl 1):S5–S8.
18. Seidell JC, Visscher TLS. Body weight and weight change and their health implications for the elderly. Eur J Clin Nutr 2000; 54(suppl 3):S33–S39.
19. Molarius A, JC Seidell, S Sans, J Tuomilehto, K Kuulasmaa. Educational level and relative body weight and changes in their associations over ten years—an international perspective from the WHO MONICA project. Am J Public Health 2000; 90:1260–1268.
20. Pomerleau J, Pudule I, Grinberga D, Kadziauskiene K, Abaravicius A, Bartkeviciute R, Vaask S, Robertson A, McKee M. Patterns of body weight in the Baltic Republics. Public Health Nutr 2000; 3:3–10.
21. Doak CM, Popkin BM. The emerging problem of obesity in developing countries. In: Semba RD, Bloem MW, eds. Nutrition and Health in Developing Countries. Totowa, New Jersey: Humana Press, 2001:447–464.
22. Mokhtar N, Elati J, Chabir R, Bour A, Elkari K, Schlossman NP, Cballero B, Aguenaou H. Diet, culture and obesity in Northern Africa. J Nutr 2001; 131:887S–892S.
23. WHO. The World Health Report 1998. Life in the 21st Century—A Vision for All. Geneva: WHO, 1998.
24. Prentice AM, Black AE, Coward WA, Cole TL. Energy expenditure in overweight and obese adults in affluent societies: an analysis of 319 doubly labelled water measurements. Eur J Clin Nutr 1996; 50:93–97.
25. Egger G, Swinburn B. An ecological approach to the obesity pandemic. Br Med J 1997; 315:477–480.
26. Katzmarzyk P, Davis C. Thinness and body shape of Playboy centrefolds from 1978 to 1998. Int J Obes 2001; 25:590–592.
27. Dawson DA. Ethnic differences in female overweight: data from the 1985 National Health Interview Survey. Am J Public Health 1988; 78:1326–1329.
28. Mvo Z, Dick J, Steyn K. Perceptions of overweight African women about acceptable body size of women and children. Curationis 1999; 22:27–31.
29. Doak CM, Adair LS, Monteiro C, Popkin BM. Overweight and underweight coexist within households in Brazil, China and Russia. J Nutr 2000; 2965–2971.
30. Olson CM. Nutrition and health outcomes associated with food insecurity and hunger. J Nutr; 129(suppl 2): 521S–524S.

5

Fetal Origins of Obesity

David J. P. Barker

University of Southampton, Southampton, England

I INTRODUCTION

Obese children tend to become obese adults, especially if their parents are obese (1,2). One study showed that 80% of children who were overweight at ~12 years of age were obese at ~30 years (3). Among a group of elderly men and women in Helsinki, those who were obese, defined by a body mass index (weight/height^2) of >30 kg/m^2, had had above average body mass indices at the age of 7 years (4). Such findings indicate that adult obesity may be initiated or "entrained" during early life (5). There may be critical periods of development when this occurs. Critical periods, during which changes tend to be irreversible, may be distinguished from high-risk periods which occur throughout life and are associated with reversible increases in body weight. Pregnancy and times of emotional stress are examples of high-risk periods. There is evidence for three critical periods for body weight—prenatal, childhood, and adolescence. This chapter focuses on the prenatal period, describing how this may influence later obesity and how it interacts with obesity in childhood and adult life to determine later disease.

II BODY SIZE AT BIRTH AND LATER BODY COMPOSITION

People who had high birth weight or were heavy during the first year after birth are at increased risk of obesity in later life (6,7). The effect, however, is small. In a study of military conscripts in Denmark, for example, mean body mass index rose from 22.7 kg/m^2 in men whose birth weights were <2500 g to 24.9 kg/m^2 in men whose birth weights were >4500 g (8).

People who had low birth weight tend to accumulate fat on the trunk and abdomen, a pattern of adiposity found in the insulin resistance syndrome in which central obesity, impaired glucose tolerance, hypertension, and altered blood lipid concentrations occur in the same patient (9). This disorder is associated with an increased risk of coronary heart disease (10). In two studies in the United Kingdom men who had low birth weight had high ratios of waist-to-hip circumference after allowing for adult body mass index (Table 1) (11). This association with low birth weight has been replicated in a study of men in Sweden (12). In the Swedish study birth weight was also associated with truncal fat, as measured by a high ratio of subscapular to triceps skinfold thickness. After allowing for current body mass index truncal fat increased by 0.30 standard deviations with each kilogram decrease in birth weight.

In one of the U.K. studies placental weight was also available (Table 1). Its association with the waist-hip ratio was in the opposite direction to birth weight so that the highest ratios of waist-to-hip circumference were in men who had had a high placental weight in relation to birth weight. High placental weight to birth weight ratios are a known marker of fetal hypoxia or undernutrition (13–15). The association with placental weight has not been examined in other studies, and may be inconstant because placental hypertrophy is only one

Table 1 Simultaneous Effects, Regression Coefficients (95% CI) of Birth Weight, Placental Weight, and Adult Body Mass Index on Waist-Hip Ratio (%) in Two Samples of Men in the United Kingdom

	Preston (men aged 51)	Hertfordshire (men aged 64)
Adult body mass index (kg/m^2)	0.70 (0.54–0.86)	0.83 (0.75–0.91)
Birth weight (lbs)	−0.83 (−1.50 to −0.15)	−0.29 (−0.52 to −0.05)
Placental weight (lbs)	1.76 (−0.73 to 4.24)	

of the fetus's responses to undernutrition. It depends on the timing of undernutrition and the mother's nutritional state (14).

Low birth-weight has been shown to be associated with truncal fat in young people. This association occurs across the normal range of birth weight. Among 30-year-old Mexican and non-Hispanic Americans low birth weight was associated with truncal fat but not with a high waist-to-hip ratio (16). Among English girls aged 14–16 years, those who were smallest at birth but fattest as teenagers also had the highest ratio of subscapular to triceps skinfold (17). Among children aged 7–12 years in Philadelphia, there was a similar association between low birth weight and truncal fat deposition with partial correlations between birth weight and the ratio of subscapular to triceps skinfolds of ~0.20, after allowing for body mass index (18). In 8-year-old Indian children the subscapular-to-triceps skinfold ratio fell from 84.8 to 77.7 across what is the normal range of birth weight in India, from 2.0 kgs or less to 3.25 kgs. Above 3.25 pounds the ratio rose to 82.2, which may reflect macrosomia at birth and persisting overweight in the offspring of mothers with gestational diabetes or impaired glucose tolerance (19). No association between birth weight and truncal fat was found in a comparison between 15-year-olds who had low birthweight, < 5.5 lbs, and controls within the normal birth weight range (20). This could reflect aspects of body composition specific to babies weighing < 5.5 lbs, since as adolescents these low–birth weight babies were markedly thinner than the controls.

High waist-hip ratio and high truncal fat may reflect different aspects of body composition, hormonal status, and metabolism (12). In the Swedish study low birth weight predicted a smaller hip but not a larger waist and therefore did not reflect abdominal obesity. A study of young American men applying for military service led to the same conclusion (21). Birth weight was linearly associated with body mass index and with the area of thigh muscle but not with subcutaneous fat on the thigh. The association between birth weight and body mass index may therefore have reflected an association with lean tissue rather than fat. Waist-hip ratio and truncal fat also have different metabolic associations. Waist-hip ratio is more strongly associated with serum triglyceride and HDL cholesterol concentrations than is the subscapular-triceps skinfold ratio (22). The associations between low birth weight and these two measures of body composition are likely to reflect influences in the intrauterine environment that are either different or act at different times.

III FETAL NUTRITION AND LATER BODY COMPOSITION

Nutrition has a central role in the regulation of fetal growth (15). Cross-breeding and embryo transplant experiments in animals show that size at birth is largely determined by the intrauterine environment, with only a small effect from parental genotype (23). The major hormonal mediators of fetal growth are insulin and the insulinlike growth factors (24). These in turn are regulated by fetal nutrient supply (15,25). It is important that "fetal nutrition," which defines the supply of metabolic substrata to the fetus, is distinguished from maternal dietary intake because the mammalian fetus grows at the end of a long and sometimes precarious supply line, which includes the mother's body composition, metabolic and endocrine status, uterine blood flow, and placental function (15). Notwithstanding this complexity, it is clear from the effects of wartime famine that a mother's diet in pregnancy can influence the body composition of her offspring through their lives.

A Undernutrition

Famine began abruptly in western Holland in November 1944 and ended with the liberation by the Allied armies in May 1945. In the early months of 1945 official rations varied between 400 and 800 calories per day. A study of ~300,000 young military conscripts who were born around that time showed that those who were conceived during the famine had higher rates of obesity than those who were either in utero or born when the famine began, or those who were never exposed to famine (26). By the time the men and women exposed to famine in utero reached 50 years of age, the picture had changed (27). The men conceived in famine were no longer more obese than other men, but the women conceived in famine were on average 7.9 kg heavier than women not exposed to famine; their body mass indices were 7.4% higher, and their waist circumference was 7.4 cm greater. These associations did not depend on their body size at birth: indeed, their birth weights were similar to those of unexposed children—presumably because their mothers became well nourished in the second half of pregnancy.

These fascinating observations suggest that high body mass index and high abdominal fat, for which waist circumference is a validated indicator (28), can originate through fetal undernutrition. The sex differences in response to undernutrition suggest that the processes underlying its association with later obesity are more likely to involve alterations in central hormonal regulatory mechanisms rather than changes at the level of the fat cell.

B Overnutrition

Studies of the children of women with diabetes during pregnancy provide some of the clearest evidence that obesity may be linked to metabolic experience in utero. Figure 1 shows the change in body mass index from birth to 17 years in a group of 139 children born to diabetic mothers (29). They are compared with standard growth curves in the United States. Having been heavy and macrosomic at birth, the children's body mass indices became similar to those of other children at the age of 1 year. They remained similar until ~4 years of age, after which they began to increase. They remained overweight up to the age of 17 years. At 14–17 years of age their mean body mass index was 24.6 kg/m^2, compared with 20.9 kg/m^2 in a group of control children. The degree of overweight was not related to birth weight or to the level of macrosomia at birth. Because the children were similar to other children at 1 year, their overweight cannot reflect persistence of excessive fat accumulated in utero. Some form of "metabolic programming" is implied. Overweight was related to the concentration of insulin in the amniotic fluid, which suggests that premature activation of the pancreatic beta cells in the offspring of diabetic mothers could be linked to their later development of obesity.

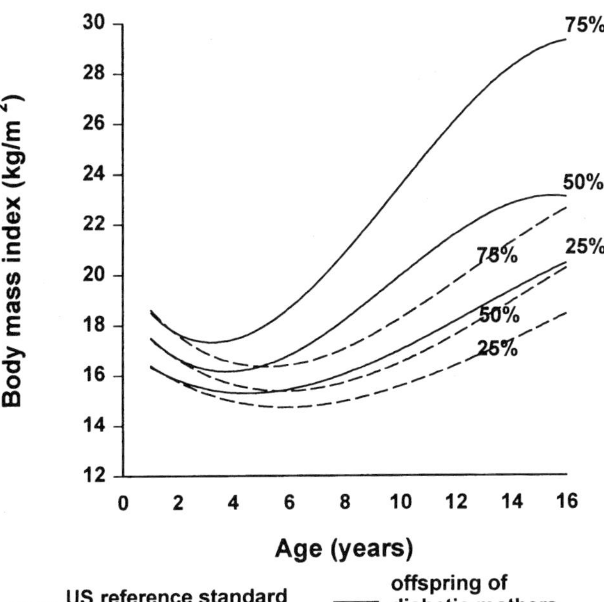

Figure 1 Change in body mass index from birth to 17 years in 139 children born to diabetic mothers. (From Ref. 29.)

The effects of intrauterine exposure to the metabolic consequences of maternal diabetes could be confounded, however, by genetic influences. To address this, 52 families of Pima Indians were studied in which at least one sibling was born after the mother was found to have diabetes (30). The mean body mass index in these siblings was 2.6 kg/m^2 higher than in their siblings from nondiabetic pregnancies. Since siblings born before and after diabetes are at the same risk of inheriting genes determining obesity, the difference in body mass index is likely to reflect the effect of intrauterine exposure to diabetes.

IV INFANT FEEDING AND OBESITY

A recent study of 15,000 children aged 9–14 years found that in those who had been only or mostly fed breast milk, the odds ratio for being overweight was 0.78 (95% CI 0.66–0.91) compared with children who had been only or mostly fed infant formula (31). This apparent protective effect of breastfeeding against obesity persisted after adjustment for energy intake, physical activity, mother's body mass index, and other variables. The same association has not been found consistently in younger children, and there may be a latent period during childhood before it is manifest. A mechanistic explanation of the association is that breastfed babies have greater control of their intake than bottle-fed babies, and therefore develop better self-regulatory mechanisms. Another possibility is that hormones and growth factors in breast milk permanently change the baby's metabolism. There is no specific evidence for this, but breastfeeding has been shown to be associated with lower levels of cardiovascular risk factors including lower low-density lipoprotein concentrations (32). It seems likely that associations between breastfeeding and later adiposity will prove to be complex.

V FETAL GROWTH AND OBESITY-RELATED DISEASE INTERACTIONS BETWEEN FETAL GROWTH AND CHILDHOOD BODY MASS

Studies of the fetal and infant origins of obesity are part of a wider field of research on the early origins of adult diseases (33) It is now known that people who had low birth weight, or who were thin or stunted at birth, are at increased risk of type 2 diabetes, coronary heart disease, and hypertension (34–40). These diseases, especially type 2 diabetes, are associated with obesity (41). Their association with small body size at birth has led to the conclusion that they originate in persisting changes in the body's structure, physiology, and metabolism that result from fetal undernutrition and are associated with slow growth in utero (15,33).

Figure 2 shows the path of growth of boys who as adults were either admitted to hospital with coronary heart disease or died from the disease. They belong to a cohort of 4630 boys born in Helsinki (40). Their body size is expressed as mean standard deviation or Z scores. The Z score for the cohort is set at zero, and a boy maintaining a steady position as large or small in relation to other boys would follow a horizontal path on the figure. Boys who later developed coronary heart disease, however, having been small at birth and during infancy, had accelerated gain in weight and body mass index thereafter. A 1-unit increase in standard deviation score for body mass index between 1 and 12 years was associated with a hazard ratio of 1.20 (95% CI 1.08–1.33). The effect of increase in body mass index, however, was conditioned by birthweight and, more strongly, by ponderal index at birth (birth weight/length^3), a measure of fatness.

Table 2 shows that at any body mass index at 12 years, the latest age for which there are data, the risk of coronary heart disease was greater in boys who were thin at birth. Findings at younger ages in childhood were similar. In animals accelerated or "compensatory" growth after a period of undernutrition during development can have long-term costs, including reduced life span (42). Whether this general biological phenomenon is related to the association between rapid childhood weight gain and human disease is not known.

The same general pattern of growth, small size at birth and during infancy followed by compensatory growth in childhood, is associated with type 2 diabetes and hypertension (38,39). There are differences in detail

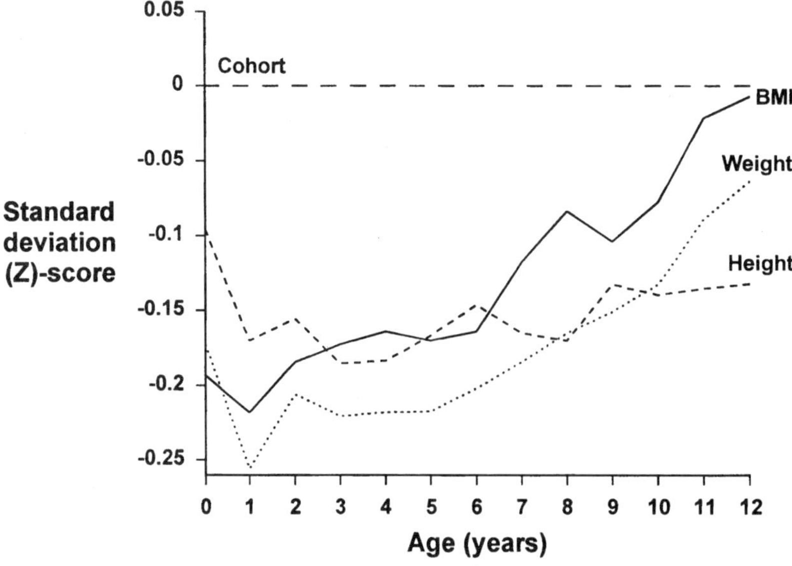

Figure 2 Growth of 357 boys who later developed coronary heart disease in a cohort of 4630 boys born in Helsinki.

Table 2 Hazard Ratios for Deaths from Coronary Heart Disease According to Ponderal Index at Birth (birth weight/length^3) and Body Mass Index at 12 Years

Ponderal index at birth (kg/m^3)	Body mass index at 12 years (kg/m^2)			
	–16	–17	–18	>18
≤25	547[a]	426	288	233
–27	618	692	507	424
–29	458	614	475	436
>29	225	317	317	279
≤25	2.0 (0.9–4.4)[b]	2.1 (1.0–4.7)	2.8 (1.2–6.2)	4.3 (1.9–9.5)
–27	1.3 (0.6–2.9)	2.5 (1.2–5.2)	2.5 (1.1–5.3)	2.2 (1.0–4.8)
–29	1.3 (0.6–3.0)	1.5 (0.7–3.2)	1.6 (0.7–3.6)	2.1 (0.9–4.6)
>29	1.0	1.1 (0.4–2.6)	1.9 (0.8–4.4)	1.5 (0.6–3.5)

[a] No. of men.
[b] 95% confidence intervals in parentheses.

between the diseases and between the two sexes (43), but the overall picture is the same. Disease is related to the rate of increase in body mass index as well as to body mass index attained at any particular age (38,39). The diseases are therefore related to the tempo of weight gain in childhood as well as to the state of being obese or overweight in adult life. The data from Helsinki can be used to estimate the number of cases of disease that are statistically attributable to fetal, infant, and childhood growth. If, for example, each man and woman in the cohort had had (1) a birth weight above the median for the cohort, 3.4 kg, (2) weight at 1 year above the median, 10.0 kg, and (3) an increase in body mass index between 3 and 12 years below the median increase, 0.5 kg/m^2, there would have been a 44% (95% CI 27–59) reduction in hospital admissions and deaths from coronary heart disease, a 62% (95% CI 43–79) reduction in the incidence of type 2 diabetes, and a 31% (95% CI 19–43) reduction in the incidence of hypertension.

There are a number of possible processes by which, in humans, undernutrition and small size at birth followed by rapid childhood weight gain could lead to cardiovascular disease and type 2 diabetes in later life (38–40). Babies who are thin at birth, having a low ponderal index, lack muscle, a deficiency which will persist as the critical period for muscle growth is ~30 weeks in utero and there is little cell replication after birth (44). If they develop a high body mass index in childhood, they may have a disproportionately high fat mass. This may be associated with the development of insulin resistance, as children and adults who had low birth weight but are currently heavy are insulin resistant (19,45), and the adults have high rates of the insulin resistance syndrome (46,47).

VI INTERACTIONS BETWEEN FETAL GROWTH AND ADULT BODY MASS

The effects of birth weight interact with the effects of body mass index in adult life as well as in childhood. Table 3 shows that the effect of increasing birth weight on reducing systolic pressure is greater among men who have a high body mass index (48). This interaction

Table 3 Slope of Relation of Systolic Pressure (mmHg) at Age 50 per Kilogram Increase in Birth Weight by Thirds of Distribution of Body Mass Index Among 1333 Men in Uppsala, Sweden

Men	Body mass index (kg/m^2)		
	<23.5 Difference (95% CI)	23.5 to 25.9 Difference (95% CI)	≥26 Difference (95% CI)
All	–1.3 (–4.3 to 1.7)	–3.9 (–7.1 to –0.6)	–4.1 (–7.6 to –0.5)
Born at term (38–41 weeks' gestation)	–1.4 (–7.6 to 4.7)	–3.5 (–10.1 to 3.1)	–9.1 (–16.4 to –1.9)
Height >176 cm	–2.1 (–6.8 to 2.5)	–2.3 (–7.1 to 2.5)	–9.3 (–14.8 to –3.8)

between birth weight and body mass index was stronger in men who were born at term, and whose low birth weight is therefore due to slow fetal growth rather than premature birth. It was strongest in men who were tall, so that in men who were born at term, who were in the top third of body mass index, and of above median height, a 1-kg increase in birth weight was associated with a 15.9 mm Hg (95% CI 5.2–26.5) fall in systolic pressure. The authors suggested that tall men who had low birth weight had sustained a greater failure to realize growth potential in utero, and this failure that led to a greater increase in blood pressure. Another possibility is that these men had staged more rapid compensatory growth and had therefore sustained higher long-term metabolic costs.

A mechanism other than insulin resistance by which the effects of birth weight and body mass index may interact is through their effects on plasma cortisol concentrations. A recent study showed that fasting plasma cortisol concentrations in adult men and women fell by 23.9 nmol (95% CI 9.6–8.2) with each kilogram increase in birth weight (49). This is thought to reflect persistingly increased cortisol secretion in people who grew slowly in utero, and who may have enhanced their glucocorticoid secretion in order to accelerate maturation of key organs including, importantly, the lung (50).

Although obesity is associated with a reduction in plasma cortisol concentrations (51), Table 4, which combines studies in the United Kingdom and Australia (49), shows that the association between high plasma cortisol and raised blood pressure is stronger in people who are overweight or obese. This suggests the existence of a group of men and women who, while becoming overweight, paradoxically maintain elevated plasma cortisol concentrations. It is this group that has the highest blood pressures. This requires further study, but it is part of a framework of ideas that may explain the consistent finding that obesity amplifies the influence of low birth weight on cardiovascular and metabolic disease.

Table 4 Systolic Blood Pressure in 845 Men and Women According to Fasting Plasma Cortisol Concentrations and Current Body Mass Index

Plasma cortisol (nmol/L)	Body mass index (kg/m^2)			
	−25	−30	>30	All
≤300	146 (127)	147 (152)	152 (42)	148 (321)
−400	147 (98)	151 (105)	157 (31)	150 (234)
>400	150 (145)	154 (110)	166 (35)	153 (290)
All	148 (370)	150 (367)	158 (108)	150 (845)

VII CONCLUSIONS

Around the world the transition from chronic malnutrition to adequate nutrition, the so-called nutritional transition (52), is characterized by accelerated childhood weight gain and the emergence of adult obesity in people who were undernourished in utero and during infancy. This is the path of growth that leads to cardiovascular disease and type 2 diabetes. The WHO study of the global burden of disease found that, contrary to the preconception that these diseases are "diseases of affluence," the probability of death from them and other noncommunicable diseases is higher in low-income regions than in high-income regions such as established marked economies (53). One resolution of this apparent paradox is that the high rates of maternal and perinatal disorders, nutritional deficiencies and infective disease which characterize low-income regions lead to poor fetal and infant growth and therefore enhanced susceptibility to the effects of rapid weight gain and obesity.

Although the epidemic of obesity in Western countries is linked to the epidemics of type 2 diabetes and coronary heart disease, the paths of childhood growth that lead to obesity and to these diseases differ. In the Helsinki studies, children who became obese in later life tended to be born with above average birthweight and to continue to have above-average weight in childhood (4). Children who developed obesity-related disorders had below-average body size at birth and at 1 year, and thereafter had accelerated weight gain so that their body mass index reached the average at some point in childhood and thereafter exceeded it (38,39,54). This dissociation in the paths of growth that lead to them may help to explain why despite an increasing prevalence of obesity in Western countries (55) coronary heart disease is declining (56).

To understand the origins of obesity and the disorders to which it is related, we may need to direct our attention away from the lifestyles of adults, however important these may be, to growth and development in utero, and during infancy and childhood. We need to understand how nutrition in early life establishes metabolic and endocrine pathways that lead to obesity and premature death (14). Strategies to prevent obesity-related disorders should include improvements of fetal growth and the prevention of obesity in childhood.

REFERENCES

1. Whitaker RC, Wright JA, Pepe MS, Seidel KD, Dietz WH. Predicting obesity in young adulthood from childhood and parental obesity. N Engl J Med 1997; 337:869–873.
2. Parsons TJ, Power C, Logan S, Summerbell CD. Childhood predictors of adult obesity: a systematic review. Int J Obes 1999; 23(suppl 8):S1–S107.
3. Abraham S, Nordseick M. Relationship of excess weight in children and adults. Public Health Rep 1960; 75:263–273.
4. Eriksson J, Forsen T, Tuomilehto J, Osmond C, Barker D. Size at birth, childhood growth and obesity in adult life. Int J Obes 2001; 25:735–740.
5. Dietz WH. Early influences on body weight regulation. In: Bouchard C, Bray GA, eds. Regulation of Body Weight. Chichester: John Wiley, 1996.
6. Charney E, Chamblee Goodman H, McBride M, Lyon B, Pratt R. Childhood antecedents of adult obesity. Do chubby infants become obese adults? N Engl J Med 1976; 295:6–9.
7. Seidman DS, Laor A, Gale R, Stevenson DK, Danon YL. A longitudinal study of birth weight and being overweight in late adolescence. Am J Dis Child 1991; 145:782–785.
8. Sorensen HT, Sabroe S, Rothman KJ, Gillman M, Fischer P, Sorensen TIA. Relation between weight and length at birth and body mass index in young adulthood: cohort study. BMJ 1997; 315:1137
9. Reaven GM. Banting Lecture 1988. Role of insulin resistance in human disease. Diabetes 1988; 37:1595–1607.
10. Larsson B, Svardsudd K, Welin L, Wilhelmsen L, Bjorntorp P, Tibblin G. Abdominal adipose tissue distribution, obesity, and risk of cardiovascular disease and death: 13 year follow up of participants in the study of men born in 1913. BMJ 1984; 288:1401–1404.
11. Law CM, Barker DJP, Osmond C, Fall CHD, Simmonds SJ. Early growth and abdominal fatness in adult life. J Epidemiol Community Health 1992; 46: 184–186.
12. Byberg L, McKeigue PM, Zethelius B, Lithell HO. Birth weight and the insulin resistance syndrome: association of low birth weight with truncal obesity and raised plasminogen activator inhibitor-1 but not with abdominal obesity or plasma lipid disturbances. Diabetologia 2000; 43:54–60.
13. McCrabb GJ, Egan AR, Hosking BJ. Maternal undernutrition during mid-pregnancy in sheep; variable effects on placental growth. J Agric Sci 1992; 118:127–132.
14. Barker DJP. Mothers, Babies and Health in Later Life, 2nd ed. Edinburgh: Churchill Livingstone, 1998.
15. Harding JE. The nutritional basis of the fetal origins of adult disease. Int J Epidemiol 2001; 30:15–23.
16. Valdez R, Athens MA, Thompson GH, Bradshaw BS, Stern MP. Birthweight and adult health outcomes in a biethnic population in the USA. Diabetologia 1994; 37:624–631.
17. Barker ME, Robinson S, Osmond C, Barker DJP. Birthweight and body fat distribution in adolescent girls. Arch Dis Child 1997; 77:381–338.
18. Malina RM, Katzmarzyk PT, Beunen G. Birth weight and its relationship to size attained and relative fat distribution at 7 to 12 years of age. Obes Res 1996; 4: 385–390.
19. Bavdekar A, Chittaranjan S, Fall CHD, Bapat S, Pandit AN, Deshpande V, Bhave S, Kellingray SD, Joglekar C. Insulin resistance syndrome in 8-year-old Indian children. Small at birth, big at 8 years, or both? Diabetes 1999; 48:2422–2429.
20. Matthes JWA, Lewis PA, Davies DP, Bethel JA. Body size and subcutaneous fat patterning in adolescence. Arch Dis Child 1996; 75:521–523.
21. Kahn HS, Narayan KMV, Williamson DF, Valdez R. Relation of birth weight to lean and fat thigh tissue in young men. Int J Obes 2000; 24:667–672.
22. Haffner SM, Stern MP, Hazuik HP, Pugh J, Patterson J-K. Do upper body and centralised obesity measure different aspects of regional body fat distribution? Relationship to non-insulin-dependent diabetes mellitus, lipids and lipoproteins. Diabetes 1987; 36:43–51.
23. Snow MHL. Effects of genome on fetal size at birth. In: Sharp F, Fraser RB, Milner RDG, eds. Fetal Growth: Proceedings of the 20th Study Group. London: Royal College of Obstetricians and Gynaecologists, 1989: 1–11.
24. Fowden AL. The role of insulin in prenatal growth. J Dev Physiol 1989; 12:173–182.
25. Oliver MH, Harding JE, Breier BH, Evans PC, Gluckman PD. Glucose but not a mixed amino acid infusion regulates plasma insulin-like growth factor-1 concentrations in fetal sheep. Pediatr Res 1993; 34(l):62–65.
26. Ravelli GP, Stein ZA, Susser MW. Obesity in young men after famine exposure in utero and early infancy. N Engl J Med 1976; 295:349–353.
27. Ravelli ACJ, Van der Meulen JHP, Osmond C, Barker DJP, Blecker OP. Obesity at the age of 50y in men and women exposed to famine prenatally. Am J Clin Nutr 1999; 70:811–816.
28. Pouliot MC, Despres JP, Lemieux S, et al. Waist circumference and abdominal sagittal diameter: best simple anthropometric indexes of abdominal visceral adipose tissue accumulation and selected cardiovascular risk in men and women. Am J Cardiol 1994; 73:460–468.
29. Silverman BL, Cho NH, Rizzo TA, Metzger BE. Long-term effects of the intrauterine environment. Diabetes Care 1998; 21:B142–B149.
30. Dabelea D, Hanson RL, Lindsay RS, Pettitt DJ, Imperatore G, Gabir MM, Roumain J, Bennett PH,

Knowler WC. Intrauterine exposure to diabetes conveys risks for type 2 diabetes and obesity. A study of discordant sibships. Diabetes 2000; 49:2208–2211.

31. Gillman MW, Rifas-Shiman SL, Camargo CA, Berkey CS, Frazier AL, Rockett HRH, Field AE, Colditz GA. Risk of overweight among adolescents who were breastfed as infants. JAMA 2001; 285:2461–2467.
32. Ravelli ACJ, Van der Meulen JHP, Osmond C, Barker DJP, Bleker OP. Infant feeding and adult glucose tolerance, lipid profile, blood pressure and obesity. Arch Dis Child 2000; 82:248–252.
33. Barker DJP. Fetal origins of coronary heart disease. BMJ 1995; 311:171–174.
34. Barker DJP, Osmond C, Winter PD, Margetts B, Simmonds SJ. Weight in infancy and death from ischaemic heart disease. Lancet 1989; 2:577–580.
35. Rich-Edwards JW, Stampfer MJ, Manson JE, Rosner B, Hankinson SE, Colditz GA, Willett WC, Hennekens CH. Birth weight and risk of cardiovascular disease in a cohort of women followed up since 1976. BMJ 1997; 315:396–400.
36. Leon DA, Lithell HO, Vagero D, Koupilova I, Mohsen R, Berglund L, Lithell UB, McKeigue PM. Reduced fetal growth rate and increased risk of death from ischaemic heart disease: cohort study of 15 000 Swedish men and women born 1915–29. BMJ 1998; 317:241–5.
37. Huxley RR, Shiell AW, Law CM. The role of size at birth and postnatal catch-up growth in determining systolic blood pressure: a systematic review of the literature. J Hypertens 2000; 18:815–831.
38. Forsen T, Eriksson J, Tuomilehto J, Reunanen A, Osmond C, Barker D. The fetal and childhood growth of persons who develop type 2 diabetes. Ann Intern Med 2000; 133:176–182.
39. Eriksson J, Forsen T, Tuomilehto J, Osmond C, Barker D. Fetal and childhood growth and hypertension in adult life. Hypertension 2000; 36:790–794.
40. Eriksson JG, Forsen T, Tuomilehto J, Osmond C, Barker DJP. Early growth and coronary heart disease in later life: longitudinal study. BMJ 2001; 322:949–953.
41. Willett WC, Dietz WH, Colditz GA. Guidelines for healthy weight. N Engl J Med 1999;341:427–434.
42. Morgan IJ, Metcalfe NB. Deferred costs of compensatory growth after autumnal food shortage in juvenile salmon. Proc R Soc Lond B 2001; 268:295–301.
43. Forsen T, Eriksson JG, Tuomilehto J, Osmond C, Barker DJP. Growth in utero and during childhood among women who develop coronary heart disease: longitudinal study. BMJ 1999; 319:1403–1407.
44. Widdowson EM, Crabb DE, Milner RDG. Cellular development of some human organs before birth. Arch Dis Child 1972;47:652–655.
45. Phillips DIW. Insulin resistance as a programmed response to fetal undernutrition. Diabetologia 1996; 39:1119–1122.
46. Barker DJP, Hales CN, Fall CHD, Osmond C, Phipps K, Clark PMS. Type 2 (non-insulin-dependent) diabetes mellitus, hypertension and hyperlipidaemia (syndrome X): relation to reduced fetal growth. Diabetologia 1993; 36:62–67.
47. Mi J, Law CM, Zhang KL, Osmond C, Stein CE, Barker DJP. Effects of infant birthweight and maternal body mass index in pregnancy on components of the insulin resistance syndrome in China. Ann Intern Med 2000; 132:253–260.
48. Leon DA, Koupilova I, Lithell HO, Berglund L, Mohsen R, Vagero D, Lithell UB, McKeigue PM. Failure to realise growth potential in utero and adult obesity in relation to blood pressure in 50 year old Swedish men. BMJ 1996; 312:401–406.
49. Phillips DIW, Walker BR, Reynolds RM, Flanaghan DEH, Wood PJ, Osmond C, Barker DJP, Whorwood CB. Low birth weight predicts elevated plasma cortisol concentrations in adults from 3 populations. Hypertension 2000; 35:1301–1306.
50. Fowden AL. Endocrine regulation of fetal growth. Reprod Fertil Dev 1995; 7:351–363.
51. Kopelman PG. Hormones and obesity. Baillières Clin Endocrinol Metab 1994; 8:549–575.
52. Popkin BM. The nutrition transition and its implications for the fetal origins hypothesis In: Barker DJP, ed. Fetal Origins of Cardiovascular and Lung Disease. New York: Marcel Dekker, 2001.
53. Murray CJL, Lopez AD. Mortality by cause for eight regions of the world: global burden of disease study. Lancet 1997; 349:1269–1276.
54. Eriksson JG, Forsen T, Tuomilehto J, Winter PD, Osmond C, Barker DJP. Catch-up growth in childhood and death from coronary heart disease: longitudinal study. BMJ 1999; 318:427–431.
55. Mokdad AH, Serdula MK, Dietz WH, Bowman BA, Marks JS, Koplan JP. The continuing epidemic of obesity in the United States. JAMA 2000; 284:1650–1651.
56. Pisa Z, Uemura K. Trends of mortality from ischaemic heart disease and other cardiovascular diseases in 27 countries, 1968–1977. World Health Stat Q 1982; 35: 11–47.

6

Pediatric Overweight: An Overview

Bettylou Sherry and William H. Dietz

Centers for Disease Control and Prevention, Atlanta, Georgia, U.S.A.

I INTRODUCTION

Overweight is one of the most prevalent nutritional problems affecting children in developed countries. In this chapter, we briefly describe the public health importance of pediatric overweight as well its identification, definition, and prevalence. We then address the physiologic changes of adiposity with age, the critical periods for the development of overweight, the associations and potential risk factors in the physical and behavioral environment, and implications for clinical practice. The data reviewed support the assertion that effective prevention and treatment of childhood overweight will have a major impact on the prevalence of adult overweight and obesity and their complications.

Although the intent of this chapter is to provide a perspective of childhood obesity, we will avoid the term "obesity," instead using the term "overweight," Calling children obese may have undesirable sequelae, including various types of psychosocial dysfunction. Thus, we will follow the more preferred terminology.

Today, the diagnosis of overweight connotes a state of ill health and the potential for serious consequences in childhood, adulthood, or both. In the past, it was believed rare for overweight boys and girls to suffer serious health consequences while they were still children or adolescents, and much less was known about the "tracking" of childhood overweight into adulthood or about the consequences for adult health of having been overweight in childhood. Psychosocial dysfunction, such as poor self-esteem (1,2), was considered the primary reason that parents and pediatricians should be concerned about the overweight child. Now that we know that overweight children commonly have adverse lipid, insulin, and blood pressure levels (3), elevated C-reactive protein (4), type 2 diabetes (5), increased linear growth and advanced bone age (6), hepatic steatosis (7), cholelithiasis (8), as well as a variety of less common disorders such as sleep apnea (9), and that overweight tracks increasingly with advancing age in childhood into adulthood (10,11), we must accord overweight much greater importance among the problems with which pediatricians and families must deal. When we improve our understanding of the consequences of childhood overweight, the dramatic increase in prevalence compels us to give this issue a high priority among our public health concerns.

The adverse consequences of pediatric overweight during childhood warrant more discussion. Of particular concern are the dramatic increase in the incidence of type 2 diabetes in children and adolescents and the fact that this disease is strongly associated with overweight children. In one study of 10- to 19-year-old children in Cincinnati, the incidence of type 2 diabetes increased from 0.7 per 100,000 in 1982 to 7.2 per 100,000 in 1994, and studies from several developed and developing countries document the emergence of type 2 diabetes among children (5). Freedman et al. found that compared to non-overweight children [body mass index (BMI) < 85th centile], overweight children (BMI > 95th centile) had a significantly increased risk of having elevated fasting insulin levels [odds ratio (OR) = 12.1, 95%, confidence interval (CI) = 10–16], elevated triglycerides (OR = 7.1, 95% CI = 5.8–8.6), elevated systolic blood pressure (OR = 4.5, 95% CI = 3.6–5.8), low levels of high-density lipoprotein (HDL) cholesterol (OR = 3.4, 95% CI = 2.8–4.2), high levels of low-density lipoprotein (LDL) cholesterol (OR = 3.0, 95% CI = 2.4–3.6), and elevated diastolic blood pressure (OR = 2.4, 95% CI = 1.8–3.0) (3). Fifty-eight percent of the overweight children were found to have at least one risk factor, and using overweight as their screening tool allowed them to identify 50% of the children who had two or more risk factors (3).

There is evidence of adverse consequences of child-onset overweight in adulthood as well. In a 55-year follow-up study of adults who were overweight as adolescents, the relative risks of coronary heart disease and atherosclerosis were increased relative to adults who had not been overweight during adolescence (12). These analyses were adjusted for BMI and smoking status at age 53 years. Among the men in this study, there was a significantly greater risk of all-cause mortality and death from coronary heart disease, atherosclerotic cerebrovascular disease, and colorectal cancer (12).

In a second study examining the consequences of child-onset overweight in adulthood, we demonstrated that overweight present in older adolescents and young adults had a substantial adverse impact on a variety of psychosocial outcomes (13). As shown in Table 1, obesity present in young women was associated with an adverse impact on educational attainment, rates of marriage, household income, and poverty status. The persistence of these effects after controlling for a variety of baseline measures, including self-esteem, parental education, and the income of the family of origin, suggests that obesity is an important determinant rather than a consequence of socioeconomic status in women. Short stature, however, appeared to play a role in men comparable to the role of obesity in women on the social and economic indicators examined. These results suggest that discrimination against obese women is widespread, with grave social and economic consequences. However, although we anticipated that the effects of discrimination would have an adverse impact on the self-esteem of the women included in the study, no such effect could be demonstrated.

Table 1 Effects of Obesity[a] in Young Women on Psychosocial Outcomes

Outcome	Adjusted difference (95% CI)
School	−0.3 year (−0.1 year, −0.6 year)
Marriage	−20% (−13%, −27%)
Household income	−$6710 (−$3942, −$9478)
Poverty	+10% (+4%, +16%)

[a] Obesity was defined as a BMI greater than the 95th centile for women of the same age studied in NHANES I. The data represent the differences in the outcomes and the confidence intervals of the differences between obese and nonobese women. Results controlled for baseline income, parental education, chronic health condition, height, self-esteem, age, and ethnicity.
Source: Ref. 13.

Few long-term studies have examined the degree to which excess adiposity in childhood predicts obesity in adulthood. Fatness and fat distribution determined by anthropometric measures in early childhood do not correlate well with fatness and fat distribution present at puberty (14). Retrospective data suggest that ~30% of obese women were overweight in adolescence, but only 10% of obese men were overweight during the same period (14). A review of the literature suggests that almost 40% of overweight children become obese adults, but only 15–20% of obese adults were overweight as children (14–16). However, there is a dose-response effect. Children who are severely overweight are more likely to remain obese as adults than are children who are moderately overweight (17). Because studies differ widely in design, populations considered, definition of overweight, the age at which subjects were measured, and the duration of follow-up, reports of the percent of overweight children who became obese adults vary from 26% to 63% (17).

More recent work on the tracking of overweight from childhood to age 21–29 years shows that for overweight young children, the risk of adult obesity is strongly influenced by obesity in one or both parents. Indeed, parental overweight has consistently been identified as a risk factor for adult obesity (10,11,18–22). Whitaker et al. (10) found among children < 3 years of age that the major predictor of obesity in young adulthood was their parents' obesity status. Compared to children < 3 years old whose parents were not obese, those with both parents obese were nearly 14 times as likely to be obese as an adult (OR = 13.6, 95% CI = 3.7–50.4). The < 3-year-old child's weight status irrespective of BMI was not predictive of adult obesity. As children aged, however, their BMI became more predictive: by age 6, the child's overweight status had become a significant predictor, and by age 15–17 an obese adolescent was 17.5 times as likely to become an obese young adult than was a nonoverweight adolescent (95% CI = 7.7–39.5) (10).

Lake and colleagues found that children with two obese parents were more likely to be overweight as children and showed the strongest tracking of any group with an elevated BMI from 7 years to age 33 years (19). In another study, changes in childhood BMI appeared to be more related to adult obesity in females than in males (11). Overweight Japanese school children became heavier adults than the general population (20).

Evidence is still inconclusive as to whether it is childhood overweight per se, the persistence of overweight, the length of time one is overweight, or being obese as an adult that increases the risk of adult morbidity and mortality (17). We have ample information from the Bogalusa Heart Study (3,23) that childhood overweight has direct implications for adverse lipid, insulin, and blood pressure levels. In this study, excess truncal fat during childhood was associated with these risk factors as well (23). Tracking studies demonstrate that ~40% of overweight children will be obese as adults (9,15,16), and the tracking of overweight is stronger at about age 18 than during early childhood and early adolescence (10,11). Overweight in childhood is associated in adulthood with early mortality, primarily due to coronary heart disease (17), type 2 diabetes mellitus, colon cancer, gestational hypertension, gout, arthritis, hip fractures, and menstrual problems (15,16).

II IDENTIFICATION AND DEFINITION

Adiposity, or the amount of body fat measured directly or indirectly, is used to determine overweight status. There are three key issues regarding the identification of overweight children: (1) whether the same measures of adiposity should be used for clinical and research purposes; (2) whether indirect measures of adiposity are adequate for screening purposes; and (3) the recommended cutoff points for defining overweight. From the point of view of those in epidemiology and public health, measures of overweight should be internationally standardized and accepted to ensure comparability of prevalence estimates within and between studies. The measures should have reasonable predictive value for morbidity and mortality, and should be easily and inexpensively obtained, especially in the clinical practice setting. In addition, if the assessment tool is not a direct measure of body fat, it should correlate well with a child's total fat.

Clinicians would no doubt share some of these preferences and would likely add that the measure should be highly specific. Having a specific measure is probably more important than having one that is highly sensitive (24) because of the great concern of psychosocial dysfunction associated with the diagnosis of overweight and the high prevalence of eating disorders among certain subsets of the pediatric population, such as adolescent girls. Thus, clinicians are likely to favor a measure that minimizes false positives, even if it does not detect all children who are overweight.

Pediatricians commonly used an indirect measure of adiposity, a weight-for-height index, to screen for overweight in children. Previously, weight-for-height was used. However, the new Centers for Disease Control and Prevention (CDC) growth charts provide weight-for-height^2, or BMI, percentiles for children ages 2–20 years, allowing a single screening tool to be used (and compared) throughout the life span after 2 years of age (25). For children < 2 years of age, weight-for-height is still the screening tool of choice to assess weight status (25). With the exception of 3- to 5-year-olds, BMI is more correlated with body fat than is weight-for-height. Among children and adolescents ages 3–19 years, the correlation coefficients between BMI and percentage of body fatness defined by pooled dual-energy x-ray absorptiometry (DXA), a direct measure of adipostiy, range from 0.78 to 0.88, which are higher than those found between DXA and weight-for-height (26). This indicates that BMI-for-age is better than weight-for-height for predicting both underweight and overweight, except among 2- to 5-year-olds, for whom the two approaches are equivalent (26). Thus, for indirectly assessing overweight, BMI can be used for all children ages 2 years and above, although weight-for-height might be substituted for those aged 2–5 years.

More direct assessment of adiposity is possible by several methods including DXA (27,28), underwater weighing, bioelectrical impedance analyses, total body water, and measurement of triceps skinfold thickness. With the exception of triceps skinfold thickness, these methods are still primarily used for research, because they are more complex to obtain and require expensive equipment. Each of these measurement techniques has different assumptions and limitations, yet the percent fat values derived from the methods are highly correlated (28–30). Unfortunately, measurement of triceps skinfold thickness requires calipers, which are not commonly available in pediatrician's offices. More importantly, reproducible skinfold measurements may be a problem. Obtaining reliable triceps skinfold measurements requires practice, and between-observer measurements are not as reproducible as measurements of height and weight. Furthermore, skinfold measurement may become less reliable as body fatness increases. Because skinfold measurements are currently the only practical direct measure of adiposity available to most clinical practice settings, we recommend using triceps skinfold measurements as the primary diagnostic method for confirming that those overweight are overfat. However, adequate staff training and monitoring of the accuracy of their measurements is crucial to obtain accurate results.

Although both triceps skinfold measures and BMI are correlated with morbidity (3,23), BMI is easier to use as an initial screening tool. BMI and weight-for-height also predict the persistence of obesity into adulthood (10,11). Thus, given all their attributes, the use of BMI (10,11,25,31) for children ages 2–20 years or weight-for-height (25,26,32) for those ages from birth to 5 years appears well suited to estimating the risks for chronic diseases, persistent obesity, or other long-term sequelae of childhood overweight.

These observations led the International Obesity Task Force (33–35) to suggest that the internationally accepted scheme of BMI cutpoints for adult morbidity be used for children and adolescents. Cole et al. (36) used these criteria to create centile curves based on the centile values identified by the adult cutpoints of 25 and 30 kg/m^2 at age 18 years. These standards have been further refined and clarified by an Expert Committee on Pediatric Obesity established by the Maternal and Child Health Bureau (37), which recommended that children and adolescents with a BMI ≥85th centile be screened for complications such as the presence of additional risk factors, including family history, blood pressure, cholesterol, and be evaluated and possibly treated (Fig. 1).

This committee recommended the following defining criteria: children with a BMI ≥85th centile and <95th centile for the same age and gender be categorized as at risk for overweight and those with a BMI ≥95th centile for the same age and gender be defined as overweight. Among children ages 2–20 years, if BMI is at or exceeds the 95th centile for the same age and gender, the diagnosis of excess adipose tissue should be confirmed by triceps skinfold thickness. In addition, it is also useful for selecting intervention strategies to know if the child or adolescent is concerned about his or her weight. Although these cutpoints were originally based on BMI cutpoints for adult morbidity, Freedman et al. (3) found these cutpoints were able to identify adverse lipid, insulin, and blood pressure in childhood as well.

III PREVALENCE

Prevalence estimates based on BMI and on triceps skinfolds have shown substantial increases in the prevalence of obesity in the United States since the 1960s (21,21a). The prevalence estimates of overweight summarized in Table 2 were based on the new CDC growth chart reference, using the gender- and age-specific 95th weight-for-length and BMI percentile cutoffs to define overweight. In 1999–2000 approximately 12% of 6–23 month olds, 10% of 2–5 yr olds, and 15% of 6–19 yr olds were overweight. For the 2–19 yr olds, there were no significant differences by gender in 1999–2000. Available data indicate that the greatest increases occurred between 1976–1980 and 1988–1994 except for 6–23 month old girls, 2–5 yr old boys, and 12–19 yr old girls, all of whom had greater increases between 1988–1994 and 1999–2000 (21a). Significant increases in the prevalence of overweight between 1988–1994 and 1999–2000 were found for non-Hispanic blacks and Mexican

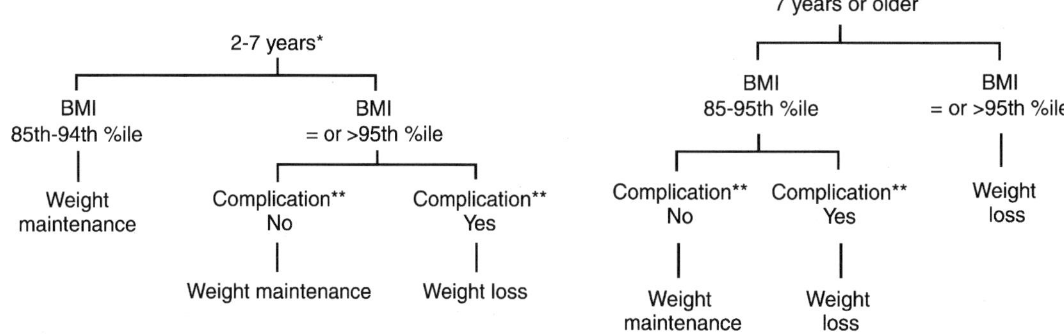

Figure 1 Recommendations for weight goals. Patients with acute complications, such as pseudotumor cerebri, sleep apnea, obesity hypoventilation syndrome, or orthopedic problems, should be referred to a pediatric obesity center. *Children younger than 2 years should be referred to a pediatric obesity center for treatment. **Complications such as mild hypertension, dyslipidemias, and insulin resistance. (From Ref. 37.)

Table 2 Prevalence of Overweight (BMI ≥95th percentile for age and gender) Between 1963 and 2000 in the United States: Children Aged 6 Months to 19 Years[a]

		Prevalence of overweight (percent)					
Age	Gender	1963–1965[b]	1966–1970[c]	1971–1974[d]	1976–1980[e]	1988–1994[f]	1999–2000[g]
6–23 mo[h]	Boys				8.2	9.9	9.8
	Girls				6.1	7.9	14.3
2–5 yr	Boys			5.0	4.7	6.1	9.9
	Girls			4.9	5.3	8.2	11.0
6–11 yr	Boys	4.0		4.3	6.6	11.6	16.0
	Girls	4.5		3.6	6.4	11.0	14.5
12–19 yr	Boys		4.5	6.1	4.8	11.3	15.5
	Girls		4.7	6.2	5.3	9.7	15.5

[a] BMI percentiles based on the CDC growth charts.
[b] National Health Examination Survey (NHES) II.
[c] NHES III.
[d] National Health and Nutrition Examination Survey I (NHANES I).
[e] NHANES II.
[f] NHANES III.
[g] NHANES.
[h] Weight-for-length ≥95th percentile is considered overweight.
Source: Ref. 21a.

American 12–19 yr olds: their prevalence of overweight increased from 13.4% to 23.6% and from 13.8% to 23.4% respectively (21a). The changes in the thickness of the triceps skinfold were of the same order of magnitude as those seen for BMI (21). Further analyses of BMI and triceps skinfold data indicated that the distributions of these data at least through 1988–1994 have become more right skewed (21,22). There were minor increases in stature between NHANES II and III, but these were not likely to have accounted for the trends seen in BMI (22). Similar analyses of low-income preschool children using the 95th percentile of weight-for-height as the cutoff documented an increase in overweight from 8.5% in 1983 to 10.2% in 1995; using the 85th percentile, the increase was from 18.6% to 21.6% (38). In addition to evidence from these large national survey data, secular increases in relative weight and adiposity have occurred among children in the Bogalusa Heart Study (39).

Racial/ethnic and socioeconomic characteristics affect the prevalence of overweight in children and adolescents. For children and adolescents from 6 months to 19 yrs old, the prevalence of overweight was greater among non-Hispanic blacks and Mexican Americans than for non-Hispanic whites, with the exception of 2–5 yr olds (21a). The presumed lower acculturation of Mexican American children may be associated with their higher prevalence of overweight, as this association defined as adopting the language of a culture in the first two generations has been observed in Mexican American women (40). Native American children appear at particularly high risk for overweight (41,42): among Navajo 6 to 12 year-olds the prevalence of overweight was 15.2% for boys and 21.1% for girls (43). In contrast to adults, the prevalence of overweight in NHANES III in childhood varied less consistently with socioeconomic status than in previous national surveys. In NHANES III, the only significant association with socioeconomic status was an inverse relationship between family income for non-Hispanic white adolescents and the prevalence of overweight (21).

International comparisons of the prevalence of overweight (weight-for-height >2.0 SD above the NCHS/WHO reference median) showed that preschool children in Australia and Canada had a higher prevalence of overweight than their counterparts in the United States, while preschoolers in Japan and the United Kingdom had a lower prevalence than did those in the United States (44). A study of the prevalence and trends of overweight among preschool children in 94 countries found a global prevalence of 3.3% with wide variation (44). Developing countries with the highest prevalence were in the Middle East (Qatar), North Africa (Algeria, Egypt, Morocco), and Latin America (Argentina, Chile, Bolivia, Peru, Uruguay, Costa Rica, and Jamaica). Other countries with a high prevalence that were not included in these regions were Armenia, Kiribati, Malawi, South Africa, and Uzbekistan (44).

In Africa and Asia, the prevalence of wasting (weight-for-height <2 SD below the NCHS/WHO reference median) was 2.5–3.5 times higher than that of overweight (44). Other country reports found that mean BMI appeared to be increasing rapidly among children and adolescents in Denmark (45), Italy (46), Bahrain (47), and Brazil (48).

In the 94-country study cited above, the prevalence of overweight increased in 16 of 38 countries for which trend data were available (44). In Latin American and Caribbean countries, however, no increased trend in the prevalence of overweight among preschool children was apparent (49). Canadian researchers documented even greater secular trends in the increase in prevalence of overweight among children than has been reported in the United States (50) (Table 3). Between 1981 and 1996, the prevalence of overweight (BMI >95th centile) among 13- to 17-year-old Canadians increased from 5% in both boys and girls to 13.5% in boys and 11.8% in girls (50). In contrast, between 1976 and 1994, the prevalence of overweight (BMI >95th centile) among 12- to 17-year-old Americans increased from 4.6% to 12.2% in white boys and from 4.2% to 9.4% in white girls (21). Changes in prevalence over time are reported

Table 3 International Secular Trends in the Prevalence Overweight and at Risk for Overweight Among Children and Adolescents

Country	Reference	Age	Samples	Indices	Change in prevalence
Canada (national)	50	7–13 yr	1981: 4176 1996: 7847	BMI >85th	Boys: 15 to 28.8% Girls: 15 to 23.6%
				>95th	Boys: 5 to 13.5% Girls: 5 to 11.8%
Great Britain (region, Wirral Health Authority)	51	2 yr 11 mo to 4 yr	1989: 2728 1998: 2633	BMI >85th >95th	Children: 14.7 to 23.6% Children: 5.4 to 9.2%
France (national)	52	5–19 yr	1980: NA 1991: NA	BMI >85th	1980: children 15% 1991: boys 18%, girls, 20%
Germany (city, Jena)	53	7–14 yr	1985: 1536 1995: 1901	BMI for French children >90th	Boys: 11.8 to 16.3% Girls: 13.0 to 20.7%
				>97th	Boys: 6.1 to 8.2% Girls: 5.3 to 9.9%
Spain (region, Aragón)	54	6–7 yr 13–14 yr	1985 to 1996 6–7 yr = 90997 13–14 yr = 106284	BMI >85th	Boys 6–7: ~6 to ~14% Girls 6–7: ~10 to ~18% 13–14 Boys: ~3 to ~6% 13–14 Girls: ~1 to ~1.5%
Chile (national)	55	5–8 yr	1987: NA 1996: NA	Weight-for-height (WHO) >2 SD	Boys: 6.5 to 13.1% Girls: 7.7 to 14.7%
Bolivia (national)	56	1–5 yr	1989: NA 1997: 4860	Weight-for-height >85th >95th	 Children: 15.9 to 22.7% Children: 2.1 to 4.6%
Dominican Republic (national)	56	1–5 yr	1986: NA 1996: 2984	Weight-for-height >85th >95th	 Children: 12.3 to 15.3% Children: 2.6 to 4.6%
Guatemala (national)	56	1–5 yr	1981: NA 1996: 6477	Weight-for-height >85th >95th	 Children: 4.9 to 10.0% Children: 0.5 to 2.0%
Peru (national)	56	1–5 yr	1992: NA 1996: 11796	Weight-for-height >85th >95th	 Children: 20.6 to 23.9% Children: 3.9 to 4.7%
United States (national)	56	1–5 yr	1975: NA 1988–1994: 4112	Weight-for-height >85th >95th	 Children: 12.5 to 15.3% Children: 2.8 to 3.1%

NA = Not available.

in Table 3 for a sample of developed and developing countries.

IV CHANGES IN ADIPOSITY WITH AGE

Adiposity changes dramatically in childhood and adolescence. In an early and important series of studies of the body composition of children and adolescents, Cheek described their changes in body fat, determined by measuring body composition with deuterium oxide (57). Based on Cheek's data, body fat as a percentage of body weight in boys increases in the prepubertal phase of growth, then declines coincident with the growth spurt. In contrast, fat as a percentage of body weight remains relatively constant in girls prior to adolescence but increases during the adolescent growth spurt. Between the ages of 10 and 15 years, Cheek estimated that body fat as a percentage of body weight declined from 17.8% to 11.2% in boys but rose from 16.6% to 23.5% in girls. Similar changes were subsequently described by other investigators (58).

Studies of adipocyte size and number in infancy and childhood demonstrate substantial age-dependent variations in their contribution to body fat mass (59,60). Cross-sectional and longitudinal studies of adipocyte numbers indicate that adipocyte numbers increase modestly throughout infancy and childhood in nonoverweight children, but that a pronounced and significant increase occurs after age 10 years. In contrast, the size of fat cells increases to adult levels in late infancy, after which it decreases to the level observed in early infancy in nonoverweight children (59), then remains constant until adolescence. Fat cell size in overweight children continues to increase to adult levels coincident with the development of overweight, after which the cells do not increase in size again until adolescence. In addition, overweight children have more adipocytes than do nonoverweight children, regardless of the age at which they are studied. These data indicate that in late infancy, increases in body fat in nonoverweight children may be primarily attributable to increases in adipocyte size, whereas after age 10 years, increases in body fat in these children reflect an increase in both adipocyte size and number. Among overweight children, both adipocyte size and number are increased from the time they become overweight, irrespective of their age. Weight loss reduces adipocyte size, but does not affect adipocyte number (61).

Changes in the thickness of triceps skinfold parallel the changes in body fat described by Cheek (62). Beginning at age 4–5 years, the triceps skinfold begins to increase slightly in girls, subsequently increasing more rapidly coincident with the increases in body fat that accompany their growth spurt. In boys, skinfold thickness decreases around age 4 years, increases 1 or 2 years before adolescence, and subsequently decreases coincident with the increase in fat-free mass and decrease in fat mass that accompanies the male adolescent growth spurt.

BMI increases over the first year of life in both boys and girls, then declines to its nadir at age 4–7 years. Thereafter, the BMI begins to increase again in both males and females (63). Clinicians can use the triceps skinfold to clarify whether an increased BMI reflects an increase in frame size and muscle mass or an increase in body fat.

Changes in the distribution of body fat begin immediately prior to adolescence and continue to change throughout this period of rapid growth (14,64). In both genders, body fat shifts from a peripheral to a central distribution. In girls, cross-sectional studies have found that ratios of trunk-to-extremity skinfold thicknesses begin to increase at ~8 years of age and plateau by about age 12 years. In comparable studies of boys, the increase in the trunk:extremity skinfold ratio begins between 10 and 11 years of age, perhaps coincident with their preadolescent increase in fatness. In contrast to girls, no plateau in these ratios appears to occur in boys. By late adolescence, body fat distribution becomes more centralized in males than in females.

The limited studies available suggest that visceral fat deposition also changes substantially through childhood and adolescence. Visceral fat occupies ~50% of the cross-sectional abdominal fat area in 11- to 13-year-old children (65–67), but between adolescence and adulthood, this area increases four- to fivefold (68). However, these measurements are probably not as relevant metabolically as the ratio of intra-abdominal adipose tissue to total body fat. As Goran et al. have pointed out, the ratio of intra-abdominal adipose tissue to total body fat almost triples from early childhood to adulthood (65). Longitudinal or cross-sectional studies to examine the interrelationships between visceral and total body fat in adolescents, and the relationship of changes in the ratio of intra-abdominal to visceral fat to the timing of puberty, have not yet been done.

Although the foregoing studies do not encompass the entire range of childhood and adolescence, they suggest that the most rapid increases in visceral fat occur in late adolescence. In adults, body fatness relates directly to the quantity of visceral fat deposition, and the relationship between total and visceral fat differs by gender (68).

No such data are yet available for adolescents, but a similar relationship would be expected. The mechanisms that control the location and quantity of fat deposited, as well as those that control the changes in body fat that occur at adolescence, remain unclear. As for observed differences in relative weight and overweight between black and white, adolescents (21), analyses of the Bogalusa Heart Study data have shown that after controlling for height, mean relative weight of black girls was consistently greater than that of white girls after the age of 13, and that sexual maturation was a stronger correlate of relative weight among black girls than white girls (69), but we don't know if the higher weight is due to increased adiposity, lean body mass, or heavier bones.

V CRITICAL PERIODS FOR THE DEVELOPMENT OF OVERWEIGHT

The likelihood that childhood overweight will persist, and therefore the likelihood of adverse consequences of childhood obesity in adulthood, may be related to its age of onset (70). There is a growing body of evidence that two periods and possibly a third appear to constitute specific periods of increased risk for persistence and subsequent disease: the prenatal period, "adiposity rebound," and the period of adolescence. At present, the mechanisms entrained at these periods to promote the increased risk of persistence of obesity or its complications remain poorly understood. In addition, stunting during childhood appears to put children at risk for the development of overweight; this will briefly be discussed in this section.

The most compelling data to suggest that the prenatal period constitutes a period of increased risk for persistent adiposity derive from studies of infants of mothers who had diabetes during pregnancy. Regardless of whether their diabetes was gestational, insulin-dependent, or non-insulin-dependent, these infants tend to be fatter at birth than those whose mothers were nondiabetic or prediabetic during pregnancy (71). Long-term follow-up of infants whose mothers had diabetes suggests they have an increased prevalence of obesity at later ages that extends through adolescence (72). Shorter-term studies further suggest that body weight in such infants normalizes by about 1 year of age but subsequently begins to be higher than the norm between ages 5 and 7 years (73). Pregravid overweight status of the mother has been associated with macrosomia independent of maternal age, smoking status, race/ethnicity, height, parity, gestational age, and sex of infant (74). In turn, children who were large for gestational age at birth have greater and progressively increasing adiposity through 3–6 years of age than do their normal-size counterparts (75).

The argument that fetal life represents a critical period for adiposity has not been totally resolved, the evidence from the infants of mothers with diabetes notwithstanding. Several large studies have shown an association between high birth weight and child adiposity (75–78) or adult adiposity after controlling for gestational age (77,78), but most did not adjust for confounding variables such as parental fatness, maternal smoking, gestational diabetes, or socioeconomic status (79). Conversely, low birth weight may be associated with an increase in intra-abdominal fat deposition that may in turn account for an increased likelihood of risk factors for cardiovascular disease, including hypertension, diabetes, and hyperlipidemia (80). However, the association between lower birth weight and the development of overweight has not been clearly demonstrated. Although babies with lower birth weight have been shown to have an increased risk of syndrome X and of heart and pulmonary disease in adulthood (81), it is not clear that these consequences are mediated by excess adiposity.

The second period of apparent increased risk for later obesity, "adiposity rebound," involves early acceleration of the BMI after its nadir at 4–7 years of age. This phenomenon appears to be associated with an increased risk of later obesity (82,83). That infants of mothers with gestational or insulin-dependent diabetes during pregnancy also appear to have onset of overweight during this period (74) raises questions as to whether early acceleration of the BMI after its nadir is a risk for later obesity. Other research shows that parental obesity is also associated with early adiposity rebound (84) and that early rebound may reflect overweight associated with maternal diabetes. Thus, whether there exists a true period of risk for the development of overweight at this time, independent of maternal diabetes and/or parental overweight, remains unclear.

Although adiposity rebound has been associated with adult adiposity, this may only be an epiphenomenon (85). Increased BMI at rebound has not yet been associated with higher body fat, nor do we know whether the increased BMI observed in adults who have had early rebound is attributable to greater body fat. In addition, whether age at rebound or the size of the BMI at rebound has the greater influence on adult BMI remains unclear. New evidence shows that the BMI at age 7 years and age at rebound both predict adult BMI (86), and a positive association has been found between childhood height at age 5 years and adult BMI (87).

The final developmental stage of increased risk, adolescence, may be much more of a concern for females than for males. Females, who mature earlier, are at increased risk for greater BMIs as adults (88,89); the relationship for males is less clear. In addition, while ~30% of obesity present in 36-year-old-women may begin in adolescence, only about 10% may begin then in males (32).

Some evidence from developing countries indicates an increase in overweight among stunted children, but this may be a spurious finding due to limitations in the indices used to define overweight and metabolic differences. As indicated in the first section of this chapter, indices used for evaluating relative weight, such as BMI and weight-for-height, do not directly measure body fat. In the case of stunted children, those with increased BMIs may have an excess of body fat, heavier bones, or larger muscles. On the other hand, metabolic defects may contribute. In Brazil, mild stunting was associated with the percentage of energy from fat and weight gain, suggesting that stunted children may be more susceptible to the effects of a high-fat diet than other children (90). Still another possibility is that stunted children may be more likely to have impaired fat oxidation (91). Evidence from a longitudinal study in Guatemala has shown that severely stunted children have increased abdominal fatness as adults, after controlling for fatness and other confounders (92).

VI ENVIRONMENTAL ASSOCIATIONS

Most of the variables associated with childhood and adolescent obesity can be categorized under the physical, behavioral, or social environment.

A The Physical Environment

A U.S. study published in 1984 found that childhood overweight (defined as triceps >95th centile among those included in the study) was associated with region, season, and population density (93), with each of these variables doubling or tripling risk. Compared to the West, the odds ratios for overweight adjusted for region and season of were 3.0 in the Northeast, 2.6 in the Midwest, and 1.2 in the South. Within each region, rates of obesity increased in the winter and spring and decreased in the summer and fall. Also in each region, obesity was more prevalent in highly urbanized areas than in those less densely populated. The mechanisms that accounted for the environmental associations were not clear.

B The Behavioral Environment

Dietary intake and the energy spent on activity represent the only discretionary components of energy intake and expenditure. Over the past 30 years, important changes have occurred in family eating patterns, including greater consumption of fast food, carbonated beverages, and preprepared meals. At the same time, some children are less physically active because of increased use of cars, concern for neighborhood safety, and decreased opportunity for physical activity at school or on the way to school. Children's time spent watching television and playing video games has increased. Both the food intake and physical activity of young children are strongly influenced by their parents. Although the literature that examines the effect of the potential risk factors for overweight in children is growing, as yet there are few longitudinal studies of adequate duration and rigor that have identified causal factors.

1 Breastfeeding

Breastfeeding may protect against subsequent overweight in childhood. Two review papers on this topic published in 1999 and in 2001 both failed to find conclusive evidence of a significant positive effect of breastfeeding (79,94). Nonetheless, well-designed studies with large samples that controlled for potential confounders have demonstrated a protective effect of breastfeeding against overweight in childhood. Von Kries et al. (95) found that infants who were ever breastfed were 0.75 (95% Confidence Interval [CI] = 0.57–0.98) times as likely to be overweight (BMI >90th centile German schoolchildren) at 5–6 years of age. Gillman et al. (96) found that infants who were exclusively or mostly breastfed were 0.78 (95% CI = 0.66–0.81) times as likely to be overweight (BMI >95th centile NCHS/CDC reference) at 9–14 years of age. Both studies found a dose-response effect: breastfeeding of at least 6 or 7 months was more protective than <3 months. Although the Hediger et al. study (NHANES III) found an insignificant protective effect (odds ratio for mostly breastfeeding was 0.84, 95% CI = 0.62–1.13) (97), the small sample size of overweight children in this study may have influenced their ability to document a protective effect. Only ~300 of ~2700 children were overweight by 3–5 years of age (97).

2 Dietary Practice

The behavior and practices of parents strongly influences the dietary intake of their children. During childhood, parental intake of carbohydrate, fat, and energy appears to account for 23–97% of the variance in children's intakes of these nutrients (98). However, family resemblances in nutrient intake may reflect familial resemblances only in body size, since we do not know from this study whether actual BMIs were comparable. This possibility is strengthened by the observation that the relationship between the preferences of parents and children for specific sets of foods does not differ substantially from the relationship between the preferences of children and unrelated adults (99). Resemblances in nutrient intake, when they occur, appear to reflect a common environment rather than a genetically mediated preference for macronutrients (100).

The family environment has the potential to promote healthy eating. For example, children who eat meals with their family consume more fruits and vegetables, have a more nutritionally dense diet with less of their energy intake derived from fat, and drink fewer carbonated and sugared beverages than do children who do not eat with their families (101). A recent summary of the intakes of youth ages 2–19 years, based on the U.S. Department of Agriculture's 1989–1991 Continuing Surveys of Food Intakes by Individuals, documented that American children have a widespread need for improvement in their diets (102). Indeed, the authors found that only 1% of youth met their recommended intake of nutrients, and membership in this small group was associated with excess intake, especially of fat (102). Daily consumption of three meals of approximately equal energy content may be another potential strategy to reduce adiposity in children (103). Further evidence that food patterns may contribute to overweight is the association between incident overweight and the consumption of sugar-sweetened drinks in school children (104). Interestingly, the available trend data on energy intake among children suggest that it has not changed over ~20 years: total energy intake did not change between 1973 and 1994 among 10-year-old children in the Bogalusa Heart Study (105).

3 Child Feeding Practices

Children appear quite capable of self-regulating their dietary intake in unsupervised settings. Their meal-to-meal variation in energy intake is substantial, but variation in day-to-day energy intake is considerably lower (106). Certain parent-child interactions at feeding may disrupt the ability of the child to regulate intake; the more parents encourage the consumption of certain foods, the less likely children are to eat them (107). Conversely, restricting access to certain foods appears to encourage their consumption when children have access to them (107). In a setting in which the ability of children to adjust their food intake in response to the caloric density of the diet was measured, children whose mothers were more controlling of their food intake were less capable of self-regulation of food intake, and these children had greater body fat stores (108). However, whether the lack of self-regulation is a cause or a consequence of the mother's control remains uncertain. At least two longitudinal studies of children suggest that parental control of child intake is not associated with energy intake and the development of overweight (109,110).

Interestingly, lack of knowledge about a child's intake is also associated with impairment of self-regulation. As a recent Danish study showed (111), the risk of subsequent overweight among 9- to 10-year-old children was not increased by their frequency of consuming sweets or when the mother accepted the child's consumption of sweets, but it was increased significantly if the mother lacked knowledge about her offspring's sweet-eating habits independent of their degree of fatness in childhood, their gender, and their social background.

Parental neglect has predicted overweight in young adulthood independent of gender, age, socioeconomic status, and childhood BMI (112). Additional observations have suggested that psychosocial stress is associated with rapid rates of weight gain (113,114). The greater effects of stress on weight gain in girls may emphasize both their biologic susceptibility to obesity in early puberty, as well as the adverse social effects that obesity imposes on them. In the studies cited, the retrospective collection of data represents a potential source of bias. In addition, these observations do not eliminate the possibility that rapid weight gain caused an increase in psychosocial problems rather than the reverse.

4 Physical Activity and Sedentary Behavior

Both activity and inactivity appear to affect the risk of obesity and its complications in childhood and adolescence. In preschoolers, for example, the energy spent on activity appears inversely related to fatness (115). Whether decreased nonbasal energy expenditure on physical activity increases the risk for developing childhood or adolescent overweight has not been clearly established. As shown in Table 4, the proportion of energy spent on activity, expressed as a ratio of total energy expenditure, appears to increase from infancy and early childhood to adolescence. One explanation for this intuitively unlikely result is that lower nonbasal energy expenditure of early childhood may reflect increased time spent sleeping rather than a decrease in the energy spent on activity.

Not surprisingly, the prevalence of physical activity and sedentary behavior, as well as factors associated with activity levels and overweight in children and adolescents, has varied by study. Unfortunately, the lack of consistency in measures or categories of physical activity and sedentary activity and differences in the samples or populations studied make comparing them difficult. In general, physical activity among children appears to have decreased significantly. For example, research in the United Kingdom among 0- to 14-year-old children found that between 1985 and 1992 the average distance walked annually decreased by 20% and the distance cycled by 26%, while the distance traveled by car increased 40% (121). In their review of studies, Parsons et al. found no association between activity before children are old enough to walk and later fatness; no consistent association was found between activity after children could walk and subsequent fatness (79). Analyses of the NHANES III data found that 80% of 8- to 16-year-old children participated in three or more episodes of vigorous activity each week; rates were lower in non-Hispanic black and Mexican-American girls (122). The Youth Risk Behavior Survey for 1999 and the National Longitudinal Study of Adolescent Health data for 1996 found that approximately two-thirds of youths in grades 7–12 participated in three or more episodes of vigorous activity each week, and minority females other than Asians had lower levels (123,124). One objective for Healthy People 2010 is to increase vigorous physical activity episodes of 20 minutes or more to at least 3 days per week for 85% of adolescents (125). The survey data above demonstrate that non-Hispanic black and Hispanic (or Mexican-American) females are not meeting this objective.

Table 4 Ratio (SD) of Mean Energy Expenditure of Activity to Mean Resting Energy Expenditure for Children and Adolescents. Data Expressed as the Ratio of Total Energy Expenditure (kcal/day)/Resting or Sleeping Energy Expenditure (kcal/day) Metabolic Rate[a]

Age group (Ref.)	Males	Combined[b]	Females
Infants (116)		1.35 (.29)	
5 years (117)	1.36 (.13)		1.40 (.17)
9–12 years (118)	1.61 (.23)		1.53 (.28)
12–18 years (119)	1.79 (.20)		1.69 (.28)

[a] All studies measured total energy expenditure using the doubly labeled water method. The infant study (116) predicted basal energy expenditure from body weight based on the equation from Schofield (120). The other three studies used ventilated-hood indirect calorimetry to determine basal or resting energy expenditure.
[b] Data not differentiated by gender.

A recent review of studies (126) conducted between 1970 and 1998 found consistent positive correlations of physical activity in children (4–12 years old) with gender (male), having overweight parents, healthy diet, previous physical activity, intention to be physically active, preference for physical activity, access to facilities, and time spent outdoors. The only consistent negative correlate in this review was perceived barriers to physical activity (126). No associations were found between physical activity and socioeconomic status, race/ethnicity, body image, self-esteem, perceived benefits, attitudes toward sweating, other after-school activity, alcohol use, smoking, caloric intake, neighborhood safety, or parents providing transportation (126). In the same review, among adolescents 13–18 years old, physical activity correlated with gender (male), race/ethnicity (white), perceived competence in the activity, intentions to be physically active, previous physical activity, community sports, sensation seeking, parental support, support from others, sibling physical activity, direct help from parents, and opportunities to exercise. The only consistently negative correlates were depression and sedentary activities after school and on weekends (126). In 1996, the Surgeon General's Report (Physical Activity and Health), which reviewed the literature through 1995, found slightly different associations (127). To verify that the potential determinants listed are causally related to physical activities, they need to be examined prospectively and in concert with other potentially associated variables.

Evidence is now available from cross-sectional studies that strongly suggest that television watching is a risk factor for overweight (128,129). In their recent examination of the association among television watching, energy intake, and overweight in U.S. children based on the nationally representative NHANES III, Crespo et al. found that the prevalence of overweight (BMI > 95th centile in NHANES II and III data) was lowest among children who watched ≤1 hr of television per day and highest among those who watched ≥4 hr daily (128). Further analyses of the NHANES III data showed that among the 26% of children who watched ≥4 hr of television per day, body fat and BMI were higher than among those who watched <2 hr (122). Data from the Framingham Children's Study showed that when age, television viewing, energy intake, baseline triceps, and parents' BMI were controlled, inactive children were 3.8 times as likely to have increasing triceps skinfold measurements between age 4 years and entry into the first grade than were active children (130).

Activity levels seem to have a strong familial component. The higher familial correlations for activity within than across generations suggest that the environment is more important than genetics (131). Intensive analyses of a large cohort representing almost 400 families confirmed the observation that stronger correlations of physical activity occurred within the same generation (132), but they also demonstrated a heritability of 29% for level of habitual physical activity. No genetic effect was found for exercise participation (132). In recent studies in which we compared parent and child patterns of activity (personal communication, William H. Dietz, May 25, 2001), measures of vigorous activity were better correlated between spouses than between mother-daughter or father-daughter pairs. In contrast, time watching television was better correlated within families. These results suggest that patterns of inactivity, but not patterns of activity, are correlated within families.

C Social Environment

Socioeconomic status has not been consistently associated with overweight in childhood, but two studies that controlled for parental fatness found negative associations between parental education and childhood BMI (133,134). In contrast, there is a strong consistent, positive relationship between low socioeconomic status in childhood and fatness in adulthood (79). If women change social class as adults, they are likely to reflect the prevalence of obesity in the social class they join (32,135).

VII SCREENING OVERWEIGHT

Now that we have an accepted standardized screening tool for identifying overweight and risk of overweight in children, it is important that all infants and children be evaluated for their weight status by their primary care physician. As mentioned previously, Figure 1 gives recommendations for weight goals and referrals to pediatric obesity centers recommended by the Expert Committee on Pediatric Obesity (37).

The evidence that childhood overweight increases the risk of comorbidity in both childhood and in adulthood emphasizes the need to identify overweight children with other risk factors as early as possible. The Expert Committee (37) also recommends that all children and adolescents with a BMI ≥85th centile be screened for complications, evaluated, and possibly treated, depending on the findings. The complications that should be sought include hypertension, dyslipidemias, orthopedic disorders, sleep disorders, gallbladder disease, and insulin resistance. In addition, a recent large change in a child's BMI should also be evaluated. The Expert Committee emphasized that clinicians should also seek signs of exogenous obesity such as genetic syndromes, endocrinologic disease, and psychologic disorders. In addition to screening, the committee advocated that an in-depth medical assessment be done for all children and adolescents with a BMI ≥95th centile.

This committee also recommended early treatment that involved the family as much as possible. The family's readiness to make changes in diet and lifestyle should determine the pace and intensity of treatment. The family's ability to take responsibility for the lifestyle changes is key to progress and success.

VIII SUMMARY AND IMPLICATIONS FOR CLINICAL PRACTICE AND PUBLIC HEALTH

In the past two decades, obesity has become one of the most prevalent nutritional diseases among children and adolescents in North America. Comparable international data demonstrate that the prevalence of overweight is also increasing rapidly in developed and developing countries outside of North America. The substantial effects of childhood overweight on morbidity and mortality indicate that effective prevention and therapy for this problem may well have a large impact on the incidence of adult disease. Programs aimed at treatment of overweight children appear to have a substantially better long-term success rate than similar programs in adults (136). Effective interventions to prevent childhood overweight, greater allocation of health care resources, and reimbursement for the treatment of obesity are needed for primary care practitioners to be effective in preventing overweight during childhood. Intervention strategies need to include interventions that address the range of potential risk factors and critical periods. For example, improved understanding of the incentives that promote the initiation and extended duration of breastfeeding, and the elimination of the barriers that lead to early termination of breastfeeding, must become high priorities. Work site facilities and policies that allow mothers who must return to work to continue to provide breast milk for their infants may represent one of the policy shifts necessary to help address the overweight epidemic (137).

In the public health sector, states are developing state obesity plans that include targeting their high-risk populations and testing intervention programs in these groups. Fresh new ideas for increasing physical activity need to be included at the community level. For example, community planners need to consider opportunities for family physical activity, such as sidewalks, neighborhoods with stores and schools within walking distance, and community parks. Efforts must be directed toward the identification of children who are overweight or at risk for overweight in childhood and toward the propagation of successful treatment and prevention strategies.

REFERENCES

1. Strauss RS. Childhood obesity and self-esteem. Pediatrics 2000; 105(1). URL: http://www.pediatrics.org/cgi/content/full/full/105/1/e15.
2. Davison KK, Birch LL. Weight status, parent reaction, and self-concept in five-year-old girls. Pediatrics 2001; 107:46–53.
3. Freedman DS, Dietz WH, Srinivasan SR, Berenson GS. The relation of overweight to cardiovascular risk factors among children and adolescents: the Bogalusa Heart Study. Pediatrics 1999; 103:1175–1182.
4. Ford ES, Galuska DA, Gillespie C, Will JC, Giles WH, Dietz WH. C-reactive protein and body mass index: findings from the Third National Health and Nutrition Examination Survey, 1988–1994. J Pediatr 2001; 138:486–492.
5. American Diabetes Association. Type 2 diabetes in children and adolescents. Pediatrics 2000; 105:671–680.
6. Garn SM, Clark DC. Nutrition, growth, development, and maturation: findings from the ten-state nutrition survey of 1968–1970. Pediatrics 1975; 56:306–319.
7. Kinugasa A, Tsunamoto K, Furukawa N, et al. Fatty liver and its fibrous changes found in a simple obesity of children. J Pediatr Gastroenterol Nutr 1984; 3:408–414.
8. Crichlow RW, Seltzer MH, Jannetta PJ. Cholecystitis in adolescents. Dig Dis 1972; 17:68–72.
9. Dietz WH. Health consequences of obesity in youth: childhood predictors of adult disease. Pediatrics 1998; 101(suppl 3):518S–525S.
10. Whitaker RC, Wright JA, Pepe MS, Seidel KD, Dietz WH. Predicting obesity in young adulthood from childhood and parental obesity. N Engl J Med 1997; 337:869–873.
11. Guo SS, Huang C, Maynard KM, et al. Body mass index during childhood, adolescence and young adulthood in relation to adult overweight and adiposity: the Fels Longitudinal Study. Int J Obes Relat Metab Disord 2000; 24:1628–1635.
12. Must A, Jacques PF, Dallal GE, Bajema CJ, Dietz WH. Long-term morbidity and mortality of overweight adolescents. A follow-up of the Harvard Growth Study of 1922 to 1935. N Engl J Med 1992; 327:1350–1355.
13. Gortmaker SL, Must A, Perrin JM, Sobol AM, Dietz WH. Social and economic consequences of overweight in adolescence and young adulthood. N Engl J Med 1993; 329:1008–1012.
14. Roche AF, Baumgartner RN. Tracking in fat distribution during growth. In: Bouchard C, Johnston FE, eds. Fat Distribution During Growth and Later Health Outcomes. New York: Alan R. Liss, Inc., 1988.
15. Must A, Strauss RS. Risks and consequences of childhood and adolescent obesity. Int J Obes Relat Metab Disord 1999;23(suppl2):S2–S11.
16. Power C, Lake JK, Cole TJ. Measurement and long-term health risks of child and adolescent fatness. Int J Obes Relat Metab Disord 1997;21:507–526.
17. Freedman DS, Serdula MK, Kettel Khan L. The adult consequences of childhood obesity. In: Chen C and Dietz WH, eds. Obesity in Childhood and Adolescence. Nestlé Nutrition Workshop Series. Vol 49. Vevey, Switzerland: Nestec Ltd., and Philadelphia, PA: Lippincott Williams & Wilkins, 2002.
18. Serdula MK, Ivery D, Coates RJ, Freedman DS, Williamson DF, Byers T. Do obese children become obese adults? A review of the literature. Prev Med 1993; 22:167–177.
19. Lake JK, Power C, Cole TJ. Child to adult body mass index in the 1958 British birth cohort: associations with parental obesity. Arch Dis Child 1997; 77:376–381.
20. Kotani K, Nishida M, Yamashita S, et al. Two decades of annual medical examinations in Japanese obese children: do obese children grow into obese adults? Int J Obes Relat Metab Disord 1997;21:912–921.
21. Troiano RP, Flegal KM. Overweight children and adolescents: description, epidemiology, and demographics. Pediatrics 1998;101:497–504.

21a. Ogden CL, Flegal KM, Carroll MD, Johnson CL. Prevalence and trends in overweight among U.S. children and adolescents, 1999–2000. JAMA 2002; 288: 1728–1732.

22. Flegal KM, Troiano RP. Changes in the distribution of body mass index of adults and children in the U.S.

population. Int J Obes Relat Metab Disord 2000;24: 807–818.

23. Freedman DS, Serdula MK, Srinivasan SR, Berenson GS. Relation of circumferences and skinfold thicknesses to lipid and insulin concentrations in children and adolescents: the Bogalusa Heart Study. Am J Clin Nutr 1999;69:308–317.
24. Himes JH, Bouchard C. Validity of anthropometry in classifying youths as obese. Int J Obes 1989;13: 183–193.
25. Kuczmarski RJ, Ogden CL, Guo SS, et al. 2000 CDC growth charts for the United States: methods and development. National Center for Health Statistics. Vital Health Stat 11(246), 2002.
26. Mei A, Grummer-Strawn LM, Peitrobelli A, Goulding A, Goran MI, Dietz WH. Validity of the body mass index compared to other body composition screening indices in the assessment of body fatness for children and adolescents. Am J Clin Nutr 2002; 75:978–985.
27. Goran MI, Driscoll P, Johnson R, Nagy TR, Hunter G. Cross-calibration of body-composition techniques against dual-energy x-ray absorptiometry in young children. Am J Clin Nutr 1996; 63:299–305.
28. Gutin B, Litaker M, Islam S, Manos T, Smith C, Treiber F. Body-composition measurement in 9-11-year-old children by dual-energy x-ray absorptiometry, skinfold-thickness measurements, and bioimpedance analyses. Am J Clin Nutr 1996;63:287–292.
29. Maynard LM, Wisemandle W, Roche AF, Chumlea WC, Guo SS, Siervogel RM. Childhood body composition in relation to body mass index. Pediatrics 2001;107:344–350.
30. Cohn SH, Ellis KJ, Vartsky D, Sawitsky A, Gartenhaus W, Yasumura S, Vaswani AN. Comparison of methods of estimating body fat in normal subjects and cancer patients. Am J Clin Nutr 1981;34:2839–2847.
31. Must A, Dallal GE, Dietz WH. Reference data for obesity: 85th and 95th percentiles of body mass index (wt/ht^2) and triceps skinfold thickness—a correction. Am J Clin Nutr 1991;54:773.
32. Braddon FEM, Rodgers B, Wadsworth MEJ, Davies JMC. Onset of obesity in a 36 year birth cohort. BMJ 1986;293:299–303.
33. Himes JH, Dietz WH. Guidelines for overweight in adolescent preventive services: recommendations from an expert committee. The Expert Committee on Clinical Guidelines for Overweight in Adolescent Preventive Services. Am J Clin Nutr 1994;59:307–316.
34. Dietz WH, Robinson TN. Use of the body mass index (BMI) as a measure of overweight in children and adolescents. J Pediatr 1998;132:191–193.
35. Bellizzi MC, Dietz WH. Workshop on childhood obesity: summary of the discussion. Am J Clin Nutr 1999; 70:173S–175S.
36. Cole TJ, Bellizzi MC, Flegal KM, Dietz WH. Establishing a standard definition for child overweight and obesity worldwide: international survey. BMJ 2000;320: 1240–1243.
37. Barlow SE, Deitz WH. Obesity evaluation and treatment: Expert Committee recommendations. The Maternal and Child Health Bureau, Health Resources and Services Administration and the Department of Health and Human Services. Pediatrics 1998;102(3). URL: http://www.pediatrics.org/cgi/content/full/102/3/e29.
38. Mei Z, Scanlon KS, Grummer-Strawn LM, Freedman DS, Yip R, Trowbridge FL. Increasing prevalence of overweight among US low-income preschool children: the Centers for Disease Control and Prevention pediatric nutrition surveillance, 1983 to 1995. Pediatrics 1998; 101(1). URL: http://www.pediatrics.org/cgi/content/full/101/l/el2.
39. Freedman DS, Srinivasan SR, Valdez RA, Williamson DF, Berenson GS. Secular increases in relative weight and adiposity among children over two decades: the Bogalusa Heart Study. Pediatrics 1997;99: 420–426.
40. Khan LK, Sobal J, Martorell R. Acculturation, socioeconomic status, and obesity in Mexican Americans, Cuban Americans, and Puerto Ricans. Int J Obes Relat Metab Disord 1997;21:91–96.
41. Broussard BA, Sugarman JR, Bachman-Carter K, et al. Toward comprehensive obesity prevention programs in Native American communities. Obes Res 1995;3(suppl 2):289S–297S.
42. Freedman DS, Serdula MK, Percy CA, Ballew C, White L. Obesity, levels of lipids and glucose, and smoking among Navajo adolescents. J Nutr 1997; 127: 2120S–2127S.
43. Eisenmann JC, Katzmarzyk PT, Arnall DA, Kanuho V, Interpreter C, Malina RM. Growth and overweight of Navajo youth: secular changes from 1955 to 1997. Int J Obes Relat Metab Disord 2000; 24:211–218.
44. De Onis M, Blössner M. Prevalence and trends of overweight among preschool children in developing countries. Am J Clin Nutr 2000;72:1032–1039.
45. Thomsen BL, Ekstrom C. Sorensen TIA. Changes in the distribution of weight, height and body mass index ($BMI = W/H^2$) at ages 7 to 14 years in a population of Danish boys born 1930 through 1966. Int J Obes Relat Metab Disord 1995;19(suppl 2):52.
46. Marelli G, Colombo E. Six years of epidemological monitoring of childhood obesity. Int J Obes Relat Metab Disord 1995;19(suppl 2):52.
47. Musaiger AO, Matter AM, Alekiri SA, Mahdi AR. Obesity among secondary school students in Bahrain. Nutr Health 1993;9:25–32.
48. Sichieri R, Recine E, Everhart JE. Growth and body mass index of Brazilians ages 9 through 17 years. Obes Res 1995;3(suppl 2):117s–121s.

49. Martorell R, Khan LK, Hughes ML, Grummer-Strawn LM. Obesity in Latin American women and children. J Nutr 1998;128:1464–1473.
50. Tremblay MS, Willms JD. Secular trends in the body mass index of Canadian children. CMAJ 2000;163: 1429–1433.
51. Bundred P, Kitchiner D, Buchan I. Prevalence of overweight and obese children between 1989 and 1998: population based series of cross sectional studies. BMJ 2001;322:326–328.
52. Charles MA. Update on the epidemiology of obesity and type 2 diabetes in France. (in French) Diabetes Metab 2000; 26(suppl 3):17–20.
53. Kromeyer-Hauschild K, Zellner K, Jaeger U, Hoyer H. Prevalence of overweight and obesity among school children in Jena (Germany). Int J Obes Relat Metab Disord 1999;23:1143–1150.
54. Moreno LA, Sarría A, Fleta J, Rodríguez G, Bueno M. Trends in body mass index and overweight prevalence among children and adolescents in the region of Aragón (Spain) from 1985 to 1995. Int J Obes Relat Metab Disord 2000;24:925–931.
55. Kain J, Uauy R, Diaz M. Increasing prevalence of obesity among school children in Chile, 1987–1996. Int J Obes Relat Metab Disord 1998;22(suppl 4): Abstract 7.
56. Martorell R, Khan LK, Hughes ML, Grummer-Strawn LM. Overweight and obesity in preschool children from developing countries. Int J Obes Relat Metab Disord 2000;24:959–967.
57. Cheek DB. Human Growth. Philadelphia: Lea & Febiger, 1968.
58. Malina RM, Bouchard C. Models and methods for studying body composition. In: Malina RM, Bouchard C, eds. Growth, Maturation, and Physical Activity. Champaign IL: Human Kinetics, 1991.
59. Knittle JL, Timmers K, Ginsberg-Fellner F, Brown RE, Katz DP. The growth of adipose tissue in children and adolescents. Cross-sectional and longitudinal studies of adipose tissue cell number and size. J Clin Invest 1979;63:239–246.
60. Poissonnet CM, LaVelle M, Burdi AR. Growth and development of adipose tissue. J Pediatr 1988;113:1–9.
61. Knittle JL, Ginsberg-Fellner F. Effect of weight reduction on in vitro adipose tissue lipolysis and cellularity in obese adolescents and adults. Diabetes 1972;21:754–761.
62. Garn SM, Clark DC. Trends in fatness and the origins of obesity. Ad Hoc Committee to Review the Ten-State Nutrition Survey. Pediatrics 1976;57:443–456.
63. Rolland-Cachera MF, Deheeger M, Guilloud-Bataille M, Avons P, Patois E, Sempe M. Tracking the development of adiposity from one month of age to adulthood. Ann Hum Biol 1987;14:219–229.
64. Malina RM, Bouchard C. Subcutaneous fat distribution during growth. In: Bouchard C, Johnston FE, eds. Fat Distribution During Growth and Later Health Outcomes. New York: Alan R. Liss, 1988.
65. Goran MI, Kaskoun M, Shumman WP. Intra-abdominal adipose tissue in young children. Int J Obes Relat Metab Disord 1995;19:279–283.
66. Fox K, Peters D, Armstrong N, Sharpe P, Bell M. Abdominal fat deposition in 11-year-old children. Int J Obes Relat Metab Disord 1993;17:11–16.
67. De Ridder CM, De Boer RW, Seidell JC, et al. Body fat distribution in pubertal girls quantified by magnetic resonance imaging. Int J Obes Relat Metab Disord 1992;16:443–449.
68. Lemieux S, Prud'homme D, Bouchard C, Tremblay A, Després JP. Sex differences in the relation of visceral adipose tissue accumulation to total body fatness. Am J Clin Nutr 1993;58:463–467.
69. Freedman DS, Kettel-Khan L, Srinivasan SR, Berenson GS. Black/white differences in relative weight and obesity among girls: the Bogalusa Heart Study. Prev Med 2000; 30:234–243.
70. Dietz WH. Critical periods in childhood for the development of obesity. Am J Clin Nutr 1994;59: 955–959.
71. Whitaker RC, Dietz WH. Role of the prenatal environment in the development of obesity. J Pediatr 1998;132:768–776.
72. Pettit DJ, Baird HR, Aleck KA, Bennett PH, Knowler WC. Excessive obesity in offspring of Pima Indian women with diabetes during pregnancy. N Engl J Med 1983;308:242–245.
73. Vohr BR, Lipsitt LP, Oh W. Somatic growth of children of diabetic mothers with reference to birth size. J Pediatr 1980;97:196–199.
74. Larsen CE, Serdula MK, Sullivan KM. Macrosomia: influence of maternal overweight among a low-income population. Am J Obstet Gynecol 1990;162: 490–494.
75. Hediger ML, Overpeck MD, McGlynn A, Kuczmarski RJ, Maurer KR, Davis WW. Growth and fatness at three to six years of age of children born small- or large-for-gestational age. Pediatrics 1999;104(3). URL: http//www.pediatrics.org/cgi/content/full/104/3/e33.
76. O'Callaghan MJ, Williams GM, Andersen MJ, Bor W, Najman JM. Prediction of obesity in children at 5 years: a cohort study. J Paediatr Child Health 1997;33: 311–316.
77. Rasmussen F, Johansson M. The relation of weight, length and ponderal index at birth to body mass index and overweight among 18-year-old males in Sweden. Eur J Epidemiol 1998;14:373–380.
78. Sorensen HT, Sabroe S, Rothman KJ, Gillman M, Fischer P, Sorensen TI. Relation between weight and length at birth and body mass index in young adulthood: cohort study. BMJ 1997; 315:1137.
79. Parsons TJ, Power C, Logan S, Summerbell CD. Childhood predictors of adult obesity: a systematic

review. Int J Obes Relat Metab Disord 1999; 23 (suppl 8): S1–S107.
80. Law CM, Barker DJ, Osmond C, Fall CH, Simmonds SJ. Early growth and abdominal fatness in adult life. J Epidemiol Community Health 1992; 46:184–186.
81. Barker DJ, Hales CN, Fall CH, Osmond C, Phipps K, Clark PM. Type 2 (non-insulin-dependent) diabetes mellitus, hypertension and hyperlipidaemia (syndrome X): relation to reduced fetal growth. Diabetologia 1993;36:62–67.
82. Rolland-Cachera MF, Deheeger M, Bellisle F, et al. Adiposity rebound in children: a simple indicator for predicting obesity. Am J Clin Nutr 1984; 39:129–135.
83. Siervogel RM, Roche AF, Guo S, Mukherjee D, Chumlea WC. Patterns of change in weight/stature^2 from 2 to 18 years: findings from long-term serial data for children in the Fels longitudinal growth study. Int J Obes Relat Metab Disord 1991; 15:479–485.
84. Dorosty AR, Emmett PM, Cowin IS, Reilly JJ, ALSPAC Study Team. Factors associated with early adiposity rebound. Pediatrics 2000; 105:1115–1118.
85. Dietz WH. "Adiposity rebound": reality or epiphenomenon? Lancet 2000; 356:2027–2028.
86. Williams S, Davie G, Lam F. Predicting BMI in young adults from childhood data using two approaches to modelling adiposity rebound. Int J Obes Relat Metab Disord 1999; 23:348–354.
87. Freedman DS, Kettel Khan L, Serdula MK, Srinivasan SR, Berenson GS. BMI rebound, childhood height and obesity among adults: the Bogalusa Heart Study. Int J Obes Relat Metab Disord 2001; 25:543–549.
88. Guo SS, Chumlea WC, Roche AF, Siervogel RM. Age- and maturity-related changes in body composition during adolescence into adulthood: the Fels longitudinal study. Int J Obes Relat Metab Disord 1997;21:1167–1175.
89. Garn SM, LaVelle M, Rosenberg KR, Hawthorne VM. Maturational timing as a factor in female fatness and obesity. Am J Clin Nutr 1986;43:879–883.
90. Sawaya AL, Grillo LP, Verreschi I, Da Silva AC, Roberts SB. Mild stunting is associated with higher susceptibility to the effects of high fat diets: studies in a shantytown population in São Paulo, Brazil. J Nutr 1998; 128(2 suppl):415S–420S.
91. Hoffman DJ, Sawaya AL, Verreschi I, Tucker KL, Roberts SB. Why are nutritionally stunted children at increased risk of obesity? Studies of metabolic rate and fat oxidation in shantytown children from São Paulo, Brazil. Am J Clin Nutr 2000;72:702–707.
92. Schroeder DG, Martorell R, Flores F. Infant and child growth and fatness and fat distribution in Guatemalan adults. Am J Epidemiol 1999;149:177–185.
93. Dietz WH Jr, Gortmaker SL. Factors within the physical environment associated with childhood obesity. Am J Clin Nutr 1984;39:619–624.
94. Butte NF. Breastfeeding 2001, Part I. The evidence for breastfeeding. The role of breastfeeding in obesity. Pediatr Clin North Am 2001;48:189–198.
95. Von Kries R, Koletzko B, Sauerwald T, et al. Breast feeding and obesity: crosssectional study. BMJ 1999; 319:147–150.
96. Gillman MW, Rifas-Shiman SK, Camargo CA Jr, et al. Risk of overweight among adolescents who were breastfed as infants. JAMA 2001; 285:2461–2467.
97. Hediger ML, Overpeck MD, Kuczmarski RJ, Ruan WJ. Association between infant breastfeeding and overweight in young children. JAMA 2001; 285:2453–2460.
98. Laskarzewski P, Morrison JA, Khoury P, et al. Parent-child nutrient intake interrelationships in school children ages 6 to 19: the Princeton School District Study. Am J Clin Nutr 1980;33:2350–2355.
99. Birch LL. The relationship between children's food preferences and those of their parents. J Nutr Ed 1980; 12:14–18.
100. Perusse L, Tremblay A, LeBlanc C, et al. Familial resemblance in energy intake: contribution of genetic and environmental factors. Am J Clin Nutr 1988; 47: 629–635.
101. Gillman MW, Rifas-Shiman SL, Frazier AL, et al. Family dinner and diet quality among older children and adolescents. Arch Fam Med 2000; 9:235–240.
102. Muñoz KA, Krebs-Smith SM, Ballard-Barbash R, Cleveland LE. Food intakes of US children and adolescents compared with recommendations. Pediatrics 1997; 100:323–329.
103. Maffeis C, Provera S, Filippi L, et al. Distribution of food intake as a risk factor for childhood obesity. Int J Obes Relat Metab Disord 2000;24:75–80.
104. Ludwig DS, Peterson KE, Gortmaker SL. Relation between consumption of sugar-sweetened drinks and childhood obesity: a prospective, observational analysis. Lancet 2001;357:505–508.
105. Nicklas TA, Elkasabany A, Srinivasan SR, Gerenson G. Trends in nutrient intake of 10-year-old children over two decades (1973–1994): the Bogulasa Heart Study. Am J Epidemiol 2001;153:969–977.
106. Birch LL, Johnson SL, Andresen G, Peters JC, Schulte MC. The variability of young children's energy intake. N Engl J Med 1991;324:232–235.
107. Fisher JO, Birch LL. Restricting access to palatable foods affects children's behavioral response, food selection, and intake. Am J Clin Nutr 1999;69:1264–1272.
108. Johnson SL, Birch LL. Parents' and children's adiposity and eating style. Pediatrics 1994;94:653–661.
109. Montgomery C, MacRitchie J, Jackson D, Reilly J. Relationship between parental control over child feeding and energy intake prior to the adiposity rebound. Obes Res 1999;7(suppl 1):49S.
110. Robinson TN, Kiernan M, Matheson DM, Haydel KF. Is parental control over children's eating asso-

ciated with childhood obesity? Results from a population-based sample of third graders. Obes Res 2001; 9:306–312.

111. Lissau I, Breum L, Sorensen TI. Maternal attitude to sweet eating habits and risk of overweight in offspring: a ten-year prospective population study. Int J Obes Relat Metab Disord 1993;17:125–129.

112. Lissau I, Sorensen TI. Parental neglect during childhood and increased risk of obesity in young adulthood. Lancet 1994;343:324–327.

113. Mellbin T, Vuille JC. Rapidly developing overweight in school children as an indicator of psychosocial stress. Acta Paediatr Scand 1989; 78:568–575.

114. Mellbin T, Vuille JC. Further evidence of an association between psychosocial problems and increase in relative weight between 7 and 10 years of age. Acta Paediatr Scand 1989;78:576–580.

115. Davies PS, Gregory J, White A. Physical activity and body fatness in pre-school children. Int J Obes Relat Metab Disord 1995;9:6–10.

116. Davies PS, Wells JC, Fieldhouse CA, Day JM, Lucas A. Parental body composition and infant energy expenditure. Am J Clin Nutr 1995;61:1026–1029.

117. Fontvieille AM, Harper IT, Ferraro RT, Spraul M, Ravussin E. Daily energy expenditure by five-year-old children, measured by doubly labeled water. J Pediatr 1993;123:200–207.

118. Livingstone MB, Coward WA, Prentice AM, et al. Daily energy expenditure in free-living children: comparison of heart rate monitoring with the doubly labeled water ($^2H_2{}^{18}O$) method. Am J Clin Nutr 1992; 56:343–352.

119. Bandini LG, Schoeller DA, Dietz WH. Energy expenditure in obese and nonobese adolescents. Pediatr Res 1990;27:198–203.

120. Schofield WN. Predicting basal metabolic rate, new standards and review of previous work. Hum Nutr Clin Nutr 1985;39c(suppl):5–41.

121. DiGuiseppi C, Roberts I, Li L. Influence of changing travel patterns on child death rates from injury: trend analysis. BMJ 1997;314:710–713 [published erratum appears in BMJ 1997;314:1385].

122. Anderson RE, Crespo CJ, Bartlett SJ, Cheskin KJ, Pratt M. Relationship of physical activity and television watching with body weight and level of fatness among children: results from the Third National Health and Nutrition Examination Survey. JAMA 1998;279:938–942.

123. Centers for Disease Control and Prevention. CDC Surveillance Summaries, June 9, 2000. MMWR 2000; 49(No. SS-5).

124. Gordon-Larsen P, McMurray RG, Popkin BM. Adolescent physical activity and inactivity vary by ethnicity: the National Longitudinal Study of Adolescent Health. J Pediatr 1999; 35:301–306.

125. U.S. Department of Health and Human Services. Healthy People 2010, 2nd ed. With Understanding and Improving Health and Objectives for Improving Health. Vol 2. Washington: Government Printing Office, 2000, chap 22, p 19.

126. Sallis JF, Prochaska JJ, Taylor WC. A review of correlates of physical activity of children and adolescents. Med Sci Sports Exerc 2000;32:963–975.

127. U.S. Department of Health and Human Services. Physical Activity and Health: A Resport of the Surgeon General. Atlanta: Centers for Disease Control and Prevention, National Center for Chronic Disease Prevention and Health Promotion, 1996:234–236.

128. Crespo CJ, Smit E, Troiano RP, Bartlett SJ, Macera CA, Anderson RE. Television watching, energy intake, and obesity in US children: results from the third National Health and Nutrition Examination Survey, 1988–1994. Arch Pediatr Adolesc Med 2001; 155:360–365.

129. Dietz WH, Gortmaker SL. Do we fatten our children at the television set? Obesity and television viewing in children and adolescents. Pediatrics 1985;75: 807–812.

130. Moore LL, Nguyen US, Rothman KJ, Cupples LA, Ellison RC. Preschool physical activity level and change in body fatness in young children: the Framingham Children's Study. Am J Epidemiol 1995;142:982–988.

131. Perusse L, LeBlanc C, Bouchard C. Familial resemblance in lifestyle components: results from the Canada Fitness Survey. Can J Public Health 1988; 79:201–205.

132. Perusse L, Tremblay A, LeBlanc C, Bouchard C. Genetic and environmental influences on level of habitual physical activity and exercise participation. Am J Epidemiol 1989;129:1012–1022.

133. Agras WS, Kraemer HC, Berkowitz RI, Hammer LD. Influence of early feeding style on adiposity at 6 years of age. J Pediatr 1990;116:805–809.

134. Kramer MS, Barr RG, Pless IB, et al. Determinants of weight and adiposity in early childhood. Can J Public V Health 1986;77(suppl 1):98–103.

135. Goldblatt PB, Moore ME, Stunkard AJ. Social factors in obesity. JAMA 1965;192:97–101.

136. Epstein LH, Valoski A, Wing RR, McCurley J. Ten-year follow-up of behavioral, family-based treatment for obese children. JAMA 1990;264: 2519–2523.

137. Dietz WH. Breastfeeding may help prevent childhood overweight. JAMA 2001;285:2506–2507.

7

Obesity in the Elderly: Prevalence, Consequences, and Treatment

Robert S. Schwartz

University of Colorado Health Sciences Center, Denver, Colorado, U.S.A.

I INTRODUCTION

In young and middle-aged individuals, obesity is an important metabolic and cardiovascular risk factor that is associated with highly prevalent disorders such as hypertension, diabetes, hyperinsulinemia, dyslipidemia, and atherosclerosis (1). While older individuals may not appear to be obese, they frequently suffer from these obesity-related disorders. This has led some investigators in the field of aging to consider many older individuals as having a "covert" form of obesity. Because the elderly are the fastest-growing segment of our population and contribute disproportionately to overall health care utilization and cost (2), the problem of obesity and obesity-related diseases in this older population could have staggering repercussions to our health care system as a whole, as well as to the lives of many older individuals and their families (3).

This chapter will discuss the scope of the problem of obesity in the elderly, define the body composition and fat distribution changes that normally occur with aging, outline possible etiologic factors in aging-associated obesity and, finally, consider potential treatments.

II PREVALENCE OF OBESITY IN THE ELDERLY

A Age-Related Changes in Weight and Body Composition

Data from the NHANES III study demonstrate that the prevalence of overweight reaches a maximum for both men (42%, with a mean body mass index [BMI] of 27.6) and women (52%, with a mean BMI of 28.5) between the ages of 50 and 59 (4). In this cross-sectional study (which had no upper age limit for subject entry and specifically oversampled older individuals), both the prevalence of overweight and the mean BMI tended to drop in older age groups, falling to 18% in men (mean BMI 24.7) and 26% in women (mean BMI 24.6) over age 80. There were notable differences in the effects of age on obesity in different racial/ethnic groups. African-American men had the highest prevalence of overweight in the 20–29 age range, but their weight tended to increase relatively less in the older age cohorts when compared to either Caucasians or Hispanics. Hispanic subjects had the highest prevalence of obesity in the 40- to 69-year-old males ($\approx$ 50–55%). In women a different picture emerged. Caucasian women had the lowest prevalence of obesity in each age group, with a peak ($\approx$ 50%) at 50–59 years. Hispanic women had their highest prevalence of obesity ($\approx$ 55%) at a slightly younger age (40–49 years). African-American women had their peak prevalence of obesity ($\approx$ 60%) at a later age (60–69 years) and had the highest prevalence of obesity overall when compared to the other racial/ethnic groups.

However, these findings may reflect a common problem in interpreting cross-sectional data, a bias due to disproportionately higher death rates in middle-aged obese subjects (5,6), leaving a thinner group of subsequent survivors. A truer understanding of the complex age-related changes in weight or BMI requires longitudinal data. A 15-year follow-up study of seven different age cohorts of men (21–80 yr at entry) demonstrated a significant difference in the effect of aging on weight or BMI in the different age cohorts (7). The men who were the oldest at entry weighed the least and tended to remain stable or lose a small amount of weight over the period of follow-up, while the younger cohorts were heavier at baseline and continued to gain weight with time. Thus, there was a substantial cohort effect on the relation between aging and body weight. More consistent (and possibly more important) were the changes observed in fat distribution, with all cohorts showing increments in central distribution of fat during the period of follow-up (see below).

The observed changes in weight and BMI with aging are accompanied by profound changes in body composition that can substantially influence the interpretation of data. Studies have consistently demonstrated clinically important losses of fat-free mass (FFM) with age in both men and women. More recent studies have used dual-energy x-ray absorptiometry (DXA) techniques to show that these changes appear to be predominantly accounted for by the loss of muscle mass as represented by reductions in appendicular lean mass (8). This phenomenon has received the appellation "sarcopenia" (9). When defined as an appendicular lean mass (kg/ht in m^2) of > 2 SD below that for a young reference group, sarcopenia occurs in 24% of older individuals under age 70 and >50% of individuals over age 80 (10).

While the loss of FFM influences many important geriatric care issues, such as strength, endurance and overall functional ability (9–14), here we will consider only how it might affect the determination of "obesity" in older individuals. Because FFM declines by as much as 40% between the ages of 30 and 70 (15–20), at any given body weight or BMI, older persons will be considerably fatter (8,21). Since the content of fat within lean tissues such as muscle is also greater with aging, even the standard measurements of body composition by methods such as computed tomography (CT), magnetic resonance imaging (MRI), and DXA might underestimate actual total body adiposity.

Stature frequently declines (0.5–1.5 cm/decade) with age (15), owing to decrements in the height of the vertebral bodies and shrinkage of intervertebral disk spaces. Therefore, the use of measured present height commonly causes an overestimate of BMI in the elderly (especially in women). This can be corrected by using maximal historical height, but one must be concerned with the usual caveats regarding recall data. A preferred method is the use of knee height as suggested by Chumlea (22), but, in fact, such corrections for loss of height are seldom used.

Skinfold thickness correlates less well with total adiposity in older individuals (23), making assessment of adiposity by skinfold measurements also difficult to interpret. Furthermore, the change in fat distribution with age makes determination of most peripheral subcutaneous skin fold measures less clinically relevant.

Well-known age-related changes in the composition of FFM can significantly affect the determination of body density and, therefore, body composition using the "gold standard" hydrodensitometry method (24). While the density of fat changes little with aging (0.9 g/mL), variation in hydration state and in bone mineral can distort the actual density of FFM from the value usually assumed in prediction equations (1.10 g/mL). Tissue dehydration would increase the true density of FFM while loss of bone mineral would produce the opposite effect. The loss of total body water with aging would have the more profound effect, and, for any given total body density measure, the established prediction equations would underestimate the amount of adiposity (25). However, studies are not consistent in finding a decline in the hydration state of lean tissue in older subjects (26,27). Whereas one study found no signifficant change in hydration of lean tissue between young and older women (26), a subsequent study by the same investigators (10) found that total body water declined over a 5-year follow-up period with a trend toward a greater loss in men (−0.04 vs. −0.01 kg/yr). In another study, not correcting for the measured total body water produced a 4% underestimation of percent body fat (%BF) in older women but no significant difference in older men when compared to multicompartmental methods (27). In the latter study, the variation in the measurement of %BF between the two- and four-compartment models was inversely related to the hydration state of the FFM. A recent cross-sectional study found that while total body water declined in both men and women between ages 60 and 80 the decline was significant only in the women (15). The loss of water appeared to be mainly from intracellular fluid. This cross-sectional study found that men lost FFM twice as quickly as women (0.22 vs. 0.10 kg/yr), a rate much greater than that observed in their prospective study (10). Any observed changes in body water with aging may also affect estimates of body composition using total body water or bioelectrical impedance, the latter being a measure that is exquisitely sensitive to hydration state (28).

While there is some disagreement, it appears that significant declines in total body hydration state occur in healthy older persons and may affect estimates of adiposity. The direction of these changes would tend to produce an underestimate of adiposity.

B Age-Related Changes in Fat Distribution

It has been well demonstrated that many of the metabolic abnormalities associated with obesity are strongly and independently related to a central distribution of adiposity (29–34). However, what is less well recognized is that aging is associated with an increasingly more central distribution of adiposity in both men and women (7,35–38). At any given level of adiposity, more fat will be centrally distributed in older individuals. Of interest, a cross-sectional study found no age-related change in fat distribution in men or women between the ages of 60 and 80, suggesting this accumulation may reach its maximum in middle age and early old age (15). Again, the preferential drop out of more obese subjects may bias the interpretation of data from such a cross-sectional study.

Intra-abdominal fat accumulation, known to be independently related to the metabolic concomitants of obesity (39–44), has also been demonstrated to be greater at any given BMI or %BF in older individuals (45–47). While the accumulation of intra-abdominal fat with aging may be progressive in men, it appears to greatly accelerate in women following menopause (62,48).

Although there are racial/ethnic differences in fat distribution (see Chap. 3), relatively little is known about how these are affected by aging. It appears that African-American women have greater central fat distribution than Caucasian women before menopause (50) but that the slope of the increase with age is not different between the two groups. Of interest, NHANES I also noted that central adiposity conferred relatively less risk for cardiovascular disease in black women (51). This finding agrees with earlier reports that central adiposity was not a strong risk factor for the development of non-insulin-dependent diabetes (NIDDM) or atherosclerotic cardiovascular disease in black women (52). Similarly, the Charleston Heart Study determined that central fat distribution did not predict all-cause or coronary heart disease deaths in black women (53). Other studies have found that while Hispanics have a greater central distribution of fat, this was not associated with excess all-cause mortality in subject over age 45 (54). Studies in Japanese-Americans have demonstrated relatively greater amounts of central and intra-abdominal fat when compared to Caucasians, and a strong relationship exists between intra-abdominal fat and the development of insulin resistance and NIDDM frequently observed in this population (43,44,55).

C Menopause and Obesity in Women

There are relatively few data on changes in adiposity and fat distribution associated with menopause in women. This is an important issue because of the relationships that have been noted between obesity and cardiovascular disease (5), and obesity and certain cancers (56,57) in postmenopausal women. As noted above, body weight reaches its maximum in women very near the time of menopause, and there is an increase in relative adiposity for any given weight or BMI. While some studies find that the increase in weight accompanying menopause is more related to age than menopause itself (58,59), others have noted specific menopause-related increases in BMI, overall adiposity, central adiposity and intra-abdominal adiposity (60–64). A recently published longitudinal study that followed 35 women aged 44–48 for 6 years (65) found that those women who experienced menopause during the period of follow-up lost significantly more FFM (−3 vs. −0.5 kg), and had greater increases in fat mass (FM; 2.5 vs. 1.0 kg), waist-to-hip ratio (WHR; 0.04 vs. 0.01) and insulin (11 vs. −2 pmol/L). The changes were associated with greater reductions in physical activity and resting energy expenditure in the postmenopausal women. In two randomized, placebo-controlled studies in which postmenopausal women were prospectively studied for 2–3 years, hormone replacement therapy prevented the accumulation of abdominal adiposity while having no effect on FFM (63,66).

III CAUSES OF OBESITY IN OLDER PERSONS

A Intake Versus Expenditure

The accumulation of excess calories stored as adipose tissue requires an imbalance in the usually tight relationship between caloric intake and expenditure. While adiposity has a tendency to increase with age, total caloric intake either is unchanged (67) or declines (68) when assessed in longitudinal studies. Furthermore, the increment in adiposity with aging cannot be blamed on increased relative fat intake in the diet (69), since this too appears to decline with aging (67,68). However, one must always be careful interpreting data on reporting of calorie intake. As compared to doubly labeled water determination of calories intake, underreporting of calorie intake has been found in both male and female older subjects, with greater underreporting in heavier individuals (70). The ability to appropriately detect and respond to a change in body weight also appears to be impaired in older subjects. Two well-controlled feeding trials strongly suggest that in older subjects the regulation of energy intake is impaired in response to either an imposed increase or decrease in weight. After weight loss, older subjects did not appropriately increase their intake, and following weight gain they did not properly reduce their intake when compared to younger controls (71).

It is also likely that the age-related increase in obesity is in some way related to deficits in energy expenditure. This topic has been carefully reviewed (72), and the relationship between resting metabolic rate (RMR) and age appears to be curvilinear if sufficient numbers of older individuals are included. While three-fourths of this decline in RMR can be accounted for by decrements in FFM, one-fourth remains unexplained. Poehlman has suggested that this decline in RMR may be related to inactivity and has demonstrated normalization in older men after endurance training (73). Others have not been able to demonstrate an endurance training-related improvement in RMR in older subjects (74). While the thermic effect of feeding (TEF) may decline with age (75), this may be more related to inactivity than to age itself (72). Furthermore, variability in TEF does not predict subsequent weight gain (76).

B Inactivity

The component of daily energy expenditure that is most variable among individuals is the thermic effect of exercise (TEE), the energy expended with physical activity. Older individuals are usually less active than their younger counterparts (77,78), and several investigators have proposed that this difference in activity level may account for much of the age-associated gain in adiposity (79). This is supported by 10-year follow-up data from the NHANES-I study, which looked at the relationship between recreational physical activity and subsequent weight gain (80). Both at baseline and at follow-up, physical activity was inversely related to body weight. Low physical activity at follow-up was strongly associated with major weight gain (> 13 kg), and the relative risk of major weight gain, comparing the low- and high-activity groups, was 3.1 in men and 3.8 in women. This activity component can best be measured by evaluating free-living energy expenditure using the doubly labeled water technique (81). Using this method, reduced physical activity levels are associated with increased %BF (82).

C Fat Oxidation

Another possible mechanism that could be associated with obesity with aging is abnormal fat oxidation. Indeed, recent studies have demonstrated that fat oxidation is reduced in older individuals at baseline, with exercise, and following a meal (83). It is not clear whether the decrement in fat oxidation is due to the absolute loss of lean mass, a reduced capacity for fat oxidation by aging lean mass, or abnormal hormonal regulation of fat oxidation by estrogen, testosterone, growth hormone, and/or dihydroepiandrosterone (DHEA).

IV CONSEQUENCES OF OBESITY IN OLDER PERSONS

A Metabolic

Many of the common obesity-related metabolic abnormalities found in young and middle-aged individuals appear to be related to insulin resistance and hyperinsulinemia, what has come to be called the "insulin resistance" or "metabolic" syndrome (84). While the exact components of this syndrome vary among different populations (85,86), in general it is made up of central obesity (39,87); insulin resistance and hyperinsulinemia (88); abnormal glucose metabolism (89); dyslipidemias (41,90) such as high triglycerides, low high-density lipoprotein (HDL) cholesterol and small, dense, low-density lipoprotein (LDL) particles (91), hypertension (84), and atherosclerosis (92).

These same metabolic disorders are extremely prevalent in older populations. For example, it is well known that glucose tolerance worsens with age, with a 1–2 mg/dL increase in fasting glucose and a 10–20 mg/dL increase in postprandial glucose for each decade after age 30 (93). NIDDM is the fifth most common chronic disease in the elderly, affecting > 20% of individuals over age 65, with approximately half of these being undiagnosed (94). Diabetes has profound effects on health care utilization and costs, with up to one-seventh of all health care dollars being spent caring for diabetics (95). While in the past this high frequency of diabetes and glucose intolerance has been considered to be attributable to aging, more recent studies strongly suggest that most, if not all, of the "age-related" changes in insulin sensitivity and glucose tolerance can be accounted for by changes in body composition, fat distribution, and inactivity (45,96–100).

Similarly, there is an exceedingly high prevalence of hypertension in older individuals (101). It is estimated that between 30% and 50% of all persons over age 65 have hypertension (either systolic-diastolic or isolated systolic), with somewhat lower prevalence rates in studies that require multiple readings to make the diagnosis and higher rates in African-Americans.

Dyslipidemia is commonly noted in obese individuals, especially those with a central or intra-abdominal distribution of fat (41,102). The most commonly described abnormalities include elevations in triglyceride and reductions in HDL cholesterol levels. While similar abnormalities have been detected in older subjects (103,104), these abnormalities occur in both obese and "nonobese" older individuals (105). In two prospective studies, plasma insulin level was found to predict the development of dyslipidemia after either 3.5 or 8 years of follow-up. Apolipoprotein abnormalities have also been described in older subjects, such as increases in Apo B, reductions in Apo AI and the development of dense LDL particles (106). These abnormalities are all similar to those noted with central adiposity (102) and are associated with an elevated risk for atherosclerosis (92).

The relationship between obesity and overall mortality in older individuals has been a point of major controversy for a number of years. Many studies demonstrate that obesity is related to increased mortality in young and middle-aged individuals. The relationship between body weight and mortality was initially noted to be U-shaped, with excess mortality at both extremes of the body weight range. It now seems likely that this curvilinear relationship was due to confounders such as excess cigarette smoking and illness-related weight loss in the lowest weight group. More recent analyses that controlled for these variables have found no increase in mortality in the lowest weight group (5,6).

Andres has suggested that the weight associated with the lowest mortality increases with age (107), while others suggest this is not the case when the data are corrected for smoking and early deaths (108,109). This latter interpretation of the data is expressed in a new review of guidelines for healthy weight (110). Nonetheless, it appears that the relationship between obesity and mortality changes considerably in the oldest age groups. In a recent evaluation of the very large Cancer Prevention Study I (111), crude death rates (12-year follow-up) did not rise with increasing BMI in subjects over age 75 years who had never smoked and had no evidence of heart disease, stroke, or cancer at baseline. In these subjects, the BMI associated with the lowest risk of all-cause mortality or cardiovascular death was ~28, compared to 20 in the younger age groups. The relative risk (RR) of death from cardiovascular disease was 1.08–1.10 in 30- to 44-year-olds compared to 1.02–1.03 in 65- to 74-year-olds. The interaction between BMI and age was significant for both overall and cardiovascular mortality. When these authors calculated the BMI associated with 20% and 50% excess all-cause and cardiovascular mortality, a sharp rise in the computed BMI was noted after age 65 in both men and women. A decline in the effect of obesity on mortality was also detected by these authors when they calculated other measures of effect such as rate ratio, attributable deaths, excess years of life lost, and the time period by which the rate of death was advanced owing to obesity (112).

There are few data on ethnic differences in the relationship between obesity and mortality in older individuals, but one large prospective study found the lowest mortality in the 60–84th centiles for weight in white men compared to the 40–59th centiles in black men (113). The opposite was true for women, with the lowest mortality in the 40–59th centiles for weight in white women and in the 60–84th centiles for the black women. This study demonstrated a U-shaped curve, with excess mortality at both the lowest and highest centiles for body weight, even when corrected for smoking or when only nonsmokers were included. It was suggested that the added mortality at very low weights in these older subjects might be accounted for by osteoporosis and excess hip fractures.

B Functional

Functional status is of critical importance in assessing and treating older individuals, and frailty has been closely related to major health outcome measures including mortality in several large prospective studies (114). Therefore, it is reasonable to consider how obesity might affect functional status in older patients. While some studies show that low weight is a risk for frailty (114), obesity has also been related to arthritis (115) and functional decline in older subjects (116).

There are also new data relating both baseline waist circumference and gain in waist circumference over 30 years of follow-up predicted severity of sleep-disordered breathing in older men (117).

V TREATMENT OF OBESITY IN OLDER PERSONS

A Effects of Voluntary Weight Fluctuation on Mortality

There is compelling evidence supporting the association of obesity and weight gain with heart disease (118), diabetes (119), and excess all-cause mortality (5). Less clear, however, is the impact associated with losing excess weight.

Several large studies in both middle-aged and older adults find that weight fluctuations, either up or down, are associated with excess cardiovascular and all-cause mortality (120–122), with similar findings in two separate Asian populations (123,124). However, these studies have mostly relied on self-reported weights. In a recent study of 648 Caucasian women aged 65–69, weight change was measured over three assessment periods (baseline, 1 year, and 2 years), and then the subjects were followed for an additional 4 years (125). As with other studies, subjects who experienced weight variability or "cycling" were found to have excess mortality (20% vs. 11 % in weight-stable subjects). Deaths were higher in the low-baseline BMI group (22%) than in the average-weight BMI group (13%). Subjects who lost 4.5% over the measurement period had 25% deaths, and this mortality rate was not greatly affected by the baseline BMI. Weight variability has also been related to the incidence of specific diseases, with higher relative risks found for myocardial infarction, stroke, diabetes, lung cancer, and hip fractures, with greater weight variability in the 33,834 women age 55–69 participating in the Iowa Women's Health Study (126).

These studies have been rightfully criticized because they often did not distinguish between intentional and unintentional weight loss (127) or failed to take into account important preexisting disease (128). An important study by Williamson et al. (129) has specifically attempted to obviate these problems by evaluating the effects of "intentional" weight loss in >43,000 nonsmoking, *middle-age* (40–64 yr) Caucasian women followed prospectively for 12 years. Early deaths, within the first 3 years, were excluded. The data were stratified by preexisting obesity-related illness, and adjusted for age, baseline BMI, alcohol use, physical activity, and overall health. This study demonstrated that any amount of weight loss in subjects with obesity-related illness was associated with a 20% decrement in all-cause mortality, due to both a 40–50% fall in cancer deaths and a 30–40% reduction in diabetes-related deaths. The data were much less clear in women without preexisting obesity-related disease who intentionally lost weight.

While it appears that there are potential long-range benefits to weight loss, especially in those in young and middle-age patients with obesity-related disorders, a caveat must be emphasized for the elderly, as weight loss is a common part of the failure-to-thrive syndrome frequently observed in older patients (130). A study by Wallace in a group of outpatient veterans over age 65 demonstrated that involuntary weight loss of ≥4% in 1 year was associated with a 2.5-fold greater risk of dying within the next 2 years of follow-up when compared to non-weight-losers. This was despite a decrement in central distribution of fat in the weight losers. These results were not affected by adjusting for age, BMI, tobacco, and health status. Surprisingly, the relative risk of dying was almost identical in subjects whose weight loss was apparently "voluntary."

A more recent study evaluated weight loss in 4714 community-dwelling men and women over age 65 as part of the Cardiovascular Health Study (131). Over the first 3 years of examination, 16–19% of subjects met the 5% criteria for losing weight, while 11–16% gained 5% of weight. The hazard ratio for all-cause mortality during a 4-year follow-up period was ~2.0 for those who lost ≥5% of body weight during the initial 3 years of observation. Baseline weight or health status did not affect this hazard ratio. The risks for weight loss included older age, multiple drugs, disability, slow gait, weakness, and death of a spouse. Furthermore, the hazard ratio was not affected by the reasons for the weight loss (intentional versus unintentional). The survival curves during the follow-up period were not different for those who were weight stable and those who gained weight.

Another study evaluated 5-year weight change and the 10- and 15-year mortality in 2628 Swedish men and women who were 70 years old at the baseline examination (132). The BMI associated with the lowest 15-year mortality in this older population was 27–29 for men and 25–27 for women. After excluding deaths during the initial 5-year period, the relationship between BMI and mortality was flat in men and U-shaped in women. Weight loss of ≥10% during the first 5-year period was associated with higher mortality at 10 and 15 years even when adjusted for smoking status.

Together, these data strongly suggest that while dietary weight loss in middle-aged patients with obesity-related illness may positively impact outcomes, weight cycling may produce deleterious effects. In addition, physicians should be very cautious prescribing weight loss in otherwise healthy obese older patients. Some of the discrepancies among studies in the relationship between obesity and mortality may be due to the lack of measurement of body composition. It is likely that loss of fat is associated with improvements in health while the loss of weight alone may be deleterious (133). This concept is especially important in older people where, under some circumstances, substantial loss of lean mass may accompany weight loss.

B Dietary Weight Loss Studies in Older Individuals

There have been few published reports of dietary weight loss interventions specifically in older subjects. While the study by Williamson (129) supports a benefit to intentional weight loss in middle-aged subjects, it is possible that exacerbation of the usual age-related loss of lean mass could be worsened by a weight loss diet. However, in a recently published study of otherwise healthy obese older men (mean of 60 yr) who underwent a 10-month calorie restriction, only 23% of the 9.3 kg of weight that was lost, was lost as FFM (134). This is similar to studies in our laboratory (135) in which 16 healthy obese older men (mean 66 yr) lost 10 kg on a 1200-kcal dietary restriction (Phase I American Heart Association Diet.). In this study only 20% of weight loss was as FFM. The percentages of weight lost as FFM in these relatively healthy older individuals is similar to that found in younger subjects. In both of the above studies, weight loss produced a small but significant improvement in the waist-to-hip ratio. However, in our study, despite a decrement WHR and in intra-abdominal adiposity measured by CT, there was no preferential loss of intra-abdominal fat compared to fat from more peripheral depots. It must be emphasized that subjects in both of these studies were highly screened to be healthy despite their moderate obesity and that these findings may not be generalizable to the population of older individuals who suffer from various clinical disease states.

A recent randomized controlled study compared the effect of a 9-month hypocaloric (AHA Phase I) diet on insulin action and glucose tolerance in middle-aged and older subjects (mean age 60 ± 8 yr) with either normal or impaired glucose tolerance (136). After an average weight loss of 9 kg, there was a significant fall in the glucose area (−22%) following an oral glucose challenge. This reduction in glucose area was related to the decrease in waist circumference. In fact, almost half of the subjects who initially had impaired glucose tolerance normalized following weight loss. In a subgroup of eight subjects, the weight loss was found to induce a fall in both the first and second phase insulin response to a hyperglycemic clamp and an improvement in insulin action. Early (unpublished) analysis of data from the Diabetic Prevention Program study appears to also suggest that lifestyle-related (diet and exercise) loss of weight of ~ 5% is associated with less progression to diabetes in a high-risk (mostly middle-aged) population with glucose intolerance at baseline.

In a study by Dengel et al., weight loss was associated with improvement in the lipoprotein profile, reductions in the LDL/HDL cholesterol ratio and triglyceride concentration and increments in the HDL_2 cholesterol (137). We have noted similar improvements in HDL and triglyceride concentrations but no change in the concentration of total or LDL cholesterol (135). However, there was a 22% decline in hepatic lipase consistent with less dense and less atherogenic LDL particles. Six of the seven subjects who initially had the more atherogenic, small, dense LDL phenotype pattern B reverted to a more favorable LDL pattern A following weight loss. No change was noted in the subjects with pattern A at baseline. Thus, while the concentration of LDL failed to change with weight loss, the size and composition of the LDL particles became more favorable.

There is considerable interest in the potential benefits of chronic calorie restriction to extend life and reduce morbidity (138). This hypothesis that has been proven in rodents is now being tested in nonhuman primates and humans.

C Exercise Training in Older Individuals

Many important benefits of exercise training for older persons have now been documented (139). Exercise alone is not associated with large reductions in adipose tissue mass in intervention studies (140), and it has been estimated that a 6-month period of exercise training alone would reduce fat mass by only 2.6 kg and %BF by only 3%. However, in large population studies, greater physical activity is associated with lower body weight, and higher fitness levels are inversely related to all-cause mortality in subjects at any BMI level (141). Interestingly, the most impressive effect on mortality occurs in subjects with BMIs ≥ 30. There is also good evidence that physical activity is associated with lower blood pressure (142) as well as diabetes (143), dyslipidemia and atherosclerosis (144), all disorders that are common in obesity. In addition, exercise has been demonstrated to be essential in the successful maintenance of weight loss after dietary restriction (145,146).

There are considerably fewer data on the metabolic effects of an exercise intervention in older subjects, but this has become an area of great interest in recent years. As in other groups, endurance exercise training in older subjects is associated with only modest losses in weight and fat (147,148), consistent with the estimates by Wilmore (140). However, recent studies suggest that the fat lost comes preferentially from intra-abdominal depots (145,146). This may appear to be different from the more general loss of adipose mass with caloric restriction (135). Associated with this preferential loss of central adipose tissue following exercise are improvements in lipid, glucose, and insulin metabolism (97,149,150). For example, after 6 months of intensive endurance exercise subjects lost only 2.5 kg of weight and a similar amount of fat. This was associated with a 20% loss of intra-abdominal adipose tissue area on CT. With these changes, insulin sensitivity improved by >33% despite no improvement in oral glucose metabolism (97). There was a 23% reduction in triglyceride and an almost 70% increment in HDL_2 cholesterol (149).

Recent evidence suggests that most if not all of the metabolic effects of exercise require weight loss and that metabolic improvements are greatly lessened if body weight is purposely maintained (151). Since energy intake has been noted to be increased in free-living subjects who are training (73,147), weight loss is felt to be due to enhanced energy expenditure. While both the thermic effect of exercise and RMR are increased with exercise training (73), it is of interest that 24-hr energy expenditure does not appear to increase in older men with endurance training (152). This suggests that they were more sedentary at other times of the day when they were not exercising. Therefore, the true etiology of the fat loss is unclear but may be related to enhancement of sympathetic nervous system activity (153) or lipid oxidation (154) associated with exercise training.

There are considerably fewer data on the effects of resistance training on adiposity and metabolism in older subjects. While it is now well known that the elderly can improve both their FFM and strength with resistance training (9,155), only recently has it been demonstrated that there are also reductions in both fat mass and intra-abdominal fat mass (156). Newer studies suggest that resistance training may also have positive effects, similar to endurance training on insulin action (157,158), but little or no improvement in lipoprotein profile seems to occur (159).

Numerous studies strongly indicate that both endurance and resistance exercise are beneficial in the elderly. While the amount of weight loss associated with training is small, it may preferentially come from the most critical intra-abdominal depots and thus be associated with substantial metabolic improvement. In addition, exercise is associated with the maintenance or an increment in lean body mass and may be required to maintain dietary weight loss long term.

D Drug Treatment for Obesity in the Elderly

The use of appetite suppressants to treat obesity in older patients will not be discussed here, and the reader is referred to Chapters 55–59. However, because of the continued interest in the use of trophic factor supplementation in the elderly, it is reasonable to discuss briefly how these factors may affect adiposity and fat distribution.

Ample evidence confirms an age-related decrement in the growth hormone (GH)/insulinlike growth factor-I (IGF-I) axis. These changes have been implicated in the decline in FFM with aging, and may also account for the increase in central adiposity found in the elderly (160). Indeed, studies in both growth hormone-deficient adults replaced with GH and healthy older subjects supplemented with GH demonstrate reductions in both total and central adiposity. It should be noted, however, that supplementation of older subjects with GH is not without significant side effects, and long-term positive effects on lean mass, bone mass, fat mass, and, most importantly, strength and function, remain unproved is (161).

A newly published study found that GH and GH plus testosterone supplementation in healthy older men caused within-group reductions in total, visceral, and subcutaneous abdominal fat. Only the changes in subcutaneous fat and total abdominal fat were significantly different from placebo. There were no similar declines in women treated with GH with or without estrogen (162).

Testosterone concentrations also decline with aging in men. There is no consensus about the role that this may play in aging-related obesity or the effects of testosterone supplementation alone on adiposity in older men (163). While one study found no change in weight, body fat, or WHR, another found no change in total fat but a 10% decline in intra-abdominal adiposity after 9 months of testosterone supplementation. As noted above, there are also some data that suggest that estrogen replacement in women can prevent the postmenopausal accumulation of central fat.

Dehydroepiandrosterone sulfate (DHEAS) is the most abundant steroid hormone is humans. Peak levels are typically reached in the third decade of life and decline steadily thereafter (164). Because it can be converted to testosterone and aromatized to estradiol, DHEAS level may be a determinant of sex hormone–mediated changes in fat accumulation and distribution that occur with aging. There have been few studies of DHEA replacement in people with low DHEAS levels, but there is some evidence for a fat-reducing effect in a controlled trial of DHEA replacement (50 mg/d) for 6 months in 18 women and men, aged 64–82 yr (165). In this study, fat mass was reduced by −1.4 kg in response to DHEA supplementation, and assessment by DXA indicated that the reduction occurred entirely within central body regions in both women and men. Larger clinical trials of trophic factor supplementation in older subjects should be completed in the next 2–3 years.

ACKNOWLEDGMENTS

Dr. Schwartz is supported in part by NIH grant RO-1 AG 10943, NIH grant RO-1 DK 48152, NIH grant UO-1 DK 48413, and NIH grant P-30 DK 35816.

REFERENCES

1. Pi Sunyer FX. Medical hazards of obesity. Ann Intern Med 1993; 119:655–660.
2. Mittelmark MB. The epidemiology of aging. In: Hazzard WR, Bierman EL, Blass JP, Ettinger WHJ, Halter JB, eds. The Principles of Geriatric Medicine and Gerontology. New York: McGraw-Hill, 1994: 135–152.
3. Colditz GA. Economic costs of obesity. Am J Clin Nutr 1992; 55:503S–507S.
4. Kuczmarski RJ, Flegal KM, Campbell SM, Johnson CL. Increasing prevalence of overweight among US adults. The National Health and Nutrition Examination Surveys, 1960 to 1991 [see comments]. JAMA 1994; 272:205–211.
5. Manson JE, Willett WC, Stampfer MJ, Colditz GA, Hunter DJ, Hankinson SE, Hennekens CH, Speizer FE. Body weight and mortality among women [see comments]. N Engl J Med 1995; 333:677–685.
6. Lee IM, Manson JE, Hennekens CH, Paffenbarger RS Jr. Body weight and mortality. A 27-year follow-up of middle-aged men [see comments]. JAMA 1993;270: 2823–2828.
7. Grinker JA, Tucker K, Vokonas PS, Rush D. Body habitus changes among adult males from the normative aging study: relations to aging, smoking history and alcohol intake. Obes Res 1995; 3:435–446.
8. Gallagher D, Ruts E, Visser M, Heshka S, Baumgartner, RN, Wang J, Pierson RN, Pi-Sunyer FX, Heymsfield SB. Weight stability masks sarcopenia in elderly men and women. Am J Physiol Endocrinol Metab 2000; 279:E366–E375.
9. Evans WJ, Campbell WW. Sarcopenia and age-related changes in body composition and functional capacity. J Nutr 1993; 123:465–468.
10. Baumgartner RN, Koehler KM, Gallagher D, Romero L, Heymsfield SB, Ross RR, Garry PJ, Lindeman RD. Epidemiology of sarcopenia among the elders in New Mexico. Am J Epidemiol 1998; 147:755–763.
11. Frontera WR, Meredith CN, O'Reilly KP, Knuttgen HG, Evans WJ. Strength conditioning in older men: skeletal muscle hypertrophy and improved function. J Appl Physiol 1988; 64:1038–1044.
12. Fiatarone MA, Marks EC, Ryan ND, Meredith CN, Lipsitz LA, Evans WJ. High-intensity strength training in nonagenarians. Effects on skeletal muscle. JAMA 1990; 263:3029–3034.
13. Buchner DM, Beresford SA, Larson EB, LaCroix AZ, Wagner EH. Effects of physical activity on health status in older adults. II. Intervention studies. Annu Rev Public Health 1992; 13:469–488.
14. Buchner DM, Cress ME, Wagner EH, De Lateur BJ, Price R, Abrass IB. The Seattle FICSIT/MoveIt study: the effect of exercise on gait and balance in older adults. J Am Geriatr Soc 1993; 41:321–325.
15. Baumgartner RN, Stauber PM, McHugh D, Koehler KM, Garry PJ. Cross-sectional age differences in body composition in persons 60+ years of age. J Gerontol 1995; 50A:M307–M316.
16. Evans WJ. What is sarcopenia? J Gerontol 1995; 50A:5–8.
17. Flynn MA, Nolph GB, Baker AS, Martin WM, Krause G. Total body potassium in aging humans: a longitudinal study. Am J Clin Nutr 1989; 50:713–717.
18. Novak LP. Aging, total body potassium, fat-free mass, and cell mass in males and females between ages 18 and 85 years. J Gerontol 1972; 27:438–443.
19. Tzankoff SP, Norris AH. Longitudinal changes in basal metabolism in man. J Appl Physiol 1978; 45:536–539.
20. Cohn SH, Vartsky D, Yasumura S, Savitsky A, Zanzi I, Vaswani A, Ellis KJ. Compartmental body composition based on total-body potassium and calcium. Am J Physiol 1980; 239:E524–E530.
21. Baumgartner RN, Heymsfield SB, Roche AF. Human body composition and the epidemiology of chronic disease. Obes Res 1995; 3:73–95.
22. Chumlea WC, Guo SS, Steinbaugh ML. Prediction of stature from knee height for black and white adults and children with application to mobility-impaired or handicapped persons. J Am Diet Assoc 1994; 94:1385–1388.

23. Chumlea WC, Roche AF, Webb P. Body size, subcutaneous fatness and total body fat in older adults. Int J Obes 1984; 8:311–317.
24. Baumgartner RN, Stauber PM, McHugh D, Wayne S, Garry PJ, Heymsfield SB. Body composition in the elderly using multicompartmental methods. Basic Life Sci 1993; 60:251–254.
25. Baumgartner RN, Heymsfield SB, Lichtman S, Wang J, Pierson RN, Jr. Body composition in elderly people: effect of criterion estimates on predictive equations. Am J Clin Nutr 1991; 53:1345–1353.
26. Mazariegos M, Wang ZM, Gallagher D, Baumgartner RN, Allison DB, Wang J, Pierson RN Jr, Heymsfield SB. Differences between young and old females in the five levels of body composition and their relevance to the two-compartment chemical model. J Gerontol 1994; 49:M201–M208.
27. Hewitt MJ, Going SB, Williams DP, Lohman TG. Hydration of the fat-free body mass in children and adults: implications for body composition assessment. Am J Physiol 1993; 265:E88–E95.
28. Chumlea WC, Guo SS. Bioelectrical impedance and body composition: present status and future directions [see comments]. Nutr Rev 1994; 52:123–131.
29. Lapidus L, Bengtsson C, Hallstrom T, Bjorntorp P. Obesity, adipose tissue distribution and health in women—results from a population study in Gothenburg, Sweden. Appetite 1989; 13:25–35.
30. Larsson B, Seidell J, Svardsudd K, Welin L, Tibblin G, Wilhelmsen L, Bjorntorp P. Obesity, adipose tissue distribution and health in men—the study of men born in 1913. Appetite 1989; 13:37–44.
31. Ohlson LO, Larsson B, Svardsudd K, Welin L, Eriksson H, Wilhelmsen L, Bjorntorp P, Tibblin G. The influence of body fat distribution on the incidence of diabetes mellitus. 13.5 years of follow-up of the participants in the study of men born in 1913. Diabetes 1985; 34:1055–1058.
32. Larsson B, Svardsudd K, Welin L, Wilhelmsen L, Bjorntorp P, Tibblin G. Abdominal adipose tissue distribution, obesity, and risk of cardiovascular disease and death: 13 year follow up of participants in the study of men born in 1913. Br Med J Clin Res Ed 1984; 288:1401–1404.
33. Krotkiewski M, Bjorntorp P, Sjostrom L, Smith U. Impact of obesity on metabolism in men and women. Importance of regional adipose tissue distribution. J Clin Invest 1983; 72:1150–1162.
34. Kissebah AH, Vydelingum N, Murray R, Evans DJ, Hartz AJ, Kalkhoff RK, Adams PW. Relation of body fat distribution to metabolic complications of obesity. J Clin Endocrinol Metab 1982; 54:254–260.
35. Stevens J, Knapp RG, Keil JE, Verdugo RR. Changes in body weight and girths in black and white adults studied over a 25 year interval. Int J Obes 1991; 15: 803–808.
36. Carmelli D, McElroy MR, Rosenman RH. Longitudinal changes in fat distribution in the Western Collaborative Group Study: a 23-year follow-up. Int J Obes 1991; 15:67–74.
37. Shimokata H, Tobin JD, Muller DC, Elahi D, Coon PJ, Andres R. Studies in the distribution of body fat. I. Effects of age, sex, and obesity. J Gerontol 1989; 44:M66–M73.
38. Vague J. The degree of masculine differentiation of obesities: a factor determining predisposition to diabetes, atherosclerosis, gout and uric calculous disease. Am J Clin Nutr 1956; 4:20–34.
39. Despres JP. Abdominal obesity as important component of insulin-resistance syndrome. Nutrition 1993; 9:452–459.
40. Bouchard C, Despres JP, Mauriege P. Genetic and nongenetic determinants of regional fat distribution. Endocr Rev 1993; 14:72–93.
41. Pouliot MC, Despres JP, Nadeau A, Moorjani S, Prud'Homme D, Lupien PJ, Tremblay A, Bouchard C. Visceral obesity in men. Associations with glucose tolerance, plasma insulin, and lipoprotein levels. Diabetes 1992; 41:826–834.
42. Matsuzawa Y, Shimomura I, Nakamura T, Keno Y, Tokunaga K. Pathophysiology and pathogenesis of visceral fat obesity. Ann NY Acad Sci 1995; 748:399–406.
43. Boyko EJ, Leonetti DL, Bergstrom RW, Newell Morris L, Fujimoto WY. Visceral adiposity, fasting plasma insulin, and blood pressure in Japanese-Americans. Diabetes Care 1995; 18:174–181.
44. Fujimoto WY, Bergstrom RW, Leonetti DL, Newell Morris LL, Shuman WP, Wahl PW. Metabolic and adipose risk factors for NIDDM and coronary disease in third-generation Japanese-American men and women with impaired glucose tolerance. Diabetologia 1994; 37:524–532.
45. Cefalu WT, Wang ZQ, Werbel S, Bell Farrow A, Crouse JRr, Hinson WH, Terry JG, Anderson R. Contribution of visceral fat mass to the insulin resistance of aging. Metabolism 1995; 44:954–959.
46. Schwartz RS, Shuman WP, Bradbury VL, Cain KC, Fellingham GW, Beard JC, Kahn SE, Stratton JR, Cerqueira MD, Abrass IB. Body fat distribution in healthy young and older men. J Gerontol 1990; 45:M181–M185.
47. Borkan GA, Hults DE, Gerzof SG, Robbins AH, Silbert CK. Age changes in body composition revealed by computed tomography. J Gerontol 1983; 38:673–677.
48. Lemieux S, Prud'Homme D, Bouchard C, Tremblay A, Despres JP. Sex differences in the relation of visceral adipose tissue accumulation to total body fatness. Am J Clin Nutr 1993; 58:463–467.
49. Baumgartner RN, Rhyne RL, Garry PJ, Chumlea WC. Body composition in the elderly from magnetic

resonance imaging: associations with cardiovascular disease risk factors. Basic Life Sci 1993; 60:35–38.
50. Gasperino JA, Wang J, Pierson RN Jr, Heymsfield SB. Age-related changes in musculoskeletal mass between black and white women. Metabolism 1995; 44:30–34.
51. Freedman DS, Williamson DF, Croft JB, Ballew C, Byers T. Relation of body fat distribution to ischemic heart disease. The National Health and Nutrition Examination Survey I (NHANES I) Epidemiologic Follow-up Study. Am J Epidemiol 1995; 142:53–63.
52. Dowling HJ, Pi Sunyer FX. Race-dependent health risks of upper body obesity. Diabetes 1993; 42: 537–543.
53. Stevens J, Keil JE, Rust PF, Tyroler HA, Davis CE, Gazes PC. Body maps index and body girths as predictors of mortality in black and white women [see comments]. Arch Intern Med 1992; 152:1257–1262.
54. Stern MP, Patterson JK, Mitchell BD, Haffner SM, Hazuda HP. Overweight and mortality in Mexican Americans. Int J Obes 1990; 14:623–629.
55. Fujimoto WY, Newell Morris LL, Grote M, Bergstrom RW, Shuman WP. Visceral fat obesity and morbidity: NIDDM and atherogenic risk in Japanese American men and women. Int J Obes 1991; 2:41 44.
56. Colditz GA. Epidemiology of breast cancer. Findings from the Nurses' Health Study. Cancer 1993; 71: 1480–1489.
57. Austin H, Austin JM Jr, Partridge EE, Hatch KD, Shingleton HM. Endometrial cancer, obesity, and body fat distribution. Cancer Res 1991; 51:568–572.
58. Wing RR, Matthews KA, Kuller LH, Meilahn EN, Plantinga PL. Weight gain at the time of menopause. Arch Intern Med 1991; 151:97–102.
59. Wang Q, Hassager C, Ravn P, Wang S, Christiansen C. Total and regional body-composition changes in early postmenopausal women: age-related or menopause-related? Am J Clin Nutr 1994; 60:843–848.
60. Svendsen OL, Hassager C, Christiansen C. Age- and menopause-associated variations in body composition and fat distribution in healthy women as measured by dual-energy x-ray absorptiometry. Metabolism 1995; 44:369–373.
61. Ley CJ, Lees B, Stevenson JC. Sex- and menopause-associated changes in body-fat distribution. Am J Clin Nutr 1992; 55:950–954.
62. Kotani K, Tokunaga K, Fujioka S, Kobatake T, Keno Y, Yoshida S, Shimomura I, Tarui S, Matsuzawa Y. Sexual dimorphism of age-related changes in whole-body fat distribution in the obese. Int J Obes Relat Metab Disord 1994; 18:207–202.
63. Espeland MA, Stefanick ML, Kritz-Silverstein D, Fineberg SE, Waclawiw MA, James MK, Greenfield M. Effect of postmenopausal hormone therapy on body weight and waist and hip girths. J Clin Endocrinol Metab 1997; 82:1549–1556.
64. Pasquali R, Casimirri F, Labate AM, Tortelli O, Pascal G, Anconetani B, Gatto MR, Flamia R, Capelli M, Barbara L. Body weight, fat distribution and the menopausal status in women. The VMH Collaborative Group. Int J Obes Relat Metab Disord 1994; 18:614–621.
65. Poehlman ET, Toth MJ, Gardner AW. Changes in energy balance and body composition at menopause: a controlled longitundinal study. Ann Intern Med 1995; 123:673–675.
66. Haarbo J, Marslew U, Gotfredsen A, Christiansen C. Postmenopausal hormone replacement therapy prevents central distribution of body fat after menopause. Metabolism 1991; 40:1323–1326.
67. Garry PJ, Hunt WC, Koehler KM, VanderJagt DJ, Vellas BJ. Longitundinal study of dietary intakes and plasma lipids in healthy elderly men and women. Am J Clin Nutr 1992; 55:682–688.
68. Hallfrisch J, Muller D, Drinkwater D, Tobin J, Andres R. Continuing diet trends in men: the Baltimore Longitudinal Study of Aging (1961–1987). J Gerontol 1990; 45:M186–M191.
69. Swinburn B, Ravussin E. Energy balance or fat balance? Am J Clin Nutr 1993; 57:766S–770S.
70. Tomoyasu NJ, Toth MJ, Poehlman ET. Misreporting of total energy intake in older men and women. J Am Geriatr Soc 1999; 47:710–715.
71. Roberts S. Energy regulation and aging: recent findings and their implications. Nutr Rev 2000; 58:91–97.
72. Poehlman ET. Regulation of energy expenditure in aging humans. J Am Geriatr Soc 1993; 41:552–559.
73. Poehlman ET, Gardner AW, Goran MI. Influence of endurance training on energy intake, norepinephrine kinetics, and metabolic rate in older individuals. Metabolism 1992; 41:941–948.
74. Schulz LO, Nyomba BL, Alger S, Anderson TE, Ravussin E. Effect of endurance training on sedentary energy expenditure measured in a respiratory chamber. Am J Physiol 1991; 260:E257–E261.
75. Schwartz RS, Jaeger LF, Veith RC. The thermic effect of feeding in older men: the importance of the sympathetic nervous system. Metabolism 1990; 39: 733–737.
76. Tataranni PA, Larson DE, Snitker S, Ravussin E. Thermic effect of food in humans: methods and results from use of a respiratory chamber. Am J Clin Nutr 1995; 61:1013–1039.
77. Wagner EH, LaCroix AZ, Buchner DM, Larson EB. Effects of physical activity on health status in older adults. I. Observational studies. Annu Rev Public Health 1992; 13:451–468.
78. Poehlman ET, Copeland KC. Influence of physical activity on insulin-like growth factor-I in healthy younger and older men. J Clin Endocrinol Metab 1990; 71:1468–1473.
79. Vaughan L, Zurlo F, Ravussin E. Aging and energy expenditure. Am J Clin Nutr 1991; 53:821–825.
80. Williamson DF, Madans J, Anda RF, Kleinman JC,

Kahn HS, Byers T. Recreational physical activity and ten-year weight change in a US national cohort. Int J Obes Relat Metab Disord 1993; 17:279–286.
81. Goran MI, Calles-Escandon J, Poehlman ET, O'Connell M, Danforth E Jr. Effects of increased energy intake and/or physical activity on energy expenditure in young healthy men. J Appl Physiol 1994; 77: 366–372.
82. Rising R, Harper IT, Fontvielle AM, Ferraro RT, Spraul M, Ravussin E. Determinants of total daily energy expenditure: variability in physical activity. Am J Clin Nutr 1994; 59:800–804.
83. Calles-Escandon J, Poehlman ET. Aging fat oxidation and exercise. Aging (Milano) 1997; 9:57–63.
84. DeFronzo RA, Ferrannini E. Insulin resistance. A multifaceted syndrome responsible for NIDDM, obesity, hypertension, dyslipidemia, and atherosclerotic cardiovascular disease. Diabetes Care 1991; 14: 173–194.
85. Chaiken RL, Banerji MA, Huey H, Lebovitz HE. Do blacks with NIDDM have an insulin-resistance syndrome? Diabetes 1993; 42:444–449.
86. Morales PA, Mitchell BD, Valdez RA, Hazuda HP, Stern MP, Haffner SM. Incidence of NIDDM and impaired glucose tolerance in hypertensive subjects. The San Antonio Heart Study. Diabetes 1993; 42:154–161.
87. Bjorntorp P. Abdominal obesity and the metabolic syndrome. Ann Med 1992; 24:465–468.
88. Ferrannini E. The insulin resistance syndrome. Curr Opin Nephrol Hypertens 1992; 1:291–298.
89. Lemieux S, Despres JP. Metabolic complications of visceral obesity: contribution to the aetiology of type 2 diabetes and implications for prevention and treatment. Diabete Metab 1994; 20:375–393.
90. Mitchell BD, Haffner SM, Hazuda HP, Valdez R, Stern MP. The relation between serum insulin levels and 8-year changes in lipid, lipoprotein, and blood pressure levels. Am J Epidemiol 1992; 136:12–22.
91. Austin MA, Mykkanen L, Kuusisto J, Edwards KL, Nelson C, Haffner SM, Pyorala K, Laakso M. Prospective study of small LDLs as a risk factor for non-insulin-dependent diabetes mellitus in elderly men and women. Circulation 1995; 92:1770–1778.
92. Despres JP, Marette A. Relation of components of insulin resistance syndrome to coronary disease risk. Curr Opin Lipidol 1994; 5:274–289.
93. Kahn SE, Schwartz RS, Porte DJ, Abrass IB. The glucose intolerance of aging: implications for intervention. Hosp Prac 1991; 26:29–38.
94. Harris MI. Epidemiology of diabetes mellitus among the elderly in the United States. Clin Geriatr Med 1990; 6:703–719.
95. Rubin RJ, Altman WM, Mendelson DN. Health care expenditures for people with diabetes mellitus. J Clin Endocrinol Metab 1992; 78:809A–809F.
96. Meyers DA, Goldberg AP, Bleecker ML, Coon PJ, Drinkwater DT, Bleecker ER. Relationship of obesity and physical fitness to cardiopulmonary and metabolic function in healthy older men. J Gerontol 1991; 46: M57–M65.
97. Kahn SE, Larson VG, Beard JC, Cain KC, Fellingham GW, Schwartz RS, Veith RC, Stratton JR, Cerqueira MD, Abrass IB. Effect of exercise on insulin action, glucose tolerance, and insulin secretion in aging. Am J Physiol 1990; 258:E937–E943.
98. Coon PJ, Rogus EM, Drinkwater D, Muller DC, Goldberg AP. Role of body fat distribution in the decline in insulin sensitivity and glucose tolerance with age. J Clin Endocrinol Metab 1992; 75:1125–1132.
99. Shimokata H, Muller DC, Fleg JL, Sorkin J, Ziemba AW, Andres R. Age as independent determinant of glucose tolerance. Diabetes 1991; 40:44–51.
100. Kohrt WM, Kirwan JP, Staten MA, Bourey RE, King DS, Holloszy JO. Insulin resistance in aging is related to abdominal obesity. Diabetes 1993; 42:273–281.
101. Applegate WB. High blood pressure treatment in the elderly. Clin Geriatr Med 1992; 8:103–117.
102. Despres JP. Dyslipidaemia and obesity. Baillieres Clin Endocrinol Metab 1994; 8:629–660.
103. Katzel LI, Busby Whitehead MJ, Goldberg AP. Adverse effects of abdominal obesity on lipoprotein lipids in healthy older men. Exp Gerontol 1993; 28:411–420.
104. Chumlea WC, Baumgartner RN, Garry PJ, Rhyne RL, Nicholson C, Wayne S. Fat distribution and blood lipids in a sample of healthy elderly people. Int J Obes Relat Metab Disord 1992; 16:125–133.
105. Mykkanen L, Laakso M, Pyorala K. Association of obesity and distribution of obesity with glucose tolerance and cardiovascular risk factors in the elderly. Int J Obes Relat Metab Disord 1992; 16:695–704.
106. Mykkanen L, Kuusisto J, Haffner SM, Pyorala K, Laakso M. Hyperinsulinemia predicts multiple atherogenic changes in lipoproteins in elderly subjects. Arterioscler Thromb 1994; 14:518–526.
107. Andres R. Mortality and obesity: the rationale for age-specific height-weight tables. In: Bierman EL, Blass JP, Ettinger WHJ, Halter JB, eds. Principles of Geriatric Medicine and Gerontology. New York: McGraw-Hill, 1994:847–853.
108. Harris T, Cook EF, Garrison R, Higgins M, Kannel W, Goldman L. Body mass index and mortality among nonsmoking older persons. The Framingham Heart Study. JAMA 1988; 259:1520–1524.
109. Garrison RJ, Castelli WP. Weight and thirty-year mortality of men in the Framingham Study. Ann Intern Med 1985; 103:1006–1009.
110. Willett WC, Dietz WH, Colditz GA. Primary care: guidelines for healthy weight. N Engl J Med 1999; 341:427–434.
111. Stevens J, Cai J, Pamuk ER, Williamson DF, Thun MJ, Wood JL. The effect of age on the association

between body-mass index and mortality. N Engl J Med 1998; 338:1–7.

112. Stevens J, Cai J, Juhaeri, Thun MJ, Williamson DF, Wood JL. Cosequences of the use of different measures of effect to determine the impact of age on the association between obesity and mortality. Am J Epidemiol 1999; 150:399–407.
113. Comoni Huntley JC, Harris TB, Everett DF, Albanes D, Micozzi MS, Miles TP, Feldman JJ. An overview of body weight of older persons, including the impact on mortality. The National Health and Nutrition Examination Survey I—Epidemiologic Follow-up Study. J Clin Epidemiol 1991; 44:743–753.
114. Fried LP, Kronmal RA, Newman AB, Bild DE, Mittlemark MB, Polak JF, Robbins JA, Gardin JM. Risk factors for 5-year mortality in older adults: the Cardiovascular Health Study. JAMA 1998; 279:585–592.
115. Hochberg MC, Lethbridge-Cejku M, Scott WW, Reichle R, Plato CC, Tobin JD. The association of body weight, body fatness and body fat distribution with oseoarthritis of the knee: data from the Baltimore Longitudinal Study of Aging. J Rheumatol 1995; 22:488–493.
116. Sarkisian CA, Liu H, Gutierrrez PR, Seeley DG, Cummings SR, Mangione CM. Modifiable risk factors predict functional decline among older women: a prospectively validated clinical prediction tool. J Am Geriatr Soc 2000; 48: 170–178.
117. Carmelli D, Swan GE, Bliwise DL. Relationship of 30-year changes in obesity to sleep-disordered breathing in the Western Collaborative Group Study. Obes Res 2000; 632–637.
118. Willett WC, Manson JE, Stampfer MJ, Colditz GA, Rosner B, Speizer FE, Hennekens CH. Weight, weight change, and coronary heart disease in women. Risk within the 'normal' weight range [see comments]. JAMA 1995; 273:461–465.
119. Colditz GA, Willett WC, Rotnitzky A, Manson JE. Weight gain as a risk factor for clinical diabetes mellitus in women [see comments]. Ann Intern Med 1995; 122:481–486.
120. Blair SN, Shaten J, Brownell K, Collins G, Lissner L. Body weight change, all-cause mortality, and cause-specific mortality in the Multiple Risk Factor Intervention Trial [see comments]. Ann Intern Med 1993; 119:749–757.
121. Lee IM, Paffenbarger RS Jr. Change in body weight and longevity [see comments]. JAMA 1992; 268:2045–2049.
122. Andres R, Muller DC, Sorkin JD. Long-term effects of change in body weight on all-cause mortality. A review [see comments]. Ann Intern Med 1993; 119:737–743.
123. Ho SC, Woo J, Sham A. Risk factor change in older persons, a perspective from Hong Kong: weight change and mortality. J Gerontol 1994; 49:M269–M272.
124. Iribarren C, Sharp DS, Burchfiel CM, Petrovitch H. Association of weight loss and weight fluctuation with mortality among Japanese American men [see comments]. N Engl J Med 1995; 333:686–692.
125. Reynolds MW, Fredman L, Langenberg P, Magaziner J. Weight, weight change and mortality in a random sample of older community-dwelling women. J Am Geriatr Soc 1999; 47:1409–1414.
126. French SA, Folsom AR, Jeffery RW, Zheng W, Mink PJ, Baxter JE. Weight variability and incident disease in older women: the Iowa Women's Health Study. Int J Obes 1997; 21:217–223.
127. Williamson DF, Pamuk ER. The association between weight loss and increased longevity. A review of the evidence. Ann Intern Med 1993; 119:731–736.
128. Pamuk ER, Willianmson DF, Serdula MK, Madans J, Byers TE. Weight loss and subsequent death in a cohort of U.S. adults. Ann Intern Med 1993; 119:744–748.
129. Williamson DF, Pamuk E, Thun M, Flanders D, Byers T, Heath C. Prospective study of intentional weight loss and mortality in never-smoking overweight US white women aged 40–64 years [published erratum appears in Am J Epidemiol 1995; 142(3):369]. Am J Epidemiol 1995; 141:1128–1141.
130. Verdery RB. Clinical evaluation of failure to thrive in older people. Clin Geriatr Med 1997; 13:769-778.
131. Newman, AB, Yanez D, Harris T, Duxbury A, Enright PL, Fried LP. Weight change in old age and its association with mortality. J Am Geriatr Soc 2001; 49:1309–1318.
132. Dey DK, Rothenberg E, Sundh V, Bosaeus I, Steen B. Body mass index, weight change and mortality in the elderly. A 15 y longitudinal population study of 70 y olds. Eur J Clin Nutr 2001; 55:482–492.
133. Allison DB, Zannolli R, Faith MS. Weight loss increases and fat loss decreases all-cause mortality rate: results from two independent cohort studies. Int J Obes Relat Metab Disord 1999; 23:603–611.
134. Dengel DR, Hagberg JM, Coon PJ, Drinkwater DT, Goldberg AP. Effects of weight loss by diet alone or combined with aerobic exercise on body composition in older obese men. Metabolism 1994; 43:867–871.
135. Purnell JQ, Kahn SE, Albers JJ, Nevin DN, Brunzell JD, Schwartz RS. Effect of weight loss with reduction of intra-abdominal fat on lipid metabolism in older men. J Clin Endocrinol Metab 2000; 85:977–982.
136. Colman E, Katzel LI, Rogus E, Coon P, Muller D, Goldberg AP. Weight loss reduces abdominal fat and improves insulin action in middle-aged and older men with impaired glucose tolerance. Metabolism 1995; 44:1502–1508.
137. Dengel DR, Hagberg JM, Coon PJ, Drinkwater DT, Goldberg AP. Comparable effects of diet and exercise on body composition and lipoproteins in older men. Med Sci Sports Exerc 1994; 26:1307–1315.

138. Barzilai N, Bupta G. Revisiting the role of fat mass in the life extension induced by caloric restriction. J Gerontol 1999; 54:B89–B96.
139. Schwartz RS, Buchner DM. Exercise in the elderly: physiologic and functional effects. In: Hazzard WR, Bierman EL, Blass JP, Ettinger WHJ, Halter JB, eds. Principles of Geriatric Medicine and Gerontology, Vol 3. New York: McGraw-Hill, 1994:91–105.
140. Wilmore JH. Variations in physical activity habits and body composition. Int J Obes Relat Metab Disord 1995; 19:S107–S112.
141. Barlow CE, Kohl HW, Gibbons LW, Blair SN. Physical fitness, mortality and obesity. Int J Obes Relat Metab Disord 1995; 19:S41–S44.
142. Schwartz RS, Hirth VA. The effects of endurance and resistance training on blood pressure. Int J Obes Relat Metab Disord 1995; 19:S52–S57.
143. Helmrich SP, Ragland DR, Leung RW, Paffenbarger RS, Jr. Physical activity and reduced occurrence of non-insulin-dependent diabetes mellitus [see comments]. N Engl J Med 1991; 325:147–152.
144. Despres JP, Lamarche B, Bouchard C, Tremblay A, Prud'Homme D. Exercise and the prevention of dyslipidemia and coronary heart disease. Int J Obes Relat Metab Disord 1995; 19:S45–S51.
145. Pavlou KN, Krey S, Stefffee WP. Exercise as an adjunct to weight loss and maintainence in moderately obese subjects. Am J Clin Nutr 1989; 49:1115–1123.
146. Ewbank PP, Darga LL, Lucas CP. Physical activity as a predictor of weight maintenance in previously obese subjects. Obes Res 1995; 3:257–263.
147. Schwartz RS, Shuman WP, Larson V, Cain KC, Fellingham GW, Beard JC, Kahn SE, Stratton JR, Cerqueira MD, Abrass IB. The effect of intensive endurance exercise training on body fat distribution in young and older men. Metabolism 1991; 40:545–551.
148. Kohrt WM, Obert KA, Holloszy JO. Exercise training improves fat distribution patterns in 60- to 70-year-old men and women. J Gerontol 1992; 47:M99–M105.
149. Schwartz RS, Cain KC, Shuman WP, Larson V, Stratton JR, Beard JC, Kahn SE, Cerqueira MD, Abrass IB. Effect of intensive endurance training on lipoprotein profiles in young and older men. Metabolism 1992; 41:649–654.
150. Kirwan JP, Kohrt WM, Wojta DM, Bourey RE, Holloszy JO. Endurance exercise training reduces glucose-stimulated insulin levels in 60- to 70-year-old men and women. J Gerontol 1993; 48:M84–M90.
151. Katzel LI, Bleecker ER, Colman EG, Rogus EMS, Goldberg AP. Effects of weight loss vs. aerobic exercise training on risk factors for coronary disease in healthy, obese, middle-aged and older men. JAMA 1995; 274:1915–1921.
152. Goran MI, Poehlman ET. Endurance training does not enhance total energy expenditure in healthy elderly persons. Am J Physiol 1992; 263:E950–E957.
153. Poehlman ET, Danforth E Jr. Endurance training increases metabolic rate and norepinephrine appearance rate in older individuals. Am J Physiol 1991; 261: E233–E239.
154. Poehlman ET, Gardner AW, Arciero PJ, Goran MI, Calles-Escandon J. Effects of endurance training on total fat oxidation in elderly persons. J Appl Physiol 1994; 76:2281–2287.
155. Treuth MS, Ryan AS, Pratley RE, Rubin MA, Miller JP, Nicklas BJ, Sorkin J, Harman SM, Goldberg AP, Hurley BF. Effects of strength training on total and regional body composition in older men. J Appl Physiol 1994; 77:614–620.
156. Treuth MS, Hunter GR, Kekes Szabo T, Weinsier RL, Goran MI, Berland L. Reduction in intra-abdominal adipose tissue after strength training in older women. J Appl Physiol 1995; 78:1425–1431.
157. Miller JP, Pratley RE, Goldberg AP, Gordon P, Rubin M, Treuth MS, Ryan AS, Hurley BF. Strength training increases insulin action in healthy 50- to 65-yr-old men. J Appl Physiol 1994; 77:1122–1127.
158. Smutok MA, Reece C, Kokkinos PF, et al. Aerobic versus strength training for risk factor intervention in middle-aged men at high risk for coronary heart disease. Metabolism 1993; 42:177–184.
159. Kokkinos PF, Hurley BF, Smutok MA, et al. Strength training does not improve lipoprotein-lipid profiles in men at risk for CHD. Med Sci Sports Exerc 1991; 23:1134–1139.
160. Schwartz RS. Trophic factor supplementation: effect on age-associated changes in body composition. J Gerontol 1995; 50A:151–156.
161. Papadakis MA, Grady D, Black D, Tierney MJ, Gooding GAW, Schambelan M, Grunfeld C. Growth hormone replacement in healthy older men improves body composition but not functional ability. Ann Intern Med 1996; 124:708–716.
162. Munzer T, Harman SM, Hees P, Shapiro E, Christmas C, Bellantoni MF, Stevens TE, O'Connor KG, Pabst KM, St Clair C, Sorkin JD, Blackman MR. Effects of GH and/or sex steroid administration on abdominal subcutaneous and visceral fat in healthy aged women and men. J Clin Endocrinol Metab 2001; 86:3604–3610.
163. Bhasin S, Bagatell CJ, Bremner WJ, Plymate SR, Tenover JL, Korenman SG, Nieschlag E. Issues in testosterone replacement in older men. J Clin Endocrinol Metab 1998; 83:3435–3448.
164. Labrie F, Belanger A, Cusan L, Gomez JL, Candas B. Marked decline in serum concentrations of adrenal C19 sex steroid precursors and conjugated androgen metabolites during aging. J Clin Endocrinol Metab 1997; 82:2396–2402.
165. Villareal DT, Holloszy JO, Kohrt WM. Effects of DHEA replacement on bone mineral density and body composition in elderly women and men. Clin Endocrinol 2000; 53:561–568.

8

Economic Costs of Obesity

Ian D. Caterson

University of Sydney, Sydney, New South Wales, Australia

Janet Franklin

Royal Prince Alfred Hospital, Sydney, New South Wales, Australia

Graham A. Colditz

Harvard Medical School and Brigham & Women's Hospital, Boston, Massachusetts, U.S.A.

I INTRODUCTION

Everyone working in the obesity area wants to know the cost of obesity. They want a magic number, and feel it must be a high dollar cost, which can be used in advocacy with governments and health authorities. The reason for this need is to "raise the profile" of obesity on the health agenda. This, it is hoped, will enable obesity to be treated more appropriately (in proportion to the true public health impact), and for increased resource allocation to obesity prevention. The expected outcome of these invigorated treatment and prevention approaches will reduce future health expenditures on obesity and its related diseases. However, in most countries or health areas, the amount of money available for health care is finite and limited. Given constraints of health care funding, allocation of additional resources to obesity prevention and treatment requires that effective programs must be available. A trade-off therefore exists between prevention of weight gain and obesity and the future health consequences of weight gain. We emphasize both the use and the limitations of calculating or knowing the costs of obesity. While a costing can be used for advocacy, a change in the costs of obesity may not be the most appropriate or desirable end point of such advocacy. Rather it may be better to aim for changes in such things as disability-adjusted life years (DALYs), quality-of-life measures, or changes in incidence or prevalence of obesity-associated diseases.

This chapter will therefore concentrate on a number of aspects of the economic costs of obesity. Firstly a broad outline of the types of costs will be considered and then a brief review of the reported costs undertaken. Subsequent sections will highlight difficulties in the present reported methods and then the major section will suggest a practical, yet thorough, way to establish the economic costs. It needs to be emphasised at this stage that because of the nature of this Handbook of Obesity, this chapter cannot be a definitive text of all health economics theory and applications, nor can it give exhaustive discussion of all theories. It is our aim to give a summary of reported costs and a practical approach to the methods and requirements to develop one's own systematic approach to determining the costs of obesity.

II TYPES OF COSTS

When one is considering the economic cost of obesity in direct monetary terms, there are three types of Costs to be considered. These are direct, indirect, and intangible costs.

A Direct Costs

Direct costs are the health care resources applied to obesity and its attributable conditions. In general these are prevalence studies, with knowledge of the cost within a defined time period. Such studies are often possible to perform given the usual data collection of health departments and authorities. Others will argue that incidence-based studies, which depend on calculating the cost of obesity and diseases occurring within a defined time are preferable. Such studies are more difficult to perform, the data may not be available without a special collection study, and the information they give in terms of monetary cost is no more robust than that from prevalence studies. Most cost-of-obesity studies in the literature are prevalence studies.

B Indirect Costs

Indirect costs are the reduction in the level of economic activity due to the illness and premature death attributable to obesity. The economic activity is generally considered to be that captured by the gross domestic product (GDP) statistic. Examples are the wages and productivity lost due to sickness and absenteeism produced by obesity or the loss of productivity due to the mechanical difficulties caused by obesity which reduce the efficiency of performing a task. Other factors contributing to the indirect costs of obesity are the disability pensions which are paid because of obesity or its associated conditions and the loss of productivity produced by the premature deaths due to obesity. There are several ways to calculate this cost and it is more difficult to do and more varied in outcome than the health care (or direct) costs.

C Intangible (Personal) Costs

These are the social and personal costs or losses associated with obesity. While some of these may be relatively easy to estimate, for example, the amount spent on commercial weight loss programs, other aspects are more difficult, variable, and subject to the whim of the individual health economist. An example of the latter would be an estimation of the monetary value of the reduced quality of life experienced because of obesity. This will require both quality-of-life measures in individuals and populations and an estimate of what is the usual cost of a life-year. In addition, the degree of obesity will have an effect. While there are suppositions and estimations with the other type of economic costs, such factors are probably greater and more variable for intangible costs.

There are also other ways of looking at the economic costs of obesity. These include years lost to disability (YLDs) or disability-adjusted life years (DALYs), or quality-adjusted life years. An example of the use of this type of "cost" may be found in Mathers et al. (1), and this can be contrasted with the "monetary cost" approach by the same authors (2). These different approaches will be discussed later in this chapter. Initially the concentration will be on the economic or monetary costs of obesity. These too must be contrasted with the costs of disease treatment itself. For example Brown et al. (3) have described the treatment costs of type 2 diabetes in this way contrasting diet treatment alone with drug treatment and the treatment of complications. This is a further approach and will be discussed later.

III REPORTED COSTS OF OBESITY

There are a large number of obesity cost or burden of illness studies. Table 1 gives a summary of those recently published from a variety of different countries and continents. The range of direct costs reported is between US$77 million for New Zealand (14), a country in which the prevalence of obesity is now 19%, and US$70 billion in the United States (15), where the prevalence of obesity is some 25% of the adult population. Recently it has been suggested that the direct cost of obesity in Australia is now US$630 million (S. Crowley, personal communication). The differences in costs reported may reflect different obesity prevalence in the various countries or different absolute health costs in the treatment of obesity and its related diseases. More likely, however, are differences in the methodology of performing the study. Some of these differences (e.g., the body mass index [BMI] cut point used, the diseases included in the costs) will be discussed in the following section.

As a general comment, it appears that the direct cost of obesity in many countries is between 1% and 5% of their health care budget (16). It appears that this cost may be greater in the United States [most recently reported to be 7% of the health care expenditure (15)]. We note that these costs are likely conservative as the

Table 1 Recently Reported Costs of Obesity from Several Countries[a]

Country	Year (Ref.)	Type of cost	Amount	% Health care expenditure
United States	1995 (4)	Direct	US$ 70 billion	7
	1995 (5)	Direct	US$51.6 billion	5.7
		Indirect	US$47.6 billion	
	1990 (6)	Direct	US$45.8 billion	6.8
		Indirect	US$23 billion	
	1993 (7)	Direct		6
Canada	1997 (8)	Direct	C$829.4 million– C$3.4 billion	
The Netherlands	1981–89 (9)	Direct	DG1 billion	2.4
France	1992 (10)	Direct	FF5.8 billion	4
		Indirect	FF0.58 billion	
	1992 (11)	Direct	FF4.2-8.7 billion	2
United Kingdom	1990–91 (12)	Direct & Indirect	GBP130 million	0.7–1.5
Australia	1989–90 (13)	Direct	AU$464 million	
		Indirect	AU$272 million	
New Zealand	1991 (14)	Direct	NZ$135 million	> 2

[a] These studies used a variety of BMI cut points for obesity and methods for obtaining costs. These are all prevalence studies.

range of conditions included in these estimates has been somewhat limited. In Germany it was found that obesity was associated with more visits to medical care, more prescriptions, and therefore greater health care costs, but obesity was "underreported" or underutilized as a diagnosis in medical records and so the costs of obesity were underestimated (17).

Fewer studies report the indirect costs of obesity, and there is greater variation in these reported costs. Again this reflects both the factors included in indirect costs and the GDP of the country. It appears that indirect costs are generally less than the direct health care costs and vary between US$140 million for Australia in 1989–90 (13) and US$47.6 billion for the United States in 1995 (5). While acknowledging that good economic analysis had yet to be performed, Seidell reports that there is good data linking obesity with increased sick leave and disability pensions in Finland, Sweden, and the Netherlands (16). In studies in U.S. organizations, obesity has been shown to be directly linked to absenteeism and therefore increased costs (18,19). Obesity was associated with 1.74 times more "high" absenteeism and 1.61 times "moderate" absenteeism. Interestingly, Burton reported that the BMI range that was the nadir of absenteeism was BMI 25–27 (18). Jeffrey (20) has looked at work site intervention programs and their effect on absenteeism. Over 2 years, smoking cessation programs reduced absenteeism, but weight control programs did not.

There are obviously many problems in calculating the indirect costs of obesity and proper standardized analyses need to be performed and reported so that comparisons can be made. Difficulties in calculating this cost include getting the average wage lost, the time of absenteeism, the productivity lost, and the number of instances.

A number of incidence studies have been performed. Simply put, these studies take a cohort and follow them for a number of years and document the obesity-related costs of that time period. As the cohort is presumed to be representative of the country or area the costs can be extrapolated. As one example, Thompson and coworkers (21) estimated the lifetime costs of being at various BMI levels. In men at a BMI of 22.5 the lifetime cost of obesity was estimated to be US$ 19,300; at a BMI of 37.5, the costs were US$35,200. In women the costs varied between US$18,600 and $34,700 for the same range of BMIs. Clearly there is an increase in cost as an individual or group of individuals has or develops a greater BMI. In this study the costs over a period were documented and then extrapolated to obtained lifetime costs (future costs were discounted at an annual rate of 3%). In another incidence study, using a slightly different approach, Allison (22) calculated, using the data from Wolf and Colditz (5), the direct health care costs of obesity over the age range 20–85 with and without accounting for obesity-related deaths. They found the cost of obesity would be 0.89–4.32% of the U.S. health care budget. It is interesting to note that in the U.S. Navy, the cost of hospitalizations for obesity-related diseases was over US$5 million annually (23).

IV PROBLEMS WITH STUDY COMPARISON

There are difficulties and inconsistencies in the reported studies, which make comparisons of the direct costs of obesity in different countries difficult. Some of these problems are:

1. The use of different BMI cut points for overweight and obesity
2. Different obesity-associated diseases used in the analysis
3. Lack of reliable data sets which enable relative risks for obesity related diseases, in the specific community, to be calculated
4. Which cost centers are available (or used) for cost analysis
5. Great differences in the cost of the health care system in different countries (in the United States treatment costs far more than in other countries)

There is even more variation in the factors or items used for the calculation of indirect and intangible costs, and a far greater variation in the health economics methodology. While it may be possible to use a standard approach and standard items for the calculation of direct costs which will allow better comparison (and one such approach is given below in this chapter), it is far less likely that a standard approach to indirect or intangible costs will be developed in the near future.

In the studies described in Table 1 there is variation in the BMI cut points used. For example, in the study by Seidell from the Netherlands (16), the costs were calculated for both overweight and obesity, i.e., for a BMI > 25. It is interesting to note that this study estimated that three-quarters of the costs incurred were for the BMI range 25–30. One percent of health care costs was due to obesity (BMI > 30) itself. In other studies where a BMI > 30 was used, it was found that up to 7% of health care expenditure (15) could be attributed to the direct costs of obesity. In the recent Canadian study, obesity was defined as a BMI > 27 (8). In the incidence study of Thompson (21), several different BMI values were utilized as representing the midpoint of the ranges recommended by the WHO (BMIs of 22.5, 27.5, 32.5, and 37.5 were used). It is difficult to compare costs unless a standard definition of obesity is utilized. It is to be hoped that with the recent publication of the WHO Technical Report on obesity (24), the standard cut points for overweight (called "preobese" in the WHO report) and obesity suggested therein will be utilized.

Different studies use different obesity related diseases. Examples of the diseases included in some of the studies are given in Table 2. Of course costs will vary with the number of diseases included as obesity-associated and studies, which have chosen, for example, not to include musculoskeletal diseases will have lower overall health costs. It is interesting to note than none of the recent studies have included costs due to nonalcoholic steatohepatitis (NASH), which it is estimated

Table 2 Diseases Used for Calculation of Costs of Obesity in Various Studies

Disease	United States (25)	Canada (8)	France (10)	United Kingdom (12)	New Zealand (14)	Australia (13)
Type 2 diabetes mellitus	X	X	X	X	X	X
Coronary heart disease	X		X		X	
Hypertension	X	X	X		X	X
Dyslipidemia		X	X	X		
Vascular disease			X			X
Stroke		X	X	X		
Gallbladder disease	X	X	X		X	X
NASH						
Cancer						
Colon	X	X	X		X	X
Breast (postmenopausal)	X	X	X		X	X
Endometrial	X	X	X	X		X
Osteoarthritis	X		X	X		
Venous thrombosis and pulmonary embolism		X	X			
Overweight and obesity				X		
Gout			X			

may be the cause of 10% of the cirrhosis in some societies. The reasons for excluding diseases may be practical (no data available, or it is difficult to calculate a local relative risk) or because the disease is not considered important or costly in a specific locality. Still, unless a similar list of obesity-associated disorders is utilized, it will continue to be difficult to compare studies directly. As research continues and the impact of obesity on an increasing range of conditions becomes clearly documented, the evolution of this list of diseases will continue to create problems in looking at the costs of obesity either over time or even over publications from different years. Recent data from the follow-up of the Cancer Prevention Survey II at the American Cancer Society indicate that at least 10% of cancer mortality among men and 15% among women can be attributed to obesity (BMI 30 or greater) (E. Calle, personal communication December 2000). This is a far higher proportion of cancer than previously allocated to obesity in cost estimates.

One of the problems with doing any cost-of-illness study is the calculation of the relative risk of any particular disease in a community. To obtain this there needs to have been a large population-based study with both disease presence and BMI recorded. Even better would be the availability in a community of a number of such data collections over a period of time. This would allow the incidence of disease and relationship to obesity to be determined, which would allow the relative risk of any particular disease to obesity to be calculated. This relative risk is important, because it allows the population attributable fraction (PAF) to be calculated. This latter factor is used in any determination of direct costs. While the United States has many of these data available (admittedly mainly from studies with Caucasian populations), other countries and communities do not have these data readily available. There is therefore a tendency in studies of the costs of obesity to use relative risks obtained in communities other than the one being studied. This does lead to inaccuracy. The costs obtained can be swayed by the use of a conservative relative risk (RR), or of a higher one. For example, the RR of type 2 diabetes mellitus that has been used in studies ranges between 2.9 and 27.6 (see Table 3). The choice of a particular RR will obviously influence the population attributable fraction and hence the final cost calculated.

The risk of any disease caused by obesity may vary according to the composition of the population, such as the ethnic makeup. It appears that the risk of metabolic disease such as diabetes, hypertension, and dyslipidemia is particularly influenced by ethnic origin. This may be due to a greater propensity for abdominal fat distribution in a given group, or to a specific difference in the relationship between obesity and the particular disease in a given population. For example, it appears that the Chinese population has a greater risk of diabetes, nonalcoholic steatohepatitis (NASH), and dyslipidemia at BMI in the preobese range (BMI 25–29.9) than does the Caucasian population (26). Similarly, the Japanese population has a far greater risk for hypertension. At a BMI of 24.9 (in the healthy weight range) the risk for diabetes is 3.0 and the nadir of risk appears to be at a BMI of 22.6 (27). Until relative risks of obesity related diseases are available for more communities, ethnic groups, and countries, the standard Caucasian RRs will

Table 3 Relative Risk Values for the Obese Population Used in Recent Studies (see Tables 1, 2)

Disease	U.S.	Canada	France	New Zealand	Australia
Type II diabetes	27.6	4.37	2.9	16.7	16.7
Coronary heart disease	3.5	1.72	—	3.3	3.3
Endometrical Ca	2	2.19	2	2	2
Hypertension	3.9	2.51	2.9	4.3	4.3
Gallstones/gallbladder disease	3.2	1.85	2	10	10
PM breast cancer	1.3	1.31	1.2	1.3	1.3
Colon cancer	1.5	1.16	1.3	1.3	—
Myocardial infarction	—	—	1.9	—	—
Stroke	—	1.14	3.1	—	—
Venous thrombosis	—	—	1.5	—	—
Hyperlipidemia	—	1.41	1.5	—	—
Gout	—	—	2.5	—	—
Osteoarthritis	—	—	1.8	—	—
Pulmonary embolism	—	2.39	—	—	—

Ca, cancer; PM, postmenopausal.

continue to be used, probably with an underestimation of the true cost of obesity.

Another obvious problem is what cost centers to include in direct costs. There are a number of obvious possibilities such as visits to physicians and dietitians, hospital and laboratory costs, and drug costs. A list of potential inclusions is given in Table 4. Again, reported costs of obesity will vary depending on which cost centers are included and whether appropriate costings are available in the specific community or country.

There is one final thing that needs to be considered in any comparison of the costs of obesity. The cost of health care varies from country to country. That is, the cost of identical drugs, numbers of physician visits, days in hospital, and so on, will vary. The populations of countries also vary. The absolute cost of obesity will therefore be different in different countries. This is well shown by comparing the United States with New Zealand (Table 1). There is a difference in expenditure of $45 billion! One way of reducing this difference is to consider the direct cost of obesity as a percentage of health care expenditure, but even this will not totally eliminate discrepancies and differences. Unless there is identical methodology, the use of appropriate relative risks and the cost is expressed per head of population, it will continue to be difficult to compare the cost of obesity in one country with the cost in another.

DALYs are another possible way of looking at potential "costs" of obesity. They can be calculated as the number of years lost due to the premature mortality caused by obesity plus the number of years of healthy life lost due to the diseases associated with obesity. The years of healthy life lost requires the estimation of the incidence of the obesity related health conditions in a specified time period. The methodology has been described by Murray and Lopez (28). In a recent Australian analysis, obesity itself accounted for 4.3 DALYs, and when this is added to the effect of associated risk factors, physical inactivity (~6.8 DALYs), and lack of fruit and vegetables (~2.7 DALYs), the obesity associated cluster becomes a disease risk (and cost) to rival cigarette smoking (12.1 DALYs in men and 6.8 in women) (29).

Table 4 Cost Centers Used in Determination of Direct Costs

Personal health care
Hospital care
Inpatient and outpatient
Public and private
Medical services
GP/primary care consultations
Physicians' consultations
Dietitians' consultations
Other allied health professionals' consultation
Drugs
Laboratory services
Other professional services
Nursing home care

V REQUIREMENTS FOR COST OF OBESITY STUDIES

From the above discussion it can be seen that there are a number of prerequisites before a meaningful cost of obesity study can be performed. There needs to be a good study of the prevalence of obesity (defined using the WHO's suggested BMI cut points). In addition, a standard group of obesity-associated disorders should be included and it is optimal if there are known local RRs of these disorders from previous studies. Such estimates of RR will account for details of ethnic variation that may otherwise not be fully detailed in an analysis. If there are no local RRs, then it would be appropriate to use published values from other countries, trying as best as possible to match ethnic groupings and perhaps using a conservative risk factor as well as a high value. This approach assumes that the physiological and pathologic consequences of obesity are consistent across communities, which is not unreasonable. There also needs to be a standard approach to cost centers used for direct costs. In this way, it will become easier to compare costs across countries and perhaps a little easier to perform the studies themselves if the type of data utilized is standardized and collected.

To estimate the proportion of disease that could be prevented by eliminating obesity, we calculate the population-attributable risk percent (PAR%) or the population attributable fraction. This is the maximum proportion of disease attributable to the specific exposure (such as obesity). PAR% is based on the incidence of disease in the exposed (i.e., obese group) as compared with the nonexposed, taking relative risks from analyses that control for confounders (e.g., age, smoking, dietary intake, etc.). PAR% is calculated using

$$P(RR - 1)/1 + P(rr - 1)$$

where P is the prevalence of exposure in the population and RR the relative risk for disease.

A key issue in estimates of the proportion of disease due to obesity is the reference group. Is the disease burden estimated compared to those with a BMI < 25, who are considered average weight, or is a BMI such as 22 used as the reference for estimation. The choice of reference group has a substantial impact on the magnitude of the relative risk, and hence the estimate of the proportion of disease due to obesity. As one compares across studies, the distribution of BMI within the normal range will thus have influence on the observed RR. For example, as more of the population approaches overweight, the comparison of obese versus normal weight is not as extreme a comparison as when most of the population is in the lean end of normal weight. Further, for many obesity-related conditions, even within the normal weight range there is evidence of increased risk with increasing BMI in the normal range. [See figures in Willett et al. (30).] For example, in the prospective Nurses' Health Study, 10-year risk of being diagnosed with diabetes for obese women (30–34.9 kg/m^2) is 10 (8.4–11.8) times that of women in the average BMI range (< 25). However, when BMI of 18.5–21.9 is used as the comparison, the relative risk among obese women is 17.8 (13.4–23.7). In sum, using average weight (BMI < 25) as the reference for estimating the burden of obesity will underestimate the true proportion of disease that is attributable to excess adiposity.

Costs of services must also be estimated. As noted earlier in this chapter these include direct, indirect, and intangible costs. For the direct costs of health services it is important to distinguish true resource costs from typical charges. In countries with systems of health care that use cost accounting and document resource allocation, estimates for the resources used to treat obesity and its consequences are more readily available than in health systems that use mixed models of care including fee for service.

Indirect costs represent the values of lost rather than diverted resources as a result of temporary illness, permanent disability, or premature death. Thus they represent the value of productivity that is lost forever. To estimate these costs one requires the earnings of individuals, the level of labor force participation, and the level of premature mortality according to level of BMI or obesity. These labor force data are typically generated by government agencies.

For both direct and indirect costs, comparisons across nations will again be confounded by the value of resources allocated to health care and the relative earnings of individuals and labor force participation. However, despite these limitations, the percentage of the health expenditures consumed by obesity-related conditions still represents a more intuitive measure than the actual costs of obesity in a given country. The use of the percentage of health expenditures helps control for the population size.

VI CONCLUSION

The obesity epidemic is continuing to increase in magnitude globally. Estimates of the costs of obesity provide one measure that integrates the public health burden of this preventable condition and its health consequences. Two factors drive the economic burden of obesity—the prevalence of obesity, and the range of conditions that arise as a consequence of obesity. Uniform classification of obesity will lead to more consistent estimation of the costs of obesity. The prevalence of obesity is, however, expected to rise in many countries given the recent global trends. While published estimates may considerably underestimate the true burden of obesity, the substantial proportion of health expenditures consumed by conditions that arise as a consequence of obesity indicates that perhaps greater priority should be placed on prevention of excess weight gain and the development of obesity. Future studies of the costs of obesity should strive to adhere to the methodologic points summarized in this chapter. However, as new conditions become clearly linked to obesity as our understanding of the health consequences of obesity continue to broaden, the costs of disease will likely also increase purely as a consequence of these new insights, regardless of the proportion of the population who are obese.

REFERENCES

1. Mathers C, Vos T, Stevenson C. The Burden of Disease and Injury in Australia. Canberra: Australian Institute of Health and Welfare, 1999.
2. Mathers C, Penn R. Health System Costs of Cardiovascular Diseases and Diabetes in Australia 1993–94. Canberra: Australian Institute of Health and Welfare, 1999.
3. Brown JB, Nichols GA, Glauber HS, Bakst AW, Schaeffer M, Kelleher CC. Health care costs associated with escalation of drug treatment in type 2 diabetes mellitus. Am J Health System Pharmacol 2001; 58:151–157.
4. Colditz GA. Economic costs of obesity and inactivity. Med Sci Sports Exerc 1999; 31:S663–S667.
5. Wolf AM, Colditz GA. Current estimates of the economic cost of obesity in the United States. Obes Res 1998; 6:97–106.
6. Wolf AM, Colditz GA. The cost of obesity: the US perspective. Pharmacoeconomics 1994; 5:34–37.
7. Quesenberry C, Caan B, Jacobsen A. Obesity, health

services use and health care costs among members of a health maintenance organisation. Arch Intern Med 1998; 158:466–472.
8. Birmingham CL, Muller JL, Palepu A, Spinelli JJ, Anis AH. The cost of obesity in Canada. Can Med Assoc J 1999; 160:503–506.
9. Seidell JC. The impact of obesity on health status: some implications for health care costs. Int J Obes 1995; 19:S13–S16.
10. Levy E, Levy P, LePen C, Basdevant A. The economic cost of obesity: the French situation. Int J Obes 1995; 19:788–792.
11. Detourmay B, Fagnani F, Phillippo M, Pribil C, Charles MA, Sermet C, Basdevant A, Eschwege E. Obesity morbidity and health care costs in France: an analysis of the 1991–1992 Medical Care Household Survey. Int J Obes 2000; 24:151–155.
12. West, R. Obesity. In: Office of Health Economics Monographs on Current Health Issues. London: Office of Health Economics, 1994:38–42.
13. Segal L, Carter R, Zimmet P. The cost of obesity: the Australian perspective. Pharmacoeconomics 1994; 5:45–52.
14. Swinburn, B, Ashton T, Gillespie J, Cox B, Menon A, Simmons D, Birbeck J. Health care costs of obesity in New Zealand. Int J Obes 1997; 21:891–896.
15. Colditz G, Mariani A. The cost of obesity and sedentarism in the United States. In: Bouchard C, ed. Physical Activity and Obesity. Champaign, IL: Human Kinetics, 2000:55–66.
16. Seidell JC. Societal and personal costs of obesity. Exp Clin Endocrinol Diabetes 1998; 106:7–9.
17. Hauner, H, Koster I, Von Ferber L. Frequency of "obesity" in medical records and utilisation of out-patient health care by "obese" subjects in Germany. An analysis of health insurance data. Int J Obes 1996; 20:820–824.
18. Burton WN, Chen CY, Schultz AB, Edington DW. The economic costs associated with body mass idex in a workplace. J Occup Environ Med 1998; 40:786–792.
19. Tucker LA, Friedman GM. Obesity and absenteeism: an epidemiologic study of 10,825 employed adults. Am J Health Promot 1998; 12:202–207.
20. Jeffery RW, Forster JL, Dunn BV, French SA, McGovern PG, Lando HA. Effects of work-site health promotion on illness-related absenteeism. J Occup Med 1993; 35:1142–1146.
21. Thompson D, Edelsberg J, Colditz G, Bird A, Oster G. Lifetime health and economic consequences of obesity. Arch Intern Med 1999; 159:2177–2183.
22. Allison D, Zannolli R, Narayan K, Venkay M. The direct health care costs of obesity in the United States. Am J Clin Nutr 1999; 89:1194–1199.
23. Bradham DD, South BR, Saunders HJ, Hauser MD, Pane KW, Dennis KE. Obesity-related hospitalization costs to the US Navy, 1993 to 1998. Milit Med 2001; 166:1–10.
24. Obesity: preventing and managing the global epidemic. Report of a WHO consultation. World Health Org Tech Rep Ser 894, 2000.
25. Wolf AM, Colditz GA. Social and economic costs of body weight in the United States. Am J Clin Nutr 1996; 63:466S–469S.
26. Pan W-H. Epidemiology of obesity and dyslipidaemia. In: Third World Congress of International Society for Apheresis, Taipei, 56, 2001:A52.
27. Zimmet P, Inoue S, eds. The Asia-Pacific perspective: redefining obesity and its treatment. WHO, IASO, IOTF, 2000. Available from the International Association for the Study of Obesity (IASO), London. www.iaso.org.
28. Murray CJ, Lopez AD. The global burden of disease: a comprehensive assessment of mortality and disability from diseases, injuries and risk factors in 1990 and projected to 2020. Global Burden of Disease and Injury Series. Cambridge: Harvard School of Public Health, Vol 1, 1996.
29. Mathers C, Vos T, Stevenson C. The burden of disease and injury in Australia. Canberra: Australian Institute of Health and Welfare, 2000.
30. Willett WC, Dietz WH, Colditz GA. Guidelines for healthy weight. N Engl J Med 1999; 341:427–434.

9

Genetics of Human Obesity

Claude Bouchard

Pennington Biomedical Research Center, Baton Rouge, Louisiana, U.S.A.

Louis Pérusse

Laval University, Saìnte-Foy, Quebec, Canada

Treva Rice and D. C. Rao

Washington University School of Medicine, St. Louis, Missouri, U.S.A.

I INTRODUCTION

There are about 250 million adults who are obese and at least 500 million who are overweight in the world at the moment (1). Given these numbers, it is not surprising that the genetics of human obesity is receiving increasing attention. The interest in the causes of the present epidemic of obesity in the Western world and the promise of finding new potentially prophylactic and therapeutic means are largely responsible for this new interest. Excess weight has also become the most important public health problem in the United States and Canada, and this has contributed enormously to the present interest for the molecular and genetic causes of the problem. Several lines of research are currently being explored in the effort to identify the genes involved in causing obesity, rendering someone susceptible to obesity, or determining the metabolic response to an obese state.

This chapter will cover the following major topics: (1) the obesity phenotypes; (2) the findings from genetic epidemiology studies; (3) specific genes and association or linkage with obesity; (4) genotype-environment interaction effects; and (5) a brief discussion on useful strategies to undertake the genetic dissection of human obesity. The evidence for a role of genetic factors in energy and macronutrient intake as well as in the various energy expenditure components (resting metabolic rate, thermic response to food, nutrient partitioning, and energy expenditure associated with physical activity) will not be reviewed in any detail here. Two other chapters are dealing with topics of relevance for the understanding of the role played by genetic differences in obesity. One is Chapter 11 by York that reviews the rodent models, including the evidence from transgenics and knockouts. The other is Chapter 10 by Chua et al., which covers in detail the current understanding of the biology of single gene defects leading to obesity in rodents and humans.

II THE PHENOTYPES

Interest in the genetics of human obesities has increased considerably over the past decade partly because of the realization that some forms of obesity were associated with higher risks than others for various morbid conditions and mortality rate. Obesity can no longer be seen as a homogeneous phenotype.

Obesity is characterized by excess body mass or body fat without any particular reference to the concentration of fat in a given area of the body. Many obese individuals are characterized by an excess amount of subcutaneous fat on the trunk, particularly in the abdominal area, the so-called android obesity, or male type of fat deposition. Another type is characterized by an excessive amount of fat in the abdominal visceral area and has been labeled abdominal visceral obesity. The last is known as gluteofemoral obesity and is observed primarily in women (gynoid obesity). Thus, excess fat can be stored primarily in the truncal-abdominal area or in the gluteal and femoral area. This implies that a given body fat content, say, 30% or 30 kg, may exhibit different anatomical distribution characteristics.

Strictly speaking, one should therefore talk about the obesities rather than obesity. But the situation is even more complex as the phenotypes are not of the simple Mendelian kind. Segregation of the genes is not readily perceived, and whatever the role of the genotype in the etiology, it is generally attenuated or exacerbated by nongenetic factors. In other words, variation in human body fat is caused by a complex network of genetic, nutritional, metabolic, energy expenditure, psychological, and social variables, all playing a role in the modulation of energy balance and nutrient partitioning. Figure 1 depicts the key determinants and suggests how genetic differences can lead to obesity over time.

It is important to recognize that these phenotypes are not fully independent of one another, as shown by the data of Figure 2. The level of covariation among the various body fat phenotypes ranges from ~30% to ~50% and perhaps more in some circumstances. One implication of the above is that studies designed to investigate the causes of the individual differences in the various body fat phenotypes, including genetic causes, should control for these levels of covariation.

In clinical settings, the body mass index (BMI), measured in kg/m^2, is commonly used to assess the normality of body weight in patients. This is perfectly reasonable as most of the evidence from large-scale prospective studies that have associated obesity with morbidities and premature death is based on the BMI. The correlation between the BMI and total body fat or percent body fat is high in large and heterogeneous samples. The predictive value of the BMI is, however, much less impressive in a given individual, especially when the BMI is <30 kg/m^2 or so. Thus, the BMI is an indicator of heaviness and only indirectly of body fat (2,3). Any estimate of the genetic effect on BMI should not necessarily be considered valid for adiposity, as it is influenced in unknown proportions by the contribution of the genotype to fat mass, muscle mass, skeletal mass, and other components as well. Nevertheless, the BMI is worth considering because of its clinical validity, simplicity to measure, and widespread use.

The data summarized in Table 1 indicate why the BMI is only a partially acceptable surrogate measure of body fat content. The variance explained by BMI in percent body fat derived from underwater weighing in large samples of adult men and women, 35–54 years of age, attains only ~40%. At the extremes of the body fat content distribution, BMI is more closely associated with percent body fat; that is, the variance explained may reach 60% and more. This is not

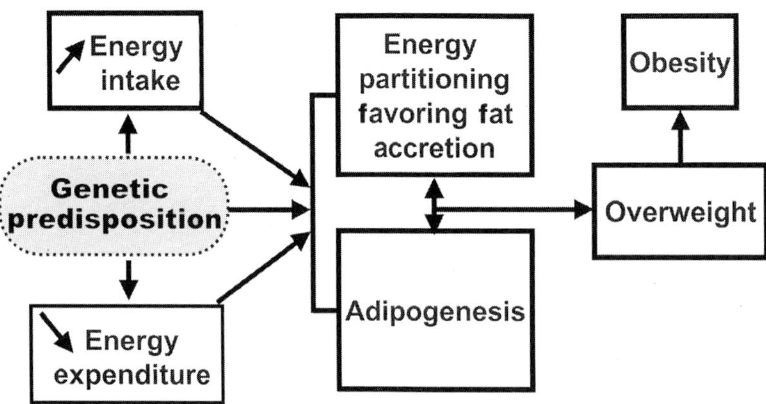

Figure 1 Diagram of the determinants of positive energy balance and fat deposition with indication about the sites of action of a genetic predisposition.

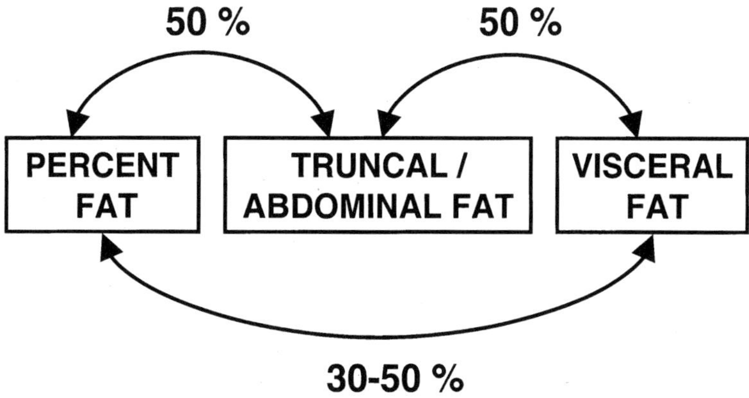

Figure 2 Common variance between three body fat phenotypes. Percent fat estimated from underwater weighing: truncal-abdominal fat assessed from skinfolds or CT scans; abdominal visceral fat estimated by CT scan at the L4/L5 vertebrae. (From Ref. 219.)

entirely satisfactory as genetic studies deal with individual differences in the phenotype of interest and, for them to be successful, the phenotype of a complex multifactorial trait must be measured with a reasonable degree of precision.

That percent body fat remains quite heterogeneous at any level of BMI is further illustrated in Table 2, based on data from middle-aged adult males. For instance, in 27 men with a BMI of 28–30, the mean percent body fat was 28, but the range varied from 15% to 41%. We have observed the same phenomenon and with as much heterogeneity in women at all levels of BMI.

The same point can be made for regional fat distribution phenotypes. Thus the correlation between the waist-to-hip circumferences ratio (WHR) and abdominal visceral fat is positive and generally significant in various populations, but the association is characterized by a wide scatter of scores. For instance, in a study of 51 adult obese women, the correlation between WHR and CT-assessed abdominal visceral fat reached 0.55 (4). However, for a WHR of ~0.80, the visceral fat area at the L4-L5 level ranged from a low of ~50 cm^2 to a high of ~200 cm^2. Even though the covariation between total body fat and abdominal visceral fat is statistically significant, the relationship is also characterized by a high degree of heterogeneity. As shown in Table 3, when BMI and percent body fat (%BF) are constrained to narrow ranges, one finds generally a threefold range for the amount of CT-assessed abdominal visceral fat in adult males. Thus in 16 men with BMI values of 30 or 31 and a percentage of body fat ranging from 30 to 33, mean abdominal visceral fat was 153 cm^2 with a range from 77–261 cm^2. Again, the same lack of coupling among BMI, %BF, and abdominal visceral fat was observed in adult women.

Table 1 Percent Variance ($r^2 \times 100$) Explained by BMI in Body Composition in Adults, 35–54 Years of Age

	BMI in 342 males	BMI in 356 females
Percent fat	41	40
Fat-free mass	37	25
Sum 6 skinfolds	58	67
TER	10	8

Percent fat and fat-free mass were derived from underwater weighing assessment of body density. TER = ratio of trunk to extremity skinfolds. Trunk skinfolds are the sum of subscapular, suprailiac, and abdominal skinfolds. Extremity skinfolds are the sum of triceps, biceps, and medial calf skinfolds.
Source: Ref. 219.

Table 2 Heterogeneity of Body Fat Content for a Given BMI Class in Males, 35–54 Years of Age

		Percent body fat[a]		
N	BMI	Mean	Min.	Max.
27	20–22	17	8	32
76	23–25	22	11	35
46	26–27	26	16	40
27	28–30	28	15	41

[a] From underwater weighing.
Source: Ref. 219.

Table 3 Variation in Amount of Abdominal Visceral Fat for Given BMI and %BF Classes in Males, 35–54 Years of Age

			Visceral fat in cm^2		
N	BMI	% Fat (range)	Mean	Min.	Max.
15	21–22	14–18	58	31	84
19	24–25	19–24	89	50	140
18	27–28	25–29	133	63	199
16	30–31	30–33	153	77	261

Abdominal visceral fat measured by CT scan at the L4–L5 level. Percent fat derived from underwater weighing.
Source: Ref. 219.

The above data suggest that even though it may be necessary to use the BMI or waist circumference for the prediction of abdominal visceral fat in clinical settings, such practice is not desirable in the context of scientific research designed to understand the causes and metabolic consequences of variation in body fat content or in fat topography.

In summary, useful data for the understanding of the genetics of obesity are likely to be obtained if the phenotype falls into one of the following categories: affected (obese) vs. unaffected (nonobese); BMI; indicators of adiposity (fat mass, percentage body fat, sum of several skinfolds); indicators of leanness (fat-free mass); indicators of abdominal obesity (abdominal fat, abdominal visceral fat, waist girth, sagittal diameter).

III GENETIC EPIDEMIOLOGY OF HUMAN OBESITY

There are several considerations in genetic epidemiological studies of obesity (5). First, obesity is not a simple Mendelian trait. For example, expression of genetic propensities may depend on appropriate environmental stimulation (i.e., gene-by-environment interaction), or developmental stage (i.e., age dependency), or sex (i.e., sex limited). Second, obesity is not a homogeneous trait stemming from a unique gene or set of genes. Third, the trait measured may index other traits such as bone and muscle mass, which also may have separate genetic determinants.

Genetic epidemiological methods are useful for addressing specific questions in human obesity, such as determining if there are genetic factors underlying an obesity phenotype, characterizing the sources of the genetic influence through maternal vs. paternal transmission, and whether the trait is sex limited or age dependent, or if there is assortative mating, etc. Other strategies include documenting the presumptive causes of obesity (e.g., energy intake or energy expenditure), and considering their complex biological and behavioral interactions in a network design (i.e., multivariate genetic epidemiological studies). Here, we briefly describe the types of data and analytical methods commonly used by genetic epidemiologists, and then review the findings for several human obesity traits.

A Review of Methods

1 Multifactorial

Genetic epidemiological studies of human obesity use a variety of family designs and a variety of statistical methods to partition the underlying phenotypic variance of a trait into genetic and environmental sources. In multifactorial studies (i.e., with polygenic and common environmental effects), the basic model is:

$$V_P = V_G + V_C + V_E$$

where the phenotypic variance (V_P) is due to the additive genetic variance (V_G), common (shared) environmental variance (V_C), and the residual or nonshared environmental variance (V_E). These factors can be partitioned, in turn, into more specific environmental (sibling vs. spouse vs. between generations) and genetic (gene-by-environment and gene-by-gene interactions, dominance deviations) components. The genetic heritability of a trait is expressed as the percent of total phenotypic variance due to the additive genetic effects ($h^2 = V_G/V_P$), and the common environmental component is the percent due to the common environment ($c^2 = V_C/V_P$).

The specific parameters that can be estimated depend on the study design, with typical designs including family (i.e., parents and their biological offspring), twin, and adoption studies. Design issues have been extensively covered elsewhere (e.g., 6–10), so we will only briefly review them here. For each study design, analytical methods range from relatively simple ones such as computing the familial correlations to more complex model-fitting using path or variance components analysis (11). Each design allows for estimation of specific types of familial effects, although each has underlying assumptions that must be recognized. For example, in the traditional family study (12,13) parents and offspring share both genes and familial environments to some degree, so it is difficult to separate G and C components (see 7). However, results from family studies are more easily generalized to the population at large, and other sources of familial variance (e.g., spouse resemblance and additional sibship resemblance) can be investigated. Twin studies (14–16) allow for separation of the G component since monozygotic (MZ) twins share 100% of their genes while dizygotic (DZ) twins share half on the average. Major concerns with twin data are that MZ twins may share more common environmental effects (and they do share more dominance deviations) than do DZ twins that can inflate the genetic component (see 6). The correlation between MZ twins reared apart is a relatively unbiased estimate of the broad-sense heritability (additive + dominance), although one must assume that the twins were reared in uncorrelated environments. Full adoption studies (see 17) are useful in separating common environmental effects since adoptive parents and their adopted offspring (and adopted sibling pairs) share only environmental sources of variance while the adoptees and their biological parents share only genetic sources of variance. Assumptions underlying adoption designs include no selective (or late) placement into the adoptive home and that adoptive families are representative of the general population.

Longitudinal assessment (i.e., repeated measures across time) can be applied to any of the family, twin, or adoption designs (see 18–20). Longitudinal study designs are particularly important in obesity research since it is generally recognized that fat accumulates with time, and trends in the familial effect may arise through secular environmental effects, or through age-limited developmental effects of genes as for example the growth spurt at puberty (21). Even more importantly, with body fat accretion up to a new body mass level (e.g., a given obesity level), the causes of the positive energy balance leading to obesity may be progressively masked over time. For instance, an apparent deficit in resting energy expenditure is compensated by an increase in the metabolic mass associated with weight gain (22), similarly for an apparent deficit in lipid oxidation rate which is eliminated when the gain in fat mass has been large enough to ensure a greater reliance on lipid oxidation (23). It adds a dimension to the complex task of understanding the causes of obesity and defining the role of genes. To unmask the true susceptibilities to be in positive energy balance, one has to rely on longitudinal data that will make it possible to define the relevant predictors of obesity and to specify their genetic and molecular basis.

Multivariate assessment is another important design issue in the study of obesity since there are likely to be multiple relevant predictors, each having unique determinants. Multivariate genetic epidemiology studies simultaneously examine several traits and determine the extent to which the separate measures may be influenced by unique and common genes and environment. The fundamental concept underlying multivariate studies is cross-trait resemblance between pairs of relatives; for example, trait 1 in parents with trait 2 in offspring (see 24). These methods are useful in documenting the complex behavioral and biological interactions in a network design.

2 Major Gene

Multifactorial effects typically arise from the action of many genes each having a small and additive influence on the phenotype (i.e., polygenic) that lead to a single normal distribution. However, other types of genetic effects are not necessarily additive (i.e., major gene) and are characterized as a mixture of distributions. Segregation analysis is used to determine whether the trait is due to a major gene that is segregating in families according to Mendelian expectations. In the mixed model (25), the phenotype is composed of the independent and additive contributions from a major gene effect, a multifactorial background, and a unique environmental component (residual). The major effect is assumed to result from the segregation at a single locus, and the transmission pattern from parents to offspring is tested to verify if the gene is segregating according to Mendelian expectations. Some models also allow for genotype-dependent covariate effects [e.g., PAP (26,27), and REGRES (28)]. For example, the major gene effect may depend on the age of the individual (i.e., genes turning on or off over time) or may have different effects depending on sex. Pleiotropic (i.e., single gene influencing multiple traits) and oligogenic (i.e., multiple genes) models also can be tested with multilocus-multitrait segregation models (e.g., 29).

3 Combined Models

Complex traits such as obesity involve multiple intercorrelated phenotypes, and it is highly unlikely that we will discover anything close to "the gene" which explains most of the variation for the phenotype. Instead, we expect genetic effects in the oligogenic (few genes) to polygenic (many genes) range, with an elaborate interplay between many factors, including gene-gene and gene-environmental interactions. While a lot of analytic progress has been made using the strategies discussed so far, a combined approach (see 30) is potentially much more powerful and holds great promise for these traits. Combined approaches describe models that include multiple sources of variance, as for example combined multifactorial and segregation models (31–33) and combined segregation and linkage models (28,34,35). Indeed, a combined approach may be the only way to disentangle the interplay of the multiple underlying processes for obesity traits.

B Review of Findings

1 Excess Body Mass or Body Fat

While most multifactorial studies of the BMI show significant familial resemblance, the relative importance of genes and common familial environments varies. Some studies place more importance on the familial environment as compared to polygenic effects (36–40), and others suggest that genetic effects outweigh those of the familial environment (41–49). For example, in MZ twins reared apart (44,48,50), the correlations were very similar to those for MZ twins reared together, suggesting that the shared familial environment had little or no effect. Two of the larger studies of the BMI [Norwegian sample of ~75,000 individuals (51) and > 9000 individuals in Tecumseh, Michigan] (40), suggest that the total additive familial effect may be between 30% and 40% in families. A somewhat higher estimate (69%) was reported in the large Virginia study of adult twins and their families (nearly 30,000 indviduals) (52).

Table 4 describes the trends in the heritability levels based upon a large number of studies (53). The results are generally quite heterogeneous. The heritability level is highest with twin studies, intermediate with nuclear family data, and lowest when derived from adoption data. When several types of relatives are used jointly in the same design, the heritability estimates typically cluster around 25–40% of the age- and gender-adjusted phenotype variance. There is no clear evidence for a specific maternal or paternal effect, and the common familial environmental effect is marginal. The table is based on the trends in ~50 different studies. In most of these studies, the BMI was the phenotype considered. In some cases, skinfolds or estimates of %BF or fat mass were used.

Table 4 Overview of the Genetic Epidemiology of Human Body Fat/Obesity

	Heritability/ transmission	Maternal/ patenal	Familial environment
Nuclear families	30–50	No	Minor
Adoption studies	10–30	Mixed results	Minor
Twin studies	50–80	No	No
Combined strategies	25–40	No	Minor

Source: Ref. 53.

Temporal trends (or age effects) in the familial resemblance for BMI have also been explored (54). Recent studies suggest that age trends in the familial effects of BMI may be primarily genetic in nature and that the trends diverge in different directions between childhood and adulthood. Two studies using path analysis techniques (20,55) suggested that the familiality increased from birth to adulthood, which Cardon (55), using adoptive and biological families measured longitudinally, attributed to genetic rather than environmental factors. In studies assessing familiality in adults (56–59), there was a general decrease in the genetic heritability during adulthood. Fabsitz et al. (57) suggested that there were two major genetic effects in male twins, one increasing at or prior to age 20, the other decreasing after age 20. Similarly, a longitudinal analysis of Polish twins suggested a peak additive genetic effect at age ~18 in males and ~14 in females (60). In fact, the largest estimates of genetic heritability for BMI (>80%) are reported in twins during this age range (e.g., 61). These and other studies (e.g., 62) suggest that although some of the same genes are active across time, there are unique genetic factors active as well.

Different genes may also be responsible for adiposity in the normal or moderate range as versus those leading to massive obesity (63 for review). A common observation is that the obese cases in familial studies of obesity is, on the average, 10–15 BMI units heavier than his/her mother, father, brothers, or sisters (64–66). Such a large difference between a proband and his/her first-degree relative is suggestive of the contribution of a recessive gene having a large effect. In further support, the risk for obesity when a first-degree relative is extremely obese (BMI $\geq$ 40) is higher than when a relative is moderately obese (BMI $\geq$ 30). For example, Price and Lee (67) reported risks of five to nine times higher when there was an extremely obese relative, as compared to a risk of ~2 if the relative was moderately obese. This supports not only a major gene hypothesis, but also that the genetic factors leading to extreme obesity may not be the same as those leading to moderate obesity. These hypotheses can be tested by complex segregation analysis.

While there is a great deal of heterogeneity among the major gene studies for the BMI (or some measure of height-adjusted weight) using segregation analysis (see Table 5), support for a major gene generally resulted when studies incorporated very large sample sizes (68–70), used samples selected for obesity (7,72), or allowed for genotype-dependent effects in the major gene component (73).

The mixed evidence for a major gene for BMI may be related to several factors, including gene-environment or gene-gene (epistasis) interactions. Gene-environment interactions occur when some genotypes are more susceptible than others; i.e., expression may depend on having an "obesity" gene and exposure to the relevant environmental conditions. Evidence of this is suggested in the experiments on MZ twins' response to overfeeding (see next section). Major gene effects may also depend on ethnicity (68,74–77). For example, Price and Lee (67) reported higher familial risks for extreme obesity in Caucasians (5–9 times higher) than in African-Americans (3–5 times higher). Evidence for major genes also varies depending whether age and/or sex are factored into the model (78). For example, in one family study the major gene evidence for BMI was ambiguous (79) until genotype-dependent effects of age and sex were considered (73). It is also noted that somewhat different modes of inheritance result among the different studies. For example, while some studies reported no evidence for a major gene (77,79–81), most suggested a recessive locus and a few supported a codominant effect (76). In fact, Price et al. (78) reported a recessive mode when pre– vs. post–WW II–born sibships were analyzed together, but found that a codominant mode best characterized each cohort when analyzed separately. This finding further supports temporal trends (as discussed above) due to cohorts.

Multiple genes, or gene-gene interactions, may also account for the mixed evidence for BMI. For example, Hasstedt et al. (82) and Borecki et al. (83,84) both reported evidence consistent with at least two loci underlying BMI, one leading to extreme obesity and the other for adiposity in the normal-to-moderate range. These findings are appealing given the nature of the BMI measurements; that is, the BMI is a general measure of body build and incorporates fat mass, muscle mass, and skeletal mass. Evidence suggests that there may be major gene effects for fat mass (85,86) and skeletal tissue (87). Moreover, other studies (88) suggest that the major effect of the gene for BMI may be mediated by energy intake and energy expenditure of activity that may also have underlying major gene influences (89). Further, Mitchell et al. (90) and Kaplan et al. (91) suggested that exercise or activity levels had the potential to suppress the (polygenic) heritability of BMI. Whether the same major gene affects several of these traits (i.e., genetic pleiotropy) or the gene primarily affects one trait (e.g., fat mass or energy metabolism) that in turn affects the BMI, remains to be investigated. Another indicator of overall fatness that is correlated with the BMI is the waist circumference (e.g., 92). Heritability for waist circumference ranged from 46% to 51% in two family studies (93,94), but dropped to <30% after adjusting for BMI in the former study. Thus, similar to BMI, waist circumference appears to index both overall fatness as well as some degree of fat distribution.

Relatively less is known about direct measures of general obesity (i.e., fat mass [FM] and %BF). In Utah families, Ramirez (95) reported that the familiality for %BF (measured with bioelectrical impedance) was ~25%. In the Quebec Family Study (QFS), the familiality for %BF (measured with underwater weighing) was 40% and dropped slightly to 36% after adjusting for energy intake and energy expenditure (96,97). In Quebec twins and adopted and biological families, the genetic heritability for each of %BF and FM was ~25%, with an additional 30% due to familial environmental effects (98). Together, these studies suggest that between 25% and 40% of the variance in total fat mass may be genetic due to additive genetic effects.

Somewhat more variance in total fat is accounted for when both multifactorial and major gene effects are included in the models. In the QFS (86), the HERITAGE Family Study (99) and the San Antonio Family Heart Study (85), ~60% of the variance in FM was attributable to familial factors. In the QFS and the San Antonio studies, a recessive locus accounted for up to 45% of the variance (depending on sex), with an additional 22–26% of the phenotypic variance due to (additive) multifactorial effects. However, in the HERITAGE study, the entire familial effect of about 60% was due to a recessive locus with little additional variance due to other familial sources. One of the primary differences among these studies was that in HERITAGE all subjects were selected to be sedentary at baseline (i.e., "environmental" effects due to habitual activity levels were controlled for) while the QFS and San Antonio studies presumably included a range of habitual activity levels among the subjects. Thus, a comparison among these three studies with a greater impact of the major gene in the sedentary sample indirectly supports contentions by Mitchell et al. (90)

Table 5 Segregation Studies of Obesity

Source	Sample	Individuals (families)	Phenotype	% Variance for major gene	% Variance for multi-factor	Notes
BMI or body fat						
Karlin (81)	LRC	1167 (123)	BMI	No		Ascertained[a]
Zonta (77)	Italian	(179)	BMI	No		Ascertained[b]
Price (69)	LRC	2935 (961)	BMI[c]	14%	34%	Ascertained[a]
Province (70)	Tecumseh	9226 (3281)	BMI	20%	41%	Offspring
					20%	Parents
Ness (68)	LRC white	3925 (861)	BMI	14%	34%	
	LRC black	231 (60)		No	50%	
Moll (71)	Muscatine	1302 (284)	BMI	35%	42%	Ascertained[d]
Tiret (76)	French	2534 (629)	BMI[e]	No	35–40%	
Rice (79)	QFS	1223 (301)	BMI	No	42%	
Borecki (73)	QFS	1223 (301)	BMI	Yes[f]	30%	Genotype-dependent
Price (78)	PIMA Indians	2625 (618)	BMI	Yes[g]		Recessive (combined cohorts) vs. codominant (separately by cohorts)
Price (75)	LRC white	(403)	BMI	12%	66%	
	LRC black	(29)		34%	53%	
Hasstedt (82)	Utah	616 (42)	BMI	33%		2 Loci, extreme vs. moderate obesity, ascertained[h]
				35%		
Ginsburg (74)	Kirghizian	397 (74)	BMI	17%	No	
	Turkmenian	558 (197)		40%	No	
	Chuvashian	516 (135)		40%	No	
	Israeli	672 (165)		30%	No	
	Mexican	1742 (87)		14%	19%	
Borecki (84)	NHLBI-FHS random	2461 (541)	BMI	44%	30%	Genetic heterogeneity[i]
Rice (72)	SOS	11204 (2580)	BMI	8–34% (age)[l]	17–24% (age)	Ascertained[j] age = genotype-dependent
Ginsburg (115)	Kirghizian	335 (71)	PC2 (~BMI)	37%	0	Principal components of anthropometrics
	Turkmenian	607 (201)		44%	0	
	Chuvashian	493 (134)		40%	9%	

Feitosa (88)	India	1691 (432)	BMI	37%	53–8%	Offspring-parents
			BMI-ee, ei[k]	No	80%–14%	Offspring-parents
Colilla (220)	Am. black	315 (95)	BMI	52%	0	Codominant
	Nigerian	1159 (400)		42%[l]	0	
Rice (86)	QFS	619 (175)	%BF	45%	22%	
			FM	45%	26%	
Comuzzie (85)	Mexican-Am.	543 (26)	FM	35–42%	20–35%	Males-females
Rice (99)	HERITAGE white	438 (86)	FM	64%	0	Baseline
Lecomte (221)	French	913 (220)	FM-ht	No	47%	Sex-dependent
Borecki (83)	QFS	1630 (300)	BMI	64%		2 Pleiotropic/oligogenic loci—78% of covariance
			FM	47%		
Rice (120)	HERITAGE white	440 (98)	FM	31%	No	Training response dominant
Upper or lower body fat						
Paganini-Hill (222)	S-leut	784 (89)	Triceps SF	83%		
			Subscapular	26%		
Zonta (77)	Italian	(179)	Discriminant score[m]	Yes		Ascertained[b] dominant
Hasstedt (35)	Utah	744 (59)	RFPI	42%	10%	Ascertained[n]
Province (70)	Tecumseh	(3281)	TER	No		
Borecki (54)	QFS	1223 (301)	TER-fm	37%	39%	
			SF6-fm	34%	36%	
			Trunk SF-fm	No	—%	
Feitosa (114)	India	1691 (432)	TER	34%	25%	Parent-offspring
			TER-ee,ei	34%	25%	
			TER-sf	35–51%[l]	61–17%	
Ginsburg (115)	Kirghizian	335 (71)	PC1	55%	9%	Principal components of anthropometrics
	Turkmenian	607 (201)	(~SF)	50%	No	
	Chuvasnian	493 (134)		44%	No	
Ginsburg (115)	Kirghizian	335 (71)	PC3 (~internal upper vs. lower)	57%	4%	Principal components of anthropometrics
	Turkmenian	607 (201)		33%	No	
	Chuvasnian	493 (134)		35%	No	
Ginsburg (115)	Kirghizian	335 (71)	PC4 (~subcutaneous upper vs. lower)	60%	No	Principal components of anthropometrics
	Turkmenian	607 (201)		30%	No	
	Chuvasnian	493 (134)		30%	No	

Table 5 (continued)

Source	Sample	Individuals (families)	Phenotype	% Variance for major gene	% Variance for multi-factor	Notes
An (105)	HERITAGE	482 (99)	SF6	47%	30%	
			TER	54%	17%	Additive
			TER-sf	56%	18%	Additive
			WHR	48%	No	Additive
			WHR-sf	No	50%	
Feitosa (106)	NHLBI-FHS random	2713 (1038)	WHR	35%	No	Additive
			WHR-BMI	No	35%	
Abdominal visceral fat						
Bouchard (118)	QFS phase 2	382 (100)	AVF	51%	21%	Random + obese
			AVF-fm	No	44%	
Rice (99)	HERITAGE white	438 (86)	AVF	54%	17%	Baseline
			AVF-fm	No	42%	
Rice (120)	HERITAGE white	440 (98)	AVF	18%	No	Training responses
			AVF-fm	26%	No	

Note: Major gene effect is recessive unless otherwise noted.

Abbreviations: ATF (abdominal total fat), BMI (body mass index), ee and ei (energy expenditure and energy intake), %BF (percent body fat, underwater weighing), FM (fat mass, underwater weighing or DXA scan), RFPI (regional fat pattern index), SF (skinfolds) TER (trunk-extremity skinfold ratio), WHR (waist-hip circumference ratio), AVF (abdominal visceral fat, computed tomography scan), PC (principal component), RQ (respiratory quotient), TER-sf or TER-fm or TER-ee,ei (TER adjusted for SF or FM or energy expenditure/energy intake), WHR-BMI (WHR adjusted for BMI), AVF-fm (AVF adjusted for FM), LRC (Lipid Research Center), QFS (Quebec Family Study), NHLBI-FHS (National Heart, Lung, and Blood Institute, Family Heart Study), SOS (Swedish Obese Subjects).

[a] Both random and ascertained (for high lipid value of probands) samples.

[b] Ascertained for obese and nonobese schoolchildren.

[c] BMI adjusted for social class and LRC clinic.

[d] Four ascertained groups: random, lean, heavy, and gain groups of schoolchildren. The gain group includes families of students who gained at least two quartiles of relative weight between two surveys.

[e] BMI is height (linear and quadratic)-adjusted weight using regression analysis.

[f] Multifactorial effect inferred by doubling average residual familial (sibling and parent-offspring) correlations; the major gene effect is genotype dependent on age and sex, and percent of variance accounted for was not reported.

[g] Pre– vs. post–WW cohorts, nuclear families vs. sibship analysis, transformed vs. untransformed; % variance due major gene not reported.

[h] Ascertained via NIDDM sibs.

[i] 2nd maxima was obtained but non-Mendelian, depending on field center.

[j] Ascertained via massively obese probands.

[k] BMI adjusted for energy intake and energy expenditure of activities.

[l] Major non-Mendelian effect. That is, results cannot rule out major gene whose effect is masked by other factors (i.e., another gene, genotype-dependent effects, etc.).

[m] Discriminant score (obese vs. nonobese) of weight, subscapular skinfold, chest depth and adjusted for age, sex, height.

[n] Ascertained through pedigrees with various cardiovascular, coronary heart, and hypertensive disease.

and Kaplan et al. (91) that activity may suppress the heritability levels for total fat.

2 Upper Body Fat (Android Obesity)

For the WHR, familiality estimates varied from 28% in adoptive and biological families (100) to 40–50% in traditional nuclear families (101,102) to over 60% in longitudinal family data (Fels Longitudinal Study) (103) In two other studies (95,104) the familial correlations were either nonsignificant or inconsistent across different family pairs. Two segregation studies of the WHR were recently reported (105,106). In both, a major additive locus was detected accounting for 35–48% of the variance with no additional familial sources of variance detected. However, after removing the effects of total body fat the familial variance was due to multifactorial (polygenic and/or familial environmental) rather than major gene sources, suggesting that the major gene component for WHR may be pleiotropic with respect to total body fat.

Comparison of results across studies for fat distribution using measures of skinfolds is complicated by the fact that different skinfolds are measured in different studies. One of the more widely used measures of fat distribution is the trunk-to-extremity subcutaneous skinfold ratio (TER). Most often, the simple ratio of trunk sum to extremity sum is used, although a few studies use principal components analysis to extract the relevant factors underlying a set of skinfolds. The first component derived from such analysis is generalized fat with nearly equal loading across all skinfold measures. The second component is usually a trunk-to-extremity contrast, and the third (not often reported) is an upper-to-lower contrast. The familiality for the second (33–52%) and third (31–49%) components (107,108) was likely to be due to genetic factors since spouse correlations were not significant. Path analysis of the second component in French-Canadian biological and adoptive families (109) accounted for ~40% of the familial variance, of which 18% was genetic in origin. After adjusting the second component for BMI (107,108) or total body fat content (110), the genetic heritability increased to 30–50%.

In another study, the phenotypic, genetic, and nongenetic correlation matrices extracted from an analysis of eight skinfold measures in Mexican-American families were analyzed using principal components analysis (111). The results suggested that the pattern of central vs. peripheral fat distribution was largely a function of the genetic correlation structure and was interpreted as evidence for global genetic pleiotropy among the skinfolds. Familial estimates for the TER using the ratio of simple skinfold sums is ~37% (100) in a large survey of the Canadian population (>18,000 individuals from >11,000 households). As with the principal component, after adjusting TER for percent body fat, the total familiality increased to >63%, of which 28% was genetic in origin. Similar results were obtained in the sample of twins and adoptive and biological families of the QFS (98).

These results for regional fat distribution suggest that there is a significant familial influence on the pattern of subcutaneous fat distribution and that adjusting for total body fat usually results in an increased familiality. This implies that for a given level of fatness, some individuals generally store fat on the trunk or abdominal area (android) while others store primarily on the lower body (gynoid). This pattern is consistent with a hypothesis of both genetic pleiotropy (i.e., similar genes affecting both fat distribution and total body fat) and oligogenic (an additional major genetic system specific to fat distribution). This question was more specifically addressed in the QFS using a trivariate familial correlation model (112). In that study, cross-trait familial resemblance (e.g., trait 1 in parents with trait 2 in offspring, or interindividual cross-trait correlations) was examined among %BF, BMI, and TER. The results suggested that although all three measures were significantly correlated within individuals, the interindividual (familial) cross-trait resemblance was significant for BMI with each of %BF and TER (bivariate heritabilities of 10% and 18%, respectively), but %BF and TER showed no cross-trait familial resemblance. Similarly, in another multivariate study using twins, a common genetic component for BMI and WHR accounted for >50% of the covariation (113). The latter study also reported that the genetic correlation between WHR and a skinfold ratio (subscapular to triceps) was not significant, suggesting multiple dimensions of fat patterning. Together, these results support the hypotheses that 1) the BMI may index both total body fat and fat distribution to some degree, 2) some of the same genes may influence total fat and fat distribution (pleiotropic), 3) each of total fat and fat distribution also may be influenced by unique genes and/or environmental factors (oligogenic), and 4) there may be multiple fat topography dimensions.

Relatively few segregation studies have been reported for fat distribution measures. For the TER, no support for a major gene was found in the large Tecumseh sample (70) or in the QFS (54). However, after adjusting the fat distribution measure for overall level of fatness (54), a recessive locus accounted for 37% of the variance with an additional 29% due to a multifactorial component. These findings are consistent with the hypothesis that there is more than one genetic factor underlying fat distribution, and that removal of the "gene" for total fat allows for a second locus specific to fat distribution to be detected. However, in the HERITAGE study (105), an additive major gene accounting for >50% of the variance was found, but total fat adjustment had no effect on the major gene inference. This was in contrast to results for WHR in the same study (previously discussed), in which total fat adjustment reduced the major gene inference. Together, these studies support the previous multifactorial studies suggesting that both pleiotropic and oligogenic loci underlie body composition. A putative major locus was also reported in Utah pedigrees (35) for a relative fat pattern index [RFPI = subscapular/(subscapular + suprailiac)], and two recent studies also support major gene effects for fat distribution in other ethnic groups from India (114) and Eastern Europe (115).

3 Abdominal Visceral Fat

We are aware of only two family studies investigating abdominal visceral fat—the QFS and the HERITAGE Family Study. Familial correlations in the QFS (116) for abdominal total, abdominal visceral, and abdominal subcutaneous fat tissue were ~0.35, with somewhat lower spouse correlations for total (0.30) and subcutaneous (0.21) and higher spouse correlations for abdominal visceral fat (0.36). The heritability was ~70% for each of the three measures. The effect of adjusting each of these measures for total body fat was to reduce the magnitude of the familial correlations and thus the heritability estimates (>55% for total and visceral abdominal fat and 42% for subcutaneous abdominal fat). This suggests that some of the same multifactorial factors (polygenic and/or familial environmental) impact similarly on total body fat and visceral fat. Similar results were obtained in the HERITAGE Family Study (117).

A major gene hypothesis for abdominal visceral fat was examined in the QFS (118) and the HERITAGE (99). In each study, a putative recessive locus accounted for about 50% of the variance, with an additional 20% due to a multifactorial component. However, after adjusting for fat mass, support for a major gene was reduced; although the major effect was significant, the Mendelian and no-transmission (i.e., environmental) models were not resolved. It was suggested that the major gene previously noted for fat mass in these data (86) was also responsible for the major gene detected for abdominal visceral fat. In other words, genetic pleiotropy was inferred, where the same major gene affected both fat mass and the abdominal visceral fat traits. A cross-trait study conducted between fat mass and abdominal visceral fat (119) supported the pleiotropy hypothesis. The bivariate (cross-trait) familiality was 29–50% (with sex differences), indicating genetic pleiotropy. Moreover, since the univariate familiality for each trait was even higher (55–77% for fat mass and 55–65% for abdominal visceral fat), each trait was assumed to be influenced by additional familial factors that were specific to each (i.e., oligogenic). Given the significant spouse cross-trait correlations, at least some of the bivariate familial effect may be environmental in origin. Finally, the visceral fat response to exercise training was also a function of a recessive major gene accounting for 20–25% of the variance (120). However, in this case, adjusting for total fat did not change the major gene inference. This suggests that the genes for visceral fat response to exercise training may be independent from those affecting total level of fatness.

4 Lower Body Fat (Gynoid Obesity)

All studies reviewed in the section on android obesity as assessed from WHR, TER, or principal components of sets of skinfolds apply equally well to the evaluation of the genetic components of gynoid obesity. In addition, one other study purported to measure gluteofemoral fat. In a study based on the Danish Adoption Register, participants were asked to match their (and other relatives') body types to one of nine silhouette pictures that ranged from very thin to obese (121). While this measure correlated with the BMI (ranging from 0.63 to 0.88) and with the sum of several skinfolds (ranging from 0.39 to 0.66), the authors suggested that it favored the gynoid type of fat distribution. Relatives were placed in four classes as determined by weight of the adoptee. The mean silhouette score of the adoptees' biological mothers and siblings increased significantly across weight classes, while no mean differences were observed for adoptive relatives, suggesting primarily a genetic control for this measure.

5 Relationship Between Total Fat and Fat Topography

The genetic epidemiological studies reported in this chapter regarding total fat and fat topography suggest a complex relationship underlying the etiological causes of their covariation. Most of the evidence comes from studies comparing the multifactorial and major gene evidence for fat distribution phenotypes both prior to and after adjusting for total fat (using multiple regression). In general, total fat adjustment alters the familial inferences for topographical measures. These studies suggest substantial shared major gene and multifactorial determinants between total fat and abdominal visceral fat, but only the major gene component for total fat mass appears to influence subcutaneous fat distribution.

Regarding the major gene component for subcutaneous fat distribution, prior to adjustment for total fat there was evidence for a major (non-Mendelian) effect for TER, but only after adjustment did the transmission appear to be Mendelian. In other words, the TER may be both a pleiotropic and oligogenic trait, in that removal of the effects due to a putative major locus for total fat leads to the detection of a secondary locus specific to fat distribution. In contrast, adjusting abdominal visceral fat for total fat reduces the evidence for a putative major locus. Together, these results suggest at least two putative major loci underlying obesity phenotypes, one determining total and abdominal visceral fat, and the other determining how subcutaneous adipose tissue is distributed.

Regarding the multifactorial (polygenic and/or common environmental) causes of the covariation between the traits, similar patterns are noted. For subcutaneous fat distribution, the generalized heritabilities increase after total fat adjustment, while bivariate studies find no evidence for a genetic correlation. Together, these results suggest that there are entirely different multifactorial causes for the variations in total fat and subcutaneous fat distribution. For abdominal visceral fat, however, total fat adjustment leads to decreased generalized heritability estimates, with bivariate studies suggesting a substantial bivariate heritability. Thus, total fat and abdominal visceral fat may share many of the same polygenic and/or common environmental factors.

IV GENES AND MOLECULAR MARKERS OF HUMAN OBESITY

A Review of Methods

This section focuses on association studies with candidate genes and on the results of genomic scans designed to identify genomic regions that harbor genes of importance for obesity. The molecular dissection of complex phenotypes such as obesity is based on two strategies: linkage and association studies. Both rely on the same principle, i.e., the coinheritance of adjacent DNA markers, with the difference that linkage focuses only on recent and usually observable generations, while association relies on the fact that particular DNA markers can remain together on ancestral haplotypes for several generations, leading to a phenomenon known as linkage disequilibrium (122,123). Reviews of methods and strategies to identify genes underlying complex phenotypes can be found elsewhere (123–126). The number of genes and DNA sequence variations that have been shown to be associated and/or linked with obesity has increased considerably since the first edition of this volume. The yearly updates of the obesity gene map published since 1996 (127–134) provide a good indication of the progress accomplished in the past several years in the search for genes determining human obesity. Other topics of relevance for the understanding of the molecular basis of human obesities can be found in Chapter 10 by Chua et al. All the gene symbols, names, and chromosomal locations of the genes listed in this section are given in the Appendix found at the end of this chapter.

B Review of Findings

1 Association Studies

The search for genes influencing overweight and obesity in humans has been thus far mostly based on association studies with *candidate genes*, those with known chromosomal locations that are metabolically or physiologically relevant for the phenotype under study (functional candidate genes). They could also be genes targeted because of their position in a region of the genome (positional candidate gene), near a Mendelian obesity syndrome, within a quantitative trait locus homologous to a locus linked to obesity in animal models (see below) or identified through genome-wide scans of human obesity (see below). The genes showing positive evidence of association with obesity-related phenotypes are listed in Table 6, which provides the chromosomal location of the gene, the phenotypes that were shown to be associated with the gene, and the range of *P* values from the various studies. This list shows that a total of 51 candidate genes have been shown to be associated with obesity-related phenotypes. It should be noted that the table does not include the results of early association studies performed with the ABO (9q34) blood group and the human leukocyte antigen (HLA) system on chromosome 6p21.3. A review of these studies (135) revealed that the results were

Table 6 Evidence for the Presence of an Association Between Markers of Candidate Genes with BMI, Body Fat, and Other Obesity-Related Phenotypes

Gene	Location	Phenotype	*P* value	Ref.
TNFRSF1B	1p36.3-p36.2	BMI, overweight, leptin	$<.05$	(223,224)
LEPR	1p31	%Fat, fat mass, fat-free mass, obesity, BMI, abdominal fat, weight loss, hip girth, leptin	$.003 < P < .05$	(225–231)
HSD3B1	1p13.1	Subcutaneous fat	.04	(232)
LMNA	1q21.2-q21.3	Leptin, BMI, WHR, lipodystrophy	$.0001 < P < .05$	(233–235)
ATP1A2	1q21-q23	%Fat, respiratory quotient	$.0001 < P < .05$	(236,237)
AGT	1q42-q43	WHR, fat mass	$.007 < P < .02$	(238,239)
ACP1	2p25	BMI	$.002 < P < .02$	(240,241)
APOB	2p24-p23	BMI, %fat, abdominal fat	$.005 < P < .05$	(242,243)
POMC	2p23.3	Leptin, early-onset obesity	$<.01$	(170,244)
ADRA2B	2p13-q13	Basal metabolic rate	.01	(245)
IRS1	2q36	BMI, leptin	$.03 < P < .05$	(246–248)
PPARG	3p25	Leptin, BMI, body weight, fat-free mass, fat mass, waist and hip girths, obesity, overweight	$.001 < P < .05$	(249–258)
APOD	3q26.2-qter	BMI	.006	(259)
CCKAR	4p15.2-p15.1	%Fat, leptin	.003–.041	(260)
FABP2	4q28-q31	Abdominal fat, BMI, %fat, fat oxidation	$.008 < P < .01$	(261–263)
UCP1	4q28-q31	High fat gainers, weight, BMI	$.001 < P < .05$	(264–266)
NPY5R	4q31-q32	Morbid obesity	$<.05$	(267)
CART	5q	WHR in men	.0021	(268)
GRL	5q31-q32	Abdominal visceral fat, BMI, WHR, leptin	$.001 < P < .039$	(269–271)
ADRB2	5q31-q32	BMI, fat mass, fat cell volume, body weight, waist and hip girths, WHR, obesity, leptin	$.001 < P < .05$	(154,254,272–279)
TNFA	6p21.3	%Fat, BMI, obesity	$.004 < P < .035$	(224,280–284)
ESR1	6q25.1	Android obesity	.0001	(285)
GCK	7p15.3-p15.1	Birth weight	.002	(286)
NPY	7p15.1	Birth weight, BMI, WHR	$.03 < P < .04$	(287,288)
PON2	7q21.3	Birth weight	$<.05$	(289)
LEP	7q31.3	Weight loss, body weight, leptin, BMI, obesity, overweight	$.005 < P < .05$	(290–297)
LPL	8p22	BMI (leanness)	.05	(298)
ADRB3	8p12-p11.2	Weight gain, weight, WHR, BMI, obesity, abdominal fat, fat mass, hip and waist girths, fat mass	$.002 < P < .05$	(136–156)
CBFA2T1	8q22	%Fat, BMI, waist and hip girths	$.0002 < P < .02$	(299)
ADRA2A	10q24-q26	Abdominal fat, TER	$.002 < P < .012$	(154,300)
SUR1	11p15.1	Morbid obesity	.02	(301)
IGF2	11p15.5	BMI	.02	(302)
INS	11p15.5	Birth weight, WHR, BMI	$.0002 < P < .009$	(302–304)
UCP2	11q13	Obesity, BMI, body weight, energy expenditure, fat oxidation, respiratory quotient, percent fat, fat mass	$.001 < P < .05$	(305–311)
UCP3	11q13	BMI, body weight, fat oxidation, respiratory quotient, WHR	$.0037 < P < .04$	(312–316)
APOA4	11q23	BMI, WHR, %fat	$.004 < P < .023$	(317,318)
DRD2	11q23	Relative weight, subcutaneous fat, obesity, BMI	$.002 < P < .05$	(319–321)
GNB3	12p13	BMI, body weight, waist and hip girths, subcutaneous fat, birth weight	$.001 < P < .05$	(322–326)

Table 6 (continued)

Gene	Location	Phenotype	*P* value	Ref.
IGF1	12q22-q23	%Fat, fat mass, fat-free mass, changes in fat-free mass after 20-week endurance training	<.05	(327)
CD36L1	12q24.1-q24.3	BMI in lean women	.004–.03	(328)
HTR2A	13q14-q21	Total energy, carbohydrate, and alcohol intake in obese subjects	.028–.047	(329)
HSPA2	14q21	Obesity	$<10^{-6}$	(330)
NMB	15q22-qter	Obesity, body weight	.03	(331)
MC5R	18p11.2	BMI in females	.003	(332)
MC4R	18q22	Fat mass, %fat, fat-free mass in females	$.0022 < P < .004$	(332)
INSR	19p13.3-p.13.2	Obesity (BMI >26) in hypertensives	.05	(333)
LDLR	19p13.3	BMI in hypertensives and normotensives, obesity, subcutaneous fat	$.001 < P < .04$	(197,334–337)
LIPE	19q13.1-q13.2	Obesity	.002	(338)
GYS1	19q13.3	Obesity	.03	(339)
ADA	20q12-q13.11	BMI in diabetic subjects	.0004–.01	(340)
HTR2C	Xq24	BMI > 28 kg/m^2	.0009–.02	(341)

See Table 5 legend for definitions.

rather ambiguous, some studies finding associations with obesity, while others did not.

Despite the large number of positive findings reported in Table 6, it is important to keep in mind that for most of these genes, very few replications in independent populations have been reported and that for many of these genes, there are as many negative as positive results that have been reported. A good example of this is the results obtained with the beta-3-adrenergic receptor (ADRB3) gene. The ADRB3 gene is probably the candidate gene that has been the most widely tested for association with obesity-related phenotypes with positive findings reported for weight gain (137–139), obesity, BMI, and/or body fatness (140–155), and various indicators of abdominal fat (139,146,148,151,154,156) and changes in BMI during pregnancy (137). Despite these positive findings, a whole series of negative results, reviewed elsewhere (129,157,158) has also been reported for the ADRB3 gene. Finally, three independent meta-analyses yielded contradictory results, one concluding that the ADRB3 gene has no effect on obesity (159), another one finding an effect (160), while a third one based only on Japanese studies concluded that the mutation in ADRB3 was associated with obesity (161).

Among the genes listed in Table 6, a few have been shown to be associated with obesity-related phenotypes in at least five different studies. These include the LEPR gene, the PPARG gene, the ADRB2 gene, the TNFA gene, the LEP gene, the UCP2 and UCP3 genes, the GNB3 gene, and the LDLR gene. Other genes that were found to be associated with obesity phenotypes include the TNFRSF1B, HSD3B1, LMNA, ATP1A2, AGT, ACP1, APOB, POMC, ADRA2B, IRS1, APOD, CCKAR, FABP2, UCP1, NPY5R, CART, GRL, ESR1, GCK, NPY, PON2, LPL, CBFA2T1, SUR1, IGF2, INS, APOA4, DRD2, IGF1, CD36L1, HTR2A, HSPA2, NMB, MC5R, MC4R, INSR, LIPE, GYS1, ADA, and HTR2C genes.

2 QTLs from Cross-Breeding Experiments

The molecular signature of complex traits such as obesity can also be investigated using experimental crosses among various animal strains. Crosses between two inbred strains of animals diverging for a quantitative trait will create linkage disequilibrium between loci that differ between the two strains, which results in associations between marker loci and linked segregating quantitative trait loci (162). A quantitative trait locus (QTL), thus, simply refers to a locus at which segregation contributes to a quantitative trait. Since the homology between human and several animal genomes is increasingly well characterized, QTL mapping offers a powerful strategy to begin characterizing the molecular basis of complex traits in humans as the QTL identified in animals can lead to the identification of a target human chromosomal region. Reviews of the methodology underlying QTL mapping in animals can be found elsewhere (125,162–164).

The number of obesity QTLs identified using this strategy has expanded considerably in the past 5 years. In the first edition of this chapter, eight obesity QTLs, all identified from mice crosses, were mapped. The results reviewed in the 2000 update of the obesity gene map (133) reveal that the number of obesity QTLs reached 115. These QTLs have been identified from 19 different mice crosses (81 QTLs), eight different rat crosses (21 QTLs), eight different pig crosses (12 QTLs), and one chicken cross (1 QTL). These QTLs were found to affect a wide variety of phenotypes, including body weight, weight gain, total adiposity, specific fat depots, percentage body fat, heat loss, and food intake and their human homologs are distributed over all human chromosomes, except the Y chromosome. Details about the chromosomal locations of these QTLs and their human homologs can be found in the review paper (133).

3 Linkage Studies

Several studies have tested linkage with obesity-related phenotypes. These linkage studies were performed with candidate gene markers or with a variety of anonymous polymorphic markers such as microsatellites. Most of the linkage studies are performed with a large number of polymorphic markers selected to cover the whole genome and test for linkage with a variety of obesity phenotypes in order to detect QTLs. The obesity QTLs uncovered in such genomewide scans provides the identification of chromosomal regions, or in some cases of positional candidate genes, that can be further investigated for their role in the phenotype of interest. The methodology underlying the identification of human obesity QTLs can be found elsewhere (124). The results of the genomewide scans for obesity are reviewed in detail here (Table 7).

C Linkages from Genomewide Scans of Obesity

1 Pima Indians

The first genomewide scan for obesity was performed in Pima Indians and used percent body fat as the phenotype (165). A total of 674 genetic markers with an average intermarker distance of 8.3 cM were tested for linkage with percent body fat measured by underwater weighing in 283 sibling pairs from 88 Pima Indian families. Significant evidence of linkage was reported on 11q2l-q22 with a peak LOD score of 2.8 between markers D11S2000 and D11S2366. Another genomic scan for obesity (451 sibpairs from 127 families) and energy metabolism (236 sibpairs from 82 families) was performed in the same population using 576 markers with a mean spacing of 6.4 cM (166). The phenotypes investigated included, in addition to percent body fat, the ratio of waist-to-high circumference (WTR), 24-hr energy expenditure (EE) and 24-hr respiratory quotient (RQ) measured in a respiratory chamber. For percent body fat, the strongest linkages were detected at llq21-q22 with marker D11S2366 (LOD = 2.1) and 18q21 with marker D18S877 (LOD = 2.3). No strong evidence of linkage was observed for WTR with all multipoint LOD scores < 1.5. For 24-hr EE, the strongest linkage was observed at llq23 with marker D11S976 (LOD = 2.0), while for 24-hr RQ linkages were found at 1p3l-p21 (LOD = 2.8 with D1S550) and 20q11.2 (LOD = 3.0 with D20S601). Another genomic scan for phenotypes related to diabetes revealed evidence of linkage to BMI (LOD = 3.6) between markers D11S4464 and D11S912 at 11q24 (167) near the dopamine D2 receptor gene. Finally, a fourth genomewide linkage scan based on 770 subjects from 239 famines revealed evidence of linkage between plasma leptin levels near marker D6S271 (LOD = 2.1) at 6p21-p12 (168).

2 San Antonio Family Heart Study

The results of the genome scans for obesity-related phenotypes in the San Antonio Family Heart Study (SAFHS) has been reported in three papers (169–171). The phenotypes investigated in SAFHS include BMI, body fat mass measured by bioelectric impedance, and plasma leptin levels measured in a sample of up to 470 Mexican-Americans from 10 large multigenerational families. The first study based on a 20-cM map (169) revealed strong evidence of linkage at 2p21 between marker D2S1788 and fat mass (LOD = 2.8) as well as plasma leptin levels (LOD = 4.9). Evidence of linkage with leptin was also observed at 8q11.1. In a second study in which six additional markers were typed around the peak linkage for leptin at 2p21, in addition to the 15 that were already available in the first study, the LOD score for leptin was increased to 7.5 (170). The QTL for leptin identified in SAFHS at 2p21 was partly replicated in a study performed in African-Americans (172). Finally, a genome scan of BMI performed using a 10 cM map revealed evidence of linkage at 6q25, 8p12-p11.2 near the ADRB3 gene and 17q11 (171).

3 Paris-Lille French Study

A genome scan for obesity was undertaken in 158 French families from the Hôtel-Dieu Hospital in Paris

Table 7 Summary of Genome Scan Studies for Obesity-Related Phenotype

Location	Trait	Markers	LOD score	Candidate gene
Pima Indians (165–168)				
1p31-p21	24-h RQ	D1S550	2.8	LEPR
6p21-p12	Leptin	D6S271	2.1	TNFA
11q21-q22	%fat	D11S200–D11S2366	2.8	
11q23	24-h EE	D11S976	2.0	
11q24	BMI	D11S4464–D11S912	3.6	DRD2
16q21	Leptin	D16S265	2.0	
18q21	%fat	D18S877	2.3	MC4R
20q11.2	24-h RQ	D20S601	3.0	ASIP
San Antonio Family Heart Study (169–171)				
2p21	Fat mass	D2S1788	2.8	POMC
	Leptin	D2S1788	4.9–7.5	
6q25	BMI	D6S1008	1.5	
8p12-p11.2	BMI	D8S1121	3.2	ADRB3
8q11.1	Leptin	D8S1110	2.2	
17q11	BMI	D17S1293	2.3	
Paris-Lille French Study (173)				
2p21	Leptin	D2S165–D2S367	2.4–2.7	POMC
5p11	Leptin	D5S426	2.9	
10p12	Obesity (BMI > 27)	D10S197	4.9	
University of Pennsylvania Family Study (176)				
20q13	Obesity (BMI > 30)	D20S476, 211, 149	1.5–3.2	ASIP, GNAS1, MC3R
Quebec Family Study (177,178)				
1p11.2	ASF	D1S534	2.3	NHLH2, HSDB3
4q32.1	ASF	D4S2417	1.8	NPY2R
4p15.1	ASF	D4S2397	2.3	PPARGC1
7p15.3	FFM	D7S1808	2.7	NPY, GHRHR
7q31.1	ASF	D7S1875	2.0	LEP, CAV2
9q22.1	ASF	D9S1122,257	2.1–2.3	HSD17B3
12q22-q23	ASF	IGF1	1.9	IGF1
12q24.3	ASF	D12S2078, 1045	1.5–2.9	TCF1
13q34	ASF	D13S285	1.9	NA
15q25-q26	FFM	IGF1R	3.6	IGF1R
17q21.1-q21.3	ASF	D17S2180, 1290, 1302	1.5–2.2	HSD17B1, PYY, PYY
18q12	FFM	D18S535	3.6	
Finnish Families (179)				
18q21	Obesity (BMI ≥ 30)	D18S1155	2.4	MC4R
Xq24	Obesity (BMI ≥ 30)	DX6799–DX6804	3.5	HTR2C
TOPS Family Study (180)				
3q27	BMI, waist circumference	D3S2427	2.4–3.3	SLC2A2, APM1
17p12	Leptin	D17S947	5.0	SLC2A4
HERITAGE Family Study (181,182)				
2p14	ASF	D2S441	1.88	
2q22.1	AVF	D2S1334, D2S1399	1.97–2.33	
2q36.1-q36.3	AVF	D2S434, IRS1	1.87–2.49	IRS1

Table 7 (continued)

Location	Trait	Markers	LOD score	Candidate gene
3p26.3	ASF	D3S2387	2.16	
3q29	ASF	D3S1311	2.45	
4q31.22	ASF	D4S2431	2.34	CPE
5q31.2-q31.3	ASF, ATF	D5S658, D5S1480	1.84–2.06	
7q36.2-q36.3	ASF, ATF	D7S3070, NOS3, D7S559	1.74–2.53	NOS3
8q23.3	BMI	D8S556	2.0	
9q34.3	BMI	D9S158	2.3	
10p15.3-p15.1	BMI, FM	D10S1435, 189	2.1–2.7	
11p15.2-p14.1	ASF	C11P15_3, GATA34E08	1.75–1.85	SUR, CCKBR, TUB
12p12.1	BMI, FM	D12S1042	2.1–2.2	
14q24.1	ASF	D14S588	2.38	
14q11-q11.2	BMI, FM, FFM	D14S283, 742, 1280	1.7–2.4	ANG
19p13	Leptin	LDLR	$P = .0009$	LDLR
22q11.23	ASF	D22S264	1.96	
Old Order Amish (183)				
3p25.2	%fat	D3S3608	1.6	PPARG
7q31-q36	Leptin-BMI	D7S640, 636	1.8	LEP
10p12-p11	Leptin-BMI	D10S220	2.7	
14q22-q31	Waist circumference	D14S276	1.8	
	Leptin-BMI	D14S74, 280	2.5	
16p	BMI	D16S510	1.7	
	Leptin	D16S407	1.7	

ASF, abdominal subcutaneous fat; AVF, abdominal visceral fat; FFM, fat-free mass; RQ, 24-hr respiratory quotient.

and the Institut Pasteur in Lille with a morbidly obese (BMI $\geq$ 40 kg/m^2) proband (173). Strong evidence of linkage with obesity (defined as a BMI > 27 kg/m^2) was found at 10p12 (LOD = 4.9 with marker D10S197) and with leptin at 2p21 (LOD = 2.7 between markers D2S165 and D2S367) and 5p11 (LOD = 2.9). Two independent studies attempted to replicate the linkage found on 10p12 with obesity in the French population. The first study was performed in 386 subjects from 93 German families with at least two obese children using 11 markers spanning a 23-cM region on chromosome 10 (174). Although the linkage with marker D10S197 was not as strong (LOD = 1.7) as in the French families, evidence of linkage with obesity was observed with 4 other markers (LODs ranging from 1.1 to 2.4) located within 5 cM of the peak linkage found in the French population. The second study investigated linkage between obesity and 13 markers spanning ~110 cM on chromosome 10 in two cohorts: one comprising 862 subjects from 170 Caucasian families, the other comprising 212 individuals from 43 black families (175). Evidence of linkage was found with markers located on 10p in both Caucasians ($P = .03$ with marker D10S208) and blacks ($P = .01$ with marker D10S582) as well as in the combined cohort ($P = .0005$ with D10S197).

4 University of Pennsylvania Family Study

The fourth genomic scan for obesity was undertaken in 513 individuals from 92 families ascertained through a morbidly obese proband as part of an ongoing linkage study at the University of Pennsylvania (176). Several obesity phenotypes were measured in these subjects including BMI, percent body fat measured by bioelectric impedance, the waist-to-hip circumference ratio and plasma leptin levels. The strongest evidence of linkage reported in that study was between obesity, defined as a BMI $\geq$ 30 kg/m^2, and three markers spanning 12 cM on chromosome 20q13 (176).

5 Quebec Family Study

The QFS is an ongoing longitudinal family study aimed at the identification of genes associated with obesity and its various metabolic complications in French-Canadian families. Two genomic scans for phenotypes related to obesity were published from this population. One investigated linkage with fat-free mass (FFM) derived from body density measurements obtained from underwater weighing in 748 subjects from 194 families (177), while the other investigated linkage with abdominal fat assessed by computed tomography in 521 subjects from 156 families (178). Results of the study with FFM revealed evidence of linkage on three different regions: 7p15.3 with marker D7S1808 (LOD = 2.7), 15q25-q26 with a polymorphism within the insulinlike growth factor 1 receptor (LOD = 3.6) and 18q12 with marker D18S535 (LOD = 3.6). In the other genome scan, CT-assessed abdominal fat was adjusted for total body fatness and tested for linkage with 293 markers with a mean spacing of 11.9 cM. A total of nine QTLs, all affecting abdominal subcutaneous fat, were uncovered (178). Two of these QTLs were found to be close to genes involved in the regulation of food intake (4q32 and 17q21), while three others (1p11.2, 9q22 and 17q21) were found close to genes influencing sex steroids. No significant linkage with abdominal visceral fat was uncovered.

6 Finnish Families

Another genome scan performed in 367 obese individuals from 166 Finnish families revealed evidence of 2 QTLs influencing obesity, defined as a BMI ≥ 30 kg/m^2 (179). The strongest evidence of linkage was uncovered on chromosome Xq24 between markers DX6799 and DX6804 (LOD = 3.5) in a region where the serotonin 2C receptor (HTR2C) gene is located. Evidence of linkage with obesity was also observed in a region of chromosome 18q21 (LOD = 2.4 with D18S1155) flanking the MC4R gene.

7 TOPS Family Study

In an attempt to identify QTLs influencing phenotypes associated with the metabolic syndrome, Kissebah et al. (180) tested 2209 individuals distributed over 507 Caucasian families recruited from the TOPS (Take Off Pounds Sensibly) membership. A total of 387 markers, including 17 X-linked and four Y-linked markers, with an average genetic spacing of 10 cM were tested for linkage with seven phenotypes including the following obesity phenotypes: BMI, waist circumference, and plasma leptin levels. The peak LOD scores for BMI (LOD = 3.3) and waist circumference (LOD = 2.4) were found on the same region of chromosome 3 (3q27) close to the marker D3S2427. The candidate genes located in this region of chromosome 3 include glucose transporter 2 (GLUT2) and the adipose tissue–secreted protein adiponectin. Plasma leptin levels showed its strongest linkage signal on chromosome 17p12 (LOD = 5.0) near marker D17S947 in a region where the glucose transporter 4 (GLUT4) and the peroxisome proliferative-activated receptor-alpha (PPARA) genes are located.

8 HERITAGE Family Study

In an attempt to identify genes associated with body composition phenotypes and their response to exercise training, Chagnon et al. (181) measured BMI, subcutaneous fat, %BF, fat mass (FM), FFM, and plasma leptin levels in 522 subjects from 99 Caucasian families of the HERITAGE Family Study cohort before and after 20 weeks of endurance training, and performed a genome scan of the baseline and response (difference between pre- and posttraining values) phenotypes using 344 autosomal markers. Only results from the baseline analyses are presented in Table 7. The strongest multipoint linkages were found on chromosomes 8q23.3 (BMI), 9q34.3 (BMI), 10p15.3-p15.1 (BMI and FM), 12p12.1 (BMI and FM), 14q11-q11.2 (BMI, FM, and FFM). For plasma leptin level evidence of singlepoint linkage was found on chromosome 19p13 with the LDL receptor gene ($P = .0009$). From the same study, a genomic scan focusing on abdominal subcutaneous fat and abdominal visceral fat has also been published. For pretraining abdominal fat measures assessed with computed tomography, promising linkages were noted for AVF on 2q22 and 2q36, and for ASF on several different chromosomes as shown in Table 7 (182). However, the results for ASF on 4q and 11p are considered strongest since they replicate those from the only other genome scan of these abdominal phenotypes (the QFS). For the abdominal fat training responses, promising results were limited to ASF on 7q36.2 (including NOS3), with suggestive findings ($P < .01$) on 1q21.2-q24.1 (S100A, ATP1A2, ATP1B1), 10q25.2 (ADRA2A), and 11p15.5 (IGF2).

9 Old Order Amish Population

A genomewide scan of obesity-related traits was also performed in the Old Order Amish population, a rural-living population characterized by considerable homogeneity in lifestyle (183). BMI, waist circumference, %BF estimated by bioelectric impedance and serum leptin concentrations were measured in 672 individuals from 28 extended families ranging in size from three to 69 subjects. Linkage between 357 autosomal markers with average intermarker distance of 10.2 cm and the obesity phenotypes and between leptin concentrations adjusted for BMI (leptin-BMI) was tested using a variance component method. Peak linkages were found on chromosomes 3p25.2, near the PPARG gene, for %BF, 7q31-q36 and 10p12-p11 for leptin-BMI, 14q22-q31 for waist circumference and leptin-BMI, and 16p for BMI and leptin concentrations. The strongest linkage for leptin-BMI on 10p12-p11 (LOD = 2.7) was ~10–20 cM telomeric to the obesity QTL reported in the French population (173) and replicated in other studies (174,175).

In summary, nine genomewide scans relevant to obesity have been reported to date. They were undertaken among many different ethnic groups. The sampling strategy varies from study to study. The density of the markers used for the genomic scans is also quite variable. Phenotypes and analytical strategies are also different across the nine studies. As is evident from the preceding review, a large number of QTLs have been observed with considerable differences across family cohorts. The latter should not be surprising, considering how little the cohorts, experimental designs, panels of markers, and analytical strategies have in common.

Table 8 Genomic Regions with Obesity QTLs from at Least Two Studies

Gene	Studies	Ref.
1p11-31	Pima Family Study	(165,166)
	Quebec Family Study	(177,178)
2p21	Paris-Lille Family Study	(173)
	San Antonio Family Heart Study	(169–171)
7q31	Old Order Amish Family Study	(183)
	Quebec Family Study	(177,178)
8q11-23	HERITAGE Family Study	(181,182)
	San Antonio Family Heart Study	(169–171)
9q22-34	HERITAGE Family Study	(181,182)
	Quebec Family Study	(177,178)
10p12-15	HERITAGE Family Study	(181,182)
	Old Older Amish Family Study	(183)
	Paris-Lille Family Study	(173)
14q11-31	HERITAGE Family Study	(181,182)
	Old Order Amish Family Study	(183)
17q11-21	Quebec Family Study	(177,178)
	San Antonio Family Heart Study	(169–171)
18q12-21	Finnish Family Study	(179)
	Pima Family Study	(165–168)
	Quebec Family Study	(177,178)
20q11-13	Pima Family Study	(165–168)
	University of Pennsylvania Family Study	(176)

What is of great interest, however, is that in 10 cases, two or three of the nine studies have detected evidence for a QTL in the same chromosomal regions. Table 8 lists these 10 regions and identifies the studies with convergent findings in each case. Two of these regions (10p12-15 and 18q12-21) are each supported by the results of three family studies. Overall, these observations suggest that there are probably some common genes and sequence variants involved in the genetic predisposition to obesity among a whole variety of populations or ethnic groups. Further, they suggest that the predisposition to obesity could also be influenced by other genes and alleles whose prevalences and effect sizes vary from population to population.

D Linkages with Candidate Genes and Other Markers

Besides the genomewide scans, others have reported evidence of linkage for obesity-related traits with polymorphisms within or around candidate genes. A summary of the positive findings is given in Table 9. The genes involved in the positive finding of linkages are: PGD, LEPR, ATP1B1, ATP1A2, ACP1, POMC, IGKC, GYPA, ISL1, GRL, ADRB2, BF, TNFA, GLO1, NPY, LEP, KEL, ADRB3, ORM1, AK1, SUR1, CCKBR, UCP2 and UCP3, IGF1, ESD, MC5R, MC4R, ADA, MC3R, and P1 genes. None of these linkages was replicated in independent studies.

V GENE-ENVIRONMENT AND GENE-GENE INTERACTIONS

Genotype-environment interaction (G × E) arises when the response of a phenotype (e.g., fat mass) to environmental changes (e.g., dietary restriction) depends on the genotype of the individual. Although it is well known that there are interindividual differences in the responses to various dietary interventions, whether in terms of serum cholesterol changes to high-fat diet (184) or in terms of body weight gains following chronic overfeeding (185), very few attempts have been made to test whether these differences are genotype dependent. Most of the genetic epidemiology studies of human obesity have assumed the absence of genotype-environment interactions simply because of the difficulty in handling such interaction effects in quantitative genetic models. Methods from both genetic epidemiology (unmeasured genotype approach) and from molecular epidemiology (measured genotype

Table 9 Evidence for the Presence of Linkage with Obesity-Related Phenotypes

Gene[a]	Markers	Location	Phenotypes	*P* or LOD value	Ref.
PGD		1p36.2-p36.13	Subcutaneous fat	.03	(341)
	D1S193, 200, 476	1p35-p31	BMI, subcutaneous fat, fat mass	$.009 < P < .02$	(157)
LEPR	Q223R, CA (IVS 3), CTTT (IVS 16)	1p31	BMI, subcutaneous fat, fat mass, fat free mass	$.005 < P < .05$	(225)
ATP1B1		1q22-q25	Respiratory quotient	.04	(236)
ATP1A2		1q21-q23	Respiratory quotient	.02	(343)
ACP1		2p25	BMI, subcutaneous fat	$.004 < P < .02$	(341,344)
POMC	D2S2337	2p23.3	Leptin	LOD = 2.0	(244)
IGKC		2p12	Subcutaneous fat	.03	(342)
GYPA		4q28.2-q31.1	TER	.02	(345)
ISL1		5q22.3	Obesity, BMI, leptin	$.0004 < P < .03$	(346)
GRL		5q31-q32	BMI > 27	.009	(347)
ADRB2		5q31-q32	TER	.02	(300)
BF		6p21.3	Subcutaneous fat	$.01 < P < .03$	(342)
TNFA	TNFir24, D6S273,291	6p21.3	%Fat	$.002 < P < .05$	(283)
GLO1		6p21.3-p21.1	Subcutaneous fat, relative weight	$.004 < P < .05$	(342)
NPY		7p15.1	Principal component of height, weight, skinfolds, abdominal and hip circumferences, obesity	$.04 < P < .05$	(348)
LEP	D7S680,514, 530, 504, 1875, 495	7q31.3	Obesity, fat mass, BMI, subcutaneous fat, waist circumference, WHR	$.0001 < P < .04$	(343,348–353)
KEL		7q33	BMI, subcutaneous fat, trunk to extremity skinfolds ratio	$.0001 < P < .04$	(345)
ADRB3	D8S1121	8p12-p11.2	BMI	LOD = 3.2	(171)
ORM1		9q31-q32	Subcutaneous fat	.03	(342)
AK1		9q34.1	Subcutaneous fat	.01	(342)
	D10S204,193,178 1 and TCF8	10p11.22	Obesity	$1.1 < LOD < 2.5$	(174)
SUR1	D11S419	11p15.1	BMI	.003	(301)
CCKBR		11p15.4	Leptin	.01	(346)
UCP2/UCP3		11q13	Resting metabolic rate	.000002	(354)
IGFI		12q22-q23	Visceral fat	.02	(327)
ESD		13q14.1-q14.2	Subcutaneous fat, % fat	< .04	(345)
MC5R		18p11.2	BMI, subcutaneous fat, fat mass, %fat, fat-free mass, resting metabolic rate	$.001 < P < .02$	(332)
MC4R		18q22	Respiratory quotient, obesity	$.001 < P < .04$	(332)
ADA	D20S17,120	20q12-q13.11	BMI, subcutaneous fat, fat mass, %fat	$.004 < P < .02$	(345,355)
MC3R		20q13.2-q13.3	BMI, subcutaneous fat, fat mass	$.008 < P < .02$	(355)
P1		22q11.2-qter	Relative weight	.03	(342)

[a] The absence of gene symbol indicates that the linkage study involved a targeted chromosomal region.
See Table 5 legend for definitions.

approach) can now be used to detect $G \times E$ effects in humans. These methods will first be briefly reviewed followed by a summary of our current knowledge about the importance of $G \times E$ effects for phenotypes related to obesity.

A Review of Methods

An epidemiologic approach was proposed by Ottman (186) to investigate the relationship between genetic predisposition and associated risk factors and determine if there is support for a $G \times E$ interaction, and if so, the form it may take. For example, Figure 3 illustrates five plausible models as described by Ottman (186). These models are not path diagrams, but rather are more similar to metabolic paths, and the direction of the arrows denotes direction of causality. The model in Figure 3(A) posits that the genotype increases the expression of the risk factor. In Figure 3(B), the genotype exacerbates the effect of the risk factor. In both cases, only the presence of the risk factor is necessary for disease expression, although the genotype will have some additional effect. Figure 3(C) is the reverse of 3(B), where the risk factor exacerbates the effect of the genotype; only the latter is "required" for disease expression. In Figure 3(D), both the genotype and the risk factor are required to raise risk, and in Figure 3(E), the genotype and the risk factor each influence risk of disease individually.

The basic approach involves classifying individuals into four groups based on the presence or absence of genetic susceptibility and presence or absence of the risk factor (186). Genetic susceptibility can be measured directly if the susceptibility gene is known or if there are closely linked markers. Even in the absence of any molecular data, however, family history of the disease can be used to develop indicators of genetic susceptibility. In the most simplistic analysis, the pattern of hits and misses in the four groups (assessed with odds ratios) suggests whether or not a particular type of $G \times E$ interaction (as illustrated in Fig. 3) is consistent. The basic method has been expanded to include assessing relative risks in affected twin pairs with known exposure (187), and in assessing the preventive effects of targeted environmental exposures to genetically susceptible persons in population studies (188). Familial aggregation of disease was also examined within strata based on classifying probands with respect to their relative risks (189). However, none of these methods have been applied to the study of obesity.

Several other genetic approaches can be used to detect $G \times E$ effects. Two of these strategies are of the unmeasured-genotype approach. The first one would be to incorporate $G \times E$ effects in the statistical genetic

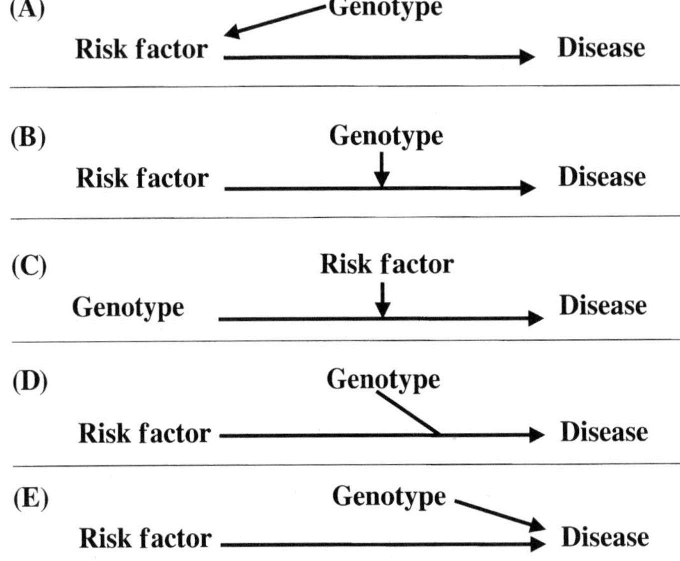

Figure 3 Five hypothetical relationships between genetic susceptibility to disease and risk factors for disease. The genetic susceptibility may be either polygenic or due to a dominant, recessive, or X-linked major locus. The risk factor may be only one of many factors associated with disease risk, and may itself have either genetic or nongenetic origins. (From Ref. 186.)

models (190–193). Ignoring such interaction effects when they exist has been shown to reduce the power to detect major gene effects (73,194). Second, using intervention studies we have proposed that one way to test for the presence of a G × E effect in humans is to challenge several genotypes in a similar manner by submitting both members of MZ twin pairs to a standardized treatment (environment) and compare the within- and the between-pair variances of the response to the treatment (195). This comparison can be done using a two-way analysis of variance (ANOVA) for repeated measures on one factor (the treatment effect), in which the genotype effect is random, the treatment effect is fixed and twins are nested within pairs. Using this ANOVA, F ratios for the treatment effect and for genotype-treatment effect can be easily obtained. The intraclass correlation can be computed from the within- and between-pair mean squares. The finding of a significantly higher variance in the response between pairs than within pairs suggest that the changes induced by the treatment are more heterogeneous in genetically dissimilar individuals, which will translate into a higher intrapair resemblance in the response.

Some of the conditions that are important to fulfill in this intervention design include (195): (1) determine the twin zygosity as precisely as possible; (2) keep age variation at a minimum; (3) use same-sex twin pairs or control for sex differences if both male and female twin pairs are involved; (4) apply the treatment in exactly the same manner to all twins under rigorously controlled conditions; (5) select phenotypes that are not greatly influenced by prior exposure to the treatment used in the study. In a series of experiments conducted on male MZ twins over the last 10 years in our laboratory, we used either exercise training or overfeeding as treatments to investigate G × E effects in obesity-related phenotypes (results described below). Although the design is useful to detect G × E effects, there are some important limitations associated with it. First, for obvious ethical reasons, there are limitations regarding the experimental treatments that can be undertaken with human subjects regarding the severity of the nutritional stress imposed and the duration of the treatment. Second, even though it is possible to exert a satisfactory experimental control and reach full standardization over energy intake, it is not possible to fully standardize energy expenditure in positive or negative energy balance studies. Indeed, because of individual differences in resting metabolic rate, thermic effect of food, fidgeting, or variations in the energy cost of weight maintenance associated with changes in body mass, subjects will invariably differ in their levels of energy expenditure. Third, such intervention studies, in addition to being very expensive to undertake, are very difficult to conduct over a long period of time on a large number of subjects.

Four methods can be used to provide evidence for G × E effects in humans when molecular markers are available. The first is to compare the influence of a gene on a given phenotype between populations of different ethnic and cultural backgrounds. An example of this approach is provided by the study of Hallman et al. (196), who showed that the effect of apolipoprotein-E polymorphism on total cholesterol levels varied among populations with different amounts of fat in their diet. The cholesterol-raising effect of the ε_4 allele, for example, was found to be highest in populations on high-fat diets like Tyrolea and Finland, and lowest in populations on low fat diets like Japan and Sudan, which provides evidence of gene-diet interaction. The second method consists of comparing the effect of a gene between subgroups of individuals within the same population, but categorized on the basis of variables that can potentially affect the phenotype under study (e.g., sex, age, race, disease status, etc.). An example of this approach could be found in the results of Zee et al. (197), who reported an association between a polymorphism in the LDL receptor gene and hypertension, but only in overweight or obese subjects. In the third method, the response to an environmental stimulus (diet, exercise training, medication, or others) is investigated among individuals with different genotypes at a given gene or marker locus. For example, using an approach similar to the MZ twin experimental design described above, but with singletons instead of twins, it would be possible to study the response to chronic alterations in energy balance as a function of genetic characteristics at specific candidate genes or marker loci. A fourth method is based on the "variability gene" concept introduced by Berg (198). Compared to a "level gene," which influences the level of a phenotype, a "variability gene" is one that contributes to the framework within which environmental factors cause phenotypic variation or, in other words, to the susceptibility to changes in the environment. To detect this G × E effect, it has been proposed that phenotypic differences between members of MZ twins of various genotypes at the genetic locus be compared (199).

An important advantage of the measured genotype approach over the unmeasured genotype approach in the study of G × E is that it makes possible the identification of the responsible genes, thereby providing a means of recognizing individuals at higher risk of disease because of differences in susceptibility to risk factors.

B Review of Findings

Evidence from both the unmeasured and measured genotype approaches is available regarding the presence of G × E effects in obesity-related phenotypes. Using appropriate statistical modeling, three studies reported major gene effects for measures of height-adjusted weight, but only after accounting for age and/or gender effects in the model (73,76,86), suggesting that the effect of this putative gene on body mass is dependent on the sex and the age of the individual, which is a special case of genotype-environment effect.

Using the unmeasured genotype approach, we studied the role of the genotype in determining the response to changes in energy balance by submitting both members of MZ twin pairs to either positive energy balance induced by overfeeding (200,201) or negative energy balance induced by exercise training (202–204). The objective of these studies was to determine whether the sensitivity of individuals to gain fat when exposed to positive energy balance or to lose fat when exposed to negative energy balance was modulated by the genotype. The results of these studies (reviewed below) revealed the presence of significant genotype-energy balance interaction effects for body weight, body fat, and fat distribution phenotypes, suggesting that genetic factors are important in determining how an individual will respond to alterations in energy balance.

1 Positive Energy Balance Experiments

It is generally recognized that there are some individuals prone to excessive accumulation of fat, for which losing weight represents a continuous battle, and others who seem relatively well protected against such a menace. We have tried to test whether such differences could be accounted for by inherited differences. In other words, we asked whether there were differences in the sensitivity of individuals to gain fat when chronically exposed to short- and long-term positive energy balance and whether such differences were dependent or independent of the genotype.

Twelve pairs of male MZ twins ate a 2.4 MJ/day (1000 kcal/day) caloric surplus, 6 days a week, during a period of 100 days (201). Significant increases in body weight and fat mass were observed after the period of overfeeding. Data showed that there were considerable interindividual differences in the adaptation to excess calories and that the variation observed was not randomly distributed, as indicated by the significant within pair resemblance in response. For instance, there was at least three times more variance in response between pairs than within pairs for the gains in body weight, fat mass, and fat-free mass (Fig. 4, left panel). These data, and those of the response to

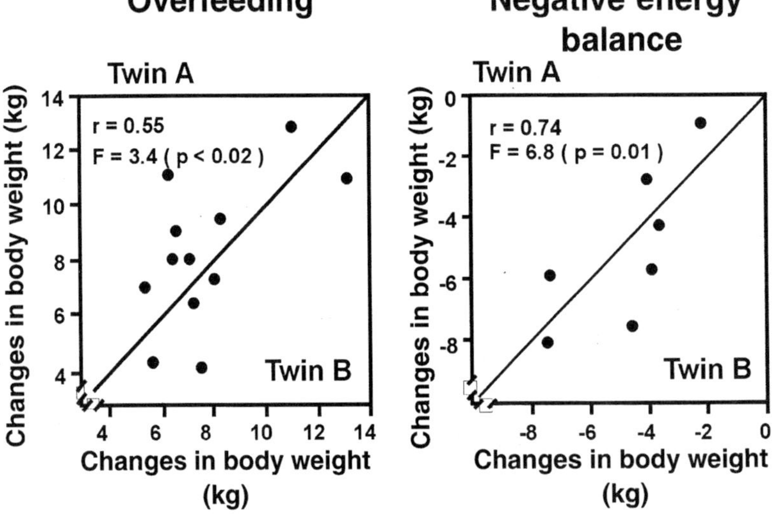

Figure 4 Intrapair resemblance in the response of identical twins to long-term changes in energy balance. Left panel: 12 pairs of identical twins were submitted to an 84,000-kcal energy intake surplus over 100 days. Right panel: 7 pairs were subjected to a negative energy balance protocol caused by exercise. The energy deficit was 58,000 kcal over 93 days. (From Refs. 201 and 204.)

short-term overfeeding, demonstrate that some individuals are more at risk than others to gain fat when energy intake surplus is clamped at the same level for everyone and when all subjects are confined to a sedentary lifestyle. The within-identical-twin-pair response to the standardized caloric surplus suggests that the amount of fat stored is likely influenced by the genotype. Similar results were essentially obtained in a shorter (22 days) overfeeding experiment (200).

The long-term overfeeding study also revealed that there was six times more variance between pairs than within pairs for the changes in upper body fat and in CT-determined abdominal visceral fat when both were adjusted for the gain in total fat mass. These observations indicate that some individuals are storing fat predominantly in selected fat depots primarily as a result of undetermined genetic characteristics. It also suggests that variations in regional fat distribution are more closely related to the genotype of the individuals than variations in body mass and in overall body composition.

At the beginning of the overfeeding treatment, almost all the daily caloric surplus was recovered as body energy gain, but the proportion decreased to 60% at the end of the 100-day protocol (205). The weight gain pattern followed an exponential with a half-duration of ~86 days. We have estimated that the weight gain attained in the experiment would have reach about 55% of the anticipated maximal weight gain had the overfeeding protocol been continued indefinitely (205). The mean body mass gain for the 24 subjects of the 100-day overfeeding experiment was 8.1 kg, of which 5.4 kg was fat mass and 2.7 kg was fat-free mass. Assuming that the energy content of body fat is ~22 MJ/kg (9300 kcal/kg, assuming a 100% triglyceride content) and that of fat-free tissue is 2.42 MJ/kg (1020 kcal/kg), then about 63% of the excess energy intake was recovered on the average as body mass changes. This proportion is of the same order as that reported by other investigators (206,207), i.e., between 60% and 75% of total excess energy intake. There were, however, individual differences among the 24 subjects with respect to the amount of fat and fat free tissue gained.

Resting metabolic rate in absolute terms increased by ~10% with overfeeding. However, the increase was only marginal when expressed by unit of fat-free mass (208,209). The intrapair resemblance for the changes in resting metabolic rate brought about by overfeeding was significant but became nonsignificant when the changes in body mass or body composition were taken into account. The thermic response to food, as assessed by indirect calorimetry for a period of 4 hours following the ingestion of a 2.4 MJ (1000 kcal) meal of mixed composition, did not increase with overfeeding when resting metabolic rate was subtracted from postprandial energy expenditure (208). In contrast, postprandial energy expenditure and the total energy cost of weight maintenance increased significantly but the increments were mostly due to the gain in body mass. Interestingly, resting metabolic rate and thermic response to a standardized meal did not correlate with the body mass and adiposity changes just as they did not in a separate overfeeding protocol conducted with singletons (210).

Attempts have been made to identify genetic variants that could account for the differences in response to overfeeding among the 12 pairs of twins. No associations were seen between markers in UCP1, UCP2, and UCP3 genes and body weight or body fatness increases (211). On the other hand, the Gln223Arg polymorphism in the LEPR gene was related to plasma leptin induced changes in response to the long-term overfeeding protocol, with the Gln/Glu genotypes experiencing the largest increases, but it was not associated with body mass and adiposity changes (212). In contrast, Gln27Gln twins at the ADRB2 gene gained more weight and subcutaneous fat than other genotypes with exposure to 100 days of overfeeding (213). Finally, the GG twins at an ApaI (restriction enzyme) polymorphism in the IGF2 gene gained more fat mass and subcutaneous fat with overfeeding than the AA and AG twins (214). These exploratory studies with a small sample size suggest that it may be possible to eventually identify the genes and sequence variants responsible for the genotype-overfeeding interaction effects observed in the 100-day overfeeding experiment with identical twins.

2 Negative Energy Balance Experiment

Seven pairs of young adult male identical twins completed a negative energy balance protocol during which they exercised on cycle ergometers twice a day, 9 out of 10 days, over a period of 93 days while being kept on a constant daily energy and nutrient intake (204). The mean total energy deficit caused by exercise above the estimated energy cost of body weight maintenance reached 244 MJ. Baseline energy intake was estimated over a period of 17 days preceding the negative energy balance protocol. Mean body weight loss was 5.0 kg and was entirely accounted for by the loss of fat mass. Fat-free mass was unchanged. Body energy losses reached 191 MJ, which represented ~78% of the estimated energy deficit. Decreases in metabolic rates and in the energy expenditure of activity not associated with the cycle ergometer protocol must have occurred to explain the difference between the estimated energy deficit and the body energy losses. Subcutaneous fat loss was slightly more pronounced on the trunk than on the limbs as estimated from skinfolds, circumferences, and computed tomography.

The reduction in abdominal visceral fat area was quite striking, from 81 cm^2 to 52 cm^2. At the same submaximal power output level, subjects oxidized more lipids than carbohydrates after the program as indicated by the changes in the respiratory exchange ratio. Intrapair resemblance was observed for the changes in body weight (Fig. 4, right), fat mass, percent fat, body energy content, sum of 10 skinfolds, abdominal visceral fat, and respiratory exchange ratio during submaximal work. Even though there were large individual differences in response to the negative energy balance and exercise protocol, subjects with the same genotype were more alike in responses than subjects with different genotypes particularly for body fat, body energy, and abdominal visceral fat changes. High lipid oxidizers and low lipid oxidizers during submaximal exercise were also seen despite the fact that all subjects had experienced the same exercise and nutritional conditions for ~3 months.

Thus, changes in body mass, body fat, and body energy content were characterized by more heterogeneity between twin pairs than within pairs. These results are remarkably similar to those we reported earlier for body mass, body fat, and body energy gains with 12 pairs of twins subjected to a 100-day overfeeding protocol.

VI RECOMMENDATIONS

The evidence reviewed herein suggests a significant genetic component in human obesity. However, the nature of the evidence and the magnitude of the genetic component varied a great deal depending on the phenotype, and the particular type of genetic epidemiological method used. A picture that is clearly emerging from the diverse findings is that multiple genetic loci are involved in human obesity.

In the present context, it may be helpful to distinguish between *primary* and *secondary* obesity genes, which collectively contribute to and determine the variability in obesity. We define *primary genes* as those whose effect sizes may be large enough to be detected. Likewise, the *secondary genes* for human obesity are those whose effects are likely much smaller and their detection in the context of obesity may be very difficult. The combined effects of the primary genes may be characterized as oligogenic (few genes each with a large enough effect), and the aggregate effects of the secondary obesity genes may be regarded as polygenic (many genes, each with a small effect). Regardless of the terminology, it is commonly recognized that human obesity involves multiple genes, some with large and some with small effects.

While the model-fitting approaches in genetic epidemiology have been largely successful in demonstrating the underlying complexity in the transmission of human obesity, there are limitations in such studies that necessitate alternatives. One limitation arises because most model-fitting approaches are based on largely untestable assumptions. However realistic some of these assumptions may be, there is always some degree of uncertainty. Second, analysis of multilocus traits like obesity requires more advanced and complex models that are mostly lacking or highly specialized (see 29). For example, when segregation analysis based on single-locus models is applied to a trait determined by two genes, it fails to characterize either gene accurately [even though it can sometimes succeed in inferring a gene with a large effect (215)]. Finally, such model-fitting approaches alone are inadequate for evaluating the specific genetic determinants of human obesity, although they are useful in suggesting possible genetic mechanisms. DNA sequence variants in targeted genes are essential.

We believe that an optimum strategy for complex multifactorial traits such as obesity should combine the strengths of three companion methods so as to maximize our chances of finding the primary genes. Only after finding the primary genes can specialized methods be fruitful in finding the secondary genes.

A Genetic Epidemiological Model-Fitting Approach

While this approach alone is unlikely to yield major findings, the results can guide our subsequent inquiries, especially when multivariate models and longitudinal studies are employed. This approach could be even more useful after finding specific obesity genes using the molecular approaches discussed below. They will aid in evaluating gene-gene and gene-environment interactions and in characterizing the gene effects. They will also enable investigation as to whether any additional familial (genetic) component exists, after accounting for all known obesity genes, something that can motivate the search for additional genes.

B Genomewide Explorations

A useful method involves nonparametric sibpair linkage using evenly spaced anonymous markers. To maximize the power, we propose that full sibships be used for this purpose. Each sibship should contain at least two sibs, and at least one of them must be obese or very obese. Sampling from the upper tail is known to be more powerful, and hence requires smaller sample sizes (216). Variance components linkage methodology can then be used to exploit the full variability within sibships [e.g., SOLAR (217) and SEGPATH (218)].

For a trait with a sibling correlation of 0.25, to detect a gene with 80% power that explains 27% of phenotypic variance, one needs a sample of 110 sibpairs (220 subjects) where each pair contains at least one sib whose BMI is in the upper decile. One can attain 90% power with 146 such sibpairs (292 subjects). One can also attain 80% power with 47 sibling triplets (141 subjects) or 90% power with 64 triplets (192 subjects), where each triplet contains at least one sib whose BMI is in the upper decile. These calculations are based on single gene models and zero recombination between the trait and marker loci. Multiple trait loci and nonzero recombination both require considerably larger samples. A sample of ~300 sibships of varying sizes, each with at least two sibs and at least one of them above the 90th centile, may be regarded as a minimal design.

Since the gene effects are quite likely mediated by a host of lifestyle and other metabolic factors, it is desirable to obtain as much information on each subject as possible, including detailed phenotypic characterizations. That way, the possible role of these covariates can be incorporated in the data analysis. Also, even though the sampling may be based on BMI, the QTL analysis should be performed for each of the correlated phenotypes (e.g., BMI, %BF, etc.). This will maximize the yield, since different genes may primarily contribute to different components of obesity.

C Implicating Specific Genes and Mutations

The ultimate goal of the studies designed to understand the genetic and molecular basis of human variation in a trait such as obesity is to resolve the issue in terms of the specific genes and DNA sequence variants. As a result of the advances in the sequencing of the human genome by the public and private institutions, ~55% of the sequence is now said to be complete and highly reliable. In addition, a draft sequence is also available for >90% of the human genome. For a substantial fraction of the genome, a reasonably reliable physical map can thus be defined. For some chromosome regions, a complete and fully reliable sequence map exists.

These advances together with the progress in the development of large panels of single nucleotide polymorphisms (SNPs), the availability of efficient high throughput sequencing technologies, and the large repertoire of mapped expressed sequences (ESTs) have increased the ability of investigators to resolve genetic effects in terms of genes and sequence differences. The investigator is typically confronted with two different situations. In the first case, a strong candidate gene has been identified through a variety of strategies, e.g., based on physiopathological reasoning, evidence from a knockout mouse, etc. The goal then becomes one of establishing whether DNA sequence variation in this gene contributes to human heterogeneity in the trait of interest. Informative SNPs and sequencing of targeted regions of the gene such as exons, intronic splicing sequences, short and long promoter regions among affected and nonaffected carefully matched subjects would be the methods of choice. Alternatively, one could apply the same technologies to a large sample of unrelated subjects exhibiting considerable heterogeneity in phenotype and test for genotype differences using a variety of statistical tools.

In the second case, a candidate chromosomal position (for instance, a QTL from a genomic scan) is the starting point. The inventory of genes and ESTs encoded in the region covered by the QTL does not yield strong candidate genes or generate a number of candidate genes, but none with compelling evidence to justify taking it to the next step (see first case). This case is decidedly more complex. The strategy described below will clearly work best when a valid physical map of the region is available.

Increasing the density of polymorphic markers to narrow the size of the DNA fragment underlying the QTL is a critical first step. Adding such markers may typically reduce the size of the chromosomal segment of interest to about one or two megabases. Further decrease in the size of the region can often be achieved by typing a number of SNPs to cover the entire QTL. A combination of single SNP and haplotype studies are then conducted, using association analytical strategies as well as quantitative TDT analysis (QTDT). Constant comparisons between the results of such studies and the features of the physical map and panels of candidate genes and ESTs are absolutely necessary, the goal being to evolve toward one or a few candidate genes or a fragment size amenable to sequencing studies. The success of this complex process is highly dependent on the quality and informativeness of the populations of normal weight and obese subjects upon which the project is anchored.

Finally, when some obesity genes are found, it would be very useful to type these genes in a large random sample. This will enable estimation of the relevant gene frequencies in the underlying population. More importantly, detailed phenotypic characterization and studies of additional covariates will enable characterization of the gene effects and investigations of gene-gene and gene-environment interactions. This can be achieved through one of several means, for example, by regression of a phenotype (say %BF) on all covariates, measured genotypes, and interactions among them.

This chapter summarizes the data pertaining to the heritability and the contribution of major genes for phenotypes of total body fat and fat topography based on the genetic epidemiology methods. The evidence for a contribution of genetic-environment interaction effects to variation in body mass, body fat, and fat distribution was also considered. The current status of associated and linkage studies conducted on human samples was reviewed. Finally, the chapter suggests a variety of strategies to optimize the search for the genes associated with the susceptibility to obesity and to define the inheritance patterns. This overview of the available evidence highlights the need for the development of longitudinal databases that will increase the chance of untangling causes versus effects of positive energy balance.

APPENDIX Symbols, Full Names, and Cytogenetic Location of Genes and Loci Listed in this Chapter*

Gene or locus	Name	Location
A		
ACP1	Acid phosphatase 1, soluble	2p25
ADA	Adenosine deaminase	20q12-q13.11
ADRB2	Adrenergic, beta-2-, receptor, surface	5q31-q32
ADRA2A	Adrenergic, alpha-2A-, receptor	10q24-q26
ADRA2B	Adrenergic, alpha-2B-, receptor	2p13-q13
ADRB3	Adrenergic, beta-3-, receptor	8p12-p11.2
AGT	Angiotensinogen	1q42-q43
AK1	Adenylate kinase 1	9q34.1
ANG	Angiogenin, ribonuclease, RNase A family, 5	14q11.1-q11.2
APM1	Adipose most abundant gene transcript 1, adiponectin	3q27
APOA4	Apolipoprotein A-IV	11q23
APOB	Apolipoprotein B (including Ag (x) antigen)	2p24-p23
APOD	Apolipoprotein D	3q26.2-qter
ASIP	Agouti (mouse) signaling protein	20q11.2-q12
ATP1A2	ATPase, Na^+ K^+ transporting, alpha 2 (+) polypeptide	1q21-q23
ATP1B1	ATPase, Na^+ K^+ transporting, beta 1 polypeptide	1q22-q25
ATRN	Attractin (with dipeptidylpeptidase IV activity)	20p13
B, C		
BBS2	Bardet-Biedl syndrome 2 gene	16q21
BBS4	Bardet-Biedl syndrome 4 gene	15q22.3-q23
BF	B-factor, properdin	6p21.3
BSCL2	Berardinelli-Siep congenital lipodystrophy 2 gene	11q13
CART	Cocaine- and amphetamine-regulated transcript	5q
CAV2	Caveolin 2	7q31.1
CBFA2T1	Core-binding factor, runt domain, alpha subunit 2; translocated to, 1; cyclin D-related	8q22
CCKAR	Cholecystokinin A receptor	4p15.2-p15.1
CCKBR	Cholecystokinin B receptor (or gastrin receptor)	11p15.4
CD36L1	CD36 antigen (collagen type I receptor, thrombospondin receptor)-like 1	12q24.1-q24.3
CPE	Carboxypeptidase E	4q32
D–F		
DRD2	Dopamine receptor D2	11q23
ESD	Esterase D/formylglutathione hydrolase	13q14.1-q14.2

Gene or locus	Name	Location
ESR1	Estrogen receptor 1	6q25.1
FABP2	Fatty acid binding protein 2, intestinal	4q28-q31
FBS	Fanconi-Bickel syndrome	3q26.1-q26.3
FGR3	Fibroblast growth factor receptor 3 (achondroplasia, thanatophoric dwarfism)	4p16.3
FGF13	Fibroblast Growth Factor 13	Xq26
G–I, K		
GCK	Glucokinase (hexokinase 4, maturity onset diabetes of the young 2	7p15.3-p15.1
GHRH	Growth hormone releasing hormone	20q11.2
GHRHR	Growth hormone releasing hormone receptor	7p14
GLO1	Glyoxalase I	6p21.3-p21.1
GNAS1	Guanine nucleotide binding protein (G protein), alpha stimulating activity polypeptide 1	20q13.2-q13.3
GNB3	Guanine nucleotide binding protein (G protein), beta polypeptide 3	12p13
GPC3	Glypican 3	Xq26.1
GPC4	Glypican 4	Xq26.1
GRL	Glucocorticoid receptor	5q31-q32
GYPA	Glycophorin A (includes MN blood group)	4q28.2-q31.1
GYS1	Glycogen synthase 1 (muscle)	19q13.3
HSD3B1	Hydroxy-delta-5-steroid dehydrogenase, 3 beta- and steroid delta-isomerase 1	1p13.1
HSD17B1	11-Hydroxysteroid (17-beta) dehydrogenase 1	17q11-q21
HSD17B3	11-Hydroxysteroid (17-beta) dehydrogenase 3	9q22
HSPA2	Heat shock 70kD protein 2	14q21

Gene or locus	Name	Location
HTR2A	5-hydroxytryptamine (serotonin) receptor 2A	13q14-q21
HTR2C	5-hydroxytryptamine (serotonin) receptor 2C	Xq24
IGF1	Insulin-like growth factor 1 (somatomedin C)	12q22-q23
IGF1R	Insulin-like growth factor 1 receptor	15q25-q26
IGF2	Insulin-like growth factor 2 (somatomedin A)	11p15.5
IGKC	Immunoglobulin kappa constant	2p12
INS	Insulin	11p15.5
INSR	Insulin receptor	19p13.3-p13.2
IRS	Insulin Resistance syndromes	19p13.3
IRS1	Insulin receptor substrate 1	2q36
ISL1	ISL1 transcription factor, LIM/homeodomain (islet-1)	5q22.3
KEL	Kell blood group	7q33
L		
LDLR	Low-density lipoprotein receptor (familial hypercholesterolemia)	19p13.3
LEPR	Leptin receptor	1p31
LEP	Leptin (murine obesity homolog)	7q31.3
LIPE	Lipase, hormone sensitive	19q13.1-q13.2
LMNA	Lamin A/C	1q21.2-q21.3
LPL	Lipoprotein lipase	8p22
M–O		
MC3R	Melanocortin 3 receptor	20q13.2-q13.3
MC4R	Melanocortin 4 receptor	18q22
MC5R	Melanocortin 5 receptor	18p11.2
MKKS	McKusick-Kaufman syndrome	20p12
NDN	Necdin(mouse) homolog	15q11.2-q12
NHLH2	Nescient helix loop helix 2	1p12-p11
NMB	Neuromedin B	15q22-qter
NOS3	Nitric oxide synthase 3 (endothelial cell)	7q36.2
NPY	Neuropeptide Y	7p15.1
NPY2R	Neuropeptide Y receptor Y2	4q31

Gene or locus	Name	Location
NPY5R	Neuropeptide Y receptor Y5	4q31-q32
ORM1	Orosomucoid 1	9q31-q32
P, S		
P1	P blood group (P one antigen)	22q11.2-qter
PCSK1	Proprotein convertase subtilisin/kexin type 1	5q15-q21
PGD	Phosphogluconate dehydrogenase	1p36.2-p36.13
PMM2	Phosphoman-nomutase 2	16p13.3-p13.2
POMC	Proopiomelanocortin	2p23.3
PON2	Paraoxonase 2	7q21.3
PPARG	Peroxisome proliferative activated receptor, gamma	3p25
PPARGC1	Peroxisome proliferative activated receptor, gamma, coactivator 1	4p15.1
PPCD	Posterior Polymorphous Corneal dystrophy	20q11
PPY	Pancreatic polypeptide	17q21
PROP1	Prophet of Pit 1, paired-like homeodomain transcription factor	5q
PYY	Peptide YY	17q21.1
SIM1	Single-minded (Drosophila) homolog 1	6q16.3-q21
SLC2A2	Solute carrier family 2 (facilitated glucose transporter), member 2	3q26.1-q26.2
SLC2A4	Solute carrier family 2 (facilitated glucose transporter), member 4	17p13
SNRPN	Small nuclear ribo-nucleoprotein polypeptide N	15q12
SUR1	Sulfonylurea receptor 1	11p15.1
T, U, W		
TBX3	T-box3 (ulnar mammary syndrome)	12q24.1
TCF1	Transcription factor 1, hepatic; hepatic nuclear factor (HNF1)	12q24.2
TCF8	Transcription factor 8 (represses inter-leukin 2 expression)	10p11.2
THRB	Thyroid hormone receptor, beta	3p24.3
TNFA	Tumor necrosis factor	6p21.3
TNFRSF1B	Tumor necrosis factor receptor superfamily member 1B	1p36.3-p36.2
TUB	Tubby (mouse) homolog	11p15.5
UCP1	Uncoupling protein 1 (mitochondrial, proton carrier)	4q28-q31
UCP2	Uncoupling protein 2 (mitochondrial, proton carrier)	11q13
UCP3	Uncoupling protein 3 (mitochondrial, proton carrier)	11q13

* The gene symbols, names and cytogenetic locations are from the Locus Link Web site (*http//www.ncbi.nlm.nih.gov/LocusLink*) available from the National Center for Biotechnology Information

REFERENCES

1. Seidell JC. Obesity: a growing problem. Acta Paediatr Suppl 1999; 88:46–50.
2. Bouchard C. Human obesities: chaos or determinism? In: Ailhaud G, Guy-Grand B, Lafontan M, Ricquier C, eds. Obesity in Europe 91. Proceedings of the 3rd European Congress on Obesity. Paris: John Libbey, 1992:7–14.
3. Garn SM, Leonard WR, Hawthorne VM. Three limitations of the body mass index. Am J Clin Nutr 1986; 44:996–997.
4. Ferland M, Després JP, Tremblay A, Pinault S, Nadeau A, Moorjani S, Lupien PJ, Thériault G, Bouchard C. Assessment of adipose tissue distribution by computed axial tomography in obese women: association with body density and anthropometric measurements. Br J Nutr 1989; 61:139–148.
5. Bouchard C. Genetics of body fat, energy expenditure and adipose tissue metabolism. In: Berry EM, Blondheim SH, Eliahou HE, Shafrir E, eds. Recent Advances in Obesity Research. London: Libbey, 1987: 16–25.
6. Hopper JL. The epidemiology of genetic epidemiology. Acta Genet Med Gemellol 1992; 41:261–273.
7. Rice TK, Borecki IB. Familial resemblance and heritability. Adv Genet 2001; 42:35–44.
8. Schull WJ, Weiss KM. Genetic epidemiology : Four strategies. Epidemiol Rev 1980; 2:1–18.

9. Susser M, Susser E. Indicators and designs in genetic epidemiology: separating heredity and environment. Rev Epidemiol Sante Publ 1987; 35:54–77.
10. Thompson EA. Genetic epidemiology: a review of the statistical basis. Stat Med 1986; 5:291–302.
11. Rao DC, McGue M, Wette R, Glueck CJ. Path analysis in genetic epidemiology. In: Chakravarti A, ed. Human Population Genetics: The Pittsburgh Symposium. Stroudsburg, PA: Van Nostrand-Reinhold, 1984:35–81.
12. Rao DC, Wette R. Environmental index in genetic epidemiology: an investigation of its role, adequacy, and limitations. Am J Hum Genet 1990; 46:168–178.
13. Rice J, Cloninger CR, Reich T. Multifactorial inheritance with cultural transmission and assortative mating. I. Description and basic properties of the unitary models. Am J Hum Genet 1978;30: 618–643.
14. Boomsma DI, Martin NG, Neale MC. Genetic analysis of twin and family data: structural modeling using LISREL. Behav Genet 1989; 19:5–161.
15. DeFries JC, Fulker DW. Multiple regression analysis of twin data. Behav Genet 1985; 15:467–473.
16. Jöreskog KG, Sörbom D. LISREL: Analysis of Linear Structural Relationships by the Method of Maximum Likelihood. Chicago: National Educational Resources, 1986.
17. Plomin R, DeFries JC, McClearn GE. Behavioral Genetics: A Primer, 2nd ed. New York: W.H. Freeman, 1990:341–360.
18. Bouchard C. Transient environmental effects detected in sibling correlations. Ann Hum Biol 1980; 7:89–92.
19. Mueller WH. Transient environmental changes and age-limited genes as causes of variation in sib-sib and parent-offspring correlations. Ann Hum Biol 1978; 5: 395–398.
20. Province MA, Rao DC. Path analysis of family resemblance with temporal trends: applications to height, weight, and Quetelet index in northeastern Brazil. Am J Hum Genet 1985; 37:178–192.
21. Malina RM, Bouchard C. Subcutaneous fat distribution during growth. In: Bouchard C, Johnston FE, eds. Fat Distribution During Growth and Later Health Outcomes. Current Topics in Nutrition and Disease, Vol 17. New York: Alan R. Liss, 1988:63–84.
22. Ravussin E, Lillioja S, Knowler WC, Christin L, Freymond D, Abbott WGH, Boyce V, Howard BV, Bogardus C. Reduced rate of energy expenditure as a risk factor for body-weight gain. N Engl J Med 1988; 318:467–472.
23. Zurlo F, Lillioja S, Esposito-Del Puente A, Nyomba BL, Raz I, Saad MF, Swinburn BA, Knowler WC, Bogardus C, Ravussin E. Low ratio of fat to carbohydrate oxidation as predictor of weight gain: study of 24-h RQ. Am J Physiol 1990; 259:E650–E657.
24. Vogler GP, Fulker DW. Human behavior genetics. In: Nesselroade JR, Cattell RB, eds. Handbook of Multivariate Experimental Psychology, 2nd ed. New York: Plenum, 1988:475–503.
25. Lalouel JM, Morton NE. Complex segregation analysis with pointers. Hum Hered 1981; 31:312–321.
26. Hasstedt SJ. PAP: Pedigree Analysis Package, Rev 3. Salt Lake City: Department of Human Genetics, University of Utah, 1989.
27. Konigsberg LW, Blangero J, Kammerer CM, Mott GE. Mixed model segregation analysis of LDL-C concentration with genotype-covariate interaction. Genet Epidemiol 1991; 8:69–80.
28. Bonney GE, Lathrop GM, Lalouel JM. Combined linkage and segregation analysis using regressive models. Am J Hum Genet 1988; 43:29–37.
29. Blangero J, Konigsberg LW. Multivariate segregation analysis using the mixed model. Genet Epidemiol 1991; 8:299–316.
30. Rao DC, Province MA. The future of path analysis, segregation analysis, and combined models for genetic dissection of complex traits. Hum Hered 2000; 50:34–42.
31. Li Z, Bonney GE, Lathrop GM, Rao DC. Genetic analysis combining path analysis with regressive models: the TAU model of multifactorial transmission. Hum Hered 1994; 44:305–311.
32. Li Z, Bonney GE, Rao DC. Genetic analysis combining path analysis with regressive models: the BETA path model of polygenic and familial environmental transmission. Genet Epidemiol 1994; 11:431–442.
33. Province MA, Rao DC. General purpose model and a computer program for combined segregation and path analysis (SEGPATH): automatically creating computer programs from symbolic language model specifications. Genet Epidemiol 1995; 12:203–219.
34. Borecki IB, Lathrop GM, Bonney GE, Yaouanq J, Rao DC. Combined segregation and linkage analysis of genetic hemochromatosis using affection status, serum iron, and HLA. Am J Hum Genet 1990; 47: 542–550.
35. Hasstedt SJ, Ramirez ME, Kuida H, Williams RR. Recessive inheritance of a relative fat pattern. Am J Hum Genet 1989; 45:917–925.
36. Annest JL, Sing CF, Biron P, Mongeau JG. Familial aggregation of blood pressure and weight in adoptive families. III. Analysis of the role of shared genes and shared household environment in explaining family resemblance for height, weight and selected weight/height indices. Am J Epidemiol 1983; 117:492–506.
37. Garn SM, Bailey SM, Cole PE. Similarities between parents and their adopted children. Am J Phys Anthrop 1976; 45:539–543.
38. Hartz A, Giefer E, Rimm A. Relative importance of the effect of family environment and heredity on obesity. Ann Hum Genet 1977; 41:185–193.
39. Khoury P, Morrison JA, Laskarzewski PM, Glueck CJ. Parent-offspring and sibling body mass index associations during and after sharing of common

household environments: the Princeton School District Family Study. Metabolism 1983; 32:82–89.
40. Longini IM Jr, Higgins MW, Hinton PC, Moll PP, Keller JB. Genetic and environmental sources of familial aggregation of body mass in Tecumseh, Michigan. Hum Biol 1984; 56:733–757.
41. Biron P, Mongeau J-G, Bertrand D. Familial resemblance of body weight and weight/height in 374 homes with adopted children. J Pediatr 1977; 91:555–558.
42. Heller R, Garrison RJ, Havlik RJ, Feinleib M, Padgett S. Family resemblances in height and relative weight in the Framingham Heart Study. Int J Obes 1984; 8:399–405.
43. Price RA, Cadoret RJ, Stunkard AJ, Troughton E. Genetic contributions to human fatness: an adoption study. Am J Psychiatry 1987; 144:1003–1008.
44. Price RA, Gottesman II. Body fat in identical twins reared apart: roles for genes and environment. Behav Genet 1991; 21:1–7.
45. Sørensen TIA, Price RA, Stunkard AJ, Schulsinger F. Genetics of obesity in adult adoptees and their biological siblings. BMJ 1989; 298:87–90.
46. Stunkard AJ, Foch TT, Hrubec Z. A twin study of human obesity. JAMA 1986; 256:51–54.
47. Stunkard AJ, Sørensen TIA, Hanis C, Teasdale TW, Chakraborty R, Schull WJ, Schulsinger F. An adoption study of human obesity. N Engl J Med 1986; 314:193–198.
48. Stunkard AJ, Harris JR. Pedersen NL, McClearn GE. The body-mass index of twins who have been reared apart. N Engl J Med 1990; 322:1483–1487.
49. Vogler GP, Sørensen TIA, Stunkard AJ, Srinivasan MR, Rao DC. Influences of genes and shared family environment on adult body mass index assessed in an adoption study by a comprehensive path model. Int J Obes 1995; 19:40–45.
50. MacDonald A, Stunkard J. Body mass indexes of British separated twins. N Engl J Med 1990; 322:1530.
51. Tambs K, Moum T, Eaves L, Neale M, Midthjell K, Lund-Larsen PG, Ness S, Holmen J. Genetic and environmental contributions to the variance of the body mass index in Norwegian sample of first- and second-degree relatives. Am J Hum Biol 1991; 3:257–267.
52. McLaughlin JA. The inheritance of body-mass index in the Virginia 30,000. Behav Genet 1991; 21:581 (abstract).
53. Bouchard C. Genetics of obesity: overview and research directions. In: Bouchard C. ed. The Genetics of Obesity, Boca Raton, FL: CRC Press, 1994:223–233.
54. Borecki IB, Rice T, Pérusse L, Boulard C, Rao DC. Major gene influence on the propensity to store fat in trunk versus extremity depots: evidence from the Quebec Family Study. Obes Res 1995; 3:1–8.
55. Cardon LR. Developmental analysis of the body mass index in the Colorado Adoption Project. Behav Genet 1991; 21:563–564 (abstract).
56. Fabsitz R, Feinleib M, Hrubec Z. Weight changes in adult twins. Acta Genet Med Gemellol 1980; 29:273–279.
57. Fabsitz RR, Carmelli D, Hewitt JK. Evidence for independent genetic influences on obesity in middle age. Int J Obes 1992; 16:657–666.
58. Fabsitz RR, Sholinsky P, Carmelli D. Genetic influences on adult weight gain and maximum body mass index in male twins. Am J Epidemiol 1994; 140:711–720.
59. Korkeila M, Kaprio J, Rissanen A, Koskenvuo M. Effects of gender and age on the heritability of body mass index. Int J Obes 1991; 15:647–654.
60. Huggins RM, Hoang NH, Loesch DZ. Analysis of longitudinal data from twins. Genet Epidemiol 2000; 19:345–353.
61. Pietiläinen KH, Kaprio J, Rissanen A, Winter T, Rimpelä A, Viken RJ, Rose RJ. Distribution and heritability of BMI in Finnish adolescents aged 16y and 17y: a study of 4884 twins and 2509 singletons. Int J Obes 1999; 23:107–115.
62. Rice T, Pérusse L, Bouchard C, Rao DC. Familial aggregation of body mass index and subcutaneous fat measures in the longitudinal Quebec Family Study. Genet Epidemiol 1999; 16:316–334.
63. Pérusse L, Chagnon YC, Bouchard C. Etiology of massive obesity: Role of genetic factors. World J Surg 1998; 22:907–912.
64. Adams TD, Hunt SC, Mason LA, Ramirez ME, Fisher AG, Williams RR. Familial aggregation of morbid obesity. Obes Res 1993; 1:261–270.
65. Lissner L, Sjöström L, Bengtsson C, Bouchard C, Larsson B. The natural history of obesity in an obese population and associations with metabolic aberrations. Int J Obes 1994; 18:441–447.
66. Reed DR, Bradley EC, Price RA. Obesity in families of extremely obese women. Obes Res 1993; 1:167–172.
67. Price RA, Lee JH. Risk ratios for obesity in families of obese African-American and Caucasian women. Hum Hered 2001; 51:35–40.
68. Ness R, Laskarzewski P, Price RA. Inheritance of extreme overweight in black families. Hum Biol 1991; 63:39–52.
69. Price RA, Ness R, Laskarzewski P. Common major gene inheritance of extreme overweight. Hum Biol 1990; 62:747–765.
70. Province MA, Arnqvist P, Keller J, Higgins M, Rao DC. Strong evidence for a major gene for obesity in the large, unselected, total Community Health Study of Tecumseh. Am J Hum Genet 1990; 47(suppl):A143.
71. Moll PP, Burns TL, Lauer RM. The genetic and environmental sources of body mass index variability: the Muscatine Ponderosity Family Study. Am J Hum Genet 1991; 49:1243–1255.
72. Rice T, Sjöström CD, Pérusse L, Rao DC, Sjöström L, Bouchard C. Segregation analysis of body mass index

in a large sample selected for obesity: the Swedish Obese Subjects study. Obes Res 1999; 7:246–255.

73. Borecki IB, Bonney GE, Rice T, Bouchard C, Rao DC. Influence of genotype-dependent effects of covariates on the outcome of segregation analysis of the body mass index. Am J Hum Genet 1993; 53:676–687.
74. Ginsburg E, Livshits G, Yakovenko K, Kobyliansky E. Major gene control of human body height, weight and BMI in five ethnically different populations. Ann Hum Genet 1998; 62:307–322.
75. Price RA. Within birth cohort segregation analyses support recessive inheritance of body mass index in white and African-American families. Int J Obes 1996; 20:1044–1047.
76. Tiret L, André J-L, Ducimetière P, Herbeth B, Rakotovao R, Guegen R, Spyckerelle Y, Cambien F. Segregation analysis of height-adjusted weight with generation- and age-dependent effects: the Nancy Family Study. Genet Epidemiol 1992; 9:389–403.
77. Zonta LA, Jayakar SD, Bosisio M, Galante A, Pennetti V. Genetic analysis of human obesity in an Italian sample. Hum Hered 1987; 37:129–139.
78. Price RA, Charles MA, Pettitt DJ, Knowler WC. Obesity in Pima Indians: genetic segregation analyses of body mass index complicated by temporal increases in obesity. Hum Biol 1994; 66:251–274.
79. Rice T, Borecki IB, Bouchard C, Rao DC. Segregation analysis of body mass index in an unselected French-Canadian sample: The Quebec Family Study. Obes Res 1993; 1:288–294.
80. Fain PR. Characteristics of simple sibship variance tests for the detection of major loci and application to height, weight and spatial performance. Ann Hum Genet 1978; 42:109–120.
81. Karlin S, Williams PT, Jensen S, Farquhar JW. Genetic analysis of the Stanford LRC Family Study data. I. Structured exploratory data analysis of height and weight measurements. Am J Epidemio] 1981; 113:307–324.
82. Hasstedt SJ, Hoffman M, Leppert MF, Elbein SC. Recessive inheritance of obesity in familial non-insulin-dependent diabetes mellitus, and lack of linkage to nine candidate genes. Am J Hum Genet 1997; 61:668–677.
83. Borecki IB, Blangero J, Rice T, Pérusse L, Bouchard C, Rao DC. Evidence for at least two major loci influencing human fatness. Am J Hum Genet 1998; 63: 831–838.
84. Borecki IB, Higgins M, Schreiner PJ, Arnett DK, Mayer-Davis E, Hunt SC, Province MA. Evidence for multiple determinants of the body mass index: the National Heart, Lung, and Blood Institute Family Heart Study. Obes Res 1998; 6:107–114.
85. Comuzzie AG, Blangero J, Mahaney MC, Mitchell BD, Hixson JE, Samollow PB, Stern MP, MacCluer JW. Major gene with sex-specific effects influences fat mass in Mexican Americans. Genet Epidemiol 1995; 12:475–488.
86. Rice T, Borecki IB, Bouchard C, Rao DC. Segregation analysis of fat mass and other body composition measures derived from underwater weighing. Am J Hum Genet 1993; 52:967–973.
87. Jouanny P, Guillemin F, Kuntz C, Jeandel C, Pourel J. Environmental and genetic factors affecting bone mass: similarity of bone density among members of healthy families. Arth Rheum 1995; 38:61–67.
88. Feitosa MF, Rice T, Nirmala A, Rao DC. Major gene effect on body mass index: the role of energy intake and energy expenditure. Hum Biol 2000; 72: 781–799.
89. Rice T, Tremblay A, Dériaz O, Pérusse L, Rao DC, Bouchard C. A major gene for resting metabolic rate unassociated with body composition: results from the Quebec Family Study. Obes Res 1996; 4:441–449.
90. Mitchell LE, Nirmala A, Rice T, Reddy PC, Rao DC. The impact of energy intake and energy expenditure of activity on the familial transmission of adiposity in an Indian population. Am J Hum Biol 1993; 5:331–339.
91. Kaplan RM, Patterson TL, Sallis JF Jr, Nader PR. Exercise suppresses heritability estimates for obesity in Mexican-American families. Addict Behav 1989; 14: 581–588.
92. Lean MEJ, Han TS, Morrison CE. Waist circumference as a measure for indicating need for weight management. BMJ 1995; 311:158–161.
93. Katzmarzyk PT, Malina RM, Pérusse L, Rice T, Province MA, Rao DC, Bouchard C. Familial resemblance in fatness and fat distribution. Am J Hum Biol 2000; 12:395–404.
94. Pérusse L, Rice T, Province MA, Gagnon J, Leon AS, Skinner JS, Wilmore JH, Rao DC, Bouchard C. Familial aggregation of amount and distribution of subcutaneous fat and their responses to exercise training in the HERITAGE Family Study. Obes Res 2000; 8:140–150.
95. Ramirez ME. Familial aggregation of subcutaneous fat deposits and the peripheral fat distribution pattern. Int J Obes 1993; 17:63–68.
96. Bouchard C. Inheritance of fat distribution and adipose tissue metabolism. In: Vague J, Björntorp P, Guy-Grand B, Rebuffé-Scrive M, Pague P, eds. Metabolic Complications of Human Obesities. Amsterdam: Elsevier Science, 1985:87–96.
97. Savard R, Bouchard C, Leblanc C, Tremblay A. Familial resemblance in fatness indicators. Ann Hum Biol 1983; 10:111–118.
98. Bouchard C, Pérusse L, Leblanc C, Tremblay A, Thériault G. Inheritance of the amount and distribution of human body fat. Int J Obes 1988; 12:205–215.
99. Rice T, Després JP, Pérusse L, Gagnon J, Leon AS, Skinner JS, Wilmore JH, Rao DC, Bouchard C. Segregation analysis of abdominal visceral fat: the HERITAGE Family Study. Obes Res 1997; 5:417–424.

100. Pérusse L, Leblanc C, Bouchard C. Inter-generation transmission of physical fitness in the Canadian population. Can J Sport Sci 1988; 13:8–14.
101. Donahue RP, Prineas RJ, Gomez O, Hong CP. Familial resemblance of body fat distribution: the Minneapolis Children's Blood Pressure Study. Int J Obes 1992; 16:161–167.
102. Sellers TA, Drinkard C, Rich SS, Potter JD, Jeffery RW, Hong C-P, Folsom AR. Familial aggregation and heritability of waist-to-hip ratio in adult women: The Iowa Women's Health Study. Int J Obes 1994; 18:607–613.
103. Towne B, Roche AF, Chumlea WC, Guo S, Siervogel RM. No evidence of pleiotropy for either body mass index or waist/hip circumference ratio and plasma cholesterol concentration. Obes Res 1993; 1:1105 (abstract).
104. Esposito-Del Puente A, Scalfi L, De Filippo E, Peri MR, Caldara A, Caso G, Contaldo F, Valerio G, Franzese A, Di Maio S, Rubino A. Familial and environmental influences on body composition and body fat distribution in childhood in southern Italy. Int J Obes 1994; 18:596–601.
105. An P, Rice T, Borecki IB, Pérusse L, Gagnon J, Leon AS, Skinner JS, Wilmore JH, Bouchard C, Rao DC. Major gene effect on subcutaneous fat distribution in a sedentary population and its response to exercise training: the HERITAGE Family Study. Am J Hum Biol 2000; 12:600–609.
106. Feitosa MF, Borecki I, Hunt SC, Arnett DK, Rao DC, Province M. Inheritance of the waist-to-hip ratio in the National Heart, Lung, and Blood Institute Family Heart Study. Obes Res 2000; 8:294–301.
107. Mueller WH, Reid RM. A multivariate analysis of fatness and relative fat patterning. Am J Phys Anthrop 1979; 50:199–208.
108. Li Z, Rice T, Pérusse L, Bouchard C, Rao DC. Familial aggregation of subcutaneous fat patterning: principal components of skinfolds in the Quebec Family Study. Am J Hum Biol 1996; 8:535–542.
109. Bouchard C. Inheritance of human fat distribution. In: Bouchard C, Johnston FE, eds. Fat Distribution During Growth and Later Health Outcomes. Current Topics in Nutrition and Disease, Vol 17. New York: Alan R. Liss, 1988:103–125.
110. Bouchard C. Genetic and environmental influences on regional fat distribution. In: Oomura Y, Tarui S, Inoue S, Shimazu T, eds. Progress in Obesity Research 1990. London: Libbey, 1991:303–308.
111. Comuzzie AG, Blangero J, Mahaney MC, Mitchell BD, Stern MP, MacCluer JW. Genetic and environmental correlations among skinfold measures. Int J Obes 1994; 18:413–418.
112. Rice T, Bouchard C, Pérusse L, Rao DC. Familial clustering of multiple measures of adiposity and fat distribution in the Quebec Family Study: a trivariate analysis of percent body fat, body mass index, and trunk-to-extremity skinfold ratio. Int J Obes 1995; 19:902–908.
113. Cardon LR, Carmelli D, Fabsitz RR, Reed T. Genetic and environmental correlations between obesity and body fat distribution in adult male twins. Hum Biol 1994; 66:465–479.
114. Feitosa MF, Rice T, Nirmala-Reddy A, Reddy PC, Rao DC. Segregation analysis of regional fat distribution in families from Andhra Pradesh, India. Int J Obes 1999; 23:874–880.
115. Ginsburg E, Livshits G, Yakovenko K, Kobyliansky E. Genetics of human body size and shape: evidence for an oligogenic control of adiposity. Ann Hum Biol 1999; 26:79–87.
116. Pérusse L, Després JP, Lemieux S, Rice. T, Rao DC, Bouchard C. Familial aggregation of abdominal visceral fat level: results from the Quebec Family Study. Metabolism 1996; 45:378–382.
117. Rice T, Després JP, Daw EW, Gagnon J, Borecki IB, Pérusse L, Leon AS, Skinner JS, Wilmore JH, Rao DC, Bouchard C. Familial resemblance for abdominal visceral fat: the HERITAGE Family Study. Int J Obes 1997; 21:1024–1031.
118. Bouchard C, Rice T, Lemieux S, Després JP, Pérusse L, Rao DC. Major gene for abdominal visceral fat area in the Quebec Family Study. Int J Obes 1996; 20:420–427.
119. Rice T, Pérusse L, Bouchard C, Rao DC. Familial clustering of abdominal visceral fat and total fat mass: the Quebec Family Study. Obes Res 1996; 4: 253–261.
120. Rice T, Hong Y, Pérusse L, Després J-P, Gagnon J, Leon AS, Skinner JS, Wilmore JH, Bouchard C, Rao DC. Total body fat and abdominal visceral fat response to exercise training in the HERITAGE Family Study: evidence for major locus but no multifactorial effects. Metabolism 1999; 48:1278–1286.
121. Sørensen TIA, Stunkard AJ. Does obesity run in families because of genes? An adoption study using silhouettes as a measure of obesity. Acta Psychiatr Scand 1993; 370(suppl):67–72.
122. Borecki IB, Suarez BK. Linkage and association: basic concepts. Adv Genet 2001; 42:45–66.
123. Cardon LR, Bell JI. Association study designs for complex diseases. Nat Rev Genet 2001; 2:91–99.
124. Comuzzie AG, Williams JT, Martin LJ, Blangero J. Searching for genes underlying normal variation in human adiposity. J Mol Med 2001; 79:57–70.
125. Flint J, Mott R. Finding the molecular basis of quantitative traits: successes and pitfalls. Nat Rev Genet 2001; 2:437–445.
126. Risch NJ. Searching for genetic determinants in the new millennium. Nature 2000; 405:847–856.
127. Bouchard C, Pérusse L. Current status of the human obesity gene map. Obes Res 1996; 4:81–90.

128. Chagnon YC, Pérusse L, Bouchard C. The human obesity gene map: the 1997 update. Obes Res 1998; 6:76–92.
129. Chagnon YC, Pérusse L, Weisnagel SJ, Rankinen T, Bouchard C. The human obesity gene map: the 1999 update. Obes Res 2000; 8:89–117.
130. Pérusse L, Bouchard C. Identification of genes contributing to excess body fat and fat distribution. In: Angel A, Anderson H, Bouchard C, Lau D, Leiter L, Mendelson R, eds. Seventh International Congress on Obesity. Progress in Obesity Research. Toronto: John Libbey, 1996:281–289.
131. Pérusse L, Chagnon YC, Dionne FT, Bouchard C. The human obesity gene map: the 1996 update. Obes Res 1997; 5:49–61.
132. Pérusse L, Chagnon YC, Weisnagel J, Bouchard C. The human obesity gene map: the 1998 update. Obes Res 1999; 7:111–129.
133. Pérusse L, Chagnon YC, Weisnagel SJ, Rankinen T, Snyder E, Sands J, Bouchard C. The human obesity gene map: the 2000 update. Obes Res 2001; 9:135–169.
134. Rankinen T, Pérusse L, Weisnagel SJ, Snyder EE, Chagnon YC, Bouchard C. The human obesity gene map: the 2001 update. Obes Res. In press.
135. Pérusse L, Chagnon YC. Summary of human linkage and association studies. Behav Genet 1997; 27:359–372.
136. Clément K, Vaisse C, Manning BSJ, Basdevant A, Guy-Grand B, Ruiz J, Silver KD, Shuldiner AR, Froguel P, Strosberg AD. Genetic variation in the β_3-adrenergic receptor and an increased capacity to gain weight in patients with morbid obesity. N Engl J Med 1995; 333:352–354.
137. Festa A, Krugluger W, Shnawa N, Hopmeier P, Haffner SM. Schernthaner G. Trp64Arg polymorphism of the beta3-adrenergic receptor gene in pregnancy: association with mild gestational diabetes mellitus. J Clin Endocrinol Metab 1999; 84:1695–1699.
138. Nagase T, Aoki A, Yamamoto M, Yasuda H, Kado S, Nishikawa M, Kugai N, Akatsu T, Nagata N. Lack of association between the Trp64 Arg mutation in the beta 3-adrenergic receptor gene and obesity in Japanese men: a longitudinal analysis. J Clin Endocrinol Metab 1997; 82:1284–1287.
139. Widén E, Lehto M, Kanninen T, Walston J, Shuldiner AR, Groop LC. Association of a polymorphism in the β_3-adrenergic-receptor gene with features of the insulin resistance syndrome in Finns. N Engl J Med 1995; 333:348–351.
140. Endo K, Yanagi H, Hirano C, Hamaguchi H, Tsuchiya S, Tomura S. Association of Trp64Arg polymorphism of the beta3-adrenergic receptor gene and no association of Gln223Arg polymorphism of the leptin receptor gene in Japanese schoolchildren with obesity. Int J Obes Relat Metab Disord 2000; 24:443–449.
141. Fujisawa T, Ikegami H, Yamato E, Takekawa K, Nakagawa Y, Hamada Y, Oga T, Ueda H, Shintani M, Fukuda M, Ogihara T. Association of Trp64Arg mutation of the beta 3-adrenergic-receptor with NIDDM and body weight gain. Diabetologia 1996; 39:349–352.
142. Higashi K, Ishikawa T, Ito T, Yonemura A, Shige H, Nakamura H. Association of a genetic variation in the beta 3-adrenergic receptor gene with coronary heart disease among Japanese. Biochem Biophys Res Commun 1997; 232:728–730.
143. Hoffstedt J, Poirier O, Thorne A, Lonnqvist F, Herrmann SM, Cambien F, Arner P. Polymorphism of the human beta 3-adrenoceptor gene forms a well-conserved haplotype that is associated with moderate obesity and altered receptor function. Diabetes 1999; 48:203–205.
144. Jeyasingam CL, Bryson JM, Caterson ID, Yue DK, Donnelly R. Expression of the beta 3-adrenoceptor gene polymorphism (Trp64Arg) in obese diabetic and non-diabetic subjects. Clin Exp Pharmacol Physiol 1997; 24:733–735.
145. Kadowaki H, Yasuda K, Iwamoto K, Otabe S, Shimokawa K, Silver K, Walston J, Yoshinaga H, Kosaka K, Yamada N. A mutation in the beta 3-adrenergic receptor gene is associated with obesity and hyperinsulinemia in Japanese subjects. Biochem Biophys Res Commun 1995; 215:555–560.
146. Kim-Motoyama H, Yasuda K, Yamaguchi T, Yamada N, Katakura T, Shuldiner AR, Akanuma Y, Ohashi Y, Yazaki Y, Kadowaki T. A mutation of the beta 3-adrenergic receptor is associated with visceral obesity but decreased serum triglyceride. Diabetologia 1997; 40:469–472.
147. McFarlane-Anderson N, Bennett F, Wilks R, Howell S, Newsome C, Cruickshank K, Forrester T. The Trp64Arg mutation of the beta3-adrenergic receptor is associated with hyperglycemia and current body mass index in Jamaican women. Metabolism 1998; 47:617–621.
148. Mitchell BD, Blangero J, Comuzzie AG, Almasy LA, Shuldiner AR, Silver K, Stern MP, MacCluer JW, Hixson JE. A paired sibling analysis of the beta-3 adrenergic receptor and obesity in Mexican Americans. J Clin Invest 1998; 101:584–587.
149. Oksanen L, Mustajoki P, Kaprio J, Kainulainen K, Jänne O, Peltonen L, Kontula K. Polymorphism of the beta 3-adrenergic receptor gene in morbid obesity. Int J Obes Relat Metab Disord 1996; 20:1055–1061.
150. Ongphiphadhanakul B, Rajatanavin R, Chanprasertyothin S, Piaseu N, Chailurkit L, Komindr S, Bunnag P, Puavilai G. Relation of beta3-adrenergic receptor gene mutation to total body fat but not percent body fat and insulin levels in Thais. Metabolism 1999; 48:564–567.
151. Sakane N, Yoshida T, Umekawa T, Kondo M, Sakai Y, Takahashi T. Beta 3-adrenergic-receptor poly-

morphism: a genetic marker for visceral fat obesity and the insulin resistance syndrome. Diabetologia 1997; 40:200–204.

152. Shima Y, Tsukada T, Nakanishi K, Ohta H. Association of the Trp64Arg mutation of the beta3-adrenergic receptor with fatty liver and mild glucose intolerance in Japanese subjects. Clin Chim Acta 1998; 274:167–176.
153. Thomas GN, Tomlinson B, Chan JC, Young RP, Critchley JA. The Trp64Arg polymorphism of the beta3-adrenergic receptor gene and obesity in Chinese subjects with components of the metabolic syndrome. Int J Obes Relat Metab Disord 2000; 24:545–551.
154. Ukkola O, Rankinen T, Weisnagel SJ, Sun G, Perusse L, Chagnon YC, Despres JP, Bouchard C. Interactions among the alpha2-, beta2-, and beta3-adrenergic receptor genes and obesity-related phenotypes in the Quebec Family Study. Metabolism 2000; 49: 1063–1070.
155. Urhammer SA, Clausen JO, Hansen T, Pedersen O. Insulin sensitivity and body weight changes in young white carriers of the codon 64 amino acid polymorphism of the beta3-adrenergic receptor gene. Diabetes 1996; 45:1115–1120.
156. Strazzullo P, Iacone R, Siani A, Cappuccio F, Russo O, Barba G, Barbato A, D'Elia L, Trevisan M, Farinaro E. Relationship of the Trp64Arg polymorphism of the beta3-adrenoceptor gene to central adiposity and high blood pressure: interaction with age. Cross-sectional and longitudinal findings of the Olivetti Prospective Heart Study. J Hypertens 2001; 19:399–406.
157. Chagnon YC, Pérusse L, Bouchard C. Familial aggregation of obesity, candidate genes and quantitative trait loci. Curr Opin Lipidol 1997; 8:205–211.
158. Mauriège P, Bouchard C. Trp64Arg mutation in beta 3-adrenoceptor gene of doubtful significance for obesity and insulin resistance. Lancet 1996; 348: 698–699.
159. Allison DB, Heo M, Faith MS, Pietrobelli A. Meta-analysis of the association of the Trp64Arg polymorphism in the beta3 adrenergic receptor with body mass index. Int J Obes 1998; 22:559–566.
160. Fujisawa T, Ikegami H, Kawaguchi Y, Ogihara T. Meta-analysis of the association of Trp64Arg polymorphism of beta 3-adrenergic receptor gene with body mass index. J Clin Endocrinol Metab 1998; 83: 2441–2444.
161. Kurokawa N, Nakai K, Kameo S, Liu ZM, Satoh H. Association of BMI with the beta3-adrenergic receptor gene polymorphism in Japanese: meta-analysis. Obes Res 2001; 12:741–745.
162. Lynch M, Walsh B. Genetics and Analysis of Quantitative Traits. Sunderland, MA: Sinauer Associate, 1998.
163. Darvasi A. Experimental strategies for the genetic dissection of complex traits in animal models. Nat Genet 1998; 18:19–24.
164. Frankel WN. Taking stock of complex trait genetics in mice. Trends Genet 1995; 11:471–477.
165. Norman RA, Thompson DB, Foroud T, Garvey WT, Bennett PH, Bogardus C, Ravussin E. Genome-wide search for genes influencing percent body fat in Pima Indians: suggestive linkage at chromosome 11q21-q22. Am J Hum Genet 1997; 60:166–173.
166. Norman RA, Tataranni PA, Pratley R, Thompson DB, Hanson RL, Prochazka M, Baier L, Ehm MG, Sakul H, Foroud T, Garvey WT, Burns D, Knowler WC, Bennett PH, Bogardus C, Ravussin E. Autosomal genomic scan for loci linked to obesity and energy metabolism in Pima Indians. Am J Hum Genet 1998; 62:659–668.
167. Hanson RL, Ehm MG, Pettitt DJ, Prochazka M, Thompson DB, Timberlake D, Foroud T, Kobes S, Baier L, Burns DK, Almasy L, Blangero J, Garvey WT, Bennett PH, Knowler WC. An autosomal genomic scan for loci linked to type II diabetes mellitus and body-mass index in Pima Indians. Am J Hum Genet 1998; 63: 1130–1138.
168. Walder K, Hanson RL, Kobes S, Knowler WC, Ravussin E. An autosomal genomic scan for loci linked to plasma leptin concentration in Pima Indians. Int J Obes Relat Metab Disord 2000; 24:559–565.
169. Comuzzie AG, Hixson JE, Almasy L, Mitchell BD, Mahaney MC, Dyer TD, Stern MP, MacCluer JW, Blangero J. A major quantitative trait locus determining serum leptin levels and fat mass is located on human chromosome 2. Nat Genet 1997; 15: 273–276.
170. Hixson JE, Almasy L, Cole S, Birnbaum S, Mitchell BD, Mahaney MC, Stern MP, MacCluer JW, Blangero J, Comuzzie AG. Normal variation in leptin levels is associated with polymorphisms in the proopiomelanocortin gene, POMC. J Clin Endocrinol Metab 1999; 84:3187–3191.
171. Mitchell BD, Cole SA, Comuzzie AG, Almasy L, Blangero J, MacCluer JW, Hixson JE. A quantitative trait locus influencing BMI maps to the region of the beta-3 adrenergic receptor. Diabetes 1999; 48:1863–1867.
172. Rotimi CN, Comuzzie AG, Lowe WL, Luke A, Blangero J, Cooper RS. The quantitative trait locus on chromosome 2 for serum leptin levels is confirmed in African-Americans. Diabetes 1999; 48:643–644.
173. Hager J, Dina C, Francke S, Dubois S, Houari M, Vatin V, Vaillant E, Lorentz N, Basdevant A, Clément K, Guy-Grand B, Froguel P. A genome-wide scan for human obesity genes reveals a major susceptibility locus on chromosome 10. Nat Genet 1998; 20:304–308.
174. Hinney A, Ziegler A, Oeffner F, Wedewardt C, Vogel M, Wulftange H, Geller F, Stubing K, Siegfried W,

Goldschmidt HP, Remschmidt H, Hebebrand J. Independent confirmation of a major locus for obesity on chromosome 10. J Clin Endocrinol Metab 2000; 85: 2962–2965.

175. Price RA, Li WD, Bernstein A, Crystal A, Golding EM, Weisberg SJ, Zuckerman WA. A locus affecting obesity in human chromosome region 10p12. Diabetologia 2001; 44:363–366.
176. Lee JH, Reed DR, Li WD, Xu W, Joo EJ, Kilker RL, Nanthakumar E, North M, Sakul H, Bell C, Price RA. Genome scan for human obesity and linkage to markers in 20q13. Am J Hum Genet 1999; 64: 196–209.
177. Chagnon YC, Borecki IB, Perusse L, Roy S, Lacaille M, Chagnon M, Ho-Kim MA, Rice T, Province MA, Rao DC, Bouchard C. Genome-wide search for genes related to the fat-free body mass in the Quebec Family Study. Metabolism 2000; 49:203–207.
178. Pérusse L, Rice T, Chagnon YC, Després JP, Lemieux S, Roy S, Lacaille M, Ho-Kim MA, Chagnon M, Province MA, Rao DC, Bouchard C. A genome-wide scan for abdominal fat assessed by computed tomography in the Quebec Family Study. Diabetes 2001; 50: 614–621.
179. Ohman M, Oksanen L, Kaprio J, Koskenvuo M, Mustajoki P, Rissanen A, Salmi J, Kontula K, Peltonen L. Genome-wide scan of obesity in Finnish sibpairs reveals linkage to chromosome Xq24. J Clin Endocrinol Metab 2000; 85:3183–3190.
180. Kissebah AH, Sonnenberg GE, Myklebust J, Goldstein M, Broman K, James RG, Marks JA, Krakower GR, Jacob HJ, Weber A, Martin L, Blangero J, Comuzzie AG. Quantitative trait loci on chromosomes 3 and 17 influence phenotypes of the metabolic syndrome. Proc Natl Acad Sci USA 2000; 97:14478–14483.
181. Chagnon YC, Rice T, Perusse L, Borecki IB, Ho-Kim MA, Lacaille M, Pare C, Bouchard L, Gagnon J, Leon AS, Skinner JS, Wilmore JH, Rao DC, Bouchard C. Genomic scan for genes affecting body composition before and after training in Caucasians from HERITAGE. J Appl Physiol 2001; 90:1777–1787.
182. Rice T, Chagnon YC, Pérusse L, Borecki IB, Ukkola O, Rankinen T, Gagnon J, Leon AS, Skinner JS, Wilmore JH, Bouchard C, Rao DC. A genomewide linkage scan for abdominal subcutaneous and visceral fat in Black and White Families: the HERITAGE Family Study. Diabetes 2002; 51:848–855.
183. Hsueh WC, Mitchell BD, Schneider JL, St Jean PL, Pollin TI, Ehm MG, Wagner MJ, Burns DK, Sakul H, Bell CJ, Shuldiner AR. Genome-wide scan of obesity in the Old Order Amish. J Clin Endocrinol Metab 2001; 86:1199–1205.
184. Beynen AC, Katan MB, Van Zutphen LF. Hypo- and hyperresponders: individual differences in the response of serum cholesterol concentration to changes in diet. Adv Lipid Res 1987; 22:115–171.
185. Sims EA, Goldman RF, Gluck CM, Horton ES, Kelleher PC, Rowe DW. Experimental obesity in man. Trans Assoc Am Phys 1968; 81:153–170.
186. Ottman R. An epidemiologic approach to gene-environment interaction. Genet Epidemiol 1990; 7: 177–185.
187. Ottman R. Epidemiologic analysis of gene-environment interaction in twins. Genet Epidemiol 1994; 11: 75–86.
188. Khoury MJ, Wagener DK. Epidemiological evaluation of the use of genetics to improve the predictive value of disease risk factors. Am J Hum Genet 1995; 56:835–844.
189. Ottman R, Susser E, Meisner M. Control for environmental risk factors in assessing genetic effects on disease familial aggregation. Am J Epidemiol 1991; 134:298–309.
190. Blangero J. Statistical genetic approaches to human adaptability. Hum Biol 1993; 65:941–966.
191. Eaves LJ. The resolution of genotype × environment interaction in segregation analysis of nuclear families. Genet Epidemiol 1984; 1:215–228.
192. Eaves LJ. Including the environment in models for genetic segregation. J Psychiatr Res 1987; 21:639–647.
193. Plomin R, DeFries JC, Loehlin JC. Genotype-environment interaction and correlation in the analysis of human behavior. Psychol Bull 1977; 84:309–322.
194. Tiret L, Abel L, Rakotovao R. Effect of ignoring genotype-environment interaction on segregation analysis of quantitative traits. Genet Epidemiol 1993; 10:581–586.
195. Bouchard C, Pérusse L, Leblanc C. Using MZ twins in experimental research to test for the presence of genotype-environment interaction effect. Acta Genet Med Gemellol 1990; 39:85–89.
196. Hallman DM, Boerwinkle E, Saha N, Sandholzer C, Menzel HJ, Csazar A, Utermann G. The apolipoprotein E polymorphism: a comparison of allele frequencies and effects in nine populations. Am J Hum Genet 1991; 49:338–349.
197. Zee RYL, Griffiths LR, Morris BJ. Marked association of a RFLP for the low density lipoprotein receptor gene with obesity in essential hypertensives. Biochem Biophys Res Commun 1992; 189: 965–971.
198. Berg K. Twin studies of coronary heart disease and its risk factors. Acta Genet Med Gemellol 1984; 33: 349–361.
199. Berg K, Borresen AL, Nance WE. Apparent influence of marker genotypes on variation in serum cholesterol in monozygotic twins. Clin Genet 1981; 19:67–70.
200. Poehlman ET, Tremblay A, Després JP, Fontaine E, Perusse L, Theriault G, Bouchard C. Genotype-controlled changes in body composition and fat morphology following overfeeding in twins. Am J Clin Nutr 1986; 43:723–731.

201. Bouchard C, Tremblay A, Després JP, Nadeau A, Lupien PJ, Theriault G, Dussault J, Moorjani S, Pinault S, Fournier G. The response to long-term overfeeding in identical twins. N Engl J Med 1990; 322:1477–1482.
202. Poehlman ET, Tremblay A, Nadeau A, Dussault J, Thériault G, Bouchard C. Heredity and changes in hormones and metabolic rates with short-term training. Am J Physiol 1986; 250:E711–E717.
203. Poehlman ET, Tremblay A, Marcotte M, Pérusse L, Thériault G, Bouchard C. Heredity and changes in body composition and adipose tissue metabolism after short-term exercise training. Eur J Appl Physiol 1987; 56:398–402.
204. Bouchard C, Tremblay A, Després JP, Thériault G, Nadeau A, Lupien PJ, Moorjani S, Prudhomme D, Fournier G. The response to exercise with constant energy intake in identical twins. Obes Res 1994; 2: 400–410.
205. Dériaz O, Tremblay A, Bouchard C. Nonlinear weight gain with long term overfeeding in man. Obes Res 1993; 1:179–185.
206. Norgan NG, Durnin JVGA. The effect of 6 weeks of overfeeding on the body weight, body composition, and energy metabolism of young men. Am J Clin Nutr 1980; 33:978–988.
207. Ravussin E, Schutz Y, Acheson KJ, Dusmet M, Bourquin L, Jéquier E. Short-term, mixed-diet overfeeding in man: no evidence for "Luxuskonsumption." Am J Physiol 1985; 249:E470–E477.
208. Tremblay A, Després JP, Thériault G, Fournier G, Bouchard C. Overfeeding and energy expenditure in humans. Am J Clin Nutr 1992; 56:857–862.
209. Dériaz O, Fournier G, Tremblay A, Després JP, Bouchard C. Lean-body-mass composition and resting energy expenditure before and after long-term overfeeding. Am J Clin Nutr 1992: 56:840–847.
210. Levine JA, Eberhardt NL, Jensen MD. Role of nonexercise activity thermogenesis in resistance to fat gain in humans. Science 1999; 283:212–214.
211. Ukkola O, Tremblay A, Sun G, Chagnon YC, Bouchard C. Genetic variation at the uncoupling protein 1, 2 and 3 loci and the response to long-term overfeeding. Eur J Clin Nutr. 2001; 55:1008–1015.
212. Ukkola O, Tremblay A, Despres JP, Chagnon YC, Campfield LA, Bouchard C. Leptin receptor Gln223Arg variant is associated with a cluster of metabolic abnormalities in response to long-term overfeeding. J Intern Med 2000; 248:435–439.
213. Ukkola O, Tremblay A, Bouchard C. Beta-2 adrenergic receptor variants are associated with subcutaneous fat accumulation in response to long-term overfeeding. Int J Obes Relat Metab Disord 2001; 25:1604–1608.
214. Ukkola O, Sun G, Bouchard C. Insulin-like growth factor 2 (IGF2) and IGF-binding protein 1 (IGFBP1) gene variants are associated with overfeeding-induced metabolic changes. Diabetologia 2001; 44:2231–2236.
215. Dizier MH, Bonaïti-Pellié C, Clerget-Darpoux F. Conclusions of segregation analysis for family data generated under two-locus models. Am J Hum Genet 1993; 53:1338–1346.
216. Cardon LR, Fulker DW. The power of interval mapping of quantitative trait loci, using selected sib pairs. Am J Hum Genet 1994; 55:825–833.
217. Almasy L, Blangero J. Multipoint quantitative-trait linkage analysis in general pedigrees. Am J Hum Genet 1998; 62:1198–1211.
218. Province MA, Rice T, Borecki IB, Gu C, Rao DC. A multivariate and multilocus variance components approach using structural relationships to assess quantitative linkage via SEGPATH. Genet Epidemiol 2003; 24(2):128–138.
219. Bouchard C. Genetics of human obesities: introductory notes. In: Bouchard C, ed. The Genetics of Obesity. Boca Raton, FL: CRC Press, 1994:1–15.
220. Colilla S, Rotimi C, Cooper R, Goldberg J, Cox N. Genetic inheritance of body mass index in African-American and African families. Genet Epidemiol 2000; 18:360–376.
221. Lecomte E, Herbeth B, Nicaud V, Rakotovao R, Artur Y, Tiret L. Segregation analysis of fat mass and fat-free mass with age- and sex-dependent effects: The Stanislas Family Study. Genet Epidemiol 1997; 14: 51–62.
222. Paganini-Hill A, Martin AO, Spence MA. The S-leut anthropometric traits: Genetic analysis. Am J Phys Anthrop 1981; 55:55–67.
223. Benjafield AV, Wang XL, Morris BJ. Tumor necrosis factor receptor 2 gene (TNFRSF1B) in genetic basis of coronary artery disease. J Mol Med 2001; 79: 109–115.
224. Fernandez-Real JM, Gutierrez C, Ricart W, Casamitjana R, Fernandez-Castaner M, Vendrell J, Richart C, Soler J. The TNF-alpha gene Nco I polymorphism influences the relationship among insulin resistance, percent body fat, and increased serum leptin levels. Diabetes 1997; 46:1468–1472.
225. Chagnon YC, Chung WK, Pérusse L, Chagnon M, Leibel RL, Bouchard C. Linkages and associations between the leptin receptor (LEPR) gene and human body composition in the Quebec Family Study. Int J Obes Relat Metab Disord 1999; 23:278–286.
226. Chagnon YC, Wilmore JH, Borecki IB, Gagnon J, Perusse L, Chagnon M, Collier GR, Leon AS, Skinner JS, Rao DC, Bouchard C. Associations between the leptin receptor gene and adiposity in middle-aged Caucasian males from the HERITAGE family study. J Clin Endocrinol Metab 2000; 85:29–34.
227. Mammes O, Aubert R, Betoulle D, Pean F, Herbeth B, Visvikis S, Siest G, Fumeron F. LEPR gene polymorphisms: associations with overweight, fat

mass and response to diet in women. Eur J Clin Invest 2001; 31:398–404.
228. Rosmond R, Chagnon YC, Holm G, Chagnon M, Perusse L, Lindell K, Carlsson B, Bouchard C, Bjorntorp P. Hypertension in obesity and the leptin receptor gene locus. J Clin Endocrinol Metab 2000; 85:3126–3131.
229. Roth H, Korn T, Rosenkranz K, Hinney A, Ziegler A, Kunz J, Siegfried W, Mayer H, Hebebrand J, Grzeschik K. Transmission disequilibrium and sequence variants at the leptin receptor gene in extremely obese German children and adolescents. Hum Genet 1998; 103:540–546.
230. Thompson DB, Ravussin E, Bennett PH, Bogardus C. Structure and sequence variation at the human leptin receptor gene in lean and obese Pima Indians. Hum Mol Genet 1997; 6:675–679.
231. Wauters M, Mertens I, Chagnon M, Rankinen T, Considine RV, Chagnon YC, Van Gaal LF, Bouchard C. Polymorphisms in the leptin receptor gene, body composition and fat distribution in overweight and obese women. Int J Obes Relat Metab Disord 2001; 25:714–720.
232. Vohl MC, Dionne FT, Pérussc L, Dériaz O, Chagnon M, Bouchard C. Relation between BglII polymorphism in 3β-hydroxysteroid dehydrogenase gene and adipose tissue distribution in humans. Obes Res 1994; 2:444–449.
233. Hegele RA, Anderson CM, Wang J, Jones DC, Cao H. Association between nuclear lamin A/C R482Q mutation and partial lipodystrophy with hyperinsulinemia, dyslipidemia, hypertension, and diabetes. Genome Res 2000; 10:652–658.
234. Hegele RA, Cao H, Harris SB, Zinman B, Hanley AJ, Anderson CM. Genetic variation in LMNA modulates plasma leptin and indices of obesity in aboriginal Canadians. Physiol Genomics 2000; 3:39–44.
235. Hegele RA, Cao H, Huff MW, Anderson CM. LMNA R482Q mutation in partial lipodystrophy associated with reduced plasma leptin concentration. J Clin Endocrinol Metab 2000c; 85:3089–3093.
236. Dériaz O, Dionne F, Pérusse L, Tremblay A, Vohl MC, Cote G, Bouchard C. DNA variation in the genes of the Na,K-adenosine triphosphatase and its relation with resting metabolic rate, respiratory quotient, and body fat. J Clin Invest 1994; 93:838–843.
237. Katzmarzyk PT, Rankinen T, Pérusse L, Deriaz O, Tremblay A, Borecki I, Rao DC, Bouchard C. Linkage and association of the sodium potassium-adenosine triphosphatase alpha2 and beta1 genes with respiratory quotient and resting metabolic rate in the Quebec Family Study. J Clin Endocrinol Metab 1999; 84:2093–2097.
238. Hegele RA, Brunt JH, Connelly PW. Genetic variation on chromosome 1 associated with variation in body fat distribution in men. Circulation 1995; 92: 1089–1093.
239. Rankinen T, Gagnon J, Pérusse L, Rice T, Leon AS, Skinner JS, Wilmore JH, Rao DC, Bouchard C. Body fat, resting and exercise blood pressure and the angiotensinogen M235T polymorphism: the HERITAGE family study. Obes Res 1999; 7:423–430.
240. Lucarini N, Finocchi G, Gloria-Bottini F, Macioce M, Borgiani P, Amante A, Bottini E. A possible genetic component of obesity in childhood. Observations on acid phosphatase polymorphism. Experientia 1990; 46:90–91.
241. Lucarini N, Antonacci E, Bottini N, Gloria-Bottini F. Low-molecular-weight acid phosphatase (ACP1), obesity, and blood lipid levels in subjects with non-insulin-dependent diabetes mellitus. Hum Biol 1997; 69: 509–515.
242. Rajput-Williams J, Knott TJ, Wallis SC, Sweetnam P, Yarnell J, Cox N, Bell GI, Miller NE, Scott J. Variation of apolipoprotein-B gene is associated with obesity, high blood cholesterol levels, and increased risk of coronary heart disease. Lancet 1988; 2: 1442–1446.
243. Saha N, Tay JSH, Heng CK, Humphries SE. DNA polymorphisms of the apolipoprotein B gene are associated with obesity and serum lipids in healthy Indians in Singapore. Clin Genet 1993; 44:113–120.
244. Miraglia del Guidice E, Cirillo G, Santoro N, D'Urso L, Carbone MT, Di Toro R, Perrone L. Molecular screening of the proopiomelanocortin (POMC) gene in Italian obese children: report of three new mutations. Int J Obes Relat Metab Disord 2001; 25:61–67.
245. Heinonen P, Koulu M, Pesonen U, Karvonen MK, Rissanen A, Laakso M, Valve R, Uusitupa M, Scheinin M. Identification of a three-amino acid deletion in the alpha2B-adrenergic receptor that is associated with reduced basal metabolic rate in obese subjects. J Clin Endocrinol Metab 1999; 84:2429–2433.
246. Celi FS, Negri C, Tanner K, Raben N, De Pablo F, Rovira A, Pallardo LF, Martin-Vaquero P, Stern MP, Mitchell BD, Shuldiner AR. Molecular scanning for mutations in the insulin receptor substrate-1 (IRS-1) gene in Mexican Americans with type 2 diabetes mellitus. Diabetes Metab Res Rev 2000; 16:370–377.
247. Krempler F, Hell E, Winkler C, Breban D, Patsch W. Plasma leptin levels: interaction of obesity with a common variant of insulin receptor substrate-1. Arterioscler Thromb Vasc Biol 1998; 18:1686–1690.
248. Lei HH, Coresh J, Shuldiner AR, Boerwinkle E, Brancati FL. Variants of the insulin receptor substrate-1 and fatty acid binding protein 2 genes and the risk of type 2 diabetes, obesity, and hyperinsulinemia in African-Americans: the Atherosclerosis Risk in Communities Study. Diabetes 1999; 48:1868–1872.
249. Cole SA, Mitchell BD, Hsueh WC, Pineda P, Beamer BA, Shuldiner AR, Comuzzie AG, Blangero J, Hixson JE. The Pro12Ala variant of peroxisome proliferator-activated receptor-gamma2

(PPAR-gamma2) is associated with measures of obesity in Mexican Americans. Int J Obes Relat Metab Disord 2000; 24:522–524.
250. Deeb SS, Fajas L, Nemoto M, Pihlajamaki J, Mykkanen L, Kuusisto J, Laakso M, Fujimoto W, Auwerx J. A Pro12Ala substitution in PPARgamma2 associated with decreased receptor activity, lower body mass index and improved insulin sensitivity. Nat Genet 1998; 20:284–287.
251. Ek J, Urhammer SA, Sorensen TI, Andersen T, Auwerx J, Pedersen O. Homozygosity of the Pro12Ala variant of the peroxisome proliferation-activated receptor-gamma2 (PPAR-gamma2): divergent modulating effects on body mass index in obese and lean Caucasian men. Diabetologia 1999; 42:892–895.
252. Hsueh WC, Cole SA, Shuldiner AR, Beamer BA, Blangero J, Hixson JE, MacCluer JW, Mitchell BD. Interactions between variants in the beta 3-adrenergic receptor and peroxisome proliferator-activated receptor-gamma 2 genes and obesity. Diabetes Care 2001; 24:672–677.
253. Lei HH, Chen MH, Yang WS, Chiu MC, Chen MC, Tai TY, Chuang LM. Peroxisome proliferator-activated receptor gamma 2 Pro12Ala gene variant is strongly associated with larger body mass in the Taiwanese. Metabolism 2000; 49:1267–1270.
254. Meirhaeghe A, Fajas L, Helbecque N, Cottel D, Auwerx J, Deeb SS, Amouyel P. Impact of the peroxisome proliferator activated receptor gamma2 Pro12Ala polymorphism on adiposity, lipids and non-insulin-dependent diabetes mellitus. Int J Obes Relat Metab Disord 2000; 24:195–199.
255. Meirhaeghe A, Fajas L, Helbecque N, Cottel D, Lebel P, Dallongeville J, Deeb S, Auwerx J, Amouyel P. A genetic polymorphism of the peroxisome proliferator-activated receptor gamma gene influences plasma leptin levels in obese humans. Hum Mol Genet 1998; 7:435–440.
256. Ristow M, Müller-Wieland D, Pfeiffer A, Krone W, Kahn CR. Obesity associated with a mutation in a genetic regulator of adipocyte differentiation. N Engl J Med 1998; 339:953–959.
257. Vaccaro O, Mancini FP, Ruffa G, Sabatino L, Colantuoni V, Riccardi G. Pro12Ala mutation in the peroxisome proliferator-activated receptor gamma2 (PPARgamma2) and severe obesity: a case-control study. Int J Obes Relat Metab Disord 2000; 24:1195–1199.
258. Valve R, Sivenius K, Miettinen R, Pihlajamaki J, Rissanen A, Deeb SS, Auwerx J, Uusitupa M, Laakso M. Two polymorphisms in the peroxisome proliferator-activated receptor-gamma gene are associated with severe overweight among obese women. J Clin Endocrinol Metab 1999; 84:3708–3712.
259. Vijayaraghavan S, Hitman GA, Kopelman PG. Apolipoprotein-D polymorphism: a genetic marker for obesity and hyperinsulinemia. J Clin Endocrinol Metab 1994; 79:568–570.
260. Funakoshi A, Miyasaka K, Matsumoto H, Yamamori S, Takiguchi S, Kataoka K, Takata Y, Matsusue K, Kono A, Shimokata H. Gene structure of human cholecystokinin (CCK) type-A receptor: body fat content is related to CCK type-A receptor gene promoter polymorphism. FEBS Lett 2000; 466: 264–266.
261. Hegele RA, Harris SB, Hanley AJG, Sadikian S, Connelly PW, Zinman B. Genetic variation of intestinal fatty acid-binding protein associated with variation in body mass in Aboriginal Canadians. J Clin Endocrinol Metab 1996; 81:4334–4337.
262. Kim CH, Yun SK, Byun DW, Yoo MK, Lee KU, Suh KI. Codon 54 polymorphism of the fatty acid binding protein 2 gene is associated with increased fat oxidation and hyperinsulinemia, but not with intestinal fatty acid absorption in Korean men. Metabolism 2001; 50:473–476.
263. Yamada K, Yuan X, Ishiyama S, Koyama K, Ichikawa F, Koyanagi A, Koyama W, Nonaka K. Association between Ala54Thr substitution of the fatty acid-binding protein 2 gene with insulin resistance and intra-abdominal fat thickness in Japanese men. Diabetologia 1997; 40:706–710.
264. Fumeron F, Durack-Bown I, Betoulle D, Cassard-Doulcier AM, Tuzet S, Bouillaud F, Melchior JC, Ricquier D, Apfelbaum M. Polymorphisms of uncoupling protein (UCP) and beta 3 adrenoreceptor genes in obese people submitted to a low calorie diet. Int J Obes Relat Metab Discord 1996; 20:1051–1054.
265. Heilbronn LK, Kind KL, Pancewicz E, Morris AM, Noakes M, Clifton PM. Association of −3826 G variant in uncoupling protein-1 with increased BMI in overweight Australian women. Diabetologia 2000; 43: 242–244.
266. Kogure A, Yoshida T, Sakane N, Umekawa T, Takakura Y, Kondo M. Synergic effect of polymorphisms in uncoupling protein 1 and beta 3-adrenergic receptor genes on weight loss in obese Japanese. Diabetologia 1998; 41:1399.
267. Jenkinson CP, Cray K, Walder K, Herzog H, Hanson R, Ravussin E. Novel polymorphisms in the neuropeptide-Y Y5 receptor associated with obesity in Pima Indians. Int J Obes Relat Metab Disord 2000; 24:580–584.
268. Challis BG, Yeo GS, Farooqi IS, Luan J, Aminian S, Halsall DJ, Keogh JM, Wareham NJ, O'Rahilly S. The CART gene and human obesity: mutational analysis and population genetics. Diabetes 2000; 49: 872–875.
269. Buemann B, Vohl MC, Chagnon M, Chagnon YC, Gagnon J, Pérusse L, Dionne FT, Despres JP, Tremblay A, Nadeau A, Bouchard C. Abdominal visceral fat is associated with a BclI restriction

fragment length polymorphism at the glucocorticoid receptor gene locus. Obes Res 1997; 5:186–192.
270. Dobson MG, Redfern CP, Unwin N, Weaver JU. The N363S polymorphism of the glucocorticoid receptor: potential contribution to central obesity in men and lack of association with other risk factors for coronary heart disease and diabetes mellitus. J Clin Endocrinol Metab 2001; 86:2270–2274.
271. Rosmond R, Chagnon YC, Holm G, Chagnon M, Perusse L, Lindell K, Carlsson B, Bouchard C, Bjorntorp P. A glucocorticoid receptor gene marker is associated with abdominal obesity, leptin, and dysregulation of the hypothalamic-pituitary-adrenal axis. Obes Res 2000; 8:211–218.
272. Bengtsson K, Orho-Melander M, Melander O, Lindblad U, Ranstam J, Rastam L, Groop L. beta2-adrenergic receptor gene variation and hypertension in subjects with type 2 diabetes. Hypertension 2001; 37: 1303–1308.
273. Ehrenborg E, Skogsberg J, Ruotolo G, Large V, Eriksson P, Arner P, Hamsten A. The Q/E27 polymorphism in the beta2-adrenoceptor gene is associated with increased body weight and dyslipoproteinaemia involving triglyceride-rich lipoproteins. J Intern Med 2000; 247:651–656.
274. Ishiyama-Shigemoto S, Yamada K, Yuan X, Ichikawa F, Nonaka K. Association of polymorphisms in the beta 2-adrenergic receptor gene with obesity, hypertriglyceridaemia, and diabetes mellitus. Diabetologia 1999; 42:98–101.
275. Large V, Hellstrom L, Reynisdottir S, Lonnqvist F, Eriksson P, Lannfelt L, Arner P. Human beta-2 adrenoceptor gene polymorphisms are highly frequent in obesity and associate with altered adipocyte beta-2 adrenoceptor function. J Clin Invest 1997; 100:3005–3013.
276. Meirhaeghe A, Helbecque N, Cottel D, Amouyel P. Beta2-adrenoceptor gene polymorphism, body weight, and physical activity. Lancet 1999; 353:896.
277. Mori Y, Kim-Motoyama H, Ito Y, Katakura T, Yasuda K, Ishiyama-Shigemoto S, Yamada K, Akanuma Y, Ohashi Y, Kimura S, Yazaki Y, Kadowaki T. The Gln27Glu beta2-adrenergic receptor variant is associated with obesity due to subcutaneous fat accumulation in Japanese men. Biochem Biophys Res Commun 1999; 258:138–140.
278. Rosmond R, Ukkola O, Chagnon M, Bouchard C, Bjorntorp P. Polymorphisms of the beta2-adrenergic receptor gene (ADRB2) in relation to cardiovascular risk factors in men. J Intern Med 2000; 248: 239–244.
279. Yamada K, Ishiyama-Shigemoto S, Ichikawa F, Yuan X, Koyanagi A, Koyama W, Nonaka K. Polymorphism in the 5′-leader cistron of the beta2-adrenergic receptor gene associated with obesity and type 2 diabetes. J Clin Endocrinol Metab 1999; 84:1754–1757.
280. Herrmann SM, Ricard S, Nicaud V, Mallet C, Arveiler D, Evans A, Ruidavets JB, Luc G, Bara L, Parra HJ, Poirier O, Cambien F. Polymorphisms of the tumour necrosis factor-alpha gene, coronary heart disease and obesity. Eur J Clin Invest 1998; 28:59–66.
281. Hoffstedt J, Eriksson P, Hellstrom L, Rossner S, Ryden M, Arner P. Excessive fat accumulation is associated with the TNF alpha-308 G/A promoter polymorphism in women but not in men. Diabetologia 2000; 43:117–120.
282. Kamizono S, Yamada K, Seki N, Higuchi T, Kimura A, Nonaka K, Itoh K. Susceptible locus for obese type 2 diabetes mellitus in the 5′-flanking region of the tumor necrosis factor-alpha gene. Tissue Antigens 2000; 55:449–452.
283. Norman RA, Bogardus C, Ravussin E. Linkage between obesity and a marker near the tumor necrosis factor-α locus in Pima Indians. J Clin Invest 1995, 96:158–162.
284. Pausova Z, Deslauriers B, Gaudet D, Tremblay J, Kotchen TA, Larochelle P, Cowley AW, Hamet P. Role of tumor necrosis factor-alpha gene locus in obesity and obesity-associated hypertension in French Canadians. Hypertension 2000; 36:14–19.
285. Speer G, Cseh K, Winkler G, Vargha P, Braun E, Takacs I, Lakatos P. Vitamin D and estrogen receptor gene polymorphisms in type 2 diabetes mellitus and in android type obesity. Eur J Endocrinol 2001; 144:385–389.
286. Hattersley AT, Beards F, Ballantyne E, Appleton M, Harvey R, Ellard S. Mutations in the glucokinase gene of the fetus result in reduced birth weight. Nat Genet 1998; 19:268–270.
287. Bray MS, Boerwinkle E, Hanis CL. Sequence variation within the neuropeptide Y gene and obesity in Mexican Americans. Obes Res 2000; 8:219–226.
288. Karvonen MK, Koulu M, Pesonen U, Uusitupa MI, Tammi A, Viikari J, Simell O, Ronnemaa T. Leucine 7 to proline 7 polymorphism in the preproneuropeptide Y is associated with birth weight and serum triglyceride concentration in preschool aged children. J Clin Endocrinol Metab 2000; 85:1455–1460.
289. Busch CP, Ramdath DD, Ramsewak S, Hegele RA. Association of PON2 variation with birth weight in Trinidadian neonates of South Asian ancestry. Pharmacogenetics 1999; 9:351–356.
290. Butler MG, Hedges L, Hovis CL, Feurer ID. Genetic variants of the human obesity (OB) gene in subjects with and without Prader-Willi syndrome: comparison with body mass index and weight. Clin Genet 1998; 54:385–393.
291. Hager J, Clement K, Francke S, Dina C, Raison J, Lahlou N, Rich N, Pelloux V, Basdevant A, Guy-Grand B, North M, Froguel P. A polymorphism in the 5′ untranslated region of the human ob gene is associated with low leptin levels. Int J Obes Relat Metab Disord 1998; 22:200–205.

292. Le Stunff C, Le Bihan C, Schork NJ, Bougneres P. A common promoter variant of the leptin gene is associated with changes in the relationship between serum leptin and fat mass in obese girls. Diabetes 2000; 49:2196–2200.
293. Li WD, Reed DR, Lee JH, Xu W, Kilker RL, Sodam BR, Price RA. Sequence variants in the 5′ flanking region of the leptin gene are associated with obesity in women. Ann Hum Genet 1999; 63:227–234.
294. Mammes O, Betoulle D, Aubert R, Giraud V, Tuzet S, Petiet A, Colas-Linhart N, Fumeron F. Novel polymorphisms in the 5′ region of the LEP gene: Association with leptin levels and response to low-calorie diet in human obesity. Diabetes 1998; 47:487–489.
295. Mammes O, Betoulle D, Aubert R, Herbeth B, Siest G, Fumeron F. Association of the G-2548A polymorphism in the 5′ region of the LEP gene with overweight. Ann Hum Genet 2000; 64:391–394.
296. Oksanen L, Ohman M, Heiman M, Kainulainen K, Kaprio J, Mustajoki P, Koivisto V, Koskenvuo M, Janne OA, Peltonen L, Kontula K. Markers for the gene ob and serum leptin levels in human morbid obesity. Hum Genet 1997; 99:559–564.
297. Shintani M, Ikegami H, Yamato E, Kawaguchi Y, Fujisawa T, Nakagawa Y, Hamada Y, Ueda H, Miki T, Ogihara T. A novel microsatellite polymorphism in the human OB gene: a highly polymorphic marker for linkage analysis. Diabetologia 1996; 39:1398–1401.
298. Jemaa R, Tuzet S, Portos C, Betoulle D, Apfelbaum M, Fumeron F. Lipoprotein lipase gene polymorphisms: associations with hypertriglyceridemia and body mass index in obese people. Int J Obes 1995; 19:270–274.
299. Wolford JK, Bogardus C, Prochazka M. Polymorphism in the 3′ untranslated region of MTG8 is associated with obesity in Pima Indian males. Biochem Biophys Res Commun 1998; 246:624–626.
300. Oppert JM, Tourville J, Chagnon M, Mauriège P, Dionne FT, Pérusse L, Bouchard C. DNA polymorphisms in the α_2 and β_2 adrenoceptor genes and regional fat distribution in humans: association and linkage studies. Obes Res 1995; 3:249–255.
301. Hani EH, Clement K, Velho G, Vionnet N, Hager J, Philippi A, Dina C, Inoue H, Permutt MA, Basdevant A, North M, Demenais F, Guy-Grand B, Froguel P. Genetic studies of the sulfonylurea receptor gene locus in NIDDM and in morbid obesity among French Caucasians. Diabetes 1997; 46:688–694.
302. O'Dell SD, Bujac SR, Miller GJ, Day IN. Associations of IGF2 ApaI RFLP and INS VNTR class I allele size with obesity. Eur J Hum Genet 1999; 7:821–827.
303. Dunger DB, Ong KKL, Huxtable SJ, Sherriff A, Woods KA, Ahmed ML, Golding J, Pembrey ME, Ring S, Bennett ST, Todd JA. Association of the INS VNTR with size at birth. Nat Genet 1998; 19: 98–100.
304. Weaver JU, Kopelman PG, Hitman GA. Central obesity and hyperinsulinaemia in women are associated with polymorhism in the 5′ flanking region of the human insulin gene. Eur J Clin Invest 1992; 22:265–270.
305. Astrup A, Toubro S, Dalgaard LT, Urhammer SA, Sorensen TIA, Pedersen O. Impact of the v/v 55 polymorphism of the uncoupling protein 2 gene on 24-h energy expenditure and substrate oxidation. Int J Obes Relat Metab Disord 1999; 23:1030–1034.
306. Cassell PG, Neverova M, Janmohamed S, Uwakwe N, Qureshi A, McCarthy MI, Saker PJ, Albon L, Kopelman P, Noonan K, Easlick J, Ramachandran A, Snehalatha C, Pecqueur C, Ricquier D, Warden C, Hitman GA. An uncoupling protein 2 gene variant is associated with a raised body mass index but not type II diabetes. Diabetologia 1999; 42:688–692.
307. Esterbauer H, Schneitler C, Oberkofler H, Ebenbichler C, Paulweber B, Sandhofer F, Ladurner G, Hell E, Strosberg AD, Patsch JR, Krempler F, Patsch W. A common polymorphism in the promoter of UCP2 is associated with decreased risk of obesity in middle-aged humans. Nat Genet 2001; 28: 178–183.
308. Evans D, Minouchehr S, Hagemann G, Mann WA, Wendt D, Wolf A, Beisiegel U. Frequency of and interaction between polymorphisms in the beta3-adrenergic receptor and in uncoupling proteins 1 and 2 and obesity in Germans. Int J Obes Relat Metab Disord 2000; 24:1239–1245.
309. Nordfors L, Heimburger O, Lonnqvist F, Lindholm B, Helmrich J, Schalling M, Stenvinkel P. Fat tissue accumulation during peritoneal dialysis is associated with a polymorphism in uncoupling protein 2. Kidney Int 2000; 57:1713–1719.
310. Walder K, Norman RA, Hanson RL, Schrauwen P, Neverova M, Jenkinson CP, Easlick J, Warden CH, Pecqueur C, Raimbault S, Ricquier D, Silver MH, Shuldiner AR, Solanes G, Lowell BB, Chung WK, Leibel RL, Pratley R, Ravussin E. Association between uncoupling protein polymorphisms (UCP2-UCP3) and energy metabolism/obesity in Pima Indians. Hum Mol Genet 1998; 7:1431–1435.
311. Yanovski JA, Diament AL, Sovik KN, Nguyen TT, Li H, Sebring NG, Warden CH. Associations between uncoupling protein 2, body composition, and resting energy expenditure in lean and obese African American, white, and Asian children. Am J Clin Nutr 2000; 71:1405–1420.
312. Argyropoulos G, Brown AM, Willi SM, Zhu J, He Y, Reitman M, Gevao SM, Spruill I, Garvey WT. Effects of mutations in the human uncoupling protein 3 gene on the respiratory quotient and fat oxidation in severe obesity and type 2 diabetes. J Clin Invest 1998; 102:1345–1351.
313. Cassell PG, Saker PJ, Huxtable SJ, Kousta E, Jackson AE, Hattersley AT, Frayling TM, Walker

M, Kopelman PG, Ramachandran A, Snehelatha C, Hitman GA, McCarthy MI. Evidence that single nucleotide polymorphism in the uncoupling protein 3 (UCP3) gene influences fat distribution in women of European and Asian origin. Diabetologia 2000; 43: 1558–1564.
314. Halsall DJ, Luan J, Saker P, Huxtable S, Farooqi IS, Keogh J, Wareham NJ, O'Rahilly S. Uncoupling protein 3 genetic variants in human obesity: the c-55t promoter polymorphism is negatively correlated with body mass index in a UK Caucasian population. Int J Obes Relat Metab Disord 2001; 25:472–477.
315. Otabe S, Clement K, Dubois S, Lepretre F, Pelloux V, Leibel R, Chung W, Boutin P, Guy-Grand B, Froguel P, Vasseur F. Mutation screening and association studies of the human uncoupling protein 3 gene in normoglycemic and diabetic morbidly obese patients. Diabetes 1999; 48:206–208.
316. Otabe S, Clement K, Dina C, Pelloux V, Guy-Grand B, Froguel P, Vasseur F. A genetic variation in the 5′ flanking region of the UCP3 gene is associated with body mass index in humans in interaction with physical activity. Diabetologia 2000; 43: 245–249.
317. Fisher RM, Burke H, Nicaud VV, Ehnholm C, Humphries SE. Effect of variation in the apo A-IV gene on body mass index and fasting and postprandial lipids in the European Atherosclerosis Research Study II. J Lipid Res 1999; 40:287–294.
318. Lefevre M, Lovejoy JC, DeFelice SM, Keener JW, Bray GA, Ryan DH, Hwang DH Greenway FL. Common apolipoprotein A-IV variants are associated with differences in body mass index levels and percentage body fat. Int J Obes Relat Metab Disord 2000; 24:945–953.
319. Jenkinson CP, Hanson R, Cray K, Wiedrich C, Knowler WC, Bogardus C, Baier L. Association of dopamine D2 receptor polymorphisms Ser311Cys and TaqIA with obesity or type 2 diabetes mellitus in Pima Indians. Int J Obes Relat Metab Disord 2000; 24:1233–1238.
320. Spitz MR, Detry MA, Pillow P, Hu YH, Amos CI, Hong WK, Wu XF. Variant alleles of the D2 dopamine receptor gene and obesity. Nutr Res 2000; 20:371–380.
321. Thomas GN, Tomlinson B, Critchley JA. Modulation of blood pressure and obesity with the dopamine D2 receptor gene TaqI polymorphism. Hypertension 2000; 36:177–182.
322. Gutersohn A, Naber C, Muller N, Erbel R, Siffert W. G protein beta3 subunit 825 TT genotype and post-pregnancy weight retention. Lancet 2000; 355:1240–1241.
323. Hegele RA, Anderson C, Young TK, Connelly PW. G-protein beta3 subunit gene splice variant and body fat distribution in Nunavut Inuit. Genome Res 1999; 9:972–977.
324. Hocher B, Slowinski T, Stolze T, Pleschka A, Neumayer HH, Halle H. Association of maternal G protein beta3 subunit 825T allele with low birth-weight. Lancet 2000; 355:1241–1242.
325. Siffert W, Forster P, Jockel KH, Mvere DA, Brinkmann B, Naber C, Crookes R, Du P Heyns A, Epplen JT, Fridey J, Freedman BI, Muller N, Stolke D, Sharma AM, Al Moutaery K, Grosse-Wilde H, Buerbaum B, Ehrlich T, Ahmad HR, Horsthemke B, Du Toit ED, Tiilikainen A, Ge J, Wang Y, Yang D, Husing J, Rosskopf D. Worldwide ethnic distribution of the G protein beta3 subunit 825T allele and its association with obesity in Caucasian, Chinese, and black African individuals. J Am Soc Nephrol 1999; 10:1921–1930.
326. Siffert W, Naber C, Walla M, Ritz E. G protein beta3 subunit 825T allele and its potential association with obesity in hypertensive individuals. J Hypertens 1999; 17:1095–1098.
327. Sun G, Gagnon J, Chagnon YC, Perusse L, Despres JP, Leon AS, Wilmore JH, Skinner JS, Borecki I, Rao DC, Bouchard C. Association and linkage between an insulin-like growth factor-1 gene polymorphism and fat free mass in the HERITAGE family study. Int J Obes Relat Metab Disord 1999; 23:929–935.
328. Acton S, Osgood D, Donoghue M, Corella D, Pocovi M, Cenarro A, Mozas P, Keilty J, Squazzo S, Woolf EA, Ordovas JM. Association of polymorphisms at the SR-BI gene locus with plasma lipid levels and body mass index in a white population. Arterioscler Thromb Vasc Biol 1999; 19:1734–1743.
329. Aubert R, Betoulle D, Herbeth B, Siest G, Fumeron F. 5-HT2A receptor gene polymorphism is associated with food and alcohol intake in obese people. Int J Obes Relat Metab Disord 2000; 24:920–924.
330. Chouchane L, Danguir J, Beji C, Bouassida K, Camoin L, Sfar H, Gabbouj S, Strosberg AD. Genetic variation in the stress protein hsp70-2 gene is highly associated with obesity. Int J Obes Relat Metab Disord 2001; 25:462–466.
331. Oeffner F, Bornholdt D, Ziegler A, Hinney A, Gorg T, Gerber G, Goldschmidt HP, Siegfried W, Wright A, Hebebrand J, Grzeschik KH. Significant association between a silent polymorphism in the neuromedin B gene and body weight in German children and adolescents. Acta Diabetol 2000; 37:93–101.
332. Chagnon YC, Chen WJ, Pérusse L, Chagnon M, Nadeau A, Wilkison WO, Bouchard C. Linkage and association studies between the melanocortin receptors 4 and 5 genes and obesity-related phenotypes in the Quebec Family Study. Mol Med 1997; 3:663–673.
333. Zee RYL, Lou YK, Morris BJ. Insertion variant in intron 9, but not microsatellite in intron 2, of the insulin receptor gene is associated with essential hypertension. J Hypertens 1994; 12(suppl):S13–S22.

334. Griffiths LR, Nyholt DR, Curtain RP, Gaffney PT, Morris BJ. Cross-sectional study of a microsatellite marker in the low density lipoprotein receptor gene in obese normotensives. Clin Exp Pharmacol Physiol 1995; 22:496–498.

335. Mattevi VS, Coimbra CE Jr, Santos RV, Salzano FM, Hutz MH. Association of the low-density lipoprotein receptor gene with obesity in Native American populations. Hum Genet 2000; 106:546–552.

336. Rutherford S, Nyholt D, Curtain RP, Quinlan SR, Gaffney PT, Morris BJ, Griffiths LR. Association of a low density lipoprotein receptor microsatellite variant with obesity. Int J Obes Relat Metab Disord 1997; 21:1032–1037.

337. Zee RYL, Schrader AP, Robinson BG, Griffiths LR, Morris BJ. Association of HincII RFLP of low density lipoprotein receptor gene with obesity in essential hypertensives. Clin Genet 1995; 47:118–121.

338. Magré J, Laurell H, Fizames C, Antoine PJ, Dib C, Vigouroux C, Bourut C, Capeau J, Weissenback J, Langin D. Human hormone-sensitive lipase. Genetic mapping, identification of a new dinucleotide repeat, and association with obesity and NIDDM. Diabetes 1998; 47:284–286.

339. Orho-Melander M, Almgren P, Kanninen T, Forsblom C. Groop L. A paired-sibling analysis of the XbaI polymorphism in the muscle glycogen synthase gene. Diabetologia 1999; 42:1138–1145.

340. Bottini E, Gloria-Bottini F. Adenosine deaminase and body mass index in non-insulin-dependent diabetes mellitus. Metabolism 1999; 48:949–951.

341. Yuan X, Yamada K, Ishiyama-Shigemoto S, Koyama W, Nonaka K. Identification of polymorphic loci in the promoter region of the serotonin 5-HT2C receptor gene and their association with obesity and type II diabetes. Diabetologia 2000; 43:373–376.

342. Wilson AF, Elston RC, Tran LD, Siervogel RM. Use of the robust sib-pair method to screen for single-locus, multiple-locus, and pleiotropic effects: application to traits related to hypertension. Am J Hum Genet 1991; 48:862–872.

343. Onions KL, Hunt SS, Rutkowski MP, Klanke CA, Su YR, Reif M, Menon AG. Genetic markers at the leptin (OB) locus are not significantly linked to hypertension in African Americans. Hypertension 1998; 31:1230–1234.

344. Bailey-Wilson JE, Wilson AF, Bamba V. Linkage analysis in a large pedigree ascertained due to essential familial hypercholesterolemia. Genet Epidemiol 1993; 10:665–669.

345. Borecki IB, Rice T, Pérusse L, Bouchard C, Rao DC. An exploratory investigation of genetic linkage with body composition and fatness phenotypes: the Quebec Family Study. Obes Res 1994; 2:213–219.

346. Clément K, Dina C, Basdevant A, Chastang N, Pelloux V, Lahlou N, Berlan M, Langin D, Guy-Grand B, Froguel P. A sib-pair analysis study of 15 candidate genes in French families with morbid obesity: indication for linkage with islet 1 locus on chromosome 5q. Diabetes 1999; 48:398–402.

347. Clément K, Philippi A, Jury C, Pividal R, Hager J, Demenais F, Basdevant A, Guy-Grand B, Froguel P. Candidate gene approach of familial morbid-obesity-linkage analysis of the glucocorticoid receptor gene. Int J Obes Relat Metab Disord 1996; 20: 507–512.

348. Bray MS, Boerwinkle E, Hanis CL. Linkage analysis of candidate obesity genes among the Mexican-American population of Starr County, Texas. Genet Epidemiol 1999; 16:397–411.

349. Clément K, Garner C, Hager J, Philippi A, LeDuc C, Carey A, Harris TJR, Jury C, Cardon LR, Basdevant A, Demenais F, Guy-Grand B, North M, Froguel P. Indication for linkage of the human OB gene region with extreme obesity. Diabetes 1996; 45:687–690.

350. Duggirala R, Stern MP, Mitchell BD, Reinhart LJ, Shipman PA, Uresandi OC, Chung WK, Leibel RL, Hales CN, O'Connell P, Blangero J. Quantitative variation in obesity-related traits and insulin precursors linked to the OB gene region on human chromosome 7. Am J Hum Genet 1996; 59:694–703.

351. Lapsys NM, Furler SM, Moore KR, Nguyen TV, Herzog H, Howard G, Samaras K, Carey DG, Morrison NA, Eisman JA, Chisholm DJ. Relationship of a novel polymorphic marker near the human obese (OB) gene to fat mass in healthy women. Obes Res 1997; 5:430–433.

352. Reed DR, Ding Y, Xu W, Cather C, Green ED, Price RA. Extreme obesity may be linked to markers flanking the human OB gene. Diabetes 1996; 45:691–694.

353. Roth H, Hinney A, Ziegler A, Barth N, Gerber G, Stein K, Bromel T, Mayer H, Siegfried W, Schafer H, Remschmidt H, Grzeschik KH, Hebebrand J. Further support for linkage of extreme obesity to the obese gene in a study group of obese children and adolescents. Exp Clin Endocrinol Diabetes 1997; 105: 341–344.

354. Bouchard C, Pérusse L, Chagnon YC, Warden C, Ricquier D. Linkage between markers in the vicinity of the uncoupling protein 2 gene and resting metabolic rate in humans. Hum Mol Genet 1997; 6: 1887–1889.

355. Lembertas AV, Pérusse L, Chagnon YC, Fisler JS, Warden CH, Purcell-Huynh DA, Dionne FT, Gagnon J, Nadeau A, Lusis AJ, Bouchard C. Identification of an obesity quantitative trait locus on mouse chromosome 2 and evidence of linkage to body fat and insulin on the human homologous region 20q. J Clin Invest 1997; 100:1240–1247.

10

Molecular Genetics of Rodent and Human Single Gene Mutations Affecting Body Composition

Streamson Chua, Jr., Kathleen Graham Lomax, and Rudolph L. Leibel

Columbia University College of Physicians and Surgeons, New York, New York, U.S.A.

I INTRODUCTION

The existence of a biological basis for the regulation of body composition was established by the characterization of rodent models of obesity caused by single gene mutations and experimental hypothalamic lesions (1). Obesity induced by hypothalamic lesions clearly demonstrated the major impact of the central nervous system and the neuroendocrine system in regulating ingestive behavior and energy expenditure. The identifications of the leptin/leptin receptor and the melanocortin systems by molecular genetics and positional cloning methodologies provided clear molecular and cellular substrates for the interactions between peripheral tissues (adipocytes in the case of leptin, and pancreatic beta cells in the case of insulin) and the brain. Other elements of the neuroendocrine system such as growth hormone, cortisol, thyroid hormone, and sex steroids/gonadotropins influence the disposition of ingested calories toward expenditure or storage in various tissues as specific molecules ("partitioning"). This chapter reviews the insights regarding the control of energy homeostasis that have come from the identification and functional characterization of the monogenic mouse obesities and their human orthologs.

Obesity is the presence of excessive adipose tissue. The excess can be absolute, relative to lean tissue, or (in most clinical instances) both. Excess absolute fat mass can be achieved only by a chronic positive imbalance between energy intake and expenditure. In humans and animals in which such imbalance is induced by manipulation of diet or the central nervous system (CNS), the increments of body fat are usually greater (out of proportion) to gains in lean body mass, resulting in increased absolute and relative fat mass. It is possible, however, to preferentially affect body composition (vs. mass) by metabolic shunting (partitioning) of ingested calories to fat (by virtue of metabolic "steal" or deficient fatty acid oxidation in muscle), hyper- or hypoplastic development of adipose tissue (SREBP) or muscle (myogenin). Rodent obesities due to primary derangements of energy intake, expenditure, and partitioning have been identified and are described below. Our discussion of rodent obesities is focused primarily on those occurring as a result of spontaneous mutations in single genes. Induced mutations and studies of quantitative trait loci (QTLs) modifying body composition have been extremely important in helping to understand the molecular physiology of weight regulation. Several of these are discussed here when they shed light on major pathways affected by the spontaneous mutations. Otherwise, these genes are described elsewhere in this handbook.

II NATURALLY OCCURRING SINGLE GENE OBESITY MUTATIONS IN RODENTS

A Agouti-Yellow (Dominant Yellow Allelic Series)

The yellow mutation (A^y) is a dominant allele, as are the other alleles that produce yellow pigmentation and obesity (MGI accession ID 87853). The original yellow mutation is descended from a mutation that arose in the so-called Japanese "mouse fancy" that involved collection and display of unusual-looking mice. Other dominant yellow mutations have been collected as part of an interesting allelic series. Mice carrying any one of these dominant yellow mutations are obese (2). The degree of obesity correlates with the amount of yellow pigmentation, suggesting that the degree of expression of the agouti protein is directly responsible for producing obesity. The yellow obese mice exhibit increased linear growth, reflecting an auxotrophic effect of their increased caloric intake. Obesity is not clearly manifest until the mice are adults (6–8 weeks), although hyperphagia is present prior to the development of obesity. The hyperphagia is a major factor in the development of obesity since pair-feeding yellow mutant mice to wild type mice produces yellow mice of near normal body fat content (3). Diabetes and glucose intolerance are associated with the obesity of yellow mice. The yellow mice are mildly insulin resistant, with elevated fasting insulin levels. The diabetes syndrome is clearly regulated by other genetic factors, as genetic background controls diabetes risk. On the C57BL/6J background, obese yellow mice are nearly euglycemic and mildly glucose intolerant. With the yellow mutation on the KK background, obese yellow mice are hyperglycemic (4). Both sexes of the yellow mice are fertile, although fertility is reduced as the obesity increases (Table 1).

The original A^y mutation is due to a large deletion of the 5′ region of the agouti gene and a neighboring gene, *Raly* (hnRNP-associated with lethal yellow). The deletion juxtaposes the ubiquitously and strongly expressed *Raly* promoter to the agouti coding sequence, causing expression of agouti mRNA in all tissues (5,6). The other dominant yellow alleles arise owing to insertion of retroviral sequences (6,7) that juxtapose the promoter elements of their long terminal repeats (LTRs) to drive expression of the agouti coding sequence. Presumably, either the specific LTR sequence or the insertion site determines the strength of expression of the agouti allele. Indeed, the A^{vy} allele displays variable expression such that pseudo-agouti individuals are observed that are lean and nonyellow. Whereas the A^y mutation is lethal in the homozygous state because the *Raly* gene product is required during embryogenesis, the other yellow alleles are viable in the homozygous state since the *Raly* locus has not been affected.

A large number of dominant yellow mutations have been described, and almost all are due to retroviral insertions between the agouti coding sequences and its various promoters. The large (> 100 kbp) distance, between the proximal hair cycle-specific promoters and the ventral hair-specific promoter is probably responsible for the frequency of insertional mutations within the agouti gene. The agouti gene's large size also makes it a good target in x-irradiation mutagenesis screens that have produced numerous agouti alleles. In fact, it was the availability of numerous deletions and rearranged alleles of agouti that aided in its initial identification by positional cloning.

1 Molecular Clues to the Identification of *Agouti* (agouti signaling protein = ASP)

The large number of dominant and recessive alleles, comprising deletions, insertions, and inversions, were extremely helpful in the eventual cloning of *Agouti* (8,9). At the time of agouti's identification, genomics tools such as detailed chromosomal maps and large insert clone libraries were either crude or nonexistent. The task was made easier by fortuitous events, such as the discovery of a large inversion that simultaneously produced two new alleles of *Agouti* and *limb deformity*. This allele provided a molecular breakpoint that was within the *Agouti* gene and allowed the accurate mapping of molecular probes to *Agouti* and the eventual realization that the A^y mutation was due to a large deletion. The application of electrophoretic separation of DNA fragments in the 100 kbp to 1 Mbp by pulsed-field gel electrophoresis was instrumental in this discovery. However, most deletions result in a loss-of-function mutation, and further work was needed to account for the dominant nature of some agouti mutations. The eventual identification of the molecular basis of the gain-of-function mutation was foreshadowed by the identification of a ubiquitously expressed fusion transcript that was the result of splicing the 5′ untranslated region of an ubiquitously expressed gene (*Raly*) to a gene that was normally expressed exclusively in skin (*Agouti*) (10,11) (Fig. 1).

Ectopic Agouti (ASP) overexpression causes obesity mainly by causing hyperphagia. ASP is an antagonist of melanocortin receptors with an affinity in the nanomolar range (12). The melanocortin receptors are a family of G protein coupled receptors that cause intracellular accumulation of cAMP upon binding of melanocyte-stimulating hormone (MSH). ASP inhibits the accumulation of cAMP by MSH stimulation. Since the loss of melanocortin receptor 4 (MC4R) causes hyperphagia and obesity (13), ASP overexpression in the brain leads to inhibition of MC4R, simulating the syndrome of MC4R deficiency. Single ICV injections of agouti-related protein (AGRP) increase food intake for up to 7 days (14), indicating the powerful antagonistic effect of this protein on MC4R activity. In addition, the relative binding affinities of agouti and MSH for MC4R differ by nearly an order of magnitude: ASP binds to MC4R in the low nanomolar range while MSH binds to MC4R between 20 and 40 nM (15). This discrepancy highly favors the inhibitory effect of agouti on MC4R and the induction of hyperphagia.

It has been suggested that ASP acts as an inverse agonist at the melanocortin receptors. Inverse agonists are ligands that suppress spontaneous receptor signaling. In the case of inducing hyperphagia, it is possible that ASP acts by suppressing spontaneous activity of melanocortin receptors, MC3R and MC4R, in addition to antagonizing MSH stimulation.

2 Normal Action of *Agouti* and Various Alleles of *Agouti*

The agouti gene (ASP) is normally expressed only in the skin, acting as a paracrine factor on melanocytes. The intermittent expression of ASP and the continuous expression of MSH are responsible for the alternate bands of eumelanin (black pigment produced during MSH action) and pheomelanin (yellow pigment under ASP control/lack of MSH stimulation) on hair follicles of agouti-pigmented rodents (16). Eumelanin is a brown/black pigment produced by the combined action on tyrosine of at least three enzymes: tyrosinase, TRP1 (tyrosinase-related protein 1), and TRP2 (17). Pheomelanin is a yellowish pigment also derived from the action of tyrosinase on tyrosine. Only tyrosinase, in the presence of cysteine, is required to produce pheomelanin. ASP action reduces total melanin content through inhibition of tyrosinase, and near complete inhibition of TRP1 and TRP2 activity. The actual ratio of eumelanin to pheomelanin is altered by ASP such that more pheomelanin than eumelanin is produced. This is an important point to consider since reductions of tyrosinase activity, as seen in hypomorphic mutations of tyrosinase, result in a reduction of eumelanin content without significant alterations in pheomelanin content. An understanding of this capacity of agouti could be relevant to the various actions of ASP, AGRP (see below), and MSH within the hypothalamus and their effects on food intake and energy balance.

In the A^{w} (Agouti white belly) allele, an upstream skin-specific promoter causes increased ASP expression in ventral (abdominal) skin which causes a further decrease in pigment deposition, resulting in a light cream to white pigmentation (16). Interestingly, black mice of the C57 strains and other derivatives are due to a retroviral insertion before the first coding exon of agouti such that no Agouti mRNA is detected (7). It has not been determined whether the inserted VL30 element interferes with transcription of the agouti gene or splicing of the agouti transcript, or both. Several embryonic lethal *a* alleles are the result of large deletions that span the *Agouti* and *Raly* genes. Agouti expression is normally restricted to skin in rodents, although human adipocytes express ASP at low levels.

3 Pigmentation Phenocopies of Agouti Alleles Generated by Alleles at *Mc1r*

So-called recessive yellow is another mutation in mice that produces yellow fur. It is a recessive allele of an allelic series at the *Extension* locus that encodes a skin-specific MSH receptor, MC1R. The recessive yellow allele inactivates the *Mc1r* gene, producing a pigmentation phenocopy of the dominant yellow mutation, without producing obesity (18). This observation also suggested that the brain melanocortin receptors were primarily responsible for the obesity resulting from ectopic overexpression of agouti. Interestingly, semidominant point mutations that produce constitutively active MCIR alleles of *Mc1r* produce darkening of pigmentation such that homozygotes are indistinguishable from nonagouti mice (*a/a*).

4 Modifiers of *Agouti* Action—*Mahogany* (*Attractin*) and *Mahoganoid Mahogunin*

Two genes modifying Agouti action have been identified by virtue of their ability to darken agouti pigmentation—*mahogany* and *mahoganoid*. Both of these loci appear to act as codominants; homozygosity produces a dark coat that is dissimilar to pure black (*a/a*) coloration due to the persistence of yellow pigment (19). The *mahogany* locus results from inactivating mutations of *Attractin* (20), whereas *mahoganoid* remains to be characterized in molecular terms. Attractin was initially described as a human serum glycoprotein that caused the spreading of monocytes that attract nonproliferat-

Table 1 Human and Mouse Single Gene and Syndromic Obesities[a]

Gene	Gene product	Location/mouse and human	Nature of mutation	Knockout model, rodent phenotype	Human phenotype	Refs.
ASIP (mouse: *Agouti*, A^y	Agouti signaling protein	Mouse: 2 at 89; human: 20q11.2	Deletion	In mice with "lethal yellow" A^y and "viable yellow" A^{vy} mutations, agouti is ectopically overexpressed; yellow coat, obesity, hyperphagia, hyperinsulinemia, increased linear growth.	None reported	(11,49)
BRS3	Bombesinlike receptor 3	Mouse: X; human: Xq26-q28	Generated *Brs3*-null mice by rendering male mice hemizygous for deletion of *Brs3* by homologous recombination in embryonic stem cells	Mice without *Brs3* develop obesity due to hyperphagia and have slight decrease in physical activity and reduced metabolic rate.	None reported	(273)
CCKAR	Cholecystokinin receptor	Mouse: 5 at 34; human: 4p15.2-p15.1	Deletion of, promoter and 1st 2 exons, prevents synthesis of mature transcript	Spontaneously mutant OLETF rat with adult-onset obesity, hyperphagia, males with impaired glucose tolerance.	1. het Gly21Arg in obese, NIDDM African-American; 2. Val365Ile obese African-American; 3. aberrant splicing of exon 3, predicted to result in a nonfunctional receptor, in 1 obese patient with cholesterolgallstone disease	(274,275)
Callipyge locus		Not reported locus/gene	Polar overdominance where paternally imprinted mutant allele only produces effect in heterozygous state	Spontaneous mutation in sheep associated with increased muscle mass in hindquarters of sheep	None reported	(276)
CEBP (alpha, beta, gamma)	CCAAT/enhancer binding protein	*Cebpα*: mouse: Chr. 7 at 12; human: 19q13.1 *Cebpβ*: mouse: Chr. 2 at 95.5; human: 20q13.1 *Cebpγ*: mouse: not reported *Cebpε*: mouse: Chr. 14 at 20.5; human: 14q11.2	Targeted deletions	*Cebpα* homozygous KO mice die hours after birth. Mice doubly homozygous for KO of *Cebpβ/γ* also have increased neonatal mortality and reduced fat pad weight. Decreased fat content likely due to impaired differentiation of preadipocytes.	None reported (mutations in CEBPα have been found in humans with acute myeloid leukemia)	(277)
CPE	Carboxy peptidase E	Mouse: Chr. 8 at 32.6; human: 4q32	S202P mutation abolishes activity of enzyme	Knockout mice have missorting and unregulated secretion of POMC; late-onset, moderate obesity, early and severe hyperproinsulinemia, transient hyperglycemia.	None reported with *CPE*. See *PCSK1* (i.e., *PC1*) that acts just proximal to CPE in posttranslational processing of proinsulin, POMC, GH, CCK, neurotensin, MCH, and gastrin.	(49,149,278)

DGAT	Diacylglycerol acyltransferase (i.e., *ARGP1*)	Mouse: 15 at 46.9; human: 8qter	Targeted disruption	*Dgat*-deficient mice are viable and still synthesize triglycerides; are lean and resistant to diet-induced obesity. The obesity resistance involved increased energy expenditure and increased activity.	None reported	(279)
Dopamine		Selective loss of DA only w/in DA neurons obtained by knock-in using homologous recombination. 1st: TH locus inactive by homologous recombination; TH activity reconstituted in noradrenergic cells by insertion of functional TH construct within DBH locus		DA-deficient mice hypoactive, aphagic, adipsic several weeks after birth; similar to aphagic/adipsia syndrome caused by bilateral lesions of lateral hypothalamus. Near-normal growth achieved with L-DOPA treatment.	Similar phenotype in subjects with bilateral lesions of lat hypothalamus	(280)
DBH	Dopamine beta hydroxylase	Mouse: 2 at 15.5; human: 9q34	Targeted gene inactivation (unable to synthesize noradrenaline or adrenaline)	These mice were cold intolerant (impaired peripheral vasoconstriction); unable to induce thermogenesis in BAT (brown adipose tissue) through uncoupling protein (UCP); increased food intake but not obese because BMR (basal metabolic rate) was also elevated. (Increased BMR not due to hyperthyroidism, compensation by UCP2, or shivering.)	None reported	(280,281)
FGF13	Fibroblast growth factor 13 (i.e., FHF2)	Mouse: X at 18; human: Xq26.3	Gene within duplication breakpoint interval	None reported.	Borjeson-Forssman-Lehmann: mental retardation, obesity, short stature, epilepsy	(232)
GNAS1	Guanine nucleotide-binding protein, alpha stimulating activity polypeptide 1	Mouse: 2 at 104; human: 20q13.2	16 Mutations described in AHO patients; some create premature stop codons, others increase GDP (guanosine diphosphate) release	Homozygous deficiency is lethal in embryonic period. Evidence for imprinting as heterozygotes with maternal null allele have different phenotypes from heterozygotes with paternal null allele.	1. Albright Hereditary Osteodystrophy (AHO): skeletal and developmental abnormalities, mental retardation, obesity; 2. McCune Albright syndrome; 3. pituitary tumors	(282)
GPC3	Glypican 3	Mouse: not reported; human: Xq26	1. 13 bp del NT391 2. exon 2 del 3. Trp296Arg 4. IVS5, G-T, +1 (premature stop) 5. Arg199Ter	None reported.	Simpson-Golabi-Behmel 1: obesity, X-linked overgrowth syndrome with associated visceral and skeletal abnormalities	(253)
GPC4	Glypican 4	Mouse: X at 16; human: Xq26	Deletion of last 2 exons *GPC3* and entire *GPC4* gene	None reported.	Simpson-Golabi-Behmel 1: obesity, X-linked overgrowth syndrome with associated visceral and skeletal abnormalities	(283)

Table 1 (continued)

Gene	Gene product	Location/mouse and human	Nature of mutation	Knockout model, rodent phenotype	Human phenotype	Refs.
GHRHR	Growth hormone–releasing hormone receptor	Mouse: 6 at 26; human: 7p15-p14	Spontaneous mutation in "lit" mice; inactivating mutation	*lit/lit* mice have increased adipose tissue at weaning despite normal intake—partitioning preferentially into fat.	Glu72TER and IVS1, G-A, +1; in 2 first cousins from a consanguineous Indian Muslim family; extremely short and no GH secretion in response to provocative stimulation	(284–287)
HMGIC	High mobility group protein isoform I-C	Mouse: 10 at 67.5; human: 12q15	Inactivation in pygmy (pg) mice	Homozygous KO mice have dwarfing phenotype corresponding to reduced cell replication during fetal development; partially resistant to obesity-inducing effects of leptin deficient and high fat diet.	Mutations found in several benign and malignant tumors; especially found in lipomas	(288–290)
IGF2	Insulin-like growth factor 2	Mouse: 7 at 69.1; human: 11p15.5	Transactivation in mouse model of Sun; targeted disruption in mouse model of DeChiara	**Sun model**: mice with overexpression of *Igf2* developed most of the signs of Beckwith-Wiedemann syndrome, including prenatal overgrowth, polyhydramnios, fetal/neonatal lethality, disproportionate organ overgrowth (including tongue) and skeletal abnormalities. **DeChiara model**: Transmission paternally: heterozygotes were growth deficient. When transmitted maternally, heterozygotes phenotypically normal. Only the paternal allele was expressed in embryos (except in the choroid plexus and leptomeninges) where both alleles transcribed).	Overexpressed in Wilms' tumor and in some cases of Beckwith-Wiedemann syndrome; regulated by genomic imprinting, with maternal allele inactive in most normal tissues	(291,292)
LEP	Leptin	Mouse: 6 at 10.5; human: 7q31.3	1. guanine deletion, codon 133 (G_{398}) 2. C→T, codon 105, exon 3; R105W	*Lep*^{ob} mice; early-onset, severe obesity, hyperphagia, hypercorticosteronemia, defective thermogenesis.	Early-onset, severe obesity, hypogonadotropic hypogonadism in 4 individuals (2 consanguineous families each with 2 affecteds)	(49,166,170,278, 293,294)

LEPR	Leptin receptor	Mouse: 4 at 46.7; human: 1p31	G→A in 3' splice donor site of exon 16	*Lep*^{db} mice; early-onset, severe obesity, hyperphagia, hypercorticosteronemia, defective thermogenesis.	Early-onset, severe obesity, hypogonadotropic hypogonadism moderately growth hormone deficient, central hypothyroidism in 3 sisters of highly consanguineous family	(49,180,278,293, 294)
MC4R	Melanocortin 4 receptor	Mouse: not reported; human: 18q21.3	27 Different mutations in humans published; most are missense (for example Ser30Phe) with 2 frameshift (GATT insertion in codon 244; CTCT deletion codon 211), 1 nonsense (Tyr35 STOP), 1 loss of function (deletion of 18q)	*Mc4r* −/−mice; late-onset dominant obesity, hyperphagia, hyperinsulinemia, hyperglycemia; −/−mice don't respond to anorectic actions of MSH agonist; do not respond to inhibitory effects of leptin on feeding. Do respond to orexigenic actions of NPY and PYY and to anorectic actions of CNTF and CRF.	Majority of reported cases in morbidly obese subjects with childhood onset hyperphagia. In some studies, up to 5% of subjects with BMI > 40 were heterozygous for *MC4R* mutations.	(13,49,189,190,192, 278,293,294)
MCH	Melanocyte concentrating hormone (i.e., *PMCH*)	Mouse: Chr. 10 at 47; human: 12q23-q24	Targeted deletion	MCH-deficient mice had reduced body weight and leanness due to hypophagia, inappropriately increased metabolic rate, reduced amount of both leptin and arcuate nucleus POMC mRNA. MCH is critical regulator of feeding and energy balance, acts downstream of leptin and the melanocortin system.	None reported	(295)
MKKS	McKusick-Kaufman syndrome gene	Mouse: not reported; human: 20p12 BBS6 mutations: compound heterozygote for Leu277Pro and 280delT; cmp'd het for Gly52Asp and 1679 T→A, Tyr264toter, Y264STOP; homo for 2 deletions 1316delC and 1324-1326 delGTA; Tyr264Ter; 1bp del, 280T; Thr57Ala	**Barde-Biedl syndrome type 6:** patients with complete loss of function mutations: **MKKS** subjects with variety and missense mutations	None reported.	**BBS6:** mental retardation, obesity, postaxial polydactyly, retinopathy, renal malformations **MKKS:** developmental anomalies include hydrometrocolpos postaxial polydactyly, congenital heart disease	(223,224,228,296–299)
MYO9A	Myosin IX A	Mouse: 9 at 33; human: 15q22-q23	None reported, but gene within region of BBS4	None reported.	Bardet-Biedl syndrome type 4 (**BBS4**): mental retardation, obesity, postaxial polydactyly, retinopathy, renal disease	(300)

Table 1 (continued)

Gene	Gene product	Location/mouse and human	Nature of mutation	Knockout model, rodent phenotype	Human phenotype	Refs.
MYOD1	Myogenin (MYOD regulates skeletal muscle differentiation; essential for repair of damaged tissue)	Mouse: 7 at 23.5; human: 11p15.4	KO	Myogenin-deficient mice are born alive but immobile; die perinatally due to lack of skeletal muscle.	None reported	(301,302)
GDF8/ aka *MSTN*	Growth differentiation factor 8; i.e., Myostatin	Mouse: 1 at 27.8; human: 2q32.1	Gene targeted disruption; deletion (double muscled cattle); autosomal recessive (*cmpt* mice)	**Gdf8-null mice** are significantly larger than wildtype or with large and widespread increase in skeletal muscle mass; (individual muscles of mutants weigh 2–3× more than wt), and the increase in mass appears to result from a combination of muscle cell hyperplasia/hypertrophy—*Gdf8* may function as a negative regulator of skeletal muscle growth. -**'compact' (Cmpt) mice** are hypermuscular; caused by deletion in the myostatin gene. -**double muscled cattle** have 20% increased muscle mass due to general skeletal muscle hyperplasia—mutation in Gdf8.	None reported	(303–305)
Nhlh2	Nescient helix-loop-helix 2; also known as *HEN2* and *NSCL2*	Mouse: Chr. 3 (syntenic); human: 1p12-p11	Targeted deletion	Homozygotes exhibit progressive adult-onset obesity and hypogonadism; male *Nhlh2*−/− mice are microphallic, hypogonadal, and fertile. Female *Nhlh2*−/− mice reared alone are hypogonadal; when reared with males, their ovaries and uteri develop normally and they are fertile.	None reported	(306)
NPY	Neuropeptide Y/receptors	Mouse: Chr. 6; human: 7p15.1	Double mutant mice; NYP-null, leptin-null	*ob/ob* mice deficient in NPY; mice were less obese due to reduced food intake and increased energy expenditure, and were less severely affected by diabetes, sterility, and somatotropic defects.	None reported	(307)

PCSKI	Proprotein convertase subtilisin/kexin type 1; also known as PC1	Mouse: 13 at 44; human: 5q15-q21	Compound heterozygote: Gly483Arg, A→C^{+4}, exon 5 donor splice site	None reported.	One woman with extreme childhood-onset obesity, hypogonadotropic hypogonadism, low ACTH/low cortisol	(293,308)
PLIN	Perilipin	Mouse: Chr. 7 is syntenic; human: 15q26	Targeted disruption; KO	**Plin null mice** consumed more food than controls but were leaner, more muscular and had normal body weight. Also, null mice were resistant to diet-induced obesity. **KO mice:** 30% less adipose tissue mass in null mice than wt with equal food intake; isolated adipocyte of perilipin null mice exhibited elevated basal lipolysis and dramatically attenuated stimulated lipolytic activity; plasma leptin in null animals greater than expected for the reduced fat mass. Null mice had greater lean body mass and increased metabolic rate but they also showed an increased tendency to glucose intolerance and peripheral insulin resistance. When fed high-fat diet, the perilipin null mice were resistant to diet-induced obesity but not to glucose intolerance.	None reported	(309,310)
PMM2	Phosphomannomutase 2	Mouse: Chr. 16 (syntenic); human: 16p13.3-p13.2	Nearly 60 mutations described, most in exons 5 and 8; 90% accounted for by F119L and R141H	None reported.	Congenital disorder of glycosylation type 1a: psychomotor retardation, growth retardation, moderate obesity, serum glycoprotein abnormalities	(311)
POMC	Pro-opiomelanocortin	Mouse: Chr. 12 at 4; human: 2p23.3	16 Published mutations in humans; half are silent	Hyperphagia, obesity, hypoplastic adrenal cortex due to low ACTH, light skin and hair pigmentation.	3 yo female, 30 kg; 7 yo boy, 50 kg; early-onset obesity, red hair pigmentation, ACTH deficiency	(40,194)
PPAR gamma 2	Peroxisome proliferator activated receptor gamma 2	Mouse: Chr. 6 at 52.7; human: 3p25	5 Published mutations related to obese phenotype: Pro115Gln missense mutation; Pro12Ala; His478His; helix 12 destablizing mutations	*Pparg2* heterozygote mice (homozygous KO is lethal) have improved insulin sensitivity, overexpress and hypersecrete leptin, have smaller adipocytes and reduced fat mass.	4 cases of Pro115Gln mutation in adults with marked obesity	(278,293,312)

Table 1 (continued)

Gene	Gene product	Location/mouse and human	Nature of mutation	Knockout model, rodent phenotype	Human phenotype	Refs.
Prader-Willi syndrome (PWS)		Mouse: P: 7 at 28 *Ipw*: Chr. 7 at 28; *Snrpn*: Chr. 7 at 29; *Ndn*: Chr. 7 at 28; human: 15q11.2-q12	PWS is a contiguous gene syndrome presumably resulting from deletion or disruption of the paternal copies of the imprinted *SNRPN* gene, the necdin (*NDN*) gene, and possibly other genes. PWS can also be caused by maternal uniparental disomy.	***Snrpn* KO:** mice with only intragenic deletion—normal. Mice heterozygous for paternally inherited deletion (putative imprinting center [*Ipw*]) appeared normal at birth except underweight and unable to support selves on hind feet; these mice died as neonates. ***Ndn* KO:** postnatal lethality associated with loss of paternal gene strain dependent; viable mice had reduced oxytocin and LHRH neurons.	Severe early-onset obesity (from ~ 1–2 years of age), hypotonia, mental retardation, short stature, hypogonadotropic hypogonadism	(313–318)
SIM1 (dimerizes with *ARNT2)*	SIM1 is human homolog of *Drosophila Sim*: ("single-minded"), bHLH-PAS transcription factor involved in midline neurogenesis	Mouse: Chr. 10 at 26.5; human: 6q16.3-q21	Translocation which disrupts *SIM1* gene on 6q	Haploinsufficient mouse is obese (mouse *Sim1* is expressed in developing kidney and CNS; is essential for development of several neuroendocrine lineages in supraoptic and PVN nuclei of the hypothalamus [arginine vasopressin, oxytocin, corticotropin-releasing hormone, thyrotropin releasing hormone]).	One young girl with early-onset obesity (67 months, 47.5 kg), normal energy expenditure; translocation between 1p22.1 and 6q16.2. Phenotype resembles heterozygous *MC4R* mutation.	(218–220)
SOX3	SRY-BOX 3	Mouse: Chr. X at 24.5; human: Xq26-q27	Deletion	None reported.	Borjeson-Forssman-Lehman: mental retardation, obesity, short stature, epilepsy	(233)
STAT5A	Signal transducer and activator of transcription 5A	A and B: mouse: Chr. 11 at 60.5; B: human: 17q11.2	KO	***Stat 5a/5b* KO:** small, not fat, severely anemic. ***Stat5a***: small, fat. ***Stat5b***: similar to GHR-deficient subjects; proportionate dwarfism, obese, elevated GH, low IGFI.	None reported	(319)

TBX3	T-box 3	Mouse: Chr. 5 at 65; human: 12q24.1	1. 1-bp del 227T, premature stop codon; 2. IVS 2ds, G-C, +1; predicted to alter gene splicing	None reported.	Ulnar mammary syndrome: complex malformations of ulnar ray, teeth, axillary apocrine glands, urogenital system; obesity	(256)
THRB	Thyroid hormone receptor beta	Mouse: not reported; human: 3p24.3	Nearly 40 documented mutations leading to generalized thyroid hormone resistance	Resistant to thyroid hormone, severe dysfunction of pituitary-thyroid axis, impaired growth/weight gain, advance bone age.	Many cases of generalized thyroid hormone resistance, for example:15 yo female, BMI 26.3; combined hypothyroid and hyperthyroid symptoms	(165,320)
TUB	Tubby transcription factor	Mouse: Chr. 7 at 51.5; human: 11p15.5	Larger transcript in tubby mice due to G- to T-transversion in single splice donor site, leading to substitution of 44 amino acid C-terminus	Tubby mice: late-onset, mild obesity, hyperinsulinemia, retinal degeneration, progressive deafness.	None reported, see *TULP1*	(153,157,158, 321)
TULP1	Tubby-like gene expressed in retina	Mouse: not reported; human: 6p21.3	Compound heterozygotes, 3 mutations in conserved carboxy terminal region; 4th mutation affects donor splice site upstream of carboxy terminal region	Tulp1 −/− mice have early-onset retinal degeneration but normal hearing and normal body weight.	Recessive retinitis pigmentosa	(155,322)

[a] Single-gene mutations that produce obesity in humans are well documented: e.g., Bardet-Biedl, and more recently, genes that are components of the "leptin axis." Intensive screening of human populations for mutations in orthologs of the spontaneous rodent obesity mutations have shown that such mutations (*LEP*, *LEPR*) exist, thereby confirming the role(s) of these genes in the control of human body weight. However, such mutations are extremely rare in humans. Other genes, known by virtue of physiology or the phenotypes of knockout animals to participate in energy homeostasis, have been implicated in human obesity: pro-opiomelanocortin (*POMC*), melanocortin-4 receptor (*MC4R*), and prohormone convertase 1 (*PCSK1*). Of these, *MC4R* mutations are highly prevalent, and are found in 3–5% of patients with BMI > 40. However, not all individuals with these mutations are obese, suggesting that obesity is contingent on the presence of genetic variation in other genes in these individuals and/or on specific developmental or environmental factors. For rare types of "syndromic" human obesity (e.g., Prader-Willi, Bardet-Biedl, Alstrom, Biemond, Cohen), specific regions of the genome have been implicated.

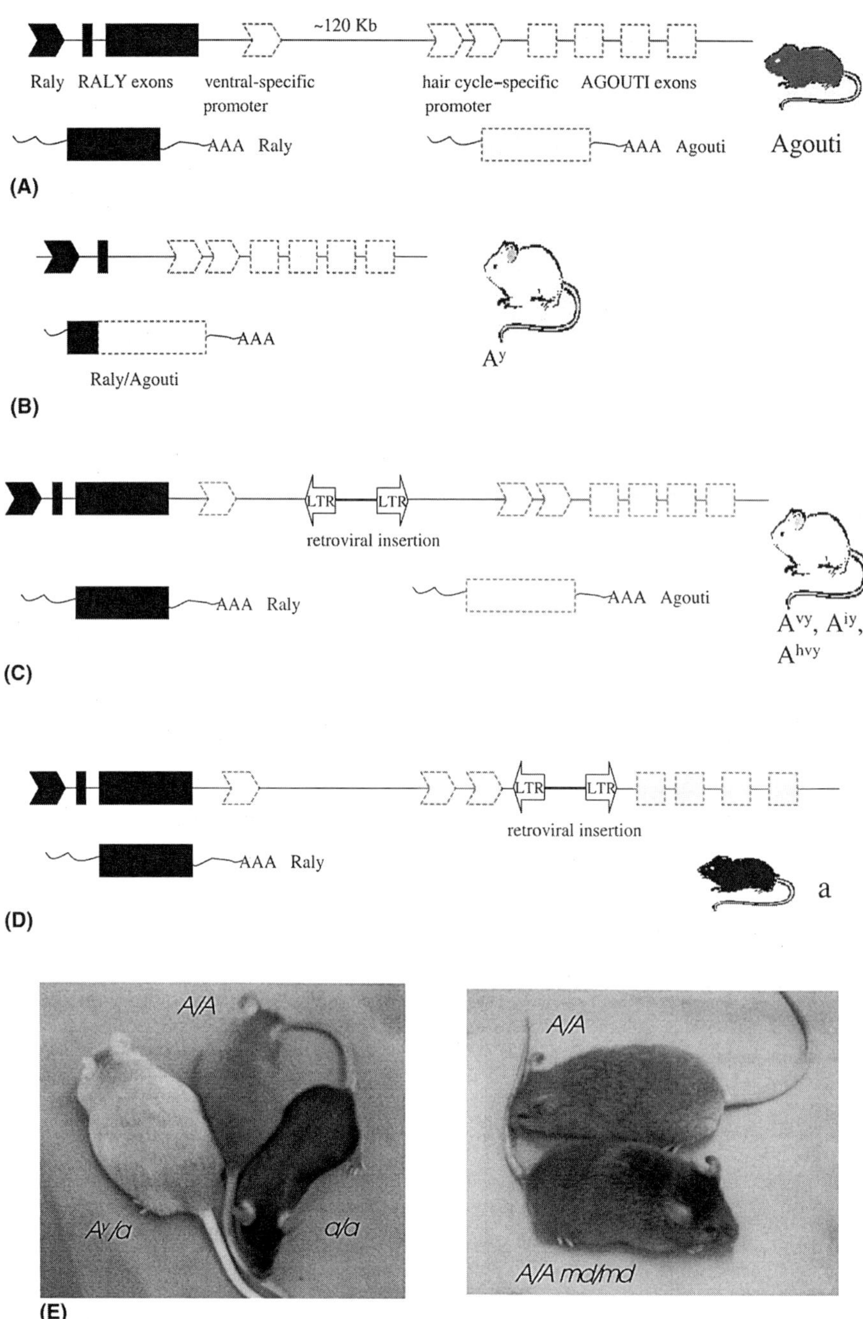

Figure 1 Structure of Agouti locus. (A) Gene structure of Raly and Agouti in normal mice, including resulting transcripts and appearance of mice with normal brown coat color. (B) Structure of Agouti locus in Ay mice, with altered transcript and obese mice with yellow coat color. (C) Structure of Agouti locus, transcripts, and mouse appearance for A^{vy}, A^{iy}, A^{hvy} mice. (D) Structure of Agouti locus, transcripts, and mouse appearance (normal weight, black coat color) for *a* mice. (E) Photographs of wild-type mice (a/a), agouti mice (A/A), heterozygous mouse for yellow mutation (Ay/a), and double homozygous mouse for agouti and mahoganoid (A/A, md/md).

ing T-lymphocytes (21). The two mRNA species, 8.5 kb and 4 kb, correspond to proteins that encode membrane-bound and soluble forms of attractin. The membrane-bound form is found in the brain, skin, heart, kidney, liver, and lung, while the soluble form is specific to hematopoietic tissues. The protein has several putative motifs: serine protease, EGF-like regions, a CUB domain, c-type lectin domain, and a ligand-binding domain for gamma chain cytokines. Mahogany mouse mutants are hyperphagic but remain lean, perhaps owing to increased energy expenditure. The mahogany mutation was also able to prevent the obesity and the yellow pigmentation caused by the dominant Yellow mutation. Surprisingly, *mahogany* is unable to prevent the obesity resulting from transgenic overexpression of AGRP, a peptide clearly related to ASP (see below). However, the identification of an *Attractin* mutation in the rat neurological mutation *zitter* suggests that a reassessment of the *mahogany* phenotype may be necessary (20,22,23). Transgenic complementation with the membrane bound form of attractin corrected the neurological defect as well as the abnormal pigmentation of *zitter* rats, whereas the soluble attractin did not affect either phenotype. All of the rodent *Attractin* mutations cause spongiform encephalopathy and hypomyelination. Thus, the lean phenotype of *Attractin* mutants might be due to a wasting syndrome caused by encephalopathy and/or the movement disorder caused by hypomyelination rather than being due to a specific effect on Agouti (ASP) or AGRP action.

The *mahoganoid* mutation was recently cloned and identified as a 54 kDa RING-containing protein with E3 ubiquitin ligase activity. The gene has been named Mahogunin (gene symbol, *Mgrn1*). The allelic series is due mostly to spontaneous IAP (intracisternal particle) insertions; the $Mgrn1^{nc}$ *(nonagouti curly)*, a chemically-induced mutation, may be due to a T→A mutation in intron 9. Based on the failure of overexpression of *Attractin* (*Atrn*) to rescue the phenotype of *md* animals, *Atrn* is placed proximal to *Mgrn1* in a pathway that operates at or proximal to the melanocortin receptor 1 and possibly 3/4. Levels of *Mgrn*1 expression are not affected by *Atrn*, and vice versa. Like *Atrn*, *Mgrn1* is widely expressed in adult tissues, with similar expression patterns throughout the brain. The patterns of spongiform degeneration in brain (hippocampus, thalamus, stem and cerebellum) are similar in *md* and *mg* affecteds, and are proportionate to the apparent degree of inactivation of gene expression. For example, both $Atrn^{mg\text{-}L}$ and $Mgrn1^{md}$ mutants (apparent hypomorphic alleles) show no evidence of brain degeneration up to 8 and 12 months, respectively, whereas the $Mgrn1^{md\text{-}nc}$, $Atrn^{mg}$, and $Atrn^{mg3J}$ (putative nulls) do (23a; 23b). The mechanisms by which *mg* and *md* rescue the obesity phenotype of A^y, may be related to anatomic effects within the hypothalamus and/or to effects on increased energy expenditure due to tremor. However, neither *mg* (23c) or *md* (unpublished data) appears to rescue the obese phenotype of the Lep^{ob} mouse, creating the possibility that, as implied by the coat color effects conveyed via MC1R, that the *mg* and *md* mutations are quite specific to the melanocortin pathway with regard to effects on energy homeostasis, and/or that the magnitude of the aberration in the Lep^{ob} overwhelms any compensation provided by *md* or *mg*.

5 Agouti Gene-Related Peptide (*Agrp*) [Agouti Related Transcript (*Art*)]

The cloning of the agouti gene and understanding of the effects of its protein product, ASP, on food intake led to the proposal that an endogenous ligand/receptor system existed that was being modulated by the overexpression of ASP. As agouti protein is not normally expressed within the brain, an endogenous ligand(s) and its cognate receptor(s) was postulated to mediate the obesity-producing effects of agouti overexpression. Homology searches through a cDNA database and an actual cDNA library identified a transcript that is expressed in the ventral hypothalamus and adrenal gland, as well as in testis and kidney (24,25). The gene, "agouti-related peptide" (*Agrp*), encodes a peptide that has 25% overall homology to agouti protein, with a higher degree of homology within the carboxyl terminus. The bioactive peptide may be a smaller cleavage product of AGRP, as the peptide derived from the carboxyl terminus (26) is equipotent to the full-length AGRP in evoking feeding, and hypothalamic extracts contain this smaller peptide rather than the full-length AGRP. The putative protease and the steps in processing and secretion of AGRP remain to be elucidated.

6 Regulation of *Agrp* Expression by Fasting and Leptin

AGRP mRNA concentrations in the hypothalamus are regulated by nutritional state: fasting increases AGRP mRNA (about four- to 10-fold increases in the mouse and about two- to four-fold increases in the rat), and refeeding promptly reduces these levels to the basal state. These nutritional effects may be mediated partially by leptin since, ad libitum–fed leptin- and leptin receptor–deficient mice have elevated concentrations of AGRP in the hypothalamus. This may not be a universal phenomenon, however, since leptin receptor–deficient rats do not show the elevated hypothalamic AGRP mRNA levels seen in mice. Since nonmutant rats do show fasting-induced increases in AGRP mRNA, it is possible that other factors influence AGRP expression. Since AGRP/NPY neurons bearing MC3R are responsive to melanocortins, it is probable that Agrp expression is regulated by melanocortin agonists, such as MSH peptides, and antagonists, such as AGRP itself. In A^y mice, hypothalamic AGRP mRNA is considerably suppressed, presumably due to the inhibitory effect of high levels of ASP on melanocortin receptors. It is quite possible that there exists an ultrashort feedback autoregulatory loop for *Agrp* expression. For example, AGRP, upon its release and inhibition of melanocortin receptors on AGRP/NPY neurons, inhibits its own synthesis and release (Fig. 2).

Overexpression of an *Agrp* transgene behind an actin promoter for ubiquitous expression simulates the obesity (24) produced by overexpression of agouti (ASP) as well as the obesity syndrome of melanocortin receptor-4 deficiency (see MC4R below). Both ASP and AGRP are antagonists of MSH peptides at the melanocortin receptors. However, AGRP does not bind to MC1R, the MSH receptor in skin, explaining the inability of AGRP to affect pigmentation. AGRP and ASP bind well to melanocortin receptors found in the brain (both MC3R and MC4R), and both prevent the accumulation of intracellular cAMP that normally occurs with binding of MSH.

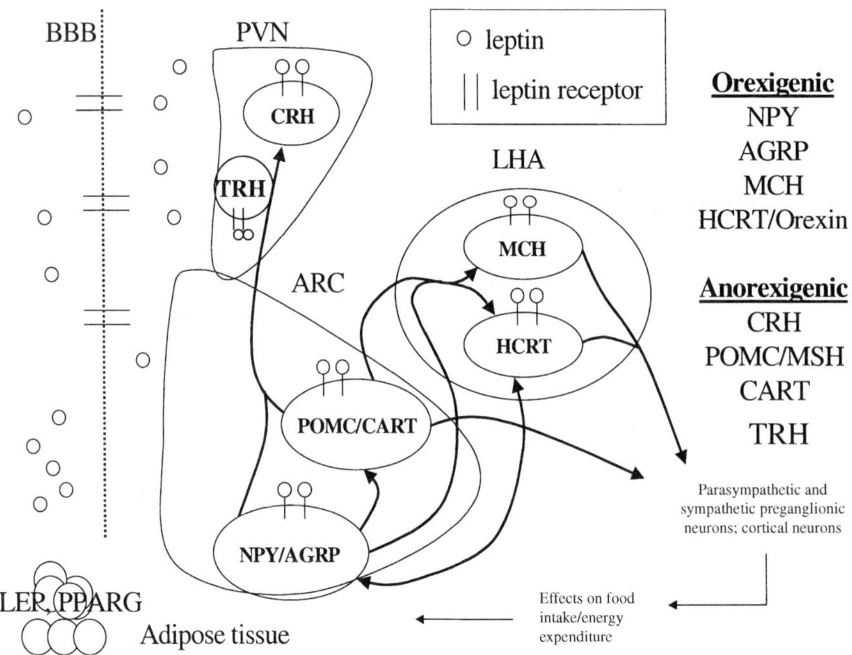

Figure 2 Genes regulating body fat. This figure includes only some of the genes known to participate in regulating body fat. The genes in **boldface** have been shown by mutation and pedigree analysis to be capable of causing human obesity. See Table 1 for other candidate genes (272): ARCuate, ParaVentricular Nucleus, Lateral HypothAlamus. The receptors for the various peptides are not shown, but are also candidate genes in the context of this proposal. For example, **POMC** is processed to **aMSH**, ACTH, and various opioid peptides. aMSH is a ligand for the **MC4 receptor (MC4R)** that it engages to reduce food intake and energy expenditure. **AGRP** interferes with the action of aMSH at this receptor, and hence has the effect of increasing food intake and energy expenditure. **PCSK1** is a processing enzyme for many of these peptides, and **PPARg** is a transcription factor that affects adipocyte differentiation. Genes such as the *ADRB3* and members of the *UCP* family may play roles in energy expenditure. *Symbols*: aMSH (a melanocyte stimulating hormone); *ADRB3* (β 3 adrenergic receptor), *AGRP* (agouti-related peptide); ARC (arcuate nucleus); BBB (blood-brainbarrier); *CART* (cocaine-amphetamine related transcript); *CRH* (corticotropin releasing hormone); *HCRT*/orexin (hypocretin); *LEP* (leptin); *LEPR* (leptin receptor); LHA (lateral hypothalamus); *MC4R* (melanocortin 4 receptor); *MCH* (melanocyte-concentrating hormone); *NPY* (neuropeptide Y); *PCSK1* (pro-protein convertase); *POMC* (pro-opiomelanocortin); *PPARg* (peroxisome proliferator activated receptor gamma); *PVN* (paraventricular nucleus); *TRH* (thyrotropin-releasing hormone); *UCP* (uncoupling protein).

7 Modifier of AGRP Action—Syndecan-3

Obesity was present in a transgenic mouse expressing syndecan-1 (27). Syndecans are extracellular heparan sulfate glycoproteins that bind a variety of macromolecules, including extracellular matrix proteins and cytokines (28). Transgenic syndecan-1 expression was found within the brain and hypothalamus, and binding studies showed a strong interaction between syndecan-1 and AGRP. As syndecan-3 is expressed within the brain, whereas syndecan-1 is not found in the brain, the role of syndecan-3 in energy balance and ingestive behavior was tested. Syndecan-3 protein is induced in the hypothalamus severalfold by a prolonged fast. Syndecan-3 knockout mice were tested for abnormal energy homeostasis. The mice had normal body weights and appeared to be healthy. However, when challenged with a prolonged fast, the syndecan-3 mutants did not show the anticipated hyperphagic response. Thus, it is likely that syndecan-3 modulates AGRP action and ingestive behavior within the brain.

8 Coexpression of AGRP with Neuropeptide Y in the Arcuate Nucleus of the Hypothalamus

The discrete expression of AGRP within the medial area of the arcuate nucleus in the rodent hypothalamus led to the finding that two orexigenic peptides, AGRP and NPY, were coexpressed, defining a unique population of neurons (29). This finding is remarkable since NPY was the most potent orexigenic neuropeptide known until the characterization of AGRP. Neuropeptide Y was initially isolated from pig brain extracts as an amidated peptide of unknown function and high abundance (30). Intracranial injections of NPY into male rats resulted in increased food intake and a decided preference of the rats to ingest chow, even when exposed to sexually receptive females (31). Neuropeptide Y has been shown to elicit ingestive behavior in numerous mammalian and avian species. In a manner similar to *Agrp*, *Npy* gene expression in the hypothalamus is regulated by nutritional state and overall energy balance; increases of hypothalamic NPY or its mRNA are observed during fasting (32), insulinopenic diabetes (33), pregnancy/lactation (34), and cold exposure (35). The correction of the negative energy balance restores NPY mRNA concentrations to the basal state. These alterations are probably mediated by ambient leptin concentrations since leptin receptor–deficient ad libitum–fed rats and mice show equivalent increases in hypothalamic NPY mRNA (36,37), unlike the situation for *Agrp* (38) in rats. However, NPY is widely distributed in neural tissues, as well as the adrenal medulla and vasa vasorum, unlike the discrete neuroanatomical localization of *Agrp* expression in the medial arcuate hypothalamus.

9 Proopiomelanocortin (POMC)

The function of POMC-derived peptides in ingestive behavior and energy balance was not well appreciated until the characterization of naturally occurring and induced obesity-producing mutations of genes within the melanocortin system and the development of potent agonists and antagonists for melanocortin receptors. Well known as the precursor for adrenocorticotropin, endorphin, and melanocyte-stimulating hormone, *Pomc* expression in the hypothalamus results primarily in the synthesis and release of alpha MSH, gamma MSH, and endorphin as the processing enzymes cleave the ACTH sequence to produce alpha MSH (39). Inactivation of *Pomc* using gene-targeting methodology produced homozygous mutant mice unable to produce POMC and its peptides (40). The mutation acted as a recessive allele. The initial report describes the effects of POMC deficiency on energy balance and pigmentation. Surprisingly, the mutant mice did not exhibit a lethal phenotype, given the predicted lack of ACTH and adrenal steroid secretion. However, some early mortality was described, presumably due to adrenal insufficiency. Indeed, the mutants have aplastic/hypoplastic adrenal glands, suggesting a critical role for POMC peptides in adrenal development. The surviving mutant mice exhibited hyperphagia and early onset obesity. The mutants, bearing agouti coloration, exhibited a somewhat lighter coat (less eumelanin) than wild-type agouti controls and the pigmentation could be darkened by MSH injections (Fig. 3).

The phenotypes of the *Pomc* knockout mouse can be understood through analysis of the various melanocortin receptors: (1) MC1R, the MSH receptor found in skin; (2) MC2R, the ACTH receptor in the adrenal cortex; (3) MC3R, a brain melanocortin receptor; (4) MC4R, a brain melanocortin receptor; and (5) MC5R, a melanocortin receptor in exocrine glands (including lacrimal and sebaceous) (41,42). The loss of alpha MSH causes a decrease in stimulation of MC1R and increased synthesis of pheomelanin. However, the mice are not completely yellow, as is the case with inactivating mutations of MC1R, and as might have been expected by the intermittent expression of agouti during mouse hair follicle development. The adrenal aplasia is a somewhat unexpected phenotype, considering the lack of proliferation induced by ACTH on adrenal cortical cells. However, gamma MSH stimulates adre-

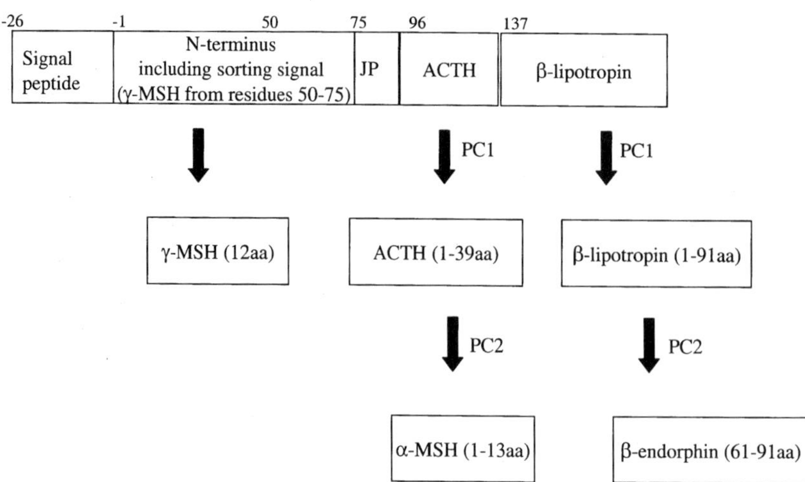

Figure 3 POMC posttranslational processing. POMC is a 267–amino acid length precursor molecule which is processed in the pituitary to several peptides, the major peptides being ACTH (39 amino acids), α-MSH (13 amino acids), and β-endorphin (30 amino acids). The POMC precursor has basic residue cleavage sites listed above the diagram showing sites at which processing of the prohormone occurs. PC1 cleaves POMC into ACTH and β-lipotropin, whereas PC2 cleaves POMC into β-endorphin and α-MSH. Carboxypeptidase E (CPE) is a proprotein processing exopeptidase, cleaving at C-terminal basic residues, and may function as a regulated secretory pathway sorting receptor, using a sorting signal sequence in the N-terminal region of the POMC precursor molecule. JP, joining peptide.

nal cortical cells to proliferate and an adrenal secretory protease that specifically cleaves gamma MSH from the POMC precursor has been identified. Moreover, expression of adrenal secretory protease is induced in the proliferative zone of the adrenal cortex after unilateral adrenalectomy. However, there may be an unidentified member of the MC receptor family since knockout alleles of MC1R to MC5R have been generated but none have the phenotype of adrenal aplasia. The lack of MSH stimulation at MC3R and MC4R is responsible for the obesity and hyperphagia of POMC-deficient mice since mice deficient for either MC3R or MC4R exhibit obesity. The POMC-deficient mouse was not tested for the exocrine gland secretory deficiency of MC5R-null mice.

10 Melanocortin Receptors—MC4R and MC3R

The discovery of melanocortin receptors unique to the brain provided strong evidence for functions of melanocortins that were mediated via the central nervous system. The melanocortin receptors form a gene family that encodes G-protein coupled receptors that are coupled to Gs, having the traditional seven transmembrane domains. However, at the time of their discovery, the nature of these functions was unclear. There were some indications that MSH and melanocortin receptors might be involved in regulating ingestion, based on the information about agouti and the dominant yellow mutation. The task of providing conclusive evidence regarding the functions of central melanocortin receptors fell to mice with targeted mutations of *Mc3r* (43,44) and *Mc4r* (13). Mice that are homozygous for the knockout allele of *Mc4r* develop adult onset obesity accompanied by diabetes, a phenotype very similar to the obesity/diabetes syndrome observed in dominant Yellow mice. The mutants also have increased linear growth as seen in A^y mice. Indeed, heterozygous $Mc4r^{+/-}$ mice have a mild degree of obesity, suggesting a degree of haploinsufficiency that may be considered a semidominant phenotype.

Mice that are homozygous for the knockout allele of *Mc3r* develop late onset, mild obesity that appears to be mediated by metabolic aberrations rather than changes in ingestive behavior. The obesity is exacerbated by providing a high fat diet that is calorically denser than regular chow, and the increased adiposity is attained without an apparent increase in caloric intake. Therefore, metabolic alterations mediated by the loss of

MC3R are responsible for the obesity of the mutant mice. It remains to be determined whether the alteration is mediated via a specific expansion of adipose tissue or differential utilization of caloric stores ("partitioning").

As both of these receptors bind MSH and AGRP, it is reasonable to propose that both of these receptors mediate the functions of MSH and AGRP. The exact nature of the interactions between the receptors and their ligands remains to be fully explored. Since the melanocortin receptors are found presynaptically and postsynaptically, short and long feedback loops must be present that are made more intricate by the reciprocal innervations of NPY/AGRP and POMC/CART neurons (45) (see Fig. 2).

Superpotent agonists (NDP-MSH and Melanotan II/MTII) and antagonists (SHU9119) are relatively poor discriminators between MC3R and MC4R, and the results of intracranial injections of these compounds reflect this nondiscriminatory behavior. Effects are observed on both ingestive behavior as well as nutrient partitioning (46,47). The data are also consistent with the phenotypes of the two knockout mouse models, showing that obesity is produced via hyperphagia as well as preferential fat deposition, although the metabolic effects result in much smaller amounts of excess fat accumulation.

III LEPTIN (*OBESE*)

The *obese* mutation was initially identified in an outbred colony of mice ("stock V") carrying the waltzer (v) mutation (48). The recessive mutation causes hyperphagia with early-onset obesity, insulin resistance with glucose intolerance, cold intolerance, and infertility (49). Almost all of these phenotypes are modified by other downstream effectors and have proven to be an extremely rich area of investigation (see Fig. 1). Positional cloning of the *obese* mutation revealed a gene, later called *Leptin*, that encodes a novel, adipocyte-specific hormone (50) that belongs to the cytokine superfamily. The hormone is processed to a mature form that circulates in a form bound to serum proteins that include a soluble form of the leptin receptor (51). The concentrations of leptin in blood are directly related to the amount of fat in the body and show an extremely good correlation to total fat mass (52). Most of the leptin found in blood is derived from white adipose tissue; smaller amounts of leptin are derived from brown adipose tissue. In neonatal rodents, initially all circulating leptin comes from BAT since rodent pups have no white adipose tissue at birth.

A Mechanisms Causing Obesity in Leptin Deficiency

1 Hyperphagia and Obesity

Leptin-deficient mice (Lep^{ob}) exhibit early-onset hyperphagia and obesity, being obese to inspection at the time of weaning at postnatal day 21 or up to a week later. After weaning, the mutant mice ingest up to twice the calories of lean littermates and rapidly gain weight and adipose tissue. On the C57BL/6J strain, mutant mice of both sexes are twice the weight of lean siblings at 8 weeks. The mutants maintain this extreme adiposity as long as circulating insulin concentrations are sufficiently elevated above physiological concentrations. In some strains of mice (such as C57BLKS/J), leptin deficiency leads to insulinopenia and severe hyperglycemia with persistent insulin resistance (53). In this state of absolute and relative insulin deficiency, the mutant mice rapidly lose weight and adipose tissue. The importance of hyperphagia in the development of the obese state is shown by pair-feeding studies in which *obese* mice are fed the amount of food taken spontaneously by genetically lean mice. In such studies, the *obese* animals still gain slightly more weight than the lean animals, but a much higher fraction of the additional weight is adipose tissue (54). Thus, the increased body fat of the *obese* mice reflects the confluence of leptin's effects on energy intake, expenditure and partitioning.

2 Glucose Intolerance

Leptin-deficient mice are glucose intolerant and this is readily evident upon weaning onto standard laboratory chow that is carbohydrate rich (55). The mutant mice develop hyperglycemia when ingesting standard rodent chow; a prolonged fast reduces blood glucose concentrations to the normal range. The hyperglycemia is caused by insulin insensitivity, probably due in part to hypothalamic defects in the regulation of autonomic nervous system outflow.

As the tissues of mutant mice are insulin resistant, it is counterintuitive to think that adipose tissue, which is dependent on insulin for its growth and maintenance, would be greatly expanded. However, the insulin concentrations that are attained in mutant mice can be > 100-fold elevated over lean mice, providing sufficient stimulation of insulin pathways to maintain adipose tissue mass. This proposition is supported by the extreme fat mass loss of mutants that are insulinopenic, for example, C57LBKS/J mice. Furthermore, the loss of calories by glycosuria is probably offset by the massive caloric intake of these mutants.

The role of leptin in modulating carbohydrate metabolism remains to be fully described. While humans with leptin and leptin receptor deficiencies do not show overt glucose intolerance, humans and mice with lipodystrophy show extreme glucose intolerance and diabetes. Moreover, in some lipodystrophic mice, diabetes is reversed by transplantation of adipose tissue, leptin injections, or expression of a leptin transgene (see Modifiers of Leptin Action).

3 Cold Intolerance

In rodents, leptin deficiency results in hypothermia and cold intolerance (56). Mutant mice usually display basal hypothermia when raised under standard vivarium temperatures (~22°C). The mutant mice are also unable to maintain core temperature during a moderate cold challenge (4°C over 1–2 hr). This thermal defect can be partially corrected by prolonged rearing under mild cold challenges (12–14°C) over a period of several weeks (57,58). Upon examination of the physiological response to a cold challenge, the leptin deficient mice are able to shiver but fail to activate brown adipose tissue via the sympathetic nervous system. Prolonged cold rearing allows a direct trophic effect on BAT since BAT from mutants raised under cold thermal challenge is nearly normal in mass and function. In conventionally reared mutants, the BAT is atrophic with a severe reduction in mitochondrial content and uncoupling protein 1, showing morphology reminiscent of white adipose tissue. Therefore, there appear to be two deficiencies in the mutants—an acute inability to activate BAT via the sympathetic nervous system (SNS), and the absence of a trophic stimulation on BAT. The prolonged cold rearing probably activates BAT via direct stimulation from cold sensitive neurons in the peripheral nervous system.

Rearing *obese* mice at thermoneutrality (~35°C) does not prevent the appearance of obesity (59). In addition, as mentioned above, cold rearing to induce the development of BAT in *obese* mice does not significantly affect the development of obesity. Thus, the thermogenic defect does not contribute substantially to the obesity of these mice.

4 Caloric Partitioning

Hyperphagia per se should not lead to obesity in a continuously growing animal such as mice and rats during their rapid postweaning growth phase. Increased caloric intake can lead to symmetric expansion of all body compartments, leading to a larger organism. There are apparent developmental and genetic factors in the regulation of growth of various tissue compartments, such as preferential expansion of white adipose tissue, to lead to obesity. Body composition analyses in mice consistently show that leptin deficiency causes an excessive absolute and relative accumulation of white adipose tissue, with a reduction in skeletal muscle, diminished linear growth, and reduced brain weights. There are several candidate mechanisms for this effect, each of which has been observed in leptin deficient mice: (1) defective growth hormone axis; (2) defective thyroid hormone axis; (3) hypothalamic hypogonadism; and (4) reduced physical activity. The caloric partitioning effect is dramatically demonstrated during pair-feeding studies in which the ingested calories of mutant mice are yoked to genetically lean control mice (60). After a period of such restricted feeding, the mutant mice attain slightly greater body weights than lean mice. However body composition analysis shows that the mutant mice have increased absolute fat content (about twofold) (55). Therefore, the obesity of leptin deficiency is due to both hyperphagia and to preferential deposition of stored calories as fat.

5 Infertility and Hypothalamic Hypogonadism

It is well known that hypogonadism alters body composition and increases fat accumulation in both sexes. Leptin deficiency, in most of the strains tested (C57BL/6J, C57BLKS/J, DBA/2V, and V), causes hypothalamic hypogonadism and infertility (53). The low sex hormone levels probably contribute to the adiposity of the mutant mice. However, the original strain of leptin receptor deficient rats (Zucker fatty strain) can be selected for fertility in mutant males. Recently, the Lep^{ob} mutation has been transferred to the BALB/cJ strain (61). Both male and female mutants of this strain are obese, yet fertile and produce normal pups. This striking strain difference between C57BL/6J, the standard obese inbred strain host, and BALB/cJ could be utilized to identify allelic variants of genes that modify leptin effects on the integrity of the gonadal axis.

B Leptin Effects on Normal and *obese* Mice

The production of synthetic leptin led to the rapid evaluation of leptin's actions on normal and mutant mice (62–64). When injected either into the periphery or into the brain, leptin can correct all of the abnormalities of obese mice. Indeed, if treated for a sufficient period of time, the mutant mice become phenotypically lean and reproduce in a normal fashion. Treatment of rodents with leptin that maintains leptin concentrations in the high physiological range actually depletes adipose tissue depots, resulting in leaner animals (65). Similar responses occur if leptin is delivered either via an adenovirus (66) or a transgene (67), indicating that normal mice can respond to elevations in leptin concentrations and reduce adipose depots. In addition, these results indicate that it is unlikely hyperleptinemia per se causes leptin resistance. However, diet-induced obese rodents are hyperleptinemic and resistant to the effects of leptin. Therefore, the hyperleptinemia of diet-induced obesity may reflect effects of increased adiposity as well as leptin insensitivity. The factors that are involved in causing the leptin resistance of diet-induced obesity should prove to be an interesting area of research.

C Regulation of Leptin in Adipose Tissue

Leptin secretion and blood levels are regulated by nutritional factors, in addition to their correlation to fat mass. Leptin is secreted via the constitutive synthetic and secretory pathway that is highly sensitive to adipocyte volume (68). The mechanism for this sensitivity to adipocyte volume is not known, but provides an explanation for the correlation of circulating leptin concentrations with adipose tissue mass. Insulin has a stimulatory effect on leptin gene transcription and translation, and causes release of a leptin from a pool of stored leptin (69). Glucocorticoids have a similar stimulatory effect on leptin gene transcription and synthesis of leptin, although glucocorticoids do not stimulate the release of stored leptin.

The insulin-mediated stimulation of leptin transcription could be mediated directly, via stimulation of the phosphorylation cascades initiated by the insulin receptor, or indirectly, via metabolites produced during glucose metabolism, such as UDP-glucosamine (70). Initial characterization of the leptin promoters from man and mouse indicated the presence of a CCAAT enhancer-binding protein (C/EBP) site (71) that could stimulate transcription in preadipocytes and that C/EBP alpha could stimulate leptin transcription (72). Subsequent studies have indicated that C/EBP alpha is downregulated during insulin treatment of fully differentiated adipocytes, suggesting that stimulation of C/EBP alpha activity is not the mechanism for insulin-mediated stimulation of leptin transcription (73). These results need to be more fully explored in order to reconcile the discrepancies (see Fig. 4).

Treatment of rodents and adipocytes with a class of drugs called thiazolidinediones (TZDs; used as insulin-sensitizing agents in type 2 diabetes mellitus) have been found to suppress leptin gene expression. In addition, TZDs can increase fat accumulation, probably by stimulating adipocyte proliferation and differentiation. TZDs activate PPAR gamma, a transcription factor that positively regulates adipocyte differentiation.

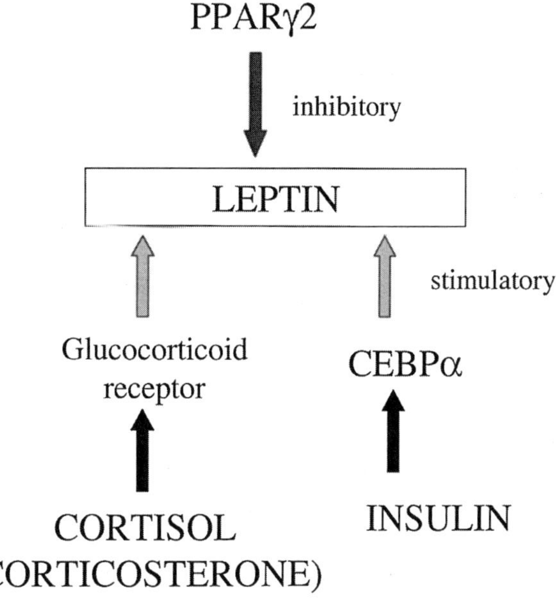

Figure 4 Regulation of leptin synthesis. Insulin and glucocorticoids stimulate leptin gene transcription and synthesis, whereas fatty acids that activate PPARγ are inhibitory to leptin synthesis.

However, in contrast to its stimulatory effect on some adipose-specific genes, PPAR gamma inhibits leptin gene transcription (74). While PPAR gamma does not appear to bind directly to the site of the leptin promoter responsible for the inhibitory effect of TZDs on leptin transcription nor to C/EBP alpha, it is possible that the two transcription factors compete for a critical cofactor (75).

D Leptin Expression in Nonadipose Tissues

Leptin has been reported to be expressed in numerous tissues in addition to adipose tissue. Leptin mRNA and/or protein have been reported in the stomach (76), skeletal muscle (70), and the trophoblast of the developing embryo (77). Leptin secreted from the stomach during or after a meal might contribute to inhibit further feeding. Among other postulated roles of gastric leptin is a cytoprotective effect against the formation of mucosal ulcers (78). Within skeletal muscle, leptin gene expression is induced by increased leptin concentrations and glucosamine, a metabolic intermediate of a proposed nutrient-sensing pathway in skeletal muscle and adipose tissue. Leptin has been found in the preimplantation embryo, and it is derived from maternal leptin mRNA. Leptin is found in a gradient and eventually localizes to outside cells of the morula that are destined to become trophoblastic cells. However, leptin is not absolutely necessary for ontogenesis since embryos from leptin-deficient dams develop into normal fetuses and pups.

E Circulating Leptin and Soluble Leptin Receptor

Leptin circulates in a bound form in most lean individuals. The leptin binding protein in humans is probably a proteolytically shed form of membrane bound leptin receptor since the 3′ terminal exon for the soluble leptin receptor isoform is nonfunctional in humans, due to absence of a polyadenylation signal (79). In rodents, a transcript (LEPR-E) directly encodes a soluble leptin receptor. In obese individuals, circulating leptin concentrations are higher and the ratio of bound leptin to free leptin is altered in favor of free leptin, presumably due to independent mechanisms that modulate leptin and soluble leptin receptor (51,80).

Leptin is cleared primarily by the kidneys. In end stage renal disease, leptin concentrations are elevated, owing to diminished leptin clearance (81). These elevated leptin levels could be partially responsible for the anorexia and wasting associated with renal failure. Interestingly, the kidneys and the lungs are organs with high levels of expression of LEPR-A isoform, suggesting that LEPR-A might be involved in leptin clearance and degradation.

Circulating leptin is extremely elevated during pregnancy in the mouse (82), whereas a modest twofold elevation is seen during pregnancy in rats (83,84) and humans (77,85). In the mouse, the soluble leptin receptor is produced via a placental-specific promoter driving synthesis of the soluble LEPR-E isoform. This increase in LEPR-E leads to increased amounts of LEPR-bound leptin and diminished clearance of leptin. An interesting difference between the hyperleptinemic states of pregnancy and obesity accounts for the increased leptin concentrations. Increased adipose tissue mass produces increased amounts of leptin, leading to increased free leptin. During pregnancy, the increased amounts of soluble leptin receptor bind leptin, increasing the amount of bound leptin and decreasing the clearance of leptin. The evolutionary advantage of such leptin accumulation could be related to the extreme energy demands of gestation and lactation in a small homeotherm, the mouse. Maintaining the health of the pregnant dam and the developing fetuses requires a constant, high level of caloric intake and prolonged caloric deficits would be deleterious to both the dam and the developing pups. Therefore, it is reasonable to argue that the decreased availability of free leptin during pregnancy is a mechanism to drive feeding even in the face of increasing adipose depots and increased leptin biosynthesis. Apparently, the rat and human *LEPR* genes do not have such a strong placental promoter, leading to the much more modest increases in circulating leptin during gestation in rats and humans.

F Effects of Leptin Outside of the Brain and Neuroendocrine System

Leptin receptors are found in numerous tissues outside of the brain. Leptin receptors, particularly LEPR-B, are found in abundance in developing long bones and cartilage (86). Moreover, leptin-deficient mice have increased cortical bone thickness and leptin treatment of *ob/ob* mice normalizes bone thickness (87), although it has also been reported that leptin promotes bone growth in *ob/ob* mice (88). Moreover, leptin deficiency causes mild growth hormone deficiency with associated decreased linear growth. Thus, the effects of leptin on the skeletal system remain to be further elucidated.

Leptin-deficient mice have a mild immune system deficiency, and LEPR-B is expressed in lymphocytes at levels equivalent to the hypothalamus (89). Because leptin is a cytokinelike molecule, it is not surprising that immune cells respond to leptin (90). Since fasting and caloric restriction produce a mild repression of immune function, it is possible that the decreased leptin concentration associated with negative energy balance is partly responsible. High turnover of circulating immune cells is energy costly and might be dispensable under conditions of nutritional deficit and might have evolved as a means of maximizing metabolic fuel efficiency.

Leptin has angiogenic properties, stimulating the growth of new capillaries (91). LEPR-B is expressed in human endothelial cells, and the control of capillary growth could be important to the delivery of metabolic substrates to various tissues—in particular, adipose tissue. It is possible that differential blood flow to various adipose depots could be responsible for the substantial metabolic differences between subcutaneous and visceral adipose depots.

G Mutant Alleles of Leptin

The leptin transcript is remarkable for a long 3′ untranslated region. The transcript comprises two exons, and the first Lep^{ob} mutation is a point mutation in the second exon that generates a premature termination codon (50). Since the mutation occurs in the 3′ terminal exon, the mutant transcript is not susceptible to nonsense-mediated mRNA decay and accumulates at much higher concentrations than the wild-type allele. Although cytoplasmic concentrations of Lep^{ob} leptin have not been measured, the protein is certainly not secreted from the adipocyte. In humans, a similar mutation generating a premature termination codon has been described. In these individuals, mutant leptin remains within the cytoplasm of adipocytes and is not secreted (see below). While such accumulation might be attributable to high levels of stimulation due to high concentrations of insulin, it is also possible that there is an autoregulatory feedback loop for leptin gene expression in the adipocyte and that the lack of leptin autoinhibition leads to increased leptin gene transcription.

The Lep^{ob2J} mutation is due to an insertion of a transposon element within the proximal promoter of the leptin gene (92). Very little if any leptin transcript is observed with this mutation. The mutation arose on the SM/J strain and the mutant mice of this strain are not severely hyperglycemic, suggesting the presence of alleles that are protective against type 2 diabetes (see Fig. 5).

H Mediators and Modifiers of Leptin Action in the Hypothalamus

The proximal mediators of leptin action relevant to energy balance are leptin-sensitive neurons within the hypothalamus and their constituent neurotransmitters (93). This is highlighted by the fact that intracerebroventricular injections of small doses of leptin are

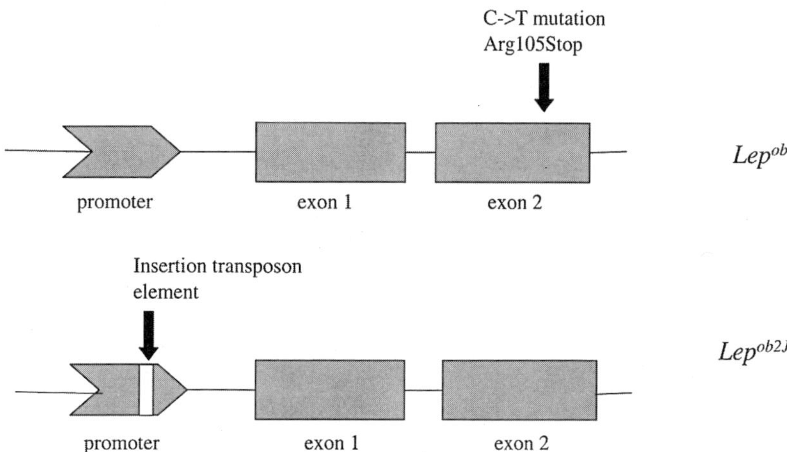

Figure 5 Genetic structure of the Lep^{ob} and Lep^{ob2J} loci. Lep^{ob} contains a point mutation in the second exon, R105X, that leads to premature chain termination. Lep^{ob2J} has a transposon element inserted into the promoter. This transposon element is from the ETn family of transposons and contains multiple splice-acceptor sites that interfere with normal splicing.

sufficient to correct the obese phenotype, as noted previously (62). In addition, these leptin injections into the brain can correct the glucose intolerance prior to the appearance of the effects on feeding (94), suggesting that there may be different thresholds for the various actions of leptin. A large number of leptin-sensitive neurons have been identified, and each type contributes to the obesity/diabetes syndrome of leptin deficiency. Upon binding to its receptor, activation of the JAK/STAT pathway is responsible for leptin's effects (89,95,96), although the stimulatory and inhibitory effects on specific neuropeptide genes remain to be fully explained. The genes encoding orexigenic peptides (NPY, AGRP, MCH [melanocyte-concentrating hormone]) are downregulated by leptin while the genes encoding anorectic peptides (POMC and CART [cocaine- and amphetamine-regulated transcript] in arcuate nucleus neurons) are upregulated [reviewed by Spiegelman and Flier (93)]. Leptin also can hyperpolarize hypothalamic neurons (97), an effect perhaps mediated by the activation of ATP-sensitive potassium channels, probably contributing to decreased release of the orexigenic peptides. However, this action would not be expected to be correlated with leptin's effect on POMC neurons since hyperpolarization would inhibit release of POMC-derived peptides. Indeed, leptin depolarizes POMC neurons directly and relieves GABA-mediated inhibition (45). Thus, leptin can have directly opposite actions on resting potential, depending on neuronal cell type. This action will require much farther investigation to elucidate its mechanism.

These actions of leptin appear to orchestrate a coordinated response to alterations in circulating leptin concentration. Under conditions of negative energy balance and decreased leptin concentrations, the neurons secreting orexigenic peptides, such as NPY (98) and MCH, are activated and increase release of their orexigenic peptides. Simultaneously, the decreased leptin concentrations stimulate the transcription of the same neuropeptide genes to allow for increased synthesis of the neuropeptides being released. The POMC/CART neuron is controlled in a reciprocal fashion to maximize the drive to feed. Decreased leptin concentrations decrease POMC and CART synthesis (99–101). Correction of the leptin concentrations to the basal state normalizes neuronal activity and neuropeptide gene transcription/translation.

In normal rodents, exogenous leptin administration via leptin infusion or gene transfer techniques (viral vectors or transgenes) causes hypophagia and diminished adipose tissue mass. Leptin infusions that increase leptin concentrations at the high end of physiological concentrations (10 ng/mL) do not appear to cause alterations in NPY mRNA, but other neuropeptides remain to be studied. It is remarkable that the lack of adipose tissue in these leptin-treated animals does not lead to insulin resistance and diabetes usually associated with lipodystrophy, a syndrome characterized by diminished adipose depots. In fact, leptin transgenic mice are exceptionally lean and have increased glucose tolerance, implying that high leptin concentrations in normal lean organisms cause enhanced glucose metabolism. The paradox remains as to the lack of efficacy of leptin in correcting obesity and insulin resistance in diet-induced obesity.

IV LEPTIN RECEPTOR (*DIABETES* AND *FATTY*)

The *diabetes* mutation arose in the C57BLKS/J strain; obese mice of this strain are susceptible to developing insulinopenia and severe diabetes (102). The phenotypes of young *db/db* mice are strikingly similar to that of young *ob/ob* mice: early-onset hyperphagia and obesity with the attendant thermogenic defect. In addition, both mutations cause early onset hyperglycemia and hyperinsulinemia that diverge only later in life, with *db* C57BLKS/J mice developing severe insulinopenia and early mortality. When the *ob* and *db* mutations were both transferred to the C57BL/6J strain, the two mutations showed identical phenotypes, suggesting that the diabetes susceptibility of C57BLKS/J *db* mice was due to a strain-specific combination of allelic variants (103,104). These similarities in phenotypes led Douglas Coleman to perform parabiosis studies to test the hypothesis that the normal *ob* and *db* gene products constituted a ligand-receptor system (105). Coleman found that *ob:ob* pairs and *db:db* pairs showed no differences in the partners of the pairs. However, in *ob:db* pairs, the *ob* partners lost weight and occasionally succumbed to starvation. While this might be a strong indication that the *ob* gene product was a diffusible substance and that the *db* gene product was its receptor (as later shown by molecular cloning of both genes), parabiosis between *ob* and lean animals did not produce such clear-cut results. Both partners of the *ob*:lean pairs thrived and gained weight in nearly the same fashion as singleton animals of the same genotypes. One would have predicted that the *ob* partners of *ob*:lean pairs should have lost weight upon exposure to the diffusible substance provided by the lean partner.

Remarkably, two rat mutations, *fatty* [Zucker (106)] and *fatty-f* [Koletsky (107)], caused a nearly identical obesity/diabetes phenotype as *obese* and *diabetes* mouse mutants. The mutations were recessive and caused early onset obesity with hyperphagia, cold intolerance, hyperglycemia and insulin resistance, and infertility. The similarities of the phenotypes suggested that diabetes and fatty might be molecular orthologs. This was confirmed upon the mapping of the *fatty* mutation to a segment of rat chromosome 1 (108) that was orthologous to a segment of mouse chromosome 5 that contained *diabetes*.

A Molecular Clues to the Identification of *diabetes*

Various approaches were combined to provide the conclusive evidence that mutations of the leptin receptor gene and *diabetes* and *fatty* alleles were one and the same. Mapping studies had shown that the mouse *diabetes* mutations and the rat *fatty* alleles were orthologs. A positional cloning approach by two groups had narrowed the critical chromosomal interval to ~1 Mbp (109,110). A leptin-binding protein expression cloned from the choroid plexus mapped to this critical interval (111). However, analysis of the most frequently studied alleles of *diabetes* and *fatty* initially proved to be uninformative in terms of providing the evidence that mutations were present in the leptin receptor gene. It fell to the infrequently studied db^{Pas} allele to provide the proof. Genomic analysis of the leptin receptor in db^{Pas} showed the presence of a partial duplication, eventually shown to be a duplication of four exons, which eliminated all leptin receptor transcripts (110,112). While the original *db* allele was found to have a mutation that generated a new splice donor site in one of the alternative 3′ terminal exons (109,113), preventing the translation of one of the isoforms ("Rb"), the mutation did not eliminate three other membrane-bound leptin receptor isoforms, providing a puzzle that could only be explicated with further studies of the molecular properties of the leptin-leptin receptor signaling system.

The homology of the leptin receptor to cytokine receptors was not surprising, given the structural similarity of leptin to cytokines (111). Given this structural similarity, the *diabetes* mutation's elimination of the STAT signaling-competent isoform. LEPR-B, proved to be a critical element in highlighting the importance of LEPR-B function and the hypothalamus in the obesity/diabetes syndrome (89,95), given the normal expression of the other LEPR isoforms in *db/db* mice.

B Alternative 3′ Terminal Exons Provide a Variety of Leptin Receptor Isoforms

The leptin receptor gene has multiple 3′ terminal exons (79) that may be alternatively spliced in a tissue-specific manner (89) (Fig. 6). Each of these 3′ terminal exons contains a stop codon and a polyadenylation signal. Two of the exons, 14′ and 17′, are extensions of the preceding exons and start with a canonical splice donor site, an arrangement for 3′ terminal exons that is not uncommon in genes that are differentially spliced in cells that undergo differentiation and maturation, such as the gene encoding the heavy chains of immunoglobulins. The presence of multiple 3′ terminal exons was a complication in the initial identification of disruptive mutations of *Lepr* (109,110,113). However, the identification of the single nucleotide alteration for $Lepr^{db}$ was highly instructive regarding the singular critical role of the membrane-bound B isoform of LEPR. Analysis of cDNA clones indicated that there was heterogeneity in the 3′ terminus of transcripts that *Lepr* encoded. All of the transcripts contain the same ligand-binding domain (present in exons 8, 9, 10, and 11) so that all of the LEPR isoforms should bind leptin equally. There is a short transcript that includes coding exons 1–14 and the 3′ terminal exon that has been called exon 14′ This soluble receptor (LEPR-E) is found in the circulation and its production is strikingly increased during pregnancy in the mouse due to a placenta-specific promoter (82), resulting in extreme hyperleptinemia (10-fold elevation of total leptin in the blood). However, the hyperleptinemia in pregnant rats or humans is only twofold, suggesting that any advantages conferred by the extreme hyperleptinemia of pregnancy in the mouse may not be necessary for satisfactory gestations in other species (114). In fact, the human gene does not contain a functional exon 14′, since it lacks a polyadenylation site. The human *LEPR* does not produce LEPR-E mRNA although there is soluble LEPR in the circulation. Human LEPR-E is produced by proteolytic cleavage of membrane bound LEPR isoforms; this phenomenon is seen frequently amongst members of the cytokine receptor superfamily (79).

There are several membrane-bound LEPR isoforms, all of which include coding exons 1–17 and one of several 3′ terminal exons. Exon 16 encodes the transmembrane domain while exon 17 encodes a membrane proximal segment containing the JAK activation region to which JAK and SOCS3 bind. Two of the alternative terminal exons, 17′ and 18a, encode short cytoplasmic tails that do not appear to have functional motifs. The number of these 3′ terminal exons and LEPR isoforms

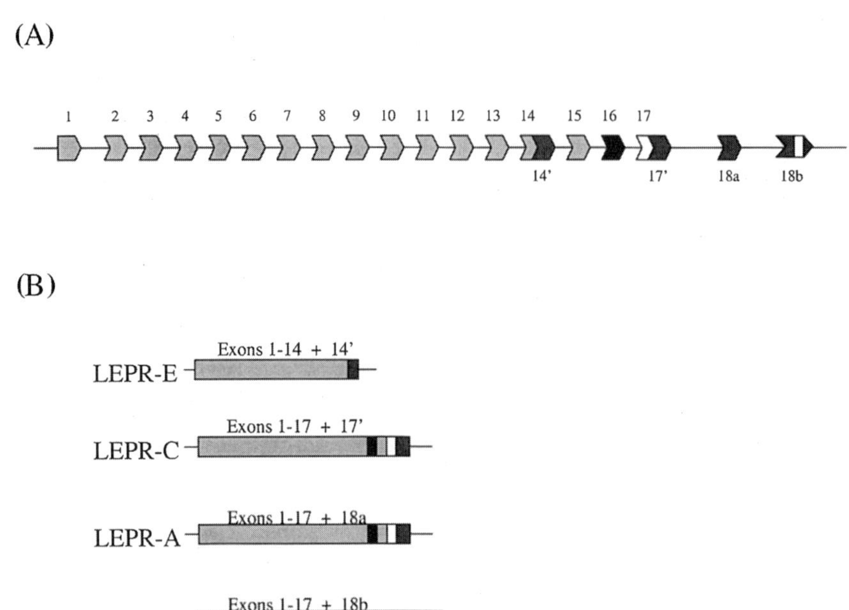

Figure 6 Genomic structure of *Lepr* and alternative transcripts. (A) Genomic structure of *Lepr*. Coding exons are in blocks and numbered. Terminal exons are denoted by numbers under the exons while coding exons are numbered above the exons (exon 16 bears a transmembrane domain). Colored blocks within exons represent sequence motifs: yellow represents a JAK box, white represents a STAT box, while a black block represents the single transmembrane domain. (B) Alternative transcripts of Lepr. Four isoforms of LEPR are represented. LEPR-E is a soluble receptor, terminating at exon 14′ and excluding the transmembrane domain (black) in exon 16. All of the membrane bound receptors (LEPR-A, LEPR-B, LEPR-C) include exon 17, which has a JAK box. The LEPR-B isoform is the sole receptor that contains the STAT box.

is species dependent; rats and humans have at least four of membrane-bound isoforms (rat LEPR-D and human B219, in addition to the ones described in detail) as opposed to the three isoforms in the mouse. Interestingly, only one LEPR isoform, LEPR-B, has a long cytoplasmic tail (accounting for its common designation as the "long-form" leptin receptor) that can activate STAT (signal transduction and transactivation) proteins. The sole loss of LEPR-B caused by the $Lepr^{db}$ mutation produces an obesity/diabetes/infertility syndrome that is identical to the loss of all LEPR isoforms by the other *Lepr* mutations (112,115), such as $Lepr^{dbPas}$ and $Lepr^{db3J}$, indicating the crucial role performed of STAT activation by the LEPR-B isoform. LEPR-B is the major isoform only in some tissues, such as in neurons of the hypothalamus and lymphocytes (89). The nature of the tissue specificity of splicing of the terminal exons remains obscure, although any investigations that suggest regulation of specific LEPR isoforms need to address this issue. Specific alterations in the ratios of LEPR isoforms are probably mediated via splicing rather than regulation via effects on transcription rates.

Another surprising aspect of LEPR isoforms is that studies have failed to detect heterodimer formation in cells transfected with two different membrane-bound LEPR isoforms—LEPR-A and LEPR-B. LEPR appears to form homodimers prior to ligand binding (116), and one can postulate that the cytoplasmic tails of the isoforms dictate preferential self-dimerization or differential sorting to various subcellular compartments.

C LEPR-B, a STAT-Competent Signaling Isoform, Is Critical for Leptin Signaling

Complete loss of LEPR mRNA results in an obesity/diabetes syndrome that is identical to that produced by the loss of the LEPR-B mRNA. This finding indicates that LEPR-B is necessary and sufficient to mediate all of leptin's actions regarding energy regulation. However, the other LEPR isoforms may perform functions outside of this context that remain to be more fully explored. LEPR-B is the only isoform that bears a STAT-activating motif (111), indicative of the critical function of STAT3 in transducing leptin receptor activation. All membrane-bound LEPR isoforms (A, B, C, and D) can bind and activate JAK. Interestingly, leptin activates

STAT3 within the hypothalamus (95), whereas leptin can activate STAT3 and STAT5 in vitro (89).

D Alleles of *Lepr* in Mice and Rats

Several additional diabetes alleles have been detected since the initial identification of *db*. The large size of *Lepr* (> 100 kbp) and easy phenotypic discrimination (severe obesity) may produce an ascertainment bias contributing to the apparent high frequency of mutations. All of the *Lepr* mutations are recessive and cause a similar phenotype, minor differences being attributable to the strain on which the specific allele is characterized. The variety of the nature of the mutations also suggests that the size of the gene provides a large target for mutational mechanisms. A relatively large number of potentially significant sequence variants have also been described in humans (see below).

1 *db*

The nature of the *db* allele has been described above. The molecular consequences of this allele are relatively minor in terms of its effects on amount of RNA. The mutation's major impact lies in the prevention of the translation of the LEPR-B isoform through the interposition of the 3′ terminal exon for the LEPR-A isoform in the LEPR-B transcript. Originally arising in the C5BLKS/J strain, this allele has been subsequently transferred to multiple strains (117). The variation in severity of diabetes in obese animals of different strains has been exploited to look for modifiers of diabetes.

2 db^{3J}

A 17-bp deletion within an exon disrupts the reading frame (118,119). As the exon is within the middle of the coding sequence and prior to the transmembrane spanning region, any leptin receptor that is produced is found as a soluble protein. Owing to the premature termination, a considerable reduction in LEPR mRNA results. The *db3J* mutation arose on the 129/J strain and showed a unique phenotype of extreme hyperinsulinemia so severe that older mutant mice were found to be hypoglycemic.

3 db^{Pas}

A large interstitial duplication exists of coding exons 3, 4, 5, and 6 (112,120). The disruption of the coding sequence probably leads to an unstable transcript and a significant reduction in LEPR mRNA. The duplication occurs prior to the putative ligand-binding domain and any LEPR produced would be predicted to be unable to bind leptin. This allele was discovered in the DW strain maintained at the Pasteur Institute.

4 db^{NCSU}

A single basepair deletion in an exon reduces LEPR mRNA and shifts the reading frame of all LEPR isoforms (121). No membrane bound isoforms are expressed by this mutant allele. This mutation occurred in an outbred population of CD1 mice maintained at North Carolina State University. The stock is directly descended from Swiss albino mice and is genetically unrelated to most of the mouse stocks on which *ob* and *db* have been analyzed. The severe diabetic phenotype of these mice highlights the importance of strain background in determining diabetes susceptibility in rodents.

5 $Lepr^{Tg(Mth11)1Aig}$

This is a mutation due to a transgenic insertion coupled with deletion of all exons 3′ to coding exon 17′ (122,123). This mutation illustrates some of the difficulties encountered with molecular analysis due to transgenesis. The insertion of the transgene would probably have been sufficient to inactivate Lepr transcription. However, additional molecular events, such as large-scale deletions or rearrangements, are possible and compound the analysis of the effects of the mutational event.

E Extinct $Lepr^{db}$ Mutations

Two documented alleles for *db* were described although no DNA is available for molecular analysis. The two alleles are db^{ad} and db^{2J}. The db^{ad} allele was described in 1959 and demonstrated to be allelic to *db* (124). Interestingly, this allele was also discovered in mouse lines that were being selected for large size and increased growth, similar to the background for discovery of *fatty* and the $Socs2^{hg}$ mutations. The db^{2J} mutation was discovered at Jackson Laboratories as indicated by its allelic designation and found to be allelic to the first *db* mutation (104). This was the mutation with which some of the initial comparisons of strain effects on the obesity-diabetes syndrome were performed.

1 *fatty*

The *fatty* mutation arose in an outbred population of rats that had been generated to study genetic effects on nutrition and body weight regulation (106). The 13M stock was made heterogeneous by outcrosses of at least four different rat strains at the outset of the experiment to maximize diversity in the gene pool. The spontaneous recessive *fatty* mutation produced the obese phenotype. Obese rats of the outbred Zucker stock are obese and mildly glucose intolerant but never develop overt hyperglycemia and glycosuria. In keeping with the minimal pathology associated with obesity in the Zucker stock, obese males are occasionally fertile. This trait can be selected for and the proportion of fertile obese males can be significantly enhanced by this procedure. This is in contrast to two inbred rat strains derived from the original 13M fatty stock—the Zucker Diabetic Fatty [ZDF (125)] and the Wistar Diabetic Fatty [WDF (126,127)]. The ZDF rats were derived by initial selection of the 13M stock for pairs that produced obese diabetic progeny, and subsequent inbreeding to fix the diabetic trait. The WDF rats were produced simply by transferring the *fatty* mutation to the WKY/N inbred strain. The resulting co-isogenic WDF strain produced obese rats with severe diabetes. Obese males of the ZDF and WDF strains are much more severely affected in terms of diabetes than obese females, following a trend of some protective effect of female sex found in most obese mice. It has been proposed that sulfurylation of estrogens by sulfotransferases differentially expressed between the sexes might be responsible for this effect (128).

The *fatty* mutation is a point mutation that substitutes a proline for glutamine at residue 269 (129,130). The effect of this mutation on RNA abundance and protein abundance is negligible. In fact, the mutant protein binds leptin with an affinity equal to the native receptor. Thus, the mutation was not helpful in the initial attempts to show that leptin receptor mutations were responsible for the obese phenotype. However, the mutant protein fails to be expressed at the cell surface, presumably owing to misfolding and inappropriate subcellular sorting. Thus, the mutation abrogates leptin-dependent STAT3 activation. However, the mutant protein has constitutive STAT activating activity, although at a much lower level than the native receptor.

2 $fatty^f$

This mutation arose in a cross between Sprague-Dawley and spontaneously hypertensive rats (SHR). The mutation was given a provisional symbol "*f*" by its discoverer, Koletsky (107). The stock has been maintained as such and has been duly named the Koletsky mutation (fa^K). Owing to the SHR background, obese rats showed profound pathology associated with obesity, hyperglycemia, hyperlipidemia, and hypertension. Subsequently, the mutation was transferred to two other inbred strains (131,132), LA/N and SHR/N, and was given another name, *corpulent*. The obese LA rats are mildly hyperglycemic and are quite similar in phenotype to obese C57BL/6J mice, whereas obese SHR rats are obese and overtly hyperglycemic, suffering early mortality due to the diabetes and hypertension imposed by the strain background. In order to limit the profusion/confusion of names, and to comply with terminology precedents, it is preferable to use the initial symbol given, $fatty^f$.

The $fatty^f$ mutation is a single base substitution that generates a premature termination codon prior to the transmembrane domain (133,134). The amount of LEPR mRNA is greatly reduced by the mutation, probably due to degradation of the mutant transcript by nonsense-mediated decay. However, sufficient amounts of LEPR mRNA remain to permit amplification and subsequent sequence analysis as the mutation was identified from amplified cDNA.

F Critical Tissues and Cells That Mediate Leptin's Actions

All of leptin's actions on hyperphagia and glucose metabolism appear to be mediated by the brain since small intracranial infusions of leptin can normalize ingestive behavior and glucose tolérance in *ob* mice. However, it remains to be determined whether all of leptin's actions on metabolism and ingestion are mediated by the brain. Due to the specific actions of leptin on lymphocytes and vascular endothelium, which are not mediated by the brain, it is possible that adipocytes, hepatocytes, pancreatic beta cells, and muscle cells can be directly affected by leptin. However, these extrahypothalamic contributions toward energy homeostasis must be of a small magnitude since LEPR-B expression within the brain is sufficient to correct most or all of the obesity/diabetes syndrome of leptin receptor deficiency (135).

LEPR-B is expressed in many of the critical hypothalamic neuronal populations that regulate energy balance—NPY/AGRP, POMC/CART, TRH, CRH, and MCH. Moreover, leptin regulates the expression of these neuropeptide genes (via STAT-mediated transcription effects) and modulates their release (probably by effects on membrane potential). These effects of leptin occur over a longer time interval than most effectors, taking ~20–30 min to attain maximal effect (45,97). However, these effects are also long-lasting and take up to an hour to dissipate after the initial stimulus. While the stimulatory effect of leptin on POMC activity can be explained by stimulatory effects of STAT3 on *Pomc* transcription, it is more difficult to relate STAT3 activation to the suppression of *Npy* and *Agrp* transcription. There is no doubt regarding the effects of leptin on these genes (136) since leptin can reverse the fasting-induced changes in *Pomc* (leptin reverses fasting-related inhibition) and *Npy* (leptin reverses fasting-related induction).

Since it has been identified that leptin, upon binding to its receptor, activated STAT3 in the hypothalamus, it was interesting to note that ciliary neurotrophic factor (CNTF), another cytokine, could mimic the anorexigenic effects of leptin (137). Similar to leptin, CNTF and its analogs activate STAT3 within the hypothalamus by a mechanism that is not dependent upon LEPR, since the effect is seen in *db/db* animals. Presumably, there is considerable overlap between the distributions of LEPR and CNTFR, although this has not been directly determined. The drug axokine, which activates CNTFR, is under trial as a weight-reducing agent.

G Modulation of the Hyperglycemia and Insulinopenia of C57BLKS-*db* Mice

The severe diabetic syndrome of *db/db* C57BLKS/J mice is not an irremediable phenotype. Food restriction can ameliorate the diabetes and prevent early mortality although the mutant mice still develop hyperglycemia (138). The diabetes is not an autoimmune phenomenon although some autoimmune markers can be observed, such as islet immunoreactive antibodies (139). An intact immune system, either T-cells, B-cells, or both, is not necessary for the development of the diabetes. However, a simple nutritional modification, substitution of all carbohydrate sources in the diet with protein, can prevent the development of hyperglycemia, insulinopenia, and pancreatic beta-cell loss (138). There appears to be a critical period for this protective effect of dietary manipulation since it is most effective within the first 1 or 2 weeks after weaning. Mutant mice that are older cannot be rescued by this diet, suggesting that there has been a depletion of precursor stem cells or that a block in capacity for differentiation has occurred. The molecular bases of this diabetes susceptibility remains to be further explored since there are numerous well-characterized inbred strains that differ in their diabetes susceptibility. While it is possible that a simple two-allele system is responsible for this diabetes susceptibility, it is just as likely that a large set of genes and their allelic variants are responsible for differential diabetes susceptibility among different rodent strains. These genes may affect beta-cell development and function, and insulin sensitivity in muscle, liver, and adipose tissue.

H Adrenal Steroids Affect the Progression of Obesity

Adrenalectomy can halt or reverse the development of obesity in virtually all genetically obese rodents. Obese *ob* and *db* mice have supraphysiological circulating concentrations of corticosterone, the main glucocorticoid in rodents (140,141). After adrenalectomy, subphysiological replacement doses of corticosterone allow the full expression of the obesity (142). Thus, these mutant animals are apparently hypersensitive to these effects of corticosterone. The full physiological impact of glucocorticoids requires further exploration. However, it has been shown that many of the neuropeptide genes within the hypothalamus are modulated by glucocorticoids. Whether it is all of these genes that are affected by adrenal steroids or a select few remains to be determined.

V CARBOXYPEPTIDASE E (*fat*)

The *fat* mutation was identified in a colony of HRS/J mice (carrying the *hairless* mutation) and subsequently transferred to the C57BLKS/J strain for ease of propagation and comparative studies with other obesity mutations (143). The obesity develops in adult animals and is obvious at approximately a similar age as in A^y mice. Mutant mice of both sexes are infertile, as has been found for many of the recessive obese mutations maintained on the C57BL strains. The mutants are also glucose intolerant with hyperinsulinemia of a sort that is unlike that seen in any of the other mouse obesity mutants. The insulin found in the blood is primarily proinsulin produced from the two insulin genes of the mouse genome (144). This remarkable observation, coupled with the chromosomal mapping of the mutation, was crucial to the eventual identification of the *fat* mutation.

The gene that is mutated in *fat* mice was, at the time of the identification of the mutation, a well-characterized enzyme, carboxypeptidase E, a member of a family of carboxypeptidases that have similar and overlapping activities (145). The carboxypeptidases cleave the carboxyl residues from proteolytically cleaved substrates of proprotein convertases. Some substrates can be cleaved by multiple carboxypeptidases, such as carboxypeptidase D cleaving similar substrates as CPE. CPE is found in many secretory tissues (islet beta cells and salivary glands among them) as well as the brain and neuroendocrine organs. While the activity of CPE was well known, it remained for studies of the CPE mutation to highlight the central role of CPE in processing of many hormones and neuropeptides.

A Molecular Clues to the Identification of the *Cpe*^{fat} Mutation

As previously mentioned, Ed Leiter had observed the profound hyperproinsulinemia of *fat* mutants. He had also mapped the *fat* mutation to chromosome 8 within an interval that contained the *Cpe* locus. Further characterization of the nature of the circulating proinsulin indicated that the proinsulins were extended by an amino acid at the carboxy terminus, a defect that was consistent with a lack of carboxypeptidase processing. The identification of the *fat* mutation highlights the value of key observations regarding the basic pathological processes affected by a mutation combined with relatively crude genetic mapping—an excellent candidate gene was immediately identified.

B Nature of the *fat* Mutation

These observations led to the direct test for mutations of the *Cpe* gene in *fat* mutants and the identification of a point mutation in the *Cpe* coding sequence that causes a Ser202Pro substitution. Although the mutation did not alter mRNA abundance or protein levels, there was a complete loss of CPE enzymatic activity. The simple amino acid substitution would not be predicted to alter transcript size or abundance or to affect translation. However, the amino acid substitution presumably affects the three dimensional structure of the protein so that the protein is misfolded leading to either an inactive conformation or defective sorting to the appropriate subcellular compartments.

C CPE Functions as a Sorting Enzyme in the Regulated Secretory Pathway

A characterization of the proteolytic products and the secretory pathways of protein in CPE-deficient cells and tissues led to discovery of another previously unknown function of CPE. There are two major cellular pathways for protein secretion: the constitutive secretory pathway, and the regulated secretory pathway (146). The constitutive pathway secretes proteins continuously and these proteins are mainly minimally processed in terms of proteolytic cleavage and other posttranslational modifications. The regulated secretory pathway is used by many secretory cells, including neuroendocrine cells, to control the timing and rate of secretion of many extensively processed hormones and neuropeptides, e.g., POMC (147) and preproinsulin. CPE-deficient cells constitutively secrete neuropeptides and hormones in their partially processed states that are usually inactive or retained only partial activity (148). It was discovered that CPE has a membrane-bound form that is the sorting protein that funnels prohormones to the regulated secretory pathway by recognizing sequence motifs within the prohormones. This function could be the major defect in fat mice, since other carboxypeptidases could compensate for proteolytic deficiency. The inability to sort most peptide hormones and neuropeptides to the appropriate secretory pathway would effectively inactivate regulated secretion of neurons, neuroendocrine and endocrine cells, preventing effective regulation of the intricate networks that rely on cosecretion and feedback stimuli (both positive and negative).

D Defective Neuropeptide Processing Probably Underlies the Obesity of *fat* Mutants

As would be expected, the brains of fat mice show numerous abnormalities in neuropeptide content. Almost all neuropeptides are processed via the regulated secretory pathway and require CPE function, both for proteolytic cleavage and for sorting (149). Chief among these defects are deficiencies in the processing of POMC and CCK (150) that might be predicted to lead to a loss of inhibition of food intake. Orexigenic peptides such as MCH are also improperly processed in *fat* mice, perhaps muting somewhat the increase in food intake that might occur if only anorexiant peptides were affected. However, the action of the extremely potent orexiant, AGRP, may actually be enhanced by CPE deficiency. In the AGRP transgenic mouse, constitutive expression of unprocessed AGRP is sufficient to promote hyperphagia and obesity. Thus, the net effect of CPE deficiency on anorexigenic and orexigenic peptides and neurons could result in obesity.

VI *TUBBY*

The *tubby* mutation was identified as a recessive allele that produced mild, late onset obesity in C57BL/6J mice (143). Subsequently, the mice were also found to suffer from vision and hearing loss, owing to retinal degeneration and the loss of cochlear hair cells, respectively, by apoptosis (151). The identification of the gene and the mutation were achieved through positional cloning approaches by two groups (152,153). The gene encodes the founding member of a novel gene family that includes TULP1, TULP2, and TULP3. TULP1 mutations are responsible for some forms of retinitis pigmentosa in nonobese humans (154), suggesting that there may be common features and functions between members of this family. The *tubby* mutation alters 3′ splice donor site causing the loss of 44 carboxyl terminal amino acids and their replacement by 22 intron-encoded amino residues. Thus, the carboxyl terminus is essential for the function of tubby protein.

A Molecular Clues to the Identification of the *Tubby* Mutation

The *Tubby* gene was isolated by positional cloning (152,153). A physical contig was generated that was analyzed by exon trapping and direct sequencing. Putative exons were found that hybridized to a transcript that was increased in size by ~ 400 bp (7.5 kb in tubby brain vs. 7 kb in normal brain) and was increased in amount in the mutant. The eventual identification of the splice donor site mutation in the penultimate exon (exon 11 of a total of 12 exons) fully explained the anomalous mutant transcript's size and quantity. The loss of the donor splice site prevented the excision of the last intron (~ 400 bp in length), leading to the increased transcript size. The increased transcript amount could be explained by lack of possible feedback inhibition, and the premature termination codon in the now terminal exon that protected the mutant transcript from nonsense-mediated mRNA decay that usually acts on mutations occurring prior to the terminal exon.

B Tubby Encodes a Transcriptional Transactivator Activated by Gq-Coupled Receptors

The tubby protein is expressed in neural tissues, primarily in the hypothalamus (arcuate, PVN, and VMN) and other regions of the brain, as well as the retina and cochlea. Within neuronal cells, the tubby protein is localized to the nucleolus (155). While increased apoptosis has been implicated as a causal mechanism for the loss of hearing and vision, this is unlikely to be the case for the obesity and hypothalamic neurons. Expression studies show that *tubby* mRNA is increased in the hypothalamus of mutant mice. This would be unlikely to be the case if neurons were being eliminated via apoptosis. A selective reduction of a subpopulation of neurons is possible since there is a small reduction of NPY mRNA in the arcuate nucleus of *tubby* mice with a concomitant induction of NPY expression in the VMN and the DMN (156). This is very similar to the pattern of expression of NPY mRNA in A^y mice, suggesting that altered neuropeptide gene expression, as a result of faulty TUBBY transactivation, might be the responsible obesity-producing mechanism. Also, POMC mRNA is greatly reduced in mature, obese *tubby* mutants although this has not been observed in young, preobese mutant mice. In favor of selective apoptosis of a neuronal subpopulation is that a similar phenomenon of ectopic induction of NPY mRNA is observed in mice with lesions of the hypothalamic arcuate nucleus generated by gold thioglucose (GTG treatment of adult mice) and glutamate (MSG treatment of neonates). Therefore, the mechanism causing obesity in *tubby* mice remains to be determined, at both the molecular and cellular levels.

In a novel approach to understanding the function of tubby protein, structural analyses were conducted to determine the conformation of the protein (157,158). The amino terminus has a simple sequence that is a characteristic of transactivating domains while the carboxyl terminus bears a large groove lined with positively charged amino acids that binds and bends double stranded DNA, a characteristic of DNA binding domains of transcriptional transactivators. An interesting feature of the tubby protein is its dual localization to the plasma membrane and the nucleus, having a sequence motif in its carboxyl terminus that binds phosphotidylinositides, anchoring it to the plasma membrane as well as a nuclear localization sequence near the carboxyl end.

Tubby is functionally coupled to Gq protein and Gq-coupled receptors. HTR2C is such a receptor (see below). Activation of HTR2C and Gq-coupled receptors causes the release of tubby protein from its plasma membrane anchor resulting in translocation into the nucleus, presumably to function as a transcriptional transactivator of target genes that remain to be identified. Given the similarities in the obese phenotypes of *tubby* and *Htr2c* knockout mice, it is quite possible that the functional coupling described in vitro faithfully reflects the situation in the brain.

There have been no studies of the ingestive behavior of *tubby* mice, and it remains to be resolved whether the mild obesity is due to hyperphagia or increased metabolic efficiency. However, the late-onset obesity and degree of adiposity are similar to the phenotype of *Htr2c* knockout mice, which have been reported to be purely hyperphagic. One can surmise that tubby mutant mice develop obesity due to mild hyperphagia, but it remains to be determined whether there is a metabolic component to the weight gain.

C Modifier of Tubby Hearing—*Moth1*

In outcross progeny, Tubby homozygotes are not uniformly deaf. A modifier gene, *moth1*, for modifier of tubby hearing, was localized to chromosome 2 (155). Analysis of the mode of inheritance indicated that the B6 allele was recessive suggesting that a loss-of-function mutation is present in the C57BL/6J strain that is only manifest in the absence of tubby protein. Because no other phenotypes were analyzed, it is not known whether the modifier affects the degree of obesity and the retinal degeneration. However, since retinal degeneration due to *TULP1* mutations (humans and mice) is the only phenotype, and the mutations do not produce obesity or deafness, it is quite possible that tissue-specific expression of *moth1* would only manifest as an effect on hearing.

VII CCK AND CCK RECEPTORS

Cholecystokinin has satiety-producing effects during the ingestion of a meal (159). Exogenous CCK will limit meal size, and the prevention of intestinal CCK release will lead to continuous ingestion, as modeled in rats with gastric cannulae during sham-feeding studies. The action of intestinal CCK appears to be mediated by CCK receptors on afferent vagal neurons, although a direct action of CCK in the brain has also been suggested.

A spontaneous mutation of the CCK-A receptor has been identified in a rat model of adult-onset obesity and diabetes, the Otsuka Long-Evans Takashima Fatty rat (OLETF) (160). The recessive mutation is due to a deletion of a large segment of the *CCKAR* gene. The affected rats ingest larger meals, consistent with a defect in satiation mediated by the CCK receptor (161,162). However, mutant mice with a knockout of the *Cck* (163) or the *Cckbr* (164) genes do not develop obesity, although they are resistant to the satiety effects of CCK. In addition, humans with apparent inactivating mutations of CCKAR are not obese.

It appears that the role of CCK differs among mice, rats, and humans. CCK appears to play a more central role in satiation in rats. Alternatively, the OLETF rat may have another mutation in another locus that interacts with the CCKAR deficiency to produce obesity. This is quite possible since a diabetes phenotype in OLETF rats is dependent on two loci. This rat obesity model suggests that mutations at multiple loci can interact to produce an obese phenotype that mimics the effects of single gene mutations.

VIII HUMAN SINGLE-GENE OBESITIES

Human orthologs for all of the spontaneous rodent single gene obesities have been identified. Mutations in human orthologs of *Lep*, *Lepr*, and *Cpe* (*PC1* in human) that result in obesity have been described (see below). These important instances confirm the role of these genes and their constituent pathways in the regulation of body fat in humans. However, such mutations, and other single-gene obesities, account for only a small number of instances of human obesity (165)]. Association and linkage studies, as well as physiological data, indicate that most instances of human obesity are not due to mutations in a single gene. However, such instances are of great importance for the insights they provide with regard to the molecular physiology of weight regulation.

A Orthologs of Single-Gene Obesities in Rodents

1 Leptin. *LEP* (7q31.3)

a. LEP G398→Del

Montague et al. (166) reported a consanguineous Pakistani family with two children who were homozygous for an inactivating G398→Del leptin mutation. The children (8-year-old girl, BMI 45.8; 2-year-old boy, BMI 36.6) were identified because of their extreme obesity and hyperphagia; both had heights at the 75th centile for their ages. The mutation creates a frameshift resulting from the deletion of a guanine nucleotide at position 398, codon 133. Fourteen amino acids are introduced into the reading frame of the mutant protein, followed by a premature stop codon. Transient transfection experiments of CHO cells with the mutant protein demonstrated the presence of mutant leptin in the cell lysates but none was secreted, suggesting abnormal protein transport within the cell. Western blot analysis of the sera of the affected children showed no serum leptin, supporting the prediction that the mutation prevented protein secretion. In this sense, the functional effect of this human mutation closely resembles that of Lep^{ob}.

Similar to *ob/ob* mice with inactivating leptin mutations, these children developed early-onset, severe hyperphagia and obesity. These children had few associated endocrine abnormalities, mainly mild euglycemic hyperinsulinemia. The older child had much higher insulin concentrations than the younger child, suggesting an increase of insulin resistance with age. Of note, however, the. mild hyperinsulinemia was much less than the striking elevations seen in *ob*/*ob* mice. The young children also had gonadal axis profiles consistent with a pre-pubertal state. In distinction to the *ob*/*ob* mice, both children had normal plasma cortisol and body temperature; the older child responded normally to a 1-mg dexamethasone suppression test. Both children showed slight elevations of TSH, in contrast to the mild hypothalamic hypothyroidism of the *ob*/*ob* mouse. Growth hormone was not studied, though the older child's growth velocity was normal and she had an advanced bone age (at age 9 years, bone age was 12.5 years) (167). As indicated earlier, *ob*/*ob* mice display hypogonadotropic hypogonadism, as have human subjects found to have inactivating *LEP* and *LEPR* mutations. However, at least one female with an inactivating *LEPR* mutation has entered spontaneous puberty at age 21 years (personal communication, K. Clement). Thus, as for the effects of *ob* on sexual maturation in mice (see above) (168,169), there may be important genetic modifiers of leptin actions on the gonadal axis in humans. The older child was subsequently treated with a 12-month course of daily subcutaneous recombinant leptin, 0.028 mg/kg lean body mass (167). This dose was chosen to achieve peak serum leptin concentrations of 10% of the predicted normal leptin for this obese child (70 ng/mL). She experienced a 16.4-kg weight loss during the 12-month treatment period; 95% of the weight loss was due to loss of body fat. She also had a significant and rapid change in her eating behavior (within 1 week of initiating leptin injections): she ate much less food, at a slower rate, and did not seek or request food between meals. The reduction in food intake was sustained throughout the study. She had similar total energy expenditure before and after 12 months of therapy, so the leptin therapy primarily affected her energy intake, not her energy expenditure. At the start of therapy, the subject had endocrinologic studies consistent with a prepubertal state; after 1 year of therapy (at age 10), she had a profile consistent with early puberty: nocturnal, pulsatile gonadotropin secretion.

b. LEP Arg105Trp C→T

A second family with an inactivating missense leptin mutation was described by Strobel et al. (170). Two homozygous subjects were members of a highly consanguineous Turkish family. The mutation was a C→T missense mutation leading to Arg105Trp, which is similar to *ob* mice that have an Arg105STOP mutation. COS-1 expression studies showed the presence of immunoreactive protein in cell lysates but no secretion, similar to the G398→Del mutation in the Pakistani kindred. One subject was a 22-year-old male, BMI 55.8, and the second was a 24-year-old female, BMI 46.9. Both had early-onset hyperphagia and obesity. The affected woman had primary amenorrhea, and the male had evidence of hypothalamic hypogonadism. The adult male subject also had evidence of reduced sympathetic autonomic nervous system tone (low systolic blood pressure in response to cold pressor test, reduced sympathetic skin response, and mild orthostatic hypotension). The homozygous Arg105Trp C→T mutation was found in three additional obese relatives of these individuals. Family members heterozygous for the *LEP* mutation were said to be of normal body weight and to have normal plasma leptin concentrations. Subsequent studies of three nominally unrelated Pakistani families segregating for a del G133 (glycine deletion) mutation in *LEP* have found increased body fat and low circulating leptin in heterozygous individuals (171). These findings are remarkably similar to those reported earlier in mice heterozygous for the Lep^{ob} and $Lepr^{db}$ mutations (172), and support the idea that moderate deficiency of leptin may have physiological consequences (173). While several large studies have demonstrated the rarity of major *LEP* mutations in obese humans (174,175), minor differences in *LEP* coding or regulatory sequences could contribute to variation in body fat in humans (Table 2). As possible evidence of such effects, among humans with the same body fat, serum leptin concentrations vary considerably, either higher or lower than expected given the subject's degree of adiposity (176,177). Also, molecular markers in the region of *LEP* (7q31.3) have been linked to skinfold thickness using a sibship database of Mexican-American probands with type 2 diabetes (178), and a *LEP* polymorphism (A19G in first [untranslated] exon) has been associated with severe obesity in some studies (179). And, finally, that humans, mice, and rats heterozygous for mutations in leptin or the leptin receptor are fatter than wild-type individuals indicates that the systems regulating body composition are sensitive to partial deficiencies of these molecules (173).

2 Leptin Receptor. *LEPR* (1p31-p22)

Clement et al. (180) described three sisters from a consanguineous Algerian family (Berbers) who were homozygous for an inactivating *LEPR* mutation: IVS16, G→A, +1. The mutation is in the 3′ donor splice site

Table 2 *LEP* Mutations in Human Subjects

Mutation	Association with obesity	Refs.
G398→Del	Yes	(166)
Arg105Trp C→T	Yes	(170)
A19G	Variable association	(323–325)
−2548 G→A	Effects on BMI in response to diet; polymorphism more frequent in obese population	(323,326)
−2437 T→G	Effects on BMI in response to diet	(323)
−1887 C→T	Effects on BMI in response to diet	(323)
−1823 C→T	Effects on BMI in response to diet	(323)
−1387 G→A	Effects on BMI in response to diet	(323)
−633 C→T	Effects on BMI in response to diet	(323)
−188 C→A	Effects on BMI in response to diet	(323,327)
Gln25Gln (nucleotide 131)	None	(328)
G144A	Decreased leptin concentration in 2 subjects	(324)
G328A; Ala110Met	Decreased leptin concentration in 2 subjects	(324)
C538T	None; silent mutation	(324)

of exon 16 and results in skipping of this exon. The resulting protein is truncated (831 amino acids) and lacks the transmembrane and intracellular domains. Accordingly, the long form of the leptin receptor (1162 amino acids with STAT binding domain) is completely absent in these subjects, similar to the *db/db* mouse. The three affected sisters had early-onset obesity and severe hyperphagia. At ages 13, 19, and 19 (now deceased) years, they had BMIs of 71.5, 65.5, and 52.5, respectively, and had heights considered low for their degree of obesity (25–50th centile for age) (181). Leptin concentrations were much higher than predicted based on their degree of adiposity (670 and 600 ng/mL, respectively). The five heterozygous family members had intermediate levels of circulating leptin and were moderately obese (BMI range 26.5–31). Interestingly, in both homozygous and heterozygous individuals, 80% of circulating leptin was in a high molecular weight (MW) complex (~450 kDa), whereas in nonmutant individuals, only 5–20% of circulating leptin is present in the high MW form (51,182).

Endocrine studies of the surviving homozygous subjects showed absence of a nighttime GH surge with reduced GH release in response to secretagogues. IGF-1 concentration was low, but increased after GH administration, a response also characteristic of GH-deficient subjects. The affecteds had no physical changes suggestive of puberty and had low estradiol, LH, and FSH levels consistent with central hypogonadism. However, as indicated above, one of the females has entered puberty spontaneously at age 21 years.

Besides this Berber family reported by Clement et al. (180), several studies of obese humans have found a high frequency of sequence variation in the coding sequences of *LEPR* but none which unequivocally lead to obesity (183). Also, several association studies showed no connection between *LEPR* allelic variation and adiposity (184–186), and a Danish study found no association between *LEPR* variations and early-onset obesity (187). A recent meta-analysis of data from nine independent studies (3263 individuals) also showed no significant linkage of these sequence variants to BMI (188) (Table 3).

3 Melanocortin 4 Receptor. *MC4R* (18q21.3-q22)

The molecular physiology of the melanocortin system is described above. Inactivating *MC4R* mutations were originally described in two nonconsanguineous families; all subjects were heterozygous for mutations that segregated in a dominant fashion (189,190). These are the only reported cases of dominantly expressed obesity in humans, similar to the codominant obesity of *Mc4r* null mice. One family had a 4-bp deletion at codon 211 (4-BP DEL, NT631), and the second family had a 4-bp insertion at codon 244 (4-BP INS, NT732). In both cases, these frameshift mutations led to truncation of the protein in either the fifth or sixth transmembrane region, respectively. Since the transmembrane regions are critical for obtaining proper receptor conformation, mutations affecting/obliterat-

Table 3 *LEPR* Mutations in Human Subjects

Mutation	Association with obesity	Ref.
Lys109Arg	Variable	(183,185,187,329,330)
Lys204Arg	No association with obesity	(187,331)
Gln223Arg	Variable	(183,185–187,329,330,332–335)
Ser343Ser	No association with BMI	(185)
Lys656Asn	Variable	(183,185–187,330)
Ser675Thr	Found in 2 subjects	(331)
Pro1019Pro	Variable	(185,332)
Codon 986 (silent)	Associated with BMI among lean subjects	(185)
IVS16, G→A, +1	Found in 3 subjects	(180)

ing specific transmembrane regions would be predicted to significantly affect receptor functioning. The affected subjects had childhood-onset hyperphagia and obesity with elevated leptin concentrations consistent with their level of adiposity.

To date, 27 mutations have been described in *MC4R*, the majority of which are associated with obesity. However, for some apparently significant deletions (191) and missense mutations (192), variable or no phenotypic impact has been reported. In some studies, 5% of morbidly obese subjects have been reported to be heterozygous for *MC4R* mutations (193).

4 Pro-opiomelanocortin. *POMC*(2p23.2)

POMC is synthesized as a large precursor molecule, pre-POMC, that is processed in the pituitary into several transcripts, including ACTH, αMSH, β-lipotropin, and β-endorphin (see Fig. 3). PC1 cleaves POMC into ACTH and β-lipotropin, whereas PC2 cleaves POMC into β-endorphin and αMSH (see Fig. 3). Krude et al. (194) described two unrelated children with inactivating *POMC* mutations. Both had severe, early-onset obesity, adrenal insufficiency, and red hair. The phenotypes are consistent with absence of the pre-POMC cleavage products: ACTH and αMSH. The functional consequences of absence of ACTH and αMSH ligand/receptor activity are discussed with regard to the relevant mouse mutations above. The light skin and hair of the children with these mutations are due to reduced MSH activity at MC1R.

One patient was a 3-year-old girl who weighed 32 kg and was a compound heterozygote for mutations in exon 3: G7013T and C7133Del (194). Both mutations in the 3-year-old led to premature termination of POMC, at codons 79 and 131, respectively, and absence of ACTH, α MSH, and β-endorphin. She had no detectable circulating ACTH or cortisol after CRH stimulation, but the other anterior pituitary hormones were in the normal range. Her older brother, who had died at 7 months, was found on autopsy to have bilateral adrenal hypoplasia, which led to recognition of his sister's similar status at 23 days of life. His newborn screening filter paper blood specimen was located after his death and used for *POMC* mutation analysis; he had the same *POMC* genotype as his sister.

The second subject was a 5-year-old boy who weighed 48 kg, had adrenal insufficiency and red hair, and was homozygous for C3804A which is 11 bp 5′ of the normal start site of the 5′UTR in exon 2 (194). This mutation adds an out-of-frame start codon within a consensus sequence for translation initiation and is thus predicted to abolish *POMC* translation. Consistent with this prediction, the subject had no detectable circulating ACTH. The obligate heterozygote parents were described as having normal body weight and dark hair.

There have been at least 14 other *POMC* mutations described, but none with complete loss of POMC cleavage products, though most are associated with obesity (except for several silent mutations) (192) (see Table 4). Linkage studies have shown that a region on chromosome 2 that includes *POMC* accounted for 32% of variation in fat mass and 47% of variation in serum leptin concentration (195,196).

5 *PC1* (5q15-q21)

Prohormone convertase 1, also called PCSK1 or PC3, is a member of the family of serine proteases of the subtilisin family that are located in acidic secretory vesicles (197). PC1 acts just proximal to carboxypeptidase E (CPE) in the posttranslational processing of many prohormones and proneuropeptides, including insulin. Specifically, PC1 cleaves proinsulin at a dibasic peptide, Arg31-Arg32, joining the B-chain and C-peptide. Thus,

Table 4 *POMC* Mutations in Human Subjects

Mutation in *POMC*; location	Mechanism (Ref.)
G7013T, C7133del exon 3	Interference with appropriate synthesis of ACTH and α-MSH (194)
C3804A exon 2	Abolishes POMC translation (194)
Nucleotide 51 (promoter) G→C	Silent (336)
Nucleotide 670 (5′UTR) G→A	
Nucleotide 4512 (codon 6) C→T, Cys/Cys	
Nucleotide 7726 (codon 116) C→T, Leu/Leu	
Nucleotide 8246 (3′UTR) C→T	
Nucleotide 8086 (codon 236) G→C, Arg/Gln	Seen in only 1 subject (336)
In-frame 9-bp insertion and 18-bp insertion between codons 73, 74	Insertion of either Ser-Ser-Gly or Ser-Ser-Gly-Ser-Ser-Gly (337)
Out-of-frame 6-bp insertion within codon 176, GGG CCC	Insertion of Arg-Ala (337)
Glu188Gly	Missense (337)
G7016A, Asp80Asn	Missense (337)
C6982T, C7285T	Silent (337)
C3832T	Silent (337)
C7111G	Silent (337)
G7316T, Glu180Stop	Premature stop codon within γ-LPH sequence (337)

PC1 is crucial to the regulation of insulin biosynthesis. In the *fat* mouse (see above for details), CPE deficiency leads to altered processing of proinsulin, POMC, GH, CCK, neurotensin, MCH, and gastrin. The Cpe^{fat} mice display a late-onset, moderate obesity (198–202).

While no *CPE* mutations leading to obesity have been described in humans, there has been one instance of obesity associated with mutations in *PC1* (203). O'Rahilly et al. (203) described a morbidly obese 43-year-old woman (89.2 kg) with childhood-onset extreme obesity (36 kg by age 3 years). She was found to be a compound heterozygote for mutations in *PC1*: G483R and A→C +4 at the donor splice site of exon 5 (IVS5DS, A-C, +4) (203). G483R prevents processing of the proPC1 molecule, and the second mutation (IVS5DS, A-C, +4) causes a frameshift and a premature stop codon. The patient's endocrine phenotype was characterized by extremely high circulating proinsulin concentration, nearly undetectable insulin, hypocortisolism, and hypogonadotropic hypogonadism, all consistent with impaired processing of the respective prohormones. Interestingly, the Cpe^{fat} mice display hyperproinsulinemia, consistent with their more distal enzymatic defect in carboxypeptidase E.

6 PPARγ (3p25)

PPARγ2 is specifically expressed in adipose tissue, is induced early in adipocyte differentiation, and, when experimentally expressed in fibroblasts, induces the fibroblasts to differentiate into adipocytes. Since PPARγ2 leads to adipocyte differentiation and thus fat cell accumulation, the more active the PPARγ2 protein (activating mutations), the higher the BMI and the higher the risk for insulin resistance. Similarly, the less active the PPARγ2 molecule is at inducing adipocyte differentiation (inactivating mutations), the lower the BMI with improved insulin sensitivity. When activated by agonists such as thiazolidinediones, PPARγ2 acts an insulin sensitizer in adipose tissue, liver, skeletal muscle, and kidney. There have been six mutations described in PPARγ2 with inconsistent associations with obesity.

In expression studies, Pro12Ala decreases TZD-mediated transcriptional activation and adipogenesis (204). Pro12Ala was associated with higher insulin sensitivity and reduced BMI (205,206), but the apparent effect on insulin sensitivity was eliminated by correction for BMI. Other studies have found an association with an increased BMI (207,208), while two studies have not found such an association (209,210). Meta-analysis indicated that Pro12Ala was associated with a decreased risk for type 2 diabetes mellitus (211). A potential explanation of these conflicting findings comes from the recent paper of Hasstedt et al. (212), in which Pro12Ala was found to act as a recessive mutation with effects on many traits associated with the insulin resistance syndrome (including BMI, blood pressure, triglyceride levels, and glucose tolerance), and had a homozygote frequency of 1–2% of the population. The varying associations with Pro12Ala found in the literature could be due to population differences in the frequency of the mutation (212).

Meirhaeghe et al. (213) examined whether a relatively common, silent polymorphism (C161T in exon 6) was associated with phenotypes related to obesity. The authors found no association between the polymorphism and BMI, body weight, leptin concentration, waist-hip ratio, but did find a statistically significant interaction between the polymorphism, BMI, and plasma leptin. At any given leptin concentration, obese subjects (BMI > 30) who were heterozygous or homozygous for the polymorphism had relatively lower BMIs than obese wild-type subjects (213). A study of the same mutation by Wang (214) also showed no association with obesity but did find a decreased risk of cardiovascular disease in heterozygous and homozygous subjects.

A Pro115Gln mutation affects phosphorylation at the adjacent Ser114, accelerating adipocyte differentiation and possibly reducing insulin responsiveness (215). Pro115Gln was studied in a cohort of 358 Germans (mean age 59 years) (215). Four markedly obese subjects were heterozygous carriers of the mutation, which was not found in any nonobese individuals. Of note, the four carriers of the mutation had BMIs greater than the obese (BMI > 29) noncarriers of the mutation: affected BMIs ranged from 37.9 to 47.3; obese, noncarriers mean BMI 33.6.

A silent mutation, C1431T in exon 6, has been linked to severe overweight and increased fat mass in obese women (207). Postmenopausal Japanese women who were either heterozygous or homozygous for the mutant T-allele were also shown to have reduced bone mineral density in comparison to individuals with the C allele (216). The same mutation was also weakly associated ($P < .03$) with circulating leptin concentration in 820 French subjects (213).

Barroso et al. (217) described two mutations, Val290-Met and Pro467Leu, which destabilize helix 12 in the ligand-binding domain and lead to transcriptional impairment by apparent dominant negative effects on the nonmutant transcripts. A mother and her son were identified who were heterozygous for Pro476Leu. Both subjects had type 2 diabetes and hypertension, but were not obese (55-year-old woman, BMI 24.9; 3l-year-old male, BMI 25.9). A 15-year-old girl was identified who was heterozygous for Val290Met. She also had type 2 diabetes and hypertension, and was not obese (BMI 25.6) (Table 5).

7 *SIM1* (6q16.3-q21)

SIM1 is the human ortholog of the *Drosophila Sim* ("single-minded") transcription factor that is involved in midline neurogenesis and is essential for development of several neuroendocrine lineages in the supraoptic nuclei and PVN in the hypothalamus, including arginine vasopressin, oxytocin, corticotropin-releasing hormone, and thyrotropin-releasing hormone (218). Haploinsufficient mice have a reduction in cell number in the PVN, and are obese (219). Holder et al. (220) described a girl with a balanced translocation between 1p22.1 and 6q16.2 that disrupted *SIM1*. She displayed hyperphagia and early-onset obesity (weight 47.5 kg at age 5 years), and had normal energy expenditure.

Table 5 *PPARγ* Mutations in Human Subjects

Mutation in *PPARγ*; location	Mechanism (reference)
Pro12Ala exon B (unique to PPARg2) C→G	Missense C→G; expression study (204) showed mutant with decreased ability to mediate transcriptional activation and adipogenesis induced by TZDs; Ala allele has decreased binding affinity to cognate promoter elements and decreased ability to transactivate responsive promoters (206); less active PPARγ: decreased BMI, improved insulin sensitivity (208,211).
C161T; exon 6 (ligand-binding domain)	Ligand-binding domain (213).
Pro115Gln; exon 6 (ligand-binding domain)	Overexpression in fibroblasts produces a protein with defective serine phosphorylation at position 114, accelerated adipocyte differentiation greater triglyceride accumulation than wildtype. More active PPARγ may result in increased BMI and increased insulin resistance (214,215).
Val290Met	Mutations destabilized helix 12 in the ligand-binding domain leading to transcriptional impairment by dominant negative effects on non-mutant transcripts (217).
Pro476Leu	
His478His, C1431T, exon 6	Silent; association between this SNP, RFLP, and bone mineral density in postmenopausal Japanese women (216).

Holder suggested that her obesity could be due to *SIM1* haploinsufficiency.

IX HUMAN GENETIC OBESITIES WITHOUT MOUSE HOMOLOGS

A Obesity Syndromes with Single or Oligo/Contiguous Gene Basis

1 Albright Hereditary Osteodystrophy

Albright hereditary osteodystrophy (AHO) (pseudo-hypoparathyroidism) is a genetically heterogeneous syndrome (generally autosomal dominant) characterized by skeletal and developmental abnormalities (short stature, brachydactyly, subcutaneous ossifications), mental retardation (in some cases), and obesity. Some instances are due to mutations in the *GNAS1* gene, a complex locus that encodes several overlapping transcripts. AHO has resulted from heterozygosity for inactivating mutations in the alpha subunit of a stimulatory G protein [G(s)alpha] encoded by *GNAS1*. Mutations in Gs may lead to obesity based on reduced function of this stimulatory G-protein in the lipolytic pathway, where Gs transduces lipolytic signals through the β-adrenergic receptor. There is evidence for genomic imprinting at the *GNAS1* locus. When the mother transmits the mutation, the phenotype is usually PHPIa (pseudo-hypoparathyroidism type Ia) with low serum calcium and elevated PTH, whereas paternally transmitted mutations lead to PPHP (pseudo-pseudo-hypoparathyroidism) with normal calcium levels and no generalized hormone resistance; all patients manifest osteodystrophy. In both PHPIa and PPHP patients, levels of Gsα expression and activity are 50% normal in the affected tissues. Almost 40 different inactivating mutations distributed throughout the *GNAS1* gene have been described in association with AHO; most are either frameshift mutations, creating premature stop codons, or missense mutations (221).

Of note, several activating mutations in *GNAS1* have also been described in association with McCune-Albright syndrome and several endocrine tumors (such as pituitary adenomas, pheochromocytomas, and thyroid carcinomas; the *GNAS1* gene is designated "gsp oncogene" in tumor tissues). Patients with McCune-Albright are somatic mosaics for gain-of-function *GNAS1* mutations and have abnormalities in bone, skin, and endocrine tissues, with widely varying symptoms depending on the tissue expressing the mosaicism. Common findings in this autosomal dominant, embryonic lethal (unless mosaic) condition include polyostotic fibrous dysplasia, large café au lait spots (irregular margins, "coast of Maine"), hyperthyroidism, and precocious puberty (due to constitutively activated gonadal LH and FSH receptors) (222).

2 Bardet Biedl Syndrome 1–6 (BBS)

BBS is a heterogeneous autosomal-recessive disorder with six different chromosomal regions implicated, termed BBS types 1–6: 11q13, 16q21, 3p12, 15q22.3-q23, 2q31, 20p12. Three genes have been identified to date as causative: *BBS2*, which encodes a protein of unknown function; myosin IX A (*MY09A*) for BBS4; and *MKKS*, a putative chaperonin, for BBS6. A recent report (223,224) described triallelic inheritance for BBS. They screened 163 BBS families for mutations in *BBS2* and *BBS6* and found three mutant alleles in 4 pedigrees of affected individuals. In one family, affected subjects had 3 mutant alleles: homozygous *BBS6* mutation, heterozygous *BBS2* mutation. In a second family, affected subjects were heterozygous for two different *BBS2* nonsense mutations and also were heterozygous for a single *BBS6* nonsense mutation. However, several pedigrees with *BBS2* mutations in this report do have a classic recessive segregation pattern, so some cases of *BBS* 2 or 6 may be due to alterations in a single gene.

The phenotype does not differ substantially among the different BBS types, and includes mental retardation, obesity, postaxial polydactyly, hypogonadism (apparently at both the hypothalamic and gonadal level), pigmentary retinopathy, and renal disease. The incidence of congenital cardiac anomalies (wide variety of lesions) is increased (225,226), as is that of type 2 diabetes mellitus and hepatic fibrosis (227). BBS1 and 4 are more prevalent in European populations while BBS2 and 3 are typically found in Arab-Bedouin families. Of note, obesity, pigmentary retinopathy, and renal disease are present in almost all patients, while polydactyly and mental retardation are present in only one-third to one-half of patients.

Myosin IX A (*MYO9A*) is implicated in BBS4. *MYO9A* is expressed throughout the nervous system, neural layer of the retina, inner ear, kidney, thyroid, and teeth. The mechanism(s) by which loss of function of this molecule produces the BBS phenotype are unclear.

The *MKKS* (BBS6) predicted protein has amino acid sequence homology to the chaperonin family of proteins that are involved in protein folding and assembly (228). Chaperonins share a common ring structure with a central cavity where incorrectly folded proteins bind (not in a sequence-specific manner), and via ATP-hydrolysis, the chaperonin enables the misfolded protein to achieve its native shape. The well-studied eukaryotic cytosolic chaperonin, CCT, is composed of two rings, each with eight dissimilar units, in a cylindrical assembly. Inactivating mutations of *MKKS* lead to BBS6, whereas less severe mutations (missense, frameshift) result in the McKusick-Kaufman syndrome (hydrometrocolpos, postaxial polydactyly, and congenital heart disease). It is possible that inactivation of *MKKS* leads to misfolding of target proteins whose resulting malfunction results in BBS. Alternatively, *MKKS* may be part of an oligomeric protein whose function is disrupted by the absence or aberrant sequence of *MKKS*.

Heterozygosity effects have been described for BBS. Croft found that heterozygous BBS subjects (type unspecified) had increased frequency of obesity, hypertension, diabetes mellitus, and renal disease (229). In a study of 34 heterozygotes, again without specifying BBS types (230), the proportion of overweight (defined as BMI > 31.1) male heterozygotes (26.7%) was significantly higher than age-matched U.S. white males (8.9%).

3 Borjeson-Forssman-Lehmann Syndrome (BFLS) (Xq26.3)

BFLS is an X-linked syndrome with incompletely recessive inheritance characterized by obesity, hypometabolism, hypogonadism, characteristic facies (swollen subcutaneous facial tissue, deep-set eyes, narrow palprebral fissures), epilepsy, and mental retardation. Although BFLS is primarily manifest in males, there have been a few cases described in females. One female with BFLS had extremely nonrandom X-inactivation, which accounted for the manifestation of this X-linked disorder (231). Gecz et al. described a male infant with BFLS-like features and a duplication: 46,Y, dup (X)(q26q28), with the duplication breakpoint containing the fibroblast growth factor-13 gene (*FGF13*) (232). In 10- to 12-week human fetal tissue, *FGF13* showed maximal expression in brain and skeletal muscle.

Another gene that localizes to the same region, *SOX3*, is also a candidate for causing BFLS. *SOX3*, SRY-related HMG-box 3, is a member of a family of genes that are related to *SRY*, the testis-determining gene. The homology between *SOX3* and *SRY* is in the region of *SRY* encoding the HMG-box class DNA-binding motif. *SOX3* is expressed in the human fetal brain and spinal cord, and the murine homolog is expressed at very high levels in neuronal tissues during development. Thus, mutation or deletion of *SOX3* could conceivably result in hypothalamic and CNS cortical dysfunction, consistent with the BFLS phenotype. Rousseau et al. described a male patient with *SOX3* deletion who had hemophilia and mental retardation, and partial primary testicular failure, recapitulating several features of BFLS (mild mental retardation, small testes) (233).

4 Congenital Disorder of Glycosylation Type 1a (CDG1a) (16p13.3-p13.2)

The CDG1a syndrome, also known as Jaeken syndrome, is a severe, multisystemic, autosomal-recessive disorder that usually presents in the neonatal period and is characterized by the defective glycosylation of glycoconjugates (especially asparagine-N-linked oligosaccharides in the ER) (234). The syndrome includes severe encephalopathy, axial hypotonia, abnormal eye movement, pronounced psychomotor retardation, peripheral neuropathy, and serum glycoprotein abnormalities. Patients have a peculiar distribution of subcutaneous fat (fat pads above buttocks, lipodystrophy), moderate obesity, and hypogonadism. *PMM2*, phosphomannomutase 2, has been implicated as the responsible gene, which is required for the synthesis of GDP-mannose (converts mannose 6-phosphate to mannose 1-phosphate). Nearly 60 mutations have been described, mostly in exons 5 and 8, with 90% accounted for by two mutations: F119L and R141H (not seen in homozygous state, mutant protein with zero activity in in vitro assay).

5 Prader-Willi Syndrome (15q11.2-q12)

Prader-Willi syndrome (PWS) is a contiguous deletion/disruption defect involving the region between 15q11.2-q12, likely due to the disruption of *SNRPN*, necdin, and potentially other genes (235). This region of chromosome 15 is imprinted. Maternal uniparental disomy (UPD) for these genes results in PWS; paternal uniparental disomy and disruption of the E6-associated protein, ubiquitin-protein ligase (*UBE3A*), results in Angelman syndrome (236).

PWS is characterized by diminished fetal activity, failure to thrive in infancy, hypotonia, followed by the onset of hyperphagia with rapid weight gain after 1 year of age, leading to massive obesity. Body composition is altered, however, even before the subjects develop obesity: PW infants have increased fractional body fat content even during their period of slow postnatal growth (237). Mental retardation, short stature, hypogonadotropic hypogonadism, relative pain insensitivity, and thick saliva are other characteristic features. Most of the features are consistent with CNS effects, but not all (narrow bitemporal diameter, almond eyes, small narrow hands, small feet, skin depigmentation) (238).

Most cases of PWS are sporadic, resulting either from spontaneous interstitial deletions (often microdeletions), de novo unbalanced translocations, or maternal uniparental disomy. Seventy percent of instances are due to microscopic 15q11 deletions, 25% to maternal UPD (often with balanced translocation), < 5% to imprinting center mutation and transmitted unbalanced translocation (235). There have been familial cases of PWS, but these are very rare. The recurrence rate in siblings of affected patients is ~ 1:1000, versus a population risk of ~ 1:25,000. Most of the instances of maternal UPD result from meiosis-1 errors, whereas paternal UPD cases of Angelman syndrome usually result from meiosis-2 or mitotic errors (239).

There are slight phenotypic differences among patients with different molecular defects leading to PWS. For example, subjects with paternal deletions manifest the classic PWS phenotype, whereas subjects with maternal UPD generally manifest a milder phenotype and have better cognitive function. Subjects with both maternal UPD and mosaic trisomy 15 are the most severely affected and also have a high incidence of congenital heart disease. Maternal age is higher in patients with disomy, in line with the expected findings of a nondisjunction event (240). Depigmentation is more frequent in subjects with deletions (77%) than in those with UPD (39%). Also, female subjects with UPD have slightly milder phenotype than those with deletions (241). The differences in phenotype point to underlying differences in the respective regions and amounts of chromosome 15 that are affected.

SNRPN (15q12) has been implicated in the pathogenesis of PWS. *SNRPN* encodes small ribonucleoprotein polypeptide N, a protein found in spliceosomes, and possibly has a role in mediating alternative splicing of CNS mRNA transcripts. Reed et al. showed there is maternal imprinting of *SNRPN* and that the maternal allele is not expressed in the human fetal brain (242). Ishikawa et al. reported two siblings with PWS who had deletions in *SNRPN* by FISH (243). Sun et al. described another PWS patient with a paternal balanced reciprocal translocation t (15; 19)(ql2; q13.41) with the breakpoint occurring between exons 0 and 1 of *SNRPN* (exons numbered −1 to 8) (244). No complete *SNRPN* mRNA transcript was identified in this patient. Similarly, Kuslich et al. described a PWS patient with a de novo balanced translocation (4; 15)(q27; q11.2) between *SNRPN* exons 2 and 3 (245). The reports by Sun and Kuslich support the inference that the region between SNRPN exons 2 and 3 is critical, and that mutations affecting this region contribute to the major phenotypic manifestations of PWS.

Dittrich et al. described a model involving an imprinting center mapping to 15q11-q13 (246). Their model proposed that the imprinting center (IC) contained an imprintor and an imprint switch initiation site (involving exon 1 of *SNRPN*), and that the imprintor is transcribed only from the paternal chromosome. There are numerous transcripts encoded in the IC that are alternatively spliced and that are only expressed from the paternal chromosome. Since some subjects with PWS (and Angelman's) have mutations affecting the IC, the transcripts are not expressed. Thus, the IC may be critical in regulating alternative RNA splicing in the *SNRPN* transcripts. Lyko et al. studied this region in *Drosophila* and showed that a 215-bp region containing the *SNRPN* promoter region has a silencer of maternal *SNRPN* (247). Lyko suggested that this silencer element may play a role in the imprinting of 15q11-13 and may repress *SNRPN* expression from the maternal allele.

Bressler et al., however, showed that a deletion of exon 1 of mouse *Snrpn* (~ 1 kb) did not elicit any obvious phenotypic change, while a 4.8-kb deletion including the same region led to a partial imprinting defect and perinatal lethality when paternally inherited (248). Also, Schulze et al. reported a PWS patient with a balanced 9:15 translocation whose breakpoint was between *SNRPN* and an adjacent gene, *PAR1*, with *SNRPN* unaffected by the translocation (249). This patient met formal criteria for PWS, including obesity (moderate), hypopigmented in relation to his family, PWS facies, and delayed puberty, but he displayed no hyperphagia (250). These data suggest that *SNRPN* may play a role in regulation of food intake, but not in the other somatic and endocrine phenotypes associated with PWS.

It is unlikely a single gene will be implicated as the cause of the diverse range of PWS phenotypic features given the sizeable deletion in most PWS patients and the number of genes (at least two) in that interval (251). *Drosophila* or mice harboring *Snprn* deletions and contiguous gene interruptions may help to clarify the molecular pathogenesis of the PWS.

6 Simpson-Golabi-Behmel 1 Syndrome (SGBS) (Xq26)

SGBS is an X-linked overgrowth-obesity syndrome. Affected subjects have weights and heights over 97th centile at birth, and manifest postnatal overgrowth, cardiac abnormalities (conduction defects, ventricular septal defects, pulmonic stenosis, transposition of the great vessels, and cardiomyopathies), risk for embryonal tumors, and in general, show significant phenotypic overlap with Beckwith-Wiedemann syndrome (neonatal exomphalos, macroglossia, and gigantism).

Two genes have been implicated, glypican 3 and 4 (*GPC3, 4*). Pilia et al. reported two SGBS patients with X/autosome translocations with breakpoints near the ends of the 500-kb *GPC3* gene at Xq26 (252). In three families, microdeletions in *GPC3* cosegregated with SGBS. Veugelers et al. reported on one of the patients initially described by Pilia and found a deletion of the last two exons of *GPC3* as well as the entire *GPC4* gene (253).

GPC3 and *GPC4* are members of a family of cell surface proteoglycans that appear to control growth and cell division, especially of embryonic mesodermal tissues. *GPC3* seems to act by forming a complex with IGF2. This is reminiscent of another overgrowth syndrome, Beckwith-Wiedemann, which appears to be caused by overexpression of *IGF2* (254).

7 Ulnar Mammary Syndrome (UMS) (12q24.1)

UMS is an autosomal-dominant syndrome characterized by obesity; delayed growth and puberty; and complex malformations of the ulnar ray, teeth, axillary apocrine glands, and urogenital system. The *TBX3* gene (12q24.1) has been implicated as causative by Bamshad et al. (255). *TBX3* encodes a transcription factor that seems to be critical to the morphogenesis of several organs. Mutations in a related gene, *TBX5*, are associated with anterior limb malformations in the Holt-Oram syndrome; *TBX3* appears to be associated with the posterior limb malformations of UMS. The affected subjects were doubly heterozygous for mutations predicted to alter DNA binding: 1 bp del 227T leading to a premature stop codon; IVS 2ds, G→C, +1. Further study by Bamshad found additional novel *TBX3* mutations in families with UMS, but identified no obvious phenotypic differences between those with missense mutations, frameshifts, or deletions (256). The molecular mechanism for the obesity in this syndrome is unknown.

8 Human Alleles of UCPs

The role of allelic variation/mutation in UCPs in human energy homeostasis remains unclear. A number of studies have reported associations with allelic variants of *UCP1* (4q31) with obesity-related phenotypes in humans (some in interaction with an allele of *B3AR*) (257) (258), while others have not found such associations (259). Because BAT is apparently not an important thermogenic organ in humans outside of the neonatal period, *UCP1* is not a particularly strong candidate for a role in human obesity. *UCP2* and *UCP3* are adjacent to each other on chromosome 11q13. Microsatellites in the region of *UCP2/UCP3* have been associated with aspects of metabolic rate and body composition (260). Three alleles of *UCP2* or *UCP3* have been associated with measures of metabolic rate in Pima Indians (261), and Esterbauer et al. (262) reported an association between a promoter polymorphism in *UCP2* (11q13) and obesity in adults. Because of its primary expression in skeletal muscle, *UCP3* is perhaps the best candidate for effects on energy expenditure in humans. Homozygosity for a V102I mutation in *UCP3* was associated with obesity in three Gullah-speaking African-Americans, and compound heterozygosity for an R143X mutation and a splice junction mutation eliminating the terminal (6) exon (IVS6, G-A, +1) was found in a morbidly obese 16-year-old with type 2 diabetes (263). However, homozygosity for the splice mutation was detected in obese and lean African-Americans, and was not associated with any abnormality in metabolic rate or skeletal muscle mitochondrial coupling (264). No association of this allele with BMI or diabetes was detected in an analysis of a large group of African-Americans (264). An Arg70Trp mutation was found in a severely obese, diabetic 15-year-old Chinese male (265,266).

B Lipodystrophy Syndromes with Single-Gene Basis

These mutations are included in this discussion because of their profound effects on adipose tissue mass. The genes and pathways involved may also have roles in obesity by virtue of reciprocal effects.

1 Berardinelli-Seip Congenital Lipodystrophy Syndrome (BSCL) (9q34)

During the neonatal period affected patients manifest generalized lipodystrophy, low fat mass, insulin-resistant diabetes mellitus, acanthosis nigricans, elevated basal metabolic rate, and hypertrigycleridemia. Some patients subsequently develop polycystic ovaries and muscular hypertrophy. BSCL is caused by mutations in *BSCL2* (11q13) and *RXRA* (9q34) (267). *BSCL2* is highly expressed in most regions of the central nervous system. All affected subjects with *BSCL2* mutations have been either homozygous or compound heterozygous for mutations that severely disrupt the protein structure (usually frameshifts with premature termination). *RXRA* encodes a nuclear receptor that can function as either a homodimer or as a heterodimer (RXRA/RAR) and has a crucial role in adipocyte differentiation. A mouse model lacking functional hepatic *Rxra* (via CRE-mediated recombination) had wide-ranging hepatic metabolic abnormalities, showing the importance of intact *Rxra* function to the regulation of cholesterol, fatty acid, bile acid, and steroid metabolism (268). As there are two genetic loci implicated in cases of BSCL, it is possible that each encodes a protein with effects on the same pathway, possibly affecting G proteins or transcription factors involved in activating genes involved in the fatty acid synthetic pathway.

2 Familial Partial Lipodystrophy Dunnigan (FPLD) (1q21.2)

Mutations in the lamin A/C gene (*LMNA*; 1q21.2) lead to an autosomal dominant form of insulin resistant diabetes mellitus. Affected patients often manifest acanthosis nigricans and pubertal-onset lipoatrophy. Once puberty commences, the patients experience a slow loss of subcutaneous fat from the extremities, buttocks, and truncal areas while simultaneously accumulating fat tissue on the face and neck, leading to a cushingoid appearance. Lamin A and Lamin C are both encoded by *LMNA*, with alternative splicing of exon 10 leading to two different transcripts for A and C. Lamins A, B, and C comprise the nuclear lamina in mammals and are highly conserved throughout evolution. The nuclear lamina is a protein-rich layer that is juxtaposed to and interacts with proteins in the inner nuclear membrane. Cao and Hegele described an *LMNA* Arg482G1n mutation in five Canadian FPLD families (269). Mutations in *LMNA* also lead to muscle wasting in the autosomal-recessive and -dominant forms of Emery-Dreifuss muscular dystrophy (270) as well as a familial dilated cardiomyopathy with conduction defects (CMD1A). Mutations in the globular C-terminal domain have been found in subjects with FPLD, mutations in the head or tail domains have been found in cases of Emery-Dreifuss muscular dystrophy, and mutations in the rod domain have been found in CMD1A subjects (271). Possibly mutations at each of the aforementioned domains uniquely alters *LMNA* interactions with different components of the inner nuclear membrane, leading to the disparate disease phenotypes.

X SUMMARY

Human obesity is an apparently simple convergent phenotype that actually resolves extremely complex genetic, developmental, and environmental processes. None of these is sufficiently well understood to be able to "fix" it experimentally in efforts to understand the others. It is now clear that the genetic contribution to human obesity is substantial, but, in most instances, strongly dependent for expression upon the other two factors. The single-gene obesities in humans and mice are the exception to this general principle, because they are phenotypically apparent in virtually all environmental and developmental circumstances. The inactivating mutations of these genes account for only a small fraction of human obesity, but the pathways that they affect must be crucial in the regulation of body fat. For this reason alone these mutations (and those yet to be identified) are of critical importance to our understanding of human energy homeostasis. And, it remains a formal and likely possibility that subtle variation in expression/function of these genes may account for much or all of the genetic contribution to body weight regulation (173).

REFERENCES

1. Bray GA, York DA. Hypothalamic and genetic obesity in experimental animals: an autonomic and endocrine hypothesis. Physiol Rev 1979; 59:719–809.
2. Wolff GL, Roberts DW, Mountjoy KG. Physiological consequences of ectopic agouti gene expression: the yellow obese mouse syndrome. Physiol Genomics 1999; 1:151–163.
3. Wolff GL, Kodell RL, Kaput JA, Visek WJ. Caloric restriction abolishes enhanced metabolic efficiency induced by ectopic agouti protein in yellow mice. Proc Soc Exp Biol Med 1999; 221:99–104.
4. Suto J, Matsuura S, Imamura K, Yamanaka H, Sekikawa K. Genetic analysis of non-insulin-dependent diabetes mellitus in kk and kk-ay mice. Eur J Endocrinol 1998; 139:654–661.
5. Michaud EJ, Bultman SJ, Stubbs LJ, Woychik RP. The embryonic lethality of homozygous lethal yellow mice *AY/AY* is associated with the disruption of a novel RNA-binding protein. Genes Dev 1993; 7:1203–1213.
6. Duhl DM, Stevens ME, Vrieling H, Saxon PJ, Miller MW, Epstein CJ, Barsh GS. Pleiotropic effects of the mouse lethal yellow *AY* mutation explained by deletion of a maternally expressed gene and the simultaneous production of agouti fusion RNAs. Development 1994; 120:1695–1708.
7. Bultman SJ, Klebig ML, Michaud EJ, Sweet HO, Davisson MT, Woychik RP. Molecular analysis of reverse mutations from nonagouti (a) to black-and-tan (a(t)) and white-bellied agouti (aw) reveals alternative

forms of agouti transcripts. Genes Dev 1994; 8:481–490.
8. Bultman SJ, Russell LB, Gutierrez-Espeleta GA, Woychik RP. Molecular characterization of a region of DNA associated with mutations at the agouti locus in the mouse. Proc Natl Acad Sci USA 1991; 88:8062–8066.
9. Woychik RP, Generoso WM, Russell LB, Cain KT, Cacheiro NL, Bultman SJ, Selby PB, Dickinson ME, Hogan BL, Rutledge JC. Molecular and genetic characterization of a radiation-induced structural rearrangement in mouse chromosome 2 causing mutations at the limb deformity and agouti loci. Proc Natl Acad Sci USA 1990; 87:2588–2592.
10. Miller MW, Duhl DM, Vrieling H, Cordes SP, Ollmann MM, Winkes BM, Barsh GS. Cloning of the mouse *Agouti* gene predicts a secreted protein ubiquitously expressed in mice carrying the lethal yellow mutation. Genes Dev 1993; 7:454–467.
11. Bultman SJ, Michaud EL, Woychik RP. Molecular characterization of the mouse Agouti locus. Cell 1992; 71:1195–1204.
12. Yang YK, Ollmann MM, Wilson BD, Dickinson C, Yamada T, Barsh GS, Gantz I. Effects of recombinant agouti-signaling protein on melanocortin action. Mol Endocrinol 1997; 11:274–280.
13. Huszar D, Lynch CA, Fairchild-Huntress V, Dunmore JH, Fang Q, Berkemeier LR, Gu W, Kesterson RA, Boston BA, Cone RD, Smith FJ, Campfield LA, Burn P, Lee F. Targeted disruption of the melanocortin-4 receptor results in obesity in mice. Cell 1997; 88:131–141.
14. Hagan MM, Rushing PA, Pritchard LM, Schwartz MW, Strack AM, Van der Ploeg LH, Woods SC, Seeley RJ. Long-term orexigenic effects of AGRP-(83–132) involve mechanisms other than melanocortin receptor blockade. Am J Physiol Regul Integr Comp Physiol 2000; 279:R47–R52.
15. Oosterom J, Garner KM, den Dekker WK, Nijenhuis WA, Gispen WH, Burbach JP, Barsh GS, Adan RA. Common requirements for melanocortin-4 receptor selectivity of structurally unrelated melanocortin agonist and endogenous antagonist, agouti protein. J Biol Chem 2001; 276:931–936.
16. Vrieling H, Duhl DM, Millar SE, Miller KA, Barsh GS. Differences in dorsal and ventral pigmentation result from regional expression of the mouse *Agouti* gene. Proc Natl Acad Sci USA 1994; 91:5667–5671.
17. Lamoreux ML, Wakamatsu K, Ito S. Interaction of major coat color gene functions in mice as studied by chemical analysis of eumelanin and pheomelanin. Pigment Cell Res 2001; 14:23–31.
18. Robbins LS, Nadeau JH, Johnson KR, Kelly MA, Roselli-Rehfuss L, Baack E, Mountjoy KG, Cone RD. Pigmentation phenotypes of variant extension locus alleles result from point mutations that alter MSH receptor function. Cell 1993; 72:827–834.
19. Miller KA, Gunn TM, Carrasquillo MM, Lamoreux ML, Galbraith DB, Barsh GS. Genetic studies of the mouse mutations mahogany and mahoganoid. Genetics 1997; 146:1407–1415.
20. Gunn TM, Inui T, Kitada K, Ito S, Wakamatsu K, He L, Bouley DM, Serikawa T, Barsh GS. Molecular and phenotypic analysis of attractin mutant mice. Genetics 2001; 158:1683–1695.
21. Duke-Cohan JS, Gu J, McLaughlin DF, Xu Y, Freeman GJ, Schlossman SF. Attractin (*Dppt-1*), a member of the CUB family of cell adhesion and guidance proteins, is secreted by activated human t lymphocytes and modulates immune cell interactions. Proc Natl Acad Sci USA 1998; 95:11336–11341.
22. Bronson RT, Donahue LR, Samples R, Kim JH, Naggert JK. Mice with mutations in the mahogany gene *Atrn* have cerebral spongiform changes. J Neuropathol Exp Neurol 2001; 60:724–730.
23. Kuramoto T, Kitada K, Inui T, Sasaki Y, Ito K, Hase T, Kawagachi S, Ogawa Y, Nakao K, Barsh GS, Nagao M, Ushijima T, Serikawa T. Attractin/mahogany/zitter plays a critical role in myelination of the central nervous system. Proc Natl Acad Sci USA 2001; 98:559–564.
24. Ollmann MM, Wilson BD, Yang YK, Kerns JA, Chen Y, Gantz I, Barsh GS. Antagonism of central melanocortin receptors in vitro and in vivo by agouti-related protein. Science 1997; 278:135–138.
25. Shutter JR, Graham M, Kinsey AC, Scully S, Luthy R, Stark KL. Hypothalamic expression of *Art*, a novel gene related to agouti, is up-regulated in obese and diabetic mutant mice. Genes Dev 1997; 11:593–602.
26. Rossi M, Kim MS, Morgan DG, Small CJ, Edwards CM, Sunter D, Abusnana S, Goldstone AP, Russell SH, Stanley SA, Smith DM, Yagaloff K, Ghatei MA, Bloom SR. A C-terminal fragment of agouti-related protein increases feeding and antagonizes the effect of alpha-melanocyte stimulating hormone in vivo. Endocrinology 1998; 139:4428–4431.
27. Reizes O, Lincecum J, Wang Z, Goldberger O, Huang L, Kaksonen M, Ahima R, Hinkes MT, Barsh GS, Rauvala H, Bernfield M. Transgenic expression of *Syndecan-1* uncovers a physiological control of feeding behavior by syndecan-3. Cell 2001; 106:105–116.
28. Bernfield M, Gotte M, Park PW, Reizes O, Fitzgerald ML, Lincecum J, Zako M. Functions of cell surface heparan sulfate proteoglycans. Annu Rev Biochem 1999; 68:729–777.
29. Hahn TM, Breininger JF, Baskin DG, Schwartz MW. Coexpression of *Agrp* and *Npy* in fasting-activated hypothalamic neurons. Nat Neurosci 1998; 1:271–272.
30. Tatemoto K, Carlquist M, Mutt V. Neuropeptide Y—a novel brain peptide with structural similarities to

peptide yy and pancreatic polypeptide. Nature 1982; 296:659–660.

31. Clark JT, Kalra PS, Kalra SP. Neuropeptide Y stimulates feeding but inhibits sexual behavior in rats. Endocrinology 1985; 117:2435–2442.
32. Chua SC Jr, Leibel RL, Hirsch J. Food deprivation and age modulate neuropeptide gene expression in the murine hypothalamus and adrenal gland. Brain Res Mol Brain Res 1991; 9:95–101.
33. White JD, Olchovsky D, Kershaw M, Berelowitz M. Increased hypothalamic content of preproneuropeptide-Y messenger ribonucleic acid in streptozotocin-diabetic rats. Endocrinology 1990; 126:765–772.
34. Wilding JP, Ajala MO, Lambert PD, Bloom SR. Additive effects of lactation and food restriction to increase hypothalamic neuropeptide Y mRNA in rats. J Endocrinol 1997; 152:365–369.
35. McCarthy HD, Kilpatrick AP, Trayhurn P, Williams G. Widespread increases in regional hypothalamic neuropeptide Y levels in acute cold-exposed rats. Neuroscience 1993; 54:127–132.
36. Jhanwar-Uniyal M, Chua SC Jr. Critical effects of aging and nutritional state on hypothalamic neuropeptide Y and galanin gene expression in lean and genetically obese Zucker rats. Brain Res Mol Brain Res 1993; 19:195–202.
37. Chua SC Jr, Brown AW, Kim J, Hennessey KL, Leibel RL, Hirsch J. Food deprivation and hypothalamic neuropeptide gene expression: effects of strain background and the diabetes mutation. Brain Res Mol Brain Res 1991; 11:291–299.
38. Korner J, Wardlaw SL, Liu SM, Conwell IM, Leibel RL, Chua SC Jr. Effects of leptin receptor mutation on agrp gene expression in fed and fasted lean and obese (LA/N fa^f) rats. Endocrinology 2000; 141:2465–2471.
39. Castro MG, Morrison E. Post-translational processing of proopiomelanocortin in the pituitary and in the brain. Crit Rev Neurobiol 1997; 11:35–57.
40. Yaswen L, Diehl N, Brennan MB, Hochgeschwender U. Obesity in the mouse model of pro-opiomelanocortin deficiency responds to peripheral melanocortin. Nat Med 1999; 5:1066–1070.
41. Cone RD, Lu D, Koppula S, Vage DI, Klungland H, Boston B, Chen W, Orth DN, Pouton C, Kesterson RA. The melanocortin receptors: agonists, antagonists, and the hormonal control of pigmentation. Recent Prog Horm Res 1996; 51:287–317.
42. Cone RD. The central melanocortin system and its role in energy homeostasis. Ann Endocrinol (Paris) (in French) 1999; 60:3–9.
43. Chen AS, Marsh DJ, Trumbauer ME, Frazier EG, Guan XM, Yu H, Rosenblum CI, Vongs A, Feng Y, Cao L, Metzger JM, Strack AM, Camacho RE, Mellin TN, Nunes CN, Min W, Fisher J, Gopal-Truter S, MacIntyre DE, Chen HY, Van der Ploeg LH. Inactivation of the mouse melanocortin-3 receptor results in increased fat mass and reduced lean body mass. Nat Genet 2000; 26:97–102.
44. Butler AA, Kesterson RA, Khong K, Cullen MJ, Pelleymounter MA, Dekoning J, Baetscher M, Cone RD. A unique metabolic syndrome causes obesity in the melanocortin-3 receptor-deficient mouse. Endocrinology 2000; 141:3518–3521.
45. Cowley MA, Smart JL, Rubinstein M, Cerdan MG, Diano S, Horvath TL, Cone RD, Low MJ. Leptin activates anorexigenic POMC neurons through a neural network in the arcuate nucleus. Nature 2001; 411:480–484.
46. Murphy B, Nunes CN, Ronan JJ, Hanaway M, Fairhurst AM, Mellin TN. Centrally administered mtii affects feeding, drinking, temperature, and activity in the Sprague-Dawley rat. J Appl Physiol 2000; 89:273–282.
47. Hwa JJ, Ghibaudi L, Gao J, Parker EM. Central melanocortin system modulates energy intake and expenditure of obese and lean Zucker rats. Am J Physiol Regul Integr Comp Physiol 2001; 281:R444–R451.
48. Ingalls AM, Dickie MM, Snell GD. Obese, a new mutation in the house mouse. Obes Res 1996; 4:101.
49. Leibel RL, Chung WK, Chua SC. The molecular genetics of rodent single gene obesities. J Biol Chem 1997; 272:31937–31940.
50. Zhang Y, Proenca R, Maffei M, Barone M, Leopold L, Friedman JM. Positional cloning of the mouse *Obese* gene and its human homologue. Nature 1994; 372:425–432.
51. Houseknecht KL, Mantzoros CS, Kuliawat R, Hadro E, Flier JS, Kahn BB. Evidence for leptin binding to proteins in serum of rodents and humans: modulation with obesity. Diabetes 1996; 45:1638–1643.
52. Frederich RC, Hamann A, Anderson S, Lollmann B, Lowell BB, Flier JS. Leptin levels reflect body lipid content in mice: evidence for diet-induced resistance to leptin action. Nat Med 1995; 1:1311–1314.
53. Coleman DL. Obese and diabetes: two mutant genes causing diabetes-obesity syndromes in mice. Diabetologia 1978; 14:141–148.
54. Tuig JG, Romsos DR, Leveille GA. Maintenance energy requirements and energy retention of young obese (*ob/ob*) and lean mice housed at 33 degrees and fed a high-carbohydrate or a high-fat diet. J Nutr 1980; 110:35–41.
55. Dubuc PU, Cahn PJ, Willis P. The effects of exercise and food restriction on obesity and diabetes in young *ob/ob* mice. Int J Obes 1984; 8:271–278.
56. Trayhurn P, James WP. Thermoregulation and non-shivering thermogenesis in the genetically obese (*ob/ob*) mouse. Pflugers Arch 1978; 373:189–193.
57. Smith CK, Romsos DR. Cold acclimation of obese (*ob/ob*) mice: effects of energy balance. Metabolism 1984; 33:853–857.

58. Smith CK, Romsos DR. Cold acclimation of obese (*ob/ob*) mice: effects on skeletal muscle and bone. Metabolism 1984; 33:858–863.
59. Rafael J, Herling AW. Leptin effect in *ob/ob* mice under thermoneutral conditions depends not necessarily on central satiation. Am J Physiol Regul Integr Comp Physiol 2000; 278:R790–R795.
60. Cox JE, Powley TL. Development of obesity in diabetic mice pair-fed with lean siblings. J Comp Physiol Psychol 1977; 91:347–358.
61. Qiu J, Ogus S, Mounzih K, Ewart-Toland A, Chehab FF. Leptin-deficient mice backcrossed to the BALB/cJ genetic background have reduced adiposity, enhanced fertility, normal body temperature, and severe diabetes. Endocrinology 2001; 142:3421–3425.
62. Campfield LA, Smith FJ, Guisez Y, Devos R, Burn P. Recombinant mouse ob protein: evidence for a peripheral signal linking adiposity and central neural networks. Science 1995; 269:546–549.
63. Halaas JL, Gajiwala KS, Maffei M, Cohen SL, Chait BT, Rabinowitz D, Lallone RL, Burley SK, Friedman JM. Weight-reducing effects of the plasma protein encoded by the *Obese* gene. Science 1995; 269:543–546.
64. Pellcymounter MA, Cullen MJ, Baker MB, Hecht R, Winters D, Boone T, Collins F. Effects of the *Obese* gene product on body weight regulation in *ob/ob* mice. Science 1995; 269:540–543.
65. Barzilai N, Wang J, Massilon D, Vuguin P, Hawkins M, Rossetti L. Leptin selectively decreases visceral adiposity and enhances insulin action. J Clin Invest 1997; 100:3105–3110.
66. Muzzin P, Eisensmith RC, Copeland KC, Woo SL. Correction of obesity and diabetes in genetically obese mice by leptin gene therapy. Proc Natl Acad Sci USA 1996; 93:14804–14808.
67. Ebihara K, Ogawa Y, Masuzaki H, Shintani M, Miyanaga F, Aizawa-Abe M, Hayashi T, Hosoda K, Inoue G, Yoshimasa Y, Gavrilova O, Reitman ML, Nakao K. Transgenic overexpression of leptin rescues insulin resistance and diabetes in a mouse model of lipoatrophic diabetes. Diabetes 2001; 50:1440–1448.
68. Zhang Y, Guo K-Y, Diaz PA, Heo M, Leibel RL. Determinants of leptin gene expression in fat depots of lean mice. Am J Physiol 2002; 282:R226–R234.
69. Bradley RL, Cheatham B. Regulation of *ob* gene expression and leptin secretion by insulin and dexamethasone in rat adipocytes. Diabetes 1999; 48:272–278.
70. Wang J, Liu R, Hawkins M, Barzilai N, Rossetti L. A nutrient-sensing pathway regulates leptin gene expression in muscle and fat. Nature 1998; 393:684–688.
71. Hwang CS, Mandrup S, MacDougald OA, Geiman DE, Lane MD. Transcriptional activation of the mouse *Obese* (*ob*) gene by ccaat/enhancer binding protein alpha. Proc Natl Acad Sci USA 1996; 93:873–877.
72. Mason MM, He Y, Chen H, Quon MJ, Reitman M. Regulation of leptin promoter function by SP1, C/EBP and a novel factor. Endocrinology 1998; 139:1013–1022.
73. Sloop KW, Surface PL, Heiman ML, Slieker LJ. Changes in leptin expression are not associated with corresponding changes in ccaat/enhancer binding protein-alpha. Biochem Biophys Res Commun 1998; 251:142–147.
74. De Vos P, Lefebvre AM, Miller SG, Guerre-Millo M, Wong K, Saladin R, Hamann LG, Staels B, Briggs MR, Auwerx J. Thiazolidinediones repress *ob* gene expression in rodents via activation of peroxisome proliferator-activated receptor gamma. J Clin Invest 1996; 98:1004–1009.
75. Hollenberg AN, Susulic VS, Madura JP, Zhang B, Moller DE, Tontonoz P, Sarraf P, Spiegelman BM, Lowell BB. Functional antagonism between CCAAT/enhancer binding protein-alpha and peroxisome proliferator-activated receptor-gamma on the leptin promoter. J Biol Chem 1997; 272:5283–5290.
76. Bado A, Levasseur S, Attoub S, Kermorgant S, Laigneau JP, Bortoluzzi MN, Moizo L, Lehy T, Guerre-Millo M, Le Marchand-Brustel Y, Lewin MJ. The stomach is a source of leptin. Nature 1998; 394:790–793.
77. Masuzaki H, Ogawa Y, Sagawa N, Hosoda K, Matsumoto T, Mise H, Nishimura H, Yoshimasa Y, Tanaka I, Mori T, Nakao K. Nonadipose tissue production of leptin: leptin as a novel placenta-derived hormone in humans. Nat Med 1997; 3:1029–1033.
78. Lewin MJ, Bado A. Gastric leptin. Microsc Res Tech 2001; 53:372–376.
79. Chua SC, Koutras IK, Han L, Liu SM, Kay J, Young SJ, Chung WK, Leibel RL. Fine structure of the murine leptin receptor gene: splice site suppression is required to form two alternatively spliced transcripts. Genomics 1997; 45:264–270.
80. Sinha MK, Opentanova I, Ohannesian JP, Kolaczynski JW, Heiman ML, Hale J, Becker GW, Bowsher RR, Stephens TW, Caro JF. Evidence of free and bound leptin in human circulation. Studies in lean and obese subjects and during short-term fasting. J Clin Invest 1996; 98:1277–1282.
81. Mantzoros CS. Leptin in renal failure. J Ren Nutr 1999; 9:122–125.
82. Gavrilova O, Barr V, Marcus-Samuels B, Reitman M. Hyperleptinemia of pregnancy associated with the appearance of a circulating form of the leptin receptor. J Biol Chem 1997; 272:30546–30551.
83. Chien EK, Hara M, Rouard M, Yano H, Phillippe M, Polonsky KS, Bell GI. Increase in serum leptin and uterine leptin receptor messenger RNA levels during pregnancy in rats. Biochem Biophys Res Commun 1997; 237:476–480.
84. Kawai M, Yamaguchi M, Murakami T, Shima K, Murata Y, Kishi K. The placenta is not the main

source of leptin production in pregnant rat: gestational profile of leptin in plasma and adipose tissues. Biochem Biophys Res Commun 1997; 240:798–802.

85. Schubring C, Kiess W, Englaro P, Rascher W, Dotsch J, Hanitsch S, Attanasio A, Blum WF. Levels of leptin in maternal serum, amniotic fluid, and arterial and venous cord blood: relation to neonatal and placental weight. J Clin Endocrinol Metab 1997; 82:1480–1483.
86. Chen SC, Cunningham JJ, Smeyne RJ. Expression of *ob* receptor splice variants during prenatal development of the mouse. J Recept Signal Transduct Res 2000; 20:87–103.
87. Ducy P, Amling M, Takeda S, Priemel M, Schilling AF, Beil FT, Shen J, Vinson C, Rueger JM, Karsenty G. Leptin inhibits bone formation through a hypothalamic relay: a central control of bone mass. Cell 2000; 100:197–207.
88. Steppan CM, Crawford DT, Chidsey-Frink KL, Ke H, Swick AG. Leptin is a potent stimulator of bone growth in *ob/ob* mice. Regul Pept 2000; 92:73–78.
89. Ghilardi N, Ziegler S, Wiestner A, Stoffel R, Heim MH, Skoda RC. Defective stat signaling by the leptin receptor in diabetic mice. Proc Natl Acad Sci USA 1996; 93:6231–6235.
90. Lord GM, Matarese G, Howard JK, Baker RJ, Bloom SR, Lechler RI. Leptin modulates the t-cell immune response and reverses starvation-induced immunosuppression. Nature 1998; 394:897–901.
91. Sierra-Honigmann MR, Nath AK, Murakami C, Garcia-Cardena G, Papapetropoulos A, Sessa WC, Madge LA, Schechner JS, Schwabb MB, Polverini PJ, Flores-Riveros JR. Biological action of leptin as an angiogenic factor. Science 1998; 281:1683–1686.
92. Moon BC, Friedman JM. The molecular basis of the obese mutation in *ob2j* mice. Genomics 1997; 42:152–156.
93. Spiegelman BM, Flier JS. Obesity and the regulation of energy balance. Cell 2001; 104:531–543.
94. Schwartz MW, Baskin DG, Bukowski TR, Kuijper JL, Foster D, Lasser G, Prunkard DE, Porte D Jr, Woods SC, Seeley RJ, Weigle DS. Specificity of leptin action on elevated blood glucose levels and hypothalamic neuropeptide Y gene expression in *ob/ob* mice. Diabetes 1996; 45:531–535.
95. Vaisse C, Halaas JL, Horvath CM, Darnell JE, Jr., Stoffel M, Friedman JM. Leptin activation of STAT3 in the hypothalamus of wild-type and *ob/ob* mice but not *db/db* mice. Nat Genet 1996; 14:95–97.
96. Banks AS, Davis SM, Bates SH, Myers MG Jr. Activation of downstream signals by the long form of the leptin receptor. J Biol Chem 2000; 275:14563–14572.
97. Spanswick D, Smith MA, Groppi VE, Logan SD, Ashford ML. Leptin inhibits hypothalamic neurons by activation of atp-sensitive potassium channels. Nature 1997; 390:521–525.
98. Stephens TW, Basinski M, Bristow PK, Bue-Valleskey JM, Burgett SG, Craft L, Hale J, Hoffmann J, Hsiung HM, Kriauciunas A. The role of neuropeptide *y* in the antiobesity action of the obese gene product. Nature 1995; 377:530–532.
99. Thornton JE, Cheung CC, Clifton DK, Steiner RA. Regulation of hypothalamic proopiomelanocortin mrna by leptin in *ob/ob* mice. Endocrinology 1997; 138:5063–5066.
100. Schwartz MW, Seeley RJ, Woods SC, Weigle DS, Campfield LA, Burn P, Baskin DG. Leptin increases hypothalamic pro-opiomelanocortin mrna expression in the rostral arcuate nucleus. Diabetes 1997; 46:2119–2123.
101. Korner J, Chua SC Jr, Williams JA, Leibel RL, Wardlaw SL. Regulation of hypothalamic proopiomelanocortin by leptin in lean and obese rats. Neuroendocrinology 1999; 70:377–383.
102. Hummel KP, Dickie MM, Coleman DL. Diabetes, a new mutation in the mouse. Science 1966; 153:1127–1128.
103. Coleman DL, Hummel KP. The influence of genetic background on the expression of the *Obese* (*ob*) gene in the mouse. Diabetologia 1973; 9:287–293.
104. Hummel KP, Coleman DL, Lane PW. The influence of genetic background on expression of mutations at the diabetes locus in the mouse. I. C57BL/KsJ and C57BL/6J strains. Biochem Genet 1972; 7:1–13.
105. Coleman DL, Hummel KP. Effects of parabiosis of normal with genetically diabetic mice. Am J Physiol 1969; 217:1298–1304.
106. Zucker TF, Zucker LM. Fat accretion and growth in the rat. Obes Res 1996; 4:102–108.
107. Koletsky S. Obese spontaneously hypertensive rats—a model for study of atherosclerosis. Exp Mol Pathol 1973; 19:53–60.
108. Truett GE, Bahary N, Friedman JM, Leibel RL. Rat obesity gene fatty (*fa*) maps to chromosome 5: evidence for homology with the mouse gene diabetes (*db*). Proc Natl Acad Sci USA 1991; 88:7806–7809.
109. Lee GH, Proenca R, Montez JM, Carroll KM, Darvishzadeh JG, Lee JI, Friedman JM. Abnormal splicing of the leptin receptor in diabetic mice. Nature 1996; 379:632–635.
110. Chua SC Jr, Chung WK, Wu-Peng XS, Zhang Y, Liu SM, Tartaglia L, Leibel RL. Phenotypes of mouse *diabetes* and rat *fatty* due to mutations in the *ob* (leptin) receptor. Science 1996; 271:994–996.
111. Tartaglia LA, Dembski M, Weng X, Deng N, Culpepper J, Devos R, Richards GJ, Campfield LA, Clark FT, Deeds I. Identification and expression cloning of a leptin receptor, *ob-r*. Cell 1995; 83:1263–1271.
112. Liu SM, Leibel RL, Chua SC. Partial duplication in the $Lepr^{dbPas}$ mutation is a result of unequal crossing over. Mamm Genome 1998; 9:780–781.

113. Chen H, Charlat O, Tartaglia LA, Woolf EA, Weng X, Ellis SJ, Lakey ND, Culpepper J, Moore KJ, Breitbart RE, Duyk GM, Tepper RI, Morgenstern JP. Evidence that the *diabetes* gene encodes the leptin receptor: identification of a mutation in the leptin receptor gene in *db/db* mice. Cell 1996; 84: 491–495.
114. Laivuori H, Kaaja R, Koistinen H, Karonen SL, Andersson S, Koivisto V, Ylikorkala O. Leptin during and after preeclamptic or normal pregnancy: its relation to serum insulin and insulin sensitivity. Metabolism 2000; 49:259–263.
115. Lee G, Li C, Montez J, Halaas J, Darvishzadeh J, Friedman JM. Leptin receptor mutations in 129 db^{3j}/db^{3j} mice and NIH fa^{cp}/fa^{cp} rats. Mamm Genome 1997; 8:445–447.
116. Devos R, Guisez Y, Van der Heyden J, White DW, Kalai M, Fountoulakis M, Plaetinck G. Ligand-independent dimerization of the extracellular domain of the leptin receptor and determination of the stoichiometry of leptin binding. J Biol Chem 1997; 272:18304–18310.
117. Leiter EH. The genetics of diabetes susceptibility in mice. FASEB J 1989; 3:2231–2241.
118. Leiter EH, Coleman DL, Eisenstein AB, Strack I. A new mutation (db^{3j}) at the diabetes locus in strain 129/j mice. I. Physiological and histological characterization. Diabetologia 1980; 19:58–65.
119. Li C, Ioffe E, Fidahusein N, Connolly E, Friedman JM. Absence of soluble leptin receptor in plasma from db^{Pas}/db^{Pas} and other *db/db* mice. J Biol Chem 1998; 273:10078–10082.
120. Aubert R, Herzog J, Camus MC, Guenet JL, Lemonnier D. Description of a new model of genetic obesity: the db^{Pas} mouse. J Nutr 1985; 115:327–333.
121. Brown JA, Chua SC Jr, Liu SM, Andrews MT, Vandenbergh JG. Spontaneous mutation in the *db* gene results in obesity and diabetes in *Cd-1* outbred mice. Am J Physiol Regul Integr Comp Physiol 2000; 278:R320–R330.
122. Reichart U, Renner-Muller I, Hoflich A, Muller OJ, Franz WM, Wolf E, Muller M, Brem G, Aigner B. Contrasting obesity phenotypes uncovered by partial leptin receptor gene deletion in transgenic mice. Biochem Biophys Res Commun 2000; 269:502–507.
123. Reichart U, Kappler R, Scherthan H, Wolf E, Muller M, Brem G, Aigner B. Partial leptin receptor gene deletion in transgenic mice prevents expression of the membrane-bound isoforms except for *ob-rc*. Biochem Biophys Res Commun 2000; 269:496–501.
124. Falconer DS, Isaacsom JH. Adipose, a new inherited obesity of the mouse. J Hered 1959; 50:290–292.
125. Friedman JE, De Vente JE, Peterson RG, Dohm GL. Altered expression of muscle glucose transporter glut-4 in diabetic *fatty* Zucker rats (*ZDF/drt-fa*). Am J Physiol 1991; 261:E782–E788.
126. Turkenkopf IJ, Kava RA, Feldweg A, Horowitz C, Greenwood MR, Johnson PR. Zucker and Wistar diabetic *fatty* rats show different response to adrenalectomy. Am J Physiol 1991; 261:R912–R919.
127. Kava RA, West DB, Lukasik VA, Wypijewski C, Wojnar Z, Johnson PR, Greenwood MR. The effects of gonadectomy on glucose tolerance of genetically obese (*fa/fa*) rats: Influence of sex and genetic background. Int J Obes Relat Metab Disord 1992; 16:103–111.
128. Leiter EH, Chapman HD. Obesity-induced diabetes (diabesity) in C57BL/KsJ mice produces aberrant trans-regulation of sex steroid sulfotransferase genes. J Clin Invest 1994; 93:2007–2013.
129. Chua SC Jr, White DW, Wu-Peng XS, Liu SM, Okada N, Kershaw EE, Chung WK, Power-Kehoe L, Chua M, Tartaglia LA, Leibel RL. Phenotype of fatty due to GLN269PRO mutation in the leptin receptor (*Lepr*). Diabetes 1996; 45:1141–1143.
130. Takaya K, Ogawa Y, Isse N, Okazaki T, Satoh N, Masuzaki H, Mori K, Tamura N, Hosoda K, Nakao K. Molecular cloning of rat leptin receptor isoform complementary dnas—identification of a missense mutation in Zucker *fatty* (*fa/fa*) rats. Biochem Biophys Res Commun 1996; 225:75–83.
131. Ellwood KC, Michaelis OEt, Emberland JJ, Bhathena SJ. Hormonal and lipogenic and gluconeogenic enzymatic responses in LA/N-corpulent rats. Proc Soc Exp Biol Med 1985; 179:163–167.
132. Michaelis OEt, Ellwood KC, Judge JM, Schoene NW, Hansen CT. Effect of dietary sucrose on the SHR/N-corpulent rat: a new model for insulin-independent diabetes. Am J Clin Nutr 1984; 39:612–618.
133. Wu-Peng XS, Chua SC Jr, Okada N, Liu SM, Nicolson M, Leibel RL. Phenotype of the obese Koletsky (*f*) rat due to TYR763STOP mutation in the extracellular domain of the leptin receptor (*Lepr*): evidence for deficient plasma-to-CSF transport of leptin in both the Zucker and Koletsky obese rat. Diabetes 1997; 46:513–518.
134. Takaya K, Ogawa Y, Hiraoka J, Hosoda K, Yamori Y, Nakao K, Koletsky RJ. Nonsense mutation of leptin receptor in the obese spontaneously hypertensive Koletsky rat. Nat Genet 1996; 14:130–131.
135. Kowalski TJ, Liu SM, Leibel RL, Chua SC Jr. Transgenic complementation of leptin-receptor deficiency. I. Rescue of the obesity/diabetes phenotype of *Lepr*-null mice expressing a *Lepr-b* transgene. Diabetes 2001; 50:425–435.
136. Ahima RS, Kelly J, Elmquist JK, Flier JS. Distinct physiologic and neuronal responses to decreased leptin and mild hyperleptinemia. Endocrinology 1999; 140:4923–4931.
137. Xu B, Dube MG, Kalra PS, Farmerie WG, Kaibara A, Moldawer LL, Martin D, Kalra SP. Anorectic effects of the cytokine, ciliary neurotropic

factor, are mediated by hypothalamic neuropeptide Y: comparison with leptin. Endocrinology 1998; 139:466–473.

138. Leiter EH, Coleman DL, Eisenstein AB, Strack I. Dietary control of pathogenesis in C57BL/KsJ *db/db* diabetes mice. Metabolism 1981; 30:554–562.
139. Leiter EH, Prochazka M, Shultz LD. Effect of immunodeficiency on diabetogenesis in genetically diabetic (*db/db*) mice. J Immunol 1987; 138:3224–3229.
140. Solomon J, Mayer J. The effect of adrenalectomy on the development of the obese-hyperglycemic syndrome in *ob/ob* mice. Endocrinology 1973; 93:510–512.
141. Makimura H, Mizuno TM, Roberts J, Silverstein J, Beasley J, Mobbs CV. Adrenalectomy reverses obese phenotype and restores hypothalamic melanocortin tone in leptin-deficient *ob/ob* mice. Diabetes 2000; 49:1917–1923.
142. Chen HL, Romsos DR. Dexamethasone rapidly increases hypothalamic neuropeptide y secretion in adrenalectomized *ob/ob* mice. Am J Physiol 1996; 271:E151–E158.
143. Coleman DL, Eicher EM. Fat (*fat*) and tubby (*tub*): two autosomal recessive mutations causing obesity syndromes in the mouse. J Hered 1990; 81:424–427.
144. Naggert JK, Fricker LD, Varlamov O, Nishina PM, Rouille Y, Steiner DF, Carroll RJ, Paigen BJ, Leiter EH. Hyperproinsulinaemia in obese *fat/fat* mice associated with a carboxypeptidase E mutation which reduces enzyme activity. Nat Genet 1995; 10:135–142.
145. Fricker LD. Carboxypeptidase E. Annu Rev Physiol 1988; 50:309–321.
146. Blazquez M, Shennan KI. Basic mechanisms of secretion: sorting into the regulated secretory pathway. Biochem Cell Biol 2000; 78:181–191.
147. Shen FS, Aguilera G, Loh YP. Altered biosynthesis and secretion of pro-opiomelanocortin in the intermediate and anterior pituitary of carboxypeptidase *e*-deficient, Cpe^{fat}/Cpe^{fat} mice. Neuropeptides 1999; 33:276–280.
148. Zhang CF, Snell CR, Loh YP. Identification of a novel prohormone sorting signal-binding site on carboxypeptidase E, a regulated secretory pathway-sorting receptor. Mol Endocrinol 1999; 13:527–536.
149. Cool DR, Normant E, Shen F, Chen HC, Pannell L, Zhang Y, Loh YP. Carboxypeptidase *e* is a regulated secretory pathway sorting receptor: genetic obliteration leads to endocrine disorders in Cpe^{fat} mice. Cell 1997; 88:73–83.
150. Beinfeld MC. CCK biosynthesis and processing: recent progress and future challenges. Life Sci 1997; 61:2359–2366.
151. Ohlemiller KK, Hughes RM, Mosinger-Ogilvie J, Speck JD, Grosof DH, Silverman MS. Cochlear and retinal degeneration in the *tubby* mouse. Neuroreport 1995; 6:845–849.
152. Noben-Trauth K, Naggert JK, North MA, Nishina PM. A candidate gene for the mouse mutation *tubby*. Nature 1996; 380:534–538.
153. Kleyn PW, Fan W, Kovats SG, Lee JJ, Pulido JC, Wu Y, Berkemeier LR, Misumi DJ, Holmgren L, Charlat O, Woolf EA, Tayber O, Brody T, Shu P, Hawkins F, Kennedy B, Baldini L, Ebeling C, Alperin GD, Deeds J, Lakey ND, Culpepper J, Chen H, Glucksmann-Kuis MA, Moore KI. Identification and characterization of the mouse obesity gene *Tubby*: a member of a novel gene family. Cell 1996; 85:281–290.
154. Lewis CA, Batlle IR, Batlle KG, Banerjee P, Cideciyan AV, Huang J, Aleman TS, Huang Y, Ott J, Gilliam TC, Knowles JA, Jacobson SG. Tubby-like protein 1 homozygous splice-site mutation causes early-onset severe retinal degeneration. Invest Ophthalmol Vis Sci 1999; 40:2106–2114.
155. Ikeda A, Zheng QY, Rosenstiel P, Maddatu T, Zuberi AR, Roopenian DC, North MA, Naggert JK, Johnson KR, Nishina PM. Genetic modification of hearing in tubby mice: evidence for the existence of a major gene (*Moth1*) which protects tubby mice from hearing loss. Hum Mol Genet 1999; 8:1761–1767.
156. Guan XM, Yu H, Van der Ploeg LH. Evidence of altered hypothalamic pro-opiomelanocortin/neuropeptide Y MRNA expression in *tubby* mice. Brain Res Mol Brain Res 1998; 59:273–279.
157. Santagata S, Boggon TJ, Baird CL, Gomez CA, Zhao J, Shan WS, Myszka DG, Shapiro L. G-protein signaling through *tubby* proteins. Science 2001; 292:2041–2050.
158. Boggon TJ, Shan WS, Santagata S, Myers SC, Shapiro L. Implication of *tubby* proteins as transcription factors by structure-based functional analysis. Science 1999; 286:2119–2125.
159. Smith GP, Gibbs J. Satiating effect of cholecystokinin. Ann NY Acad Sci 1994; 713:236–241.
160. Miyasaka K, Kanai S, Ohta M, Kawanami T, Kono A, Funakoshi A. Lack of satiety effect of cholecystokinin (CCK) in a new rat model not expressing the *Cck-a* receptor gene. Neurosci Lett 1994; 180:143–146.
161. Moran TH, Katz LF, Plata-Salaman CR, Schwartz GJ. Disordered food intake and obesity in rats lacking cholecystokinin A receptors. Am J Physiol 1998; 274:R618–R625.
162. Moran TH. Cholecystokinin and satiety: current perspectives. Nutrition 2000; 16:858–865.
163. Lacourse KA, Swanberg LJ, Gillespie PJ, Rehfeld JF, Saunders TL, Samuelson LC. Pancreatic function in *Cck*-deficient mice: adaptation to dietary protein does not require CCK. Am J Physiol 1999; 276:G1302–G1309.
164. Miyasaka K, Shinozaki H, Suzuki S, Sato Y, Kanai S, Masuda M, Jimi A, Nagata A, Matsui T, Noda T, Kono A, Funakoshi A. Disruption of cholecystokinin *Cckb* receptor gene did not modify bile or pancreatic

secretion or pancreatic growth: a study in *Cckb* receptor gene knockout mice. Pancreas 1999; 19:114–118.

165. Perusse L, Chagnon YC, Weisnagel SJ, Rankinen T, Snyder E, Sands J, Bouchard C. The human obesity gene map: the 2000 update. Obes Res 2001; 9:135–169.
166. Montague CT, Farooqi IS, Whitehead JP, Soos MA, Rau H, Wareham NJ, Sewter CP, Digby JE, Mohammed SN, Hurst JA, Cheetham CH, Earley AR, Barnett AH, Prins JB, O'Rahilly S. Congenital leptin deficiency is associated with severe early-onset obesity in humans. Nature 1997; 387:903–908.
167. Farooqi IS, Jebb SA, Langmack G, Lawrence E, Cheetham CH, Prentice AM, Hughes IA, McCamish MA, O'Rahilly S. Effects of recombinant leptin therapy in a child with congenital leptin deficiency. N Engl J Med 1999; 341:879–884.
168. Chehab FF, Lim ME, Lu R. Correction of the sterility defect in homozygous obese female mice by treatment with the human recombinant leptin. Nat Genet 1996; 12:318–320.
169. Chehab FF. Mounzih K, Lu R, Lim ME. Early onset of reproductive function in normal female mice treated with leptin. Science 1997; 275:88–90.
170. Strobel A, Issad T, Camoin L, Ozata M, Strosberg AD. A leptin missense mutation associated with hypogonadism and morbid obesity. Nat Genet 1998; 18:213–215.
171. Farooqi IS, Keogh JM, Kamath S, Jones S, Gibson WT, Trussell R, Jebb SA, Lip GY, O'Rahilly S. Partial leptin deficiency and human adiposity. Nature 2001; 414:34–35.
172. Chung WK, Belfi K, Chua M, Wiley J, Mackintosh R, Nicolson M, Boozer CN, Leibel RL. Heterozygosity for Lep^{ob} or $Lepr^{db}$ affects body composition and leptin homeostasis in adult mice. Am J Physiol 1998; 274:R985–R990.
173. Leibel RL. The role of leptin in the control of body weight. Nutr Reviews 2002; 60:s15–s19.
174. Considine RV, Considine EL, Williams CJ, Nyce MR, Magosin SA, Bauer TL, Rosato EL, Colberg J, Caro JF. Evidence against either a premature stop codon or the absence of obese gene mRNA in human obesity. J Clin Invest 1995; 95:2986–2988.
175. Maffei M, Stoffel M, Barone M, Moon B, Dammerman M, Ravussin E, Bogardus C, Ludwig DS, Flier JS, Talley M. Absence of mutations in the human *ob* gene in obese/diabetic subjects. Diabetes 1996; 45:679–682.
176. Lonnqvist F, Arner P, Nordfors L, Schalling M. Overexpression of the *Obese (ob)* gene in adipose tissue of human obese subjects. Nat Med 1995; 1:950–953.
177. Lonnqvist F, Wennlund A, Arner P. Relationship between circulating leptin and peripheral fat distribution in obese subjects. Int J Obes Relat Metab Disord 1997; 21:255–260.
178. Duggirala R, Stern MP, Mitchell BD, Reinhart LJ, Shipman PA, Uresandi OC, Chung WK, Leibel RL, Hales CN, O'Connell P, Blangero J. Quantitative variation in obesity-related traits and insulin precursors linked to the ob gene region on human chromosome 7. Am J Hum Genet 1996; 59:694–703.
179. Clement K, Garner C, Hager J, Philippi A, LeDuc C, Carey A, Harris TJ, Jury C, Cardon LR, Basdevant A, Demenais F, Guy-Grand B, North M, Froguel P. Indication for linkage of the human *ob* gene region with extreme obesity. Diabetes 1996; 45:687–690.
180. Clement K, Vaisse C, Lahlou N, Cabrol S, Pelloux V, Cassuto D, Gourmelen M, Dina C, Chambaz J, Lacorte JM, Basdevant A, Bougneres P, Lebouc Y, Froguel P, Guy-Grand B. A mutation in the human leptin receptor gene causes obesity and pituitary dysfunction. Nature 1998; 392:398–401.
181. Rosenbaum M, Leibel RL. Pathophysiology of childhood obesity. Adv Pediatr 1988; 35:73–137.
182. Diamond FB Jr, Eichler DC, Duckett G, Jorgensen EV, Shulman D, Root AW. Demonstration of a leptin binding factor in human serum. Biochem Biophys Res Commun 1997; 233:818–822.
183. Chung WK, Power-Kehoe L, Chua M, Chu F, Aronne L, Huma Z, Sothern M, Udall JN, Kahle B, Leibel RL. Exonic and intronic sequence variation in the human leptin receptor gene *(LEPR)*. Diabetes 1997; 46:1509–1511.
184. Matsuoka N, Ogawa Y, Hosoda K, Matsuda J, Masuzaki H, Miyawaki T, Azuma N, Natsui K, Nishimura H, Yoshimasa Y, Nishi S, Thompson DB, Nakao K. Human leptin receptor gene in obese Japanese subjects: evidence against either obesity-causing mutations or association of sequence variants with obesity. Diabetologia 1997; 40:1204–1210.
185. Gotoda T, Manning BS, Goldstone AP, Imrie H, Evans AL, Strosberg AD, McKeigue PM, Scott J, Aitman TJ. Leptin receptor gene variation and obesity: lack of association in a white british male population. Hum Mol Genet 1997; 6:869–876.
186. Silver K, Walston J, Chung WK, Yao F, Parikh VV, Andersen R, Cheskin LJ, Elahi D, Muller D, Leibel RL, Shuldiner AR. The Gln223Arg and Lys656Asn polymorphisms in the human leptin receptor do not associate with traits related to obesity. Diabetes 1997; 46:1898–1900.
187. Echwald SM, Sorensen TD, Sorensen TI, Tybjaerg-Hansen A, Andersen T, Chung WK, Leibel RL, Pedersen O. Amino acid variants in the human leptin receptor: lack of association to juvenile onset obesity. Biochem Biophys Res Commun 1997; 233:248–252.
188. Heo M, Leibel RL, Gropp E, Boyer BB, Chung WK, Koulu M, Karvonen MK, Pesonen U, Rissanen A, Laakso M, Uusitupa M, Chagnon Y, Bouchard C,

Dononoue PA, Burns TL, Shuldiner AR, Silver K, Andersen RE, Pedersen O, Echwald S, Sorensen TIA, Behn P, Permutt MA, Jacobs KB, Elston RC, Hoffman DJ, Allison DB. Brief report: a meta-analytic investigation of linkage and association of common leptin receptor polymorphisms with body mass index and waist. Submitted.

189. Heo M, Leibel RL, Fontaine KR, et al. A meta-analytic investigation of linkage and association of common leptin receptor (*LEPR*) polymorphisms with body mass index and waist circumference. Intl Jnl of Obesity 2002; 26:640–646.

190. Vaisse C, Clement K, Guy-Grand B, Froguel P. A frameshift mutation in human *MC4R* is associated with a dominant form of obesity. Nat Genet 1998; 20:113–114.

191. Cody JD, Reveles XT, Hale DE, Lehman D, Coon H, Leach RJ. Haplosufficiency of the melancortin-4 receptor gene in individuals with deletions of 18q. Hum Genet 1999; 105:424–427.

192. Hinney A, Schmidt A, Nottebom K, Heibult O, Becker I, Ziegler A, Gerber G, Sina M, Gorg T, Mayer H, Siegfried W, Fichter M, Remschmidt H, Hebebrand J. Several mutations in the melanocortin-4 receptor gene including a nonsense and a frameshift mutation associated with dominantly inherited obesity in humans. J Clin Endocrinol Metab 1999; 84:1483–1486.

193. Wardlaw SL. Clinical review 127: obesity as a neuroendocrine disease: Lessons to be learned from proopiomelanocortin and melanocortin receptor mutations in mice and men. J Clin Endocrinol Metab 2001; 86:1442–1446.

194. Krude H, Biebermann H, Luck W, Horn R, Brabant G, Gruters A. Severe early-onset obesity, adrenal insufficiency and red hair pigmentation caused by *pomc* mutations in humans. Nat Genet 1998; 19:155–157.

195. Comuzzie AG, Hixson JE, Almasy L, Mitchell BD, Mahaney MC, Dyer TD, Stern MP, MacCluer JW, Blangero J. A major quantitative trait locus determining serum leptin levels and fat mass is located on human chromosome 2. Nat Genet 1997; 15:273–276.

196. Hixson JE, Almasy L, Cole S, Birnbaum S, Mitchell BD, Mahaney MC, Stern MP, MacCluer JW, Blangero J, Comuzzie AG. Normal variation in leptin levels in associated with polymorphisms in the proopiomelanocortin gene, *POMC*. J Clin Endocrinol Metab 1999; 84:3187–3191.

197. Davidson HW, Peshavaria M, Hutton JC. Proteolytic conversion of proinsulin into insulin. Identification of a Ca^{2+}-dependent acidic endopeptidase in isolated insulin-secretory granules. Biochem J 1987; 246:279–286.

198. Normant E, Loh YP. Depletion of carboxypeptidase e, a regulated secretory pathway sorting receptor, causes misrouting and constitutive secretion of proinsulin and proenkephalin, but not chromogranin *a*. Endocrinology 1998; 139:2137–2145.

199. Rovere C, Viale A, Nahon J, Kitabgi P. Impaired processing of brain proneurotensin and promelanin-concentrating hormone in obese *fat/fat* mice. Endocrinology 1996; 137:2954–2958.

200. Udupi V, Gomez P, Song L, Varlamov O, Reed JT, Leiter EH, Fricker LD, Greeley GH Jr. Effect of carboxypeptidase *e* deficiency on progastrin processing and gastrin messenger ribonucleic acid expression in mice with the *fat* mutation. Endocrinology 1997; 138:1959–1963.

201. Shen FS, Loh YP. Intracellular misrouting and abnormal secretion of adrenocorticotropin and growth hormone in Cpe^{fat} mice associated with a carboxypeptidase E mutation. Proc Natl Acad Sci USA 1997; 94:5314–5319.

202. Cain BM, Wang W, Beinfeld MC. Cholecystokinin (CCK) levels are greatly reduced in the brains but not the duodenums of Cpe^{fat}/Cpe^{fat} mice: a regional difference in the involvement of carboxypeptidase E (CPE) in Pro-CCK processing. Endocrinology 1997; 138:4034–4037.

203. O'Rahilly S, Gray H, Humphreys PJ, Krook A, Polonsky KS, White A, Gibson S, Taylor K, Carr C. Brief report: impaired processing of prohormones associated with abnormalities of glucose homeostasis and adrenal function. N Engl J Med 1995; 333:1386–1390.

204. Masugi J, Tamori Y, Kasuga M. Inhibition of adipogenesis by a COOH-terminally truncated mutant of PPARgamma2 in 3T3-L1 cells. Biochem Biophys Res Commun 1999; 264:93–99.

205. Koch M, Rett K, Maerker E, Volk A, Haist K, Deninger M, Renn W, Haring HU. Thc PPARgamma2 amino acid polymorphism Pro12Ala is prevalent in offspring of type II diabetic patients and is associated to increased insulin sensitivity in a subgroup of obese subjects. Diabetologia 1999; 42:758–762.

206. Deeb SS, Fajas L, Nemoto M, Pihlajamaki J, Mykkanen L, Kuusisto J, Laakso M, Fujimoto W, Auwerx J. A Pro12Ala substitution in PPARgamma2 associated with decreased receptor activity, lower body mass index and improved insulin sensitivity. Nat Genet 1998; 20:284–287.

207. Valve R, Sivenius K, Miettinen R, Pihlajamaki J, Rissanen A, Deeb SS, Auwerx J, Uusitupa M, Laakso M. Two polymorphisms in the peroxisome proliferator-activated receptor-gamma gene are associated with severe overweight among obese women. J Clin Endocrinol Metab 1999; 84:3708–3712.

208. Beamer BA, Yen CJ, Andersen RE, Muller D, Elahi D, Cheskin LJ, Andres R, Roth J, Shuldiner AR. Association of the Pro12Ala variant in the peroxisome

proliferator-activated receptor-gamma2 gene with obesity in two Caucasian populations. Diabetes 1998; 47:1806–1808.
209. Ringel J, Engeli S, Distler A, Sharma AM. Pro12ala missense mutation of the peroxisome proliferator activated receptor gamma and diabetes mellitus. Biochem Biophys Res Commun 1999; 254:450–453.
210. Oh EY, Min KM, Chung JH, Min YK, Lee MS, Kim KW, Lee MK. Significance of Pro12Ala mutation in peroxisome proliferator-activated receptor-gamma2 in Korean diabetic and obese subjects. J Clin Endocrinol Metab 2000; 85:1801–1804.
211. Altshuler D, Hirschhorn JN, Klannemark M, Lindgren CM, Vohl MC, Nemesh J, Lane CR, Schaffner SF, Bolk S, Brewer C, Tuomi T, Gaudet D, Hudson TJ, Daly M, Groop L, Lander ES. The common PPARgamma Pro12Ala polymorphism is associated with decreased risk of type 2 diabetes. Nat Genet 2000; 26:76–80.
212. Hasstedt SJ, Ren QF, Teng K, Elbein SC. Effect of the peroxisome proliferator-activated receptor-gamma 2 Pro12Ala variant on obesity, glucose homeostasis, and blood pressure in members of familial type 2 diabetic kindreds. J Clin Endocrinol Metab 2001; 86:536–541.
213. Meirhaeghe A, Fajas L, Helbecque N, Cottel D, Lebel P, Dallongeville J, Deeb S, Auwerx J, Amouyel P. A genetic polymorphism of the peroxisome proliferator-activated receptor gamma gene influences plasma leptin levels in obese humans. Hum Mol Genet 1998; 7:435–440.
214. Wang XL, Oosterhof J, Duarte N. Peroxisome proliferator-activated receptor gamma C161→T polymorphism and coronary artery disease. Cardiovasc Res 1999; 44:588–594.
215. Ristow M, Muller-Wieland D, Pfeiffer A, Krone W, Kahn CR. Obesity associated with a mutation in a genetic regulator of adipocyte differentiation. N Engl J Med 1998; 339:953–959.
216. Ogawa S, Urano T, Hosoi T, Miyao M, Hoshino S, Fujita M, Shiraki M, Orimo H, Ouchi Y, Inoue S. Association of bone mineral density with a polymorphism of the peroxisome proliferator-activated receptor gamma gene: PPARgamma expression in osteoblasts. Biochem Biophys Res Commun 1999; 260:122–126.
217. Barroso I, Gurnell M, Crowley VE, Agostini M, Schwabe JW, Soos MA, Maslen GL, Williams TD, Lewis H, Schafer AJ, Chatterjee VK, O'Rahilly S. Dominant negative mutations in human PPARgamma associated with severe insulin resistance, diabetes mellitus and hypertension. Nature 1999; 402:880–883.
218. Michaud JL, Rosenquist T, May NR, Fan CM. Development of neuroendocrine lineages requires the *BLLH-PAS* transcription factor SIM1. Genes Dev 1998; 12:3264–3275.
219. Michaud JL, DeRossi C, May NR, Holdener BC, Fan CM. *Arnt2* acts as the dimerization partner of *Sim1* for the development of the hypothalamus. Mech Dev 2000; 90:253–261.
220. Holder JL, Butte NF, Zinn AR. Profound obesity associated with a balanced translocation that disrupts the *Sim1* gene. Hum Mol Genet 2000; 9:101–108.
221. Aldred MA, Trembath RC. Activating and inactivating mutations in the human *Gnas1* gene. Hum Mutat 2000; 16:183–189.
222. de Sanctis C, Lala R, Matarazzo P, et al. McCune-Albright syndrome: a longitudinal clinical study of 32 patients. J Pediat Endocr Metab 1999; 12:817–826.
223. Katsanis N, Ansley SJ, Badano JL, Eichers ER, Lewis RA, Hoskins BE, Scambler PJ, Davidson WS, Beales PL, Lupski JR. Triallelic inheritance in Bardet-Biedl syndrome, a Mendelian recessive disorder. Science 2001; 293:2256–2259.
224. Burghes AH, Vaessin HE, De La Chapelle A. Genetics: the land between Mendelian and multifactorial inheritance. Science 2001; 293:2213–2214.
225. Kwitek-Black AE, Carmi R, Duyk GM, Buetow KH, Elbedour K, Parvari R, Yandava CN, Stone EM, Sheffield VC. Linkage of Bardet-Biedl syndrome to chromosome 16q and evidence for non-allelic genetic heterogeneity. Nat Genet 1993; 5:392–396.
226. Elbedour K, Zucker N, Zalzstein E, Barki Y, Carmi R. Cardiac abnormalities in the Bardet-Biedl syndrome: echocardiographic studies of 22 patients. Am J Med Genet 1994; 52:164–169.
227. Green JS, Parfrey PS, Harnett JD, Farid NR, Cramer BC, Johnson G, Heath O, McManamon PJ, O'Leary E, Pryse-Phillips W. The cardinal manifestations of Bardet-Biedl syndrome, a form of Laurence-Moon-Biedl syndrome. N Engl J Med 1989; 321:1002–1009.
228. Slavotinek AM, Biesecker LG. Unfolding the role of chaperones and chaperonins in human disease. Trends Genet 2001; 17:528–535.
229. Croft JB, Swift M. Obesity, hypertension, and renal disease in relatives of Bardet-Biedl syndrome sibs. Am J Med Genet 1990; 36:37–42.
230. Croft JB, Morrell D, Chase CL, Swift M. Obesity in heterozygous carriers of the gene for the Bardet-Biedl syndrome. Am J Med Genet 1995; 55:12–15.
231. Kubota T, Oga S, Ohashi H, Iwamoto Y, Fukushima Y. Borjeson-Forssman Lehmann syndrome in a woman with skewed X-chromosome inactivation. Am J Med Genet 1999; 87:258–261.
232. Gecz J, Baker E, Donnelly A, Ming JE, McDonald-McGinn DM, Spinner NB, Zackai EH, Sutherland GR, Mulley JC. Fibroblast growth factor homologous factor 2 (fhf2): gene structure, expression and mapping to the Borjeson-Forssman-Lehmann syndrome region in *xq26* delineated by a duplication breakpoint in a *bfls*-like patient. Hum Genet 1999; 104:56–63.
233. Rousseau F, Vincent A, Rivella S, Heitz D, Triboli C,

Maestrini E, Warren ST, Suthers GK, Goodfellow P, Mandel JL. Four chromosomal breakpoints and four new probes mark out a 10-cm region encompassing the fragile-X locus (*fraxa*). Am J Hum Genet 1991; 48:108–116.

234. Matthijs G, Schollen E, Van Schaftingen E, Cassiman JJ, Jaeken J. Lack of homozygotes for the most frequent disease allele in carbohydrate-deficient glycoprotein syndrome type 1a. Am J Hum Genet 1998; 62:542–550.
235. Nicholls RD, Saitoh S, Horsthemke B. Imprinting in Prader-Willi and Angelman syndromes. Trends Genet 1998; 14:194–200.
236. Kishino T, Lalande M, Wagstaff J. *UBE3A/E6-AP* mutations cause Angelman syndrome. Nat Genet 1997; 15:70–73.
237. Eiholzer U, Blum WF, Molinari L. Body fat determined by skinfold measurements is elevated despite underweight in infants with Prader-Labhart-Willi syndrome. J Pediatr 1999; 134:222–225.
238. Cassidy SB, Schwartz S. Prader-Willi and Angelman syndromes. Disorders of genomic imprinting. Medicine (Baltimore) 1998; 77:140–151.
239. Robinson WP, Bernasconi F, Mutirangura A, Ledbetter DH, Langlois S, Malcolm S, Morris MA, Schinzel AA. Nondisjunction of chromosome 15: origin and recombination. Am J Hum Genet 1993; 53:740–751.
240. Robinson WP, Bottani A, Xie YG, Balakrishman J, Binkert F, Machler M, Prader A, Schinzel A. Molecular, cytogenetic, and clinical investigations of Prader-Willi syndrome patients. Am J Hum Genet 1991; 49:1219–1234.
241. Mitchell J, Schinzel A, Langlois S, Gillessen-Kaesbach G, Schuffenhauer S, Michaelis R, Abeliovich D, Lerer I, Christian S, Guitart M, McFadden DE, Robinson WP. Comparison of phenotype in uniparental disomy and deletion prader-willi syndrome: sex specific differences. Am J Med Genet 1996; 65:133–136.
242. Reed ML, Leff SE. Maternal imprinting of human snrpn, a gene deleted in Prader-Willi syndrome. Nat Genet 1994; 6:163–167.
243. Ishikawa T, Kibe T, Wada Y. Deletion of small nuclear ribonucleoprotein polypeptide *n* (*snrpn*) in Prader-Willi syndrome detected by fluorescence in situ hybridization: two sibs with the typical phenotype without a cytogenetic deletion in chromosome 15q. Am J Med Genet 1996; 62:350–352.
244. Sun Y, Nicholls RD, Butler MG, Saitoh S, Hainline BE, Palmer CG. Breakage in the *SNRPN* locus in a balanced *46*,XY,*t(15;19)* Prader-Willi syndrome patient. Hum Mol Genet 1996; 5:517–524.
245. Kuslich CD, Kobori JA, Mohapatra G, Gregorio-King C, Donlon TA. Prader-Willi syndrome is caused by disruption of the *SNRPN* gene. Am J Hum Genet 1999; 64:70–76.
246. Dittrich B, Buiting K, Korn B, Rickard S, Buxton J, Saitoh S, Nicholls RD, Poustka A, Winterpacht A, Zabel B, Horsthemke B. Imprint switching on human chromosome 15 may involve alternative transcripts of the *SNRPN* gene. Nat Genet 1996; 14:163–170.
247. Lyko F, Buiting K, Horsthemke B, Paro R. Identification of a silencing element in the human 15q11-q13 imprinting center by using transgenic Drosophila. Proc Natl Acad Sci USA 1998; 95:1698–1702.
248. Bressler J, Tsai TF, Wu MY, Tsai SF, Ramirez MA, Armstrong D, Beaudet AL. The *SNRPN* promoter is not required for genomic imprinting of the Prader-Willi/Angelman domain in mice. Nat Genet 2001; 28:232–240.
249. Schulze A, Hansen C, Skakkebaek NE, Brondum-Nielsen K, Ledbetter DH, Tommerup N. Exclusion of *snrpn* as a major determinant of Prader-Willi syndrome by a translocation breakpoint. Nat Genet 1996; 12:452–454.
250. Holm VA, Cassidy SB, Butler MG, Hanchett JM, Greenswag LR, Whitman BY, Greenberg F. Prader-Willi syndrome: consensus diagnostic criteria. Pediatrics 1993; 91:398–402.
251. De los Santos T, Schweizer J, Rees CA, Francke U. Small evolutionarily conserved RNA, resembling C/D box small nucleolar RNA, is transcribed from *PWCRL*, a novel imprinted gene in the Prader-Willi deletion region, which is highly expressed in brain. Am J Hum Genet 2000; 67:1067–1082.
252. Pilia G, Hughes-Benzie RM, MacKenzie A, Baybayan P, Chen EY, Huber R, Neri G, Cao A, Forabosco A, Schlessinger D. Mutations in *GPC3*, a glypican gene, cause the Simpson-Golabi-Behmel overgrowth syndrome. Nat Genet 1996; 12:241–247.
253. Veugelers M, Cat BD, Muyldermans SY, Reekmans G, Delande N, Frints S, Legius E, Fryns JP, Schrander-Stumpel C, Weidle B, Magdalena N, David G. Mutational analysis of the *GPC3/GPC4* glypican gene cluster on Xq26 in patients with Simpson-Golabi-Behmel syndrome: identification of loss-of-function mutations in the *GPC3* gene. Hum Mol Genet 2000; 9:1321–1328.
254. Weksberg R, Shen DR, Fei YL, Song QL, Squire J. Disruption of insulin-like growth factor 2 imprinting in Beckwith-Wiedemann syndrome. Nat Genet 1993; 5:143–150.
255. Bamshad M, Lin RC, Law DJ, Watkins WC, Krakowiak PA, Moore ME, Franceschini P, Lala R, Holmes LB, Gebuhr TC, Bruneau BG, Schinzel A, Seidman JG, Seidman CE, Jorde LB. Mutations in human *TBX3* alter limb, apocrine and genital development in ulnar-mammary syndrome. Nat Genet 1997; 16:311–315.
256. Bamshad M, Le T, Watkins WS, Dixon ME, Kramer BE, Roeder AD, Carey JC, Root S, Schinzel A, Van Maldergem L, Gardner RJ, Lin RC, Seidman CE,

Seidman JG, Wallerstein R, Moran E, Sutphen R, Campbell CE, Jorde LB. The spectrum of mutations in *TBX3*: genotype/phenotype relationship in ulnar-mammary syndrome. Am J Hum Genet 1999; 64:1550–1562.

257. Oppert JM, Vohl MC, Chagnon M, Dionne FT, Cassard-Doulcier AM, Ricquier D, Perusse L, Bouchard C. DNA polymorphism in the uncoupling protein (*UCP*) gene and human body fat. Int J Obes Relat Metab Disord 1994; 18:526–531.
258. Clement K, Ruiz J, Cassard-Doulcier AM, Bouillaud F, Ricquier D, Basdevant A, Guy-Grand B, Froguel P. Additive effect of A→G (−3826) variant of the uncoupling protein gene and the Trp64Arg mutation of the beta 3-adrenergic receptor gene on weight gain in morbid obesity. Int J Obes Relat Metab Disord 1996; 20:1062–1066.
259. Urhammer SA, Fridberg M, Sorensen TI, Echwald SM, Andersen T, Tybjaerg-Hansen A, Clausen JO, Pedersen O. Studies of genetic variability of the uncoupling protein 1 gene in caucasian subjects with juvenile-onset obesity. J Clin Endocrinol Metab 1997; 82:4069–4074.
260. Bouchard C, Perusse L, Chagnon YC, Warden C, Ricquier D. Linkage between markers in the vicinity of the uncoupling protein 2 gene and resting metabolic rate in humans. Hum Mol Genet 1997; 6:1887–1889.
261. Walder K, Norman RA, Hanson RL, Schrauwen P, Neverova M, Jenkinson CP, Easlick J, Warden CH, Pecqueur C, Raimbault S, Ricquier D, Silver MH, Shuldiner AR, Solanes G, Lowell BB, Chung WK, Leibel RL, Pratley R, Ravussin E. Association between uncoupling protein polymorphisms (*UCP2-UCP3*) and energy metabolism/obesity in Pima Indians. Hum Mol Genet 1998; 7:1431–1435.
262. Esterbauer H, Schneitler C, Oberkofler H, Ebenbichler C, Paulweber B, Sandhofer F, Ladurner G, Hell E, Strosberg AD, Patsch JR, Krempler F, Patsch W. A common polymorphism in the promoter of *UCP2* is associated with decreased risk of obesity in middle-aged humans. Nat Genet 2001; 28:178–183.
263. Argyropoulos G, Brown AM, Willi SM, Zhu J, He Y, Reitman M, Gevao SM, Spruill I. Garvey WT. Effects of mutations in the human uncoupling protein 3 gene on the respiratory quotient and fat oxidation in severe obesity and type 2 diabetes. J Clin Invest 1998; 102:1345–1351.
264. Chung WK, Luke A, Cooper RS, Rotini C, Vidal-Puig A, Rosenbaum M, Chua M, Solanes G, Zheng M, Zhao L, LeDuc C, Eisberg A, Chu F, Murphy E, Schreier M, Aronne L, Caprio S, Kahle B, Gordon D, Leal SM, Goldsmith R, Andreu AL, Bruno C, DiMauro S, Leibel RL. Genetic and physiologic analysis of the role of uncoupling protein 3 in human energy homeostasis. Diabetes 1999; 48:1890–1895.
265. Brown AM, Willi SM, Argyropoulos G, Garvey WT. A novel missense mutation, R70W, in the human uncoupling protein 3 gene in a family with type 2 diabetes. Hum Mutat 1999; 13:508.
266. Brown AM, Dolan JW, Willi SM, Garvey WT, Argyropoulos G. Endogenous mutations in human uncoupling protein 3 alter its functional properties. FEBS Lett 1999; 464:189–193.
267. Garg A, Wilson R, Barnes R, Arioglu E, Zaidi Z, Gurakan F, Kocak N, O'Rahilly S, Taylor SI, Patel SB, Bowcock AM. A gene for congenital generalized lipodystrophy maps to human chromosome 9q34. J Clin Endocrinol Metab 1999; 84:3390–3394.
268. Wan YJ, An D, Cai Y, Repa JJ, Hung-Po Chen T, Flores M, Postic C, Magnuson MA, Chen J, Chien KR, French S, Mangelsdorf DJ, Sucov HM. Hepatocyte-specific mutation establishes retinoid X receptor alpha as a heterodimeric integrator of multiple physiological processes in the liver. Mol Cell Biol 2000; 20:4436–4444.
269. Cao H, Hegele RA. Nuclear lamin A/C R482Q mutation in Canadian kindreds with Dunnigan-type familial partial lipodystrophy. Hum Mol Genet 2000; 9:109–112.
270. Raffaele Di Barletta M, Ricci E, Galluzzi G, Tonali P, Mora M, Morandi L, Romorini A, Voit T, Orstavik KH, Merlini L, Trevisan C, Biancalana V, Housmanowa-Petrusewicz I, Bione S, Ricotti R, Schwartz K, Bonne G, Toniolo D. Different mutations in the lmna gene cause autosomal dominant and autosomal recessive Emery-Dreifuss muscular dystrophy. Am J Hum Genet 2000; 66:1407–1412.
271. Speckman RA, Garg A, Du F, Bennett L, Veile R, Arioglu E, Taylor SI, Lovett M, Bowcock AM. Mutational and haplotype analyses of families with familial partial lipodystrophy (Dunnigan variety) reveal recurrent missense mutations in the globular C-terminal domain of lamin a/c. Am J Hum Genet 2000; 66:1192–1198.
272. Schwartz MW, Woods SC, Porte D, Seeley RJ, Baskin DG. Central nervous system control of food intake. Nature 2000; 404:661–671.
273. Ohki-Hamazaki H, Watase K, Yamamoto K, Ogura H, Yamano M, Yamada K, Maeno H, Imaki J, Kikuyama S, Wada E, Wada K. Mice lacking bombesin receptor subtype-3 develop metabolic defects and obesity. Nature 1997; 390:165–169.
274. Inoue H, Iannotti CA, Welling CM, Veile R, Donis-Keller H, Permutt MA. Human cholecystokinin type a receptor gene: cytogenetic localization, physical mapping, and identification of two missense variants in patients with obesity and non-insulin-dependent diabetes mellitus (NIDDM). Genomics 1997; 42:331–335.
275. Miller LJ, Holicky EL, Ulrich CD, Wieben ED. Abnormal processing of the human cholecystokinin

receptor gene in association with gallstones and obesity. Gastroenterology 1995; 109:1375–1380.

276. Duckett SK, Snowder GD, Cockett NE. Effect of the callipyge gene on muscle growth, calpastatin activity, and tenderness of three muscles across the growth curve. J Anim Sci 2000; 78:2836–2841.
277. Wang ND, Finegold MJ, Bradley A, Ou CN, Abdelsayed SV, Wilde MD, Taylor LR, Wilson DR, Darlington GJ. Impaired energy homeostasis in *c/ebp* alpha knockout mice. Science 1995; 269:1108–1112.
278. Comuzzie AG, Allison DB. The search for human obesity genes. Science 1998; 280:1374–1377.
279. Smith SJ, Cases S, Jensen DR, Chen HC, Sande E, Tow B, Sanan DA, Raber J, Eckel RH, Farese RV Jr. Obesity resistance and multiple mechanisms of triglyceride synthesis in mice lacking *Dgat*. Nat Genet 2000; 25:87–90.
280. Thomas SA, Matsumoto AM, Palmiter RD. Noradrenaline is essential for mouse fetal development. Nature 1995; 374:643–646.
281. Thomas SA, Palmiter RD. Thermoregulatory and metabolic phenotypes of mice lacking noradrenaline and adrenaline. Nature 1997; 387:94–97.
282. Yu S, Yu D, Lee E, Eckhaus M, Lee R, Corria Z, Accili D, Westphal H, Weinstein LS. Variable and tissue-specific hormone resistance in heterotrimeric GS protein alpha-subunit (GS alpha) knockout mice is due to tissue-specific imprinting of the GS alpha gene. Proc Natl Acad Sci USA 1998; 95:8715–8720.
283. Veugelers M, Vermeesch J, Watanabe K, Yamaguchi Y, Marynen P, David G. *GPC4*, the gene for human K-Glypican, flanks *GPC3* on Xg26: Deletion of the *GPc3-GPc4* gene cluster in one family with, Simpson-Golabi-Behmel syndrome. Genomics 1998; 53:1–11.
284. Lin SC, Lin CR, Gukovsky I, Lusis AJ, Sawchenko PE, Rosenfeld MG. Molecular basis of the little mouse phenotype and implications for cell type–specific growth. Nature 1993; 364:208–213.
285. Wajnrajch MP, Gertner JM, Harbison MD, Chua SC, Leibel RL. Nonsense mutation in the human growth hormone-releasing hormone receptor causes growth failure analogous to the *little (lit)* mouse. Nat Genet 1996; 12:88–90.
286. Netchine I, Talon P, Dastot F, Vitaux F, Goossens M, Amselem S. Extensive phenotypic analysis of a family with growth hormone (GH) deficiency caused by a mutation in the GH-releasing hormone receptor gene. J Clin Endocrinol Metab 1998; 83:432–436.
287. Maheshwari HG, Silverman BL, Dupuis J, Baumann G. Phenotype and genetic analysis of a syndrome caused by an inactivating mutation in the growth hormone–releasing hormone receptor: dwarfism of *SINDH*. J Clin Endocrinol Metab 1998; 83:4065–4074.
288. Anand A, Chada K. In vivo modulation of hmgic reduces obesity. Nat Genet 2000; 24:377–380.
289. Arlotta P, Tai AK, Manfioletti G, Clifford C, Jay G, Ono SJ. Transgenic mice expressing a truncated form of the high mobility group I-C protein develop adiposity and an abnormally high prevalence of lipomas. J Biol Chem 2000; 275:14394–14400.
290. Mine N, Kurose K, Nagai H, Doi D, Ota Y, Yoneyama K, Konishi H, Araki T, Emi M. Gene fusion involving *HMGIC* is a frequent aberration in uterine leiomyomas. J Hum Genet 2001; 46:408–412.
291. DeChiara TM, Robertson EJ, Efstratiadis A. Parental imprinting of the mouse insulin-like growth factor II gene. Cell 1991; 64:849–859.
292. Sun FL, Dean WL, Kelsey G, Allen ND, Reik W. Transactivation of *IGF2* in a mouse model of Beckwith-Wiedemann syndrome. Nature 1997; 389:809–815.
293. Perusse L, Chagnon YC, Weisnagel J, Bouchard C. The human obesity gene map: the 1998 update. Obes Res 1999; 7:111–129.
294. Clement K. Leptin and the genetics of obesity. Acta Paediatr Suppl 1999; 88:51–57.
295. Shimada M, Tritos NA, Lowell BB, Flier JS, Maratos-Flier E. Mice lacking melanin-concentrating hormone are hypophagic and lean. Nature 1998; 396:670–674.
296. Katsanis N, Beales PL, Woods MO, Lewis RA, Green JS, Parfrey PS, Ansley SJ, Davidson WS, Lupski JR. Mutations in mkks cause obesity, retinal dystrophy and renal malformations associated with Bardet-Biedl syndrome. Nat Genet 2000; 26:67–70.
297. Stone DL, Slavotinek A, Bouffard GG, Banerjee-Basu S, Baxevanis AD, Barr M, Biesecker LG. Mutation of a gene encoding a putative chaperonin causes McKusick-Kaufman syndrome. Nat Genet 2000; 25: 79–82.
298. Slavotinek AM, Biesecker LG. Phenotypic overlap of McKusick-Kaufman syndrome with Bardet-Biedl syndrome: a literature review. Am J Med Genet 2000; 95:208–215.
299. Slavotinek AM, Stone EM, Mykytyn K, Heckenlively JR, Green JS, Heon E, Musarella MA, Parfrey PS, Sheffield VC, Biesecker LG. Mutations in *MKKS* cause Bardet-Biedl syndrome. Nat Genet 2000; 26:15–16.
300. Gorman SW, Haider NB, Grieshammer U, Swiderski RE, Kim E, Welch JW, Searby C, Leng S, Carmi R, Sheffield VC, Duhl DM. The cloning and developmental expression of unconventional myosin *IXA* (*MYO9A*) a gene in the Bardet-Biedl syndrome (*BBS4*) region at chromosome 15q22-q23. Genomics 1999; 59:150–160.
301. Hasty P, Bradley A, Morris JH, Edmondson DG, Venuti JM, Olson EN, Klein WH. Muscle deficiency and neonatal death in mice with a targeted mutation in the myogenin gene. Nature 1993; 364:501–506.
302. Nabeshima Y, Hanaoka K, Hayasaka M, Esumi E, Li S, Nonaka I. Myogenin gene disruption results in perinatal lethality because of severe muscle defect. Nature 1993; 364:532–535.

303. Szabo G, Dallmann G, Muller G, Patthy L, Soller M, Varga L. A deletion in the myostatin gene causes the compact (*cmpt*) hypermuscular mutation in mice. Mamm Genome 1998; 9:671–672.
304. Gonzalez-Cadavid NF, Taylor WE, Yarasheski K, Sinha-Hikim I, Ma K, Ezzat S, Shen R, Lalani R, Asa S, Mamita M, Nair G, Arver S, Bhasin S. Organization of the human myostatin gene and expression in healthy men and HIV-infected men with muscle wasting. Proc Natl Acad Sci USA 1998; 95:14938–14943.
305. McPherron AC, Lee SJ. Double muscling in cattle due to mutations in the myostatin gene. Pros Natl Acad Sci USA 1997; 94:12457–12461.
306. Good DJ, Porter FD, Mahon KA, Parlow AF, Westphal H, Kirsch IR. Hypogonadism and obesity in mice with a targeted deletion of the *Nhlh2* gene. Nat Genet 1997; 15:397–401.
307. Erickson JC, Hollopeter G, Palmiter RD. Attenuation of the obesity syndrome of *ob/ob* mice by the loss of neuropeptide *Y*. Science 1996; 274:1704–1707.
308. Jackson RS, Creemers JW, Ohagi S, Raffin-Sanson ML, Sanders L, Montague CT, Hutton JC, O'Rahilly S. Obesity and impaired prohormone processing associated with mutations in the human prohormone convertase 1 gene. Nat Genet 1997; 16:303–306.
309. Martinez-Botas J, Anderson JB, Tessier D, Lapillonne A, Chang BH, Quast MJ, Gorenstein D, Chen KH, Chan L. Absence of perilipin results in leanness and reverses obesity in *Lepr(db/db)* mice. Nat Genet 2000; 26:474–479.
310. Tansey JT, Sztalryd C, Gruia-Gray J, Roush DL, Zee JV, Gavrilova O, Reitman ML, Deng CX, Li C, Kimmel AR, Londos C. Perilipin ablation results in a lean mouse with aberrant adipocyte lipolysis, enhanced leptin production, and resistance to diet-induced obesity. Proc Natl Acad Sci USA 2001; 98:6494–6499.
311. Van Schaftingen E, Jaeken J, Phosphomannomutase deficiency is a cause of carbohydrate-deficient glycoprotein syndrome type I. FEBS Lett 1995; 377:318–320.
312. Miles PD, Barak Y, He W, Evans RM, Olefsky JM. Improved insulin-sensitivity in mice heterozygous for PPAR-gamma deficiency. J Clin Invest 2000; 105:287–292.
313. MacDonald HR, Wevrick R. The necdin gene is deleted in Prader-Willi syndrome and is imprinted in human and mouse. Hum Mol Genet 1997; 6:1873–1878.
314. Butler MG. Hypopigmentation: a common feature of Prader-Labhart-Willi syndrome. Am J Hum Genet 1989; 45:140–146.
315. Nicholls RD, Knoll JH, Butler MG, Karam S, Lalande M. Genetic imprinting suggested by maternal heterodisomy in nondeletion Prader-Willi syndrome. Nature 1989; 342:281–285.
316. Buiting K, Dittrich B, Gross S, Greger V, Lalande M, Robinson W, Mutirangura A, Ledbetter D, Horsthemke B. Molecular definition of the Prader-Willi syndrome chromosome region and orientation of the *snrpn* gene. Hum Mol Genet 1993; 2:1991–1994.
317. Muscatelli F, Abrous DN, Massacrier A, Boccaccio I, Le Moal M, Cau P, Cremer H. Disruption of the mouse *Necdin* gene results in hypothalamic and behavioral alterations reminiscent of the human Prader-Willi syndrome. Hum Mol Genet 2000; 9:3101–3110.
318. Yang T, Adamson TE, Resnick JL, Leff S, Wevrick R, Francke U, Jenkins NA, Copeland NG, Brannan CI. A mouse model for Prader-Willi syndrome imprinting-centre mutations. Nat Genet 1998; 19:25–31.
319. Socolovsky M, Fallon AE, Wang S, Brugnara C, Lodish HE. Fetal anemia and apoptosis of red cell progenitors in *Stat5a-/-5b-/-* mice: a direct role for *Stat5* in *Bcl-x(1)* induction. Cell 1999; 98:181–191.
320. Kaneshige M, Kaneshige K, Zhu X, Dace A, Garrett L, Carter TA, Kazlauskaite R, Pankratz DG, Wynshaw-Boris A, Refetoff S, Weintraub B, Willingham MC, Barlow C, Cheng S. Mice with a targeted mutation in the thyroid hormone beta receptor gene exhibit impaired growth and resistance to thyroid hormone. Proc Natl Acad Sci USA 2000; 97:13209–13214.
321. Stubdal H, Lynch CA, Moriarty A, Fang Q, Chickering T, Deeds JD, Fairchild-Huntress V, Charlat O, Dunmore JH, Kleyn P, Huszar D, Kapeller R. Targeted deletion of the tub mouse obesity gene reveals that *tubby* is a loss-of-function mutation. Mol Cell Biol 2000; 20:878–882.
322. Hagstrom SA, North MA, Nishina PL, Berson EL, Dryja TP. Recessive mutations in the gene encoding the *tubby*-like protein *Tulpl* in patients with retinitis pigmentosa. Nat Genet 1998; 18:174–176.
323. Mammes O, Betoulle D, Aubert R, Giraud V, Tuzet S, Petiet A, Colas-Linhart N, Fumeron F. Novel polymorphisms in the 5′ region of the *Lep* gene: association with leptin levels and response to low-calorie diet in human obesity. Diabetes 1998; 47:487–489.
324. Hager J, Clement K, Francke S, Dina C, Raison J, Lahlo N, Rich N, Pelloux V, Basdevant A, Guy-Grand B, North M, Froguel P. A polymorphism in the 5′ untranslated region of the human *ob* gene is associated with low leptin levels. Int J Obes Relat Metab Disord 1998; 22:200–205.
325. Lucantoni R, Ponti E, Berselli ME, Savia G, Minocci A, Calo G, de Medici C, Liuzzi A, Di Blasio AM. The a19g polymorphism in the 5′ untranslated region of the human *Obese* gene does not affect leptin levels in severely obese patients. J Clin Endocrinol Metab 2000; 85:3589–3591.
326. Mammes O, Betoulle D, Aubert R, Herbeth B, Siest G, Fumeron F. Association of the G-2548A polymorphism in the 5′ region of the *LEP* gene with overweight. Ann Hum Genet 2000; 64:391–394.

327. Oksanen L, Kainulainen K, Heiman M, Mustajoki P, Kauppinen-Makelin R, Kontula K. Novel polymorphism of the human *OB* gene promoter in lean and morbidly obese subjects. Int J Obes Relat Metab Disord 1997; 21:489–494.
328. Shigemoto M, Nishi S, Ogawa Y, Isse N, Matsuoka N, Tanaka T, Azuma N, Masuzaki H, Nishimura H, Yoshimasa Y, Hosoda K, Nakao K. Molecular screening of both the promoter and the protein coding regions in the human *OB* gene in japanese obese subjects with non-insulin-dependent diabetes mellitus. Eur J Endocrinol 1997; 137:511–513.
329. Thompson DB, Ravussin E, Bennett PH, Bogardus C. Structure and sequence variation at the human leptin receptor gene in lean and obese Pima Indians. Hum Mol Genet 1997; 6:675–679.
330. Wauters M, Mertens I, Chagnon M, Rankinen T, Considine RV, Chagnon YC, Van Gaal LF, Bouchard C. Polymorphisms in the leptin receptor gene, body composition and fat distribution in overweight and obese women. Int J Obes Relat Metab Disord 2001;25:714–720.
331. Roth H, Korn T, Rosenkranz K, Hinney A, Ziegler A, Kunz J, Siegfried W, Mayer H, Hebebrand J, Grzeschik KH. Transmission disequilibrium and sequence variants at the leptin receptor gene in extremely obese German children and adolescents. Hum Genet 1998; 103:540–546.
332. De Silva AM, Walder KR, Aitman TJ, Gotoda T, Goldstone AP, Hodge AM, De Courten MP, Zimmet PZ, Collier GR. Combination of polymorphisms in *OB-R* and the *OB* gene associated with insulin resistance in Nauruan males. Int J Obes Relat Metab Disord 1999; 23:816–822.
333. Chagnon YC, Chung WK, Perusse L, Chagnon M, Leibel RL, Bouchard C. Linkages and associations between the leptin receptor (*LEPR*) gene and human body composition in the quebec family study. Int J Obes Relat Metab Disord 1999; 23:278–286.
334. Yiannakouris N, Yannakoulia M, Melistas L, Chan JL, Klimis-Zacas D, Mantzoros CS. The Q223R polymorphism of the leptin receptor gene is significantly associated with obesity and predicts a small percentage of body weight and body composition variability. J Clin Endocrinol Metab 2001; 86:4434–4439.
335. Rand L, Winchester EC, Millwood IY, Penny MA, Kessling AM. Maternal leptin receptor gene variant Gln223Arg is not associated with variation in birth weight or maternal body mass index in UK and South Asian populations. Int J Obes Relat Metab Disord 2001; 25:753–755.
336. Echwald SM, Sorensen TI, Andersen T, Tybjaerg-Hansen A, Clausen JO, Pedersen O. Mutational analysis of the proopiomelanocortin gene in Caucasians with early onset obesity. Int J Obes Relat Metab Disord 1999; 23:293–298.
337. Hinney A, Becker 1, Heibult O, Nottebom K, Schmidt A, Ziegler A, Mayer H, Siegfried W, Blum WF, Remschmidt H, Hebebrand J. Systematic mutation screening of the pro-opiornelanocortin gene: identification of several genetic variants including three different insertions, one nonsense and two missense point mutations in probands of different weight extremes. J Clin Endocrinol Metab 1998; 83:3737–3741.

11

Rodent Models of Obesity

David A. York

Pennington Biomedical Research Center, Louisiana State University, Baton Rouge, Louisiana, U.S.A.

I INTRODUCTION

Since publication of the initial chapter on animal models in 1998 (1), there has been an explosive increase in the number of animal models in mice. This has arisen from two major avenues of research—the use of transgenic and gene-targeting approaches for proof of function for several genes that were thought to alter energy balance or through the use of similar approaches to study genes that had not previously been associated with obesity but in which a phenotype of altered body composition and/or food intake has emerged. These genes (Table 1) have a wide range of functions including effects on food intake, energy expenditure and physical activity, tissue metabolism, and adipose tissue differentiation. Further important developments have been the identification of the tub gene as an insulin-signaling molecule expressed in the nervous system and the elucidation of the signaling pathways associated with leptin activation of its long form of receptor in the hypothalamus. Thus, the identity of all of the spontaneous single gene mutations that cause obesity is now known. While these models were a major focus of the previous review, this chapter will concentrate on new information that has been published in the interim period. Readers are referred to the original chapter (1) and other chapters in the present edition of the Handbook of Obesity for more detailed information on the single gene models and other nonrodent models of obesity.

Until the recent past, the animal models that were available for the study of obesity either were of spontaneous origin or were the result of experimental manipulation of the environment or the hypothalamic centers that regulate food intake and energy balance (2–4). Much emphasis has been placed recently on dietary obesity in which a wide species-dependent variability has been described. Indeed, body weight gain when fed a high-fat diet has become a standard "test phenotype" for mice with experimentally altered gene expression. Interest in virally mediated obesities has also been renewed in recent years.

The research to date with animal models has provided substantive insight into the hypothalamic control systems and physiological disturbances that can lead to obesity. However, the recognition that so many gene manipulations can alter body composition and energy balance emphasizes the complexity of the systems involved and the research effort needed to obtain a fuller understanding of the role each of these genes play. Nevertheless, we can be encouraged by the human research that is establishing the relevance of many of the genes identified from studies of rodent models to human obesity.

Historically, the animal models have been subdivided into three groups, genetic, dietary, and neuroendocrine, according to the origin of the disorder. The explosion of information that has come from genetic and molecular studies of the obese models has emphasized the inappropriateness of this classification

Table 1 Transgenic (Tg) and Gene Knockout (KO) Models That Affect Energy Balance and/or Body Composition

Gene	Name	Position (Chr, cM)	Transgenic (Tg) or knockout (KO)	Comment	Effect
I. Receptors/transporters					
MC3	Mc3r	2,100	KO		Obesity without hyperphagia, hyperactivity
MC4	Mc4r	unknown	KO		Hyperphagia and obesity
MC3/MC4			KO	Double-knockout	Greater obesity than MC3 or MC4 knockouts
Syndecan 1	Sdc1	12, 1	Tg		Maturity onset obesity that resembles agouti-related obesity
Syndecan 3	Sdc3	15, 12.4	KO		Impaired feeding response to food deprivation
NPY Y1	Npy1r	8, 33	KO		Mild obesity with aging
NPY Y2	Npy2r	3, 36	KO		Obesity on HF diets
NPY Y5	Npy5r	8, 32.5	KO		Mild obesity with aging
GRII antisense			Tg		Cushingoid-type obesity
GRII	Nr3c1	18, 20	KO	Target to brain	Cushingoid-type obesity
Insulin receptor	Insr	8, 1	KO	Neuron-specific knockout	Obesity on a high-fat diet
CCKA	Cckar	5, 34	KO		Natural OLETF rats
TNF_2P75	Tnfrsf1b	4, 75.5	KO		Lower weight gain on high-fat diet
TNF_2P55	Tnfrsf1a	6, 60.55	KO		Attenuated cachetic response
Bombesin BRS-3	Brs3	X	KO		Mild obesity, altered food preferences
Estrogen Rα	Esr1	10, 12	KO		Develop obesity after puberty
FSH-R	Fshr	unknown	KO		Obesity, skeletal abnormalities
Muscarinic M3R	Chrm3	13, 7.0	KO		Hypophagic and reduced body weight
Histamine H1	H1r	6, 49	KO		Increased weight gain on high fat diet
5HT2C	Htr2c	X, 66.15	KO		Obese on HF diet/attenuates response to D-fenfluramine
5HT1B	Htr1b	9,46	KO		Reduced anorectic response to D-fenfluramine
Dopamine D_1	Drd1a	13, 32	KO		Reduced body weight, hyperactive
Dopamine D_2	Drd2	9, 28	KO		Reduced body weight, hypoactive
Dopamine D_3R	Drd3	16, 23.3	KO		Hyperphagic and obese on high-fat diet
β_3-adrenergic	$Adrb_3$	8, 10	KO		No obesity but loss of anorectic response to β_3-agonists
GABA transporter I	Gabt1	3, 50.4	Tg		Obesity with altered feeding pattern
II. Hormones/peptides					
Agouti	a	2, 89	Tg	β-Actin promoter	Reproduces obesity syndrome of $A^y/_a$ mice
AgRP	Agrp	8	Tg	β-Actin promoter	Obesity without coat color changes
POMC	Pomc	12, 4	KO		Obesity
Mahogany (mg)	Atrn	2, 73.9	KO	Several mutations	Increased food intake, variable obesity
Mahogonoid (Md)	Md	16, 2	KO	Single mutation	Like mg but increased activity
β-endorphin	Pomc41	12, 4	KO	POMC knockout/β-endorphin-deleted knockin	Small increase in weight
MCH	Pmch	10, 47	TG & KO		KO thin, smaller mice; overexpression causes obesity

Orexin (hypocretin)	Hcrt	11, 61	KO		Narcolepsy, late-onset obesity
Tyrosine hydroxylase	Th	7, 69.2	KO	Lethal unless NE synthesis restored	Dopamine-deficient mice are aphagic and hypoactive
Leptin	Lep	6, 10.5	Tg		Lean mouse
Insulin-like growth factor 1 binding protein	Igfbp1	11, 1.3	Tg		Attenuates dietary obesity and preadipocyte differentiation
Growth hormone	Gh	11, 65	Tg		Increased body mass, decreased body fat
Growth hormone	Gh	11, 65	KO		Obese "little" mice
Growth hormone	Gh	11,65	Tg	On metallothionin promoter	Cessation of expression leads to obesity
GHRH	Ghrh	2, 89	Tg		Obesity despite increased GH levels
CRH	Crh	3, 8	Tg	Metallothionin promoter	Cushingoid-type obesity
CHR binding protein	Crhbp	13, 52	Tg	Metallothionin promoter	Sexually dimorphic obesity
CRH binding protein	Crhpb	13, 52	KO		Hyperphagia and reduced weight
Pancreatic polypeptide	Ppy	11, syntenic	Tg	cmv-βactin promoter	Reduced weight, food intake, and food consumption
Amylin	Iapp	6, 62	KO		Increase in body weight and fat
IL6	Il6	5, 17	KO		Absence of tumor-induced cachexia
TNFα	Tnf	17, 19.1	KO		No effect or weight loss
TNF receptor P75	Tnfrsf1b	4,75.5	KO		Resistant to high-fat diet obesity
TNF receptor P55	Tnfrsf1a	6,60.55	KO		Attenuated cachectic response
IL 1 receptor antagonist	Il1rn	2, 10	Tg		Reduced weight
TGF1β	Tgfb1	7, 6.5	Tg	PEPCK promoter	Reduced weight and adipose tissue mass
III. Metabolic					
Acetyl CoA carboxylase 2	Acc2	unknown	KO	Muscle mitochondrial enzyme	Obesity without hyperphagia
Perilipin	Plin	unknown	KO		Resistant to high fat diet–induced obesity, increased lean body mass; reverses obesity of $Lepr^{ob/ob}$ mice
HSL	Lipe	7, 5.5	KO		Normal body weight, increased fat cell size but increased brown adipose tissue mass
aP2	Fabp4	6, 56	KO	Fatty acid binding protein	Obesity when fed a high-fat diet
DGAT	Dgat	15, 46.9	KO		Resistant to dietary obesity
Glut4	Slc2a4	11, 40	KO		Decreased body weight and body fat
Glut4	Slc2a4	11, 40	Tg	Effect depends on promoter used	Obesity on normal high-fat diet
Glutamine:fructose-6-phosphate amino transferase	Gfptl	6, 35.5	Tg	Increased hepatic exosamine flux	Obesity and insulin resistance in older mice
Aromatase	Cyp19	Unknown	KO		Increase in intra-abdominal adipose tissue
IL1β converting E.	Casp1	9, 1	KO		Resistant to lipopolysaccharide-induced anorexia
7B2	Sgne1	2, 64	KO	Necessary for synthesis of proconvertase 2	Cushingoid-type of obesity
G3PDH	Gapd	6, 56	Tg		Normal body weight, no adipose tissue

Table 1 (continued)

Gene	Name	Position (Chr, cM)	Transgenic (Tg) or knockout (KO)	Comment	Effect
7B2	Sgne1	2, 64	KO	Necessary for synthesis of proconvertase 2	Cushingoid-type of obesity
G3PDH	Gapd	6, 56	Tg		Normal body weight, no adipose tissue
G3PDH	Gapd	6, 56	KO		Reduced body weight
UCP1	Ucpl	8, 38	Tg	aP2 Promoter/myosin light chain promoter	Resistance to diet-induced obesity with both promoters
UCP1	Ucp1	8, 38	KO		Not obese but cold sensitive
UCP2	Ucp2	7, 50	KO		No obese phenotype
UCP3	Ucp3	7/50	KO/Tg		KO no phenotype. High overexpression in muscle gives lean mice
UCP1-Dta			KO	UCP1 promoter linked to diptheria toxin chain	Obesity and hyerphagia
UCP1/UCP3	Ucp1/Ucp3	8, 38/7, 50	KO	Double knockout	Same phenotype as UCP1 branch out
Metallothionein I & II	Mt	8, 45	KO		Moderate obesity and hyperphagia
ASP	C3	17, 34.3	KO		Reduced body fat, but body weight only reduced in females
IV. Signaling proteins					
PKARIIβ	Pkar2b	unknown	KO		Normal weight but 50% decrease in white adipose tissue, increased metabolic rate
Gsα	Gnas	2, 104	KO	Homozygous lethal	Heterozygote with maternal null allele obese, paternal null allele lean
PTP1B	Ptprb	5, 58	KO	MTI and MTII	Increased insulin sensitivity and resistance to high fat diet–induced obesity
STAT5	Stat5	11, 60.5	KO	Both a and b genes	Decreased weight and body fat in young, obesity in old mice
V. Transcription factors/nuclear proteins					
Lipin	Lipin1	12, 1	KO		Mutations cause lipodystrophy
PPARα	Ppara	15, 48.8	KO		Sexually dimorphic late-onset obesity
SREB-1C and 1a	Srebf1/Srebf2	8, 33/15, 48.5	Tg	1a Liver and 1c adipose tissue	Lipodystrophy, enlarged brown adipose tissue
AZIP/F			Tg	Overexpression on aP2	No adipose tissue, hyperphagia
CEBPα, CEBPβ, and CEBPγ	Cebp	7, 12/14, 20.5	KO	Many die	Surviving animals, little fat stored
Nhlh2	Nhlh2	3, syntenic	KO		Obesity at 10–15 weeks of age
VgF	Vgf		KO		Small, reduced body fat from birth, hyperactive
VI. Structural					
Hmgic	Hmga2	10, 67.5	KO		Reduced body fat, reduces obesity of $Lepr^{ob/ob}$ mice
ICAM-1	Icam1	9,7	KO		Late onset obesity

as we have identified the peripheral and central mechanisms for controlling energy balance and their interdependence. While identification of the five single genes (A^y, lep^{ob}, $lepr^{db}$, $lepr^{fa}$, Cpe^{fat}, and tub) that cause obesity in rodents provided the catalyst that promoted the research focus on obesity, the wide range of experimental genetic manipulations that have been shown to alter the susceptibility to develop obesity emphasize the multicausational nature of the disease. While the spontaneous single gene rodent models emphasize the overriding effects of single genes, numerous experimental genetic manipulations have been shown only to cause obesity with the appropriate environment, such as a high-fat diet. Rat and mouse strains vary greatly in their sensitivity to this form of obesity (5), and this characteristic has facilitated genomewide linkage studies of this response. Another example is the obesity that develops in desert rodents when they are fed a laboratory chow diet.

The animal models also vary in the age of onset and in the severity of the obesity. More importantly, they illustrate the importance of the background genome on the phenotype that results from any particular gene mutation. Likewise, within primate colonies there are wide-ranging individual differences in responses (6). The multigenic factors that predispose animals to this form of obesity make them probably the closest models for the study of human obesity.

The neurochemical explanations for the hyperphagia and obesity that results from lesions of the ventromedial hypothalamus and the paraventricular nucleus and for the aphagia and leanness that follows lesions of the lateral hypothalamus (3,4,7) has become apparent in recent years. Studies with these models have illustrated the inextricable links between regulation of feeding behavior and autonomic regulation of peripheral metabolism and endocrine activity. The effects of these lesions may now be mimicked by infusions of specific neuropeptides or manipulations of the expression of specific genes. This provides the functional neurochemical links to the anatomical circuitry that had been previously identified. The mechanisms through which endocrine, e.g., insulin and leptin manipulations, alter feeding behavior and body composition are also now becoming clearer as their interactions with the central neuropeptide circuits are identified. Finally, it is becoming evident that the natural seasonal and migratory changes observed in several species may well be explained by changes in the activity of the peripheral and central pathways that have been identified from studies of laboratory animal models (8).

A Advantages and Disadvantages of Animal Models for the Study of Human Obesity

The advantages and disadvantages of animal models for the study of human obesity were discussed in our previous review (1). What has become evident in the intervening years is the relevance of these animal models to human disease. Thus while mutations in the leptin gene or leptin receptor gene are rare, linkages of several indices relating obesity to chromosomal regions of these genes have been documented (9). Further, a number of mutations in either the proopiomelanocortin gene or in the melanocortin receptors have been linked with morbid obesity in humans (10), emphasizing the importance of this system to human energy balance. We are confident that, as the polygenic nature of the susceptibility of human subjects to obesity (9) is further explored, many of the genes that have been shown to cause or prevent animal obesity will also be implicated in human obesity.

In this chapter, we shall review the recent developments in our understanding of obesity that has been obtained through the study of the wide range of rodent models and review the many new experimental genetic manipulations that have provided insight into the function of known, or heretofore unknown gene products. The chapter will not be a comprehensive review of the literature in this field, but rather an update of animal models with a focus on the genetic basis of obesity.

II GENETIC MODELS OF OBESITY

A Single-Gene Obesities

1 Genes of the Leptin Signaling Pathway

Mutations in both the leptin gene and the leptin receptor gene underlie the phenotype of three single-gene obesity models. The obese mouse (lep^{ob}/lep^{ob}) inherits its obesity as a result of a C428T mutation of the leptin gene which changes an arginine codon (CGA) to a stop codon (TGA) at codon 105, resulting in a shortened nonfunctional product (11). Despite very high levels of expression of the lep^{ob} gene in adipose tissue of the lep^{ob}/lep^{ob} mouse, no leptin can be detected in the serum of these mice. A second mutation ob^{2j}/ob^{2j} has been mapped 7 kb upstream of the 4.5-kb ob RNA start site and is assumed to be the result of a structural alteration or a mutation in the promoter region.

As predicted from the classical parabiotic studies of Coleman (12) and Hervey et al. (13), the mutations responsible for the obesity phenotype of the diabetes mouse ($lepr^{db}/lepr^{db}$) and the Zucker fatty ($lepr^{fa}/lepr^{fa}$) rat are both in the leptin receptor. The long intracellular signaling domain of the leptin receptor is not translated in lepr^{db}/lepr^{db} mice since a G-to-T mutation (14,15) introduces a novel consensus splice donor site (AGGGAAA sequence to an AGGTAAA sequence). As a result of this mutation, a 106-base sequence of the terminal exon of the short form of the receptor is spliced into the long form of the receptor mRNA. This introduces a stop codon that prevents translation of the long intracellular domain of the receptor. In contrast the mutations in the Zucker rat (16,17) and the Koletsky rat (18) are both in the extracellular domain of the leptin receptor; in the lepr^{fa}/lepr^{fa} rat an A880C (G1n269Pro) mutation reduces the localization of the receptor in the cell membrane (19), whereas in the Koletsky rats a T2349A nonsense mutation results in no expression of the gene (18).

It is thus not surprising that these animals share a similar phenotype, the variation appearing to result mainly from the background genome on which the mutation is expressed. The phenotype is of an early-onset form of obesity associated with hyperphagia, impaired sympathetic activation of brown adipose tissue (BAT) thermogenesis, an enhanced insulin secretory activity, overactivity of the hypothalamic-pituitary-adrenal axis, decreased growth hormone secretion, stunted growth, impaired thyroid hormone metabolism, and infertility together with some immune function deficits. The reader is referred to our previous review for a fuller description (1). The phenotype of lepr^{db}/lepr^{db} mice can be partially corrected by transgenic expression of the long form, but not the short form, of the leptin receptor (20).

The severity and temporal characteristics of diabetes vary with the background strain in these obese mice models; hyperglycemia and hypertension are significant phenotypic variations across the rat mutations with strain. By introducing the Koletzky (fa^{cp}) gene onto an inbred strain of rats derived from the hypertensive Okamoto strain (SHR/N) and further crossing onto other strains, e.g., LA/N, a variety of strains exhibiting various aspects of the Syndrome X metabolic profile have been developed (21). By transferring the lepr^{fa} gene from its Brown-Norway background strain, on which diabetes is normally absent, to other backgrounds, long-lasting severe diabetes may become characteristic, e.g., diabetic fatty (ZDF/Drt-fa), the Wistar Kyoto fatty (WKY/NDrt-fa), or the Wistar Kyoto diabetic (WDF/TA-fa). Transgene insertion to prevent the expression of the long form of the leptin receptor in an outbred strain of mice led to wide divergence in the diabetes phenotype and provides another model for studies of the interactions of the leptin system with the background genome (22).

The other major difference across these models is the obvious one that those with mutations in the leptin receptor are partially or totally resistant to the effects of leptin whereas the obese mouse has a supersensitivity to exogenous leptin (23–25). Treatment of the lep^{ob}/lep^{ob} mouse with leptin reverses all of the phenotypic characteristics, reducing body fat, food intake, insulin secretion, and corticosterone levels and restoring sympathetic activity and brown adipose tissue thermogenesis to yield a lean mouse that is also fertile (23–25). Likewise, transgenic overexpression of leptin in normal mice leads to a very lean animal (26).

2 The Fat Mouse (fat/fat or Cpe^{fat}/Cpe^{fat})

The fat mouse, unlike the lep^{ob}/lep^{ob} and lepr^{db}/lepr^{db} mice and the lepr^{fa}/lepr^{fa} rat, is an example of a late-onset form of obesity (27). The obesity may be severe (60–70 g body weight at 24 weeks) and is expressed in all adipose depots. In this mutant the obesity is not normally evident until 8–12 weeks of age and is not pronounced until 16–20 weeks of age. It arose out of an inbred HRS/J strain of mice and has been crossed onto the C57BLKS/J background strain to facilitate comparison with the obese and diabetes mutations. The fat mouse is characterized by massive hyperinsulinemia without significant hyperglycemia from weaning, suggestive of extreme insulin resistance, but does not display the pancreatic failure and severe diabetes that are evident in older lep^{ob}/lep^{ob} and lepr^{db}/lepr^{db} mice (27). When the mutation is transferred to the C57BLKS/J(HKS) background strain, the fat/fat mouse is diabetic, but the diabetes is still less severe than that seen with lep^{ob}/lep^{ob} and lepr^{db}/lepr^{db} mice on the same background. Indeed, the mouse remains extremely sensitive to exogenous insulin. This paradox has been explained by the recognition that the apparent hyperinsulinemia is in fact a hyperproinsulinemia (2). The fat gene, located on chromosome 8 codes for carboxypeptidase E (2). A single base mutation that results in a ser202pro substitution severely reduces or completely abolishes the activity of carboxypeptidase E in the pancreatic islet, hypothalamus, pituitary, gastrointestinal tract, and other tissues (28). The functional effect of this mutation was confirmed by site-specific mutagenesis of the Cpe gene and its expression in a baculovirus system. Indeed immunoreactive carboxypeptidase E protein is undetectable in pancreas and pituitary of fat/fat mice, suggesting that the mutation affects either transcriptional or translational activity or stability of the mRNA or protein.

Carboxypeptidase E (also known as carboxypeptidase H) is required for cleavage of two arginine residues from the B-chain of insulin during its processing from proinsulin. The impairment in enzyme activity in Cpe^{fat}/Cpe^{fat} mice explains their 10-fold increased proinsulin to insulin ratios in the pancreas and the very high level of proinsulin rather than insulin in the circulation. The obesity, however, results from the role of carboxypeptidase E in the posttranslational processing of numerous neuropeptides including pro-opiomelanocortin to α-MSH, β-endorphin and β-lipotropin, proenkephalins, preproNPY, vasopressin, oxytocin, gastrin, and CCK. While Naggert et al. (2) suggest that the obesity of Cpe^{fat}/Cpe^{fat} mouse is likely to result from a complex pattern of alterations in neuropeptide activity and secretion within the hypothalamic-pituitary system rather than the hyperproinsulinemia, it is not surprising that it has many similarities to the obesity of the MC4 receptor knockout mouse (29). The mutation also appears to have differential effects on postranslational processing in the CNS and the periphery. The processing of procholecystokinin provides an example of this. In Cpe^{fat}/Cpe^{fat} mice bioactive CCK was reduced in neural tissue but not in gastrointestinal endocrine cells, although the level of the enzyme substrate glycylarginine-extended CCK was greatly elevated in both tissues (30).

3 Tubby (*tub/tub*) Mouse

This mutation was first reported by Coleman and Eicher in 1990 (27). It is an autosomal-recessive mutation on chromosome 7 in the gene coding for the tubby protein, one of a family of four proteins that also includes TULPs 1–3. A characteristic of these proteins is the ~260–amino acid domain at the carboxyl terminus that forms a helix barrel structure that binds avidly to DNA. The tubby mutation introduces a splice site at the junction of the 3′-coding sequence that leads to the loss of this carboxyl terminus domain (31). Knockout of tub confirmed that the tubby gene mutation is a loss of function mutation (32).

The wild-type tub protein is expressed in the hypothalamus and other brain regions, where it is localized to plasma membranes, released by activation of Gαq protein, and translocated into the nucleus (33). This process may be activated by 5HT2c receptor activity. Studies of CHO cells expressing the human insulin receptor have shown an insulin-dependent phosphorylation of tyrosine residues on the tub protein. This has led to the suggestion that tub acts as an adapter protein linking the insulin receptor to protein tyrosine kinases and may function as part of a neural insulin signaling mechanism (34).

On the C57BL/6J background, Tubby mice are phenotypically very similar to 5HT2c receptor knock out mice and to fat mice except that the obesity in fat mice develops more slowly, not being visually apparent until 9–12 weeks of age. All fat depots are enlarged. The tub mutation is associated with distinct sexual dimorphism in blood glucose, serum insulin, islet hypertrophy and hyperplasia, and β-cell degranulation, all changes being more pronounced in male mice. The hyperinsulinemia, mild at weaning, progressively increases with age. Morphological changes in the pancreatic islets occur earlier and are more pronounced in males. However, the tub mice remain mildly hypoglycemic, indicating the absence of the pronounced insulin resistance common to other mouse models of obesity. This insulin resistance appears to be centrally expressed since NPY mRNA levels are massively elevated in *tubby* mice (35). Infertility is also a feature of this mouse when severe obesity develops.

4 The Yellow (A^y/a) Obese Mouse

The agouti gene of the Yellow (A^y/a) obese mouse was the first single-gene mutation for obesity to be identified in mice (see (36) for review). The Yellow (A^y/a) obese mouse and the KK mouse (37) discussed below are the only models of dominant inheritance of obesity so far described. The obesity of the yellow mouse is inherited as a mutation in the agouti protein coded on chromosome 2, and is associated with a moderate obesity and a high incidence of tumor growth. Although the homozygous (A^y/A^y) mouse is lethal in utero, there are a number of different alleles (A^{vy}/A^{vy}, A^{iy}/A^{iy}) at the agouti locus in which the defects are less severe and in which the degree of obesity is linked directly to the level of yellow pigmentation in the coat (38). The obesity of the yellow mice is less pronounced than in the obese and diabetes micc and is of later onset (8–12 weeks of age). While these animals share many of the characteristics common to all rodent obesities, they do differ in the clear sexual dimorphism of the associated hyperglycemia (39) and in the apparently normal activity of the hypothalamic-pituitary-adrenal axis (39,40). The A^y/a mouse is extremely leptin resistant. This appears to be mainly of central focus since transgenic overexpression of leptin in A^y/a mice improves the diabetes but does not ameliorate the obesity (24).

The agouti (a) gene encodes a 131–amino acid protein that is normally uniquely expressed in the hair follicle where it acts to inhibit eumelanin synthesis in response to stimulation by α-melanophore-stimulating hormone (α-MSH). In the Yellow mouse exon 1 of the agouti gene is replaced by a unique sequence, but exons

2–4, which contain the full coding sequence, are normal. The result of this mutation is the ubiquitous expression of the agouti gene in a wide range of tissues including white adipose tissue and brain (41). Transgenic mice expressing agouti unregulated and ubiquitously driven by the human β-actin promoter also develop yellow coat color and become obese (42–44), confirming that ectopic expression of normal agouti protein results in the obese yellow phenotype.

Two potential actions of agouti protein have been identified. Its ability to increase intracellular calcium levels may promote insulin resistance (45). Intracellular calcium levels are related to the level of expression of agouti protein and to body weight and degree of coat color. Using a murine melanoma cell line, Lu et al. (46) were able to demonstrate that agouti protein inhibited the stimulation of adenylyl cyclase by α-MSH, shifting the dose required for half-maximal stimulation from 1.7 to 13.4 nM by acting as a potent antagonist of the melanocortin-4 receptor (MC4-R). However, agouti had no effects on MC1, MC2, MC3, or MC5 receptors.

Identification of agouti and its interactions with the melanocortin 4 receptor led to the cloning of a natural MC4 receptor antagonist, agouti-related protein (AgRP) (47) that is expressed in the hypothalamus. Transgenic and gene-knockout studies have provided new insight into the role of this melanocortin pathway in regulating energy balance. A fuller description is provided in Section B.1.

5 KK Mice

Since the original description of the KK mouse (48), several different strains have been identified (see 19, 35 for review). While the obesity and diabetes were originally thought to be inherited as a polygenic trait, the KK gene is now regarded as a dominant gene with low (25%) penetrance (37). The obesity and hyperinsulinemia are relatively mild, although the hyperglycemia may be severe. The KK mice are, however, very sensitive to diet, and obesity may be prevented by dietary restriction. The temporal changes in this mouse are also very different from the other mouse models in that changes to or toward normality of body composition, insulin secretion, and insulin resistance may be evident in older (>6 months) animals. In these mice the pancreas appears to have the ability to increase insulin secretion without the subsequent necrosis seen in ob/ob and db/db mice. Once again there are major variations across the different strains of KK mice.

B Transgenic and Gene Knockout Models

During the past four years extensive use of transgenic and knockout approaches has identified 60 genes that modulate energy balance, either increasing energy storage and obesity, or reducing or eliminating energy storage in white adipose tissue (Table 1). While many of these studies have aimed to substantiate a function which prior experimental data had suggested for the gene product on energy balance, other studies were designed primarily to identify a function for the specific gene.

To help in reviewing the large number of animal models, I have subdivided the genes into those that can be related to receptors and transporters, hormone and neuropeptide systems, metabolic genes, signaling proteins, transcription factors/nuclear proteins, and finally to structural genes.

1 Hormones and Neuropeptide Systems

a. The Melanocortin System

Studies of the Yellow obese syndrome (A^y/a, A^{vy}/a, etc.) led to the identification of the important role of α-MSH, an anorectic peptide (49) derived from the precursor pro-opiomelanocortin (POMC), and the antagonist AgRP peptide as the major regulators of this system (47, 50–52),which affects feeding behavior, energy expenditure, and insulin secretion. Several genetic models have been used to illustrate the functionality of this system. Transgenic mice ectopically expressing agouti recapitulate the obese yellow syndrome of the A^y/a mouse (43). Likewise, expression of the hypothalamic homolog protein AgRP produces a similar obesity but without the coat color changes associated with antagonism of the MC1 receptor (53). α-MSH, a product cleaved from the POMC precursor protein, is an agonist for all melanocortin receptors except MC2. Knockout of the precursor POMC gene produces obesity (54). Knockout of the 7B2 gene (Sgne1), which prevents the production of proconvertase 2 and the cleavage of ACTH and α-MSH, also produces obesity (55). The effect of α-MSH on energy balance appears to result from actions at both the MC4 and MC3 receptors. MC4 receptor knockout mice (29) are hyperphagic and obese, whereas MC3 receptor knockout mice become obese in the absence of significant hyperphagia (56) while exhibiting decreased locomotor activity and an atypical increase in respiratory quotient on a high fat diet (57). These observations suggest that α-MSH may primarily inhibit feeding through MC4 receptors and enhance energy expenditure and influence energy partitioning through MC3 receptors. Indeed, the double knockout Mc3r−/−/Mc4r−/− becomes more obese than either of the individual receptor knockouts.

The expression of the agouti gene in humans differs from that in mice, where it is only transiently expressed in hair follicles. In humans, agouti is also expressed in a variety of peripheral tissues, including adipose tissue. To develop a model of human agouti, Mynatt and colleagues (58,59) have created transgenic mice expressing agouti in adipose tissue. These transgenic mice develop a mild obesity and show an enhanced sensitivity of adipose tissue to insulin.

Neural tracing and immunohistochemical approaches have been used to identify the functional neuroanatomy of the melanocortin system. Two subsets of neurons in the arcuate nucleus, coexpressing either POMC and CART or NPY and AgRP, send axonal projections to both the PVN and LH to synapse with cell bodies that express either MC3 or MC4 receptors, and may regulate secretion of melanin-concentrating hormone and orexin. The presence of leptin receptors on the arcuate POMC and AgRP neurons provides the link among leptin, the melanocortin system, feeding behavior, and energy expenditure. Of all the animal models, the natural mutations and the experimental manipulations of this melanocortin system appear to be most relevant to human obesity, where a number of mutations have also been linked to severe obesity and changes in hair color (9,10).

In addition to the agouti mutation, two other genes, mahogany (mg) and mahoginoid (md) (60) have effects on both body weight and coat color. Several mutations have been identified at the mg locus giving total or partial loss of function but, to date, only a single md mutation has been reported. The phenotypes of these mutant animals are similar, although the degree of obesity is variable. Both md and mg mutations inhibit agouti-related obesity and its associated changes in linear growth and insulin secretion, but do not alter the hyperphagia. Mg and md (Atrn) mutations appear to enhance food intake, and mg also increases physical activity.

Mahogany, a transmembrane protein, has been identified as a member of the Attractin (Atrn) gene family (61). It is expressed widely in the CNS, including the major regions known to be important for the regulation of energy balance (62). The site of action of mg is unknown. Since the mg mutation has no effect on energy balance in MC4R knockout mice or in $lepr^{db}/lepr^{db}$, tub/tub, or Cpe^{fat}/Cpe^{fat} mice, it is thought to act upstream of the MC4 and MC1 receptors. However, mg can suppress diet-induced obesity (63).

b. The Syndecans

Syndecans are a family of cell surface heparin sulphate proteoglycans that show differential tissue distribution. The extracellular domains of the syndecans are released from the cell surface and may act as either positive or negative paracrine regulators. Transgenic overexpression of Syndecan I (Sdc1) using the CMV promoter (64) led to a maturity-onset type of obesity that was phenotypically very similar to the obesities associated with agouti or agouti-related protein. While Syndecan I is not normally expressed in the brain, Syndecan III null mice (a neural syndecan), while of normal body phenotype, show an impaired feeding response to fasting (64). Reizes et al. (64) propose that the released ectodomains of the syndecans modulate the interactions between α-MSH and agouti-related protein with the MC4 receptor, and that the hypothalamic Syndecan III levels are physiological modulators of feeding behavior.

c. The NPY System

Neuropeptide Y (NPY) is recognized as the most powerful orexigenic peptide yet to be identified. Physiological and pharmacological evidence support a role for NPY in the regulation of feeding behavior. However, experimental genetic manipulations of the NPY system have failed to show that it is essential for normal feeding. Recently, however, NPY knockout mice have been shown to have an attenuated response to fasting (65). When obob mice are made Npy−/−, there is an attenuation of the level of obesity (66). However, Npy−/− mice grow normally, and knockout of NPY1, Y2, and Y5 receptors does not attenuate food intake or weight gain as would have been predicted from pharmacological studies. Indeed, surprisingly, both Y1 and Y5 receptor-deficient mice develop a mild obesity with aging, and Y2 receptor-deficient mice become obese when provided with a high-fat diet.

Pancreatic polypeptide, another member of the NPY family, is expressed at high levels in the pancreas and gut. Overexpression regulated by a cytomegalovirus β-actin promoter was lethal to many of the transgenic mice, but surviving animals were characterized by reduced growth, lower body fat, and lower food intake and oxygen consumption (67).

d. The CRH/Urocortin-Glucocorticoid System

In addition to a role in regulation of pituitary-adrenal function, CRH and Urocortin inhibit food intake and promote energy expenditure, particularly the sympathetically mediated BAT thermogenesis. Numerous models, targeting specific components of this system, have identified the ability to alter homeostasis. These models generally produce a cushingoid-type of central adiposity. The models include the transgenic overexpression of antisense cDNA to the brain type II glucocorticoid receptor (GR) (68,69), knockout of the brain type II GR, and transgenic expression of CRH (70,71). The concentration of free CRH in the CNS is affected by the levels of the CRH-binding protein. Knockout of this gene results in a hypophagic small mouse whereas overexpression regulated by the metallothionin promoter caused obesity (72,73). Despite these effects, knockout of CRH1 and CRH2 receptors does not have any major phenotypic effects on body weight or food intake although the response to exogenous urocortin or CRH may be absent or diminished (74–77).

e. Melanin Concentrating Hormone (MCH)

This peptide is synthesized in lateral hypothalamic neurons that are innervated by POMC/CART or NPY/AgRP axons from the arcuate nucleus. Although MCH has only a modest orexigenic effect when given intracerebroventricularly, MCH knockout mice have reduced body weight and are hypophagic and lean (78). Absence of MCH release could explain the effects of lateral hypothalamic lesions. In contrast, transgenic overexpression of MCH increases body weight of mice fed a chow diet and induces obesity in mice fed a high fat diet (79).

f. Orexin

Orexin is also expressed in the LH. While orexin appears to have moderate orexigenic effects, mutations in this receptor appear to be related to narcolepsy (80), suggesting that orexin has a primary role in arousal rather than energy homeostasis. However, ablation of orexigenic neurons by specific expression of a truncated Machado-Joseph disease product Ataxin-3 produced a late-onset obesity in addition to a narcoleptic phenotype (81).

g. Insulin/Insulinlike Growth Factor (IGF)-1 and Amylin

Like leptin, insulin has been proposed as a long-term signal to the brain on the status of the energy reserves of the body. When given ICV, it may reduce food intake and body weight, although, like leptin, this effect is absent in obese rats. Strong evidence for the importance of this regulatory system comes from the neuron-specific knock out of the insulin receptor. These mice become obese when given a high fat diet and develop mild insulin resistance and hypertriglyceridemia. Hyperphagia was only evident in female mice (82). The importance of insulin sensitivity in muscle for the prevention of obesity is emphasized by the observation that transgenic overexpression of dominant-negative insulin receptors in muscle, which causes muscle insulin resistance, results in a major increase in body fat (22–38%) and a loss of lean body mass (83).

Amylin is a 361–amino acid protein cosecreted with insulin from pancreatic β-cells. It has been shown to have multiple effects including suppression of food intake and inhibition of gastric emptying. Amylin knockout mice of both sexes show an approximate 20% increase in body weight and body fat (84).

Transgenic mice overexpressing the IGF-1-binding protein in adipose tissue have been used to explore the effects of IGF-1 on adipocyte differentiation (85). IGF-1-binding protein overexpression attenuated the weight gain and increase in adipose tissue mass and fat cell size of mice provided a sucrose-enriched diet. These data, together with some in vitro studies, suggest that IGF-1 has a critical role in the differentiation of preadipocytes and in the development of obesity.

h. Cholecystokinin (CCK)

CCK is expressed both in the gastrointestinal tract and in the CNS. When given both peripherally and centrally, CCK inhibits food intake through actions mediated by CCKA receptors (86). A natural mutation which prevents the expression of CCKA receptors has been identified in OLETF rats (87). These are hyperphagic and heavier than the wild-type LETO rats. Further, they fail to suppress food intake normally in response to a dietary supplement of fat (88). In contrast, knockout of CCKA receptors in mice does not appear to have any effects on energy balance (89,90).

i. Bombesin

Bombesin is one member of a family of peptides that are also expressed widely in the CNS and GI tract. They inhibit food intake and stimulate sympathetic-related energy expenditure. Of the three receptors identified, the bombesin receptor subtype 3 (BRS-3) appears to be important for energy balance, since BRS-3 knockout mice develop mild obesity, hypertension, and impaired glucose tolerance (91). BRS-3-deficient mice also show changes in sensitivity to nutrient stimuli, showing an enhanced preference for saccharin solutions but also a stronger aversive response to LiCl (92).

j. Growth Hormone (GH)

Both overexpression and knockout approaches have been used to study the effects of GH on energy balance and body composition. GH deficiency, as in "little" mice, is associated with decreased somatic growth but increased body fat (93) despite normophagia (per gram body weight). In contrast, overexpression of GH is associated with increased somatic growth and decreased body fat (94), which has been related to a severe insulin resistance of adipose tissue (95). Overexpression of an ovine GH transgene driven by a metallothionein promoter (96) leads, as expected, to larger mice. However, when expression of this transgene is switched off by removal of dietary zinc, significant obesity results, suggesting downstream effects in the GH pathway. Overexpression of GHRH, which results in elevated GH levels, results in hyperphagic mice of increased body mass but, unexpectedly, also increased body fat (97). The reason for the increased body fat is unclear but may be related to a dysregulation of the leptin receptor system in the hypothalamus.

k. TNFα and Other Cytokines

With the recognition of adipose tissue as an endocrine organ and the suggestion that TNFα secretion was linked to insulin resistance (98), attention has focused on the possibility that TNFα and other cytokines may have an important role in the physiological control of energy balance as well as their pathological role in cancer cachexia. Divergent results have been reported. TNFα-null mice either may be of normal weight or even gain weight normally when fed a high-fat diet (99) or they may be characterized by a significant reduction in body weight (100). To date, two receptor subtypes (P55 and P75) have been identified. Mice that are P75−/− have lower body weight than wild type mice (101) when fed a high fat diet whereas P55−/− mice exhibit an attenuated cachectic response to tumors (102). Similarly, mice lacking the IL6 gene do not exhibit the tumor related reduction in food intake (103). Genetic studies in which the expression of IL1 receptor antagonist (Il1ra) is manipulated also suggest a role for IL1 in energy regulation and cancer cachexia. Transgenic overexpression of IL1ra, which blocks the binding of IL1 to its receptor, promotes weight reduction as would be anticipated (104).

l. Adrenergic Receptors (β_3AR and $\alpha 2AR$)

β_3-AR knockout mice do not become obese despite the role of this receptor in signaling sympathetically mediated BAT thermogenesis (105). This may result from a number of compensatory changes. However, of particular interest with these mice has been the ability to show, using tissue-specific knockins of β_3AR in β_3-AR knockout mice, that the β_3-adrenergic suppression of food intake is mediated by white adipose tissue β_3ARs (106). The chemical mediator(s) of this response have yet to be identified. Transgenic overexpression of α_2-adrenergic receptors in β3-AR-null mice leads to obesity and adipocyte hyperplasia in mice fed a high-fat diet (107). This model emphasizes the importance of α_2ARs in the stimulation of adipocyte hyperplasia.

m. Neurotransmitters

The anorectic response of 5HT is diminished in both 5HT2c and 5HT1b receptor knockout mice. This suggests that both receptor subtypes are necessary for this activity. The 5HT2c knockout mice become obese with age and show a greater sensitivity to high-fat diets than wild-type mice (108,109). These mice also appear to have an enhanced preference for dietary fat (Brenda Richards, personal communication). However, 5HT1b null mice are indistinguishable from wild-type mice in body weight and daily food intake.

Dopamine appears to be essential for the motor components of feeding. Knockout of tyrosine hydroxylase (an enzyme necessary for dopamine and norepinephrine synthesis) is lethal (110). However, when norepinephrine synthesis is restored, the dopamine-deficient mice live to ~4 weeks of age. They are aphagic and hypoactive (111). Both D1 receptor and D2 receptor knockout mice have reduced body weight, and the latter mice are hypoactive (111–113). In contrast, the D3 receptor knockout mouse is hyperphagic on a high-fat diet and becomes obese (Stephen Woods, personal communication).

Histamine also appears to be an important neurotransmitter for feeding behavior. Knockout of the H1 receptor has no effect in mice fed a regular chow diet, but is associated with excessive weight gain on a high-fat diet and a reduced response to ICV leptin (114). Acetylcholine is widely distributed in the central and autonomic nervous systems. Mice that are deficient in the M3 muscarinic receptors are hypophagic and have a reduced body weight (115).

Gamma-aminobutyric acid (GABA) is a major inhibitory neurotransmitter within the CNS. Ubiquitous overexpression of the GABA transporter I gene caused a moderate obesity that was characterized by an altered feeding pattern and a small reduction in physical activity (116).

n. Other Hormone Receptors

Estrogens have been recognized to have significant effects in feeding behavior. Knockout of the estradiol α-receptor is associated with increased white but not brown adiposity, which appears to develop after the onset of puberty (117) in both males and females (118). As in aromatase-deficient mice, the obesity appears to be associated with a decrease in energy expenditure rather than hyperphagia. Similarly, knockout of the FSH receptor, which causes severe estrogen deficiency from an early age, induces obesity and skeletal abnormalities that give a hunchback appearance to the mice (119).

2 Metabolic Genes

a. Lipid Metabolism

1 Acetyl CoA carboxylase 2 (Acc2) Acc2 is predominantly expressed in heart and muscle as opposed to the hepatic and adipose tissue expression of acetyl CoA carboxylase 1. Knockout of the muscle ACC2 results in lean mice that had reduced tissue malonyl CoA levels and enhanced muscle fatty acid oxidation rates by 30% (120). Adipose tissue depot size of the Acc2-null mice was only 50% of that on the wild type. This occurred despite a 20–30% increase in food intake that might be either associated with the low leptin levels or a direct effect of the reduced levels of malonyl CoA in hypothalamic centers (121).

2 Perilipin Although only a single gene codes for perilipin, there are multiple tissue-specific isoforms as the result of alternative splicing. Perilipin A coats the trigylceride droplets in adipose tissue, where it protects the lipid from hydrolysis by hormone sensitive lipase. Activation of perilipin by protein kinase A is necessary for hormone-sensitive lipase activity. The perilipin (plin)-null mice have enhanced basal lipolysis but severely impaired stimulated lipolytic activity. Perilipin-null mice have normal body weight but a greatly reduced adipose tissue mass, an increased lean body mass, an increased metabolic rate, and a tendency to develop insulin resistance (122,123). Food intake may be normal or increased, and the mice are resistant to high-fat diet–induced obesity. A similar phenotype has been reported for the protein kinase A RIIβ subunit (Pkar2b) null mouse (124), suggesting that failure to activate perilipin might also explain the phenotype of this mouse, although PKA activity is increased. Transferring the perilipin (plin)-null mutation into the diabetes mouse ($Lepr^{db}$ /$Lepr^{db}$) dramatically attenuates their obesity (122,123).

3 Hormone-sensitive lipase (Lipe) This enzyme catalyzes the initial stage of the hydrolysis of stored triglycerides to fatty acids and glycerol. Its activity is regulated by numerous endocrine and neural inputs to the adipose tissue. Lipe-null mice did not become obese, although fat cells in white and brown adipose tissue were significantly enlarged by two- and fivefold, respectively (125). Brown adipose tissue mass was increased. No differences in metabolic rate or response to a cold environment could be detected in Lipe-null mice where the major phenotype was male sterility.

4 Adipocyte binding protein (aP2; Fabp4) This protein is expressed mainly in adipose tissue and binds intracellular fatty acids. Its promoter is frequently used to target gene expression to adipose tissue. Fabp4-null mice grow normally but show an exaggerated obesity when placed on a high-fat diet. This obesity is unique in that insulin resistance does not develop (126). Transfer of the Fabp4 null allele onto the lep^{ob}/lep^{ob} mouse increases its level of obesity yet enhances the insulin sensitivity compared to lep^{ob}/lep^{ob} mice expressing the Fabp4 gene (127).

5 Acyl COA: diacylglycerol acyl transferase (Dgat) This enzyme transfers a fatty acid to convert diglycerides into triglycerides. Dgat-null mice have normal body weight, but lower body fat when fed a standard chow diet. Despite the absence of enzyme activity, the Dgat-null mice gain significant weight and body fat when fed a high-fat diet to reach levels similar to those in wild-type mice (128).

b. Carbohydrate Metabolism

1 Glucose transporters Glut4 is an insulin-regulated glucose transporter expressed in adipose tissue and muscle. In adipose tissue glucose carbon is required for glyceride synthesis and for fatty acid synthesis. Overexpression of the Glut4 gene (Slc2a4) in adipose tissue using the aP_2 promoter results in an obese mouse with enhanced glucose clearance that is not further exaggerated by feeding a high-fat diet (129). Expressing Glut4 in muscle with the myosin light chain promoter has no effects on body weight or body composition, but does again improve insulin-stimulated glucose disposal (130,131). In contrast, Glut4 (Slc2a4)-null mice have little white adipose tissue and have a lower body weight but decreased sensitivity to insulin (132).

2 *Glutamine:fructose-6-phosphate amidotransferase (GFAT)* GFAT is the rate-limiting enzyme for hexosamine synthesis in the liver. Transgenic overexpression of the GFAT gene (Gfptl) using the PEPCK promoter resulted in mice that appear to have enhanced or normal insulin sensitivity and elevated hepatic glycogen when young, but which become obese when old (133).

c. Converting Enzymes

1 *Aromatase* Aromatase is responsible for the final step in estrogen biosynthesis from C_{19} steroids. Human mutations in the aromatase gene have been associated with visceral obesity, insulin resistance, and the metabolic syndrome. The aromatase gene (Cyp19) knockout mouse of either sex likewise accumulates excess abdominal fat deposits. This phenotype occurs despite a reduction in food intake and normal metabolic rate, and reflects the 50% reduction in the level of spontaneous physical activity (134).

2 *Interleukin 1β converting enzyme* This enzyme is responsible for the production of biologically active IL1β. Mice lacking the enzyme fail to demonstrate the hypophagic response to lipopolysaccharide (135).

3 *7B2* The 7B2 protein is necessary for the expression of proconvertase 2. Obesity that occurs in 7B2 (Sgne)-null mice probably reflects their inability to process POMC into α-MSH (54).

d. Thermogenic Pathways

1 *α-Glycerol phosphate dehydrogenase (αGPDH)* This enzyme forms part of a substrate cycle that effectively shuttles protons from NADH to FADH so releasing the equivalent of 1ATP energy as heat, in addition to its role in the supply of glycerophosphate for triglyceride synthesis. Over-expression of the αGPDH gene (Gapd) at high levels leads to a lean mouse devoid of white adipose tissue (136) and resistant to both dietary-induced obesity and gold thioglucose–induced obesity (137). Knockout of the αGPDH gene also leads to a small mouse, possibly by impairing lipid deposition and phospholipid biosynthesis (138).

2 *Uncoupling proteins (UCPs)* Multiple approaches have been used to alter the expression of genes coding for UCPs. Targeted expression of a diptheria toxin A chain gene has been used to selectively knock out tissue functional activity. By coupling the gene to uncoupling protein gene expression, brown adipose tissue thermogenic function was abolished, and mice became obese (139) and developed hyperphagia. This model not only illustrates the importance of BAT thermogenesis to energy balance in rodents but also emphasizes that BAT may reciprocally affect food intake (140), probably through a sympathetically mediated signal, e.g., heat (141). This approach appears to be more successful than knockout of the β_3-adrenergic receptor gene in white and brown adipose tissue (142), as this yields only a moderate form of obesity in which BAT remained morphologically normal and responded normally to cold acclimation. This questions the relationship between BAT thermogenesis and feeding behavior proposed by Himms-Hagen (141). Surprisingly, however, Ucpl knockouts do not induce obesity although they do induce an impaired thermogenic response to a cold environmental stimulus (143). This suggests that other thermogenic mechanisms can replace the dietary thermogenic needs but not the greater thermogenic requirement imposed by cold temperatures.

Targeted overexpression of Ucp 1 to adipose tissue using the aP_2 promoter had no phenotypic effect until mice were placed on a high-fat diet on which they were resistant to becoming obese (144). Likewise, targeting Ucpl gene expression to muscle with the rat myosin light chain 2 promoter reduces body size and confers resistance to high-fat dietary obesity (145), but the physiological significance of high expression of this gene in muscle has to be questioned.

The identification of other members of the uncoupling family of genes promised the possibility of multiple approaches to manipulate thermogenesis. This promise is largely unfulfilled and it does not appear that the major physiological role of UCP2 and UCP3 is regulation of body temperature or diet induced thermogenesis. Ucp2 knockout mice do not become obese and have a normal response to both cold exposure and high-fat diets (146).

Ucp3 gene expression is primarily in muscle. However, while knockout of the Ucp3 gene reduces the mitochondrial proton leak in muscle, null mutation mice remain lean (147), and the double-null mutation of Ucpl and Ucp3 retains the phenotype of the UCP1 knockout mouse. While massive overexpression of Ucp3 in muscle induces hypophagia and leanness (148), it is doubtful that this reflects any physiological role of UCP 3 on energy balance.

e. Other

1 Metallothionein I and II (MtI and MtII) Targeted disruption of both MtI and MtII genes leads to a moderate obesity that first becomes evident at 5–6 weeks of age (149). However, the mechanism through which proteins associated with copper and zinc homeostasis and free radical metabolism induce changes in energy balance is not clear at this time.

2 Acylation-stimulating protein (ASP) This protein is a product of the cleavage of complement C3. ASP gene (C3) null mice exhibit sexual dimorphism in body weight, male null mice being of normal weight whereas female null mice are smaller than wild-type females. Body fat is reduced in both sexes but food intake is increased, suggesting that there is also an increase in either basal metabolic rate or physical activity (150).

3 Signaling Proteins

a. PKARIIβ

Protein kinase A (PKA) is a multiunit complex enzyme consisting of two catalytic and two enzymatic subunits. Mice lacking the PKARIIβ subunit, normally expressed in both white and brown adipose tissue, have greatly reduced levels of white adipose tissue when fed a normal chow diet. Additionally, PKARIIβ (Pkar2b) null mice are resistant to the development of obesity when placed on a high-fat diet (151,152). The lean phenotype may arise from multiple effects that include enhanced brown adipose tissue thermogenesis (124) and enhanced basal levels of lipolysis (153). In contrast, targeted knockout of protein kinase Bβ or the Pkakt gene has no apparent effect on growth and development but induces an insulin resistant state (154).

b. G Protein Alpha Subunit (Gnas)

Previously known as Gsα, Gnas is a stimulatory G protein linked with receptor-mediated activation of adenyl cyclase and other membrane-related proteins. The phenotype associated with knockout of the Gnas gene depends on the parental origin of the mutation. Homozygous null mice die in utero. Obesity is associated with maternal origin of the heterozygote null allele, but leanness is the result with paternal origin of the mutation. The changes in body composition are related to alterations in energy expenditure rather than food intake. Male Gnas−/+ mice have increased basal metabolic rate and physical activity whereas female Gnas−/+ mice have low metabolic rate and decreased physical activity (155).

c. Protein Tyrosine Phosphatase 1B (PTRB)

Activity of this enzyme appears to attenuate the metabolic response to insulin. The mice null for the PTRB gene (Ptrb) mutation have increased insulin sensitivity of muscle and liver but not adipose tissue, and are resistant to development of a high-fat diet–induced obesity (156). Both heterozygote Ptrb−/+ and homozygous null Ptrb−/− mice are similarly resistant to the development of obesity, indicating the need for full activity of PTR1B for the development of obesity. Food intake is unaltered in −/− mice suggesting that the obesity of the knockout mice results from changes in energy expenditure.

d. Signal Transducers and Activators of Transcription (STATs)

The STATs are a family of proteins that mediate the transcriptional responses to cytokines such as growth hormone and leptin. STAT5 is phosphorylated in response to numerous signals including growth hormone, prolactin, and IL2. Knockout of the STAT5 gene (Stat5) results in a phenotype of growth hormone deficiency that includes reduced longitudinal growth, decreased adiposity in young, but obesity in older mice (157).

4 Transcription Factors

a. Lipin (fld)

Lipin is an 891–amino acid protein predominantly localized in the nucleus that appears to be necessary for adipose tissue development and metabolism.

Natural mutations in the gene (Lpin 1) that encodes the protein have been described in BALB/c and C3H mouse strains and are associated with a lipodystrophic phenotype, fatty liver, and neuropathy of peripheral nerves (158).

b. PPARα

The peroxisome proliferator-activated receptors (PPARs) are a family of transactivating proteins related to the steroid/thyroid/retinoid receptors. PPARγ is essential for adipose tissue development (159). PPARα gene (Ppara)-null mice develop a late-onset obesity that shows a sexual dimorphism in the temporal development, females becoming obese at a much younger age than males (160). The cause of this obesity remains unclear since investigators have been unable to identify changes in either food intake (160) or metabolic rate (161). Pparb null mice also have reduced adipose tissue stores (162).

c. SREBP-1c

The sterol regulatory element binding proteins (SPEBPs) are expressed in multiple tissues. Overexpression of a truncated form of the adipose tissue form (SREPB-1c) gene (Srebf1) from the aP2 promoter leads to a mouse of similar phenotype to the A-ZIP/F-1 mouse described below, with a general lipodystrophy, severe diabetes, and liver engorged with lipid (163). Leptin treatment normalizes insulin and glucose levels (164). Transgenic overexpression of the liver form protein (SREBP-1a) gene (Srebf2) on the PEPCK promoter results in a similar but less severe phenotype (165).

d. A-ZIP/F-1

A-ZIP/F is a protein that prevents the binding of B-ZIP transcription factors to both C/EBP and Jun DNA binding sites. Transgenic expression of the A-ZIP/F gene under the control of the aP2 promoter results in a mouse devoid of white adipose tissue that is severely diabetic, has enlarged internal organs and reduced fecundity, and often dies prematurely. Body weight is normal (males) or increased (females) despite the absence of white adipose tissue (166). It has been proposed as a model of human lipoatrophic diabetes. Transplantation of adipose tissue and transgenic leptin overexpression reverses the metabolic phenotype (167,168), illustrating again the role of adipose tissue and or leptin in the control of insulin sensitivity and glucose metabolism.

e. C/EBP

The CCAAT enhancer-binding proteins (CEBPs) are a family of transcriptional regulator proteins. At least two of these, CEBPα and CEBPβ, are thought to be important regulators of preadipocyte differentiation. CEBPα gene (Cebpa) knockout has high lethality, but surviving mice are devoid of white adipose tissue (169), consistent with the observations described above for the transgenic overexpression of A-ZIP-F. Further, mice with the double knockout of Cebpa and Cebpb genes also have a partial lipodystrophy (170).

f. Nhlh2

This transcription factor gene is expressed in neural tissue particularly in those hypothalamic areas that have been implicated in the regulation of energy balance, the arcuate nucleus, and the ventomedial and lateral hypothalamus. Both homozygous and heterozygous knockout mice develop a severe maturity-onset obesity yet do not develop diabetes on the 129 × C56BL/6J background. Hypogonadism is also characteristic (171).

g. Vgf

The function of the protein encoded by the Vgf gene is unknown at this time. However, it is expressed in neural tissue and particularly in the hypothalamus. Null mutations of this gene are particularly interesting since they cause a phenotype of increased physical activity, increased basal metabolic rate, relative hyperphagia related to their reduced body weight and decreased adipose tissue stores (172).

5 Structural Genes

a. Hmgic

Hmgic are a family of 3 proteins that function as structural components of the enhancesome. Hmgic is expressed in undifferentiated cells during proliferation, and is expressed highly and selectively in adipose tissue. Both heterozygote Hmgic gene (Hmga2)−/+ and null mutant Hmga2−/− are completely resistant to obesity induced by a high-fat diet, while Hmgic deficiency attenuated the obesity of obese lep^{ob}/lep^{ob} and diabetes $lepr^{db}/lepr^{db}$ mice in a gene-dosage-dependent manner (173). This effect results from an inability of Hmgic-deficient preadipocytes to differentiate into mature adipocytes.

b. Intercellular adhesion molecule 1 (ICAM-1)

ICAM-1 is a membrane protein that interacts with β-integrins to facilitate the migration of leucocytes. ICAM-1 gene (Icaml)-null mice develop a late-onset moderate form of obesity, where excess adipose tissue is predominantly deposited in subcutaneous depots (174). Food intake appears to be similar to that of wild-type mice.

C Obesity and Related Phenotypes Associated with Multiple Genes

The polygenic forms of obesity provide a particular challenge to identify the individual genes and their contributions to the phenotype. In general, polygenic obesity has been related to those mouse strains that will develop obesity either spontaneously or in response to a dietary influence, although there are also numerous examples in rats and other animal species (175). The Sand Rat (*Psammomys obesus*) becomes obese when it is transferred from its usual herbivorous desert diet to a high-carbohydrate laboratory chow. A similar murine obesity and diabetes has been reported in the Spiny Mouse (*Acomys caharinus*) (176). There is a relatively low frequency of diabetes and large variance in the severity of the syndrome in those animals affected. The NZO mouse, originally described by Bielschowsky and Bielschowsky (177), develops a moderate form of obesity from early life and has many of the features of the metabolic syndrome (hypertension, elevated blood lipids, hyperglycemia) (178). While these mice have a variant leptin receptor (A720T/T1044I), that alone does not explain the obesity. However, interaction with other genes (eg Nob1 on chromosome 5) may be a significant contributor to the obesity (179).

More recently, the variation in susceptibility to become obese in the offspring of crosses of individual inbred strains that differed in their propensity to become obese, has become a popular form of polygenic obesity to study. BSB mice, derived from a backcross of *Mus spretus* and C57BL/6J strains, have a body fat content that shows individual variation from 1% to 50% (180,181). Backcrosses between AKR/J and C57BL/J mice likewise give a variation in body fat that has allowed the identification of linked chromosomal regions (182). The full range of linkages gained from genomewide scans in crosses of different mouse strains has been summarized elsewhere (9,10).

The susceptibility to dietary-induced obesity has been a popular model for the identification of genetic linkages. We described the wide range of dietary manipulations that can induce the development of obesity in our previous review (1). A prominent feature of all of the dietary manipulations is the variability of response across individuals and strains of rodents (5,183,184), indicating a strong interaction between genotype and diet. This characteristic may be particularly relevant to the current epidemic of obesity in humans. The strain variability also provides the experimental opportunity for genetic analysis of these differences (185,186).

Several laboratories have mapped quantitative trait loci (QTLs) that influence body fat, particularly after feeding a high-fat diet. Numerous linkages on multiple chromosomes have been identified, many in regions not known to contain an obesity gene (180–182,185–187). Congenic mice or radiation-induced chromosomal deletions have been used to try to narrow the DNA region and identify the specific gene. This approach has successfully identified a novel ATPase coded on chromosome 7 as a potential obesity-related gene (188), although no functional studies have yet been made for proof of function.

D Hypothalamic Obesity

The use of animal models to study the causes and consequences of obesity really began with the destructive lesioning of specific hypothalamic areas (3,4). Since that time a wide range of methods have been used to damage or activate specific brain sites including selective knife cuts and electrical, chemical (gold thioglucose, bipiperidyl mustard, monosodium glutamate, ibotenic acid, neurotransmitters, neuropeptides), or viral routes. These models were reviewed extensively previously (1,3,4). During the past few years, the possibility of a viral cause of obesity has received increased attention.

Four animal viruses and one human virus have been shown to induce obesity or some degree of additional adiposity in animal models. These are the canine distemper virus in mice (189), the Rous-associated virus in chickens (190,191), the Borna disease virus in rats (192), the adenovirus SMAM-1 in chickens (193), and the related human adenovirus Ad-36 in chicken and mice (194). These have been reviewed recently (195).

In general, there is variability in the level of obesity and the metabolic changes that depend on the age of infection and the animal model. The demonstration that a human adenovirus can induce obesity has raised interest particularly since antibodies to the virus have been reported to be linked to higher body weight in small numbers of humans (196). However, the effect size is small, and has been linked with an atypical reduction in serum cholesterol, making it unlikely to be a major cause of human obesity. Similarly, in mice and chicken the increase in body fat in response to adenoviral infection is small, $< 10\%$ (194). While the mechanisms of action of all of the viruses has not been demonstrated, evidence of neuronal damage supports the hypothesis that the virus may have their effects through changes in the activity of the hypothalamic neuropeptide circuits that are modulated by leptin (197,198).

The hypothalamic models of obesity have led to the recognition of the different but overlapping functions of specific hypothalamic regions in the control of energy balance. The VMH is recognized as a primary center regulating the autonomic outflow in response to dietary related signals (3,4,199). The lateral hypothalamus has opposing actions to the VMH on the autonomic nervous system, but also is responsible for feeding behavior. In contrast the PVN region has less to do with sympathetic regulation of brown adipose tissue and vagal regulation of insulin secretion, but is a powerful site for the regulation of feeding behavior. It is only in recent years, with the benefit of molecular and genetic studies, that the neurochemical basis for the activities of these centers has been identified. In particular, the two subpopulations of neurons in the arcuate-PVN pathway (NPY/AGRP neurons and POMC/CART neurons) and the identification of MCH and Orexin (hypocretin) in LH neurons have provided neurochemical insight into function of these sites.

E Endocrine Obesity

Endocrine manipulations have long been known to influence feeding behavior and body composition (1,3,4). These include peripheral injections of insulin (200), excessive glucocorticoid activity (70), and ovariectomy (201–204). The use of transgenic and gene knockout approaches (see Sec. B above) to manipulate hormone and receptor levels has helped to study the role of insulin, adrenal, and gonadal steroids. In addition, these approaches have identified effects of numerous other endocrine influences including pancreatic polypeptide, amylin, IGF-1, CRH, growth hormone, and CCK on energy balance.

F Features Common to Many Models of Obesity

In our previous review we identified numerous features that were common to virtually all animal models of obesity. These included the hypersecretion of insulin and the development of insulin resistance, the hyperphagia and/or autonomic dysfunction, and the glucocorticoid dependence of the obesities (1). It is not our intent to review these characteristics again. However, it is appropriate to identify some significant advances in these areas.

Serum leptin levels are closely related to body fat. Increased levels of leptin gene expression have been reported in all obese models, including the Zucker fa/fa rat (205,206), the diabetes db/db mouse (11), and rats made obese by VMH lesions (207), in rats fed a high-fat diet (208), in the obesity associated with aging (209), and in nonhuman primates (207). The coincidence of hyperleptinemia and obesity is indicative of a failure of leptin to modulate food intake and energy expenditure appropriately, a state of leptin resistance.

A number of studies have sought to identify the site of this leptin resistance by comparison of the responses to peripheral and centrally administered leptin. The loss of response to peripheral leptin, but not to central leptin, has been noted in high-fat diet–induced obesity in both mouse and rat models (210–213) and in CCKA receptor-deficient rats (214), suggesting that transport of leptin across the blood brain barrier is reduced in obesity. This has been confirmed by direct measurement of leptin transport in high-fat-fed obese mice (215). However, this effect may be related to the dietary fat rather than the obesity, since we (216) have shown that the response to peripheral leptin is lost within 24 hr of feeding a high-fat diet. It is likely, though, that the temporal sequence and magnitude of this response are variable across animal models (212).

Leptin resistance is probably manifest at multiple sites in addition to transport across the blood brain barrier. It is now clear that there are significant changes within the signaling pathways in the hypothalamus that also contribute to leptin resistance. Leptin appears to express its biological activity through regulation of the expression and release of several neuropeptides within specific hypothalamic neurons known to affect energy balance. This includes NPY, α-MSH, AgRP, CART, and CRH. The reduced inhibition of arcuate neurons by leptin in overfed rats has been directly demonstrated by electrical recording of nerve activity (217). Decreases in either message or protein levels of the long form of the leptin receptor have been documented (208,218,219), including attenuated transport of leptin across the blood brain barrier as well as reduced activity of the signaling pathways (JAK-STAT, MAP kinase, K-dependent ATPase) or enhanced activity of the suppressors of cytokine signaling (SOCS3) that regulate the release and synthesis of these neuropeptides (210,220). This central leptin resistance might result from effects of leptin itself (221), from downregulation in response to insulin (222), or from the effects of glucocorticoids (223). Readers are referred to other chapters for a full description of these signaling pathways.

III SUMMARY

Obesity is now recognized as the major nutritionally related disease in the Western world. The rapid development in our understanding of the causes and consequences of obesity owes much to the intensive studies of a wide range of animal models, ranging from rodents to nonhuman primate colonies. In rodents, the application of transgenic and gene knockout technologies has created many new models and provided the tools for proof of function of particular genes in causing obesity, affecting adipocyte development or altering feeding behavior and energy expenditure. These models have provided tools for investigation and identification of the hypothalamic pathways and neuropeptidergic systems that regulate feeding behavior and the autonomic nervous system control of energy expenditure. Genetic studies increasingly show the relevance of these animal models to human obesity.

The genes causing a number of spontaneous obesities have been identified; identification of the agouti gene in the Yellow Obese mouse has led to the discovery of the melanocortin pathways; identification of the carboxypeptidase E gene mutation in the Fat (Cpe^{fat}/Cpe^{fat}) mouse has identified the importance of posttranslational processing of peptides; and the identification of the mutations in the Obese and the Diabetes mice and in the Zucker rat led to the discovery of leptin and its signaling pathway. The interaction of environment and genes and its importance for the development of obesity has been studied in crosses of mouse strains and after genetic manipulations that enhance or attenuate the sensitivity to induction of obesity on a high-fat diet. Linkage analysis has identified other gene loci that can be linked to obesity. Age and sex may also be important factors in determining the degree of obesity and the intensity of the associated disorders, particularly diabetes. The possibility of a viral cause of obesity has also been raised.

The application of imaging systems to identify specific mRNA or proteins has linked the genetic and molecular studies to the neuroanatomical networks that had previously been demonstrated to regulate feeding behavior and autonomic control of thermogenesis and insulin secretion. They have also identified abnormalities in these systems that promote obesity.

By study of such divergent experimental models, it has become clear that there may be many different causes of the obesity, but also that there are a number of features that are common to all obesities. Further, it has illustrated the potential for significant gene × gene interactions to enhance or reduce the susceptibility to obesity. The new insight that has been gained from genetic manipulations in mice and from the identification of the function of those genes responsible for the genetically inherited obesities has led to the identification of new targets for the therapeutic prevention and treatment of obesity. The continuing use of genetic manipulations in animals and the identification of genes responsible for linkage traits in animals and humans is likely to identify even more genes that will affect energy balance. Understanding the interactions of these multiple systems is a challenge for the next decade.

REFERENCES

1. York DA, Hansen B. Animal models of obesity. In: Bray GA, Bouchard C, James WP, eds. Handbook of Obesity. New York: Marcel Dekker, 1997:191–221.
2. Naggert JK, Fricker LD, Varlamov O, Nishina PM, Rouille Y, Steiner DF, Carroll RJ, Paigen BJ, Leiter EH. Hyperproinsulinaemia in obese fat/fat mice associated with a carboxypeptidase E mutation which reduces enzyme activity. Nat Gene 1995; 10:135–142.
3. Bray GA, York DA, Fisler JS. Experimental obesity: a homeostatic failure due to defective nutrient stimulation of the sympathetic nervous system. Vitam Horm 1990; 45:1–125.
4. Bray GA, Fisler JS, York DA. Neuroendocrine control of the development of obesity: understanding gained from studies of experimental models of obesity. Prog Neuroendocrinol 1990; 4:128–181.
5. Schemmel R, Mickelson O, Gill J. Dietary obesity in rats: body weight and fat accretion in seven strains of rat. J Nutr 1970; 100:1041–1048.
6. Hansen BC, Bodkin NL, Jen K-LC, Ortmeyer, HK. Primate Models of Diabetes. In: Rifkin H, Colwell JA, Taylor SI, eds. Diabetes. Amsterdam: Elsevier Science, 1991:587–590.
7. Hansen BC. Obesity and diabetes in monkeys. In: Bjorntorp P, Brodoff BN, eds. Obesity. Philadelphia: Lippincott, 1992:256–265.
8. Morrison P, Galster W. Patterns of hibernation in the arctic ground squirrel. Can J Zool 1975; 53:1345–1355.
9. Perusse L, Chagnon YC, Weisnagel SJ, Rankinen T, Snyder E, Sands J, Bouchard C. The human obesity gene map: the 2000 update. Obes Res 2001; 9(2):135–169.
10. Barsh GS, Farooqi IS, O'Rahilly S. Genetics of body-weight regulation. Nature 2000; 404:644–651.
11. Zhang Y, Proenca R, Maffei M, Barone M, Leopold L, Friedman JM. Positional cloning of the mouse obese gene and its human homologue. Nature (Lond) 1994; 372:425–432.
12. Coleman DL. Obesity and diabetes: two mutant genes causing diabetes-obesity syndromes in mice. Diabetologia 1978;14:141–148.
13. Harris RB, Hervey E, Hervey GR, Tobin G. Body composition of lean and obese Zucker rats in parabiosis. Int J Obes 1987; 11:275–283.
14. Chen H, Charlat O, Tartaglia LA, Woolf EA, Weng X, Ellis SJ, Lakey ND, Culpepper J, Moore KJ, Breitbart RE, Duyk GM, Tepper RI, Morgenstern JP. Evidence that the diabetes gene encodes the leptin

receptor: identification of a mutation in the leptin receptor gene in db/db mice. Cell 1996; 84:491–495.
15. Lee G-H, Proenca R, Montez JM, Carol KM, Darvishzadeh JG, Lee JI, Friedman JM. Abnormal splicing of the leptin receptor in diabetic mice. Nature (Lond) 1996; 379:632–635.
16. Phillips MS, Liu Q, Hammond HA, Dugan V, Hey PJ, Casker CT, Hess JF. Leptin receptor missense mutation in the fatty Zucker rat. Nat Genet 1996; 13(1):18–19.
17. Iida M, Muraakami T, Ishida K, Mizuno A, Kuwajima M, Shima K. Phenotype-linked amino acid alteration in leptin receptor cDNA from Zucker fatty (fa/fa) rat. Biochem Biophys Res Commun 1996; 222:19–26.
18. Crouse JA, Elliott GE, Burgess TL, Chiu L, Bennett L, Moore J, Nicolson M, Pacifici RE. Altered cell surface expression and signaling of leptin receptors containing the fatty mutation. J Biol Chem 1998; 273:18365–18373.
19. Takaya K, Ogawa Y, Hiraoka J, Hosoda K, Yamori Y, Nakao K, Koletsky RJ. Nonense mutation of leptin receptor in the obese spontaneously hypertensive Koletsky rat. Nat Genetics 1996; 14:130–131.
20. Kowalski TJ, Liu SM, Leibel RL, Chua SC Jr. Transgenic complementation of leptin-receptor deficiency. I. Rescue of the obesity/diabetes phenotype of LEPR-null mice expressing a LEPR-B transgene. Diabetes 2001; 50:425–435.
21. Shafrir E. Animal models of non-insulin-dependent diabetes. Diabetes Metab Rev 1992; 8:179–208.
22. Reichart U, Renner-Muller I, Hoflich A, Muller OJ, Franz WM, Wolf E, Muller M, Brem G, Aigner B. Contrasting obesity phenotypes uncovered by partial leptin receptor gene deletion in transgenic. Biochem Biophy Res Commun 2000; 269:502–507.
23. Campfield LA, Smith FJ, Guisez Y, Devos R, Burn P. Recombinant mouse ob protein: evidence for a peripheral signal linking adiposity and central neural networks. Science 1995; 269:546–549.
24. Halaas JL, Gajiwala KS, Maffei M, Cohen SL, Chait BT, Rabinowitz D, Lallone RL, Burley SK, Friedman JM. Weight-reducing effects of the plasma protein encoded by the obese gene. Science 1995; 269:543–546.
25. Pelleymounter MA, Cullen MJ, Baker MB, Hecht R, Winters D, Boone T, Collins F. Effects of the obese gene product on body weight regulation in ob/ob mice. Science 1995; 269:540–543.
26. Masuzaki H, Ogawa Y, Aizawa-Abe M, Hosoda K, Suga J, Ebihara K, Satoh N, Iwai H, Inoue G, Nishimura H, Yoshimasa Y, Nakao K. Glucose metabolism and insulin sensitivity in transgenic mice overexpressing leptin with lethal yellow agouti mutation: usefulness of leptin for the treatment of obesity-associated diabetes. Diabetes 1999; 48:1615–1622.
27. Coleman DL, Eicher EM. Fat (fat) and Tubby (tub): two autosomal recessive mutations causing obesity syndromes in the mouse. J Hered 1990; 81:424–427.
28. Udupi V, Gomez P, Song L, Varlamov O, Reed JT, Leiter EH, Fricker LD, Greeley GH Jr. Effect of carboxypeptidase E deficiency on progastrin processing and gastrin messenger ribonucleic acid expression in mice with the fat mutation. Endocrinology 1997; 138:1959–1963.
29. Huszar D, Lynch CA, Fairchild-Huntress V, Dunmore JH, Fang Q, Berkemeier L, Gu W, Kesterson RA, Boston BA, Cone RD, Smith FJ, Campfield LA, Burn P, Lee F. Targeted disruption of the melanocortin-4 receptor results in obesity in mice. Cell 1997; 88:131–141.
30. Lacourse KA, Friis-Hansen L, Samuelson LC, Rehfeld JF. Altered processing of procholecystokinin in carboxypepidase E-deficient fat mice: differential synthesis in neurons and endocrine cells. FEBS Lett 1998; 436(1):61–66.
31. Kleyn PW, Fan W, Kovats SG, Lee JJ, Pulido JC, Wu Y, Berkemeier LR, Misumi DJ, Holmgren L, Charlat O, Woolf EA, Tayber O, Brody T, Shu P, Hawkins F, Kennedy B, Baldini L, Ebeling C, Alperin GD, Deeds J, Lakey ND, Culpepper J, Chen H, Glucksmann-Kuis MA, Moore KJ. Identification and characterization of the mouse obesity gene tubby: a member of a novel gene family. Cell 1996; 85:281–290.
32. Stubdal H, Lynch CA, Moriarty A, Fang Q, Chickering T, Deeds JD, Fairchild-Huntress V, Charlat O, Dunmore JH, Kleyn P, Huszar D, Kapeller R. Targeted deletion of the tub mouse obesity gene reveals that tubby is a loss-of-function mutation. Mol Cell Biol 2000; 20:878–882.
33. Santagata S, Boggon TJ, Baird CL, Gomez CA, Zhao J, Shan WS, Myszka DG, Shapiro L. G-protein signaling through tubby proteins. Science 2001; 292:2041–2050.
34. Kapeller R, Moriarty A, Strauss A, Stubdal H, Theriault K, Siebert E, Chickering T, Morgenstern JP, Tartaglia LA, Lillie J. Tyrosine phosphorylation of tub and its association with Src homology 2 domain-containing proteins implicate tub in intracellular signaling by insulin. J Biol Chem 1999; 274:24980–24986.
35. Guan XM, Yu H, Van der Plog LH. Evidence of altered hypothalamic pro-opiomelanocortin/neuropeptide Y mRNA expression in tubby mice. Brain Res 1998; 59:273–279.
36. Bray GA, York DA. Hypothalamic and genetic obesity in experimental animals. Physiol Rev 1979; 59:719–809.
37. Butler L, Gerritsen GC. A comparison of the modes of inheritance of diabetes in the Chinese hamster and KK mouse. Diabetologia 1970; 6:163–167.
38. Wolff GC. Body composition and coat colour

correlation in different phenotypes of "viable yellow" mice. Science 1965; 147:1145–1147.
39. Gill AM, Leiter EH, Powell JG, Chapman HD, Yen TT. Dexamethasone-induced hyperglycemia in obese A^{vy}/a (viable yellow) female mice entails preferential induction of hepatic estrogen sulfotransferase. Diabetes 1994; 43:999–1004.
40. Wolff GL, Flack JD. Genetic regulation of plasma corticosterone concentration and its response to castration and allogenic tumor growth in the mouse. Nat New Biol 1971; 232:181–182.
41. Bultman SJ, Michaud EJ, Woychik RP. Molecular characterization of the mouse agouti locus. Cell 1992; 71:1195–1204.
42. Perry W, Hustad C, Swing D, Jenkins N, Copeland N. A transgenic mouse assay for agouti protein activity. Genetics 1995; 140:267–274.
43. Klebig ML, Wilkinson JE, Geisler, JG, Woychik RP. Ectopic expression of the agouti gene in transgenic mice causes obesity, features of type II diabetes, and yellow fur. Proc Natl Acad Sci USA 1995; 92:4728–4732.
44. Wilson BD Ollman MM Kany L, Stoffer M, Bell GI, Barsch GS. Structure and function of ASP, the human homolog of the mouse agouti gene. Hum Mol Genet 1995; 4:223–230.
45. Zemel MB, Kim JH, Woychik RP, et al. Agouti regulation of intracellular calcium: role in the insulin resistance of viable yellow mice. Proc Natl Acad Sci USA 1995; 92:4733–4737.
46. Lu D, Willard D, Patel IR, Kadwell S, Overton L, Kost T, Luther M, Chen W, Woychik RP, Wilkison WO, Cone RD. Agouti protein is an antagonist of the melanocyte-stimulating hormone receptor. Nature (Lond) 1994; 371:799–802.
47. Ollman MM, Wilson BD, Yang Y-K, Kerns JA, Chen Y, Gantz I, Barsh GS. Antagonism of central melanocortin receptors in vitro and in vivo by agouti-related protein. Science 1997; 278:135–138.
48. Nakamura M, Yamada K. Studies on a diabetic (KK) strain in the mouse. Diabetologia 1967; 3:212–221.
49. Shimizu H, Shargill NS, Bray GA, Yen FT, Geselchen PD. Effects of MSH on food intake, body weight and coat color of the yellow obese mouse. Life Sci 1989; 45:543–552.
50. Fan W, Boston BA, Kesterson RA, Hruby VJ, Cone RD. Role of melanocortinergic neurons in feeding and the agouti obesity syndrome. Nature 1997; 385:165–168.
51. Fan W, Dinulescu DM, Butler AA, Zhou J, Marks DL, Cone RD. The central melanocortin system can directly regulate serum insulin levels. Endocrinology 2000; 141:3072–3079.
52. Flier JS, Harris M, Hollenberg AN. Leptin, nutrition, and the thyroid: the why, the wherefore, and the wiring. J Clin Invest 2000; 105:859–861.
53. Graham M, Shutter JR, Sarmiento U, Sarosi I, Stark KL. Overexpression of Agrt leads to obesity in transgenic mice. Nat Genet 1997; 17:273–274.
54. Yaswen L, Diehl N, Brennan MB, Hochgeschwender U. Obesity in the mouse model of pro-opiomelanocortin deficiency responds to peripheral melanocortin. Nat Med 1999; 5:1066–1117.
55. Westphal CH, Muller L, Zhou A, Zhu X, Bonner-Weir S, Schambelan M, Steiner DF, Lindberg I, Leder P. The neuroendocrine protein 7B2 is required for peptide hormone processing in vivo and provides a novel mechanism for pituitary Cushing's disease. Cell 1999; 96:689–700.
56. Chen AS, Marsh DJ, Trumbauer ME, Frazier EG, Guan X-M, Yu H, Rosenblum CI, Vongs A, Feng Y, Cao L, Metzger JM, Strack AM, Camacho RE, Mellin TN, Nunes CN, Min W, Fisher J, Gopal-Truter S, MacIntyre DE, Chen HY, Van der Ploeg LHT. Inactivation of the mouse melanocortin-3 receptor results in increased fat mass and reduced lean body mass. Nat Genet 2000; 26:97–102.
57. Butler AA, Kesterson RA, Khong K, Cullen MJ, Pelleymounter MA, Dekoning J, Baetscher M, Cone RD. A unique metabolic syndrome causes obesity in the melanocortin-3 receptor-deficient mouse. Endocrinology 2000; 141:3518–3521.
58. Mynatt RL, Stephens JM. Agouti regulates adipocyte transcription factors. Am Physiol Cell Physiol 2001; 280:C954–C961.
59. Mynatt RL, Miltenberger RJ, Klebig ML, Zemel MB, Wilkinson JE, Wilkinson WO, Woychick RP. Combined effects of insulin treatment and adipose tissue-specific agouti expression on the development of obesity. Proc Natl Acad Sci USA 1997; 94:919–922.
60. Miller KA, Gunn TM, Carrasquillo MM, Lamoreaux ML, Galbraith DB, Barsh GS. Genetic studies of the mouse mutations mahogany and mahoganoid. Genetics 1997; 146:1407–1415.
61. Gunn TM, Miller KA, He L, Hyman RW, Davis RW, Azarani A, Schlossman SF, Duke-Cohan JS, Barsh GS. The mouse mahogany locus encodes a transmembrane form of human attractin. Nature 1999; 398:152–156.
62. Lu X., Gunn TM, Shieh K, Barsh GS, Akil H, Watson SJ. Distribution of mahogany/attractin mRNA in the rat central nervous system. FEBS Lett 1999, 462:101–107.
63. Nagle DL, McGrail SH, Vitale J, Woolf EA, Dussault BJ Jr, DiRocco L, Holmgren L, Montagno J, Bork P, Huszar D, Fairchild-Huntress V, Ge P, Keilty J, Ebeling C, Baldini L, Gilchrist J, Burn P, Carlson GA, Moore KJ. The mahogany protein is a receptor involved in suppression of obesity. Nature 1999; 398:148–152.
64. Reizes O, Lincecum J, Wang Z, Goldberger O, Huang

L, Kaksonen M, Ahima R, Hinkes MT, Barsh GS, Rauvala H, Bernfield M. Transgenic expression of syndecan-1 uncovers a physiological control of feeding behavior by syndecan-3. Cell 2001; 106:105–116.
65. Bannon AW, Seda J, Carmouche M, Francis JM, Norman MH, Karbon B, McCaleb ML. Behavioral characterization of neuropeptide Y knockout mice. Brain Res 2000; 868:79–87.
66. Erickson JC, Hollopeter G, Palmiter JD. Attenuation of the obesity syndrome of ob/ob mice by the loss of neuropeptide Y. Science 1996; 274:1704–1707.
67. Ueno N, Inui A, Iwamoto M, Kaga T, Asakawa A, Okita M, Fujimiya M, Nakajima Y, Ohmoto Y, Ohnaka M, Nakaya Y, Miyazaki JI, Kasuga M. Decreased food intake and body weight in pancreatic polypeptide-overexpressing mice. Gastroenterology 1999; 17:1427–1432.
68. Pepin M-C, Barden N. Decreased glucocorticoid receptor activity following glucocorticoid receptor antisense RNA gene fragment transfection. Mol Cell Biol 1991; 1647–1653.
69. Richard D, Chapdelaine S, Deshaies Y, Pepin M-C, Barden N. Energy balance and lipid metabolism in transgenic mice bearing an antisense GCR gene construct. Am J Physiol 1993; R146–R150
70. Stenzel-Poore MP, Cameron VA, Vaughan J, Sawchenko PE, Vale W. Development of Cushing's syndrome in corticotropin-releasing factor transgenic mice. Endocrinology 1992; 130:3378–3386.
71. Tronche F, Kellendonk C, Kretz O, Gass P, Anlag K, Orban PC, Bock R, Klein R, Schutz G. Disruption of the glucocorticoid receptor gene in the nervous system results in reduced anxiety. Nat Genet 1999; 23:99–103.
72. Karolyi IJ, Burrows HL, Ramesh TM, Nakajima M, Lesh JS, Seong E, Camper SA, Seasholtz AF. Altered anxiety and weight gain in corticotropin-releasing hormone-binding protein-deficient mice. Proc Natl Acad Sci USA 1999; 96:11595–11600.
73. Lovejoy DA, Aubry JM, Turnbull A, Sutton S, Potter E, Yehling J, Rivier C, Vale WW. Ectopic expression of the CRF-binding protein: minor impact on HPA axis regulation but induction of sexually dimorphic weight gain. J Neuroendocrinol 1998; 10:483–491.
74. Coste SC, Kesterson RA, Heldwein KA, Stevens SL, Heard AD, Hollis JH, Murray SE, Hill JK, Pantely GA, Hohimer AR, Hatton DC, Phillips TJ, Finn DA, Low MJ, Rittenberg MB, Stenzel P, Stenzel-Poore MP. Abnormal adaptations to stress and impaired cardiovascular function in mice lacking corticotropin-releasing hormone receptor-2. Nat Genet 2000; 24:403–409.
75. Bale L, Contarino A, Smith GW, Chan R, Gold LH, Sawchenko PE, Koob GF, Vale WW, Lee KF. Mice deficient for corticotropin-releasing hormone receptor-2 display anxiety-like behaviour and are hypersensitive to stress. Nat Genet 2000; 24:410–414.
76. Bradbury MJ, McBurnie MI, Denton DA, Lee KF, Vale WW. Modulation of urocortin-induced hypophagia and weight loss by corticotropin-releasing factor receptor I deficiency in mice. Endocrinology 2000; 141:2715–2724.
77. Kishimoto T, Radulovic J, Radulovic M, Lin CR, Schrick C, Hooshmand F, Hermanson O, Rosenfeld MG, Spiess J. Deletion of crhr2 reveals an anxiolytic role for corticotropin-releasing hormone receptor-2. Nat Genet 2000; 24:415–419.
78. Shimada M, Tritos NA, Lowell BB, Flier JS, Maratos-Flier E. Mice lacking melanin-concentrating hormone are hypophagic and lean. Nature 1998; 396:670–674.
79. Ludwig DS, Tritos NA, Mastaitis JW, Kulkarni R, Kokkotou E, Elmquist J, Lowell B, Flier JS, Maratos-Flier E. Melanin-concentrating hormone overexpression in transgenic mice leads to obesity and insulin resistance. J Clin Investigation 2001; 107: 379–386.
80. Chemelli RM, Willie JT, Sinton CM, Elmquist JK, Scammell T, Lee C, Richardson JA, Williams SC, Xiong Y, Kisanuki Y, Fitch TE, Nakazato M, Hammer RE, Saper CB, Yanagisawa M. Narcolepsy in orexin knockout mice: molecular genetics of sleep regulation. Cell 1999; 98:437–451.
81. Hara J, Beuckmann CT, Nambu T, Willie JT, Chemelli RM, Sinton CM, Sugiyama F, Yagami K, Goto K, Yanagisawa M, Sakurai T. Genetic ablation of orexin neurons in mice results in narcolepsy, hypophagia, and obesity. Neuron 2001; 30:345–354.
82. Bruning JC, Gautam D, Burks DJ, Gillette J, Schubert M, Orban PC, Klein R, Krone W, Muller-Wieland D, Kahn CR. Role of brain insulin receptor in control of body weight and reproduction. Science 2000; 289:2122–2125.
83. Moller DE, Change PY, Yaspelkis BB 3rd, Flier JS, Wallberg-Henriksson H, Ivy JL. Transgenic mice with muscle-specific insulin resistance develop increased adiposity, impaired glucose tolerance, and dyslipidemia. Endocrinology 1996; 137:2397–2405.
84. Devine E, Young AA. Weight gain in male and female mice with amylin gene knockout. Diabetes 1998; 47:A317 (abstract).
85. Rajkumar K, Modric T, Murphy LJ. Impaired adipogenesis in insulin-like growth factor binding protein-1 transgenic mice. J Endocrinol 1999; 162:457–465.
86. Baldwin BA, Parrott RF, Ebenezer IS. Food for thought: a critique on the hypothesis that endogenous cholecystokinin acts as a physiological satiety factor. Prog Neurobiol 1998; 55:477–507.
87. Fumakoshi A, Miyassaka K, Shinozaki H, Masada M, Kawanami T, Takata Y, Komo A. An animal

model of congenital defect of gene expression of cholecystokinin (CCK)-A receptor. Biochem Biophys Res Commun 1993; 210:787–796.
88. Schwartz GJ, Whitney A, Skoglund C, Castonguay TW, Moran TH. Decreased responsiveness to dietary fat in Otsuka Long-Evans Tokushima fatty rats lacking CCK-A receptors. Am J Physiol 1999; 277:R1144–R1151.
89. Kopin AS, Mathes WF, McBride EW, Nguyen M, Al-Haider, Schmitz F, Bonner-Weir S, Kanarak S, Beinbom M. The cholecystokinin-A receptor mediates inhibition of food intake yet is not essential for the maintenance of body weight. J Clin Invest 1999; 103:383–391.
90. Lacourse KA, Swanbert LJ, Gillespie PJ, Rehfeld JF, Saunders TL, Samuelson LC. Pancreatic function in CCK-deficient mice: adaptation to dietary protein does not require CCK. Am J Physiol 1999; 276:G1302–G1309.
91. Ohki-Hamazaki H, Watase K, Yamamoto K, Ogura H, Yamano M, Yamada K, Maeno H, Imaki J, Kikuyama S, Wada E, Wada K. Mice lacking bombesin receptor subtype-3 develop metabolic defects and obesity. Nature 1997; 390:165–169.
92. Yamada K, Wada E, Imaki J, Ohki-Hamazaki H, Wada K. Hyperresponsiveness to palatable and aversive taste stimuli in genetically obese (bombesin receptor subtype-3-deficient) mice. Physiol Behav 1999; 66:863–867.
93. Donahue LR, Beamer WG. Growth hormone deficiency in 'little' mice results in aberrant body composition, reduced insulin-like growth factor-I and insulin-like grown factor–binding protein-3 (IGFBP-3), but does not affect IGFBP-2, -1 or -4. J Endocrinol 1993; 136:91–104.
94. Searle TW, Murray JD, Baker PJ. Effect of increased production of growth hormone on body composition in mice: transgenic versus control. J. Endocrinol 1992; 132:285–291.
95. Chen XL, Lee K, Hartzell DL, Dean RG, Hausman GJ, McGraw RA, Della-Ferra MA, Baile CA. Adipocyte insensitivity to insulin in growth hormone-transgenic mice. Biochem Biophys Res Commun 2001; 283:933–937.
96. Oberbauer AM, Runstadler JA, Murray JD, Havel PJ. Obesity and elevated plasma leptin concentration in oMT1A-o growth hormone transgenic mice. Obes Res 2001; 9:51–58.
97. Cai A, Hyde JF. The human growth hormone-releasing hormone transgenic mouse as a model of modest obesity: differential changes in leptin receptor (OBR) gene expression in the anterior pituitary and hypothalamus after fasting and OBR localization in somatotrophs. Endocrinology 1999; 140: 3609–3614.
98. Hotamisligil GS, Shargill NS, Spiegelman BM. Adipose expression of tumor necrosis factor-alpha: direct role in obesity-linked insulin resistance. Science 1993; 259:87–91.
99. Uysal KT, Wiesbrock SM, Marino MW, Hotamisligil GS. Protection from obesity-induced insulin resistance in mice lacking TNF-alpha function. Nature 1997; 389:610–614.
100. Ventre J, Doebber T, Wu M, MacNaul K, Stevens K, Pasparakis M, Kollias G, Moller DE. Targeted disruption of the tumor necrosis factor-alpha gene: metabolic consequences in obese and nonobese mice. Diabetes 1997; 46:1526–1531.
101. Schreyer SA, Chua SC Jr, LeBoeuf RC. Obesity and diabetes in TNF-alpha receptor-deficient mice. J Clin Invest 1998; 102:402–411.
102. Llovera M, Garcia-Martinez C, Lopez-Soriano J, Carbo N, Agell N, Lopez-Soriano FJ, Argiles JM. Role of TNF receptor 1 in protein turnover during cancer cachexia using gene knockout mice. Mol Cell Endocrinol 1998; 142:183–189.
103. Molotkov A, Satoh M, Tohyama C. Tumor growth and food intake in interleukin-6 gene knock-out mice. Cancer Lett 1998; 132:187–192.
104. Hirsch E, Irikura VM, Paul SM, Hirsh D. Functions of interleukin 1 receptor antagonist in gene knockout and overproducing mice. Proc Natl Acad Sci USA 1996; 93:11008–11013.
105. Susulic VS, Frederich RC, Lawitts J, Tozzo E, Kahn BB, Harper ME, Himms-Hagen J, Flier JS, Lowell BB. Targeted disruption of the beta 3-adrenergic receptor gene. J Biol Chem 1995; 270:29483–29492.
106. Grujic D, Susulic VS, Harper ME, Himms-Hagen J, Cunningham BA, Corkey BE, Lowell BB. Beta3-adrenergic receptors on white and brown adipocytes mediate beta3-selective agonist-induced effects on energy expenditure, insulin secretion, and food intake. A study using transgenic and gene knockout mice. J Biol Chem 1997; 272:17686–17693.
107. Valet P, Grujic D, Wade J, Ito M, Zingaretti MC, Soloveva V, Ross SR, Graves RA, Cinti S, Lafontan M, Lowell BB. Expression of human alpha 2-adrenergic receptors in adipose tissue of beta 3-adrenergic receptor-deficient mice promotes diet-induced obesity. J Biol Chem 2000; 275:34797–34802.
108. Nonogaki K, Strack AM, Dallman MF, Tecott LH. Leptin-independent hyperphagia and type 2 diabetes in mice with a mutated serotonin 5-HT2C receptor gene. Nat Med 1998; 4:1152–1156.
109. Lucas JJ, Yamamoto A, Scearce-Levie K, Saudou F, Hen R. Absence of fenfluramine-induced anorexia and reduced c-fos induction in the hypothalamus and central amygdaloid complex of serotonin 1B receptor knock-out mice. J Neurosci 1998; 18:5537–5544.
110. Zhou QY, Quaife CJ, Palmiter RD. Targeted disruption of the tyrosine hydroxylase gene reveals that catecholamines are required for mouse fetal development. Nature 1995; 374:640–643.

111. Zhou QY, Palmiter RD. Dopamine-deficient mice are severely hypoactive, adipsic, and aphagic. Cell 1995; 83:1197–1209.
112. Drago J, Gerfen CR, Lachowicz JE, Steiner H, Hollon TR, Love PE, Ooi GT, Grinberg A, Lee EJ, Huang SP. Altered striatal function in a mutant mouse lacking D1A dopamine receptors. Proc Natl Acad Sci USA 1994; 91:12564–12568.
113. Xu M, Moratalla R, Gold LH, Hiroi N, Koob GF, Graybiel AM, Tonegawa S. Dopamine D1 receptor mutant mice are deficient in striatal expression of dynorphin and in dopamine-mediated behavioral responses. Cell 1994; 79:729–742.
114. Masaki T, Yoshimatsu H, Chiba S, Watanabe T, Sakata T. Targeted disruption of histamine H1-receptor attenuates regulatory effects of leptin on feeding, adiposity, and UCP family in mice. Diabetes 2001; 50:385–391.
115. Yamada M, Miyakawa T, Duttaroy A, Yamanaka A, Moriguchi T, Makita R, Ogawa M, Chou CJ, Xia B, Crawley JN, Felder CC, Deng CX, Wess J. Mice lacking the M3 muscarinic acetylcholine receptor are hypophagic and lean. Nature 2001; 410:207–212.
116. Ma YH, Hu JH, Zhou XG, Zeng RW, Mei ZT, Fei J, Guo LH. Transgenic mice overexpressing gamma-aminobutyric acid transporter subtype I develop obesity. Cell Res 2000; 10:303–310.
117. Heine PA, Taylor JA, Iwamoto GA, Lubahn DB, Cooke PS. Increased adipose tissue in male and female estrogen receptor-knockout mice. Proc Natl Acad Sci USA 2000; 97:12729–12734.
118. Cooke PS, Heine PA, Tyalor JA, Lubahn DB. The role of estrogen and estrogen receptor-alpha in male adipose tissue. Mol Cell Endocrinol 2001; 178:147–154.
119. Danilovich N, Babu PS, Xing W, Gerdes M, Krishnamurthy H, Sairam MR. Estrogen deficiency, obesity, and skeletal abnormalities in follicle-stimulating hormone receptor knockout (FORKO) female mice. Endocrinology 2000; 141:4295–4308.
120. Abu-Elheiga L, Matzuk MM, Abo-Hashema KAH, Wakil SJ. Continuous fatty acid oxidation and reduced fat storage in mice lacking acetyl-co-A carboxylase 2. Science 2001; 291:2613–2616.
121. Loflus TM, Jaworsky DE, Frehywot GL, Townsend CA, Ronnett GV, Lane MD, Kuhajda FP. Reduced food intake and body weight in mice treated with fatty acid synthase inhibitors. Science 2000; 288: 2379–2381.
122. Martinez-Botas J, Anderson JB, Tessier D, Lapillonne A, Change BH-J, Quast MJ, Gorenstein D, Chen K-H, Chan L. Absence of perilipin results in leanness and reverses obesity in Lepr$^{db/db}$ mice. Nat Gen 2000; 26:474–479.
123. Tansey JT, Sztalryd C, Gruia-Gray J, Roush DL, Zee JV, Gavrilova O, Reitman ML, Deng C-X, Li C, Kimmel AR, Londos C. Perilipin ablation results in a lean mouse with aberrant adipocyte lipolysis, enhanced leptin production, and resistance to diet-induced obesity. Proc Natl Acad Sci USA 2001; 6494–6499.
124. Cummings DE, Brandon EP, Planas JV, Motamed K, Idzerda RL, McKnight GS. Genetically lean mice result from targeted disruption of the RII beta subunit of protein kinase A. Nature 1996; 382:622–626.
125. Osuga J, Ishibashi S, Oka T, Yaguy H, Tozawa R, Fujimoto A, Shionoiri F, Yahagi N, Kraemer FB, Tsutsumi O, Yamada N. Targeted disruption of hormone-sensitive lipase results in male sterility and adipocyte hypertrophy, but not in obesity. Proc Natl Acad Sci USA 2000; 97:787–792.
126. Hotamisligil GS, Johnson RS, Distel RJ, Ellis R, Papaioannou VE, Spiegelman BM. Uncoupling of obesity from insulin resistance through a targeted mutation in aP2, the adipocyte fatty acid binding protein. Science 1996; 274:1377–1379.
127. Uysal KT, Scheja L, Wiesbrock SM, Bonner-Weir S, Hotamisligil GS. Improved glucose and lipid metabolism in genetically obese mice lacking aP2. Endocrinology 2000; 141:3388–3396.
128. Smith SJ, Cases S, Jensen DR, Chen HC, Sande E, Tow B, Sanan DA, Raber J, Eckel RH, Farese RV Jr. Obesity resistance and multiple mechanisms of triglyceride synthesis in mice lacking Dgat. Nat Genet 2000; 25:87–90.
129. Shepherd PR, Gnudi L, Tozzo E, Yang H, Leach F, Kahn BB. Adipose cell hyperplasia and enhanced glucose disposal in transgenic mice overexpressing GLUT4 selectively in adipose tissue. J Biol Chem 1993; 268:22243–22246.
130. Ikemoto S, Thompson KS, Takahashi M, Itakura H, Lane MD, Ezaki O. High fat diet–induced hyperglycemia: prevention by low level expression of a glucose transporter (GLUT4) minigene in transgenic mice. Proc Natl Acad Sci USA 1995; 92:3096–3099.
131. Tsao TS, Burcelin R, Katz EB, Huang L, Charron MJ. Enhanced insulin action due to targeted GLUT4 overexpression exclusively in muscle. Diabetes 1996; 45:28–36.
132. Stenbit AE, Tsao TS, Li J, Burcelin R, Geenen DL, Factor SM, Houseknecht K, Katz EB, Charron MJ. GLUT4 heterozygous knockout mice develop muscle insulin resistance and diabetes. Nat Med 1997; 3:1080–1081.
133. Veerababu G, Tang J, Hoffman RT, Daniels MC, Hebert LF Jr, Crook ED, Cooksey RC, McClain DA. Overexpression of gluatamine: fructose-6-phosphate amidotransferase in the liver of transgenic mice results in enhanced glycogen storage, hyperlipidemia, obesity, and impaired glucose tolerance. Diabetes 2000; 49:2070–2078.
134. Jones MEE, Thorburn AW, Britt KL, Hewitt KN, Wreford NG, Proietto J, Oz OK, Leury BJ, Robertson

KM, Yao S, Simpson ER. Aromatase-deficient (ArKO) mice have a phenotype of increased adiposity. Proc Natl Acad Sci USA 2000; 97:12735–12740.

135. Yao JH, Ye SM, Burgess W, Zachary JF, Kelley KW, Johnson RW. Mice deficient in interleukin-1beta converting enzyme resist anorexia induced by central lipopolysaccharide. Am J Physiol 1999; 277:R1435–R1443.

136. Kozak LP, Kozak UC, Clarke GT. Abnormal brown and white fat development in transgenic mice overexpressing glycerol 3-phosphate dehydrogenase. Genes 1991; 5:2256–2264.

137. Ookuma K, Bray GA, York DA. The effect of goldthioglucose on the feeding response to CL 316,243 in transgenic mice overexpressing glycerophosphate dehydrogenase or uncoupling protein. Int J Obes 1998; 22(suppl 3):S16 (abstract).

138. Eto K, Tsubamoto Y, Terauchi Y, Sugiyama T, Kishimoto T, Takahashi N, Yamauchi N, Kubota N, Murayama S, Aizawa T, Akanuma Y, Kasai H, Yazaki Y, Kadowaki T. Role of NADH shuttle system in glucose-induced activation of mitochondrial metabolism and insulin secretion. Science 1999; 283:981–985.

139. Lowell BB, S-Susulic V, Hamann A, Lawitts JA, Himms-Hagen J, Boyers BB, Kozak LP, Flier JS. Development of obesity in transgenic mice after genetic ablation of brown adipose tissue. Nature (Lond) 1993; 366:740–742.

140. Bray GA. Reciprocal relation between the sympathetic nervous system and food intake. Brain Res Bull 1991; 27:517–520.

141. Himms-Hagen J. Role of brown adipose tissue termogenesis in control of thermoregulatory feeding in rats. A new hypothesis that links thermostatic and glucostatic hypotheses for control of food intake. Proc Soc Exp Biol Med 1995; 208:159–169.

142. Ross SR, Graves RA, Spiegelman BM. Targeted expression of a toxin gene to adipose tissue: transgenic mice resistant to obesity. Genes Dev 1993; 7:1318–1324.

143. Enerback S, Jacobsson A, Simpson EM, Guerra C, Yamashita H, Harper M-E, Kozak LE. Mice lacking mitochondrial uncoupling protein are cold-sensitive but not obese. Nature 1997; 387:90–94.

144. Kopecky J, Hodny Z, Rossmeisl M, Syrovy I, Kozak LP. Reduction of dietary obesity in aP2-Ucp transgenic mice: physiology and adipose tissue distribution. Am J Physiol 1996; 270(5 Pt 1):E768–E775.

145. Li B, Nolte LA, Ju JS, Han DH, Coleman T, Holloszy JO, Semenkovich CF. Skeletal muscle respiratory uncoupling prevents diet-induced obesity and insulin resistance in mice. Nat Med 2000; 6(10): 1115–1120.

146. Arsenijevic D, Onuma H, Pecqueur C, Raimbault S, Manning BS, Mirous B, Couplan E, Alves-Guerra MC, Goubern M, Surwit R, Bouillaud F, Richar D, Collins S, Ricquier D. Disruption of the uncoupling protein-2 gene in mice reveals a role in immunity and reactive oxygen species production. Nat Genet 2000; 26(4):387–388.

147. Gong D-W, Monemdjou S, Gavrilova O, Leon LR, Marcus-Samuels B, Chou CJ, Everett C, Kozak LP, Li C, Deng C, Harper M-E, Reitman ML. Lack of obesity and normal response to fasting and thyroid hormone in mice lacking uncoupling protein-3. J Biol Chem 2000; 275:16251–16257.

148. Clapham JC, Arch JR, Chapman H, Haynes A, Lister C, Moore GB, Piercy V, Carter SA, Lehner I, Smith SA, Beeley LJ, Godden RJ, Herrity N, Skehel M, Changani KK, Hockings PD, Reid DG, Squires SM, Hatcher J, Trail B, Latcham J, Rastan S, Harper AJ, Cadenas S, Buckingham JA, Brand MD, Abuin A. Mice overexpressing human uncoupling protein-3 in skeletal muscle are hyperphagic and lean. Nature 2000; 406:415–418.

149. Beattie JH, Wood AM, Newman AM, Bremner I, Choo KHA, Michalska AE, Duncan JS, Trayhurn P. Obesity and hyperleptinemia in metallothionein (-I and -II). Proc Natl Acad Sci USA 1998; 95:358–363.

150. Murray SE, Coste SC, Lindberg I, Stenzel–Poore MP. Genetic mutants with dysregulation of corticotropin pathways. In: Castro M, ed. Transgenic Models of Endocrinology. New York: Kluwer, 2000.

151. McKnight SL. WAT-free mice: diabetes without obesity. Genes Dev 1998; 12:3145–3148.

152. McKnight GS, Cummings DE, Amieux PS, Sikorski MA, Brandon EP, Planas JV, Motamed K, Idzerda RL. Cyclic AMP, PKA, and the physiological regulation of adiposity. Recent Prog Horm Res 1998; 53: 139–159.

153. Planas JV, Cummings DE, Idzerda RL, McKnight GS. Mutation of the RIIbeta subunit of protein kinase A differentially affects lipolysis but not gene induction in white adipose tissue. J Biol Chem 1999; 274:36281–36287.

154. Cho H, Mu J, Kim JK, Thorvaldsen JL, Chu Q, Crenshaw EB III, Kaestner KH, Bartolomei MS, Shulman GI, Birnbaum MJ. Insulin resistance and a diabetes mellitus–like syndrome in mice lacking the protein kinase Akt2 (PKBβ). Science 2001; 292:1728–1731.

155. Yu S, Gavrilova O, Chen H, Lee R, Liu J, Pacak K, Parlow AF, Quon MJ, Reitman ML, Weinstein LS. Paternal versus maternal transmission of a stimulatory G-protein alpha subunit knockout produces opposite effects on energy metabolism. J Clin Invest 2000; 105:615–623.

156. Elchebly M, Payette P, Michaliszyn E, CromLish W, Collins S, Loy AL, Normandin D, Cheng A, Himms-Hagen J, Chan C-C, Ramachandran C, Gresser MJ, Tremblay ML, Kennedy BP. Increased insulin sensi-

tivity and obesity resistance in mice lacking the protein tyrosine phosphatase-1B gene. Science 1999; 283: 1544–1548.
157. Udy GB, Towers RP, Snell RG, Wilkins RJ, Park SH, Ram PA, Waxman DJ, Davey HW. Requirement of STAT5b for sexual dimorphism of body growth rates and liver gene expression. Proc Natl Acad Sci USA 1997; 94:7239–7244.
158. Peterfy M, Phan J, Xu P, Reue K. Lipodystrophy in the f/d mouse results from mutation of a new gene encoding a nuclear protein, lipin. Nat Genet 2001; 27:121–124.
159. Barak Y, Nelson MC, Ong ES, Jones YZ, Ruiz-Lozano P, Chien KR, Koder A, Evans RM. PPAR gamma is required for placental, cardiac, and adipose tissue development. Mot Cell 1999; 4:585–595.
160. Costet P, Legendre C, More J, Edgar A, Galtier P, Pineau T. Peroxisome proliferator-activated receptor alpha-isoform deficiency leads to progressive dyslipidemia with sexually dimorphic obesity and steatosis. J Biol Chem 1998; 273:29577–29585.
161. Kersten S, Seydoux J, Peters JM, Gonzalez FJ, Desvergne B, Wahli W. Peroxisome proliferator-activated receptor alpha mediates the adaptive response to fasting. J Clin Invest 1999; 103:1489–1498.
162. Peters JM, Lee SS, Li W, Wand JM, Gavrilova O, Everetet C, Reitman ML, Hudson LD, Gonzalez FJ. Growth, adipose, brain, and skin alterations resulting from targeted disruption of the mouse peroxisome proliferator-activated receptor beta (delta). Mol Cell Biol 2000; 20:5119–5128.
163. Shimomura I, Hammer RE, Richardson JA, Ikemoto S, Bashmakov Y, Goldstein JL, Brown MS. Insulin resistance and diabetes mellitus in transgenic mice expressing nuclear SREBP-lc in adipose tissue: model for congenital generalized lipodystrophy. Genes Dev 1998; 12:3182–3194.
164. Shimomura I, Hammer RE, Ikemoto S, Brown MS, Goldstein JL. Leptin reverses insulin resistance and diabetes mellitus in mice with congenital lipodystrophy. Nature 1999; 401:73–76.
165. Shimano H, Horton JD, Hammer RE, Shimomura I, Brown MS, Goldstein JL. Overproduction of cholesterol and fatty acids causes massive liver enlargement in transgenic mice expressing truncated SREBP-la. J Clin Invest 1996; 98:1575–1584.
166. Moitra J, Mason MM, Olive M, Krylov D, Gavrilova O, Marcus-Samuels B, Feigenbaum L, Lee E, Aoyama T, Eckhaus M, Reitman ML, Vinson C. Life without white fat: a transgenic mouse. Genes Dev 1998; 12:3168–3181.
167. Reitman ML, Gavrilova O. A-ZIP/F-l mice lacking white fat: a model for understanding lipoatrophic diabetes. Int J Obes Rel Metab Disord 2000; 24 (suppl4):S11–S14.
168. Ebihara K, Ogawa Y, Masuzaki H, Shintani M, Miyanaga F, Aizawa-Abe M, Hayashi T, Hosoda K, Inoue G, Yoshimasa Y, Gavrilova O, Reitman ML, Nakao K. Transgenic overexpression of leptin rescues insulin resistance and diabetes in a mouse model of lipoatrophic diabetes. Diabetes 2001; 50:1440–1448.
169. Wang ND, Finegold MJ, Bradley A, Ou CN, Abdelsayed SV, Wilde MD, Taylor LR, Wilson DR, Darlington GJ. Impaired energy homeostasis in C/EBP alpha knockout mice. Science 1995; 269:1108–1112.
170. Tanaka T, Yoshida N, Kishimoto T, Akira S. Defective adipocyte differentiation in mice lacking the C/EBPbeta and/or C/EBPdelta gene. EMBO J 1997; 16:7432–7443.
171. Good DJ, Porter FD, Mahon KA, Parlow AF, Westphal H, Kirsch JR. Hypogonadism and obesity in mice with a targeted deletion of the Nhih2 gene. Nat Genet 1997; 15:397–401.
172. Hahm S, Mizuno TM, Wu TJ, Wisor JP, Priest CA, Kozak CA, Boozer CN, Peng B, McEvoy RC, Good P, Kelley KA, Takahashi JS, Pintar JE, Roberts JL, Mobbs CV, Salton SR. Targeted deletion of the Vgf gene indicates that the encoded secretory peptide precursor plays a novel role in the regulation of energy balance. Neuron 1999; 23:537–548.
173. Anand A, Chada K. In vivo modulation of Hmgic reduces obesity. Nat Genet 2000;24:377–380.
174. Dong ZM, Gutierrez-Ramos JC, Coxon A, Mayadas TN, Wagner DD. A new class of obesity genes encodes leukocyte adhesion receptors. Proc Natl Acad Sci USA 1997;4:7526–7530.
175. Pomp D. Animal models of obesity. Mol Med Today 1999; 5:459–460.
176. Gonet AE, Stauffacher W, Pictet R, Renold AE. Obesity and diabetes mellitus with striking congenital hyperplasia of the islets of Langerhans in spiny mice (*Acomys cahirinus*). I. Histological findings and preliminary metabolic observations. Diabetologia 1965; 1:162–171.
177. Bielschowsky M, Bielschowsky F. A new strain of mouse with hereditary obesity. Proc Univ Otago Med School 1953; 31:29–31.
178. Ortlepp JR, Kluge R, Giesen K, Plum L, Radke P, Hanrath P, Joost HG. A metabolic syndrome of hypertension, hyperinsulinaemia and hypercholesterolaemia in the New Zealand obese mouse. Eur J Clin Invest 2000; 30:195–202.
179. Kluge R, Giesen K, Bahrenberg G, Plum L, Ortlepp JR, Joost HG. Quantitative trait loci for obesity and insulin resistance (Nob 1, Nob2) and their interaction with the leptin receptor allele (LeprA720T/T10441) in New Zealand obese mice. Diabetologia 2000; 43:1565–1572.
180. Warden CH, Fisler JS, Shoemaker SM, Ping-Zi W, Svenson KL, Pace M, Lusis AJ. Identification of four

chromosomal loci determining obesity in a multifactorial mouse model. J Clin Invest 1995; 95:1545–1552.
181. Warden CH, Fisler JS, Pace MJ, Svenson L, Lusis AJ. Coincidence of genetic loci for plasma cholesterol levels and obesity in a multifactorial mouse model. J Clin Invest 1993; 92:773–779.
182. Taylor BA, Phillips SA. Detection of of obesity QTLs on mouse chromosomes 1 and 7 by selective DNA pooling. Genomics 1996; 34:389–398.
183. West DB, Boozer CN, Moody DC, Atkinson RL. Dietary obesity in nine inbred mouse strains. Am J Physiol 1992; 262:R1025–R1032.
184. Fisler JS, Bray GA. Dietary obesity: effects of drugs on food intake in S5B/Pl and Osborne-Mendel rats. Physiol Behav 1985; 34:225–231.
185. West DB, Waguespack J, York B, Goudey-Lefevre J, Price RA. Genetics of dietary obesity in AKR/J × SWR/J mice: segregation of the trait and identification of a linked locus on chromosome 4. Mamm Genome 1994; 5:546–552.
186. West DB, Goudey-Lefevre J, York B, Truett GE. Dietary obesity linked to genetic loci on chromosomes 9 and 15 in a polygenic mouse model. J Clin Invest 1994; 94:1410–1416.
187. York B, Truett AA, Monteiro MP, Barry SJ, Warden CH, Naggert JK, Maddatu TP, West DB. Gene-environment interaction: a significant diet-dependent obesity locus demonstrated in a congenic segment on mouse chromosome 7. Mamm Genome 1999; 10:457–462.
188. Dhar M, Webb LS, Smith L, Hauser L, Johnson D, West D. A novel ATPase on mouse chromosome 7 is a candidate gene for increased body fat. Physiol Genomics 2000; 4:93–100.
189. Lyons MJ, Faust IM, Hemmes RB, Buskirk DR, Hirsch J, Zabriskie JB. A virally induced obesity syndrome in mice. Science 1982; 216:82–85.
190. Carter JK, Ow CL, Smith RE. Rous-associated virus type 7 induces a syndrome in chickens characterized by stunting and obesity. Infect Immun 1983; 39:410–422.
191. Carter JK, Garlich JD, Donaldson WE, Smith RE. Influence of diet on a retrovirus-induced obesity and stunting syndrome. Avian Dis 1983; 27:317–322.
192. Gosztonyi G, Ludwig H. Borna disease—neuropathology and pathogenesis. Curr Top Microbiol Immunol 1995; 190:39–73.
193. Dhurandhar NV, Kulkarni P, Ajinkya SM, Sherikar A. Effect of adenovirus infection on adiposity in chicken. Vet Microbiol 1992; 31:101–107.
194. Dhurandhar NV, Israel BA, Kolear JM, Mayhew GF, Cook ME, Atkinson RL. Increased adiposity in animals due to a human virus. Int J Obes 2000; 24:989–996.
195. Dhurandhar NV, Atkinson RL. Viruses and obesity. Curr Opin Endocrinol Diabetes 2000; 7:247–251.
196. Dhurandhar NV, Kulkarni PR, Ajinkya SM, Sherikar AA, Atkinson RL. Association of adenovirus infection with human obesity. Obes Res 1997; 5:464–469.
197. Bernard A, Zwingelstein G, Meister R, Wild TF. Hyperinsulinemia induced by canine distemper virus infection of mice and its correlation with the appearance of obesity. Comp Biochem Physiol B 1988; 91:691–696.
198. Bernard A, Cohen R, Khuth ST, Vedrine B, Verlaeten O, Akaoka H, Giraudon P, Belin MF. Alteration of the leptin network in late morbid obesity induced in mice by brain infection with canine distemper virus. J Virol 1999; 73:7317–7327.
199. Rohner-Jeanrenaud F. A neuroendocrine reappraisal of the dual-centre hypothesis: its implications for obesity and insulin resistance. Int J Obes 1995; 19:517–534.
200. Lotter FC, Wards SC. Injections of insulin and changes of body weight. Physiol Behav 1977; 18:293–297.
201. Mook DG, Kenney NJ, Robert S, Nussbaum AI, Rodier WI III. Ovarian-adrenal interactions in regulation of body weight by female rats. J Comp Physiol Psychol 1972; 81:198–211.
202. Beatty WW, Briant DA, Vilberg TR. Effect of ovariectomy and estradiol injections on food intake and body weight in rats with hypothalamic lesions. Pharmacol Biochem Behav.1975; 3:539–544.
203. Jones AP, McElroy JF, Crnic L, Wades GN. Effects of ovariectomy on thermogenesis in brown adipose tissue and liver in Syrian hamsters. Physiol Behav 1991; 50:41–45.
204. Hausberger FX, Hausberger BC. Castration-induced obesity in mice. Body composition, histology of adrenal cortex and islets of Langerhans in castrated mice. Acta Endocrinol 1966; 53:571–583.
205. Murakami T, Shima K. Cloning of rat obese cDNA and its expression in obese rats. Biochem Biophys Res Commun 1995; 209:944–952.
206. Lin X, York DA, Harris RBS, Bray GA, Bruch RL. The effect of adrenalectomy and glucocorticoid replacement on Ob mRNA levels in adipose tissue of obese Zucker fa/fa rats. Obes Res 1995; 3:339s.
207. Funahashi T, Shimomura I, Hiraoka H, Arai T, Takahashi M, Nakamura T, Nozaki S, Yamashita S, Takemura K, Tokunaga K, Matsuzawa Y. Enhanced expression of rat obese (ob) gene in adipose tissues of ventromedial hypothalamus (VMH)-lesioned rats. Biochem Biophys Res Commun 1995; 211: 469–475.
208. Madiehe AM, Schaffhauser AO, Braymer DH, Bray GA, York DA. Differential expression of leptin receptor in high- and low-fat fed Osborne-Mendel and S5B/PI rats. Obes Res 2000; 8:467–474.
209. Scarpace PH, Matheny M, Moore RL, Turner N. Impaired leptin responsiveness in aged rats. Diabetes 2000; 49:431–435.

210. El-Haschimi K, Pierroz DD, Hileman SM, Bjorbaek C, Flier JS. Two defects contribute to hypothalamic leptin resistance in mice with diet-induced obesity. J Clin Invest 2000; 105:1827–1832.
211. Van Heek M, Compton DS, France CF, Tedesco RP, Fawzi AB, Graziano MP, Sybertz EJ, Strader CD, Davis HR Jr. Diet-induced obese mice develop peripheral, but not central, resistance to leptin. J Clin Invest 1997; 99:385–390.
212. Lin S, Thomas TC, Storlien LH, Huang XF. Development of high fat diet–induced obesity and leptin resistance in C57B1/6J mice. Int J Obes Relat Metab Disord 2000; 24:639–646.
213. Lin X, Chavez MR, Bruch RC, Kilroy GE, Simmons LA, Lin L, Braymer HD, Bray GA, York DA. The effects of a high fat diet on leptin mRNA, serum leptin and the response to leptin are not altered in a rat strain susceptible to high fat diet-induced obesity. J Nutr 1998; 128:1606–1613.
214. Niimi M, Sato M, Yokote R, Tada S, Takahara J. Effects of central and peripheral injection of leptin on food intake and on brain Fos expression in the Otsuka Long-Evans Tokushima Fatty rat with hyperleptinaemia. J Neurobiol 1999; 11:605–611.
215. Banks WA, DiPalma CR, Farrell CL. Impaired transport of leptin across the blood-brain barrier in obesity. Peptides 1999; 20:1341–1345.
216. Lin L, Martin R, Schaffhauser AO, York DA. Acute changes in the response to peripheral leptin with alteration in the diet composition. Am J Physiol Regul Integr Comp Physiol 2001; 280: R504–R509.
217. Davidowa H, Plagemann A. Decreased inhibition by leptin of hypothalamic arcuate neurons in neonatally overfed young rats. Neuroreport 2000; 11:2795–2798.
218. Martin RL, Perez E, He YJ, Dawson R Jr, Millar WJ. Leptin resistance is associated with hypothalamic leptin receptor mRNA and protein downregulation. Metabolism 2000; 49:1479–1484.
219. Scarpace PJ, Matheny M, Shek EW. Impaired leptin signal transduction with age-related obesity. Neuropharmacology 2000; 39:1872–1879.
220. Bjorbaek C, El-Haschimi K, Frantz JD, Flier JS. The role of SOCS-3 in leptin signaling and leptin resistance. J Biol Chem 1999; 274:3059–3065.
221. Hikita M, Bujo H, Hirayama S, Takahashi K, Morisaki N, Saito Y. Differential regulation of leptin receptor expression by insulin and leptin in neuroblastoma cells. Biochem Biophy Res Commun 2000; 271:703–709.
222. Dunbar JC, Lu H. Chronic intracerebroventricular insulin atttenuates the leptin-mediated but not alpha melanocyte stimulating hormone increase in sympathetic and cardiovascular responses. Brain Res Bull 2000; 52:123–126.
223. Madiehe AM, Lin L, White C, Braymer HD, Bray GA, York DA. Constitutive activation of STAT-3 and down-regulation of SOCS-3 expression induced by adrenalectomy. Am J Phys 2001; 281:R2048–R2058.

12

Primates in the Study of Aging-Associated Obesity

Barbara C. Hansen

University of Maryland, Baltimore, Maryland, U.S.A.

I AGING-ASSOCIATED NATURALLY OCCURRING SPONTANEOUS OBESITY IN NONHUMAN PRIMATES

Within the class Mammalia, obesity has been identified in a number of orders, including the Rodentia, the Carnivora (e.g., dogs, bears), the Artoidactyla (pigs, cattle), and the order Primates (which includes, for example, lemurs, monkeys, apes, and humans, a total of ~200 primate species), as well as in other orders which include such mammals as the whale, walrus, manatee, hedgehog, and rhinoceros. Within the suborder Anthropoidea, obesity has been described in two of three superfamilies: Cercopithecoidea (Old World monkeys, including many species of macaques) and Hominoidea (including orangutans, chimpanzees and gorillas—with specimens of this last sometimes found to weigh >180 kg 400 lb). Obesity may also occur in the third superfamily Ceboidea (New World monkeys); however, to date it has not been well documented. Most commonly, within the genus *Macaca*, obesity has been described in the species *Macaca fascicularis* (cynomolgus monkeys), *Macaca nigra* (misnomered the Celebes ape), and most of all, in *Macaca mulatta* (rhesus monkeys)(1–3).

Spontaneous, naturally occurring obesity is common both in free-ranging and in laboratory or zoo-maintained nonhuman primates and has been described in a wide range of primate species. In addition, primate models of obesity have been experimentally induced. Previous reviews have described the various measures used to produce experimental obesity in primates (4,5), including the production of hypothalamic lesions to induce weight gain and diabeteslike syndromes, drug and hormonal approaches, and diet manipulations (6) or forced overfeeding (7,8) to produce weight gain. These methods have received little use in the past 10 years, probably because, as monkeys have been held longer under laboratory conditions, well into middle age, more and more spontaneously obese animals have been identified, thus reducing the need to experimentally create obese primate models. Further, the induced obese models may deviate significantly from the "normal" naturally occurring form(s), both in underlying mechanisms and in responses to treatment. The present review will, therefore, focus on spontaneous obesity in both free-ranging and laboratory-maintained monkeys.

One of the first surveys aimed at identifying the prevalence of obesity in a colony of group-housed monkeys examined the medical records of >800 pig-tailed macaques (*Macaca nemestrina*) in a large breeding facility (9). Tritiated water was then used to determine the relative body composition of those selected on the basis of heavy body weight for age. Several spontaneously obese individuals were identified; however, the incidence appeared to be very low. Retrospective consideration of this study, based on further understanding of obesity in primates gained over the past 20 years, suggests that the reason for the finding of a very low number of obese animals was the relatively young age distribution of the breeding colony. It is, in fact, unusual to find monkeys of either sex over the age of 15 years in a breeding colony, as they are usually moved before reaching such an age.

The obesity of nonhuman primates is clearly of adult onset, with no cases of obesity having yet been identified in an animal under the age of 7 years. For reference, sexual maturity is reached in the female between 3 and 5 years (10) with completion of growth at 6–7 years of age, while in the male the corresponding ages are 4–6 years (11) and 8 years. The obese monkeys, identified in a survey of a free-ranging chow-provisioned colony living on the island of Cayo Santiago, ranged in age from 9 to 16 years (12,13). Peak body weight on average is reached around the age of 15 years in *Macaca mulatta.*

Obesity in male monkeys has been associated with abnormal androgen metabolism, with obese males having lower serum testosterone and lower dihydrotestosterone than leans (5). Females had lower serum androgen levels than males, but there were no differences between obese and lean females. Gonadectomy in male and in female monkeys reduced body weight relative to intact animals; however, replacement therapy with testosterone propionate or dihydrotestosterone propionate resulted in an increase in lean body mass, but not in adiposity (14).

No early markers for the propensity to develop obesity at a later age have yet been found that could be used to identify in young adult monkeys (or in, for that matter, humans) the predisposition toward obesity—with the exception of family history (and an unconstraining environment).

II DIET, FOOD INTAKE, ACTIVITY, AND ENERGY EXPENDITURE IN NONHUMAN PRIMATE OBESITY

In spontaneously obese male rhesus monkeys ranging from 10 to 17 kg, no differences in food intake were observed between the most obese and the least obese groups, suggesting that differences in energy expenditure may contribute principally to the development of obesity. Obese animals showed reduced physical activity (15); however, it has not been possible to document reduced activity in advance of the development of obesity (16). In some studies obese monkeys have been found to ingest fewer calories than lean monkeys (17), thus providing no evidence for hyperphagia as an important contributor to the development of obesity or its sustaining. Prevention of obesity by restraint of calories neither increased nor decreased physical activity relative to similar-weight animals (15). Energy expenditure per kg lean body mass was significantly reduced by a degree of calorie restriction sufficient only to prevent the development of obesity (15).

Although several studies have involved dietary manipulations thought to facilitate the development of obesity, where these dietary regimens have been tested in young animals, obesity has not developed (18). Some very high fat diets, for example, 60% fat, have been found to produce weight gain in young monkeys. High-fat diets have been used to alter lipoprotein composition (19). The usual dietary regimen of laboratory monkeys, primate chow, would be expected to be optimal in the prevention of obesity, as it is high in fiber, low in fat (17%), and relatively low in caloric density (4 kcal/g). In colonies where the calorie allocation to each monkey is strictly controlled, that is, restricted below ad libitum levels, obesity does not develop. Under conditions of ad libitum feeding (food continuously available for 8–24 hr/d), obesity will eventually develop in perhaps 50% or more of the laboratory-maintained animals, despite the presumed optimal diet composition. As discussed below, long-term experimental limitation of calories, adjusted on an individual basis to prevent body weight increase, can prevent the development of this middle-age-onset obesity (20).

III MEASUREMENT OF ADIPOSITY IN MONKEYS

The assessment of obesity in monkeys can be made by body weight alone, since, in adult animals, body weight and percent fat are highly correlated (within each sex) ($r = .62$, $p < .01$)(21). The body mass index, or Quetelet index (weight/height^2), was adapted for use in monkeys by substitution of the crown-rump length (in cm) for height (21). This body mass index, termed the Obesity Index Rh (for rhesus monkeys), was shown to be highly correlated with percent weight as fat ($r = .80$, $p < .01$), midgirth circumference ($r = .82$, $p < .001$), and body weight ($r = .80$, $p < .001$), but not with height, and is therefore the best simple measurement of body fatness in monkeys. Total height is not readily or accurately measured in monkeys, particularly as they age, and thus the usual body mass index used for humans is not sufficiently reliable. All rhesus monkeys over the body weight of 15 kg had >25% of weight as fat. In obese male rhesus monkeys, body fat can reach 50% of body weight. The tritiated water dilution method has also been reliably used to estimate total body fat content, and is highly correlated with the body mass index for monkeys.

Computed tomography has been used to assess abdominal fat distribution, with the observation in *Macaca fascicularis* of very strong positive correlations between body mass index and intra-abdominal fat, subcutaneous fat, and total abdominal fat (r's > .89)(22). Sharma et al. (23) compared magnetic resonance imaging (MRI) and various anthropometric measures in *Macaca fascicularis*, and found significant heterogeneity in the amounts of intra-abdominal and subcutaneous fat. Body weight correlated with intra-abdominal fat in these male cynomolgus monkeys. Although little has yet been published on the use of the DXA (dual-energy x-ray absorptiometry) method in non-human primates, it is likely with careful standardization to become the "gold standard" for assessing body composition. Female cynomolgus monkeys have been examined by DXA for body composition against a standard, with the observation that percent body fat of soft tissue mass is a better index of obesity than body weight and/or anthropometry (24).

IV FEATURES COMMON TO MANY PRIMATE MODELS OF OBESITY

Obese rhesus monkeys, followed longitudinally, show a gradual slow decline in glucose tolerance, many years before the development of overt diabetes (25), and this has been observed in cynomolgus monkeys as well (26–29). This deterioration takes place at the same time as pancreatic insulin output is increased both basally and under stimulated conditions. β-cell hyperresponsiveness to a glucose load has been shown to be a very early defect in obesity, possibly preceding the development of significant insulin resistance and hyperinsulinemia (30). In obese monkeys, prior to the development of overt diabetes, deKoning et al. (31) found beginning changes in pancreatic β-cells, with proliferation of β-cell mass, and small deposits of islet-associated polypeptide as islet amyloid, as also noted in cynomolgus (28).

The insulin resistance is not a requirement for the development of obesity in rodents or primates. Furthermore, the hepatic insulin resistance as evidenced by the failure of insulin to suppress hepatic glucose production is not associated with obesity per se, but has been directly related to the subsequent development of overt type 2 diabetes mellitus in monkeys (32).

Reduced hepatic extraction of insulin has also been shown to be involved in the sustaining of hyperinsulinemia (33). Nevertheless, this reduction does not appear to be primary, occurring only as insulin levels increase above a portal insulin level of 700–1000 pmol/L (peripheral insulin level of >350 pmol/L). Thus at the early stages in the development of both obesity and hyperinsulinemia, there appears to be no defect in hepatic insulin uptake (34).

V IN VIVO METABOLIC AND ENDOCRINE DEFECTS ASSOCIATED WITH OBESITY AND DIABETES IN PRIMATES

Abdominal obesity in humans, as well as in monkeys, has been shown to be associated with diabetes mellitus. Monkeys with central or abdominal obesity could be classified as insulin-sensitive or insulin-resistant and showed a strong linear relationship between abdominal circumference and fasting plasma insulin and an inverse relationship with insulin resistance. Within the obese group there was, however, a diversity of degrees of insulin resistance (33).

In primates, spontaneous obesity has been shown to be associated with an increased frequency of dyslipidemia. Monkeys, like humans, show individual variability in susceptibility to diet-induced or spontaneous atherosclerosis (35), and these primates develop atherosclerotic lesions similar to humans (36). There was, however, no significant relationship in this study between abdominal circumference and various lipoprotein fractions. Hannah et al. (37) showed that obese hyperinsulinemic normoglycemic monkeys have beginning increases in VLDL triglycerides, small reductions in HDL cholesterol, and no change in LDL cholesterol. This dyslipidemia was significantly exacerbated in those monkeys with type 2 diabetes mellitus.

As previously described, many but not all obese monkeys go on to develop impaired glucose tolerance and then progress to overt type 2 diabetes mellitus (4,20). This longitudinal process was first described by Hamilton and Ciaccia (38) as a period of middle-aged obesity and normal glucose tolerance associated with hyperinsulinemia, followed by glucose intolerance and frank diabetes. The progressive process was further defined as a series of successive phases leading from normal lean young animals to older monkeys with or without obesity (39). Among the obese, some then progress through successive phases of increasing hyperinsulinemia and insulin resistance, progressive impairment of glucose tolerance, and finally overt diabetes (39). Glucose tolerance, one measure of this progressive process, has been calculated using a number of different formulas, the optimal of which is defined by the slope of the time points 5 and 20 min of an IV glucose tolerance test using a glucose load of 0.25 g/kg body weight. This time period was determined to be optimally applicable to monkeys across the entire range of tolerance from young normal to severe diabetic (12). Kemnitz et al. (5,14) showed that during pregnancy, a deterioration of glucose tolerance and an increase in fasting plasma insulin levels occur in the rhesus monkeys in the highest preconception tertile of adiposity. Wagner et al. (40) also showed a similar effect in cynomolgus monkeys.

VI GENETICS OF OBESITY IN PRIMATES

A Gene-Environment Interactions

Nonhuman primates provide excellent models for examining gene-environment interactions and for seeking the mechanisms underlying the development of aging-associated non-dietary-induced obesity, and possible mechanisms for its mitigation (41). Both the induction and the remission of obesity require cellular events involving overall energy balance (42). As in humans, several studies have documented a familial association in the development of obesity. A mother and daughter pair was identified in the 1977 survey of *Macaca nemestrina* mentioned above (9), and Schwartz et al. (13,43,44) noted several primary familial relationships among the obese animals of the Cayo Santiago colony. Environmental factors, principally ready access to food, also influence the incidence of obesity, which has been reported to range from 7% among the free-ranging Cayo Santiago troops ranging up to age 16, to 50% or more in individually housed animals in an age range up to 40 years.

Further support for a genetic basis of nonhuman primate obesity comes by inference from studies of groups of *Macaca mulatta* held under identical and constant environmental and dietary conditions, in which some animals have become significantly obese, while others have remained lean throughout their lives (44a).

B Candidate Genes for Obesity

No single-gene induced cases of obesity have been reported in nonhuman primates. Examination of the genetics of obesity in nonhuman primates has, to date, focused on a wide range of candidate genes, some specific to adipose tissue, and others potentially involved in insulin action and insulin sensitivity. Several candidate genes have, however, recently received special attention for their possible roles in obesity. Both human and mouse sequence data have assisted in the characterization of the molecular features of nonhuman primate obesity, and physiologic and molecular data from monkeys have assisted in the evaluation of the relevance of these genes and their products to human obesity. Although many candidate genes have been considered, we will deal specifically here with leptin and the *ob* gene, adiponectin, the β-3 receptor, the peroxisome proliferator-activated receptors, insulin and its insulin receptor, and the newest adipose specific protein, galectin-12.

Adipose tissue is now known to be the largest of the endocrine organs, secreting many different products into the circulation, including, for example, leptin, adiponectin, interleukin-6, TNFα, angiotensinogen, plasminogen activator-inhibitor 1(PAI-1), adipsin (complement factor D), sex steroids, and glucocorticoids. In addition, some adipocyte products apparently act in a paracrine manner. Prior to 1994, several such products were known, but despite efforts to do so, they were not successfully connected to the pathophysiology of obesity or to causal mechanisms (45). Recent reviews have summarized the expanding knowledge of adipose tissue as an endocrine organ and its role in the regulation of energy balance and obesity (42,46).

C Leptin, the Circulating Protein, the OB Gene, and the OB Receptor

Evidence for the existence of one or more circulating factors emanating from adipose tissue and playing a role in regulating body weight came first from the parabiosis experiments of Coleman and colleagues more than 30 years ago (47,48). Mice with genetic forms of diabetes (47) and with genetic forms of obesity (48) were parabiosed with normal mice, with the results suggesting that the obese mice lacked a substance secreted by normal mice and that the diabetic mice lacked the ability to respond to this factor. Much later the *ob* gene was cloned and characterized by Zhang et al. (49), and shown to be located on human chromosome 7q31.3. The product of this gene, leptin, is an adipocyte-derived 16-KDa circulating protein that clearly is involved in body weight regulation. Administration of this product, now called leptin, to obese *ob/ob* mice reversed many of the consequences of the *ob/ob* gene mutation, including reducing food intake and decreasing body weight (50). The *db* gene was subsequently shown by Tartaglia et al. to encode the ob receptor, OB-R, which is the receptor for leptin (51,52), and was found to be highly expressed in the central nervous system.

With the discovery of the gene responsible for obesity in the *ob/ob* mouse, and the identification of the circulating protein that it encodes (leptin) and its receptor, exploration of the possible role of leptin in the spontaneous obesity of monkeys was pursued. Interestingly, cross-circulation experiments in monkeys (53), carried out about the same time as the parabiosis studies in mice, did not lead to a prediction of any abnormal circulating factor or receptor regulating short-term feeding behavior in the monkey. The absence of such an abnormal gene or gene product in monkeys was subsequently proved to be true (see below). Cross-circulation studies in nonhuman primates accurately predicted the absence of a powerful circulating factor controlling short term energy regulation and short-term food intake (53). In these studies, various paradigms were tested, but the most informative one was the sustaining of pairs of monkeys for 4+ days in complete rapid cross-circulation, with one but not the other of the pair of monkeys allowed free access to food. It was anticipated that, in making the equivalent of one monkey "pregnant" with a whole second monkey's body, that the first monkey would regulate to "eat for two." This did not happen, despite the lack of any gastrointestinal limitations on increased chow consumption. On the contrary, the "feeding" monkey ate normally, ignoring the presence of the second monkey in his circulatory bed. (And by short-term tests, the nonfeeding monkey remained acutely hungry, even during the postmeal period of its partner.) This cross-circulation was engineered to be femoral artery to femoral vein, and thus, only the GI tract and the liver of the feeding monkey "saw" a different environment (the absorption of nutrients). The neural signals to the CNS from the gut of the feeding monkey undoubtedly differed from those of the parabiosed monkey, while the circulating signals were undoubtedly shared by both. We interpret this to mean that the humoral signals, whatever they may be, are relatively weak in controlling short-term feeding. Alternatively, those humoral or bloodborne signals must be received in the CNS in concert with the gut neural signals. Given contradictory information (fed state in the circulation and fasted state in the gut), the humoral signals were insufficient to produce satiety in the nonfeeding monkey. Further, in the feeding monkey, the signals (both humoral and neural) from the GI tract and liver were strong enough to overcome any such signals. The feeding animal lost a small amount of weight, but despite this, did not increase feeding to "eat for two."

The ob cDNA of the monkey was cloned from adipose tissue and shown to have at least 47 bp of 5′ noncoding region, 501 bp of coding region, and 219 bp of 3′ noncoding region (54). The ob mRNA is 0.8 kb long, which is shorter than that of rodents or humans due principally to a shorter 3′ noncoding region. The ob protein is 167 amino acids in length, as in humans and rodents, and has 91% amino acid similarity to the human ob protein. The *ob* mRNA was only expressed in adipose tissue (55).

Among a group of normal weight 7-year-old monkeys, the level of ob mRNA in adipose tissue was correlated to body weight and body fat. In a larger group of older animals, plasma leptin levels were correlated to obesity (% body fat), as shown in Figure 1;

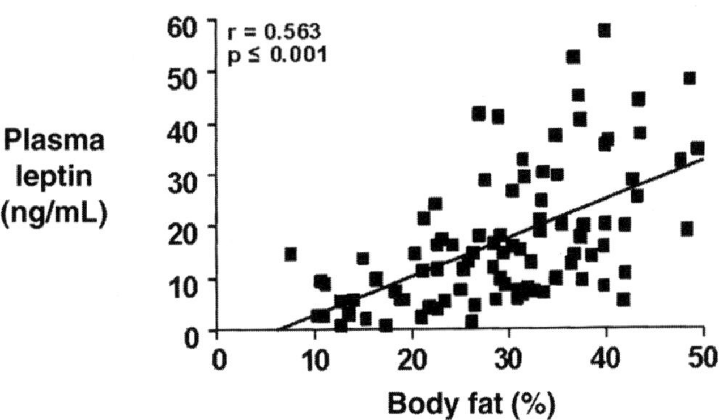

Figure 1 Relationship between fasting plasma leptin levels and percent body fat in rhesus monkeys varying in degree of adiposity. (From Ref. 56.)

however, this association was found to be reduced due to a subgroup of animals showing no relation between body weight and leptin. In 10 of 13 older monkeys examined during the development of increasing body weight and increasing adiposity, an increase in circulating leptin was positively associated with the increase in body weight (56). There was a tendency for ob mRNA to be increased in the hyperinsulinemic obese group of monkeys and reduced relative to normals in a group of diabetic animals that had previously lost body weight.

Figure 2 shows leptin levels across a longitudinal study period for two monkeys. The data shown in the top 4 panels represent a monkey that "tracked" body weight with leptin level changes very closely. On the bottom 4 panels, however, is another example, a monkey that, despite a similar degree of obesity, showed no elevation of leptin at all. These extremes are also seen across humans (57) and suggest that leptin is not solely an indicator of the amount of adipose tissue, but that other factors must also significantly alter its levels. Since the two animals shown in Figure 2 were maintained and studied under identical laboratory, diet, and environmental conditions, one must speculate on other genetic influences as contenders for inducing such differences.

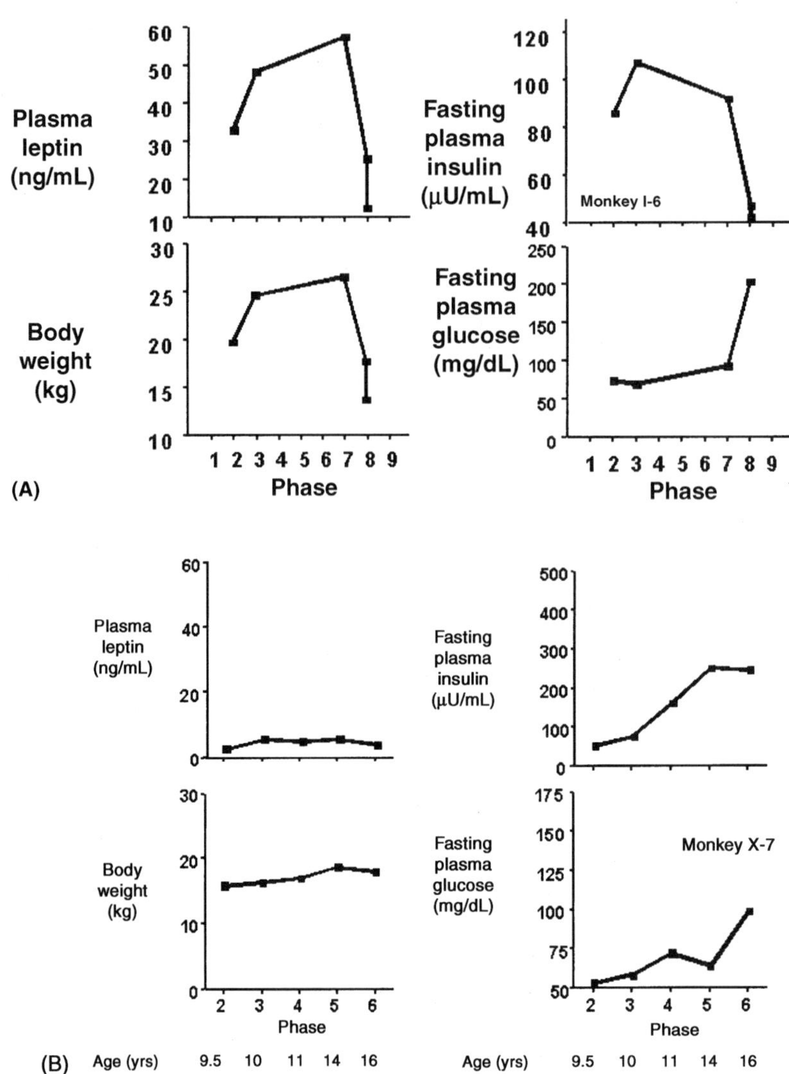

Figure 2 Longitudinal changes in plasma leptin levels compared to changes in plasma insulin, plasma glucose, and body weight in two monkeys. Panel A shows a monkey in which leptin and body weight changes are highly related, while panel B shows a monkey that is equally obese but shows no elevation in plasma leptin levels.

Indeed, we now know that leptin plays a role in a wide range of physiologic processes, and that while its absence (no leptin production or no functional receptor) has profound effects to increase body fatness in rodents and in humans, its presence in varying amounts in individuals with normal receptors appears to be without consequence. It has been suggested that leptin may play a role in puberty; however, a longitudinal analysis of male rhesus monkeys found no significant fluctuations in leptin levels prior to or during the puberty associated rise in testosterone secretion (58).

The ob or leptin receptor, primarily acting through its obRb form in the arcuate nucleus, seems to transduce leptin signals to two sets of neurons—one set with properties leading to feeding inducing (which are reduced by leptin), and another set with appetite suppressing properties (which are induced by leptin) (42). The monkey leptin receptor cDNA has been cloned and its sequence analyzed (59). Two alternatively spliced variants were identified, one with homology to the mouse obRb (long form) and the other a short form homologous to the mouse obRa. The long form in the rhesus monkey was found to be 96% homologous to the human long form (59). The receptor was expressed in liver and in kidney as in humans, suggesting that leptin may act not only through the CNS, but also through various peripheral tissues. The mRNA levels of the leptin receptor in the monkey were not related to obesity, hyperinsulinemia, or type 2 diabetes.

D Effects of the Administration of Leptin

The pharmacokinetics of human leptin administered to monkeys indicates a half-life of ~96 min after IV administration, and >8 hr after SC dosing, and was similar to that observed in humans (60). Attempts to alter feeding regulation and fatness via peripheral administration of leptin to monkeys (61,62) and to humans (63) had little if any effect on body weight. Although there was no acute effect of centrally administered leptin to lower food intake in monkeys, a day after the central leptin administration, food intake was reduced by 40–50% (61). The cause of this effect was not readily discerned.

The failure of peripheral leptin administration in monkeys and humans to alter food intake and body weight significantly may be due to the absence of a defect in the leptin molecule of these subjects. Clearly in children with congenital leptin deficiency, leptin treatment can reduce body weight and adiposity and improve reproductive hormone activity (64). Leptin administration to monkeys had no effect on the fasting-induced acute changes in growth hormone, luteinizing hormone, or cortisol secretion, although the fasting-induced fall in leptin was prevented (65). Leptin also did not have effects to acutely regulate either basal or ACTH-stimulated adrenal cortisol secretion (66). During food restriction, leptin levels (67) and reproductive hormones (68) are acutely suppressed. Replacement of leptin, however, had no effect on the other hormones; therefore, leptin does not mediate the effect of food deprivation on reproductive hormones (68).

What, if any, physiological signal is produced by the relatively high leptin levels frequently seen in obese humans and in obese monkeys is unknown. Further, while the concept of "leptin resistance" has been proposed, there is, to date, no evidence to support such a phenomenon other than its inference from the absence of apparent consequences of high leptin. Thus, the original view of leptin as the "adipostat," sensing the amount of adipose tissue in the body and signaling that information to the brain, thus acting as a mediator of food intake and body weight, does not appear to be the case.

We conclude that the leptin pathway may not serve as a simple "servomechanism/feedback loop" for regulating obesity or food intake, and should be considered not for a primary role in obesity for most humans, but as a far more complex hormone interacting with many systems, as yet not fully understood.

E Adiponectin (Acrp3, AdipoQ, apM1, GBP 28)

In searching an adipose specific cDNA library for novel genes expressed abundantly in fat tissue, Maeda et al. (69) identified an adipose specific collagenlike factor that was termed apM1 for AdiPoseMost abundant gene transcript 1. The protein expressed by this gene was separately identified in plasma by Nakano et al. (70) as GBP28, a novel gelatin-binding protein of 244 amino acids with a secretory signal sequence at the amino terminal. The gene was located on chromosome 3q27 and consists of three exons and two introns. Two polymorphisms have been identified in humans, but neither was associated with obesity (71). This protein, specifically secreted by adipose tissue, was subsequently named adiponectin, and was initially thought to function in lipid metabolism and fat storage. Unlike leptin, adiponectin is lower in obesity. In cultured cell lines, adiponectin inhibits the phagocytic activity of macrophages and the production of TNFα, thus raising the possibility that adiponectin plays a role in ending inflammatory responses (72).

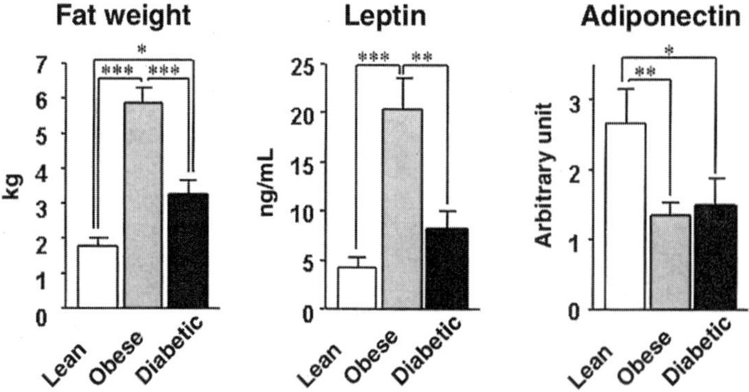

Figure 3 Comparison of fat weight, plasma leptin levels, and plasma adiponectin levels in three groups of monkeys—lean, obese with insulin resistance, and obese with type 2 diabetes. $*P<.05$, $**P<.01$, $***P<.001$. (From Ref. 74.)

Adiponectin also suppressed macrophage to foam cell transformation (73).

Monkey adiponectin was cloned and sequenced and shown to be ~ 96% homologous to human adiponectin and specifically expressed in adipose tissue, as it is in humans (69,74). Body fat weight was determined by the tritiated water method for three groups of monkeys—lean, obese with insulin resistance, and overt type 2 diabetes. Fat weight was then compared to plasma leptin levels and plasma adiponectin levels for the three groups, as shown in Figure 3. We also sought to determine the longitudinal changes in plasma adiponectin levels during the progression from normal to insulin resistant/obese to overtly diabetic in nonhuman primates with a high predisposition to type 2 diabetes and dyslipidemia. Plasma adiponectin levels declined as insulin sensitivity declined, and then remained at low levels as insulin resistant animals progressed to overt diabetes (74), as shown in Figure 4. The glucose uptake rate during a euglycemic hyperinsulinemic clamp was highly correlated to plasma adiponectin levels ($r=.66$, $P<.001$). There was no clear association between the plasma adiponectin levels and the mRNA expression in adipose tissue, nor were these related to total body fat mass.

Low levels of adiponectin have been associated in humans with cardiovascular disease (75) and with diabetes (76) and insulin resistance (77). Adiponectin has been administered to rodents with promising results; however, there are not yet reports of its administration to nonhuman primates. It is hypothesized that changes in metabolism induced by this hormone would

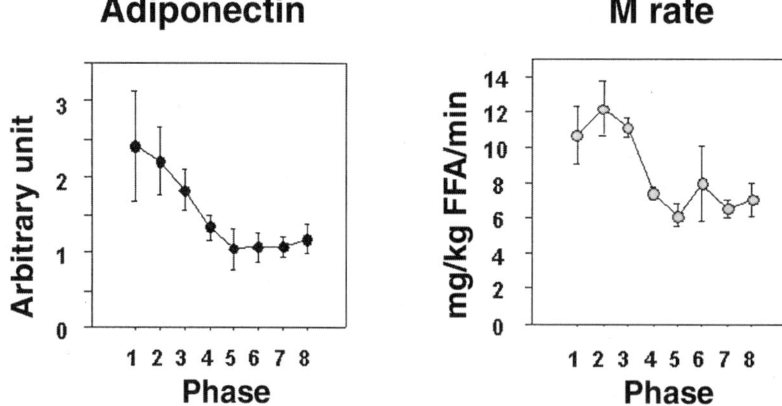

Figure 4 Longitudinal changes in plasma adiponectin levels (left panel) and insulin sensitivity as measured by a euglycemic hyperinsulinemic clamp (M rate, glucose uptake rate) as monkeys progress from normal/lean (phase 1) to obese with increasing insulin resistance (phases 3–6), to impaired glucose tolerance (phase 7), to overt type 2 diabetes mellitus (phase 8).

reduce markers of the metabolic syndrome and potentially mitigate the risk of cardiovascular disease and diabetes.

VII ENERGY EXPENDITURE AND THE ADRENERGIC RECEPTORS IN PRIMATES

A The β-3 Adrenergic Receptor and Agonists

On the energy expenditure side, attempts have been made to increase energy output selectively in the adipose tissue by activation of the β-3 adrenergic receptor. The β-3 adrenergic receptor, which is specifically expressed in adipose tissue, has been sequenced in the rhesus monkey (78). It shows 95% amino acid identity with the human β-3 receptor, differing between the two species in 22 of 408 amino acids. The rhesus monkey receptor contains an arginine at position 64, an amino acid that has been found in greater frequency in several groups of humans with a high propensity to obesity. Because of the similarity of the monkey to the human β-3 receptor, nonhuman primates have been used to examine the potential of β-3-specific agonists to alter the metabolism of adipose tissue, with the goal of producing adipose tissue specific weight loss in humans (79). Early agents, such as BRL-37344, CL-316243, ICI-D7114, and SR58611A, were found to be lipolytic in rat and dog adipocytes, but proved to be only weakly lipolytic or not at all active in baboon, macaque, and human cells. L757,793 and GR5261X are human selective β-3-specific agonists that stimulate lipolysis and show other metabolic effects. In nonhuman primates, chronic dosing produced no change in food intake and no decline in body weight, despite evidence of lowering of nonesterified fatty acids, triglycerides, and plasma insulin levels (79). While the theory remains seductive, as yet, there is no β-3-specific agonist that has been reported to have strong clinical potential for use in humans. Further, it is recognized that with weight loss itself, energy expenditure may be disproportionately reduced, thus potentially limiting further weight loss.

B Other Means of Sympathetic Activation

Other methods to increase energy expenditure are based on the hypothesis that a contributing factor in obesity is low sympathetic nervous system activity (SNS). One study has attempted to promote weight loss in obese monkeys using this approach (17). The agents used were ephedrine (6 mg) and caffeine (50 mg) three times per day. Food intake was reduced and energy expenditure increased with the net effect of a reduction in body weight of ~7% over 8 weeks in the obese monkeys. These effects too may be mediated via the β-adrenergic receptors. Weight was regained within 5 weeks of the end of the study.

VIII PEROXISOME PROLIFERATOR-ACTIVATED NUCLEAR RECEPTORS AND THEIR AGONISTS

A family of nuclear receptors termed the peroxisome proliferator-activated receptors has been identified, initially on the basis of the identification of pharmacological ligands. They are of three subtypes, PPARα, PPARγ, and PPARδ, and they are the products of different genes on different chromosomes. They were first cloned as "orphan" receptors, but the past 10 years has shown a proliferation of papers on the PPARs, and with those, a growing understanding of their diverse roles, particularly in the areas of insulin sensitizing and amelioration of dyslipidemias. Concerning obesity, these PPARs have not been found to be causally involved; however, the association of obesity with insulin insensitivity and dyslipidemia has made the agonists of these receptors particularly of interest for addressing the pathophysiology associated with obesity. Nonhuman primates have been used effectively in the examination of ligands for each of the three subtypes, and have been shown to be predictive of the effects in humans (80).

Species specificity has proved to be important, since many of the PPAR agonists act at the human and nonhuman primate receptors, but not at the rodent receptors (or have different effects at the rodent receptor). Thus, human cell lines have been used to predict activity in primates.

A PPARα Receptor and Agonists

The PPARα receptor gene has been mapped to chromosome 22q12-q13.1, and its tissue distribution shows increased expression in metabolically active tissues such as heart, liver, kidney, and muscle. No single high-affinity natural ligand for the PPARα receptor has been found, but this receptor may sense the flux of free fatty acids in the tissues where it is expressed. Among the known activators of this receptor are the fibrates. Although compounds that activate these receptors in rodents induce peroxisome proliferation and hepatomegaly in man following years of extensive use of the fibrates, PPARα ligands are not believed to have these effects. Thus, there appear to be functional and physiological differences that are species specific. In humans and nonhuman primates, the PPARα ligands generally function in lipid and fatty acid homeostasis. In addition to pharmaceutical agents, these receptors are probably activated by fatty acids and their metabolites. Monkeys share with humans 97% cDNA identity, and 99% identity with the putative protein of the PPARα receptor (81).

The fibrates were developed before the receptor was known, based on their lipid-lowering properties, and include such agents as fenofibrate, clofibrate, and bezafibrate. Fenofibrate, for example, is a dual activator of both PPARα and PPARγ, but has 10-fold higher selectivity for PPARα, while bezafibrate acts at all three receptor types. Fenofibrate has been shown to lower triglycerides (50%), to lower LDL cholesterol (27%), and to increase HDL cholesterol (35%). Apoproteins B-100 and CIII were also lowered (70% and 29%, respectively). Elevated plasma insulin levels were reduced by 40% in monkeys, supporting a role as an insulin sensitizer (81). Thus, this PPARα agent improved features of the metabolic syndrome including reducing the insulin resistance of obesity, but did not produce weight loss.

We have termed another PPARα activator, BM 17.0744, a calorie restriction mimetic agent as, in obese insulin-resistant monkeys, it appears to exert many of the positive features associated with-long-term calorie restriction (see below). This agent is not in the fibrate class [it is 2,2-dichlorophenyl dodecanoic acid, and its general features have been described (82)]; however, it seems to carry significant PPARα activity, acting as both an antidyslipidemic and antidiabetic agent. In overweight insulin-resistant male rhesus monkeys, body weight was significantly reduced in a dose-related manner across six of six subjects, an effect not observed with other PPARα agents. Hyperinsulinemia declined, although it was not normalized, and insulin sensitivity was greatly improved. Triglycerides were substantially reduced, particularly the VLDL triglycerides. While total cholesterol and LDL cholesterol were not significantly affected, HDL cholesterol was nearly doubled, suggesting improvement in the lipid profile of these monkeys (83).

B PPARγ Receptor and Agonists

Since 1994, when a ligand class of insulin sensitizers called the thiazolidinediones were recognized to interact with the PPARγ receptor, and the three classes of PPARs clearly delineated, great attention has been given to finding better ligands for this receptor (84). The role of PPARγ has been particularly of interest in the field of obesity because this nuclear transcription regulator is essential to adipocyte differentiation. The PPARγ protein is well conserved across species, and its gene has been mapped to chromosome 3p25. There are two principal isoforms, PPARγ1 and PPARγ2. This receptor, and particularly its PPARγ2 isoform, is found primarily in adipose tissue, but also is expressed in the colon and in macrophages. The monkey PPARγ2 protein showed 99% identity with the human protein. PPARγ2 is a critical transcription factor in adipose cell differentiation. This adipogenesis appears to require the coordinated expression of other transcription factors including C/EBP and ADD-1/SREBP-1. ADD-1/SREBP-1 are known to control several enzymes of fatty acid metabolism (85). PPARγ1 mRNA was shown to be most abundant in adipose tissue, but it is expressed in various other tissues, while PPARγ2 is primarily in adipose tissue. The mRNA levels of C/EBPα, LPL, and GLUT4 were highly correlated to that of total PPARγ mRNA and these appear to be coordinately regulated (86). (Note that Total was not related to the amount of adipose tissue.) The ratio of the expression of the two isoforms apparently changes in obesity, with the ratio of PPARγ2 to total PPARγ showing a high correlation to degree of obesity both in humans and in monkeys (86,87).

Several polymorphisms have been identified in the PPARγ gene of humans (88), with much attention focused upon the Pro12Ala missense mutation. This mutation may in fact convey some diabetes protective feature, as at least in some human groups insulin sensitivity is improved (89).

The ligands for the PPARγ receptor include fatty acids, especially those of the eicosinoids such as prostaglandin J2, and the glitazones or thiazolidinediones. PPARγ plays an important role in adipogenesis, and, in fact, without PPARγ, no fat cells are made. Separately, and perhaps at another developmental stage, PPARγ agonists show antidiabetic and insulin-sensitizing properties that do not appear to be directly related to the adipogenic properties, probably by influencing the expression of a different cohort of genes.

Several thiazolidinediones have been reported to be active in nonhuman primates. Pioglitazone administration to rhesus monkeys resulted in a reduction in plasma insulin levels of 64% at a dose of 3.0 mg/kg/d. Triglycerides in this study were lowered by 44% (90). Another thiazolidinedione, R-102380, lowered glucose in those monkeys with moderate increases in plasma glucose, but did not affect glucose in those with initially normal glycemia. Similarly, those with the greatest elevations of plasma triglycerides showed the greatest triglyceride-lowering effects. This agent showed evidence of direct effects on insulin sensitizing of skeletal muscle, even though at the whole-body level, the insulin sensitivity as measured by a euglycemic hyperinsulinemic clamp was not significantly altered (91).

Rosiglitazone (BRL49653) has also been used in nonhuman primates, and is in clinical use in humans as an insulin sensitizer. In monkeys, this PPARγ agonist significantly reduced plasma insulin levels as well as plasma triglycerides, and increased *in vivo* insulin action on skeletal muscle. Rosiglitazone induced an increase in the insulin-induced activation of glycogen synthase, without change in glycogen content (92).

Another PPARγ agonist, GI262570, has been shown to be highly potent in nonhuman primates and in humans. In monkeys, this agent produced a 63% reduction in plasma insulin levels and a 54% reduction in plasma triglycerides, while raising HDL cholesterol by 23% (93).

C PPARδ

The PPARδ receptor is ubiquitously expressed, and until recently was of unknown function, there being no known ligand for it until the presentation of a highly specific δ agonist in monkeys (80). Interestingly, despite its wide tissue distribution, it has shown highly specific lipid regulating properties.

PPARδ has been mapped to chromosome 6p21.1-p21.2 and is widely expressed in all tissues that are involved in lipid metabolism (94). The eicosinoid PGA1 and PGD2 have been found to activate PPARδ.

New agonists selective for the PPARδ receptor subtype are under study in nonhuman primates to examine the potential for development for human applications (80). GW501516 is such an agent, and has been shown in human cell lines to increase the expression of the reverse cholesterol transporter ATP-binding cassette, and to induce apolipoprotein A1-specific cholesterol efflux. Although inactive in rodent models, this agent caused a dose-dependent rise in HDL cholesterol, lowered small dense LDL cholesterol, lowered fasting VLDL triglycerides, and reduced fasting plasma insulin levels (80). These results suggest a potential for addressing the Metabolic Syndrome, and potentially reducing the risk of cardiovascular disease with such a PPARδ receptor subtype agonist.

IX INSULIN AND THE INSULIN RECEPTOR

Defects in the insulin molecule, the insulin receptor, and/or its variants have long been considered possible candidates for the underlying cause of insulin resistance and obesity. The insulin molecule of the monkey is identical in structure to that of human, and the proinsulin differs in only one amino acid (95). The monkey insulin receptor has been cloned and sequenced and found to have 99% amino acid identity to that of human (96). The two identified nonconservative amino acid changes have been examined by site-directed mutagenesis of the human insulin receptor, and found to have no effect on insulin receptor affinity or autophosphorylation, thus indicating that these are not responsible for the heightened insulin resistance of monkeys relative to humans (97).

Since obesity has not been shown to be associated with any defect in the insulin receptor structure, nor with a defective insulin molecule in most humans or monkeys (although there are a few well-documented cases of each of these defects in extreme cases of insulin resistance in humans), the possibility of a defect in expression of the major insulin receptor variants was considered. Differential expression of the two primary naturally occurring variants of the insulin receptor has been proposed to be involved in insulin resistance. Huang et al. (96) studied the relative expression of the type A insulin receptor isoform lacking exon 11 and of the type B isoform containing exon 11 in muscle of monkeys. Increased expression of the type A (higher-affinity) isoform in obese hyperinsulinemic monkeys was observed compared to either normal or diabetic animals, indicating that alterations in the insulin receptor mRNA splicing may be involved in the mechanisms of insulin resistance.

X GALECTIN-12

Another new gene that has been recently cloned and sequenced is galectin-12, a member of the galectin family of beta-galactoside-binding lectins. The galectins are involved in the regulation of a variety of processes, including cell adhesion, cell migration, cell growth (98), and apoptosis (99,100). While many galectins are widely expressed, galectin-12 is specifically expressed in adipose tissue. The cDNA coded for a 336–amino acid protein.

Galectin-12 mRNA levels were examined in monkey subcutaneous and omental adipose tissue (100). There were no differences between the mRNA levels of normal, obese, or type 2 diabetic monkeys, nor were there differences between subcutaneous and omental adipose tissue. Galectin-12 expression levels were increased by treatment with troglitazone, an insulin sensitizer. This treatment in rats was paralleled by an increase in the number of apoptotic cells. Another treatment that increases insulin sensitivity in both rodents and monkeys is sustained calorie restriction. Comparison of long-time calorie-restricted monkeys to ad libitum–fed animals showed a significant increase in the number of apoptotic cells, suggesting that galectin-12 may be involved in regulating adipose tissue growth, as shown in Figure 5.

XI OTHER CANDIDATE GENES

Other specific candidate genes, including adipose-specific genes (101), are being identified and studied in nonhuman primates (102), and their ongoing study in spontaneously obese primates should offer insights into their roles in obesity.

In addition, the development of new antiobesity compounds directed toward new target genes or their receptors suggests further possibilities for the mitigation of obesity. The GLP-1 receptor is one such target, with at least two new long-acting agents having been examined in monkeys (103,104). We had previously shown the ability of GLP-1 to raise insulin levels; however, GLP-1 itself is too short-acting to be considered an attractive therapeutic agent (79).

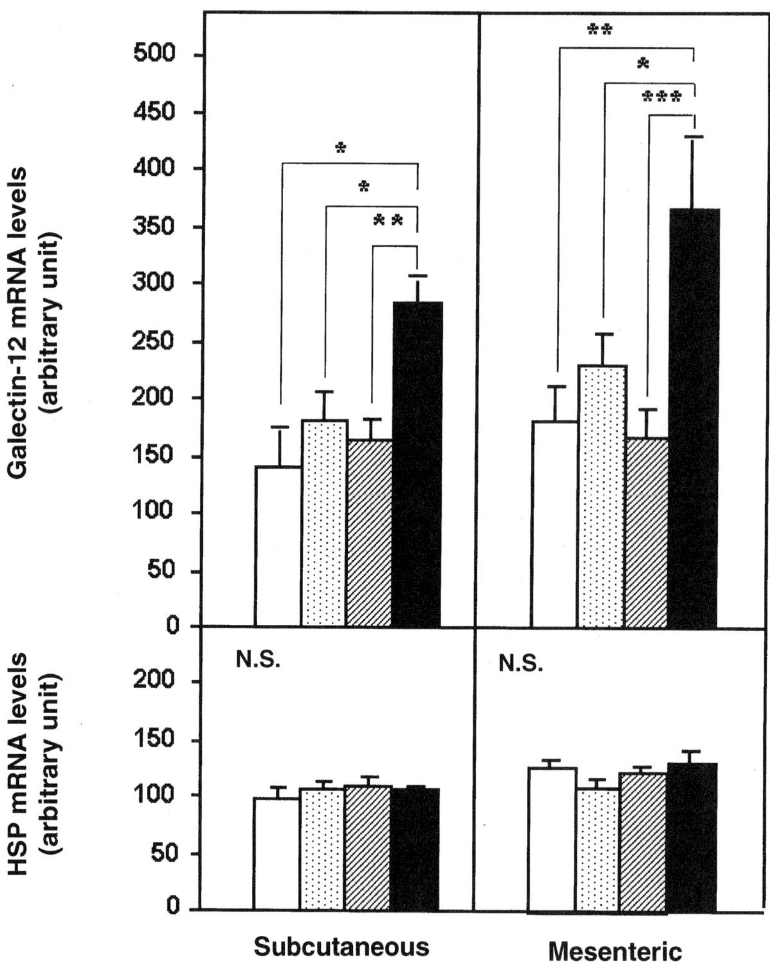

Figure 5 Expression of Galectin-12 in the subcutaneous and omental adipose tissue of four groups of rhesus monkeys: lean, obese, type 2 diabetic, and long-time calorie restricted. (From Ref. 100.)

XII PREVENTION OF OBESITY IN NONHUMAN PRIMATES HAVING A HIGH PROPENSITY TO DEVELOP OBESITY

Obesity is well recognized to be closely associated with the development of type 2 (non-insulin-dependent) diabetes mellitus (NIDDM) in human and nonhuman primates. A long-term study, still ongoing, has attempted to prevent the development of adult-onset obesity in a group of monkeys through a calorie titration regimen in which calories have been adjusted weekly on an individual animal basis to prevent the development of obesity or weight gain. Thus, under this protocol, any gain of weight in fully adult monkeys was met with a reduction in allocated calories, and conversely, weight loss was the trigger for increasing the calories allowed to each adult animal.

Primary prevention of obesity in adult rhesus monkeys has been shown to powerfully and completely prevent the development of type 2 diabetes mellitus (105). At the least, the onset of overt diabetes has been indefinitely delayed. Chronic long-term restriction of calories to prevent the development of obesity appears to have major effects on several metabolic pathways of insulin action. The development of insulin resistance has been shown to be mitigated (105), and plasma insulin levels were reduced by calorie restriction (106). Basal glycogen synthase activity was greatly increased above the levels of normal lean young monkeys, and the normal effect of insulin to activate glycogen synthase was absent in the calorie-restricted monkeys (107). The change in glycogen synthase activity was inversely related to the change in glycogen phosphorylase activity (108). Nevertheless, despite prevention of the development of obesity, calorie restriction appeared to unmask some early defects potentially associated with the propensity to ultimately develop obesity.

REFERENCES

1. Hamilton CL, Brobeck JR. Control of food intake in normal and obese monkeys. Ann NY Acad Sci 1965; 131:583–592.
2. Hansen BC, Bodkin NL, Jen K-LC, Ortmeyer HK. Primate models of diabetes. In: Rifkin H, Colwell JA, Taylor SI, eds. Diabetes. Amsterdam: Elsevier Science, 1991:587–590.
3. Hansen BC. Animal models of the aging-associated metabolic syndrome of obesity. In: Bouchard C, Bray G, eds. Regulation of Body Weight: Biological and Behavioral Mechanisms. Chichester: John Wiley & Sons, 1996:45–60.
4. Hansen BC. Obesity and diabetes in monkeys. In: Bjorntorp P, Brodoff BN, eds. Obesity. New York: J.B. Lippincott, 1992:256–265.
5. Kemnitz JW, Goy RW, Flitsch TJ, Lohmiller JJ, Robinson JA. Obesity in male and female rhesus monkeys: fat distribution, glucoregulation, and serum androgen levels. J Clin Endocrinol Metab 1989; 69: 287–293.
6. Hamilton CL, Kuo PT, Feng L. The effects of high carbohydrate diets on hyperinsulinemic monkeys (*Macaca mulatta*). J Med Primatol 1974; 3:276–284.
7. Hansen BC. Induction of obesity in nonhuman primate models of human obesity. In: Hayes KC, ed. Primates in Nutritional Research. New York: Academic Press, 1979:291–314.
8. Jen K-LC, Hansen BC. Feeding behavior during experimentally induced obesity in monkeys. Physiol Behav 1984; 33:863–869.
9. Walike BC, Goodner CJ, Koerker DJ. Assessment of obesity in pigtailed monkeys (*Macaca nemestrina*). J Med Primatol 1977; 6:151–162.
10. Wilson ME, Gordon TP, Blank MS, Collins DC. Timing of sexual maturity in female rhesus monkeys (*Macaca mulatta*) housed outdoors. J Reprod Fertil 1984; 70:625–633.
11. Wolfe L. Age and sexual behavior of Japanese macaques (*Macaca fuscata*). Arch Sex Behav 1978; 7:55–68.
12. Howard CF, Kessler MJ, Schwartz S. Carbohydrate impairment and insulin secretory abnormalities among *Macaca mulatta* from Cayo Santiago. J Med Primatol 1986; 11:147–146.
13. Schwartz SM, Kemnitz JW. Age- and gender-related changes in body size, adiposity, and endocrine and metabolic parameters in free-ranging rhesus macaques. Am J Phys Anthropol 1992; 89:109–121.
14. Kemnitz JW, Sladky KK, Flitsch TJ, Pomerantz SM, Goy RW. Androgenic influences on body size and composition of adult rhesus monkeys. Am J Physiol 1988; 255:E857–864.
15. DeLany JP, Hansen BC, Bodkin NL, Hannah J, Bray GA. Long-term calorie restriction reduces energy expenditure in aging monkeys. J Gerontol A Biol Sci Med Sci 1999; 54:B5–B11.
16. Kemnitz J, Francken G. Characteristics of spontaneous obesity in male rhesus monkeys. Physiol Behav 1986; 38:477–483.
17. Ramsey JJ, Colman RJ, Swick AG, Kemnitz J. Energy expenditure, body composition, and glucose metabolism in lean and obese rhesus monkeys treated with ephedrine and caffeine. Am J Clin Nutr 1998; 68:42–51.
18. Jen K-LC, Bodkin N, Metzger BL, Hansen BC.

Nutrient composition: effects on appetite in monkeys with oral factors held constant. Physiol Behav 1985; 34:655–659.
19. Gray DS, Sharma RC, Chin HP, Jiao Q, Kramsch DM. Body fat and fat distribution by anthropometry and the response to high-fat cholesterol-containing diet in monkeys. Exp Mol Pathol 1993; 58:53–60.
20. Hansen BC. Primate animal models of non-insulin dependent diabetes mellitus. In: LeRoith D, Taylor SI, Olesfky JM, eds. Diabetes Mellitus: A Fundamental and Clinical Text. Philadelphia: Lippincott-Raven, 1996:595–603.
21. Jen K-LC, Hansen BC, Metzger BL. Adiposity, anthropometric measures, and plasma insulin levels of rhesus monkeys. Int J Obes 1985; 9:213–224.
22. Laber-Laird K, Shively CA, Karstaedt N, Bullock BC. Assessment of abdominal fat deposition in female cynomolgus monkeys. Int J Obes 1991; 15:213–220.
23. Sharma RC, Kramsch DM, Lee PL, Colletti P, Jiao Q. Quantitation and localization of regional body fat distribution-a comparison between magnetic resonance imaging and somatometry. Obes Res 1996; 4:167–178.
24. Narita H, Ohkubo F, Yoshida T, Cho F, Yoshikawa Y. Measuring bone mineral content and soft tissue mass in living the cynomolgus monkey. Jikken Dobutsu (Exp Anim) 1994; 43:261–265.
25. Metzger BL, Hansen BC, Speegle LM, Jen K-LC. Characterization of glucose intolerance in obese monkeys. J Obes Weight Regul 1985; 4:153–167.
26. Wagner JD, Cline JM, Shadoan MK, Bullock BC, Rankin SE, Cefalu WT. Naturally occurring and experimental diabetes in cynomolgus monkeys: a comparison of carbohydrate and lipid metabolism and islet pathology. Toxicol Pathol 2001; 29:142–148.
27. O'Brien TD, Wagner JD, Litwak KN, Carlson CS, Cefalu WT, Jordan K, Johnson KH, Butler PC. Islet amyloid and islet amyloid polypeptide in cynomolgus macaques (*Macaca fascicularis*): an animal model of human non-insulin-dependent diabetes mellitus. Vet Pathol 1996; 33:479–485.
28. Wagner JD, Carlson CS, O'Brien TD, Anthony MS, Bullock BC, Cefalu WT. Diabetes mellitus and islet amyloidosis in cynomolgus monkeys. Lab Anim Sci 1996; 46:36–41.
29. Cefalu WT, Wagner JD, Bell-Farrow AD. Role of glycated proteins in detecting and monitoring diabetes in cynomolgus monkeys. Am Assoc Lab Anim Sci 1993; 43:73–77.
30. Hansen BC, Bodkin NL. β-Cell hyperresponsiveness: earliest event in development of diabetes in monkeys. Am J Physiol 1990; 259:R612–R617.
31. deKoning EJP, Bodkin NL, Hansen BC, Clark A. Diabetes mellitus in *Macaca mulatta* monkeys is characterized by islet amyloidosis and reduction in beta-cell population. Diabetologia 1993; 36:378–384.
32. Bodkin NL, Metzger BL, Hansen BC. Hepatic glucose production and insulin sensitivity preceding diabetes in monkeys. Am J Physiol 1989; 256:E676–E681.
33. Bodkin NL, Hannah JS, Ortmeyer HK, Hansen BC. Central obesity in rhesus monkeys: association with hyperinsulinemia, insulin resistance, and hypertriglyceridemia? Int J Obes 1993; 17:53–61.
34. Hansen BC, Bodkin NL. Primary prevention of diabetes mellitus by prevention of obesity in monkeys. Diabetes 1993; 42:1809–1814.
35. Kritchevsky D. Diet in heart disease and cancer. Adv Exp Med Biol 1995; 369:201–209.
36. Clarkson TB, Koritnik DR, Weingand KW. Nonhuman primate models of atherosclerosis: potential for the study of diabetes mellitus. Diabetes 1985; 31:51–59.
37. Hannah JS, Verdery RB, Bodkin NL, Hansen BC, Ngoc AL, Howard BV. Changes in lipoprotein concentrations during the development of noninsulin dependent diabetes mellitus in obese rhesus monkeys (*Macaca mulatta*). J Clin Endocrinol Metab 1991; 72:1067–1072.
38. Hamilton CL, Ciaccia P. The course of development of glucose intolerance in the monkey (*Macaca mulatta*). J Med Primatol 1978; 7:165–173.
39. Hansen BC, Bodkin NL. Heterogeneity of insulin responses: phases in the continuum leading to non-insulin-dependent diabetes mellitus. Diabetologia 1986; 29:713–719.
40. Wagner JD, Jayo MJ, Bullock BC, Washburn SA. Gestational diabetes mellitus in a cynomolgus monkey with group A streptococcal metritis and hemolytic uremic syndrome. J Med Primatol 1992; 21:371–374.
41. Bray GA, Tartaglia LA. Medicinal strategies in the treatment of obesity. Nature 2000; 404:672–677.
42. Spiegelman BM, Flier JS. Obesity and the regulation of energy balance. Cell 2001; 104:531–543.
43. Schwartz SM, Kemnitz JW, Howard CF. Obesity in free-ranging rhesus macaques. Int J Obes 1993; 17:1–10.
44. Schwartz SM. Characteristics of spontaneous obesity in the Cayo Santiago rhesus macaque: preliminary report. P R Health Sci J 1989; 8:103–106.
44a. Hansen BC, Ortmeyer HK. Obesity, diabetes, and aging: lessons from lifetime studies in monkeys. In: Guy-Grand B, ed. Progress in Obesity Research. London: John Libbey Eurotext, 1999:525–544.
45. White RT, Damm D, Hancock N, Rosen BS, Lowell BB, Usher P, Flier JS, Spiegelman BM. Human adipsin is identical to complement factor D and is expressed at high levels in adipose tissue. J Biol Chem 1992; 267:9210–9213.
46. Ahima RS, Flier JS. Adipose tissue as an endocrine organ. Trends Endocrinol Metab 2000; 11:327–332.

47. Coleman DL, Hummel KP. Effects of parabiosis of normal with genetically diabetic mice. Am J Physiol 1969; 217:1298–1304.
48. Coleman DL. Effects of parabiosis of obese with diabetes and normal mice. Diabetologia 1973; 9:294–298.
49. Zhang Y, Proenca R, Maffei M, Barone M, Leopold L, Friedman JM. Positional cloning of the mouse *obese* gene and its human homologue. Nature 1994; 372:425–432.
50. Pelleymounter MA, Cullen MJ, Baker MB, Hecht R, Winters D, Boone T, Collins F. Effects of the obese gene product on body weight regulation in *ob/ob* mice. Science 1995; 269:540–543.
51. Tartaglia LA, Dembski M, Weng X, Deng N, Culpepper J, Devos R, Richards GJ, Campfield LA, Clark FT, Deeds J. Identification and expression cloning of a leptin receptor, OB-R. Cell 1995; 83:1263–1271.
52. Chua SC Jr, Chung WK, Wu-Peng XS, Zhang Y, Liu SM, Tartaglia L, Leibel RL. Phenotypes of mouse diabetes and rat fatty due to mutations in the OB (leptin) receptor. Science 1996; 271:994–996.
53. Walike BC, Smith OA. Regulation of food intake during intermittent and continuous cross circulation in monkeys (*Macaca mulatta*). J Comp Physiol Psychol 1972; 80:372–381.
54. Hotta K, Gustafson TA, Ortmeyer HK, Bodkin NL, Nicolson MA, Hansen BC. Regulation of *obese (ob)* mRNA and plasma leptin levels in rhesus monkeys: effects of insulin, body weight and diabetes. J Biol Chem 1996; 271:25327–25331.
55. Hotta K, Gustafson TA, Ortmeyer HK, Bodkin NL, Hansen BC. Structure and expression of the monkey *obese (ob)* mRNA. FASEB J 1996; 10:A186.
56. Bodkin NL, Nicolson M, Ortmeyer HK, Hansen BC. Hyperleptinemia: relationship to adiposity and insulin resistance in the spontaneously obese rhesus monkey. Horm Metab Res 1996; 28:674–678.
57. Considine RV, Considine EL, Williams CJ, Nyce MR, Magosin SA, Bauer TL. Evidence against either a premature stop codon or the absence of obese gene mRNA in human obesity. J Clin Invest 1995; 95:2986–2988.
58. Mann DR, Akinbami MA, Gould KG, Castracane VD. A longitudinal study of leptin during development in the male rhesus monkey: the effect of body composition and season on circulating leptin levels. Biol Reprod 2000; 62:285–291.
59. Hotta K, Gustafson TA, Ortmeyer HK, Bodkin NL, Hansen BC. Monkey leptin receptor mRNA: sequence, tissue distribution, and mRNA expression in the adipose tissue of normal, hyperinsulinemic and type 2 diabetic rhesus monkeys. Obese Res 1998; 6:353–360.
60. Ahren B, Baldwin RM, Havel PJ. Pharmacokinetics of human leptin in mice and rhesus monkeys. Int J Obes Relat Metab Disord 2000; 24:1579–1585.
61. Tang-Christensen M, Havel PJ, Jacobs R, Larsen PJ, Cameron JL. Central administration of leptin inhibits food intake and activates the sympathetic nervous system in rhesus macaques. J Clin Endocrinol Metab 1999; 84:711–717.
62. Wagner JD, Jayo MJ, Cefalu WT, Hardy VA, Rankin SE, Toombs CF. Recombinant human leptin (rHu-Leptin) reduces body weight and body fat and improves insulin sensitivity in nonhuman primates. Obes Res 1996; 4:27S.
63. Heymsfield SB, Greenberg AS, Fujioka K, Dixon RM, Kushner R, Hunt T, Lubina JA, Patane J, Self B, Hunt P, McCamish M. Recombinant leptin for weight loss in obese and lean adults: a randomized, controlled, dose-escalation trial. JAMA 1999; 282:1568–1575.
64. Farooqi IS, Jebb SA, Langmack G, Lawrence E, Cheetham CH, Prentice AM, Hughes IA, McCamish MA, O'Rahilly S. Effects of recombinant leptin therapy in a child with congenital leptin deficiency. N Engl J Med 1999; 341:879–884.
65. Lado-Abeal J, Hickox JR, Cheung TL, Veldhuis JD, Hardy DM, Norman RL. Neuroendocrine consequences of fasting in adult male macaques: effects of recombinant rhesus macaque leptin infusion. Neuroendocrinology 2000; 71:196–208.
66. Lado-Abeal J, Mrotek JJ, Stocco DM, Norman RL. Effect of leptin on ACTH-stimulated secretion of cortisol in rhesus macaques and on human adrenal carcinoma cells. Eur J Endocrinol 1999; 141:534–538.
67. Colman RJ, Ramsey JJ, Roecker EB, Havighurst T, Hudson JC, Kemnitz JW. Body fat distribution with long-term dietary restriction in adult male rhesus macaques. J Gerontol A Biol Sci Med Sci 1999; 54:B283–B290.
68. Lado-Abeal J, Lukyanenko YO, Swamy S, Hermida RC, Hutson JC, Norman RL. Short-term leptin infusion does not affect circulating levels of LH, testosterone or cortisol in food-restricted pubertal male rhesus macaques. Clin Endocrinol (Oxf) 1999; 51:41–51.
69. Maeda K, Okubo K, Shimomura I, Funahashi T, Matsuzawa Y, Matsubara K. cDNA cloning and expression of a novel adipose specific collagen-like factor, apM1 (AdiPose Most abundant Gene transcript 1). Biochem Biophys Res Commun 1996; 221:286–289.
70. Nakano Y, Tobe T, Choi-Miura NH, Mazda T, Tomita M. Isolation and characterization of GBP28, a novel gelatin-binding protein purified from human plasma. J Biochem (Tokyo) 1996; 120:803–812.
71. Takahashi M, Arita Y, Yamagata K, Matsukawa Y, Okutomi K, Horie M, Shimomura I, Hotta K, Kuriyama H, Kihara S, Nakamura T, Yamashita S,

Funahashi T, Matsuzawa Y. Genomic structure and mutations in adipose-specific gene, adiponectin. Int J Obes Relat Metab Disord 2000; 24:861–868.

72. Yokota T, Oritani K, Takahashi I, Ishikawa J, Matsuyama A, Ouchi N, Kihara S, Funahashi T, Tenner AJ, Tomiyama Y, Matsuzawa Y. Adiponectin, a new member of the family of soluble defense collagens, negatively regulates the growth of myelomonocytic progenitors and the functions of macrophages. Blood 2000; 96:1723–1732.
73. Ouchi N, Kihara S, Arita Y, Nishida M, Matsuyama A, Okamoto Y, Ishigami M, Kuriyama H, Kishida K, Nishizawa H, Hotta K, Muraguchi M, Ohmoto Y, Yamashita S, Funahashi T, Matsuzawa Y. Adipocyte-derived plasma protein, adiponectin, suppresses lipid accumulation and class A scavenger receptor expression in human monocyte-derived macrophages. Circulation 2001; 103:1057–1063.
74. Hotta K, Funahashi T, Bodkin NL, Ortmeyer HK, Arita Y, Hansen BC, Matsuzawa Y. Circulating concentrations of the adipocyte protein adiponectin are decreased in parallel with reduced insulin sensitivity during the progression to type 2 diabetes in rhesus monkeys. Diabetes 2001; 50:1126–1133.
75. Zoccali C, Mallamaci F, Tripepi G, Benedetto FA, Cutrupi S, Parlongo S, Malatino LS, Bonanno G, Seminara G, Rapisarda F, Fatuzzo P, Buemi M, Nicocia G, Tanaka S, Ouchi N, Kihara S, Funahashi T, Matsuzawa Y. Adiponectin, metabolic risk factors, and cardiovascular events among patients with end-stage renal disease. J Am Soc Nephrol 2002; 13:134–141.
76. Hotta K, Funahashi T, Arita Y, Takahashi M, Matsuda M, Okamoto Y, Iwahashi H, Kuriyama H, Ouchi N, Maeda K, Nishida M, Kihara S, Sakai N, Nakajima T, Hasegawa K, Muraguchi M, Ohmoto Y, Nakamura T, Yamashita S, Hanafusa T, Matsuzawa Y. Plasma concentrations of a novel, adipose-specific protein, adiponectin, in type 2 diabetic patients. Arterioscler Thromb Vasc Biol 2000; 20:1595–1599.
77. Weyer C, Funahashi T, Tanaka S, Hotta K, Matsuzawa Y, Pratley RE, Tataranni PA. Hypoadiponectinemia in obesity and type 2 diabetes; close association with insulin resistance and hyperinsulinemia. J Clin Endocrinol Metab 2001; 86:1930–1935.
78. Walston J, Lowe A, Silver K, Yang Y, Bodkin NL, Hansen BC, Shuldiner AR. The β3-adrenergic receptor in the obesity and diabetes prone rhesus monkey is very similar to human and contains arginine at codon 64. Gene 1997; 188:207–213.
79. Hansen BC. Primates in the experimental pharmacology of obesity. In: Lockwood D, Heffner TG, eds. Handbook of Experimental Pharmacology: Obesity—Pathology and Therapy. Heidelberg: Springer-Verlag, 2000:416–489.
80. Oliver WR Jr, Shenk JL, Snaith MR, Russell CS, Plunket KD, Bodkin NL, Lewis MC, Winegar DA, Sznaidman ML, Lambert MH, Xu HE, Sternbach DD, Kliewer SA, Hansen BC, Willson TM. A selective peroxisome proliferator-activated receptor delta agonist promotes reverse cholesterol transport. Proc Natl Acad Sci USA 2001; 98: 5306–5311.
81. Winegar DA, Brown PJ, Wilkison WO, Lewis MC, Ott RJ, Tong WQ, Brown HR, Lehmann JM, Kliewer SA, Plunket KD, Way JM, Bodkin NL, Hansen BC. Effects of fenofibrate on lipid parameters in obese rhesus monkeys. J Lipid Res 2001; 42:1543–1551.
82. Pill J, Kuhnle HF. BM 17.0744: a structurally new antidiabetic compound with insulin-sensitizing and lipid-lowering activity. Metabolism 1999; 48:34–40.
83. Pill J, Nakayama M, Bodkin NL, Hansen BC. Effects of BM 17.0744 on lipid and carbohydrate metabolism in various animal models of insulin resistance. Perfusion 2001; 14:81.
84. Kliewer SA, Forman BM, Blumberg B, Ong ES, Borgmeyer U, Mangelsdorf DJ, Umesono K, Evans RM. Differential expression and activation of a family of murine peroxisome proliferator-activated receptors. Proc Natl Acad Sci USA 1994; 91:7355–7359.
85. Mandrup S, Lane MD. Regulating adipogenesis. J Biol Chem 1997; 272:5367–5370.
86. Hotta K, Gustafson TA, Yoshioka S, Ortmeyer HK, Bodkin NL, Hansen BC. Relationships of PPARγ and PPARγ2 mRNA levels to obesity, diabetes and hyperinsulinemia in rhesus monkeys. Int J Obes 1998; 22: 1000–1010.
87. Hotta K, Gustafson TA, Yoshioka S, Ortmeyer HK, Bodkin NL, Hansen BC. Age-related adipose tissue mRNA expression ADD1, PPARγ, lipoprotein lipase and GLUT4 glucose transporter in rhesus monkeys. J Gerontol Biol Sci 1999; 54A:B1–B8.
88. Yen CJ, Beamer BA, Negri C, Silver K, Brown KA, Yarnall DP, Burns DK, Roth J, Shuldiner AR. Molecular scanning of the human peroxisome proliferator activated receptor gamma (hPPAR gamma) gene in diabetic Caucasians: identification of a Pro12Ala PPAR gamma 2 missense mutation. Biochem Biophys Res Commun 1997; 241:270–274.
89. Ek J, Andersen G, Urhammer SA, Hansen L, Carstensen B, Borch-Johnsen K, Drivsholm T, Berglund L, Hansen T, Lithell H, Pedersen O. Studies of the Pro12Ala polymorphism of the peroxisome proliferator-activated receptor-gamma2 (PPAR-gamma2) gene in relation to insulin sensitivity among glucose tolerant caucasians. Diabetologia 2001; 44:1170–1176.
90. Kemnitz JW, Elson DF, Roecker EB, Baum ST, Bergman RN, Meglasson MD. Pioglitazone increases insulin sensitivity, reduces blood glucose, insulin, and lipid levels, and lowers blood pressure, in obese, insulin-resistant rhesus monkeys. Diabetes 1994; 43:204–211.
91. Ortmeyer HK, Bodkin NL, Haney J, Yoshioka S,

Horikoshi H, Hansen BC. A thiazolidinedione improves in vivo insulin action on skeletal muscle glycogen synthase in insulin-resistant monkeys. Int J Exp Diabetes Res 2000; 1:195–202.

92. Hansen BC, Bodkin NL, Shashkin PN, Smith SA, Ortmeyer HK. Rosiglitazone alters insulin secretion, glycogen metabolism and triglycerides in prediabetic monkeys. Diabetes Res 2000; 50:S391.
93. Hansen BC, Oliver WR. The PPARγ agonist, GI262570, improves the prediabetic features of the metabolic syndrome X in insulin resistance primates. Diabetologia 2000; 43:269.
94. Willson TM, Brown PJ, Sternbach DD, Henke BR. The PPARs: from orphan receptors to drug discovery. J Med Chem 2000; 43:527–550.
95. Naithani VK, Steffens GJ, Tager HS. Isolation and amino-acid sequence determination of monkey insulin and proinsulin. Hoppe-Seylers Z Physiol Chem 1984; 365:571–575.
96. Huang Z, Bodkin NL, Ortmeyer HK, Hansen BC, Shuldiner AR. Hyperinsulinemia is associated with altered insulin receptor mRNA splicing in muscle of the spontaneously obese diabetic rhesus monkey. J Clin Invest 1994; 94:1289–1296.
97. Fan Z, Kole H, Bernier M, Huang Z, Accilli D, et al. Molecular mechanism of insulin resistance in the spontaneously obese and diabetic rhesus monkey: site directed mutagenesis of the insulin receptor. Endocrinology 1995; 77:180.
98. Barondes SH, Castronovo V, Cooper DN, Cummings RD, Drickamer K, Feizi T, Gitt MA, Hirabayashi J, Hughes C, Kasai K. Galectins: a family of animal beta-galactoside-binding lectins. Cell 1994; 76:597–598.
99. Hadari YR, Arbel-Goren R, Levy Y, Amsterdam A, Alon R, Zakut R, Zick Y. Galectin-8 binding to integrins inhibits cell adhesion and induces apoptosis. J Cell Sci 2000; 113(pt 13):2385–2397.
100. Hotta K, Funahashi T, Matsukawa Y, Takahashi M, Nishizawa H, Kishida K, Matsuda M, Kuriyama H, Kihara S, Nakamura T, Tochino Y, Bodkin NL, Hansen BC, Matsuzawa Y. Galectin-12, an adipose-expressed galectin-like molecule possessing an activity to induce apoptosis. J Biol Chem 2001; 276:34089–34097.
101. Yang R, Braileanu G, Hansen BC, Shuldiner AR, Gong D-W. Analysis of 10,437 expressed sequence tags from human omental adipose tissue. Endocrinology 2002; 536:3.
102. Angeloni SV, Hansen B. Molecular features of insulin resistance, obesity, and type II diabetes in non human primates. In: Hansen BC, Shafrir E, eds. Insulin Resistance and Insulin Resistance Syndrome. London: Harwood Academic Publishing, 2002:89–123.
103. Young AA, Gedulin BR, Bhavsar S, Bodkin N, Jodka C, Hansen B, Denaro M. Glucose-lowering and insulin-sensitizing actions of exendin-4: studies in obese diabetic (*ob/ob*, *db/db*) mice, diabetic fatty Zucker rats and diabetic monkeys (*Macaca mulatta*). Diabetes 1999; 48:1026–1034.
104. Hansen BC, Izuka M, Bjenning C, Knudsen LB. Obese rhesus monkeys show reduced food intake and weight loss during treatment with NN2211, a long-acting GLP-1 derivative. Obes Res 2002; 10:104.
105. Bodkin NL, Ortmeyer HK, Hansen BC. Long-term dietary restriction in older-aged rhesus monkeys: effects on insulin resistance. J Gerontol Biol Sci 1995; 50:B142–B147.
106. Kemnitz JW, Roecker EB, Weindruch R, Elson DF, Baum ST, Bergman RT. Dietary restriction increases insulin sensitivity and lowers blood glucose in rhesus monkeys. Am J Physiol 1994; 266:E540–E547.
107. Ortmeyer HK, Bodkin NL, Hansen BC. Chronic caloric restriction alters glycogen metabolism in rhesus monkeys. Obes Res 1994; 2:549–555.
108. Ortmeyer HK, Bodkin NL, Hansen BC. In vivo insulin regulates glycogen synthase and glycogen phosphorylase reciprocally in liver of young lean rhesus monkeys. FASEBJ 1995; 9:A554.

13

Behavioral Neuroscience and Obesity

Sarah F. Leibowitz

The Rockefeller University, New York, New York, U.S.A.

Bartley G. Hoebel

Princeton University, Princeton, New Jersey, U.S.A.

I INTRODUCTION

An animal's brain monitors energy in the environment and within the body and then adjusts eating behavior, energy utilization, and fat stores to maintain a balance. This chapter will discuss how the brain performs this life-giving task. The brain integrates energy-related sensory information from the eyes, ears, nose, tongue, gastrointestinal tract, liver, pancreas, and blood. In many parts of the body and brain, there are specialized receptors to detect nutrient-rich molecules. The hypothalamus is one of the areas that use this information to adjust physiological functions for storing or utilizing energy at appropriate times. The hypothalamus also contributes to the control of food intake by interacting with mechanisms for voluntary behavior that are essential for obtaining food. This physiological and behavioral control involves connections to the pituitary for endocrine regulation and feedback actions of hormones impacting on the brain. It also involves connections to the hindbrain, which subserve essential feeding reflexes and gut responses. The whole system is integrated by circuits extending to forebrain systems for choosing, instigating and reinforcing food choices. These circuits allow the brain to adjust its physiology and behavior to meet the economic demands of the ecological niche in which the animal lives. This introductory section briefly summarizes the different hormones, neurochemicals and brain areas that are required to perform these functions. These are listed in Table 1, together with the abbreviations used in the sections below.

A Hormones

An important function of the hypothalamus is to synthesize neuropeptides, which control hormone secretion from the pituitary that, in turn, influences hormone synthesis in target organs. Hypothalamic neurosecretory cells produce peptides that are delivered to the portal blood vessels and transported to the anterior pituitary. These brain peptides include corticotropin-releasing hormone (CRH), luteinizing hormone-releasing hormone (LHRH), and thyrotropin-releasing hormone (TRH). They regulate the release of three pituitary hormones—adrenocorticotropic hormone (ACTH), luteinizing hormone, and thyroid-stimulating hormone (TSH). These pituitary hormones, then, travel in the bloodstream and impact on target glands to stimulate the production, respectively, of the adrenal steroid, corticosterone (CORT), the gonadal steroids, estradiol (E_2), progesterone (P), and the thyroid hormone, thyroxine. In addition, there are other

Table 1 Abbreviations of Hormones and Neurochemicals Reviewed in This Chapter

Hormones involved in eating and body weight regulation
- ACTH, adrenocorticotropic hormone
- CORT, corticosterone
- E_2, estradiol
- GH, growth hormone
- Glucose
- HPA, hypothalamo-pituitary-adrenal
- Insulin
- Leptin
- Lipids
- P, progesterone

Peptides that increase eating and body weight
- AGRP, agouti-related protein
- Amandamide
- Beacon
- DYN, dynorphin
- GAL, galanin
- GALP, galaninlike peptide
- Ghrelin
- GHRH, growth hormone–releasing hormone
- GHRP, growth hormone–releasing peptide
- GnRH, gonadotrophin-releasing hormone
- MCH, melanin-concentrating hormone
- NPY, nueropeptide Y
- Opioid peptides
- ORX, orexin
- PRL, prolactin
- PYY, peptide YY
- VGF (nonacronym)

Peptides that reduce eating and body weight
- α-MSH, alpha-melanocyte-stimulating hormone
- aFGF, acidic fibroblast growth factor
- Amylin
- apo A-1V, apolipoprotein A-IV
- apo D, apolipoprotein D
- AVP, arginine vasopressin
- BBS, bombesin
- Calcitonin
- CART, cocaine- and amphetamine-regulated transcript
- CCK, cholecystokinin
- CGRP, calcitonin gene-related peptide
- CNTF, ciliary neurotropic factor
- CRH, corticotropin-releasing hormone
- Cyclo(his-Pro)
- Cytokines
- ENT, enterostatin
- GLP-1, glucagon-like peptide 1
- Glucagon
- IL, interleukin
- Melanocortins
- MSH, melanocyte-stimulating hormone
- NMU, neuromedin U
- NT, neurotensin
- OT, oxytocin
- POMC, pro-opiomelanocortin
- PrRP, prolactin-releasing peptide
- TNFα, tumor necrosis factor-alpha
- TRH, thyrotropin-releasing hormone

Biogenic amines in the control of eating behavior and metabolism
- 5HIAA, 5-hydroxy-3-indole acetic acid
- 5HT, serotonin
- AMPH, amphetamine
- DA, dopamine
- Histamine
- NE, norepinephrine

Acetylcholine and amino acids in feeding-related circuits
- ACh, acetylcholine
- GABA, gamma-aminobutyric acid
- GLUT, glutamate

Receptors
- $\alpha_{1,2}$ -noradrenergic receptors
- $\beta_{1,2}$ -adrenergic receptors
- 5HT1B/2C receptors, serotonin receptor subtype 1B/2C
- CCK_A receptor, cholecystokinin receptor subtype A
- CRH_1 receptor, corticotropin-releasing hormone receptor subtype 1
- CRH_2 receptor, corticotropin-releasing hormone receptor subtype 2
- D_1 receptor, dopamine receptor subtype 1
- D_2 receptor, dopamine receptor subtype 2
- GHS receptor, growth hormone secretagogue receptor
- GALR1 receptor, galanin receptor subtype 1
- GALR2 receptor, galanin receptor subtype 2
- H_1 receptor, histamine receptor subtype 1
- M_5 receptor, muscarinic receptor subtype 5
- MC1,3,4-R, melanocortin receptor subtype 1,3,4
- Ob-Ra, short leptin receptor isoform
- Ob-Rb, long leptin receptor isoform
- Y_1 receptor, neuropeptide Y receptor subtype 1
- Y_5 receptor, neuropeptide Y receptor subtype 5

Signaling factors
- ATP, adenosine triphosphate
- JAK, Janus kinase
- K^+, potassium
- K-ATP, potassium adenosine triphosphate
- mRNA, messenger ribonucleic acid
- SHP-2, SH2 domain-containing tyrosine phosphatase type 2
- SOCS-3, suppressor of cytokine signaling-3
- STAT, signal transducer and activator of transcription

Brain areas
- ARC, arcuate nucleus
- DMN, dorsomedial nucleus
- GP, globus pallidus
- LH, lateral hypothalamus
- ME, median eminence
- MH, medial hypothalamus
- MPO, medial preoptic area
- NAc, nucleus accumbens
- NTS, nucleus tractus solitarius
- PBN, parabrachial nucleus
- PFC, prefrontal cortex
- PFLH, perifornical lateral hypothalamus
- PVN, paraventricular nucleus
- SCN, suprachiasmatic nucleus
- VMH, ventromedial hypothalamus
- VTA, ventral tegmental area

hypothalamic neurons that synthesize the peptides, arginine vasopressin (AVP) and oxytocin (OT), and send axons to the posterior pituitary. Here, they end in close proximity to the vascular bed of the gland to store and release these neurosecretory products directly into the bloodstream.

Each of these hormones, controlled by the hypothalamus and released by the pituitary, has potent metabolic actions in peripheral tissues that affect body fat. In addition, they have direct impact on the brain, where they produce complex behavioral and physiological responses related to the intake and metabolism of nutrients. These responses are believed to be mediated through the feedback actions of these hormones on brain peptides and monoamines. In addition to the adrenal and gonadal hormones, the pancreatic hormone, insulin, and the adipocyte hormone, leptin, also have important effects on central and peripheral neurochemical systems that are involved in energy and nutrient balance.

Section II below, on circulating hormones, provides a general overview of our current understanding of these peptide and steroid hormones. It also includes a discussion of the metabolic fuels, glucose and triglycerides, which like hormones are greatly altered by food ingestion and weight gain and, in turn, have marked effects on both peripheral and central tissues. It is energy-rich molecules such as these that provide the fuel for living. Thus, a major function of the body and brain is to obtain and regulate these metabolites and keep them in balance with other physiological and neurochemical processes.

B Neurochemicals

Recent investigations of neurochemical mechanisms underlying obesity focus on a variety of peptides that modulate nutrient balance and body weight. As illustrated in Figure 1, these peptides include the original feeding-stimulatory peptides, neuropeptide Y (NPY) and galanin (GAL), which have cell bodies in the hypothalamus.

A newly discovered "feeding peptide," agouti-related protein (AGRP), which colocalizes with NPY, is also depicted with a plus sign in Figure 1. In addition to acting as an agonist for the feeding system, AGRP is an endogenous receptor antagonist, which blocks the inhibitory action of the "satiety peptide," alpha-melanocyte stimulating hormone (α-MSH). As shown in Figure 1, α-MSH is colocalized with a more recently discovered satiety peptide, cocaine- and amphetamine-regulated transcript (CART). These "satiety peptides"

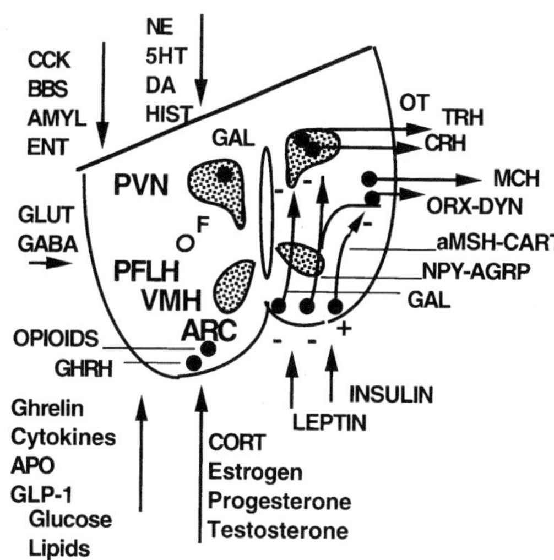

Figure 1 Diagram of selected neurochemical features of the hypothalamus. Note that insulin and leptin have effects in the ARC indicated by plus and minus signs. These hormones are shown as inhibiting (minus sign) feeding-stimulatory peptides, such as GAL and NPY-AGRP pathways in the ARC, which thereby disinhibits the TRH and CRH satiety outputs of the PVN. The α-MSH-CART pathway, on the other hand, is activated by insulin and leptin (plus sign), which thereby inhibits the ORX-DYN or MCH feeding outputs of the PFLH. Thus, satiation is promoted in both cases. The diagram also illustrates the projection to the PFLH, where AGRP acts as an endogenous receptor antagonist to block α-MSH and thereby promote feeding. This diagram includes, and the text discusses, additional steroid and protein hormones (Sec. II), peptides for feeding (Sec. III) and for satiation (Sec. IV), the monoamines (Sec. V), acetylcholine and amino acids (Sec. VI), behavioral systems (Sec. VII), and relationships to the autonomic nervous system (Sec. VIII). Abbreviations are given in Table 1.

are shown in Figure 1 as inhibiting a lateral hypothalamic feeding system that uses the feeding-stimulatory peptides, orexin and DYN. Also listed in Figure 1 are additional satiety peptides. The classic example is cholecystokinin (CCK), which inhibits feeding through its actions in the gut as well as the brain. Recent research links both the feeding and satiety peptide systems to the powerful endocrine influences mentioned above: insulin, leptin, CORT, and the gonadal steroids, E_2 and P. The interactions of these hormones with brain neurotransmitters and neuromodulators are critical in determining specific states of nutrient balance and weight gain. This is illustrated in Figure 1, by insulin and leptin inhibiting the production of the feeding-stimulatory peptides, NPY and AGRP, while stimulating the feeding-inhibitory peptides, α-MSH and CART. These and other neuropeptide systems are reviewed in detail in Sections III and IV below. These sections summarize our present knowledge of different peptides that stimulate or inhibit eating behavior and body weight.

In addition to these peptides, there is considerable evidence to suggest a role for the biogenic amines, norepinephrine (NE), serotonin (5-HT), dopamine (DA), and histamine, in the control of food intake and related behaviors. A DA pathway is illustrated in Figure 2.

In Section V below, these neurotransmitters are discussed in terms of their roles in modulating the peptide systems as a function of states of sleep, arousal, selective attention, and stress. This is followed by Section VI, which reviews evidence supporting two different roles for acetylcholine (ACh) in the reinforcement of feeding (Fig. 2). Specifically, the release of ACh is necessary to arouse a DA motivation system in the midbrain, whereas ACh interneurons inhibit eating by counteracting DA when it is released in the forebrain. The amino acid neurotransmitters, glutamate and gamma-amino butyric acid (GABA) also have interest-

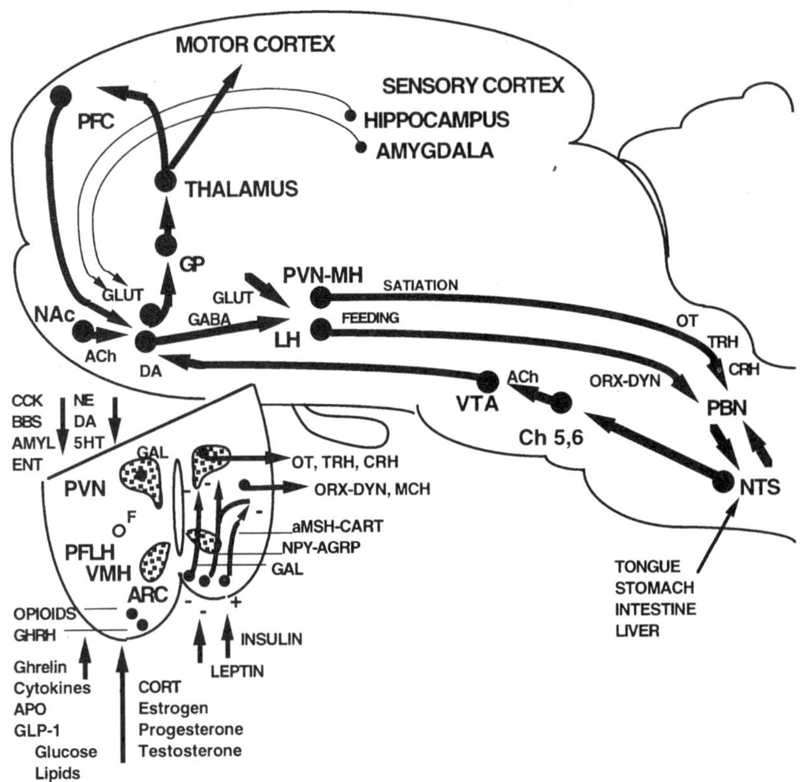

Figure 2 Schematic side view of the brain with emphasis on the hypothalamic area (in the expanded cross section) and the two neural circuits (shown with bold arrows). The expanded view of the hypothalamus indicates some of the local feeding and satiety neurons and their inputs (see Fig. 1). The hypothalamus is part of a much larger feeding circuit. Starting in the lower right corner, signals from the tongue and gut enter the brainstem. The hypothalamus also senses chemical information and sends it to the brainstem. The NTS output goes to the PBN and from there, via the thalamus, projects to the areas labeled, sensory cortex, amygdala, and hippocampus. Here chemosensory information is combined with other sense modalities, such as sights, sounds, locations, and codes for safe nutrition vs. toxic foods. The arrows from the hippocampus (place memory), amygdala (emotion memory), and prefrontal cortex (complex choice memory) sweep into the nucleus accumbens (NAc) and hypothalamus on GLUT neurons (input to NAc is shown). The NAc is a sensorimotor interface in the cognitive/limbic loop drawn in bold lines from PFC to NAc then GP and back to the PFC via the thalamus, with commands branching off to motor output circuits. The ACh interneurons in the NAc may act as gates that counteract DA input from the VTA. Other monoamines and opioid peptides that act in this circuit are discussed in the text (Secs. V–VII). The medial and lateral hypothalamus help control the NAc via the pathways shown descending from the hypothalamus to the brainstem, including an ORX/DYN output for feeding and a CRH pathway for satiation. The circuit ascends via cholinergic cell groups 5 and 6, to the VTA where DA cells project to the NAc and to the rest of the limbic system. The NAc projects back to the hypothalamus. By this route, feeding and satiety signals generated in the hypothalamus can influence DA/ACh balance in the NAc to reinforce or inhibit instrumental behavior and motivation.

ing functions, as described in Section VI. Glutamate in the hypothalamus stimulates feeding, whereas GABA rises as the meal progresses and brings it to a close (Fig. 2).

C Brain Areas

In studying brain neurochemicals that control appetite, it is essential to identify and examine the different brain areas and hypothalamic nuclei that are critical for their effects on eating behavior and body weight regulation. In addition to the hormones and neurochemicals, Table 1 lists the areas and nuclei, together with their abbreviations, that are discussed in the chapter. Studies of the hypothalamus in laboratory animals reveal specific nuclei that have a direct role in maintaining energy or nutrient balance. Figure 1 illustrates a few of these nuclei and gives specific examples of interactions that occur between circulating hormones and hypothalamic neurochemicals. The nuclei in the medial hypothalamus (MH) include the paraventricular nucleus (PVN), arcuate nucleus (ARC), ventromedial hypothalamus (VMH) and dorsomedial nucleus (DMN), which control both nutrient intake and metabolism. The figure displays nerves that synthesize the peptides, OT, CRH, and TRH, which have satiety functions (1). The medial preoptic area (MPO) anterior to the PVN is involved in reproductive physiology, which shifts with metabolic fuels and body weight most notably at puberty and during pregnancy. The suprachiasmatic nucleus (SCN) is the master controller of circadian rhythms for both physiological and behavioral processes. The ARC and median eminence (ME) in the basomedial hypothalamus control the secretion of anterior pituitary hormones in relation to nutrient balance. The ARC and ME also transport leptin and insulin across the blood brain barrier and bring these hormones into contact with hypothalamic peptide systems that control eating and satiety. These hormones, then, inhibit such peptides as NPY and AGRP to reduce the tendency to excite the feeding outputs.

Along with these MH nuclei, there is the lateral hypothalamus (LH), which is like a city train station with a welter of nerve fibers passing through local circuitry and sensory cell groups. The complexity of the LH is reflected in the scientific history of this region, which Stellar characterized as a feeding center (2). The LH contains glucose-sensitive cells, feeding-related neurons with monoamine and peptide receptors, nerve fibers involved in feeding reward, and fibers of passage subserving motive functions. The perifornical (PF) area along the medial aspect of the LH, together referred to as the PFLH, may be specialized for potentiating feeding reflexes and reinforcing voluntary motor functions of ingestive behavior. Cells that synthesize orexins and MCH lie at the heart of this PFLH area (1), which has long been allied with stimulation-induced eating and a site where self-stimulation varies with appetite (3).

Section VII takes the hypothalamic systems portrayed in Figure 1 and places them in the larger context of the whole brain, as shown in Figure 2. Some LH fibers are part of a reinforcement circuit from the PFLH to brainstem nuclei, such as the parabrachial nucleus (PBN) and nucleus of the solitary tract (NTS). These nuclei integrate descending information with primary taste input and ascending autonomic signals from the gut (4). Part of the brainstem output goes to cortical sensory areas, whereas another part goes to midbrain ACh neurons that connect to midbrain DA fibers in the ventral tegmental area (VTA). These DA fibers ascend forward through the LH on their way to the entire limbic system, including the nucleus accumbens (NAc). The NAc is one of the limbic areas projecting to the LH thus forming the loop through the hypothalamus shown in Figure 2.

Complex "cognitive" sensory information about food is funneled into the NAc from several higher brain regions, such as the cortex, hippocampus and amygdala. These areas also project directly to the hypothalamus, but for the sake of clarity, the diagram is simplified and only depicts the inputs to the NAc. The prefrontal cortex (PFC) takes cortical sensory taste information, transforms it to reflect sensory specific satiety (5), and probably sends it in part to the LH and NAc (6). The anterior piriform cortex has a region specialized to respond to repletion of indispensable amino acid imbalance by sending signals to the LH and NAc (7). The NAc also receives multimodal sensory information from the amygdala and hippocampus, reflecting good and bad experiences with tastes, smells, sights, sounds, and important places in the environment. The NAc output courses its way to motor command systems, with a prominent component for feeding.

As seen in Figure 2, part of the NAc output goes via the globus pallidus (GP), and another part descends to the hypothalamus. The GP instructs the motor system and feeds back in the loop shown going to the PFC. Thus, the NAc lies at the intersection of the hypothalamic and PFC loops. It serves as a sensorimotor interface for appetitive motivation, and it is gated, in part, by signals from the hypothalamus (8).

The NAc is also known to be involved with addiction to drugs of abuse. Since it is at the crossroads of systems controlling the motivation to eat, there is the hypothetical possibility of becoming addicted to certain foods. In fact, the addiction process may have evolved for that purpose. Various brain opioids are released by starvation and by palatable foods. Thus, intermittent fasting and bingeing may release sufficient endogenous opioids to create signs of addiction in rats, with similarities to human eating disorders. These circuits, together with evidence for sugar dependency, are described in greater detail in Section VII.

Section VIII deals in broad strokes with the peripheral and central components of the autonomic nervous system in regulatory physiology and regulatory behavior. Low sympathetic tone in the system controlling brown adipose tissue, for example, is associated with many types of obesity. Apparently, it causes the potential to overeat until such time as the animal becomes sufficiently obese to counteract the process. Leptin and other adipocyte hormones may play a role in curbing the motivation to eat, by inhibiting the feeding-reinforcement pathway, as the animal gains weight. It is interesting that the sympathetic system, itself, may strongly influence leptin production. This discussion is followed by Section IX, which provides a brief summary and overview of the different systems that are involved in maintaining energy homeostasis.

II HORMONES INVOLVED IN EATING AND BODY WEIGHT REGULATION

Many peptides, proteins, steroids, metabolites, and other molecules circulating in the blood are likely to have a role in energy balance. There are a few, however, that have received greatest attention, particularly in terms of their impact on neurochemical systems in the brain. These are the pancreatic and adipocyte hormones, insulin and leptin, and the adrenal and gonadal steroids. A subsequent section discusses the metabolites, glucose and lipids, which are also believed to have impact on the brain.

A Insulin

Insulin is the major hormone that enables tissues to remove glucose from the blood. Thus, its secretion from pancreatic β-cells is directly responsive to circulating glucose levels (9). Insulin secretion also varies in proportion to body adiposity, with a heavier individual secreting proportionally more insulin to a given increase in glucose. Thus, insulin levels reflect both ongoing metabolic needs and level of body fat accrual. The importance of insulin as an adiposity signal to the brain is revealed by evidence that insulin-deficient animals are hyperphagic, an effect reversed by administration of insulin (10–14).

To control body weight, insulin is believed to gain access to the brain through areas with a reduced blood brain barrier and by a saturable, receptor-mediated mechanism that transports insulin through the blood-brain barrier and into the interstitial fluid (14,15). In the brain, it acts as a humoral feedback regulator of food intake and energy balance. Insulin injections into the brain reduce food intake, meal size, and weight gain and stimulate the sympathetic nervous system. Consistent with these observations, the *tubby* mouse, characterized by hyperphagia and obesity, is found to have a mutation in the intracellular insulin-signaling pathway within the ventral hypothalamus (16). One site of insulin's action is the hypothalamus, where insulin receptors and intracellular signaling molecules, e.g., insulin receptor substrate-1, are concentrated and where insulin-specific antibodies have opposite effects to insulin itself.

This metabolic hormone may act, in part, through its effects on the production of brain neurochemicals (10,11,17–19), as described in Sections III and IV. For example, insulin inhibits gene expression of peptides, such as NPY and GAL, that enhance food ingestion and exert anabolic effects. The insulinlike growth factor 2, which has anorexic actions, also reduces NPY release in vitro. Conversely, insulin stimulates the activity of peptides, such as CCK, CRH, and α-MSH, which have satiety or catabolic actions. Thus, overall insulin secretion may link short-term changes in energy intake and expenditure with long-term body weight regulation (11). Obese states are invariably associated with hyperinsulinemia and insulin resistance, which produce marked disturbances in the expression and production of these hypothalamic peptides.

B Leptin

Leptin, a product of the *ob* gene, is mutated in the obese *ob/ob* mouse and is produced almost exclusively in fat cells (20). The leptin receptor, found in various peripheral tissues as well as the brain, has also been cloned (21), and a mutation of this receptor produces the syndrome of the diabetic *db/db* mouse (22). This structure belongs to the class I cytokine receptor family, and one of the binding proteins may be the extracellular domain analogous to the growth hormone–binding protein, another member of the cytokine family (23). Leptin produces its biological effects by acting on the long-form receptor isoform, which contains intracellular motifs required for activation of the JAK-STAT signal transduction pathway (see Table 1). Whereas a primary defect in leptin expression may lead to human disease, as shown in studies of consanguineous kindreds with extreme obesity, mutations of the genes that produce leptin or its receptor are rare in humans (22,24).

Leptin expression is influenced by the status of energy stores in body fat, with adipocyte size an important determinant of leptin synthesis (25). Whereas leptin levels in blood correlate strongly with total body fat stores, it is unknown whether leptin expression is influence by triglyceride levels, lipid metabolites, or mechanical factors associated with increased adipocyte size (22,23). Since changes in leptin expression after fasting and feeding do not necessarily correspond with changes in body fat, leptin may serve as a mediator of energy balance, as well as an indicator of energy stores. Regulation of leptin expression by nutrition may be mediated, in part, by insulin, which is positively related to leptin levels, and also to glucocorticoids, which are negatively related (22,23,26). Cytokines also stimulate the synthesis of leptin, which may contribute to the anorexia and weight loss in response to inflammation.

Anatomical and functional studies suggest that leptin exerts its effects on energy balance primarily by acting in the brain. This protein is secreted into the circulation and enters the brain through a saturable transport mechanism (9,22,27,28). Peripheral leptin injection activates neurons in hypothalamic feeding-regulatory areas that have dense concentrations of leptin receptors. Peripheral as well as central injection of leptin reduces food intake, insulin secretion and adiposity (28), with centrally administered leptin producing more potent effects. Leptin also increases energy expenditure and normalizes blood glucose concentrations in obese mice (29). Hyperleptinemia, produced in normal-weight rats through adenovirus gene transfer of the *ob* gene, causes loss of virtually all body fat, an effect that is absent in rats with MH lesions (30).

Leptin-sensitive neurons in the hypothalamic nuclei express neuropeptides and neurotransmitters that are implicated in the central regulation of energy balance and, thus, may mediate leptin's actions (1,22,31). The long-form leptin receptor in the ARC is coexpressed with peptides that stimulate feeding, as well as with those that inhibit feeding. In general, the expression or synthesis of neurochemicals that potentiate feeding behavior is inhibited by leptin injection and elevated in leptin-deficient or food-deprived rodents. Diametrically opposite changes, in contrast, are seen with neurochemicals that suppress food intake. By modulating these peptides in the ARC, leptin may also influence feeding by controlling the expression of orexigenic peptides in other hypothalamic sites, such as the PVN and LH, which are possibly controlled by projections from the ARC. To understand the physiological significance of these findings obtained with leptin injections or gene mutations, further studies of this hormone performed under natural feeding conditions are needed. A fall in leptin levels during fasting, accompanied by a rise in feeding-stimulatory peptides, has been suggested to signal starvation (1). However, a reevaluation of leptin's physiological functions and its relationship to specific peptides has been encouraged by specific evidence, for example, that leptin corrects the neuroendocrine abnormalities of *ob/ob* mice at considerably lower doses than those required to reverse the overeating and obesity (32). Moreover, its effects in intact mice may not be altered by targeted mutations of the feeding-regulatory peptide gene (33).

The evidence that leptin injection produces feeding suppression and weight loss restricted to adipose tissue, while increasing energy expenditure and lipid oxidation (22,34–36), supports a role for this hormone as an antiobesity hormone. However, this is inconsistent with the finding that circulating leptin concentrations rise in direct proportion to the amount of adipose tissue (31). This rise in leptin with obesity has been interpreted as an indication of "leptin resistance" (22), possibly resulting from a dysregulation of leptin synthesis and secretion or from abnormalities of brain leptin transport, leptin receptors, and/or postreceptor signaling. Potential molecular mediators of leptin resistance may include SOCS-3, a member of the suppressors of cytokine signaling family, as well as SH2-containing tyrosine phosphatase, SHP-2, and molecules downstream from the initial step of receptor interaction (see Table 1 for abbreviations). Evolutionarily, it is extremely important to be efficient in the storage of energy when food is available.

Thus, the common occurrence of leptin-resistant obesity suggests that the predominant function of this hormone in energy balance is not to reduce body fat but is to mediate physiological processes of adaptation during fasting and promotion of energy conservation (22,37). Starvation triggers complex neural, metabolic, hormonal, and behavioral adaptations to maintain energy substrates, protect lean mass, and promote survival. This is accomplished by switching from a carbohydrate- to fat-based metabolism, mediated by a decline in insulin and rise in counterregulatory hormones. Starvation also involves suppression of energy utilization, reproductive function, and growth through a decline in gonadal and thyroid hormones and rise in adrenal glucocorticoids. The main effect of these adaptations is to stimulate gluconeogenesis, to supply glucose for vital cellular function and fatty acids for use by skeletal muscle. These endocrine and metabolic adaptations are accompanied by a reduction in leptin caused, in part, by an increase in sympathetic nervous system activity (38). That this decrease in leptin during starvation mediates many of the adaptive responses to fasting is supported by evidence that this state can be reversed or prevented by exogenous leptin, in the absence of a change in adiposity (22). Moreover, leptin restores fertility in female *ob/ob* mice independent of any effect on weight gain, and it advances the time of first estrus in normal mice (39). This may reflect the close relationship between fat accumulation at puberty and activation of the hypothalamic-pituitary-gonadal axis, with leptin informing the brain of the adequacy of fat stores needed for reproduction.

Thus, independent of its role in long-term weight regulation, leptin exerts acute effects on metabolism (22,38,40,41). These include an increase in gluconeogenesis, glucose metabolism, and lipolysis, as well as thermogenesis in brown adipose tissue. Also, leptin prevents triglyceride overload in skeletal muscle and stimulates fatty acid metabolism in liver and sympathetic nervous system activity. Evidence presented in Sections III and IV below provides strong support for the idea that these effects of leptin, while involving direct actions on peripheral tissues, are also mediated through its modulatory actions on the hypothalamic neuropeptide circuitry.

C Adrenal Steroid Hormones

There is a vast literature on the adrenal steroids and their role in controlling feeding and body weight. This literature, which has been extensively reviewed (42–46), leads to the conclusion that, at normal physiological levels, the steroids CORT and aldosterone have specific functions in maintaining carbohydrate and fat stores across the daily light/dark cycle. This process is accomplished through behavioral and metabolic actions, which involve the mediation of both the type I and type II steroid receptors. These receptors exist in the brain and act, in part, through their permissive interactions with neurochemical systems that modulate nutrient balance. Under conditions of obesity and repeated stress, the adrenal steroids are elevated, resulting in chronic disturbances in the steroid-neurochemical interactions. In the absence of these steroids, such as after adrenalectomy, all forms of obesity are attenuated (46).

1 Type I and Type II Steroid Receptors

Studies of the natural light/dark cycle in normal-weight animals have led to the proposal that distinct functions are performed by the different steroid receptors (42). The type I receptor is activated under conditions of low levels of circulating CORT (0.5–2.0 μg/dL), and it functions tonically throughout the daily cycle to sustain feeding, particularly fat intake, and enhance fat deposition. Fat intake occurs at a fairly constant level across the feeding cycle in almost every meal, although it rises toward the second half of the active phase. This stable behavioral pattern provides a continuous supply of a high-caloric nutrient, which can be readily stored in the gastrointestinal tract or adipose tissue for short- or long-term use, respectively. This tonic control of fat intake, possibly mediated through hypothalamic type I receptors, may be analogous to their function in the basal forebrain for maintaining salt balance (47) and in lower brainstem for monitoring blood pressure (48).

The type II receptor, in contrast, is activated under conditions of somewhat higher or moderate levels of CORT. This receptor may function phasically during the early hours of the active cycle when CORT normally rises to levels of 3–10 μg/dL, and it also comes into play also during periods of stress when even higher levels are achieved (42). A primary function of the type II receptor at the onset of the feeding cycle is to replenish and defend the body's carbohydrate stores through both ingestion and storage. This immediate defense is required to prevent the hypoglycemia that may develop after periods of little eating and continued utilization of carbohydrate stores. This defense provides adequate supplies to the brain to stabilize neuronal processes (49,50). The phasic, anabolic effect of moderate levels of CORT may be contrasted with the type II receptor actions of high CORT levels, such as after severe stress or starvation. In addition to stimulating nutrient ingestion, unusually high CORT concentrations actually have catabolic actions on the body's fat and protein stores to provide additional substrates for maintaining normal carbohydrate balance. Under stable conditions, however, the type II receptor subtype is very likely inactive at times of the circadian cycle or in physiological states when glycogen stores are plentiful, cellular glucose uptake is normal, and circulating CORT levels are low.

Thus, these two receptor subtypes work towards a common goal in maintaining the body's nutrient stores from day to day. Through ingestion and metabolism, they provide the nutrients essential for maintaining the body's carbohydrate stores under different environmental conditions. As circulating CORT levels rise, the priorities of nutrient partitioning favor the actions of type II receptors, which restore carbohydrate through behavioral and metabolic processes. Thus, at any moment across the light/dark cycle, but particularly during the initial phase of the feeding cycle, there exists an inverse relation between the carbohydrate and fat content of a meal (51). The differential functions of the receptor subtypes, however, are most evident under conditions of abnormally high CORT levels, when type II receptor activation exerts catabolic effects on certain tissues to shift essential nutrients towards carbohydrate replenishment and storage. Transgenic mice with disturbed expression of the type II glucocorticoid receptors exhibit increased food intake, weight gain, and body fat accrual and a characteristic phenotype of a hyperactive hypothalamopituitary-adrenal axis (HPA) (52).

2 Corticosterone Interactions with Hypothalmic Peptides

Receptors mediating these actions of the adrenal steroids across the circadian cycle are located in the brain (42). As described below, they are particularly responsive in the hypothalamic PVN, which plays a primary role in controlling CORT release as well as nutrient balance. Neurons in the ARC are similarly responsive to CORT. In maintaining carbohydrate stores, the type II receptors act in part through central neurochemical systems that synthesize NPY in the ARC and NE in the brainstem. Circulating CORT enhances gene expression, transport, and receptor activity, ultimately potentiating the action of NPY and NE released in the medial PVN, and it very likely determines the circadian rhythm of endogenous NPY and noradrenergic activity detected in the hypothalamus. Natural rhythms of circulating steroids and their receptor subtypes are critical in maintaining normal control of physiological processes (53,54). These rhythms allow for necessary shifts in phases of priming, activation and rest. Without these rhythms, a chronic state of activation, which constitutes a stress to the organism, will eventually result in pathology. In the control of nutrient balance, the dual-control receptor systems involving type I and type II receptors provide a mechanism that responds to shifts in circulating CORT and assists in coordinating metabolic processes appropriate for specific circadian periods or environmental challenges. The loss of these rhythms in states of obesity has clear negative consequences on cellular and physiological functions. Evidence indicates that the obesity-promoting effects of NPY require the presence of glucocorticoids (55).

3 Corticosterone Interactions with Insulin and Leptin

In evaluating the anabolic and catabolic effects of CORT, it is important to consider its actions in relation to the primary metabolic hormone, insulin (42,43). Corticosterone and insulin are well known for their antagonistic actions, particularly in their effects on glucose uptake and metabolism in the periphery. This antagonism is also evident in their behavioral actions, whereby insulin is released in proportion to the body's fat mass, reduces food intake, and attenuates the steroid's stimulatory action on feeding. This antagonistic interaction between CORT and insulin may occur within the brain as well as in peripheral tissues, possibly involving differential effects on brain neurochemicals, such as NPY. It may differ, however, in other tissues, such as the liver, where CORT and insulin act synergistically to increase lipogenesis and glycogen synthesis. It may also vary at different times of the daily cycle, such as at the onset of the natural feeding cycle when both hormones normally peak, with CORT potentiating eating and insulin allowing efficient postprandial storage of the ingested carbohydrates. In states of obesity, the antagonism between CORT and insulin becomes exaggerated when circulating CORT levels are abnormally and chronically high. There occurs a compensatory rise in insulin secretion along with increased insulin resistance. The resulting chronic hyperinsulinemia and hypercortisolemia increase hepatic lipogenesis, while reducing gluconeogenesis, and they produce catabolic effects within muscle where CORT's actions outweigh those of inselin.

In addition to insulin, there is an antagonistic interaction between leptin and CORT (56,57). Leptin's inhibitory effect on food intake and body weight is markedly enhanced in adrenalectomized rats. Moreover, it is attenuated after glucocorticoid administration. As indicated above, this antagonism between leptin and CORT is evident in terms of their opposing effects on NPY production in the ARC. There is evidence that the obesity syndrome produced by chronic central infusion of glucocorticoids may be attributed, in part, to an increase in hypothalamic NPY, as well as a decline in CRH, effects that may result from a steroid-induced reduction in leptin's actions (57).

D Gonadal Steroid Hormones

Reproductive physiology and behavior depend on the availability of oxidizable metabolic fuels. Energetic factors that affect reproduction, such as food availability, ambient temperature, exercise, and storage and mobilization of fatty acids, all affect the availability of metabolic fuels (58,59). These changes in metabolic fuels influence reproduction through actions at multiple sites. These include key sites in the brain and involve alterations in the activity of neurons that synthesize gonadotrophin-releasing hormone (GnRH) and growth hormone-releasing hormone (GHRH) or have steroid receptor binding sites. The ovarian steroids, E_2 and P, play a major role in this process, producing changes in nutrient ingestion, partitioning and utilization of fuels that differ markedly from the anabolic actions of testosterone.

Estradiol is associated with a reduction in eating behavior, adiposity, and body weight in adult rats (58). Ovariectomy produces the opposite effect, such that animals gain weight in an E_2-reversible manner. As described in subsequent sections, these effects of E_2 may be mediated through its influence on hypothalamic peptide systems, such as NPY, CRH, and CCK (60–63). For example, E_2 replacement after ovariectomy reduces NPY gene expression in the ARC and NPY release in the PVN, which is likely to result in a decline in food intake and loss of body weight.

The reverse pattern is seen with steroid effects on CRH and CCK. Estradiol stimulates the production or function of these peptides, which normally act to inhibit feeding and decrease weight gain. This combination of hypothalamic events, enhanced catabolic signaling combined with impaired compensatory activation of anabolic pathways, leads to body weight loss during chronic high levels of E_2 in adults. There is recent evidence that estradiol cyclically increases the activity of the CCK and glucagon satiation-signaling pathways, causing a reduction in meal size and food intake during the estrous phase of the ovarian cycle (64,65).

In understanding the role of gonadal steroids in feeding and metabolism, one must additionally consider the impact of P, which has diverse actions that may involve an early enhancing effect followed by an inhibition. Thus, while E_2 inhibits NPY, P actually stimulates this peptide's production in E_2-primed animals (66), suggesting an antagonism between the two steroids. In contrast, GAL is activated by E_2 alone, and this effect is enhanced by administration of P (67,68). The resulting pattern, of increased NPY and GAL production under the influence of the two steroids together, may explain the finding of increased caloric intake and body weight that occurs in females at puberty, when the gonadal steroids and peptides rise to peak levels (69–71). Thus, the role of P contrasts with that of E_2. It builds energy stores through behavioral as well as metabolic actions, in contrast to the anorexic and lipolytic actions of E_2 (58,59). The precise nature and site of the steroid-neurochemical interactions underlying these physiological effects remain to be characterized.

E Glucose

The brain is among the most metabolically active tissues. It is dependent almost exclusively on plasma glucose, rather than alternative substrates, such as fatty acids and ketone bodies, and it is responsive to changes in glucose levels (73,713). In the brain, there exist neurons that sense a dangerous decline in circulating glucose levels and utilization and perform the function of reducing neuronal activity and, consequently, metabolic demand. In addition, the brain appears to respond to physiological changes in blood glucose and its utilization. These changes can either stimulate or inhibit the activity of neuroendocrine neurons with integrative metabolic functions, including counterregulatory responses, food intake, and metabolic rate. These neurons, largely confined to the hypothalamus, are referred to as "glucose-responsive" or "glucose-sensitive" if stimulated, respectively, by a rise or fall in glucose levels. The physiological relevance of glucose-responsive neurons is underscored by the observation that they cease firing just before a meal and, then, begin to fire once again as the meal progress (72). It is suggested that local concentrations of glucose to which neuroendocrine hypothalamic neurons are exposed may be higher than those to which other neurons are exposed, owing to the presence of specialized hypothalamic glucose transporters (73).

Evidence has accumulated to suggest that glucose-sensing mechanisms of glucose-responsive neurons and pancreatic endocrine cells share common features. In addition ATP-sensitive K^+ (K-ATP) channels, a key element in this mechanism is the presence of glucokinase (73). This enzyme has properties that allow cells to metabolize glucose in proportion to plasma levels of glucose in the physiological range. It may serve as a glucose transduction mechanism, which links the effects of small changes in glucose to ATP generation. There is recent evidence showing that neurons in the ARC that synthesize the feeding-stimulatory peptide, NPY (see below), colocalize glucokinase mRNA as well as Kir6.2 mRNA, the pore-forming subunit of the

ATP-sensitive K^+ channel (74). The mechanisms underlying the response of glucose-sensitive neurons, which are more concentrated in the LH, remain to be characterized (75).

Both obesity and diabetes are associated with alterations in brain glucose sensing (76). Rats with diet-induced obesity, hyperinsulinemia, or insulin-dependent diabetes have abnormalities in glucose-responsive neurons. These include disturbances in neurotransmitter systems, specific peptides, monoamines, and amino acids that are involved in glucose sensing. A functional relationship between circulating glucose and central neurochemical systems is suggested by the finding that glucose-responsive neurons in the ARC are hyperpolarized by the actions of both leptin and insulin on the K-ATP channel (76). Further, the expression and production of brain peptides, such as NPY in the ARC, or ligand binding to specific α_2-noradrenergic receptors in the PVN, for example, are stimulated by the injection or ingestion of glucose (77,78), suggesting the involvement of glucose-responsive neurons.

F Lipids

In addition to glucose, there is evidence that circulating lipids have impact on the brain (79). Except for adipose tissue, the brain has a higher lipid content and greater diversity of lipid species than any other organ. Although many fatty acid constituents of the brain can be synthesized de novo, essential fatty acids must be transported into the brain from the plasma. Albumin is considered the physiological vehicle for taking fatty acids into target tissues. Ingested fatty acids bind to albumin in several forms, including triglycerides, which are incorporated into chylomicrons or are bound to lysophosphotidylcholine.

In order to enter the brain, triglycerides are rapidly hydrolyzed in capillary endothelial cells. They are transported, possibly via specific transporters, to astrocytes surrounding the endothelium and, then, to neurons and other cells. Brain microvessel endothelial cells, astrocytes, and neurons readily take up polyunsaturated fatty acids. Radiolabeled lipids injected into the carotid artery are found in the brain within 15 mins, and they remain for up to 17 days (80). Ingested fatty acids are also found in the adult brain (81). Whereas lipids can enter the brain through passive diffusion, protein-mediated transport mechanisms have also been proposed (79). This latter model implies that lipid membranes introduce permeability barriers to fatty acids and that selective transport of fatty acids into brain is accomplished by specific protein transporters.

There is evidence that extracellular fatty acids affect neuronal function in the brain. For example, they inhibit the reuptake of glutamate in synaptosomes (82). They also activate a novel type of K^+ channel in neurons (83). Consumption of a high-fat diet is found to stimulate the expression and production of the feeding-stimulatory peptide, GAL, in the PVN (84), in addition to the opioid peptide, DYN (85). Recent evidence demonstrates a strong, positive correlation between PVN GAL mRNA and circulating triglyceride levels in several different animal models (86). Thus, in addition to certain hormones, circulating lipids may have impact on neurochemical systems in the hypothalamus that control eating and body weight.

III PEPTIDES THAT INCREASE EATING AND BODY WEIGHT

Through pharmacological and biochemical studies, specific peptides and neurotransmitters have been identified within the hypothalamic areas and implicated in physiological and behavioral processes that impact on body weight. It is now clear that there is great redundancy involving multiple neurochemicals and actions, both stimulatory and inhibitory, on eating and metabolism. These systems are activated under diverse physiological states and environmental conditions that affect an organism during its lifetime. This section reviews evidence obtained with peptides that have stimulatory effects on eating behavior and weight gain and are implicated in the development of obesity (Table 1).

A Neuropeptide Y

Neuropeptide Y (NPY) is a 36–amino acid member of a highly conserved group of peptides. It is one of the most abundant peptides in the mammalian brain and a very potent stimulator of feeding that, with repeated injection, stimulates weight gain (31,57,87). The available evidence demonstrates that NPY neurons are highly responsive to states of energy deficiency, increased metabolic demand, and disturbed glucoregulation (88). When enhanced, this peptide helps to reverse these disturbances and maintain glucose homeostasis by stimulating processes of carbohydrate ingestion and utilization that gear substrates toward fat synthesis (69,89,90). The neurocircuit underlying this neurochemical action involves a dense NPY projection, which originates in neurons of the ARC, projects to the PVN and PFLH (Fig. 1), and function through NPY receptors of the Y_1 and Y_5 subtype that are concentrated in these areas (31,91).

The effects produced by hypothalamic NPY injections support the proposed role of this peptide in maintaining carbohydrate balance. These actions of exogenous NPY, summarized in greater detail in various reviews (69,89,90,92), include a stimulatory effect on feeding behavior, with a preferential effect on carbohydrate intake. The endocrine effects of NPY (56,93,94) involve enhanced release of CORT, which favors the availability and utilization of glucose, and increased pancreatic secretion of insulin, which functions together with CORT to promote lipogenesis (95). These behavioral and endocrine effects of NPY are accompanied by metabolic changes effecting enhanced parasympathetic nervous system activity and reduced sympathetic activity (93,96). The effects include a reduction in energy expenditure and thermogenesis, decreased glucose uptake in muscle, and a diversion of excess energy and glucose towards fat synthesis in white adipose tissue.

Pharmacological and anatomical studies (31,91) suggest that these effects of NPY, involving the neurocircuit from the ARC to the PVN, may be mediated, in part, through connections with other neural systems involved in energy homeostasis (Fig. 1). These include reciprocal connections with systems that inhibit feeding, such as CRH in the PVN, melanocortin neurons in the ARC, and 5HT in the midbrain. They also involve peptides that stimulate feeding, including MCH and orexin in the PFLH. The demonstration that NPY neurons in the ARC also express the peptide AGRP, an endogenous antagonist of the feeding-inhibitory melanocortin system, provides evidence for another avenue of communication between NPY and other neuropeptides modulating feeding (91,97–99).

Endogenous NPY has a role in mediating natural feeding. With acute administration, injections of NPY antisera, receptor antagonists, and antisense oligodeoxynucleotides to NPY mRNA invariably reduce food intake (100–102). Moreover, with repeated injections, NPY produces overeating, obesity, and related endocrine and metabolic disturbances (56,87). Antisense oligodeoxynucleotides to NPY mRNA reduce endogenous NPY levels in the ARC and suppress body weight gain (102). In light of these findings, it was surprising that NPY knockout mice and NPY overexpressing mice showed little change in eating or body weight (33,88). The ability of NPY-deficient mice to maintain normal eating patterns may be attributed, in part, to a compensatory increase in the production of other peptides, such as AGRP and GAL, which also enhance food intake and weight gain (103). There is evidence, however, that a knockout of the NPY gene can reduce weight gain in mice that have a mutation of the leptin gene or diabetes, indicating a role for endogenous NPY in mediating some effects of leptin or insulin deficiency (104). Moreover, a recent genetic study demonstrates that, in homozygous mice, NPY overexpression in the brain leads to an obese phenotype on a sucrose-loaded diet, accompanied by overeating, hyperglycemia, and hyperinsulinemia (105).

A variety of endocrine signals feed back to regulate NPY synthesis in the ARC-PVN neural projection. This is reflected in measures of gene expression or translation, in addition to peptide synthesis, transport, release, and receptor activity. In these hypothalamic areas, the adrenal steroid CORT acts through glucocorticoid type II receptors to stimulate NPY gene expression, synthesis, and receptor activity (42,106–109). Moreover, the behavioral action of NPY is similarly enhanced by CORT, while antagonized by a glucocorticoid receptor blocker. These effects of CORT on NPY may be direct as well as indirect via the CRH system (109). This suggests that NPY helps to integrate the activities of the hypothalamic feeding systems and the HPA axis, which are important for the circadian rhythmicity of physiological processes (109). A different pattern becomes evident with the gonadal steroids, E_2 and P. Administration of E_2 inhibits NPY gene expression in the ARC and its release in the PVN, and E_2 deficiency increases NPY in the PVN. This suggests a role for this peptide in the anorexic action of E_2 (31). In contrast, administration of P has a stimulatory effect on NPY in E_2-primed animals (60,110–112). This evidence obtained with P, similar to CORT, suggests that both steroids promote weight gain and body fat accrual through their stimulatory effect on NPY in the ARC (108,113).

In contrast to these steroids are the hormones insulin and leptin, which are released in relation to the amount of body fat. These hormones have a potent, inhibitory effect on NPY gene expression in the ARC, NPY peptide levels in the PVN, and feeding induced by NPY injection (1,114). These suppressive effects may explain the enhanced expression of NPY after food deprivation, which reduces levels of insulin and leptin and, conversely, the satiety-producing effects seen with injections of these hormones (11). Further support for this close relationship between NPY neurons and the circulating hormones is obtained from the findings that leptin and insulin receptors are densely expressed in the ARC. A subpopulation of NPY neurons coexpresses the leptin receptor. The expression of NPY in these neurons is invariably elevated in rats deficient in insulin, leptin, or the leptin receptor (31,91,97).

Studies of physiological or pathological states reveal associations between dietary macronutrients, circulating hormones, metabolic processes, and hypothalamic NPY (10,115–118). For example, the relationships among carbohydrate intake, circulating CORT levels, lipogenic processes, and NPY levels are evident in adult rats given a choice of macronutrient diets. They exhibit strong, positive correlations among NPY, CORT levels, and spontaneous intake of carbohydrate, as opposed to fat or protein (42,51,108,119,120). These relationships are seen at the start of the active feeding period. Carbohydrate is the preferred dietary nutrient at this time, when CORT levels and NPY gene expression naturally peak, and both gluconeogenesis and glycogenolysis are elevated to support the utilization of carbohydrate. Dietary and pharmacological manipulations also reveal enhanced NPY expression and CORT under conditions of diet-induced insulin resistance or after 2-deoxy-D-glucose blockade of glucose utilization (121–123). In fact, in weanling animals, both the NPY system and the HPA axis reach peak development at an age when carbohydrate accounts by choice for >65% of the animals' diet and lipogenesis is elevated (70,71,124,125).

Similar to CORT, a possible stimulatory effect of P on NPY is evident across the 4-day female cycle. Proestrus reveals peak levels of NPY in the MPO, as well as the ARC and PVN. This occurs with a rise in circulating levels of P, subsequent to E_2 priming, and an increase in lipogenesis (112,126,127). The inhibitory relationship between NPY and both leptin and insulin is clearly evident in studies of obesity-prone rats (128–130). In a preobese state, when leptin and insulin levels are relatively low, NPY mRNA is elevated in the obesity-prone subjects, sugesting a role for this peptide in the early stages of weight gain. This is in contrast to a reduction in NPY detected in the postobese state, when leptin and insulin levels rise significantly with body fat accrual in the obesity-prone subjects. A strong, inverse relationship between NPY and circulating leptin or insulin is underscored by the findings that NPY is reduced in a variety of obese states, such as those produced by a high-fat or high-energy diet, VMH lesions, neurotoxins, or a mutation of the *tubby* gene (131–134). These findings lead one to question the function of NPY in the maintenance of obesity and contrast with those obtained for other feeding-stimulatory peptides, such as GAL and the endorphins. These latter peptides are elevated in different states of obesity and are less responsive or even stimulated by the elevation of leptin or insulin, suggesting their role in promoting obesity in already obese subjects (31,88,132,135).

B Galanin and Galaninlike Peptide

Galanin (GAL) is widely distributed through the brain and has a number of physiological and behavioral effects that are mediated via distinct GAL receptor subtypes (136). Similar to NPY, GAL stimulates feeding behavior and has a variety of endocrine and metabolic effects. Although these peptide systems may overlap anatomically (31), an abundance of evidence indicates that they are functionally distinct (69). In addition to the ARC where NPY neurons are concentrated, GAL-expressing neurons also exist in the PVN, in both its medial parvocellular and lateral magnocellular areas, and in the PFLH and MPO (Fig. 1). The behavioral, endocrine, and metabolic actions of GAL in the PVN, mediated by two receptor subtypes, GALRI and GALR2, are very different from those of NPY (69,137–140). The GAL-induce feeding response is smaller and shorter-lasting than that of NPY, although it may involve the release of endogenous NPY (141).

Although GAL has little effect on an animal's preference for carbohydrate or fat, a variety of evidence links this peptide's feeding-stimulatory response to dietary fat (142–144). In contrast to NPY, GAL-elicited feeding is stronger and more prolonged in subgroups or strains of rats that naturally prefer fat or in subjects maintained on a high-fat compared to low-fat diet. Further, GAL but not NPY is suppressed by the pentapeptide enterostatin, which selectively reduces the consumption of fat (145). It is also blocked by the GAL antagonist M40, which reduces fat intake (146,147). Repeated PVN injections of antisense oligonucleotides to GAL mRNA produce a marked reduction in fat ingestion and weight gain, in conjunction with a decline in PVN GAL levels (148,149). Whereas both GAL and NPY reduce energy expenditure and inhibit sympathetic nervous system activity (150,151), GAL's endocrine and gastrointestinal effects are, in some cases, diametrically opposite to those of NPY (42,152,153). They include a suppression of CORT, insulin, and AVP release, and an increase in gastric acid secretion. In contrast to NPY, GAL has little impact specifically on carbohydrate or fat metabolism (150).

Differences between these two peptide systems are also evident in their responsiveness to endocrine and physiological feedback signals. In contrast to the robust stimulatory effect of CORT on NPY expression and feeding response, this steroid has little impact or transiently inhibits GAL gene expression in PVN neurons, and has no effect on GAL's feeding behavioral action in this nucleus (42,154,155). Moreover, E_2 alone or in combination with P has a potent stimulatory effect on GAL in the PVN, MPO, and ME (67,156–158), which is not seen with NPY in the ARC. Insulin suppresses both GAL and NPY (18), but these peptides in the ARC show a markedly different response to leptin. This hormone has a potent inhibitory effect on NPY but produces no change in basal GAL expression in the ARC, only a small suppression of PVN GAL, and little change in GAL-induced release of CRH (141,159). This differential responsiveness to leptin, possibly due to the low concentration of leptin receptors on GAL neurons (159), may explain their different responses to food restriction, which reduces leptin levels and markedly enhances NPY in the ARC while having little impact on GAL (160). It may also be related to the finding that GAL, but not NPY, is suppressed by an inhibitor of fat oxidation (161), and NPY but not GAL is stimulated by an antagonist of carbohydrate oxidation (162).

These differences between NPY and GAL, in both their physiological actions and feedback regulation, suggest that they may function through distinct mechanisms and in different physiological states or conditions. The clearest finding, demonstrated in a number of studies and animal models (143,163–165), is that GAL gene expression and peptide production in the PVN, but not the ARC, are positively related to amount of dietary fat, and they also rise in direct proportion to body fat. This is in contrast to NPY, which is reduced by fat consumption and declines in relation to body fat, possibly owing to an increase in leptin to which GAL in less responsive (128,166). In recent studies, GAL in the PVN is strongly, positively related to circulating levels of triglycerides, in addition to measures of fat oxidation in muscle (86). This relationship is robust, seen in different models of dietary obesity but also under conditions of acute exposure (2–24 hr) to a high-fat diet, indicating its independence of changes in body fat and leptin (86). Fat-preferring, obesity-prone rats exhibit higher levels of GAL mRNA and production in the PVN, while NPY in the ARC is reduced (128,142). They are also more responsive to the feeding-stimulatory effects of GAL, but not NPY (167). Circulating levels of GAL are found to be significantly elevated in obese women (168).

The biological rhythms of GAL also differ from NPY (69,137). Across the light/dark cycle, PVN GAL neurons show peak levels during the middle of the feeding cycle, when fat ingestion spontaneously rises. Levels of GAL also rise during proestrous in the MPO and PVN, in association with a rise in circulating E_2 and P and a preferential increase in fat ingestion (126,156,158,169). A marked increase in GAL is also seen at puberty, specifically in the ARC of male rats, possibly attributed to a rise in testosterone and growth hormone (GH). An increase occurs in the PVN and MPO of females, attributed to an elevation of E_2 and P levels and accompanied by a rise in fat ingestion and body fat accrual (70,71,170–172). A genetic study shows that GAL-deficient mice feed and grow normally and have unaltered NPY in the hypothalamus (173), suggesting that GAL is not an essential peptide in the early stages of development.

A 60–amino acid, GAL-like peptide (GALP), was recently isolated from the porcine hypothalamus (174). This peptide shares sequence homology with GAL and binds with high affinity to GAL receptors. However, studies to date reveal clear differences between these two peptides. In contrast to GAL, GALP is expressed almost exclusively in the ARC (175), and these GALP-synthesizing neurons do not project to the ME (176). Whereas GAL mRNA in this nucleus is not altered by leptin administration, GALP mRNA in the ARC is markedly reduced in leptin-deficient *ob/ob* mice, while stimulated by intracerebroventricular infusion of leptin (177). Moreover, GALP is similarly decreased by fasting, an effect reversed by leptin injection (177). While GAL acts via both receptor subtypes, GALR1 and GALR2, GALP appears to be selective for GALR2 (175). Further studies are needed to determine the physiological effects and hormone regulation of this peptide.

C Agouti-Related Protein

Agouti-related protein (AGRP) is a naturally occurring antagonist that binds to a receptor to prevent its response to another molecule (178). This protein inhibits the activity of melanocortins, small peptides derived from a large precursor, pro-opiomelanocortin (POMC), which also gives rise to β-endorphin. As described in Section IV, the melanocortins have an inhibitory effect on feeding and body weight, and AGRP, while having little intrinsic signaling activity, binds directly to melanocortin receptors primarily to inhibit melanocortin binding.

A variety of evidence suggests a close relationship between AGRP and the NPY neurocircuit. AGRP colocalizes almost 100% with NPY in neurons of the ARC (98,179). As with NPY, AGRP is a very potent stimulant of feeding behavior, and it promotes body fat accrual. In fact, this peptide is even more potent than

NPY over the long term, because its actions outlast the drug itself and increase eating for days (180). The endocrine profile for AGRP is similar to that for NPY, including an increase in insulin levels (181,182). There is evidence that AGRP and NPY send similar types of signals that reinforce one another, possibly through the inhibition of a Gs-coupled receptor by AGRP and the activation of Gi-coupled receptor by NPY (183). The possibility that these two peptides represent redundant components of a parallel circuit may help to explain why NPY-deficient animals show only minor defects in eating behavior and leptin signaling (33). However, some differences between the AGRP and NPY neurocircuits appear to exist. The stimulatory effect of AGRP on food intake is longer-lasting than, and additive with, that of NPY, and it is accompanied by a somewhat different pattern of c-Fos immunoreactivity in extrahypothalamic areas (184,185).

That the endogenous peptides function in a similar manner is supported by evidence revealing similar changes in endogenous AGRP and NPY expression under physiological conditions (186,187). For example, both peptides in the ARC are stimulated by conditions of negative energy balance and reduced leptin levels. This is evident in leptin-deficient or streptozotocin-induced diabetic mice, after food deprivation or on a carbohydrate-rich diet, and in response to glucopenia induced by 2-deoxy-D-glucose (122,181,188,189). Further, these peptides are both suppressed under conditions of positive energy balance or enhanced leptin levels. This is evident in obese or leptin-injected rodents (187,188), in adrenalectomized rats with reduced glucocorticosteroid levels (190,191), or after insulin injection in streptozotocin-induced diabetes (189). As described in sections below, these patterns observed with endogenous NPY and AGRP expression are opposite to those seen with measurements of POMC and α-MSH. This supports the idea that the NPY/AGRP and melanocortin systems interact antagonistically in the control of eating and body weight.

D Orexins

The orexins are a recently identified class of neuropeptides, also described as hypocretins (192,193). Orexin A and orexin B, sharing 46% identity, are coded by the same gene, and are localized in neurons of the PFLH. Administration of orexin A stimulates feeding behavior more effectively than orexin B, possibly through activation of orexin-1 and orexin-2 receptors (192). This effect, localized to the PFLH and PVN (31), is considerably smaller and of shorter duration than that produced by NPY or AGRP. In addition to this feeding-stimulatory effect, orexin A injection increases energy metabolism and vagal nerve–dependent gastric acid acid secretion (194,195). The importance of the orexins in feeding behavior is suggested by evidence from genetic studies, revealing an increase in food intake in orexin-overexpressing mice and a decrease in orexin-deficient mice (196).

Neuroanatomical studies demonstrate reciprocal synaptic contacts between orexin cells in the PFLH and leptin-responsive neurons in the ARC that express NPY, AGRP, POMC (197–199). This suggests that orexin may function as a downstream effector molecule of these peptide systems. Orexin-containing axons also contact other orexin cells that express leptin receptors, indicating possible autoregulation of orexin function (199). These orexin-expressing neurons in the PFLH lie adjacent to, but do not overlap, another cell population, described below, that produces a different feeding-stimulatory peptide, melanin-concentrating hormone (197,198,200).

Despite their close anatomical relationship, it is clear that the orexins in the PFLH function differently from other feeding-stimulatory systems in the ARC, suggesting that the regulatory mechanisms of these peptides differ (201). Whereas the PFLH and ARC systems may be upregulated by food deprivation (192,202,203), diametrically opposite results are obtained in genetically obese mice, which show a decrease in hypothalamic orexin mRNA (204,205) but an increase in NPY and AGRP (204,205). Further, in contrast to the ARC peptides that are inhibited by leptin and invariably elevated when leptin is low (see above), functional evidence for a direct interaction between leptin and orexin neurons in the PFLH is lacking, despite the presence of leptin receptors (199,201). Orexin mRNA or peptide level is reduced both when leptin is deficient and when it is injected (204,206). Moreover, the orexins remain stable in conditions or states with markedly altered leptin levels, including overfeeding, dietary obesity, or food restriction with leptin treatment (203, 205–207).

Whereas leptin may not be a key regulator of the orexins, there is evidence suggesting that the orexin neurons are controlled by changes in circulating glucose and may stimulate feeding specifically under conditions of hypoglycemia. Prepro-orexin mRNA in the PFLH is elevated when plasma glucose falls and food is withheld (203,208), and it is reduced by food ingestion (209), suggesting a role in short-term feeding behavior. Some neurons in the LH are known to be glucose sensitive, that is, stimulated by a decline in glucose (75). These glucose-sensitive cells include orexin neurons, which are stimulated by insulin-induced hypoglycemia (208,210). Recent evidence (211) indicates that the orexin neurons are the same as those identified as containing "prolactinlike immunoreactivity" that are also activated by hypoglycemia. In addition to being stimulated by hypoglycemia following insulin injection, the orexin neurons are inhibited by signals related to nutrient ingestion and are functionally linked to neuronal activity in the hindbrain (209).

It is unclear whether the orexin neurons have a role in obesity. Knockout of the orexin gene, while reducing food intake, actually leads to obesity (196). This may reflect an underlying reduction in energy expenditure due to decreased motor activity, lower basal metabolic rate, or both. That the orexins have a role in controlling energy metabolism is suggested by studies showing that orexin A injection stimulates metabolic rate in mice independently of an increase in food intake or activity (194). In freely feeding mice, this orexin-induced increase in metabolic rate is accompanied by a decrease in respiratory quotient, indicating the use of lipids as energy substrates. This is in contrast to the increase in respiratory quotient and carbohydrate metabolism produced by food deprivation. Consistent with a role for the orexins in lipid metabolism, recent findings show that orexin gene expression is stimulated by consumption of a high-fat diet compared to a low-fat diet, and orexin mRNA rises even further in association with obesity on a high-fat diet. This increase in orexins is closely associated with circulating triglycerides, leading to the proposal that the orexins, like GAL, belong to a class of fat-stimulated peptides (212,213).

In addition to controlling feeding and energy homeostasis, the orexins act at different levels of the neuroaxis to modulate hypothalamic regulatory systems involved in arousal, neuroendocrine, and autonomic processes. This is supported by the extensive projections of orexin fibers to many areas of the brain and spinal cord (200,214–216). The importance of the orexins in the sleep-wake cycle is underscored by the discoveries that a knockout of the mouse *orexin* gene or a mutation affecting the *orexin-2 receptor* gene in dogs induces narcolepsy (196,217–219). Moreover, orexin injections produce an increase in locomotor activity, grooming, and searching behaviors, suggesting a role for the orexins in vigilance and regulation of arousal states (220). A possible relationship between these effects and those of orexin on energy balance is supported by evidence showing obesity in narcoleptic animals (201). Orexin is localized with DYN in neurons that may perform a function in feeding behavior based on opioid effects in the PBN. This is discussed in the opioid peptide section below and is illustrated in Figures 1 and 2.

There is further evidence indicating the involvement of an orexin peptide system in neuroendocrine and autonomic functions. This is demonstrated by the stimulatory effect of orexin A injection on blood pressure and heart rate, on autonomic efferent nerve activity and gastric acid secretion, and on luteinizing hormone secretion, at lower doses than those required to stimulate feeding (221–223). This pressor response to orexin A is accompanied by an increase in renal sympathetic nerve activity and plasma catecholamines in conscious rats (224). The finding that orexins act on medullary neurons to increase sympathetic nerve activity to the heart and blood vessels (225) raises the possibility that this peptide system underlies the increased sympathetic activation and risk of high blood pressure associated with obesity (226).

E Melanin-Concentrating Hormone

In addition to the orexins, other neurons in the LH and zona incerta produce melanin-concentrating hormone (MCH), a cyclic 19–amino acid neuropeptide originally isolated from salmon pituitaries (227,228). This peptide acts via a specific receptor with a typical seven-transmembrane domain region seen with G-protein-coupled receptors (229,230). The involvement of MCH in the control of feeding behavior was first suggested by studies showing that central administration of MCH potentiates food intake (231,232). This MCH-induced feeding response is relatively small and of short duration compared to the responses induced by NPY and AGRP. Also, long-term administration of this peptide has little effect on daily food intake and body weight (232).

Studies of endogenous MCH provide support for its role in feeding and body weight regulation. The expression of MCH is stimulated by fasting, augmented in *ob/ob* mice with leptin deficiency, and decreased by leptin (56,231,232). This peptide is potentiated by insulin-induced hypoglycemia, similar to the orexins in the PFLH but contrary to the ARC NPY/AGRP system, as described above. MCH is also increased by compounds that block glucose and fatty acid oxidation, suggesting that it responds to changes in the availability of immediate fuel sources, perhaps by stimulating food intake. Further, the expression of MCH is responsive to E_2, which inhibits hypothalamic MCH expression in ovariectomized rats and blocks deprivation-induced increase in MCH (233,234). This suggests that decreased MCH signaling may contribute to the pathogenesis in certain types of anorexia.

A physiological role for MCH in energy homeostasis is strongly supported by genetic studies. For example, targeted ablation of the MCH gene leads to a thin phenotype associated with hypophagia and an inappropriate increase in metabolic rate (235). Moreover, trasgenic mice that overexpress MCH in the LH exhibit hyperphagia, hyperleptinemia, hyperglycemia, and insulin resistance on a high-fat diet compared to wild-type animals (236). The finding that MCH-deficient mice show low levels of leptin and POMC mRNA is unexpected, given the anorexia in this strain. The leanness in mice with deletion of the MCH gene, despite other intact orexigenic systems, suggests that this peptide acts downstream of leptin as well as the NPY/AGRP and POMC/melanocortin signaling cascades. This is supported by the immunohistochemical demonstration of a projection from the ARC neurons, which synthesize NPY/AGRP or melanocortins, to MCH neurons in the LH (197,198). It also agrees with the finding that leptin administration decreases MCH expression as well as MCH-induced feeding (56,237).

F Opioid Peptides

The opioid system is composed of three families of biologically active peptides—DYN, β-endorphin, and enkephalin. One of the many functions of opioid peptides is their role in mediating the component of food intake control that is enhanced by both food palatability and food deprivation. Therefore, opioid systems may be important in binge eating and diet-induced obesity. Systemic morphine increases food ingestion, and the opioid receptor antagonist naloxone reduces intake of palatable food (238,239). When macronutrient diets are available, opioid agonists preferentially enhance ingestion of fat-rich diets (240). Patterns of ingesting sweet solutions under the influence of morphine or naloxone suggest that opioids inhibit aversive components of overeating and, thereby, increase the amount of food ingested (241–243). Opioids released in the nervous system by eating palatable food can also cause analgesia in rats and humans (244–246). Therefore, eating may occur to suppress pain or discomfort.

1 Opioid Subsystems

It has been difficult using systemic injections to unravel the roles of various mu, kappa, and delta systems and their multiple receptors. Progress is being made, however, as summarized in several reviews (238,247–249). The opioid peptides DYN, β-endorphin, and enkephalin act primarily via kappa, mu, and delta receptors, respectively (238,250–253). When labeling the brain for opioid peptides and their receptors, the regions involved with taste, autonomic control, feeding, and reward stand out. Evidence suggests that mu_1 receptors affect body weight and alter physiological responses of the glucostatic and lipostatic systems, whereas some of the kappa receptor systems stimulate food palatability and promote feeding by blocking satiety (254,255).

Early work involving local brain injection in the PVN-MH region showed that β-endorphin, DYN, or an enkephalin analog each induces feeding (256,257). If one starts with the hypothalamus in Figure 2 and follows the hypothalamic loop to the PBN, NTS, VTA, and back to the hypothalamus, there are opioid influences at each step of the way and in the amygdala as well. There may be a specific opioid pathway involved in feeding and its reinforcement (250). The threshold for feeding induced by LH stimulation is raised by specific antibodies against DYN-A (258). Naloxone also raises the threshold for stimulation-induced eating, and this effect, unlike the classic anorexic action of amphetamine (AMPH) and phenylpropanolamine, is potentiated by eating. A site where naloxone exerts its anorexic effect via kappa or mu receptors lies in the PBN, a brainstem region that relays taste and vagal information to and from the forebrain. Thus, an identified DYN path from LH to PBN may potentiate eating for taste and by inhibiting satiation (250,259,260). In addition, food intake and decreased sympathetic activity produced by PVN injection of NPY is blocked by naloxone in the NTS. Thus, NPY-induced feeding depends, in part, on opioids in the NTS (238,261). One or more opioid systems may be involved in GAL-induced eating as well (262). In the VTA, local injection of morphine has a potent feeding-stimulatory effect that is mimicked by DYN (263). A mu opioid antagonist injected in the VTA blocks food-induced release of DA in the NAc, but not in the PFC, and it reduces the animal's appetite (264). This result may depend on the palatability of the food (265). In the NAc, a specific mu opioid agonist induces eating of preferred foods (266,267). A mu agonist in the amygdala also stimulates eating, and this effect is blocked by an opiate antagonist in the NTS (239,268). Studies of feeding with transgenic animal models of opioid abnormalities have also been reviewed (56,97,269).

2 Opioid Reward and Eating

The next question is whether the LH-PBN opioid-related path is involved in self-stimulation and feeding reinforcement, as well as in the prolongation of a meal. In support of this proposal electrodes in the LH that induce feeding also support self-stimulation (3). Opiate antagonists sometimes decrease self-stimulation (270). The self-stimulation rate at eating sites in the LH is inhibited by a meal. This clearly reflects loss of appetite, as long as control is used for motor effects on bar press rate (3,270–272). In a majority of such studies, the converse is also true, whereby food deprivation increases the LH self-stimulation rate or lowers the threshold (250,273). This effect is reversed by ventricular infusion of naltrexone (250). Therefore, opioids potentiate the behavior reinforcement system,which is defined by LH self-stimulation in the PFLH, when it is a stimulation-induced eating site.

It is hypothesized that a natural incentive mechanism for eating is stimulated by palatable tastes via an opioid system, which is sensitized by the metabolic needs imposed by weight loss (250). This appetite enhancement mechanism seems to involve several limbic regions, including the DYN pathway that starts in or near the PFLH and projects to the PBN (259). This may be part of the feeding reinforcement system that is modulated by food intake, food deprivation, and insulin (271). It is potentiated by DYN release and sensitized by an opioid process in response to weight loss or diabetes (250). Therefore, DYN can be envisioned in Figure 2 as part of the feeding and reinforcement system drawn from the LH to the PBN. In light of recent evidence for orexin-expressing cells in the PFLH region that project axons to the hindbrain as well as the prefrontal cortex (216), the orexins may also be excellent candidates for part of the feeding reinforcement circuit. In fact, DYN and orexin coexist in cells of the LH (274).

Opiates are behavior reinforcers in the VTA, as shown by morphine self-injection, conditioned place preference, and potentiation of self-stimulation (270, 275–278). In the NAc, rats self-inject morphine or enkephalin (279,280). From a clinical point of view, it is conceivable that this feeding reinforcement system depicted in Figure 2 is the metabolism-modulated, taste-activated appetitive system that drives bingeing behavior (281). Enterostatin, a peptide released by a fatty meal, may suppress food intake by inhibiting a kappa opioid feeding component (282), which may also be linked to GAL. Logically, enterostatin may inhibit the LH-PBN orexin/DYN pathway of the feeding reinforcement system, but this is yet to be demonstrated.

3 Inhibition of Opioid Reward and Feeding

Kappa agonists have either stimulatory or inhibitory effects on feeding in different parts of the brain. As reviewed above, food deprivation potentiates behavior in part by releasing DYN-A in the PBN (250). On the other hand kappa agonists in the VTA or NAc inhibit the mesolimbic DA system (283) and may play a role in stopping food intake or generating aversion. Thus, there seems to be more than one kappa opioid system involved in the circuitry for eating (284). Naloxone injected locally in the NAc to block opioid receptors, probably the mu subtype, can release ACh, and the ACh can inhibit feeding. Naloxone works in the NAc when something has been done to release endogenous opioids, such as food deprivation or morphine treatment (285). After a week of daily morphine injections, local or systemic naloxone precipitates withdrawal, and in the NAc, the release of DA decreases while ACh increases (285). The same response occurs with systemic naloxone injection after a few weeks of drinking excessive amounts of sugar in the binge-eating model described in Section VII below.

G Amandamide

The endogenous cannabinoid, amandamide, can induce eating and may interact with opioid systems (286). Tetrahydrocannabinol (THC) induces accumbens DA release that can be blocked by an opioid antagonist in the VTA. Thus, marijuana reinforces behavior, in part, by releasing DA via an opioid system. This may also be the mechanism through which marijuana induces appetite for food (287). A cannabinoid receptor antagonist reduces food intake in rats (288). The same drug causes a small but significant decrease in body weight in people (289).

H Growth Hormone-Releasing Hormone

Growth hormone regulates overall body and cell growth, in addition to nutrient metabolism (290). Its release is stimulated by GHRH, while inhibited by somatostain. Evidence suggests a stimulatory role for GHRH in feeding behavior (Fig. 1) (291–294). Central injections of GHRH enhance food intake in rats and sheep. The hypothalamic regions most responsive to this peptide effect are in the area of the MPO and SCN, which have a high concentration of GHRH-containing terminals. This feeding-stimulatory action is centrally mediated and independent of the growth hormone-promoting properties.

From injection studies at different times of the circadian cycle, it seems that endogenous GHRH may contribute to the burst of feeding exhibited at the start of the active cycle (292–294). This proposal receives support from experiments with antiserum raised against GHRH, which suppresses spontaneous feeding. Injections of GHRH stimulate intake of protein, having little impact on carbohydrate or fat intake. Moreover, an antiserum against GHRH preferentially inhibits protein consumption at the onset of the natural feeding cycle. This may reflect a role for endogenous GHRH, in the MPO/SCN area, in stimulating both growth and the ingestion of the nutrients important for growth.

There is evidence that growth hormone–releasing peptides (GHRP), acting within the brain, mimic an unidentified native GH-releasing hormone-amplifying hormone. Systemic administration of GHRP-6 induces c-Fos protein in the ARC (295). Further, intracerebroventricular administration of low doses of the GHRP, KP-102, stimulates feeding in rats, while having no effect after systemic administration, and it amplifies the feeding-stimulatory effect of GHRH through a specific GHRP receptor, possibly in the hypothalamus (296). There is also evidence that GHRH may interact with other neurochemical systems in the brain to control eating and body weight. For example, the GHRH system is closely associated with, and may depend on, the opioid system in the PVN. Opiate agonists stimulate the ingestion of protein as well as fat, an effect blocked by GHRH antiserum, and the action of GHRH is antagonized by PVN injections of opioid receptor antagonists (291,297). Also, GHRH-expressing neurons in the ARC coexpress GAL, which stimulates feeding and increases adiposity after chronic administration (see above). Studies demonstrate that, in these ARC neurons, GAL expression is induced by GH and reduced in the absence of GH, suggesting that the pattern of GHRH and GH release may, in turn, be shaped by GAL (172). In a recent study, double-labeling immunohistochemistry indicates that orexin-containing, but not MCH-containing, neurons in the LH are activated by central administration of GHRP-6 (298).

In obesity, GH secretion is impaired, secondary to the rise in body fat and circulating lipids, and treatment with GH decreases adiposity, reduces triglyceride accumulation, and enhances lipolysis (290,299). A role for GH in body fat accumulation is confirmed by the observation that mice overexpressing GH have increased abdominal fat (300). They are larger and exhibit hyperphagia and increased levels of insulin and leptin, in association with reduced responsiveness of the leptin receptor to fasting. Whereas the physiological mechanisms underlying this obese state remain to be defined, this mouse model points to the importance of GHRH in the regulation of body composition.

I Ghrelin

Recent evidence suggests that, in addition to GHRH, there exists another peptide, ghrelin, which stimulates the release of GH (301). Ghrelin is a 28–amino acid peptide, and its mRNA is expressed in the stomach. It is secreted into blood vessels to act directly on pituitary cells to stimulate GH release (302). Although ghrelin content in the brain is low, a population of ghrelin-containing neurons exists in the ARC. In addition to producing a dose-dependent rise in GH, intracerebroventricular administration of ghrelin potentiates food intake (303–306) and stimulates gastric acid secretion and motility (307). In contrast to the other feeding-stimulatory peptides described above, ghrelin also stimulates eating when administered peripherally, although the response is not as strong or sustained as that seen with central ghrelin. Antighrelin antibodies suppress feeding behavior with central as well as peripheral administration, supporting a role for endogenous ghrelin in this behavioral response. The feeding-stimulatory effect of ghrelin is independent of this peptide's ability to stimulate GH secretion (305). Ghrelin may stimulate feeding to ensure the provision of calories that GH requires for growth and repair (308).

Ghrelin acts through the growth hormone secretagogue (GHS) receptor. This receptor is expressed at high levels in the ARC. Systemically administered ghrelin increases the electrical activity and *c-fos* gene expression in ARC neurons (309), suggesting that it reaches these receptors through the general circulation. The GHS receptor mRNA is found in essentially all neurons expressing NPY, but it exists in only a small percentage of POMC- or GHRH-expressing neurons. Ghrelin injection increases NPY as well as AGRP mRNA, while having no effect on POMC mRNA (303,304,306,310). Further, NPY antagonists inhibit ghrelin-induced feeding (298). Whereas these findings suggest a role for NPY in mediating ghrelin's action, this peptide is not essential, since ghrelin can increase feeding and body weight in NPY-deficient mice (305).

There is some evidence indicating the involvement of ghrelin in obesity. With chronic subcutaneous injections in mice, ghrelin increases body weight, with a significant gain in fat mass but no change in lean body mass (305). This is accompanied by an increase in respiratory quotient, reflecting a decrease in fat metabolism. Whereas one study shows that ghrelin mRNA in the stomach is stimulated by chronic administration of leptin (311), other evidence reveals a competitive interaction between ghrelin and leptin. Ghrelin concentrations in the blood and mRNA in the stomach are increased by fasting that reduces leptin, and ghrelin is suppressed by feeding (303,305). Further, ghrelin mRNA is elevated in leptin-deficient *ob/ob* mice and reduced by acute leptin injection (308). The role of ghrelin in weight gain is suggested by evidence that the obese phenotype of *ob/ob* mice is partially reversed by antighrelin antiserum (303). Also, the reduction in weight gain induced by a pro-inflammatory cytokine is attenuated by ghrelin administation (303). Circulating ghrelin levels are decreased in states of obesity in humans (308). Ghrelin is also reduced by carbohydrate diets and glucose in rodents (303,305). This suggests the involvement of this peptide in physiological mechanisms of glucose homeostasis.

J Beacon

The *beacon* gene was recently identified by differential display polymerase hypothalamic mRNA from a polygenic animal model of obesity and type II diabetes (312). This gene is overexpressed in the hypothalamus of obese animals, and its mRNA level is positively correlated with body fat content. Immunohistochemical studies localize beacon mRNA to the retrochiasmatic area of the hypothalamus. Central administration of beacon stimulates food intake and increases NPY expression in the ARC (312). Repeated injections of beacon increase feeding behavior and weight gain, primarily owing to an increase in body fat accrual (313). With no detectable effect of beacon on nutrient partitioning, physical activity, or energy expenditure, the accumulation of body fat is attributed primarily to the changes in food ingestion (313). This contrasts with other feeding-stimulatory peptides, described above, which have potent and diverse effects on metabolic processes.

K VGF

VGF was originally identified as a nerve growth factor–regulated transcript, which is rapidly stimulated by neurotrophins (314). Its mRNA and encoded protein are selectively synthesized in neuroendocrine and neuronal cells, and VGF is stored and released from dense core vesicles through the regulated secretory pathway. The VGF polypeptide sequence is rich in paired basic amino acids, potential sites for proteolytic processing. A range of low-molecular-weight VGF peptides have been identified that are preferentially released by nerve terminals upon stimulation (315). This suggests that VGF is the precursor of one or more biologically active peptides and that it may play a role in the regulated release of other peptides from secretory vesicles (314).

While widely expressed through the central and peripheral nervous systems, VGF mRNA is particularly abundant in the hypothalamus (316). In the suprachiasmatic nucleus, VGF mRNA is induced by light and exhibits a circadian rhythm in animals kept in constant light (314). An investigation of VGF knockout mice (317) suggests the involvement of VGF in energy homeostasis. Mice lacking the protein display markedly reduced body weight, body fat, and leptin, indicating a possible stimulatory role for this protein in weight regulation. The major defect in these mice is excess energy expenditure and locomotor activity, rather than reduced food intake. Fasting stimulates VGF mRNA in the ARC (314). Further, the VGF knockout mice exhibit altered expression of hypothalamic peptides in the ARC that affect feeding and metabolism. Whereas VGF-deficient mice have elevated NPY and AGRP mRNA, they show a reduction in POMC expression. Thus, VGF's mechanism of action may involve an effect on the synthesis and release of these peptides known to be involved in energy homeostasis.

L Prolactin

Prolactin (PRL) is a peptide hormone, which is elevated during lactation, a physiological culmination of the reproductive cycle in female mammals (58). This hormone is synthesized in the anterior pituitary gland but is also expressed, albeit in low concentrations, by cells in the brain, notably the medial basal hypothalamus (318). As the mammary tissue develops the capacity for milk production, there occurs an increase in demand for nutrients, leading the lactating female to look to both metabolic and behavioral adaptations to meet these demands (58). These adaptations include hyperphagia, conservation of energy by reduced activity, decreased rates of nonshivering thermogenesis, lipid synthesis, triglycerol turnover, and more efficient use of nutrients through a change in insulin responsiveness.

Injection studies reveal multiple behavioral as well as physiological actions of PRL related to reproduction. In addition to its well-known actions of enhancing milk production and stimulating growth, PRL acts on behavioral systems. It increases grooming, facilitates sexual receptivity, and promotes maternal behavior (319). Prolactin also stimulates eating behavior in mammals and birds. Lactation in rodents is characterized by marked hyperphagia. Prolactin levels and hyperphagia are directly proportional to litter size, suggesting a causal relationship (58,320,321). An increase in food intake is also seen after systemic administration of PRL in female rats. Interestingly, a protein-rich diet is preferred after PRL injections, as well as during lactation (58,320,322). Prolactin is effective when administered into the brain, where it functions independently of ovarian hormones (323). Sites of action include nuclei of the MH where PRL receptors are concentrated (319,324). A feedback loop may involve the eating-stimulatory peptide GAL, which is synthesized in PVN neurons and stimulates the release of PRL from the pituitary (325). A hypothalamic β-endorphin-containing circuit may also play a role (326).

The possibility that PRL controls fat synthesis is suggested by the findings that the PRL receptor exists in mouse adipocytes (327) and that DA-induced inhibition of PRL secretion decreases fat stores and blocks lipogenic responsiveness to insulin (328). In addition, fat deposition in migrating species is promoted or inhibited in close relation to circulating levels of PRL as well as CORT. An increase in plasma prolactin is seen in females following puberty, a time of fat deposition (329). Responses to PRL and the circadian rhythm of PRL release are altered in adult obesity, perhaps owing to hyperinsulinemia, and these disturbances are normalized by weight reduction. In obese men, a strong, positive correlation is evident between fasting levels of leptin and prolactin (330).

IV PEPTIDES THAT REDUCE EATING AND BODY WEIGHT

Many peptides have been discovered that have inhibitory effects on feeding and weight gain (Table 1). An important question addressed in the investigation of these substances is whether their behavioral or physiological effects are both specific and meaningful in the overall control of energy balance. Discussed below are most of the satiety peptides that have sufficient evidence to support their role in the control of feeding and metabolism. In most cases, the peptides are synthesized in the brain to act through local neurocircuits. In others, these substances are synthesized in peripheral organs and send signals to the brain via the circulation, vagus nerve, or sympathetic afferents.

A Melanocortins

Pro-opiomelanocortin (POMC) is a 267–amino acid precursor protein that is synthesized in the ARC as well as the anterior pituitary. The posttranslational processing of POMC results in a number of peptides with very different biological activities. In the anterior pituitary, it is processed predominantly to ACTH as well as to β-lipoprotein. In the ARC, ACTH is further processed to produce α-MSH, whereas β-lipoprotein is cleaved to β-endorphin. Pharmacological studies show that central injections of α-MSH and other MSH agonists suppress food intake and reduce body weight (331). Mice with a mutation in the coding region for the POMC-derived peptides have defective adrenal development and lack corticosteroids (332). They also develop hyperphagia and obesity, which are reversed by injections of α-MSH (332). A similar phenotype is seen in humans with a genetic POMC mutation resulting in a deficiency of α-MSH (333).

The biological actions of the MSH peptides are mediated by interactions with at least five G-protein-coupled receptors, with the MC3-R and MC4-R heavily expressed in the brain. Whereas the MC3-R is localized to the hypothalamus and limbic system and is richly expressed in the ARC including in POMC neurons, the MC4-R is more widely distributed throughout the brain and, within the hypothalamus, is highly expressed specifically in the PVN and PFLH (334). Pharmacological blockade or targeted disruption of MC4-R in rodents produces hyperhagia, increased fat mass, and hyperinsulinemia (24,335,336), and spontaneous MC4-R mutations have been linked to morbid obesity in humans (24,337). The additional importance of the MC3-R in energy homeostasis is indicated by the finding that mice lacking this receptor have increased fat mass but not hyperphagia, whereas mice lacking both the MC3-R and MC4-R weigh more than mice lacking only the MC4-R (338). A recent study in MC4-R-null mutant mice suggests a role for this receptor, independent of leptin, in mediating high-fat diet–induced thermogenesis and increase in physical activity (339).

Two naturally occurring MSH antagonists, agouti protein and AGRP (see Section III), have been identified. Agouti, which is normally expressed in hair follicles, antagonizes the effects of α-MSH at the MC1-R and, consequently, blocks the synthesis of pigments, resulting in a lighter coat color (334). Ectopic expression of agouti seen in the yellow mouse obesity syndrome, similar to that seen with targeted disruption of the MC4-R (340), leads to the blockade of MC4-R in the brain, and this causes a phenotype of hyperphagia, hyperinsulinemia and obesity (341). In transgenic mice, the overexpression of AGRP in ARC neurons also causes hyperphagia, hyperinsulinemia, and obesity (178,182). Injections of AGRP, as well as other synthetic melanocortin receptor antagonists, can block the inhibition of food intake induced by α-MSH and, by themselves, can stimulate feeding, indicating a role for endogenous α-

MSH in food intake control (342). The interaction of these melanocortin antagonists with the melanocortin receptors may be mediated or facilitated by the protein mahogany. This neuroactive protein may increase the concentration of agouti/AGRP antagonists in the vicinity of the MC1-R or MC4-R or affect the process of receptor desensitization via posttranslational modifications or cellular internalization (343).

A complex neuronal system involves a variety of downstream MC4-R- and MC3-R-containing neurons in the ARC. The endogenous antagonist AGRP is expressed in separate neurons medial to those expressing POMC, and AGRP-immunoreactive fibers form a projection that is separate from, but overlaps, the α-MSH fibers (183). This indicates that the melanocortin system may function either through agonists released by POMC neurons or through an endogenous antagonist released from non-POMC neurons (Fig. 1). Despite this dissociation, the α-MSH and AGRP peptides very likely interact at the hypothalamic MC4-R in their role in maintaining energy homeostasis. These peptides are modulated in a reciprocal fashion by various manipulations, such as leptin or food deprivation, and also in obese, leptin-deficient, or leptin receptor–deficient mice (183,344). Although this reciprocal relationship between the agonist and antagonist is not apparent under all conditions (344), the evidence generally suggests that leptin can regulate the melanocortin system either by increasing levels of the agonist, α-MSH, or by decreasing levels of the antagonist, AGRP. The importance of the melanocortin system in the signaling cascade of leptin in the brain is further revealed by evidence that antagonists of the melanocortin receptor block the feeding-inhibitory and metabolic-stimulatory actions of leptin (345,346). There is electrophysiological evidence that leptin increases the frequency of action potentials in the anorexigenic POMC neurons, either by depolarization or by reducing the inhibitory effect of local orexigenic NPY neurons (347).

As indicated above, the melanocortin system and NPY neurocircuit are closely related. The POMC and NPY neurons are concentrated in the ARC and project to similar nuclei of the hypothalamus, including the PVN where MC4-R immunoreactivity is dense (334). Moreover, pharmacological studies demonstrate a complete suppression of NPY's orexigenic effect with injection of the melanocortin agonist, MTII (348). Electrophysiolocal studies provide evidence supporting a cellular basis for this interaction (24). The melanocortin antagonist, AGRP , which colocalizes with NPY in ARC neurons (98,179), is a potent stimulant of feeding behavior. As described in Section III, injection of AGRP, like NPY, promotes body fat accrual and increases insulin levels (181). Moreover, measurements of endogenous NPY and AGRP expression reveal opposite patterns to those detected with measurements of POMC and α-MSH (349). This evidence supports the idea that the melanocortin and NPY systems interact antagonistically in the control of eating and body weight.

B Cytokines

Cytokines are protein molecules released by lymphocytes and/or monocyte macrophages during various disease states, such as infection and cancer. Several proinflammatory cytokines, most notably tumor necrosis factor-alpha (TNFα), interleukin (IL)-1, IL-6, and ciliary neurotropic factor (CNTF), induce anorexia and body weight loss (88,350,351). Evidence suggests that the anorexia is mediated by central neural mechanisms, most notably in the hypothalamus where the receptors for most cytokines are particularly dense (352). Peripherally administered TNFα and IL-1B produce anorexia in rats at doses estimated to yield pathophysiological concentrations in the cerebrospinal fluid of animal models or patients with wasting disorders (353). These peripheral cytokines are released into the circulation and, through the blood brain barrier and circumventricular organs, are transported into the brain, where they exert their effects via the vagus nerve or second messengers, such as nitric oxide and prostanoids in the brain vasculature. Cytokines are also produced by neurons and glia within the brain, including the hypothalamus, in response to microbial and inflammatory products or peripheral cytokines. Whereas the absence of TNFα does not prevent the development of obesity, targeted mutation of the TNFα gene or its type 1 and 2 receptor subtypes improves insulin sensitivity, supporting a role for TNFα as a mediator of insulin resistance in obesity-diabetes models (88,354). Furthermore, IL-1B and IL-6 mutant mice resist anorexia, body weight loss, and fever caused by inflammatory-inducing agents, and IL-1 receptor antagonist–null mice have reduced body weight (88).

The idea that circulating signals generated in proportion to body fat mass influence appetite and energy expenditure through central mechanisms has been clearly demonstrated with the cloning of the leptin gene (20) and the finding that leptin, which is positively related to body fat mass, reduces food intake through leptin receptors in the hypothalamus (22). Leptin is a member of the IL-6 superfamily of proteins, with many biochemical features of a cytokine molecule (20), and the leptin receptor is most closely related to glycoprotein 130, a common signal transducer among receptors for members of the IL-6 superfamily (355,356). Evidence suggests that leptin increases hypothalamic production of cytokines (357) and activates cytokinelike signal transduction pathways, by stimulating JAK-STAT via the leptin receptor (358–360) (see Table 1 for abbreviations). Leptin also activates SOCS-3, which reduces intracellular signaling by inhibiting JAK activity, a potential mechanism underlying leptin resistance (360). Thus, excessive leptin or leptinlike signaling, resulting from increased inflammatory cytokines in overlapping and redundant cytokine networks, may contribute to the anorexia and weight loss in wasting illnesses (361), although it is not essential to this response (362).

In light of the inhibitory effect of leptin on NPY expression in the ARC described above, it is not surprising to find a similar relationship between circulating cytokines and the NPY feeding system in the development of anorexia (361). Cytokines such as IL-1 and CNTF antagonize NPY gene expression in the ARC and reduce NPY-induced feeding as well as Y_1 receptor abundance (363,364). Whereas this effect may occur indirectly via stimulation of leptin secretion (361), a direct action is supported by the finding that a CNTF derivative corrects the obesity and metabolic disorders of mice deficient in leptin or its receptor and also of diet-induced obesity models unresponsive to leptin (358). Further evidence supporting the involvement of NPY in cytokine effects is obtained in anorexic, tumor-bearing rats, which show a reduction in NPY levels or release, NPY-induced feeding, and NPY receptor affinity in association with anorexia and weight loss (353,365).

Whereas cytokine-induced anorexia may also involve other neurochemicals, such as CRH, CCK, and 5HT, that suppress feeding and modulate NPY (88,361,366), there is compelling evidence supporting a key role for the melanocortin system that provides a bidirectional tuning necessary to maintain energy stability under different conditions (367,368). This includes the finding that anorexia and weight loss induced by sarcoma growth are both reversed and prevented by administration of AGRP, the endogenous melanocortin antagonist. Further, both genetic and pharmacologic blockade of central melanocortin receptor signaling prevents the complex cytokine response and the weight loss that accompanies lipopolysaccharide injection. Whereas a close relationship is known to exist between leptin and the melanocortin system, the effects of melanocortin blockade occur independently of this hormone.

Since the discovery that CNTF produces severe anorexia and weight loss in rodents and humans, further studies have been conducted to more fully characterize this effect (358,366). A CNTF derivative, $CNTF_{Ax15}$, is highly effective in correcting obesity and resulting metabolic disorders in mice, apparently with minimal side effects. It is believed to act by penetrating the blood brain barrier and impacting on the alpha subunit of the CNTF receptor complex in the hypothalamus. It mobilizes intracellular signal transduction pathways that are similar to those activated by leptin, but not the prototype cytokine, IL-1. Like leptin, CNTF reduces NPY-induced feeding and NPY mRNA and peptide in the ARC and PVN. However, it functions independently of leptin, as well as the melanocortin system. In fact, it is effective in diet-induced obesity models that are resistant to leptin (358). The ability of CNTF to produce weight loss and improve insulin sensitivity in humans makes this compound an attractive agent for obesity treatment, given that certain side effects can be controlled (366,369).

C Cocaine- and Amphetamine-Regulated Transcript

Cocaine- and amphetamine-regulated transcript (CART) was originally identified by differential display polymerase chain reaction as a novel mRNA stimulated after acute administration of psychomotor stimulants (370). The predicted protein product of CART mRNA has a leader sequence and several pairs of basic amino acids, suggesting that it is processed and secreted. The mature peptide contains several cleavage sites, indicating that CART may be posttranscriptionally processed into long and short fragments, with both forms of CART peptides found in the rat and only the short-form peptide found in humans (370,371). In the rat, CART mRNA and the short-form CART peptide (amino acids 42–89) are found in various nuclei of the hypothalamus, including the ARC, PVN, and LH, as well as in extrahypothalamic areas (372–374). Moreover, CART coexists with peptides involved in the control of energy balance. Virtually all CART neurons in the ARC also express POMC (375), as well as the long-form leptin receptor (376). Hypothalamic CART neurons outside the ARC coexpress DYN and MCH and, as in the ARC, are direct targets of leptin (376). Further, in the PVN, 25–50% of CART-expressing neurons express GAL (377,378), and CART coexists with GAL or MCH in neurons of the PFLH (377,379).

A number of studies suggest that CART has a role in eating behavior and obesity. Administration of this peptide produces a dose-dependent decrease in food intake and reduces feeding stimulated by NPY (380,381). Moreover, antibodies that block CART increase nocturnal feeding, suggesting that this peptide has a tonic inhibitory effect on food intake (382). Other effects of CART include a stimulation of uncoupling proteins (383) and inhibition of gastric acid secretion (384). Chronic administration of CART leads to a marked decrease in body weight in rats (385).

Investigations of the endogenous peptide show that CART expression is regulated by leptin (380). It is stimulated by leptin administration and is reduced in genetically obese *fa/fa* rats, leptin-deficient *ob/ob* mice, and food-deprived rats. Whereas this decline in CART may contribute to the hyperphagia characteristic of these animals, overeating and obesity induced by a high-fat diet is similarly associated with elevated levels of leptin, together with CART in the hypothalamus (386), in particular the ARC and PVN (387). Since obesity induced by a high-fat diet is less marked than that of genetically obese rodents, this higher expression of CART on a fat-rich diet may function in limiting the level of body fat accrual. Supporting this idea are recent studies showing that targeted deletion of the *CART* gene in mice on a high-fat diet induces hyperphagia and increased body weight and fat mass compared to wild-type mice on the same diet (388). Other genetic studies provide further evidence that variation in the *CART* locus may influence fat distribution and variables related to syndrome X (389).

D Corticotropin-Releasing Hormone

A well-known role of corticotropin-releasing hormone (CRH) is to control the HPA axis, exerting powerful regulatory effects on the release of ACTH and glucocorticoids. In addition, however, this peptide has been implicated in the mediation of the integrated physiological and behavioral responses of stress, which are largely independent of the activation of the HPA axis and involve a direct action of CRH on brain receptors.

Included in the responses of endogenous CRH are changes in eating behavior and metabolism, involving a constellation of effects favoring a state of negative energy balance (88,390–394). The specific effects observed with CRH injections into the MH or PVN include a marked suppression of spontaneous or fasting-induced feeding. This is coupled with stimulation of sympathetic outflow, which increases lipolysis and energy expenditure and raises blood glucose, while inhibiting any increase in insulin secretion. Chronic central CRH administration causes a sustained reduction in food intake and body weight. Urocortin, an endogenous peptide related to CRH, is considerably more potent than CRH in suppressing feeding, and is more selective in binding to the CRH_2 receptor subtype, which may mediate the anorexic and thermogenic responses (395). Studies in knockout mice suggest that the feeding-suppressive effect induced by urocortin may actually have two phases, with the early phase mediated by the CRH_1 receptor and the long-term phase by the CRH_2 receptor (394).

A role of endogenous CRH or urocortin in energy balance is suggested by evidence showing an increase in feeding after pharmacological blockade of CRH receptors, expression, or synthesis (88,394,396). This receives further support from the finding that food intake is reduced by chronic administration of a CRH-binding protein inhibitor, which increases CRH/urocortin availability in the hypothalamus (397). In states of glucocorticoid insufficiency induced by adrenalectomy, CRH expression in the PVN is enhanced, and this neurochemical change is associated with a decline in eating and body weight, impaired recovery of weight loss after food deprivation, and the prevention of experimentally induced obesity (392). Circulating glucocorticoids normally released by CRH may provide the feedback signal for inhibition of CRH and regulation of adipose tissue. Other studies have suggested the involvement of CRH or urocortin in the anorexic effects induced by restraint stress, treadmill running, E_2, and caffeine and in the thermogenic actions of 5HT agonists (394). Possible sites of action include the PVN and MPO (31,398). The finding that MC4-R-deficient mice are hypersensitive to the anorexic effects of CRH provides evidence for crosstalk between the melanocortin and CRH pathways (399,400).

There is further evidence supporting the possibility that CRH has a role in the development of obesity. Chronic injections of CRH or an inhibitor of the CRH-binding protein reduce weight gain in genetically obese rats with normally reduced CRH content in the hypothalamus (397). Moreover, the expression of the CRH_2 receptor in the VMH is reduced in obese rats, and leptin suppresses the synthesis and release of CRH (394). A variety of evidence focuses attention on CRH as an important mediator of the actions of leptin. The behavioral and metabolic effects of CRH are similar to those produced by leptin, and the anorexic effects of leptin are attenuated by CRH antagonists (394,401). In addition, central injection of leptin increases hypothalamic CRH content (401).

A variety of evidence demonstrates a close, inverse relationship between CRH and the feeding-stimulatory peptide NPY (396,402,403). Administration of CRH reduces NPY-elicited feeding as well as NPY gene expression in the ARC (404), and CRH antagonists enhance NPY feeding (396,402). In addition, adrenalectomy, which enhances CRH expression in the PVN, suppresses NPY mRNA in the ARC, and these effects are reversed by glucocorticoids (405,406). Thus, conditions associated with changes in eating behavior and body weight have opposite effects on CRH and NPY. These studies support the possibility that the effects of CRH may be mediated, in part, by inhibition of endogenous NPY, whereby a reduction in CRH release mediates the stimulatory effect of glucocorticoids on NPY. A role for leptin in this relationship between CRH and NPY is suggested by the evidence demonstrating a negative feedback loop between leptin and glucocorticoids (406).

Central CRH blockade also inhibits anorexia evoked by stress, such as physical restraint, suggesting a direct relation between endogenous CRH and stress-related changes in feeding (407,408). The actions of CRH on metabolism and energy balance, as well as gastric emptying, may also involve alterations in immune signals, particularly cytokines (393,409). This is reflected in the similarity of their effects, in the stimulatory effect of cytokines, such as IL-1, on CRH release and HPA axis, and in the essential role of CRH in the hypophagic effect of IL-1 and its impact on fever, thermogenesis, and ACTH release. The possibility of bidirectional communication is suggested by the influence of CRH on immune and inflammatory responses. Thus, the role of this peptide in energy balance must be evaluated in a broader context, as an integrator of the physiological responses to stress in relation to immunity and infection.

E Enterostatin

Enterostatin (ENT) is the intestinal amino-terminal pentapeptide that is released from pancreatic procolipase in response to fat intake, with the remaining colipase serving as an essential cofactor for pancreatic lipase during the digestion of fat (410). Procolipase gene transcription and ENT release into the lymph and circulation are increased by high-fat diets. Also, systematically or centrally injected ENT selectively inhibits voluntary intake of fat as opposed to carbohydrate. This pentapeptide acts through sites in the brain as well as the periphery, and peripheral responses to ENT are dependent on an afferent vagal signaling pathway to the brain (145,411,412). Systemically administered ENT activates neurons in the PVN, where injections of this peptide also reduce food intake, performing a function that parallels its actions in the gut (413).

An ENT circuit in the brain causes satiety through both serotonergic and opioid interactions in the brain (410). It inhibits the opioid system that promotes fat ingestion (282). Enterostatin antagonizes kappa agonists that stimulate fat intake, and, conversely, a kappa agonist (U50488) at low doses can interfere with the suppression of fat intake normally caused by ENT. Also, both ENT and kappa antagonists suppress an animal's choice of fatty food. Thus, York and Lin (413) propose the existence of a kappa opioid system in the PVN that controls appetite for fat and that is inhibited by ENT. They also demonstrate that ENT reduces the consumption of a fat-rich diet induced by GAL, whereas it has no effect on NPY-elicited feeding (414). This is consistent with the evidence showing endogenous GAL to be stimulated by high-fat diet consumption, while NPY expression is reduced (see Sec. III). As described below, the GAL-ENT-kappa system supported by this evidence may control the balance between DA and ACh in the NAc for the promotion and inhibition of instrumental responses for fatty food (see Sec. VI).

A possible role for ENT in obesity is indicated by evidence that chronically administered ENT reduces fat intake and body fat accrual (415). This effect may result from multiple metabolic actions of ENT. These include a decrease in insulin secretion, activation of the sympathetic nervous system and stimulation of the HPA axis. Studies show low ENT production or responsiveness in rats that are fat preferring and become obese. In humans, there is some evidence that obesity is associated with reduced secretion of pancreatic procolipase (410) or ENT (416) after a test meal.

F Neurotensin

Neurotensin (NT), a 13–amino acid peptide, increases in the plasma of humans after eating a meal, and the increase is significantly larger if the meal is hot and palatable rather than cold and poorly accepted (417). When NT is injected peripherally in rats, there is no compelling evidence that it causes satiety by itself (418), although large doses are reported to inhibit feeding and grooming behaviors (419). Peripheral NT may act physiologically in synergy with other satiety peptides normally released at the same time.

When injected into the PVN-MH region, NT decreases food intake, provided the active portion of the peptide chain is used (418,420). It also inhibits the orexigenic effect of MCH, but has no impact on NPY (421). Neurotensin is expressed and synthesized in the ARC, PVN and DMN. Its expression in the hypothalamus is elevated in rats consuming a high-carbohydrate diet (422) and is reduced in association with the development of obesity in *ob/ob* mice and *fa/fa* rats (423,424). There is evidence that NT may be involved in mediating the central effect of leptin on feeding. Both NT antiserum and NT receptor antagonist completely block the inhibitory effect of leptin on food intake (425). Further, leptin injection stimulates NT expression in the hypothalamus (426) and potentiates NT's satiety-producing effect (427). In fat-preferring rats, NT concentrations in the PVN are increased and positively correlated with elevated levels of leptin (427).

This peptide interacts closely with the monoamines, which are reviewed in more detail in Section V below. Neurotensin modulates hypothalamic NE release (428) and inhibits feeding induced by NE (420). In the mesolimbic system, NT is colocalized with DA in neurons that project from the VTA to the NAc. Neurotensin iontophoresed into the VTA increases DA cell firing rate. These clues have led to the demonstration that rats self-inject NT into the VTA (429). Repeated NT injections in the VTA sensitize animals to the hyperactivity produced by subsequent injections, due to increased responsiveness of DA neurons (430). In the posterior, medial NAc where NT is coreleased with DA, injections of NT are like CCK in potentiating self-stimulation (431). On the other hand, NT in parts of the NAc can prevent dopaminergic effects and, thus, alter motivation. Glucocorticoids may also affect motivation by acting on peptide expression in the NAc (432).

G Apolipoproteins

Apolipoprotein A-IV (apo A-IV) is a glycoprotein produced by the small intestine and released into the blood in response to a lipid meal (433–436). The increased synthesis of apo A-IV in response to fat absorption, rather than related to the uptake or reesterification of fatty acids to triglycerides, is induced by the formation of chylomicrons. It may also be responsive to a factor from the ileum, probably peptide tyrosine-tyrosine (PYY). The evidence that other apolipoproteins in the intestine are unresponsive to fat consumption indicates a specific role for apo A-IV in relation to dietary fat. After systemic or central administration, apo A-IV causes a significant, dose-dependent suppression of feeding. Since the secretion of apo A-IV is rapid, this protein may play a role in the short-term control of food intake, acting as a circulating satiety signal produced specifically by a high-fat meal. Apo A-IV may also be involved in the long-term regulation of food intake and body weight. Chronic ingestion of a high-fat diet blunts the intestinal apo A-IV response to lipid feeding, in conjunction with a rise in leptin. This suggests a possible mechanism whereby a high-fat diet promotes obesity. Pharmacological studies show that apo A-IV synthesis is reduced by leptin administration (436).

De novo synthesis of apo A-IV in the brain is under investigation (437). Studies support the possibility that apo A-IV released by the small intestine traverses the blood brain barrier, enters the cerebrospinal fluid, and is taken up by astrocytes (436). A recent investigation, however, has revealed apo A-IV mRNA in the hypothalamus, particularly in the ARC, and has demonstrated an increase in expression after consumption of a high-fat diet (438). The existence of apo A-IV in the ARC suggests a possible relationship with neuropeptides, such as NPY, in the control of feeding. This receives support from the finding that NPY injection stimulates the expression of ap A-IV in the hypothalamus (438). This is interesting in light of the evidence (436) that apo A-IV synthesis and secretion in the intestine are stimulated by PYY, a member of the peptide family that includes NPY. This peptide is believed to mediate the stimulatory effect of a high-fat diet on apo A-IV and possibly to act centrally by sending signals through the vagus nerve.

There is evidence that another apolipoprotein, apo D, may also have a role in body weight regulation. In contrast to other apolipoproteins, apo D is heavily expressed in the brain, most abundantly in the hypothalamus, and it exists at low levels in peripheral tissues (438). To clone genes that regulate food ingestion and body fat accrual, a recent study (438) used both representational difference analysis to identify genes responsive to dietary fat and the yeast two-hybrid system to isolate proteins that interact with the leptin receptor, Ob-Rb. This report demonstrates that apo D mRNA in the hypothalamus is stimulated by consumption of a high-fat diet. Moreover, this protein interacts with the cytoplasmic portion of Ob-Rb and not with the short-form receptor, Ob-Ra. Anatomical studies show that apo D and Ob-Rb are coexpressed in neurons and other cell types in the ARC and PVN (438). In addition to being stimulated by dietary fat, hypothalamic apo D mRNA is elevated in rats and inbred mice that become obese on a high-fat diet. This phenomenon may occur in response to changes in leptin and body fat, which are also increased and strongly, positively correlated with apo D mRNA. This positive association with body fat, however, is lost in obese *ob/ob* and *db/db* mice, which exhibit markedly reduced levels of hypothalamic apo D mRNA compared to that of wild-type mice. This suggests a role for apo D in obesity on a high-fat diet.

Although designated an "apolipoprotein," apo D is atypical in that it actually belongs to the lipocalin family of proteins that bind and transport small hydrophobic ligands (5,439–441). However, the specific ligand to which apo D binds has not been unequivocally identified. Numerous reports suggest that it may bind to a variety of small molecules (5,442). That apo D binds with progesterone in breast cyst fluid (443) and with an axillary odorant in apocrine glands (444) suggests that the ligand may be specific to the tissue or cell type where apo D is expressed. In hypothalamic neurons, apo D may have a specific ligand where it exerts signaling functions similar to that of other apolipoproteins (445). This putative ligand may be produced as a consequence of the leptin stimulation of Ob-Rb. In fact, previous work has suggested the existence of a ligand generated following the activation of Ob-Rb (446). This apo D–specific ligand may be either a small molecule that functions as a paracrine signal within particular hypothalamic nuclei or a hormone that enters the circulation, possibly via the pituitary, where both apo D and Ob-Rb are expressed in moderate levels. Pregnenolone may be one such candidate that deserves further investigation as a specific ligand that binds apo D in the hypothalamus and participates in body weight regulation. This steroid is present in the brain and associates with apo D with high affinity (447,448). Further, its production is modulated by leptin (449), and high plasma levels of pregnenolone are associated with hyperphagia in rats (450) and obesity in humans (451). Taken together, this evidence suggests that apo D in the hypothalamus is involved in the leptin/Ob-Rb signal transduction pathway and that a deficiency of apo D protein contributes to the development of obesity, particularly on a high-fat diet (438). This proposed function of hypothalamic apo D is consistent with previous reports that a T*aq* I apo D polymorphism is linked to obesity and hyperinsulinemia, as well as to non-insulin-dependent diabetes mellitus, a condition commonly associated with obesity in animals and humans (438).

H Glucagon

Glucagon is released from the pancreas during a meal (452,453). Pharmacological studies indicate that portal vein administration of glucagon reduces the size of spontaneous meals, whereas highly specific glucagon antibodies increase meal size, suggesting a physiological role in controlling food intake. The mechanism for glucagon's satiety action may involve signals within the liver, as well as the hepatic branch of the abdominal vagus. Further studies are needed to determine whether glucagon acts via stimulation of hepatic glucose production or fatty acid oxidation. The finding that this pancreatic peptide interacts synergistically with other gut-brain peptides, such as CCK, suggests that it may contribute in a complex manner to the array of peripheral signals controlling meal size. There is evidence that hyperglucagonemia in the tumor-bearing state may be the most important hormonal alteration causing anorexia and abnormal carbohydrate metabolism, effects reversed by inhibiting glucagon secretion (88).

I Glucagon-like Peptide 1

The peptide hormone, glucagon-like peptide 1 (GLP-1), results from posttranslational processing of proglucagon in the gastrointestinal tract (454). It is secreted into the circulation, in a vagal-dependent manner, in response to the ingestion of meals, primarily fat and carbohydrates. This peptide, functioning through several diverse but complementary physiological systems, plays an important role in the control of blood glucose levels (454). It lowers circulating glucose by stimulating insulin secretion and inhibiting glucagon secretion, thereby decreasing hepatic glucose production. It also inhibits gastric emptying and gastric acid secretion.

Whereas circulating GLP-1 may have central effects through receptors in the area postrema and subfornical organs, recent studies indicate that GLP-1 is also synthesized in the brain (454–456). Neurons expressing GLP-1 exist in the brainstem, mainly the solitary tract, and send projections to different nuclei of the hypothalamus, where its receptors are concentrated. Central administration of GLP-1 inhibits feeding, while a GLP-1 antagonist stimulates feeding, enhances NPY-elicited feeding, and blocks leptin-induced inhibition of food intake, suggesting a physiological role (457, 458). A possible site of action is the PVN, where the peptide's receptors are concentrated and the immediate early gene, *c-fos*, is stimulated by GLP-1 (457,459). This and other evidence has led to the hypothesis that GLP-1 is a natural mediator of satiety, possibly responding to the postmeal rise in circulating glucose levels. This idea is supported by the finding that the feeding-suppressive effect of this peptide is strongest in rats fed a high-carbohydrate diet, which raises glucose levels (460). In addition, acute onset of anorexia occurs in animals receiving transplantable glucagonoma tumor lines, which produce highly elevated levels of proglucagon mRNA and plasma GLP-1 and glucagon (461).

A possible role for GLP-1 in obesity is suggested by evidence that chronic administration of GLP-1 reduces feeding and body weight, and a GLP-1 antagonist produces the opposite effect (409,456,462). Also, obese subjects exhibit lower levels of GLP-l in response to a meal (463). However, the involvement of this peptide in normal body weight regulation is not substantiated by genetic studies (454,464). Targeted disruption of the GLP-1 receptor gene has little effect on feeding and weight gain in mice, even after several months on a high-fat diet, despite fasting hyperglycemia and reduced insulin secretion. Moreover, a combined disruption of leptin and GLP-1 action produces mice of comparable body weight to those with leptin deficiency alone. Also, transgenic mice with sustained elevations in circulating exendin-4, a potent GLP-1 agonist, eat normally.

An alternative possibility is that GLP-1 acts on neurons involved in the stress response (454,465). Central administration of GLP-1 produces conditioned taste aversion and has aversive side effects. It induces similar patterns of neuronal *c-fos* activation to that caused by lithium chloride, which can be blocked by a GLP-1 receptor antagonist. Further, deletion of the GLP-1 receptor gene results in an exaggerated CORT response to restraint stress. The available evidence indicates that different central pathways mediate GLP-1 induced satiety and taste aversion (465). This peptide is a likely candidate in mediating cancer-induced anorexia (88).

J Cholecystokinin

As an integrative peptide for satiety, CCK has parallel functions in the gut and certain brain regions, such as the PVN-MH (466–471). This peptide also has roles in the mesolimbic DA system, which provides a challenge to any simple overall explanation of function (472).

Although CCK-8 is the form of the active peptide that is typically studied in paracrine and neurotransmitter research, CCK-33 is more effective in the periphery due to its endocrine actions at distant sites including the liver (473). This peptide can stimulate the release of OT, which in rats is involved in nausea (474,475). However, CCK satiety without nausea has also been demonstrated (461,472,476,477). The overall effect of CCK at an appropriate dose in humans is to suppress food intake without nausea (478,479). As further evidence for CCK satiety, CCK antagonists can increase food intake when given peripherally or locally in regions, such as the PVN-MH (480).

Functioning as a paracrine hormone, CCK is released from secretory cells and nerve fibers in the upper intestine, where it works locally to stimulate pancreatic secretion and gallbladder contraction. The peptide also inhibits gastric emptying by constricting the pyloric sphincter (470). Receptors for CCK involved in feeding suppression exist, for example, in the pyloric sphincter, the sensory vagus nerve where they are transported to vagal nerve terminals, and the PBN and PVN. These sites may all be part of a CCK pathway involved in the control of feeding. The sequence of events after a meal to promote satiety may include the release of peripheral CCK, which acts on vagal nerve endings in the gut, followed by signals to the hindbrain and hypothalamus through central CCK neurons.

To suppress feeding, CCK in the PVN may act by counteracting the α_2-noradrenergic feeding response, synergizing with 5HT (481,482) or leptin (14,471), and interacting with E_2 during the estrous period (439,483). There is evidence that CCK's satiating action increases during estrus in female rats (484) and is attenuated by consumption of a high-fat diet (485). The hypothalamic output under the influence of CCK is presumably biased to adjust the hindbrain centers to stop feeding reflexes. The PVN projects back to the vagal motor nucleus, where there are cells excited by CCK. This may involve a hindbrain DA-CCK interaction (486). The vagal output, in turn, projects back to the gastrointestinal tract. Technical approaches used to demonstrate this circuit include CCK suppression of sham eating, sphincter extirpation, selective vagotomy, CCK receptor binding, local CCK brain injections, receptor antagonists, c-Fos immunoreactivity, and electrophysiological recording (469,470,487–490). Thus, CCK acts in both the body and the brain, and it sends neural information from one to the other but does not seem to cross the blood brain barrier. The primary receptor for CCK satiety is the CCK_A subtype, which has the same sequence and overall function in the brain and body (491,492). Mice lacking the CCK_A receptor are hyperphagic, diabetic, and obese (493). An antagonist of the CCK_A receptor can attenuate satiety without affecting preference conditioning, suggesting separate mechanisms (494).

Cholecystokinin can inhibit the learning of food incentives (495). Rats perform fewer responses for food if they have prior experience performing the response under the influence of CCK injections. Apparently,

CCK can devalue the incentive properties of food in hungry animals, and this is manifest later when the animals work for less of that food. Similarly, CCK is more effective at suppressing the intake of a flavored solution if the flavor is linked to a caloric reward, ethanol (496). Given that a flavor paired with calories can release DA in the NAc (497), CCK through the circuitry of Figure 2 may inform the brain of "nutritive expectations" (496). The hypothalamus may be one region where CCK can inhibit conditioned mesolimbic DA release. When injected into the PVN, CCK inhibits DA release in the NAc. It also synergizes with 5HT to release accumbens ACh, which apparently contributes to satiation by counteracting DA (498).

Some of the mesolimbic DA neurons contain CCK as a cotransmitter. Thus, CCK is a neurotransmitter in some DA projection sites, such as the NAc (499). The NAc has intrinsic CCK neurons as well. There are studies showing the effects of satiety peptides on dopaminergic reinforcement processes, as reflected in hypothalamic self-stimulation (500). Ventricular injection of CCK-8 decreases self-stimulation as one might predict for a satiety factor when self-stimulation is related to appetite. However, the same dose of CCK increases self-stimulation rate when injected into the posterior, medial NAc, where CCK is a DA cotransmitter. One may speculate that CCK potentiates some of the reinforcing effects of DA when the two are released together in the NAc. Thus, CCK in the posterior, medial shell of the NAc is probably involved in locomotion and in some aspects of the primary or secondary reinforcement of eating (501).

K Bombesin

Soon after bombesin (BBS) was found in the mammalian gut, the satiety properties of this peptide were discovered (502). The evidence suggests that BBS-like peptides fit most of the criteria for an integrative peptide with parallel functions in the body and brain (503). Peripheral BBS shortens meals and lengthens the time to the next meal, without behavioral or subjective signs of illness (504). Central injection of BBS into different sites of the hypothalamus and forebrain also reduces feeding (505,506). There exist several BBS-like peptides, such as gastrin-releasing peptide and forms of neuromedin, which may act within the brain or body (507). Peripherally administered BBS can stimulate the release of gastrin, CCK, insulin, and other gut peptides that contribute to satiety. When given chronically on an appropriate schedule, BBS can cause weight loss (508). Evidence that BBS receptor knockout mice become obese (509) suggests a role for this peptide in body weight regulation.

L Neuromedin U

Neuromedin U (NMU) is a neuropeptide that is distributed throughout the gut and brain (510). Peripheral activities of NMU include regulation of adrenocortical function and stimulation of smooth muscle. Two NMU receptors have recently been identified. These are G-protein-coupled receptors, with NMU1R expressed predominantly in peripheral tissues and NMU2R in specific regions of the brain, including the PVN and the ependymal layer of the third ventricle (510). Neuromedin U is expressed in the VMH, and fasting downregulates NMU mRNA. Moreover, intracerebroventricular injection of NMU markedly suppresses food intake and body weight in rats (510,511), while anti-NMU antiserum increases feeding (512). Central injection of NMU also stimulates activity level, body temperature, and heat production (511). These findings suggest that NMU, a potent anorexic peptide, is a catabolic signaling molecule in the brain, possibly involving neural mechanisms in the ventromedial region of the hypothalamus.

M Amylin

Amylin, also known as islet amyloid polypeptide, is a 37–amino acid peptide with extensive sequence overlap with calcitonin gene-related peptide (513). It is coreleased with insulin from pancreatic β-cells in response to a variety of stimuli. These include meal ingestion and elevated blood concentrations of glucose, arginine, and β-hydroxybutyrate.

Amylin has multiple biologic actions related to glucose (513,514). Although it is coreleased with insulin, it inhibits insulin secretion and counteracts insulin's metabolic actions. In vivo studies indicate that amylin alone stimulates glycogenolysis, decreases glucose uptake, enhances blood glucose and lactate levels, and induces insulin resistance, although these effects generally require supraphysiological concentrations. In addition to altering glucose homeostasis, peripheral injections of amylin reduce food intake in rodents (514). Unlike the satiety actions of CCK, this effect of amylin is not altered by abdominal vagotomy, nor is it mediated by a change in gastric emptying. Precise meal pattern analyses reveal a specific action of amylin on the satiety processes at the end of a meal, rather than on feeding rate or on the size and duration of subsequent meals (515). Amylin and insulin, cosecreted by pancreatic β-cells in response to a nutrient stimulus, interact to reduce food intake and, ultimately, body weight (516).

Amylin, like insulin and leptin, is synthesized peripherally and is rapidly and efficiently transported across the blood brain barrier into discrete brain regions, including the hypothalamus, where amylin binding sites are located (517–519). Central injection of amylin suppresses feeding behavior (520,521). Moreover, repeated intracerebroventricular injections of this peptide potently and dose-dependently reduce daily food intake, weight gain, and body fat accrual (522).Insulin and amylin combine synergistically to reduce food intake, leading to the proposal that amylin, like insulin and leptin, is a circulating adiposity signal to the brain (520). Systemic administration of amylin causes a rise in hypothalamic concentrations of 5HT, and it reduces forebrain DA metabolism (523). Thus, amylin may act centrally, through these and other neurochemical changes, in the long-term regulation of food intake and energy balance. This hypothesis receives further support from the finding that repeated injections of an amylin antagonist into the third ventricle increase feeding, adiposity, and circulating insulin levels (522). In addition, targeted deletion of the amylin gene, resulting in amylin deficiency, also stimulates weight gain (524).

Amylin function is disturbed in both type I insulin-dependent and type II insulin-independent diabetic conditions (513). This peptide is the predominant component of the amyloid deposits in the pancreatic islets of type II diabetic patients. These excess peptide concentrations may contribute to disordered glucose homeostasis, e.g., glucose intolerance and insulin resistance, suggesting that amylin antagonists may be potential therapeutic agents in these patients. Type I diabetes, however, is associated with decreased production of amylin and decreased release after a meal. In this condition of insulin insufficiency, intravenous infusion of an amylin analog may help to reduce postprandial hyperglycemia.

N Calcitonin

Calcitonin belongs to a family of peptides that include calcitonin gene-related peptide (CGRP), adrenomedullin, and islet amyloid polypeptide. These peptides are each found to reduce food intake when centrally injected (521,525–528). The hypothalamus is a main targe site for calcitonin-induced anorexia, and it contains high concentrations of calcitonin receptors. As indicated above, CGRP is structurally similar to amylin, and these peptides have similar biological effects, including feeding suppression. Consumption of a high-fat meal causes a significant rise in circulating CGRP levels. In obese women, plasma CGRP concentrations are found to be elevated (529).

O Prolactin-Releasing Peptide

Until recently, the hypothalamic peptide hormone regulating the secretion of PRL from the anterior pituitary was unknown. A new peptide, prolactin-releasing peptide (PrRP), has been identified which is proposed to perform this function (530). This peptide, however, is not found in the external layer of the ME, precluding its role as a classical hypophysiotropic hormone. Additional studies, however, suggest that this peptide has other functions related to energy homeostasis. The expression of PrRP is concentrated in the DMN and brainstem, with PrRP receptor mRNA highest in the DMN and PVN (531). A recent study shows that PrRP and mRNA is reduced in obese Zucker rats (532) and in situations of negative energy balance, including fasting and lactation (516), when leptin levels are low. Moreover, central administration of PrRP reduces food intake and weight gain, producing its strongest effect after injection into the DMN (516,533). Further, in vitro studies demonstrate a stimulatory effect of PrRP on the release of α-MSH and NT, two feeding-inhibitory peptides (533), suggesting possible mechanisms through which this peptide may act to control feeding behavior.

P Oxytocin and Vasopressin

An oxytocinergic pathway for the inhibition of feeding has been suggested (474,534). Pituitary OT in rats inhibits food intake under conditions other than normal satiety, e.g., in states of nausea or dehydration. Central OT injections reduce food intake as well as sodium appetite (535–537). Also, OT receptor antagonists stimulate feeding (538). Arginine vasopressin replaces OT for these functions in primates and, like OT, inhibits feeding in rats (539,540). This feeding-suppressive effect of AVP is not affected by vagotomy, indicating that its peripheral mechanisms of action are different from those of CCK and ENT (541).

Evidence suggests the involvement of other neuromodulators in OT's action. These include 5HT, which has a stimulatory effect on the release of OT. d-Fenfluramine increases pituitary OT release via the PVN and inhibits it via the DMN (542), suggesting a possible function of OT in the action of this serotonergic anorexic compound. The peptide CRH also stimulates OT, which may be an additional factor underlying its feeding-suppressive effect (543). Conversely, brain GAL, which stimulates feeding, plays a role in inhibiting pituitary OT release (544).

Q Acidic Fibroblast Growth Factor

Acidic fibroblast growth factor (aFGF) is one of several growth factor peptides that do more than promote mitosis and tissue repair (545). It facilitates learning and memory and, in addition, inhibits eating behavior (546). Proof of a role in satiety comes from an increase in nighttime eating in rats given aFGF antibodies. This peptide is found in both the body and brain, where it is synthesized and released from storage sites in ependymal cells of the gut and ventricular walls. When aFGF is released into the CSF by a meal, it permeates the hypothalamic structures and inhibits the same glucose-sensitive cells in the LH that are inhibited by glucose itself. Evidence suggests that blood glucose stimulates both insulin release from the pancreas and aFGF release from the ventricular lining, with both cooperating in the inhibition of eating via hypothalamic mechanisms. There is evidence that an aFGF increases the release of CRH which, in turn, activates sympathetic outflow after feeding (547). This idea is consistent with the fact that exogenous and endogenous aFGF both induce reactions similar to the integrated physiological responses induced by CRH (see above).

R Cyclo(His-Pro)

Cyclo(His-Pro) is a dipeptide derived from TRH. It is distributed widely throughout the brain and gastrointestinal tract (548). This dipeptide at high doses reduces food intake and causes a reduction in body weight (548). Levels of cyclo(His-Pro) are increased in the LH of obese Zucker rats, and these elevated levels are reduced by dehydroepiandrosterone, which itself reduces feeding and weight gain (549). Plasma levels are altered by oral glucose ingestion, and administration of cyclo(His-Pro) causes higher insulin levels, possibly by decreasing hepatic insulin clearance (550). There is evidence (551) that decreased levels of cyclo(His-Pro) may contribute to the hyperinsulinemia of obesity.

V BIOGENIC AMINES IN THE CONTROL OF EATING BEHAVIOR AND METABOLISM

The peptide systems in the hypothalamus, reviewed in Sections III and IV, are modulated by the biogenic amines. Apparently, the monoamines potentiate or "prime" different systems at different times. For example, one major role is to impose a circadian rhythm on the feeding systems. Biogenic amines may also selectively potentiate subsystems for selection of specific macronutrients, which vary across the light-dark cycle. Norepinephrine has another feature of particular interest. This monoamine can modulate opposing systems depending on which noradrenergic pathway is active and which receptors are upregulated at the time. Remarkably, changes in receptor binding and gene expression can occur in a matter of hours and perhaps minutes. These and other mechanisms of action are reviewed below.

A Norepinephrine

There is support for a strong circadian rhythm of hypothalamic norepinephrine (NE) and its receptors, suggesting that it plays an important role in the animal's overall state of arousal. Measurements of NE release, receptor activity, and neuronal firing demonstrate a peak at the onset of the natural feeding cycle (420,552). The more excited the animal becomes, the faster noradrenergic neurons fire (553). While this suggests a general role for NE in brain arousal and selective attention, NE additionally modulates specific types of motivation, such as food consumption.

Hypothalamic injections of NE can have very specific behavioral effects (554–556). When injected into the PVN, it enhances lab chow intake, and when a choice of macronutrients is allowed, NE causes a preferential increase in the ingestion of carbohydrate, compared to fat or protein. This catecholamine induces feeding via α_2-noradrenergic receptors concentrated in the PVN. Local injections of antagonists of α_2 receptors reduce feeding. The strongest effect of NE can be seen at the onset of the natural feeding cycle, showing that natural rhythms are critical in understanding its function. The same is true for peptides, notably NPY, with which NE coexists.

The arousal effect of NE is consistent with its close interaction with the adrenal steroid, CORT (42,556). Blood levels of this glucocorticoid rise just prior to the active cycle when it has an important role in arousal. It also activates the NE system in the PVN by potentiating α_2-receptor binding and increasing NE-induced feeding responses. The rise in circulating CORT coincides with a natural rise in extracellular NE in the PVN at the onset of the active period (552,557), in association with an increase in appetite for carbohydrate (51). Also, CORT fosters a rise in blood glucose as it potentiates carbohydrate intake (42), which in turn has a stimulatory effect on α_2-receptor-binding sites in the PVN (558).

As a consequence of this relationship with CORT and perhaps other feeding-stimulatory neurochemicals, NE injections in the MH region have effects that are similar to those produced by lesions in this region, including increased food intake, parasympathetic activity, and body weight gain. Therefore, it appears that NE inhibits, and MH lesions destroy, various satiety signals (559) and sympathetic functions (560). The dorsal noradrenergic bundle may be a source of the NE that acts via α_2-receptor sites to inhibit satiety and increase eating (559).

There are several studies suggesting that NE stimulation of hypothalamic α_2 receptors contributes to the development of obesity. Norepinephrine increases body weight in rats after repeated injections into the PVN, which cause hyperphagia for carbohydrate (561). Moreover, in a recent study (562), chronic NE infusion in the VMH produces a full set of changes characteristic of obese, insulin-resistant animal models. Norepinephrine increases feeding and body fat accrual, causes marked endocrine changes, including hyperinsulinemia, hyperleptinemia, and hypertriglyceridemia, and affects metabolism, producing increases in white adipocyte activities, whole body fat oxidation, and glucose intolerance. In obesity-prone Sprague-Dawley rats, a variety of disturbances in the hypothalamic noradrenergic system are evident, supporting its role in obesity (563,564). Obesity-prone subjects have higher levels of circulating NE, reflecting a decline in NE turnover and low sympathetic nervous activity, an increase in glucose-stimulated NE, and an altered ratio of α_2/α_1 noradrenergic receptors in the hypothalamus (565). In an animal model of the Dutch famine during World War II, male rats born of mothers deprived of food early in pregnancy grew up to be overweight and have increased NE in the PVN (566). Distubances in the hypothalamic noradrenergic system are also detected in genetically obese *ob/ob* or *fa/fa* rodents. Compared to their wild-type controls, they have higher levels of medial hypothalamic NE, reduced NE turnover, increased α_2-receptor binding, and greater responsiveness to the feeding-stimulatory effect of NE or the α_2-agonist, clonidine (567–571). Increased VMH noradrenergic activities are also associated with other glucose-intolerant conditions that accompany seasonal, genetic or experimentally induced obesity (562).

In contrast to NE's feeding-stimulatory action on α_2-noradrenergic receptors, the α_1-receptor subtype in the PVN mediates feeding suppression (555,572). Injections of α_1 agonists reduce food consumption, while specific α_1-receptor antagonists stimulate feeding. A notable example of a drug that acts on these receptors is phenylpropanolamine. It is effective in the short term in reducing body weight (573) and inhibiting feeding by acting on α_1 receptors in the PVN (574). The density of both α_1 and α_2 receptors can vary with body weight (565), which provides support for their role in weight regulation. Radiolabeled anorexic drugs can be used to mark sites in the brain where they bind (575). AMPH and mazindol bind particularly well in the PVN and VMH. This binding is reduced by food deprivation in association with a decline in blood glucose.The phenomenon is similar to a glucose-dependent decline reported for α_2-receptor binding in the PVN (78). Based on this, it was hypothesized that anorexic drug binding inhibits α_2 receptors, thereby reducing carbohydrate intake (575). AMPH is also effective in the LH via other monoamine receptors, as discussed below.

Whereas the focus of these studies has been on NE's action on α_1- and α_2-noradrenergic receptors in the MH, there is evidence that the LH responds differently. In the PFLH, NE or epinephrine suppresses feeding behavior via β-adrenergic receptors (576,577). Destruction of a subset of noradrenergic and adrenergic neurons, which project in part to the hypothalamus, causes hyperphagia and body weight gain (573,578). This selective lesion of the ventral noradrenergic bundle also disinhibits LH self-stimulation and reduces AMPH-induced anorexia (579). Thus, adrenergic inputs can have different effects on feeding depending on the site of innervation and the receptors that predominate. As a general rule, α_2 receptors foster feeding, while α_1- and β-adrenergic receptors reduce feeding. This pattern of control in the brain may have its counterpart in the periphery, where the net lipolytic effect of catecholamines is dependent on a similar functional balance between α_2- and β-adrenergic receptors in fat cells (580). Whereas genetically obese rodents show greater responsiveness to the feeding-suppressive effects of a β_3-agonist, they exhibit reduced activity of the β_2-adrenergic receptors that decrease feeding (571).

B Serotonin

As with NE, circadian changes in the firing rate of serotonergic neurons suggest that they also play an important role in the animal's overall state of arousal and feeding pattern. An animal's level of excitement rises as 5HT neurons fire faster (553). Serotonergic activation is most evident at the onset of the natural feeding cycle. Central injection studies show that 5HT, specifically at this time, suppresses food intake, preferentially carbohydrate intake, by an action on MH nuclei, including the PVN and VMH (581,582). There is evidence that serotonergic drug treatment can also reduce intake of dietary fat (583). Microdialysis studies show a significant increase in extracellular 5HT release during the meal (584), as well as before the meal in response to the sight and smell of food (584,585). Additional 5HT is released as the animal consumes the food, but it declines over the next 30 min to baseline levels. This time course is consistent with an anticipatory and short postingestive satiety effect for 5HT, rather than a long-lasting action.

Evidence strongly suggests that 5HT potentiates systems that respond to postingestive signals. Microdialysis in the PVN/VMH region demonstrates that a carbohydrate meal is particularly effective in releasing 5HT, whereas a protein or fat meal has the opposite effect (586). Serotonin and DA release are related to satiety in normal rats and Zucker rats (587–589). A conditioned aversive taste releases hypothalamic 5HT as part of a life-saving reaction to poisonous food (584). Hypothalamic 5HT also increases in response to peripheral tryptophan, d-fenfluramine, fluoxetine, and a low-dose AMPH challenge after lithium treatment. The results indicate roles for 5HT in pharmacotherapy for appetite, depression, and bipolar disorder (590–592). Disturbances in the serotonergic system in relation to overeating and obesity are indicated by the finding that obese rodents have decreased hypothalamic levels of the 5HT metabolite, 5-hydroxy-3-indole acetic acid and they exhibit decreased responsiveness to 5HT administration (567–570,593,594).

Biogenic amines often have effects that depend on other local neurochemical signals. Hypothalamic 5HT may act in synergy with other peptides that produce satiety (595), acting when postingestive signals are present to release cofactors, such as CCK, in the hypothalamus. This peptide may come from serotonergic neurons as a cotransmitter and have longer-lasting effects on feeding than the monoamine alone. CCK may also be released in the hypothalamus in response to vagal inputs that are relayed from the stomach to the hypothalamus (578). The proposal that 5HT and CCK work together is further supported by the finding that 5HT receptor blockers antagonize CCK's anorexic effect (439,472), and conversely, a CCK antagonist blocks 5HT's effect (596). Serotonin and CCK injected together into the PVN have a superadditive effect in the NAc by releasing ACh that inhibits eating behavior (498).

The compound d-fenfluramine is an anorexic drug that is a 5HT reuptake blocker at low doses and a releaser of 5HT at higher doses (597–599). Consistent with results obtained with 5HT, the feeding-suppressive effect of d-fenfluramine is attenuated by various 5HT receptor antagonists (600). Thus, the actions of d-fenfluramine, or its active metabolite nor-fenfluramine, may involve specific 5HT receptors that provide some degree of behavioral specificity. d-Fenfluramine additionally increases background metabolism by enhancing utilization of the body's fuels (601). This increased metabolism contributes to weight loss. Owing to the toxicity of d,l-fenfluramine in combination with phentermine (602), attention has shifted to sibutramine. This NE and 5HT reuptake blocker fosters the sympathetic state, while attenuating NPY production and affecting the melanocortin system (603).

Serotonin may act, in part, via an inhibitory action on the α_2-noradrenergic system of the MH (447,555). Serotonin and d-fenfluramine reduce the hyperphagic actions of NE in the PVN. This may explain why serotoneric drugs are used to treat carbohydrate craving and related obesity (448). The interaction between NE and 5HT may also be a mechanism through which these drugs inhibit a component of the self-stimulation system related to feeding reinforcement (449), thereby contributing to their appetite-reducing properties (450). However, in hamsters, long-term excess of NE and 5HT in the VMH leads to hyperinsulinimia and insulin resistance (604).

It is clear that there are other sites, besides the MH and LH regions, where 5HT acts in the control of feeding behavior and metabolism. For example, diets with an amino acid imbalance cause primary anorexia and conditioned taste aversion. This effect, which is blocked by 5HT antagonists, is mediated in part through actions in the piriform cortex (451). Serotonin also contributes to postingestive onset of satiety through brainstem structures (605), as well as through its potent actions in the periphery (606). In a genetic model of obesity, 5HT2C mutant mice overeat and gain weight in adulthood (97) and display reduced sensitivity to d-fenfluramine (607). Confirmation by pharmacological studies (608) has focused attention on this 5HT receptor subtype as a therapeutic target. However, there is abundant evidence that attacking multiple DA, NE and 5HT targets affords a better strategy for suppression of the appetite for food and drugs, if a safe combination can be found.

C Dopamine

Dopamine and AMPH-related compounds have long been known to suppress feeding through their action in the hypothalamus. However, the full story of DA's actions in the brain is only beginning to unfold. Dopamine has effects in the LH and MH. It also has powerful actions related to feeding behavior in other brain regions, notably the NAc where it is a behavior reinforcer and generates incentive motivation (Fig. 2).

1 Dopamine in the Hypothalamus

Hypothalamic DA contributes to AMPH-induced anorexia (609–611). This is of renewed interest due to the recent upsurge in the use of phentermine, which is a dopaminergic and noradrenergic drug (612). A variety of DA-related effects may occur in the hypothalamus, depending on the site of intervention and experimental technique used. Hypothalamic DA is released, in part, from an incertohypothalamic cell group, also MH neurons intimately involved in the control of pituitary functions (613), and from one or more DA cell groups (A8, A9, A10) with branches that ascend from the midbrain. Injections of DA in the LH suppress food intake, an action blocked specifically by DA receptor antagonists (609,610). Anorexic doses of AMPH injected in the LH increase extracellular DA, although NE and 5HT are also increased (614). All three monoamines may suppress feeding and mediate the actions of AMPH under different conditions (559, 577,584,611,615).

As further evidence of a DA satiety function in the LH, some compounds that block DA receptors stimulate eating behavior. This was demonstrated with the nonspecific receptor antagonist chlorpromazine and with the specific D_2 receptor antagonist sulpiride (559,616). Chronic peripheral injections of sulpiride cause hyperphagia and obesity in rats, analogous to the effect sometimes seen in schizophrenic patients undergoing antipsychotic treatment with D_2 antagonists (610,616). This effect may be due, in part, to dopaminergic control of pituitary functions, such as E_2 release (617), or to disinhibition of a behavior reinforcement system that leads to overeating. Sulpiride in the LH has locomotor and reward effects. Remarkably, rats will even self-inject sulpiride into their own LH (616). This suggests that DA agonists can act at hypothalamic D_2 receptors to inhibit instrumental responses, including responses involved in the reinforcement of eating.

In studies using microdialysis, the release of DA in the MH is positively correlated with eating behavior (618). It is proposed that taste and smell may enhance the release of hypothalamic DA at the start of a meal, to organize autonomic reflexes for receiving food (619). Diabetic rats that are hyperphagic also exhibit enhanced DA turnover in the VMH (620). Thus, DA release may influence eating as well as satiety, depending on which DA system is activated and the state of their multiple receptor subtypes.

Recording studies in monkeys find taste-responsive cells in the hypothalamus that are sensitive to DA (621). Some of these cells are tuned to features of the animal's external environment. Other cells that are glucose sensitive are for monitoring the internal state (621). Cells in the hypothalamus, some of which are responsive to DA, influence feeding via an output that connects to the mesolimbic DA system. The mesolimbic system passes through the hypothalamus on its way to the NAc (Fig. 2). As a clear demonstration of this, a DA antagonist, sulpiride, injected in the LH causes the release of DA in the NAc (622).

2 Dopamine as a Behavior Reinforcer in the Mesolimbic System

Neurons projecting from the VTA to the NAc can reinforce behavior and are involved in generating the incentive to eat (622–626). This seems to be based on a dual role in instrumental and classical conditioning. Dopamine is released in the NAc by behavior, such as self-stimulation, psychostimulant self-administration, and eating (275,627–630). Self-stimulation or stimulation-induced feeding in the LH releases DA in the NAc, with or without food present (631). When food-deprived rats eat a meal, DA release in the NAc may be especially salient because the DA baseline level is low (382,386,632). In addition, DA can be released in the NAc by classically conditioned stimuli, as discussed below. As a meal continues, DA release diminishes, suggesting that it plays a larger role in initiating the meal and responding to food novelty than in maintaining a meal (264,633).

An increase in extracellular DA in the NAc can be a positive reinforcer. This is shown in rats with NAc cannulas for self-injection of AMPH or DA directly into that region (634,635). When rats self-administer cocaine intravenously, they respond in a manner that raises extracellular DA whenever it falls to a trigger level (636). Neurochemicals are reinforcers if they stimulate DA cells in the VTA, the prime examples being opiates, nicotine, and NT (637–640). This means that the mesolimbic DA system activates a reinforcement process (by definition, a reinforcer increases instrumental responding). Therefore, DA is probably a reinforcer when it is released by self-stimulation, drugs, or natural behavior such as eating, mating, aggression, and associated stimuli. It appears from a teleological point of view that animals perform voluntary behavior in order to get the effects of DA release in the NAc and perhaps in other forebrain sites such as the PFC (641). Recording from VTA cells in the awake monkey suggests that neural activity signals a salient change in the environment (642). The debate as to whether DA creates a simple error signal, a reward (pleasure and liking), or an incentive (motivation and wanting) seems to hinge on which component of the ascending DA system is being addressed. Evidence is accumulating to indicate that DA in the NAc shell region generates "wanting," or what in the feeding field is usually referred to as appetite (625,643).

Dopamine in the NAc is also involved in reinforcing behavior to escape an aversive stimulus. Extracellular DA increases during MH stimulation escape behavior, but not during the same stimulation when it is inescapable (622). Thus, DA may be a negative reinforcer for active escape, as well as a positive reinforcer for active approach in feeding situations. Its role in these reinforcement processes could be incentive motivation.

3 Taste Reactions and Dopamine

Dopamine antagonists administered systemically or directly into the NAc block locomotion, instrumental behavior, and sucrose intake (241). Results with the DA antagonist raclopride are particularly interesting. An animal drinking sucrose, with a fistula so it never gets full, acts as if the sucrose has been diluted when treated with this DA blocker. The avidity for sweet taste diminishes when raclopride is given systemically or locally into the NAc (644). Reinforcement may involve both D_1 and D_2 receptors. The literature is not clear on this, due to the discovery of new receptor subtypes, the nonspecificity of some pharmaceutical agents, multiple facets of reinforcement, and multiple actions in many brain regions such as the hypothalamus and NAc (645).

A definitive role for mesolimbic DA has been demonstrated by neural recordings from DA cells in the VTA of awake monkeys. Some of the neurons that project to the NAc increase their firing rate during eating (646). As the monkey gains practice at the feeding task, neural activity precedes food presentation, coinciding with discriminative stimuli that are a sign of forthcoming food. Thus, with experience, DA release becomes allied with conditioned stimuli and perhaps with secondary reinforcers. This suggests that mesolimbic DA in primates is involved in learning what, where, and when to eat, more than in the act of eating. Dopamine is an anticipatory signal that reflects novelty, and it may be one factor that makes satiety "sensory specific." A new taste can reinitiate eating with the help of renewed DA release (647). The taste and anticipation may release DA in the NAc shell and core differentially (648).

4 Body Weight and Dopamine

Microdialysis shows that basal extracellular DA may be as low as half normal in rats at 80% of free-feeding body weight (382,386). Given the demonstration that rats respond for cocaine when accumbens DA decreases to a certain level (636), it is quite possible that animals also respond for food when DA reaches a low level. Drug self-administration, self-stimulation, and eating are all potentiated by food deprivation (273,649,650), and they all can increase extracellular DA in the NAc. It is therefore likely that animals or people with diminished amounts of DA, for any reason, may have a tendency to take foods or drugs that restore synaptic DA.

Although DA depletion in the nigrostriatal pathway causes aphasia and weight loss (651), rats can still eat when DA is depleted in the NAc. For example, 6-hydroxydopamine was used to deplete accumbens DA to 16% of normal, but the rats could still swallow a normal amount of sucrose when delivered directly into the mouth (486). Dopamine-depleted animals eat normally when the food is easy to get, but they opt not to perform difficult tasks (652). Rats that bar-press for cocaine and food pellets in alternation stop responding for the dopaminergic drug when DA is depleted, but they still bar-press for food (653). Apparently, accumbens DA serves partly as a priming signal that activates the systems needed for difficult tasks, for learning or switching behavior (654,655). For simple tasks, other areas such as the striatum, hypothalamus, midbrain, and brainstem may be sufficient. A decerebrate rat, with no forebrain at all, can still swallow food put in its mouth and reject it when full. Thus, the caudal brainstem participates strongly in neural control of feeding (656).

5 Classical Conditioning of Neurotransmitter Release

Dopamine that is released by a conditioned stimulus, such as a taste, a special place or even an advertisement, may prime instrumental behavior leading to more DA release. When DA is low, as during food restriction, a conditioned stimulus is needed to release the initial DA and help start the behavior. Dopamine release in the NAc can be conditioned with food flavors. A flavor associated with intragastric feeding becomes a preferred flavor (657) that releases DA in the NAc (585). Conversely, a flavor that reminds the animal of lithium-induced nausea causes extracellular DA to decrease (658). Thus conditioned DA release in the NAc may play an important role in the animal's decision to approach or avoid food.

There are several components to behavior reinforcement. These include the facets people think of as motivation, drive, wanting, incentive, or willingness to work. In addition, they include the hedonic aspect involved in liking and pleasure and other related concepts, such as satisfaction. Researchers are currently engaged in the fascinating enterprise of dissecting out the roles of DA, as well as opioid peptides and other neurotransmitters, in these different aspects of the total reinforcement process (623,624,641,659–661).

D Histamine

Histamine, which is synthesized from histidine, is well known for its role in regulating body temperature and stimulating drinking (662,663). Neuronal histamine, in addition, is involved in the regulation of feeding, mastication, and circadian rhythms (662,664–667). Peripheral histidine injections which increase brain histamine levels cause a concomitant decrease in food intake. Peripheral or ventricular administration of drugs which block histamine receptors enhance feeding. In the hypothalamus, food-deprived rats show increased levels of endogenous histamine, and obese rats exhibit reduced levels (668,669). Pharmacological activation of hypothalamic histamine suppresses feeding through the H_1 receptor subtype. Sites of action include the PVN and VMH, areas richest in histamine and H_1 receptors. Iontophoretic application of H_1 antagonists suppress neuronal activity in these areas.

Sakata et al. (670,671) propose a role for hypothalamic histamine in the homeostatic control of energy stores. Fasting and 2-deoxy-D-glucose, as well as insulin-induced hypoglycemia, all stimulate the turnover of histamine. The essential stimulant is a reduction in glucose utilization and a consequent histamine-dependent decrease in brain glycogen to maintain brain glucose availability. A further role for histamine may be reflected in the impact of high ambient temperatures, which elevate hypothalamic histamine and suppress food intake (669). Histamine injected into the preoptic area reduces body temperature (672). This process of histaminergic thermoregulation raises the possibility that this biogenic amine is also involved in the changes in ingestive behavior and body temperature induced by EL-1β, which is released in response to infection, injury and inflammation (669). Ventricular injection of the cytokine suppresses food intake and induces thermogenesis (673,674). These responses, which are accompanied by a rise in histamine turnover, are attenuated by depletion of neuronal histamine in the hypothalamus (675). Histamine may mediate the anorexic action of some peptides, such as amylin (676). The finding that Zucker fatty rats have lower hypothalamic levels of this biogenic amine and are unresponsive to the feeding-stimulatory actions of histamine receptor antagonists (668,677) provides support for a role of central histamine in obesity.

VI ACETYLCHOLINE AND AMINO ACIDS IN FEEDING-RELATED CIRCUITS

It has long been known that nicotine in cigarettes suppresses appetite, and smoking cessation leads to increased body weight. Thus, acetylcholine, acting on nicotinic receptors, is particularly relevant to the discussion of obesity. Amino acids are very important in several contexts, including neurotransmission that controls meal size in the hypothalamus. In addition to their direct actions, new evidence suggests that the brain can detect amino acid imbalance in the diet and, thereby, affect food choice.

A Acetylcholine

Acetylcholine (ACh) has several roles at nicotinic as well as muscarinic receptors in the circuits that control eating. In the LH, the muscarinic agonist carbachol potentiates eating and drinking (395,678–680), and cholinergic drugs influence locomotion related to eating (681). Hypothalamic stimulation that supports self-stimulation or stimulation-bound eating causes the release of ACh in the VTA (682). Figure 2 shows this circuit by which cholinergic cells of the midbrain project onto DA cell bodies of the VTA. When injected into the VTA, antisense to the M5 muscarinic receptor blocks LH self-stimulation, and atropine also suppresses self-stimulation and feeding (682,683). Nicotine in the VTA, as well as the NAc, stimulates the release of DA in the NAc (639,640,684,685), showing that the VTA has nicotinic as well as muscarinic receptors. Thus, cigarettes have a double dopaminergic action, by activating the mesolimbic DA projection at both its origin and terminals.

Acetylcholine interneurons in the NAc may contribute to the inhibition of eating behavior. Most, if not all, of the ACh in the NAc comes from interneurons that play a special role in gating motivated behavior output. As a working hypothesis, it is suggested that these ACh interneurons act as gates that control instrumental behavior for reinforcers such as food (686). Just as striatal DA/ACh balance is a factor in Parkinson's disease and Huntington's chorea, accumbens DA/ACh balance may be a factor in disorders of motivated behavior, such as anorexia and binge eating. Measurements of ACh during a meal show that the highest levels coincide with the slowing of eating (686). Neostigmine infused into the NAc to elevate endogenous ACh can stop an ongoing meal. This suggests that accumbens ACh is involved in a "no-go" command that counters the DA "go" signal.

A conditioned taste aversion releases ACh in the NAc when the taste stops the animal from ingesting a flavor associated with nausea. Thus, the conditioned stimulus raises extracellular ACh at the same time as it lowers the release of DA (687). This may contribute to inhibition of behavior output such as eating. The DA/ACh imbalance, with low DA and high ACh release, is very different from what occurs with a normal satiating meal that can raise first extracellular DA and then ACh at the same time (686). A nicotinic antagonist injected in the NAc can block the conditioned taste aversion caused by a cholinergic agonist (688). This supports the hypothesis that ACh in the posterior, medial NAc, through nicotinic receptors, can contribute to stopping eating behavior.

ACh in the major projection system to the neocortex and hippocampus is probably involved in all kinds of cognitive behaviors, including memory formation and retrieval, foraging, and social factors in eating (689, 690). Four ACh system components have been described above, in the hypothalamus, midbrain, accumbens, and cortex. The hypothalamic and midbrain components may have similar cells of origin, whereas the others are totally separate systems. This is one reason that systemic cholinergic drugs have not yet found a use in treating eating disorders, other than nicotine, which is addictive.

B Amino Acids

The metabolism of energy in the brain is coupled to the formation of several amino acids, including glutamate and GABA, which serve neurotransmitter roles. This may confer on them a special role in brain mechanisms for eating and body weight regulation. Obese Zucker rats have disturbances in brain GABA that may contribute to their overeating (691). They are refractory to the anorexic effects of the GABA-transaminase inhibitor EOS, which elevates GABA levels in the brain. Moreover, transgenic mice that ubiquitously overexpress GABA transporter subtype I exhibit heritable obesity, which features increased body weight and fat deposition (692).

The role of GABA in feeding varies in different brain areas. The PVN is the most sensitive site to the feeding-stimulatory effects induced by injections of GABA agonists and the feeding-inhibitory effect of a GABA antagonist (693–695). In the VMH, mixed results with injections of GABA agonists have been obtained (693–696). GABA is released during hypoglycemia (697). There may be a metabolically distinct GABA-ergic system that exerts inhibitory control over feeding (696). This is based on the finding that levels of endogenous GABA are high in the VMH during the light phase when natural feeding is low (698). Other conditions associated with decreased feeding also cause enhanced levels of VMH GABA (699). The release of GABA in the LH correlates with the end of a meal and may have a very different function than in the PVN (700).

As indicated in Figure 2, complex sensory inputs to the NAc arrive on glutamate pathways from the PFC, amygdala, and hippocampus. Output signals leave the NAc on GABA pathways of the extrapyramidal motor system to the VTA, GP, and LH. Glutamate projections to the NAc shell stimulate feeding that can be blocked by GABA antagonists in the LH (701,702). There are also glutamate inputs directly to the LH that stimulate feeding (703–705), and these may be inhibited by GABA agonists (702). Microdialysis coupled to capillary electrophoresis was used to measure glutamate and GABA simultaneously in the LH every 30 sec during a meal. Glutamate peaked near the start of the meal and then decreased, while GABA peaked at meal's end. This strongly supports the hypothesis that glutamate helps start the meal, and GABA participates in satiation (700). In the NTS, glutamate has been implicated in the suppression of feeding by CCK and by glucose-induced satiety (706). A benzodiazepine-GABA system is involved in responses to palatable tastes (707).

Further evidence demonstrates that the anterior piriform cortex can detect and respond to indispensable amino acid imbalance. One of the responses to threonine injection in the piriform cortex of threonine-depleted rats is an increase in neural activity in the

LH. Under natural conditions, this may initiate life-saving ingestive behavior (7).

VII BRAIN AND BEHAVIOR: REINFORCEMENT SYSTEMS AND OVEREATING

Motivation to eat is a major factor in the development and maintenance of obesity. Neural mechanisms have evolved to anticipate the animal's energy needs and to avoid past mistakes. The brain learns and remembers a myriad of responses for finding, storing, and rationing food supplies. The animal is both consciously and unconsciously aware of fuel sources within its ecological niche and its own body. It uses innate reflexes plus classical and instrumental conditioning to get food, to know how hard to work for it, and to know how much to eat. Responses that engage the environment are particularly clever when they involve motivation and learning of complex and arbitrary motor sequences that must be chained together from the animal's repertoire of simpler responses. To survey the chemical neuroanatomy of classical and instrumental conditioning of feeding behavior in a few pages is to leave out most of the available information. Nonetheless, some basic principles can be drawn from the above discussion during a brief tour of the feeding reinforcement circuit, as we now know it (578,641,708).

An overview of Figure 2 indicates that sensory signals from vision, audition, somesthesis, and the chemosenses are entered separately or as multimodal signals into the inputs of two major circuits or loops. One loop from PFC to NAc (the vertical oval) uses sensory information to generate motor output patterns. Thus, the NAc is often referred to as a sensorimotor interface (709). The other loop from the LH to the NAc (the horizontal oval) reinforces output from the sensorimotor interface.

A Sensory Inputs

Chemosensory inputs for taste, olfaction, metabolism, and fuel storage are fed into the NTS, PBN (710,711), hypothalamus, and amygdala (239). Glucoreceptors are widespread in a network throughout much of the brain (712,713). The prime example of chemosensory processing is the taste signal that has been traced from the tongue to NTS, where some of it combines with hepatic vagal inputs representing glucose and amino acids in the liver (714). This signal travels on to the PBN and thalamus (directly to the hypothalamus in rodents) and, then, taste sensory cortex, where more cells respond to stimuli on the tongue. Electrophysiological studies in monkeys follow this trace from the classic taste cortex to the orbital PFC, where cells respond to tastes as a function of appetite and satiety. As a monkey eats a flavorful food and gradually becomes satiated, the PFC cells gradually stop responding to the flavor. This effect is specific for the flavor of a particular food (6). The animal, like the cells in its PFC, no longer responds to one food when satiated, but it still responds to another. This neurological phenomenon corresponds to sensory-specific satiety.

B Behavior Generator System

As shown in Figure 2, complex sensory information that enters the NAc on glutamate neurons is gated by ACh neurons and leaves the NAc on the GABA neurons of the motor systems. The PFC is involved in making choices, including choices of foods. It projects strongly via glutamate neurons to the NAc and other parts of the striatum. The NAc has various rostral-caudal and shell-core inputs and outputs with functionally distinct neuronal ensembles (715,716). Acetylcholine interneurons in the NAc may act as gates that stop instrumental motor output (686,687). These gating neurons are modulated by DA and other transmitters, including 5HT (717) and certain opioids (53) as well as other peptides. Excitatory influences on the GABA output neurons cause downstream excitation of the instrumental motor output. The output from the NAc goes, in part, to the ventral GP, then to the thalamus, and out to motor systems (718,719). The information also loops back from the thalamus to the PFC (75,720), as shown in Figure 2.

C Behavior Reinforcement and Inhibition Systems

The hypothalamus is part of a system that evaluates the sensory outcomes of behavior and, then, reinforces behavior. These functions are important for maintaining a normal body weight. As indicated in the lower center of Figure 2, cells sensitive to insulin and leptin in the ARC influence feeding-related cells in the PVN. Figure 2 further suggests that the PFLH feeding reinforcement path descends (260,627,721) and connects to the VTA, PBN, and NTS. Recording studies show that PFLH stimulation, which is capable of inducing eating and brain stimulation reward, has effects on NTS cells that mimic the effects of palatable tastes on the tongue (722). The descending components of these systems may connect to the ascending ACh path that stimulates the

VTA cells of the mesolimbic DA system, as discussed above (682,723). The VTA projects to forebrain limbic structures, including the NAc, ventral globus pallidus, amygdala, hippocampus, and PFC, which have inputs back to the LH (702,724). Overall, these projections can be viewed as a behavior reinforcement circuit that increases the rate or force of ongoing behavior and recruits responses to associated signals for incentive motivation (623). Both positive and negative reinforcement of behavior can release DA, as shown by the increased extracellular DA in the NAc during LH self-stimulation or stimulation escape (725,726). This is a major portion of the system for reinforcing eating behavior and for appetitive and aversive motivation. Thus, it is very likely to play important roles in eating disorders (8,727).

In the NAc, DA helps to reinforce behavior in a variety of ways (623,728,729). The time course of DA release in the NAc fails to fit a simple notion of a feeding reward. Microdialysis experiments have found both DA release and decrease while the animal is still eating but often DA remains elevated for up to an hour after the meal is over (631,730). The synaptic overflow of DA into the extracellular space revealed by microdialysis is functional DA. It can have synaptic actions on dopaminergic receptors and at uptake sites some distance from the release site in the manner of "volume transmission" (731). Sometimes DA is released in anticipation of eating, as reflected in a conditioned rise in extracellular DA before a meal (497,732). This agrees with recording studies in monkeys, showing that "naïve" DA cells in the VTA fire during eating but later "learn" to fire during the presentation of discriminative stimuli that signal forthcoming food (646). Therefore, as described in the section above, these cells can release DA in response to conditioned discriminative stimuli that predict food.

D Hypothalamic Control of Reinforcement

It has been known for 30 years that the hypothalamus influences complex responces for food, but only now is the mechanism becoming clear. The above discussion depicts a pathway from the LH to the NAc by which the hypothalamus influences operant eating responses. As evidence for this idea, GAL injections into the PVN cause a significant increase in DA release in the NAc (733). This occurs in the absence of food and only in animals that, in a separate test with food present, exhibit a GAL induced-feeding response. Thus, it is feeding behavior that is likely to be reinforced by the DA-activated circuit in the NAc. Eating or associated stimuli can release more DA, which further reinforces the behavior. This positive feedback may contribute to bingeing on the kinds of foods, rich in fat and carbohydrate, which are enhanced by GAL (69). As mentioned in the earlier dopamine section of this review, hypothalamic injection of GAL not only releases DA that may accelerate eating; it also decreases extracellular ACh in the NAc. This is thought to disinhibit eating (733). Conversely, CCK and 5HT injected in the PVN cause satiation and, in separate tests, inhibit accumbens DA while synergizing to release ACh (498).

Hypothalamic injection of the D_2 antagonist sulpiride is another way to induce eating (734). When injected in the LH, sulpiride causes the release of DA in the NAc in the absence of food, much like GAL. In this case, we have direct evidence of the reinforcing effect, as rats self-inject sulpiride into their own hypothalamus (616). Perhaps any hypothalamic manipulation that releases accumbens DA, without also releasing accumbens ACh, can motivate the animal to repeat its behavior. This may contribute to hyperphagia when there is no natural satiety factor sufficient to stop it.

In the course of eating a meal, a rise in ACh release in the NAc very likely contributes to the stopping or switching behaviors (735). When hypothalamic stimulation is aversive, one finds that stimulation releases ACh in the NAc. If the rats are allowed to work to escape the stimulation, they succeed in lowering the ACh (725). Apparently, ACh not only inhibits feeding, but, if ACh is excessive relative to DA, this creates an aversive state. This condition is seen under natural conditions when experiencing a conditioned taste aversion or drug withdrawal (285,687,736). It also occurs during withdrawal from sugar in the animal model of sugar addiction described below.

E Models of Food Addiction

The neural systems for reinforcing eating are the same as those involved in addiction (8,625,737–739). This suggests that certain foods might be addictive under appropriate conditions. There are remarkable overlaps between the effects of palatable foods and addictive drugs. Food deprivation potentiates consumption of food and self-administration of drugs (740,741). Hypothalamic self-stimulation that is sensitive to hunger and appetite also responds to drugs of abuse (3,740,742). In a model in which young rats undergo periods of deprivation-induced weight loss and refeeding (743), there is a proclivity to drug self-administration (744). Animals will even substitute a sweet flavor for an addictive drug that is in short supply (745,746). There are also "gateway effects" such as motivation for sugar that is engendered by sensitization to AMPH (747). Some animals are born with a proclivity to drink sweet fluids and take drugs of abuse (748,749). Dopamine release in the NAc is clearly one of the underlying substrates that is common to the reinforcement of food and drug intake (750). Opioid receptor activation is another. Sweet flavors can suppress pain (751) and potentiate morphine-induced analgesia (427). Likewise, morphine can potentiate ingestion of sweet foods, and naloxone blocks it (239). Naloxone can also precipitate withdrawal with somatic symptoms, such as teeth chattering and shakes, in rats fed a cafeteria diet or a sugar-enhanced diet (422,752,753).

This suggested that some foods might have addictive properties under certain conditions. It has been hypothesized that long-lasting changes occur in the brains of rats on a cycle of fasting and refeeding. These may be similar to the changes caused by intermittent intake of drugs of abuse. To test this hypothesis, rats were deprived for half of each day and given highly palatable glucose to drink with chow a few hours after they would normally have started eating. With this paradigm, they gradually double their daily sugar intake and develop a binge pattern of glucose ingestion. This excessive sugar intake results in increased D_1 receptor and mu receptor binding in the NAc shell (422). Moreover, opioid receptor blockade with naloxone causes withdrawal symptoms, including teeth chattering, anxiety, and disruption of DA and ACh balance. During withdrawal, extracellular DA is low and ACh is high, similar to withdrawal from morphine. These animals also show signs of craving, such as reinstatement of excessive sugar intake after 3 months of sugar abstinence (unpublished). Given this evidence for three stages of addiction, namely, sensitization with receptor changes, withdrawal with neurochemical imbalance, and craving in terms of memorized motivation, one can conclude that animals may become addicted to highly palatable food, as hypothesized earlier (8,752).

This may apply to some cases of binge-eating disorder or bulimia in humans (754–759). Sugar-dependent rats and obese people both show decreased D_2 receptor binding in the striatum (422,760). Binge eaters also have decreased 5HT transporter binding (761). Opioid antagonists have been tested in humans with obesity, binge-eating disorder, or bulimia, with limited success in certain cases (762–767). The therapeutic paradox in using opioid antagonists lies in blocking the motivation to abuse palatable food, without precipitating withdrawal symptoms that promote relapse.

VIII SYMPATHETIC AND PARASYMPATHETIC NERVOUS SYSTEMS

The sympathetic nervous system is defined as primarily an energy output system that is activated in times of stress ("fight and flight"). The parasympathetic system, in contrast, is considered on the input side of the equation ("rest and digest"). It is not a simple matter to classify feeding, which involves both energy output to find food and energy input during ingestion. The proper distinctions may come with full understanding of these systems, which have many components that can be activated separately or all together. For example, the sympathetic system has a subdivision for the body extremities and another for the visceral region that, in turn, is further subdivided (768). The subcomponents can be activated by the appropriate spinal sympathetic afferents, and the larger units can be activated by adrenal catecholamine hormones, epinephrine, and DA. For the sake of clarity, this discussion focuses primarily on the sympathetic system; although as a general rule the parasympathetic system plays an equally important and opposite role.

A Three Components of Sympathetic Output

Sympathetic energy output on a given food ration can be divided into the thermic effect of food (body heat production), physical exercise, and metabolic rate, all of which affect body weight. A person or animal that is eating normally but gaining weight might have low levels of any of these three outputs. The thermic effect of food refers to the amount of heat produced (thermogenesis) above and beyond the basal metabolic rate (769). This changes with the animal's weight and is closely related to body fat. When a normal animal or person gains weight by overeating and depositing fat, the thermic effect of a meal increases. This allows the subject to adapt to the extra fat by squandering heat and curtailing further weight gain. Prostaglandin-E1 is partially responsible for activating the sympathetic system and causing thermogenesis via the VMH (770). During the dynamic phase of overeating after VMH lesions, the thermic effect of food remains low, while the animals gains weight rapidly. This low heat production may signal an impaired sympathetic state that occurs in cases of impending obesity (771). High body temperature not only gets rid of unneeded calories; it also inhibits food intake via a histaminergic system in the hypothalamus (772). A hot rat usually eats less (773), and histamine and its receptors may play a role in producing this response, providing a pharmacological avenue to control appetite.

Second, physical activity accounts for a large amount of energy expenditure. Low physical activity is a major factor in obesity (774). Hyperactivity contributes to weight loss, whereas a sedentary life can lead to obesity. Food-restricted rats conserve energy by becoming less active and more reactive (775). With the availability of a running wheel, underweight rats may display hyperactivity that exacerbates their weight loss (776). When food is restricted to achieve ~80% of normal body weight, rats exhibit marked changes in the brain, such as a decline in basal levels of DA in the NAc (382,386), leading them to engage in behaviors that release DA. Low basal DA is also observed in the NAc of genetically obese Zucker rats (777). Both the underweight rat without the opportunity to run and the obese rat are hypoactive compared to normal rats.

The third factor on the output side is basal metabolic rate. With a computerized metabolism cage that corrects for temperature and activity, a decline in background metabolism can be detected just before a meal (601). Blood glucose also falls before a meal, and as the body's metabolism changes and glucose levels start to rise, the animal initiates the meal (778). Under controlled conditions, the nadir in blood glucose level is so reliable as a predictor of a meal that one must assume the brain can respond to glucose dynamics or, more likely, to the chemical factors that reverse the decline in glucose. This is a revival of Mayer's glucostatic theory (779). However, the liver plays a powerful role in responding to fat, as well as glucose, and it creates "metabolic sensations" via vagal signals that are transformed into brain perceptions (780). Ghrelin, a newly discovered peptide from the stomach wall, varies in the bloodstream in accordance with meals; it predicts meals accurately and is closely associated with insulin and glucose metabolism (303,305,781). Measurements of the immediate early gene product, *c-fos*, as an indication of cellular activity, confirm that the hypothalamus is one of several brain areas that change their activity in response to decreased utilization of either glucose or fat (782). In an attempt encompass both glucostasis and lipostasis, it is proposed that fuels for the brain are monitored in the hypothalamus as a microcosmic representation of the whole body (601). The LH may sense its own intermediary metabolism, and this may be related to the DMN, which is an important locus of the CRH output pathway that is part of the sympathetic system (75,783). It is clear that the hypothalamus exerts control over the various components of the multifaceted sympathetic nervous system.

B High Symphatetic (Low Parasympathetic) Tone

High sympathetic tone in the brown adipose tissue system is associated with loss of the urge to eat. In the MH, electrical stimulation can increase sympathetic neural output to brown adipose tissue and stimulate glucose uptake in skeletal muscles (784). Stimulation tends to be aversive, and it inhibits or interrupts eating. Lesions in the LH have some of the same effects as stimulation of the MH. Depending on the exact size and location, LH can cause various aspects of the well-known syndrome of aphagia, sensory neglect, and motor impairment (440,785) and can disinhibit sympathetic signs, such as peripheral NE release. Leptin from the adipose tissue has similar effects to MH stimulation or some excitotoxic LH lesions. This hormone heightens some facets of satiation and stimulates the component of the sympathetic system that projects to brown adipose tissue. It does this, in part, by indirectly exciting and disinhibiting the CRH and/or TRH satiety output, as shown in Figure 1. It also tends to indirectly inhibit a feeding system. It is interesting that regulation of leptin release may itself be a function of the sympathetic system, as well as of the amount of adipose fat (38). The hypothalamic peptide components of this sympathetic satiation system include a variety of satiety-producing peptides, namely, CRH, CART, CCK, BBS, ENT, and α-MSH (768). Bombesin, for example, acts via the CRH system to promote activation of the HPA axis to cause a rise in plasma ACTH, CORT, epinephrine, and glucose (786). Also, sympathetic activity and satiation are potentiated by 5HT, acting at 5HT1B/2C receptors, and by NE, acting at β_2- and β_3-adrenergic receptors. These influences cause lipolysis and provide fuel while augmenting sympathetic tone (787).

C Low Sympathetic Tone

Lesions of the MH region or PVN do the opposite of MH stimulation and leptin. The MH lesions cause overeating and an elevated plateau for body weight maintenance (561,788), with low sympathetic activity occurring during the dynamic weight gain phase. Ventromedial hypothalamic damage may also destroy neurons necessary for inhibition of peripheral insulin secretion (789). This leads to hyperinsulinemia that is proportional to the elevated level of body weight (790). Thus, these lesions unsettle the autonomic nervous system by creating an animal with low sympathetic tone, which is accompanied by an increase in parasympathetic tone (443). A similar state of parasympathetic dominance occurs in the obese state, as shown in animals that are genetically obese (791) and in obese men (792). They deposit excess fat with or without overeating, although they generally do overeat, and this hyperphagia further exacerbates their obesity. Spontaneous food intake is usually inversely correlated with the sympathetic activity that is measured in terms neural activation of brown adipose tissue (560). Paradoxically, low sympathetic tone can be found in both underweight and overweight animals. One possible explanation is that the "overweight" animals may actually be "underweight" in relation to their weight plateau. This is the familiar description of VMH-lesioned animals, which in their dynamic phase are overeaters and gain weight but are actually underweight relative to their own eventual weight level (788). Thus, low sympathetic activity in brown adipose tissue and related systems reflects not only high food intake but also the tendency or "potential" to eat (771). Perhaps any animal that is under its preferred weight level for a given diet can have a large feeding potential coupled with low sympathetic activity. This may include food-deprived animals, VMH-lesioned animals in the dynamic phase, genetically obese animals, or dietary obese animals that are denied their palatable diet.

Some of these effects can be seen with electrical stimulation of the PFLH region. Self-stimulation of this site can promote eating to the extent of causing obesity (793). Stimulation also causes parasympathetic functions in peripheral tissues, as evidenced by increased cholinergic tone (442–444,784). The LH stimulation site most relevant to this discussion is in the PFLH, where orexin and MCH cell bodies are located. Orexin neurons extend, in part, to medullary sympathetic outputs and may play a role in the control of cardiovascular sympathetic responses (225,794). However, this pressor response system is different than the brown adipose thermogenesis system, even though both are part of the sympathetic nervous system. Thus, the complex orexin system may be involved in both parasympathetic feeding processes as well as sympathetic arousal via the spinal cord. There is evidence that CCK, bombesin and leptin can inhibit the self-stimulation reward system (795,796). This may occur through the connection to the orexin/DYN system shown in Figures 1 and 2.

IX CONCLUSION

As evident from the new references in this review, the study of ingestive behavior and obesity from the neuroscience perspective is a burgeoning field. There are many exciting discoveries, including the revelation of peptides for eating and satiation that were hitherto unknown. Two examples serve to illustrate the panoply of interactions that are described above. The first "feeding peptide" discovered was NPY. This peptide not only induces a strong appetite; it causes vital metabolic adjustments. A variety of endocrine signals feed back to regulate NPY and its receptors. For example, leptin and insulin control the production of NPY, and CORT controls NPY receptors. Now, NPY is known to be colocalized with AGRP, which acts as an endogenous antagonist to block a CART/α-MSH satiety system and induce increased food intake over a period of several days. This long-lasting effect, which may occur through some yet-to-be-discovered change in gene expression, involves the newly discovered orexin pathway, which induces feeding with its axons that travel from the LH to both the hindbrain and frontal cortex. Orexin is colocalized with the opioid peptide DYN. Therefore, this orexin-DYN path may be a major component of the classic LH feeding systems that subserve appetite and reinforcement, as displayed in stimulation-induced eating and self-stimulation.

The behavior reinforcement pathway is a circuit that includes both the hindbrain centers for the taste and visceral integration, and the forebrain centers for cognitive integration. For example, in the NAc, DA potentiates eating, and ACh potentiates satiation. Release of these neurotransmitters is part of a learning process that allows the animal to plan ahead to acquire nutritious food, coded as palatable, and avoid poisonous items coded as unpalatable. The output is motivation to eat, conditioned cephalic reflexes for eating, and adjustments of the autonomic nervous system for energy homeostasis. The most palatable and, therefore, preferred foods cause the release of opioids that prolong a meal and may even create signs of dependency.

The remarkable aspect of all that is reviewed above is the wealth of information about neural mechanisms that extend all the way from the gut and liver that send signals to the hindbrain and then to the motivational centers for feeding in the accumbens and the cognitive processes in the frontal cortex. The hypothalamus serves as "base of operations" that receives much of this neural information, plus its own hormonal signals and energy-rich molecules, and coordinates an output that sustains the energy needs for life. A major miscalculation at any step can lead to starvation or obesity. The unfolding beauty and intricacy of the neural and hormonal systems is a thing of awe. However, its application in modern times is impossible without parallel appreciation of the enormous impact of the environment, food availability, and food taste. The neural-hormonal system of energy homeostasis evolved in an environment of scarcity. It needs sociopolitical help in coping with problems created by refugee migrations on the one hand, and advertised superabundance on the other. An understanding of the neuroscience of ingestive behavior and obesity must bring with it a sensible food distribution and education system. Otherwise, it will just be science for the sake of treatment, without all the benefits that could accrue from prevention of starvation and overeating.

ACKNOWLEDGMENTS

Some of the research described in this review has been supported by U.S. Public Health Service grants MH 43422 (S.F.L.) and MH 30697 and DA 10608 (B.G.H.). We thank Ms. Kate Sepiashvili, Henrietta Enninful-Eghan, and Nicole Avena for their assistance in the preparation of this review chapter.

REFERENCES

1. Schwartz MW, Woods SC, Porte D Jr, Seeley RJ, Baskin DG. Central nervous system control of food intake. Nature 2000; 404:661–671.
2. Teitelbaum P, Stricker EM. Compound complementarities in the study of motivated behavior. Psychol Rev 1994; 101:312–317.
3. Hoebel BG. Brain-stimulation reward and aversion in relation to behavior. In: Wauquier A, Rolls ET, eds. Brain-Stimulation Reward. Amsterdam: Elsevier/North-Holland, 1976:335–372.
4. Berthoud H-R, Seeley RJ. Neural and metabolic control of macronutrient intake. Boca Raton: CRC Press, 2000.
5. Rolls ET. Neuronal activity related to the control of feeding. In: Ritter RC, Ritter S, Barnes CD, eds. Feeding Behaviour Neural and Humoral Controls. Orlando: Academic Press, 1986:163–190.
6. Rolls ET. Taste, olfactory, visual, and somatosensory representations of the sensory properties of foods in the brain, and their relation to the control of food intake. In: Berthoud HR, Seeley RJ, eds. Neural and Metabolic Control of Macronutrient Intake. Boca Raton: CRC Press, 2000:247–262.
7. Gietzen DW. Amino acid recognition in the central nervous system In: Berthoud HR, Seeley RJ, eds. Neural and Metabolic Control of Macronutrient Intake. Boca Raton; CRC Press, 2000:339–360.
8. Hoebel BG, Rada PV, Mark GP, Pothos EN. Neural systems for reinforcement and inhibition of behavior: relevance to eating, addiction and depression. In: Kahneman D, Diener E, Shwarz N, eds. Well Being: The Psychological Foundations of Hedonism. New York: Russel Sage Foundation 1999:560–574.
9. Woods SC, Chavez M, Park CR, Riedy C, Kaiyala K, Richardson RD, et al. The evaluation of insulin as a metabolic signal influencing behavior via the brain. (Review) Neurosci Biobehav Rev 1996; 20:139–144.
10. Schwartz MW, Sipols AJ, Marks JL, Sanacora G, White JD, Scheurink A, et al. Inhibition of hypothalamic neuropeptide Y gene expression by insulin. Endocrinology, 1992; 130:3608–3616.
11. Kaiyala KJ, Woods SC, Schwartz MW. New model for the regulation of energy balance and adiposity by the central nervous system. (Review) Am J Clin Nutr 1995; 62:1123S–1134S.
12. McGowan MK, Andrews KM, Kelly J, Grossman SP. Effects of chronic intrahypothalamic infusion of insulin on food intake and diurnal meal patterning in the rat. Behav Neurosci 1990; 104:373–385.
13. Vanderweele DA. Insulin is a prandial satiety hormone. Physiol Behav 1994; 56:619–622.
14. Woods SC, Schwartz MW, Baskin DG, Seeley RJ. Food intake and the regulation of body weight. Annu Rev Psychol 2000; 51:255–277.
15. Baura GD, Foster DM, Porte D Jr, Kahn SE, Bergman RN, Cobelli C, et al. Saturable transport of insulin from plasma into the central nervous system of dogs in vivo. A mechanism for regulated insulin delivery to the brain. J Clin Invest 1993; 92:1824–1830.
16. Kapeller R, Moriarty A, Strauss A, Stubdal H, Theriault K, Siebert E, et al. Tyrosine phosphorylation of tub and its association with Src homology 2 domain-containing proteins implicate tub in intracellular signaling by insulin. J Biol Chem 1999; 274:24980–24986.
17. Schwartz MW, Figlewicz DP, Baskin DG, Woods SC, Porte D Jr. Insulin in the brain: a hormonal regulator of energy balance. (Review) Endocr Rev 1992; 13:387–414.
18. Tang C, Akabayashi A, Manitiu A, Leibowitz SF. Hypothalamic galanin gene expression and peptide levels in relation to circulating insulin: possible role in energy balance. Neuroendocrinology 1997; 65:265–275.
19. Sahu A, Dube MG, Phelps CP, Sninsky CA, Kalra PS, Kalra SP. Insulin and insulin-like growth factor II suppress neuropeptide Y release from the nerve terminals in the paraventricular nucleus: a putative hypothalamic site for energy homeostasis. Endocrinology 1995; 136:5718–5724.
20. Zhang Y, Proenca R, Maffei M, Barone M, Leopold L, Friedman JM. Positional cloning of the mouse obese gene and its human homologue. Nature 1994; 372:425–432.
21. Tartaglia LA, Dembski M, Weng X, Deng N, Culpepper J, Devos R, et al. Identification and expression

cloning of a leptin receptor, OB-R. Cell 1995; 83:1263–1271.

22. Ahima RS, Flier JS. Leptin. Annu Rev Physiol 2000; 62:413–437.
23. Harris BS. Leptin—much more than a satiety signal. Annu Rev Nutr 2000; 20:45–75.
24. Marks DL, Cone RD. Central melanocortins and the regulation of weight during acute and chronic disease. Recent Prog Horm Res 2001; 56:359–375.
25. Hamilton BS, Paglia D, Kwan AY, Deitel M. Increased obese mRNA expression in omental fat cells from massively obese humans. Nat Med 1995; 1:953–956.
26. Buyse M, Viengchareun S, Bado A, Lombes M. Insulin and glucocorticoids differentially regulate leptin transcription and secretion in brown adipocytes. FASEB J 2001; 15:1357–1366.
27. Banks WA, Kastin AJ, Huang W, Jaspan JB, Maness LM. Leptin enters the brain by a saturable system independent of insulin. Peptides 1996; 17:305–311.
28. Caro JF, Sinha MK, Kolaczynski JW, Zhang PL, Considine RV. Leptin: the tale of an obesity gene. Diabetes 1996; 45:1455–1462.
29. Campfield LA, Smith FJ, Guisez Y, Devos R, Burn P. Recombinant mouse OB protein: evidence for a peripheral signal linking adiposity and central neural networks. Science 1995; 269:546–549.
30. Koyama K, Shimabukuro M, Chen G, Wang MY, Lee Y, Kalra PS, et al. Resistance to adenovirally induced hyperleptinemia in rats. Comparison of ventromedial hypothalamic lesions and mutated leptin receptors. J Clin Invest 1998; 102:728–733.
31. Kalra SP, Dube MG, Pu S, Xu B, Horvath TL, Kalra PS. Interacting appetite regulating pathways in the hypothalamic regulation of body weight. (Review) Endocr Rev 1999; 20:68–100.
32. Ioffe E, Moon B, Connolly E, Friedman JM. Abnormal regulation of the leptin gene in the pathogenesis of obesity. Proc Natl Acad Sci USA 1998; 95:11852–11857.
33. Erickson JC, Clegg KE, Palmiter RD. Sensitivity to leptin and susceptibility to seizures of mice lacking neuropeptide Y. Nature 1996; 381:415–421.
34. Halaas JL, Boozer C, Blair-West J, Fidahusein N, Denton DA, Friedman JM Physiological response to longterm peripheral and central leptin infusion in lean and obese mice. Proc Natl Acad Scl USA 1998; 94: 8878–8883.
35. Shimabukuro M, Koyama K, Chen G, Wang MY, Trieu F, Lee Y, et al. Direct antidiabetic effect of leptin through triglyceride depletion of tissues. Proc Natl Acad Sci USA 1997; 94:4637–4641.
36. Quian H, Azani MJ, Compton MM, Hartzell D, Hausman GH, Baile CA. Brain adminstration of leptin causes deletion of adipocytes by apoptosis, Endocrinology 1997; 139:791–794.
37. Ahima RS, Prabakaran D, Mantzoros C, Qu D, Lowell B, Maratos-Flier E, et al. Role of leptin in the neuroendocrine response to fasting. Nature 1996; 382: 250–252.
38. Rayner DV, Trayhurn P. Regulation of leptin production: sympathetic nervous system interactions. J Mol Med 2001; 79:8–20.
39. Barash IA, Cheung CC, Weigle DS, Ren H, Kabigting EB, Kuijper JL, et al. Leptin is a metabolic signal to the reproductive system. Endocrinology 1996; 137: 3144–3147.
40. Unger RH. Leptin physiology: a second look. Regul Pept 2000; 92:87–95.
41. Baile CA, Della-Fera MA, Martin RJ. Regulation of metabolism and body fat mass by leptin. Annu Rev Nutr 2000; 20:105–127.
42. Tempel DL, Leibowitz SF. Adrenal steroid receptors: interactions with brain neuropeptide systems in relation to nutrient intake and metabolism. (Review) J Neuroendocrinol 1994; 6:479–501.
43. Dallman MF, Strack AM, Akana SF, Bradbury MJ, Hanson ES, Scribner KA, et al. Feast and famine: critical role of glucocortoticoids with insulin in daily energy flow. (Review) Front Neuroendocrinol 1993; 14:303–347.
44. Devenport L, Knehans A, Sundstrom A, Thomas T. Corticosterone's dual metabolic actions. Life Sci 1989; 45:1389–1396.
45. King BM. Glucocorticoids and hypothalamic obesity. (Review) Neurosci Biobehav Rev 1988; 12:29–37.
46. Bray GA, Fisler JS, York DA. Neuroendocrine control of the development of obesity: understanding gained from studies of animal models. Front Neuroendocrinol 1996; 11:128–181.
47. Epstein AN. Neurohormonal control of salt intake in the rat. (Review) Brain Res Bull 1991; 27:315–320.
48. Gomez-Sanchez EP, Fort C, Thwaites D. Central mineralocorticoid receptor antagonism blocks hypertension in Dahl S/JR rats. Am J Physiol 1992; 262: E96–E99.
49. Virgin CE Jr, Ha TP, Packan DR, Tombaugh GC, Yang SH, Horner HC, et al. Glucocorticoids inhibit glucose transport and glutamate uptake in hippocampal astrocytes: implications for glucocorticoid neurotoxicity. J Neurochem 1991; 57:1422–1428.
50. Sapolsky RM, Krey LC, McEwen BS. The neuroendocrinology of stress and aging: the glucocorticoid cascade hypothesis. (Review) Endocr Rev 1986; 7:284–301.
51. Shor-Posner G, Ian C, Brennan G, Cohn T, Moy H, Ning A, et al. Self-selecting albino rats exhibit differential preferences for pure macronutrient diets: characterization of three subpopulations. Physiol Behav 1991; 50:1187–1195.
52. Richard D, Chapdelaine S, Deshaies Y, Pepin MC, Barden N. Energy balance and lipid metabolism in

transgenic mice bearing an antisense GCR gene construct. Am J Physiol 1993; 265:R146–R150.
53. McEwen BS. Non-genomic and genomic effects of steroids on neural activity. (Review) Trends Pharmacol Sci 1991; 12:141–147.
54. Born J, DeKloet ER, Wenz H, Kern W, Fehm HL. Gluco- and antimineralocorticoid effects on human sleep: a role of central corticosteroid receptors. Am J Physiol 1991; 260:E183–E188.
55. Jeanrenaud B, Rohner-Jeanrenaud F. CNS-periphery relationships and body weight homeostasis: influence of the glucocorticoid status. Int J Obes Relat Metab Disord 2000; 24(suppl 2):S74–S76.
56. Jeanrenaud B, Rohner-Jeanrenaud F. Effects of neuropeptides and leptin on nutrient partitioning: dysregulations in obesity. Annu Rev Med 2001; 52:339–351.
57. Rohner-Jeanrenaud F. Hormonal regulation of energy partitioning. Int J Obes Relat Metab Disord 2000; 24(suppl 2):S4–S7.
58. Wade GN, Schneider JE. Metabolic fuels and reproduction in female mammals. (Review) Neurosci Biobehav Rev 1992; 16:235–272.
59. Wade GN, Schneider JE, Li H. Control of fertility by metabolic cues. Am J Physiol 1996; 270:1–20.
60. Bonavera JJ, Dube MG, Kalra PS, Kalra SP. Anorectic effects of estrogen may be mediated by decreased neuropeptide-Y release in the hypothalamic paraventricular nucleus. Endocrinology 1994; 134:2367–2370.
61. Baskin DG, Norwood BJ, Schwartz MW, Koerker DJ. Estradiol inhibits the increase of hypothalamic neuropeptide Y messenger ribonucleic acid expression induced by weight loss in ovariectomized rats. Endocrinology 1995; 136:5547–5554.
62. Swanson LW, Simmons DM. Differential steroid hormone and neural influences on peptide mRNA levels in CRH cells of the paraventricular nucleus: a hybridization histochemical study in the rat. J Comp Neurol 1989; 285:413–435.
63. Butera PC, Xiong M, Davis RJ, Platania SP. Central implants of dilute estradiol enhance the satiety effect of CCK-8. Behav Neurosci 1996; 110:823–830.
64. Geary N. Estradiol, CCK and satiation. Peptides 2001; 22:1251–1263.
65. Geary N, Asarian L. Estradiol increases glucagon's satiating potency in ovariectomized rats. Am J Physiol Regul Integr Comp Physiol 2001; 281:R1290–R1294.
66. Laferrere B, Wurtman RJ. Effect of d-fenfluramine on serotonin release in brain of anaesthetized rats. Brain Res 1989; 504:258–263.
67. Gabriel SM, Washton DL, Roncancio JR. Modulation of hypothalamic galanin gene expression by estrogen in peripubertal rats. Peptides 1992; 13:801–806.
68. Merchenthaler I, Lennard DE, Lopez FJ, Negro-Vilar A. Neonatal imprinting predetermines the sexually dimorphic, estrogen-dependent expression of galanin in luteinizing hormone–releasing hormone neurons. Proc Natl Acad Sci USA 1993; 90:10479–10483.
69. Leibowitz SF. Brain peptides and obesity: pharmacologic treatment. (Review) Obes Res 1995; 3(suppl 4):573S–589S.
70. Alexander JT, Akabayashi A, Gabriel SM, Thomas BE, Leibowitz SF. Galanin and neuropeptide Y immunoreactivity in brain nuclei of female and male rats in relation to puberty. Soc Neurosci Abstr 1994; 20:99.
71. Leibowitz SF, Lucas DJ, Leibowitz KL, Jhanwar YS. Developmental patterns of macronutrient intake in female and male rats from weaning to maturity. Physiol Behav 1991; 50:1167–1174.
72. Ono T, Sasaki K, Shibata R. Feeding- and chemical-related activity of ventromedial hypothalamic neurones in freely behaving rats. J Physiol 1987; 394:221–237.
73. Mobbs CV, Kow LM, Yang XJ. Brain glucose-sensing mechanisms: ubiquitous silencing by aglycemia vs. hypothalamic neuroendocrine responses. Am J Physiol Edocrinol Metab 2001; 281:E649-E654.
74. Lynch RM, Tompkins LS, Brooks HL, Dunn-Meynell AA, Levin BE. Localization of glucokinase gene expression in the rat brain. Diabetes 2000; 49:693–700.
75. Bernardis LL, Bellinger LL. The lateral hypothalamic area revisited: ingestive behavior. Neurosci Biobehav Rev 1996; 20:189–287.
76. Levin BE, Dunn-Meynell AA, Routh VH. Brain glucose sensing and body energy homeostasis: role in obesity and diabetes. Am J Physiol 1999; 276:R1223-R1231.
77. Wang J, Dourmashkin JT, Yun R, Leibowitz SF. Rapid changes in hypothalamic neuropeptide Y produced by carbohydrate-rich meals that enhance corticosterone and glucose levels. Brain Res 1999; 848:124–136.
78. Jhanwar-Uniyal M, Papamichael MJ, Leibowitz SF. Glucose-dependent changes in alpha 2-noradrenergic receptors in hypothalamic nuclei. Physiol Behav 1988; 44:611–617.
79. Watkins PA, Hamilton JA, Leaf A, Spector AA, Moore SA, Anderson RE, et al. Brain uptake and utilization of fatty acids: applications to peroxisomal biogenesis diseases. J Mol Neurosci 2001; 16:87–92.
80. Drew PA, Smith E, Thomas PD. Fat distribution and changes in the blood brain barrier in a rat model of cerebral arterial fat embolism. J Neurol Sci 1998; 156: 138–143.
81. Brossard N, Croset M, Lecerf J, Pachiaudi C, Normand S, Chirouze V, et al. Metabolic fate of an oral tracer dose of [^{13}C]docosahexaenoic acid triglycerides in the rat. Am J Physiol 1996; 270:R846-R854.
82. Volterra A, Trotti D, Cassutti P, Tromba C, Salvaggio A, Melcangi RC, et al. High sensitivity of glutamate uptake to extracellular free arachidonic acid levels in

rat cortical synaptosomes and astrocytes. J Neurochem 1992; 59:600–606.
83. Horimoto N, Nabekura J, Ogawa T. Arachidonic acid activation of potassium channels in rat visual cortex neurons. Neuroscience 1997; 77:661–671.
84. Leibowitz SF, Akabayashi A, Wang J. Obesity on a high-fat diet: role of hypothalamic galanin in neurons of the anterior paraventricular nucleus projecting to the median eminence. J Neurosci 1998; 18:2709–2719.
85. Tsujii S, Nakai Y, Fukata J, Nakaishi S, Takahashi H, Usui T, et al. Effects of food deprivation and high fat diet on immunoreactive beta-endorphin levels in brain regions of Zucker rats. Endocrinol Jpn 1987; 34:903–909.
86. Leibowitz SF, Dourmashkin JT, Chang GQ, Hill JD, Gayles EC, Fried SK, Wang J. Acute high-fat diet links hypothalamic peptide to triglycerides and lipid metabolism. Physiol Behav 2003. Submitted.
87. Stanley BG, Kyrkouli SE, Lampert S, Leibowitz SF. Neuropeptide Y chronically injected into the hypothalamus: a powerful neurochemical inducer of hyperphagia and obesity. Peptides 1986; 7:1189–1192.
88. Inui A. Transgenic approach to the study of body weight regulation. Pharmacol Rev 2000; 52:35–61.
89. Dryden S, Frankish H, Wang Q, Williams G. Neuropeptide Y and energy balance: one way ahead for the treatment of obesity. (Review) Eur J Clin Invest 1994; 24:293–308.
90. Billington CJ, Briggs JE, Harker S, Grace M, Levine AS. Neuropeptide Y in hypothalamic paraventricular nucleus: a center coordinating energy metabolism. Am J Physiol 1994; 266(Pt 2):R1765–R1770.
91. Williams G, Harrold JA, Cutler DJ. The hypothalamus and the regulation of energy homeostasis: lifting the lid on a black box. Proc Nutr Soc 2000; 59:385–396.
92. Stanley BG. Neuropeptide Y in multiple hypothalamic sites controls eating behavior, endocrine and autonomic systems for body energy balance. In: Colmers WF, Wahlestedt C, eds. The Biology of Neuropeptide Y and Related Peptides. Totowa, NJ: Humana Press, 1993:457–509.
93. Palou A, Serra F, Bonet ML, Pico C. Obesity: molecular bases of a multifactorial problem. Eur J Nutr 2000; 39:127–144.
94. Parikh R, Marks JL. Metabolic and orexigenic effects of intracerebroventricular neuropeptide Y are attenuated by food deprivation. J Neuroendocrinol 1997; 9:789–795.
95. Minshull M, Strong CR. The stimulation of lipogenesis in white adipose tissue from fed rats by corticosterone. Int J Biochem 1985; 17:529–532.
96. Egawa M, Yoshimatsu H, Bray GA. Neuropeptide Y suppresses sympathetic activity to interscapular brown adipose tissue in rats. Am J Physiol 1991; 260:R328–R334.
97. Robinson SW, Dinulescu DM, Cone RD. Genetic models of obesity and energy balance in the mouse. Annu Rev Genet 2000; 34:687–745.
98. Broberger C, Johansen J, Johansson C, Schalling M, Hokfelt T. The neuropeptide Y/agouti gene-related protein (AGRP) brain circuitry in normal, anorectic, and monosodium glutamate-treated mice. Proc Natl Acad Sci USA 1998; 95:15043–15048.
99. Chen P, Li C, Haskell-Luevano C, Cone RD, Smith MS. Altered expression of agouti-related protein and its colocalization with neuropeptide Y in the arcuate nucleus of the hypothalamus during lactation. Endocrinology 1999; 140:2645–2650.
100. Stanley BG, Magdalin W, Seirafi A, Nguyen MM, Leibowitz SF. Evidence for neuropeptide Y mediation of eating produced by food deprivation and for a variant of the Y1 receptor mediating this peptide's effect. Peptides 1992; 13:581–587.
101. Leibowitz SF, Xuereb M, Kim T. Blockade of natural and neuropeptide Y–induced carbohydrate feeding by a receptor antagonist PYX-2. Neuroreport 1992; 3: 1023–1026.
102. Akabayashi A, Wahlestedt C, Alexander JT, Leibowitz SF. Specific inhibition of endogenous neuropeptide Y synthesis in arcuate nucleus by antisense oligonucleotides suppresses feeding behavior and insulin secretion. Brain Res 1994; 21:55–61.
103. Leibowitz SF. Differential functions of hypothalamic galanin cell grows in the regulation of eating and body weight. (Review) Ann NY Acad Sci 1998; 863:206–220.
104. Erickson JC, Hollopeter G, Palmiter RD. Attenuation of the obesity syndrome of ob/ob mice by the loss of neuropeptide Y. Science 1996; 274:1704–1707.
105. Kaga T, Inui A, Okita M, Asakawa A, Ueno N, Kasuga M, et al. Modest overexpression of neuropeptide Y in the brain leads to obesity after high-sucrose feeding. Diabetes 2001; 50:1206–1210.
106. Larsen PJ, Jessop DS, Chowdrey HS, Lightman SL, Mikkelsen JD. Chronic administration of glucocorticoids directly upregulates prepro-neuropeptide Y and Y1-receptor mRNA levels in the arcuate nucleus of the rat. J Neuroendocrinol 1994; 6:153–159.
107. White BD, Dean RG, Edwards GL, Martin RJ. Type II corticosteroid receptor stimulation increases NPY gene expression in basomedial hypothalamus of rats. Am J Physiol 1994; 266:R1523–R1529.
108. Akabayashi A, Watanabe Y, Wahlestedt C, McEwen BS, Paez X, Leibowitz SF. Hypothalamic neuropeptide Y, its gene expression and receptor activity: relation to circulating corticosterone in adrenalectomized rats. Brain Res 1994; 665:201–212.
109. Krysiak R, Obuchowicz E, Herman ZS. Interactions between the neuropeptide Y system and the hypothalamic- pituitary-adrenal axis. Eur J Endocrinol 1999; 140:130–136.

110. Urban JH, Bauer-Dantoin AC, Levine JE. Effects of steroid replacement on neuropeptide-Y (NPY) gene expression in the arcuate nucleus (ARC) of ovariectomized (OVX) rats. Soc Neurosci Abstr 1992; 18:110.
111. Brann DW, McDonald JK, Putnam CD, Mahesh VB. Regulation of hypothalamic gonadotropin-releasing hormone and neuropeptide Y concentrations by progesterone and corticosteroids in immature rats: correlation with luteinizing hormone and follicle-stimulating hormone release. Neuroendocrinology 1991; 54:425–432.
112. Kalra SP, Crowley WR. Neuropeptide Y: a novel neuroendocrine peptide in the control of pituitary hormone secretion, and its relation to luteinizing hormone. (Review) Front Neuroendocrinol 1992; 13:1–46.
113. Leibowitz SF, Akabayashi A, Alexander JT, Wang J. Gonadal steroids and hypothalamic galanin and neuropeptide Y: role in eating behavior and body weight control in female rats. Endocrinology 1998; 139:1771–1780.
114. Wang J, Leibowitz KL. Central insulin inhibits hypothalamic galanin and neuropeptide Y gene expression and peptide release in intact rats. Brain Res 1997; 777: 231–236.
115. Leibowitz SF. Brain neuropeptide Y: an integrator of endocrine, metabolic and behavioral processes. (Review) Brain Res Bull 1991; 27:333–337.
116. Sahu A, Sninsky CA, Phelps CP, Dube MG, Kalra PS, Kalra SP. Neuropeptide Y release from the paraventricular nucleus increases in association with hyperphagia in streptozotocin-induced diabetic rats. Endocrinology 1992; 131:2979–2985.
117. Beck B, Stricker-Krongrad A, Burlet A, Nicolas JP, Burlet C. Specific hypothalamic neuropeptide Y variation with diet parameters in rats with food choice. Neuroreport 1992; 3:571–574.
118. Jhanwar-Uniyal M, Beck B, Jhanwar YS, Burlet C, Leibowitz SF. Neuropeptide Y projection from arcuate nucleus to parvocellular division of paraventricular nucleus: specific relation to the ingestion of carbohydrate. Brain Res 1993; 631:97–106.
119. Larue-Achagiotis C, Martin C, Verger P, Louis-Sylvestre J. Dietary self-selection vs. complete diet: body weight gain and meal pattern in rats. Physiol Behav 1992; 51:995–999.
120. Jhanwar-Uniyal M, Beck B, Burlet C, Leibowitz SF. Diurnal rhythm of neuropeptide Y–like immunoreactivity in the suprachiasmatic, arcuate and paraventricular nuclei and other hypothalamic sites. Brain Res 1990; 536:331–334.
121. Kanarek RB, Marks-Kaufman R, Ruthazer R, Gualtieri L. Increased carbohydrate consumption by rats as a function of 2-deoxy-D-glucose administration. Pharmacol Biochem Behav 1983; 18:47–50.
122. Sergeyev V, Broberger C, Gorbatyuk O, Hokfelt T. Effect of 2-mercaptoacetate and 2-deoxy-D-glucose administration on the expression of NPY, AGRP, POMC, MCH and hypocretin/orexin in the rat hypothalamus. Neuroreport 2000; 11:117–121.
123. Giraudo SQ, Kim EM, Grace MK, Billington CJ, Levine AS. Effect of peripheral 2-DG on opioid and neuropeptide Y gene expression. Brain Res 1998; 792: 136–140.
124. Allen JM, McGregor GP, Woodhams PL, Polak JM, Bloom SR. Ontogeny of a novel peptide, neuropeptide Y (NPY) in rat brain. Brain Res 1984; 303:197–200.
125. Sutton SW, Mitsugi N, Plotsky PM, Sarkar DK. Neuropeptide Y (NPY): a possible role in the initiation of puberty. Endocrinology 1988; 123:2152–2154.
126. Alexander JT, Akabayashi A, Gabriel SM, Baskin LE, Owen CJ, Leibowitz SF. Galanin and neuropeptide-Y immunoreactivity in hypothalamic nuclei in relation to the estrous cycle. Soc Neurosci Abstr 1995; 21.
127. Bauer-Dantoin AC, Urban JH, Levine JE. Neuropeptide Y gene expression in the arcuate nucleus is increased during preovulatory luteinizing hormone surges. Endocrinology 1992; 131:2953–2958.
128. Levin BE. Arcuate NPY neurons and energy homeostasis in diet-induced obese and resistant rats. Am J Physiol 1999; 276:R382–R387.
129. Levin BE, Dunn-Meynell AA. Dysregulation of arcuate nucleus preproneuropeptide Y mRNA in diet-induced obese rats. Am J Physiol 1997; 272:R1365–R1370.
130. Wang J, Chang G.Q., Dourmashkin J, Yun R, Gayles EC, Hill J. Neuropeptide Y in models of dietary obesity: stimulation by conditions that promote lipogenesis and inhibition by elevated leptin and body fat. Obes Res 2003. Submitted.
131. Dube MG, Xu B, Kalra PS, Sninsky CA, Kalra SP. Disruption in neuropeptide Y and leptin signaling in obese ventromedial hypothalamic-lesioned rats. Brain Res 1999; 816:38–46.
132. Guan XM, Yu H, Van Der Ploeg LH. Evidence of altered hypothalamic pro-opiomelanocortin/ neuropeptide Y mRNA expression in tubby mice. Mol Brain Res 1998; 59:273–279.
133. Bergen HT, Mobbs CV. Ventromedial hypothalamic lesions produced by gold thioglucose do not impair induction of NPY mRNA in the arcuate nucleus by fasting. Brain Res 1996; 707:266–271.
134. Widdowson PS, Upton R, Henderson L, Buckingham R, Wilson S, Williams G. Reciprocal regional changes in brain NPY receptor density during dietary restriction and dietary-induced obesity in the rat. Brain Res 1997; 774:1–10.
135. McMinn JE, Seeley RJ, Wilkinson CW, Havel PJ, Woods SC, Schwartz MW. NPY-induced overfeeding suppresses hypothalamic NPY mRNA expression: potential roles of plasma insulin and leptin. Regul Pept 1998; 75–76:425–431.
136. Gundlach AL, Burazin TC, Larm JA. Distribution,

regulation and role of hypothalamic galanin systems: renewed interest in a pleiotropic peptide family. Clin Exp Pharmacol Physiol 2001; 28:100–105.
137. Tempel DL, Leibowitz SF. Diurnal variations in the feeding responses to norepinephrine, neuropeptide Y and galanin in the PVN. Brain Res Bull 1990; 25:821–825.
138. Chae HJ, Hoebel BG, Tempel DL, Paredes M, Leibowitz SF. Neuropeptide-Y, galanin and opiate agonists have differential effects on nutrient ingestion. Soc Neurosci Abstr 1995; 21:696.
139. Kyrkouli SE, Stanley BG, Hutchinson R, Seirafi RD, Leibowitz SF. Peptide-amine interactions in the hypothalamic paraventricular nucleus: analysis of galanin and neuropeptide Y in relation to feeding. Brain Res 1990; 521:185–191.
140. Leibowitz SF. Macronutrient and brain peptides: what they do and how they respond. In: Berthoud HR, Seeley RJ, eds. Neural and Metabolic Control of Macronutrient Intake. Boca Raton: CRC Press, 2000: 389–406.
141. Bergonzelli GE, Pralong FP, Glauser M, Cavadas C, Grouzmann E, Gaillard RC. Interplay between galanin and leptin in the hypothalamic control of feeding via corticotropin-releasing hormone and neuropeptide Y. Diabetes 2001; 50:2666–2672.
142. Leibowitz SF. Hypothalamic galanin, dietary fat, and body fat. In: Bray G, Ryan D, eds. Nutrition, Genetics and Obesity. Baton Rouge: Louisiana State University Press, 1999: 338–381.
143. Akabayashi A, Koenig JI, Watanabe Y, Alexander JT, Leibowitz SF. Galanin-containing neurons in the paraventricular nucleus: a neurochemical marker for fat ingestion and body weight gain. Proc Natl Acad Sci USA 1994; 91:10375–10379.
144. Barton C, Lin L, York DA, Bray GA. Differential effects of enterostatin, galanin and opioids on high-fat diet consumption. Brain Res 1995; 702(1–2):55–60.
145. Lin L, Bray G, York DA. Enterostatin suppresses food intake in rats after near-celiac and intracarotid arterial injection. Am J Physiol Regul Integr Comp Physiol 2000; 278:R1346–R1351.
146. Corwin RL, Rowe PM, Crawley JN. Galanin and the galanin antagonist M40 do not change fat intake in a fat-chow choice paradigm in rats. Am J Physiol 1995; 269: R511–R518.
147. Koegler FH, Ritter S. Feeding induced by pharmacological blockade of fatty acid metabolism is selectively attenuated by hindbrain injections of the galanin receptor antagonist, M40. Obes Res 1996; 4:329–336.
148. Leibowitz SF, Kim T. Impact of a galanin antagonist on exogenous galanin and natural patterns of fat ingestion. Brain Res 1992; 599:148–152.
149. Corwin RL, Robinson JK, Crawley JN. Galanin antagonists block galanin-induced feeding in the hypothalamus and amygdala of the rat. Eur J Neurosci 1993; 5:1528–1533.
150. Menendez JA, Atrens DM, Leibowitz SF. Metabolic effects of galanin injections into the paraventricular nucleus of the hypothalamus. Peptides 1992; 13:323–327.
151. Nagase H, Bray GA, York DA. Effect of galanin and enterostatin on sympathetic nerve activity to interscapular brown adipose tissue. Brain Res 1996; 709: 44–50.
152. Koenig JI, Hooi SC, Maiter DM. On the interaction of galanin within the hypothalamopituitary axis of the rat. In: Hokfelt T, Bartfai T, Jacobowitz T, Ottson DT, eds. Galanin—A New Multifunctional Peptide in the Neuroendocrine System. New York: Macmillan, 1991:331–342.
153. Kondo K, Murase T, Otake K, Ito M, Oiso Y. Centrally administered galanin inhibits osmotically stimulated arginine vasopressin release in conscious rats. Neurosci Lett 1991; 128:245–248.
154. Hedlund PB, Koenig JI, Fuxe K. Adrenalectomy alters discrete galanin mRNA, levels in the hypothalamus and mesencephalon of the rat. Neurosci Lett 1994; 170:77–82.
155. Akabayashi A, Watanabe Y, Gabriel SM, Chae HJ, Leibowitz SF. Hypothalamic galanin-like immunoreactivity and its gene expression in relation to circulating corticosterone. Mol Brain Res 1994; 25:305–312.
156. Merchenthaler I, Lopez FJ, Negro-Vilar A. Anatomy and physiology of central galanin-containing pathways. (Review) Prog Neurobiol 1993; 40:711–769.
157. Bloch GJ, Eckersell C, Mills R. Distribution of Galanin-immunoreactive cells within sexually dimorphic components of the medial preoptic area of the male and female rat. Brain Res 1993; 620:259–268.
158. Brann DW, Chorich LP, Mahesh VB. Effect of progesterone on galanin mRNA levels in the hypothalamus and the pituitary: correlation with the gonadotropin surge. Neuroendocrinology 1993; 58:531–538.
159. Cheung CC, Hohmann JG, Clifton DK, Steiner RA. Distribution of galanin messenger RNA-expressing cells in murine brain and their regulation by leptin in regions of the hypothalamus. Neuroscience 2001; 103: 423–432.
160. Beck B, Burlet A, Nicolas JP, Burlet C. Galanin in the hypothalamus of fed and fasted lean and obese Zucker rats. Brain Res 1993; 623:124–130.
161. Manitiu A, Nascimento J, Akabayashi A, Leibowitz SF. Inhibition of fatty acid oxidation via injection of mercaptoacetate. Int Behav Neurosci Abstr 1994; 3:67.
162. Akabayashi A, Zaia CT, Silva I, Chae HJ, Leibowitz SF. Neuropeptide Y in the arcuate nucleus is modulated by alterations in glucose utilization. Brain Res 1993; 621:343–348.

163. Dube MG, Kalra SP, Kalra PS. Hypothalamic galanin is up-regulated during hyperphagia and increased body weight gain induced by disruption of signaling in the ventromedial nucleus. Peptides 2000; 21:519–526.
164. Odorizzi M, Max JP, Tankosic P, Burlet C, Burlet A. Dietary preferences of Brattleboro rats correlated with an overexpression of galanin in the hypothalamus. Eur J Neurosci 1999; 11:3005–3014.
165. Mercer JG, Speakman JR. Hypothalamic neuropeptide mechanisms for regulating energy balance: from rodent models to human obesity. Neurosci Biobehav Rev 2001; 25:101–116.
166. Wang J, Akabayashi A, Dourmashkin J, Yu H-J, Alexander JT, Chae HJ, et al. Neuropeptide Y in relation to carbohydrate intake, corticosterone and dietary obesity. Brain Res 1998; 802:75–88.
167. Lin L, York DA, Bray GA. Comparison of Osborne-Mendel and S5B/PL strains of rat: central effects of galanin, NPY, beta-casomorphin and CRH on intake of high-fat and low-fat diets. Obes Res 1996; 4:117–124.
168. Baranowska B, Radzikowska M, Wasilewska-Dziubinska E, Roguski K, Borowiec M. Disturbed release of gastrointestinal peptides in anorexia nervosa and in obesity. Diabetes Obes Metab 2000; 2:99–103.
169. Marks DL, Smith MS, Vrontakis M, Clifton DK, Steiner RA. Regulation of galanin gene expression in gonadotropin-releasing hormone neurons during the estrous cycle of the rat. Endocrinology 1993; 132:1836–1844.
170. Gabriel SM, Kaplan LM, Martin JB, Koenig JI. Tissue-specific sex differences in galanin-like immunoreactivity and galanin mRNA during development in the rat. Peptides 1989; 10:369–374.
171. Rossmanith WG, Marks DL, Clifton DK, Steiner RA. Induction of galanin gene expression in gonadotropin-releasing hormone neurons with puberty in the rat. Endocrinology 1994; 135:1401–1408.
172. Hohmann JG, Clifton DK, Steiner RA. Galanin: analysis of its coexpression in gonadotropin-releasing hormonc and growth hormonc-rclcasing hormonc neurons. Ann NY Acad Sci 1998; 863:221–235.
173. Wynick D, Small CJ, Bloom SR, Pachnis V. Targeted disruption of the murine galanin gene. Ann NY Acad Sci 1998; 863:22–47.
174. Ohtaki T, Kumano S, Ishibashi Y, Ogi K, Matsui H, Harada M, et al. Isolation and cDNA cloning of a novel galanin-like peptide (GALP) from porcine hypothalamus. J Biol Chem 1999; 274:37041–37045.
175. Larm JA, Gundlach AL. Galanin-like peptide (GALP) mRNA expression is restricted to arcuate nucleus of hypothalamus in adult male rat brain. Neuroendocrinology 2000; 72:67–71.
176. Cunningham MJ, Krasnow SM, Jureus A, Li D, Carlson AE, Teklemichael DN, et al. Galanin-like peptide (GALP) as a potential regulator of pituitary hormone secretion. 31st Annual Meeting of the Society for Neurosciences, San Diego, CA, Nov 10–15, 2001.
177. Jureus A, Cunningham MJ, Li D, Johnson LL, Krasnow SM, Teklemichael DN, et al. Distribution and regulation of galanin-like peptide (GALP) in the hypothalamus of the mouse. Endocrinology 2001; 142: 5140–5144.
178. Ollmann MM, Wilson BD, Yang YK, Kerns JA, Chen Y, Gantz I, et al. Antagonism of central melanocortin receptors in vitro and in vivo by agouti-related protein. Science 1997; 278:135–138.
179. Baskin DG, Hahn TM, Schwartz MW. Leptin sensitive neurons in the hypothalamus. Horm Metab Res 1999; 31:345–350.
180. Hagan MM, Rushing PA, Pritchard LM, Schwartz MW, Strack AM, Van der Ploeg LH, et al. Long-term orexigenic effects of AgRP-(83-132) involve mechanisms other than melanocortin receptor blockade. Am J Physiol Regul Integr Comp Physiol 2000; 279:R47–R52.
181. Wortley KE, Davydova Z, Leibowitz SF. Agouti-related peptide (AGRP), like NPY is stimulated in the arcuate nucleus by a high-carbohydrate diet and, after injection, increases levels of hormones that promote lipogenesis. Obes Res 2002; 10(1):65–67.
182. Graham M, Shutter JR, Sarmiento U, Sarosi I, Stark KL. Overexpression of Agrt leads to obesity in transgenic mice. Nat Genet 1997; 17:273–274.
183. Wilson BD, Bagnol D, Kaelin CB, Ollmann MM, Gantz I, Watson SJ, et al. Pysiological and anatomical circuitry between Agouti-related protein and leptin signaling. Endocrinology 1999; 140:2387–2397.
184. Hagan MM, Benoit SC, Rushing PA, Pritchard LM, Woods SC, Seeley RJ. Immediate and prolonged patterns of Agouti-related peptide-(83-132)-induced c-Fos activation in hypothalamic and extrahypothalamic sites. Endocrinology 2001; 142:1050–1056.
185. Wirth MM, Giraudo SQ. Agouti-related protein in the hypothalamic paraventricular nucleus: effect on feeding [in process citation]. Peptides 2000; 21:1369–1375.
186. Mizuno TM, Mobbs CV. Hypothalamic agouti-related protein messenger ribonucleic acid is inhibited by leptin and stimulated by fasting. Endocrinology 1999; 140:814–817.
187. Ziotopoulou M, Mantzoros CS, Hileman SM, Flier JS. Differential expression of hypothalamic neuropeptides in the early phase of diet-induced obesity in mice. Am J Physiol Endocrinol Metab 2000; 279:E838–E845.
188. Ebihara K, Ogawa Y, Katsuura G, Numata Y, Masuzaki H, Satoh N, et al. Involvement of agouti-related protein, an endogenous antagonist of hypothalamic melanocortin receptor, in leptin action. Diabetes 1999; 48:2028–2033.
189. Qu SY, Yang YK, Li JY, Zeng Q, Gantz I. Agouti-

related protein is a mediator of diabetic hyperphagia. Regul Pept 2001; 98:69–75.

190. Makimura H, Mizuno TM, Roberts J, Silverstein J, Beasley J, Mobbs CV. Adrenalectomy reverses obese phenotype and restores hypothalamic melanocortin tone in leptin-deficient ob/ob mice. Diabetes 2000; 49:1917–1923.

191. Arvaniti K, Huang Q, Richard D. Effects of leptin and corticosterone on the expression of corticotropin-releasing hormone, agouti-related protein, and proopiomelanocortin in the brain of ob/ob mouse. Neuroendocrinology 2001; 73:227–236.

192. Sakurai T, Amemiya A, Ishii M, Matsuzaki I, Chemelli RM, Tanaka H, et al. Orexins and orexin receptors: a family of hypothalamic neuropeptides and G protein–coupled receptors that regulate feeding behavior. Cell 1998; 92:573–585.

193. De Lecea L, Kilduff TS, Peyron C, Gao X, Foye PE, Danielson PE, et al. The hypocretins: hypothalamus-specific peptides with neuroexcitatory activity. Proc Natl Acad Sci USA 1998; 95:322–327.

194. Lubkin M, Stricker-Krongrad A. Independent feeding and metabolic actions of orexins in mice. Biochem Biophys Res Commun 1998; 253:241–245.

195. Takahashi N, Okumura T, Yamada H, Kohgo Y. Stimulation of gastric acid secretion by centrally administered orexin-A in conscious rats. Biochem Biophys Res Commun 1999; 254:623–627.

196. Hara J, Beuckmann CT, Nambu T, Willie JT, Chemelli RM, Sinton CM, et al. Genetic ablation of orexin neurons in mice results in narcolepsy, hypophagia, and obesity Neuron 2001; 30:345–354.

197. Broberger C, De Lecea L, Sutcliffe JG, Hokfelt T. Hypocretin/orexin-and melanin-concentrating hormone-expressing cells form distinct populations in the rodent lateral hypothalamus: relationship to the neuropeptide Y and agouti gene-related protein systems. J Comp Neurol 1998; 402:460–474.

198. Elias CF, Saper CB, Maratos-Flier E, Tritos NA, Lee C, Kelly J, et al. Chemically defined projections linking the mediobasal hypothalamus and the lateral hypothalamic area. J Comp Neurol 1998; 402:442–459.

199. Horvath TL, Diano S, Van den Pol AN. Synaptic interaction between hypocretin (orexin) and neuropeptide Y cells in the rodent and primate hypothalamus: a novel circuit implicated in metabolic and endocrine regulations. J Neurosci 1999; 19:1072–1087.

200. Peyron C, Tighe DK, Van den Pol AN, De Lecea L, Heller HC, Sutcliffe JG, et al. Neurons containing hypocretin (orexin) project to multiple neuronal systems. J Neurosci 1998; 18:9996–10015.

201. Willie JT, Chemelli RM, Sinton CM, Yanagisawa M. To eat or to sleep? Orexin in the regulation of feeding and wakefulness. Annu Rev Neurosci 2001; 24:429–458.

202. Mondal MS, Nakazato M, Date Y, Murakami N, Yanagisawa M, Matsukura S. Widespread distribution of orexin in rat brain and its regulation upon fasting. Biochem Biophys Res Commun 1999; 256: 495–499.

203. Cai XJ, Widdowson PS, Harrold J, Wilson S, Buckingham RE, Arch JR, et al. Hypothalamic orexin expression: modulation by blood glucose and feeding. Diabetes 1999; 48:2132–2137.

204. Mondal MS, Nakazato M, Matsukura S. Orexins (hypocretins): novel hypothalamic peptides with divergent functions. Biochem Cell Biol 2000; 78:299–305.

205. Yamamoto Y, Ueta Y, Date Y, Nakazato M, Hara Y, Serino R, et al. Down regulation of the prepro-orexin gene expression in genetically obese mice. Mol Brain Res 1999; 65:14–22.

206. Beck B, Richy S. Hypothalamic hypocretin/orexin and neuropeptide Y: divergent interaction with energy depletion and leptin. Biochem Biophys Res Commun 1999; 258:119–122.

207. Taheri S, Mahmoodi M, Opacka-Juffry J, Ghatei MA, Bloom SR. Distribution and quantification of immunoreactive orexin A in rat tissues. FEBS Lett 1999; 457:157–161.

208. Griffond B, Risold PY, Jacquemard C, Colard C, Fellmann D. Insulin-induced hypoglycemia increases preprohypocretin (orexin) mRNA in the rat lateral hypothalamic area. Neurosci Lett 1999; 262:77–80.

209. Cai XJ, Evans ML, Lister CA, Leslie RA, Arch JR, Wilson S, et al. Hypoglycemia activates orexin neurons and selectively increases hypothalamic orexin-B levels: responses inhibited by feeding and possibly mediated by the nucleus of the solitary tract. Diabetes 2001; 50:105–112.

210. Moriguchi T, Sakurai T, Nambu T, Yanagisawa M, Goto K. Neurons containing orexin in the lateral hypothalamic area of the adult rat brain are activated by insulin-induced acute hypoglycemia. Neurosci Lett 1999; 264:101–104.

211. Risold PY, Griffond B, Kilduff TS, Sutcliffe JG, Fellmann D. Preprohypocretin (orexin) and prolactin-like immunoreactivity are coexpressed by neurons of the rat lateral hypothalamic area. Neurosci Lett 1999; 259:153–156.

212. Leibowitz SF, Wortley K.E., Chang G.Q. Prepro-orexin expression in hypothalamic neurons is potentiated by a high-fat diet and elevated in obesity-prone rats maintained on a high-fat diet. Obes Res 2000; 8(suppl 1):1.

213. Wortley KE, Chang GQ, Davydova Z, Leibowitz SF. Orexin gene expression is increased during states of hypertriglyceridemia. Am J Physiol Regul Integr Comp Physiol 2003. In press.

214. Cutler DJ, Morris R, Sheridhar V, Wattam TA, Holmes S, Patel S, et al. Differential distribution of

orexin-A and orexin-B immunoreactivity in the rat brain and spinal cord. Peptides 1999; 20:1455–1470.
215. Date Y, Ueta Y, Yamashita H, Yamaguchi H, Matsukura S, Kangawa K, et al. Orexins, orexigenic hypothalamic peptides, interact with autonomic, neuroendocrine and neuroregulatory systems. Proc Natl Acad Sci USA 1999; 96:748–753.
216. Nambu T, Sakurai T, Mizukami K, Hosoya Y, Yanagisawa M, Goto K. Distribution of orexin neurons in the adult rat brain. Brain Res 1999; 827:243–260.
217. Chemelli RM, Willie JT, Sinton CM, Elmquist JK, Scammell T, Lee C, et al. Narcolepsy in orexin knockout mice: molecular genetics of sleep regulation. Cell 1999; 98:437–451.
218. Lin L, Faraco J, Li R, Kadotani H, Rogers W, Lin X, et al. The sleep disorder canine narcolepsy is caused by a mutation in the hypocretin (orexin) receptor 2 gene. Cell 1999; 98:365–376.
219. Siegel JM. Narcolepsy: a key role for hypocretins (orexins). Cell 1999; 98:409–412.
220. Ida T, Nakahara K, Katayama T, Murakami N, Nakazato M. Effect of lateral cerebroventricular injection of the appetite-stimulating neuropeptide, orexin and neuropeptide Y, on the various behavioral activities of rats. Brain Res 1999; 821:526–529.
221. Pu S, Jain MR, Kalra PS, Kalra SP. Orexins, a novel family of hypothalamic neuropeptides, modulate pituitary luteinizing hormone secretion in an ovarian steroid-dependent manner. Regul Pept 1998; 78:133–136.
222. Samson WK, Gosnell B, Chang JK, Resch ZT, Murphy TC. Cardiovascular regulatory actions of the hypocretins in brain. Brain Res 1999; 831:248–253.
223. Chen CT, Hwang LL, Chang JK, Dun NJ. Pressor effects of orexins injected intracisternally and to rostral ventrolateral medulla of anesthetized rats. Am J Physiol Regul Integr Comp Physiol 2000; 278:R692–R697.
224. Shirasaka T, Nakazato M, Matsukura S, Takasaki M, Kannan H. Sympathetic and cardiovascular actions of orexins in conscious rats. Am J Physiol 1999; 277: R1780–R1785.
225. Dun NJ, Le Dun S, Chen CT, Hwang LL, Kwok EH, Chang JK. Orexins: a role in medullary sympathetic outflow. Regul Pept 2000; 96:65–70.
226. Rumantir MS, Vaz M, Jennings GL, Collier G, Kaye DM, Seals DR, et al. Neural mechanisms in human obesity-related hypertension. J Hypertens 1999; 17: 1125–1133.
227. Vaughan JM, Fischer WH, Hoeger C, Rivier J, Vale W. Characterization of melanin-concentrating hormone from rat hypothalamus. Endocrinology 1989; 125:1660–1665.
228. Nahon JL. The melanin-concentrating hormone: from the peptide to the gene. Crit Rev Neurobiol 1994; 8: 221–262.
229. Saito Y, Nothacker HP, Wang Z, Lin SH, Leslie F, Civelli O. Molecular characterization of the melanin-concentrating-hormone receptor. Nature 1999; 400: 265–269.
230. Chambers J, Ames RS, Bergsma D, Muir A, Fitzgerald LR, Hervieu G, et al. Melanin-concentrating hormone is the cognate ligand for the orphan G-protein-coupled receptor SLC-1. Nature 1999; 400: 261–265.
231. Qu D, Ludwig DS, Gammeltoft S, Piper M, Pelleymounter MA, Cullen MJ, et al. A role for melanin-concentrating hormone in the central regulation of feeding behaviour. Nature 1996; 380:243–247.
232. Rossi M, Choi SJ, O'Shea D, Miyoshi T, Ghatei MA, Bloom SR. Melanin-concentrating hormone acutely stimulates feeding, but chronic administration has no effect on body weight. Endocrinology 1997; 138:351–355.
233. Mystkowski P, Seeley RJ, Hahn TM, Baskin DG, Havel PJ, Matsumoto AM, et al. Hypothalamic melanin-concentrating hormone and estrogen-induced weight loss. J Neurosci 2000; 20:8637–8642.
234. Murray JF, Baker BI, Levy A, Wilson CA. The influence of gonadal steroids on pre-pro melanin-concentrating hormone mRNA in female rats. J Neuroendocrinol 2000; 12:53–59.
235. Shimada M, Tritos NA, Lowell BB, Flier LS, Maratos-Flier E. Mice lacking melanin-concentrating hormone are hypophagic and lean. Nature 1998; 396: 670–674.
236. Ludwig DS, Tritos NA, Mastaitis JW, Kulkarni R, Kokkotou E, Elmquist J, et al. Melanin-concentrating hormone overexpression in transgenic mice leads to obesity and insulin resistance. J Clin Invest 2001; 107:379–386.
237. Sahu A. Leptin decreases food intake induced by melanin-concentrating hormone (MCH), galanin (GAL) and neuropeptide Y (NPY) in the rat. Endocrinology 1998; 139:4739–4742.
238. Gosnell BA, Levine AS. Stimulation of ingestive behaviour by preferential and selective opiod agonists. In: Cooper SJ, Clifton PG, eds. Drug Receptor Subtypes and Ingestive Behaviour. London: Academic Press, 1996:147–166.
239. Glass MJ, Billington CJ, Levine AS. Opioids, food reward, and macronutrient selection. In: Berthoud HR, Seeley RJ, eds. Neural and Metabolic Control of Macronutrient Intake. Boca Raton: CRC Press, 2000: 407–424.
240. Leibowitz SF. Opioid, α-noradrenergic and adrenocorticotropin systems of hypothalamic paraventricular nucleus. In: Weiner H, Baum A, eds. Perspective in Behavioral Medicine, Eating Regulation and Discontrol. Hillsdale, NJ: Lawrence Elbaum, 1987:113–136.
241. Sclafani A, Aravich PF, Xenakis S. Dopaminergic and endorphinergic mediation of a sweet reward. In:

Hoebel BG, Novin D, eds. The Neural Basis of Feeding and Reward. Brunswick, ME: Haer Inst., 1982:507–515.
242. Siviy SM, Calcagnetti DJ, Reid LD. A temporal analysis of naloxone's suppressant effect on drinking. Pharmacol Biochem Behav 1982; 16:173–175.
243. Rudski JM, Billington CJ, Levine AS. Naloxone's effects on operant responding depend upon level of deprivation. Pharmacol Biochem Behav 1994; 49:377–383.
244. Cooper SJ. Sweetness, reward and analgesia. Trends Pharmacol Sci 1984; 322–323.
245. Kanarek RB, White ES, Biegen MT, Marks-Kaufman R. Dietary influences on morphine-induced analgesia in rats. Pharmacol Biochem Behav 1991; 38:681–684.
246. Blass EM, Hoffmeyer LB. Sucrose as an analgesic for newborn infants. Pediatrics 1991; 87:215–218.
247. Bodnar RJ. Opioid receptor substype antagonists and ingestion. In: Cooper SJ, Clifton PG, eds. Drug Receptor Subtypes and Ingestive Behaviour. San Diego: Academic Press, 1996:127–166.
248. Nencini P. Sensitization to the ingestive effects of opioids. In: Cooper SJ, Clifton PG, eds. Drug Receptor Subtypes and Ingestive Behaviour. San Diego: Academic Press, 1996:193–218.
249. Vaccarino FJ. Dopamine-opioid mechanisms in ingestion. In: Cooper SJ, Clifton PG, eds. Drug Receptor Subtypes and Ingestive Behaviour. San Diego: Academic Press, 1996:219–232.
250. Carr KD. Opioid receptor subtypes and stimulation-induced feeding. In: Cooper SJ, Clifton PG, eds. Drug Receptor Subtypes and Ingestive Behavior. San Diego: Academic Press, 1996:167–192.
251. Reid LD. Endogenous opioid peptides and regulation of drinking and feeding (Review) Am J Clin Nutr 1985; 42:1099–1132.
252. Morley JE, Levine AS, Gosnell BA, Kneip J, Grace M. The kappa opioid receptor, ingestive behaviors and the obese mouse (ob/ob). Physiol Behav 1983; 31:603–606.
253. Cooper SJ. Evidence for opioid involvement in controls of drinking and water balance. In: Rodgers RJ, Cooper SJ, eds. Endorphins, Opiates and Behavioural Processes. New York: John Wiley & Sons, 1988: 187–216.
254. Bodnar RJ, Beczkowska IW, Koch JE. Opioid receptor subtypes differentially alter palatable fluid intake in rats. Appetite 1993; 21:165.
255. Badiani A, Rajabi H, Nencini P, Stewart J. Modulation of food intake by the kappa opioid U-50,488H: evidence for an effect on satiation. Behav Brain Res 2001; 118:179–86.
256. Leibowitz SF, Hor L. Endorphinergic and alpha-noradrenergic systems in the paraventricular nucleus: effects on eating behavior. Peptides 1982; 3:421–428.
257. McLean S, Hoebel BG. Feeding induced by opiates injected into the paraventricular hypothalamus. Peptides 1983; 4:287–292.
258. Carr KD, Bak TH, Simon EJ, Portoghese PS. Effects of the selective kappa opioid antagonist, nor-binaltorphimine, on electrically-elicited feeding in the rat. Life Sci 1989; 45:1787–1792.
259. Zardetto-Smith AM, Moga MM, Magnuson DJ, Gray TS. Lateral hypothalamic dynorphinergic efferents to the amygdala and brainstem in the rat. Peptides 1988; 9:1121–1127.
260. Carr KD, Aleman DO, Bak TH, Simon EJ. Effects of parabrachial opioid antagonism on stimulation-induced feeding. Brain Res 1991; 545:283–286.
261. Levine AS, Grace M, Billington CJ. The effect of centrally administered naloxone on deprivation and drug-induced feeding. Pharmacol Biochem Behav 1990; 36:409–412.
262. Barton C, York DA, Bray GA. Opioid receptor subtype control of galanin-induced feeding. Peptides 1996; 17:237–240.
263. Hamilton ME, Bozarth MA. Feeding elicited by dynorphin (1–13) microinjections into the ventral tegmental area in rats. Life Sci 1988; 43:941–946.
264. Tanda G, Di Chiara G. A dopamine-mul opioid link in the rat ventral tegmentum shared by palatable food (Fonzies) and non-psychostimulant drugs of abuse. Eur J Neurosci 1998; 10:1179–1187.
265. Taber MT, Zernig G, Fibiger HC. Opioid receptor modulation of feeding-evoked dopamine release in the rat nucleus accumbens. Brain Res 1998; 785:24–30.
266. Ragnauth A, Moroz M, Bodnar RJ. Multiple opioid receptors mediate feeding elicited by mu and delta opioid receptor subtype agonists in the nucleus accumbens shell in rats. Brain Res 2000; 876:76–87.
267. Zhang M, Kelley AE. Enhanced intake of high-fat food following striatal mu-opioid stimulation: microinjection mapping and fos expression. Neuroscience 2000; 99:267–277.
268. Levine B, Smialek JE. Considerations in the interpretation of urine analyses in suspected opiate intoxications. J Forensic Sci 1998; 43:388–389.
269. Inui A. Cancer anorexia-cachexia syndrome: are neuropeptides the key? Cancer Res 1999; 59:4493–4501.
270. Wise RA. Opiate reward: sites and substrates. (Review.) Neurosci Biobehav Rev 1989; 13:129–133.
271. Hernandez L, Hoebel BG. Hypothalamic reward and aversion: a link between metabolism and behavior. In: Veal WL, Lederis K, eds. Current Studies of Hypothalamic Function, Vol 2. Metabolism and Behavior. Basel: Karger, 1978:72–92.
272. Wise RA. The brain and reward. In: Liebman JM, Cooper SJ, eds. The Neuropharmacological Basis of Reward. New York: Oxford University Press, 1989: 377–424.
273. McClelland RC, Hoebel BG. d-Fenfluramine and self-

stimulation: loss of fenfluramine effect on underweight rats. Brain Res Bull 1991; 27:341–345.
274. Chou TC, Lee CE, Lu J, Elmquist JK, Hara J, Willie JT, et al. Orexin (hypocretin) neurons contain dynorphin. J Neurosci 2001; 21:RC168.
275. Koob GF, Goeders NE. Neuroanatomical substrates of drug self-administration. In: Liebman JM, Cooper SJ, eds. The Neuropharmacological Basis of Reward. New York: Oxford University Press, 1989:214–263.
276. DeWitte P, Heidbreder C, Roques BP. Kelatorphan, a potent enkephalinase inhibitor, and opioid receptor agonists DAGO and DTLET, differentially modulate self-stimulation behaviour depending on the site of administration. Neuropharmacology 1989; 28:667–676.
277. Glimcher PG, Giovino AA, Margolin DH, Hoebel BG. Endogenous opiate reward induced by an enkephalinase inhibitor, thiorphan, injected into the ventral midbrain. Behav Neurosci 1984; 98:262–268.
278. Carr GD, Fibiger HC, Phillips GD. Conditioned place preference as a measure of drug reward. In: Liebman JM, Cooper SJ, eds. The Neuropharmacological Basis of Reward. New York: Oxford University Press, 1989: 264–319.
279. Goeders NE, Lane TD, Smith JE. Self-administration of methionine enkephalin into the nucleus accumbens. Pharmacol Biochem Behav 1984; 20:451–455.
280. Olds ME. Reinforcing effects of morphine in the nucleus accumbens. Brain Res 1982; 237:429–440.
281. Colantuoni C, Schwenker J, McCarthy J, Rada P, Ladenheim B, Cadet JL, et al. Excessive sugar intake alters binding to dopamine and mu-opioid receptors in the brain. Neuroreport 2001; 12:3549–3552.
282. Lin L, Okada S, York DA, Bray GA. Structural requirements for the biological activity of enterostatin. Peptides 1994; 15:849–854.
283. Shippenberg TS, Bals-Kubik R. Involvement of the mesolimbic dopamine system in mediating the aversive effects of opioid antagonists in the rat. Behav Pharmacol 1995; 6:99–106.
284. Cooper SJ. Interactions between endogenous opiods and dopamine: implications for reward and aversion. In: Willner P, Scheel-Kruger J, eds. The Mesolimbic Dopamine System: From Motivation to Action. New York: John Wiley & Sons, 1991:331–366.
285. Rada PV, Mark GP, Taylor KM, Hoebel BG. Morphine and naloxone, i.p. or locally, affect extracellular acetylcholine in the accumbens and prefrontal cortex. Pharmacol Biochem Behav 1996; 53:809–816.
286. Kirkham TC, Williams CM. Synergistic efects of opioid and cannabinoid antagonists on food intake. Psychopharmacology (Berl) 2001; 153:267–270.
287. Tanda G, Pontieri FE, Di Chiara G. Cannabinoid and heroin activation of mesolimbic dopamine transmission by a common mul opioid receptor mechanism. Science 1997; 276:2048–2050.
288. Arnone M, Maruani J, Chaperon F, Thiebot MH, Poncelet M, Soubrie P, et al. Selective inhibition of sucrose and ethanol intake by SR 141716, an antagonist of central cannabinoid (CB1) receptors. Psychopharmacology (Berl) 1997; 132:104–106.
289. Heshmati HM, Fatourechi V, Dagam SA, Piepgras DG. Hypopituitarism caused by intrasellar aneurysms. Mayo Clin Proc 2001; 76:789–793.
290. Dieguez C, Carro E, Seoane LM, Garcia M, Camina JP, Senaris R, et al. Regulation of somatotroph cell function by the adipose tissue. Int J Obes Relat Metab Disord 2000; 24(suppl 2):S100–S103.
291. Dickson PR, Vaccarino FJ. GRF-induced feeding: evidence for protein selectivity and opiate involvement. Peptides 1994; 15:1343–1352.
292. Dickson PR, Feifel D, Vaccarino FJ. Blockade of endogenous GRF at dark onset selectively suppresses protein intake. Peptides 1995; 16:7–9.
293. Vaccarino FJ, Feifel D, Rivier J, Vale W. Antagonism of central growth hormone–releasing factor activity selectively attenuates dark-onset feeding in rats. J Neurosci 1991; 11:3924–3927.
294. Vaccarino FJ, Hayward M. Microinjections of growth hormone-releasing factor into the medial preoptic area/suprachiasmatic nucleus region of the hypothalamus stimulate food intake in rats. Regul Pept 1988; 21:21–28.
295. Luckman SM, Rosenzweig I, Dickson SL. Activation of arcuate nucleus neurons by systemic administration of leptin and growth hormone–releasing peptide-6 in normal and fasted rats. Neuroendocrinology 1999; 70:93–100.
296. Okada K, Ishii S, Minami S, Sugihara H, Shibasaki T, Wakabayashi I. Intracerebroventricular administration of the growth hormone-releasing peptides KP-102 increases food intake in free-feeding rats. Endocrinology 1996; 137:5155–5158.
297. Vaccarino FJ, Taube MR. Intra-arcuate opiate actions stimulate GRF-dependent and protein-selective feeding. Peptides 1997; 18:197–205.
298. Lawrence CB, Snape AC, Baudoin FM, Luckman SM. Acute central ghrelin and GH secretagogues induce feeding and activate brain appetite centers. Endocrinology 2002; 143:155–162.
299. Scacchi M, Pincelli AI, Cavagnini F. Growth hormone in obesity. Int J Obes Relat Metab Disord 1999; 23: 260–271.
300. Cai A, Hyde JF. The human growth hormone-releasing hormone transgenic mouse as a model of modest obesity: differential changes in leptin receptor (OBR) gene expression in the anterior pituitary and hypothalamus after fasting and OBR localization in somatotrophs. Endocrinology 1999; 140:3609–3614.
301. Kojima M, Hosoda H, Date Y, Nakazato M, Matsuo H, Kangawa K. Ghrelin is a growth-hormone-releasing acylated peptide from stomach. Nature 1999; 402:656–660.

302. Kojima M, Hosoda H, Matsuo H, Kangawa K. Ghrelin: discovery of the natural endogenous ligand for the growth hormone secretagogue receptor. Trends Endocrinol Metab 2001; 12:118–122.
303. Inui A. Ghrelin: an orexigenic and somatotrophic signal from the stomach. Nat Rev Neurosci 2001; 2:551–560.
304. Nakazato M, Murakami N, Date Y, Kojima M, Matsuo H, Kangawa K, et al. A role for ghrelin in the central regulation of feeding. Nature 2001; 409: 194–198.
305. Tschop M, Smiley DL, Heiman ML. Ghrelin induces adiposity in rodents. Nature 2000; 407:908–913.
306. Shintani M, Ogawa Y, Ebihara K, Aizawa-Abe M, Miyanaga F, Takaya K, et al. Ghrelin, an endogenous growth hormone secretagogue, is a novel orexigenic peptide that antagonizes leptin action through the activation of hypothalamic neuropeptide Y/Y1 receptor pathway. Diabetes 2001; 50:227–232.
307. Masuda Y, Tanaka T, Inomata N, Ohnuma N, Tanaka S, Itoh Z, et al. Ghrelin stimulates gastric acid secretion and motility in rats. Biochem Biophys Res Commun 2000; 276:905–908.
308. Horvath TL, Diano S, Sotonyi P, Heiman M, Tschop M. Minireview: ghrelin and the regulation of energy balance–a hypothalamic perspective. Endocrinology 2001;142:4163–4169.
309. Hewson AK, Dickson SL. Systemic administration of ghrelin induces Fos and Egr-1 proteins in the hypothalamic arcuate nucleus of fasted and fed rats. J Neuroendocrinol 2000; 12:1047–1049.
310. Kamegai J, Tamura H, Shimizu T, Ishii S, Sugihara H, Wakabayashi I. Central effect of ghrelin, an endogenous growth hormone secretagogue, on hypothalamic peptide gene expression. Endocrinology 2000; 141: 4797–4800.
311. Toshinai K, Mondal MS, Nakazato M, Date Y, Murakami N, Kojima M, et al. Upregulation of ghrelin expression in the stomach upon fasting, insulin-induced hypoglycemia, and leptin administration. Biochem Biophys Res Commun 2001; 281:1220–1225.
312. Collier GR, McMillan JS, Windmill K, Walder K, Tenne-Brown J, De Silva A, et al. Beacon: a novel gene involved in the regulation of energy balance. Diabetes 2000; 49:1766–1771.
313. Walder K, McMillan JS, Lee S, Civitarese A, Zimmet P, Collier GR. Effects of beacon administration on energy expenditure and substrate utilisation in *Psammomys obesus* (Israeli sand rats). Int J Obes Relat Metab Disord 2001; 25:1281–1285.
314. Salton SRJ, Ferri GL, Hahm S, Snyder SE, Wilson AJ, Possenti R, et al. VGF: a novel role for this neuronal and neuroendocrine polypeptide in the regulation of energy balance. Front Neuroendocrinol 2000; 21:199–219.
315. Trani E, Ciotti T, Rinaldi AM, Canu N, Ferri GL, Levi A, et al. Tissue-specific processing of the neuroendocrine protein VGF. J Neurochem 1995; 65:2441–2449.
316. Snyder SE, Salton SR. Expression of VGF mRNA in the adult rat central nervous system. J Comp Neurol 1998; 394;91–105.
317. Hahm S, Mizuno TM, Wu TJ, Wisor JP, Priest CA, Kozak CA, et al. Targeted deletion of the Vgf gene indicates that the encoded secretory peptide precursor plays a novel role in the regulation of energy balance [see comments]. Neuron 1999; 23:537–548.
318. Dutt A, Kaplitt MG, Kow LM, Pfaff DW. Prolactin, central nervous system and behavior: a critical review. Neuroendocrinology 1994; 59:413–419.
319. Crumeyrolle-Arias M, Latouche J, Jammes H, Djiane J, Kelly PA, Reymond MJ, et al. Prolactin receptors in the rat hypothalamus: autoradiographic localization and characterization. Neuroendocrinology 1993; 57: 457–466.
320. Dial J, Avery DD. The effects of pregnancy and lactation on dietary self-selection in the rat. Physiol Behav 1991; 49:811–813.
321. Noel MB, Woodside B. Effects of systemic and central prolactin injections on food intake, weight gain, and estrous cyclicity in female rats. Physiol Behav 1993; 54:151–154.
322. Heil S.H, Cramer CP. Prolactin injections result in dose-dependent protein consumption in rats. International Society for Developmental Psychobiology 1993.
323. Sauve D, Woodside B. The effect of central administration of prolactin on food intake in virgin female rats is dose-dependent, occurs in the absence of ovarian hormones and the latency to onset varies with feeding regimen. Brain Res 1996; 729:75–81.
324. Hnasko RM, Buntin JD. Functional mapping of neural sites mediating prolactin-induced hyperphagia in doves. Brain Res 1993; 623:257–266.
325. Koshiyama H, Kato Y, Inoue T, Murakami Y, Ishikawa Y, Yanaihara N, et al. Central galanin stimulates pituitary prolactin secretion in rats: possible involvement of hypothalamic vasoactive intestinal polypeptide. Neurosci Lett 1987; 75:49–54.
326. Horvath TL, Kalra SP, Naftolin F, Leranth C. Morphological evidence for a galanin-opiate interaction in the rat mediobasal hypothalamus. J Neuroendocrinol 1995; 7:579–588.
327. Ling C, Billig H. PRL receptor-mediated effects in female mouse adipocytes: PRL induces suppressors of cytokine signaling expression and suppresses insulin-induced leptin production in adipocytes in vitro. Endocrinology 2001; 142:4880–4890.
328. Cincotta AH, Meier AH. Reduction of body fat stores by inhibition of prolactin secretion. Experientia 1987; 43:416–417.
329. Kopelman PG. Physiopathology of prolactin secretion

in obesity. Int J Obes Relat Metab Disord 2000; 24(suppl 2):S104-S108.
330. Kohsaka A, Watanobe H, Kakizaki Y, Habu S, Suda T. A significant role of leptin in the generation of steroid-induced luteinizing hormone and prolactin surges in female rats. Biochem Biophys Res Commun 1999; 254:578–581.
331. Vergoni AV, Bertolini A. Role of melanocortins in the central control of feeding. Eur J Pharmacol 2000; 405: 25–32.
332. Yaswen L, Diehl N, Brennan MB, Hochgeschwender U. Obesity in the mouse model of pro-opiomelanocortin deficiency responds to peripheral melanocortin. Nat Med 1999; 5:1066–1070.
333. Krude H, Biebermann H, Luck W, Horn R, Brabant G, Gruters A. Severe early-onset obesity, adrenal insufficiency and red hair pigmentation caused by POMC mutations in humans. Nat Genet 1998; 19: 155–157.
334. Cone RD. The central melanocortin system and energy homeostasis. Trends Endocrinol Metab 1999; 10:211–216.
335. Skuladottir GV, Jonsson L, Skarphedinsson JO, Mutulis F, Muceniece R, Raine A, et al. Long-term orexigenic effect of a novel melanocortin 4 receptor selective antagonist. Br J Pharmacol 1999; 126:27–34.
336. Fan W, Dinulescu DM, Butler AA, Zhou J, Marks DL, Cone RD. The central melanocortin system can directly regulate serum insulin levels. Endocrinology 2000; 141:3072–3079.
337. Vaisse C, Clement K, Durand E, Hercberg S, Guy-Grand B, Froguel P. Melanocortin-4 receptor mutations are a frequent and heterogeneous cause of morbid obesity. J Clin Invest 2000; 106:253–262.
338. Chen AS, Marsh DJ, Trumbauer ME, Frazier EG, Guan XM, Yu H, et al. Inactivation of the mouse melanocortin-3 receptor results in increased fat mass and reduced lean body mass. Nat Genet 2000; 26:97–102.
339. Butler AA, Marks DL, Fan W, Kuhn CM, Bartolome M, Cone RD. Melanocortin-4 receptor is required for acute homeostatic responses to increased dietary fat. Nat Neurosci 2001; 4:605–611.
340. Huszar D, Lynch CA, Fairchild-Huntress V, Dunmore JH, Fang Q, Berkemeier LR, et al. Targeted disruption of the melanocortin-4 receptor results in obesity in mice. Cell 1997 88:131–141.
341. Moussa NM, Claycombe KJ. The yellow mouse obesity syndrome and mechanisms of agouti-induced obesity. Obes Res 1999; 7:506–514.
342. Rossi M, Kim MS, Morgan DG, Small CJ, Edwards CM, Sunter D et al. A C-terminal fragment of Agouti-related protein increases feeding and antagonizes the effect of alpha-melanocyte stimulating hormone in vivo. Endocrinology 1998; 139:4428–4431.
343. Dinulescu DM, Cone RD. Agouti and agouti-related protein: analogies and contrasts. J Biol Chem 2000; 275:6695–6698.
344. Harrold JA, Williams G, Widdowson PS. Changes in hypothalamic agouti-related protein (AGRP), but not alpha-MSH or pro-opiomelanocortin concentrations in dietary-obese and food-restricted rats. Biochem Biophys Res Commun 1999; 258:574–577.
345. Seeley RJ, Yagaloff KA, Fisher SL, Burn P, Thiele TE, Van Dijk G, et al. Melanocortin receptors in leptin effects. Nature 1997; 390:349.
346. Haynes WG, Morgan DA, Djalali A, Sivitz WI, Mark AL. Interactions between the melanocortin system and leptin in control of sympathetic nerve traffic. Hypertension 1999; 33:542–547.
347. Cowley MA, Smart JL, Rubinstein M, Cerdan MG, Diano S, Horvath TL, et al. Leptin activates anorexigenic POMC neurons through a neural network in the arcuate nucleus. Nature 2001; 411:480–484.
348. Fan W, Boston BA, Kesterson RA, Hruby VJ, Cone RD. Role of melanocortinergic neurons in feeding and the agouti obesity syndrome. Nature 1997; 385:165–168.
349. Elmquist JK, Elias CF, Saper CB. From lesions to leptin: hypothalamic control of food intake and body weight. Neuron 1999; 22:221–232.
350. Plata-Salaman CR. Leptin (OB protein), neuropeptide Y, and interleukin-1 interactions as interface mechanisms for the regulation of feeding in health and disease [editorial]. Nutrition 1996; 12:718–719.
351. Sternberg EM. Neural-immune interactions in health and disease. J Clin Invest 1997; 100:2641–2647.
352. Hopkins SJ, Rothwell NJ. Cytokines and the nervous system. I. Expression and recognition. Trends Neurosci 1995; 18:83–88.
353. Sonti G, Ilyin SE, Plata-Salaman CR. Anorexia induced by cytokine interactions at pathophysiological concentrations. Am J Physiol 1996; 270:R1394–R1402.
354. Sethi JK, Hotamisligil GS. The role of TNF alpha in adipocyte metabolism. Semin Cell Dev Biol 1999; 10: 19–29.
355. Bessesen DH, Faggioni R. Recently identified peptides involved in the regulation of body weight. Semin Oncol 1998; 25:28–32.
356. Friedman JM, Halaas JL. Leptin and the regulation of body weight in mammals. (Review) Nature 1998; 395: 763–770.
357. Luheshi GN, Gardner JD, Rushforth DA, Loudon AS, Rothwell NJ. Leptin actions on food intake and body temperature are mediated by IL-1. Proc Natl Acad Sci USA 1999; 96:7047–7052.
358. Lambert PD, Anderson KD, Sleeman MW, Wong V, Tan J, Hijarunguru A, et al. Ciliary neurotrophic factor activates leptin-like pathways and reduces body fat, without cachexia or rebound weight gain, even in leptin-resistant obesity. Proc Natl Acad Sci USA 2001; 98:4652–4657.

359. Gloaguen I, Costa P, Demartis A, Lazzaro D, Di Marco A, Graziani R, et al. Ciliary neurotrophic factor corrects obesity and diabetes associated with leptin deficiency and resistance. Proc Natl Acad Sci USA 1997; 94:6456–6461.
360. Bjorbaek C, El Haschimi K, Frantz JD, Flier JS. The role of SOCS-3 in leptin signaling and leptin resistance. J Biol Chem 1999; 274:30059–30065.
361. Inui A. Neuropeptide Y: a key molecule in anorexia and cachexia in wasting disorders? Mol Med Today 1999; 5:79–85.
362. Faggioni R, Fuller J, Moser A, Feingold KR, Grunfeld C. LPS-induced anorexia in leptin-deficient (ob/ob) and leptin receptor-deficient (db/db) mice. Am J Physiol 1997; 273:R181-R186.
363. Xu B, Dube MG, Kalra PS, Farmerie WG, Kaibara A, Moldawer LL, et al. Anorectic effects of the cytokine, ciliary neurotropic factor, are mediated by hypothalamic neuropeptide Y: comparison with leptin. Endocrinology 1998; 139:466–473.
364. Pu S, Dhillon H, Moldawer LL, Kalra PS, Kalra SP. Neuropeptide Y counteracts the anorectic and weight reducing effects of ciliary neurotropic factor. J Neuroendocrinol 2000; 12:827–832.
365. Gayle D, Ilyin SE, Plata-Salaman CR. Central nervous system IL-1 beta system and neuropeptide Y mRNAs during IL-1 beta–induced anorexia in rats. Brain Res Bull 1997; 44:311–317.
366. Kalra SP. Circumventing leptin resistance for weight control. Proc Natl Acad Sci USA 2001; 98:4279–4281.
367. Marks DL, Ling N, Cone RD. Role of the central melanocortin system in cachexia. Cancer Res 2001; 61:1432–1438.
368. Huang QH, Hruby VJ, Tatro JB. Role of central melanocortins in endotoxin-induced anorexia. Am J Physiol 1999; 276:R864-R871.
369. Ahima RS, Osei SY. Molecular regulation of eating behavior: new insights and prospects for therapeutic strategies. Trends Mol Med 2001; 7:205–213.
370. Douglass J, McKinzie AA, Couceyro P. PCR differential display identifies a rat brain mRNA that is transcriptionally regulated by cocaine and amphetamine. J Neurosci 1995; 15:2471–2481.
371. Douglass J, Daoud S. Characterization of the human cDNA and genomic DNA encoding CART: a cocaine- and amphetamine-regulated transcript. Gene 1996; 169:241–245.
372. Koylu EO, Couceyro PR, Lambert PD, Ling NC, DeSouza EB, Kuhar MJ. Immunohistochemical localization of novel CART peptides in rat hypothalamus, pituitary and adrenal gland. J Neuroendocrinol 1997; 9:823–833.
373. Dun NJ, Dun SL, Kwok EH, Yang J, Chang J. Cocaine- and amphetamine-regulated transcript-immunoreactivity in the rat sympatho-adrenal axis. Neurosci Lett 2000; 283:97–100.
374. Hurd YL, Fagergren P. Human cocaine- and amphetamine-regulated transcript (CART) mRNA is highly expressed in limbic- and sensory-related brain regions. J Comp Neurol 2000; 425:583–598.
375. Elias CF, Lee C, Kelly J, Aschkenasi C, Ahima RS, Couceyro PR, et al. Leptin activates hypothalamic CART neurons projecting to the spinal cord. Neuron 1998; 21:1375–1385.
376. Elias CF, Lee CE, Kelly JF, Ahima RS, Kuhar M, Saper CB, et al. Characterization of CART neurons in the rat and human hypothalamus. J Comp Neurol 2001; 432:1–19.
377. Chang GQ, Leibowitz SF. CART and galanin coexist in hypothalamic neurons: high-fat diet increases the number of double-labeled neurons exclusively in the PVN. 31st Annual Meeting of the Society for Neurosciences, San Diego, CA, Nov 10–15, 2001.
378. Vrang N, Larsen PJ, Clausen JT, Kristensen P. Neurochemical characterization of hypothalamic cocaine-amphetamine-regulated transcript neurons. J Neurosci 1999; 19:RC5.
379. Broberger C. Hypothalamic cocaine- and amphetamine-regulated transcript (CART) neurons: histochemical relationship to thyrotropin-releasing hormone, melanin-concentrating hormone, orexin/hypocretin and neuropeptide Y. Brain Res 1999; 848:101–113.
380. Kristensen P, Judge ME, Thim L, Ribel U, Christjansen KN, Wulff BS, et al. Hypothalamic CART is a new anorectic peptide regulated by leptin. Nature 1998; 393: 72–76.
381. Lambert PD, Couceyro PR, McGirr KM, Dall Vechia SE, Smith Y, Kuhar MJ CART peptides in the central control of feeding and interactions with neuropeptide Y. Synapse 1998; 29:293–298.
382. Pothos EN, Creese I, Hoebel BG. Restricted eating with weight loss selectively decreases extracellular dopamine in the nucleus accumbens and alters dopamine response to amphetamine, morphine and food intake. J Neurosci 1995; 15:6640–6650.
383. Wang C, Billington CJ, Levine AS, Kotz CM. Effect of CART in the hypothalamic paraventricular nucleus on feeding and uncoupling protein gene expression. Neuroreport 2000; 11:3251–3255.
384. Okumura T, Yamada H, Motomura W, Kohgo Y. Cocaine-amphetamine-regulated transcript (CART) acts in the central nervous system to inhibit gastric acid secretion via brain corticotropin-releasing factor system. Endocrinology 2000; 141:2854–2860.
385. Larsen PJ, Vrang N, Petersen PC, Kristensen P. Chronic intracerebroventricular administration of recombinant CART(42-89) peptide inhibits and causes weight loss in lean and obese Zucker (fa/fa) rats. Obes Res 2000; 8:590–596.
386. Pothos EN, Hernandez L, Hoebel BG. Chronic food deprivation decreases extracellular dopamine in the nucleus accumbens: implications for a possible neuro-

chemical link between weight loss and drug abuse. Obes Res 1995; 3(suppl 4):525S-529S.
387. Wortley KE, Chang GQ, Zarayskaya E, Akabayashi A, Leibowitz SF. CART expression in hypothalamic neurons, in association with leptin, is increased by consumption of a high-fat diet and is elevated in rats that exhibit obesity on a high-fat diet. Oral presentation at the annual meeting of the Society for Neuroscience, 2000.
388. Asnicar MA, Smith DP, Yang DD, Heiman ML, Fox N, Chen YF, et al. Absence of cocaine- and amphetamine-regulated transcript results in obesity in mice fed a high caloric diet. Endocrinology 2001; 142:4394–4400.
389. Challis BG, Yeo GS, Farooqi IS, Luan J, Aminian S, Halsall DJ, et al. The CART gene and human obesity: mutational analysis and population genetics. Diabetes 2000; 49:872–875.
390. Arase K, York DA, Shimizu H, Shargill N, Bray GA. Effects of corticotropin-releasing factor on food intake and brown adipose tissue thermogenesis in rats. Am J Physiol 1988; 225:255–259.
391. Egawa M, Yoshimatsu H, Bray GA. Effect of corticotropin releasing hormone and neuropeptide Y on electrophysiological activity of sympathetic nerves to interscapular brown adipose tissue. Neuroscience 1990; 34:771–775.
392. Glowa JR, Barrett JE, Russell J, Gold PW. Effects of corticotropin releasing hormone on appetitive behaviors. (Review) Peptides 1992; 13:609–621.
393. Rothwell NJ. Central effects of CRF on metabolism and energy balance. (Review) Neurosci Biobehav Rev 1990; 14:263–271.
394. Richard D, Huang Q, Timofeeva E. The corticotropin-releasing hormone system in the regulation of energy balance in obesity. Int J Obes Relat Metab Disord 2000; 24:S36–S39.
395. Spina M, Merlo-Pich E, Chan RK, Basso AM, Rivier J, Vale W, et al. Appetite-suppressing effects of urocortin, a CRF-related neuropeptide. Science 1996; 273: 1561–1564.
396. Heinrichs SC, Menzaghi F, Pich EM, Hauger RL, Koob GF. Corticotropin-releasing factor in the paraventricular nucleus modulates feeding induced by neuropeptide Y. Brain Res 1993; 611:18–24.
397. Heinrichs SC, Lapsansky J, Behan DP, Chan RK, Sawchenko PE, Lorang M, et al. Corticotropin-releasing factor-binding protein ligand inhibitor blunts excessive weight gain in genetically obese Zucker rats and rats during nicotine withdrawal. Proc Natl Acad Sci USA 1996; 93:15475–15480.
398. Wang C, Mullet MA, Glass MJ, Billington CJ, Levine AS, Kotz CM. Feeding inhibition by urocortin in the rat hypothalamic paraventricular nucleus. Am J Physiol Regul Integr Comp Physiol 2001; 280:R473–R480.
399. Coste SC, Kesterson RA, Heldwein KA, Stevens SL, Heard AD, Hollis JH, et al. Abnormal adaptations to stress and impaired cardiovascular function in mice lacking corticotropin-releasing hormone receptor-2. Nat Genet 2000; 24:403–409.
400. Bradbury MJ, McBurnie MI, Denton DA, Lee KF, Vale WW. Modulation of urocortin-induced hypophagia and weight loss by corticotropin-releasing factor receptor 1 deficiency in mice. Endocrinology 2000; 141:2715–2724.
401. Uehara Y, Shimizu H, Ohtani K, Sato N, Mori M. Hypothalamic corticotropin-releasing hormone is a mediator of the anorexigenic effect of leptin. Diabetes 1998; 47:890–893.
402. Menzaghi F, Heinrichs SC, Pich EM, Tilders FJ, Koob GF. Functional impairment of hypothalamic corticotropin-releasing factor neurons with immunotargeted toxins enhances food intake induced by neuropeptide Y. Brain Res 1993; 618:76–82.
403. Bchini-Hooft van Huijsduijnen OB, Rohner-Jeanrenaud F, Jeanrenaud B. Hypothalamic neuropeptide Y messenger ribonucleic acid levels in pre-obese and genetically obese (fa/fa) rats; potential regulation thereof by corticotropin-releasing factor. J Neuroendocrinol 1993; 5:381–386.
404. Bchini-Hooft van Huijsduijnen OB, Rohner-Jeanrenaud F, Jeanrenaud B. Hypothalamic neuropeptide Y messenger ribonucleic acid levels in pre-obese and genetically obese (fa/fa) rats; potential regulation thereof by corticotropin-releasing factor. J Neuroendocrinol 1993; 5:381–386.
405. Halford JC, Blundell JE. Separate systems for serotonin and leptin in appetite control. Ann Med 2000; 32:222–232.
406. Cavagnini F, Croci M, Putignano P, Petroni ML, Invitti C. Glucocorticoids and neuroendocrine function. Int J Obes Relat Metab Disord 2000; 24(suppl 2):S77–S79.
407. Krahn DD, Gosnell BA, Grace M, Levine AS. CRF antagonist partially reverses CRF- and stress-induced effects on feeding. Brain Res Bull 1986; 17:285–289.
408. Uehara A, Habara Y, Kuroshima A, Sekiya C, Takasugi Y, Namiki M. Increased ACTH response to corticotropin-releasing factor in cold-adapted rats in vivo. Am J Physiol 1989; 257:E336-E339.
409. Inui A. Feeding and body-weight regulation by hypothalamic neuropeptides—mediation of the actions of leptin. Trends Neurosci 1999; 22:62–67.
410. Erlanson-Albertsson C, York D. Enterostatin—a peptide regulating fat intake. Obes Res 1997; 5:360–372.
411. Okada S, York DA, Bray GA, Mei J, Erlanson-Albertsson C. Diffferential inhibition of fat intake in two strains of rat by the peptide enterostatin. Am J Physiol 1992; 262(Pt 2):R1111–R1116.
412. Lin L, McClanahan S, York DA, Bray GA. The peptide enterostatin may produce early satiety. Physiol Behav 1993; 53–789–794.

413. York DA, Lin L. Enterostatin: a peptide regulator of fat ingestion. In: Bray GA, Ryan DH, eds. Molecular and Genetic Aspects of Obesity. Baton Rouge: Louisiana State University Press, 1996: 281–297.
414. Lin L, Gehlert DR, York DA, Bray GA. Effect of enterostatin on the feeding response to galanin and NPY. Obes Res 1993; 1(3):186–192.
415. Lin L, Chen J, York DA. Chronic ICV enterostatin preferentially reduced fat intake and lowered body weight. Peptides 1997; 18:657–661.
416. Prasad C, Imamura M, Debata C, Svec F, Sumar N, Hermon-Taylor J. Hyperenterostatinemia in premenopausal obese women. J Clin Endocrinol Metab 1999; 84:937–941.
417. Plata-Salaman CR, Borkoski JP. Chemokines/intercrines and central regulation of feeding. Am J Physiol 1994; 266:R1711–R1715.
418. Stanley BG, Hoebel BG, Leibowitz SF. Neurotensin: effects of hypothalamic and intravenous injections on eating and drinking in rats. Peptides 1983; 4:493–500.
419. Sandoval SL, Kulkosky PJ. Effects of peripheral neurotensin on behavior of the rat. Pharmacol Biochem Behav 1992; 41:385–390.
420. Stanley BG, Leibowitz SF, Eppel N, St-Pierre S, Hoebel BG. Suppression of norepinephrine-elicited feeding by neurotensin: evidence for behavioral, anatomical and pharmacological specificity. Brain Res 1985; 343:297–304.
421. Tritos NA, Vicent D, Gillette J, Ludwig DS, Flier ES, Maratos-Flier E. Functional interactions between melanin-concentrating hormone, neuropeptide Y, and anorectic neuropeptides in the rat hypothalamus. Diabetes 1998; 47:1687–1692.
422. Colantuoni C, McCarthy J, Hoebel BG. Evidence for food addiction. Appetite 1997; 29:391–392.
423. Beck B, Burlet A, Nicolas JP, Burlet C. Neurotensin in microdissected brain nuclei and in the pituitary of the lean and obese Zucker rats. Neuropeptides 1989; 13:1–7.
424. Wilding JP, Gilbey SG, Bailey CJ, Batt RA, Williams G, Ghatei MA, et al. Increased neuropeptide-Y messenger ribonucleic acid (mRNA) and decreased neurotensin mRNA in the hypothalamus of the obese (ob/ob) mouse. Endocrinology 1993: 132:1939–1994.
425. Sahu A, Carraway RE, Wang YP. Evidence that neurotensin mediates the central effect of leptin on food intake in rat. Brain Res 2001; 888:343–347.
426. Sahu A. Evidence suggesting that galanin (GAL), melanin-concentrating hormone (MCH), neurotensin (NT), proopiomelanocortin (POMC) and neuropeptide Y (NPY) are targets of leptin signaling in the hypothalamus. Endocrinology 1998; 139:795–798.
427. Kanarek RB, White ES, Biegen MT, Marks-Kaufman R. Dietary influences on morphine-induced analgesia in rats. Pharmacol Biochem Behav 1991; 38:681–684.
428. Lee TF, Rezvani AH, Hepler JR, Myers RD. Neurotensin releases norepinephrine differentially from perfuse hypothalamus of sated and fasted rat. Am J Physiol 1987; 252:E102–E109.
429. Glimeher PG, Giovino AA, Hoebel BG. Neurotensin self-injection in the ventral tegmental area. Brain Res 1987; 403:147–150.
430. kalivas PW, Taylor S. Behavioral and neurochemical effect of daily injection with neurotensisn into the ventral tegmental area. Brain Res 1985; 358:70–76.
431. Rompre P-P, Gratton A. Mesencephalic microinjections of neurotensin-(1-13) and its C-terminal fragment neurotensin-(8-13), potentiate brain stimulation reward. Brain Res 1993; 616:154–162.
432. Angulo JA, McEwen BS. Molecular aspects of neuropeptide regulation and function in the corpus striatum and nucleus accumbens. Brain Res Rev 1994; 19:1–28.
433. Hayashi H, Nutting DF, Fujimoto K, Cardelli JA, Black D, Tso P. Transport of lipid and apolipoproteins A-I and A-IV in intestinal lymph of the rat. J Lipid Res 1990; 31:1613–1625.
434. Fujimoto K, Fukagawa K, Sakata T, Tso P. Suppression of food intake by apolipoprotein A-IV is mediated through the central nervous system in rats. J Clin Invest 1993; 91:1830–1833.
435. Okumura T, Fukagawa K, Tso P, Taylor IL, Pappas TN. Mechanism of action of intracisternal apolipoprotein A-IV in inhibiting gastric acid secretion in rats. Gastroenterology 1995; 109:1583–1588.
436. Tso P,.Liu M, Kalogeris TJ, Thomson AB. The role of apolipoprotein. A-IV in the regulation of food intake. Annu Rev Nutr 2001; 21:231–254.
437. Elshourbagy NA, Walker DW, Paik YK, Boguski MS, Freeman M, Gordon JI, et al. Structure and expression of the human apolipoprotein A-IV gene. J Biol Chem 1987; 262:7973–7981.
438. Liu Z, Leibowitz SF. Apolipoprotein D interacts with the long form leptin receptor: a hypothalamic function in control of energy homeostasis. FASEB J 2001.
439. Smith GP, Gibbs J. Satiating effect of cholecystokinin. Ann NY Acad Sci 1994; 713:236–241.
440. Lenard L, Jando G, Karadi Z, Hajnal A, Sandor P. Lateral hypothalamic feeding mechanisms; iontophoretic effects of kainic acid ibolenic acid and 6-hydroxydopamine. Brain Res Bull 1988; 20:847–856.
441. Rassart E, Bedirian A, Do CS, Guinard O, Sirois J, Terisse I, et al. Apolipoprotein D [in process citation]. Biochim Biophys Acta 2000; 1482:185–198.
442. Bernardis LL, Bellinger LL. The lateral hypothalamic area revisited: neuroanatomy, body weight regulation, neuroendocrinology and metabolism. Neurosci Biobehav Rev 1993; 17:141–193.
443. Powley TL, Opsahl CA. Autonomic components of the hypothalamic feeding syndromes. In: Novin D, Wyrwicka W, Bray GA, eds. Hunger: Basic Mecha-

nisms and Clinical Implications. New York: Raven Press. 1976; 313–326.

444. Steffens AB, Strubbe JH, Scheurink AJ, Balkan B. Neuroendocrine activity during food intake modulates secretion of the endocrine pancreas and contributes to the regulation of body weight. In: Friedman MI, Tordoff MG, Kare MR, eds. Chemical Senses: Appetite and Nutrition New York: Marcel Dekker, 1991; 405–425.
445. Gibson EL, Kennedy AJ, Curzon G. d-Fenfluramine- and d-norfenfluramine-induced hypophagia: differential mechanisms and involvement of postsynaptic 5-HT receptors. Eur J Pharmacol 1993; 242:83–90.
446. Grignaschi G, Sironi F, Samanin R. The 5-HT1B receptor mediates the effect of d-fenfluramine of eating caused by intra-hypothalamic injection of neuropeptide Y. Eur J Pharmacol 1995; 274:221–224.
447. Leibowitz SF, Weiss GF, Suh IS. Medial hypothalamic nuclei mediate serotonin's inhibitory effect on feeding behavior. Pharmacol Biochem Behav 1990; 37:735–742.
448. Wurtman RJ, Wurtman JJ. Carbohydrate craving, obesity and brain serotonin. Appetite 1986; 7(suppl): 99–103.
449. McClelland RC, Sarfaty T, Hernandez L, Hoebel BG. The appetite suppressant, d-fenfluramine, decreases self-stimulation at a feeding site in the lateral hypothalamus. Pharmacol Biochem Behav 1989; 32:411–414.
450. Blundell JE, Rogers PJ, Hunger, hedonics and the control of satiation and satiety. In: Friedman MI, Tordoff MG, Kare MR, eds Chemical Senses: Appetite and Nutrition. New York: Marcel Dekker, 1991:127–148.
451. Hammer VA, Gietzen DW, Beverly JL, Rogers QR. Serotonin3 receptor antagonists block anorectic responses to amino acid imbalance. Am Physiol Soc 1990; 259:R627–R636.
452. Geary N. Pancreatic glucagon signals postprandial satiety. (Review) Neurosci Biobehav Rev 1990; 14: 323–338.
453. Geary N, Le Sauter J, Noh U. Glucagon acts in the liver to control spontaneous meal size in rats. Am J Physiol 1993; 264:R116–R122.
454. Drucker DJ. Minireview; the glucagon-like peptides. Endocrinology 2001; 142:521–527.
455. Kreymann B, Ghatei MA, Burnet P, Williams G, Kanse S, Diani AR, et al. Characterization of glucagon-like peptide-1-(7-36)amide in the hypothalamus. Brain Res 1989; 502:325–331.
456. Small CJ, Rossi M, Bloom SR. Glucagon like peptide-1 (GLP-1), neuropeptide Y (NPY) and melanin concentrating hormone (MCH) in the hypothalamic regulation of food intake. In: Guy-Grand B, Ailhaud G, eds. Progress in Obesity Research. London: John Libbey, 1999:279–288.
457. Turton MD, O'Shea D, Gunn I, Beak SA, Edwards CM, Meeran K, et al. A role for glucagon-like peptide-1 in the central regulation of feeding. Nature 1996; 379:69–72.
458. Goldstone AP, Mercer JG, Gunn I, Moar KM, Edwards CM, Rossi M, et al. Leptin interacts with glucagon-like peptide-1 neurons to reduce food intake and body weight in rodents. FEBS Lett 1997; 415: 134–138.
459. Shughrue PJ, Lane MV, Merchenthaler I. Glucagon-like peptide-1 receptor (GLP1-R) mRNA in the rat hypothalamus. Endocrinology 1996; 137:5159–5162.
460. Choi YH, Anderson GH. An interaction between hypothalamic glucagon-like peptide-1 and macronutrient composition determines food intake in rats. J Nutr 2001; 131:1819–1825.
461. Madsen OD, Karlsen C, Blume N, Jensen HI, Larsson LI, Holst JJ. Transplantable glucagonomous derived from pluripotent rat islet tumor tissue cause severe anorexia and adipsia. Scand J Clin Lab Invest Suppl 1995; 220:27–35.
462. Bray GA, Greenway FL. Current and potential drugs for treatment of obesity . Endocr Rev 1999; 20:805–875.
463. Verdich C, Toubro S, Buemann B, Lysgard MJ, Juul HJ, Astrup A. The role of postprandial releases of insulin and incretin hormones in meal-induced satiety—effect of obesity and weight reduction. Int J Obes Relat Metab Disord 2001; 25:1206–1214.
464. Scrocchi LA, Brown TJ, MaClusky N, Brubaker PL, Auerbach AB, Joyner AL, et al. Glucose intolerance but normal satiety in mice with a null mutation in the glucagon-like peptide I receptor gene. Nat Med 1996; 2:1254–1258.
465. Van Dijk G, Thiele TE. Glugagon-like peptide-1 (7-36) amide: a central regulator of satiety and interoceptive stress. Neuropeptides 1999; 33:406–414.
466. Hoebel BG. Integrative peptides. Brain Res Bull 1985; 14:525–528.
467. Gibbs J, Smith GP. Gut peptides and feeding behavior: The model of cholecystokinin. In: Ritter RC, Ritter S, Barnes CD, eds. Feeding Behavior Neural and Humoral Controls, Orlando: Academic Press, 1986:329–352.
468. Galef JBG, Beck M. Diet selection and poison avoidance by mammals individually and in social groups. In: Stricker EM, ed. Handbook of Behavioral Neurobiology: Vol 10. New York: Plenum Press, 1990: 329–349.
469. Schwartz DH, Dorfman DB, Hernandez L, Hoebel BG, Cholecystokinin. 1. CCK antagonists in the PVN induce feeding. 2. Effects of CCK in the nucleus accumbens on extracellular dopamine turnover. In: Wang RY, Schoenfeld R, eds. Neurology and Neurobiology: Cholecystokinin Antagonists. New York: Alan R. Liss. 1988:285–305.
470. Moran TH. Receptor subtype and affinity state under-

lying the satiety actions of cholecystokinin (CCK). In: Cooper SJ, Clifton PG, eds. Drug Receptor Subtypes and Ingestive Behaviour. London: Academic Press, 1996:1–18.

471. Moran TH. Cholecystokinin and satiety: current perspectives. Nutrition 2000; 16:858–865.

472. Crawley JN, Corwin RL. Biological actions of cholecystokinin. Peptides 1994; 15:731–755.

473. Smith GP, Dorre D, Melville L. CCK-33 inhibits food intake after intraportal and intravenous administration. Soc Neurosci Abstr 1996:22.

474. Verbalis JG, McCann MJ, McHale CM, Stricker EM. Oxytocin secretion in response to cholecystokinin and food: differentiation of nausea from satiety. Science 1986; 232:1417–1419.

475. Deutsch JA, Hardy WT. Cholecystokinin produces bait shyness in rats. Nature 1977; 266:196.

476. Mueller K, Hsaie S. Specificity of cholecystokinin satiety effect: reduction of food but not water intake. Pharmacol Biochem Behav 1977; 6:643–646.

477. Flood JF, Silver AJ, Morley JE. Do peptide-induced changes in feeding occur because of changes in motivation to eat? Peptides 1990; 11:265–270.

478. Degen L, Matzinger D, Drewe J, Beglinger C. The effect of cholecystokinin in controlling appetite and food intake in humans. Peptides 2001; 22:1265–1269.

479. Melton PM, Kissileff HR. Pi-Sunyer FX. Cholecystokinin (CCK-8) affects gastric pressure and ratings of hunger and fullness in women. Am J Physiol 1992; 263:452–456.

480. Dourish CT. Behavioral analysis of the role of CCK-A and CCK-B receptors in the control of feeding in rodents. In: Dourish CT, Cooper SJ, Inverson SD, Iverson LL, eds. Multiple Cholecystokinin Receptors in the CNS. Oxford: Oxford University Press, 1992: 234–253.

481. Zippel U, Heidel E, Davidowa H. Action of cholecystokinin and serotonin on lateral hypothalamic neurons of rats. Eur J Pharmacol 1999; 379:135–140.

482. Burton-Freeman B, Gietzen DW, Schneeman BO. Cholecystokinin and serotonin receptors in the regulation of fat- induced satiety in rats. Am J Physiol 1999; 276:429–434.

483. Geary N, Trace D, McEwen B, Smith GP. Cyclic estradiol replacement increases the satiety effect of CCK- 8 in ovariectornized rats. Physiol Behav 1994; 56:281–289.

484. Eckel LA, Geary N. Endogenous cholecystokinin's satiating action increases during estrus in female rats. Peptides 1999; 20:451–456.

485. Covasa M. Ritter RC. Rats maintained on high-fat diets exhibit reduced satiety in response to CCK and bombesin. Peptides 1998; 19:1407–1415.

486. Sodersten P, Bednar I, Qureshi GA, Carrer H, Qian M, Mamoun H, Kaplan JM, Johnson AE. Cholecystokinin-dopamine interactions in satiety. In: Cooper SJ, Clifton PG, eds. Drug Receptor Subtypes and Ingestive Behaviour. London: Academic Press, 1996: 19–38.

487. Corp ES, McQuade J, Moran TH, Smith GP. Characterization of type A and type B CCK receptor binding sites in rat vagus nerve. Brain Res 1993; 623: 161–166.

488. Crawley JN. Cholecystokinin modulates dopamine dediated behaviors: differential actions in medial posterior versus anterior nucleus accumbens. Ann NY Acad Sci 1994; 713:138–142.

489. Gibbs J, Smith GP, Greenberg D. Cholecystokinin: a neuroendocrine key to feeding behavior. In: Schulkin J, ed. Hormonally Induced Changes in Mind and Brain. Orlando: Academic Press, 1993:51–69.

490. Li B-H, Rowland NE. Effects of vagotomy on cholecystokinin- and dexfenfluramine-induced fos-like immunoreactivity in the rat brain. Brain Res Bull 1995; 37:589–593.

491. Glatzle J, Kreis ME, Kawano K, Raybould HE, Zittel TT. Postprandial neuronal activation in the nucleus of the solitary tract is partly mediated by CCK-A receptors. Am J Physiol Regul Integr Comp Physiol 2001; 281:222–229.

492. Broberger C, Holmberg K, Shi TJ, Dockray G, Hokfelt T. Expression and regulation of cholecystokinin and cholecystokinin receptors in rat nodose and dorsal root ganglia. Brain Res 2001; 903:128–140.

493. Schwartz GJ, Whitney A, Skoglund C, Castonguay TW, Moran TH. Decreased responsiveness to dietary fat in Otsuka Long-Evans Tokushima fatty rats lacking CCK-A receptors. Am J Physiol 1999; 277: 1144–1151.

494. Perez C, Lucas F, Sclafani A. Devazepide, a CCK(A) antagonist, attenuates the satiating but not the preference conditioning effects of intestinal carbohydrate infusions in rats. Pharmacol Biochem Behav 1998; 59:451–457.

495. Balleine B, Davies A, Dickinson A. Cholecystokinin attenuates incentive learning in rats. Behav Neurosci 1995; 109:312–319.

496. Fedorchak PM, Bolles RC. Nutritive expectancies mediate cholecystokini's suppression-of-intake effect. Behav Neurosci 1988; 102:451–455.

497. Mark GP, Smith SE, Rada PV, Hoehel BG. An appetitively conditioned taste elicits a preferential increase in mesolimbic dopamine release. Pharmacol Biochem Behav 1994; 48:651–660.

498. Helm KA, Rada PV, Hoebel BG. Cholecystokinin combined with serotonin in the hypothalamus limits accumbens dopamine release while increasing acetylcholine: a possible satiation mechanism. Brain Res 2003; 963:290–297.

499. Hokfelt T, Skirboll L, Rehfeld JF, Goldstein M, Markey K, Dann 0. A subpopulation of mesencephalic dopamine neurons projecting to limbic areas contains

a cholecystokinin-like peptide: evidence from immunohistochemistry combined with retrograde tracing. Neuroscience 1980; 5:2093–2124.

500. Heidbreder C, Gewiss M, De Mott B, Mertens I, De Witte P. Balance of glutamate and dopamine in the nucleus accumbens modulates self-stimulation behavior after injection of cholecystokinin and neurotensin in the rat brain. Peptides 1992; 13:441–449.
501. Tanganelli S, Fuxe K, Antonelli T, O'Connor WT, Ferraro L. Cholecystokinin/dopamine/GABA interactions in the nucleus accumbens: biochemical and functional correlates. Peptides 2001; 22:1229–1234.
502. Gibbs J, Fauser DJ, Row EA, Rolls BJ, Rolls ET, Maddison SP. Bombesin suppresses feeding in rats. Nature 1979; 282:208–210.
503. McCoy JG, Avery DD. Bombesin: potential integrative peptide for feeding and satiety. Peptides 1990; 11:595–607.
504. Kulkosky PJ, Gray L, Gibbs J, Smith GP. Feeding and selection of saccharin after injections of bombesin, LiCl, and NaCl. Peptides 1981; 2:61–64.
505. Merali Z, McIntosh J, Anisman H. Role of bombesin-related peptides in the control of food intake. Neuropeptides 1999; 33:376–386.
506. Vigh J, Lenard L, Fekete E, Hernadi I. Bombesin injection into the central amygdala influences feeding behavior in the rat. Peptides, 1999; 20:437–444.
507. Lee MC, Schiffman SS, Pappas TN. Role of neuropeptides in the regulation of feeding behavior: a review of cholecystokinin, bombesin, neuropeptide Y, and galanin. Neurosci Biobehav Rev 1994; 18:313–323.
508. West DB, Williams RH, Bragert DJ, Woods SC. Bombesin reduces food intake of normal and hypothalamically obese rats and lowers body weight when given chronically. Peptides 1982; 3:61–67.
509. Yamada K, Wada E, Wada K. Bombesin-like peptides: studies on food intake and social behaviour with receptor knock-out mice. Ann Med 2000; 32:519–529.
510. Howard AD, Wang R, Pong SS, Mellin TN, Strack A, Guan XM, et al. Identification of receptors for neuromedin U and its role in feeding. Nature 2000; 406:70–74.
511. Nakazato M, Hanada R, Murakami N, Date Y, Mondal MS, Kojima M, et al. Central effects of neuromedin U in the regulation of energy homeostasis. Biochem Biophys Res Commun 2000; 277:191–194.
512. Kojima M, Haruno R, Nakazato M, Date Y, Murakami N, Hanada R, et al. Purification and identification of neuromedin U as an endogenous ligand for an orphan receptor GPR66 (FM3). Biochem Biophys Res Commun 2000; 276:435–438.
513. Cooper GJ. Amylin compared with calcitonin gene-related peptide: structure, biology, and relevance to metabolic disease. (Review) Endocr Rev 1994; 15:163–201.
514. Edwards BJ, Morley JE. Amylin. Life Sci 1992; 51:1899–1912.
515. Lutz TA, Geary N, Szabady MM, Del Prete E, Scharrer E. Amylin decreases meal size in rats. Physiol Behav 1995; 58:1197–1202.
516. Lawrence CB, Celsi F, Brennand J, Luckman SM. Alternative role for prolactin-releasing peptide in the regulation of food intake. Nat Neurosci 2000; 3:645–646.
517. Banks WA, Kastin AJ, Maness LM, Huang W, Jaspan JB. Permeability of the blood-brain barrier to amylin. Life Sci 1995; 57:1993–2001.
518. Sexton PM, Paxinos. G, Kenney MA, Wookey PJ, Beaumont K. In vitro autoradiographic localization of amylin binding sites in rat brain. Neuroscience 1994; 62:553–567.
519. Banks WA, Kastin AJ. Differential permeability of the blood-brain barrier to two pancreatic peptides: insulin and amylin. Peptides 1998; 19:883–889.
520. Woods SC, Seeley RJ. Adiposity signals and the control of energy homeostasis. Nutrition 2000; 16:894–902.
521. Chance WT, Balasubramaniam A, Zhang FS, Wimalawansa SJ, Fischer JE. Anorexia following the intrahypothalamic administration of amylin. Brain Res 1991; 539:352–354.
522. Rushing PA, Hagan MM, Seeley RJ, Lutz TA, D'Alessio DA, Air EL, et al. Inhibition of central amylin signaling increases food intake and body adiposity in rats. Endocrinology 2001; 142:5035.
523. Chance WT, Balasubramaniam A, Stallion A, Fischer JE. Anorexia following the systemic injection of amylin. Brain Res 1993; 607:185–188.
524. Gebre-Medhin S, Mulder H, Pekny M, Westermark G, Tornell J, Westermark P, et al. Increased insulin secretion and glucose tolerance in mice lacking islet amyloid polypeptide (amylin). Biochem Biophys Res Commun. 1998; 250:271–277.
525. Chait A, Suaudeau C, De Beaurepaire R. Extensive brain mapping of calcitonin-induced anorexia. Brain Res Bull 1995; 36:467–472.
526. Krahn DD, Gosnell BA, Levine AS, Morley JE. Effects of calcitonin gene-related peptide on food intake. Peptides 1984; 5:861–864.
527. Freed WJ, Perlow MJ, Wyatt RJ. Calcitonin: inhibitory effect on eating in rats. Science 1979; 206:850–852.
528. Taylor GM, Meeran K, O'Shea D, Smith DM, Ghatei MA, Bloom SR. Adrenomedullin inhibits feeding in the rat by a mechanism involving calcitonin gene-related peptide receptors. Endocrinology 1996; 137: 3260.
529. Zelissen PM, Koppeschaar HP, Lips CJ, Hackeng WH. Calcitonin gene-related peptide in human obesity. Peptides 1991; 12:861–863.

530. Hinuma S, Habata Y, FuJii R, Kawamata Y, Hosoya M, Fukusumi S, et al. A prolactin-releasing peptide in the brain. Nature 1998; 393:272–276.
531. Roland BL, Sutton SW, Wilson SJ, Luo L, Pyati J, Huvar R, et al. Anatomical distribution of prolactin-releasing peptide and its receptor suggests additional functions in the central nervous system and periphery. Endocrinology 1999; 140:5736–5745.
532. Ellacott KL, Lawrence CB, Rothwell NJ, Luckman SM. The novel anorexigenic prolactin-releasing peptide (PrRP) interacts with leptin to reduce food intake. Society for Neuroscience Abstracts 2001.
533. Seal LJ, Small CJ, Dhillo WS, Stanley SA, Abbott CR, Ghatei MA, et al. PRL-releasing peptide inhibits food intake in male rats via the dorsomedial hypothalamic nucleus and not the paraventricular hypothalamic nucleus. Endocrinology 2001; 142:4236–4243.
534. Verbalis JG, Blackburn RE, Hoffman GE, Stricker EM. Establishing behavioral and physiological functions of central oxytocin: insights, from studies of oxytocin and ingestive behaviors. Adv Exp Med Biol 1995; 395:209–225.
535. Olson BR, Drutarosky MD, Chow MS, Hruby VJ, Stricker EM, Verbalis JG. Oxytocin and an oxytocin agonist administered centrally decrease food intake in rats. Peptides 1991; 12:113–118.
536. Verbalis JG, Blackburn RE, Olson BR, Stricker EM. Central oxytocin inhibition of food and salt ingestion: a mechanism for intake regulation of solute homeostasis. Regul Pept 1993; 45:149–154.
537. Blackburn RE, Samson WK, Fulton RJ, Stricker EM, Verbalis JG. Central oxytocin inhibition of salt appetite in rats: evidence for differential sensing of plasma sodium and osmolality. Proc Natl Acad Sci USA 1993; 90:10380–10384.
538. Olson BR, Drutarosky MD, Stricker EM, Verbalis JG. Brain oxytocin receptor antagonism blunts the effects of anorexigenic treatments in rats: evidence for central oxytocin inhibition of food intake. Endocrinology 1991; 129:785–791.
539. Langhans W, Delprete E, Scharrer E. Mechanisms of vasopressin's anorectic effect. Physiol Behav 1991; 49:169–176.
540. Reghunandanan V, Badgaiyan RD, Marya RK, Maini BK. Suprachiasmatic injection of a vasopressin antagonist modifies the circadian rhythm of food intake. Behav Neur Biol 1987; 48:344–351.
541. Bray GA. Afferent signals regulating food intake. Proc Nutr Soc 2000; 59:373–384.
542. Van de Kar LD, Rittenhouse PA, Li Q, Levy AD, Brownfield MS. Hypothalamic paraventricular, but not supraoptic neurons, mediate the serotonergic stimulation of oxytocin secretion. Brain Res Bull 1995; 36: 45–50.
543. Olson BR, Drutarosky MD, Stricker EM, Verbalis JG. Brain oxytocin receptors mediate corticotropin-releasing hormone–induced anorexia. Am J Physiol 1991; 260:R448–R452.
544. Bjorkstrand E, Hulting A-L, Meister B, Uvnas-Moberg K. Effect of galanin on plasma levels of oxytocin and cholecystokinin. Neuroreport 1993; 4:10–12.
545. Hanai K, Oomura Y, Kai Y, Nishikawa K, Shimizu N, Morita H, et al. Central action of acidic fibroblast growth factor in feeding regulation. Am J Physiol 1989; 256:R217–R223.
546. Oomura Y, Sasaki K, Li AJ. Memory facilitation educed by food intake. Physiol Behav 1993; 54:493–498.
547. Matsumoto I, Niijima A, Oomura Y, Sasaki K, Tsuchiya K, Aikawa T. Acidic fibroblast growth factor activates adrenomedullary secretion and sympathetic outflow in rats. Am J Physiol 1998; 275:R1003-RI012.
548. Prasad C. Neurobiology of cyclo(His-Pro). (Review.) Ann NY Acad Sci 1989; 553:232–251.
549. Prasad C, Mizuma H, Brock JW, Porter JR, Svec F, Hilton C. A paradoxical elevation of brain cyclo(His-Pro) levels in hyperphagic obese Zucker rats. Brain Res 1995; 699:149–153.
550. Mizuma H, Svec F, Prasad C, Hilton C. Cyclo(His-Pro) augments the insulin response to oral glucose in rats. Life Sci 1997; 60:369–374.
551. Peiris AN, Mueller RA, Smith GA, Struve MF, Kissebah AH. Splanchnic insulin metabolism in obesity. Influence of body fat distribution. J Clin Invest 1986; 78:1648–1657.
552. Paez X, Stanley BG, Leibowitz SF. Microdialysis analysis of norepinephrine levels in the paraventricular nucleus in association with food intake at dark onset. Brain Res 1993; 606:167–170.
553. Jacobs BL. Brain monoaminergic unit activity in behaving animals. In: Epstein AN, Morrison AR, eds. Progress in Psychobiology and Physiological Psychology. New York: Academic Press, 1987:171–206.
554. Leibowitz SF, Weiss GF, Yee F, Tretter JB. Noradrenergic innervation of the paraventricular nucleus: specific role in control of carbohydrate ingestion. Brain Res Bull 1985; 14:561–567.
555. Currie PJ. Medial Hypothalamic α_2-Adrenergic and serotenergic effects on ingestive behaviour. In: Cooper SJ, Clifton PG, eds. Dopamine Receptor Subtype and Ingestive Behaviour. London: Academic Press, 1996: 285–300.
556. Leibowitz SF. Neurochemical-neuroendocrine systems in the brain controlling macronutrient intake and metabolism. (Review) Trends Neurosci 1992; 15:491–497.
557. Stanley BG, Schwartz DH, Hernandez L, Hoebel BG, Leibowitz SF. Patterns of extracellular norepinephrine in the paraventricular hypothalamus: relationship to circadian rhythm and deprivation-induced eating behavior. Life Sci 1989; 45:275–282.
558. Jhanwar-Uniyal M, Leibowitz SF. Impact of circulating corticosterone on alpha I- and alpha 2-noradren-

ergic receptors in discrete brain areas. Brain Res 1986; 368:404–408.

559. Hoebel BG, Leibowitz SF. Brain monoamines in the modulation of self-stimulation, feeding, and body weight. Assoc Res Nerv Ment Dis 1981; 59:103–142.
560. Bray GA. Hypothalamic and genetic obesity: an appraisal of the autonomic hypothesis and the endocrine hypothesis. In: Sullivan AC, Garattini S, eds. Novel Approaches and Drugs for Obesity. London: John Libbey, 1985:119–137.
561. Leibowitz SF, Roossin P, Rosenn M. Chronic norepinephrine injection into the hypothalamic paraventricular nucleus produces hyperphagia and increased body weight in the rat. Pharmacol Biochem. Behav 1984; 21:801–808.
562. Cincotta AH, Luo S, Zhang Y, Liang Y, Bina KG, Jetton TL, et al. Chronic infusion of norepinephrine into the VMH of normal rats induces the obese glucose-intolerant state. Am J Physiol Regul Integr Comp Physiol 2000; 278:R435-R444.
563. Levin BE, Planas B. Defective glucoregulation of brain alpha 2-adrenoceptors in obesity-prone rats. Am J Physiol 1993; 264(Pt 2):R305–R311.
564. Levin BE. Reduced norepinephrine turnover in organs and brains of obesity-prone rats. Am J Physiol 1995; 268:R389–R394.
565. Wilmot CA, Sullivan AC, Levin BE. Effects of diet and obesity on brain alpha 1- and alpha 2-noradrenergic receptors in the rat. Brain Res 1988; 453:157–166.
566. Jones AP, Olster DH, States B. Maternal insulin manipulations in rats organize body weight and noradrenergic innervation of the hypothalamus in gonadally intact male offspring. Brain Res Dev Brain Res 1996; 97:16–21.
567. Currie PJ, Wilson LM. Central injection of 5-hydroxytryptamine reduces food intake in obese and lean mice. Neuroreport 1992; 3:59–61.
568. Currie PJ, Wilson LM. Yohimbine attenuates clonidine-induced feeding and macronutrient selection in genetically obese (ob/ob) mice. Pharmacol Biochem Behav 1992; 43:1039–1046.
569. Currie PJ. Differential effects of NE, CLON, and 5-HT on feeding and macronutrient selection in genetically obese (ob/ob) and lean mice. Brain Res Bull 1993; 32:133–142.
570. Routh VH, Murakami DM, Stern JS, Fuller CA, Horwitz BA. Neuronal activity in hypothalamic nuclei of obese and lean Zucker rats. Int J Obes 1990; 14:879–891.
571. Tsujii S, Bray GA. Food intake of lean and obese Zucker rats following ventricular infusions of adrenergic agonists. Brain Res 1992; 587:226–232.
572. Morien A, McMahon L, Wellman PJ. Effects on food and water intake of the alpha 1-adrenoceptor agonists amidephrine and SK&F-89748. Life Sci 1993; 53:169–174.
573. Hoebel BG. Brain neurotransmitters in food and drug reward. Am J Clin Nutr 1985; 42:1133–1150.
574. Wellman PJ, Davies BT. Reversal of phenylpropanolamine anorexia in rats by the alpha-1 receptor antagonist benoxathian. Pharmacol Biochem Behav 1991; 38:905–908.
575. Angel I. Central receptors and recognition sites mediating the effects of monoamines and anorectic drugs on feeding behavior. Clin Neuropharmacol 1990; 13:361–391.
576. Leibowitz SF. Reciprocal hunger-regulating circuits involving alpha- and beta-adrenergic receptors located, respectively, in the ventromedial and lateral hypothalamus. Proc Natl Acad Sci USA 1970; 67: 1063–1070.
577. Margules DL. Beta-adrenergic; receptors in the hypothalamus for learned and unlearned taste aversions. J Comp Physiol Psychol 1970; 73:13–21.
578. Hoebel BG. Neuroscience and motivation: pathways and peptides that define motivation. In: Atkinson RC, Herrnstein RJ, Lindzey G, Luce RD, eds. Steven's Handbook of Experimental Psychology. New York: John Wiley & Sons, 1988:547–625.
579. Hoebel BG. Hypothalamic self-stimulation and stimulation escape in relation to feeding and mating. Fed Proc 1979; 38:2454–2461.
580. Lafontan M, Berlan M. Fat cell adrenergic receptors and the control of white and brown fat cell function. J Lipid Res 1993; 34:1057–1091.
581. Leibowitz SF, Weiss GF, Shor-Posner G. Hypothalamic serotonin: pharmacological, biochemical, and behavioral analyses of its feeding-suppressive action. Clin Neuropharmacol 1988; 11(suppl 1):S51–S71.
582. Leibowitz SF, Alexander JT. Hypothalamic serotonin in control of eating behavior, meal size and body weight. Biol Psychiatry 1998; 44(9):851–864.
583. Smith BK, York DA, Bray GA. Chronic d-fenfluramine treatment reduces fat intake independent of macronutrient preference. Pharmacol Biochem Behav 1998; 60:105–114.
584. Schwartz DH, Hernandez L, Hoebel BG. Serotonin release in lateral and medial hypothalamus during feeding and its anticipation. Brain Res Bull 1990; 25: 797–802.
585. Mark GP, Schwartz DH, Hernandez L, West HL, Hoebel BG. Application of microdialysis to the study of motivation and conditioning: measurements of dopamine and serotonin in freely-behaving rats. In: Robinson TE, Justice JB, eds. Microdialysis in the Neurosciences. Amsterdam: Elsevier Science, 1991: 369–385.
586. Orosco M, Gerozissis K, Nicolaïdis S. Effects of pure micronutrient diets on 5-HT release in the rat hypothalamus: relationship to insulin secretion and possible mechanism for feedback control of fat and carbohydrate ingestion. In: Berthoud HR, Seeley RJ, eds.

Neural and Metabolic Control of Macronutrient Intake. Boca Raton: CRC Press, 2000:447–454.
587. Fetissov SO, Meguid MM, Chen C, Miyata G. Synchronized release of dopamine and serotonin in the medial and lateral hypothalamus of rats. Neuroscience 2000; 101:657–663.
588. De Fanti BA, Hamilton JS, Horwitz BA. Meal-induced changes in extracellular 5-HT in medial hypothalamus of lean (Fa/Fa) and obese (fa/fa) Zucker rats. Brain Res 2001; 902:164–170.
589. Mori RC, Guimaraes RB, Nascimento CM, Ribeiro EB. Lateral hypothalamic serotonergic responsiveness to food intake in rat obesity as measured by microdialysis. Can J Physiol Pharmacol 1999; 77:286–292.
590. Hernandez L, Parada M, Baptista T, Schwartz D, West HL, Mark GP, et al. Hypothalamic serotonin in treatments for feeding disorders and depression as studied by brain microdialysis. J Clin Psychiatry 1991; 52:32–40.
591. Schwartz DH, Hernandez L, Hoebel BG. Tryptophan increases extracellular serotonin in the lateral hypothalamus of food-deprived rats. Brain Res Bull 1990; 25:803–807.
592. Schwartz D, Hernandez L, Hoebel BG. Fenfluramine administered systemically or locally increases extracellular serotonin in the lateral hypothalamus as measured by microdialysis. Brain Res 1989; 482:261–270.
593. Shimizu H, Uehara Y, Negishi M, Shimomura Y, Takahashi M, Fukatsu A, et al. Altered monoamine metabolism in the hypothalamus of the genetically obese yellow (Ay/a) mouse. Exp Clin Endocrinol 1992; 99:45–48.
594. Garthwaite TL, Kalkhoff RK, Guansing AR, Hagen TC, Menahan LA. Plasma free tryptophan, brain serotonin, and an endocrine profile of the genetically obese hyperglycemic mouse at 4–5 months of age. Endocrinology 1979; 105:1178–1182.
595. Cooper SJ, Dourish CT, Barber DJ. Reversal of the anorectic effect of (+)-fenfluramine in the rat by selective cholecystokinin receptor antagonist MK-329. Br J Pharmacol 1990; 99:65–70.
596. Stallone D, Nicolaidis S, Gibbs J. Cholecystokinin-induced anorexia depends on serotoninergic function. Am J Physiol 1989; 256:1138–1141.
597. Campbell DB. Dexfenfluramine: an overview of its mechanisms of action. Rev Contemp Pharmacother 1991; 2:93–113.
598. Rowland NE, Carlton J. Tolerance to the effects of D-fenfluramine in rats, hamsters and mice. In: Ferrari E, Brambilla F, eds. Disorders of Eating Behaviour: A Psychoneuroendocrine Approach. Oxford: Pergamon Journals, 1986:367–374.
599. Samanin R, Garattini S. The Neurophamacology of obesity: experimental studies. Rev Contemp Pharmacother 1991; 2:53–59.
600. Lawton CL, Blundell JE. 5-HT and carbohydrate suppression: effects of 5-HT antagonists on the action of d-fenfluramine and DOI. Pharmacol Biochem Behav 1993; 46:349–360.
601. Nicolaidis S, Even P. Metabolic rate and feeding behavior. (Review) Ann NY Acad Sci 1989; 575:86–104.
602. Wellman PJ, Maher TJ. Synergistic interactions between fenfluramine and phentermine. Int J Obes Relat Metab Disord 1999; 23:723–732.
603. Levin BE, Dunn-Meynell AA. Sibutramine alters the central mechanisms regulating the defended body weight in diet-induced obese rats. Am J Physiol Regul Integr Comp Physiol 2000; 279:2222–2228.
604. Luo S, Luo, J, Cincotta AH. Chronic ventromedial hypothalamic infusion of norepinephrine and serotonin promotes insulin resistance and glucose intolerance. Neuroendocrinology 1999; 70:460–465.
605. Li BH, Spector AC, Rowland NE. Reversal of dexfenfluramine-induced anorexia and c-Fos/c-Jun expression by lesion in the lateral parabrachial nucleus. Brain Res 1994; 640:255–267.
606. Simansky KJ, Jakubow J, Sisk FC, Vaidya AH, Eberle-Wang K. Peripheral serotonin is an incomplete signal for eliciting satiety in sham-feeding rats. Pharmacol Biochem Behav 1992; 43:847–854.
607. Vickers SP, Clifton PG, Dourish CT, Tecott LH. Reduced satiating effect of d-fenfluramine in serotonin 5-HT(2C) receptor mutant mice. Psychopharmacology (Berl) 1999; 143:309–314.
608. Clifton PG, Lee MD, Dourish CT. Similarities in the action of Ro 60–0175, a 5-HT2C receptor agonist and d-fenfluramine on feeding patterns in the rat. Psychopharmacology (Berl) 2000; 152:256–267.
609. Leibowitz SF, Brown LL. Histochemical and pharmacological analysis of catecholaminergic projections to the perifornical hypothalamus in relation to feeding inhibition. Brain Res 1980; 201:315–345.
610. Leibowitz SF, Rossakis C. Pharmacological characterization of perifornical hypothalamic dopamine receptors mediating feeding inhibition in the rat. Brain Res 1979; 172:115–130.
611. Leibowitz SF. Midbrain-hypothalamic catecholamine projection systems mediating feeding stimulation and inhibition in the rat. In: Usher P, Kopin IJ, Barchas J, eds. Catecholamines: Basic and Clinical Frontiers. New York: Pergamon Press, 1979:1675–1677.
612. Garattini S, Borroni E, Mennini T, Samanin R. Differences and similarities among anorectic agents. In: Garattini S, Samanin R, eds. Central Mechanisms of Anorectic Drugs. New York: Raven Press, 1978: 127–143.
613. Moore KE, Demarest KT, Lookingland KJ. Stress, prolactin and hypothalamic dopaminergic neurons. (Review.) Neuropharmacology 1987; 26:801–808.
614. Parada M, Hernandez L, Schwartz D, Hoebel BG.

Hypothalamic infusion of amphetamine increases extracellular serotonin, dopamine and norepinephrine. Physiol Behav 1988; 44:607–610.
615. Wellman PJ. A review of the physiological bases of the anorexic action of phenylpropanolamine (d,l-norephedrine). (Review) Neurosci Biobehav Rev 1990; 14:339–355.
616. Parada MA, Puig de Parada M, Hoebel BG. Rats self-inject a dopamine antagonist in the lateral hypothalamus where it acts to increase extracellular dopamine in the nucleus accumbens. Pharmacol Biochem Behav 1995; 52:179–187.
617. Parada MA, Hernandez L, Paez X, Baptista T, Puig de Parada M, et al. Mechanism of the body weight increase induced by systemic sulpiride. Pharmacol Biochem Behav 1989; 33:45–50.
618. Orosco M, Nicolaidis S. Spontaneous feeding-related monoaminergic changes in the rostromedial hypothalamus revealed by microdialysis. Physiol Behav 1992; 52:1015–1019.
619. Meguid MM, Yang Z-J, Bellinger LL, Gleason JR, Koseki M, Laviano A, et al. Innervated liver plays an inhibitory role in regulation of food intake. Surgery 1996; 119:202–207.
620. Shimizu H. Alteration in hypothalamic monoamine metabolism of freely moving diabetic rat. Neurosci Lett 1991; 131:225–227.
621. Karadi Z, Oomura Y, Nishino H, Scott TR, Lenard L, Aou S. Responses of lateral hypothalamic glucose-sensitive and glucose-insensitive neurons to chemical stimuli in behaving rhesus monkeys. J Neurophysiol 1992; 67:389–400.
622. Hoebel BG, Rada PV, Mark GP, Parada M, Puig de Parada, M, Pothos E, Hernandez L. Hypothalamic control of accumbens dopamine: a system for feeding reinforcement. In: Bray GA, Ryan D, eds. Molecular and Genetic Aspects of Obesity. Baton Rouge: LSU Press, 1995.
623. Berridge KC. Food reward: brain substrates of wanting and liking. Neurosci Biobehav Rev 1996; 20:1–25.
624. Salamone JD, Cousins MS, McCullough LD, Carriero DL, Berkowitz RJ. Nucleus accumbens dopamine release increases during instrumental lever pressing for food but not free food consumption. Pharmacol Biochem Behav 1994; 49:25–31.
625. Berridge KC, Robinson TE. What is the role of dopamine in reward: hedonic impact, reward learning, or incentive salience. Brain Res Rev 1998; 28:309–369.
626. Wyvell CL, Berridge KC. Intra-accumbens amphetamine increases the conditioned incentive salience of sucrose reward: enhancement of reward "wanting" without enhanced "liking" or response reinforcement. J Neurosci 2000; 20:8122–8130.
627. Wise RA. Common neural basis of brain stimulation reward, drug reward, and food reward. In: Hoebel BG, Novin D, eds. The Neural Basis of Feeding and Reward. Brunswick, ME: Haer Institute, 1982:445–454.
628. Fibiger HC, Phillips AG. Reward, motivation, cognition: psychobiology of mesotelencephalic dopamine system. In: Bloom FE, ed. Handbook of Physiology. Vol. IV. Intrinsic Regulatory Systems of the Brain. Bethesda: American Physiological Society 1986:647–675.
629. Hoebel BG, Hernandez L, Mark GP, Schwartz DH, Pothos E, Steckel JM, Stone EH. Brain microdialysis as a molecular approach to obesity: serotonin, dopamine, cyclic-AMP. In: Bray G, Ricquier D, Spiegleman B, eds. Obesity: Towards a Molecular Approach. New York: Alan R. Liss, 1990:45–61.
630. Kornetsky C, Porrino LJ. Brain mechanisms of drug-induced reinforcement. In: O'Brien CP, Jaffee JH, eds. Addictive States: Association for Research in Nervous and Mental Diseases. New York: Raven Press, 1992: 59–77.
631. Hernandez L, Hoebel BG. Feeding and hypothalamic stimulation increase dopamine turnover in the accumbens. Physiol Behav 1988; 44:599–606.
632. Wilson C, Nomikos. GG, Collu M, Fibiger HC. Dopaminergic correlates of motivated behavior: importance of drive. J Neurosci 1995; 15:5169–5178.
633. Di Chiara G, Tanda. G. Blunting of reactivity of dopamine transmission to palatable food: a biochemical marker of anhedonia in the CMS model? Psychopharmacology (Berl) 1997; 134:351–353.
634. Hoebel BG, Monaco AP, Hernandez L, Aulisi EF, Stanley BG, Lenard L. Self-injection of amphetamine directly into the brain. Psychopharmacology 1983; 81:158–163.
635. Guerin B, Goeders NE, Dworkin SI, Smith JE. Intracranial self-administration of dopamine into the nucleus accumbens. Soc Neurosci Abstr 1984; 10:1072.
636. Wise RA, Newton P, Leeb K, Burnette B, Pocock D, Justice JB Jr. Fluctuations in nucleus accumbens dopamine concentration during intravenous cocaine self-administration in rats. Psychopharmacology 1995; 120:10–20.
637. Bozarth MA. The mesolimbic dopamine system as a model reward system. In: Wellner P, Scheel-Kruger J, eds. The Mesolimbic Dopamine System: From Motivation to Action. New York: John Wiley and Sons, 1991:301–333.
638. Glimcher PW, Giovino AA, Hoebel BG. Neurotensin selfinjection in the ventral tegmental area. Brain Res 1987; 403:147–150.
639. Mifsud J-C, Hernandez L, Hoebel BG. Nicotine infused into the nucleus accumbens increases synaptic dopamine as measured by in vivo microdialysis. Brain Res 1989; 478:365–367.
640. Schilstrom. B, Svensson HM, Svensson TH, Nomikos GG. Nicotine and food induced dopamine release in the nucleus accumbens of the rat: putative role of

alpha7 nicotinic receptors in the ventral tegmental area. Neuroscience 1998; 85:1005–1009.

641. Kalivas PW, Barnes CD. Limbic Motor Circuits and Neuropsychiatry. Boca Raton: CRC Press, 1993.
642. Schultz W, Dayan P, Montague PR. A neural substrate of prediction and reward. Science 1997; 275: 1593–1599.
643. Berridge KC. Measuring hedonic impact in animals and infants: microstructure of affective taste reactivity patterns. Neurosci Biobehav Rev 2000; 24:173–198.
644. Smith GP. Dopamine and food reward. In: Fluharty S, Morrison AM, eds. Progress in Psychobiology and Physiological Psychology. New York: Academic Press, 1995:83–144.
645. Terry P. Dopamine receptor subtypes and ingestive behaviour. In: Cooper SJ, Clifton PG, eds. Drug Receptor Subtypes and Ingestive Behaviour. London: Academic Press, 1996:233–266.
646. Schultz W, Apicella P, Ljungberg T. Responses of monkey dopamine neurons to reward and conditioned stimuli during successive steps of learning a delayed response task. J Neurosci 1993; 13:900–913.
647. Ahn S, Phillips AG. Dopaminergic correlates of sensory-specific satiety in the medial prefrontal cortex and nucleus accumbens of the rat. J Neurosci 1999; 19:RC29.
648. Bassareo V, Di Chiara G. Differential responsiveness of dopamine transmission to food-stimuli in nucleus accumbens shell/core compartments. Neuroscience 1999; 89:637–641.
649. Carr KD, Papadouka V. The role of multiple opioid receptors in the potentiation of reward by food restriction. Brain Res 1994; 639:253–260.
650. Carroll ME, France CP, Meisch RA. Food deprivation increases oral and intravenous drug intake in rats. Science 1979; 205:319–321.
651. Stricker EM, Zigmond MJ. Recovery of function after damage to central catecholamine-containing neurons: a neurochemical model for the lateral hypothalamic syndrome. In: Sprague JM, Epstein AN, eds. Progress in Psychobiology and Physiological Psychology. New York: Academic Press, 1978:121–188.
652. Cousins MS, Salamone JD. Nucleus accumbens dopamine depletions in rats affect relative response allocation in a novel cost/benefit procedure. Pharmacol Biochem. Behav 1994; 49:85–91.
653. Koob GF, Robledo P, Markou A, Caine SB. The mesocorticolimbic circuit in drug dependence and reward—a role for the extended amygdala? In: Kalivas PW, Barnes CD, eds. Limbic Motor Circuits and Neuropsychiatry. Boca Raton: CRC Press, 1996: 289–310.
654. Kelley AE, Delfs JM. Dopamine and conditioned reinforcement. Psychopharmacology 1991; 103:187–196.
655. Weiss FMT, Lorang MT, Bloom FE, Koob GF. Oral alcohol self-administration stimulates dopamine release in the rat nucleus accumbens: genetic and motivational determinants. J Pharmacol Exp Ther 1993; 267:250–258.
656. Grill HJ, Kaplan JM. Caudal brainstem participates in the distributed neural control of feeding. In: Stricker EM, ed. Handbook of Behavioral Neurobiology. New York: Plenum Press, 1990: 125–149.
657. Sclafani A. Nutritionally based learned flavor preferences in rats. In: Capaldi ED, Powley TL, eds. Taste, Experience and Feeding. Washington: Psychological Association, 1990: 139–156.
658. Mark GP, Blander DS, Hoebel BG. A conditioned stimulus decreases extracellular dopamine in the nucleus accumbens after the development of a learned taste aversion. Brain Res 1991; 551:308–310.
659. Horvitz JC, Richardson WB, Ettenberg A. Dopamine receptor blockade and reductions in thirst produce differential effects on drinking behavior. Pharmacol Biochem Behav 1993; 45:725–728.
660. Leibman JM, Cooper SJ, eds. The Neuropharmacological Basis of Reward. New York: Clarendon Press, 1989.
661. McGinty JF, ed. Advancing from the ventral striatum to the extended amygdala. Annals NY Acd Sci 1999. Vol. 877. New York: New York Acad of Sci. Vol. 877.
662. Sakata T, Kurokawa M, Oohara A, Yoshimatsu H. A physiological role of brain histamine during energy deficiency. Brain Res Bull 1994; 35:135–139.
663. Leibowitz SF. Histamine: modification of behavioral and physiological components of body fluid homeostasis. In: Yellin TO, ed. Histamine Receptors. New York: SP Medical and Scientific Books, 1977:219–253.
664. Sheiner JB, Morris P, Anderson GH. Food intake suppression by histidine. Pharmacol Biochem Behav 1985; 23:721–726.
665. Ookuma K, Yoshimatsu H, Sakata T, Fujimoto K. Hypothalamic sites of neuronal histamine action on food intake by rats. Brain Res 1989; 490:268–275.
666. Ookuma K, Sakata T, Fukagawa K, Yoshimatsu H, Kurokawa M, Machidori H, et al. Neuronal histamine in the hypothalamus suppresses food intake in rats. Brain Res. 1993; 628:235–242.
667. Morimoto T, Yamamoto Y, Yamatodani A. Brain histamine and feeding behavior. Behav Brain Res 2001; 124:145–150.
668. Machidori H, Sakata T, Yoshimatsu H, Ookuma K, Fujimoto K, Kurokawa M. Zucker obese rats: defect in brain histamine control of feeding. Brain Res 1992; 590:180–186.
669. Sakata T. Histamine receptor and its regulation of energy metabolism. Obes Res 1995; 3(suppl 4): 541S–548S.
670. Sakata T. Glucose transport and energy metabolism regulated by brain histamine. Jpn J Physiol 1997; 47(suppl 1): S32–S34.

671. Yoshimatsu H, Chiba S, Tajima D, Akehi Y, Sakata T. Histidine suppresses food intake through its conversion into neuronal histamine. Exp Biol Med (Maywood) 2002; 227:63–68.
672. Brezenoff HE, Lomax P. Temperature changes following microinjection of histamine into the thermoregulatory centers of the rat. Experientia 1970; 26:51–52.
673. Hashimoto M. Characterization and mechanism of fever induction by interleukin-1 beta. Pflugers Arch 1991; 419:616–621.
674. Plata-Salaman CF, Oomura Y, Kai Y. Tumor necrosis factor and interleukin-1 beta: suppression of food intake by direct action in the central nervous system. Brain Res 1988; 448:106–114.
675. Kang M, Yoshimatsu H, Oogawa R, et al. Hypothalamic neuronal histamine modulates ingestive behavior and thermogenesis induced by interleukin-1 beta. Am J Physiol 1995; 269:R1308–1313.
676. Mollet A, Lutz TA, Meier S, Riediger T, Rushing PA, Scharrer E. Histamine H(l) receptors mediate the anorectic action of the pancreatic hormone amylin. Am J Physiol Regul Integr Comp Physiol 2001; 281:1442–1448.
677. Yoshimatsu H, Sakata T, Machidori H, Fujimoto K, Yamatodani A, Wada. H. Ginsenoside Rg1 prevents histaminergic modulation of rat adaptive behavior from elevation of ambient temperature. Physiol Behav 1993; 53:1–4.
678. Chance WT, Lints CE. Eating following cholinergic stimulation of the hypothalamus. Physiol Psych 1977; 5:440–444.
679. Fukuda M, Ono T, Nakamura K, Tamura R. Dopamine and ACh involvement in plastic learning by hypothalamic neurons in rats. Brain Res Bull 1990; 25:109–114.
680. Singer G, Kelly J. Cholinergic and adrenergic interaction in the hypothalamic control of drinking and eating behavior. Physiol Behav 1972; 8:885–890.
681. De Parada MP, Parada MA, Rada P, Hernandez L, Hoebel BG. Dopamine-acetylcholine interaction in the rat lateral hypothalamus in the control of locomotion. Pharmacol Biochem Behav 2000; 66:227–234.
682. Rada PV, Mark GP, Yeomans JJ, Hoebel BG. Acetylcholine release in ventral tegmental area by hypothalamic self-stimulation, eating, and drinking. Pharmacol Biochem Behav 2000; 65:375–379.
683. Yeomans J, Forster G, Blaha C. M5 muscarinic receptors are needed for slow activation of dopamine neurons and for rewarding brain stimulation. Life Sci 2001; 68:2449–2456.
684. Museo E, Wise RA. Place preference conditioning with ventral tegmental injections of cytisine. Life Sci 1994; 55:1179–1186.
685. Nisell M, Nomikos GG, Svensson TH. Infusion of nicotine in the ventral tegmental area or the nucleus accumbens of the rat differentially affects accumbal dopamine release. Pharmacol Toxicol 1994; 75:348–352.
686. Mark G, Rada P, Pothos E, Hoebel BG. Effects of feeding and drinking on acetylcholine release in the nucleus accumbens striatum and hippocampus of freely-behaving rats. J Neurochem 1992; 58:2269–2274.
687. Mark GP, Weinberg JB, Rada PV, Hoebel BG. Extracellular acetylcholine is increased in the nucleus accumbens following the presentation of an aversively conditioned taste stimulus. Brain Res 1995; 688:184–188.
688. Shoaib MM, Stolerman II. Conditioned taste aversions in rats after intracerebral administration of nicotine. Behav Pharmacol 1995; 6:375–385.
689. Berger-Sweeney J, Stearns NA, Frick KM, Beard B, Baxter MG. Cholinergic basal forebrain is critical for social transmission of food preferences. Hippocampus 2000; 10:729–738.
690. Miranda MI, Ramirez-Lugo L, Bermudez-Rattoni F. Cortical cholinergic activity is related to the novelty of the stimulus. Brain Res 2000; 882:230–235.
691. Coscina DV, Castonguay TW, Stern JS. Effects of increasing brain GABA on the meal patterns of genetically obese vs. lean Zucker rats. Int J Obes Relat Metab Disord 1992; 16:425–433.
692. Ma YH, Hu JH, Zhou, XG, Zeng RW, Mei ZT, Fei J, et al. Transgenic mice overexpressing gamma-aminobutyric acid transporter subtype I develop obesity. Cell Res 2000; 10:303–310.
693. Tsujii S, Bray GA. GABA-related feeding control in genetically obese rats. Brain Res 1991; 540:48–54.
694. Kelly J, Rothstein J, Grossman SP. GABA and hypothalamic feeding systems. I. Topographic analysis of the effects of microinjections of muscimol. Physiol Behav 1979; 23:1123–1134.
695. Kelly J, Grossman SP. GABA and hypothalamic feeding systems. II. A comparison of GABA, glycine and actylcholine agonists and their antagonists. Pharmacol Biochem Behav 1979; 11:647–652.
696. Panksepp J, Meeker RB. The role of GABA in the ventromedial hypothalamic regulation of food intake. Brain Res Bull 1980; 5:453–460.
697. Beverly JL, De Vries MG, Bouman SD, Arseneau LM. Noradrenergic; and GABAergic systems in the medial hypothalamus are activated during hypoglycemia. Am J Physiol Regul Integr Comp Physiol 2001; 280:563–569.
698. Cattabeni F, Maggi A, Monduzzi M, De Angelis L, Racagni G. GABA: circadian fluctuations in rat hypothalamus. J Neurochem 1978; 31:565–567.
699. Meeker RB, Myers RD. GABA and glutamate: possible metabolic intermediaries involved in the hypothalamic regulation of food intake. Brain Res Bull 1980; 5:253–259.
700. Rada P, Mendialdua A, Hernandez L, Hoebel BG.

Extracellular glutamate increases in the lateral hypothalamus during meal initiation, and GABA peaks during satiation: microdialysis measurements every 30 sec. Behavioral Neuroscience. In press.

701. Khan AM, Curras MC, Dao J, Jamal FA, Turkowski CA, Goel RK, et al. Lateral hypothalamic NMDA receptor subunits NR2A and/or NR2B. mediate eating: immunochemical/behavioral evidence. Am J Physiol 1999; 276:880–891.
702. Maldonado-Irizarry CS, Swanson CJ, Kelley AE. Glutamate receptors in the nucleus accumbens shell control feeding behavior via the lateral hypothalamus. J Neurosci 1995; 15:6779–6788.
703. Stanley BG. Glutamate and its receptors in lateral hypothalamic stimulation of eating In: Cooper SJ, Clifton PG, eds. Dopamine Receptor Subtypes and Ingestive Behaviour. London: Academic Press, 1996:301–322.
704. Stanley BG, Willett VL, Donias HW, Ha LH, Spears LC. The lateral hypothalamus: a primary site mediating excitatory amino acid-elicited eating. Brain Res 1993; 630:41–49.
705. Stanley BG, Ha LH, Spears LC, Dee MG. Lateral hypothalamic injections of glutamate, kainic acid, D, L-alpha-amino-3-hydroxy-5-methyl-isoxazole propionic; acid or N-methyl-D-aspartic acid rapidly elicit intense transient eating in rats. Brain Res 1993; 613: 88–95.
706. Bednar I, Qian M, Qureshi GA, Kallstrom L, Johnson AE, Carrer H, et al. Glutamate inhibits ingestive behaviour. J Neuroendocrinol 1994; 6:403–408.
707. Berridge KC, Pecina S. Benzodiazepines, appetite, and taste palatability. (Review) Neurosci Biobehav Rev 1995; 19:121–131.
708. Berthoud HR. An overview of neural pathways and networks involved in the control of food intake and selection. In: Berthoud HR, Seeley RJ, eds. Neural and Metabolic Control of Macronutrient Intake. Boca Raton: CRC Press, 2000:361–388.
709. Mogenson GJ, Brudzynski SM, Wu M, Yang CR, Yim CY. From motivation to action: a review of dopaminergic regulation of limbic → nucleus accumbens → ventral palladium → pedunculopontine nucleus circuitries involved in limbic-motor integration. In: Kalivas PW, Barnes CD, eds. Limbic Motor Circuits and Neuropsychiatry. Boca Raton: CRC Press, 1993:193–236.
710. Spector AC. Gustatory function in the parabrachial nuclei: implications from lesion studies in rats. Rev Neurosci 1995; 6:143–175.
711. Travers SP, Norgren R. Organization of orosensory responses in the nucleus of the solitary tract of the rat. J Neurophysiol 1995; 73:2144–2162.
712. Lennard DE, Eckert WA, Merchenthaler I. Corticotropin-releasing hormone neurons in the paraventricular nucleus project to the external zone of the median eminence: a study combining retrograde labeling with immunocytochemistry. J Neuroendocrinol 1993; 5: 175–181.
713. Lenard L, Karadi Z, Faludi B, Hernadi I. Role of forebrain glucose-monitoring neurons in the central control of feeding, I. Behavioral properties and neurotransmitter sensitivities. Neurobiology (Bp) 1995; 3:223–239.
714. Niijima A, Meguid MM. An electrophysiological study on amino acid sensors in the hepato-protal system in the rat. Obes Res 1995; 3:741S–745S.
715. Meredith GE, Blanf B, Groenewegen HJ. The distribution and compartmental organization of the cholinergic neurons in nucleus accumbens. Neuroscience 1989; 31:327–345.
716. Pennartz CMA, Groenewegen HJ, Lopes da Silva FH. The nucleus accumbens as a complex of functionally distinct neuronal ensembles: an integration of behavioral, electrophysiological and anatomical data. Prog Neurobiol 1994; 42:719–761.
717. Rada PV, Mark GP, Hoebel BG. In vivo modulation of acetylcholine in the nucleus accumbens of freely moving rats, I. Inhibition by serotonin. Brain Res 1993; 619:98–104.
718. Koob GF, Swerdlow NR. The functional output of the mesolimbic dopamine system. In: Kalivas PW, ed. The Mesocorticolimbic Dopamine System. New York: New York Academy of Sciences, 1988:216–227.
719. Olive MF, Bertolucci M, Evans CJ, Maidment NT. Microdialysis reveals a morphine-induced increase in pallidal opioid peptide release. Neuroreport 1995; 6:1093–1096.
720. Parent A, Hazrati L-N. Functional anatomy of the basal ganglia. I. The cortico-basal ganglia-thalamo-cortical loop. Brain Res Rev 1995; 20:91–127.
721. Shizgal P, Kiss I, Bielajew C. Psychophysical and electrophysiological studies of the substrate for brain stimulation reward. In: Hoebel BG, Novin D, eds. The Neural Basis of Feeding and Reward. Brunswick, ME: Haer Institute, 1982:419–430.
722. Hernandez L, Murzi E, Schwartz DH, Hoebel BG. Neuroelectrophysiological and neurochemical approach to a hierarchical feeding organization. In: Bjorntorp P, Brodoff B, eds. Obesity. Philadelphia: J.B. Lippincott, 1992:171–183.
723. Yeomans JS, Mathur A, Tampakeras M. Rewarding brain stimulation: role of tegmental cholinergic neurons that activate dopamine neurons. Behav Neurosci 1993; 107:1077–1087.
724. Heimer L, Alheid GF. Piecing together the puzzle of basal forebrain anatomy. In: Napier TC, ed. The Basal Forebrain. New York: Plenum Press, 1991:1–42.
725. Rada PV, Hoebel BG. Aversive hypothalamic stimulation releases acetylcholine in the nucleus accumbens, and stimulation-escape decreases it. Brain Res 2001; 888:60–65.

726. Rada PV, Mark GP, Hoebel BG. Dopamine release in the nucleus accumbens by hypothalamic stimulation-escape behavior. Brain Res 1998; 782:228–234.
727. Hoebel BG, Leibowitz SL, Hernandez L. Neurochemistry of anorexia and bulemia. In: Anderson H, ed. The Biology of Feast and Famine: Relevance to Eating Disorders. Oxford: Oxford University Press, 1992:21–45.
728. Salamone JD. Behavioral pharmacology of dopamine systems: a new synthesis. In: Willner P, Scheel-Kruger J, eds. The Mesolimbic Dopamine System: From Motivation to Action. Cambridge: Cambridge University Press, 1991:599–613.
729. Wise RA, Spindler J, De Wit H, Gerber GJ. Neuroleptic-induced anhedonia in rats: pimozide blocks the reward quality of food. Science 1978; 201:262–264.
730. Radhakishun FS, Van Ree JM, Westerink BH. Scheduled eating increases dopamine release in the nucleus accumbens of food-deprived rats as assessed with on-line brain dialysis. Neurosci Lett 1988; 85:351–356.
731. Agnati LF, Bjelke B, Fuxe K. Volume transmission in the brain. Am Sci 1992; 80:362–373.
732. Blackburn JR, Phillips AG, Jakubovic A, Fibiger HC. Dopamine and preparatory behavoir. II. A neurochemical analysis. Behav Neurosci 1989; 103:15–23.
733. Hoebel BG, Rada P, Mark GP, Hernandez L. The power of integrative peptides to reinforce behavior by releasing dopamine. In: Strand FL, Beckwith BE, Chronwall B, Sandman CA, eds. Models of Neuropeptide Action. New York: New York Academy of Sciences, 1994:36–41.
734. Parada MA, Hernandez L, De Parada MP, Paez X, Hoebel BG. Dopamine in the lateral hypothalamus may be involved in the inhibition of locomotion related to food and water seeking. Brain Res Bull 1990; 25:961–968.
735. Hoebel BG, Rada P, Mark GP, Parada M, Puig de Parada M, Pothos E, Hernandez L. Hypothalamic control of accumbens dopamine: a system for feeding reinforcement. In: Gray G, Ryan D, eds. Molecular and Genetic Aspects of Obesity. Baton Rouge: Louisiana State University Press, 1996:263–280.
736. Rada P, Jensen K, Hoebel BG. Effects of nicotine and mecamylamine-induced withdrawal on extracellular dopamine and acetylcholine in the rat nucleus accumbens. Psychopharmacology (Berl) 2001; 157:105–110.
737. Wise RA. Addiction becomes a brain disease. Neuron 2000; 26:27–33.
738. Koob GF. Neurobiology of addiction. Toward the development of new therapies. Ann NY Acad Sci 2000; 909:170–185.
739. Nestler EJ. Genes and addiction. Nat Genet 2000; 26:277–281.
740. Carr KD, Kim GY, Cabeza de Vaca S. Chronic food restriction in rats augments the central rewarding effect of cocaine and the delta1 opioid agonist, DPDPE, but not the delta2 agonist, deltorphin-II [in process citation]. Psychopharmacology (Berl) 2000; 152:200–207.
741. Carroll ME. The role of food deprivation in the maintenance and reinstatement of cocaine seeking behavior in rats. Drug Alcohol Depend 1985; 16:95–109.
742. Kornetsky C, Esposito RU, McLean S, Jacobson JO. Intracranial self-stimulation thresholds: a model for the hedonic effects of drugs of abuse. Arch Gen Psychiatry 1979; 36:289–292.
743. Hagan MM, Moss DE. An animal model of bulimia nervosa: opioid sensitivity to fasting episodes. Pharmacol Biochem Behav 1991; 39:421–422.
744. Specker SM, Lac ST, Carroll ME. Food deprivation history and cocaine self-administration: an animal model of binge eating. Pharmacol Biochem Behav 1994; 48:1025–1029.
745. Campbell UC, Carroll ME. Reduction of drug self administration by an alternative non-drug reinforcer in rhesus monkeys: magnitude and temporal effects. Psychopharmacology (Berl) 2000; 147:418–425.
746. Carroll ME, Lac ST. Dietary additives and the acquisition of cocaine self-administration in rats. Psychopharmacology (Berl) 1998; 137:81–89.
747. Wyvell CL, Berridge KC. Incentive sensitization by previous amphetamine exposure: increased cue-triggered "wanting" for sucrose reward. J Neurosci 2001; 21:7831–7840.
748. Dess NK, Badia-Elder NE, Thiele TE, Kiefer SW, Blizard DA. Ethanol consumption in rats selectively bred for differential saccharin intake. Alcohol 1998; 16:275–278.
749. Gosnell BA. Sucrose intake predicts rate of acquisition of cocaine self-administration.Psychopharmacology (Berl) 2000; 149:286–292.
750. Sills TL, Crawley JN. Individual differences in sugar consumption predict amphetamine-induced dopamine overflow in nucleus accumbens. Eur J Pharmacol 1996; 303:177–181.
751. Blass EM, Hoffmeyer LB. Sucrose as an analgesic for newborn infants. Pediatrics 1991; 87:215–218.
752. Le Magnen J. A role for opiates in food reward and food addiction. In: Capaldi ED, Powley TL, eds. Taste, Experience, and Feeding. Washington: American Psychological Association, 1990:241–254.
753. Hoebel BG, Hernandez L, Rada PV, Parada M, Mark GP, Taylor KM, et al. A theory of feeding motivation and its inhibition based on dopamine and acetylcholine in the nucleus acumbens. Appetite 1996; 27:281.
754. Gendall KA, Joyce PR, Abbott RM. The effects of meal composition on subsequent craving and binge eating. Addict Behav 1999; 24:305–315.
755. Tuomisto T, Hetherington MM, Morris MF, Tuomisto MT, Turjanmaa V, Lappalainen R. Psychological and physiological characteristics of sweet food "addiction." Int J Eat Disord 1999; 25:169–175.

756. Mercer ME, Holder MD. Food cravings, endogenous opioid peptides, and food intake: a review. Appetite 1997; 29:325–352.
757. Hill AJ, Weaver CF, Blundell JE. Food craving, dietary restraint and mood. Appetite 1991; 17:187–197.
758. Macdiarmid JI, Hetherington MM. Mood modulation by food: an exploration of affect and cravings in 'chocolate addicts'. Br J Clin Psychol 1995; 34(Pt 1):129–138.
759. Rozin P, Levine E, Stoess C. Chocolate craving and liking. Appetite 1991; 17:199–212.
760. Wang GJ, Volkow ND, Logan J, Pappas NR, Wong CT, Zhu W, et al. Brain dopamine and obesity. Lancet 2001; 357:354–357.
761. Kuikka JT, Tammela L, Karhunen L, Rissanen A, Bergstrom KA, Naukkarinen H, et al. Reduced serotonin transporter binding in binge eating women. Psychopharmacology (Berl) 2001; 155:310–314.
762. Marrazzi MA, Markham KM, Kinzie J, Luby ED. Binge eating disorder: response to naltrexone. Int J Obes Relat Metab Disord 1995; 19:143–145.
763. Spiegel TA, Stunkard AJ, Shrager EE, O'Brien CP, Morrison MF, Stellar E. Effect of naltrexone on food intake, hunger, and satiety in obese men. Physiol Behav 1987; 40:135–141.
764. Kaye WH, Weltzin TE. Neurochemistry of bulimia nervosa. J Clin Psychiatry 1991; 52(suppl):21–28.
765. Neumeister A, Winkler A, Wober-Bingol C. Addition of naltrexone to fluoxetine in the treatment of binge eating disorder. Am J Psychiatry 1999; 156:797.
766. Chatoor I, Herman BH, Hartzler J. Effects of the opiate antagonist, naltrexone, on bingeing antecedents and plasma beta-endorphin concentrations. J Am Acad Child Adolesc Psychiatry 1994; 33:748–752.
767. Drewnowski A, Krahn DD, Demitrack MA, Nairn K, Gosnell BA. Naloxone, an opiate blocker, reduces the consumption of sweet high-fat foods in obese and lean female binge eaters. Am J Clin Nutr 1995; 61:1206–1212.
768. Bray GA. Reciprocal relation of food intake and sympathetic activity: experimental observations and clinical implications. Int J Obes Relat Metab Disord 2000; 24(suppl 2):S8–S17.
769. Jequier E. Energy regulation and thermogenesis in humans. In: Bray GA, Spiegelman BM eds Obesity: Towards a Molecular Approach. New York: Wiley-Liss, 1990:95–106.
770. Monda M, Sullo A, De Luca B. Lesions of the ventromedial hypothalamus reduce postingestional thermogenesis. Physiol Behav 1997; 61:687–691.
771. Bray GA. Food intake, sympathetic activity, and adrenal steroids. Brain Res Bull 1993; 32:537–541.
772. Sakata T, Ookuma K, Fujimoto K, Fukagawa K, Yoshimatsu H. Histaminergic control of energy balance in rats. Brain Res Bull 1991; 27:371–375.
773. Brobeck JR. Food and temperature. Recent Prog Horm Res 1960; 16:439–459.
774. Schoeller DA. The importance of clinical research: the role of thermogenesis in human obesity. Am J Clin Nutr 2001; 73:511–516.
775. Campbell BA, Misanin JR. Basic drives. Annu Rev Psychol 1960; 20:57–84.
776. Aravich PF, Doerries LE, Stanley E, Metcalf A, Lauterio TJ. Glucoprivic feeding and activity-based anorexia in the rat. In: Schneider LH, Cooper SJ, Halmi KA, eds. The Psychobiology of Human Eating Disorders. New York: New York Academy of Sciences, 1989:490–492.
777. Shimizu H, Simomura Y, Takahashi M, Uehara Y, Fukatsu A, Sato N. Altered amublatory activity and related brain monoamine metabolism in genetically obese Zucker rats. Exp Clin Endocrinol 1991; 97:39–44.
778. Campfield LA, Smith FJ. Systemic factors in the control of food intake: evidence for patterns as signals. In: Stricker EM, ed. Handbook of Behavioral Neurobiology. New York: Plenum Press, 1990:183–206.
779. Mayer J. Glucostatic mechanism of regulation of food intake. Obes Res 1996; 4:493–496.
780. Friedman MI, Rawson NE, Tordoff MG. Control of food intake. In: Bray GA, ed. Molecular and Genetic Aspects of Obesity. Baton Rouge: LSU Press, 1996:318–339.
781. Cummings DE, Purnell JQ, Frayo RS, Schmidova K, Wisse BE, Weigle DS. A preprandial rise in plasma ghrelin levels suggests a role in meal initiation in humans. Diabetes 2001; 50:1714–1719.
782. Calingasan NY, Ritter S. Hypothalamic paraventricular nucleus lesions do not abolish glucoprivic or lipoprivic feeding. Brain Res 1992; 595:25–31.
783. Bernardis LL, Bellinger LL. The dorsomedial hypothalamic nucleus revisited: 1998 update. Proc Soc Exp Biol Med 1998; 218:284–306.
784. Shimazu T. Central nervous system regulation of energy expenditure in brown adipose tissue and skeletal muscle. In: Angel A, Anderson H, Bouchard C, Lace D, Leiter L, Mendelson R, eds. Progress in Obesity Research. London: John Libbey, 1996:193–199.
785. Steffens AB, Strubbe JH, Balkan B, Scheurink JW. Neuroendocrine mechanisms involved in regulation of body weight, food intake and metabolism. (Review.) Neurosci Biobehav Rev 1990; 14:305–313.
786. Kent P, Bedard T, Khan S, Anisman H, Merali Z. Bombesin-induced HPA and sympathetic activation requires CRH receptors. Peptides 2001; 22:57–65.
787. Ruffin M, Nicolaidis S. Electrical stimulation of the ventromedial hypothalamus enhances both fat utilization and metabolic rate that precede and parallel the inhibition of feeding behavior. Brain Res 1999; 846:23–29.
788. Hoebel BG, Teitelbaum P. Weight regulation in normal and hypothalamic hyperphagic rats. J Comp Physiol Psychol 1966; 61:189–193.

789. Inoue S. Animal models of obesity: hypothalamic lesion. In: Bjorntorp P, Brodoff BN, eds. Obesity. Philadelphia: J.B. Lippincott, 1992:266–277.
790. Woods SC, Lotter EC, McKay LD, Porte DJ. Chronic intracerebroventricular infusion of insulin reduces food intake and body weight of baboons. Nature 1979; 282:503–505.
791. York DA, Marchington D, Holt SJ, Allars J. Regulation of sympathetic activity in lean and obese Zucker (fa/fa) rats. Am J Physiol 1985; 249:E299–E305.
792. Peterson HR, Rothschild M, Weinberg CR, Fell RD, McLeish KR, Pfeifer MA. Body fat and the activity of the autonomic nervous system. N Engl J Med 1988; 318:1077–1083.
793. Hoebel BG. Brain reward and aversion systems in the control of feeding and sexual behavior. Nebr Symp Motiv 1975; 22:49–112.
794. Antunes VI?, Brailoiu GC, Kwok EH, Scruggs P, Dun NJ. Orexins/hypocretins excite rat sympathetic preganglionic neurons in vivo and in vitro. Am J Physiol Regul Integr Comp Physiol 2001; 281:R1801–R1807.
795. Fulton S, Woodside B, Shizgal P. Modulation of brain reward circuitry by leptin. Science 2000; 287:125–128.
796. Bushnik T, Bielajew C, Konkle AT, Merali Z. Influence of bombesin on threshold for feeding and reward in the rat. Acta Neurobiol Exp (Warsz) 1999; 59:295–302.

14

Experimental Studies on the Control of Food Intake

Henry S. Koopmans

University of Calgary, Calgary, Alberta, Canada

I INTRODUCTION: INTERNAL SIGNALS CONTROL FOOD INTAKE

The amount of food eaten is an essential component of the control of body weight. Food provides the chemical energy required for metabolism and for the storage of nutrients for later use. If the amount of ingested food is inadequate for the body's needs, the animal will burn its endogenous stores of fat and protein and will lose weight. If food is eaten in excess of needs, some of that food will be stored in fat, muscle, and liver for later use. Thus, the proper control of food intake is essential for maintaining a healthy body composition and avoiding obesity.

There is little doubt that daily food intake is controlled by internal signals. If rats are force-fed for a period of time until they become obese, they will reduce their food intake, when allowed to do so, and will bring their body weight back down to normal levels (1). Conversely, when the rat's food intake is restricted for a period of time so that they lose weight and become thin, they will increase their food intake, when they are allowed to do so, and will again bring their body weight up to normal levels. Although several studies clearly show that there are internal mechanisms that will adjust daily food intake following changes in body weight, they do not show how the task is accomplished. During force-feeding and partial starvation there are changes in the degree of stimulation of the gastrointestinal tract, in the internal metabolic pathways of the liver and other organs, in the nutrients present in the blood and transferred to tissue, and in the storage of nutrient in muscle and fat. When force-feeding or starvation stop, any or all of these organs could be responsible for generating an internal signal that brings cumulative food intake and body weight back to normal levels.

Since food intake is a behavior, it must be mediated by the brain. Although many regions of the brain are involved in the control of daily intake, several important studies have shown that two major regions, the paraventricular or ventromedial hypothalamus and the lateral hypothalamus, are critically involved in the control of daily food intake and body weight (2). If lesions are made in the ventromedial hypothalamus or in the paraventricular nucleus, an animal will begin to eat soon after coming out of the anesthesia, will gorge itself for several hours, and will continue overeating for weeks or months until a new level of body weight has been achieved. Thereafter, food intake is stabilized and the new level of body weight will be defended (3). As with normal rats, if these lesioned, obese rats are overfed and forced to reach a new level of body weight, they will voluntarily reduce their daily food intake and bring body weight back to the previous obese levels (see Fig. 1). If they are starved, they will subsequently increase their food intake until they again reach their previous level of obesity. These obese rats are no longer as accurate in their control of food intake: they become finicky, that is, they respond to improved food quality by overeating and to food adulteration by undereating.

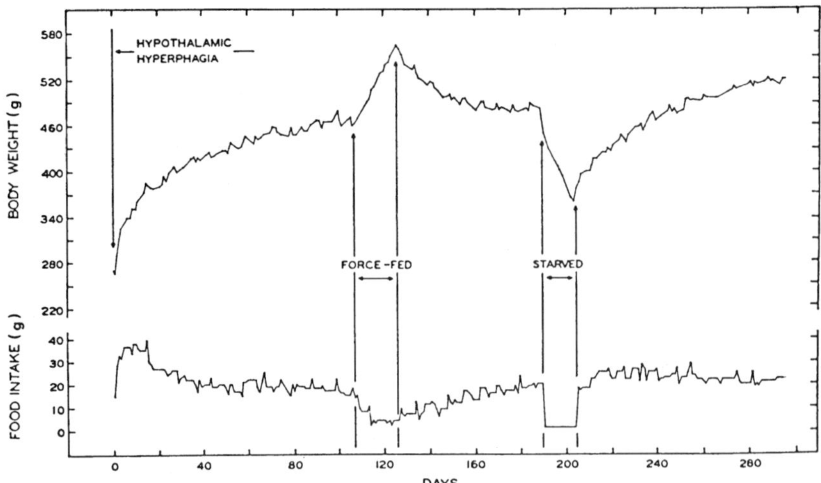

Figure 1 Body weight and food intake of rats given ventromedical hypothalamic lesions, allowed to reach a new level of body weight, and then force-fed or starved. After being force-fed or starved, the rats alter their food intake and bring their body weight back to their new obese level. (From Ref. 3.)

Thus, they are more likely to change their food intake and body weight in response to changes in the quality of their diet than are normal rats. They are also less willing to work for food: if they are required to press a lever several times to get access to food, they will eat less and lose some of their body weight.

Lesions to the lateral hypothalamus cause animals to eat less and lose weight. If the lesions are large, the rats have to be nursed back to health by feeding or intubing liquid diets (4). If the lesions are relatively small, the rats reduce their food intake for a period of time until they have arrived at a lower body weight, and then they eat to maintain that weight. Lesions that limit or inhibit food intake are difficult to interpret since the absence of a behavior can have several causes. The lesion may have damaged a regulatory center and reset body weight at a new lower level. Alternately, the lesion may have destroyed the motor capabilities that underlie feeding or a sensory quality that makes feeding attractive. The possibility that a motor or sensory deficit may result from a lesion can be explored by depriving the rat of food and lowering its body weight before the lesion is performed (5) (see Fig. 2). Rats that are starved before the lesion increase their food intake after the brain

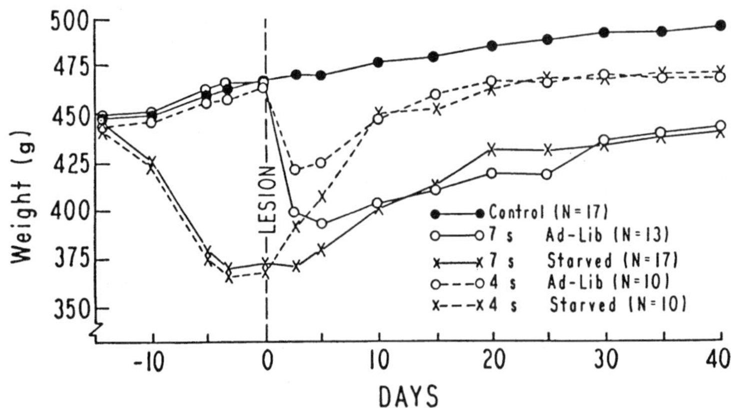

Figure 2 Body weight of rats that were free-fed or starved before being given two different sizes of lesions in the lateral hypothalamus. The rats reach a level of body weight related to the size of the lesion and the starved rats increase their food intake after lesion. (From Ref. 5.)

surgery showing that the lesion did not affect their ability to eat or the attractiveness of food. These deprived rats actually ate more than normal after the surgery and stabilized their body weight at the same lower level as nondeprived rats with the same-size lesion. These studies demonstrate that the lesion acts by changing the set point for body weight. The combination of the results from VMH and LH lesions show that there are two major regions of the brain that respond to internal signals in a way that controls daily food intake. In fact, the internal circuitry regulating food intake is quite complex (6,7). Again, it is important to remember that the relationship of these brain regions to peripheral signals generated in the gut, through metabolism or in storage organs, has not been clarified by these lesion studies. The overfeeding or underfeeding of the rats has affected all of the body's organs and all of the processes involved in digesting, absorbing, transporting, metabolizing, and storing food. It has also altered a large number of endogenous signals.

Internal regulation of food intake is also demonstrated in nature (8). Rodents that hibernate gain weight during the summer and autumn and then gradually lose weight during the winter as their body temperature drops to just above freezing. Bears also gain weight in the autumn and then retire to their dens where they lower body temperature by a few degrees and slowly lose weight. Some birds gain weight twice a year before their biannual migrations and arrive at their destinations with little body fat. Deer and walruses gain weight before mating season and then make little effort to eat and lose weight throughout their courtship period. Some birds and mammals reduce their intake during periods when they are incubating eggs or looking after young. Thus, the signals that control daily intake and the deposition of fat are under internal control and vary with external conditions. However, none of these natural experiments demonstrate which internal changes involved in causing the readily observed changes in food intake and body weight. These internal signals have been shown to be regulatory because birds incubating eggs eat very little of the food fat that is made readily available, and they continue to lose weight until the season is at an end (9). After forced starvation, they will eat more to put themselves back on a standard, predetermined pattern of weight loss.

Other types of external challenges have been shown to cause large changes in daily food intake to limit loss of body weight. When there is a large need for calories, daily food intake can be doubled. Lactating mammals more than double their food intake to provide milk for their young (10). Rats exposed to the cold show large increases in food intake to provide the heat needed to maintain body temperature (11,12).

Internal regulation of food intake can also be demonstrated in pairs of parabiotic rats in which a 30-cm segment of one rat's upper small intestine is disconnected from its own digestive tract and sewn into the intestine of its partner (see Fig. 3). This surgery requires three transections of the small intestines in two rats, but none of the major nerves or blood vessels are cut. As a result of this surgery, one rat in the pair continually loses some of its ingested food into the crossed intestinal segment and into the bloodstream of its partner. The partner, on the other hand, has its own digestive tract shortened by connecting its upper duodenum end-to-end to its lower jejunum. All of the food eaten by the partner is retained in its own gut and is absorbed into its own bloodstream. One consequence of this surgery is that the rat that loses food into its partner's small intestine

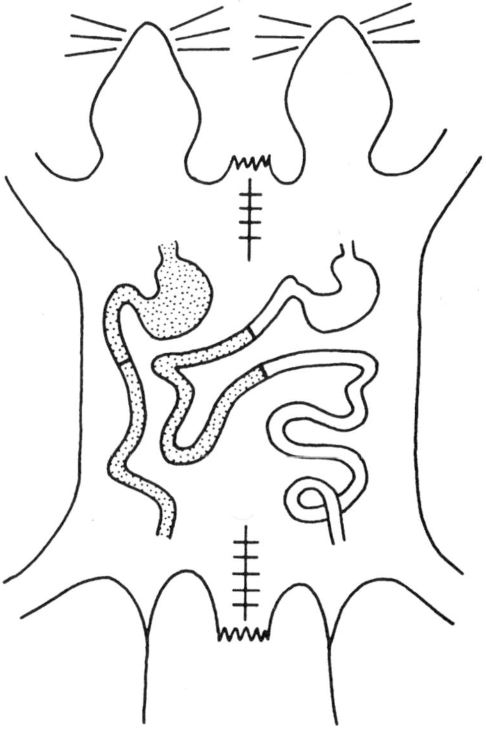

Figure 3 Diagram of a one-way crossed-intestines rat. The stippled gut belongs to the rat on the left. The right rat is continually losing food into the intestine and bloodstream of its partner. No major nerves or blood vessels are cut. (From Ref. 11.)

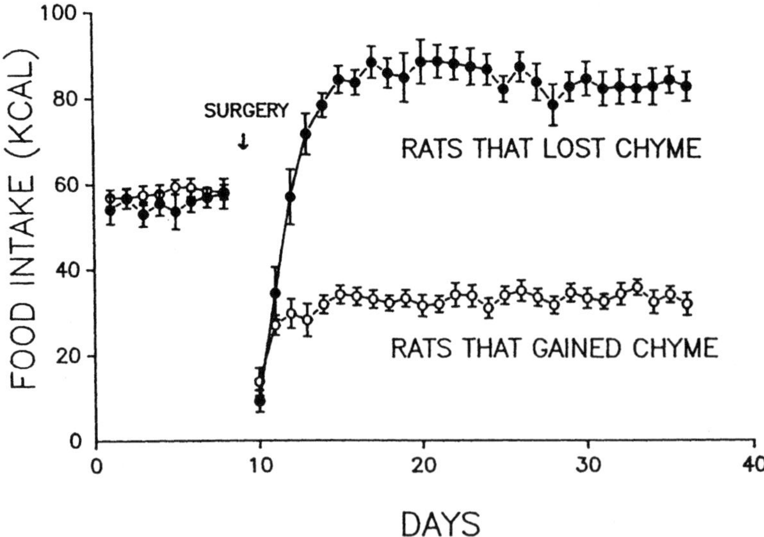

Figure 4 Daily food intake of one-way crossed-intestines rats. The surgery was done on day 9. The rat on the right in Figure 3 that lost food or chyme into the partner's crossed intestinal segment showed a large increase in daily food intake while its partner reduced its daily intake. These large changes in daily food intake are sustained for the rest of the animals' lives.

and bloodstream exhibits a large 50% increase in daily food intake, while its partner reduces its daily food intake by about the same amount (13) (see Fig. 4). The pair as a whole continues to eat the same total quantity of food and to gain weight at the same rate as controls. The threefold difference in daily food intake between the two rats in a crossed-intestines pair is sustained for the rest of these animals' lives. This study clearly shows that daily food intake is internally regulated. The rats show large and sustained changes in daily food intake due to relatively minor surgery. The surgery involves only three transections and reconnections of the small intestines, which in themselves would not cause a sustained change in food intake (14). The altered feeding results from the rerouting of food through the gut, the altered stimulation of the rats' internal organs, and the change in the amount of ingested food that has been absorbed into each animal's bloodstream.

II TYPES OF INTERNAL SIGNALS

The most convenient way to describe the possible internal signals that are involved in the control of food intake is to trace the route that the food moves through the body from the moment when it is first touches the tongue until it is excreted as waste by the kidney or rectum, or is reduced through metabolism to water and carbon dioxide, or is stored in tissues for later use. When an animal becomes hungry, it begins to search for food and often uses strategies that minimize its cost in obtaining the food (15–16). Once food is encountered, it is explored through smell and taste. Once identified, the sensory qualities of the food can be compared to previous experiences, and an estimate can be made of its satiating properties (17). If the food is found to be acceptable, it is ingested and comes into contact with the mucosa of the tongue, where it stimulates taste receptors. At the same time, volatile substances in the food excite odor receptors in the nose. When the food is swallowed, it passes from the mouth through the throat and esophagus into the stomach, and can stimulate various stretch and chemoreceptors in these organs. These neural messages may provide part of a short-term signal for the control of intake during a meal. Some of the food in the stomach passes rapidly as a small bolus into the upper small intestine (18). The presence of food in the intestine inhibits and controls stomach emptying (18–19). Within a few minutes after the beginning of a meal, glucose derived from laboratory chow is absorbed from the gut and is present in the bloodstream (20) (see Fig. 5). This leads to a shift in the release of gut hormones and, once the critically important pancreatic hormone insulin has been released (21), to the transport of some of the

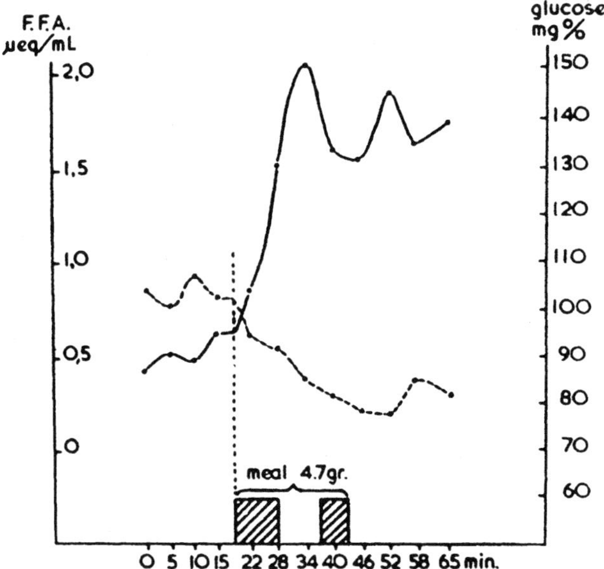

Figure 5 Changes in plasma glucose and free fatty acid levels occur within minutes of the initiation of a laboratory chow meal in 24-hr-food-deprived rats. These changes begin well before the meal has come to an end. (From Ref. 20.)

absorbed nutrient into tissues. Since most of these changes occur within the first few minutes after feeding and since animals usually require 5–30 min to complete a meal, a large number of internal changes provide possible short-term satiety signals. Our major task is to determine which of these signals are needed to cause the termination of a meal. After a meal ends, the ingested nutrients are transferred slowly from the gut to the bloodstream and then to the tissues, where they enter various metabolic pathways and provide energy for the cells. Changes in the rate of nutrient transfer may provide signals that terminate one meal or initiate another, and may control the subsequent meal patterns throughout the day. Excess nutrients are stored mainly in liver, muscle, and fat, and these tissues may provide possible long-term signals that control daily food intake and energy balance.

In short, there are three main types of internal signals that may be involved in the control of food intake. Signals will arise quickly from the gastrointestinal tract due to the stimulation of the mucosa with food and the absorption of nutrients across the gastrointestinal wall. These signals could be involved in the termination of a single meal. Both short-term and medium-term signals can arise from the presence of absorbed nutrients in the bloodstream and their deposition into tissues where they can be used for metabolism or for storage of excess food. Long-term signals that are involved in controlling food intake over several days are more likely to arise from shifts in metabolism and from the storage organs. The relative importance of all of these types of signals for the control of meal and daily food intake is still in considerable dispute. There are a wide range of theories about food intake regulation with some supporting evidence for each possibility, but there are few definitive explanations of the underlying control mechanisms.

III SIGNALS ARISING IN THE GASTROINTESTINAL TRACT—TASTE AND SMELL

The nose and mouth are the first organs to come into contact with food. The neural messages generated by the smell and taste of food are sent to the olfactory bulb or to the brainstem and are relayed up to higher centers of the brain. Taste and smell are usually thought to provide chemical messages for the decision about whether and how much to ingest, but they can become rewards in themselves and lead to overeating and obesity. While stimuli from the gut and from other internal organs are certainly involved in the control of feeding behavior, there is definitely a cognitive component. Animals need to decide when and where to feed and to remember their past encounters with food. The particular flavors and textures can then be used to guide feeding behavior. Collier and his collaborators have been the major contributors to laboratory studies that examine the decisions that are made about the cost requirements of finding food and ingesting it. They have shown that increasing the cost of obtaining food by increasing the number of lever presses needed to gain access to a food source leads to a decision to reduce the number of meals each day (22) (see Fig. 6). While meal number goes down, the size of the average meal increases so that total daily food intake is held fairly constant (22,23). If the tasks become very complex or require too much effort, the animal may choose to eat somewhat less than its normal daily portion and, thereby, trade off the amount of effort in obtaining food against its level of body weight. Daily food intake may decrease to 80–90% of its previous level. Collier has argued that there is too much emphasis upon a depletion-repletion model of the control of food intake (24). He notes that changes in external requirements cause large changes in meal patterns, but not in daily intake. He questions whether there are fixed internal

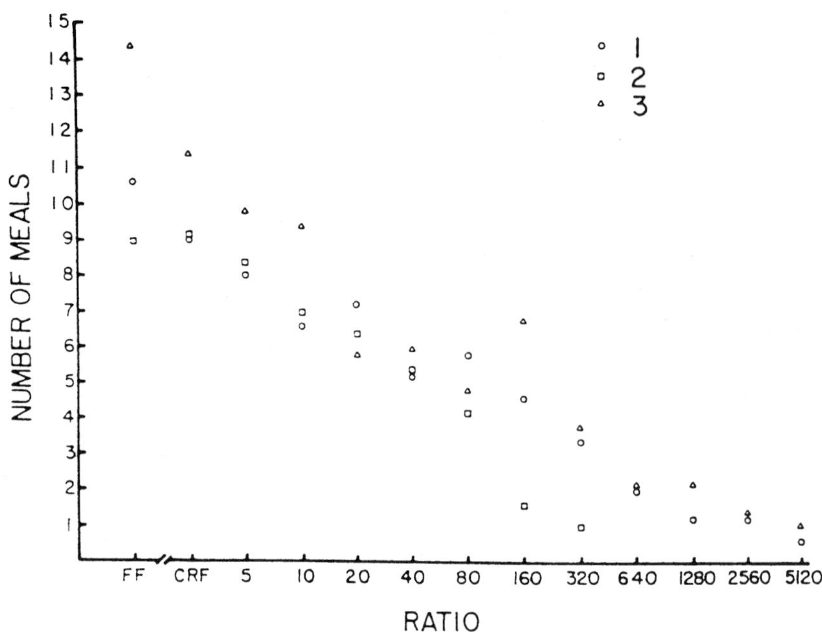

Figure 6 Number of daily meals taken by each of three rats (1, 2, 3) when they are free-feeding (FF) or when they have to press one (CRF) or more times to gain access to food. As the lever-pressing requirement increases, the rats take fewer but larger meals. They maintain their normal level of daily food intake until they reach the highest levels of bar pressing, when they reduce daily intake a little. (From Ref. 22.)

signals controlling meal intake and believes that the choice of meal size has a large cognitive component. The counterargument is that a hungry animal with free access to food will eat much more food when the food is removed at the same time from the esophagus, stomach, or intestine (13,25). Some internal signals from the gastrointestinal tract or elsewhere in the body must be involved in terminating a meal. Thus, the amount eaten may depend on cognitive estimates of the food's calorie value and availability as well as on tentative satiety signals generated in the gastrointestinal tract or beyond. The cognitive component would be influenced or conditioned by subsequent information generated by the metabolism and storage of absorbed nutrients. The cognitive component would have to be controlled by some unconditioned stimulus which, in the case of food intake, is probably the same signal that controls the amount of food eaten.

IV ESOPHAGEAL AND GASTRIC FISTULI

Once a decision has been made to swallow food, it passes down through the throat and esophagus to the stomach. The early physiologists, Bernard and Pavlov, did experiments using an esophageal fistula that allowed food that was eaten to pass out of the body before it could reach the stomach. They were trying to determine whether internal signals led to the termination of feeding behavior. They discovered that dogs and horses with esophageal fistuli greatly overate (26). These experiments have been replicated on other types of animals in more recent times and have been given clearer definition. Hull et al. (27) did an experiment on a single dog and showed that on the first and second sham feeding session, the dog greatly overate. Their 10-kg dog ate nearly its body weight in food before pausing for 5 min. This group also showed that the dog was gradually able to realize that it was losing the ingested food (sham-feeding) during the experimental test and, by the eighth day, the dog refused to eat in the experimental cage. However, when returned to its home cage and offered food, the dog sham-fed, showing that there was a cognitive component the dog's previous cessation of sham-feeding behavior. This result of excessive feeding after an esophageal fistula was confirmed by Janowitz and Grossman, who found that dogs sham fed four to five times their normal intake (28).

The sham-feeding paradigm has also been demonstrated in rats. Mook created an esophageal fistula in rats and fed them glucose, sucrose, and saline solutions (29). He found that when the nutrients were prevented from reaching the stomach, intake was greatly increased in a 1-hr test. In addition, the rats showed a preference for higher concentrations of the ingested solution. After doing a gastric fistula in rats, Smith et al. (30) found that the rats continued feeding for more than 2 hr. A rat with an open gastric fistula will eat at a normal rate for 15–20 min and, thereafter, will continue to feed over the next 100 min at a rate that is about half its previous rate (see Fig. 7). The fact that the well-trained rat continues to feed suggests that distension or chemical cues arising in the stomach, in the small intestine, or beyond are important for the inhibition of intake during a single meal. The decrease in the rate of food intake after 20 min shows that mucosal stimulation inhibits the rat's avid desire for food or that the animal tires of the motor movements involved in feeding.

There are advantages and disadvantages to the use of either esophageal or gastric fistuli. With an esophageal fistula, the esophagus is transected, usually in the neck, and both ends of the esophagus are externalized, or, alternatively, the end leading to the stomach is closed and a gastric tube is inserted. Thus, the food eaten by the animal as well as its salivary secretions pass entirely out of the animal and do not reach the stomach or intestine. Sufficient food and water can be given to the animal by putting the food into the externalized lower esophagus or through the gastric tube. The major advantage of the esophageal fistula is that one can be certain that only the mucosa of the mouth, throat, and upper esophagus is stimulated by food: none of the food can stimulate the wall of the stomach or pass into the intestine and be digested and absorbed.

The main drawbacks of the esophageal fistula preparation is that the feeding procedure is often quite messy, the animal must be fed by tube, and the fluid and electrolyte content of the saliva must be appropriately replaced. If replacement is inadequate, then subsequent intake may be affected by deficits that the animal cannot correct for itself. The gastric fistula does not suffer from these difficulties because most of the time the fistula is closed and food moves through the digestive tract in its normal fashion. Only at the time of the experiment is the fistula opened, the stomach flushed, and the experiment begun. If the animal is fed a liquid diet, most of the food will drain out of the gastric cannula, preventing the distension of the stomach and the associated neural or hormonal signals. However, two studies have shown that some of the nutrient ingested is emptied through the pylorus into the intestine and is absorbed into the bloodstream (31,32). Thus, the weakness of the gastric fistula is that the stomach and the rest of the gut will receive some stimulation of the mucosa by food which makes the results more difficult to interpret. Of course,

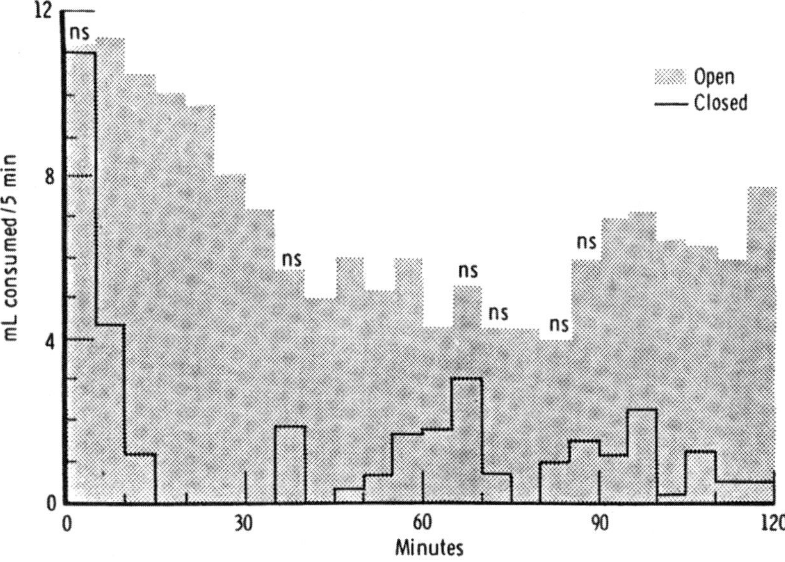

Figure 7 Food intake of rats that have a gastric fistula that is either open or closed. When the fistula is closed, a 17-hr-deprived rat will complete its meal in 15 min and then take a few small meals in the next 2 hr. When the fistula is open and the food drains out of the body, the rat will continue to feed throughout the 2-hr period. (From Ref. 30.)

the bulk of the food has been lost through the fistula, and the intensity of downstream signals is greatly reduced. The use of both the esophageal and the gastric fistula leads to considerable overfeeding, called sham-feeding. The sham-feeding animal receives taste stimuli but little or no postingestive stimuli. Sham feeding will continue well beyond the usual time when feeding ceases in an intact animal.

All of the experiments agree that signals arising from stimulation of the mucosal lining of the mouth, throat and esophagus by food are not enough to stop feeding behavior. Some additional signals must arise at the level of the stomach or the small intestine to inhibit intake during a single meal. These results are entirely consistent with the results from the crossed-intestines rats mentioned above (13). After the intestinal surgery (see Fig. 3), these rats exhibit a threefold difference in daily food intake. Since all of the food necessarily passes through the mouth, throat, and esophagus, these upper gut organs are stimulated three times as much in one rat as in its partner. If stimulation of these organs were the main signals controlling daily food intake, then the large differences in food intake would not have been seen in these rats. The large, long-term differences in food intake of these one-way crossed intestines rats show that these mucosal signals can play only a minor regulatory role in the control of daily food intake.

V SIGNALS ARISING IN THE STOMACH

The stomach has been thought to be a storage site for food and an inhibitor of food intake since the ancient Greeks understood the anatomy of the gastrointestinal tract (33). In man and large animals, the bulk of the meal eaten over a relatively short period of time remains in the stomach for more than an hour. After a short period of adjustment following the beginning of a meal, the rate of gastric emptying becomes steady, and a fixed number of calories is delivered to the small intestine per unit time (18,34,35). Because the bulk of the ingested food stays in the stomach after a meal, gastric distension is one obvious mechanism for the short-term inhibition of food intake. An assessment of the total amount of food eaten during a meal would appear to depend to a large extent upon two types of signals: (1) the degree of distension of the stomach, and (2) the activation of chemoreceptors in the gastric or intestinal wall.

Distension can not be the only signal involved in the regulation of food intake. Animals will increase their food intake when nonnutritive diluents are added to the diet. Adolph found that rats will adjust their food intake to compensate when the amount of dilution was not too large (36). At higher concentrations of diluents, the rats compromised by reducing intake. Janowitz and Grossman showed a less complete and gradual adjustment to the addition of diluents in the food of dogs and cats (37). A recent study using a liquid fiber that gels in the stomach found diminished reports of hunger in human subjects, but food intake was only slightly reduced and then only after a delay of several hours (38). Thus, gastric distension by itself, without activation of chemoreceptors, is not a major regulator of food intake. The determination of the nutritive characteristics of the food is also essential.

Davis and Campbell (25) did studies that focussed on the role of the stomach in the inhibition of food intake. They placed a tube in the stomach of 4-hr food-deprived rats fed a liquid milk or elemental diet and then withdrew the food during the time when the rats were feeding or at various times after the meal was complete. They found that on the first day of continual withdrawal of diet and sham-feeding, the rats nearly doubled their 30-min intake. Some food must have remained in the stomach to allow continued removal of the liquid diet by suction, and some may have emptied into the duodenum. On subsequent days, their intake increased even further until the rats ate four to five times their usual amount of liquid food in a 30-min period. In a second experiment, the rats ate about 17 mL of an attractive liquid diet, sweetened condensed milk. When 8–10 mL of their stomach contents were withdrawn at 10, 30, or 50 min after the meal, the rats responded by eating a nearly equivalent amount of food, which showed that the rats noticed the withdrawal of food and compensated for it by eating more. There are two difficulties with this experiment. Even though the rats were only 4 hr deprived, they ate 17 mL of this attractive, high-energy diet: an amount that should either match or exceed stomach capacity. Perhaps the animals were eating to reach full distension and they were not concerned about the number of calories ingested. Furthermore, some of the ingested food would have moved into the duodenum, making it impossible to conclude that the signals that inhibited food intake arose solely in the stomach. There may have been an added intestinal component. Nevertheless, these experiments did point to gastric distension as having an important role in the inhibition of a single meal.

Deutsch et al. (39) extended and clarified these studies through the use of a pyloric cuff which was intended to prevent the food from leaving the stomach. In addition, they added a gastric tube that could drain stomach contents so that the level of gastric pressure would not exceed the normal level after a meal. They fed 12-hr-deprived rats a milk meal while measuring gastric pressure with a water manometer. The rats drank 13.6 mL with the pyloric cuff open and 11.5 mL with the cuff closed. These values were not significantly different and showed that the rats stopped feeding on the basis of gastric distension and chemoreception and did not appear to require stimulation of the duodenum with food. However, the rats drank to stomach capacity, which was demonstrated in overflow experiments to be ~13.6 mL. Thus, it was not clear whether the intake was regulatory for calories eaten or was inhibited by the limits of gastric distension. In a subsequent study, Deutsch and his associates showed rats could eat smaller meals of a liquid diet without noticing the surreptitious delivery of saline into the stomach (40). This study showed that the calories present in the stomach were somehow sensed by the animal. Deutsch (41) claimed that there were nutrient receptors embedded in the wall of the stomach, which would become exposed to the lumenal contents as the gastric volume increased. The combination of gastric distension and the caloric concentration, as determined by exposure to the "nutrient receptors," would provide information to the brain to inhibit feeding behavior.

One difficulty with the Deutsch theory is that it pays little attention to the anatomy of the stomach when describing the hypothetical nutrient receptors. Neural receptors are not likely to be present in the lumen of the stomach or in the lumen of the gastric glands or pits. First of all, the gastric contents are highly corrosive and nerve terminals would be readily destroyed. Moreover, there is a constant turnover of mucosal cells throughout the digestive tract, and these rapidly dividing cells migrate continuously along the basement membrane. They would override nerve terminals that might be aimed toward the lumen. Furthermore, there have been no descriptions of nerve terminals beyond the lamina propria, the support tissue for the gastric mucosa. Thus, nerves would be able to sense the presence of food in the gastric lumen only if the food was absorbed into the wall of the stomach. Relatively little nutrient is absorbed through the gastric mucosa (42). It remains possible that the food could release gastric hormones from cells that have villus tufts projecting into the gastric lumen and that these hormones would stimulate vagal afferents (see below).

Recently, Kaplan et al. (43,44) have challenged the interpretation of the pyloric cuff experiments. They confirm that rats eat the same amount of food whether a pyloric cuff is open or closed, which is the fundamental observation in previous studies (31,39,45). However, they have shown that during the first meal of a food-deprived rat there is a rapid emptying of the stomach that may be as much as 25–40% of the meal (46). When they measure the amount of nutrient in the stomach after a meal with the cuff either open or closed, they find that the gastric contents were 30% greater in the rat with the cuff closed. They conclude that although the rats with a closed cuff eat the same amount of food as rats with an open cuff, they require a larger gastric distension signal to terminate a meal. In short, they believe that the amount of food in the gastrointestinal tract, not just the amount of food in the stomach, controls short-term food intake.

Phillips and Powley (47) looked more closely at whether gastric volume or nutrient sensing occurred in rats with pyloric cuffs. They found that when the cuffs were closed, the rats showed an equivalent reduction of food intake when 5 mL of either saline or 10%, 20%, or 40% glucose was delivered to the stomach before injections. Furthermore, it did not matter whether the infused substance was 40% glucose, fructose, or sucrose with different chemical structures, metabolic pathways, and caloric values. However, when the cuffs were open, the nutritional content of these sugars as well as of the more balanced liquid diet, Isocal, did inhibit food intake. They conclude that gastric distension inhibits food intake, not gastric nutrient sensing, while ingested nutrients work at the level of the intestine to inhibit gastric emptying and to limit food intake.

The role of the stomach in the inhibition of food intake has to be affected by the rate of stomach emptying. As food empties, there is less food in the stomach and less gastric distension. McHugh and Moran have done a series of experiments on gastric emptying in rats and monkeys (48–50). They have found that saline empties rapidly in an exponential way from the stomach. On the other hand, nutrients empty rapidly from the stomach for the first 4–5 min, but, thereafter, the presence of nutrient in the small intestine slows down the emptying rate to a steady state until the meal is gone. A fixed number of calories empty from the stomach per unit time regardless of the composition of the food placed in the stomach (34,48). They argue that the intestine inhibits stomach emptying and that distension of the stomach inhibits food intake. Both stomach and intestinal signals are important.

Although there is general agreement that the stomach provides part of the signal that inhibits food intake during a single meal, we still do not know the nature of the signal or how it is transmitted to the brain. Nerves are the most likely route of transmission. The information about the degree of gastric distension or the presence of nutrients in the gastrointestinal walls could be transmitted to the brain through either nerves or hormones. Paintal (51) and Iggo (52) have shown that there are vagal stretch receptors in the stomach. These nerves increase their discharge rate as a linear function of the degree of gastric distension (see Fig. 8).

In a recent review paper, Phillips and Powley (53) describe two distinctly different types of afferent receptors in the stomach wall. One type has characteristics of an "in-series" tension receptor, and the other appears to be a stretch receptor. While the current electrophysiological evidence does not establish the presence of more than one receptor type, the nerve cell anatomy strongly supports the conclusion that there are two types of receptors. In another paper, Powley has suggested that one sensor might respond to small changes in gastric volume, while the other would respond as a stretch receptor responding to large, sustained changes in gastric contents (54). Gonzalez and Deutsch have argued that vagotomy eliminates the satiety signals that results from gastric distension after a very large meal, but that gastric nutrient content of the stomach can still be sensed (55–56).

A study in which the stomach and upper intestine was transplanted from one inbred rat into another suggests that an unidentified gastric hormone may inhibit food intake (57). Four rats given multiple feeding tests showed a compensatory reduction of food intake when food was infused at the standard feeding rate into the completely denervated and supplementary stomach and upper small intestine. At the time of the feeding test, the rats' natural digetive tract was intact, empty, and normally innervated. Recently, two new peptides have been discovered in the stomach—ghrelin (58) and leptin (59). Both peptides affect food intake when given centrally (7) and may play some role in the peripheral inhibition of food intake. Ghrelin is a peptide of 28 amino acids that is a growth hormone secretagogue and is quite distinct from growth hormone–releasing hormone (GHRH) (58). Its sequence differs between rat and human by only 2 amino acids, which indicates a highly conserved structure during evolution. Its highest concentration is in the stomach, where it is found in X/A-like endocrine cells in the oxyntic mucosa (60). These cells do not make contact with the lumen of the glands (61). Serum concentrations of ghrelin are increased by fasting and reduced by refeeding (62,63), suggesting that the presence of food in the stomach may inhibit ghrelin release. Ghrelin is also found in a few cells in the arcuate nucleus of the hypothalamus and the upper small intestine. Intracranial injection of ghrelin stimulates food intake, gastric acid secretion and releases growth hormone

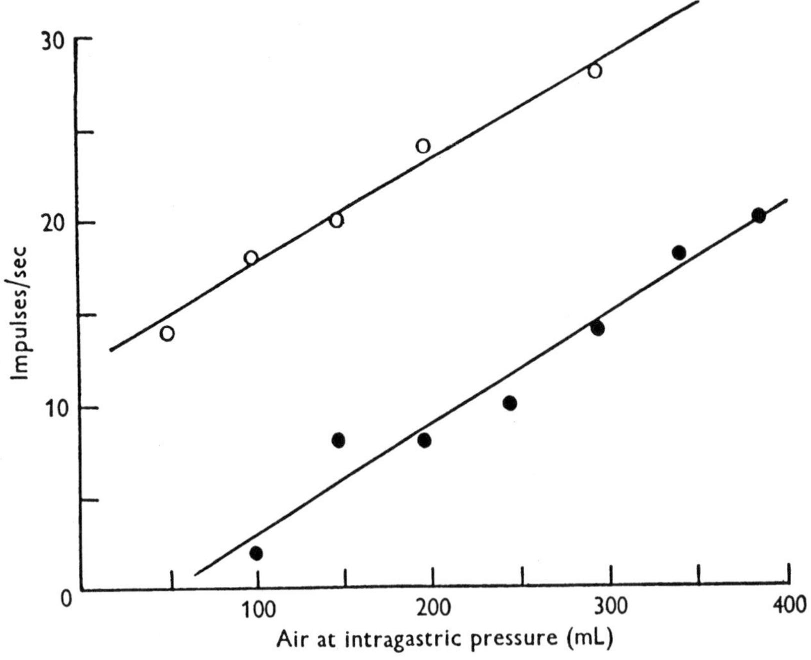

Figure 8 Rate at which single fibers isolated from the vagus nerve of a cat fire as the amount of air in an intragastric balloon is increased to the designated volume. (From Ref. 51.)

(64,65). It is possible that increasing secretion of ghrelin during fasting induces food intake and that its decreased release after feeding augments the feeling of satiety generated by other gastric and intestinal signals.

Leptin is a peptide discovered by cloning the defective gene in ob/ob mice (66). It is a secretion product of adipocytes (see section on Storage Signals) and is known to inhibit food intake and increase energy expenditure when given intraperitoneally or intraventricularly (67,69). It is also present in the gastric mucosa (59,69) and is released into the bloodstream. It appears to be present in both the chief cells which make contact with the gastric lumen and secrete pepsinogen as well as in a specialized endocrine cell, called a P-cell. Leptin is secreted into the gastric lamina propria from which it is absorbed into the bloodstream (70,71). Its plasma levels have a circadian rhythm with low levels during the day and high levels at night (63,72). Leptin levels appear to fall just after a meal and then rise gradually as the meal is digested and absorbed. The diurnal pattern is quite similar to that of ghrelin (63) with smaller changes for leptin just before and after meals. Leptin receptors have recently been found on the afferent and efferent terminals of the vagus nerve (73,74). Since IV leptin inhibits and IV ghrelin stimulates food intake, it is possible that their modulated release from the stomach might fine-tune the changes in food intake during meals.

While hormones and nerves may provide gastric signals that alter meal intake, it is unlikely that changes in intragastric pressure are major determinants of satiety since the relaxation reflex prevents an increase in pressure beyond a fixed level (75,76). However, increases in abdominal pressure may inhibit meal intake, as shown in one human study (77). Since there is relatively little absorption of food from the stomach (42), a gastric signal is unlikely to be an absorbed nutrient, but could be neural or hormonal.

There are at least two limitations to a gastric theory of the control of food intake. It is well known that most animals have a circadian rhythm of feeding behavior with meals occurring at times that are appropriate for the animals' nocturnal or diurnal orientation. Rats eat heavily during the early dark phase (78). As implied above, if food empties from the stomach at a fixed caloric rate, then repeated bouts of food intake during the early part of the dark phase should greatly distend the stomach. New meals would have to initiated while the stomach remains relatively full.

This prediction has recently been confirmed using a noninvasive technique for measuring gastric filling and emptying over a period of several hours. Van der Velde and Koopmans (79) added a radioactive tracer, technetium 99m sulfur colloid, to a standard liquid diet and were able to view three regions of interest within the rat's body every 2 min using a gamma camera. The regions were the stomach, measuring gastric nutrient filling or, indirectly, distension; the intestines, measuring gastric emptying; and the total rat, measuring cumulative food intake. They found that the rats ate five or six meals over 6.5 hr. Four meals were analyzed in detail: the first and second meal after a 7-hr fast, a meal just after the middle of the 6.5-hr period, and the last meal eaten. All meals were of approximately the same size. In accordance with Kaplan et al. and others (46,80), they found that the gastric contents emptied during feeding at more than three times the average rate and that ~25% of the ingested food emptied from the stomach during the meal. This was true not just of the first meal but of all meals analyzed over 6.5 hr. In the 10 min following a meal, there was a significant reduction of emptying rate as intestinal signals kicked in. One of their most interesting findings was that rats initiated new meals at times when the stomach was still quite full and, therefore, inhibition of food intake required even greater distension of the stomach for later meals. In the later part of the 6.5-hr feeding session, the rats initiated meals when gastric nutrient filling was greater than it was at the termination of the first meal. Thus, the degree of gastric distension necessary to provide an inhibitory signal for feeding behavior has to vary throughout the day. Most of the experiments on stomach emptying have been done on deprived rats, dogs, pigs, or monkeys at a fixed time of day. This procedure would tend to show that food intake is inhibited by gastric distension while studies done over 24 hr show that the degree of gastric distension necessary to inhibit food intake depends on the time of day. These new results using a gamma camera in conscious, free-feeding rats undoubtedly complicate the theory that gastric distension is a major inhibitor of food intake and shift attention toward the brain as an interpreter of the importance of gastric distension relative to time of day.

Another limitation of a gastric theory can be seen from the results of the one-way crossed-intestines study previously described (see Fig. 3). Following the surgery, one rat in the pair eats three times as much as its partner and this change persists for the rest of the animals' lives. This means that three times the amount of food passes through the stomach of the rat that eats more relative to its partner that eats less. If the stretch or nutrient receptors in the mucosa or in the muscular wall of the stomach were sensing the total calorie value of the food passing through the stomach and using this information to control daily food intake, then the food intake of these rats would not change after the surgery. Instead, the food-losing rat would lose weight while its partner would gain weight. Since daily food intake did change dramatically and body weight changed only a little, the stomach must not have a way of sensing the total amount of food passing through it. However, gastric distension could retain its importance in the control of food intake if there were changes in the rate of stomach emptying in these rats. If, for example, there were a threefold difference in the rate of gastric emptying for the two rats in a pair (matching the observed difference in food intake), then the degree of distension and chemical stimulation of the two rats' stomachs might remain the same. Preliminary data suggest that there are large changes in the rate of gastric emptying in these rats and, thus, gastric signals may still be partially responsible for the control of daily intake. However, the intestinal mechanisms involved in the control of gastric emptying would become important regulators of daily food intake.

The results of the crossed-intestines study show that the ultimate control of daily food intake must occur at the level of the small intestine or beyond. It is not yet clear whether intestinal or metabolic signals influence food intake by controlling stomach emptying or by some other response to the absorbed food. Neural or hormonal signals generated in the small intestine may act directly on the brain to inhibit food intake, or they may act indirectly on food intake, by changing the rate of gastric emptying. These neural or hormonal satiety signals would be generated as the food comes into contact with or is transported into the absorptive cells of the intestinal mucosa or as the absorbed nutrients or released hormones come into contact with the nerves that terminate in the wall (lamina propria) of the small intestine (54).

VI SIGNALS ARISING IN THE INTESTINE

The studies cited above indicate that gastric distension is an important short-term signal that inhibits food intake. However, it is possible that other signals are involved in the termination of a meal. Messages arising in the intestine or in other organs may also be involved in generating satiety signals. Some early studies have shown that the intestine can be a source of signals for the inhibition of food intake (81,82). These investigators found that the delivery of hyperosmotic nutritive and nonnutritive solutions to the duodenum reduced meal size in the rat. One interpretation of the results of these early infusion experiments is that the intestine is a source of satiety signals during a meal. Another interpretation is that the infusions cause some discomfort or intensify signals in an abnormal way.

Many of the recent studies of intestinal satiety have used the paradigm of the sham-feeding rat. A gastric fistula is implanted into the animal and it is opened during the feeding test. At various times before or after feeding, an infusion of glucose or some other nutrient is made into the duodenum. One rat study found that infusing 2.25 kcal of an elemental liquid diet over 6 min into the duodenum reduced sham-feeding most effectively when the infusion began 12 min after the rat began eating (83). This delay may correspond to the time when a rat normally begins to end a feeding bout. Oddly enough, the same substantial infusion of the diet 6–12 min into the duodenum before the rat began sham-feeding had no effect on its feeding behavior. This result suggests that the intestinal signal is quite transient and that oral, gastric, and intestinal signals must occur at the same time for feeding to be inhibited.

Most of the intestinal satiety studies have been done in rats and monkeys. In one rat study, Liebling et al. (84) infused a liquid diet with a caloric value of .375 kcal/mL directly into the doudenum of rats. They found a small reduction in sham feeding when 3 mL was infused over 3 min and a larger reduction when 6 mL was infused over 6 min. This rate of infusion is double the normal rate of nutrient delivery to the intestine. In a similar study in rhesus monkeys, 20, 40, and 60 mL of a liquid diet containing 1 kcal/mL was delivered into the duodenum at a rate of 5 or 7.5 mL/min (85). The 20-mL infusion produced a small significant inhibition of sham feeding, which increased with increasing doses. In most of these sham-feeding studies, feeding continues throughout the test period in part because gastric distension is not available as a signal to inhibit food intake.

Most of these studies suggest that there is an intestinal signal that inhibits food intake. Such a satiety signal could be transmitted to the brain through the peripheral nerves. Several investigators have recorded from the vagus and from mesenteric nerves. They have found that there is an increased firing rate when glucose or amino acids are placed in the lumen of the intestine (86–89). Other studies have shown that vagotomy prevents the reduced food intake caused by intestinal infusions (82,90). In recent years, Yox et al. have continued the exploration of the way in which intestinal satiety is communicated to the brain. They used an infusion rate that they determined was the equivalent of the gastric emptying rate of their rats.

The infusion of 10 cc of maltose or oleic acid at a rate of 0.13 kcal/min reduces food intake while octanoic acid and casein hydrolysate has minimal effects. The effects of maltose and oleic acid on sham-feeding can be blocked by capsaicin treatment or by vagotomy (91,92), which again shows that the intestinal signal may travel through the vagal afferents to diminish food intake.

In a very interesting study, McHugh and Moran (93) allowed monkeys to drink 150 mL of a 1 kcal/mL glucose solution and found that 21.6 mL passed into the duodenum in the first 5 min. Then, they infused the 21.6 mL into the intestine of fasted monkeys over 3–5 min and observed their feeding behavior for the next 4 hr. The monkeys with glucose infused directly into their intestine showed a substantially reduced food intake during the first hour compared to monkeys that had delivered the same amount of glucose into their own intestine through normal gastric emptying. Only after 3–4 hr did their food intake return to the same levels as the controls. Thus, the delivery of an appropriate amount of glucose directly into the intestine, but in a less than physiological way, caused an extra large suppression of food intake. The authors conclude that an intestinal infusion, without the stimuli associated with the taste and swallowing of food and without gastric distension, may have reduced food intake in an abnormal way. They question whether the infusion of nutrients into the intestine produces a normal satiety. If the delivery of food to the intestine makes the animal feel discomfort or malaise, then the reduction of food intake cannot be accurately ascribed to internal mechanisms that normally produce satiety.

What would be a physiological mode and rate of delivery of food into the small intestine? It is obvious that food normally arrives in the intestine after it has been mixed with saliva and partially digested by acid and digestive enzymes in the stomach. The release of food from the stomach is periodic and results from a pressure differential between the gastric antrum and the duodenal bulb (76). A small spurt of food is delivered into the upper doudenum at the end of some of the gastric contractions depending on local pressure levels. This food is then distributed along the upper small intestine by repeated constrictions of the intestinal circular muscles, which mix the chyme rapidly with bicarbonate and digestive enzymes secreted from the pancreas and with bile secreted from the liver and gallbladder. Thus, under normal physiological conditions, the food is already partially processed before it reaches the duodenum, and then it is immediately mixed with the current intestinal contents. The food must arrive at the duodenal bulb in a predigested state for delivery to be considered normal. Complex foods such as plant or animal tissues would be most changed by the digestive process while simplified foods, such as pure sugar or amino acid solutions, would change little. These latter simple foods are most often used in experiments but they rarely occur in nature and are even limited in the kitchen cupboard. Most importantly, the food must be delivered at a rate that is within the normal physiological range. That rate can be estimated by examining the total food intake of a rat or any other animal during a 24-hr period. Adult rats eat between 60 and 100 kcal/d depending upon the strain and the physical conditions of the experiment. If this amount of food were delivered to the duodenum at a constant rate throughout the day, then 0.04–0.07 kcal would arrive per minute. As discussed above, the rate of gastric emptying increases during a meal to a level that is three to four times the average rate between meals and then slows to about half the normal rate in the 10 min after the meal ceases. A reasonable estimate of the rate of delivery of food to the small intestines of the rat is 0.14–0.25 kcal/min during a meal and 0.02–0.04 kcal/min in the 10 min thereafter. Deliveries of liquid food to the small intestine at a much higher rate are common in the feeding behavior literature.

An important test of the value of an food intake experiment is whether the delivery of food to the intestine has approximated physiological conditions. Many studies in the literature deliver food at a rate that goes beyond normal physiological limits and, in almost all studies, the infused food has not been processed by the digestive tract. The study that comes closest to using physiological procedures to assess the importance of intestinal satiety has been done with crossed-intestines rats (94). These rats are parabiotic pairs that have a further intestinal surgery in which a 30-cm segment of lower duodenum or upper jejunum is isolated from the small intestine of each rat in the pair and then surgically connected to the intestine of its partner (see Fig. 9). After the surgery is complete, the food eaten by each rat in the pair arrives in the rat's own stomach, travels through a 5-cm segment of upper duodenum that includes the entrance of the common bile and pancreatic duct and then passes into the 30-cm crossed segment of its partner. Thus, the food ingested by these rats has been mixed with saliva and gastric secretions before entering the small intestine, where it is also mixed with pancreatic and hepatic secretions before it crosses into the intestinal segment of its partner. Some of this food is digested and absorbed in the partner's upper small intestine, and then the remaining food passes back into

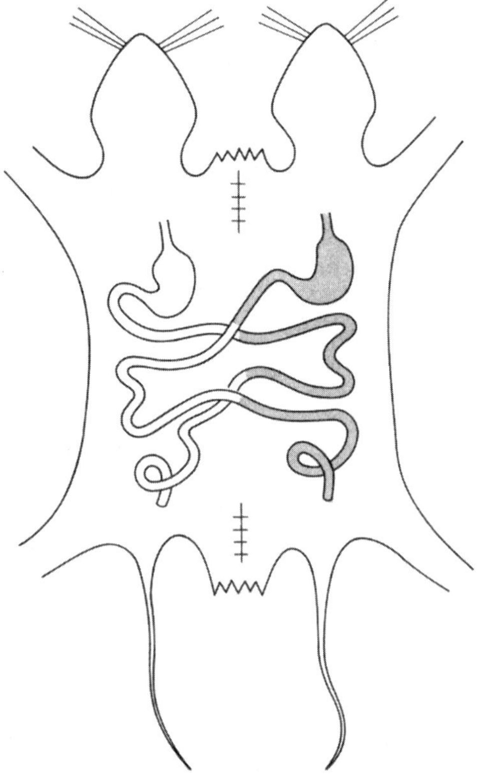

Figure 9 Diagram of two-way crossed-intestines rats. A 30-cm segment of lower duodenum and upper jejunum is isolated from the gastrointestinal (GI) tract of each rat and is connected to the intestine of its partner. The preparation is symmetrical. Each rat loses food into the upper small intestine of its partner, and some of that food returns to its own lower jejunum. The stippled GI tract belongs to the rat on the right.

the lower jejunum of the rat that fed and travels down along the rest of the length of that rat's small intestine and lower gut. The surgery is symmetrical, so that each rat loses some of the food that it eats into the upper small intestine of its partner.

The short-term experiment testing the role of the intestine in the termination of a meal, is done by feeding one rat in the pair 10 or 30 min before the partner and then measuring the partner's intake after the crossed segment has been stimulated by food. A rat will normally complete its first meal after a 7-hr fast in 6–8 min. The results of several experiments show that the food intake of both rats is not affected by having a delay of 10 or 30 min (94). The rat allowed to feed first does not overeat even through its own lower duodenum and upper jejunum have not come into contact with ingested food. The unfed partner does not reduce its food intake when allowed to eat even through the ingested food of the feeding rat can definitively be shown to be present in the crossed segment and some of it has been absorbed into the bloodstream within minutes after the beginning of the first rat's meal. Thus, endogenous signals arising in a 30-cm segment of the small intestine do not alter food intake during a meal after a 7-hr fast, especially when the food has been processed by the gut in a highly physiological way.

The major limitation of the crossed intestines experiment is that the 30-cm crossed segment is only part of the normal length of the rat's small intestine, which has a total length of 100–110 cm. Of course, the top third of the small intestine sees the ingested food more rapidly and is a major site for the absorption of nutrients (95). Nevertheless, it could be argued that it is necessary to stimulate a longer length of intestine to show "intestinal satiety." On the other hand, the experiment is exceptional in its physiological delivery of food into this critical upper intestinal segment. The food has been processed through the mouth, stomach, and upper duodenum and has been mixed with digestive enzymes and other salivary, gastric, pancreatic, and intestinal secretions. Experiments have shown that the rate of gastric emptying is slightly higher during the first 10 min after a meal in the crossed-intestines rats than in control parabiotic pairs (94). Thus, feeding one rat in the pair should have delivered slightly more food than is normal to the crossed segment of the partner. Still, there was no effect on the partner's food intake when measured at 10 or 30 min. Measurements were made of the rate of absorption of radioactive glucose and amino acid that were added to the diet, and it was found that at 10 min there was significantly more radiolabel in the bloodstream of the unfed and hungry rat than in the bloodstream of the fed and satiated rat (94). The conclusion from this experiment is that the combined signals arising in the 30-cm crossed-intestinal segment, including neural, hormonal, and metabolic signals, were insufficient to inhibit short-term food intake. Since the upper small intestine is a major site for the absorption of ingested food, these results suggest that the upper intestine may not generate signals that inhibit food intake. If intestinal signals are normally involved in the control of food intake during a meal, then it is also puzzling that a free-feeding crossed-intestines rat that lacks signals arising in its own 30-cm crossed-intestinal segment does not overeat, since "satiety" signals are missing in this animal.

The reader might be confused by the seemingly contradictory conclusions drawn between the results from the above study (94) (see Fig. 9) and from the one-way crossed-intestines experiment (13) (see Fig. 3) in which there was a large change in the daily food intake of both partners in a parabiotic pair when one rat continuously lost food into the crossed segment of its partner. It is important to note that the study described in this section used a symmetrical surgical preparation and was designed to investigate changes in short-term food intake, while the second study (Fig. 3) was designed to investigate changes in daily food intake due to the continuous loss of calories from one rat into the intestine and bloodstream of the other. The seeming contradiction about the role of the intestine in the control of short- and long-term intake can be readily investigated in the left rat of the one-way crossed-intestines model (Fig. 3). By feeding the rat on the right 30 min before or after its partner, the rat on the left, which receives nutrients into its 30-cm crossed-intestinal segment, either can have its crossed segment stimulated by predigested food when it begins to feed or the intestinal segment can remain empty during feeding. If the signals in the crossed-intestinal segment were to inhibit food intake during a meal, then the rat on the left, which has its crossed segment stimulated with food, should eat less while the same rat with an empty crossed segment should eat more. In fact, these rats ate the same amount of food whether fed before or after their partners (13). Thus, we can conclude that even in this one-way crossed-intestines preparation where the rats have dramatically changed their daily food intakes, there is still no effect of the physiological stimulation of the 30-cm crossed-intestinal segments on short-term food intake. Indeed, the two crossed-intestines experiments are consistent in providing data from which one can draw the conclusion that the physiological stimulation of the 30-cm crossed segment does not alter short-term food intake.

Another important conclusion from the one-way crossed-intestines experiment is that the short-term and the long-term controls of food intake are clearly different. In the same animals that show large and sustained changes in daily food intake, there is no effect of intestinal stimulation on short-term intake. In other words, the same surgery that alters daily food intake in a dramatic and long-lasting way has no effect on meal intake after a 7-hr fast. The results from this model strongly argue for two separate physiological mechanisms: the first involved in the control of short-term or meal intake, and the second, in the control of long-term or daily food intake.

In summary, several experiments have shown that infusion of nutrients into the small intestine can inhibit food intake during a single meal. This inhibition is often blocked by vagotomy. When nutrients are infused into the duodenum of rhesus monkeys at the same rate that it is normally released from the stomach, there is an inhibition of food intake that is much greater than when the same amount of food is delivered to the intestine by gastric emptying. In addition, when nutrients are delivered to a limited segment of the upper small intestine in a physiological way, there is little change in short-term food intake. Furthermore, most studies that deliver food directly to the intestine do so at nonphysiological rate and in a nonphysiological form. Thus, the presence of a short-term "intestinal satiety" signal during normal feeding remains possible but has not been adequately demonstrated. The results of the one-way crossed-intestine studies show that there are signals arising at the level of the upper small intestine and/or resulting from the absorption of food that have no effect on short-term food intake, but that do control daily food intake in a very large and significant way. The importance of "satiety" signals arising in the stomach and small intestine can also be assessed by observing the effect of the infusion of intravenous nutrients that bypass the gut. These studies will be reviewed in a later section of this paper on Metabolic Control of Food Intake.

VII EFFECT OF GASTROINTESTINAL HORMONES ON FOOD INTAKE

The issue of whether the stomach and small intestine are sources of short-term satiety signals also has direct implications for the role of gastrointestinal hormones in the control of food intake. If an organ generates signals that induce satiety, then the hormones it releases may also be part of the that signal.

During a normal meal, the ingested food is delivered to the stomach, which allows some food to pass rapidly into the duodenum until intestinal mechanisms inhibit gastric emptying (18). Thus, soon after the beginning of a meal, the mucosal surface of the gut from mouth to mid-ileum has been partially stimulated with nutrients. As previously mentioned, plasma glucose and fatty acid levels change within minutes after the beginning of a meal of laboratory chow (20). Plasma insulin levels also increase rapidly, in part due to cephalic insulin release (96) and in part due to the sustained absorption of glucose and the release of intestinal hormones, such as gastric inhibitory peptide (GIP) and glucagon-like peptide 1 (GLP1) (97). Thus, food has been digested and absorbed and gut hormones have been released long before the end of a meal. This fact leaves the distinct possibility that hormones released by the small intestine during the absorption of food could be part of the signal that terminates a meal.

The gut is the largest endocrine organ in the body (98). After a meal, a large number of gastrointestinal hormones are released including gastrin, somatostatin, secretin, cholecystokinin (CCK), GIP, neurotensin, GLP-1, GLP-2, and peptide YY (PYY) (99). Any of these hormones, especially those arising in the stomach or upper small intestine, would be considered prime candidates as possible gastrointestinal satiety signals. The first gut hormones to be examined for a role in the control of food intake during a meal were secretin and cholecystokinin (CCK). Glick et al. (100) injected secretin and CCK separately or together into the peritoneal cavity or into the aorta of rats and found that neither hormone produced a significant reduction of food intake. There was a tendency for the IP injection of CCK to reduced food intake, but the result with multiple tests on six rats was not significant at P = .05. Koopmans et al. (101) injected CCK into the peritoneal cavity of mice and found that the mice reduced both their food and water intake, suggesting that the dose of CCK was not specific to feeding behavior and may have been causing malaise in the animals. Thereafter, Gibbs et al. (102,103) injected CCK and its octapeptide into the peritoneal cavity of rats and found a dose-dependent reduction of food intake for both forms of CCK. Secretin alone or in conjunction with CCK had no effect on food intake. They injected an intermediate dose of CCK, 20 U/kg IP, and found no effect on water intake.

To test the possibility of malaise resulting from the CCK injection, they used a relatively weak test. A one-bottle conditioned aversion paradigm was used with the attractive substance, saccharin, added to water paired with the injection of CCK. They found that a high dose of CCK, 40 U/kg, failed to generate a conditioned taste aversion in these rats, although lithium chloride, a nauseating poison, was very effective. Deutsch and Hardy (104) challenged these results by doing a more sensitive, two-bottle conditioned aversion test with different neutral flavors associated with CCK and vehicle administration. They found that intake of the flavored water associated with the 40 U/kg CCK injection was reduced from 9.4 mL to 3.3 mL for the flavor paired with CCK injection. Thus, at the highest dose, they found a mild conditioned taste aversion which can be interpreted as due to either malaise or the aversive side of excessive satiety.

The importance of CCK as a satiety signal remains controversial. CCK injected into the peritoneal cavity causes an inhibition of gastric motility and an excitation of duodenal phasic activity (105). A meal usually generates an increase in gastric motility and an inhibition of duodenal activity. Thus, exogenous CCK could be causing unusual gut motility patterns that are communicated by nerves to the brain to inhibit food intake. It is now well established that exogenous CCK requires an intact vagus nerve to cause an inhibition of food intake (106–108). There is also evidence hat doses of CCK that inhibit food intake produce plasma levels that are an order of magnitude higher than normal postprandial CCK levels (109). Moreover, IV infusion of a monoclonal antibody to CCK blocked CCK-stimulated pancreatic enzyme secretion, but had no stimulatory effect on food intake (110).

One of the most convincing pieces of evidence that endogenous CCK acts to reduced food intake is that specific CCK antagonists cause an increase in food intake (111–113). Since these antagonists cause an increase in feeding behavior, it is unlikely that the change can be due to some nonspecific cause. There are two known types of CCK receptors: (1) CCK-A receptors that are present in the pancreas, gallbladder, pyloric sphincter, afferent vagal fibers (114,115), and specific brain regions, including the area postrema, the nucleus tractus solitarius, and the hypothalmus, and (2) CCK-B receptors that are distributed widely in the brain and in the stomach (116). Specific blockade of type A receptors, but not of type B receptors, attenuates the inhibition of food intake caused by CCK (117,118). However, these antagonists cross the blood brain barrier, are distributed throughout the body, and could have their effects either in the periphery or in the brain. Since CCK-A receptors are found in both the brain and the periphery, it is not yet clear where the antagonists act (119). It is possible that CCK-A antagonists act in the brain to increase food intake and not in the periphery. Another indication that the CCK-A receptor is involved in the inhibition of food intake is the existence of OLETF rats that have been shown to have a deletion in the CCK-A receptor that makes it nonfunctional (120). These rats are hyperphagic, have an overexpression of NPY in the dorsomedial hypothalamus, and become moderate obese (121). As mentioned above, the role of the mutant CCK-A receptor could be either central or peripheral.

The ability of the upper gut peptides gastrin, secretin, and GIP to reduce food intake has been tested using a sham-feeding paradigm on rats with open gastric fistuli (119). It was found that even at relatively high doses, none of these peptides had an inhibitory effect on feeding behavior. However, CCK and CCK octapeptide were effective in inhibiting sham feeding.

Another peptide that has been reported to reduce food intake is bombesin. Its intraperitoneal delivery induced a dose-dependent reduction of food intake (122,123) (see Fig. 10). Bombesin is isolated from amphibian skin and has some sequence homology with the mammalian neurotransmitter, gastrin-releasing polypeptide (GRP). It normally does not circulate in mammals, but its injection into the bloodstream causes the release of several pancreatic and gut hormones (124), making it difficult to asses the specific action of GRP. Injection of bombesin into the lateral ventricle reduced food intake and produced an increase in grooming and resting at a dose below that needed to inhibit food intake (125). There is controversy about the way in which bombesin inhibits food intake. One study disconnected all the nerves to the gut by doing a vagotomy and cord transection. They found that complete denervation, but not vagotomy alone, inhibited bombesin's effect on food intake (126). However, the rats were 18-hr food deprived and ate more than normal stomach capacity. This study suggests that bombesin acts peripherally to inhibit food intake. On the other hand, other studies suggest that bombesin may act on the central nervous system. Bombesin-like peptides are present in the paraventricular nucleus, drop during feeding behaviour, and rise after the meal is finished (127). In addition, the reduction of food intake induced by peripheral bombesin can be blocked by the intraventricular injection of a bombesin receptor antagonist (128). A bombesin antagonist administered at high doses had no effect on normal food intake but was able to block bombesin-induced satiety (129). It appears to act independently of CCK.

Serotonin is present in many endocrine cells in the gut (ECL cells) and is released by a wide variety of stimuli (130). Its major effect is local since serotonin is rapidly inactivated in the bloodstream. It appears to stimulate afferent vagal neurons that terminate in the intestinal mucosa and project to the brain (131). Recent work has shown that CCK and serotonin activate different vagal afferents (132) and that glucose stimulates 5HT release while peptides stimulate CCK release from endocrine cells (133). Serotonin has also been shown to inhibit the intake of all the major macronutrients when injected IP (134). Its precursor, trytophan, also reduces food intake in humans (135). Both of these studies delivered serotonin (or its precursor) to the periphery, making it difficult to determine whether the effects were central or peripheral because brain serotonin also inhibits food intake (7).

Another set of hormones are present in endocrine cells of the lower gut, and some of these have been shown to inhibit food intake. The hormones, neurotensin (NT), peptide YY (PYY) and glucagon-like peptide 1 and 2 (GLP-1 and GLP-2), are present in endocrine cells that have an increased frequency as

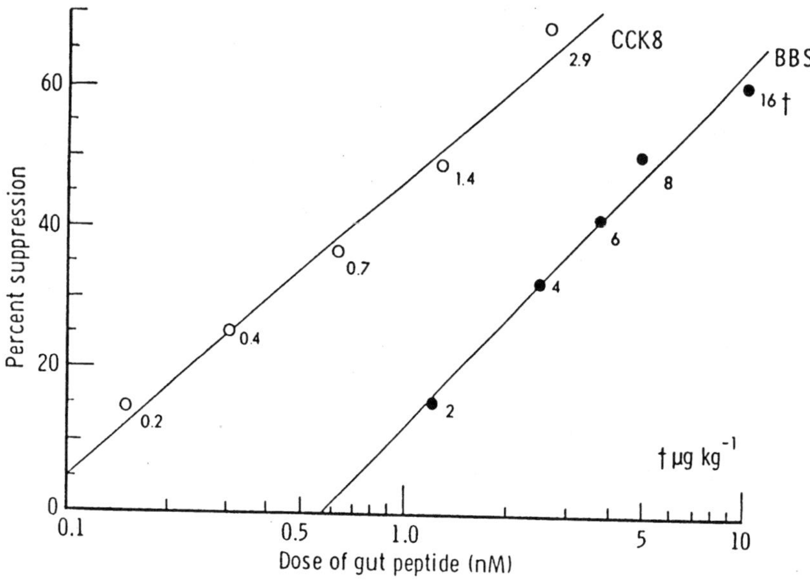

Figure 10 Percent suppression of food intake during the first 15 min of food presentation as increasing amounts of the gut peptides cholecystokinin octapeptide (CCK8) and bombesin (BBS) are injected into the peritoneal cavity of rats. (From Ref. 122.)

one moves down the small intestine (97). A description of these hormones will be presented in the section on Signals Arising in the Lower Gut (see below).

VIII EFFECT OF PANCREATIC HORMONES ON FOOD INTAKE

When nutrients stimulate the surface of the small intestine, GI hormones are released. Two hormones, one from the upper small intestine, gastric inhibitory polypeptide (GIP), and another from the lower small intestine, glucagon-like peptide 1 (GLP-1), have been shown to be incretins for the release of the pancreatic hormones, insulin and amylin, and to indirectly inhibit the release of glucagon (97). Thus, after a meal containing carbohydrate, plasma insulin and amylin levels rise and glucagon levels fall. Glucagon may continue to be released if there is protein in the diet since it helps to mediate amino acid disposal (136).

The pancreatic hormone glucagon has long been known to suppress food intake in man and rodents (137,138). This suppression can be blocked by vagotomy (139) and, more specifically, by hepatic vagotomy (140). Glucagon is the hormone of starvation and catabolism, and its plasma levels increase during a fast. It falls soon after a carbohydrate meal or an oral glucose tolerance test, but can remain elevated or even go up slowly after a meal containing protein and fat (136,141). Sometimes it even goes down after a mixed meal (142). If it has a role in satiety, it must be rather specific for the noncarbohydrate macronutrients. The most convincing piece of evidence that glucagon may be acting as a satiety agent is that the injection of glucagon antibodies causes an increase in food intake (143,144). Glucagon reduces food intake when it is infused into the portal vein (138) and is less effective when it is infused into the vena cava (145). All of these results suggest that the glucagon acts on the liver to inhibit food intake and that the information about the presence of glucagon is sent to the brain through the hepatic vagal nerve. Whether its effect is the result of normal physiology or malaise is not clear. The major difficulty with the glucagon hypothesis is that glucagon is the hormone of starvation, provoking both glycogenolysis and gluconeogenesis, and glucagon has its highest concentration in the blood during a fast when the animals are usually hungry.

Another pancreatic hormone, insulin, has long been thought to be involved in the control of food intake. Insulin rises after a meal and gradually declines as carbohydrate absorption diminishes (21). The "glucostatic" theory originated by Jean Mayer in the 1950s asserted that rats became satiated when there was an arteriovenous difference in blood glucose levels, indicating that there was a significant uptake of glucose by peripheral tissues and that they became hungry when the A-V difference disappeared (146). Since insulin is the main hormone that moves glucose out of the bloodstream into cells and, thereby, causes an A-V difference, the theory was essentially an insulin theory of the termination of food intake. Woods and Porte (147) extended this theory and claimed that the average plasma insulin level feeds back on the brain to inhibit food intake. Investigators have noted that blood insulin levels tended to increase with increasing obesity, demonstrating the phenomenon of insulin resistance (148,149). Woods and Porte postulated that these elevated blood insulin levels provide a feedback signal that informs the brain about the amount of adipose tissue and, if adipose tissue is excessive, inhibits food intake. One difficulty with this theory is that obese individuals tend to eat more, rather than less, than their lean counterparts (150), so well-documented increases in plasma insulin could not be inhibiting their food intake. The Woods and Porte theory is supported by a number of studies that have shown that insulin delivered intracranially causes a reduction of food intake and a loss of body weight (151,152).

However, the critical question is whether peripheral insulin crosses over into the brain to inhibit food intake. It has been shown in dogs that peripheral insulin crosses slowly into the brain and appears in the cerebral spinal fluid (153). Does this insulin alter food intake? There is conflicting evidence. Vanderweele et al. (154) infused 1, 2, and 6 units of insulin in the peritoneal cavity of rats by osmotic minipump and found a small reduction of daily food intake, but it was not dose dependent. In diabetic animals that had been allowed to become hyperphagic, increasing doses of insulin reduced daily food intake but failed to bring food intake back to normal levels (155). In another rat study, very low doses of insulin, either 1 or 2 mU, were infused into the hepatic portal vein during each voluntary meal throughout the daylight hours (156). Meal size decreased in a dose-dependent manner while there was no change in the number of meals. Daily intake was not measured. In contrast, Willing et al. (157,158) continuously infused 2–4 units of insulin into the vena cava of rats that had been made diabetic 1 day before infusion. The rats' food intake increased with increasing dose until it reached 30–40% above baseline levels (see Fig. 11). During this time, urinary glucose was gradually reduced to zero, showing that the insulin was

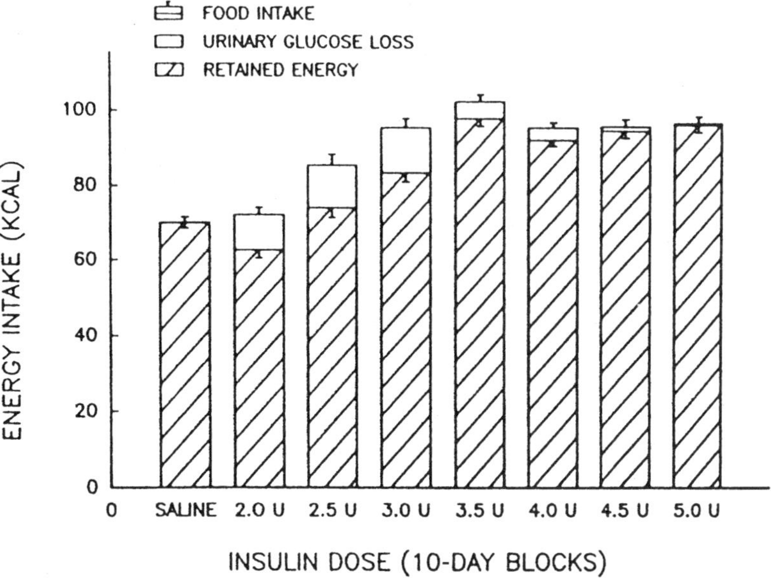

Figure 11 Daily food intake of rats made diabetic after the baseline infusion of saline and, thereafter, infused intravenously with increasing daily doses of insulin. The open bars indicate the amount of glucose lost in the urine of these rats. Daily food intake increases at the lower doses of insulin even though there is an elevated blood glucose and substantial loss of glucose through the urine.

effective in moving glucose into cells. Overfeeding occurred before glucose had been cleared from the urine and while blood glucose levels were greatly elevated. The same increases in intake were observed whether insulin was infused in the vena cava or into the portal vein. To test whether insulin might cross the blood brain barrier to affect food intake, Walls and Koopmans (159) continuously infused insulin into the carotid artery leading to the brain. Since blood flow to the brain is 2–3% of cardiac output, blood insulin levels enhanced by the infusion would be greatly elevated while passing through the brain. They found that carotid insulin was no more effective in altering food intake than vena cava insulin, and in both cases, food intake was significantly increased.

When human studies are examined, insulin infusion during a meal either produced no effect or caused an increase in food intake. Woo et al. (160) infused both insulin and glucose to mimic their postprandial levels before the meal began. They found no change in meal size even with substantially elevated insulin levels. Rodin et al. (161) infused insulin while maintaining plasma glucose levels. They recorded increased hunger ratings with a high insulin infusion and a substantially increased meal at the end of the infusion. Holt and Miller (162) tested different types of rice meals and found that those meals that allowed rapid absorption of glucose and high plasma insulin levels produced higher hunger ratings and increased food intake at the end of the 2-hr session. Most clinical studies have found that insulin infusion leads to a gain in body weight (163). In short, human studies have tended to find that insulin increases rather than inhibits food intake.

A third pancreatic hormone, amylin, is cosecreted from the beta-cells with insulin and has been shown to inhibit food intake in mice and rats (164,165). Amylin reduces basal and glucose-stimulated insulin secretion (166) and is normally released after a meal. Amylin also decreases food intake when injected intraventricularly (167,168). High-affinity binding sites have been found for amylin in several brain regions (169). Recent work has shown that peripheral amylin inhibits food intake and gastric emptying at close to physiological doses (170). Subdiaphragmatic vagotomy does not block peripheral amylin's effect (171).

Another islet hormone is somatostatin, which is a 14– or 28–amino acid peptide that was originally isolated from sheep hypothalamus (172) but is present in many of the organs of the gut, including stomach, pancreatic islets, and small intestine (97). Somatostatin (SOM) has been found in the CNS and enteric nerves as well as endocrine cells (173) and cells with short paracrine processes that terminate on other endocrine cells (174). Its main effect is to inhibit the release of other hormones or to inhibit various physiological functions, such as gastric acid and pepsin secretion (175,176), pancreatic exocrine secretion (177), endocrine secretion (178), and intestinal absorption (179). When injected IP, SOM has been shown to inhibit food intake in rats (180). This result is very hard to interpret since one would expect that SOM injection would alter the plasma levels of several brain or gut hormones, including growth hormone, gastrin, cholecystokinin, insulin, and glucagon, all of which could have effects on food intake, not to mention a lot of other changes in gut activity and function. A recent study reports that a somatostatin analog reduced the rate of gastric emptying during the period of time when the stomach was being filled (181).

IX UNUSUAL GUT-RELATED PEPTIDE HORMONES

Several unusual peptides have been shown to have an effect on food intake. These peptides are generated during the processes of digesting and absorbing food and could provide an indirect signal to the brain of the amount and type of food that has been absorbed. The previous studies on one-way crossed-intestines rats (see Fig. 3) have shown that the absorption of food provides the major signal that controls long-term food intake. The three gut-related peptides that affect food intake are enterostatin, B-casomorphin, and apo A-IV.

Enterostatin has been shown to inhibit food intake when injected into the stomach, intestine, or peritoneal cavity (182). It is a pentapeptide that is released by the cleavage of procolipse by trypsin in the lumen of the digestive tract to produce enterostatin and colipase (183). Enterostatin's amino acid sequence is well preserved across many animal species. Procolipase is secreted from the pancreas in response to CCK and specifically inhibits fat intake if animals are given a choice of diets or dietary components (184). If fat is a sustained portion of the diet, more procolipase is secreted and could inhibit feeding behavior. One difficulty with the belief that enterostatin inhibits food intake under normal circumstances is that enterostatin is degraded by membrane peptidases in the intestinal brush border (185) and is, therefore, unlikely to be absorbed intact unless some special transport mechanism exists. However, Mei and Erlanson-Albertsson (186) have shown that plasma levels of enterostatin increased significantly after a meal and respond to the fat content of the meal. An interesting finding is that mRNA for procolipase and the procolipase protein are present in endocrine cells in the fundic region of the stomach as well as in the antrum and duodenum (187). The gastric procolipase was cloned, sequenced, and found to be identical to pancreatic procolipase (188). Colipase has been found in the lumen of the stomach (189), and it is possible that cleaved enterostatin could be released into the bloodstream. Injection of small amounts of enterostatin into cereberal ventricles suppress fat intake. There is reasonably strong evidence the enterostatin inhibits the intake of fat after a fast, but the role of enterostatin in the long-term control of food and fat intake under the free-feeding conditions has been questioned (190).

Another peptide, beta-casomorphin, is a cleavage product of milk casein that stimulates food intake when delivered intraperitoneally. This septapeptide was first discovered from a digest of milk because of it's morphine-like activity (191). It has been found to increase fat intake, to inhibit intestinal motility (192,193), and to stimulate sleep in neonates (194). It appears to interact with enterostatin by preventing enterostatin's usual suppression of fat intake. Indeed, based on their feeding behavior curves, White et al. (195) hypothesize that beta-casomorphin may be an enterostatin receptor antagonist. The role of beta-casomorphin in the control of food intake has the same explanatory problem as enterostatin: How does the peptide avoid digestion and get transferred into the GI tissue or the bloodstram in order to have a systemic influence? Of course, its importance for the control of food intake is based on the presence of milk in the diet. Since beta-casomorphin stimulates food intake, it is possible that its main role is to override satiety signals in the early stages of life, when milk is a large part of the animal's diet and when rapid growth is important for survival. Indeed, it has been known for a long time that satiety signals are quite limited in neonatal rats (196).

The third gut-related peptide that affects food intake is a glycoprotein (with a molecular weight of ~ 46,000) that is attached to newly synthesized fat particles, called chylomicrons, in the intestinal absorptive cell (197). The apoproteins, apo A-I and apo A-IV, are added to the surface of the chylomicron in order to solubilize it for transport through the lamina propria of the intestine and through the intestinal lymph ducts before these chylomicrons enter the bloodstream near the heart. Apo A-IV is readily displaced from chylomicrons to other lipoproteins, such as HDL, in the bloodstream, and 80% of it circulates in the bloodstream as a free protein. Only the intestine makes Apo A-IV (198,199). Patrick Tso and colleagues have shown that Apo A-IV is effective in reducing food intake (200,201). They collected intestinal lymph before and at 6–8 hr after a meal and then infused it intravenously into rats that had been deprived of food for 24 hr. They found that postmeal lymph caused a substantial reduction of food intake in the first 30 min of feeding compared to rats that had a saline or a fasting lymph infusion. An infusion of the equivalent amount of lipid and phospholipid (2% intralipid infusion) had very little effect on short-term food intake which is consistent with the long-term lipid infusion studies (see Metabolic Signals below). However, infusion of three increasing doses of apo A-IV demonstrated a clear dose-dependent inhibition while infusion of Apo A-I had no efect on food intake. Immunoprecipitation of Apo A-IV in postmeal lymph returned food intake back to normal levels, demonstration a very specific Apo A-IV effect. Apo A-IV was also effective in inhibiting intake when infused in small amounts intracranially, while antirat Apo A-IV delivered ICV increased food intake (202). Intracisternal Apo A-IV also increased gastric acid secretion and motility (203,204). Apo A-IV or a related fragment has been found in cerebrospinal fluid (202). It is difficult to understand how such a large peptide as Apo A-IV would enter the brain unless actively transported. Although IV infused Apo A-IV has effects on short-term food intake, the normal stimulus and route of entry of Apo A-IV into the bloodstream suggest a regulatory effect on long-term food intake, which is supported by the fact that IV infusion of Apo A-IV decreases food intake in ad libitum rats (201,205).

X CYTOKINES AND INFLAMMATORY PEPTIDE REGULATORS OF FOOD INTAKE

Not only do various gastrointestinal peptides alter food intake during a meal, but cytokines released in the gut wall or elsewhere as a result of infection, inflammation, or malignancy also tend to inhibit food intake (206–208). These cytokines are released by leukocytes and surrounding tissue. The most prominent cytokines that produce anorexia are interferon-α (IFNα); interleukin 1, 6, and 8 (IL-1, IL-6, IL-8); and tumor necrosis factor-alpha (TNFα). They can have multiple peripheral effects including changes in hormone levels (209), GI motility (210), and metabolic pathways (211), as well as changes in neurotransmitter levels in the hypothalamus (212). They may also elevate temperature and induce sleep. These cytokines can act on specific receptors in the central nervous system. IFNα and IL-1b excite the glucose sensitive neurons in the ventromedial hypothalamus and suppress neuronal activity along with TNFα in the lateral hypothalamus. The intracerebral injection of a specific IL-1 receptor antagonist blocks food intake suppression induced by IL-1b (213), showing that the site of action of IL-1 was in the brain.

Cytokines rarely act alone because they stimulate the release of other cytokines (214). Often, they enhance each other's effectiveness in producing anorexia or, in more serious conditions such as cancer, in producing cachexia, a type of wasting syndrome that includes reduced food intake. Studies have shown that IL-1 and TNFα act synergistically to reduce food intake (215). There are several ways to limit anorexia. Feeding n-3 polyunsaturated fatty acids (216), giving cytokine receptor antagonists or antibodies (213), or administering hormones, such as glucocorticoids or, more specifically, megesterol acetate (217) seems to limit the mild nausea and lack of interests in food. Another peptide closely relate to IL-6, called ciliary neurotrophic factor (CNTF), has been added to the list of cytokinelike molecules that inhibit food intake (218).

Although cytokines have now been clearly shown to have direct effects on the inhibition of food intake, these effects are probably not intended to limit body weight. The more likely goal is to limit the animal's desire for food which, if acted upon, would expose the animal to the risk of predation at a time when it is not capable of peak physical activity. The long-term need for calorie balance may be temporarily set aside for the more immediate goal of survival. There may also be some benefit to recovery by having elevated temperature or a limited use of joints, muscles, and bone (219,220). The effect of these peptides on intake should not be thought of as regulators of energy balance, but as defenders from further tissue damage.

XI CROSS-CIRCULATED RATS AND GUT NERVE SECTIONS

All of the above studies show that many gut-related peptides or hormones play a role in the inhibition of food intake. Another way of testing the role of hormones in the control of food intake is to cross the circulation of two rats in a parabiotic pair. This can be done by connecting the abdominal aorta of each rat with the ascending vena cava of its partner (see Fig. 12). After this surgery, the blood of the two rats is completely mixed every minute (221). The role of blood factors in the control of feeding behavior can be tested by feeding one of the rats in a pair 10 or 30 min before its partner after a 7-hr deprivation. Rats deprived for 7 hr

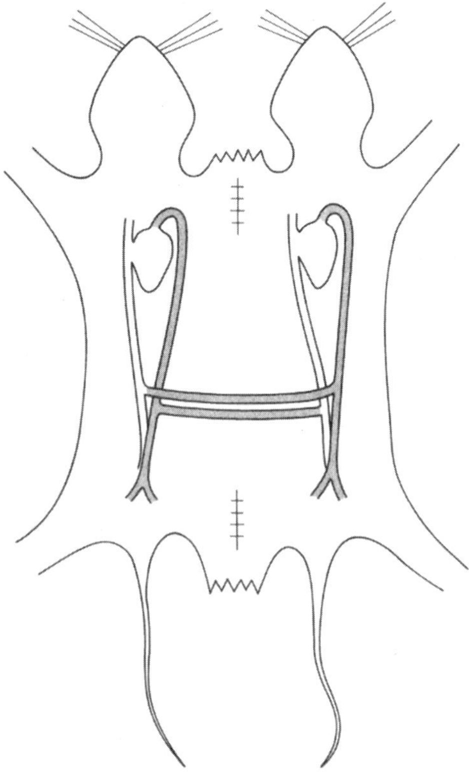

Figure 12 Diagram of conscious rats with continuous cross-circulation of the blood between the two rats. Grafts from other inbred rats are used to connect the descending aorta of one rat to the ascending vena cava of its partner. Thirty percent of cardiac output crosses in each 15-sec circulation time, and the blood is completely mixed every minute. The stippled vessels are those that carry only arterial blood.

will normally stop eating after 6–8 min based on their own internal satiety signals. The rat fed first will have all of its released hormones and absorbed nutrients diluted into twice its normal amount of blood and removed by twice the amount of tissue. This should lower the plasma levels of the hormones released by the meal and of all the absorbed nutrients. If these humoral factors are important in the control of meal intake, the rat fed first should eat a larger-than-normal meal in order to bring these humoral signals up to some specified level. On the other hand, its partner fed 10 or 30 min later will already have elevated hormones and nutrients present in its blood. If these humoral signals are important in the termination of a meal, these rats should eat a smaller meal. The results of this experiment were that the rats ate the same size meal regardless of whether they ate first, and had a low plasma level of hormones or nutrients or ate second when they were already stimulated by these humoral signals. The natural conclusion from this study is that the combination of released hormones and absorbed nutrients is not an important signal in the termination of a meal when these substances flow through the systemic circulation from one rat to the other. Hormones and nutrients may have an effect on food intake by stimulating the liver, since all gut hormones released and all water-soluble nutrients absorbed by the intestine must pass through the liver before entering the general circulation. Thus, released hormones could act on the nerves in the wall of the gut or on nerves terminating in the portal vein and liver. However, once these humoral substances have passed into the vena cava which leads to the heart, they have already been diluted by the blood of the partner which has also been arriving into the ascending vena cava. Thus, the results of this study limit the possible satiety signals derived from a meal to neural signals generated in the gastrointestinal tract and the liver. These neural signals could be generated in the gastrointestinal tract and the liver. These neural signals could be generated by the local presence of hormones, for example, the high levels of hormones released into the lamina propria of the GI tract.

The results of the cross-circulation studies do challenge many of the theories that argue that nutrients or hormones present in the blood are involved in the control of meal intake. In fact, the results show that the combination of hormones released by the meal and nutrients absorbed as a result of feeding do not affect short-term food intake. Theorists with a different point of view may argue that results from parabiotic rats are not typical of normal, single animals. While it is true that these rats are restrained in their movement by the presence of the attached partner, the parabiotic surgery is relatively minor and there is no interference with any of the rat's internal organs other than end-to-side connections to their major blood vessels. No drugs or exogenous hormones have to be given to these animals at the time of testing: there are no worries about dose, site of action, type of injection, or possible malaise. The only change is ~30% of their cardiac output is lost into their partner's bloodstream during each 15-sec recirculation time and, of course, 30% of the partner's blood returns continuously to the first rat. In short, the cross-circulated rats are normal parabiotic rats that live for more than a year without special attention. This surgical preparation has the enormous advantage of testing the role of not just one nutrient or hormone at a time, but of testing the role of all of the hormones released from the gut into the bloodstream after a meal and all of the absorbed nutrients at the same time. Since these substances are released or absorbed by normal body processes that follow a meal, their plasma levels should remain within the normal range although levels are likely to be below normal concentrations. Although these rats have some restricted movement, their daily food intake is normal and they do provide a critical test of the role of all gut hormones and absorbed nutrients on the termination of a meal.

One difficulty in interpreting the cross-circulation is that these results seem to imply that nerves provide the only signals that inhibit food intake during a single meal. In many ways, an important role for nerves in the termination of a meal is a reasonable hypothesis. The bulk of the food eaten during a meal remains in the stomach and only empties slowly into the intestine. The combination of gastric distension receptors and intestinal neural chemoreceptors would be needed to inform the brain about the amount of food ingested. Since the stomach of a free-feeding rat is rarely empty, new food eaten can only be recognized by increased gastric distention or intensified signals from intestinal chemoreceptors. Thus, the expected internal changes suggest that neural messages are involved in the termination of food intake. On the other hand, there are many studies in which vagotomies have been done with no major long-term effect on food intake. Animals with vagotomies usually lose some weight and have changes in stomach emptying depending on their diet (222,223). However, their food intake usually does return to and stabilize at near normal levels. If the vagus nerve is not essential for production of a satiety signal and humoral signals play no role in the control of intake, then how does the animal know when to stop feeding? Are the splanchnic nerves essential? Or can the animal shift its attention from one type of signal to another when the internal signals do not produce the expected changes that normally follow feeding?

Very few studies have attempted a complete gut denervation which requires extensive surgery. There are four reports that claim that all nerves to the GI tract have been severed. Grossman et al. (224) did a three-stage operation over several months on dogs that had complete section of the vagus and sympathetic nerves. After recovery of several months, food intake was measured and they found that denervated dogs ate the same-size meals as intact dogs. When the dogs were given insulin injections, food intake for both dogs increased by the same amount. Harris et al. (225) followed the same surgical procedure and confirmed that there were no lasting results of nerve section on feeding behavior, and found that amphetamine caused a similar decrease in food intake in denervated and intact dogs. Both of these studies showed that the recovered dogs ate normally and responded to substances that alter food intake in the same way as normal dogs. However, neither group of experimenters reported a postmortem confirmation that the surgery was complete and that nerve regeneration had failed to occur in the many months between surgery and behavioral testing.

More recently, Stuckey et al. (126) did a two-stage operation on rats doing dorsal rhizotomy and cord section first, allowing the rats to recover for 2–3 weeks, doing some behavioral tests and thereafter doing bilateral vagotomy with another week of recovery. The main objective of this study was to determine how bombesin affected food intake, so no data on meal pattern or daily intake were presented although the authors state that grossly normal feeding behavior was maintained. It was mentioned that the rats initially lost weight and then maintained it at a reduced level. This is not surprising since the spinal cord section would have eliminated movement in the back limbs, making both eating and exercising difficult. At postmortem, nerve section was confirmed with the aid of a dissecting microscope, but no histochemical or functional tests were done. These studies suggest that several months after complete denervation surgery, dogs and rats will feed in a grossly normal way. All of these studies required considerable recovery time.

To reexamine this important question, we have recently done a complete gut nerve section in rats (226). Four groups of rats had either bilateral vagotomy, bilateral splanchnectomy (elimination of the sympathetic nerves to the gut tissue), the combination of these two surgeries, or complete sham surgery including mobilization of the nerves and preparation for section but without an actual transection. We were determined to transect all of the accessory branches to each set of bilateral nerves. Because the nerves branch into fibers that are barely visible under a disecting microscope, our procedure included the cutting of the mesenteric membranes through which these nerves are known to travel as well as the visible nerves themselves. The rats were fed the liquid diet Ensure for 17 overnight hours per day, and the results were quite interesting. The vagotomy produced a large reduction of daily food intake (sustained at 20% below normal) and a substantial loss of body weight, which remained depressed by 25% below the level of controls at 26 days when we sacrificed the rats and took blood and tissue samples. The splanchnectomy had no effect on food intake or body weight when done alone even though we cut all of the four or five branches of the splanchnic nerve that leave the celiac and mesenteric ganglia on each side and travel toward the sympathetic ganglia and spinal cord.

Splanchnectomy combined with vagotomy was no different from vagotomy alone, showing once again that the sympathetic gut nerves did not alter energy balance, but section of the vagus nerve was very effective in lowering food intake and body weight. Our study of vagotomy produced a larger effect than that found in most other studies in the literature (222,223). We also tested the size of the first meal after a 7-hr fast and found that 15-min meal size was not different across any of the surgical groups even though vagotomy caused a large reduction in daily intake. Apparently, the section of both extrinsic afferent and efferent gut nerves had no effect on short-term intake. We also measured the rats' response to a 50% dilution of the liquid diet by water. The rats adjusted both the size of their first meal and their daily intake on the first day so that caloric intake did not change. This result suggests that vagotomized rats were somehow regulating ingested calories and not just responding to food volume.

The dramatic effect of our vagotomies on energy balance and body weight loss can be interpreted in one of two ways. Either we were very effective in cutting all the branches of the vagus nerve and the resulting complete vagotomy led to a substantial reduction in food intake and body weight relative to other studies in the literature, or our cutting of the mesenteric membranes supporting the esophagus, stomach, and liver led to changes in the rats' comfort that exacerbated the reduction in food intake and body weight after vagotomy. In the later case, the changes would be nonregulatory. We used a histochemical method at the end of the study for verifying that the nerves had been sectioned: the calcitonin gene-related peptide (CGRP) fibers disappeared from the gastric wall and the duodenal mucosa after total nerve section, showing that afferent nerves had been destroyed. The observed large decrease of food intake and body weight following vagotomy is complicated from a theoretical perspective. If transection of the nerve simply cut vagal sensory fibers that increase their firing rate to inhibit food intake [as seen in Paintal's gastric distension vagal nerve fibers (51)], then vagotomy would be anticipated to cause an increase in food intake. If, on the other hand, the transections cut nerves that stimulate food intake when activated or reduce their firing rate to signal inhibition [as found in Niijima's hepatic nerve recordings to portal glucose infusion (227)], then one would expect that food intake would decrease as has actually been found after most studies of vagotomy. These alternate explanations require further research with more selective afferent or efferent nerve sections. In fact, both vagotomies and sympathectomies cause large changes in the sensory nerve cells found, respectively, in the nodose and dorsal root ganglia. These cell bodies actually change their dominant neurotransmitters (228,229), which suggests that peripheral nerve section may be followed by a large central nervous system reorganization.

At the present time, the conflicting results from the cross-circulation and denervation studies suggest that animals may be able to shift their attention from one signal to another. The cross-circulation studies do not interfere with any of the possible communicating signals within the body because no major nerves or blood vessels are severed and blood flows continuously throughout the bodies of both rats. However, there is about a week of recovery from the time of surgery until the behavioral testing begins. During this time, the rats could learn to ignore changes in blood levels of hormones or nutrients and rely only on intact neural messages to inhibit food intake. In contrast, the denervation studies interfere with one of the major signal systems in the body, but the animals survive and recover over several weeks or months. Even with probable total gut denervation, dogs, cats, and rats are able to feed in a fairly normal way although the level of food intake and body weight may be reduced, especially after vagotomy. Perhaps during this long adjustment period, they learn to pay attention to mouth and throat signals or to the changes in the blood levels of hormones and nutrients. A possible shift over time to different internal signals seems to be one way to reconcile the two sets of studies.

Another way to reconcile the results is to examine whether some combination of signals is needed to inhibit food intake. A number of studies have shown that a combination of neural and hormonal signals may together produce an effective signal that inhibits food intake. Neither signal alone would be enough. Davison and Clarke found that there were CCK receptors on gastric afferent nerve terminals and that the combination of CCK release by the intestine and gastric distension might together produce satiety signals (230). These studies were extended to show a clear increase in nerve activity when CCK and gastric load were increased together (231). Some studies have shown that peripheral CCK and intraventricular leptin interact to produce a larger inhibition of food intake (232,233). More recently, it has been shown that intraventricular leptin enhances satiety caused by a gastric nutrient preload (234). These studies suggest that a complex combination of neural and hormonal signals may be needed to produce satiety and that focusing on just one or the other signal system independently may fail to demonstrate a major effect on short-term or daily food intake. Further investigation is needed to obtain a clear understanding of the nature of the signals that inhibit food intake after a meal. It has recently been shown that there are leptin receptors on some of the gastric afferent neurons of the vagus nerve (74). It would be interesting to know if ghrelin released into the gastric lamina propria could also inhibit food intake by attaching to receptors on vagal afferents.

XII SIGNALS ARISING IN THE LOWER GUT

Jejunoileal bypass surgery has been one of the most successful ways of causing weight loss in morbidly obese patients. In this surgery, the upper jejunum is connected to the lower ileum so that the food bypasses 80–90% of the length of the small intestine, and as a result, the ingested food is not fully digested and absorbed. Following this surgery, obese patients lose 40% of their body weight and retain this weight loss after 2–5 years (235–237). The original theory behind the surgery was that, by shortening the length of the small intestine, one would reduce the absorptive surface of the gut and prevent the absorption of much of the ingested food. The patients could eat as much as they wanted, but most of the food would pass right through the digestive tract before it could be absorbed. Presumably, patients who were unable to control their food intake would still lose weight. In fact, a major consequence of the surgery was that the patients chose to eat less which contributed to the substantial weight loss (238,239). This effect has also been observed in rats (240). In fact, the weight loss was largely caused by reduced food intake and not by malabsorption. Part of the reason for this reduction of intake may have been the discomfort of their lower gut symptoms. These jejunoileal bypass patients experienced severe diarrhea, bloating, and flatulence and were running frequently to the toilet to relieve their recurrent discomfort. Thus, there may have been some aversive conditioning that led to their reduction of food intake.

Jejunoileal bypass surgery induced a large number of medical complications due to malabsorption or to the large segment of bypassed bowel, and, because of these complications, the surgery is no longer done in major medical centers. Instead, the surgeons have focussed on gastric restriction or gastric bypass operations (241,242). These surgeries attempt to restrain food intake by producing a small gastric pouch that provides strong distension cues if the right food is eaten. Both of these operations do cause an initial major loss of body weight, but, in the case of gastroplasties or gastric vertical binding, the weight loss depends on patient compliance in food selection. If the selected foods can pass easily through the narrowed opening of the stomach pouch, as can milk shakes or blenderized meals, then the patients rapidly regain their lost weight. In recent years, obesity surgeons have returned to the gastric bypass operation (243), which combines the restriction of a stomach pouch with the stimulation of the lower gut. In the gastric bypass surgery, a small isolated pouch of upper stomach is connected through a restricted outlet to the upper jejunum. This procedure bypasses the usual controls of gastric emptying and spreads the emptied food more rapidly into the lower gut (244). Indeed, the plasma levels of lower gut hormones following a meal in gastric bypass patients (245–248) were quite similar to those found after jejunoileal bypass. The 15-fold integrated postprandial enteroglucagon response after gastric bypass was comparable to the 14-fold increase found after j-i bypass (249). Thus, the current surgery of choice, gastric bypass, has a large lower-gut component. New experimental surgeries are following the same strategy of greater stimulation of the lower gut (243).

Greater stimulation of the lower small intestine could cause reduced food intake and increased weight loss by stimulating the nerves in the ileum or by greater release of lower gut hormones. The role of ileal nerves in long-term weight loss has not yet been investigated. There are four hormones that are released from the lower small intestine and might play a role in the inhibition of food intake. Neurotensin (NT) is a tridecapeptide that was originally isolated from the hypothalamus and has the same structure in rat, dog, and human. It is found in the N-cells of the gut, which are present in increased frequency as one moves down the small intestine (250). The N-cells have microvilli that make contact with the lumen of the small intestine and may thus directly sense luminal contents. Neurotensin is released after a normal meal or after the infusion of fat into the duodenum (251). Gastric secretion and motility are inhibited by high doses of NT (97). When injected IP, neurotensin causes a reduction of food intake and grooming and an increase in drinking (252), but plasma levels were not measured and an effect on gut motility cannot be ruled out as an explanation of reduced feeding. A recent study involving the IP injection of a novel neurotensin analog also appears to inhibit food intake (253). When NT is injected into the hypothalamic paraventricular nucleus, it causes a dose-dependent reduction of food intake without associated changes in water intake, grooming, or sleeping behavior (254), but these investigators found no effect of IV infusion.

There are three other hormones originating in the lower gut, and all are found in endocrine cells, labeled L-cells, which have microvillous tufts that protrude into the intestinal lumen and, thus, could be stimulated by lower gut contents. Like N-cells, L-cells increase in number as one progresses down the small intestine, and large amounts of PYY are found in the ileum and colon (255). Pancreatic peptide YY (PYY) is a 36–amino acid peptide that was first discovered using a chemical method that detected amide groups (256). It is released after a normal meal and after oleic acid is infused into the duodenum and, in much higher amounts, after a large meal (257). It inhibits gastric acid and pancreatic enzyme secretion and causes gallbladder contraction (97). PYY also limits gastric emptying and inhibits intestinal motility, acting as an ileal brake (258). Recent work has shown that peripheral PYY acts on the dorsal vagal complex to inhibit gastrointestinal motility (259). Hormonal PYY has not been shown to alter food intake, although its close cousin, neuropeptide Y, greatly enhances food intake when injected into the cerebral ventricles or the hypothalamus (260,261). Several studies have shown that injection of PYY into the ventricles enhances food intake (262,263), in contrast to increased lower gut stimulation, which reduces food intake (264) and releases hormonal PYY. If peripheral PYY gains access to the hypothalamus, it probably works on NPY receptors in the brain to increase intake.

The two other identified lower gut hormones, the glucagonlike peptides 1 and 2 (or GLP-1 and GLP-2) are produced by alternate processing of the proglucagon gene in the small intestine and colon (265,266). When released, GLP-1 acts as an incretin in the stimulation of insulin release (267). It interacts with both glucose and GIP to enhance insulin release. GLP-1 also inhibits stomach emptying and thereby lowers blood glucose levels (268). Recent studies have shown that the intravenous infusion of GLP-1 will reduce food intake and lower plasma glucose in humans (269,270), but there is also evidence that GLP-1 may cause visceral malaise (271,272).

The other major enteroglucagon is GLP-2. GLP-1 and GLP-2 are released by the same cells in equimolar quantities (265,267). GLP-2 increases the activity of brush border enzymes and increases the rate of absorption of peptides and fats (273). It may also act as an ileal brake, inhibiting the delivery of food to the lower gut (274). The specific receptor for GLP-2 has been cloned and identified (275). It has been found only in the stomach, small intestine, hypothalamus, and brainstem. In the small intestine, the receptors appear to be present only on other endocrine cells (276). A recent study involving the central injection of GLP-2 demonstrated a small, 2-hr reduction of food intake that was not associated with conditioned aversion using a weak one-bottle saccharin aversion test (277). These authors identified the presence of GLP-2 neurons originating in the nucleus tractus solitarius of the brainstem and projecting to the dorsomedial nucleus of the hypothalamus. They argued that GLP-2 was acting as a neurotransmitter to decrease food intake, but their evidence does not exclude the possibility that peripheral GLP-2 may also act centrally as an inhibitor of food intake.

All of the lower-gut peptides can be released by glucose, 5% peptone solution, and oleic acid delivered to the lumen of the small intestine (278,279). Recent studies have shown that they all may play some role in the peripheral control of food intake, although direct evidence for a role of peripheral PYY on intake is not available. In addition, a physiological effect of NT, GLP-1, and GLP-2 on the inhibition of food intake is not yet certain. At present, the internal signals that cause the sustained lower level of daily food intake and body weight after jejunoileal and gastric bypass are not fully understood.

Another way to test the importance of the lower small intestine in the inhibition of food intake is to move a segment of the lower small intestine to the upper regions of the gut without causing any change in the length of the small intestine. In one experiment, a 10- or 20-cm segment of lower ileum was isolated from the lower small intestine and was reconnected to the mid-duodenum or upper jejunum (264,280). These rats with ileal transposition showed a decrease in food intake that led to a substantial loss of weight. The ileal transposition surgery was more effective in obese than in lean rats, although the effect was significant in both. These data suggest that overstimulation of the ileum might lead to a reduction of food intake by intensification of lower-gut signals.

The ileal transposition studies have shown that malabsorption and its associated discomfort were not the essential components of the reduction of food intake that followed jejunoileal bypass (280). Increased lower-gut stimulation was sufficient to cause a large reduction of food intake. However, these studies failed to prove that the intensification of ileal signals was reducing food intake through a normal physiological mechanism. It was still possible that the intensified signals were causing a reduction of intake by making the animal uncomfortable, that is, by generating physiological signals that were outside their usual range. One suggestion that the level of stimulation was abnormal was the large number of morphological changes that resulted from the intensified ileal stimulation. There was a 50% increase in the wet weight of the stomach, pancreas, and remaining jejunoileum, as well as a fivefold increase of the transposed ileal segment (264,281). These changes in organ size could be interpreted as an hard-wired attempt by the body to reduce ileal stimulation. In a normal rat, similar changes could increase the holding capacity of the stomach, provide more digestive enzymes for the processing of food in the upper small intestine, and increase the absorptive surface of the gut. In addition, ileal stimulation would reduce intestinal transit leading to less stimulation of the lower gut (282,283). Reduced food intake could be interpreted as another way in which the organism could prevent food from reaching the lower small intestine (281). However, all of these signals might still be outside the usual physiological range: the intense stimulation of the transposed ileal segment could be making the animal sick. After all, almost all of the ingested food had to pass through this ileal segment before it could be absorbed, which was far from the normal level of stimulation by ~3–5% of the ingested and digestible food. Was there a way to reduce the stimulation of this ileal segment and bring it closer to the normal physiological range?

The degree of the stimulation of the lower gut could be altered by using surgery on another type of parabiotic rat pair. In this surgical preparation, the small intestine of one rat in the pair was transected at the jejunoileal junction or about halfway down the lenght of the small intestine. The upper jejunal end of this rat's small intestine was connected end-to-side to the partner's small intestine at the same level (see Fig. 13). The lower ileal end was simply closed so that no more ingested food could enter into its lumen. The result of this surgery was that one rat in the pair (the rat on the right) no longer has its ileum, cecum, and colon stimulated by exogenous food, while its partner had its lower gut doubly stimulated. Instead of the 20- to 30-fold increase in the amount of ileal stimulation that might be expected in the ileal transposition rats, these rats had their full lower gut either unstimulated or doubly stimulated by chyme that had been appropriately processed for the level of intestinal stimulation (284). Of course, in this preparation, there was also a continual loss of food from the intestine of one rat into that of its partner. The rat that lost food into its partner and that had its lower gut unstimulated increased its daily food intake by 30–40% while its partner that had its lower gut doubly stimulated reduced its own intake by about the same amount. On the surface, this result would suggest that food intake is controlled by the lower small intestine, but the results need to be interpreted carefully. Is the change in daily food intake due to the loss of food from one rat to the other or due to the change in lower-gut stimulation? To answer this question, one needs to look at the changes in body weight that occur over an extended period of time. When the rats were sacrificed 24 days later, it was found that the two rats did not differ significantly in body weight or in the size of their retroperitoneal fat pads. Therefore, the adjustments of daily food intake were appropriate for the amount of food lost from one rat into the intestine of its partner. This result showed that doubling or reducing to nil the exogenous stimulation of the lower gut had no specific effect on the daily food intake of the rats. The changes that were observed could be attributed to the loss of chyme from one rat to the other. The major controller of food intake was the amount of absorbed food and not the stimulation of the lower gut. From these results, one can conclude that stimulation of the

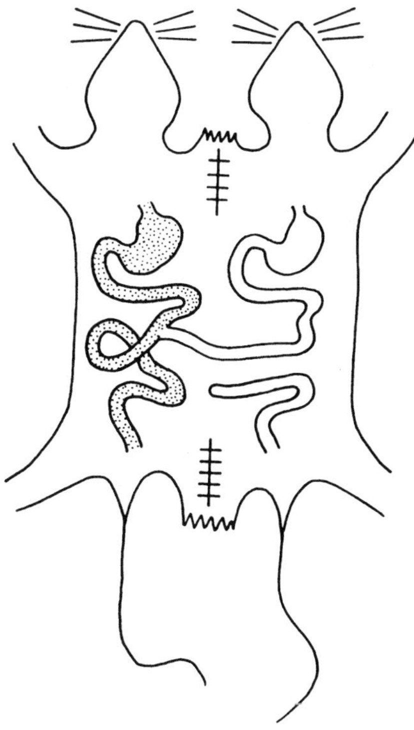

Figure 13 Diagram of rats with doubly stimulated lower guts. The rat on the right has its small intestine transected at the junction between jejunum and ileum. The jejunum is connected end-to-side to the partner's intestine at the jejunoileal junction. The stippled GI tract belongs to the rat on the left. After the surgery, the rat on the left has its lower gut doubly stimulated with chyme while the right rat has no further food enter its ileum, cecum, or colon. (From Ref. 284.)

lower gut has only a minor role in the regulatory control of food intake. At greatly elevated levels, it may be effective in causing reduced food intake and sustained weight loss, but, at near normal levels, it does not appear to be a major peripheral controller of food intake.

XIII SIGNALS ARISING IN THE LIVER

The liver originates as an outgrowth of gut tissue and plays a significant role in the secretion of bile and the absorption of fat. One of its major functions within the body is the control of the metabolism of glucose, amino acids, and fat. Therefore, the role of the liver in the control of food intake could be seen from the perspective of a gut organ coming in early contact with food or as a mediator and regulator of metabolism. It is appropriate to review its role in the control of food intake in a section that moves from gut signals to metabolic signals.

The liver is the only organ, other than the gut, that comes into direct contact with a substantial amount of the ingested food. All of the absorbed water-soluble nutrients, including sugars and amino acids, pass through the liver on their way into the general circulation. The liver removes many of these nutrients during the absorptive phase and works to control their levels in the bloodstream. Thus, the liver would be in a position to assess or monitor the total amount of carbohydrate and protein entering from outside, which could be as much as 60–90% of ingested calories. However, the liver does not come into direct initial contact with most of the absorbed fat, since ingested long-chain fatty acids are resynthesized into triglycerides and formed into fat particles called chylomicrons. These fat particles do not enter the portal vein, but instead pass into the intestinal lymphatics, travel through the thoracic duct, and enter the blood at the level of the large veins leading into the heart (285). Thus, the absorbed fat bypasses the liver before it enters the bloodstream at the heart, where it is diluted in all of the blood. Some of the absorbed fat will go directly to muscle and adipose tissue for use or for storage and never pass through the liver, making it impossible for the liver to determine the total amount of absorbed long-chain fat by direct contact. Of course, the liver could still have some indirect way to count absorbed fat calories by assessing some change in internal signals or changes in specific metabolic pathways.

Russek was the first person to propose that the liver was a major organ involved in the regulation of food intake (286). He suggested that hepatic nerves respond to changes in the metabolic activity and the resulting hyperpolarization of the hepatocyte membrane. He argued that these changes were communicated to the brain through the hepatic vagus nerve. Niijima has shown that the nerves in the hepatic branches of the vagus decrease their firing rate in an inverse relationship to the glucose concentration in the portal vein (227). Novin and his collaborators infused isotonic glucose into the portal vein of free-feeding rabbits and found that it had little effect on meal intake, but when the glucose was infused into the portal vein in 17-hr-deprived animals, it did reduce food intake over a period of 3 hr (287,288). In contrast, infusion of glucose in the duodenum reduced food intake in free-feeding rabbits but had little effect in deprived rabbits. These data are confusing because glucose infused into the duodenum should be very rapidly absorbed into the portal vein and, thus, ought to act in a similar way as direct portal vein infusion. Like portal infusion, duodenal infusion should have reduced the food intake of the deprived rabbits, unless a duodenal signal somehow blocks a later hepatic signal.

The role of the liver in the control of food intake has been more recently investigated by Tordoff and associates. They infused glucose into the portal vein and found that it was more effective than equimolar concentrations of NaCl only at the lowest concentration of 0.3 M (289,290). As the dose doubled and quadrupled, the 2-hr food intake of the rats infused with salt continued to decrease, while those infused with glucose remained at the same level (see Fig. 14). In comparison, infusion of the same amount of glucose into the jugular vein had relatively little effect on 2-hr food intake. They also found that the rats with portal glucose infusion had lower plasma glucose levels and increased hepatic glycogen compared to jugularly infused rats. This result is consistent with the fact that the infused portal glucose was altering hepatic metabolism and was being stored as glycogen. One puzzling aspect of these data was that increasing the dose of glucose caused no greater reduction of food intake even though the highest dose was the equivalent of 104 kcal/day or more than a rat would normally eat. The hepatic sensor did not seem to be measuring the amount of water-soluble nutrient passing through the liver during this short time frame. It registered the presence of glucose, but not the amount.

A more recent study has measured daily food intake over a 17-hr period when only 10 or 20 kcal of glucose (0.57 or 1.15kcal/hr) was infused into the portal or the jugular vein. It was found that using these slow infusions of relatively small amounts of glucose pro-

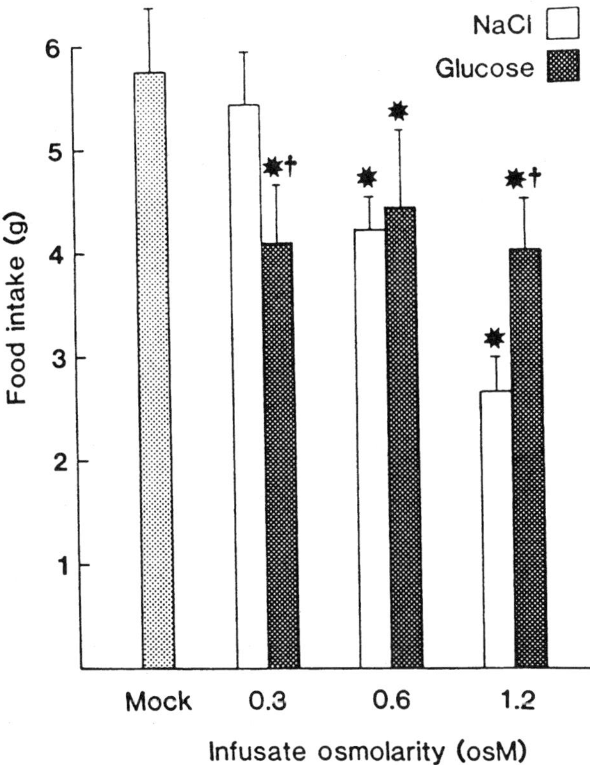

Figure 14 Food intake of rats infused with increasing concentrations of glucose and sodium chloride into the portal vein. *Food intake is significantly different from the control mock infusion. †The two treatments at a single dose differ significantly. There is no dose dependence of glucose infused into the portal vein. (From Ref. 289.)

duced a significant 5- or 10-kcal reduction of food intake but there was no difference in intake between the portal or vena cava infusions (291). Plasma levels of glucose or amino acids passing through the liver would be very different in these rats because only ~20% of cardiac output goes directly to the liver. Thus, the elevation of infused glucose passing through the liver would be five times greater in the portal than in the vena cava–infused rats. This result suggests that the liver does not sense the total amount of glucose absorbed from the intestine and use this information to control daily intake.

One way to assess the role of the liver in the control of meal intake is to allow a substantial amount of water-soluble nutrient to pass through the hepatic sinusoids and see whether the nutrient has a direct effect on food intake during a single meal. This objective can be achieved by feeding one rat in the two-way crossed-intestines rat pairs, a symmetrical preparation in which a 30-cm segment of each rat's intestine is connected to the intestine of its partner (see Fig. 9). This preparation was described above (under intestinal signals), but can be briefly described again to explore its implications for the role of the liver in the control of short-term food intake. Following this surgery, either rat in the pair has its ingested food move into its own stomach, pass through its upper duodenum, and then travel into the crossed segment of its partner's intestine at a level just below the bile duct (94,284). Some of each rat's ingested food will be digested in the partner's upper small intestine and absorbed into the partner's bloodstream, and some will continue to travel down the digestive track back into the lower jejunum of the feeding rat. Water-soluble nutrients will be digested in and absorbed from the crossed intestinal segment and will be delivered directly to the portal vein of the partner. The effect of these water-soluble nutrients on the hepatic control of food intake can be assessed in these rats by feeding only one rat of a pair after a 7-hr fast. The rat fed first has a lower delivery of absorbed nutrient into its own bloodstream and less stimulation of the liver by food during the 10 min following the beginning of a meal because its own crossed 30-cm segment of the upper intestine remains unstimulated by food. Nevertheless, its food intake does not increase, but remains at the same level as unfed control rats with no hepatic nutrient stimulation. The partner rat fed 10 or 30 min later has already had its liver stimulated by the absorbed food, but these rats ate the same amount as their partners fed earlier or as control rats without their intestines crossed. In fact, when the absorption of glucose-3H or of amino acids-3H was measured in rat pairs where one of the rats was fed a normal diet with these radioactive tracers, it was found to be significantly higher at 10 min in the rat that had not yet fed and was hungry than in the feeding partner that had completed its meal and was satiated. These results suggest that the passage of water-soluble nutrients through the liver in a physiologically controlled way does not inhibit food intake during meal. The liver does not appear to monitor the amount of absorbed nutrient passing through its sinusoids and use this information to alter meal intake.

An alternative way of testing the capacity of the liver to measure the amount of absorbed nutrient passing through its sinusoids and to use this information to alter food intake is to divert the blood coming from the gut into the systemic circulation before it reaches the liver. This can be done by use of a portacaval shunt. In this surgery, the portal vein is clamped and tied just below the liver. The vein is transected on the gut side of the tie, and the loose end is sutured end-to-side to the ascending vena cava. As a result of this surgery, all of the blood leaving the gut passes directly into the systematic circulation and does not go through the liver on its first pass into the body. The liver is supported only by blood arriving through the hepatic artery, and over the next 10 days it is diminished by 30% in wet weight (292). If the liver were monitoring the total amount of water-soluble nutrient that was entering through the gut and using this information to control food intake, one would predict that the shunted rat would overeat on its first meal after the surgery and would continue to overeat until hepatic signals to the brain had adjusted for the reduced caloric load passing through the hepatic artery. In fact, it was found that the rats ate 3.6 ± 0.7 kcal on their first meal compared to 6.2 ± 1.6 kcal for the controls ($P = .18$). These results did not change in subsequent meals. During the first night, the portacaval shunted rats ate an average meal size of 5.1 ± 2.4 kcal while the controls ate 5.5 ± 1.9 kcal ($p = .90$). The shunted rats also ate 7.4 ± 1.7 meals while the controls ate 8.1 ± 2.2 meals ($p = .80$). During the next 8 days of recovery, the shunted rats tended to eat less than controls and they lost somewhat more weight (see Figs. 15, 16). These results show that the shunted rats ate less food than controls even though their livers were deprived of contact with some of the absorbed nutrient. Some of the absorbed food would pass from gut to muscle or adipose tissue without ever coming into contact with the liver. An increase in food intake by shunted rats would be predicted by a theory that argues that the liver measures or monitors the total

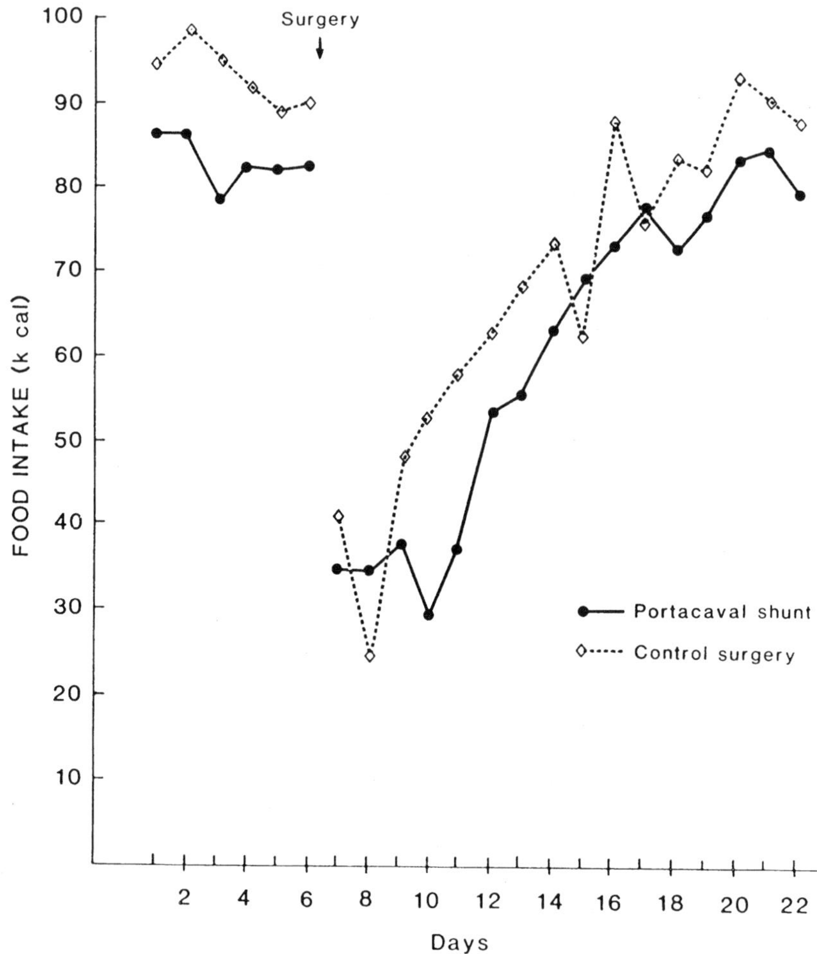

Figure 15 Daily food intake of rats provided with a portacaval shunt or given sham surgery. Measurements of meal patterns were made on the first day after surgery and during the last 6 days, when the rats had returned to the baseline intake.

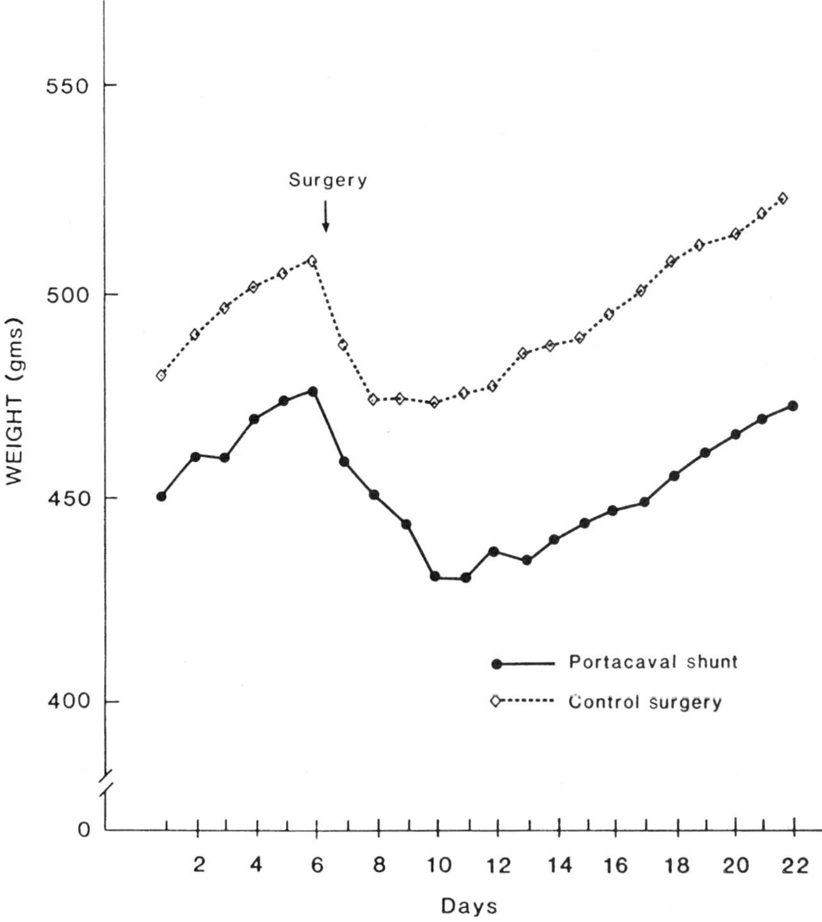

Figure 16 Body weight of rats with either portacaval shunt or sham surgery. Rats with the portacaval shunt lose more weight after surgery, but their subsequent weight gain is comparable to that of controls.

amount of exogenous water-soluble food arriving from the gut and sends a message that controls food intake.

To make sure that we were testing rats at their best performance, measurements were also made of meal patterns during the last 6 days of the study when the rat's daily food intake and rate of body weight gain had stabilized for both the shunted and controls rats (154). The rat's first meal after a 7-hr fast was 10.7 ± 1.4 kcal in shunted rats and 10.8 ± 1.2 kcal in controls (p = .98). For their average meal during the day, the shunted rats ate 5.1 ± 0.5 kcal while controls rats ate 5.9 ± 0.8 kcal (p = .26). Their number of meals were 15.8 ± 1.6 versus 14.7 ± 1.0, respectively (p = .70). Clearly, the food intake of the shunted rats was not larger than and, in fact, not significantly different from, that of controls. This results suggested that the liver does not use information that it may obtain about the amount of absorbed food passing through it to control food intake.

Russek has argued that the diversion of the blood away from the liver through the use of a portacaval shunt does not change the stimulation of the liver by absorbed food: within one circulation time, he argues, the absorbed nutrients have passed into the hepatic artery and elevated plasma levels (293). However, in shunted rats, a substantial amount of the absorbed nutrient will never pass through the liver. Some portion of the absorbed glucose and amino acids will go directly from the systematic circulation to muscle, fat, and other tissues and will be taken up by these tissues before it can ever reach the liver. Thus, the liver fails to have contact with the full amount of water-soluble nutrient absorbed from the intestine in these portacaval shunted rats and, therefore, should not be able to assess the total content of absorbed nutrient.

These last two studies show that the liver does not determine the amount of absorbed nutrient and pass this information to the brain to control food intake. In the first study, there was a physiological delivery of a substantial amount of nutrient from the upper small intestine into the portal vein leading directly to the liver. This delivery over a period of 10, 30, or 60 min did not reduce food intake and, in fact, had no effect upon the size of the first meal after a 7-hr fast. In the second study, the diversion of the nutrient-containing portal blood away from the liver did not cause an increase in the first meal after the surgery, in the meals throughout the first day, in the first meal after a 7-hr fast over the last 6 days or in the meals taken throughout a 6-day period when daily food intake and body weight gain had stabilized 10 days after the surgery. Thus, both studies show that the liver does not monitor the amount of absorbed food and convey that information to the brain to alter food intake.

Although the liver does not appear to sense the total amount of nutrient absorbed from the gut, it could be involved in relaying information to the brain about metabolic changes taking place in the body, such as the type of nutrient being used for fuel or the fasting-refeeding state. This information may influence and alter food intake. If the liver were involved in the control of food intake, it would need to send messages to the brain to produce a change. These messages would have to be sent by nerves or through the bloodstream. A partial denervation, hepatic vagotomy, has been done in free-feeding rats and produced mixed results. Friedman and Sawchenko (294) found a shift in the day/night rhythm with increased feeding during the day and reduced feeding at night. There was a small change in daily intake but only in male rats. On the other hand, Del Prete and Scharrer (295,296) have shown that hepatic vagotomy caused no change in day/night feeding but the pattern of daytime feeding was altered. These are relatively minor effects of partial denervation of the liver. When a total hepatic denervation is done, the changes in meal pattern completely disappear (297, 298, 299, 300). A recent liver transplant study showed only a small night-time decrease in daily intake in liver-denervated and transplant rats (298). Thus, hepatic denervations appear to have little effect on spontaneous food intake, and the hepatic nerves are not much involved in the control of meal patterns. On the other hand, hepatic vagotomies have been shown to affect food intake when intake is altered by external treatments, such as infusion of total parenteral nutrition (301) or glucagon (140). Thus, hepatic nerves may play a role in unusual, external challenges, but they do not have much of a role in the normal control of food intake. The other possible way in which the liver could inform the brain about peripheral changes in metabolism is by the release of some humoral factor. The type and quantity of food eaten has an effect on the release of somatomedins or insulinlike growth factors that alter metabolism and enhance growth (302). A specific inhibitor of food intake secreted from the liver has not been identified, but remains a possibility.

XIV METABOLIC SIGNALS

Although the liver does not seem to monitor the amount of water-soluble nutrient passing through it from the gut and use this information to control intake, it still responds to changes in the plasma levels of glucose, amino acids, and fats by removing or releasing these nutrients to maintain their blood levels within a well-defined range. That the liver can release glucose in the blood has been known since the days of Claude Bernard. In fact, the liver and various regulatory hormones are very effective in maintaining plasma glucose levels: they are able to substantially limit the surge in plasma glucose that follows a CHO meal and to maintain plasma glucose levels even under conditions involving extensive exercise when glucose is rapidly being used by the muscles (303). Thus, the liver could acquire some information about the flow of energy through the body without having to monitor the total amount of absorbed nutrient.

It is possible that the liver or some other tissue in the body monitors the plasma levels of the macronutrients and sends this information to the brain to alter food intake. Indeed, there are many theories that claim that plasma nutrient levels are important in the control of food intake. The early version of the "glucostatic" theory stated that elevated plasma levels of glucose inhibit food intake (304,305). When it was noted that diabetic rats had very high plasma glucose levels and were nevertheless hyperphagic, the theory was modified to claim that the use of glucose by the tissues, which produced an arteriovenous (A-V) difference in plasma glucose, controlled daily food intake (305,306). Because increased levels of plasma insulin are needed to generate an A-V difference in plasma glucose levels in peripheral tissues, the glucostatic theory has been closely associated with a theory that insulin inhibits food intake (see section on Pancreatic Hormones above). One argument against the glucostatic theory is that a meal of meat, which contains mostly protein and fat, is highly satiating, suggesting that regulation of glucose transport into cells cannot be the only mechanism involved in control of meal intake. Grossman and associates have reported that the short-term injection of glucose into veins or the peritoneal cavity in calorically significant amounts had no greater effect on the food intake of dogs than a control saline injection, but no evaluation of A-V differences was made (307,308).

In a complementary approach, the "aminostatic" theory states that increased levels of plasma amino acids are associated with decreased appetite in man (309). Amino acid levels were found to vary inversely with ratings of hunger. A major amount argument against the aminostatic theory is that increased protein content of the diet leads to substantially lower levels of plasma amino acids but no major increase in food intake (310,311). Thus, amino acid levels themselves are unlikely to control food intake. The final classic theory, the "lipostatic" theory, states that the amount of body fat controls daily food intake (312) and will be discussed in greater detail under Storage Signals.

One way of testing whether metabolic signals control food intake is to infuse nutrients directly into the bloodstream and to determine whether the infusion reduces daily food intake. Such an infusion bypasses the gut and tests the relevance of specific nutrients for the reduction of daily food intake. All relevant studies have shown that the slow, chronic infusion of nutrients into the bloodstream produces a substantial reduction of daily food intake (313–316). These studies show that the presence of these nutrients in the bloodstream or the metabolic consequences of their uptake into the body's tissues generates a signal that feeds back to the brain to inhibit feeding behavior. Each of these nutrients has its own specific effect on daily food intake (317) (see Fig. 17). If 34 kcal of glucose is infused slowly and continuously over a 17-hr feeding period, the rats show a reduction of intake in 1 day that is equivalent to 55% of the calories infused. When the infusion stops, the rats return in 1 day to their previous baseline levels of intake. In contrast, infusion of 10 or 20 kcal of an amino acid mixture causes a complete reduction of intake relative to the number of calories infused. Daily food intake is decreased during the first day of infusion and returns within a day to normal at the end of the infusion. Finally, infusion of 20 or 40 kcal of IV lipid has no significant effect on daily food intake during the first day and, then, provokes a gradual reduction over 2–3 days that stabilizes at a lower level after 4–6 days. The long-term compensation averaged only 42% of the calories infused, showing that IV lipid was the least effective in reducing voluntary food intake. When the infusion ceased, daily food

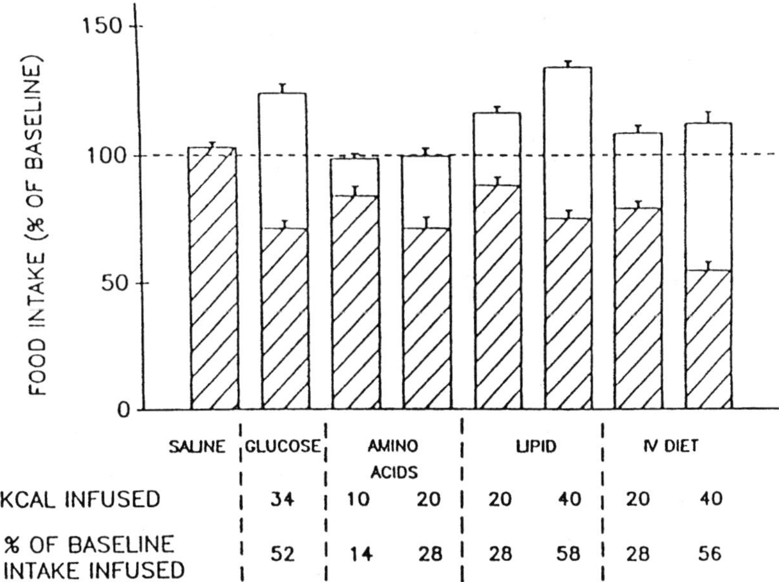

Figure 17 Average daily food and energy intake of rats infused intravenously with saline, glucose, amino acids, lipids, and an IV diet that had the same composition as the oral diet. Slashed bars are the voluntary daily food intake; open bars are the total number of calories infused. The total height of the bar is the total amount of calories ingested and infused. Rats show a 50% compensation for glucose and lipids, nearly complete compensation for amino acids, and 75–80% compensation for the IV diet. (From Ref. 317.)

intake barely increased on the first day and then rose very slowly over the next several days showing that the pattern of response to fat infusion was greatly delayed and very different from the patterns resulting from the infusion of the water-soluble macronutrients. Since the infusion of each of these macronutrients separately might lead to a less than complete compensation because of a change in the relative amounts of the macronutrients available to the tissues, we also included an infusion condition in which all of the nutrients were infused in the same proportion as the nutrients in the diet. Infusion of 20 and 40 kcal of IV diet produced reductions of daily food intake that were ~ 77% of the calories infused. In short, there was a better adjustment for all three nutrients together than for the sum of the nutrients infused separately (317,318). The body was responding partly to the altered macronutrient composition of the infusate. In addition, the infusion of all three nutrients did not produce full compensation showing that either signals originating in the gut or signals associated with the circadian pattern of food delivery were important in providing the full signal for the inhibition of food intake. One study showed that the circadian infusion pattern was important, with infusion during the normal feeding hours being the most effective in reducing daily intake (319).

All of the infusion studies show that the presence of the infused nutrients in the blood or their metabolism and storage in the tissues provides the major signal that controls daily food intake. These infusions of nutrients cause a reduction in food intake without there being a concomitant change in metabolic rate. When glucose is infused into the vena cava, the rats show an immediate reduction of daily food intake, but metabolic rate remains the same (320). There is, of course, a shift in respiratory quotient which reflects the increase in the amount of glucose that is being burned by the tissue. There is also a small increase in metabolic rate on the fourth day of glucose infusion, when there has been a sustained increase in carbohydrate calories delivered to the body, but the increase in metabolic rate was only 5% of baseline levels. On the other hand, when fat is infused in the form of an intravenous intralipid, there were gradual changes in food intake but no change in metabolic rate before, during, or after the infusion. Even if infusion of nutrients doesn't change metabolic rate, it leads to the deposit of excess calories in body fat (321).

Since the infusion of nutrients into the bloodstream is a very effective way of reducing daily food intake, there must be one or several sites within the body where the infused food is translated into a signal that is sent to the brain to alter food intake. One of the most likely sites for the measurement of plasma levels of nutrients would be the brain itself. Several studies have shown that there are neurons in the ventromedial and lateral hypothalamus that are responsive to glucose and amino acids as well as insulin and other hormones (322). These neurons could sense the plasma levels of these nutrients or hormones and use this information to initiate and control the feeding behavior of the animal. To test the role of these brain sensors in the control of daily intake, infusions of glucose or amino acids were made directly into the internal carotid artery (323). Infusions of water soluble nutrients directly into the carotid artery would greatly elevate their plasma levels during the first pass of blood through the brain, because the infused nutrients are diluted into the 2–3% of the cardiac output that goes to the rat brain. The infusions are made continuously for 24 hr. Calculations based on blood flows show that plasma glucose levels in the brain should be increased by 44 mg% above background, which was confirmed by direct glucose measurements made in the jugular vein. Once the blood with the infused nutrients has passed through the brain, it gets diluted by other blood entering from the descending and ascending vena cava and has a nutrient composition that is the same as the nutrient content after nutrient infusion directly into the vena cava, which is the control comparison condition. This study found that the rats with carotid infusions of glucose and amino acids showed the same reduction of food intake as rats with vena cava infusions. Therefore, substantially elevated glucose or amino acid levels in the blood flowing through the brain did not alter food intake any more than when the same nutrients were infused into the vena cava and diluted in the total volume of blood before reaching the brain. Plasma levels of glucose and amino acids flowing through the brain do not appear to alter food intake.

Another way to assess the effects of nutrients on the control of daily food intake is to draw nutrients that have already been absorbed out of the bloodstream. This can be done with the cross-circulated rats described above (see Fig. 12). One rat in a cross-circulated pair can be deprived of food for 4 days while the food intake of its partner is observed. If nutrients are important in the control of daily food intake, the feeding rat that loses half of its ingested food into the bloodstream and tissues of its partner should increase its daily food intake. We observed that the rats did not significantly change their food intake for 2 days and, thereafter, increased food intake on the 3rd and 4th day by ~30–40%, which was less than compensatory for the amount of food lost (221). The feeding rats should have doubled their daily food intake to sustain both animals. As a result, the rats lost weight. When food was again available to both rats, the long-term feeding rats reduced their intake to baseline levels on the first day, showing that the rats were capable of sensing increased nutrient content within 1 day.

The overall result suggests that, in cross-circulated rats, a decrease in the blood level of nutrients and the amount of nutrient transferred into tissue fails to be noticed by the mechanism that controls daily intake for 2 days. This result challenges the hypothesis that metabolism controls daily intake. However, it is in conflict with the results from studies using direct nutrient infusion where water-soluble nutrients reduce daily food intake within the first day of infusion (317,318). It is possible that nutrients are more effective in causing a reduction in food intake than in causing food intake to increase. In any case, the cross-circulation studies show that food absorbed from the gut has little effect on meal intake and that daily food intake increases only slowly when plasma metabolites are lost into the bloodstream of the partner of a cross-circulated pair.

Another way to approach the search for a metabolic signal that controls food intake is to block various metabolic pathways and see whether the blockade causes a change in food intake. Since metabolism is very central to the survival of the organism, one has to be careful to select agents that do not make the animal sick or uncomfortable. Indeed, the most convincing metabolic blockers should cause an increase in food intake showing that the agent works specifically on feeding behavior and that the animal is healthy enough to respond to the internal stimulus. A series of studies using metabolic blocking agents have suggested that there are metabolic signals that can alter food intake.

The first metabolic blocker that was shown to cause an increase in food intake was 2-deoxyglucose (2-DG), which is taken up by cells and interferes with glucose utilization (324). 2-DG causes an increase in food intake, activates the sympathoadrenal system, and substantially increases plasma glucose, FFA, epinephrine, and glucagon levels (325 326 327). Small amounts of 2-DG injected into the brain stimulate food intake (328). There are conflicting data about whether 2-DG acts on the liver to reduce food intake. Some studies claim that hepatic branch vagotomy attenuates the effect of peripherally injected 2-DG (329) while others claim that it enhances the feeding response (330). Still others find no effect of hepatic vagotomy (331,332) or total hepatic denervation (333) on 2-DG-induced feeding. The main effect, however, is that slowing down the cellular use of glucose causes increased feeding behavior.

Another blocker, 2,5-anhydro-d-mannitol (2,5-AM), also interferes with glucose metabolism and increases food intake in a dose-dependent manner (334). 2,5-AM inhibits glycogenolysis and gluconeogenesis (335). It also produces a small decrease in plasma glucose and a significant increase in plasma fatty acids, glycerol, and ketone bodies (336). It is as effective in increasing food intake in diabetic as in normal rats, suggesting that elevated blood glucose and low blood insulin levels are not detrimental to its effect. Low doses of 2,5-AM probably act in the liver. When infused intraportally, it has a faster and larger capacity to increase food intake than when infused intravenously. The effects of small doses of 2,5-AM are eliminated by hepatic vagotomy, although higher doses are still effective in increasing food intake. 2,5-AM also affects metabolism: it causes an increase in metabolic rate during the first hour after injection but has no long-lasting effect on whole body energy expenditure. It does lower RQ with a decrease in carbohydrate metabolism and an increase in fatty acid oxidation (337). 2,5-AM lowers hepatic ATP, which may provide a signal that increases food intake (338). On the other hand, infusion of 100% TPN reduces food intake by 85%, but there are no associated changes in hepatic ATP or ATP-to-Pi ratio. Thus, this ratio doesn't seem to control food intake during intravenous infusions of nutrients (339). On the 5th day of this study, voluntarily daily food intake increased considerably but there still no changes in hepatic ATP.

There are also a couple of inhibitions of fatty acid metabolism that cause an increase in food intake. Mercaptoacetate (MA) causes an increase in food intake during the day in rats fed a high-fat diet but not a low-fat diet (340). MA impairs mitochondrial beta-oxidation of fatty acids (341) and causes elevation of plasma free fatty acids, no change in plasma glucose, and a reduction of the ketone, 3-hydroxybutyrate (340). The effects of MA can be blocked by subdiaphragmatic vagotomy and by capsaicin destruction of vagal afferents (331), suggesting that the effects of MA are transmitted through the vagus nerve. MA activates the sympathetic nervous system and increases plasma levels of norepinephrine, fatty acids, and glucose (327).

Another fatty acid oxidation inhibitor, methyl palmoxirate (MP), also causes an increase in food intake (342). MP lowers fatty acid oxidation by inhibiting carnitine palmitoyltransferase I, which transports long-chain fatty acids into mitochondria (343). It elevates plasma free fatty acids and glycerol while lowering ketone bodies (344). MP also interacts with 2-DG which blocks glucose utilization to cause an increase in food intake at doses that are not effective when only MP was given (see Fig. 18). MP causes an increase in food intake when the rats are fed a high-fat diet rich in long-chain fats but not when they are fed a high-fat diet rich in medium-chain fats (345). Neither MP nor 2-DG alone or together was able to cause an increase in food intake in Syrian hamsters (346).

That these metabolic blockers are effective in increasing food intake does not necessarily imply that the metabolites with which they interfere are normally involved in the control of meal size, meal patterns, or daily food intake. It is clear from the studies cited above that several metabolic blockers act in a specific way to elevate food intake, but they also put unusual stress on the animal and, in the process, elevate stress hormones (327). It is certainly possible that these metabolic blockers could elevate food intake by activating an infrequently used escape pathway that is present only for unusual circumstances when it is necessary to rapidly boost plasma metabolite levels. Food intake may be

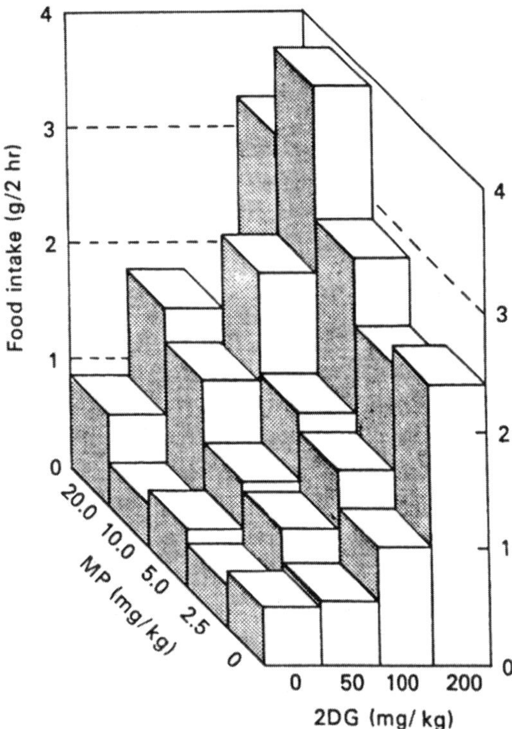

Figure 18 Two-hour food intake of rats injected with the combination of 2-deoxy-d-glucose (2-DG), an antimetabolite for glucose, and methyl palmoxirate (MP), an inhibitor of fatty acid oxidation. The drugs given together have a much larger effect than either alone on increasing food intake. (From Ref. 344.)

initiated as a last resort whenever metabolites fall to very low levels at some regulating site. After all, when other sources of metabolic fuel fail, feeding will provide some rapidly absorbed nutrient (20), and can contribute to maintaining an adequate metabolic rate. However, sudden reductions in the availability of metabolic fuels are not common in animals, and most meals are eaten in a relatively relaxed state without metabolic stress. The increase of food intake provoked by metabolic blockers may provide more of an escape from a severe metabolic deficit than a regular mechanism for the control of food intake.

XV STORAGE SIGNALS

Early studies by a number of investigators have shown that body weight is regulated. If an animal is force-fed to obesity, it will, when given free access to food, reduce its food intake and return its body weight back toward normal levels (1). In contrast, when an animal is starved or its food intake is restricted, it will slowly lose weight, but, when it is given food as lib again, it will increase its daily food intake and decrease its energy expenditure to bring its body weight back up toward normal levels (347). Since the major change in these overfed or underfed animals is the amount of stored fat, several investigators have argued that there is some internal mechanism that measures the amount of body fat and that adjusts food intake and energy expenditure to bring body fat back to its usual level. Unfortunately, these studies show only the presence of internal regulation; they do not show where or how a corrective signal is generated and transmitted. Indeed, as mentioned in the Introduction, the overfeeding or underfeeding of an animal causes changes in the stimulation of the GI tract, in delivery of soluble nutrient to the liver, in the metabolic pathways that are used by the body, and in the short- or long-term storage of nutrients in various tissues. The response to any of these changes could be responsible for bringing food intake and body weight back to normal levels.

The idea that body fat could control food intake was first proposed by Kennedy as a result of his studies on weight change after VHM lesions. The "lipostatic" theory states that the amount of body fat controls daily food intake in some way (312). However, the theory doesn't specify the nature of the signal system that brings body weight back to normal. It could be a metabolite, such as a fatty acid or glycerol, or a hormone released by adipose tissue or a chalone, defined as a negative humoral feedback signal controlling tissue size.

A number of theorists have tested the role of glycerol by injecting it subcutaneously (SC) or intracerebrally (IC). Glycerol has received considerable attention because glycerol is released by adipose tissue during lipolysis in a one-to-one relationship with the breakdown of stored triglyceride. It is also released in an amount that is directly proportional to the amount of body fat and to adipocyte size (348,349). When injected SC or IC, it causes a reduction of food intake and a decrease in body weight (350). Glycerol has been fed to rats and causes a somewhat more than compensatory reduction of food intake (351,352), but high levels of glycerol in the diet are highly unusual and adaptation to a new diet would necessarily take time. Only one study has infused glycerol into the bloodstream to try to mimic plasma levels and investigate its effect on daily intake. Glick found in 1980 that a 1-day intra-arterial infusion of glycerol caused a reduction of daily intake that was three times the amount of calories infused (351). If his results are accurate, they argue for a role for glycerol in the control of daily intake. These results, however, have not been replicated.

One way to study the role of body fat in the control of food intake is to remove some of the fat in one group of rats and see whether these rats adjust their food intake and energy expenditure to bring body fat back to normal levels. Two studies have found that lean rats that have the inguinal and epididymal fat pads removed will bring their total amount of body fat back to control levels in 3–6 weeks (353,354). Only one of these studies measured food intake under very special conditions in which Osborne-Mendel rats were fed a high-fat diet that tended to make the rats obese. The reduction in the amount of body fat did not produce an immediate increase in food intake, as one might expect if the amount of body fat were directly inhibiting food intake. Instead, the investigators found that after ~ 20 days of rapid weight gain, the lipectomized rats began to reduce their daily food intake relative to controls (353). It was clear that it took several weeks to change their food intake due to the loss of body fat. Indeed, the reduction of intake after 20 days may have resulted from a decreased capacity for storage: these high-fat-fed, lipectomized rats had large fat cells that were the same size as those of the controls on the same high-fat diet, but had less body fat at postmortem. The fat cells may have reached a maximum size which led on to an earlier reduction of food intake in lipectomized rats. Another study did lipectomy of inguinal, retroperitoneal, and epididymal fat pads or sham-surgery in ground squirrels just before they began their increase in body weight prior to hibernation (355). The authors found that 4 months later there was no difference in body composition and no significant change in cumulative food intake in the lipectomized squirrels relative to sham controls. Indeed, the lipectomized ground squirrels ate slightly less food and gained slightly more weight than their sham controls, but neither result was significant. Again, this study shows some regulation of body fat, but no necessary connection between changes in body fat and changes in food intake.

Many studies have shown that the energy balance regulating mechanism has the most difficulty recognizing the caloric content of fat: people eating high-fat diets tend to gain weight, and low-fat diets help them to diet and lose weight (356). These well-established phenomena are probably due to their body's inability to recognize fully the fat calories in their diets. The lipid infusion studies (cited above under Metabolic Signals) have shown that the adjustment to intravenous body fat is slow and incomplete with rats reducing their daily food intake by only 42% of the calories infused after 4 days of slow adjustment (317). A more recent study has shown that both intragastric and intravenous infusion of glucose was more effective in reducing food intake than the same caloric amount of fat (70% compared to 40% of calories infused, respectively) (357). Intragastric infusion caused a greater reduction of intake than intravenous infusion for both macronutrients. Control rats overate on a high-fat diet by 25 kcal/day (compared to a baseline intake of ~ 77 kcal). These studies suggest that there is not as good a satiety mechanism for the fat component of the diet as for the water-soluble macronutrients regardless of route of delivery.

Another possible way in which food intake could be disconnected from the amount of body fat is through the deposition of ingested fat into adipose tissue before it is noticed by the food intake regulating system. The ingested or infused fat could be transferred into fat or muscle by an enzyme, lipoprotein lipase (LPL), present on the capillary linings of these (358,359) and other tissues, such as mammary glands (360), before the food's caloric value has been recognized. This theory actually assumes that once circulating metabolites are moved into storage tissues, they are no longer recognized as having been ingested. It also postulates that activation of LPL should lead to overeating and obesity (358,359). The expression of LPL in adipose tissue is controlled and elevated by increased plasma insulin levels (361,362), which, in the context of this theory, suggests that insulin should increase rather than decrease food intake (see discussion in Pancreatic Hormones above). Greenwood (363) has argued that lipoprotein lipase acts as a gate keeper, directing ingested fat into adipose tissue and away from other issues. She claims that the level of adipose tissue LPL activity could alter feeding behavior in both rodents and man by sequestering some of the ingested fat away from organs that might sense the amount of ingested food. One piece of supportive evidence is that there are elevated LPL levels in young fatty (fa/fa) rats before they become hyperphagic and hyperinsulinemic (364). We now know that these rats are leptin receptor deficient. Furthermore, obese women have been found to have 3.5 times the level of adipose tissue LPL than age-matched leans (365). Even after the loss of 13 kg, or about half of their excess weight, the obese women's level of LPL in adipose tissue was still three times higher than that of their lean counterparts, suggesting that elevated LPL might move some of the ingested fat into adipose tissue and thereby maintain their obesity.

The idea that the fat component of ingested food might be moved into adipose tissue before it can be sensed by food intake regulating mechanisms has become a central component of another theory of the metabolic control of food intake (366,367). Friedman claims that the oxidation of metabolic fuels in the liver generates a signal that controls feeding behavior. If ingested food bypasses these oxidative pathways, which he believes take place in the liver, then this food will not be noticed by the regulating system. He believes that changes in the intramitochondrial oxidation of metabolic fuels govern feeding behavior (368). If fuel is partitioned so that more fuel moves into adipose tissue, less fuel will be available for oxidation and the excess fat moved into adipose tissue will thus not be noticed by the system that regulates food intake. One problem with this "oxidation" theory is that the intravenous infusion of either glucose or fat into rats produces large changes in daily food intake but no measurable changes in the overall metabolic rate (320). Both of these theories are in conflict with theory that leptin release from adipose tissue is a major controller of daily food intake and body weight (see next section).

XVI ANIMAL MODELS OF OBESITY AND NEW PEPTIDE REGULATORS

Another way to gain insight into the control of the amount of body fat is to investigate the characteristics of genetically obese mice and rats. There are several strains of obese mice including ob/ob, db/db, agouti, tubby, and fat, as well as several strains of obese rats, fatty (fa/fa), corpulent, and OLETF (120,369,370). All of these obese rodent strains occur because of the presence of a recessive gene that leads to obesity. The ob/ob and db/db mice have many characteristics in common: hyperphagia, hyperglycemia, hyperinsulinemia, and marked obesity. ob/ob mice are infertile and have difficulty maintaining body temperature under cold stress (371). The first attempt to understand the physiological signal system that was responsible for the genetic obesity that was occurring in these obese rodents was done with parabiotic mice. Coleman surgically connected combinations of ob/ob, db/db, and normal mice together into parabiotic pairs to see whether the slow exchange of blood through the parabiotic union would lead to changes in food intake and body weight (372). Parabiotic connections of two normal, two ob/ob, or two db/db mice produced pairs that grew well and exhibited no changes in intake. In contrast, when db/db mice were connected to either normal or ob/ob mice, these latter mice reduced their food intake, had reduced plasma insulin and glucose levels, and continually lost weight. Some of these normal or ob/ob partners eventually became so thin that they apparently died from malnutrition and starvation. Coleman hypothesized that the db/db mice produced a bloodborne satiety factor that the db/db mice themselves could not sense, but which inhibited the food intake of their partners and led to their slow emaciation. In addition, Coleman found that when normal mice were parabiosed with ob/ob mice, the ob/ob mice reduced their food intake and rate of growth, suggesting that normal mice also produced a satiety factor which was lacking in ob/ob mice. In short, Coleman concluded that the ob/ob mice failed to produce an effective bloodborne satiety factor and that db/db mice failed to sense its presence. With unusual prescience, Coleman thought that the genetic defect in db/db mice might be caused by a deficient sensor in the hypothalamus.

Several investigations have used molecular biology techniques to explore the character of the ob gene. These interesting studies have shown that the ob gene codes for an mRNA that is present in adipose tissue and this mRNA translates into a protein that is released into the bloodstream. Several studies have shown that when this protein, called leptin, has been injected ip into mice, there is a large reduction in food intake and body weight (see Fig. 19). These reductions are most striking in ob/ob mice that don't make a functional protein themselves, but they also occur in normal mice (67). ob/ob mice normally have a lower body temperature and lower metabolic rate, but injection of leptin brings these values back up to normal levels, showing that leptin is working

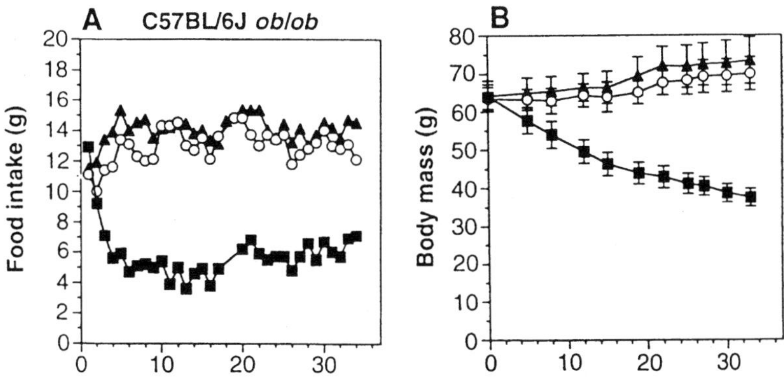

Figure 19 Food intake and body weight of ob/ob mice given a daily IP injection of ob protein for 34 days. ■, rats receiving 5 μg/g/day of ob protein; ○ and ▲, rats receiving vehicle or no treatment. Similar treatment of db/db mice produced no effect. (From Ref. 66.)

on both food intake and energy expenditure to bring body weight back to normal. Leptin also lowers serum insulin and glucose, but these effects could easily be the result of the reduced food intake.

As predicted from the parabiotic experiments of Coleman, the injection of leptin into db/db mice had no effect on food intake, showing that the db/db mice do not have a functional receptor for leptin and are thus not affected by the elevated blood leptin levels presumed to be present because of their obesity (66). Studies have shown that there is a splicing error in the processing of the gene of the leptin receptor in db/db mice (373). Leptin receptors have been isolated from the choroid plexus and from the hypothalamus which has a special long form of the receptor. Leptin is released by adipocytes and appears to act on the brain, most probably the hypothalamus. Injection of one-third of the intravenous dose of leptin into the ventricles of ob/ob mice produced similar reductions in food intake, suggesting that a brain region was sensing the presence of leptin (68).

As previously mentioned (see section on Gastric Satiety Signals), leptin has recently been found in endocrine cells of the stomach (59). Plasma leptin levels increase following a meal, and decline before the onset of the next meal (63). There is an increase in plasma leptin levels during the day, with the highest levels in man at night (63,72). The relative proportion of plasma leptin originating from stomach and adipose tissue has not been determined.

Not long after the discovery of an ob gene protein (66), researchers measured the expression of the ob gene mRNA in the adipose tissue of obese and normal human subjects and found that it was elevated in the obese (374,375). More recently, measurements of immunoreactive leptin have been made in the blood of normal and obese humans (376). These investigators found a significant fourfold increase in the serum levels of leptin-like molecules in obese individuals compared to normal weight subjects, and there was a strong positive correlation between serum concentrations of a leptinlike molecule and the percentage of body fat ($r = .85$). It is not clear whether these leptinlike molecules are restraining food intake in these obese patients or are altered and ineffective. When seven these patients were given a low-calorie diet (800 kcal/d), there was a drop in both serum leptinlike material and in the expression of ob mRNA in their adipose tissue. Both of these changes rebounded, in part, when the patients were put on a weight maintenance diet and ate more food.

The physiological triggers of leptin release have been explored by changes in the expression of the ob gene in the adipose tissues of mice and rats. Fasting led to a substantial fall in the ob mRNA in the epididymal fat pad of ob/ob mice, and refeeding brought it back toward normal levels (377). This reults was confirmed in Sprague-Dawley rats and was shown to have a circadian rhythm with the ob gene expression doubling during the 12 hr of dark when the rats were fed (378). Fasting prevented this cyclic fluctuation. A single large injection of insulin (1 IU) into fasted rats led to an increase in ob mRNA expression to the levels of fed controls. Thus, insulin may play some role in ob gene expression and leptin release. Injection of hydrocortisone also led to an increase in ob mRNA and a corresponding decrease in food intake and body weight (379). Although these studies are based only on gene expression and not on blood leptin levels, they suggest that release of leptin may be controlled by hormones as well as by absorbed food.

After the initial discovery of the leptin gene, there was tremendous excitement about the possibility of finding a medical treatment for human obesity by manufacturing a hormone analog of leptin. Some cases of leptin deficiency were discovered in England and Pakistan and were associated with severe human obesity beginning soon after birth (380). These patients were excessively hungry and highly aggressive in obtaining food. A Turkish family with three obese members was also identified with a leptin mutation, but only a small number of patients have been found worldwide with the type of leptin deficiency that occurs in ob/ob mice (381). In contrast, a French family had three female siblings with excessive morbid obesity which was caused by a mutation in the leptin receptor gene, related to the receptor gene defect in db/db mice (382). These sisters had very high plasma leptin levels, reduced growth hormone and thyrotropin levels, and no pubertal development, showing that leptin is involved in many endocrine functions. Although there are only a small number of confirmed cases of mutation of leptin or its receptor in man, leptin is effective in human subjects. In a randomized double-blind placebo-controlled human trial, subjects were given increasing doses of leptin (383). The investigators found that weight loss occurred in a dose-dependent way and that most of the loss was caused by reduced body fat.

The leptin results have provided some validation for the "lipostatic" hypothesis (312) with the identification of a possible blood factor released by adipose tissue and which also inhibits food intake. There are, in fact, several other factors released by adipose cells, but none of these have the same clear-cut relationship to food intake and energy expenditure as leptin (384). Adipose tissue releases a number of complement related factors, such as adipsin or adiponectin, as well as inflammatory cytokines, such as TNFα or IL-6, which have been shown to inhibit food intake when infused into rodents (385) (see section on Cytokine and Inflammatory Peptide Regulators of Food Intake, above). Several other factors are released by fat cells, but only leptin appears to act in a coordinated, physiological way by decreasing food intake and increasing energy expenditure, both of which limit body weight. Although leptin inhibits intake in man, a large amount of data shows elevated leptinlike material in the blood of obese human subjects, who normally eat more and exercise less than their lean counterparts. This contradictory phenomenon has been called leptin resistance and provides a challenge to the belief that leptin normally acts to regulate body weight. Whether blood levels of ob protein are a result of release from stomach or adipose tissue and whether these blood levels are involved in the day-to-day control of food intake and energy expenditure need further exploration.

XVII RELATIONSHIP OF FOOD INTAKE AND OBESITY

Obesity occurs when food intake exceeds energy expenditure for an extended period of time (386). One cause of obesity is the ready availability of a large variety of food. The alluring tastes of attractive foods seem to override the internal signals that normally inhibit food intake. Rats are known to become obese when given an attractive supermarket diet (387,388). Diets that are high in both fat and carbohydrate have been shown to cause overfeeding and weight gain (389,390). This result is also true of modern man.

Mixed meals that have a high fat content tend to cause overeating (390). Meals of high caloric value and high fat content also prevent the oxidation of the fat component of the diet. Fat oxidation is inhibited by carbohydrate-containing meals because the absorbed glucose releases insulin which, at low levels, inhibits fatty acid release (391). Insulin also activates lipoprotein lipase which moves some of the fat into adipose tissue for storage rather than allowing the fat to be transferred to tissues for oxidation (392). In addition, ingested fat is stored at a lower energy cost than is fat synthesized from carbohydrate and protein. The cost of storing fat in adipose tissue is only 3% of the ingested calories while the cost of converting carbohydrate into fat requires 23% of the calories consumed (393). When mice are given an increased percentage of their diet as fat, their body fat content increases and a larger percent of the mice have $>30\%$ of their body composition as fat (394). When human subjects have fat removed from their diet, they lose weight (395). These studies suggest that fat calories are less effective in inhibiting food intake than are carbohydrate or protein calories. This is confirmed in studies in which glucose and lipids were infused intragastrically or intravenously in rats (317,357). The lipid infusion by either route was less effective in the inhibition of daily food intake. One way to counteract a high fat content of the diet is to burn fat calories by exercising (396).

The large increase in the proportion of people in North America who have been identified as obese in the past decade (397) shows that the recent increases in the percentage of body fat are not due to our genes but to our behavior and lifestyle. These observations suggest that the ready accessibility and pleasant taste of the wide variety of foods available in developed countries and their relatively high fat content play a large role in the development of obesity. In addition, the decrease in exercise resulting from desk jobs and television viewing contributes to the reduced calorie output and to the storage of excess energy. A similar phenomenon is seen in laboratory rats that are fed a supermarket diet in a small cage that restricts activity (387). To gain weight, humans and rats must overeat, and most override the internal signals that are normally involved in the control of food intake.

ACKNOWLEDGMENTS

This chapter was supported by grants from NIH and NSERC.

REFERENCES

1. Cohn C, Joseph D. Influence of body weight and body fat on appetite of normal lean and obese rats. Yale J Biol Med 1962; 34:598–607.
2. Anand BK, Brobeck JR. Hypothalamic control of food intake in rats and cats. Yale J Biol Med 1951; 24:123–146.
3. Hoebel BG, Teitelbaum P. Weight regulation in normal and hypothalamic hyperphagic rats. J Comp Physiol Psych 1966; 61:189–193.
4. Teitelbaum P, Epstein AN. The lateral hypothalamic syndrome. Psychol Rev 1962; 69:74–90.
5. Keesey RE, Boyle PC, Kemnitz JW, Mitchel JS. The role of the lateral hypothalamus in determining the body weight set point. In: Novin D, Wyrwicka W, Bray G, ed. Hunger: Basic Mechanisms and Clinical Implications. New York: Raven Press, 1976:243–255.
6. Elmquist JK, Maratos-Flier E, Saper CB, Flier JS. Unraveling the central nervous system pathways underlying responses to leptin. Nat Neurosci 1998; 1:445–50.
7. Leibowitz SF, Hoebel BG. Central regulation of food intake. In: G. Bray and C Bouchard ed. Handbook of Obesity, 2d ed. New York: Marcel Dekker, 2003.
8. Mrosovsky N, Sherry DF. Animal anorexias. Science 1980; 207:837–842.
9. Sherry DF, Mrosovsky N, Hogan JA. Weight-loss and anorexia during incubation in birds. J Comp Physiol 1980; 94:89–94.
10. Wade GN, Schneider JE. Metabolic fuels and reproduction in female mammals. Neurosci Biobehav Rev 1992; 16:235–272.
11. Brobeck, JR. Food intake as a mechanism of temperature regulation. Yale J Biol Med 1947; 20:545–552.
12. Cottle GN, Carlson LD. Adaptive changes in rats exposed to cold. Am J Physiol 1954; 178:305–308.
13. Koopmans HS. Internal signals cause large changes in food intake in crossed-intestines rats. Brain Res Bull 1985; 14:595–603.
14. Koopmans HS, Sclafani A, Fichtner C, Aravich P. The effects of ileal transposition on food intake and body weight loss in VMH obese rats. Am J Clin Nutr 1982; 35:284–293.
15. Collier GH. Satiety: an ecological perspective. Brain Res Bull 1985; 14:693–700.
16. Johnson DF, Ackroff K, Peters J, Collier GH. Changes in the rat's meal patterns as a function of the caloric density of the diet. Physiol Behav 1986; 36:929–936.
17. Booth DA. Conditioned satiety in the rat. J Comp Physiol Psych 1972; 81:457–471.
18. McHugh PR. The control of gastric emptying. J Auton Nerv Syst 1983; 9:221–231.
19. Lin HC, Doty JE, Reedy TJ, Meyer TH. Inhibition of gastric emptying by sodium oleate depends on the length of the intestine exposed to acid. Am J Physiol 1990; 259:G1025–G1030.
20. Steffens AB. Blood glucose and FFA levels in relation to the meal pattern in the normal and the ventromedial hypothalamic lesioned rat. Physiol Behav 1969; 4:215–225.
21. Steffens AB. Plasma insulin content in relation to blood glucose level and meal pattern in the normal and hypothalamic hyperphagic rat. Physiol Behav 1970; 5:147–151.
22. Collier G. Hirsch E, Hamlin PH. The ecological determinants of reinforcement in the rat. Physiol Behav 1972; 9:705–716.
23. Kanarek RB. Availability and caloric density of the diet as determinants of meal patterns in cats. Physiol Behav 1975; 15:611–618.
24. Collier G. The dialogue between the house economist and the resident physiologist. Nutr Behav 1986; 3:9–26.
25. Davis JD, Campbell CS. Peripheral control of meal size in the rat: effect of sham feeding on meal size and drinking rate. J Comp Physiol Psych 1973; 83:379–387.
26. Rosenzweig MR. The mechanisms of hunger and thrist. In: Postman L, ed. Psychology in the Making. New York: Knopf, 1962; 73–143.
27. Hull CL, Livingston JR, Rouse RO, Barker AN. Time, sham, and esophageal feeding as reinforcements. J Comp Physiol Psych 1951; 44:236–245.
28. Janowitz HD, Grossman MI. Some factors affecting the food intake of normal dogs and dogs with esophageostomy and gastric fistulae. Amer J Physiol 1949; 159:143–148.
29. Mook DG. Oral factors in appetite and satiety. Ann NY Acad Sci 1989; 575:265–278.

30. Smith GP, Gibbs J, Young RC. Cholecystokinin and intestinal satiety in the rat. Fed Proc 1974; 33:1146–1149.
31. Scalfani A, Nissenbaum JW. Is gastric sham feeding really sham feeding? Am J Physiol 1985; 248:R387–R390.
32. Grill HJ, Berridge KC, Ganster DJ. Oral glucose is the prime elicitor of preabsorptive insulin secretion. Am J Physiol 1984; 246:R88–95.
33. Plato. The Timeaus of Plato. New York:Arno Press 1973:271.
34. Hunt JN, Stubbs DF. The volume and energy content of meals as determinants of gastric emptying. J. Physiol (Lond) 1975; 245:209–255.
35. Hunt JN. A possible relation between the regulation of gastric emptying and food intake. Am J Physiol 1980; 239:G1–G4.
36. Adolph BK. Urges to eat and drink in rats. Am J Physiol 1947; 151:110–25.
37. Janowitz HD, Grossman MI. Effects of variations in the nutritive density on intake of food in dogs and cats. Am J Physiol 1949; 258:184–193.
38. Tomlin J. The effect of the gel forming liquid fibre on feeding behavior in man. Br J Nutr 1995; 74:427–436.
39. Deutsch JA, Young WG, Kalogeris TJ. The stomach signals satiety. Science 1978; 201:165–167.
40. Deutsch JA, Gonzales MF. Gastric nutrient content signals satiety. Behav Neural Biol 1980; 30:113–116.
41. Deutsch JA. Dietary control and the stomach. Prog Neurobiol 1983; 20: 313–332.
42. Karel L. Gastric absorption. Physiol Rev 1948; 28:433–450.
43. Kaplan JM, Siemers W, Grill HJ. Ingestion, gastric fill and gastric emptying before and after withdrawal of gastric contents. Am J Physiol 1994; 267:R1257–R1265.
44. Seeley RJ, Kaplan JM, Grill HJ. Effect of occluding the pylorus on intraoral intake: a test of the gastric hypothesis of meal termination. Physiol Behav 1995; 58:245–249.
45. Kraly FS, Smith GP. Combined pregastric and gastric stimulation by food is sufficient for normal meal size. Physiol Behav 1978; 21:405–408.
46. Kaplan JM, Spector AC, Grill HJ. Dynamics of gastric emptying during and after stomach fill in the rat. Am J Physiol 1992; 263:R813–R820.
47. Phillips RJ, Powley TL. Gastric volume rather than nutrient content inhibits food intake. Am J Physiol 1996; 271:R766–R796.
48. McHugh PR, Moran TH. Calories and gastric emptying: a regulatory capacity with implications for feeding. Am J Physiol 1979; 236:R254–R260.
49. McHugh PR, Moran TH. Accuracy of the regulation of caloric ingestion in the rhesus monkey. Am J Physiol 1978; 235:R29–R34.
50. McHugh PR, Moran TH, Wirth JB. Postpyloric regulation of gastric emptying in rhesus monkeys. Am J Physiol 1982; 243:R408–R415.
51. Paintal AS. A study of gastric stretch receptors. Their role in the peripheral mechanism of satiation of hunger and thirst. J Physiol (Lond) 1954; 126:255–270.
52. Iggo A. Tension receptors in the stomach and urinary bladder. J Physiol (Lond) 1955; 128:593–607.
53. Phillips RJ, Powley TL. Tension receptors in the gastrointestinal smooth muscle: reevaluating vagal mechanoreceptors electrophysiology. Brain Res Rev 2000; 34:1–26.
54. Wang FB, Powley TL. Topographic inventories of vagal afferents in gastrointestinal muscle. J Comp Neurol 2000; 421:302–324.
55. Gonzalez MF, Deutsch JA. Vagotomy abolishes cues of satiety produced by gastric distension. Science 1981; 212:1283–1284.
56. Kraly FS, Gibbs. Vagotomy fails to block the satiating effect of food in the stomach. Physiol Behav 1990; 24:1007–1010.
57. Koopmans HS. A stomach hormone that inhibits food intake. J Auton Nerv Syst 1983; 6:157–171.
58. Kojima M, Hosoda H, Date Y, Nakazato M, Matsuo H, Kangawa K. Ghrelin is a growth-hormone-releasing acylated peptide from stomach. Nature 1999; 402:656–660.
59. Bado A, Levasseur S, Attoub S, Kermorgant S, Laigneau JP, Bortolussi MN, Moizo L, Lehy T, Guerre-Millo M, Le Marchand-Brustel Y, Lewin MJ. The stomach is a source of leptin. Nature 1998; 394;790–793.
60. Toshinai K, Mondal MS, Nakazato M, Date Y, Murakami N, Kojima M, Kangawa K, Matsukura S. Upregulation of ghrelin expression in the stomach upon fasting, insulin-induced hypoglycemia and leptin administration. Biochem Biophys Research Commun 2001; 281:1220–1225.
61. Date Y, Kojima M, Hosoda H, Sawaguchi A, Mondal A, Sugamauma T, Matsukura S, Kangawa K, Nakazato M. Ghrelin, a novel GH-releasing acylated peptide, is synthesized in a distinct endocrine cell type in the gastrointestinal tracts of rats and humans. Endocrinology 2000; 141:4255–4261.
62. Tschop M, Smiley DL, Heiman ML. Ghrelin induces adiposity in rodents. Nature 2000; 407:908–913.
63. Cummings DE, Purnell JQ, Frayo RS, Schmidova K, Wisse BE, Weigle DS. A preprandial rise in plasma ghrelin levels suggests a role in meal initiation in humans. Diabetes 2001; 50:1714–1719.
64. Wren AM, Small CJ, Ward HL, Murphy KG, Dakin CL, Taheri S, Kennedy AR, Roberts GH, Morgan DGA, Ghatei MA, Bloom SR. The novel hypothalamic peptide ghrelin stimulates food intake and growth hormone secretion Endocrine 2000; 141:4325-4328.
65. Nakazato M, Murakami N, Date Y, Kojima M, Matsuo H, Kangawa K, Matsukura S. A role for

ghrelin in the central regulation of feeding. Nature 2001; 409:194–198.
66. Halaas JL, Gajiwala KS, Maffei M, Cohen SL, Chait BT, Rabinowitz D, Lallone RL, Burley SK, Friedman JM. Weight-reducing effects of the plasma protein encoded by the obese gene. Science 1995; 269:543–546.
67. Pellymounter MA, Cullen MJ, Baker MB, Hecht R, Winters D, Boone T, Collins F. Effects of the obese gene product on body weight regulation in ob/ob mice. Science 1995; 269:540–543.
68. Campfield LA, Smith FJ, Guisez Y, Devos R, Burn P. Recombinant mouse OB protein: evidence for a peripheral signal linking adiposity and central neural networks. Science 1995; 269:546–549.
69. Konturek PC, Brozozowski T, Sulekova Z, Meixner H, Hahn EG, Konturek SJ. Enhanced expression of leptin following acute gastric injury in rat. J Physiol Pharm 1999; 50:587–595.
70. Cinti S DeMatteis R, Pico C, Cerisi E, Obrador A, Maffeis C, Oliver J, Palou A. Secretory granules of endocrine and chief cells of human stomach mucosa contain leptin. Int J Obes 2000; 24:789–793.
71. Sobhani I, Bado A, Vissuzaine C, Buyse M, Kermorgant S, Laigneau JP, Attoub S, Lehy T, Henin D, Mignon M, Lewin MJM. Leptin secretion and leptin receptor in the human stomach. Gut 2000; 47:178–183.
72. Sinha MK, Ohannesian JP, Heiman ML, Kriauciunas A, Stephens TW, Magosin S, Marco C, Caro JF. Nocturnal rise of leptin in lean, obese and non-insulin-dependent diabetes mellitus subjects. J Clin Invest 1996; 97:1344–1347.
73. Mix H, Widjaja A, Jandl O, Cornberg M, Kaul A, Goke M, Beil W, Kuske M, Brabant G, Manns MP, Wagner S. Expression of leptin and leptin receptor isoforms in the human stomach. Gut 2000; 47:481–486.
74. Buyse M, Ovesjo ML, Goiot H, Guilmeau S, Peranzi G, Moizo L, Walker F, Lewin MJM, Meister B, Bado A. Expression and regulation of leptin receptor proteins in afferent and efferent neurons of the vagus nerve. Eur J Neurosci 2001; 14:64–72.
75. Abrahamsson H, Jansson G. Elicitation of reflex vagal relaxation of the stomach from pharynx and esophagus in the cat. Acta Physiol Scand 1969; 28:267–273.
76. Mayer EA. The physiology of gastric storage and emptying. In: Johnson ER, Alpers DH, Christensen J, Jacobson ED, Walsh JH, eds. Physiology of the Gastrointestinal Tract. New York: Raven Press, 1994:929–976.
77. Geliebter A, Westriech S, Pierson RN, Van Itallie TB. Extra-abdominal pressure alters food intake, intragastric pressure and gastric emptying rate. Am J Physiol 1986; 250:R549–R552.
78. Kersten A, Strubbe JH, Spiteri N. Meal patterning of rats with changes in day length and food availability. Physiol Behav 1980; 25;953–958.
79. Van der Velde P, Koslowsky I, Koopmans HS. Measurement of gastric emptying during and between meal intake in free-feeding Lewis rats. Am J Physiol 1999; 276:R597–R605.
80. Moran TH, Knipp S, Schwartz GJ. Gastric and duodenal features of meals mediate controls of liqiud gastric emptying during fill in rhesus monkeys. Am J Physiol 1999; 277:R1282–R1290.
81. Ehman GK, Albert DJ, Jamieson JL. Injections into the duodenum and induction of satiety in the rat. Can J Psych 1971; 25:147–166.
82. Snowdon CT. Production of satiety with small intraduodenal infusions in the rat. J Comp Physiol Psych 1975; 88:231–238.
83. Antin J, Gibbs J, Smith GP. Intestinal satiety requires pregastric food stimulation. Physiol Behav 1977; 18:421–425.
84. Liebling DS, Eisner JD, Gibbs J, Smith GP. Intestinal satiety in rats. J Comp Physiol Psych 1975; 89:955–965.
85. Gibbs J, Madison SP, Rolls ET. Satiety role for the small intestine examined in sham-feeding rhesus monkeys. J Comp Physiol Psych 1981; 95:1003–1015.
86. Sharma KN, Nasset ES. Electrical activity in the mesenteric nerves after perfusion of gut lumen. Am J Physiol 1962; 202:725–730.
87. Mei N. Vagal glucoreceptors in the small intestine of the cat. J Physiol (Lond) 1978; 282:485–506.
88. Jeanningros R. Vagal unitary responses to intestinal amino acid infusions in anesthetized cat: a putative signal for protein satiety. Physiol Behav 1982; 28:9–21.
89. Mei N. Intestinal chemosensitivity. Physiol Rev 1985; 65:211–237.
90. Novin D. The integration of visceral information in the control of feeding. J Auton Nerv Syst 1983; 9:233–246.
91. Yox DP, Ritter RC. Capsaicin attenuates suppression of sham feeding induced by intestinal nutrients. Am J Physiol 1988; 255:R569–R574.
92. Yox DP, Stokesbury PH, Ritter RC. Vagotomy attenuates suppression of sham feeding induced by intestinal nutrients. Am J Physiol 1991; 260:R503–R508.
93. McHugh PR, Moran TH. The inhibition of feeding produced by direct intraintestinal infusion of glucose: is this satiety? Brain Res Bull 1986; 17:415–418.
94. Koopmans HS. The intestinal control of food intake. In: Bray G, ed. Recent Advances in Obesity Research II. London: Newman Publ Ltd, 1978: 33–43.
95. Davenport HW. Physiology of the Digestive Tract. Chicago: Year Book, 1971: 183–210.
96. Louis-Sylvestre J. Preabsorptive insulin release and hypoglycemia in rats. Am J Physiol 1976; 230:56–60.
97. Walsh JH. Gastrointestinal hormones. In: Johnson LR, Albers DH, Christenson J, Jacobson ED, Walsh JH, eds. Physiology of the Gastrointestinal Tract. New York: Raven Press, 1994:1–128.
98. Grossman MI. Trends in gut hormone research. In: Thompson JC, ed. Gastrointestinal Hormones. Austin: University of Texas Press, 1975:3–10.

99. Go VLW, Michner S, Roddy D, Koch M. Clinical relevance of regulatory gastrointestinal peptides, Clin Biochem 1984; 17:82–88.
100. Glick Z, Thomas DW, Mayer J. Absence of effect of injections of the intestinal hormones secretin and cholecystokinin-pancreozymin upon feeding behavior. Physiol Behav 1971; 6:5–8.
101. Koopsman HS, Deutsch JA, Branson PJ. The effect of cholecystokinin pancreozymin on hunger and thirst in mice. Behav Biol 1972; 7:441–444.
102. Gibbs J, Young RC, Smith GP. Cholecystokinin decreases food intake in rats. J Comp Physiol Psych 1973; 84:488–495.
103. Smith GP, Gibbs J, Young RC. Cholecystokinin and intestinal satiety in the rat. Fed Proc 1974; 33:1146–1149.
104. Deutsch JA, Hardy WT. Cholecystokinin produces bait shyness in rats. Nature 1977; 266:196.
105. Shillabeer G, Davison JS. Endogenous and exogenous cholecystokinin may reduce food intake by different mechanism. Am J Physiol 1987; 253:R379–R382.
106. Smith GP, Jerome C, Cushin BJ, Eterno R, Simansky KJ. Abdominal vagotomy blocks the satiety effect of cholecystokinin in the rat. Science 1981; 213:1036–1037.
107. Lorenz DN, Goldman SA. Vagal mediation of the cholecystokinin satiety effect in rats. Physiol Behav 1982; 29:599–604.
108. Reidelberger RD. Abdominal vagal mediation of the satiety effects of exogenous and endogenous cholecystokinin in rats. Am J Physiol 1992; 263:R1354–R1358.
109. Reidelberger RD, Kalogeris TJ, Soloman TE. Plasma CCK levels after food intake and infusion of CCK analogs that inhibit feeding in dogs. Am J Physiol 1989; 256:R1148–R1154.
110. Reidelberger RD, Varga G, Rosenquiest GL, Liehr RM, Wong H, Walsch JH. Comparative effects of CCK monoclonal antiboby on food intake and pancreatic exocrine secretion in rats. Int J Obes 1991; 15:12.
111. Hewson G, Leighton RG, Hughes J. The cholecystokinin receptor antagonist L364,718 increases food intake in the rat by attenuation of the action of endogenous cholecystokinin. Br J Pharm 1988; 93:79–84.
112. Dourish CT, Rycroft W, Iverson SD. Postponement of satiety by blockade of brain cholecystokinin (CCK-B) receptors. Science 1989; 245:1509–1511.
113. Reidelberger RD, O'Rourke MF. Potent cholecystokinin antagonist L364,718 stimulates food intake in rats. Am J Physiol 1989; 257:R1512–R1518.
114. Davison JS, Clarke GD. Mechanical properties and sensitivity to CCK of vagal gastric slowly adapting mechanoreceptors. Am J Physiol 1988; 255:G55–G60.
115. Schwartz GJ, Mchugh PR, Moran TH. Integration of vagal afferent responses to gastric loads and cholecystokinin in rats. Am J Physiol 1991; 261:R64–R69.
116. Reidelberger RD. Cholecystokinin and control of food intake. J Nutr 1994; 124:1327S–1333S.
117. Corwin RL, Gibbs J, Smith GP. Increased food intake after type A but not type B cholecystokinin receptor blockade. Physiol Behav 1991; 50:255–258.
118. Moran TH, Ameglio PJ, Schwartz GJ, McHugh PR. Blockade of type A, not type B, CCK receptors attenuates satiety actions of exogenous and endogenous CCK. Am J Physiol 1992; 262:R46–R50.
119. Lorenz DN, Kreielsheimer G, Smith GP. Effect of cholecystokinin, gastrin, secretin and GIP on sham feeding in the rat. Physiol Behav 1979, 23:1065–1072.
120. Kawano K, Hirashima T, Mori S, Saitoh Y, Kurosumi M, Natori T. Spontaneous long-term hyperglycemic rat with diabetic complications: Otsuka Long-Evans Tokushima Fatty (OLETF) strain. Diabetes 1992; 41:1422–1428.
121. Bi S, Ladenheim EE, Schwartz GJ, Moran TH. A role for NPY overexpression in the dorsomedial hypothalamus in hyperphagia and obesity of OLETF rats. Am J Physiol 2001; 281:R254–R260.
122. Gibbs J, Fauser DJ, Rowe EA, Rolls BJ, Rolls ET, Maddison SP. Bombesin suppresses feeding in rats. Nature 1979; 282:208–210.
123. Gibbs J, Kulkosky PJ, Smith GP. Effects of peripheral and central bombesin on feeding behavior in rats. Peptides 1981; 2(S2):179–183.
124. Ghatei MA, Jung RT, Stevenson JC, Hilllyard CJ, Adrian TE, Lee YC, Christofides ND, Sarson DL, Mashiter K, MacIntyre I, Bloom SR. Bombesin: action on gut hormones and calcium in man. J Clin Endocrinol Metab 1982; 54:980–985.
125. Gibbs J, Kulkosky J, Smith GP. Effects of peripheral and central bombesin on feeding behavior of rats. Peptides 1981; 2(S2):179–183.
126. Stuckey JA, Gibbs J, Smith GP. Neural disconnection of gut from brain blocks bombesin-induced satiety. Peptides 1985; 6:1249–1252.
127. Plamondon H, Merali Z. Push-pull perfusion reveals meal-dependent changes in the release of bombesin-like peptides in the rat paraventricular nucleus. Brain Res 1994; 668:54-61.
128. Motamedi F, Rashidy-Pour A, Zarrindast MR, Bavadi M. Bombesin-induced anorexia requires central bombesin receptor activation: independence from interaction with central catecholinergic systems. Psychopharmacology 1993; 110:193–197.
129. Laferrere B, Leroy F, Bonhomme G, Le Gall A, Basdevat A, Guy-Grand B. Effects of bombesin, of a new bombesin agonist (B1M187) and a new antagonist (B1M189) on food intake in rats, in relation to cholecystokinin. Eur J Pharm 1992; 215:23–28.
130. Racke K, Schworer H. Regulation of serotonin release from the intestinal mucosa. Pharm Res 1991; 23: 13–25.
131. Blackshaw LA, Grundy D. Effects of 5-hydroxytrypt-

amine on discharge of vagal mucosal receptors from the upper gastrointestinal tract of the ferret. J Auton Nerv Syst 1993; 45:41–50.

132. Hillsley K, Grundy D. Serotonin and cholecystokinin activate different populations of rat mesenteric vagal afferents. Neurosci Lett 1998; 255:63–66.
133. Zhu JX, Wu XY, Owyang C, Li Y. Intestinal serotonin acts as a paracrine substance to mediate vagal signal transmission evoked by luminal factors in the rat. J Physiol 2001; 503:431–442.
134. Bray GA, York DA. Studies on food intake of genetically obese rats. Am J Physiol 1972; 223:176–179.
135. Cangiano C, Ceci F, Cascino A, Del Ben M, Laviano A, Muscaritoli M, ntonucci F, Rossi-Fanelli F. Eating behavior and adherence to dietary prescriptions in obese adult subjects treated with 5-hydroxytryptophan. Am J Clin Nutr 1992; 56:863–867.
136. Unger RH. Alpha- and beta-cell interrelationships in health and disease. Metabolism 1974; 23:581–593.
137. Stunkard AJ, Van Itallie TB, Reis BB. The mechanism of satiety: effect of glucagon on gastric hunger contractions in man. Proc Soc Exp Biol Med 1955; 89:258–261.
138. Martin JR, Novin D. Decreased feeding in rats following hepatic-portal infusions of glucagon. Physiol Behav 1977; 19:461–466.
139. Martin JR, Novin D, Vanderweele DA. Loss of glucagon suppression of feeding after vagotomy in rats. Am J Physiol 1978; 234:E314–E318.
140. Geary N, Smith GP. Selective hepatic branch vagotomy blocks pancreatic glucagon's satiety effect. Physiol Behav 1983; 31:391–394.
141. Oppert JM, Nadeau A, Trembly A, Despres JP, Theriault G, Deriaz O, Bouchard C. Plasma glucose, insulin and glucagon before and after long-term overfeeding in identical twins. Metabolism 1995; 44:96–105.
142. Kjems LL, Kirby BM, Welsh EM, Veldhuis JD, Straume M, McIntyre SS, Yang D, Lefebvre P, Butler PC. Decrease in B-cell mass leads to impaired pulsatile insulin secretion, reduced postprandial hepatic insulin clearance, and relative hyperglucagonemia in the minipig. Diabetes 2001; 50:2001–2012.
143. Langhans W, Ziegler U, Scharrer E, Geary N. Stimulation of feeding in rats by intraperitoneal injection of antibodies to glucagon. Science 1982; 218:894–896.
144. Le Sauter J, Noh U, Geary N. Hepatic portal infusion of glucagon antibodies increases meal size in rats. Am J Physiol 1991; 261:R162–R165.
145. Geary N, Le Sauter J, Noh U. Glucagon acts in the liver to control spontaneous meal size in rats. Am J Physiol 1993; 264:R116–R122.
146. Mayer J. Regulation of energy intake and body weight: the glucostatic theory and the lipostatic hypothesis. Ann NY Acad Sci 1955; 63:15–42.
147. Woods SC, Porte D. Insulin and the set point regulation of body weight. In: Novin D, Wyrwicka W, Bray GA, eds. Hunger: Basic Mechanisms and Clinical Implications. New York: Raven Press, 1976:273–280.
148. Bagdade JD, Bierman EL, Porte DJ. The significance of basal insulin levels in the evaluation of the insulin response to glucose in diabetic and nondiabetic subjects. J Clin Invest 1967: 46:1549-1557.
149. Polonsky KS, Given BD, Van Cauter E. Twenty-four hour profiles and pulsatile patterns of insulin secretion in normal and obese subjects. J Clin Invest 1988; 81:442–448.
150. Porikos KP, Pi-Sunyer FX. Regulation of food intake in human obesity: studies with caloric dilution and exercise. Clin Endocrinol Metab 1984; 13:547–561.
151. Woods SC, Lotter EC, McKay LD, Porte D. Chronic intracerebroventricular infusion of insulin reduces food intake and body weight in baboons. Nature 1979; 282:503–505.
152. Brief DJ, Davis JD. Reduction of food intake and body weight by chronic intraventricular insulin infusion. Brain Res Bull 1984; 12:571–575.
153. Schwartz MW, Bergman RN, Kahn SE, Taborsky J, Fisher LD, Sipols AJ, Woods SC, Steil GM, Porte D. Evidence for entry of plasma insulin into cerebrospinal fluid through an intermediate compartment in dogs. J Clin Invest 1991; 88:1272–1281.
154. Vanderweele DA, Pi-Sunyer FX, Novin D, Bush MJ. Chronic insulin infusion suppresses food ingestion and body weight gain in rats. Brain Res Bull 1980; 5(S4):7–11.
155. Vanderweele DA. Insulin and satiety from feeding in pancreatic normal and diabetic rats. Physiol Behav 1993; 54:477–485.
156. Vanderweele DA. Insulin is a prandial satiety hormone. Physiol Behav 1994; 56:619–622.
157. Willing AE, Walls EK, Koopmans HS. Insulin administration leads to increased food intake in diabetic rats eating high and low fat diets. Physiol Behav 1994; 56:983–991.
158. Willing AE, Koopmans HS, Walls EK. Hepatic portal and vena cava insulin infusions lead to increased food intake in diabetic rats. Physiol Behav 1994; 56:993-1001.
159. Walls EK, Koopmans, HS. Increased food intake following carotid and systemic insulin infusions. Int J Obes 1992; 16:153–160.
160. Woo R, Kissileff HR, Pi-Sunyer FX. Elevated postprandial insulin levels do not induce satiety in normal-weight humans. Amer J Pysiol 1984; 247:R745–R749.
161. Rodin J, Wack J, Ferrannini E, DeFronzo RA. Effect of insulin and glucose on feeding behavior. Metabolism 1985; 34:826–831.
162. Holt SH, Miller JB. Increased insulin responses to ingested foods are associated with lessened satiety. Appetite 1995; 24:43–54.
163. DCCT Research Group. The effect of intensive treat-

ment of diabetes on the development and progression of long-term complications in insulin-dependent diabetes mellitus. N Engl J Med 1993; 329:977–986.
164. Morley JE, Flood JF. Amylin decreases food intake in mice. Peptides 1991; 12:865–869.
165. Chance WT, Balasubramaniam S, Stallion A, Fischer JE. Anorexia following the systemic injection of amylin. Brain Res 1993; 607:185–188.
166. Ohsawa H, Kanatsuka A, Yamaguchi T, Makino H, Yoshida S. Islet amylin polypeptide inhibits glucose-stimulated insulin secretion from isolated rat pancreatic islets. Biochem Biophys Res Commun 1989; 160:961–967.
167. Chance WT, Balasubramaniam S, Zhang FS, Wimalawamsa SJ, Fischer JE. Anorexia following intrahypothalmic administration of amylin. Brain Res 1991; 352–354.
168. Rushing PA, Hagan MM, Seeley RJ, Lutz TA, Woods SC. Amylin: a novel action in the brain to reduce body weight. Endocrine 2000; 141:850–853.
169. Sexton PM, Paxinos G, Kenney MA, Wookey PJ, Beaumont K. In vitro autoradiographic localization of amylin binding sites in rat brain. Neuroscience 1994; 62:553–567.
170. Reidelberger RD, Arnelo U, Granqvist L, Permert J. Comparative effects of amylin and cholecystokinin on food intake and gastric emptying in rats. Am J Physiol 2001; 280:R605–R611.
171. Lutz TA, Del Prete E, Scharrer E. Subdiaphragmatic vagotomy does not influence the anorexic effect of amylin. Peptides 1995; 16:457–462.
172. Brazeau P, Vale W, Burgus R, Ling N, Butcher M, Rivier J, Guillemin R. Hypothalamic polypeptide that inhibits the section of immunoreactive pituitary growth hormone. Science 1973; 179:77–79.
173. Polak JM, Pearse AGE, Grimelius L, Bloom SR, Arimura A. Growth-hormone release-inhibiting hormone in gastrointestinal and pancreatic D cells. Lancet 1975; 1:1220–1224.
174. Larsson LI, Gottermann N, De Magistris L, Rehfield J, Schwartz TW. Somatostatin cell processes as pathways for paracrine secretion. Science 1979; 205:1393–1395.
175. Konturek SJ, Kwiecien N, Obtulowicz W, Bielinski W, Olesky J, Schally AV. Effects of somatostatin-14 and somatostatin-28 on plasma hormonal and gastric sensory responses to cephalic and gastrointestinal stimulation in man. Scand J Gastroenterol 1985; 20: 31–38.
176. Park J, Chiba T, Yamada T. Mechanisms for the direct inhibition of canine gastric parietal cells by somatostatin. J Biol Chem 1987; 262:14190–14196.
177. Dollinger HC, Raptis S, Pfeiffer EF. Effects of somatostatin on exocrine and endocrine pancreatic function stimulated by intestinal hormones in man. Horm Metab Res 1976; 8:74–78.
178. Koerker DJ, Reul W, Chideckel E, Palmer J, Geodner CJ, Ensich J, Gule CC. Somatostatin: hypothalamic inhibitor of the endocrine pancreas. Science 1974; 184:482–484.
179. Schusdiarra V, Rouiller D, Harris V, Unger RH. Splanchnic somatostatin: a hormonal regulator of nutrient homeostasis. Science 1980; 207:530–532.
180. Lotter EC, Krinsky R, McKay JM, Treneer CM, Porte D, Woods SC. Somatostatin decreases food intake of rats and baboons, J Comp Physiol Psych 1981; 5:278–287.
181. Smedh U, Kaplan JM, Bjorkstrand E, Uvnas-Moberg K. Dual effects of somatostatin analog octreotide on gastric emptying during and after intragastric fill. Am J Physiol 1999; 277:R1291–R1296.
182. Erlanson-Albertsson C, Larson A. A possible physiological function of pancreatic procolipase activation peptide in appetite regulation. Biochemistry 1988; 70:1245–1250.
183. Erlanson-Albertsson C. Pancreatic colipase. Structure and physiological aspects. Biochim Biophys Acta 1992; 1125:1–7.
184. Erlanson-Albertsson C, Mei J, Okada S, York D, Bray GA. Pancreatic procolipase propeptide, enterostatin, specifically inhibits fat intake. Physiol Behav 1991; 49:1191–1194.
185. Bouras M, Huneau JF, Luengo C, Erlanson-Albertsson C, Tome D. Metabolism of enterostatin in rat intestine, brain membranes, and serum: differential involvement of proline-specific peptidases. Peptides 1995; 16:399–405.
186. Mei J, Erlanson-Albertsson C. Role of intraduodenally administered enterostatin in rats: inhibition of food intake. Obesity Res 1995; 4:161–165.
187. Sorhede M, Erlanson-Albertsson C, Mei J, Nevalainen T, Aho A, Sundler F. Enterostatin in gut endocrine cells—immunocytochemical evidence. Peptides 1996; 17:609–614.
188. Winsell MS, Lowe ME, Erlanson-Albertsson C. Rat gastric procolipase: sequence, expression and secretion during high-fat feeding. Gastroenterology 1998; 115:1179–1185.
189. Sorhede M, Mulder H, Mei J, Sundler F, Erlanson-Albertsson C. Procolipase is produced in rat stomach—a novel source of enterostatin. Biochim Biophys Acta 1996; 1301:207–212.
190. Rice HB, Corwin RL. Effects of enterostatin on the consumption of optional food in non-food-deprived rats. Obes Res 1998; 6:54–61.
191. Brantl V, Teschemacher H, Blasig J, Hneschen A, Lottspeich F. Opioid activities of b-casomorphins. Life Sci 1981; 28:1903–1909.
192. Daniel H, Vohwinkel M, Rehner G. Effect of casein and b-casomorphins on gastrointestinal motility in rats. J Nutr 1990; 120:252–257.
193. Allesher HD, Storr M, Piller C, Brantl V, Schudsd-

ziarra V. Effect of opioid active therapeutics on the ascending reflex pathway in the rat ileum. Neuropeptides 2000; 34:181–186.
194. Taira T, Hilakivi LA, Aalto J, Hilakivi I. Effect of b-casomorphin on neonatal sleep in rats. Peptides 1990; 11:1–4.
195. White CL, Bray GA, York DA. Intragastric b-casomorphin1-7 attenuates the suppression of fat intake by enterostatin, Peptides 2000; 21:1377–1381.
196. Cramer CP, Blass EM. Mechanisms of control of milk intake in suckling rats. Am J Physiol 1983; 245:154–159.
197. Hayashi H, Nutting DF, Fujimoto K, Cardell JA, Black D, Tso P. Transport of lipid and apoproteins A-I and A-IV in intestinal lymph of the rat. J Lipid Res 1990; 31:1613–1625.
198. Sherman JR, Weinberg RB. Serum apoliproprotein A-IV and lipoprotein cholesterol in patients undergoing total parenteral nutrition. Gastroenterology 1988; 95:394–401.
199. Apfelbaum TF, Davidson NO, Glickman RM. Apolipoprotein A-IV synthesis in rat intestine: regulation by dietary triglyceride. Am J Physiol 1987; 252:G662–G666.
200. Fujimoto K, Cardelli JA, Tso P. Increased apolipoprotein A-IV in rat mesenteric lymph after lipid meals acts as a physiological signal for satiation. Am J Physiol 1992; 262:G1002–G1006.
201. Liu M, Shen L, Tso P. The role of enterostatin and apolipoprotein A-IV on the control of food intake. Neuropeptides 1999; 33:425–433.
202. Fujimoto K, Fukagawa K, Sakata T, Tso P. Suppression of food intake by apolipoprotein AIV is mediated through the central nervous system in rats. J Clin Invest 1993; 91:1830–1833.
203. Okumura T, Fukagawa K, Tso P, Taylor II, Pappas TN. Mechanisms of action of intracisternal apolipoprotein AIV in inhibiting gastric acid secretion in rats. Gastroenterology 1995; 109:1583–1588.
204. Okumura T, Fukagawa K, Tso P, Taylor II, Pappas TN. Apolipoprotein AIV acts in the brain to inhibit gastric emptying in the rat . Am J Physiol 1996; 270: G49–G53.
205. Fujimoto K, Machidori H, Iwakiri R, Yamamoto K, Fukisaki J, Sakata T, Tso P. Effect of intravenous administration of apolipoprotein AIV on patterns of feeding, drinking and ambulatory activity of rats. Brain Res 1993: 608:233–237.
206. Plata-Salaman CR, Oomura Y, Kai Y. Tumor necrosis factor and interleukin-1 beta: suppression of food intake by direct action in the central nervous system. Brain Res 1988; 448:106–114.
207. Reyes-Vazquez C, Prieto-Gomez B, Dafny N. Alpha interferon suppresses food intake and neuronal activity of the lateral hypothalmus. Neuropharmacology 1994; 33:1545–1552.
208. Plata-Salaman CR, Cytokines and anorexia: a brief overview. Semin Oncol 1998; 25(S1):64–72.
209. Daun JM, McCarthy DO. The role of cholescystokinin in interleukin-1-induced anorexia. Physiol Behav 1993; 54:237–241.
210. Suto G, Kiraly A, Tache Y. Interleukin 1 beta inhibits gastric emptying in rats: mediation through prostaglandin and corticotropin-releasing factor. Gastroenterology 1994; 106:1568–1575.
211. Memon RA, Feingold KR, Grunfeld C. The effects of cytokines on intermediary metabolism. Endocrinologist 1994; 4:56-63.
212. Shintani F, Kanba S, Nakaki T, Nibuya M, Kinoshita N, Suzuki E, Yagi G, Kato R, Asai M. Interleukin-1 beta augments release of norepinephrine, dopamine, and serotonin in the rat anterior hypothalamus. J Neurosci 1993; 13:3574–3581.
213. Plata-Salamin CR, Ffrench-Mullen JMH. Intracerebroventricular administration of a specific IL-1 receptor antagonist blocks food and water intake suppression induced by interleukin-1 beta. Physiol Behav 1992; 51:1277–1279.
214. Van der Meer MJ, Sweep CG, Pesman GJ, Borm GF, Hermus RMM. Synergism between IL-1 beta TNF-alpha on the activity of the pituitary-adrenal axis and on food intake of rats. Am J Physiol 1995; 268:E551–E557.
215. Yang ZJ, Koseki M, Meguid MM, Gleason JR, Hermus RMM. Synergistic effect of rhTNF-alpha and rhIL-1 alpha in inducing anorexia in rats. Am J Physiol 1994; 267:R1056–R1064.
216. Endres S, Ghorbani R, Kelley VE, Georgilis K, Lonnemann G, Van der Meer JWM, Cannon JG, Rogers TS, Klempner MS, Weber PC, Schaefer EJ, Wolff SM, Dinarello CA. The effect of dietary supplementation with n-3 polyunsaturated fatty acids on the synthesis of interleukin-1 and tumor necrosis factor by mononuclear cells. N Engl J Med 1989; 320:265–271.
217. Ackermann M, Kirchner H, Atzpodien J. Low dose megestrol acetate can abrogate cachexia in advanced tumor patients receiving systemic interferon-alpha and/or interleukin-2 based antineoplastic therapy. Anti-Cancer Drugs 1993; 4:585–587.
218. Henderson JT, Seniuk NA, Richardson PM, Gauldie J, Roder JC. Systemic administration of ciliary neurotrophic factor induces cachexia in rodents. J Clin Invest 1994; 93:2632–2638.
219. Mackowiak PA. Fever: blessing or curse? A unifying hypothesis. Ann Intern Med 1994; 120:1037–1040.
220. Plaisance KI, Mackowiak PA. Antipyretic therapy. Physiological rationale, diagnostic implication and clinical consequences. Arch Intern Med 2000; 160:449–456.
221. Koopmans HS, Wang DM, Koslowsky I, Kloiber R. The effect of cross-circulation on food intake. Obes Res 1994; 3:331S.

222. Mordes JP, Herrera G, Silen W. Decreased weight gain and food intake in vagotomized rats. Soc Exp Biol Med 1977; 156:257–272.
223. Louis-Sylvestre J. Feeding and metabolic patterns in rats with truncular vagotomy or with transplanted B-cells. Am J Physiol 1978; 235:E119–E125.
224. Grossman MI, Cummins GM, Ivy AC. The effect of insulin on food intake after vagotomy and sympathectomy. Am J Physiol 1947; 149:100–102.
225. Harris SC, Ivy AC, Searle LM. The mechanism of amphetamine-induced loss of weight: a consideration of the theory of hunger and appetite. JAMA 1947; 134:1468–1475.
226. Furness JB, Koopmans HS, Robbins HL, Clerc N, Tobin JM, Morris MJ. Effects of vagal and splanchnic section of food intake, weight, serum leptin and hypothalamic neuropeptide Y in rat. Autonom Neurosci 2001; 92:28–36.
227. Niijima A. Glucose-sensitive afferent nerve fibers in the hepatic branch of the vagus nerve in the guinea-pig. J Physiol 1982; 332:315–323.
228. Huang FL, Zhou H, Sinclair C, Goldstein ME, McCabe JT, Helke CJ. Peripheral deafferentation alters calcitonin gene-related peptide mRNA expression in visceral sensory neurons of the nodose and petrosal ganglia. Mol Brain Res 1994; 22:290–298.
229. Zhou H, Ichikawa H, Helke CJ. Neurochemistry of the nodose ganglion. Prog Neurobiol 1997; 52:79–107.
230. Davison JS, Clarke GD. Mechanical properties and sensitivity to CCK of vagal gastric slowly adapting mechanoreceptors. Am J Physiol 1988; 255:G55–G61.
231. Schwartz GJ, McHugh PR, Moran TH. Gastric loads and cholecystokinin synergistically stimulate rat gastric afferents. Am J Physiol 1993; 265:R872–R876.
232. Barrachina MD, Martinez V, Wang L, Wei J, Tache Y. Synergistic interaction between leptin and cholecystokinin to reduce short term food intake in lean mice. Proc Natl Acad Sci USA 1997; 94:10455–10460.
233. Emond M, Schwartz GJ, Ladenheim EE, Moran TH. Central leptin modulates behavioral and neural sensitivity to CCK. Am J Physiol 1999; 276:R1545–R1549.
234. Emond M, Ladenheim EE, Schwartz GJ, Moran TH. Leptin amplifies the feeding inhibition and neural activation arising from a gastric nutrient preload. Physiol Behav 2001; 72:123–128.
235. Robinson RG, Folstein MF, McHugh PR. Reduced calorie intake following small bowel bypass surgery: a systematic study of the possible causes. Psychol Med 1979; 9:37–53.
236. Payne JH, DeWind LT. Surgical treatment of obesity. Am J Surg 1969; 118:141–146.
237. McFarland RJ, Gazet JC, Pilkington TR. A 13-year review of jejunoileal bypass. Br J Surg 1985; 72:81–87.
238. Pilkington TRE, Gazet JC Ang L, Kalucy RS, Crisp AH, Day S. Explanations for weight loss after jejunoileal bypass in gross obesity. BMJ 1976; 1:1504–1505.
239. Bray GA, Greenway FL, Barry RE. Surgical treatment of obesity: a review of our experience and an analysis of published results. Int J Obes 1977; 1:331–367.
240. Sclafani A, Koopmans HS, Vasselli JR, Reichmann M. Effects of intestinal bypass surgery on appetite, food intake and body weight in obese and lean rats. Am J Physiol 1978; 234:E389–E398.
241. Nightengale ML, Sarr MG, Kelly KA, Jensen MD, Zinsmeister AR, Palumbo PJ. Prospective evaluation of vertical banded gastroplasty as the primary operation for morbid obesity. Mayo Clin Proc 1991; 66: 773–782.
242. Mason EE, Ito C. Gastric bypass in obesity. Surg Clin North Am 1967; 47:1345–1351.
243. Balsinger BM, Murr MM, Poggio JL, Sarr MG. Bariatric surgery: surgery for weight control in patients with morbid obesity. Med Clin North Am 2000; 84:477–489.
244. Sugerman HJ, Kellum JM, Engle KM, Wolfe L, Starkey JV, Birkenhauer R, Fletcher P, Sawyer MJ. Gastric bypass for treating severe obesity. Am J Clin Nutr 1992; 55:560S–566S.
245. Lawaetz O, Blackburn AM, Bloom SR, Aritas Y, Ralphs DNL. Gut hormone profile and gastric emptying in the dumping syndrome: a hypothesis concerning the pathogenesis. Scand J Gastroenterol 1983; 18:73–80.
246. Sirinek KR, O'Dorisio TM, Howe B, McFee AS. Neurotensin, vasoactive intestinal peptide and Roux-en-Y gastrojejunostomy. Arch Surg 1985; 120:605–609.
247. Meryn S, Stein D, Strauss EW. Pancreatic polypeptide, pancreatic glucagon and enteroglucagon in morbid obesity and following gastric bypass operation. Int J Obes 1986; 10:37–52.
248. Kellum JM, Kuemmerle JF, O'Dorosio TM, Rayford P, Martin D, Engle K, Wolf L, Sugerman H. Gastrointestinal hormone responses to meals before and after gastric bypass and vertical banded gastroplasty. Ann Surg 1990; 211:763–770.
249. Sarson DL, Scopinaro N, Bloom SR. Gut hormone change after jejunoileal (JIB) or biliopancreatic bypass (BPB) for morbid obesity. Int J Obesity 1981; 5:471–480.
250. Wang XM, Thomas RP, Evers BM. Effect of gut transposition on the expression of the endocrine gene neurotensin. J Gastroenterol Surg 1998; 2:230–237.
251. Ferris CF, George JK, Eastwood G, Potegal M, Carraway RE. Plasma levels of neurotensin: methodological and physiological considerations. Peptides 1991; 12:215–220.
252. Sandoval SL, Kulkosky PJ. Effects of peripheral neurotensin on behavior of the rat. Pharm Biochem Behav 1992; 41:385–390.
253. Boules M, Cusack B, Zhao L, Fauq A, McCormick DJ, Richelson E. A novel neurotensin analog given

extracranially decreases food intake and weight in rodents. Brain Res 2000; 865:35–44.
254. Stanley BG, Hoebel BG, Leibowitz SF. Neurotensin: effects of hypothalamic and intravenous injections on eating and drinking in rats. Peptides 1983; 4:493–500.
255. Taylor IL. Distribution and release of peptide YY in dog measured by specific radioimmunoassay. Gastroenterology 1985; 88:731–737.
256. Takamoto K. Isolation and characterization of peptide YY (PYY), a candidate gut hormone that inhibits pancreatic exocrine secretion. Proc Natl Acad Sci USA 1982; 79:2514–2518.
257. Adrian TE, Savage AP, Sago GR, Allen JM, Bacarese-Hamilton AJ, Takemoto K, Polak J, Bloom Sr. Effect of peptide YY on gastric, pancreatic and biliary function in humans. Gastroenterology 1985; 89:494–499.
258. Spiller RC, Trotman IF, Higgins BE, Ghatei MA, Grimble GK, Lee YC, Bloom SR, Misiewiez JJ, Silk DBA. The ileal brake inhibition of jejunal motility after ileal fat perfusion in man. Gut 1984; 25:365–374.
259. Chen CH, Stephens RL, Rogers, RC. PYY and NPY: control of gastric motility via action on the Y1 and Y2 receptors in the DVC. Neurogastroenterol Motil 1997; 9:109–116.
260. Clark JT, Kalra PS, Crowley WR, Kalra SP. Neuropeptide Y and human pancreatic peptide stimulate feeding behavior in rats. Endocrinology 1984; 115:427–429.
261. Leibowitz SF. Hypothalamic neuropeptide Y, galanin and amines: concepts of coexistence in relation to feeding behavior. Ann NY Acad Sci 1989; 575:221–235.
262. Itoh E, Fujimiya M, Inui A. Thioperamide, an H3 receptor antagonist, powerfully suppresses peptide YY-induced food intake in rats. Biol Psychiatry 1999; 45:474–481.
263. Hagan MM, Castaneda E, Sumaya IC, Fleming SM, Galloway J, Moss DE. The effect of hypothalamic peptide YY on hippocampal acetylcholine release in vivo: implication for limbic function in binge eating behavior. Brain Res 1998; 805:20–28.
264. Koopmans HS, Ferri GL, Sarson DL, Polak J, Bloom SR. The effects of ileal transposition and jejunoileal bypass on food intake, body weight, gastrointestinal hormone levels and tissue adaptation. Physiol Behav 1984; 33:601–609.
265. Mojsov S, Heinrich G, Wilson IB, Ravazzola M, Orci L, Habener JF. Preproglucagon gene expression in pancreas and intestine diversifies at the level of post-transcriptional processing. J Biol Chem 1986; 261: 11880–11889.
266. Brubaker PL, Crivici A, Izzo A, Erlich P, Tsai CH, Drucker DJ. Circulating and tissue forms of the intestinal growth factor, glucagon-like peptide-2 Endocrin 1997; 138:4837–4843.
267. Drucker DJ. Minireview: the glucagon-like petides. Endocrinology 2001; 142:521–527.
268. Nauck MA, Niedereichholz U, Ettler R, Holst JJ, Orskov C, Ritzel R, Schmeigel WH. Glucagon-like peptide 1 inhibition of gastric emptying outweighs its insulinotropic effects in healthy humans. Am J Physiol 1997; 273:E981–E988.
269. Flint A, Raben A, Astrup A, Holst JJ. Glucagon-like peptide 1 promotes satiety and suppresses energy intake in humans. J Clin Invest 1998; 10:515–520.
270. Toft-Nielson MB, Madsbad S, Holst JJ. Continuous subcutaneous infusion of glucagon-like peptide 1 lowers plasma glucose and reduces appetite in type 2 diabetic patients. Diabetes Care 1999; 22:1137–1143.
271. Rinnaman L. A functional role for central glucagon-like peptide-1 receptors in lithium chloride–induced anorexia Am J Physiol 1999, 277:R1537–R1540.
272. Seeley RJ, Blake K, Rushing PA, Benoit S, Eng J, Woods SC, D'Allesio D. The role of the CNS glucagon-like peptide-1 (7-36) amide receptors in mediating the visceral illness effects of lithium chloride. J Neurosci 2000; 20:1616–1620.
273. Brubaker PL, Izzo A, Hill M, Drucker DJ. Intestinal function in mice with small bowel growth induced by glucagon-like peptide 2. Am J Physiol 1997; 272;E1050–E1058.
274. Wojdemann M, Wettergren A, Hartman B, Holst JJ. Glucagon-like peptide-2 inhibits centrally induced antral motility in pigs. Scand J Gastroenterol 1998; 33:828–832.
275. Thulsen J, Hartman B, Orskov G, Jeppesen PB, Holst JJ, Poulsen SS. Potential targets for glucagon-like peptide 2 (GLP-2) in the rat: distribution binding of i.v. injected (125)I-GLP-2. Peptides 2000; 21:1511–1517.
276. Yusta B, Huang L, Munroe D, Wolff G, Fantaske R, Sharma S, Demchyshyn L, Asa SL, Drucker DJ. Enteroendocrine localization of GLP-2 receptor expression in humans and rodents. Gastroenterology 2000; 119:744–755.
277. Tang-Christensen M, Larsen PJ, Thulsen J, Romer J, Vrang N. The proglucagon-derived peptide, glucagon-like peptide-2, is a neurotransmitter involved in the regulation of food intake. Nat Med 2000; 6:802–807.
278. Orskov C, Holst JJ. Radioimmunoassay for glucagon-like peptides 1 and 2 (GLP1 and GLP2). Scand J Gastroenterol 1987; 47:165–174.
279. Domoulin V, Dakka T, Plaissance P, Chayvialle JA, Cuber JC. Regulation of glucagon-like peptide-1 (7-36) amide, peptide YY and neurotensin secretion by neurotransmitters and gut hormones in the isolated vascularly perfused rat ileum. Endocrinology 1995; 136:5182–5188.
280. Atkinson RL, Brent EL, Wagner BS, Whipple JH. Energy balance and regulation of body weight after intestinal bypass in rats. Am J Physiol 1983; 243: R658–R663.

281. Koopmans HS. An integrated organismic response to lower gut stimulation. Scand J Gastroenterol 1983; 18(S82):143–153.
282. Read NW, Kinsman R. Effect of infusion of nutrient solutions into the ileum on gastrointesinal transit and plasma levels of neurotension and enteroglucagon in man. Gastoenterology 1984; 86:274–280.
283. Soper NJ, Chapman NJ, Kelly KA, Brown ML, Phillips SF, Go VL. The "ileal brake" after ileal pouch–anal anastomosis. Gastroenterology 1990; 98:111–116.
284. Koopmans HS. Endogenous gut signals and metabolites control daily food intake. Int J Obes 1990; 14(S3):93–102.
285. Tso P. Intestinal lipid absorption. In: Johnson ER, Alpers DH, Christensen J, Jacobson ED, Walsh JH, eds. Physiology of the Gastrointestinal Tract. New York: Raven Press, 1994:1867–1908.
286. Russek M. Participation of hepatic glucoreceptors in the control of the intake of food. Nature (Lond) 1963; 197:79–80.
287. Novin D, Sanderson JD, Vanderweele DA. The effect of isotonic glucose on eating as a function of feeding condition and infusion site. Physiol Behav 1974; 13: 3–7.
288. Novin D. (1976) Visceral mechanisms in the control of food intake. In: Novin D, Wyrwicka W, Bray G, eds. Hunger: Basic Mechanism and Clinical Implications. New York: Raven Press, 1976:357–367.
289. Tordoff MG, Friedman, MI. Hepatic-portal glucose infusions decrease food intake and increase food preference. Am J Physiol 1986; 251:R192–R195.
290. Tordoff MG, Tluczek JP, Friedman, MI. Effect of portal glucose concentration on food intake and metabolism. Am J Physiol 1989; 257:R1474–R1480.
291. Willing AE, Koopmans HS. Hepatic portal and vena cava glucose and amino acid infusions decrease daily food intake in rats. Neurosci Abstr 1994; 20:1226.
292. Koopmans HS. Hepatic control of food intake. Appetite 1984; 5:127–131.
293. Russek M. Reply to Koopmans' Hepatic control of food intake. Appetite 1984; 5:133–135.
294. Friedman MI, Sawchenko PE. Evidence for hepatic involvement in control of ad libitum food intake in rats. Am J Physiol 1984; 247:R106–R113.
295. Del Prete E, Scharrer E. Influence of age and hepatic branch vagotomy on the night/day distribution of food intake in rats. Zeit Ernahr 1993; 32:316–320.
296. Del Prete E, Scharrer E. Circadian effects of hepatic branch vagotomy on the feeding response to 2-deoxy-D-glucose in rats. J Auton Nerv Syst 1994; 6:27–36.
297. Bellinger LL, Mendel VE, Williams FE, Castonquay TW. The effect liver denervation on meal patterns, body weight and body composition of rats. Physiol Behav 1984; 33:661–667.
298. Bellinger LL, Williams FE. Meal patterns and plasma liver enzymes and metabolites after total liver denervations. Physiol Behav 1995; 58:625–628.
299. Louis-Sylvestre J, Servant JM, Molimard R, Le Magnen J. Effect of liver denervation on feeding pattern of rats. Am J Physiol 1980; 239:R66–R70.
300. Louis-Sylvestre J, Larue-Achagiotis C, Michel A, Houssin D. Feeding pattern in liver transplanted rats. Physiol Behav 1990; 48:321–326.
301. Beverly JL, Yang ZJ, Meguid MM. Hepatic vagotomy effects on metabolic challenges during parenteral nutrition in rats. Am J Physiol 1994; 266:R646–R649.
302. Phillips LS Nutritional regulation of somatomedin activity and growth. In: Giordano G, Van Wyk JJ, Minuto F, eds. Somatomedins and Growth. London: Academic Press, 1979; 311–323.
303. Signal RJ, Purdon C, Bilinski D, Vranik M, Marliss E. Glucoregulation during and after intense exercise: effects of beta-blockade. J Clin Endocrinol Metab 1994; 78:359–366.
304. Mayer J, Bates MW. Blood glucose and food intake in normal and hypophysectomized, alloxan-treated rats. Am J Physiol 1952; 168:812–819.
305. Mayer J. Regulation of energy intake and body weight: the glucostatic theory and the lipostatic hypothesis. Ann NY Acad Sci 1955; 63:15–42.
306. Van Itallie TB. The glucostatic theory 1953-1988: roots and branches. Int J Obes 1990; 14(S3):1–10.
307. Hanson ME, Grossman MI. The failure of intravenous glucose to inhibit food intake in dogs. Fed Proc 1948; 7:50.
308. Janowitz HD, Hanson ME, Grossman MI. Effect of intravenously administered glucose on food intake in the dog. Am J Physiol 1949; 156:87–91.
309. Mellinkoff SM, Frankland M, Boyle M, Griepel M. Relation between serum amino acid concentration and fluctuations in appetite. J Appl Psychol 1956; 8:535–538.
310. Peters JC, Harper AE. Adaptation of rats to diets containing different levels of protein: effects on food intake, plasma and brain amino acid concentrations and brain neurotransmitter metabolism. J Nutr 1985; 115:382–398.
311. Moundras C, Remesy C, Demigne C. Dietary protein paradox: decrease of amino acid availability induced by high-protein diets. Am J Physiol 1993; 264:G1057–G1065.
312. Kennedy GC. The role of depot fat in the hypothalamic control of food intake in the rat. Proc R Soc B 1952; 140:578–592.
313. Nicolaidis S, Rowland N. Metering of intravenous versus oral nutrients and the regulation of energy balance. Am J Physiol 1976; 231:661–668.
314. Woods SC, Stein LJ, McKay LD, Porte D. Suppression of food intake by intravenous nutrients and insulin in the baboon. Am J Physiol 1984; 247:R393–R401.
315. Walls EK, Koopmans HS. Effect of intravenous

nutrient infusions on food intake in rats. Physiol Behav 1989; 45:1223–1226.
316. Meguid MM, Chen TY, Yang ZJ, Campos ACL, Hitch DC, Gleason JR. Effects of continuous graded total parenteral nutrition on feeding indexes and metabolic concomitants in rats. Am J Physiol 1991; 260: E126–E140.
317. Walls EK, Koopmans HS. Differential effects of intravenous glucose, amino acids and lipid on daily food intake in rats. Am J Physiol 1992; 262:R225–R234.
318. Beverly JL, Yang ZJ, Meguid MM. Factors influencing compensatory feeding during parenteral nutrition in rats. Am J Physiol 1994, 266:R1928–R1932.
319. Walls EK, Willing AE, Koopmans HS. Intravenous nutrient-induced satiety depends on feeding-related gut signals. Am J Physiol 1991; 261:R313–R322.
320. Walls EK, Koopmans HS. Influence of intravenous nutrients on food intake and energy expenditure. Neurosci Abstr 1992; 18:1233.
321. Meguid RA, Beverly JL, Meguid MM. Surfeit calories during parenteral nutrition influences food intake and carcass adiposity in rats. Physiol Behav 1995; 57:265–269.
322. Oomura Y. Significance of glucose, insulin and free fatty acid on the hypothalamic feeding and satiety neurons. In: Novin D, Wyrwicka W, Bray G, eds. Hunger: Basic Mechanisms and Clinical Implications. New York: Raven Press, 1976:145–157.
323. Walls EK, Reinhardt PH, Willing AE, Koopmans HS. Carotid and systemic nutrient infusions reduce food intake. Soc Neurosci Abstr 1990; 16:295.
324. Smith GP, Epstein AN. Increased feeding in response to decreased glucose utilization in the rat and monkey. Am J Physiol 1969; 217:1083–1087.
325. Yamamoto H, Nagai K, Nakagawa H. Time-dependent involvement of autonomic nervous system in hyper-glycemia due to 2-deoxy-d-glucose. Am J Physiol 1988; 255:E928–E933.
326. Matsunaga H, Igucho A, Yatomi A, Uemura K, Muira H, Gotoh M, Mano T, Sakamoto S. The relative importance of nervous system and hormones to the 2-deoxy-d-glucose-induced hyperglycemia in fed rats. Endocrinology 1989; 124:1259–1264.
327. Scheurink A, Ritter S. Sympathoadrenal responses to glucoprivation and lipoprivation in rats. Physiol Behav 1993; 53:995–1000.
328. Miselis RR, Epstein AN. Feeding induced by intracerebroventricular 2-deoxy-d-glucose in the rat. Am J Physiol 1975; 229:1438–1447.
329. Del Prete E, Scharrer E. Hepatic branch vagotomy attenuates the feeding response to 2-deoxy-d-glucose. Exp Physiol 1990; 75:259–261.
330. Scharrer E, Del Prete E, Giger R. Hepatic branch vagotomy enhances glucoprivic feeding in food-deprived old rats. Physiol Behav 1993; 54:259–264.
331. Ritter S, Taylor JS. Vagal sensory neurons are required for lipoprivic but not glucoprivic feeding in rats. Am J Physiol 1990; 258:R1395–R1401.
332. Tordoff MG, Hopfenbeck, Novin D. Hepatic vagotomy (partial hepatic denervation) does not alter ingestive responses to metabolic challenges. Physiol Behav 1982; 28:417–424.
333. Bellinger CL, Williams FE. Liver denervation does not modify feeding responses to metabolic challenges or hypertonic NaCl induced water consumption. Physiol Behav 1983; 30:463–470.
334. Tordoff MG, Rafka R, DiNovi MJ, Friedman MI. 2,5-Anhydro-D-mannitol: a fructose analogue that increases food intake in rats. Am J Physiol 1988; 254:R150–R153.
335. Hanson RL, Ho RS, Wisenberg JJ, Simpson R, Younathan ES, Blair JB. Inhibition of gluconeogenesis and glycogenolysis by 2,5-anhydro-d-mannitol. J Biochem 1984; 259:218–233.
336. Tordoff MG, Rawson N, Friedman MI. 2,5-Anhydro-D-mannitol acts in liver to initiate feeding. Am J Physiol 1991; 261:R283–R288.
337. Park CR, Seeley RJ, Bentham L, Friedman MI, Woods SC. Whole body energy expenditure and fuel oxidation after 2,5-anhydro-D mannitol administration. Am J Physiol 1995; 268:R299–R302.
338. Rawson NE, Blum H, Osbakken MD, Friedman MI. Hepatic phosphate trapping decrease ATP and increase feeding after 2,5-anhydro-D-mannitol. Am J Physiol 1994; 266:R112–R117.
339. Bodoky G, Yang ZJ, Mequid MM, Laviano A, Szeverenyi N. Effects of fasting, intermittent feeding or continuous parenteral nutrition of fat liver and brain energy metabolism as assessed by ^{31}P-NMR. Physiol Behav 1995; 58:521–527.
340. Scharrer E, Langhans W. Control of food intake by fatty acid oxidation. Am J Physiol 1986; 250:R1003–R1006.
341. Bauche F, Sabourault D, Giudicelli Y, Nordmann J, Nordmann R. Inhibition in vitro of acyl-CoA-dehydrogenases by 2-mercaptoacetate in rat liver mitochondria. Biochem J 1983; 215:457–464.
342. Friedman MI, Tordoff MG, Ramirez I. Integrated metabolic control of food intake. Brain Res Bull 1986; 17:855–859.
343. Tutwiler GF, Ho W, Mohrbacher RJ. 2-Tetradeclycidic acid. Methods Enzymol 1981; 2:533–551.
344. Friedman MI, Tordoff MG. Fatty acid oxidation and glucose utilization interact to control food intake in rats. Am J Physiol 1986; 251:R840–R845.
345. Friedman MI, Ramirez I, Bowden CR, Tordoff MG. Fuel partitioning and food intake: role of mitochondrial fatty acid transport. Am J Physiol 1990; 258:R216–R221.
346. Lazzarini SJ, Schneider JF, Wade GN. Inhibition of fatty acid oxidation and glucose metabolism does not alter food intake or hunger motivation in Syrian hamsters. Physiol Behav 1988; 44:209–213.

347. Levitsky D, Faust I, Glassman M. The ingestion of food and the recovery of body weight following fasting in the naive rat. Physiol Behav 1976; 17:575–580.
348. Bjorntorp P, Bergman H, Varnas-Kas E, Lindholm B. Lipid mobilization in relation to body composition in man. Metabolism 1969; 18:112–117.
349. Goldrick RB, McLoughlin GM. Lipolysis and lipogenesis from glucose in human fat cells of different sizes. J Clin Invest 1970; 49;1213–1223.
350. Wirtshafter D, Davis JD. Body weight: reduction by long-term glycerol treatment. Science 1977; 198:1271–1273.
351. Glick Z. Food intake of rats administered with glycerol. Physiol Behav 1980; 25:621–626.
352. Grinker J, Strohmayer AJ, Horowitz J, Hirsch J, Leibel RL. The effect of the metabolite glycerol on food intake and body weight in rats. Brain Res Bull 1980; 5(S4):29–35.
353. Faust IM, Johnson PR, Hirsch J. Surgical removal of adipose tissue alters feeding behavior and the development of obesity in rats. Science 1977; 197:393–396.
354. Larson KA, Anderson DB. The effects of lipectomy on remaining adipose tissue depots in the Sprague-Dawley rat. Growth 1978; 42:469–477.
355. Dark J, Forger NG, Stern JS, Zucker I Recovery of lipid mass after removal of adipose tissue in ground squirrels. Am J Physiol 1985; 249:R73–R78.
356. Astrup A, Grunwald GK, Melanson EL, Saris WHM, Hill JO. The role of low fat diets in body weight control: a meta-analysis of ad libitum dietary intervention studies. Int J Obes 2000; 24:1545–1552.
357. Burggraf KK, Willing AE, Koopmans HS. The effects of glucose and lipid infused intravenously and intragastrically on voluntary food intake in the rat. Physiol Behav 1997; 61:787–793.
358. Schwartz RS, Brunzell JD. Increase of adipose tissue lipoprotein lipase activity with weight loss. J Clin Invest 1981; 67:1425–1430.
359. Eckel RH. Lipoprotein lipase: a multifunctional enzyme relevant to common metabolic diseases. N Engl J Med 1989; 320:1060–1068.
360. Ramos P, Martin-Hidalgo A, Herrera E. Insulin-induced up-regulation of lipoprotein lipase messenger ribonucleic acid and activity in mammary gland. Endocrinology 1999; 140:1089–1093.
361. Deshaies Y, Geloen A, Paulin A, Bukowiecki LJ. Restoration of lipoprotein lipase activity in insulin deficient rats by insulin infusion is tissue specific. Can J Physiol Pharm 1991; 69:746–751.
362. Boivin A, Deshaies Y. Contribution of hyperinsulinemia to modulation of lipoprotein lipase activity in the obese Zucker rat. Metab 2000; 49:134–140.
363. Greenwood MRC. The relationship of enzyme activity to feeding behavior in rats: lipoprotein lipase as the metabolic gatekeeper. Int J Obes 1985; 9(S1):67–70.
364. Gruen R, Hietanen E, Greenwood MRC. Increased adipose tissue lipoprotein lipase activity during development of the genetically obese rat (fafa). Metabolism 1978; 27:1955–1965.
365. Yost TJ, Eckel RH. Fat calories may be preferentially stored in reduced-obese women: a permissive pathway for resumption of the obese state. J Clin Endocrinol Metab 1988; 67:259–264.
366. Friedman MI, Ramirez I, Bowden CR, Tordoff MG. Fuel partitioning and food intake: role for mitochrondrial fatty acid transport. Am J Physiol 1990; 258:R216–R221.
367. Friedman MI. Body fat and the metabolic control of food intake. Int J Obes 1990; 14(S3):53–67.
368. Hong JI, Graczyk-Milbrandt G, Friedman MI. Metabolic inhibitors synergistically decrease hepatic energy status and increase food intake. Am J Physiol 2000; 278:1579–1582.
369. Roberts SB, Greenberg AS. The new obesity genes. Nutr Rev 1996; 54:41–49.
370. Augustine KA, Rossi RM. Rodent mutant models of obesity and their correlations to human obesity. Anat Rec 1999; 257:64–72.
371. Vinter J, Hull D, Batt RA, Tyler DD. The effect of limited feeding on thermogenesis and thermoregulation in genetically obese (ob/ob) mice during cold exposure. Int J Obes 1988; 12:111–117.
372. Coleman DL. Effects of parabiosis of obese with diabetes and normal mice. Diabetologia 1973; 9:294–298.
373. Lee G-H, Proence R, Montez JM, Carroll KM, Darvishzadeh JG, Lee JI, Friedman JM. Abnormal splicing of the leptin receptor in diabetic mice. Nature 1996; 379:632–636.
374. Lonnqvist F, Arner P, Nordfors L, Schalling M. Overexpression of the obese (ob) gene adipose tissue of human obese subjects. Nat Med 1995; 1:950–953.
375. Hamilton BS, Paglia D, Kwan AYM, Dietel M. Increased obese mRNA expression in omental fat cells from massively obese humans. Nat Med 1995; 1:953–956.
376. Considine RV, Sinha MK, Heiman ML, Kriauciunas A, Stephens TW, Nyce MR, Ohannesian JP, Marco CC, McKee LJ, Bauer TL, Caro JF. Serum immunoreactive leptin concentrations in normal-weight and obese humans. N Engl J Med 1996; 334:292–295.
377. Trayhurn P, Duncan JS, Thomas MEA, Rayner DV. Expression of the ob (obesity) gene in adipose tissue of mice. Int J Obes 1995; 19(S2):34.
378. Saladin R, De Vos P, Guerre-Millo M, Leturque A, Girard J, Steals B, Auwerx J. Transient increase in obese gene expression after food intake or insulin administration. Nature 1995; 377:527–529.
379. De Vos P, Saladin R, Auwerx J, Steals B. Induction of ob gene expression by corticosteroids is accompanied by body weight loss and reduced food intake. J Biol Chem 1995; 270:15958–15961.

380. Montague CT, Farooqi IS, Whitehead JP, Soos MA, Rau H, Wareham NJ, Sewter CP, Digby JE, Mohammed SN, Hurst JA, Cheetham CH, Earley AR, Barnett AH, Prins JB, O'Rahilly S. Congenital leptin deficiency is associated with severe early-onset obesity in humans. Nature 1997; 387:903–908.
381. Farooqi IS, O'Rahilly S. Recent advances in the genetics of severe childhood obesity. Arch Dis Child 2000; 83:31–34.
382. Clement K, Vaisse C, Lahlou N, Cabrol S, Pelloux V, Cassuto D, Gourmelem M, Dina C, Chambaz J, Lacorte JM, Basvedent A, Bougneres Y, Froguel P, Guy-Grand B. A mutation in the human leptin receptor gene causes obesity and pituitary dysfunction. Nature 1998; 392:398–401.
383. Heymsfield SB, Greenberg AS, Fujioka K, Dixon RM, Kushner R, Hunt T, Lubina JA, Patane J, Self B, Hunt P, McCamish M. Recombinant leptin for weight loss in obese and lean adults a randomized, controlled dose-escalation trial. JAMA 1999; 282:1568–1575.
384. Ahima RS, Flier JS. Adipose tissue as an endocrine organ. Trends Endocrinol Metab 2000; 11:327–332.
385. Grunfeld C, Feingold KR. Regulation of lipid metabolism by cytokines during host defense. Nutr 1996; 12:S24–S26.
386. Flatt JP, Body composition, respiratory quotient and weight maintenance. Am J Clin Nutr 1995; 62:1107S–1117S.
387. Sclafani A, Springer D. Dietary obesity in adult rats: similarities to hypothalamic and human obesity syndromes. Physiol Behav 1976; 17:461–471.
388. Rolls BJ, Van Duijvenvoorde PM, Rowe EA. Variety in the diet enhances intake in a meal and contributes to the development of obesity in the rat. Physiol Behav 1983; 31:21–27.
389. Lucas F, Sclafani A. Hyperphagia in rats produced by a mixture of fat and sugar. Physiol Behav 1990; 47:51–55.
390. Ramirez I, Friedman MI. Dietary hyperphagia in rats: role of fat, carbohydrate and energy content. Physiol Behav 1990; 47:1157–1163.
391. Umpleby Am, Sonksen, PH. The chalonic action of insulin in man. In: Garrow JS, Halliday D, eds. Substrate and Energy Metabolism, London: Libbey, 1985:169–178.
392. Eckel RH. Lipoprotein lipase: a multifunctional enzyme relevant to common metabolic diseases. N Engl J Med 1989; 320:1060–1068.
393. Flatt JP. Energetics of intermediary metabolism. In: Garrow JS, Halliday D, eds. Substrate and Energy Metabolism in Man. London: Libbey 1985:58.
394. Salmon DM, Flatt JP. Effect of dietary fat on the incidence of obesity among ad libitum fed mice. Int J Obes 1985; 9:443–449.
395. Kendall A, Levitsky DA, Strupp BJ, Lissner L. Weight loss on low-fat diet: consequence of the imprecision of the control of food intake in humans. Am J Clin Nutr 1991; 53:1124–1129.
396. Hill JO, Melby C, Johnson SL, Peters JC. Physical activity and energy requirements. Am J Clin Nutr 1995; 62:1059S–1066S.
397. Pi-Sunyer FX. The fattening of America. JAMA 1994; 272:238–239.

15

Diet Composition and the Control of Food Intake in Humans

John E. Blundell

University of Leeds, Leeds, England

James Stubbs

Rowett Research Institute, Aberdeen, Scotland

I INTRODUCTION: THE STUDY OF HUMAN FOOD INTAKE

A Context

We live in a society that is virtually obsessed with the influence of food on health, energy intake, and body weight regulation. While much of life in preindustrial societies has been concerned with locating, obtaining, or cultivating adequate quantities of appropriate foods, many people living in industrialized societies spend considerable time and effort in attempting to avoid excess food intake. For many individuals this has become an active process. The food industry in any Western society is worth billions of dollars per annum. In addition, consumers spend several billion dollars on products they hope will help them avoid excess food intake or remedy the consequences of overconsumption. Feeding and food are central to our health and well-being. Food characterizes cultural grouping and identifies social and religious occasions. The composition of the diet we eat is now considered a primary cause of morbidity and mortality [e.g., obesity, coronary heart disease (1)]. Our growing knowledge of the effect of the diet on health offers a potential means of preventing certain illnesses or alleviating the effects of others through nutritional support. The market economy has recognized the potential in this area and now "functional foods" and "nutraceuticals" are available with the promise of increased consumer longevity, health, and well-being.

A key problem, particularly for the layperson, is that it appears difficult to pinpoint the major facts that scientists have discovered about food intake. What are the salient discoveries in the area of appetite and energy balance? Researchers often find this a very difficult question to deal with. Why is this so? Is it because there are no facts (universally agreed statements)? Or is it because we are dealing with a form of *behavior* that operates according to probabilistic rather than deterministic principles? This also has implications for those seeking to unravel the specific molecular mechanisms thought to be important in controlling feeding behavior. There is a further reason why facts about food intake appear to be relatively rare. Reliable quantitative and qualitative facts about food intake appear difficult to obtain since the act of measurement may influence what is being measured. This is exemplified by current concerns over the nature and extent of misreporting of dietary intakes (2). Even more frustrating to both the scientist and the general public is the problem of communicating the results of research to a population eager to understand how to regulate their own body weight and improve health and fitness. As soon as the media reduces research results to readily digested "sound bytes" deemed fit for public consumption, the information being relayed to the public has become distorted. This is often so in science. However, the field of ingestive behavior, energy balance, and obesity is constantly the subject of media interest, so this problem of media misrepresentation of our results is more acute.

It should be kept in mind that food intake is a form of *behavior* commonly believed to be under voluntary control. This behavior can be described by terms such as amount of energy ingested, structure of dietary pattern, or macronutrient profile. But all of these terms are the consequences of behavior (food being seized by the hands and transported to the mouth). Therefore a study of food intake should concentrate on the way in which environmental, cognitive, or biological events can be translated into effects upon the act of behavior. It is also a worth mentioning that "not-eating" (one aspect of which is postingestive [PI]-satiety) is also a form of behavior. Consequently, events that prevent eating are also important. Understanding how energy balance is maintained requires an understanding of the forms of behavior that promote weight stability. Understanding the etiology of obesity and developing strategies for its treatment requires an elucidation of the mechanisms that influence the behaviors leading to weight gain and those that can bring about sustained weight loss, respectively.

It is also important to recognize that certain environmental contexts favor or constrain specific forms of behavior. For example, a calorimeter environment constrains the ability of a subject to move about and select food. In a given environmental context, eating behavior bridges the gap between the nutritional environment and the physiological/biochemical mechanisms of weight control. One view of appetite regulation is that it may be seen as the adoption of forms of behavior that ensure an appropriate supply of energy and nutrients for the optimal performance of the organism in a given environment. It follows that strategies of appetite regulation appropriate to a hunter-gatherer are not necessarily the same behavioral strategies as those of a bank clerk.

B Eating Behavior or Fuel Intake?

Food consumption is the target of scientific research for a number of different researchers including physiologists, nutritionists, psychologists, biochemists, endocrinologists, and, increasingly, molecular biologists and geneticists. All of these researchers share, as one of their primary goals, the attempt to understand the mechanisms responsible for human food consumption. However, the terminology that refers to this endpoint may appear discordant. For one group of researchers the phenomenon usually measured is called eating, human feeding, or food intake. In other scientific domains the phenomenon is called dietary intake, energy intake, or, more commonly, spontaneous energy intake. Differences are also apparent at the level of scientific practice. The first group is often concerned with qualitative aspects of eating such as food choice, preferences, and the sensory aspects of food together with subjective phenomena such as hunger, fullness, and hedonic sensations that accompany eating and which are sometimes regarded as causal agents. The second group is primarily concerned with quantitative aspects of consumption and with the energetic value of food; at the present time, particular importance is attached to the macronutrient composition of food and its impact on energy balance (3,4).

The identification of food consumption as either a form of behavior or as fuel intake is not just a semantic issue. It is fundamental to the theoretical paradigms we develop to explain the existence, nature, and strength of mechanisms concerned with the control of food intake. The study of human appetite should attempt to reconcile these different approaches to the subject. What is the relationship between the pattern of intake of meals and snacks (behavioral profile), the tastes and other sensory attributes of the foods consumed (qualitative pattern), and the total food consumed over a 24-hr period (spontaneous energy intake) together with the proportions of macronutrients (fuel balance)? How do the physiological consequences of nutrient ingestion influence subsequent feeding behavior? Is obesity brought about by enhanced feelings of hunger, weakened PI satiety, sensorily induced overconsumption, or hedonically mediated maladaptive food choices? Or is obesity a result of errors in processes governing energy balance such as inappropriate oxidation of fuels or different neuroendocrine responses to varying dietary intakes? Most critically, is energy balance truly regulated in humans and if so, under what conditions and to what extent?

If appetite research is to explain the mechanisms responsible for human food consumption, it must be multidisciplinary in nature. The outcomes of studies on feeding behavior are probabilistic rather than absolute. They are not as empirically reproducible as, for example, the behavior of molecules in solutions, or of hypothalamic peptide levels in response to changes in energy balance. This means that the experimental environment can be particularly important in determining the outcome. A specific issue or factor thought to be important in influencing feeding behavior needs to be examined in different groups of subjects and in different environments. If this factor is thought to be fundamental to biological regulation, it should be shown to operate in a number of different species.

II METHODOLOGICAL APPROACHES TO STUDIES OF HUMAN FOOD INTAKE

There are a number of key methodological issues that should be borne in mind when designing and interpreting studies of human feeding behavior.

A Precision Versus Naturalness

Since the experimental environmental itself can affect the outcome of experiments, workers involved in the study of human feeding behavior are faced with a major methodological problem. Feeding behavior can be studied either in free-living people where errors are large but subjects are behaving naturally in their usual environment, or factors affecting feeding behavior can be examined in the laboratory with great precision and accuracy, but there is a danger of creating artifacts due to the artificiality of the experimental environment. This relationship is described in Figure 1.

There has been a general shift in emphasis in recent years from qualitative studies examining factors such as eating styles, rate, and duration as potential determinants of intake, to more quantitative work based on the effects of controlled nutrient interventions on energy and nutrient intakes. A number of excellent reviews have discussed experimental techniques and methods associated with the study of feeding behavior (5–7). Various methods have their own inherent strengths and weaknesses. It is probably worth keeping in mind that neither calorimeter/cubicle environments nor free-living systems have a monopoly on scientific truth. The eating that goes on (and the nutrient and energy computations that are subsequently made) will be closely related to the nature of the research environment. For example, Shepherd (8) notes that sensory attributes of foods associated with salt, sugar, and fat may be important in influencing food choice when specific sensory measures of foods are related to nutrient intake or food consumption in the laboratory. In the real world the picture is much less clear. There is as yet little convincing evidence that the same sensory attributes determine salt, sugar and fat intake in free-living people. Other factors such as convenience, price, nutritional beliefs, availability, brand image, and cultural and social influences are likely to be more important. Thus the "noise" created by environmental influences in the real world obscures the relationships observed in the laboratory. This "noise" is important, however, since it influences food choice in the natural environment of the subjects.

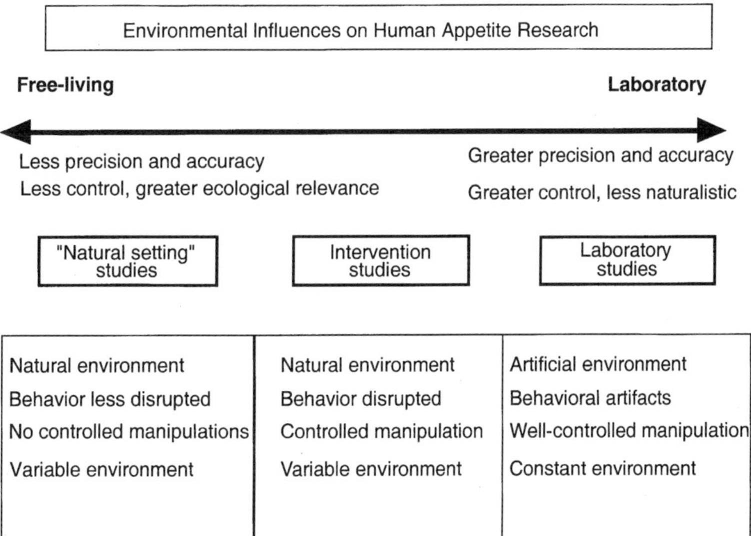

Figure 1 Constraints and limitations that the experimental environment places on studies of human feeding. In general, the environment ranges from totally free-living, which is realistic but very difficult to make measurements in, to the laboratory, where measurement are easy but may be contaminated by artifacts due to the artificiality of the laboratory surroundings.

Studies are therefore measuring not "how the biobehavioral system functions," but how it functions under different circumstances. Is any of this relevant to how the system functions when it is not in an experiment and not being measured? Currently we favor (where possible) a methodological approach which attempts to bridge the gap between the laboratory and the real world by overlapping protocols that explore the same issue in different environmental contexts. Few individual studies are likely to unequivocally resolve major issues in appetite research.

B Demand Characteristics

Although as scientists we may suppose that we can investigate the food intake of human subjects as if it were a piece of tissue in a test tube, this is unlikely to be the case. In any experimental circumstances subjects bring with them their past history of eating, beliefs, about food, and also their beliefs about what they are supposed to do to be a "good subject". These beliefs, which will influence the volitional control over responses (namely eating), are often referred to as "demand characteristics" and are widely ignored (by researchers).

Misreporting of dietary intakes is a case in point (2). It may be that the more we bombard the public with information about what we think they should eat (e.g., a low-fat diet), the more they tell us they are eating what they think we want them to eat.

C Power, Sensitivity, and Effect Size

These issues are of course relevant to all research but may assume special importance where a form of behavior is the measured variable. This is because there is likely to be large intersubject variability. As an example, attention can be drawn to short-term studies on appetite using some variant of the preload test meal paradigm. The problem concerns negative outcomes, i.e., where manipulations produce no significant effect (on the test meal intake). Negative outcomes may obviously arise from experiments conducted under low power (the type II error). This could be brought about by small numbers of subjects, small manipulations (at the border of detection threshold) and noise in the system. In certain cases an effect size of 10% may not be statistically significant. This can be contrasted with an epidemiological type of study using hundreds of subjects in which an effect size of 0.05% may be statistically significant. In these cases different arguments apply to achieve the optimum interpretation.

For those small-scale studies that fail to detect a change in the dependent variable, a problem of interpretation arises. Is the manipulated (independent) variable truly without effect, or is the experimental system insensitive? Most scientists could design a legitimate-looking experiment, whose methodology could pass peer review scrutiny, but which would inevitably lead to a negative outcome. It has been pointed out that the major problem to be overcome in biobehavioral experiments is the type II error (not the type I, which most scientists dread because they can be accused of fudging the data). The preload paradigm is vulnerable to type II errors from a number of sources such as small quantity of nutrient given or small number of subjects, or the test meal may be consumed at a time when the effects of the preload have decayed to the point where they are no longer significant. Studies conducted in the clinical setting are vulnerable to both type I and type II errors, often because of small sample sizes. Type I errors can occur due to confounding factors such as secondary complications of disease or medication.

D Relevance of Questions Asked and Veridicality of Results

Research strategies should be formulated to address key theoretical or practical issues that are important to the study of human feeding behavior. The research question asked will, in part, influence the interpretation of results. For example high-fat, energy-dense diets promote higher energy intakes than lower-fat, less energy dense diets (9–11). The common interpretation of this result is that fat is poorly recognized by the body and that dietary fat per se promotes excess energy intakes. Other studies show isoenergetically dense high- and low-fat diets to produce similar energy intakes (12,13). These observations have led to a somewhat confused debate on the role of energy density in determining energy intake. In reality dietary fat, energy density, and their effects on energy intake are interrelated (14).

There is relatively little standardization of definitions and approaches in this area of research, and this often makes comparisons of studies difficult. Furthermore, the problems of precision versus naturalness demand characteristics and of sensitivity mean that the literature is awash with studies that provide conflicting results about the same issue. It is often only possible to gain a clearer view of an issue by examining all of the studies that have addressed that issue after careful consideration has been given to methodologies employed. The literature on the influence of sweetness on appetite, and publications on the influence of dietary fat on PI satiety and the role of CCK as a PI satiety hormone are three clear examples where a number of conflicting results can be obtained from various studies in the literature. At the present time there is a considerable degree of selective presentation of research results by interested parties who aim to use the scientific literature to market products which may or may not influence human feeding behavior or energy balance. The appetite literature is a spin doctor's paradise. It is therefore important to consider all of the literature on a given area. Researchers have a responsibility to acknowledge the limitations of their own experimental designs and to avoid overgeneralizing results or drawing premature conclusions from individual studies conducted in specific experimental environments, on small numbers of subjects. Since the majority of positive results usually provide indirect support for a hypothesis, the limitations of that support should be acknowledged. The perfect experimental protocol to study human feeding behavior does not exist.

E Bottom-Up or Top-Down Research?

There is currently a tendency to view the relative "sexiness" of biological science in terms of its ability to explain biological systems at the molecular and biochemical level. However, for any mechanism to be important to feeding behavior and body weight regulation it must operate physiological conditions in the intact animal. We believe that it is useful to study human feeding by considering the way that feeding behavior operates as a system within the intact person. In addition, an understanding of how the intact system operates can be used as a reference when attempting to interpret the mechanisms underlying the development of obesity. After all, overweight and obesity now affect the majority of Western adults going about their normal lives. It is equally important to examine how changes in the key features of the system may affect its overall functioning, for example, by understanding the role of CCK in meal termination and the maintenance of PI satiety. However these components should always be viewed as parts of a more complex system, rather than the prime movers in a simple feedback loop. It is therefore necessary to attempt to understand the nature of the system and how it responds to changes in the nature in the environment.

F The Thorny Question of Regulation

It is often assumed that the "natural" state of the subject in the laboratory, when not subject to an experimentally induced manipulation, should one be one of energy and nutrient balance regulation. There is no clear reason why this should be the case, especially in short-term experiments. Indeed, given that > 50% of the adult population are now collectively overweight and obese (15), perhaps the assumed "nonmanipulated" state should be characterized by a tendency to overeat! Nevertheless, experiments that claim to address the issue of energy balance (EB) regulation should include a no-treatment control, in which subjects should be in approximate EB. If subjects are in a gross energy imbalance on such a "control," then the effect of the experiment itself on the "regulatory" system under investigation should be given serious consideration.

III THE NATURE OF THE APPETITE SYSTEM

A Behavior of the Appetite System

Feeding is determined by a redundant biological system which operates through changes in behavior (by redundant we mean the system is actually a series of overlapping subsystems, which do not all need to be fully operational or intact for the whole system to function appropriately). The physiology of appetite is therefore the physiology of feeding behavior. Anatomically, this system can be divided into the central nervous system and the neural pathways, which communicate with peripheral physiology and metabolism (Fig. 2). The whole system operates through changes in behavior in response to changes in the internal or external environment. Both central and peripheral factors operate together to evaluate and reinforce "appropriate" responses and to avoid inappropriate forms of behavior. The adaptability of this system lies in its redundancy. The fact that changes in plasma profiles of metabolites or stores of nutrients do not translate directly into feeding behavior is an important feature of a flexible system capable of adjusting to changes in the environment by learning about the sensory and physiological consequences of feeding-related actions. These aspects of feeding behavior are all too often not appreciated or even ignored by those exploring molecular mechanisms of energy balance control. In spite of the fact that there are few clear facts about food intake,

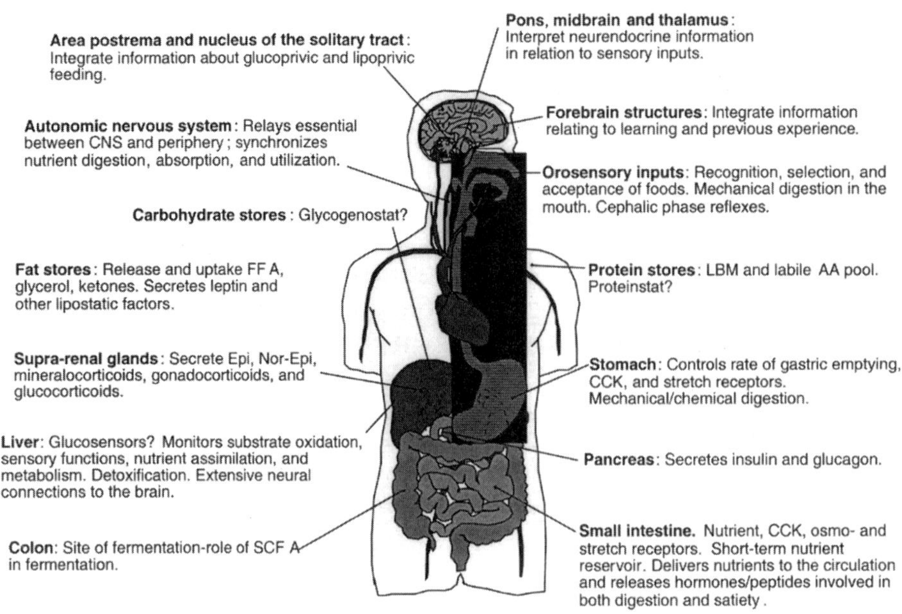

Figure 2 Anatomy of the human appetite system is represented by the relationship between peripheral physiology and the central nervous system. Only the main sites of physiological signals thought to be important in producing feedback signals that affect feeding are outlined. It is of note that all putative signals identified operate along the sequence of ingestion, absorption, metabolism, and storage. All such putative satiety signals have other primary functions.

there do appear to be a number of well-understood ways in which the system usually behaves, or its probabilistic outcomes.

1. Feeding behavior is governed by a redundant system that has numerous afferent inputs. Not all of these inputs are necessary for the system to function. Feeding behavior can change in a number of measurable ways such as meal size, frequency, and the composition of foods selected, or the rate and manner in which foods are ingested.

2. The system uses multiple sensory cues to learn about the consequences of ingesting certain foods. Mimicking the cues associated with certain foods can therefore, transiently at least, "mislead" the system.

3. The system is sensitive to certain changes in the external and internal environment (e.g., temperature or pregnancy, respectively) and to changes in the supply of energy and nutrients. With respect to energy and nutrients, the sensitivity of the system (i.e., the capacity of the system to recognize changes in the environment) can often be greater than its responsiveness (i.e., tendency to alter behavior in order to maintain the constancy of the internal environment). This may in part due to the plasticity of intermediary metabolism in response to changes in energy and nutrient intake.

4. Evolution has selected our physiology and behavior to favor overconsumption rather than underconsumption (16). This mean that the system is more responsive to deficits in energy and nutrients than to increments. Being overweight is probably the result of largely "normal" feeding responses when exposed to a Western diet under modern sedentary conditions.

5. The system tends to exist in equilibrium between energy intake and expenditure that maintains a stable body weight. This equilibrium can be disrupted in such a way that shifts body weight upward. A new equilibrium may then be achieved at a higher body weight.

6. The system is interconnected with other biological systems that influence motivation and behavior. Other external and internal influences can greatly perturb the system in such a way that food (energy and nutrient) intake patterns become maladaptive. Other biobehavioral drives can override and distort the cues associated with feeding. This is especially so in the genesis of eating disorders.

At the present time there is considerable doubt in our minds about the presence of regulatory signals that protect humans from slow, continuous weight gain. This is especially so given that over half of the adult population of the Western world are overweight and obese (15). Why does energy intake rise above energy expenditure? Why is it that a decrease in energy expenditure does not exert a restraining effect over food intake? (Are these the same questions?) Why does a positive energy balance fail to generate a negative signal to suppress food intake? Does the body contain a mechanism(s) capable of detecting a positive energy balance (or positive nutrient balances)?

Can we attribute current secular trends in body weight to a greater per capita drive to consume more food and energy, or could it be that the mechanisms concerned with resisting overconsumption are simply too weak?

B Satiety Signals

Some physiological responses which follow food consumption are believed to terminate eating and/or maintain inhibition over further intake. These responses are usually referred to as "satiety signals" (17). What are the features of foods that are believed to be monitored and which give rise to "satiety" signals? What is the status of the putative "satiety" signals?

It has been assumed or claimed that volume, weight, energy content, macronutrient proportion, and energy density may all be monitored and constitute the source of specific satiation or postingestive (PI) satiety signals. These may be divided into general factors (e.g., weight, volume) which apply to all foods, and specific factors (nutrient content, taste, and smell) which depend on the particular food consumed. Why should weight and volume appear as important features that affect food intake in some studies? (A liter of water would have weight and volume but would provide no energy or nutrients.) The ultimate function of satiation and PI satiety signals is to monitor the biological value of foods and to play a role in the processing of ingested nutrients (all physiological signals involved in satiation, e.g., rate of gastric stretch, release of CCK, gastric emptying, nutrient oxidation, etc., have functions in addition to their role in a negative feedback system). A satiety signal is a function assumed by some underlying physiological property. Given a history of food seeking and consumption, it is inevitable that weight and volume of food will have become associated with (conditioned to) the important biological components of food, namely, energy value and nutrient composition. The system has learned how to operate in a real environment, and the objective of the system is to produce a veridical response.

Brunswik's theory of perception provides a model for understanding this (18). Weight and volume are learned cues with high functional validity (proximal cues that correlate well with more distal cues such as hormone release contact with gastrointestinal receptors, etc.). This is why weight and volume often appear to be important monitored variables (rather than energy or nutrient content) when nutritional composition of food has been surreptitiously manipulated. The system is operating sensibly according to its previous experience, but it does not mean that weight is fundamentally more important than energy content. Indeed, we have recently shown that the macronutrients protein, carbohydrate, fat, and alcohol, together with water and energy density, collectively account for ~40% of the total variability in energy intake in 102 adults, self-recording their food intake for 7 days. However, each individual dietary component only explained a relatively minor proportion of variability in energy intake, suggesting that no one single dietary constituent has an overriding effect on energy intake (14).

C Satiation and Satiety

In discussing the function of "satiety signals" it would be useful to specify what aspects of eating behavior they are supposed to inhibit. Is their function to prevent weight gain? Some authors have distinguished between intrameal and intermeal satiety (19); others, such as Blundell (17), have called these process satiation and PI satiety. They distinguish between events which (i) bring eating to a halt and (ii) maintain inhibition over further eating after consumption—so-called postingestive satiety. For the purposes of this work, "satiation" refers to intrameal satiety or the process that brings a meal to an end; "postingestive satiety" (abbreviated to PI satiety) refers to the inhibition of eating between meals (intermeal satiety).

In considering the control of patterns of food intake it would seem important to distinguish between those factors (in food, in the biological system, or in the mind) that operate to adjust either the size of an eating episode as the interval between episodes. For example, CCK is often referred to as a satiety hormone; is this correct? The original studies carried out by Smith and colleagues indicated that CCK terminated eating in sham-feeding rats (20). Subsequent studies indicated that CCK reduced meal size but did not influence the frequency of meals (21). Therefore CCK should more correctly be termed a satiation hormone.

This analysis draws attention to those factors that influence food (1) while it is being eaten and (2) after it has been consumed. It would be expected that weight and volume would influence satiation, but not PI

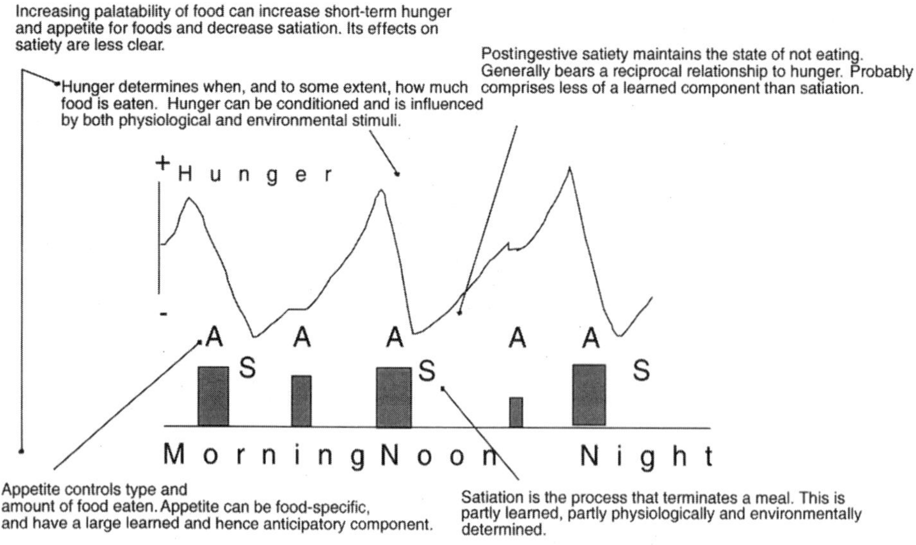

Increasing palatability of food can increase short-term hunger and appetite for foods and decrease satiation. Its effects on satiety are less clear.
Postingestive satiety maintains the state of not eating. Generally bears a reciprocal relationship to hunger. Probably comprises less of a learned component than satiation.
Hunger determines when, and to some extent, how much food is eaten. Hunger can be conditioned and is influenced by both physiological and environmental stimuli.
+ Hunger
-
A A A A A
S S S
Morning Noon Night
Appetite controls type and amount of food eaten. Appetite can be food-specific, and have a large learned and hence anticipatory component.
Satiation is the process that terminates a meal. This is partly learned, partly physiologically and environmentally determined.

Figure 3 Schematic representation (not to scale) of the relationship between the subjectively expressed constructs of motivation in relation to feeding, and their relationship to quantitative and qualitative feeding behavior.

satiety. Evidence suggests that this is so (14). Additionally, the palatability (and variety) of food would exert a major influence during consumption but less influence afterward. It may be inferred that cognitions would be markedly different during and after ingestion. Consequently, biological, environmental, and cognitive influences differ during the operation of satiation (intrameal satiety) and (intermeal) satiety. As regards overconsumption, there is little if any direct evidence that satiety signals function in a manner consistent with mechanisms geared to the tight regulation of body weight. It follows that speaking about satiety "in general" can be quite confusing. Conceptual understanding would be improved by an increase in semantic precision. A scheme illustrating the relationship among hunger, appetite, satiation, and PI satiety and their purported influence on feeding behavior is illustrated in Figure 3.

D The "Hunger State"

In 1955 Mayer pointed out that one of the key features of a short-term model of food intake is that it should be able to account for the hunger state (22). As mentioned above, this does not just have theoretical significance. There is an immense interest in pharmacological agents as tools that can be used to manipulate the hunger state (23). Parenthetically, it is of academic, and perhaps applied, interest to consider whether hunger and satiety can be dissociated. Being able to blunt the drive to eat should enhance compliance on weight-reducing programs. Being able to increase the drive to eat may increase longevity and quality of life in patients experiencing cachexia. Understanding how to manage hunger and satiety also has important implications for the nutritional support of a number of clinical conditions. One of the great benefits of using human subjects is that they can be asked about their sensations and motivations. Understanding the profile of physiological changes that attend and underlie changes in the hunger state offers key sites for intervention and manipulation of the hunger state. Both indices of carbohydrate oxidation (24) and a preprandial drop in plasma glucose have been shown to predict the onset of feeding in rats (25) and humans (26). Furthermore, in animals, abolition of the small but reproducible preprandial drop in blood glucose, by a small intravenous infusion, has been shown to inhibit eating for several hours (27). Under these conditions satiety is maintained and hunger is inhibited.

While there is little evidence that satiety signals strongly defend against overconsumption, there is ample evidence that acute (28,29) or prolonged negative energy balance (30) leads to an elevation of hunger. In extremis, significant loss of body tissue leads to an obsessive and unabating drive to eat. Understanding how the intact system operates and which physiological events underlie changes in motivation to eat and feeding behavior can help unravel and manipulate the mechanisms that influence meal size, frequency, and composition. New technological advances now enable real-time monitoring of brain activity and neurendocrine profiles (31). Bringing these approaches together with methods used to monitor human feeding behavior will provide unique insights into the physiological processes underlying normal daily fluctuations in energy and nutrient balance. By doing this it may become possible to explore how these mechanisms are perturbed in disease states. Conversely, specific disease states can shed light on the normal functioning of intact processes involved in feeding behavior. Determining the mechanisms that influence feeding behavior necessarily entails understanding how parts of the system interact (i) with the environment (especially the food component) and (ii) with each other to facilitate or inhibit eating and selection of foods.

IV COMPARTMENTS OF THE APPETITE CONTROL SYSTEM

Figure 1 illustrates the anatomy of the system, its components, and their main functions. Figure 4 illustrates the way in which physiology and behavior interact in their response to food and food-related environmental stimuli. Together, these two figures outline the nature of the system. The biobehavioral

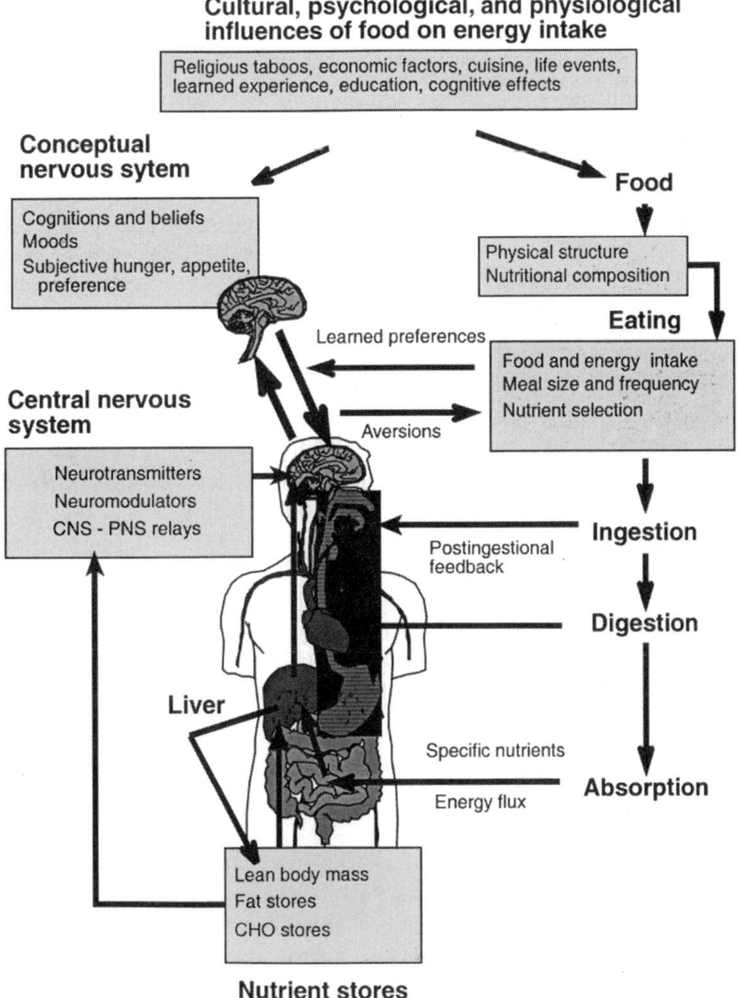

Figure 4 Interaction between physiology and behavior in their response to food and food-related environmental stimuli. It is notable that food illicits potent cognitive, learned behavioral and physiological responses which together determine the feeding strategies of an individual.

system controlling feeding can be artificially divided into the following components:

1. Orosensory components
2. Gastrointestinal components
3. Circulating factors such as hormones, peptides, cytokines, and nutrients
4. Nutrient stores—gut contents, glycogen, muscle, and adipose tissue
5. Nutrient metabolism—whole-body ATP turnover, cellular mechanisms associated with oxidation of the major metabolic fuels, e.g., sodium pump activity
6. The central and peripheral nervous systems including neurotransmitters, peptides, and other centrally acting compounds

These components of the system interact to produce facilitatory or inhibitory contributions to overall feeding patterns. Most components of the diet that are ingested are likely to act at multiple sites. Simply drinking a glass of water will influence gut motility, osmoreceptors, hormones (e.g., ADH), and the central nervous system.

A Orosensory Components

Nutrient-associated orosensory components of food are generally believed to provide facilitatory signals which increase food intake. However, it is of interest that removal of the sense of smell barely inhibits the intake of readily available food in pigs, presumably because the animals will learn to use other cues (32). Clearly, for many animals, olfaction is critical to the location and acquisition of foods. When combined with learning, olfaction is a primary cue for identifying foods as being acceptable or not. As Le Magnen (33) puts it, "The particular property of the olfactory system, compared to taste, is to individualise practically all active molecules by a discriminable odour. . . ." Taste, texture, and smell of foods warn against toxins and other damaging components of food. The strength of this mechanism is indicated by the phenomenon of conditioned aversion to foods that have produced subsequent illness (34–36). Rozin suggests that rats learn sensory preferences/aversions for diets that are adequate/deficient in micronutrients in this way only after a trial-and-error period during which they sample a variety of diets offered to them (37,38). During this time, they learn to associate the nutrient quality of the diet with its particular smell, flavor, or appearance. The same mechanisms are likely to operate in relation to dietary macronutrients. Increasing the sensory qualities and variety of these diets can lead to obesity in some strains of rats and may also be important for the maintenance of the obese state in humans (33). However, it is important to note that, while people obviously select what they like, this does not necessarily suggest that increasing the sensory quality or the variety of sensory attributes of a diet will lead to obesity. Recent evidence in humans suggests that increasing only the sensory variety of a nutritionally controlled diet leads to elevated energy intake over 7 days (39). The longer-term effects of changes in the sensory attributes of foods per se on energy balance are unknown. This may simply be due to the difficulty of conducting such an experiment. Sensory factors may interact with other factors such as diet composition or genetic predisposition to precipitate hyperphagia. Internal cues interact with sensory information to help formulate appropriate food (nutrient) selection or foraging strategies (33–37). Aspects of sensory experience have been rated by healthy, free-living adults among the top three determinants that guide their food detection and ingestion (40,41). Mattes (6) suggest that in the clinical setting where many environmental considerations are less prominent pathologically induced sensory disturbances can be important, particularly in affecting the acceptability of specific foods, e.g., clinical supplements.

B Gastrointestinal Components

The gut is known to have an important role to play in the short-term control of feeding behavior. It was initially believed that hunger sensations arose in the stomach (42). It is now accepted that a major role of the stomach is to regulate the flow of energy and nutrients into the small intestine. The stomach also places a physical constraint on the amount of food that can be consumed at a given meal. This fact has been applied, in extremis, during gastroplasty surgery as a means of obesity treatment. Stomach size adapts to the amount of food habitually eaten. This effect means that previously undernourished people have to eat small frequent meals, during the initial stage of nutritional rehabilitation, although as refeeding progresses, energy intakes can reach spectacular levels (30,43). Stretch and CCK receptors inform the CNS of the status of the stomach. The small intestine itself places a further constraint on the amount of food that can be ingested, since a certain time is taken to complete digestion and absorption. Both of these processes appear to be particularly important in releasing cascades of signals (hormones, peptides, action potentials along gastrointestinal nerves) including the nutrients themselves to the postabsorptive circulation (44). It is interesting that patients with short intestines (and few secondary complications) attempt to eat to energy requirements. This means they are hyperphagic, presumably to compensate for the decreased absorptive capacity of the shortened small intestine (M. Elia, personal communication). In addition, stretch, CCK receptors and osmoreceptors, and a variety of gastrointestinal peptides all appear to play some role in affecting short-term feeding.

C The Liver

The liver is the main organ that receives and deals with the digestion products of a meal, except for chylomicrons, which initially bypass the liver, since they are absorped through the lymphatic system. It has been suggested that this effect contributes to the delayed effects of fat in suppressing appetite (32). It has been suggested from preference-conditioning experiments using portal infusions of fructose (45) that the liver also functions as a sensory organ. This is because rats learn to prefer flavors that are paired with a glucose infusion into the hepatic portal vein. The liver possesses extensive neural connections to the brain which appear to be involved in glucoprivic and lipoprivic feeding, at least in rodents (46). Pharmacological impairment of nutrient oxidation in the liver stimulates intake (47). A detailed discussion of these links between nutrient metabolism and the CNS is given below. The liver is the main site of assimilation, metabolism, and distribution of nutrients subsequent to ingestion. The liver is most likely the central organ that communicates information about peripheral fuel status to the brain (48).

D Circulating Factors

The circulation and the peripheral nervous system together inform the brain of the overall status of energy and nutrients that are 1) in the circulation, 2) moving into the circulation from the gut (and hence indirectly of their concentration in the gut), and 3) available in nutrient stores. While the gut provides important cues which probably alert the brain to the likely influx of energy and nutrients, failure to reinforce this message by actual delivery of energy and nutrients will lead to diminished sensations of satiation and PI satiety. Thus, sham-feeding dogs (49) and rats are hyperphagic (50,51). On the other hand, nutrient infusions as lipid or glucose fail to elicit the same degree of caloric compensation as oral loads of nutrients (52).

E Monitoring of Energy and Nutrient Flux by the Nervous System

It is important to note that macronutrients exert important influences on appetite and energy intake (EI) at the preabsorptive level. These effects have been considered in detail elsewhere (6,44,53,54). Numerous models have been put forward to suggest that the stores of a single nutrient exert negative feedback on EI. These include the aminostatic (55), glucostatic (56), and lipostatic (57) hypotheses. Single nutrient based feedback models and their limitations have been described in previous discussions (see 3,58,59 for review). It is now apparent that models examining the effects of macronutrients on satiety should include the effects of all three macronutrients. Such integrative models explain a greater proportion of the variance in appetite and energy balance than single-nutrient feedback models (59).

A further development in the field of ingestive behavior in recent years has been the general acceptance that macronutrients exert multiple feedbacks on appetite and feeding behavior at the different levels of nutrient ingestion, digestion, absorption, assimilation, and metabolism (58,59). Furthermore, there is growing evidence that the major macronutrients protein, CHO, and fat simultaneously exert different effects on satiety at these different levels of organization (58,59). Thus, the effects of a given nutrient on appetite need to be considered, inter alia, in the context of (i) the presence or absence of other nutrients, (ii) the levels of physiological organization it operates at, and (iii) the metabolic state and EB profile of the subject concerned. There is now a growing body of evidence that suggests that in the fed state, increases in the oxidative disposal of recently ingested macronutrients correlate with satiety (6,7,49, 56–59). It has been suggested that nutrient oxidation in the liver influences hepatocyte membrane potentials (48). These changes apparently induce neuronal activity in vagal afferents connected to the midbrain (48,58).

Conversely, it has been shown that specific agents that competitively block carbohydrate and fat oxidation (2-deoxyglucose and methylpalmoxirate, respectively), increase food intake in rodents in a dose-dependent manner (60). 2-DG also increases hunger in man (61). The combined use of these metabolic inhibitors induces a massive emergency increase in food intake in rodents (60). These data suggest that when the oxidation of one nutrient is blocked, other energy-providing nutrients can to some extent be used. However, inhibition of the oxidation of both major energy-providing macronutrients leads the rat to seek metabolic fuels from the environment (60). This in turn suggests that the CNS is responsive to the combined effects of macronutrient metabolism rather than being driven by negative feedback from a single nutrient.

What, then, are the combined effects of nutrient oxidation on appetite and subsequent feeding likely to be? As regards diet composition, nutrient processing, and peripheral signals related to feeding, there is now sufficient evidence to provisionally link changes in diet composition to changes in the signaling systems concerned with the control of macronutrient balance. This notion is schematically illustrated in Figure 5 and summarized as follows:

1. Changes in energy and nutrient intake can influence peripheral fuel selection (62–69).
2. Peripheral changes in fuel selection are determined by physiological and thermodynamic constraints which define a hierarchy in the immediacy with which the balance of recently ingested macronutrients are autoregulated by increases in their own oxidative disposal (protein > carbohydrate > fat) (3,11,58,59).
3. This hierarchy appears to parallel a hierarchy in the satiating efficiency of the macronutrients (3,58). Thus while protein, carbohydrate, and fat each contribute to satiety, they do so to differing degrees.
4. These two hierarchies may be causatively related since a growing body of literature suggests that nutrient oxidation in the periphery is monitored by the CNS as a component of satiety (46,60). In particular, Ritter and Calingasan have provided important evidence which suggests that neural pathways monitor fat oxidation in the periphery and CHO oxidation (perhaps more precisely) in both the periphery and the CNS (46). Currently less is known about protein oxidation, except that at the level of nutrient metabolism, protein is the most satiating macronutrient (58).
5. Langhans notes that the midbrain centers, concerned with monitoring peripheral fuel utilization, are connected via extensive neural relays to the areas of the forebrain (especially the hypothalamus and the paraventricular nucleus) that are the sites of action of peptide systems concerned with the control of protein, CHO, and fat balance (70).

Thus, an integrative model is beginning to emerge which may account for the manner in which the CNS is capable of monitoring physiological signals concerned with overall macronutrient intake and fuel flux (58–60). This model accounts for the manner in which feeding behavior responds to changes in peripheral physiology and is illustrated in Figure 5. The CNS appears capable of monitoring overall fuel flux rather than responding to negative feedback from any single nutrient. In essence, feeding responses are coupled to physiological changes rather than being directly determined by them. The evolution of a flexible and adaptive system, concerned with the control of feeding behavior, is likely to have bestowed a far greater survival advantage on an opportunistic foraging species such as humans (or for that matter rodents) than a system in which behavior is an inevitable outcome of rigid physiological signals. Having considered how macronutrients and their metabolic fate influence feeding behavior, it is worth considering whether changes in macronutrient stores influence longer-term appetite and energy balance.

F Do Nutrient Stores Exert Long-Term Feedback on Energy Balance?

There has long been a belief that changes in macronutrient stores exert negative feedback on energy intake. It is interesting in this context that, despite the critical role of protein-energy relationships for survival time during under nutrition (30,68,69,71), few models have considered lean tissue changes as a major source of feedback signals that influence appetite control (see below).

Mayer proposed that peripheral CHO utilization exerts negative feedback on EI through the actions of hypothalamic glucosensors (22), which could be corrected by longer-term "lipostatic" regulation. In 1963, Russek postulated the presence of glucose receptors in the liver and formulated the hepatostatic theory of EB regulation (72). These receptors have never been localized, although it has recently been suggested that sensory vagal afferents function as hepatic glucosensors (48,70). Flatt proposed that CHO stores exert negative feedback on EI in 1987 (65). The robustness of these models has been reviewed elsewhere (58,59).

Kennedy in 1953 argued for feedback information reaching the hypothalamus from adipose tissue, which he presumed to be closely monitored in normal rats (57). The simplest way that such lipostasis could operate would be through the sensitivity of the hypothalamus to the concentration of circulating metabolites. Hervey in 1969 (73) proposed a mechanism for lipostatic regulation, based on endogenous measurement of the fat mass by means of a fat-soluble hormone. It was proposed that such a hormone would act as a physiological tracer that monitors adipose tissue mass by the dilution principle. Experiments in parabiotic rats (74,75) suggest

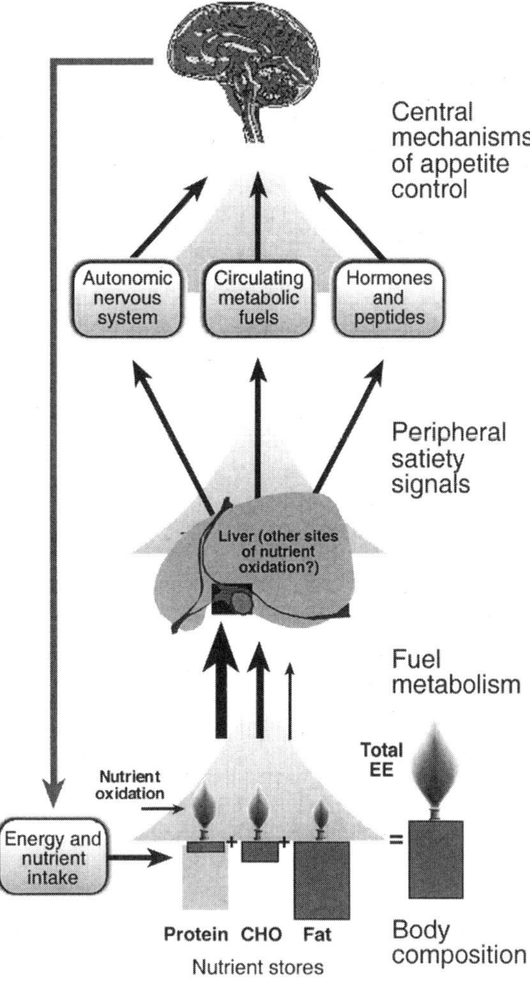

Figure 5 Schematic diagram illustrating putative connections between diet composition, fuel metabolism, peripheral satiety signals, and central control of feeding. Diet composition affects satiety. Protein is more satiating than carbohydrate, which is more satiating than fat. Diet composition also affects postingestive fuel metabolism, since increases in protein and carbohydrate, but not fat balance, are tightly modulated by autoregulatory increases in their oxidative disposal. It is known that nutrient oxidation in peripheral tissues appears to be associated with satiety. The hierarchical regulation of macronutrient balance by oxidative disposal may partially underlie the hierarchy in the satiating efficiency of the macronutrients. Indeed, high levels of protein and carbohydrate (but not fat) oxidation are indicative of the fed state. High rates of fat oxidation are usually synonymous with energy deficits. It has also been suggested that changes in peripheral fuel metabolism may act as and trigger additional peripheral satiety signals that are relayed to feeding centers of the brain believed to be concerned with the control of macronutrient balance.

there is an exchange of some bloodborne factors between lean and obese animals that affects the food intake of the lean rat.

Similar experiments in the late 1970s using genetically obese rodents (76) created the conceptual context for the studies that have led to the identification of the protein leptin (77). Since the discovery of leptin in 1994, there has been an intense focus on signals from adipose tissue as key controllers of longer-term energy balance. The importance of leptin should not be underplayed. However, the strength of negative feedback arising from adipose tissue in humans should not be overestimated. It is abundantly clear from the current prevalence of overweight and obesity (15) that adipose tissue accumulation does not exert strong negative feedback which restores energy balance, at least from the point of excess EI. There is far more evidence that loss of adipose tissue leads to its regain. For instance, the majority of people who lose weight eventually regain it (78). There is now an extensive literature on leptin and other putative feedback signals arising from adipose tissue (see 79 for a recent review). There is a minuscule literature on the extent to which changes in adipose tissue exert feedback on appetite and energy intake at the whole body level. Neither the metabolism nor size of storage of any single nutrient per se exerts a powerful unconditioned negative feedback on quantitative feeding behavior (3,4,11,14). It is therefore important to examine how changes in nutrient stores and metabolism collectively influence appetite and energy balance, longitudinally under conditions where specific components of energy balance have been perturbed. It is critical that putative physiological and molecular mechanisms of appetite control should be related where possible to the actual feeding behavior they are supposed to influence. In this context it is useful to consider the value of underfeeding studies as a means of assessing the relationship between tissue loss and subsequent feeding behavior.

As regards disturbances of this system in the development of obesity, the evidence from the human literature suggests the following.

1. In the short term, it is remarkably easy to perturb energy balance in either a positive or a negative direction. Modifications of the composition or energy density of the diet can be used to generate considerable energy imbalances (3,4,14).

2. In the medium to longer term, the evidence suggests that humans defend against induced energy deficits, regardless of body weight at the outset of the induced deficit (15,78). Over the same time window, humans are remarkably tolerant of moderate increases in energy balance. Thus American adults on average gain 0.2–2.0 kg per year (80).

3. While tolerant of excess energy balances, humans do not eat anywhere near the maximum levels of energy intake that are readily obtainable by selecting certain foods available in the Western diet. This behavior is apparent in certain pathological states such as binge eating, where intakes of up to 30 MJ/day have been reported (4).

4. It therefore seems that there is a tonic control on energy intake, which limits a very rapid weight gain in most people. There is little evidence that such tonic control operates via negative feedback loops, as for tightly regulated physiological systems. In other words, there is little evidence that, as fat mass accumulates, physiological signals become stronger and limit further gain in fat mass (81). The exact nature and strength of the mechanisms that restrain excess energy intake in humans are unclear.

5. There is greater evidence that energy deficits do induce signals that elevate appetite and energy intake. As weight loss proceeds, these signals appear to become stronger, until they become the primarily motivational forces governing an individual's behavior (82). There are a number of signaling systems in the periphery that interlink with the peptide messenger systems of the brain to increase intake when energy deficits significantly deplete tissue stores (83). The extent to which these systems are involved in the control of day-to-day feeding behavior in humans is less clear.

6. As regards depletion of body tissues during periods of energy deficit, most research has focused almost exclusively on fat (83) despite the fact that in the clinical setting a negative nitrogen balance and loss of lean tissue are known to compromise physiological function. Loss of lean tissue during therapeutic weight loss may be a major factor which signals to the brain that physiological integrity is being eroded. The signals are as yet unknown.

To explore the system determining human feeding behavior, it is appropriate to consider how central features and components of that system change under different environmental conditions. The most central feature of feeding behavior is food. Food varies in orosensory qualities and in composition. Until recently the orosensory qualities of foods acted as reliable cues that gave accurate information about the nutrient content of food and the physiological consequences of ingesting it. A growing number of advances in food technology have changed this relationship between the sensory attributes of the diet and its nutrient composi-

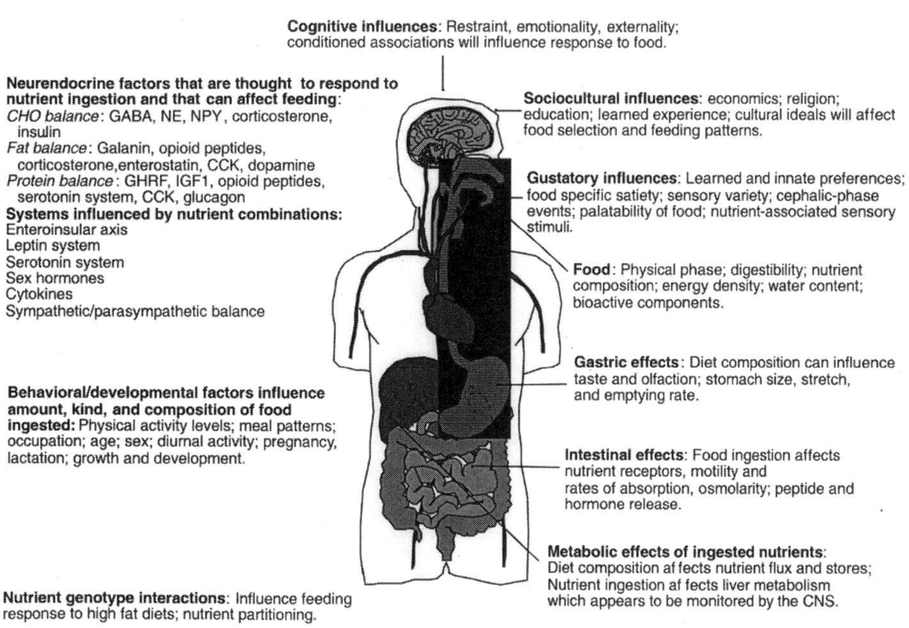

Figure 6 Primary ways in which food and nutrient ingestion influences the main compartments of the human appetite system. Food influences this system through multiple feedbacks at multiple levels which can be traced through the processes of food location, ingestion, digestion, absorption, and metabolism. Satiety is therefore maintained by a functional sequence or cascade of sequential physiological events which reinforce each other. Removing parts of a food or nutrient's effects on this sequence will therefore diminish its impact on satiety.

tion. Figure 6 summarizes the main ways in which food can affect this feeding system.

V DIET COMPOSITION AND FEEDING BEHAVIOR

Given the current prevalence of obesity worldwide and the role of overconsumption in generating a positive energy balance which is converted into weight gain, it is important to consider the composition of foods which form the basis of overconsumption. In turn, this introduces the key concept of diet composition and feeding behavior. How do the relative amounts of the energy-yielding macronutrients influence the control of food intake? There is a good deal of variation in the experimental results from research on this issue, and findings have purported to show inter alia that all macronutrients have equal power to suppress subsequent energy intake, protein exerts a greater suppressive effect on subsequent energy intake than carbohydrate or fat, carbohydrate and fat have similar effects on caloric suppression, fat generates strong signals which suppress appetite, and fat is the least effective of the macronutrients at suppressing appetite.

A Macronutrients, Satiation, and PI Satiety

1 Protein

Protein appears to be the macronutrient which suppresses energy intake to a greater extent than any of the other macronutrients. Careful retrospective analysis of food records (14,84) indicate that protein exerts postingestive action over and above the contribution from energy per se. In studies where subjects record their food intake, the percentage energy intake from protein has been found to predict decreases in intake. Percent energy intake from fat is a significant predictor of increase in energy intake and carbohydrate is very weakly related to energy intake. (14,84,85).

Protein also exerts a large influence on satiety in the laboratory. Some studies using pure macronutrient loads delivered to the stomach or solutions quickly swallowed by subjects wearing noseclips (86,87) have found that all macronutrients have equal satiating power. It is intriguing in this regard that sensory cues (especially taste) may be important in clearly identifying the effects of nutrient ingestion. Miller and Teates (88) found that male Sprague–Dawley rats were able to select from nutritionally different diets in a way that stabilized the protein energy ratio at 0.14. However, when rats were subjected to impairment of oral somatosensory input, they were unable to maintain a stable selection pattern. The authors hypothesized that selection between protein and carbohydrate (or energy) at least "involves an associative learning process in which somatosensory inputs effect feeding activity and/or the properties of the food link dietary choice behaviour to later metabolic consequences."

It also appears that there may be a critical threshold in the amount of protein required to suppress subsequent energy intake since studies that have found little effect of protein relative to other macronutrient preloads have only used small amounts of energy as protein in the preload (86,89). Hill and Blundell (90) found that a high-protein (HP) meal (31% of 2.1 MJ) produced a greater sensation of fullness and a decreased desire to eat, relative to a high-carbohydrate (HC) meal (52%) of the same energy content. Hill and Blundell (91) also found that both obese and normal-weight subjects reduced their subsequent meal intakes by 19% and 22% respectively after a HP (54% of 2 MJ) meal compared to a HC meal (63% of 2 MJ) with weight of food held constant. Barkeling et al. (92) gave 20 normal-weight women a high-protein (43% of 2.6 MJ) or a high-carbohydrate (69% of 2.6 MJ) lunch and measured the energy intake at a subsequent evening meal. They found that energy intake was depressed by 12% after consumption of the HP meal. Booth et al. (93) also found that an HP meal reduced the intake of a subsequent test meal by 26% relative to a virtually protein-free meal in normal-weight individuals. Thus, protein appears to be particularly satiating when given at moderate and large amounts.

This apparent appetite-restraining effect of protein has not yet been given a strong theoretical basis, and there has been little recent investigation of the "proteinstat." It is perhaps pertinent to note that essential amino acids when ingested in excess of requirements form a physiological stress that must be disposed of by oxidation. It is known than animals will alter feeding behavior in order to alleviate a physiological stress (94). Pigs, in particular, appear capable of learning to select a protein:energy ratio in the diet that is optimal for growth (95,96), as can rats (88). There is also evidence that the kind of animo acids ingested may influence satiety. Imbalances in single essential amino acids can greatly affect the feeding behavior of rats (97). The protein: energy ratio of foods may be important in influencing feeding. Malnourished children find it difficult to tolerate nutritional supplements whose protein:energy ratio is too high. Millward has hypothesized that lean tissue deposition may be an important factor driving appetite during catchup growth in children (98).

Stubbs and Elia have recently suggested that lean tissue depletion during weight loss may be at least as important as adipose tissue depletion in increasing appetite and driving intake upward (99). This concept has been long neglected. One seminal study has enabled the relationship between tissue loss and subsequent feeding behavior to be determined (30). The results were quiet remarkable and have recently been revisited by Dulloo (100,101). During the Minnesota semistarvation study a group of lean men were chronically underfed for 24 weeks, consuming ~40% of their normal EI throughout this period. During this time they lost ~70% of their fat mass and ~18–20% of their lean body mass. For the next 12 weeks, they were incrementally refed in a mandatory manner. By the end of this period, they were still in a deficit of ~25% for fat mass and 12–15% for lean body mass. During the final 8 weeks subjects had ad libitum access to a range of foods. During this period energy intake initially increased to 160% of requirements and gradually subsided to pre–weight loss levels. However, by this time fat mass had reached 170% of pre–weight loss values, while lean body mass had returned to pre–weight loss levels (99,100). These relationships are depicted in Figure 7A. Thus the cessation of post–weight loss hyperphagia coincided with a massive overshoot of fat mass, but precise repletion of lean body mass. There are very few datasets of this quality available, which highlights the importance of conducting more detailed longitudinal studies with this degree of precision and accuracy. If depletion of lean tissue during weight loss stimulates hunger, then increased protein intake, subsequent to significant weight loss, may replete lean tissue faster and help stabilize body weight at a new, lower level. This hypothesis is currently under test. The concept is illustrated in Figure 7B.

It can be seen from the arguments outlined in this discussion that the physiological regulation of lean tissue may be a critical factor which exerts feedback on subsequent EI. When subjects are in energy balance, excess protein intake does not increase the size of lean body mass (69). Instead, it is disposed of by transamination, deamination, and urea production. This regulation of protein balance by obligatory oxidative disposal predicts a suppression of subsequent energy intake (11). During undernutrition, lean body mass becomes depleted (30,68,69). The Keys data from the Minnesota semistarvation study suggest that when food is available ad libitum, subjects do not stop eating when fat mass is repleted but when

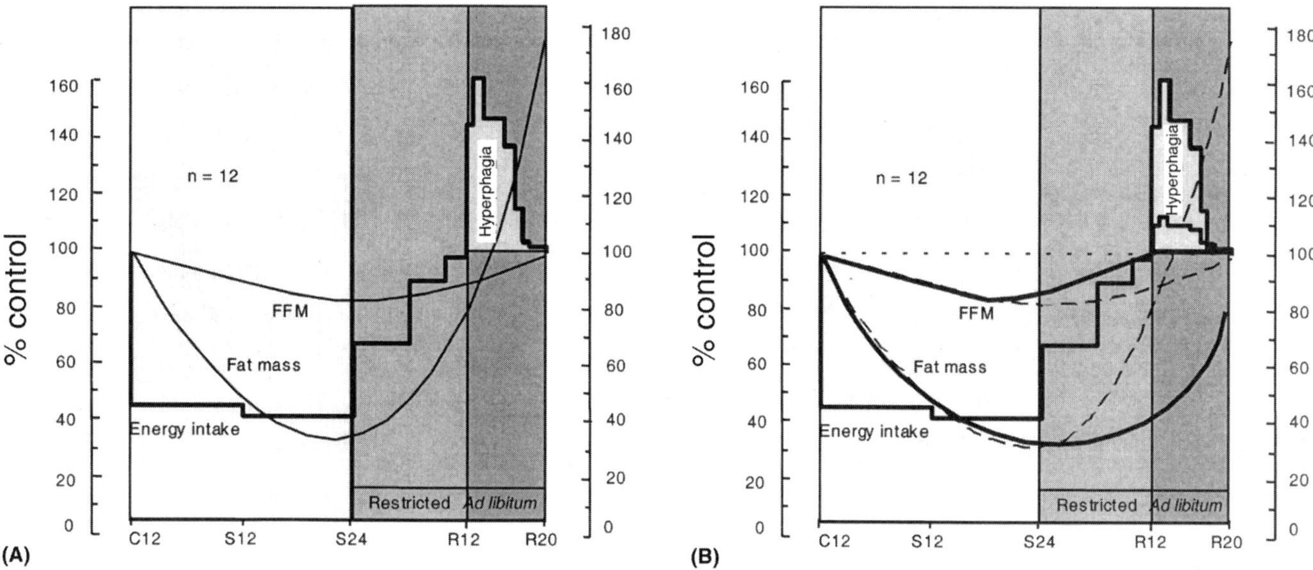

Figure 7 (A) Relationship between energy intake and tissue change during 6 months' severe undernutrition, 3 months' rehabilitation, and 2 months' ad libitum feeding in 12 of the subjects who took part in the Minnesota study. Of particular note is the fact that ad libitum energy intake returned to preunderfeeding levels at approximately the time lean tissue returned to baseline values. By this time fat mass had overshot baseline and reached ~170% of original levels. (B) predicted effects of protein supplementation on the relationship between tissue deposition and post–weight loss hyperphagia. Depletion of lean tissue may act as a signal for hyperphagia once original fat mass has been repleted. Dietary protein supplements, after weight loss, may help replete lean tissue more rapidly, diminish post–weight loss hyperphagia, and promote weight stability below pre–weight loss levels.

lean body mass is repleted. Thus there is evidence that the regulation of lean tissue (which helps maintain normal physiological function), through oxidation of excess and repletion of deficits in protein intake, may exert some negative feedback effect on longer-term energy intake (99). The role of lean tissue in this respect has been largely ignored. It is important to understand how both lean and adipose tissue changes relate to longer-term energy balance (30,99–101). This is again important in the clinical setting since loss of lean tissue in disease compromises physiological function and can complicate further the effects of disease. Understanding how loss of fat and lean tissue relate to other aspects of function, health, and well-being will be critical in improving sustained weight loss.

2 Carbohydrates

The public perception of carbohydrates has oscillated in recent decades. Throughout the 1970s there was a tendency for a number of nutritionists to view carbohydrates (especially refined forms) as conducive to weight gain. This reached its logical extreme with perceptions of sugars as "pure, white, and deadly" by Yudkin (102). Since that time the nutritional perception of carbohydrates has improved dramatically. By the mid-1990s, dietary fat had developed a reputation of near demonic proportions as the dietary villain of the late 20th century and was squarely blamed as the major dietary constituent promoting excess EI. During this time, dietary CHO was generally viewed in generic terms as a beneficial nutrient whose ingestion could promote all manner of positive outcomes with reference to weight control (103). The positive effects of carbohydrates on energy balance were enshrined in the predictions of Flatt's glycogenostatic model of energy balance control. The general perceptions about carbohydrates and energy balance at this time were as follows:

1. It was generally accepted that carbohydrates are absorbed, metabolized, and stored with less bioenergetic efficiency than dietary fat and, per MJ of energy ingested, were protective against weight gain. Indeed, a general perception was developing that because de novo lipogenesis appears limited when humans feed on Western diets, that carbohydrate ingestion does not promote fat storage (104,105).

2. At the same time, there was a renaissance of interest in carbohydrate-specific models of feeding. The notion that carbohydrate metabolism or stores exert powerful negative feedback on EI became quite firmly established in the field of energy and nutrient balance (59,81).

3. The simultaneous focus of researchers and health professionals on dietary fat as the pivotal nutrient promoting high levels of EI reinforced carbohydrate-specific models of feeding. HF hyperphagia was seen as due to the tendency for subjects to eat to carbohydrate balance rather than energy balance. Thus hyperphagia on high-fat (HF) diets (which are by definition low in the percentage of energy from carbohydrate) was seen as being driven by the need to ingest a certain level of carbohydrate (59,81).

4. By the same reasoning, diets high in carbohydrates were deemed to be more satiating, specifically because they were high in carbohydrates.

5. The extension of this logic led to the notion among some that it was difficult if not virtually impossible to overeat on a high-carbohydrate diet (104,105).

6. Finally, epidemiological observations have shown that, in subjects recording their food intakes, the percentage of EI from fat and carbohydrates are reciprocally related to each other. One form of this relationship has been termed the fat-sugar seesaw. It has been noted in one seminal study that high-sugar consumers also tend to be thinner than HF consumers are (106). This led to the suggestion that sugar displaces fat energy from the diet, and since fat is conducive to weight gain, high sugar intakes may well protect against obesity (107).

Carbohydrates had never had it so good. These messages percolated through the scientific community to governments, consumers, and industry who were (and still are) deeply concerned about diet-induced obesity in developed and developing countries. Fat reduction became the order of the day and the low-fat (LF) food market rapidly expanded (108,109). The fat reduction message has now become so strong that consumers appear to have focused on fat avoidance as a primary nutritional objective while foraging for food in local supermarkets. The food industry has gone to great lengths to diversify products in the direction of LF, lower-fat, and high-carbohydrate foods, which have sufficient sensory appeal that consumers will continue to select and ingest them. A major sensory attribute of high-carbohydrate foods, which is almost ubiquitously appealing, is sweetness.

In recent years, there have been some doubts about the paramount role of carbohydrates as the central nutrient around which energy balance is regulated and body weight controlled (59,81):

1. While there is evidence that excess carbohydrate is stored with less efficiency than fat, the relevance of these effects to free-living Western consumers has been questioned.

2. Several rigorous tests of carbohydrate specific models of feeding have suggested that carbohydrate oxidation or stores per se do not exert such powerful unconditioned negative feedback on EI (14,59,81,110). Rather, as macronutrients come in the diet (where fat is disproportionately energy dense), there appears to be a hierarchy in the satiating efficiency of the macronutrients protein, carbohydrate, and fat. Per MJ of energy ingested, protein induces supercaloric compensation, carbohydrate generates approximately caloric compensation, and fat precipitates subcaloric compensation, and hence often excess EI. Furthermore, simple statistical modeling has shown that models that include all three macronutrients explain far more of the variance in EI, either in the laboratory or among free-living subjects recording their own intakes (14). When energy density (ED) is controlled, protein is still far more satiating than carbohydrates or fats (at least when ingested in excess of 1–1.5 MJ loads). Under these conditions, differences in the satiating efficiency of carbohydrates and fats become more subtle (4,14,59) (see below).

3. HF hyperphagia can be explained by the high palatability and ED of HF foods (which facilitate greater levels of intake) and the low postabsorptive satiety value of fat (which prevents subsequent compensatory decreases in EI). While carbohydrate is more satiating than fat, excess fat intake is not necessarily driven by a need to eat to maintain carbohydrate balance.

4. There appear to be several reasons why many high-carbohydrate foods are more satiating than HF foods. First, they are usually (but not always) less energy dense that HF foods. Many high-carbohydrate foods contain dietary fiber, which limits rates of ingestion and digestion, both of which can have a limiting effect on EI. High-carbohydrate foods that are dry will tend to exert a higher osmotic load in the gut than will HF foods of similar moisture content. When the energy content and ED of high-carbohydrate and HF foods are controlled, readily assimilated carbohydrate is more satiating than fat. This difference in the satiating capacity of fat and carbohydrate can be deemed to be independent of ED or palatability. However, this effect is weaker than when HF, ED foods are compared to lower fat, less ED foods that are high in carbohydrate (103). Thus, the nutrient-specific differences in the sati-

ating effects of fats and carbohydrates need to be considered in relation to the structure and composition of the foods in which those nutrients abound (103).

5. It has frequently been stated that there is no evidence that foods high in carbohydrates promote overconsumption. This may be due to the fact that the majority of studies examining the effects of high carbohydrate and HF foods on feeding behavior, compared HF, more energy-dense foods to high-carbohydrate (LF) less energy-dense foods. The majority of studies that demonstrate the effects of fat in promoting excess EI examined how adding fat to the diet influences feeding. Very few studies have examined how *adding* carbohydrates to food affects feeding behavior or EI (103). In one study at least, increasing the ED of the diet by dramatically increasing the maltodextrin content, led to marked elevations of EI over 14 days (110).

6. While the fat-sugar seesaw has become a well-recognized phenomenon, the phenomenon itself has been harder to pin down. That fat and sugar or even fat and carbohydrate are reciprocally related to each other in the diet is almost inevitable, given that they are the main energy providing macronutrients. Indeed, we have found a strong fat-sugar seesaw in 1032 ready-to-eat foods taken from the British food tables. Gram for gram, the reciprocal relationship between fat and carbohydrate (or fat and sugar) is far less evident (4).

There is very little known about the vast range of different starches and their various structures in relation to appetite and energy balance (103). These are still uncharted landscapes on the research horizon. The foods most capable of limiting EI (both voluntary and metabolizable) are those rich in unavailable complex carbohydrates. However, there is a catch, because in general humans are not too fond of these foods, and as typified by the average Western diet, when given the choice they tend to select a diet comprising 37–42% fat, 10–20% sugar, and a variable amount of high glycemic index starches. The average Western adult's fiber intake is spectacularly low.

The evidence relating to the glycemic index of carbohdyrates cannot be interpreted owing to the heterogeneity of study designs, vehicles and treatments used, and indeed doubts as to whether the glycemic index of food is a physiological constant. This should be an area of future research. Given the range of CHO structures available to the food market and the different physicochemical properties they possess, it is particularly important to identify how these potentially beneficial effects of CHO structure can be used to enhance preabsorptive and absorptive phase satiety signals.

3 Fat

Numerous laboratory studies have now shown that when humans or animals are allowed to feed ad libitum on high-fat, energy-dense diets, they consume similar amounts (weight) of food but more energy (which is usually accompanied by weight gain) than when they feed ad libitum on lower-fat, less energy-dense diets (9–11). The ingestion of systematically manipulated HF, energy-dense diets does not appear to elicit compensatory feeding responses. Interestingly, if single midday meals are covertly manipulated, by increasing or decreasing their energy density using fat or carbohydrate, under conditions where subjects feed on range of familiar food items, compensation appears to be more precise (111,112). When experiments are conducted over similar time frames but the diet is systematically manipulated (i.e., subjects cannot select food items of differing compositions), compensation for the fat content of the diet is again poor (113). These observations further suggest that both learning and preabsorptive and absorptive-phase factors play a major role in meal to meal compensation. Furthermore, a number of prospective observational epidemiological studies show that fat consumption is a risk factor for subsequent weight gain (114). However, it is not likely to be the only risk factor, and few analyses take account of how fat may interact with other types of carbohydrates. For instance, in the short term, sweet high-fat foods have potent effect at stimulating energy intake.

We are beginning to gain insights into the effects of types of fat on appetite control, owing to the search for forms of fat which do not predispose the general population to weight gain. Fat structure varies in terms of (i) chain length, (ii) degree of saturation, (iii) degree of esterification, and (iv) by combining (i–iii), through the development of novel structured lipids. Data are scarce and fragmentary in this area, but some provisional patterns are beginning to emerge. Substitution of long-chain triglyceride (LCT) for medium-chain triglyceride (MCT) limits the high levels of energy intake that usually occurs when animals or humans ingest high-fat, energy-dense diets (115). However, very large doses of MCT are required in order to achieve these effects. MCTs may suppress appetite relative to LCT as they are more readily absorbed and oxidised. There are few data on whether short-chain fatty acids inhibit appetite in nonruminants. There is some preliminary evidence that ketone bodies (specifically beta-hydroxybutyrate) are appetite suppressants when given orally (116), and this may enhance compliance when subjects attempt to lose weight using very low calorie diets. Currently there is little evidence that degree of fatty acid esterification influences appetite and EI (117,118).

It has been suggested that polyunsaturates (PUFAs) are protective against obesity since they are more readily mobilized and oxidized and may influence gene expression of appetite-controlling peptides (119). Recent work in humans suggests that saturated fats are less satiating than mono-or polyunsaturates (120,121). An intriguing study in humans has reported that supplementation with very high levels of gamma-linolenate (at 5 g/d compared to 5 g/d olive oil) significantly reduced weight gain over 12 months after extensive weight reduction using very low calorie diets (122). Currently there are few or no reports on the effects of structured lipids on appetite and energy balance. However, it can be envisaged that structured lipids could be developed to combine some of the individually modest effects of fat type on appetite and feeding behavior. In the future, specific nutrients could be tailored to exert quantitatively significant effects on appetite control, tissue deposition, and energy balance. In this context it is of note that certain isomers of CLA can be used to influence appetite and tissue disposition in animals (123) and perhaps humans (124). The effects of conjugated linoleic acid (CLA) are not entirely understood but appear to be near pharmacological in nature.

4 The Fat Paradox

The apparently ambivalent effects of fat have generated a phenomenon referred to as the fat paradox. On the one hand, a fat such as corn oil infused into the jejunum has been shown to slow gastric emptying, increase feelings of fullness, and reduce food intake in a test meal. Infusions into the ileum bring about similar effects and also reduce feelings of hunger (125). On the other hand, similar infusions made intravenously exerted no effect on gastric emptying or measures of appetite. Lipid infusions at ~80% of resting energy requirements, over 3 days, produce only partial compensation (43%) of energy intake (126). Similar experiments have been carried out in rats where intraduodenal infusions inhibited food intake whilst intravenous infusions did not (127). These findings imply that, after the ingestion of fat, potent fat-induced satiety signals are generated by preabsorptive rather than postabsorptive physiological responses. In addition, a number of studies of short-and medium-term duration have demonstrated the existence of high intakes of energy with high-fat foods (9–11). How can these two features be reconciled? It appears that, in normal feeding, the stomach controls the rate at which nutrients are delivered to the duodenum, on an approximately caloric basis. Thus, the high levels of satiety seen in gastrointestinal infusions studies may well be due to supraphysiological saturation of satiety mechanisms arising from the small intestine.

5 Combined Effects of Macronutrients and Energy Density on Energy Intake

There has recently been a considerable debate as to whether the effects of diet composition on energy intake can be simply explained in terms of dietary energy density. Energy density should be defined in terms of the metabolizable energy per unit weight of ready to eat food. The major determinants of dietary energy density are water and fat, with water having the greatest effect. In general, the energy density of ready to eat foods is largely determined by a fat-water seesaw, with energy density falling as the water content of food rises and as the fat content of food falls. Protein and carbohydrate contribute relatively little to dietary energy density. There is considerable scope for technological developments that can alter the energy density of foods without compromising palatability. This is a major research challenge for the food industry (14).

At the present time, studies of energy density and energy intake are biased in favor of short-term interventions or longer studies where the composition of the diet is systematically altered (14). There are far fewer data from more naturalistic environments. These biases in the literature have led to an impression that energy density exerts powerful if not overriding deterministic effects on EI. Longer-term interventions are urgently needed.

As foods occur in real life, there is a hierarchy in the satiating efficiency of the macronutrients (see above discussion). The main effect of controlling energy density is to diminish the impact of differences in the satiating effects of fat and carbohydrate. Energy density exerts profound effects in constraining energy intake in short- to medium-term studies. Subjects behave differently in longer-term interventions. Energy density is a factor that at high levels can facilitate excess EI, and at low levels constrains EI (14). However, the effects that dietary energy density may exert on appetite and EI should be considered in the context of other nutritional and nonnutritional determinants of EI rather than as a substitute for those considerations.

In considering the nutritional determinants of EI in 102 free-living adults recording their food intake for 7 days, both macronutrients *and* energy density determine energy intake (14). The notion that energy density alone drives energy intake is oversimplified. Multifactor models appear more appropriate to explain nutritional determinants of feeding. This is illustrated in Figure 8. It is recommended that modeling work such as this be extended in order to better appreciate and predict the way in which the nutritional characteristics of the diet affect energy intake in people at large. Since differences between subjects can account for almost half of the variance in the relationships between food composition and energy intake (Fig. 8), models should help to identify key factors that predict a significant proportion of intersubject variation in feeding behaviour.

Drewnowski has provided evidence that energy density affects the sensory stimulation to eat (128). People tend to prefer more energy-dense foods. The implications this has for appetite control are unclear but it is our opinion that EI does not simply vary as a function of the energy density of the diet. We urgently need to understand how different types of people respond to changes in dietary energy density in the real world. The implications for consumers are that increasing consumption of foods lower in energy density may protect against weight gain but is unlikely to induce any spontaneous weight loss in subjects not attempting to control their weight. Furthermore, people appear to prefer more ED foods and so are likely to continue to select them (14,128). Psychological and possibly physiological disposition of the subjects will greatly affect their preference for and response to the energy density of foods.

6 Micronutrients

There are very few data on the effect of micronutrients on feeding behavior and body weight under normal feeding conditions. There is evidence that rodents will learn to select a diet whose ingestion will alleviate a micronutrient deficiency (38,94). It may also be supposed that the administration of a micronutrient that will, for instance, improve a deficiency-related defect in nutrient metabolism, will improve appetite for that nutrient, and perhaps appetite in general.

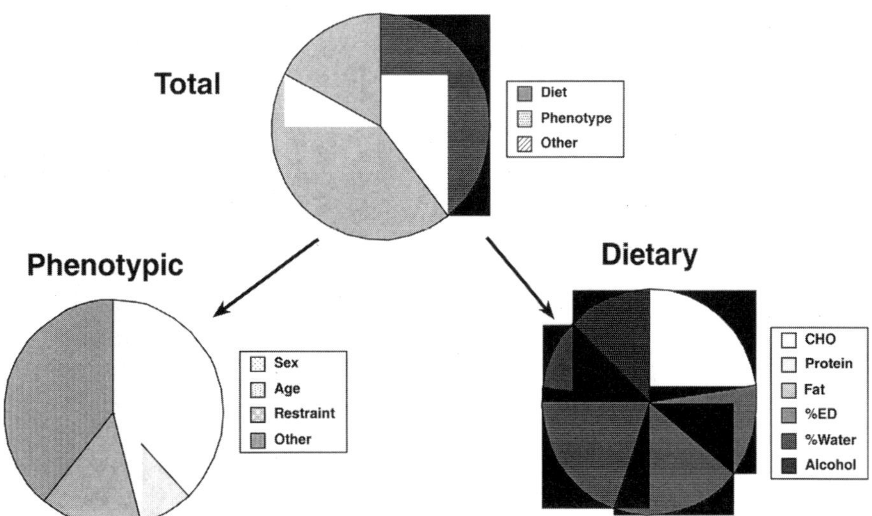

Figure 8 Pie charts illustrating the percentage of the variability in energy intake ascribable to different sources in 102 subjects recording their food intake for 7 consecutive days. Approximately 39% of the variability was due to diet and ~40% was due to intersubject variability. These two major sources of variation are subdivided further. These charts clearly illustrate that the determinants of energy intake in human adults are multifactorial.

B Issues Concerning Satiety Signals

Two further issues can be envisaged which are important and still to be resolved.

1 Postabsorptive Satiety

The pattern of food intake and the physiological events that occur at the end of a meal indicate an important role for preabsorptive signals in terminating eating and in determining the episodic nature of eating. What role is played by postabsorptive processes? The energy (fuel) balance approach to appetite control is based on the idea that the metabolic fate of nutrients in the body exerts important influences over behavior (65). Some hypotheses, such as the idea of linking food selection to serotoninergic activity (129), are based exclusively on the understanding that nutrient-induced metabolic activity exerts a directional influence on food consumption. However, some recent studies have indicated that large differences in the oxidation patterns of nutrients (fat and carbohydrate) can occur (after dietary manipulations) which do not appear to exert any influence over the quantitative aspect of food intake (130) at least for the following 24 hr. The same group has provided evidence that nutrient metabolism does exert potential influences on energy intake when these relationships are examined over a number of days (11). Logic demands that the requirement for nutrients by the body will exert an influence over the form of behavior that provides these nutrients, but what is the evidence for this, what is the nature of the mechanism involved, and what are the physiological limits within which the mechanism operates? Postabsorptive signals are probably far more effective at stimulating hunger during negative energy balance than they are at elevating satiety in the fed state. That is, tissue depletion during negative energy balance may exert a far greater physiological feedback on appetite than does tissue deposition during periods of positive energy balance.

Some studies have suggested that the rate of oxidation of fat and carbohydrate exerts an inhibitory effect on appetite (46–48,60). Specific proposals have been made by Langhans and Scharrer (48) regarding the increase in intracellular metabolism in hepatocytes. Some of this evidence is indirect. The most potent evidence relates to physiologically induced nutrient "deficits." The blockade of glucose oxidation by 2-DG or 2,5-AM (47) or fat oxidation by methylpalmoxirate or 2-mercapto acetate leads to an increase in food intake in animals (46–48,60). These phenomena have been termed glucoprivic and lipoprivic forms of feeding. These effects are strong phenomena in animals [and for 2-DG, in humans (85)] and form the basis for useful experimental models; their respective pathways through the brain can be traced by lesioning or biochemical procedures. This work by Ritter's group is extremely important since it indicates the neurochemical processing of metabolic activity (46).

Thus, decreases in nutrient oxidation appear to stimulate intake. Evidence that increases in nutrient oxidation comprise part of satiety are less direct. Considering carbohydrate metabolism, experimental results of Astrup and Raben indicate an extremely high correlation ($r = .9$) between hunger and postingestive measures of carbohydrate oxidation, AUC plasma glucose, insulin, and norepinephrine (24,104). Stubbs et al. (11) have also found statistically significant negative relationships between protein and carbohydrate stores and oxidation and the subsequent day's food intake, in normal men living in a calorimeter for 7 days at a time. The same relationships were significant for fat oxidation but not stores. Stubbs et al. (11) have interpreted these data as suggesting that the regulation of nutrient stores by increases in oxidation may partly underlie the greater capacity of protein and carbohydrate to suppress subsequent intake.

A key question here is whether or not the different profiles of nutrient oxidation arising from variations in the diet composition exert an influence over eating behavior. From a biological perspective, an animal could deal with extreme forms of diet composition through metabolic adaptation—with no consequences for behavior. There is unlikely to be any obligatory requirement to adjust behavior unless the process of metabolic adaptation incurs a physiological stress or strong benefit. It therefore seems important to establish the conditions under which nutrient-induced metabolic activity exerts either a quantitative or directional influence over eating behavior and whether it is possible to condition these effects. It seems reasonable to hypothesize that under conditions where prior learning cues are removed and extremes of metabolic adaptation are reached, then feeding behavior will be altered. Feeding behavior may subsequently be altered before such extremes are reached if the metabolic change is a cue for learning. Since the majority of Western adults are now overweight and obese, few satiety signals appear effective enough to restraint our inherent mammalian tendency to gain weight, when the environment permits.

In addition, it is possible that metabolic (postabsorptive) events only achieve biological relevance if they are accompanied (preceded) by preabsorptive signals. This would indicate that appetite control is achieved jointly by physiological responses generated at different stages in the handling of nutrients following ingestion. The organism presumably recognizes these physiological changes as sequential cues that, by reinforcing each other, cumulatively constitute the "satiety cascade" (131). Removing individual cues from the sequence may well weaken the overall impact of a food or nutrient on satiation or PI satiety.

C Specific Macronutrient Selection in Humans?

It is clear that human beings display preferences for, and selection of, different types of foods. These foods vary in taste, texture, energy density, and nutrient composition together with a host of cognitively mediated attributes. Under extreme physiological circumstances, animals and presumably humans can display a strong preference for a dietary component that is in deficit. The literature on salt appetite and on preferences of vitamin-deficient animals for foods that alleviate the deficiency are examples of this (see 94 for an introductory discussion of these phenomena). Nutrient deficits are not a necessary condition of a physiologically induced preference or aversion. To what extent can humans display a preference or aversion toward a particular macronutrient? What is the mechanism that could mediate this form of behavior? It is likely that a nutrient-based preference could develop through a process of learning. This would need a clearly defined unconditioned signal (arising from the physiological system)—a detection mechanism—linked to a particular sensory or environmental cue. For instance, rats learn to prefer flavors that are associated with fructose infusions into the portal vein (32,45). These phenomena are most likely to be best observed under conditions where a learned change in feeding behavior will alleviate some physiological stress. The metabolic handling of protein loads constitutes a greater physiological stress than the oxidation/storage of fat or carbohydrate. Under experimental conditions, a number of animal species adopt selection strategies to optimize the protein:energy ratio of their diet and avoid an intake of excess protein (32,94,95).

It is worth considering whether there is any other unconditioned physiological signal that could serve as the source of food-selecting behavior directed to a particular macronutrient under more naturalistic conditions. For instance, athletes tend to consume greater amounts of carbohydrates than the general population. Is any of this selection driven by physiological changes induced by exercise per se? The organoleptic properties of the diet may influence nutrient selection for nonphysiological reasons. It is also important to bear in mind that selection of foods can be influenced by a number of non-physiological- and non-sensory-associated factors. Examining the relative and quantitative importance of physiological versus nonphysiological determinants remains an important area for future investigation.

D Macronutrients, Appetite, and Obesity

1 Food and Macronutrient Intake in the Etiology of Obesity

Considerable attention has recently focused on the issue of how the macronutrient composition of the diet can influence the current epidemic of obesity in western society (3,4,15). Ingestion of dietary fat does appear to be a risk factor for subsequent weight gain (114), although it is possible to become obese on a high-carbohydrate diet (132). In particular, certain types of carbohydrates may interact with fat to facilitate higher levels of intake. Drenowski et al. and Mela et al. (133,134) have produced data that suggest that fatter people prefer fattier foods. There is not a great deal of direct evidence that preference per se will influence quantitative intake (i.e., how much food is eaten) to an extent that will influence body weight. It is, however, very likely that preference influences qualitative food intake—i.e., what foods are eaten. This is important because the phenomenon of passive overconsumption of energy on high-fat diets is not an issue of quantitative increases in food intake but of qualitative selection of high-fat, energy-dense foods. It has also been suggested that a genetic predisposition to store rather than oxidize fat may predispose certain individuals to rapid weight gain when they are exposed to a high-fat diet.

Lissner and Heitmann (114) have recently examined prospective data on fat intake and subsequent weight gain and have found that in women, those who exhibited a genetic susceptibility to weight gain showed the greatest tendency to gain weight when exposed to a high-fat diet. In the 1950s Jean Mayer highlighted the need to distinguish between the dynamic period of rapid weight gain and the stable plateau that body weight appears to reach in obesity. The truth is, we are remarkably ignorant of exactly how and at what rate different people gain weight. It appears from laboratory experiments that satiation, PI satiety, and hunger are influenced by food intake in obese subjects in a similar way as in lean people (90). Spitzer and Rodin (5) also note that the majority of studies on eating behavior in normal weight and overweight individuals conducted between 1969 and 1981 were "impressive in their demonstration of the lack of clear overweight-normal weight differences in eating behaviour." The situation has not changed much today. They did, however, note that in short-term studies palatability appeared to be the most consistent variable in producing overweight-normal differences in amount of food eaten.

The physiological features and psychological profiles that characterize the obese and may be involved in the maintenance of the obese state may not necessarily be the same features that led to obesity in the first place (22). Understanding the factors that produce sustained increases in energy intake over expenditure and the time course over which this occurs is crucial for understanding the etiology of obesity. It is also worth mentioning that obesity is a generic category which, like skin color, identifies an obvious recognizable feature of individuals, but explains little of the behavior of those individuals. There are likely to be a number of different factors

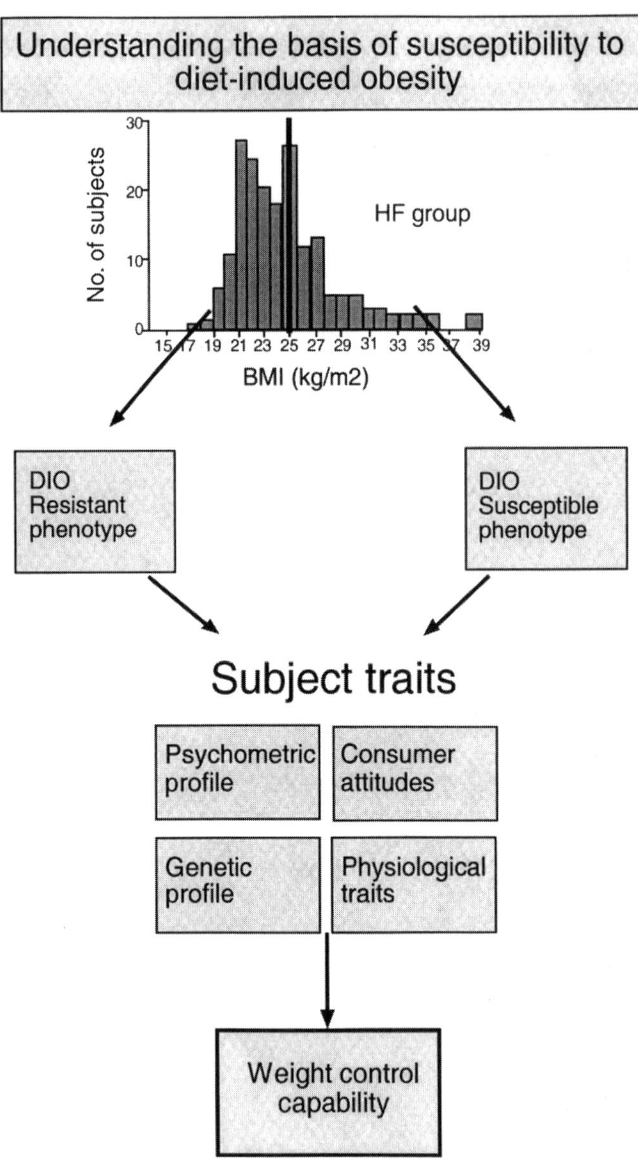

Figure 9 Scheme illustrating the selection and study of phenotypes believed to be resistant and susceptible to diet-induced obesity. At the present time it is important to characterize the differences between these phenotypes at the psychometric, behavioral, physiological, and even genetic levels.

that, individually or together, influence body weight. For instance, it is well known that not all obese subjects are restrained eaters. Similarly, not all obese subjects are insulin resistant. Since it is difficult to categorize which "type" of obesity a person belongs to or indeed how many "types" there are, it is equally difficult to identify the factors bringing about these characteristics. Thus, while there is abundant evidence that certain aspects of diet composition (e.g., dietary fat) are risk factors for weight gain, weight gain on a high-fat diet is not a biological inevitability. It should be remembered that often ~40–50% of the variance in energy intake or subjective appetite in a group of subjects is due to differences between the subjects themselves. This raises the issue of phenotypes (135,136). As regards dietary fat and phenotypes, it is becoming clear that certain high fat consumers (and high energy consumers) do not gain weight while others do so readily. We have recently begun to use these groups of subjects as models for phenotypes resistant or susceptible to diet-induced obesity (DIO). The concept is illustrated in Figure 9. This is no trivial matter. Currently the main practical solution to the current pandemic of obesity is to prevent weight gain in the preobese. How do DIO-resistant and DIO-susceptible phenotypes (the majority of us) differ? What can we understand about the psychometric, behavioral, and physiological profiles of people who are resistant to weight gain on a high-fat diet? Can this knowledge be used to benefit those who are susceptible to weight gain on Western diets?

VI PALATABILITY AND SENSORY FACTORS

A Palatability and Food Intake

In considering the capacity for energy intake to rise above energy expenditure, the weakness of inhibitory factors has to be set against the potency of facilitatory processes. The palatability of food is clearly one feature that could exert a positive influence over behavior. The logical status of palatability is that of a construct (it is not objective feature such as protein content or blood glucose) (137,138). Palatability can be influenced by a number of factors including environmental cues and the physiological state of the organism. However, palatability can be operationally defined according to the amount of food consumed, although some authors feel that this is inappropriate for animal studies (26). The independent index of palatability is usually considered to be the subjective appreciation of pleasantness. This subjective sensation is quantified by expressing it on an objective scale according to standard psychophysical procedures (139). This sensation is usually taken to reflect the hedonic dimension of food. The nature of the relationship among palatability, food consumption, and energy balance has never been systematically determined, although palatability has been invoked as a mediating principle to account for the prolongation of ingestion from a variety of foods due to sensory specific satiety operating in short-term studies.

It may be hypothesized that palatability would exert a powerful effect on intrameal satiety (while food was being consumed), but is there an enduring legacy which influences postingestive satiety? In addition, what is the effect of the expectation of getting pleasure from food on the initiation and maintenance of eating? Although almost everyone would agree that palatability exerts a powerful influence on eating behavior, there is no systematic body of data to explain the strength of the limits of the effect (140).

B Sweetness, Sucrose, and Sweeteners

For the last decade, there has been a healthy debate about the effects of sweetness, sucrose, and artificial sweeteners (141,142) on EB. The key issue relates to what effects sweetness, plus or minus carbohydrate energy, has on appetite and energy balance. There are three main hypotheses: (i) adding sweetness without calories to foods leads to lower levels of EI than when sweetness with calories are added; (ii) sweetness without calories leads to a cephalic phase stimulation to eat; and (iii) ingestion of sugars (sweetness with calories) correlates with thinness and lowers fat intake, which is itself the reason for the lower body weight. Clearly these hypotheses have enormous implications for appetite and EB control in consumers at large. Sweetness is a factor favoring the selection and subsequent ingestion of sweet foods. Most animals display a preference for sweetness at a very early age, and (until the advent of intense sweeteners) sweetness was a reliable sensory cue that a food was a source of readily available energy in the form of sugars. Conversely, different people exhibit markedly different preferences for sweetness intensities, so simply adding sweetness to foods will not stimulate everyone to eat. Assuming that sweetness does in general stimulate the selection and consumption of these foods, it is pertinent to inquire whether sweetness with or without calories affects appetite and EI.

Despite the common assumption that replacing dietary sugars with intense sweeteners will promote a more negative energy balance, there is a remarkable paucity of data to demonstrate this effect. There is certainly little epidemiological evidence to suggest that artificial sweetener consumption correlates with lower BMIs, or that increased artificial sweetener consumption in the population has contributed to any reduction in the prevalence of overweight or obesity. According to Mela (143), this effect may be accounted for by the fact that artificial sweeteners tend not to be used so much as a substitute for sugar. Rather, they are *added* to foods to enhance their appeal. The majority of studies that examine the effect of sweetness, sugars, and artificial sweeteners are short-term and therefore do not address the issue of energy balance (144).

Most authors seem to be in agreement that the purely postingestive effects of aspartame do not stimulate intake. Blundell and Rogers initially reported that artificially sweetened drinks can actually stimulate appetite. They suggested that sweetness per se provides a sensory cue for carbohydrate calories, which leads to cephalic-phase physiological changes that anticipate energy intake (145). They note that intense sweeteners have only been found to stimulate intake when a food has been sweetened with intense sweeteners or when a less sweet food has been compared with an isoenergetically equivalent food to which sweetness has been added (their "additive principle") and not when two foods of differing energy density but the same level of sweetness are compared. This they call the "substitutive principle." Again this area is bedevilled by methodological controversies, such as the appropriate drink vehicle for the sweetener (water or a familiar soft drinks), the time course of the experiment, and the subjects used. Blundell and Rogers (145) argue that the strongest experimental designs contain test of both the additive and substitutive principle. No long-term studies that address energy balance have yet achieved this dual testing.

Black and Anderson (146) report that the use of aspartame-sweetened water leads to an acute short-term increase in subjective appetite in lean men, but that aspartame-sweetened carbonated soft drinks induce a transient suppression of appetite in similar subjects over a similar time frame. The issue is complicated by the fact that satiety can be transiently conditioned by starch-containing drinks that are paired with a given sensory cue such as flavor (147). Once conditioned, similar levels of satiation can be transiently induced by the conditioning stimulus alone. Therefore, the effects of prior conditioning could influence the outcome of short-term studies using vehicles that mimic the sensory properties of similar foods.

In summary, there is little evidence that artificial sweeteners reliably decrease appetite or reduce energy intake, but they could perhaps prevent excess energy intake which would otherwise occur when calories are provided as drinks. There are conditions where artificially sweetened drinks have been found to stimulate appetite and less often energy intake, but there is little evidence to suggest that sweeteners reduce intake. Critically, the fact that intense sweeteners appear to be used as food additives rather than sugar substitutes, suggests that their current use is unlikely to promote a net reduction of energy intake in consumers at large (143). Understanding the applicability of these findings to free-living humans is an important area yet to be resolved. It is also important to bear in mind that a number of experiments examining these issues have used drinks and not solid foods. Mattes (148) has conducted a meta-analysis of feeding responses to either liquid or solid manipulations of the nutrient and energy content of the diet. The analysis suggests that the physical state of ingested CHO intake may be important in influencing subsequent caloric compensation. The reasons for this are unclear but may relate to the rate, timing, and density at which the energy is ingested. There may be a threshold in these parameters, below which energy is poorly detected.

C Fat and Fat Mimetics

There are a number of low-calorie or acaloric fat mimetics under development. These compounds are poorly absorbed across the gastrointestinal wall and are not metabolized by the calonic microflora. The most extensively studied of these are the olestras, which are a group of compounds that possess a sucrose (rather than glycerol) backbone with more than three fatty acid side chains. To date, 24 studies have examined the impact of olestra-containing foods on aspects of feeding behavior, which are published in 20 reports (see 148 for a review). The general response of human subjects to olestra-based decreases in dietary energy density (ED) is either poor caloric compensation or partial (non-macronutrient-specific) increases in EI. Averaging the degree of energy compensation across 22 studies gives a value of 27% (nonweighted mean). In studies where compensation occurred, fat intake but not energy intake was reduced (149). These effects appear to occur in lean and obese, in men and women, and under a variety of conditions ranging from the laboratory to real life. However, all but two of these studies were short-term. One study suggests that in subjects for whom weight loss is desirable, these deficits can persist for up to 3 months (150). Subjects with no wish to lose weight may compensate better over longer periods. In another 3-month study, ingestion of olestra-based foods did not induce energy deficits but limited the significant weight gain seen on a full fat control (151) The longer-term effects of olestra on body weight requires further investigation. There is evidence that restrained eaters tend to eat slightly more of olestra-based foods if they know that they are reduced in fat and energy (152,153). This is probably a general response to low-fat foods rather than to olestra *per se*. That olestra-based foods have the potential to provide the sensory qualities of real fat suggests that these foods may be particularly effective in habitual high fat consumers with a sensory preference for dietary fat.

D Variety

It has been suggested from a number of short-term studies that have been conducted (154–156), together with the cafeteria-diet model, that sensory variety of foods promotes overconsumption of energy. Furthermore, Le Magnen has shown in rats that simply increasing sensory variety can lead to excess energy intake and weight gain, provided the variety is constantly rotated. Increases and decreases in sensory variety that were stable over time had a much less pronounced effect (33). It has also been hypothesized that this effect may be pronounced in people who are more susceptible to environmental cues (157). We have recently shown that simply increasing the variety of sensorially distinguishable foods of identical nutrient content significantly elevated energy intake in men over 7 days (39). The longer-term effects of sensory factors on appetite and energy have yet to be elucidated. However, the extent to which the food industry invests in and refuses to compromise the sensory attributes of their products bears testimony to the importance of sensory factors in food choice and purchase.

There is therefore a good deal of work to do in considering the relative contribution of sensory versus nutritional determinants of feeding behavior and energy balance. This area of research is of growing importance, since the sensory qualities of the diet no longer necessarily provide reliable information regarding its nutritional content. Some individuals may be more disposed to cues such as palatability or olfactory cues associated with certain foods than to internal (physiological) cues. Disturbed sensory functioning is a major factor involved in the loss of appetite due to pathologies or side effects of the drugs used to treat certain illnesses (6).

E Meal Patterns

It has been noted that snacking and commercially available snack food are often believed to elevate EI (158–161). However, there is considerably less evidence that meal or snack patterns contribute to the development of obesity. It is important to note at this point that the relationship between a meal and a snack relates to timing and size of ingestive events in meal-feeding animals. In nonhuman species (and indeed humans) who engaged in numerous small feeding bouts throughout their diurnal cycle, there is little if any distinction between a meal and a snack. Meal-feeding animals are conditioned to ingest the majority of their energy intake in a few large ingestive events in their diurnal cycle, usually at approximately the same time points. Under these conditions, a snack can be defined as an energetically small, intermeal ingestive event (SIMIE). To avoid confusion with a common use of the word to describe a certain type of commercially available food, we use the phrase "commercially available snack foods" to described those specific foods. Commercially available snack foods tend to differ from the rest of the diet in that they are more energy dense, high in fat and carbohydrate, and low in protein and usually contain a large fraction of their edible mass as dry matter. They are by no means the only food eaten as a SIMIE in many people at large.

There are two alternative hypotheses about how snacking may influence energy intake and body weight: (i) snacking helps "fine-tune" mealtime EIs to match intake with requirements, or (ii) habitual consumption of calorific drinks and snacks between meals is a major factor driving EI up and predisposing people to weight gain and obesity (162).

The evidence in relation to meal patterns, appetite, EI, and body weight is however, indirect and fragmentary. On aggregate, cross-sectional studies tend to support no or a negative relationship between meal frequency and BMI (163–165). However, Bellisle et al. (166) convincingly argue that examinations of the relationship between snacking and energy balance in free-living subjects are extensively flawed by misreporting, misclassification of meal and snacks, and potentially by reverse causality. Under these conditions, it is difficult to draw clear conclusions about the effects of snacking in cross-sectional studies. It is therefore important to conduct controlled laboratory interventions over a number of days in humans.

It is well known in the animal literature that a variety of species can learn to adapt to meal feeding, snacking or totally ad libitum conditions in order to match EI to requirements (32,33). This suggests some flexibility in adjusting feeding behavior to feeding schedules in order to meet energy requirements. There appears to be very little direct empirical evidence in humans as to whether ingesting snacks per se affects appetite and EI. There is some evidence that people who snack frequently exhibit a greater capacity to compensate for changes in the energy content of specific meals, relative to subjects who derive most of their energy intake from fewer, larger meals (167). A recent series of studies by Mazlan have been conducted in which zero, 1.5, and 3.0 MJ of snack foods were consumed as a mandatory intake by human subjects over a week (168). The snacks were similar in taste, texture, appearance, and energy density but not composition. Whybrow has conducted a series of similar studies using commercially available snack foods. Under these conditions where snack foods are consumed as mandatory increments in intake, subjects compensated to some degree, but the net effect was an elevation of energy intake over 7 days. The longer-term effects of such interventions on energy intake and body weight is an area for urgent enquiry.

VII CONCLUSION

This present chapter aims to represent the current state of research findings in relation to diet and food intake in humans. We hope to point the reader in the direction of some major unresolved and therefore contentious issues that still surround the study of human feeding, rather than construct an uncritical list of major findings in the area. The importance of (frequently ignored) methodological differences in experimental approaches is highlighted, and these are considered in relation to the nature of the appetite system in humans. By considering these together, the strengths and limitations of whole-body human studies of diet and food intake become apparent, as does the importance of supporting these studies with animal models and epidemiological comparisons. Particular emphasis is given to the interactions between physiology and behavior, which characterize human feeding responses. Considerable attention is given to diet composition and feeding behavior, with emphasis being placed on explaining some of the apparent contradictions in the literature and discussing some perhaps premature conclusions that are becoming generally accepted. We discuss the evidence and controversies concerning the influence of dietary macronutrient composition and associated sensory stimuli on (i) quantitative intake, (ii) possible effects on subsequent nutrient selection, (iii) their influence on putative appetite signalling systems, and (iv) how macronutrient mimetics may influence feeding responses. While a number of issues are becoming resolved (e.g., the role of dietary fat vs. energy density in producing hyperphagia), other important issues emerge—for instance, the role of lean tissue depletion as a signal for post–weight loss hyperphagia and the characterization of phenotypes susceptible and resistant to diet-induced obesity. Greater progress has been made in understanding specific aspects of the appetite system and in identifying its components (through molecular and biochemical studies, often in animal models) than in understanding how these components operate and interact to influence patterns of feeding behavior linked to weight control and weight gain in humans.

The field of appetite and energy balance is becoming increasingly specialized and fragmented. Many researchers concerned with elucidating molecular and genetic mechanism of appetite control have become somewhat divorced from whole body studies of feeding behavior. In some cases, there is less evidence at the whole-body level of the phenomenon being regulated than there is for the mechanisms supposed to regulate it! Thus, the unravelling of the leptin system, believed important in regulating fat mass, proceeds apace. However, clear, direct, empirical evidence that fat mass is actually regulated in humans is embarrassingly scant. It is of critical importance that putative mechanisms of appetite and energy balance control be related to the behavior of the intact organism. Human studies of diet composition and food intake control need to be related to mechanistic work in other species, in order to assess the relevance of these mechanisms to our own species. Feeding studies of our own species in the laboratory need to be related to the general population going about their everyday lives in their natural setting. Given the current emphasis on directing research toward promoting greater human health and well-being, animal and molecular models of compartments of the appetite system provide invaluable information if related to parallel (but less invasive) protocols in human. However, these models need to be made more relevant to appetite and energy balance control in humans.

It is now more important than ever to attempt to integrate the increasingly disparate areas of research specializing in aspects of appetite and energy balance control. We still do not have a synthetic theory of feeding behavior as exists, for example, for biological evolution or quantum physics. A multidisciplinary approach to the construction of integrated models that provide a satisfactory theoretical basis for understanding mechanisms of feeding behavior and interventions that will successfully manipulate it, is now a clear necessity.

As the food we eat is changed and transformed by food producers and manufacturers for a variety of reasons, understanding the role of the diet in feeding behavior and energy balance is also more important than ever. Structured research strategies that seek to understand the mechanisms underlying quantitative and qualitative feeding behavior, within the context of energy and nutrient balance, may help us keep pace with the rapidly changing nature and effects of the diet that we eat. This knowledge will be vital for the development of successful dietary approaches to weight management, in terms of preventing weight gain in the majority of humans who are susceptible to diet-induced obesity, and developing strategies that lead to sustained weight reduction in the obese.

REFERENCES

1. Factors influencing body weight (sect 3.4.3) In: Diet Nutrition and the Prevention of Chronic Disease. A Report of a WHO Study Group. Geneva: World Health Organization, 1990.
2. Hill RJ, Davies PSW. The validity of a four day weighed food record for measuring energy intake in female classical ballet dancers. Eur J Clin Nutr 1999; 53:752–753.
3. Stubbs RJ. Macronutrient effects on appetite. Int J Obes 1995; 19(suppl 5):S11–S19.
4. Blundell JE, Stubbs RJ. High and low carbohydrate and fat intakes: limits imposed by appetite and palatability; implications for energy balance. Eur J Clin Nutr 1999; 53(suppl 1):S148–S165.
5. Spitzer L, Rodin J. Human eating behavior: a critical review of studies in normal weight and overweight individuals. Appetite 1981; 2:293–329.
6. Mattes RD. Gestation as a determinant of ingestion: methodological issues. Am J Clin Nutr 1985; 41:672–683.
7. Hill AJ, Rogers PJ, Blundell JE. Techniques for the experimental measurement of human eating behavior and food intake: a practical guide. Int J Obes 1995; 19(suppl 6):461–376.
8. Shepherd R. Sensory influences on salt, sugar and fat intake. Nutr Res Rev 1988; 1:125–144.
9. Duncan KH, Bacon JA, Weinsier RL. The effects of high and low energy density diets on satiety, energy intake, and eating time of obese and non obese subjects. Am J Clin Nutr 1983; 37:763–767.
10. Lissner L, Levitsky DA, Strupp BJ, Kalkwarf HJ, Roe DA. Dietary fat and the regulation of energy intake in human subjects. Am J Clin Nutr 1987; 46:886–892.
11. Stubbs RJ, Harbron CG, Murgatroyd PR, Prentice AM. Covert manipulation of dietary fat and energy density: effect on substrate flux and food intake in men feeding ad libitum. Am J Clin Nutr 1995; 62(suppl 2):316–330.
12. Van Stratum P, Lussenburg RN, Van Wezel LA, Vergroesen AJ, Cremer HD. The effect of dietary carbohydrate:fat ratio on energy intake by adult women. Am J Clin Nutr 1978; 31:206–212.
13. Stubbs RJ, Harbron CG, Prentice AM. The effect of covertly manipulating the dietary fat to carbohydrate ratio of isoenergetically dense diets on ad libitum food intake in free-living humans. Int J Obes 1996; 20:651–660.
14. Stubbs J, Ferres S, Horgan G. Energy density foods: effects on energy intake. Crit Rev Food Sci Nutr 2000; 40(suppl 6):481–515.
15. Obesity: preventing and managing the global epidemic. Report of a WHO consultation. World Health Organ Tech Rep Ser 2000; 894:1–253.
16. Mela DJ, Rogers PJ. Food, Eating and Obesity. The Psychobiological Basis of Appetite and Weight Control. London: Chapman and Hall, 1998.
17. Blundell JE. Hunger, appetite and satiety-constructs in search of identities. In: Turner M, ed. Nutrition and Lifestyles. London: Applied Science Publishers, 1979: 21–42.
18. Brunswick E. The Conceptual Framework of Psychology. Chicago: University of Chicago Press, 1995:80–102.
19. Van Itallie TB, Vanderweele DA. The phenomenon of satiety. In: Bjorntorp P, Cairella M, Howard AN, eds. Recent Advances in Obesity Research III. London: John Libbey, 1981:278–289.
20. Gibbs J, Young R, Smith GP. Cholecystokinin elicits in rats with open gastric fistulas. Nature 1973; 245: 323–325.
21. West DB, Greenwood MRC, Marshall KA. Lithium chloride, cholecystokinin, and meal patterns: evidence that cholecystokinin suppressess meal size in rats without causing malaise. Appetite 1987; 8:221–227.
22. Mayer J. Glucostatic mechanism of regulation of food intake. N Engl J Med 1953; 249:13–16.
23. Pharmacological treatment of obesity. Satellite Symposium to the 6th International Congress on Obesity. Am J Clin Nutr 1992; 55(suppl 1).
24. Raben A. Appetite and carbohydrate metabolism. PhD thesis, Copenhagen, Royal Veterinary and Agricultural University, 1995.
25. Campfield LA, Smith FJ. Transient declines in blood glucose signal meal initiation. Int J Obes 1990; 14(suppl 3):15–33.
26. Campfield LA, Smith FJ, Rosenbaum M, Geary N. Human hunger is there a role for blood glucose dynamics? Appetite 1992; 18:244 (letter).
27. Campfield LA, Smith FJ. Functional coupling be-

tween transient declines in blood glucose and feeding behavior: temporal relationships. Brain Res Bull 1986; 174:427–433.
28. Johnstone AM, Faber P, Clerkin D, Shannon C, Stevenson L, Gibney ER, Elia M, Reid CA and Stubbs RJ. A 36-hour fast increases fat selection in lean men. Proc Nutr Soc 2000; 59:55A.
29. Elia, M. Hunger disease. Clin Nutr 2000; 19:379–386.
30. Keys A, Brozek J, Henschel A, Mickelsen O, Longstreet-Taylor H. The Biology of Human Starvation. Minneapolis: University of Minnesota Press, 1950.
31. Mayevsky A, Doron A, Meilin S, Manor T, Ornstein E, Ouaknine GE. Brain viability and function analyzer: multiparametric real-time monitoring in neurosurgical patients. Acta Neurochir Suppl 1999; 75:63–66.
32. Forbes JM. Voluntary food intake and diet selection in farm animals. Oxon, U.K.: CAB International, 1995.
33. Le Magnen J. Neurobiology of Feeding and Nutrition. San Diego, CA: Academic Press, 1992.
34. Franke LW. The ability of rats to discriminate between diet of various degrees of toxicity. Science 1936; 83:130–135.
35. Kalat JW, Rozin P. Role of interference in taste aversion learning. J Comp Physiol Psychol 1971; 77: 53–58.
36. Bernstein IL. Development of food aversion during illness. Proc Nutr Soc 1994; 53:131–137.
37. Rozin P, Kalat JW. Specific hungers and poison avoidance as adaptive specialisations of learning. Psychol Rev 1971; 78:459–486.
38. Rozin P, Rodgers WH. Novel diet preferences in vitamin deficient in rats and rats recovering from vitamin deficiencies. J Comp Physiol Psychol 1967; 63: 421–428.
39. Stubbs RJ, Johnstone M, Mazlan N, Mbaiwa SE, Reid CA. Effect of altering the sensory variety of foods of the same macronutrient content on food intake and body weight in lean and overweight men. Eur J Clin Nutr 2000; 55:1–10.
40. Meiselman HL. Determining consumer preference in institutional food service. In: Food Service Systems. New York: Academic Press, 1979;127–153.
41. Dalton S, Linke RA, Simko MD. Reasons related to consistency between intended and actual food choice, including accuracy of and satisfaction with perceived body size. In: 67th Annual Meeting of the American Dietetic Association, Washington, 1984; 73–74. Abstract.
42. Cannon WB, Washburn AL. An explanation of hunger. Am J Physiol 1912; 29:441–454.
43. McCance RA, Widdowson EM, Dean, RFA, Thrussel RFA, Barret AM, Berridge FR, Russel Davis D, Gell PGH, Claser EM, Gunther MHD, Howarth SM, Hutchinson AO, Jones PEH, Keckwick RA, Newman MD, Prior KM, Sherlock SPV, Stanier JE, Tomson PRV, Walshie VM. Studies of Undernutrition, Wuppertal 1946–9. MRC Special Report Series No. 275. London: HMSO, 1951.
44. Read N, French S, Cunningham K. The role of the gut in regulating food intake in man. Nutr Rev 1994; 52: 1–10.
45. Tordoff MG, Ulrich PM, Sandler F. Flavour preferences and fructose: evidence that the liver detects the unconditioned stimulus for calorie based learning. Appetite 1990; 14:29–44.
46. Ritter S, Calingasan NY. Neural substrate for metabolic controls of feeding. In: Fernstrom JD, Miller GD, eds. Appetite and Body Weight Regulation: Sugar, Fat and Macronutrient Substitutes. Boca Raton, FL: CRC Press, 1994.
47. Friedman MI, Rawson NE. Fuel metabolism and appetite control. In: Fernstrom JD, Miller GD, eds. Appetite and Body Weight Regulation: Sugar, Fat and Macronutrient Substitutes. Boca Raton, FL: CRC Press, 1994.
48. Langhans W, Scharrer E. The metabolic control of food intake. World Rev Nutr Diet 1992: 70:1–68.
49. Janowitz HD, Grossman MI. Some factors affecting the food intake of normal dogs and dogs with esophagostomy and gastric fistulas. Am J Physiol 1949; 159: 143–148.
50. Young RC, Gibbs CJ, Antin J, Holt J, Smith GP. Absence of satiety during sham feeding in the rat. J Comp Physiol Psychol 1974; 87:795–800.
51. Mook DG, Culberson GR, Gelbart RJ, McDonald K. Oropharangeal control of ingestion in rats: acquisition of sham drinking patterns. Behav Neurosci 1983; 97: 574–584.
52. Walls EK, Koopmans HS. Differential effects of intravenous glucose, amino acids and lipid on daily food intake in rats. Am J Physiol 1992; 262:R225–R234.
53. Mook DG. Oral factors in appetite and satiety. Ann NY Acad Sci 1989; 575:265–280.
54. Mattes RD. Sensory influences on food intake and utilisation in humans. Hum Nutr Appl Nutr 1987; 41A:77–95.
55. Mellinkoff SM, Franklin M, Boyle D, Geipell M. Relationship between serum amino acid concentration and fluctuation in appetite. J Appl Physiol 1956; 8: 535–538.
56. Mayer J. The regulation of energy intake and the body weight. Ann NY Acad Sci 1955; 63:15–43.
57. Kennedy GC. The role of depot fat in the hypothalamic control of food intake in the rat. Proc R Soc (B) 1953; 140:578–592.
58. Stubbs RJ. Peripheral signals affecting food intake. J Nutr 1999; 15:7–8.
59. Stubbs RJ. Appetite feeding behaviour and energy

balance in human subjects. Proc Nutr Soc 1998; 57:1.

60. Friedman MI, Tordoff MG. Fatty acid oxidation and glucose utilisation interact to control food intake in rats. Am J Physiol 1986; 251:R840–R845.
61. Thompson D. Cambell R. Hunger in humans induced by 2-deoxy-d-glucose: glucoprivic control of taste preference and food intake. Science 1977; 198:1065–1068.
62. Abbot WGH, Howard BV, Christin L, Freymond D, Lillioja S, Boyce VL. Anderson TE, Bogardus C, Ravussin E, Christin L, Freymond D, Lillioja S, Boyce VL, Anderson TE, Bogardus C, Ravussin E. Short-term energy balance: relationship with protein, carbohydrate and fat balances. Am J Physiol 1988; 255:E332.
63. Acheson KJ, Jequier E. Glycogen synthesis versus lipogenesis after a 500 gram carbohydrate meal in man. Metabolism 1982; 31:1234.
64. Acheson KJ, Schutz Y, Bessard T, Anantharaman K, Flatt JP, Jequier E. Glycogen storage capacity and de novo lipogenesis during massive carbohydrate overfeeding in man. Am J Clin Nutr 1988; 48:240.
65. Flatt JP. The differences in storage capacities for carbohydrate and for fat, and its implications for the regulation of body weight. Ann NY Acad Sci 1987; 449:104.
66. Jequier E. Calorie balance versus nutrient balance. In: Kinney JM, ed. Energy Metabolism: Tissue Determinants and Cellular Corollaries. New York: Raven Press, 1992;123.
67. Hellerstein MK, Christiansen M, Kaempfer S. Measurement of de novo hepatic lipogenesis in human beings using stable isotopes. J Clin Invest 1991; 87:1841.
68. Elia M, Stubbs RJ, Henry CJ. Differences in fat, carbohydrate, and protein metabolism between lean and obese subjects undergoing total starvation. Obes Res 1999; 7:597–604.
69. Pellet PL, Young VR. The effect of different levels of energy intake on protein metabolism and of different levels of protein intake on energy metabolism: a statistical evaluation from the published literature. In: Schrimshaw NS, Schurch B, eds. Protein-Energy Interactions. Proceedings of an IDECG workshop, 1992.
70. Langhans W. Metabolic and glucostatic control of feeding. Proc Nutr Soc 1996; 55:497–515.
71. Dulloo AG, Jacquet J. The control of partitioning between protein and fat during human starvation: its internal determinants and biological significance. Br J Nutr 1999; 82:339–356.
72. Russek M. An hypothesis on the participation of hepatic glucoreceptors in the control of food intake. Nature 1963; 197:79–80.
73. Hervey GR. Regulation of energy balance. Nature 1969; 222:347–631.
74. Harris RBS, Martn RJ. Site of action of putative lipostatic factor: food intake and the peripheral pentose shunt pathway. Am J Physiol 1990; 259: R45–R52.
75. Harris RBS, Bruch RC, Martin RJ. In vitro evidence for an inhibitor of lipogenesis in serum from obese rats. Am J Physiol 1989; 257:R326–R336.
76. Coleman DL. Obese and diabetes: two mutant genes causing diabetes-obesity syndromes in mice. Diabetologia 1978; 14:141–148.
77. Zhang Y, Proenca R, Maffei M, Barone M, Leopold L, Friedman JM. Positional cloning of the mouse obese gene and its human homologue. Nature 1994; 372:425–431.
78. Garrow J. Obesity and Related Diseases. London: Churchill-Livingstone, 1988.
79. Schwartz MW, Woods SC, Porte D, Seeley RJ, Baskin DG. Central nervous system control of food intake. Nature 2000; 404:661–671.
80. Kant AK, Graubard B I, Schatzkin A, Ballard-Barbash R. Proportion of energy intake from fat and subsequent weight change in the NHANES epidemiological follow-up study. Am J Clin Nutr 1995; 61: 11–17.
81. Stubbs RJ, O'Reilly LM. Carbohydrate and fat metabolism, appetite and feeding behaviour in humans. In: Berthoud HR, Seeley RJ, eds. Neural Control of Macronutrient Selection. Boca Raton, FL: CRC Press, 1998.
82. Gill A. The Journey Back from Hell. Conversations with Concentration Camp Survivors. London: HarperCollins, 1994.
83. Mercer JG, Speakman JR. Hypothalamic neuropeptide mechanisms for regulating energy balance: from rodent models to obesity. Neurosci Biobehav Rev 2000; 25:101–116.
84. DeCastro JM. Macronutrient relationships with meal patterns and mood in the spontaneous feeding behavior of humans. Physiol Behav 1987; 39:561–569.
85. Bingham SA, Gill C, Welch A, Day K, Cassidy A, Khaw KT, Sneyd MJ, Key TJA, Roe L, Day NE. Comparison of dietary assessment methods in nutritional epidemiology: weighed records v. 24 h recalls, food-frequency questionnaires and estimated-diet records. J Nutr 1994; 72:619–643.
86. Geliebter AA. Effects of equicaloric loads of protein, fat, and carbohydrate on food intake in the rat and man. Physiol Behav 1979; 22:2647–2653.
87. De Graaf C, Schrevrs A, Blauw YH. Short term effects of different amounts of sweet and non-sweet carbohydrates on satiety and energy intake. Physiol Behav 1993; 54:833–843.
88. Miller MG, Teates JF. Acquisition of dietary self-selection in rats with normal and impaired oral sensation. Physiol Behav 1985; 34:401–408.
89. De Graaf C, Hulshof T, Westrate JA, Jas P. Short-term

effects of different amounts of protein, fat and carbohydrates on satiety. Am J Clin Nutr 1992; 55: 33–38.
90. Hill AJ, Blundell JE. Comparison of the action of macronutrients on the expression of appetite in lean and obese humans. Ann NY Acad Sci 1990.
91. Hill AJ, Blundell JE. Macronutrients and satiety: the effects of a high-protein or high-carbohydrate meal on subjective motivation to eat and food preferences. Nutr Behav 1986; 3:133–144.
92. Barkeling B, Rossner S, Bjorvell H. Efficiency of a high-protein meal (meat) and a high-carbohydrate meal (vegetarian) on satiety measured by automated computerised monitoring of subsequent food intake, motivation to eat and food preferences. Int J Obes 1990; 14:743–751.
93. Booth DA, Chase A, Campbell AT. Relative effectiveness of protein in the late stages of appetite suppression in man. Physiol Behav 1970; 5:1299–1302.
94. Lyle LD. Control of eating behavior. In: Wurtman RJ, Wurtman JJ, eds. Nutrition and the Brain. New York: Raven Press, 1977.
95. Kyriazakis I, Emmans GC, Whittemore CT. Diet selection in pigs: choices made by growing pigs given foods of different protein concentrations. Anim Prod 1990; 50:189–199.
96. Kyriazakis I, Emmans GC. Selection of a diet by growing pigs given choices between foods differing in contents protein and rapeseed meal. Appetite 1992; 19:121–132.
97. Fromentin G, Nicolaidis S. Rebalancing essential amino acids intake by self-selection in the rat. Br J Nutr 1996; 75:669–682.
98. Millward JD. A protein-stat mechanism for regulation of growth and maintenance of the lean body mass. Nutr Res Rev 1995; 8:93–120.
99. Stubbs J, Elia LM. Macronutrients and appetite control with implications for the nutritional management of the malnourished. Clin Nur 2001; 20(suppl 1):129–139.
100. Dulloo AG, Jacquet J, Girardier L. Poststarvation hyperphagia and body fat overshooting in humans: a role for feedback signals from lean and fat tissues. Am J Clin Nutr 1997; 65:717–723.
101. Dulloo AG, Jacquet J, Girardier L. Autoregulation of body composition during weight recovery in human: the Minnesota experiment revisited. Int J Obes 1996; 20:393–405.
102. Yudkin J. Pure, White and Deadly. London: Viking, 1986.
103. Stubbs, J, Mazlan N, Whybrow S. Carbohydrates, appetite and energy balance. J Nutr 2001; 131:2775S–2781S.
104. Astrup A, Raben A. Carbohydrate and obesity. Int J. Obes 1995; 19:S27–S37.
105. Hill JO. Prentice AM. Sugar and body weight regulation. Am J Clin Nutr 1995; 62:264S–274S.
106. Bolton-Smith C, Woodward M. Dietary composition and fat to sugar rations in relation to obesity. Int J Obes 1994; 18:820–828.
107. Gibney M, Sigman-Grant M, Stanton JL Jr, Keast DR. Consumption of sugars. Am J Clin Nutr 1995; 62:178S–193S.
108. International Food Information Council Foundation. Review: Uses and Nutritional Impact of Fat Reduction Ingredients. Washington: International Food International Food Information Council Foundation, 1997.
109. Leveille GA, Finley JW. Macronutrient substitutes description and uses. Ann NY Acad Sci 1997; 819: 11–22.
110. Stubbs RJ, Johnstone AM, Harbron CG, Reid C. Covert manipulation of the energy density of high-carbohydrate diets: effect on ad libitum food intake in "pseudo free-living" humans. Int J Obes 1998; 22:885–892.
111. Foltin RW, Fischman MW, Moran TH, Rolls BJ, Kelly TH. Caloric compensation for lunches varying in fat and carbohydrate contents by humans in a residential laboratory. Am J Clin Nutr 1990; 52:969–980.
112. Foltin RW, Rolls BJ, Moran TH, Kelly TH, McNelis AL, Fischman MW. Caloric, but not macronutrient compensation by humans for required eating occasions with meals and snacks varying in fat and carbohydrate. Am J Clin Nutr 1992; 55:331–342.
113. Lawton CL, Burley VJ, Wales JK, Blundell JE. Dietary fat and appetite control in obese subjects: weak effects on satiation and satiety. Int J Obes 1993; 17:409–416.
114. Lissner L, Heitmann BL. Dietary fat and obesity: evidence from epidemiology. Eur J Clin Nutr 1995; 49:79–90.
115. Stubbs RJ, Harbron CG. Covert manipulation of the ratio of medium to long-chain triglycerides in isoenergetically dense diets: effect on food intake in ad libitum feeding men. Int J Obes 1996; 20:435–444.
116. Rich AJ, Chambers P, Johnston IDA. Are ketones an appetite suppressant? J Pen 1988; 13:7S. Abstract.
117. Johnstone AM, Stubbs RJ, Reid C. Breakfasts high in monoglyceride or triglyceride: no differential effect on appetite or energy intake. Eur J Clin Nutr 1998; 52: 603–609.
118. Johnstone AM, Stubbs, RJ, Reid C. Overfeeding fat as monoglyceride or triglyceride: effect on appetite, nutrient balance and the subsequent day's energy intake. Eur J Clin Nutr 1998; 52:610–618.
119. Storlien LH. Dietary fats and insulin action. Int J Obes 1998; 22:S46, abst O174.
120. Lawton CL, Delargy HJ, Brockman J, Smith FC, Blundell JE. The degree of saturation of fatty acids influences post-ingestive satiety. Br J Nutr 2000; 83:473–482.
121. French S, Mutuma S, Francis J, Read N, Meijer G.

The effect of fatty acid composition on intestinal satiety in man. Int J Obes 1998; 22:S82, abst O299.
122. Phinney S, Schirmer M, Metz D, Tang A. Gamma linolenate reduces weight regain following weight loss by very low calorie diets in humans. Int J Obes 1998; 22:S64, abst O237.
123. Dugan MER, Aalhus JL, Schaefer AL, Kramer JKG. The effect of feeding conjugate linoleic acid on fat to lean repartitioning and feed conversion in pigs. Can J Anim Sci 1997; 77:723–725.
124. Atkinson RL, Gomez T, Clark RL, Pariza MW. Clinical implications for CLA in the treatment of obesity. Program of the Annual Meeting, National Nutritional Foods Association, San Antonio, TX, July 15–16, 1998.
125. Welch IML, Sepple CP, Read NW. Comparisons of the effects on satiety and eating behavior of infusions of lipid into the different regions of the small intestine. Gut 1988; 29:306–311.
126. Gil K, Skeie B, Kvetan V, Askanazi J, Friedman MI. Parenteral nutrition and oral intake: effect of glucose and fat infusion. J Pen 1991; 15:426–432.
127. Greenberg D, Becker DC, Gibbs J, Smith GP. Infusions of lipid into the duodenum elecit satiety in rats while similar infusions into the vena cava do not. Appetite 1989; 12:213. Abstract.
128. Drewnowski A. Energy density, palatability, and satiety: implications for weight control. Nutr Rev 1998; 56:347–353.
129. Fernstrom JD. Food induced changes in brain serotonin synthesis is there a relationship to appetite for specific macronutrients? Appetite 1987; 81:63–82.
130. Shetty PS, Prentice AM, Goldberg GR, Murgatroyd PR, McKenna APM, Stubbs RJ, Volschenk PA. Alterations in fuel selection and voluntary food intake in response to iso-energetic manipulation of glycogen stores in man. Am J Clin Nutr 1994; 60: 534–543.
131. Blundell JE. The psychobiological approach to appetite and weight control. In: Brownell KD, Fairburn CG, eds. Eating Disorders and Obesity: A Comprehensive Handbook. New York: Guildford Press, 1995.
132. Pasquet P, Apfelbaum M. Recovery of initial body weight and composition after long-term massive overfeeding in men. Am J Clin Nutr 1994; 60:861–863.
133. Drenowski A. Energy intake and sensory properties of food. Am J Clin Nutr 1995; 62:1081S–1085S.
134. Mela DJ, Sacchetti DA. Sensory preferences for fats: Relationship with diet and body composition. Am J Clin Nutr 1991; 53:908–915.
135. Cooling J, Blundell J. Are high-fat and low-fat consumers distinct phenotypes? Differences in the subjective and behavioural response to energy and nutrient challenges. Eur J Clin Nutr 1998; 52:193–201.
136. Cooling J, Blundell J. Differences in energy expenditure and substrate oxidation between habitual high fat and low fat consumers (phenotypes). Int J Obes 1998; 22:612–618.
137. Ramirez I. What do we mean when we say palatable food? Appetite 1990; 14:159–161.
138. Rogers PJ. Why a palatability construct is needed. Appetite 1990; 14:167–170.
139. Hill AJ, Blundell JE. Nutrients and behavior: research strategies for the investigation of taste characteristics food preferences, hunger sensations and eating patterns in man. J Psychol Res 1982; 17:203–212.
140. Ramirez I, Tordoff M, Friedman MI. Dietary hyperphagia and obesity: what causes them? Physiol Behav 1989; 45:163–168.
141. Booth DA, Rodin J, Blackburn GI. Sweeteners, appetite and obesity. Appetite 1988; 11(suppl 1):54–61.
142. Clydesdale FM. Nutritional and health aspects of sugars. Am J Clin Nutr 1995; 62(suppl 1):178–195.
143. Mela DJ. Impact of macronutrient-substituted foods on food choice and dietary intake. Annal NY Acad Sci 1997; 819:96–107.
144. Clydesdale FM. Nutritional and health aspects of sugars. Am J Clin Nutr 1995; 62(suppl 1):195–203.
145. Blundell JE, Rogers PJ. Sweet carbohydrate substitutes (intense sweeteners) and the control of appetite: Scientific issues. In: Fernstrom JD, Miller GD, eds. Appetite and Body Weight Regulation: Sugar, Fat and Macronutrient Substitutes. Boca Raton, FL: CRC Press, 1994.
146. Black RM, Anderson GH. Sweeteners, food intake and selection. In: Fernstrom JD, Miller GD, eds. Appetite and Body Weight Regulation: Sugar, Fat and Macronutrient Substitutes. Boca Raton, FL: CRC Press, 1994.
147. Booth DA, Rodin J, Blackburn GI. Sweeteners, appetite and obesity. Appetite 1988; 11(suppl 1):48–53; 62–72.
148. Mattes, RD, Dietary compensation by humans for supplemental energy provided as ethanol or carbohydrate in fluids. Physiol Behav 1996; 59:179–187.
149. Stubbs RJ. Olestra, appetite and energy balance in humans. Crit Rev Food Sci Nutr 2000; 41:363–386.
150. Roy H, Lovejoy M, Windhauser M, Bray G. Metabolic effects of fat substitution with olestra. Proc Fed Am Soc Exp Biol 1997; 11:2076, A358.
151. Kelly SM, Shorthouse M, Cotterell JC, Riordan AM, Lee AJ, Thurnham DI, Hanka R, Hunter JO. A 3-month, double-blind, controlled trial of feeding with sucrose polyester in human volunteers. Br J Nutr 1998; 80:41–49.
152. Westerterp-Plantenga MS, Wijckmans-Duijsens NEG, Ten Hoor F, Weststrate A. Effect of replacement of fat by nonabsorbable fat (sucrose polyester) in meals or snacks as a function of dietary restraint. Physiol Behav 1997; 61(6):939–947.
153. Miller DL, Castellanos VH, Shide DJ, Peters JC, Rolls BJ. Effect of fat-free potato chips with and without

nutrition labels on fat and energy intakes. Am J Clin Nutr 1998; 68:282–290.
154. Rolls B, Rowe E, Rolls E. Appetite and obesity: influences of sensory stimuli and external cues. In: Turner M, ed. Nutrition and Lifestyles. London: Applied Science Publishers, 1979.
155. Rolls BJ, Rolls E, Rowe EA, Kingston B, Megson A, Gunary R. Variety in a meal enhances food intake in man. Physiol Behav 1981; 26:215–221.
156. Rolls BJ, Rolls ET, Rowe EA. The influence of variety on human food selection and intake. In: Eliot Stellar AVI, ed. The Psychobiology of Human Food Selection. 1982.
157. Rodin J. Current status of the internal-external hypothesis for obesity: what went wrong. Am Psychol 1981; 36:361–372.
158. Drummond S, Crombie N, Kirk T. A critique of the effects of snacking on body weight status. Eur J Clin Nutr 1996; 50:779–783.
159. Gatenby SJ. Eating frequency: methodological and dietary aspects. Br J Nutr 1997; 77(suppl 1):S7–S20. Review.
160. Grogan SC, Bell R, Conner M. Eating sweet snacks: gender differences in attitude and behaviour. Appetite 1997; 28:19–31.
161. Nunez C, Carbajal A, Moreiras O. Body mass index and desire of weight loss in a group of young women. Nutr Hosp 1998; 13(4):172–176.
162. Booth DA. Mechanisms from models—actual effects from real life: the zero calorie drink-break option. Appetite 1988; 11:94–102.
163. Fabry P, Tepperman J. Meal frequency—a possible factor in human pathology. Am J Clin Nutr 1970; 23: 1059–1068.
164. Fabry P, Fodor J, Hejl Z, Braun T, Zvolankova K. The frequency of meals in relation to overweight, hypercholesterolaemia and decreased glucose tolerance. Lancet 1964; ii:614–615.
165. Gibney M, Lee P. Patterns of food and nutrient intake in adults consuming high and low levels of table sugar in a Dublin suburb of chronically high unemployment. Proc Nutr Soc 1989; 48: 123A.
166. Bellisle F, NcDevitt R, Prentice AM. Meal frequency and energy balance. Br J Nutr 1997; 77: S57–S70.
167. Westerterp-Plantenga MS, Wijckmans-Duysens NA, Ten Hoor F. Food intake in the daily environment after energy-reduced lunch, related to habitual meal frequency. Appetite 1994; 22:173–182.
168. Mazlan N. Effect of fats and carbohydrate on energy intake and macronutrient selection in humans. 2001, PhD thesis, University of Aberdeen, Aberdeen, Scotland.

16

Central Integration of Peripheral Signals in the Regulation of Food Intake and Energy Balance: Role of Leptin and Insulin

L. Arthur Campfield and Françoise J. Smith

Colorado State University, Fort Collins, Colorado, U.S.A.

Bernard Jeanrenaud

University of Geneva, Geneva, Switzerland

I INTRODUCTION

Recent advances in the biology of energy balance have provided a rich cast of molecular players and new pathways underlying the central and peripheral regulation of energy balance. These advances in this dynamic field have invigorated, energized, and added new foci to the obesity research agenda. Several lines of converging evidence have identified the brain integration of central and peripheral neuroendocrine, neuropeptide, and neural signals in the regulation of energy balance as an important research area. This growing area of research activity is the subject of this chapter.

In this chapter, the major peripheral and central neuroendocrine and neural signals in the regulation of energy balance will be identified and discussed. The current understanding of the brain integration of peripheral signals and central neuropeptides in the regulation of energy balance will be discussed. Specific molecules (e.g., leptin, insulin, and NPY) and pathways are then used as examples to illustrate the general principles and overall scheme. The available knowledge about the brain leptin and insulin pathways will be reviewed. This understanding is based on in vitro experiments as well as studies conducted in laboratory animals and humans. This research has revealed that leptin, by acting on diverse brain structures and mechanisms, regulates ingestive behavior, metabolism, and neuroendocrine rhythms, and controls body energy balance. These brain structures and mechanisms form the brain leptin and insulin pathways. The concept of reduced brain sensitivity to leptin in obesity is discussed.

The interaction of leptin with other brain mechanisms is then summarized. When these mechanisms are understood at the molecular level, they should provide new targets for therapeutic interventions that will reduce and maintain body fat at reduced levels and, therefore, increase metabolic fitness, reduce risk factors, and promote improved health of obese individuals (1–3).

The elucidation of the properties, target tissues, pathways, and actions of the circulating hormone leptin (also known as OB protein), which is the product of the *ob* gene, has provided a new pathway and a new context to increase our understanding of the regulation of energy balance. The circulating concentrations of leptin are proportional to adiposity and increase with increasing levels of body fat (4,5). The leptin pathway is one of the long-sought hormonal signal pathways from adipose tissue to the brain that plays a critical role in the regulation of energy balance (1,3,6–8). The brain

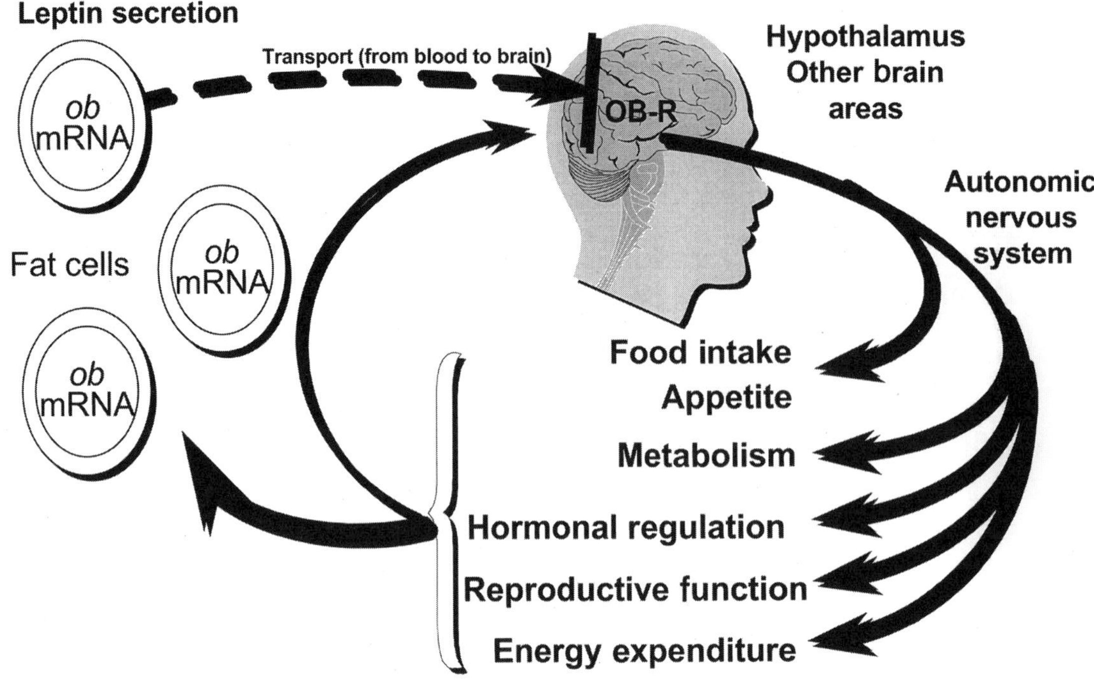

Figure 1 Schematic model of some of the important elements of the leptin signaling pathway that regulates body energy balance. See text for additional details. (From Ref. 8.)

insulin system is the other peripheral hormonal pathway from adipose tissue to the brain that is critical in the regulation of energy balance (9,10).

Leptin is a polypeptide hormone that is secreted primarily from adipose tissue, circulates in the blood, is bound to a family of binding proteins, enters the brain, binds to its receptors in hypothalamic nuclei and other brain areas, and acts on central neural networks. The *ob* gene is expressed in adipose tissue, bone marrow, and placenta, and leptin is synthesized and secreted from adipose tissue in proportion to adipocyte volume (11). Several lines of evidence suggest that leptin plays a major role in the control of body fat stores through coordinated regulation of feeding behavior, metabolism, neuroendocrine responses, autonomic nervous system, and body energy balance in rodents, primates, and humans. Leptin expresses these actions through its role in the brain integration of the central and peripheral signals involved in these responses (1,3,7,8). The key elements of the leptin pathway are shown in

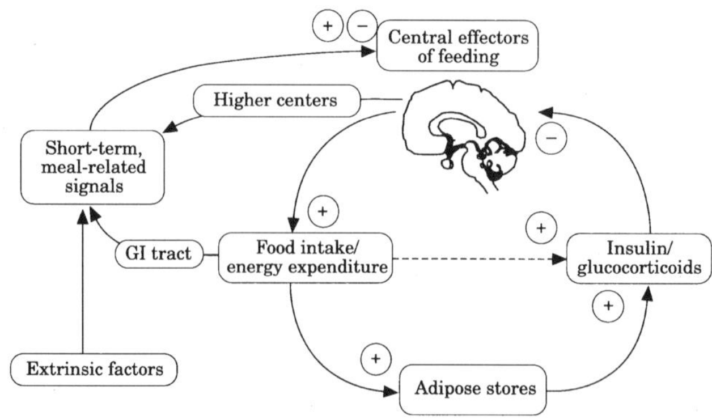

Figure 2 Schematic representation of the brain insulin hypothesis. (From Ref. 9.)

Table 1 Leptin Research Areas

1. Regulation of *ob* gene expression in adipose tissue in mice, rats, and humans
2. Characterization of the biological actions and definition of the elements of the leptin pathway in lean and obese mice and rats
3. Studies of the biology of leptin in lean and obese humans
4. Studies of the brain structures and mechanisms through which leptin acts including the interaction with other neuropeptides and pathways
5. Therapeutic use of a leptin-based molecule for the treatment of obesity

Source: Refs. 1,3,14.

Figure 1 including a transport system for leptin to enter the brain, leptin receptors in hypothalamic nuclei, and neural and neuroendocrine outputs to peripheral tissues (3,8).

Insulin is a polypeptide hormone synthesized and secreted from the pancreas. In addition to its well-known peripheral role to regulate blood glucose concentration, insulin also enters the brain, binds to its receptors in hypothalamic nuclei and other brain areas, and acts on central neural networks to regulate energy balance. The key elements of the brain insulin system are shown in Figure 2 (9).

The mechanisms in the brain responsible for determining the level at which body fat content is regulated in humans and other animals are not completely understood. A similar lack of knowledge exists for the mechanisms regulating the neuroendocrine rhythms supporting the adaptation to starvation and reproductive function in humans and other animals. Elucidation of the leptin pathway within the brain, and its interaction with the brain insulin pathway, has begun to provide important insights into these and possibly other mechanisms (1–3).

Since the cloning of the *ob* gene in December 1994 (12), leptin research has progressed along the five major parallel paths shown in Table 1.

II CONTEXT OF THE NEUROENDOCRINOLOGY OF CENTRAL INTEGRATION OF PERIPHERAL SIGNALS IN THE CONTROL OF ENERGY BALANCE IN THE OBESE STATE

Ample evidence exists that obesity is, at its basis, a disease of biological dysregulation. The integration of multiple biological factors within the brain and nervous system (including endocrine, neuroendocrine, and metabolic factors), which are at least partially genetically determined, results in the steady-state body weight of an individual. When the steady-state weight is perturbed in either direction (increased or decreased), changes in body weight are resisted and corrected by physiological mechanisms in laboratory rodents and humans (13). The physiological mechanisms that resist changes in body fat content (e.g., central neural networks, autonomic neural, metabolic, and neuroendocrine) are not completely known (1,3,14).

Obesity is characterized by the pathophysiological alterations shown in Table 2. These alterations in peripheral physiologic processes and brain pathways and their integration into coordinated responses demonstrate the critical role of central and peripheral integration in the regulation of energy balance. The signals and processes involved are hormonal (circulating hormones, neuropeptides, or neurotransmitters) and neural. They originate in the periphery or/and within the brain. In normal-weight animals or humans, all of these signals, or their representations, are detected, interpreted, and integrated within the brain, and the resulting efferent (or effector) neuroendocrine and neural components of the regulatory system act in the periphery or/and within the brain to adjust energy balance appropriately. However, in obese animals and humans, these signals and their detection, interpretation, and integration are altered owing to this biological dysregulation, leading to an inappropriate adjustment of energy balance and resulting in the augmentation or maintenance of obesity (1,3,13,14).

It is not yet completely understood how "alterations" and "errors" in the brain integration of these signals and physiological mechanisms are responsible for the weight regain that usually follows weight loss. These mechanisms are probably a combination of appropriate physiological responses to reduced body fat or energy intake together with inappropriate sensing of elevated circulating leptin and insulin concentrations

Table 2 Pathological Alterations in Obesity

1. High rates of lipid deposition in adipose tissue
2. Reduced insulin sensitivity of muscle and fat
3. Exaggerated insulin responses to meals
4. Hyperinsulinemia
5. Increased leptin and fasting insulin concentrations
6. Reduced brain and peripheral sensitivity to leptin

Source: Refs. 1,3,14,126.

and erroneous integration within the brain. However, results of available studies suggest that these alterations in general, and the brain leptin pathway in particular, play a role in this "resetting response" that is responsible for weight regain following weight loss (1,3,14).

III REGULATION OF ENERGY BALANCE: BRAIN INTEGRATION OF PERIPHERAL NEUROENDOCRINE SIGNALS

Energy balance is the result of the control of ingestive behavior, metabolism, energy expenditure, and energy storage in adipose tissues (1,3,9,14). While energy intake is a discrete process as individual meals are separated by intermeal intervals, energy expenditure and storage in adipose tissue are continuous physiological processes (15–18). The complex molecular mechanisms by which discrete ingestive behavior, continuous energy expenditure, and dynamic energy storage in adipose tissue are integrated and matched remain largely unknown. The brain insulin system and leptin pathway are two candidate signals for matching intake and expenditure (1,3,9,14). Since the *responsiveness* of both of these systems to insulin and leptin decreases markedly in obesity, appropriate and accurate matching of intake and expenditure will become more unlikely as obesity begins to develop and becomes established.

A Control of Food Intake: An Integrated Behavioral Response Dependent on Leptin, Insulin, and Central Neuropeptides

Feeding behavior is the result of the complex central nervous system integration of central and peripheral neural, hormonal, and neurochemical signals relating to brain and metabolic states. Meals are initiated, maintained, and terminated by specific sets of these central and peripheral signals several times a day separated by intermeal intervals without food intake (15–18). These signals include *patterns* of neural afferent traffic; metabolites (glucose); energy flux (fatty acid oxidation, ATP); and hormones (insulin concentrations in plasma and brain, leptin concentrations in plasma, and neuropeptide concentrations in brain) (19,20). The brain structures and mechanisms involved in the detection of these signals and the mapping of them into altered feeding behavior are beginning to emerge. One hypothesis for this integrated neural, metabolic, and hormonal control of food intake postulates the interaction of five classes of signals: (1) hypothalamic neuropeptides and neurotransmitters; (2) brain insulin; (3) leptin; (4) metabolic signals including transient declines in blood glucose concentrations; and (5) ascending and descending neural inputs (1,17,18,21). These signals interact and provide the central and peripheral integration necessary to regulate food intake and match energy intake to energy expenditure to maintain body energy balance and composition.

Many experimental studies in mice, rats, and many other species demonstrate that several neuropeptides modulate food intake when injected centrally and, in some cases, peripherally (see Chaps. 13 and 14). Among the neuropeptides that have been extensively studied and have major effects on food intake are neuropeptide Y (NPY), cholecystokinin (CCK), corticotropin-releasing hormone (CRH), and enterostatin (9,10). Synaptic concentrations of central neuropeptides and classical monoamine neurotransmitters are thought to be modulated by the central representations of peripheral metabolic state and act on postsynaptic receptors to control energy intake (1,3,9,14,17). Although some investigators still seek the identity of the "one" major neuropeptide controlling human feeding behavior, most of the field has adopted a "parallel" model in which multiple neuropeptides and hormones involved each play a role in determining human feeding behavior (1,3,8,18).

B Control of Energy Expenditure

Total daily energy expenditure can be partitioned into resting metabolic rate, dietary and cold-induced thermogenesis, and the energy cost of physical activity ((5–18,22–24) see Chaps. 23 and 24). The energy cost of various kinds of voluntary physical activity (e.g., walking, jogging, swimming) and thermogenesis due to digestion and absorption of food as well as thermogenesis induced by a cold environment have been calculated for both men and women as a function of lean body mass (or "fat-free mass"). Small repeated errors in the "matching" of energy expenditure to energy intake over individual bouts or a series of bouts of physical activity could easily lead to positive energy balance. The effects of exercise on perceptions of hunger are time dependent, complex, and highly variable. Thus, some individuals may experience hunger after exercise, while others may not (25).

The regulation of resting metabolic rate is a complex function of energy intake, energy balance, and hormonal and autonomic neural activity. Resting metabolic rate decreases when an individual reduces caloric intake and shifts into a state of negative energy balance. This regulatory adaptation appropriately reduces obligatory energy expenditure when energy intake is reduced. Adaptation to reduced caloric intake by reducing metabolic rate requires falling concentrations of both circulating insulin and leptin. However, this same adaptation causes a deceleration of weight loss following voluntary caloric restriction for the purpose of weight loss and contributes to the difficulty of maintaining weight loss, once achieved, over time (22,24).

C Control of Fat Balance

Just as energy balance is the comparison of total body energy intake and expenditure, a similar balance exists for each macronutrient. The matching of carbohydrate- and protein-derived energy flux and the rates of oxidation and storage are generally well regulated (see Chap. 28). However, fat balance is not closely regulated. Two major problems in the regulation of fat balance predispose individuals to obesity. First, it is known that excess dietary fat does not acutely increase the oxidation of fat for energy. Second, the capacity for fat storage in humans is practically unlimited. Excess calories in the form of fat are readily stored as triglyceride in adipose tissue, with a very high (>96%) efficiency (25).

It is becoming clear that positive energy balance most often results from disruptions in fat balance. However, over the long term, fat balance has to be regulated in order to achieve macronutrient and thus energy balance, and a steady-state body weight. The reestablishment of fat balance following a period of positive energy balance requires a change in the body fat mass. The rate of fat oxidation, which is related to body fat mass, must increase and eventually become equal to the rate of fat intake, and then body fat mass comes into balance and remains in steady state. It is known that fat oxidation varies directly with body fat mass (26), but the mechanisms linking these two parameters are not yet clear. If the dietary fat is increased *without a rapid change in fat oxidation*, this will produce positive fat balance and thus an increase in body fat mass. As body fat increases, fat oxidation will eventually also increase. Body fat mass will then increase to a new level at which fat oxidation matches fat intake, and the body fat stabilizes at this new, higher level (25). Another possibility is that carbohydrate oxidation may not be appropriately inhibited when some individuals are consuming a high fat diet. This would lead to positive energy balance and fat balance.

IV EXPERIMENTAL MODELS OF OBESITY DUE TO ALTERED LEPTIN PATHWAY

The obese *ob/ob* mice were discovered on the C57BL/6J background in the early 1950s; this mutation results in profound obesity (27). Mice with mutations in the *ob* gene have a premature stop signal and thus fail to synthesize and secrete leptin from their fat cells. These mice have no measurable leptin in their blood and have an early-onset, severe obese phenotype. When treated with small doses of leptin, these mice markedly reduce their food intake, lose weight, and mobilize stored triglyceride. The *db/db* mouse, which arose on the C57BL/KsJ background, is similarly obese and is also characterized by hyperglycemia. When the *ob* gene was transferred to the C57BL/KsJ background, a phenotype almost identical to that of *db/db* mice was observed (28–32). The *db/db* mice have a mutation in the gene coding for leptin receptor, *ob-r* gene, that results in a splice variant in which all the leptin receptors are in the short or nonsignaling form. These mice have high levels of leptin in their blood but are unable to respond to it.

When cross-circulation (or parabiosis) experiments were performed between *ob/ob* and *db/db* mice, the *ob/ob* partner reduced its food intake and lost weight, while the *db/db* partner maintained both its food intake and body weight. In some experiments, the *ob/ob* partner actually died when parabiosed with *db/db* mice. [However, these extreme effects have not been observed in studies with chronic leptin treatment in rodents (8).] These studies led Coleman to conclude that *ob/ob* mice fail to secrete a circulating factor (now known as leptin) from their adipose tissue, although their brain can respond to it and reduce food intake, while *db/db* mice secrete the circulating factor, but their brain cannot respond to it (28,29). Thus, an operational leptin pathway is required for the regulation of lean body composition, and the absence of functional leptin or functional leptin receptors results in obesity. Studies have also demonstrated that the mutated *ob* gene has no effect on the marked hyperglycemia seen when the mutated *ob* gene is on the diabetogenic C57BL/KsJ background; instead, hyperglycemia is thought to be the result of other genes in the KsJ background that render the pancreatic beta cell vulnerable, and eventually to fail to produce adequate amounts of insulin. Low-protein diets have been shown to prevent pancreatic failure in C57BL/KsJ mice with the mutated *ob* or *db* genes. These and other studies demonstrate that mutated *ob* or *db* genes cause obesity, which may or may not result in hyperglycemia in susceptible or resistant individuals (8).

V HOW PERIPHERAL SIGNALS GAIN ACCESS TO BRAIN PATHWAYS

One of the essential roles of peripheral signals in the regulation of energy balance is to inform the brain that it is in a body with increased fat mass. This is accomplished when peripheral signals proportional to adipose tissue mass (leptin and insulin) gain access to the brain.

A Serum Concentrations

The studies of circulating leptin concentrations in humans can be summarized as follows: When obese subjects were compared to lean individuals, it was observed that the serum leptin concentrations were higher in obese individuals, and leptin concentrations *increased* with increasing percent body fat (4,5). *Thus, most obese humans are not deficient in leptin, but rather they have elevated circulating leptin concentrations.* Women have higher leptin concentrations than men, even when corrected for the percent body fat. Subjects with NIDDM had lower leptin levels than obese subjects but higher than lean subjects. When obese subjects lost weight by caloric restriction, leptin concentration decreased and then rose slightly when the lower weight was maintained (4). Plasma leptin concentrations were correlated with subcutaneous adipose tissue mass. Serum leptin concentrations display a circadian rhythm rising from a minimum in the midmorning to a peak in the middle of the night (33,34).

Similar clinical studies of circulating insulin concentrations have established that fasting plasma insulin concentration increased with increasing percent body fat (35,36). Peak insulin or integrated insulin response to oral glucose or meals also increased with increasing percent body fat. In fact, obese individuals have elevated plasma insulin levels throughout the entire day compared to normal weight individuals. Weight loss was also associated with decreased fasting insulin concentration in both overweight and obese individuals (9,35,36).

B Brain Transport of Insulin and Leptin

Following the observation that fasting plasma insulin concentrations were proportional to adipose tissue mass, the effects of experimental elevation of brain insulin were studied. After intravenous infusion, insulin enters the brain by a saturable transport process (10,36,37). The kinetics of this process are consistent with transport mediated by insulin receptors expressed on the luminal surface of brain microvessels (10,36,37). It has been estimated that 80–90% of brain insulin uptake occurs through this insulin receptor-mediated transport process (9,10,36,37).

The transport of radiolabeled leptin into the brain of mice was reported by Banks et al. (38) and confirmed by others (39). These studies showed the presence of ^{125}I in the arcuate nucleus of the hypothalamus shortly after the injection of labeled leptin. The rate of uptake of radiolabeled leptin was decreased by coinjection of unlabeled leptin, suggesting that the transport system for leptin in mice may be saturable. A saturable transport system for leptin in isolated human brain microvessels has been discovered and reported (39). Labeled leptin bound to receptors and was translocated across the wall of isolated human brain microvessels. Furthermore, this transport was shown to be saturable.

These findings and their similarity to the saturable transport system for insulin in brain microvessels suggested a model for leptin transport in the brain (3,14, 39). This model proposes that leptin moves from binding proteins in the plasma to binding sites on the extracellular domains of its receptor located on the inside of the wall of the brain microvessels. The leptin molecule is then translocated across the microvessel wall from the lumen into the brain tissue. Once in brain tissue, it binds to long-form leptin receptors on neurons in brain regions involved in the regulation of energy balance or enters the CSF in the ventricular system. After acting at its long-form receptor, excess or degraded leptin then appears in the CSF bathing the brain. Thus, CSF leptin may not accurately reflect the transport of leptin into the brain. Just as the high density of insulin and serotonin receptors in the choroid plexus is thought to be involved in the degradation of these molecules, the high density of the short form of the leptin receptors in the choroid plexus is thought to be involved in the degradation of leptin.

VI BIOLOGICAL ACTIVITY OF LEPTIN

A Biological Activity of Leptin in Mice and Rats

To determine if the brain was a target of leptin, recombinant mouse leptin was injected into the lateral ventricle of *ob/ob* and lean*(+ /?)* mice in our first study of the biological activity of leptin (40). These mice were implanted with chronic lateral ventricle cannulas. Single injections of leptin (0.001–1 μg/mouse in 1 μL) were administered to overnight fasted *ob/ob* and lean*(+/?)* mice. Cumulative 7-hr and 24-hr food intake were suppressed in a dose-related manner. Postinjection body weight gains were also reduced in a dose-related manner compared to mice injected with vehicle control (40). Similar results have been reported in other laboratories (41,42). Several laboratories showed that peripherally administered recombinant mouse leptin significantly reduced food intake and body weight (43–45), NPY mRNA, and blood glucose concentrations (41,46). Overexpression of the leptin gene in the liver of rats resulted in a marked reduction in body fat (47).

However, when the effective dose in lean rats (3.5 μg) of leptin was placed in the third ventricle in obese Zucker rats, no behavioral effects were observed (42). In contrast, Cusin et al. (48), Rohner-Jeanrenuad et al. (49), and Lin et al. (50) reported that higher doses of leptin did suppress food intake of obese Zucker rats. Chronic treatment of Zucker rats for 3 weeks with long-acting leptin did result in suppression of daily food intake and body weight during the last week of treatment (Campfield, unpublished data). Further studies will be needed to determine the impact of the point mutation in the OB-R of the obese Zucker rats on its responsiveness to leptin. Leptin administration to obese Koletsky (corpulent) rats without leptin receptors has been shown to be without effect (51).

When a compound, peptide, or protein administered peripherally or centrally results in reduced food intake and loss of body weight, the possibility that these behavioral effects are due to nonspecific action or illness produced by the test substance must be considered. To assess this possibility for the biological effects of leptin, a conditioned taste aversion experiment was conducted (52). In these studies, lean Long-Evans rats were offered two drinking bottles containing saccharin solution or water daily for several days. The presentation of saccharin was paired with the ICV injection of leptin, the IP injection of LiCI, or no treatment. As expected, treatment with the known toxin LiCI caused striking rejection of the consumption of saccharin, the taste associated with LiCI treatment, but had no effect on the consumption of water. This decreased preference for a taste paired with a toxic substance is called a conditioned taste aversion. In contrast, ICV treatment with leptin had no effect on the consumption of saccharin or water. These studies demonstrate that leptin does not support the development of a conditioned taste aversion. These results provide strong support that the reduction in food intake and body weight observed following the administration of leptin are specific biological effects of the hormone (52).

The results of these experiments, taken together, provide further support for the hypothesis that a peripheral signal, leptin, secreted from adipose tissue, acts on central neuronal networks, and suggests that leptin plays an important role in the regulation of ingestive behavior and energy balance. The duration of action of leptin appears longer than with other neuropeptides that modulate ingestive behavior (CCK, NPY) and is similar to that of centrally administered insulin. The behavioral and physiological effects following central administration of leptin into the lateral ventricle suggest that leptin can act directly on the neural networks in the brain that regulate ingestive behavior and energy balance (1,3,14).

B Biological Activity of Leptin in Humans

Most human obesity is probably not due to a *deficiency* of leptin, but instead due to a central and/or peripheral *resistance* or *decreased responsiveness* to leptin. Support for the concept of reduced responsiveness to leptin in obesity is based on the available results in animal models and humans, summarized below (4,40). This is very similar to the case of the insulin-resistant, obese NIDDM patients. However, positive clinical experience with insulin therapy in these patients and positive results with leptin treatment of diet-induced obese mice (40) strongly suggest that therapeutic augmentation of circulating leptin levels may result in reductions of food intake, body fat mass, and body weight in many obese patients (1,3,7,8,14).

The operation of the leptin pathway in humans has now been established. First, rare mutations in the leptin and leptin receptor genes have been documented in a small number of obese humans that are similar to those in leptin-deficient and unresponsive mice (1,3,14). These humans are severely obese and have incomplete sexual maturation. Second, chronic daily subcutaneous low-dose recombinant methionyl–human leptin (met-leptin) treatment of a young very obese leptin-deficient girl with a mutated *ob* gene has been reported (53). After a life dominated by continuous weight gain, intense hunger, and food seeking, reduction of hunger, reduced food-seeking behavior, reduced body fat, and sustained weight loss were observed during the yearlong treatment. This study clearly demonstrated the biological activity of met-leptin in humans.

Third, experimental treatment of obese humans has been studied. Daily subcutaneous injections of recombinant met-leptin (0.30 mg/kg body weight) for 24 weeks in obese subjects resulted in weight loss that was significantly greater than placebo treatment. Lower doses were without effect on body weight. The majority of the weight loss was body fat, and no systemic side effects were observed, but there were significant skin irritations at the site of injection in many subjects. The rapid disappearance of leptin from the blood was described following subcutaneous dosing. Appetite was not reported in these studies (54).

A long-acting recombinant native human leptin produced by linking human leptin to polyethylene glycol (PEG) polymers to form pegylated recombinant human leptin (PEG-OB protein) has also been tested in humans. After completing safety and efficacy tests in animals (mice, rats, monkeys), Phase I and II clinical trials were conducted in obese humans. Treatment of obese men, under conditions of an energy deficit of 1–2 MJ/d, with a *weekly* subcutaneous injection of 20 mg PEG-OB protein for 12 weeks, increased serum concentrations of leptin and PEG-OB protein between weekly doses (55). The expected fall in serum leptin with weight loss did not occur in the PEG-OB protein-treated group, while in the placebo group leptin levels decreased (55). Appetite (assessed by Factor 3 [hunger] of the Three-Factor Eating Questionnaire) and hunger ratings (visual-analog scales) before breakfast were decreased in the leptin-treated group compared to the placebo group, as shown in Figure 3. The significant difference began during the first week after treatment started, and it remained constant during the next 11 weeks (56).

The observation that PEG-OB protein treatment decreased appetite under fasting conditions at a dose that did not change body weight or body composition suggests that leptin treatment acts centrally to regulate energy intake. When taken together with the results of leptin treatment of the young obese girl with a mutated *ob* gene (53) with met-leptin, these results strongly suggests that leptin treatment can suppress appetite in obese humans (53,56).

Fourth, many studies in lean and obese humans have demonstrated that weight gain is associated with an increase in serum concentrations of leptin, while weight loss is associated with a decrease in circulating leptin concentrations (3,4).

C Leptin Receptor

The leptin receptor (also known as OB-R) was rapidly identified and characterized following the demonstration of the biological activity of recombinant leptin.

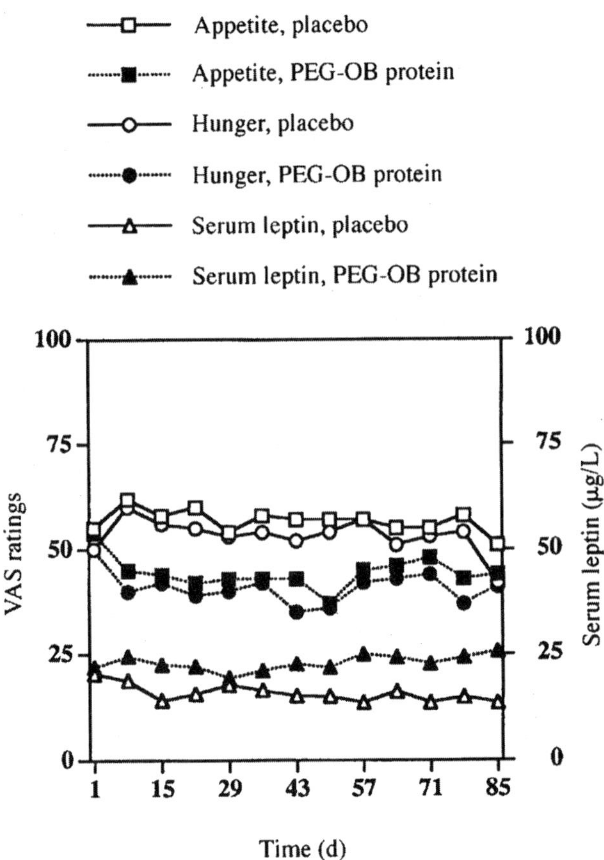

Figure 3 Visual analog scale (VAS) ratings of appetite and hunger and serum leptin levels in subjects who received 20 mg pegylated polyethylene glycol OB protein (PEG-OB protein; n = 15) or placebo (n = 15) weekly. All data were collected before breakfast. There were significant differences in changes in appetite and hunger during the treatment between the two groups (two-factor repeated measures ANOVA with interaction; $P < .01$). There were significant differences in changes in serum leptin concentrations between the two groups (two-factor repeated measures ANOVA with interaction; $P < .05$). (From Ref. 56.)

First, a central binding site for labeled leptin in the choroid plexus and pia mater in *ob/ob*, *db/db*, and lean mice as well as lean and obese Zucker rats was identified (57) and confirmed by others (38,58,59). This finding directly led to the expression cloning of the leptin receptor from the mouse choroid plexus (60).

The leptin receptor had considerable homology with the GP130 subunit of the IL-6 cytokine receptor (60). The leptin receptor was found to be expressed in the choroid plexus, the hypothalamus, and many other brain areas, as well as several peripheral tissues (61, 62). However, the leptin receptor is a low-abundance message and protein, making unambiguous detection of the receptor message and protein difficult. As a result of alternate splicing, the leptin receptor exists in multiple forms. The two major forms are a short form (OB-R_S (also known as OB-Ra) with a truncated intracellular domain), and a long form (OB-R_L (also known as OB-Rb) with the complete intracellular domain). The long form is thought to be the form that signals and mediates the biological effects of leptin (60). In situ hybridization studies have demonstrated that the mRNA for the long form of the leptin receptor is localized primarily to the hypothalamus (arcuate, lateral, ventromedial, dorsomedial nuclei) (61,63,64). Soon it was demonstrated that the *db* gene encodes the leptin receptor (65–67). Point mutations have been identified in the leptin receptor in obese *db*/*db* mice (no OB-R_L), obese Zucker (extracellular domain), and obese Koletsky (corpulent) rats (null mutation; no mRNA for OB-R) (66,68,69). The molecular biology and characterization of the leptin receptor has been reviewed (70,71).

VII THE CONCEPT OF REDUCED BRAIN RESPONSIVENESS TO LEPTIN IN OBESITY: ALTERED INTEGRATION OF PERIPHERAL SIGNALS

Strong support for the concept of *reduced responsiveness to leptin in obesity* is provided by the observation of elevated leptin concentrations in the blood of obese individuals and the experimental result that higher doses are required to affect feeding behavior, metabolism, and body fat in diet-induced obese mice (4,40) and appetite in obese humans (53–56). At one extreme of the continuum of leptin responsiveness is the obese *db*/*db* mouse, with elevated leptin levels, which is totally unresponsive to leptin: at the other end is the very responsive leptin-deficient, obese *ob*/*ob* mouse. Although these two mutant mice with defects in the leptin pathway anchor the continuum of leptin responsiveness, they have, in our opinion, little relevance to human obesity. Although diet-induced obese mice are less responsive than lean mice, they still retain a significant responsiveness to leptin (3,14,40). The leptin responsiveness of most obese humans will probably range from normal to decreased, but still responsive. Whether the reduced responsiveness to leptin is due to one or more intrinsic or regulatory defects in the postreceptor signaling pathway, downregulation of the neural network responsive to leptin, or/and decreased brain transport and uptake of leptin remains to be determined by further research (38,39).

Shifts along the continuum of leptin responsiveness as a function of adiposity have been demonstrated in studies of DIO mice. When lean AKR/J mice are fed a high-fat, energy-dense diet for several weeks, they become obese with elevated leptin and insulin concentrations. The demonstration that diet-induced obese AKR/J mice required much higher IP doses of leptin to reduce food intake contributed to the concept of leptin resistance. DIO mice also have decreased central responsiveness to leptin (72). In these studies, the suppression of food intake following ICV injection of mouse leptin in DIO mice was measured after changes in diet. Following leptin injection ICV, food intake suppression was similar in lean and nonobese mice on the same high-fat diet, but was markedly reduced in DIO mice. After being switched back to chow diet and losing weight, ICV leptin reduced food intake similarly in lean and formerly DIO mice, indicating an increase in brain responsiveness to leptin in formerly DIO mice. In contrast, decreased brain responsiveness to leptin was not observed in mice remaining lean while on a high-fat diet. Thus, these studies with DIO obese mice indicate that the brain responsiveness to leptin of the neural network in the brain controlling energy balance is decreased by weight gain and can be reversed by weight loss (72).

VIII ROLE OF THE BRAIN INSULIN IN ENERGY BALANCE

A major advance in the regulation of energy balance has been the elucidation of the brain insulin system by Woods, Porte, and their colleagues in Seattle and Cincinnati (36,37,73). Figure 2 (above) shows a schematic representation of the brain insulin hypothesis. This team made the very important observation that fasting plasma insulin was proportional to adiposity or the adipose tissue mass (9,36,37,73). Based on this observation, they performed a sequence of very ambitious, complex studies to show rigorously that central injections of small amounts of insulin into the CSF were followed by suppressed food intake and reduced body weight. The results of these studies in a variety of species including rats, birds, and monkeys provided strong experimental support for the hypothesis.

These studies clearly demonstrated that a peripheral circulating signal proportional to adiposity could act on brain mechanisms to alter feeding behavior and body energy balance. The idea that a large circulating protein like insulin provides important information to the brain; that insulin would act differently in the brain than in the periphery; that insulin in the brain could potentiate the effects of neuropeptides such as neuropeptide Y (NPY) and CCK; and that circulating steroids interact with the brain insulin in important ways, provided the basis for the paradigm of central/peripheral integration in the regulation of food intake and body energy balance (9).

The brain insulin hypothesis has also provided strong evidence for the involvement of brain neuropeptides, in addition to monoamine neurotransmitters, in the control of food intake. These investigators also demonstrated that central administration of insulin decreased the expression of NPY mRNA in the arcuate nucleus of the hypothalamus. In addition, they also showed that the central administration of insulin increased the expression of corticotropin-releasing hormone (CRH) mRNA in the paraventricular nucleus of the hypothalamus (9,37,73). Thus, central administration of insulin altered the gene expression of two major neuropeptides (decreased NPY and increased CRH mRNAs) that are important regulators of food intake and body energy regulation as well as other biological processes.

IX INTERACTION AND CENTRAL INTEGRATION OF LEPTIN AND INSULIN WITH OTHER BRAIN HORMONES AND NEUROPEPTIDES

Research on the brain mechanisms involved in leptin action has been stimulated by the long-lasting reductions in food intake and body weight of obese *ob/ob* mice observed following ICV leptin administration (40,41) together with the observation that the circulating leptin concentration was proportional to body fat in humans (4). Central administration of leptin reduced food intake and body weight, altered metabolism, and inhibited NPY-induced feeding of obese *ob/ob* mice, lean mice, and rats.

The neurotransmitters and neuropeptides that directly mediate the actions of leptin have not yet been identified, but experimental evidence is consistent with leptin acting through several brain mechanisms (NPY, AgRP, CART, POMC) to coordinate the regulation of energy balance (74–81) (see Chap. 13). In addition, leptin has been shown to interact with CRH and CRH-dependent neuronal pathways in the regulation of energy balance (63,82). Which if any neurotransmitters and neuropeptides are responsible for the decreased responsiveness to leptin in obesity is not known. However, the neuronal network controlling energy balance and the descending sympathetic nervous system following peripheral and central administration of leptin is beginning to emerge (81).

Studies of neuronal activity indicate that multiple brain regions contain neurons that are responsive to leptin and are involved in detection of its presence and in generation of its effects. Hyperpolarization of glucose-receptive ATP-sensitive potassium channels and stimulation and inhibition of firing rates have been reported in ventromedial and lateral neurons (83). Direct application of leptin to VMH and LH neurones resulting in both stimulation and inhibition of firing rates have been reported (84). Patterns of activation of brain areas in response to central or peripheral administration of leptin have been measured using c-fos immunoreactivity. Numerous studies have implicated hypothalamic nuclei (arcuate, VMH, DMH, PVN) and other brain areas thought to be involved in the control of energy balance (52,84,85). Brain administration of leptin leads to neuronal activation in many brain areas known to be involved in regulation of food intake and body energy balance including the hypothalamus, periform, and cortex. In addition, brown fat was clearly activated in the periphery. This demonstration of leptin activation of the sympathetic nervous system was consistent with norepinephrine turnover studies in brown fat (86) and c-fos studies (63,87,88). In addition, direct recording of efferent sympathetic fibers innervating multiple organs in anesthetized rats demonstrated that intravenous administration of leptin increased sympathetic nerve activity to multiple target organs (89). Colocalization studies using selective antibodies have demonstrated that leptin acts through its receptor on neurons that contain NPY, ACTH, POMC, and melanin-concentrating hormone (MCH) (87). These converging lines of evidence strongly suggest that in addition to several nuclei of the hypothalamus (ventromedial, dorsomedial, paraventricular, and arcuate), other brain areas are involved including periform cortex, brainstem, cerebellum, basal ganglia, and cortex (3,14) Thus, the biological actions of leptin to regulate energy balance are the result of a distributed leptin-responsive neural network within the brain.

Recent studies focusing on the arcuate nucleus has provided important insights into the integration of peripheral signals within the brain. Leptin and insulin have been shown to interact on specific receptors on neurons in the arcuate nucleus of the hypothalamus, and the local application of each peripheral signal within the vicinity of the arcuate has profound and predictable effects on food intake and body weight (10,74,77,78,80). Specifically, elevations of either hormone in the hypothalamus cause reduced food intake and weight loss, and reductions of the activity of either in the brain cause increased food intake and weight gain. The arcuate contains two groups of neurons sensitive to leptin and insulin. One group synthesizes neuropeptide Y (NPY) and agouti-related protein (AgRP), neurotransmitters that act throughout the hypothalamus to increase food intake and reduce energy expenditure. Both leptin and insulin inhibit the activity of these anabolic NPY/AgRP neurons. The other group of arcuate neurons synthesizes POMC, which is then processed to several small peptides, including desacetyl-MSH, which is in turn acetylated at the N-terminus to produce alpha-melanocyte-stimulating hormone (alpha-MSH) and cocaine-amphetamine-elated transcript (CART), neurotransmitters that act throughout the hypothalamus to decrease food intake and increase energy expenditures (75,76,79,90–92). Leptin and insulin stimulate activity of these alpha MSH/ CART neurons. The NPY/AgRP and the alpha-MSH/CART neurons influence many of the brain controls over the pituitary, the autonomic nervous system, and the control of food intake (10,74,76). It is very likely that similar neural substrates for the integration of peripheral signals regulating energy balance will be elucidated throughout the brain (10).

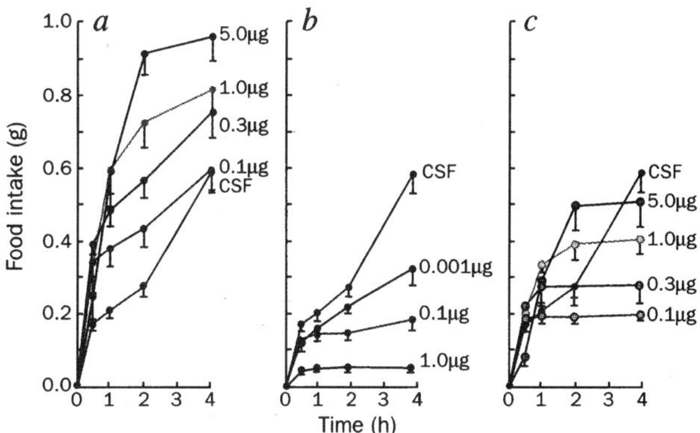

Figure 4 Effects of ICV administration of leptin on the feeding response to ICV doses of NPY in free-feeding *ob/ob* mice. Cumulative food intake during the 4 hr after the second ICV injection (time = 0) is shown. Panels show: (*a*) increased food intake after doses of NPY alone (n = 8); (*b*) decreased food intake after doses of human leptin alone (n = 7–10); (*c*) the interaction of 1 μg/mouse human leptin and increasing doses of NPY (n = 5–9). Cumulative food intake following injection of CSF (n = 25) is shown in each panel for comparison. Food, but not water, was removed from the cage during the 1-hr period between ICV injections. Values represent the mean ± SEM. Differences were tested using Student's t-test with unpaired samples with $P < .05$. (From Ref. 97.)

A Example 1: NPY and Leptin

Early in the story of leptin, it was proposed that NPY, a potent stimulator of feeding (49,93,94), was the major mediator of the actions of leptin (41,94,95). This proposal was based on the inhibitory effects of leptin on NPY gene expression (41,46,80,84) and secretion (41) observed in studies of biological activity of leptin. We examined the interaction of brain administration of leptin and NPY on the feeding behavior of *ob/ob* mice to test this hypothesis. We found that leptin inhibited the expected feeding following NPY administration as shown in Figure 4. The magnitude and time course of food intake were determined by the presence of leptin. However, at low doses of leptin, NPY was able to stimulate food intake, indicating a complex interaction exists between leptin and NPY. Similar results have been reported by others (96).

These results suggest that leptin determines the sensitivity (or gain) of the feeding response to exogenous NPY. Leptin, when placed into the lateral ventricle, may alter the binding of exogenous NPY to its receptors. These receptors are critical for feeding or/and may inhibit downstream signal transduction (97). This indicates that leptin can attenuate the actions of exogenous NPY and suggests that the receptor-mediated actions of NPY on feeding can be modulated by leptin (97). Thus, it appears that NPY interacts, particularly in the early postinjection period, with leptin or leptin-dependent signaling processes that contribute to the regulation of body energy balance. However, our results are also consistent with other mediators, besides NPY, of leptin action. This possibility has been strengthened by the report that normal-weight mice lacking NPY respond to peripheral administration of leptin (98). When both the *ob* and *npy* loci are disrupted in mice, the double knockout mice were still obese but the degree of obesity was attenuated by ~25–40%. These authors conclude that leptin-mediated antagonism of the hypothalamic NPY system is required for normal regulation of body energy balance (99). The mechanism of the functional antagonism of NPY receptors by leptin remains to be determined.

B Example 2: Circulating Glucocorticoid and Leptin

Strong evidence that NPY and glucocorticoids, acting centrally, play a major role in the development and maintenance of obesity in rodents has been provided by the work of Bernard Jeanrenaud and colleagues (48,100–105). Chronic intracerebroventricular infusions of NPY or glucocorticoids (dexamethasone) have led to an obesity syndrome: animals with increased body fat, food intake, insulin and leptin concentrations, and elevated triglycerides (103,106). In addition, ICV NPY infusions led to elevated corticosterone (104), while glucocorticoid ICV infusions led to suppressed corticosterone, increased the hypothalamic levels of NPY, decreased those of CRH, and decreased the expression of uncoupling proteins 1 and 3 (106). Adrenalectomy has been shown to completely prevent the obesity syndrome following ICV NPY infusions (101,104). Replacement of corticosterone in these rats restores the ability of ICV NPY to promote the development of obesity (103). When NPY and glucocorticoid are both infused ICV into adrenalectomized rats, an obesity syndrome was observed. Infusion of NPY or glucocorticoid alone failed to reproduce this obesity syndrome (103).

When leptin was administered into the third ventricle of the brain of lean rats, NPY gene expression in the arcuate nucleus was decreased, while corticotrophin-releasing hormone (CRH) gene expression in the paraventricular nucleus was increased in some studies (63). However, other investigators found that leptin decreased CRH gene expression in the PVN (82,92). Since CRH treatment inhibits feeding of rodents when administered ICV (9,37), these results suggest that part of the activity of leptin to inhibit feeding may be mediated through decreased NPY and increased CRH protein levels in specific hypothalamic nuclei critical for the regulation of food intake and body energy balance.

That leptin may interact with the glucocorticoid system is illustrated by (1) the finding that adrenalectomy can restore sensitivity of obese Zucker (*fa/fa*) to centrally administered insulin (9); (2) the well-established effects of glucocorticoids in animal models of obesity (100,101,107), and (3) the actions of leptin on the hypothalamic-pituitary-adrenal axis in fasted mice (108). A series of experiments were conducted in which leptin was administered centrally in adrenalectomized and sham-operated lean rats. A marked increase in potency of the leptin to reduce food intake was observed in adrenalectomized rats (102). When glucocorticoid was replaced using increasing doses, the potency of leptin to reduce food intake was decreased (100–102). Clearly, peripheral corticosterone concentrations can modulate the responsiveness of the brain to leptin. These results provide support for an important interaction between leptin and the glucocorticoid system in animals and, potentially, in humans.

C Example 3: Melanocortin and Leptin

Recent genetic and pharmaceutical research has provided strong evidence that the melanocortins and their receptors, particularly MC4-R and MC3-R, play an important role in the regulation of energy balance. In mice lacking MC4-R, late-onset obesity and altered peripheral metabolism have been observed (109). This result, combined with experiments with MC3,4-R agonists (decreased food intake) and antagonists (increased food intake) that are based on alpha-MSH, indicates that the MC4-R participates in a physiological pathway that normally inhibits food intake and fat storage, and may play an important role in late-onset obesity (91). The naturally occurring ligand for MC4-R is unknown, but is widely believed to be alpha-MSH. However, an as yet unidentified protein product of pro-opiomelanocortin (POMC) processing could also be natural ligand. Two other peptides, melanin-concentrating hormone (MCH) (110–112) and agouti-related peptide (AgRP) (92), also act to stimulate feeding.

The evidence for the interaction between leptin and the melanocortin system includes (1) central administration of leptin increases the expression of the POMC gene in the arcuate nucleus (113); (2) a nonselective peptide MC3,4-R antagonist blocked inhibition of food intake by leptin (however, the same antagonist also blocks NPY induced feeding); (3) mice lacking MC4-R responded to ICV leptin by decreasing food intake; (4) when *agouti* (A^y/a) mice and *ob/ob* mice were crossed, the combined phenotype appeared to be independent and additive (114); (5) mice lacking MC3 receptor (MC3-R) were also obese (115,116); and (6) when mice lacking MC4-R and MC3-R were crossed, mice with even greater obesity resulted (115), strongly suggesting that the MC4-R and MC3-R are involved in the regulation of energy balance (117). These studies suggest that the melanocortin signaling pathway appears to be downstream of the leptin pathway and that the two pathways converge and may interact at one or more points.

The mouse mutations mahogany (mg) and mahoganoid (md) are negative modifiers of the Agouti coat color gene, which encodes a paracrine signaling molecule that induces a switch in melanin synthesis. Both md and mg suppressed the effects of mutation A^y on both coat color and obesity. These results suggest that md and mg interfere directly with Agouti signaling, possibly at the level of protein production or receptor regulation (118).

D Example 4: CCK and Insulin and Leptin

The important role of the cholecystokinin (CCK) hypothesis in the study of ingestive behavior is widely acknowledged (119,120). The CCK hypothesis postulated that food in the intestine causes the release of CCK that acts on CCK-A receptors in the vagus nerve to provide sensory information to the brain, which causes meal termination. The critical pieces in that hypothesis were identification of the dependence on the vagus nerve, the identification of a peripheral CCK-A receptor and a receptor in the brain, initially called CCK-B but now known to be the gastrin receptor, and the demonstration that CCK-A antagonists increased food intake (121).

Evidence suggests that insulin may increase the sensitivity of the brain to signals such as CCK (20). That is, when very low amounts of insulin are slowly infused into the brain, doses of CCK that would otherwise have no effect become very effective at reducing meal size (20,122). Similar results have been reported for leptin. Hence, if an individual has lost body weight, the reduced levels of insulin in the brain make the brain less sensitive to CCK. The result is that during meals, more food will be eaten before CCK (and the other satiety signals) elicits satiety, and this will continue until body weight is restored (20).

X INTERACTION WITH OTHER NEUROENDOCRINE SYSTEMS

Leptin not only is linked to the regulation of energy balance but also may have a number of additional roles, such as maintaining the normal neuroendocrine activity that is important in the adaptation to starvation and controlling stress responses and functions such as reproduction. Starved mice and leptin-deficient *ob/ob* mice were found to have similar neuroendocrine abnormalities, including an activated hypothalamic-pituitary-adrenal response and depressed thyroid function. In addition, male mice had low levels of testosterone, and female mice had delayed ovulation. When fasted mice were treated with leptin, these neuroendocrine abnormalities were reversed (108,123). Administration of leptin to female *ob/ob* mice restored reproductive function to near normal, and the mice became pregnant and successfully carried litters to term (123). The few adult cases of human mutations in the ob-r genes present with severe obesity and incomplete sexual maturation (124,125).

XI ROLE OF THE LEPTIN PATHWAY IN THE BRAIN: A SUBSTRATE FOR INTEGRATION

One possible role for leptin is that of a modulator of gene expression and the resultant synthesis of one or more neurotransmitters and/or neuropeptides within the brain. Much of the research conducted on the leptin pathway has focused on the identification of downstream genes that are regulated by leptin. Five such genes are *npy, crh, cart, agrp*, and *POMC* because leptin has been shown to decrease NPY mRNA and AgRP mRNA levels and increase POMC and CART mRNA in arcuate nucleus and CRH mRNA levels in different areas of the hypothalamus (1–3,7).

Another possible role for leptin is that of a modulator of synaptic transmission within the brain. This could involve alteration of the release or postsynaptic action of one or more neurotransmitters and/or neuropeptides and/or states of one or more presynaptic and/or postsynaptic ion channels. Since recent electrophysiological studies have demonstrated that this hypothesis is correct, then behavioral and metabolic responses to the administration of leptin may be expected to depend on the "background" amounts of these neurotransmitters and/or neuropeptides in synapses or nerve terminals. Since the amounts of these neurotransmitters and neuropeptides change with time, variability in behavioral and/or metabolic responses to administration of leptin would be expected. However, in experiments with sequential administration of leptin and NPY, we were impressed with the very reproducible, rather than variable, nature of these interaction data (97).

Another, alternative role for leptin would be a "coordinator" or "organizer" of the seemingly disparate neurotransmitter and neuropeptide effects on, and responses to, ingestive behavior and body energy balance. The recent demonstration of "coordinated" response of NPY, POMC, CART, and AgRP gene expression to leptin administration (inhibition of NPY and AgRP mRNA, and increased POMC and CART mRNA in arcuate nucleus) provides support for this concept (92). In addition, leptin has been shown to increase CRH mRNA in the paraventricular nucleus in response to central administration of leptin and to interact with CRH-dependent neuronal pathways

(63,82). These responses were "coordinated" in both space (two different anatomical locations) and time (both changes were seen at a common time point that was correlated with the behavioral response) (1–3,7).

These three possible roles do not have to be, and are probably not, mutually exclusive. Indeed, the "coordinator" or "organizer" function of leptin within the brain may emerge from at least two distinct regulatory components mediated by the leptin receptor. One, the action of leptin to regulate gene expression within areas of the brain critical for regulation of energy balance, can be considered responsible for the "long-term" or "chronic" biological effects (e.g., critical molecules which determine the brain responsiveness to leptin, "settling point" for body fat content). Two, the action of leptin to modulate synaptic transmission within the brain by altering the release or postsynaptic action of one or more neurotransmitters and/or neuropeptides and/or states of one or more presynaptic and/or postsynaptic ion channels can be considered responsible for the "short-term," "acute," or "immediate" behavioral (suppression of food intake) and metabolic effects (decreased serum concentrations of insulin and glucose). This "dual-function" mechanism of action, regulation of gene expression and modulation of ongoing cellular function such as neurosecretion, is a common and classical property of hormones. If additional experiments support this dual-function mechanism of action for leptin, it would provide additional evidence for the concept that leptin is a hormone that plays a critical role in the regulation of brain mechanisms involved in the regulation of energy balance.

One representation of this hypothesis at the molecular levels in the hypothalamus is shown in Figure 5. Several "classes" of parallel neural pathways are represented by the five model neurons depicted. Each neuron

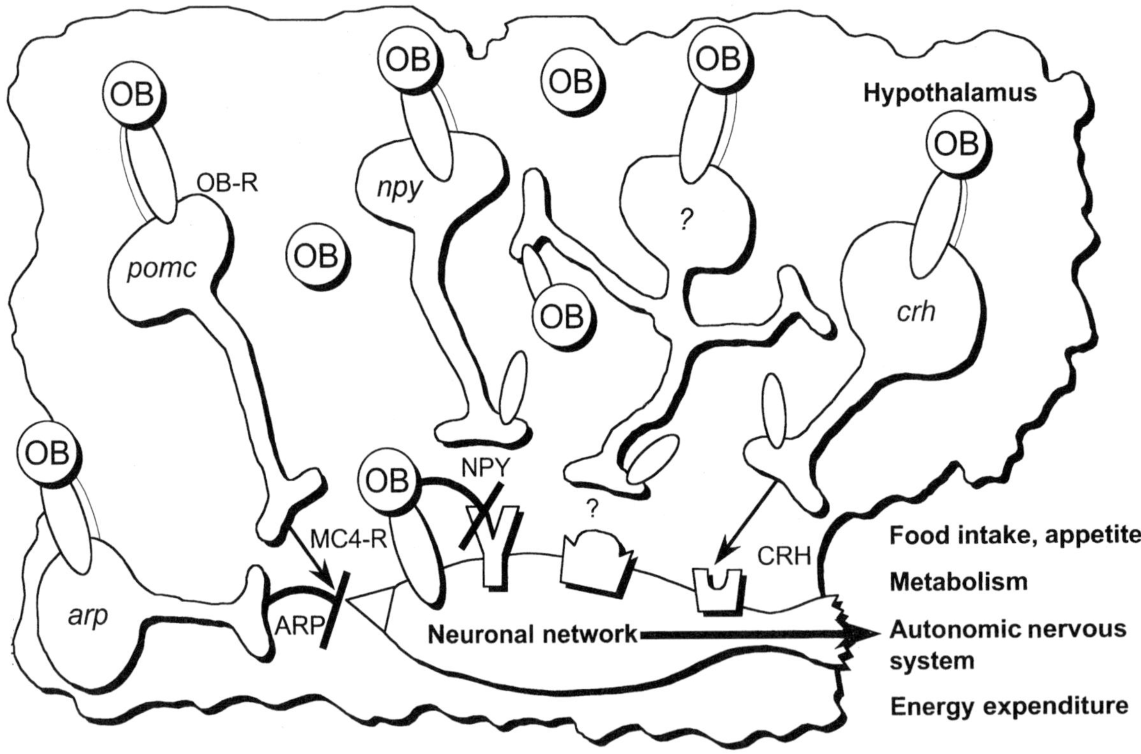

Figure 5 Schematic diagram of hypothetical neural networks controlling energy balance. Several "classes" of parallel neural pathways are represented by the four model neurons depicted. Each neuron is assumed to express the gene, synthesize and release one dominant type of neuropeptide—NPY, CRH, POMC, AgRP (ARP)? Each neuron has the long form of the OB-R receptor (ellipses) and the "final common pathway," the neuronal network controlling ingestive behavior, metabolism, and energy balance, and has distinct receptors for OB, NPY, CRH, POMC, AgRP and ? Leptin is shown as circles containing OB. Note that leptin can express its biological action through five parallel paths, each mediated by a different neuropeptide—NPY, CRH, POMC, AgRP or ? The ability of leptin to inhibit the actions of released NPY is also shown. (From Ref. 8.)

shown is assumed to have the gene and to synthesize and release one dominant type of neuropeptide—NPY, CRH, POMC, AgRP and ? Each neuron has the long form of the leptin receptor (OB-R) (ellipses), and the "final common pathway," the neuronal network controlling ingestive behavior, metabolism, and energy balance, has distinct receptors for leptin (OB), NPY, CRH, POMC, AgRP and ? The demonstrated ability of leptin to inhibit responses to NPY is shown by the heavy line blocking the NPY receptor. In this theoretical construct, leptin would fulfill the role of "conductor" integrating the distinct "sections" of the "orchestra" to behave as one while it plays the "symphony." In this analogy, the "symphony" is the integrated behavioral, neuroendocrine, and metabolic response of an individual; the "orchestra" is the spatially distributed neural network controlling ingestive behavior, metabolism, and energy balance; and the "sections" would be the elements and subsystems of this neural network. This attractive hypothesis has held up since it was proposed in 1995 but must wait further experimental testing in future studies.

ACKNOWLEDGMENTS

We thank Jack F.R. Curtis for assistance with the conceptualization and execution of some of the artwork. We also thank our many colleagues and collaborators in many laboratories throughout the world for important experiments and stimulating discussions and suggestions. Special thanks to Professor S.C. Woods for pioneering the pathway from the periphery to the brain and back again and sharing his insights.

REFERENCES

1. Campfield LA, Smith FJ. The pathogenesis of obesity. In: Bray GA, ed. Bailliere's Clinical Endocrinology and Metabolism. London: Bailliere Tindal, 1999:13–30.
2. Campfield LA, Smith FJ, Burn P. Strategies and potential molecular targets for obesity treatment. Science 1998; 280:1383–1387.
3. Campfield LA. Multiple facets of OB protein (leptin) physiology: integration of central and peripheral mechanisms in the regulation of energy balance. In: Ailhaud G, Guy-Grand B, eds. Progress in Obesity Research: 8. London: John Libbey & Company, 1999:327–335.
4. Considine RV, Sinha MK, Heiman ML, Kriauciunas A, Stephens TW, Nyce MR, Ohannesian JP, Marco CC, McKee LJ, Baur TL, Caro JF. Serum immunoreactive-leptin concentrations in normal-weight and obese humans. N Engl J Med 1996; 334:192–295.
5. Maffei M, Halaas J, Ravussin E, Pratley RE, Lee GH, Zhang Y, Fei H, Kim S, Lallone R, Ranganathan S, Kern PA, and Friedman JM. Leptin levels in human and rodent: measurement of plasma leptin and *ob* mRNA in obese and weight-reduced subjects. Nat Med 1995; 1:1155–1161.
6. Kennedy GC. The role of depot fat in the hypothalamic control of food intake in the rat. Proc R Soc Lond Ser B 1953; 140:578–592.
7. Campfield LA, Smith FJ, Burn P. The OB protein (leptin) pathway—a link between adipose tissue mass and central neural networks. Horm Metab Res 1996; 28:619–632.
8. Campfield LA, Smith FJ, Burn P. OB protein: a hormonal controller of central neural networks mediating behavioral, metabolic and neuroendocrine responses. Endocrinol Metab 1997; 4:81–102.
9. Kaiyala KJ, Woods SC, Schwartz MW. New model for the regulation of energy balance and adiposity by the central nervous system. Am J Clin Nutr 1995; 62:1123s–1134s.
10. Schwartz MW, Woods SC, Porte D Jr, Seeley RJ, Baskin DG. Central nervous system control of food intake. Nature 2000; 404:661–671.
11. De Matteis R, Dashtipour K, Ognibene A, Cinti S. Localization of leptin receptor splice variants in mouse peripheral tissues by immunohistochemistry. Proc Nutr Soc 1998; 57:441–448.
12. Zhang Y, Proenca R, Maffei M, Barone M, Leopold L, Friedman JM. Positional cloning of the mouse obese gene and its human homologue. Nature 1994; 372:425–431.
13. Leibel RL, Rosenbaum M, Hirsch J. Changes in energy expenditure resulting from altered body weight. N Engl J Med 1995; 232:621–628.
14. Campfield LA, Smith FJ. Overview: neurobiology of OB protein (leptin). Proc Nutr Soc 1998; 57:429–440.
15. Le Magnen J. The metabolic basis of the dual periodicity of feeding in rats. Behav Brain Sci 1980; 4:561–607.
16. Le Magnen J. Hunger. London: Cambridge University Press, 1985.
17. Le Magnen J. *Neurobiology of Feeding and Nutrition*. San Diego: Academic Press, 1992.
18. Campfield LA, Smith FJ. Systemic factors in the control of food intake: evidence for patterns as signals. In: Stricker EM, ed. *Handbook of Behavioral Neurobiology, Vol 10. Neurobiology of Food and Fluid Intake*. New York: Plenum Press, 1990:183–206.
19. Campfield LA. Metabolic and hormonal controls of food-intake: highlights of the last 25 year—1972–1997. Appetite 1997; 29:135–152.
20. Woods SC, Seeley RJ, Porte D Jr, Schwartz MW.

Signals that regulate food intake and energy homeostasis. Science 1998; 280:1378–1383.

21. Bray GA, Campfeld LA. Metabolic factors in the control of energy stores. Metabolism 1975; 24:99–117.
22. Bogardus C, Lillioja S, Ravussin E, Abbott W, Zawadzki JK, Young A. Familial dependence of the resting metabolic rate. N Engl J Med 1986; 315:96–100.
23. Keesey RE. Physiological regulation of body weight and the issue of obesity. Med Clin North Am 1989; 73:15–27.
24. Hill JO, Douglas HJ, Peters JC. Physical activity, fitness, and moderate obesity. In: Bouchard C, Shepard RJ, Stephens T, eds. *Physical Activity Fitness, and Health: International Proceedings and Consensus Statement*. Champaign (Illinois): Human Kinetics Publisher Inc., 1994.
25. World Health Organization. *Obesity: Preventing and Managing the Global Epidemic*. Geneva: World Health Organization, 1998.
26. Astrup A. Obesity as an adaptation to a high-fat diet: evidence from a cross-sectional study. Am J Clin Nutr 1994; 59:350–355.
27. Ingalls AM, Dickie MM, Snell GD. Obese, a new mutaion in the house mouse. J Hered 1950; 41:317–325.
28. Coleman DI. Obese and diabetes: two mutant genes causing diabetes-obesity syndromes in mice. Diabetologia 1978; 14:141–1148.
29. Coleman DL. Effects of parabiosis of obese with diabetes and normal mice. Diabetologia 1973; 9:294–298.
30. Coleman DL. Inherited obesity-diabetes syndromes in the mouse. Prog Clin Biol Res, 1981; 45:145–158.
31. Coleman DL, Hummel KP. The influence of genetic background on the expression of the obese (ob) gene in the mouse. Diabetologia 1973; 9:287–293.
32. Herberg L, Coleman DL. Laboratory animals exhibiting obesity and diabetes syndromes. Metabolism 1977; 26:59–99.
33. Sinha MK, Ohannesian JP, Heiman ML, Kriaucinunas A. Nocturnal rise in leptin in lean, obese, and non-insulin-dependent diabetes mellitus subjects. J Clin Invest 1996; 97:1344–1347.
34. Van Aggel-Leijssen DP, Van Baak MA, Tenenbaum R, Campfield LA, Saris WHM. Regulation of average 4h human plasma leptin level; the influence of exercise and physiological changes in energy balance. Int J Obes Relat Metab Disord 1999; 23:151–158.
35. Porte D Jr. Banting Lecture 1990. Beta-cells in type II diabetes mellitus. Diabetes 1991; 40:166–80.
36. Woods SC, Nolan LJ. The insulin story: a 25-year perspective. Appetite 1997; 28:281–282.
37. Schwartz MW, Figlewicz DP, Baskin DG, Woods SC, Porte D Jr. Insulin and the central regulation of energy balance: Update 1994. Endocr Rev 1994; 2:109–113.
38. Banks WA, Kastin AJ, Huang W, Jaspan JB, Maness LM. Leptin enters the brain by a saturable system independent of insulin. Peptides 1996; 17:305–311.
39. Golden PL, Maccagnan TJ, Pardridge WM. Human blood-brain barrier leptin receptor. Binding and endocytosis in isolated human brain microvessels. J Clin Invest 1997; 99:14–18.
40. Campfield LA, Smith FJ, Guisez Y, Devos R, Burn P. Recombinant mouse OB protein: Evidence for a peripheral signal linking adiposity and central neural networks. Science 1995; 269:546–549.
41. Stephens TW, Basinski M, Bristow PK, Bue-Valleskey JM, Burgett SG, Craft L, Hale J, Hoffmann J, Hsiung HM, Kriauciunas A, MacKeller W, Rosteck PR Jr, Schoner B, Smith D, Tinsley FC, Zhang X-Y, Heiman M. The role of neuropeptide Y in the antiobesity action of the obese gene product. Nature 1995; 377:530–532.
42. Seeley RJ, Van Dijk G, Campfield LA, Smith FJ, Burn P, Nelligan JA, Bell MS, Baskin DG, Woods SC, Schwartz MW. Intraventricular leptin reduces food intake and body weight of lean rats but not obese Zucker rats. Horm Metab Res 1996; 28:664–668.
43. Pelleymounter M, Cullen M, Baker M, Hecht R, Winters D, Bone T, Collins F. Effects of the obese gene product on body weight regulation in *ob/ob* mice. Science 1995; 269:540–543.
44. Rentsch J, Levens N, Chiesi M. Recombinant *ob*-gene product reduces food intake in fasted mice. Biochem Biophys Res Commun 1995; 214:131–136.
45. Halaas JL, Gajiwala KS, Maffei M, Cohen SL, Chait BT, Rabinowitz D, Lallone RL, Burley SK, Friedman JM. Weight-reducing effects of the plasma protein encoded by the obese gene. Science 1995; 269:543–546.
46. Schwartz MW, Baskin DG, Bukowski TR, Kuijper JL, Foster D, Lasser G, Prunkard DE, Porte D Jr, Woods SC, Seeley RJ, Weigle DS. Specificity of leptin action on elevated blood glucose levels and hypothalamic neuropeptide Y gene expression in *ob/ob* mice. Diabetes 1996; 45:531–535.
47. Shimabukuro M, Koyama K, Chen G. Direct effects of leptin through triglyceride depletion of tissues. Proc Natl Acad Sci USA 1997; 94:4637–4641.
48. Cusin I, Rohner-Jeanrenaud F, Stricker-Krongrad A, Jeanrenaud B. The weight-reducing effect of an intracerebroventicular bolus injection of leptin in genetically obese *fa/fa* rats. Reduced sensitivity compared with lean animals. Diabetes 1996; 1446–1450.
49. Rohner-Jeanrenaud F, Cusin I, Sainsbury A, Zakrzewska K, Jeanrenaud B. Neuropeptide Y and leptin in lean and genetically obese *fa/fa* rats. Horm Metab Res 1996; 28:642–648.
50. Lin L, Truett GE, Levans N, York DA. Central, but not peripheral administration of leptin reduced the food intake and body weight in Zucker fatty and lean rats. Obes Res 1996; 4:1S.
51. Wildman HF, Chau SCJ, Leibel RL, Smith GP.

Effects of leptin and cholecystokinin in rats with a null mutation of the leptin receptor lepr[fak]. Am J Physiol 2000; 278:R1518–R1523.
52. Thiele TE, Van Dijk G, Campfield LA, Smith FJ, Burn P, Woods SC, Bernstein IL, Seeley RJ. Central infusion of GLP-1, but not leptin, produces conditioned taste aversion in rats. Am J Physiol 1997; 272:R726–R730.
53. Farooqi IS, Jebb SA, Langmack G, Lawrence E, Cheetham CH, Prentice AM, Hughes IA, McCamish MA, O'Rahilly S. Effects of recombinant leptin therapy in a child with congenital leptin deficiency. N Engl J Med 1999; 341:879–884.
54. Heymsfield SB, Greenberg AS, Fujioka K, Dixon RM, Kushner R, Hunt T, Lubina JA, Patane J, Self B, Hunt P, McCamish M. Recombinant leptin for weight loss in obese and lean adults: a randomized, controlled, dose-escalation trial. JAMA 1999; 282:1568–75.
55. Hukshorn CJ, Saris WH, Westerterp-Plantenga MS, Farid AR, Campfield LA. Weekly subcutaneous pegylated recombinant native human leptin (PEG-OB) administration in obese men. J Clin Endocrinol Metab 2000; 85:4003–4009.
56. Westerterp-Plantenga MS, Saris WH, Hukshorn CJ, Campfield LA. Effects of weekly administration of pegylated recombinant human OB protein on appetite profile and energy metabolism in obese men. Am J Clin Nutri 2001; 74:426–434.
57. Devos R, Richards JG, Campfield LA, Tartaglia LA, Guisez Y, Van der Heyden J, Travernier J, Plaetinck G, Burn P. OB protein binds specifically to the choriod plexus of mice and rats. Proc Natl Acad Sci USA 1996; 93:5668–5673.
58. Lynn RB, Cao GY, Considine RV, Hyde TM, Caro JF. Autoradiographic localization of leptin binding in the choroid plexus of *ob/ob* and *db/db* mice. Biochem Biophys Res Commun 1996; 219:884–889.
59. Corp ES, Conze DB, Smith F, Campfield LA. Regional localization of specific [^{125}I]leptin binding sites in rat forebrain. Brain Res 1998; 789:40–47.
60. Tartaglia LA, Dembski M, Weng X, Deng N, Culpepper J, Devos R, Richards JG, Campfield LA, Clark FT, Deeds J, Muir C, Sanker S, Moriarty A, Moore KJ, Smutko JS, Mays GG, Woolf EA, Monroe CA, Tepper RI. Identification and expression cloning of a leptin receptor (OB-R). Cell 1995; 83: 1263–1271.
61. Mercer JG, Hoggard N, Williams LM, Lawrence CB, Hannah LT, Trayhurn P. Localization of leptin receptor mRNA and the long form splice variant (OB-Rb) in mouse hypothalamus and adjacent brain regions by in situ hybridization. FEBS Lett 1996; 387:113–116.
62. Ghilardi N, Ziegler S, Wiestner A, Stoffel R, Heim MH, Skoda RC. Defective STAT signaling by the leptin receptor in diabetic mice. Proc Natl Acad Sci USA 1996; 93:6231–6235.
63. Schwartz MW, Seeley RJ, Campfield LA, Burn P, Baskin DG. Identification of targets of leptin action in rat hypothalamus. J Clin Invest 1996; 98:1101–1106.
64. Elmquist JK, Bjorbaek C, Ahima RS, Flier JS, Saper CB. Distributions of leptin receptor mRNA isoforms in the rat brain. J Comp Neurol 1998; 395:535–547.
65. Lee G, Proenca R, Montez JM, Carrol KM, Darvishzadeh JG, Lee JI, Friedman JM. Abnormal splicing of the leptin receptor in diabetic mice. Nature 1996; 379:632–635.
66. Chua SC, Chung WK, Wu-Peng XS, Zhang Y, Liu S-M, Tartaglia L, Leibel RL. Phenotypes of mouse diabetes and rat *fatty* due to mutations in the OB (leptin) receptor. Science 1996; 271:994–996.
67. Chen H, Charlat O, Tartaglia LA, Woolf EA, Weng X, Ellis SJ, Lakey ND, Culpepper J, Moore KJ, Breitbart RF, Duyk GM, Tepper RI, Morgenstern JP. Evidence that the diabetes gene encodes the leptin receptor: identification of a mutation in the leptin receptor gene in *db/db* mice. Cell 1996; 84:491–495.
68. Takaya K, Ogawa Y, Hiroaka J, Hosoda K, Yamori Y, Nakao K, Koletsky RJ. Nonsense mutation of leptin receptor in the obese spontaneously hypertensive Koletsky rat. Nat Gene 1996; 14:130–131.
69. Wu-Peng XS, Chau SCJ, Okada N, Liu SM, Nicolson M, Leibel RL. Phenotype of the obese Koletsky (f) rat due to tyr763stop mutation in the extracellular domain of the leptin receptor (LEPR): evidence for deficient plasma -to-csf transport of leptin in both the Zucker and Koletsky obese rat. Diabetes 1997; 46: 513–518.
70. Tartaglia LA. The leptin receptor. J Biol Chem 1997; 272:6093–6096.
71. White DW, Tartaglia LA. Leptin and OB-R: body weight regulation by a cytokine receptor. Cytokine Growth Factor Rev 1996; 7:303–309.
72. Campfield LA, Smith FJ, Yu J, Renzetti M, Simko B, Baralt M, Mackie G, Tenenbaum R, Smith W. Dietary obesity induces decreased central sensitivity to exogenous OB protein (leptin) which is reversed by weight loss. Soc Neurosci Abstr 1997; 23:815.
73. Schwartz MW, Marks J, Sipols AJ, Baskin DB, Woods SC, Kahn SE, Prote JD. Central insulin administration reduces neuropeptide Y mRNA expression in the arcuate nucleus of food-deprived lean (*fa/fa*) but not obese (*fa/fa*) Zucker rats. Endocrinology 1991; 128:2645–2647.
74. Elmquist JK. Hypothalamic pathways underlying the endocrine, autonomic, and behavioral effects of leptin. Int J Obes Relat Metab Disord 2001; 25:S78–S82.
75. Elias CF, Lee CE, Kelly JF, Ahima RS, Kuhar M, Saper CB, Elmquist JK. Characterization of CART neurons in the rat and human hypothalamus. J Comp Neurol 2001; 432:1–19.
76. Ahima RS, Saper CB, Flier JS, Elmquist JK. Leptin

regulation of neuroendocrine systems. Front Neuroendocrinol 2000; 21:263–307.
77. Elias CF, Kelly JF, Lee CE, Ahima RS, Drucker DJ, Saper CB, Elmquist JK. Chemical characterization of leptin-activated neurons in the rat brain. J Comp Neurol 2000; 423:261–281.
78. Elmquist JK. Anatomic basis of leptin action in the hypothalamus. Front Horm Res 2000; 26:21–41.
79. Ahima RS, Kelly J, Elmquist JK, Flier JS. Distinct physiologic and neuronal responses to decreased leptin and mild hyperleptinemia. Endocrinology 1999; 140:4923–4931.
80. Elias CF, Aschkenasi C, Lee C, Kelly J, Ahima RS, Bjorbaek C, Flier JS, Saper CB, Elmquist JK. Leptin differentially regulates NPY and POMC neurons projecting to the lateral hypothalamic area. Neuron 1999; 23:775–786.
81. Elmquist JK, Maratos-Flier E, Saper CB, Flier JS. Unraveling the central nervous system pathways underlying responses to leptin. Nat Neurosci 1998; 1:445–450.
82. Huang Q, Rivest R, Richard D. Effects of leptin on corticotropin-releasing factor (CRF) synthesis and CRF neuron activation in the paraventricular hypothalamic nucleus of obese (*ob/ob*) mice. Endocrinology 1998; 139:1524–1532.
83. Spanswick D, Smith MA, Groppi VE, Logan SD, Ashford MLJ. Leptin inhibits hypothalamic neurons by activation of ATP-senstive potassium channels. Nature 1997; 390:521–525.
84. Yokosuka M, Xu B, Pu S, Karla SP. The magnocellular part of the paraventricular hypothalamic nucleus (PVN): a selective site for inhibition of NPY-induced food intake by leptin. Soc Neurosci Abstr 1997; 23: 852.
85. Van Dijk G, Theile TE, Donahey JCK, Campfield LA, Smith FJ, Burn P, Bernstein IL, Woods SC, Selley RJ. Central infusion of leptin and GLP-1(7–36) amide defferentially stimulate c-FLI in the rat brain. Am J Physiol 1996; 271:R1096–Rl100.
86. Collins S, Kuhn CM, Petro AE, Swick AG, Chrunyk BA, Surwit RS. Role of leptin in fat regulation. Nature 1996; 380:677.
87. Hakansson M-L, Brown H, Ghilardi N, Skoda RC, Meister B. Leptin receptor immunoreactivity in chemically defined target neurons of the hypothalamus. J Nueorosci 1998; 18:559–572.
88. Chen SC, Kochan JP, Campfield LA, Burn P, Smeyne RJ. Splice variants of the OB receptor gene are differentially expressed in brain and peripheral tissues of mice. J Recept Signal Transduct Res 1999; 19:245–266.
89. Haynes WG, Morgan DA, Walsh SA, Marks AL, Sivitz WI. Receptor-mediated regional sympathetic nerve by leptin. J Clin Invest 1997; 100:270–278.
90. Elias CF, Lee C, Kelly J, Aschkenasi C, Ahima RS, Couceyro PR, Kuhar MJ, Saper CB, Elmquist JK. Leptin activates hypothalamic CART neurons projecting to the spinal cord. Neuron 1998; 21:1375–1385.
91. Fan W, Boston BA, Kesterson RA, Hruby VJ, Cone RD. Melanocortinergic inhibition of feeding behavior and disruption with an agouti-mimetic. Nature 1997; 385:165–168.
92. Arvaniti K, Huang Q, Richard D. Effects of leptin and corticosterone on the expression of corticotropin-releasing hormone, agouti-related protein, and proopiomelanocortin in the brain of *ob/ob* mouse. Neuroendocrinology 2001; 73:227–236.
93. Rohner-Jeanrenaud F, Jeanrenaud B. Obesity, leptin, and the brain. N Engl J Med 1996; 334:324–325.
94. Ezzell C. Fat times for obesity research: Tons of new information, but how does it all fit together. J NIH Res 1995; 7:39–45.
95. Stanley BG, Kyrkouli SE, Lampert S, Leibowitz SF. Neuropeptide Y chronically injected into the hypothalamus: a powerful neurochemical inducer of hyperphagia and obesity. Peptides 1986; 7:189–192.
96. Stricker-Krongrad A, Chiesi M, Cumin F, Spanka C, Whitesbread S, Rentsch J, Lollman B, Hofbauer KG, Levens N. Interactions between leptin and neuropeptide Y in the control of food intake in the rat. Obes Res 1996; 4(1):37s.
97. Smith FJ, Campfield LA, Moschera JA, Bailon P, Burn P. Feeding inhibition by neuropeptide Y. Nature 1996; 382:307.
98. Erickson JC, Clegg KE, Palmiter RD. Sensitivity to leptin and susceptibility to seizures of mice lacking neuropeptide Y. Nature 1996; 381:415–418.
99. Erickson JC, Hollopetter G, Palmiter RD. Attenuation of the obesity syndrome of *ob/ob* mice by the loss of neuropeptide Y. Science 1996; 274:1704–1707.
100. Jeanrenaud B, Rohner-Jeanrenaud F. Effects of neuropeptides and leptin on nutrient partitioning: dysregulations in obesity. Annu Rev Med 2001; 52:339–351.
101. Jeanrenaud B, Rohner-Jeanrenaud F. CNS-periphery relationships and body weight homeostasis: influence of the glucocorticoid status. Int J Obes Relat Metab Disord 2000; 24:S74–S76.
102. Zakrzewska KE, Cusin I, Sainsbury A, Rohner-Jeanrenaud F, Jeanrenaud B. Glucocorticoids as counterregulatory hormones of leptin: toward an understanding of leptin resistance. Diabetes 1997; 46:717–719.
103. Zakrzewska KE, Sainsbury A, Cusin I, Rouru J, Jeanrenaud B, Rohner-Jeanrenaud F. Selective dependence of intracerebroventricular neuropeptide Y–elicited effects on central glucocorticoids. Endocrinology 1999; 140:3183–3187.
104. Sainsbury A, Cusin I, Rohner-Jeanrenaud F, Jeanrenaud B. Adrenalectomy prevents the obesity syndrome produced by chronic central neuropeptide Y infusion innormal rats. Diabetes 1997; 46:209–214.

105. Zarjevski N, Cusin I, Vettor R, Rohner-Jeanrenaud F, Jeanrenaud B. Chronic intercerebroventricular neuropeptide Y administraton to normal rats mimics hormonal and metabolic changes to obesity. Endocrinology 1993; 133:1753–1758.
106. Zakrzewska KE, Cusin I, Stricker-Krongrad A, Boss O, Ricquier D, Jeanrenaud B, Rohner-Jeanrenaud F. Induction of obesity and hyperleptinemia by central glucocorticoid infusion in the rat. Diabetes 1999; 48:365–370.
107. Bray GA, York DA. Hypothalamic and genetic obesity in experimental animals: an automonic and endocrine hypothesis. Physiol Rev 1979; 59:719–809.
108. Ahima RS, Prabakaren D, Mantzoros C, Ou D, Lowell B, Maratzoros-Flier E, Flier J. Role of leptin in the neuroendocrine responses to fasting. Nature 1996; 382:250–252.
109. Huszar D, Lynch CA, Fairchild-Huntress V, Dunmore JH, Fang Q, Berkemeier LR, Gu W, Kesterson RA, Boston BA, Cone RD, Smith FJ, Campfield LA, Burn P, Lee F. Targeted disruption of the melanocortin-4 receptor results in obesity in mice. Cell 1997; 88:131–141.
110. Ludwig DS, Tritos NA, Mastaitis JW, Kulkarni R, Kokkotou E, Elmquist J, Lowell B, Flier JS, Maratos-Flier E. Melanin-concentrating hormone overexpression in transgenic mice leads to obesity and insulin resistance. J Clin Invest 2001; 107:379–386.
111. Shimada M, Tritos NA, Lowell BB, Flier JS, Maratos-Flier E. Mice lacking melanin-concentrating hormone are hypophagic and lean. Nature 1998; 396:670–674.
112. Tritos NA, Maratos-Flier E. Two important systems in energy homeostasis: melanocortins and melanin-concentrating hormone. Neuropeptides 1999; 33:339–334.
113. Schwartz MW, Seeley RJ, Woods SC, Weigle DS, Campfield LA, Burn P, Baskin DG. Leptin increases hypothalamic pro-opiomelanocortin mRNA expression in the rostral arcuate nucleus. Diabetes 1997; 46:2119–2123.
114. Boston BA, Blaydon KM, Varerin J, Cone RD. Independent and additive effects of central POMC and leptin pathways on murine obesity. Science 1997; 278:1641–1644.
115. Chen AS, Metzger JM, Trumbauer ME, Guan XM, Yu H, Frazier EG, Marsh DJ, Forrest MJ, Gopal-Truter S, Fisher J, Camacho RE, Strack AM, Mellin TN, MacIntyre DE, Chen HY, Van der Ploeg LH. Role of the melanocortin-4 receptor in metabolic rate and food intake in mice. Transgenic Res 2000; 9:145–154.
116. Butler AA, Kesterson RA, Khong K, Cullen MJ, Pelleymounter MA, Dekoning J, Baetscher M, Cone RD. A unique metabolic syndrome causes obesity in the melanocortin-3 receptor-deficient mouse. Endocrinology 2000; 141:3518–3521.
117. Butler AA, Cone RD. Knockout models resulting in the development of obesity. Trends Genet 2001; 17:S50–S54.
118. Miller KA, Gunn TM, Carrasquillo MM, Lamoreux ML, Galbraith DB, Barsh GS. Genetic studies of the mouse mutations mahogany and mahoganoid. Genetics 1997; 146:1407–1415.
119. Gibbs J, Young RC, Smith GP. Cholecystokinin decreases food intake in rats. J Comp Physiol Pyschol 1973; 84:488–495.
120. Smith GP, Gibbs J. Satiating effect of cholecystokinin. Ann NY Acad Sci 1994; 713:236–241.
121. Moran TH, Robinson PH, Goldrich MS, McHugh PR. Two brain cholecystokinin receptor: implications for behavioral actions. Brain Res 1986; 362:175–179.
122. Riedy CA, Chavez M, Figlewicz DP, Woods SC. Central insulin enhances sensitivity to cholecystokinin. Phyiol Behav 1995; 58:755–760.
123. Chehab F, Lim M, Lu R. Correction of the sterility defect in homozygous obese female by treatment with human recombinant leptin. Nat Genet 1996; 12:318–320.
124. Clement K, Valisse C, Lahlou N, Cabrol S, Peeloux V, Cassuto D, Gourmelen M, Dina C, Chambaz J, Lacourte M, Basdevant A, Bougneres P, Lebouc Y, Froguel P, Guy-Grand B. A mutation in the human leptin receptor gene causes obesity and pituitary dysfunction. Nature 1998; 392:398–401.
125. Strobel A, Issad T, Camoin L, Ozata M, Strosberg D. A leptin missense mutation associated with hypogonadism and morbid obesity. Nat Gene 1998; 18:213–215.
126. Thomas PR, ed. *Weighing the Options: Criteria for Evaluating Weight Management Programs*. Washington: National Academy Press, 1995.

17

Development of White Adipose Tissue

Gérard Ailhaud

Centre National de la Recherche Scientifique, Nice, France

Hans Hauner

German Diabetes Research Institute, Dusseldorf, Germany

I INTRODUCTION

The development of white adipose tissue (WAT) represents a dynamic process throughout life. It was long assumed that the acquisition of fat cells was irreversible, but recent observations suggest that apoptosis may also occur in WAT, although to a much smaller extent than in brown adipose tissue (BAT). At the cellular level, there is still limited and partially contradictory information about the characteristics of the cells constituting the adipose tissue organ. This leads in turn to the question of the nature of the factors that regulate the formation of new fat cells from dormant adipose precursor cells or even multipotent mesenchymal stem cells. Once adipose tissue is formed, adipocytes represent between one-third and two-thirds of the total number of cells. The remaining cells are blood cells, endothelial cells, pericytes, adipose precursor cells of varying degree of differentiation, and, most likely, other cell types (1). The existence of very small fat cells in addition to mature adipocytes has also been documented (2). Figure 1 summarizes the various cell types present in this tissue, based on ultrastructural studies in vivo and biological studies in vitro (3).

At present, it cannot be assessed to which extent various morphological descriptions represent only different stages of the cell lineage leading to the characteristic adipocyte phenotype. From a biological perspective, all different cell types present in the whole body arise from a single fertilized egg. With development, stem cells become increasingly committed to specific lineages. The establishment of embryonic stem (ES) cell lines but also of adult stem cells has opened new experimental approaches (4). The adipose lineage originates from multipotent mesenchymal stem cells that develop into adipoblasts by largely unknown mechanisms. Commitment of adipoblasts gives rise to preadipose cells (usually termed preadipocytes), i.e., cells that have expressed early but not yet late markers and that have not yet accumulated triacylglycerol stores. However, it is becoming more and more likely that multipotent stem cells as well as adipoblasts, which are formed during embryonic development, are still present postnatally. Clearly, in vitro studies with ES cells should provide clues to answer these critical questions and to characterize the key molecular events during adipocyte formation. In vitro, lipid-free, fibroblastlike preadipose cells undergo terminal differentiation into immature adipose cells containing small lipid droplets and then into mature fat cells filled with a few or only one large lipid droplet (Fig. 1). The relationships between brown and white fat during development still remain an open question. The occurrence of brown adipocytes can be detected among all white fat pads, their proportions differ according to the localization of

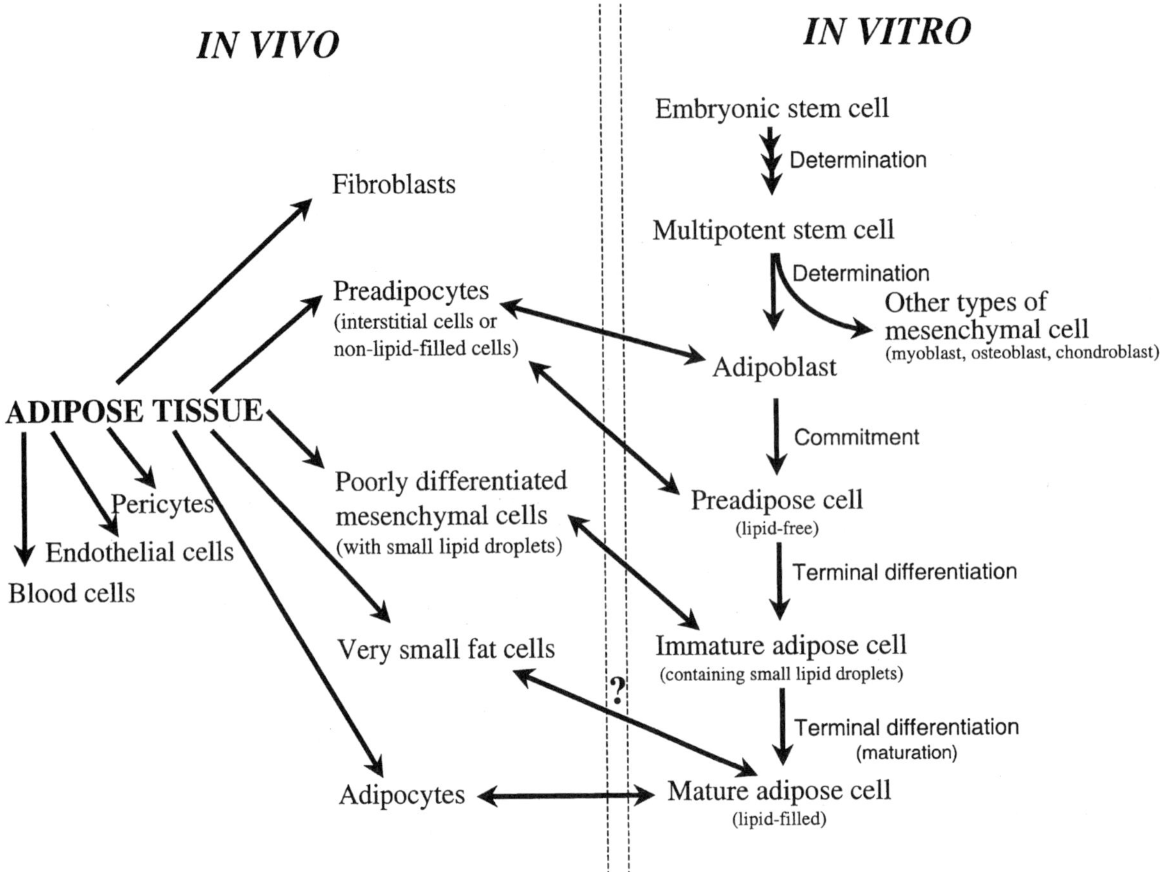

Figure 1 Relationships between morphological types in vivo and stages of cell differentiation in vitro. The adipocyte fraction corresponds to adipocytes and very small fat cells. The stromal cell fraction corresponds to a mixture of the other cell types.

the deposit, the ambient temperature, and the species. During postnatal development, the transformation of typical brown fat into white fat can occur rapidly in numerous species and deposits, suggesting a possible transformation of brown into white adipocytes. Conversely, in adult mice as well as in adult dogs, all white deposits can be rapidly and massively converted into brown fat. Using a transgenic approach, it appears that most white adipocytes, if not all, emerge independently of the brown adipocyte lineage during adipose tissue development (5).

II REGULATION OF ADIPOSE TISSUE MASS IN VIVO

A Phylogeny and Ontogeny of Adipose Tissue

Among invertebrates, adipose tissue represents an important organ in insects whereas its quantitative importance decreases in arachnids, crustaceans, and mollusks. Among vertebrates, adipose tissue develops extensively in homeotherms, although its proportion of body weight can vary greatly between species (up to 40% of body weight in cetaceans) or within a species, as is the case in migrating birds and hibernating mammals.

The development of WAT shows wide differences between species. It cannot be detected macroscopically during embryonic life or at birth in most rodents (mouse, rat), whereas it is present at birth in the guinea pig, rabbit, pig, and human. Studies of embryonic development in pigs (6) and humans (7) have emphasized the tight coordination of angiogenesis in time and space with the formation of fat cell clusters.

Histologically, WAT appears well vascularized, many adipocytes being actually in contact with a single capillary. Thus, blood supply is adequate to support the active entry and release of metabolites as well as the secretion of various peptide and nonpeptide factors (8). In the rat, the sole innervation is postganglionic, sympathetic, and noradrenergic. However, sympathetic innervation of WAT has been reported, albeit less extensively than that of BAT, where sympathetic adrenergic neurons innervate brown adipocytes directly (9).

The characterization of specific growth factors able to trigger and modulate the development of capillaries and fat cell clusters is still in its infancy. Ubiquitous angiogenesis factors have been described, some of which [transforming growth factor-β (TGF-β), prostaglandin E_2 (PGE_2), vascular endothelial growth factor (VEGF), angiopoietin-1] are synthesized and secreted by adipocytes. 1-Butyrylglycerol is solely secreted by adipocytes and appears to act as a potent angiogenesis factor only in this tissue (10). Secreted leptin also appears to act as a highly potent angiogenic factor, consistent with the presence of functional leptin receptors on the surface of endothelial cells (11,12). In addition, endothelial cells as well as fibroblasts and other cells of mesenchymal origin, including preadipocytes and adipocytes, secrete insulinlike growth factor-1 (IGF-1) and IGF-1 binding proteins. This suggests an involvement of IGF-1 in the hyperplastic development of adipose tissue during embryogenesis.

B Adipose Tissue Development in Early Life

Most studies on the early development of adipose tissue are exclusively based on morphological methods owing the lack of appropriate cell culture models. The "primitive fat organ" of Wassermann develops in the embryo from poorly defined predetermined "Anlagen" long before a visible fat deposition takes place. At this early stage, cells that later will develop into adipocytes are morphologically undistinguishable from other cell types of the connective tissue (13). Only later does fat deposition allow the retrospective identification of these cells as designated preadipocytes. Light microscopy studies in human fetuses suggest that the first traces of a fat organ are detectable between the 14th and 16th weeks of prenatal life. Aggregation of mesenchymal cells in close association with the formation of blood vessels was described as the first indication of adipogenesis in humans.

The first primitive organ structures to be identified at sites where fat accumulates characteristically are fat lobules, long before typical vacuolated fat cells are distinguishable. After the 23rd week of gestation, the number of fat lobules remains constant, while in the subsequent weeks the size of the lobules is continuously growing (14). At the sites of early fat development, a multilocular appearance of adipocytes predominates and probably reflects the early developmental stage (7). This is interesting, since the morphological development in vitro resembles the developmental steps in vivo. Preadipose cells either from clonal cell lines or from primary cultures usually exhibit a multilocular morphology, not only during early, but also during late stages of in vitro differentiation when the characteristic markers of mature fat cells are fully expressed. The available data do not provide any evidence of significant site- and sex-related differences in early development, supporting the concept that the marked regional differences in adipose tissue distribution in males and females develop later in life, presumably under the control of sex steroids and other hormones. Although some microscopic studies postulate that the second trimester may be a critical period for the development of obesity in later life, the descriptive nature of these data does not allow any firm conclusion in this respect.

At the beginning of the third trimester, adipocytes are found in the principal fat depot areas but are still rather small (7). At birth, body fat accounts for 16% of body weight as assessed by whole-body counting of ^{40}K. Analysis of biopsy samples of adipose tissue revealed that the increase in body fat during the first year of life from about 0.7 to 2.8 kg is entirely due to an increase in fat cell size, while fat cell number remains unchanged (15). Other studies on this issue gave controversial results, particularly with regard to the development of fat cell number during the first year of life. Such differences may be largely explained by variations in methodology and the general difficulties in assessing total-body fat cell number. In addition, most studies were cross-sectional, which makes interpretation of results more difficult. Longitudinal studies showed a continuous increase in fat cell weight between 1 and 12 months of age (16). It has also been pointed out that in fetal life and early infancy adipose tissue is composed of different cell populations: lipid-containing cells but also many cells that are essentially lipid-free and not readily recognized as adipocytes. Small fat cells in the early stages of fat accumulation may make an important contribution to the adipose cell mass at this age. Therefore, it is tempting to conclude that a gradual accumulation of body fat after birth is mainly reflected by increasing fat cell size (17).

C Physiology of Adipose Tissue Cellularity in Humans

Apart from species differences, the development of adipose tissue varies according to sex and age. Moreover, the ability of rodents and humans to increase the number of adipocytes also depends on the nature of the diet and the localization of the adipose depot. The formation of new fat cells following the proliferation of "dedifferentiated" cells during refeeding after a prolonged period of food deprivation, as well as the proliferation of mature adipocytes, still remain controversial events which, if present, should be of low magnitude.

Many studies during the past 25 years have been dealing with changes of adipose tissue cellularity throughout life. Based on such observations, a hypothesis was early established that postulated the existence of sensitive periods in adipose tissue development during childhood. Two peaks for accelerated adipose tissue growth were reported: one after birth, and another be-

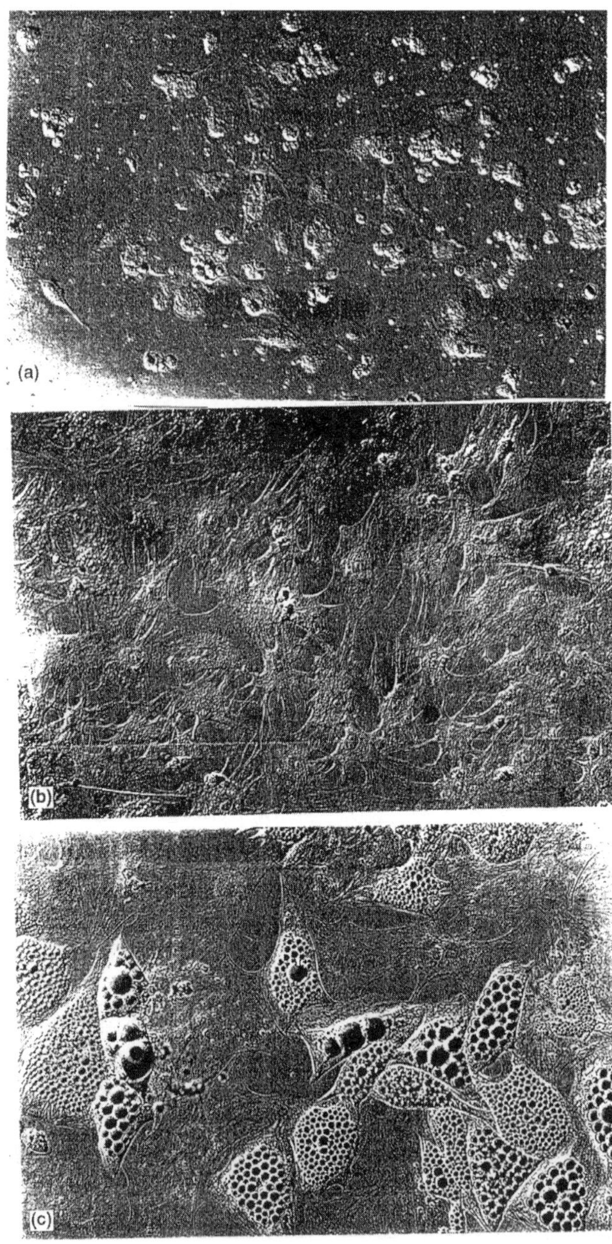

Figure 2 Human adipose precursor cells before and after terminal differentiation. Human adipose precursor cells were maintained in differentiation medium (23) for 12 hr (a), 4 days (b), and 15 days (c). Micrographs were taken with interference contrast. Magnification ×250.

tween 9 and 13 years (18). Later studies using different techniques support this hypothesis. When thymidine kinase activity was measured as an index of cellular proliferation, Baum and coworkers found that adipose tissue enzyme activity was highest in infants during the first year after birth. A second, but much smaller, peak in enzyme activity was found in the preadolescent years (19). There is only one study in which cell proliferation and differentiation were measured in cultured stromal cells isolated from adipose tissue samples of children at different ages. Despite some limitations, the results of this study also suggest that the capacity for cell proliferation and differentiation in adipose tissue is highest during the first year of life and less pronounced in the years before puberty (20). Irrespective of the debate on the existence of sensitive periods in adipose tissue growth, Knittle and coworkers demonstrated in a large cohort of children that, starting by the age of 2, children show a small but continuous increase in both cell size and number during childhood over a 4-year observation period (21).

The rate of cell proliferation in adipose tissue slows down during adolescence, and, at weight stability, fat cell number seems to remain fairly constant in adult life. An expansion of adipose tissue mass is believed to be largely due to an enlargement of existing fat cells; only in severe obesity can total fat cell number increase up to threefold (22). However, a recent in vitro study showed that adult humans are able to form new adipocytes at any age; even adipose tissue samples obtained from individuals above the age of 60 contain a significant proportion of cells that can undergo differentiation (23). In contrast to established preadipocyte cell lines from rodents, most stromal cells from human adipose tissue seem to be already in a late stage of development They obviously do not require postconfluent cell division to enter the terminal differentiation program (24). The morphological appearance of the stromal cell fraction isolated from human adipose tissue is rather homogeneous (Fig. 2). The majority of cells exhibit tiny lipid droplets arranged around the nucleus, which can be easily detected by Oil Red O staining or electron microscopy. However, a recent study suggested that these cells are not definitely committed to become adipocytes, but retain a potential to enter other developmental programs under appropriate hormonal stimulation (25).

D Hormonal Effects on Adipose Tissue Growth

Lessons learned from defined endocrine disorders indicate that hormones can affect both the adipose tissue mass and its distribution pattern. The various hormones reported to be related with dynamic changes of adipose tissue so far are summarized in Table 1. The role of some hormones that may be of particular physiological importance is described next in more detail.

1 Macrophage Colony-Stimulating Factor

Macrophage colony-stimulating factor (MCSF) has been implicated in adipocyte hyperplasia. MCSF mRNA and the protein are expressed in human adipocyte and this expression is upregulated in humans gaining weight with overfeeding. Overexpression in rabbits of MCSF by adenoviral-mediated gene transfer increases WAT growth by hyperplasia (26).

2 Thyroid Hormones

Hypothyroidism in rats induces a transient hypoplasia, whereas hyperthyroidism results in a transitory hyperplasia of retroperitoneal and epididymal fat tissues (27), which is in favor of an accelerating effect of tri-iodothyronine (T_3) on the precocious formation of mature fat cells. Interestingly, in hypophysectomized pig fetuses, but not in intact fetuses, thyroxine (T_4) profoundly enhances adipose tissue development by hyperplasia and hypertrophy, which points to a role of T_4 as an adipogenic agent, at least in early developmental stages, and suggests that growth hormone (GH) antagonizes the adipogenic potential of thyroid hormones (28).

Table 1 Effect of Selected Hormones, Cytokines, and Growth Factors on Adipose Tissue Cellularity from In Vivo and In Vitro Studies

Factor	Fat cell size	Fat cell number	Fat mass
Insulin			
Excess	↑	(↑)	↑
Cortisol			
Excess	↑	(↑)	↑
Growth hormone			
Excess	↓	↑	↓
Deficiency	↑	↓	↑
Testosterone			
Deficiency	↑	n.d.[a]	↑
Tri-iodothyronine			
Excess	↓	↑	Normal
Deficiency	Normal	↓	↓
TNFα	↓	n.d.	↓
EGF	↓	↓	↓
MCSF	Normal	↑	↑

[a] Not determined.

3 Insulin

Insulin is an anabolic hormone that potently supports lipid storage in adipose tissue, but is also a powerful growth-promoting factor. Insulin favors lipid accumulation not only via stimulation of glucose uptake and increased lipoprotein lipase (LPL) activity but also by inhibition of catecholamine-induced lipolysis. The lipogenic effect of insulin is already evident in fetal life, since hyperinsulinemia in the fetal circulation of mothers with gestational diabetes frequently results in macrosomia with an increase in fat mass. In streptozotocin-diabetic rats, insulin stimulates the in vivo cell proliferation in white adipose tissue. This growth-stimulating effect was observed in interstitial cells rather than in other cell types, including lipid-containing cells (29). In cell culture experiments, insulin was found to be both an adipogenic hormone in 3T3-L1 fibroblasts (30,31) and a positive modulator of adipose differentiation in clonal Ob17 preadipocytes (32) as well as in rat and human adipocyte precursor cells in primary culture (23,33). The growth-promoting effect of supraphysiological insulin concentrations may be exerted via the IGF-1 receptor. An interesting phenomenon in this context is insulin-induced lipohypertrophy in diabetic subjects. This clinical observation is frequently made when insulin is repeatedly injected at the same subcutaneous site, particularly in young women. Analysis of adipose tissue cellularity revealed that the mean fat cell size is only moderately increased in lipohypertrophic areas as compared to unaffected sites, strongly suggesting that, in addition, adipocyte precursor cells are recruited (Hauner and coworkers, unpublished observations).

4 Growth Hormone

Growth hormone (GH) deficiency is known to be associated with an increased body fat mass. Children with GH deficiency have enlarged fat cells but a reduced number compared to healthy children (34). Treatment with GH normalizes these disturbances of adipose tissue cellularity (34,35). The increased body fat mass in GH-deficient subjects is mainly localized in the abdominal region, and administration of GH results in preferential reduction of fat cell size in the abdomen (35). Studies using computerized tomography (CT) suggest that the visceral depots are particularly sensitive to the effect of GH. A 6-month treatment with recombinant GH of patients with adult-onset GH deficiency resulted in a 4.7-kg reduction of adipose tissue mass. Subcutaneous adipose tissue decreased by an average of 13%, whereas visceral adipose tissue was reduced by 30% (36). In contrast, in patients with acromegaly, a reduced fat mass was observed that returned to normal after treatment of the hormone excess by octreotide or pituitary surgery.

The mechanisms of the slimming effects of GH are only partially understood. Chronic administration of GH to GH-deficient children was found to induce a significant reduction in basal lipogenesis and a decreased antilipolytic action of insulin leading to a significant reduction of adipocyte size, but only in the abdominal depot (35). In cultured human adipose tissue pieces, GH counteracted the stimulatory effects of glucocorticoids on LPL activity without affecting LPL mRNA levels (37). On the other hand, recent data suggest that GH has an intrinsic lipolytic activity, which can be demonstrated in fat cells from GH-deficient adults and is even enhanced after long-term GH administration (38). As many biological actions of GH are mediated via the induction of IGF-1 synthesis, attention has been paid to the question of whether the metabolic effects of GH on adipose tissue are exerted by IGF-1. Studies in porcine preadipocyte cultures have shown that GH is able to increase IGF-1 mRNA at least twofold. Since the increase in local IGF-1 production was associated with a decrease in adipocyte development, the authors concluded that local IGF-1 may contribute to the suppression of the adipocyte phenotype (39). In contrast, IGF-1 increased adipose conversion in rabbit adipocyte precursors. The stromal-vascular cells from the perirenal adipose tissue were found to secrete large amounts of IGF-1 and IGF-binding proteins (40). In cultured human preadipocytes, GH was found to considerably reduce adipose cell differentiation. Upon stimulation by GH, stromal cells responded with an increased synthesis and release of IGF-1, which was followed by increased DNA synthesis as assessed by tritiated thymidine incorporation. It was also demonstrated in this study that human adipose cells have specific GH receptors and that the hormone exerts a variety of direct metabolic effects such as inhibition of glucose uptake and stimulation of lipolysis, which may cause a net loss of stored lipids (41).

5 Glucocorticoids

Clinical observations suggest that patients suffering from glucocorticoid excess develop an increased adipose tissue mass with a characteristic preferential accumulation of fat in the trunk and neck region. In a recent study using CT, surgical treatment of women with Cushing's disease was associated with a significant reduction of all adipose tissue depots except for leg adipose tissue. However, visceral, head, and neck adipose tissue depots were more markedly reduced than other depots (42). Studies of adipose tissue cellularity in Cushing's syndrome have shown that this expansion is primarily due to enlarged abdominal fat cells (43). This effect can be at least partly explained by the finding that fat cells from the abdominal depot exhibit more cytoplasmatic glucocorticoid receptors and higher receptor mRNA compared with adipocytes from other regions (44). In Cushing's syndrome, fat cell hypertrophy in the abdomen appears to be due to elevated adipocyte LPL activity and also to low lipolytic activity (43). Moreover, glucocorticoids are known to be potent promoters of the adipose differentiation process, a mechanism that may also contribute to adipose tissue expansion during glucocorticoid excess (23).

The role of glucocorticoids and the importance of the hypothalamic-pituitary-adrenal axis in the excessive development of adipose tissue have been documented in two models of transgenic mice. In one model (45), a reduction of the glucocorticoid receptor in the brain and also in liver and kidneys was obtained with an antisense mRNA, whereas in a second model (46) overexpression of corticotropin-releasing factor (CRF) was achieved. In both cases, the observed increase in corticotropin and corticosterone levels was accompanied by an increase in adipose tissue mass, with the development of Cushing's syndrome in CRF-overexpressing mice.

6 Sex Steroids

The role of sex steroids in the hyperplastic development of adipose tissue has not been well documented. Direct effects of sex steroids have been postulated for decades, but information on their molecular receptors in adipocytes of animals and humans remains scanty. Androgen receptors and estrogen receptors (ER) have been originally characterized in rat adipose tissue (47,48). It was recently demonstrated that both estrogen receptor subtypes are detectable in human adipocytes in a striking depot-specific distribution. The ER-β is markedly reduced in intra-abdominal adipose tissue as compared to subcutaneous adipose tissue, and the visceral adipose tissue of men contains less ER of both subtypes than the visceral fat obtained from women (49). There is some evidence for the expression of progesterone receptors by adipose cells (50), but subsequent studies found only very low levels. As adipocyte precursor cells are well known to be an important site of estrogen production, particularly after menopause, a paracrine effect of estrogens on adipocytes is rather likely.

Studies by magnetic resonance imaging (MRI) indicate that puberty in girls is associated with the preferential accumulation of adipose tissue in the gluteal and femoral region (51), suggesting that the divergence of sex steroid metabolism and serum levels among boys and girls may be responsible for the development of sex-specific fat distribution patterns at this age (52). In women, decreased ovarian estrogen production during menopause and the subsequent change in the balance between estrogens and androgens may cause a shift in fat distribution toward more abdominal pattern. Estrogen replacement therapy appears to result in a reduced amount of trunk adipose tissue as determined by dual-energy x-ray absorptiometry (53).

In men, low testosterone levels are associated with enlarged visceral adipose tissue depots (54). When middle-aged, abdominally obese men are treated with testosterone, a small decrease in visceral fat mass in conjunction with an improvement of insulin resistance and associated metabolic disturbances is observed (55). A possible explanation for this observation is that androgens are positive effectors of lipolysis in concert with GH, thereby decreasing the size of the abdominal fat cells, but may not be directly involved in the regulation of fat cell formation (54). Another interesting finding is that alcoholic men have more adipose tissue localized in the intra- and retroperitoneal depots than abstinent men, also possibly due to a lower androgen activity (56).

7 Nutrients

Long-chain fatty acids (FAs) have been shown to trigger in vitro differentiation of preadipose into adipose cells (57). In vivo, the effects of increased FA uptake on adipose tissue development have been remarkably illustrated in transgenic mice overexpressing human LPL in skeletal and cardiac muscle. Increased FA entry in both both tissues is associated with weight loss due to some loss of muscle mass and, quite strikingly, to the virtually complete disappearance of adipose tissue (58). In vivo also, the nature of FA present in triacylglycerol molecules is of importance in adipose tissue development as feeding rats a diet rich in saturated fat leads to a threefold increase in the number of adipocytes in the retroperitoneal depot compared to the number of adipocytes in animals fed a diet rich in polyunsaturated fat, which indicates that saturated FAs are more potent than unsaturated FAs in promoting mitotic clonal expansion and/or terminal differentiation of preadipose cells (59). In a recent study, Cleary and coworkers investigated the effects of diets containing either coconut oil (rich in saturated fatty acids) or safflower oil (rich in mono- and polyunsaturated fatty acids) on adipose tissue cellularity in various fat depots in Zucker rats. It turned out that feeding unsaturated fatty acids favored fat cell hyperplasia, probably through enhanced recruitment of adipocyte precursor cells, whereas saturated fatty acids preferentially promoted hypertrophy through enhanced triacylglycerol accumulation of existing adipocytes (60).

In addition to hormones, normal glucose homeostasis appears to be essential for adipose tissue development. Transgenic mice overexpressing the glucose transporter GLUT4 selectively in adipose tissue have enhanced glucose disposal in vivo and develop increased adiposity due to adipocyte hyperplasia (61). In contrast, mice deficient in GLUT4 exhibit growth retardation accompanied by a severe reduction in adipose depots despite a nearly normal glycemia (62).

E Lipectomy

Surgical removal of adipose tissue and careful observation of its regeneration is another appropriate approach to study the regulation of adipose tissue growth and body weight in vivo. To date, many studies have been performed to investigate the effect of lipectomy on adipose tissue regeneration in a variety of species and depots and under various conditions. However, the results of these studies were inconclusive, since the response to lipectomy was found to depend on various factors such as species, region of excision, time after operation, extent of removal, and type of diet. Nevertheless, in most animal studies a clear tendency for regeneration of the lost tissue was apparent at least in the perirenal and subcutaneous fat depots, but restoration at the site of excision was not always complete. In both rat and rabbit, the regenerative response was highest in the perirenal fat depot (63,64). In contrast, surgical removal of the epididymal fat pads did not lead to regeneration. These data are to some extent compatible with in vitro findings indicating that adipocyte precursor cells from the perirenal region have a higher capacity for proliferation and differentiation than stromal cells from other depots (33,65). Morphological studies in rats showed that adipose tissue regeneration at the inguinal site occurred in close association with revascularization and blood supply. Immediately after lipectomy, thymidine kinase activities are elevated at the sites of removal, but subsequently slowly drop to a level that is still above normal. Both total fat cell number and average fat cell size continuously increase during this process. Thus, the regeneration of adipose tissue resembles the processes that occur in developing adipose tissue and involves the new formation of fat cells from preadipocytes (66).

Two other aspects are of potential importance. One is related to the question whether adipose tissue regrowth after lipectomy can also occur at other sites, thereby replacing the lost tissue mass. Faust and coworkers reported a compensatory fat deposition in nonexcised tissues after removal of epididymal and inguinal fat pads in rats (63). In a recent study, lipectomy of >50% of subcutaneous adipose tissue in adult female Syrian hamsters led to similar levels of body weight after 3 months on a high-fat diet. However, there was no visible regrowth of subcutaneous adipose tissue, but an increase in the intra-abdominal fat together with higher insulin and triglyceride concentrations than in sham-operated animals. The authors concluded from the data that subcutaneous adipose tissue acts as a metabolic sink that protects against visceral obesity and its metabolic disturbances (67). In another study, in moderately obese rats, surgical removal of visceral fat resulted in improvement of hepatic insulin resistance and, interestingly, a marked decrease in gene expression of both tumor necrosis factor-α (TNFα) and leptin in subcutaneous adipose tissue (68). If these latter observations hold true in humans, surgical removal of significant amounts of subcutaneous adipose tissue could cause a redistribution of lipid stores to visceral sites, thereby favoring undesirable metabolic effects, whereas reduction of the visceral fat mass may result in an amelioration of insulin resistance and its associated metabolic disturbances.

It is largely unknown whether the site-specific differences in regenerative capacity are due to inherent characteristics of the local tissue or to differences in the local environment. Circumstantial observations in humans are apparently in favor of the former possibility; skin transplantation from the abdomen to the forearm or to the back of the hand can lead to local hypertrophy of the transplant in case of body weight gain. The cellular composition of the subcutis may vary substantially depending on the anatomical location, and some particular skin areas may lack preadipose cells, which normally excludes the development of fat cells. Systematic studies on adipose tissue regrowth are missing in humans despite the widespread application of suction lipectomy and dermolipectomy for cosmetic reasons, particularly in women. Much work needs to be done to ascertain to which degree and under which conditions adipose tissue regrowth can occur in humans.

F Regional Differences in Adipose Tissue Growth

Many studies in animals and humans indicate that various aspects of adipocyte growth and function depend on the anatomical origin of the cells (52,69). The available methodology may not always allow an accurate assessment of differences, particularly if they are only modest. Regional differences may concern not only the metabolism of adipocytes but also the capacity to form new adipocytes.

Most cell culture studies on possible regional differences in adipose tissue growth were performed in rodents. In rats, it has been repeatedly demonstrated that perirenal preadipose cells replicate more extensively under cell culture conditions than epididymal cells (65). In addition, perirenal cells differentiated more readily by morphological and biochemical criteria (33,65). In vitro differentiation of epididymal preadipocytes was also less pronounced than that of inguinal subcutaneous preadipocytes (70). These results are in good agreement with those obtained in adipose tissue cellularity studies. Available data also suggest that the composition of the preadipocyte precursor pool differs from region to region (65,71). Djian and coworkers reported that the adipocyte precursor populations derived from rat perirenal and epididymal fat are composed of cell clones that vary in capacity for replication and differentiation. Since these differences between rat perirenal and epididymal depots were still detectable during secondary culture, the authors speculated that this variation among fat depots may have an intrinsic basis (65).

It was hypothesized that regional differences in adipose tissue growth may result from variations in the distribution of hormone receptors, but there is also growing evidence that regional differences are due to differences in the local environment of the cells. Innervation and blood flow are two major determinants of the local milieu. Comparative studies have noticed that mesenteric fat cells receive more blood than subcutaneous cells (8,72). In accordance with this finding, the stromal-vascular cell fraction of omental adipose tissue contains a high proportion of endothelial cells, while the same fraction obtained from subcutaneous adipose tissue is almost free of endothelial cells. It is obvious that a better blood supply may provide greater levels of humoral factors that are involved in the regulation of adipose tissue growth and also more substrates for lipid accumulation or removal. In an elegant approach, Cousin and coworkers have recently demonstrated that a local sympathetic denervation of white adipose tissue in rats induces preadipocyte proliferation without affecting metabolic function. The surgical denervation also resulted in an accelerated recruitment of precursors as assessed by increased expression of an early marker of differentiation (73).

Only sparse data are available on site-specific differences in adipose tissue cellularity and growth in humans. They indicate that intra-abdominal fat cells are smaller than subcutaneous cells, while published results on variations in fat cell size among subcutaneous depots are inconclusive or found to be influenced by many factors, such as age, hormonal status, and diet. A comparison of adipose tissue cellularity between young and middle-aged women revealed that the latter have more body fat than the former. This difference was exclusively explained by larger fat cells in all depots, while the younger women had a significantly higher total fat cell number. The age-related increase in fat cell size was particularly pronounced in the abdominal depot. The authors conclude that abdominal fat cells are more sensitive to nutritional and/or hormonal factors than those from other regions (74).

Very limited information is available on regional differences of adipose tissue development in humans. Pettersson and coworkers compared the capacity for adipose differentiation in stromal cells from omental and subcutaneous adipose tissue. They reported that more omental than subcutaneous cells were converted into adipocytes in an enriched viscous suspension medium (75). However, in this system high serum concentrations were used, which are now known to strongly inhibit adipose differentiation in human cells due to a high mitogenic and antiadipogenic activity. In two recent studies, the relative capacities of stromal cells from subcutaneous and omental adipose tissue to undergo adipose differentiation were studied using serum-free culture conditions in the presence of thiazolidinediones, a new class of antidiabetic agents known to activate the nuclear transcription factor of peroxisome proliferator-activated receptor-γ (PPARγ). In the study by Adams and coworkers, only stromal cells from subcutaneous fat were able to develop into adipotcytes upon exposure to thiazolidinediones, although PPARγ was expressed at similar levels in both depots (76). In contrast, Van Harmelen and coworkers were unable to find a depot difference in response to thiazolidinediones between stromal cells from the two adipose tissue depots (77). This discrepancy may be partly due to differences in the methods applied as well as in the populations studied, but further investigations are required to clarify this issue. In another study, the capacity for adipose differentiation was compared in cultured stromal cells from the abdominal and femoral adipose tissue obtained from obese women by needle biopsy. Under serum-free, hormone-supplemented culture conditions, glycerol-3-phosphate dehydrogenase (GPDH) activities used as an index of adipose differentiation were significantly higher in the cells from the abdominal region, while other parameters such as number of stromal cells per gram adipose tissue were not significantly different (78).

III DEVELOPMENTAL ISSUES IN THE LEAN AND OBESE STATE

A Adipose Tissue Cellularity

An excessive amount of body fat can result from enlarged fat cells or an increase in fat cell number or both. In humans, the study of Salans and coworkers emphasized that childhood-onset obesity is characterized by a combination of fat cell hyperplasia and hypertrophy, in contrast to adulthood-onset obesity where fat cell hypertrophy is predominant (18). Indeed, studies in lean and obese children suggest that obese children exhibit more rapid and earlier elevations in both fat cell number and cell size during childhood and adolescence (21). In contrast, studies in adults indicated that obese subjects have larger adipose cells than lean subjects but no significant increase in fat cell number (18). However, further studies revealed that development of hyperplasia can also occur in adult life. During excessive weight gain, as seen in severely obese adults, both fat cell size and fat cell number increase independent of the time of onset of obesity (22). It was concluded from such studies in humans and rodents that an increase in the number of mature fat cells did not occur until existing cells reach a critical cell size (22,79). Since fat cell size is varying in different adipose tissue depots, it was speculated that this phenomenon is regulated at the local level (16,79). In addition, there is now convincing evidence that new adipocytes can be recruited throughout the whole lifetime (23).

The few studies comparing adipose tissue growth in lean and obese humans do not allow any firm conclusions concerning the main characteristics of fat cell proliferation and differentiation. Pettersson and coworkers reported that the replication rates of stromal-vascular cells isolated from adipose tissue of lean and obese subjects were similar. In addition, no difference in the capacity for differentiation was observed between cells from nonobese and obese individuals regardless of tissue site, arguing against a genetic predisposition at the cellular level (75). On the other hand, Roncari and coworkers reported an exaggerated replication and differentiation of cultured adipocyte precursor cells from massively obese subjects as compared to lean controls, which may indicate that in this particular subgroup an intrinsic defect could be responsible for fat cell hyperplasia and facilitate the development of massive obesity in humans (80). Up to now, these data await confirmation from other groups.

Apart from these limited data in humans, many in vitro studies have been performed in animal models of obesity to determine if there are significant differences in the capacities and mechanisms to form new adipocytes between obese and lean animals and, in particular, to look for intrinsic differences in genetic models of obesity. Most studies have been carried out in Zucker rats. Compared with lean rats, a decreased as well as an increased adipogenic capacity of preadipocytes derived from obese Zucker rats has been reported. However, under strictly controlled serum-free culture conditions, the only difference between lean and obese animals was that adipose conversion in cells from older obese rats was lower than from lean controls (81). It may be speculated that, owing to higher adipogenic activity, preadipose cells in advanced stages of development are recruited more extensively and rapidly in obese than in lean animals. Thus, the conclusion could be that obesity and its metabolic consequences induced by the *fa* gene cause secondary changes in the cellular composition of the stromal cell fraction. Other studies on this issue did not describe consistent differences in the capacity for preadipocyte proliferation and differentiation between obese and lean animals, arguing against an intrinsic basis for the above-mentioned differences in adipose tissue cellularity.

B Modulation of Adipose Tissue Cellularity by Diet and Weight Change

The relationship between nutrition and adipose tissue cellularity is crucial for the understanding of adipose tissue expansion. There is evidence from many studies that early nutrition can affect fat cell number in adult life. Fetal overnutrition as seen in gestational diabetes leads to larger birth weight and to subsequent obesity in childhood and later life, whereas data are inconsistent as to whether undernutrition during fetal growth is a risk factor for increased body weight later in life (82). To date, there is no information on whether early human nutrition affect fat cell development and cellularity.

In adult rats, feeding a high-fat diet can increase fat cell number (79), while energy restriction is only associated with a decrease in fat cell size but not in number, indicating that dietary manipulation in adulthood cannot reduce fat cell number. This has been elaborated in experiments where rats were overnourished for a long period of time, which resulted in an increase in both fat cell size and number. Discontinuation of the experimental diet was followed by a decline in average fat cell size until it reached the level of normal control rats. However, fat cell number remained at the high level achieved during overfeeding.

It is also uncertain whether extreme dietary restrictions can affect fat cell number. In a study of severe long-term food deprivation causing up to 99% reduction in white adipose tissue mass, there was no evidence that fat cells were lost. After refeeding, no change in fat cell number was observed despite marked changes in endothelial and nonadipocyte mesenchymal cell number adipose tissue (83). These data are not consistent with the results of some older studies that showed a decrease in fat cell number after long-term weight reduction (84). In a more recent study, induction of diabetes in rats by streptozotocin resulted not only in a marked reduction in fat cell size, but also in a decrease in white adipose tissue cellularity as assessed by quantitative cellular analysis. Interestingly, the tiny adipocytes were characterized by the presence of multilocular triglyceride droplets (85). It would also be interesting to know whether fat cell hyperplasia found in the obese state can decline during prolonged maintenance of reduced weight. Again, in most studies, the number of fat cells was not normalized in either form of obesity even after extended periods of weight reduction. Obviously, an established fat cell hyperplasia cannot be reversed by extreme nutritional intervention including extreme starvation (83,84). However, one has to keep in mind that some of the contradictory findings can be due to limitations of the applied methods. For various reasons, the classical methodological approaches for the determination of adipose tissue cellularity are inaccurate and do not allow a reliable identification of the cell populations present in adipose tissue. This makes it extremely difficult to distinguish early preadipocytes as well as tiny fat cells from other cell types in adipose tissue.

In humans, short-term studies have demonstrated that moderate weight changes are associated only with changes in fat cell weight but not in fat cell number (86,87). To date, there is only one study that investigated the long-term effects of weight change on adipose tissue cellularity. The authors reported that prolonged reduction in body weight in adult women over 6–9 years reduced the number of monolocular adipocytes (16). Other evidence for a possible reduction of fat cell number by weight loss comes from a study of morbidly obese subjects undergoing gastric surgery. After a mean weight loss of 30–40 kg, fat cell size was markedly decreased in all adipose tissue depots. In addition, the calculated fat cell number was significantly reduced (88). Irrespective of methodological limitations, these reports raise the possibility that at least some adipocytes can completely lose their lipids and regain a state of lipid depletion. This remains an important issue, since it was repeatedly hypothesized that persistence of hypercellularity may contribute to the difficulties encountered by postobese subjects to maintain a reduced body weight.

Adipose tissue growth seems to depend not only on total caloric intake but also on the composition of the diet. Older animal studies suggested that dietary fat can induce hyperplastic adipose tissue growth independent of body weight gain (89,90). This effect was also observed when strictly isocaloric diets were fed (91). This close relationship between fat intake and adipose tissue growth may be substantiated by recent in vitro data demonstrating that exogenous triglycerides via fatty acids released after hydrolysis can promote adipose differentiation. These new findings may provide a better insight at the cellular level as to why a fat-rich diet favors adipose tissue expansion in humans (57).

C Apoptosis and Dedifferentiation of White Adipose Cells

There is now abundant information on the role of cell proliferation and differentiation to determine adipose cellularity. In contrast, little is known about possible mechanisms to decrease fat cell number. Only recently evidence is emerging that white adipose cells can undergo apoptosis or programmed cell death. It was recently reported that in vitro apoptosis is enhanced by growth factor deprivation (92) and TNFα (93). Particularly, in the presence of TNFα, apoptotic cells were seen in cultures of both human preadipocytes and adipocytes at rates between 5% and 25% (93). This effect of TNFα may be partly mediated by an increased adipose expression of the proapoptotic interleukin-1β (IL-1β), as recently observed in human preadipocytes and adipocytes. In the same study, TNFα-induced apoptosis was inhibited by glucocorticoids (94).

Insulin also appears to be involved in the regulation of fat cell apoptosis. Depletion of insulin in mice led to adipose-specific cell death in obese but not in lean animals (95). Feeding a diet supplemented with conjugated linoleic acid (CLA) to mice resulted in a reduction of body fat due to apoptosis. Under these conditions, TNFα and UCP-2 expression were 12- and sixfold upregulated in adipocytes from CLA-fed mice compared to fat cells from control mice. With decreasing body fat the mice developed lipodystrophy associated with hepatomegaly and insulin resistance (96).

In humans, it has been demonstrated that patients with some malignancies exhibit signs of adipocyte apoptosis in vivo (97). This and another report (98) showed that apoptosis is higher in omental than in subcutaneous adipose cells indicating that regional fat distribution may be partly regulated by differences in apoptosis. The in vitro data currently available suggest that apoptosis is mainly found in human preadipocytes. During in vitro differentiation, preadipocytes appear to acquire a relative resistance to apoptosis due to an increasing synthesis of the cell survival proteins Bcl-2 and neuronal apoptosis inhibitory protein (99).

Other studies suggest that mature fat cells can be induced to reverse the adipocyte phenotype under certain circumstances. TNFα was found to cause a dedifferentiation of cultured human fat cells after long-term exposure leading to a complete loss of stored lipids without a change in total cell number (100). It was recently reported that adenovirus-induced hyperleptinemia in normal rats results in rapid body fat loss. The elevated leptin concentrations not only depleted adipocyte lipids but transformed the adipocytes into cells that oxidize lipids, lose characteristic adipocyte markers, and express preadipocyte markers (101).

Although the existence of apoptosis and dedifferentiation in white adipose tissue is now established the physiological importance of these phenomena is still unknown. It is also unclear whether apoptosis is involved in the pathophysiology of obesity and, if so, to what extent and by what mechanisms. The question may also arise whether this new insight can be used to develop new therapeutic strategies.

IV STUDIES OF ADIPOSE TISSUE DEVELOPMENT IN VITRO

A Cellular Models for the Study of Adipogenesis and Adipose Cell Plasticity

Cell culture techniques have the advantage that the effects of single factors can be studied under strictly defined conditions. This methodology is an ideal tool to unravel mechanisms of hormone action or cell development. However, in vivo, the physiological function of a specific cell type or organ strongly depends on its communication with the environment. As part of a complex, highly integrated organism, the adipose tissue depots are interacting with surrounding and also with distant tissues. To fully understand and corroborate the physiological importance of in vitro findings in any tissue it is essential to perform additional in vivo studies that consider the cross-talk among the various tissues. This point has been remarkably illustrated in recent years with the cloning of the *ob* gene and the various roles played by leptin.

Cells of clonal lines fall into three categories: (1) totipotent embryonic stem cells (ES cells) giving rise to embryoid bodies able to generate cells of all lineages; (2) multipotent stem cells that follow myogenic, chondrogenic, osteogenic, and adipogenic pathways; and (3) cells that have been considered as unipotent cells, termed preadipocytes (Table 2). ES cells can differentiate spontaneously into various lineages and, quite recently, conditions to induce an adipocyte lineage and adipocyte formation at a high frequency from ES cells have been described. This provides a means to identify novel regulatory genes implicated in early determination events of adipogenesis (102). So far, most studies on adipogenesis have relied on the use of supposedly unipotent adipoblastic cells and rarely on multipotent cells of mesodermal origin (Table 2). Recent evidence indicates that some preadipocyte clonal lines still exhibit multipotency. However, the gene(s) that commit progression from the multipotent mesodermal stem cell to the adipoblast stage of development have been not been identified nor have been the factors involved in self-renewal of adipoblast stem cell precursors and specific adipoblast markers.

The process of adipose cell differentiation has been primarily investigated in cells of preadipocyte clonal lines such as 3T3-L1, 3T3-F442A, Ob17, 1246, 3T3-T, and ST13, which are all aneuploid. Adipose precursor cells derived from the stromal-vascular fraction of adipose tissues from various species are diploid but have a limited life span. When transplanted into animals, cells from both sources develop into mature fat cells. In vitro they differentiate, in the presence of an appropriate hormonal milieu, to yield cells that have most characteristics of adipocytes, including hormonal responses. However, recent data indicate that one or more transcriptional programs are only activated in vivo to generate the full adipocyte phenotype (110).

One of the most exciting findings in the recent years is the possibility, on the one hand, to direct adipogenesis from multipotent cells and, on the other hand, to induce *trans*differentiation into adipocytes

Table 2 Cellular Models of Adipogenesis

Cell lines	Origin	Phenotypes	Ref.
Totipotent			
Embryonic stem cells	Mouse blastocysts	All	102
Multipotent			
10T1/2	Mouse embryo	Muscle cells, white adipocytes, chondrocytes, osteocytes	3,103
3T3-F442A	Swiss mouse embryo (3T3 cells)	White adipocytes, osteocytes	104
Unipotent			
3T3-L1	Swiss mouse embyro	White adipocytes	3,103
Ob17	Epididymal fat pad of ob/ob mice	White adipocytes	3,103
BFC-1	Mouse BAT	White adipocytes	3,103
TA1	Subclone of 10 T1/2 treated with 5-azacytidine	White adipocytes	3,103
Lisa-2	Human liposarcoma	White adipocytes	105
BIP	Bovine intramuscular WAT	White adipocytes	106
Cell strains			
Subcutaneous, epididymal, retroperitoneal WAT of newborn and adult	Rat	White adipocytes	3,103
Bone marrow	Rat	White adipocytes	3,103
Epididymal fat pad	Mouse	White adipocytes	3,103
Bone marrow	Mouse	White adipocytes	3,103
Perirenal WAT	Rabbit	White adipocytes	5,103
Subcutaneous and perirenal WAT of foetus and newborn	Pig	White adipocytes	3,103
Subcutaneous WAT	Bovine	White adipocytes	108
Subcutaneous and omental WAT	Ovine	White adipocytes	108
Subcutaneous and abdominal WAT of newborn and adult	Human	White adipocytes	3,103
Bone marrow	Human	White adipocytes	107
Subcutaneous WAT of an infant with SGB syndrome	Human	White adipocytes	109

from supposedly unipotent cells. Clonal 3T3-F442A preadipocytes can undergo osteoblastic differentiation after exposure to bone marrow morphogenetic protein-2 (104), whereas human osteosarcoma SaOS-2B10 and MG-63 cells as well as murine stromal BMS2 cells can convert to adipose cells (111,112). Cells that exhibit the characteristics of mesenchymal stem cells have been isolated from human bone marrow. These cells differentiate into the adipose chrondrocytic and osteocytic lineages, and individual stem cells retain their multilineage potential (107). Even more striking, depending on the composition of the culture medium, stromal-vascular cells from human WAT can be directed to undergo differentiation into adipogenic, chondrogenic, osteogenic and myogenic cells (25). However, it remains to be shown that the latter observations relate to the presence of individual stem cells and not to that of multiple lineage-committed cells present in the cell population. *Trans*differentiation appears also possible as both myoblasts of C2C12 clonal line and muscle satellite cells are able to convert significantly to adipose cells upon exposure of the cells to long-chain fatty acids or BRL49653, a ligand agonist of PPARγ (113).

Wnts, which are secreted signaling proteins regulating developmental processes, behave as molecular switch, likely through Wnt 10-b, which governs adipogenesis. Active Wnt signaling is required for commitment to the myocyte lineage, whereas prevention of active Wnts signaling pathway triggers adipogenesis (114). Collectively, these observations emphasize that cell plasticity is more important than anticipated and that unipotentiality should be better and more cautiously defined in vitro as the only pathway that a precursor cell can follow in response to a given hormonal milieu.

B Sequential Events of Adipogenesis

1 General Considerations

Adipogenesis is a multistep process characterized by a sequence of events during which adipoblasts divide until confluence (Fig. 3). Adipoblasts are fibroblast-like cells, and no specific markers of that stage have been identified so far. Growth arrest at the G1/S stage of the cell cycle (stage 2), rather than contact among arrested cells, is necessary to trigger the process of cell commitment to preadipocyte which is associated with the induction of genes such as those encoding $\alpha 2$ chain of collagen VI (A2COL6/pOb24), clone 5, adipocyte differentiation related protein (ADRP), lipoprotein lipase (LPL) mRNA, and LPL activity. The regulation of expression of these genes takes place primarily at a transcriptional level and does not require the various hormones which, in contrast, are required for subsequent steps. The dramatic changes observed in cell morphology are associated with alterations in extracellular matrix components. The expression of late and very late markers is associated with limited growth resumption of these committed early marker-expresssing cells. At least one round of cell division has been consistently observed in rodent cells, and this process of clonal amplification of preadipocytes (defined as postconfluent mitoses or clonal expansion) is limited both in magnitude and duration. Terminal differentiation to adipocytes (defined by the emergence of GPDH activity and triacylglycerol accumulation) then takes place, provided that cell contacts exist and that cells are exposed to the appropriate hormonal milieu. Mature fat cells then become able to secrete dozens of proteins. These observations made in vitro are consistent with those made in vivo concerning the relationships in rodent adipose tissue between cell proliferation and differentiation. Although the presence of adipoblasts cannot be excluded, the differentiation process of adipose precursor cells isolated from fat tissue corresponds primarily to the sequence: preadipose cell (preadipocyte) ➡ immature adipose cell ➡ mature adipose cell (adipocyte). When seeded at clonal densities, stromal-vascular cells from rat perirenal and epididymal fat depots show varying capacities for replication and differentiation, irrespective of donor age. At any given age, stromal-vascular cells from perirenal fat tissue showed a greater proportion of clones with a high frequency of differentiation than in epididymal fat tissue (3). Both in rat for the perirenal and epididymal adipose tissues (115) and in human for the subcutaneous adipose tissue (23), aging is associated with a decrease in the proportion of cells undergoing differentiation.

2 Receptor Equipment and Adipogenesis

Table 3 summarizes the receptor composition of adipoblasts, preadipocytes, and adipocytes. Not unexpectedly, preadipocytes express the cognate receptors of adipogenic hormones required for subsequent events to occur. The alterations in hormone responsiveness as a function of differentiation correspond to a critical "time window" of action in preadipocytes during which adipogenic hormones induce the terminal differentiation process.

Growing adipoblasts express cell surface receptors of the major prostaglandins which are produced by these cells [prostacyclin (PGI_2), prostaglandin $F_{2\alpha}$ ($PGF_{2\alpha}$), and prostaglandin E_2 (PGE_2)] as well as nuclear receptors recognizing glucocorticoids, T_3, and retinoic acid (RA). The adenosine receptor A_2 subtype, the prostacyclin IP receptor, and the PGE_2 receptor (EP4 subtype), all positively coupled to adenylate cyclase, are present in preadipocytes and then become expressed at low levels, if any, in adipocytes, consistent with the importance of the protein kinase A (PKA) pathway to trigger terminal differentiation of preadipocytes (see Sec. IV. C. 1). These observations are also consistent with those made in the comparative study of prostaglandin sensitivity of adenylate cyclase of rat primary preadipocytes and isolated adipocytes which show that G_i activity is reduced or absent in preadipocytes (116). The EP_3 subtype (α, β, and γ isoforms) of the PGE_2 receptor and the adenosine receptor A_1 subtype (118–121), all coupled negatively to adenylate cyclase, then become detectable in adipocytes, consistent with the well-known antilipolytic effects of PGE_2 and adenosine observed in mature fat cells. Commitment to preadipocytes is characterized by the emergence of the cell surface receptor of leukemia inhibitory factor (LIF) as well as that of nuclear receptor PPARδ and transcription factors C/EBPβ and δ (117).

Of growing interest are cell surface proteins which are membrane associated or potentially secreted (122,123). Pref-1 and dlk proteins are members of the EGF-like homeotic family of proteins and are polymorphic variants of the same dlk

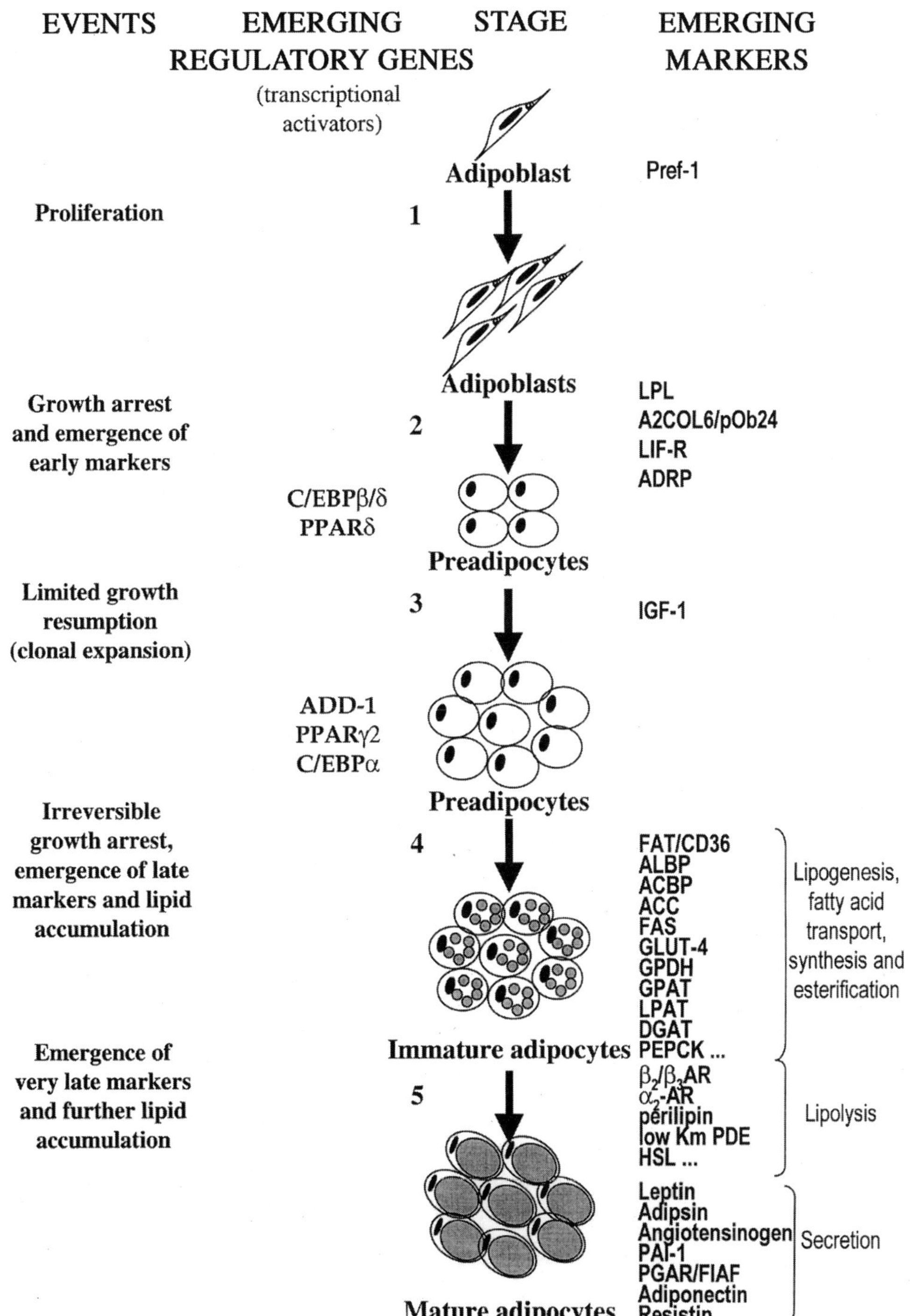

Figure 3 Multiple stages of adipose cell differentiation. The scheme is based on data obtained with 3T3-L1, 3T3-F442A, and Ob17 cells as well as with rodent adipose precursor cells. Abbreviations: Pref-1, preadipocyte factor-1; LPL, lipoprotein lipase; A2COL6/pOb24, α2-chain of collagen VI; LIF-R, leukemia inhibitory factor-receptor; ADRP, adipocyte-differentiation related protein; PGAR/FIAF, PPARγ-angiopoietin related/fasting-induced factor; C/EBP, CCAAT/enhancer-binding protein; PPAR, peroxisome proliferator–activated receptor; IGF-1, insulinlike growth factor-1; ADD-1, adipocyte determination and differentiation factor-1; FAT/CD36, fatty acid translocase; ALBP, adipocyte lipid-binding protein (aP2); ACBP, acyl CoA binding protein; ACC, acetyl-CoA carboxylase; FAS, fatty acid synthase; GLUT4, insulin-sensitive glucose transporter-4; GPDH, glycerol-3-phosphate dehydrogenase; GPAT, glycerophosphate acyltransferase; LPAT, lysophosphatidate acyltransferase; DGAT, diglyceride acyltransferase; PEPCK, phosphoenolpyruvate carboxykinase; β2-AR, β2-adrenoreceptor; β3-AR, β3-adrenoreceptor; low K_m PDE, low K_m phosphodiesterase; HSL, hormone-sensitive lipase; PAI-1 plasminogen activator inhibitor-1.

Table 3 Cell Surface Receptors, Nuclear Receptors, and Transcription Factors of Adipose Precursor Cells and Adipocytes

Markers[a]	Adipoblasts[b]	Preadipocytes[b]	Adipocytes[b]	Ref.
Cell surface receptors				
LIF-R	–	+	+	117
IP-R	++	+	(+)	118,119
FP-R	++	+	–	120
EP_1-R	++	+	(+)	119
EP_4-R	++	+	(+)	119
EP_3-R (α, β, γ isoform)	–	–	+	119
A_1-R	n.d.[c]	–	+	121
A_2-R	n.d.	+	(+)	121
GH-R	n.d.	+	+	103
IR	+	++	++	103
Pref-1/dlk	+	+	–	122,123
Nuclear receptors				
GR	+	+	+	3,103
AR	n.d.	(+)	+	47,124
ER	n.d.	(+)	+	48,49,124,125
PR	n.d.	+	(+)	50,124
RAR_α and RAR_γ	+	++	+++	126
RAR_α and RAR_β	+	++	+++	126
TR	+	+	++	127,128
PPARδ (NR1C2)	–	+	++	129
PPARγ (NR1C3)	–	(+)	++	130
AhR	+	(+)	–	131–134
Arnt	+	(+)	–	131,132
Transcription factors				
CREB	+	+	+	135
C/EBPβ and C/EBPδ	(+)	+	(+)	117,136
ADD1/SRBP-1c	–	+	+	137
C/EBPα	–	(+)	++	138,139
AP-2α	+	(+)	–	140
Id2	+	(+)	–	141,142
Id3	+	(+)	–	141,142
GATA-2&3	+	(+)	–	143

Based upon data obtained in cells of clonal lines and primary cultures.

[a] Abbreviations: LIF-R, leukemia inhibitory factor receptor; IP-R, prostacyclin receptor; FP-R, $PGF_{2}\alpha$ receptor; EP-R, PGE_2 receptor; Al-R and A2-R, adenosine (subtypes 1 and 2) receptor; GH-R, growth hormone receptor; IR, insulin receptor; pref-1/dlk, preadipocyte factor-1/delta like factor; GR, glucocorticoid receptor; AR, androgen receptor; ER estrogen receptor; PR, progesterone receptor; RAR, retinoic acid receptor; RXR, retinoic X receptor; TR, triiodothyronine receptor; PPAR, peroxisome proliferator–activated receptor; AhR, arylhydrocarbon receptor; Arnt, Ahr nuclear translocator; CREB, cAMP response element–binding protein; C/EBP, CCAAT/enhancer binding protein; ADD1/SREBP-1c, adipocyte determination and differentiation factor-1/sterol regulatory element binding protein-1c; Id, inhibitory protein of DNA binding.

[b] The signs refer to comparative levels of each mRNA or protein between adipoblasts, preadipocytes, and adipocytes, i.e., the absence (–) or the presence at very low levels (+), low levels +, or higher levels ++ and +++.

[c] Not determined.

gene. The soluble form of pref-1/dlk is present in preadipocytes and acts as a negative regulator of adipogenesis (123). In contrast, Notch-1, another transmembrane protein of the family of EGF-like homeotic genes, appears required for adipogenesis as antisense Notch-1 prevents PPARδ and PPARγ expression (144).

C Adipogenic Factors and Second-Messenger Pathways

The responsiveness of preadipose cells to external signals may vary according to differences in the stage of adipose lineage at which clonal lines have been established and that at which cells of a given line are exposed to various agents. Moreover, the requirement for adipogenic hormones shows differences between clonal and primary preadipocytes. Last but not least, serum-supplemented media are (too) often used, as many serum components are uncharacterized and thus not controllable, this renders comparisons between various studies rather difficult. The use of serum-free, chemically defined media appears more appropriate. In serum-free conditions, the most common requirements of primary preadipocytes appear to be glucocorticoids, IGF-1, and insulin. Clonal preadipocytes also require GH and T_3 and/or retinoids. A salient feature is that the required hormones have to be present simultaneously within a physiological range above threshold concentrations to trigger terminal differentiation.

1 Glucocorticoids, cAMP-Elevating Agents, and Leukemia Inhibitory Factor

Glucocorticoids, including the synthetic glucocorticoid dexamethasone, stimulate the differentiation of clonal preadipocytes and that of primary preadipocytes of various species including human, and are presumed to act via their cognate nuclear receptor GR. Dexamethasone reduces the expression of pref-1/dlk, a negative regulator of adipogenesis (145). Glucocorticoids are known to increase on a long-term basis the production confined to preadipocytes of prostacyclin, a potent adipogenic hormone (146,147). Dexamethasone is also known to upregulate the expression of C/EBPδ (148), possibly through prior production of prostacyclin, as carbacyclin—a stable analog of prostacyclin—can substitute for glucocorticoids in promoting adipogenesis (146).

Prostacyclin and carbacyclin, through binding to their cognate receptor IR-R, raise cAMP levels and induce intracellular mobilization of calcium (149). The critical role of prostacyclin as a locally produced hormone raising cAMP and Ca^{2+} levels cannot be dissociated from the developmental stage of the cells at which the effectors trigger transducing pathways. First, cAMP promotes the initiation of differentiation of 3T3-F442A preadipocytes but inhibits the late stage(s) of this process (150). Second, the Ca^{2+}-calmodulin-sensitive protein kinase II, which is required for the differentiation of 3T3-L1 preadipocytes, exhibits at an early stage within a few hours two temporally distinct phases of activity after stimulation of adipogenesis. It is likely that the time frame of exposure of clonal preadipocytes to calcium ionophores, i.e., the developmental stage at which the cells respond, explains the inhibitory or stimulatory effect previously reported (151). Synthetic cAMP analogs and methylisobutylxanthine, which increases cAMP levels, trigger adipogenesis. Enhancing cAMP levels upregulates rapidly the expression of the critical early transcription factors C/EBPβ and C/EBPδ (152).

In addition to activation of the PKA pathway, activation of leukemia inhibitory factor receptor (LIF-R) by LIF, which is exclusively produced and released by preadipocytes, upregulates also C/EBPβ and C/EBPδ via the extracellular signal-regulated kinase (ERK) pathway (117). Both pathways share CREB/ATF-1 as common downstream effectors that upregulate both C/EBPs and promote adipogenesis (153).

2 IGF-1, Insulin, and Lysophosphatidic Acid

IGF-1 has been shown to stimulate adipogenesis of clonal mouse 3T3-L1 preadipocytes and primary preadipocytes (rat, rabbit, porcine). In addition to IGF-1, clonal and primary preadipocytes also secrete insulinlike growth factor–binding proteins (IGFBPs) as a function of differentiation (39,40). The IGF-1/IGFBPs system is assumed to act in a paracrine/autocrine manner upon GH stimulation, although conflicting results have been reported with respect to the adipogenic activity of GH in vitro (see Sec. IV.C.3). In addition to its well-known effect on lipogenesis, insulin can now be considered as triggering adipogenesis, and targeted invalidation of the insulin receptor in 3T3-L1 preadipocytes impairs their ability to differentiate into adipocytes (154).

Both IGF-1 and insulin stimulate Ras, which activates the ERK pathway, consistent with the induction of adipogenesis by ectopic expression of Ras in the absence of hormonal stimulation (155). Insulin upregulates prenylation of Ras and Rho protein, and this covalent modification ensures proper phosphorylation and activation of cAMP-responsive element binding protein (CREB) which is required for adipogenesis (135,153,156). The phosphoinositide (PI)3-kinase/protein kinase B(PKB also termed Akt)/p70S6 kinase pathway is also implicated in insulin-dependent events. Ectopic expression of PKB and activation of PI-3 kinase are required for adipogenesis (157,158), consistent with the impairment of this process by inhibition of PI-3 kinase (159). Growth-arrested preadipocytes respond to IGF-1 by stimulation of the ERK pathway, and this activation disappears rapidly during terminal differentiation triggered by adipogenic factors (160). Shc, an SH2 domain-containing protein that is a direct substrate for the tyrosine kinase activity of the IGF-1 receptor, is implicated in this loss of IGF-1 response, whose relationships with postconfluent mitoses remain to be shown (161). Taken together, there is a critical and early window of time during which the ERK pathway is triggered in preadipocytes through binding of IGF-1, insulin, LIF, and prostacyclin to their cognate receptors. This time frame is critical since PPARγ, which appears after PPARδ, C/EBPβ and C/EBPδ during the differentiation process, is in contrast inhibited by direct phosphorylation of Ser112 by ERK_1 and ERK_2 (162,163). Lysophosphatidic acid (LPA) is a bioactive phospholipid which, upon release from adipocytes stimulated by α2-adrenoreceptor agonists, increased proliferation and spreading of preadipocytes through a Ca^{2+}-independent phospholipase A2 event (164,165). The endothelial differentiation gene-2 receptor appears involved in these effects through the Ras/ERK and the $p21^{rhoA}$/cytoskeleton pathway, respectively (166). Thus it is assumed that the mitogenic and paracrine effect of LPA is implicated in adipocyte hyperplasia.

3 Growth Hormone and Prolactin

Growth hormone triggers IGF-1 gene transcription, IGF-1 secretion, and adipogenesis of 3T3-F442A and Ob1771 preadipocytes (167,168). GH promotes also diacylglycerol production from phosphatidycholine breakdown and thus activates protein kinase C (PKC). PKC activators can substitute for GH in modulating cell proliferation, but the presence of IGF-1 is still required for adipogenesis (169). To add to this compexity, it appears that the Janus kinase/Signal transducers and activators of transcription (JAK-STAT) signaling pathway via STAT5 is also implicated in transducing GH-dependent signals during the initiation of 3T3-F442A preadipocyte differentiation (170). This conclusion is in agreement with the generation by homologous recombination of GH receptor–deficient mice or STAT5a- and STAT5b-deficient mice in which fat deposit was reduced (171).

Despite all these observations, the role of GH in adipogenesis remains somewhat confusing. In rat primary preadipocytes, although GH increases IGF-1 production and although IGF-1 promotes cell proliferation, GH still exhibits antiadipogenic properties independent of IGF-1 mitogenic activity (172). This inhibition appears to be due to the maintenance of high levels of pref-1 (173). To reconcile conflicting data in GH action, it is assumed that clonal and primary preadipocytes represent early and late stages of the differentiation process, respectively, as primary preadipocytes should have been previously exposed to GH and, "primed" in vivo. Prolactin stimulates in prolactin receptor–expressing fibroblasts the expression of C/EBPβ, PPARγ, and adipogenesis (174), but its adipogenic activity on authentic target cells, i.e., preadipocytes, remains to be shown.

4 Tri-iodothyronine and Retinoids

Tri-iodothyronine appears to be required for the differentiation of clonal preadipocytes (127,175). This requirement remains questionable, as no obvious requirement for T_3 is observed in primary preadipocytes isolated from pig, rat, rabbit, and human, suggesting as for GH that prior exposure to T_3 in vivo has "primed" the cells (3,176).

The ability of retinoic acid (RA) and synthetic retinoids to promote or inhibit differentiation processes has been recognized for several years. At supraphysiological concentrations, RA inhibits adipogenesis of clonal and primary preadipocytes via RA receptors (RARs). Inhibition appears to take place at an early stage, i.e., through C/EBPβ repression (177). In contrast, at concentrations close to the K_d values of RARs, RA and retinoids behave like potent adipogenic hormones in triggering the differentiation of Ob1771 preadipocytes and primary rat preadipocytes (126).

5 Fatty Acids and Metabolites

Both long-chain FA (saturated, unsaturated, nonmetabolizable) and peroxisome proliferators, which are like FA amphipatic carboxylate molecules, are able in clonal preadipocytes to act like hormones, by activating the transcription of several lipid-related genes and promoting adipogenesis in synergy with other adipogenic factors (57,178). Similar observations have been made in rat and human preadipocytes. Moreover, the main adipogenic component of serum is arachidonic acid (ARA) (179). Its adipogenic effect is blocked by cyclo-oxygenase inhibitors, suggesting that prostanoid(s) are involved. Prostacyclin (used in the form of stable carbacyclin) is the only active prostanoid in promoting adipogenesis (180), and this stimulatory effect can be extended to rat and human primary preadipocytes (149). In addition to binding to the cell surface prostacyclin receptor (IP-R), carbacyclin binds to the nuclear receptor PPARδ (181). This suggests a dual role of ARA—directly, as agonist of PPARs, and indirectly, as a precursor of prostacyclin then active via IP-R at the cell surface and via PPARδ within the nucleus. The natural ligand(s) of PPARδ may differ from prostacyclin, but this prostanoid along with PGE_2 and trace levels of $PGF_{2\alpha}$ is the only metabolite of ARA so far characterized in preadipocytes (182).

6 Angiotensin II

Angiotensin II (AngII) is secreted from WAT in vivo and also from adipocytes in vitro. WAT represents an important extrahepatic source of angiotensinogen which accumulates and is released in late differentiated cells (183,184). AngII binds to its cognate receptor(s) in adipocytes, which respond by increased lipogenesis (185) and release of prostacyclin (186). The renin-angiotensin system (RAS), which gives rise to AngII from angiotensinogen, is present in WAT and adipocytes from rodents and human, suggesting that RAS plays a role in WAT development (187). An autocrine/paracrine mechanism has been shown to operate in vivo, leading to an increased fat mass due to triglyceride accumulation in adipocytes (188).

7 Extracellular Matrix Components and the Plasminogen Cascade

Extracellular proteolysis mediated by plasma kallikrein and the substrate plasminogen is required for adipogenesis, presumably through the formation of plasmin which subsequently cleaves fibronectin. Inhibition of generated plasmin by α-2-antiplasmin but not by plasminogen-activator inhibitor-1 (PAI-1) impaired adipogenesis. Early inhibitory events are then taking place in preadipocytes, i.e., blockade of rounding up and C/EBPβ expression. Since fibronectin is a component of the preadipocyte extracellular matrix, it is assumed that activation of the plasminogen cascade induces cytoskeleton remodeling and/or bioavailability of IGF-1, which are required for later events of adipogenesis (189).

D Antiadipogenic Factors

Various factors that decrease or abolish differentiation of adipose precursor cells have been reported, including a variety of cytokines (TNFα, IL-1, IL-6), platelet-derived growth factor (PDGF), and TGFβ. The most intriguing results are those obtained in preadipose cells with TGFβ since, except for pig preadipocytes (3), terminal differentiation appears irreversibly blocked after its removal in contrast to various other factors where partial or complete recovery of the differentiated phenotype is observed (190). The situation remains unclear with regard to fibroblast growth factor (FGF) and epidermal growth factor (EGF), which have been claimed to be either inhibitory or without effect, depending on the origin of target cells. In vivo, subcutaneous administration of EGF to newborn rats results in a large decrease in the weight of inguinal fat pads, which suggests the delayed formation of adipocytes from preadipocytes (3). A downregulation of PPARγ gene expression appears to contribute to the antiadipogenic effect of TNFα (191). The inhibitory effect of TNFα on adipocyte differentiation is also observed if it is administrated at an early stage. TNFα disrupts the normal pattern of expression of p107 and p130 proteins, two members of the retinoblastoma family of proteins, and leads to a complete block in clonal expansion (192).

Among flavonoids, which are polyphenolic compounds that exist widely in plants, genistein inhibits both adipoblast proliferation and adipogenesis (193). Many fat-soluble vitamins, as well as dehydroepiandrosterone and some structural analogs, are also known to abolish terminal differentiation of clonal preadipocytes (3,194). Retinoids have been reported to inhibit differentiation, but the supraphysiological concentrations used in those studies raise serious doubt about their physiological relevance. So far, one of the most interesting antiadipogenic agent appears to be $PGF_{2\alpha}$. It inhibits differentiation of clonal and primary preadipocytes, most likely via the cognate cell surface $PGF_{2\alpha}$ receptor (FP-R) (120). Inhibition of adipogenesis by $PGF_{2\alpha}$ appears to occur through ERK-mediated phosphorylation of PPARγ, thus inhibiting its transcriptional activity (163). Nevertheless, this inhibition is rather unlikely to take place during the differentiation process, as $PGF_{2\alpha}$ is only synthesized in preadipocytes at trace levels compared to prostacyclin (182) and as its effect is fully reversed by carbacyclin (190).

V MOLECULAR MECHANISMS OF ADIPOGENESIS

A Transcriptional Activators and Repressors of Adipogenesis

Postmitotic growth arrest is followed by terminal differentiation of preadipocytes to adipocytes (stages 4 and 5) (Fig. 3), which are states of irreversible growth arrest as mature fat cells do not divide. Upon activation by FA or specific agonists, PPARδ mediates postconfluent mitoses in a cAMP-dependent manner (195,196). As PPARδ is implicated in the activation of a limited set of genes including PPARγ (196–198) and as PPARγ induces cell cycle withdrawal and irreversible growth arrest, it would appear that PPARδ and PPARγ are playing both opposite and complementary roles (199). Recent evidence indicates that PPARγ is essential for cardiac and adipose tissue development during mouse embryogenesis (200,201). Various redundant signaling pathways as well as several transcription factors are converging to upregulate PPARγ, which acts as common and essential regulator of terminal events of adipogenesis and also as a regulator of adipocyte hypertrophy (Fig. 4), emphasizing the importance of adipose tissue development to ensure physiological functions.

Forced ectopic expression of C/EBPβ in cells of various clonal lines of fibroblastic origin, which normally express very low levels of C/EBPβ, C/EBPα, and PPARγ, induces adipogenesis, with C/EBPδ acting in synergy with C/EBPβ (136). In most studies, significant adipogenesis of stable fibroblast transfectants requires the simultaneous presence of PPARγ ligands, in contrast to authentic preadipocyte target cells (3T3-L1,3T3-F442A, Ob1771 cells), suggesting that authentic differentiating cells are able to express PPARγ and simultaneously to synthesize uncharacterized PPARγ ligand(s).

Intracellular pathways that upregulate in clonal preadipocytes the expression of C/EBPβ and C/EBPδ are also able to trigger adipogenesis. It has been shown that preadipocytes have the unique capacity both (1) to synthesize and secrete LIF and prostacyclin, and (2) to express at the same time their cognate cell surface receptors LIF-R and IP-R. Binding to L1F-R and IP-R triggers the ERK and PKA pathways, respectively, which in turn activate the critical expression of C/EBPβ and C/EBPδ and promote adipogenesis (117,152). Signal transduction proteins involved in the upregulation of transcriptional activators may also regulate adipogenesis as reported for ectopic expression of the differentiation-enhancing factor-1 (DEF-1) in NIH-3T3 and

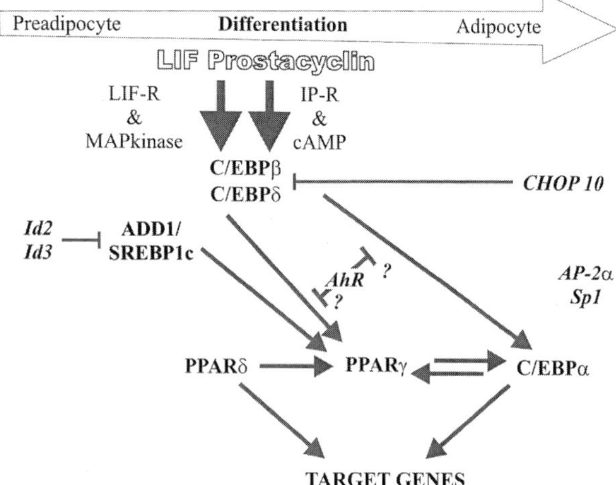

Figure 4 Transcriptional activators (bold face) and transcriptional repressors (italics) of adipogenesis. (See text for comments and abbreviations.)

BALB/c-3T3 fibroblastic cells (202). Forced expression of adipocyte determination and differentiation factor-1/sterol regulatory element binding protein-1c (ADD1/SREBP-1c) or ADD-1 403, a superactive truncated form of ADD-1, upregulates the expression of PPARγ in 3T3-L1 cells (203). This transcription factor is expressed early during adipogenesis and is part of the SREBP family, which are synthesized as membrane-bound precursors released through proteolytic processes and translocated into the nucleus. ADD-1/SREBP-1c appears to be positively controlled by insulin, thus establishing a link between this transcription factor and carbohydrate availability (204). Other stable transfectants able to express constitutively various components of the insulin signaling pathways have also been shown to trigger adipogenesis, i.e., activated Ras mutants, Raf, PI3-kinase, p70S6 kinase, and more recently PKB (c-Akt), which appears to act downstream of PI3-kinase but upstream of p70S6 kinase (205).

Taken together, these studies emphasize the existence of redundant signals of adipogenesis and the wide panoply of transcription factors and their link with the nutritional status, i.e., first PPARs and fatty acid availability and second ADD-1 and carbohydrate availability. It is important to note that heterozygous PPARγ +/− mice appear, at least in part, protected from increased fat mass upon high-fat feeding as compared to wild-type mice. Adipocyte size is significantly smaller in these mice with no change in adipocyte number (206). Thus, it cannot be excluded that subtle alterations between individuals in the activity level of some components regulating expression and/or activity of PPARγ may bring significant differences in fat tissue mass.

Transcriptional repression may involve passive mechanisms by which the negative regulator binds to activators and forms inactive heterodimers, thus playing a dominant-negative role. Alternatively, active repression may occur when the repressor binds to *cis*-acting sequences of a gene promoter and interferes with the transcriptional machinery. Both types of repression take place in preadipocytes (Fig. 4). Passive repression by Id2 and Id3 proteins (inhibitors of DNA binding) has been reported. Id2 and Id3 decrease dramatically during adipogenesis, and forced expression of Id3 protein blocks this process (141). Direct interaction of Id2 and Id3 with ADD-1 takes place, and this postulated heterodimerization decreases the functional capacity of ADD-1 to upregulate genes controlled transcriptionally by ADD-1 (142). C/EBP homologous protein-10 (CHOP-10/GADD153) is a member of the C/EBP family and acts also as a dominant-negative inhibitor

Table 4 Overexpression/Reexpression of Lipid-Related Genes in Adipose Tissue: Relationships with WAT Development

Gene	Tissue specificity	Fat depots and/or fat mass	Remarks	Refs.
Cell surface receptors and transporters				
β1-AR	Adipose tissue	↘ WAT	Resistance to HFD Adipocyte hypotrophy	210
α2-AR (β3-AR −/− background)	Adipose tissue	↗ WAT	HFD-induced obesity Adipocyte hyperplasia	211
GLUT-4	Adipose tissue	↗WAT	Low glucose levels and enhanced glucose disposal Adipocyte hyperplasia	61
Mitochondrial proteins				
UCP-1	Adipose tissue	↘ WAT	Sex dimorphism (female > male) significant at age 3 months Adipocyte hypotrophy and hyperplasia	212
Secreted proteins				
Agouti	Adipose tissue	↗ WAT with the daily insulin injections	AGOUTI expression alone insufficient for weight gain	213
Angiotensinogen	Adipose tissue	↗ WAT	Increased lipogenesis in WAT Decreased locomotor activity Adipocyte hypertrophy and hypoplasia	188
Transcription factors				
A-ZIP/F	Adipose tissue	WAT absent (lipoatrophy)	Insulin resistance Dyslipemia Increased metabolic rate	214
ADD1/SREBP-1c	Adipose tissue	↘WAT	Immature fat depots Enlargement of liver, spleen and pancreas	215
FOXC2	Adipose tissue	↘WAT) (intra-abdominal depot	Resistance to HFD UCP-1 induction in WAT BAT hypertrophy Increased sensitivity of β-adrenergic/ cAMP/PKA pathway Increased insulin sensitivity	216

UCP-1, uncoupling protein-1; α2-AR, α2-adrenoreceptor; β1-AR, β1-adrenoreceptor; GLUT-4, glucose transporter-4; ADD-1/SREB-1c, adipocyte determination and differentiation factor-1/sterol regulatory element binding protein-1c; HFD, high-fat diet.

of transcription (207). CHOP-10 sequesters C/EBPβ by heterodimerization. As preadipocytes reach the S phase, which precedes postconfluent mitoses, downregulation of CHOP-10 allows the release of C/EBPβ, which binds to C/EBPα promoter and activates C/EBPα gene expression (208). Another member of the basic helix-loop-helix (bHLH) proteins is the arylhydrocarbon receptor (AhR). Although a physiological ligand of AhR has yet to be identified, it binds 2,3,7,8-tetrachlorodibenzo-p-dioxin (TCDD) and related compounds. After ligand binding, AhR dissociates from cytosolic complex and translocates to the nucleus where it heterodimerizes with the AhR nuclear translocator (Arnt). This heterodimer then binds to xenobiotic response element (XRE) present within the promoter region of various genes. Both AhR and Arnt proteins are present in adipoblasts and disappear rapidly in differentiating preadipocytes. TCDD appears effective only when added at the adipoblast or at the early preadipocyte stage and decreases C/EBPα and PPARγ2 but not C/EBPβ and C/EBPδ levels (131).

TCDD clearly inhibits adipogenesis through the AhR pathway, as shown in AhR−/− mouse embryo fibroblasts (132). Moreover, TCDD increases phosphorylation of the repressor chicken ovalbumin upstream promoter transcription factor (COUP-TF), thus preventing PPARγ/RXRα to bind to their response element DR-1 (133). In addition, Arnt may

Table 5 Gene Invalidation Affecting WAT Development

Genes	Tissue specificity	Fat depots and/or fat mass	Remarks	Ref.
Enzymes and regulators				
HSL	—	→WAT ↗BAT	Male sterility Adipocyte hypertrophy Dispensable for lipolysis	217
Perilipin	—	↘WAT	Hyperphagy Resistance to HFD Resistance to β-AR agonist stimulation with increased basal lipolysis Adipocyte hypertrophy	218
DGAT	—	↘WAT	Resistance to HFD Increased energy expenditure	219
PTP-1B	—	↘WAT	Lean and resistance to HFD Increased energy expenditure Increased insulin sensitivity	220,221
ACC-2	—	↘WAT	Hyperphagy Increased β-oxidation in muscles Decreased hepatic fat Adipocyte hypotrophy	222
MT-I and MT-II	—	↗WAT at age 5-6 weeks	Hyperphagy	223
Tub	—	↗WAT at age 7-8 weeks	Retinal degeneration Heterozygous +/tub indistinguishable from wild-type	224
RIIβ (subunit of PKA)	—	↘WAT	Resistance to HFD Smaller length than wild-type Adipocyte hypotrophy	225
Secreted proteins				
Angiotensinogen	—	↘WAT at weaning and onwards	Decreased lipogenesis in WAT Increased locomotor activity Adipocyte hypotrophy	226
Cell surface receptors and transporters				
ICAM-1	—	↗WAT	No change in food intake	227
Mac-1		↗WAT		
GLUT-4	—	↘WAT	Growth-retarded Postprandial hyperinsulinemia	62
PRL-R	—	↘WAT (female > male)	Abdominal fat more affected than other depots	228

Table 5 Continued

Genes	Tissue specificity	Fat depots and/or fat mass	Remarks	Ref.
VLDL-R	—	↘WAT	Resistance to HFD Increased plasma triglycerides after high-fat feeding Adipocyte hypotrophy	229
Nuclear receptors and transcription factors				
PPARα (NCR1C1)	—	↗ WAT at late age (female > male)	Dyslipemia Steatosis	230
PPARδ (NR1C2)	—	↘WAT	Smaller length than wild-type Hyperphagy	231
PPARγ (NR1C3)	—	WAT absent	Lethality in utero or at birth	200,201,206
C/EBPα	—	↘WAT and BAT	Hypoglycemia due to failure of gluconeogenesis and early death	232
C/EBPβ and C/EBPδ	—	↘WAT and BAT	Adipocyte hypoplasia	233
RXRα	Excision in WAT and BAT at age 4 weeks	→ WAT on standard diet	Resistance to HFD Impaired lipolysis Adipocyte hypotrophy	234
Hmgic (architectural transcription factor)	—	WAT ↘	Resistance to HFD Smaller than wild-type Adipocyte hypoplasia	235

HSL, hormone-sensitive lipase; DGAT, diacylglycerol acyltransferase; ACC-2, acetyl-CoA carboxylase-2; MT, metallothioenia; PKA, protein kinase A; PTP-1B, protein tyrosine phosphatase-1B; ICAM-1, intercellular adhesion molecule-1; PRL-R, prolactin receptor; VLDL-R, receptor of very low density lipoproteins; PPAR, peroxisome proliferator–activated receptor; C/EBP, CCAAT/enhancer B, protein tyrosine phosphatase-1B; BP, binding protein; RXR, retinoic X receptor; HFD, high-fat diet.

play a role independent of its binding to AhR as it heterodimerizes with hypoxia inducible factor-lα (HIF-1α), which is also induced at early stage of adipogenesis (134). Active repressors which bind to regulator sequences of promoters of the C/EBPα promoter have also been reported. Two repressor-binding sites are present in the C/EBPα promoter and are recognized by an isoform of the AP-2 transcription factor family, termed C/EBPα undifferentiated protein (CUP/AP-2α1). This factor inhibits the transcriptional activation of the C/EBPα gene and thus may be implicated in the maintenance of this gene in a repressed state as well as in the maintenance of the preadipocyte stage (140). A member of the Sp family, Sp1, binds to a consensus Sp-binding site of C/EBPα unique among the promoters of adipocyte genes. By doing so, it prevents the *trans*-activation of C/EBPα gene by C/EBPs. Raising cAMP levels cause downregulation of Spl, consistent with the initial PKA-mediated events of adipogenesis (209).

The GATA family of transcription factors, i.e., GATA-2 and GATA-3 expressed in white adipocyte precursors and testis but not in BAT or other organs, are repressing adipogenesis, at least in part by inhibiting PPARγ2 gene expression through binding to consensus

DNA sequence present in its promoter. Consistently, GATA-3-deficient ES cells exhibit enhanced capacity to differentiate into adipocytes (143). It thus seems that passive mechanisms, which are functional at the time of C/EBPβ and ADD-1 expression, are reinforced by specific and active mechanisms. Both mechanisms then become nonfunctional at the onset of terminal differentiation, which leads to the adipocyte phenotype.

B WAT Development After Gain of Function or Loss of Function

The recognition of the prime importance of an adequate mass of WAT, coupled with the dramatic improvement of our understanding of regulatory mechanisms of adipogenesis, have led to numerous in vivo gain- or loss-of-function experiments.

In most cases of gain-of-function experiments (Table 4), use was made of the adipocyte-specific promoter/enhancer of the ALBP gene, which allows targeted expression in WAT and BAT of various genes of interest. Compared to wild-type control mice, and in agreement with their postulated physiological role, overexpressing the lipolytic β1-adrenoreceptor (210) or overexpressing the antilipolytic human α2-adrenoreceptor (on a β3 adrenoreceptor -/- background) (211) leads to a decreased or increased fat mass, respectively. Overexpression of agouti (213), angiotensinogen (188) (likely acting in a paracrine/autocrine manner), or the glucose transporter-4 (GLUT-4) (62) enhances fat mass. A high-fat diet magnifies this weight increase. Notably, depending on the overexpressed gene, fat mass alterations are due to change in fat cell number or in fat cell size.

The most dramatic effect of overexpression is observed in the case of genes encoding transcription factors. Mice overexpressing A-ZIP/F protein, a dominant-negative protein which binds transcription factors of the C/EBP and *c-jun* families, are fat-free and exhibit the features of human lipoatrophic diabetes (214) whereas mice overexpressing ADD-1/SREBP-1c exhibit many of the features of human congenitial generalized lipodystrophy (215). Overexpression of the transcription factor FOXC2 in adipose tissue leads to a lean and insulin sensitive phenotype. Interestingly, the sensitivity of the β-adrenoreceptor/cAMP/PKA pathway is also increased although the relative importance of β1-, β2-, and β3-adrenoreceptor remains to be investigated. As FOXC2 gene levels are upregulated by high-fat feeding and as transgenic mice exhibit resistance to diet-induced obesity, it appears that FOXC2 overexpression counteracts the major symptoms associated with obesity (216).

Adipose tissue development can be also impaired or enhanced after gene invalidation (Table 5). For the sake of clarity, genes expressed in the central nervous system have been excluded, the invalidation of which has revealed a key role in the control of body weight regulation and/or food intake. In a few cases, KO mice exhibit smaller size than wild-type mice, with a disproportionate decrease in fat mass, i.e. PPARδ -/-, Hmgic -/-, RIIβ -/-, and GLUT-4 -/- mice. Surprisingly, although lipolysis is associated with phosphorylation of hormone-sensitive lipase and that of perilipin, an adipocyte protein coating triglyceride droplets, only the invalidation of perilipin leads to resistance to diet-induced obesity (217,218). The invalidation of diacylglycerol acyltransferase gene, which encodes a key enzyme implicated in triglyceride synthesis, leads to the same phenotype but also to an unexpected increase in energy expenditure (219). An increase in energy expenditure is also observed in protein tyrosine phosphatase-1B-deficient mice which exhibit increased insulin sensitivity and resistance to diet-induced obesity (220,221). The invalidation of the gene encoding the cell surface receptor of very low density lipoproteins leads to increased plasma postprandial triglycerides and, on a long-term basis, to resistance to diet-induced obesity (229). Of interest is the invalidation of mitochondrial acetylCoA carboxylase-2, as the decrease of malonyl-CoA levels is associated with higher fatty acid oxidation in muscles and lower fat tissue mass despite hyperphagy (222).

Some rationale emerges with respect to invalidation of genes encoding C/EBPs and nuclear receptors of the PPAR family and the gene encoding Hmgic, a partner of the transcriptosome, as reduced fat mass is observed as compared to wild-type mice (230–235). That C/EBPβ -/- C/EBPδ -/- mice exhibit reduced fat mass with normal levels of C/EBPα and PPARγ strongly suggests that alternative routes to upregulate PPARγ, i.e., PPARδ and ADD-1/SREBP-1c, are functional in these double KO mice (233). Interestingly, the time-dependent specific excision of RXRα from WAT and BAT leads to impaired lipolysis and resistance to diet-induced obesity (234). Despite this wealth of information, data from these various investigations are rather difficult to compare, as WAT cellularity, food intake, energy expenditure and resistance to high-fat diet have not been systematically reported. In summary, it is clear from the data in Tables 4 and 5 that WAT mass can be altered by predicted but also by rather unexpected ways. This situation adds further complexity to devise well-defined molecular targets at the peripheral level, which will prove ultimately to be efficient in treating obese patients.

REFERENCES

1. Johnson PR, Greenwood MRC. Adipose tissue. In: Weiss L, ed. Cell and Tissue Biology—A Textbook of Histology. Munich: Urban & Schwarzenberg, 1988: 191–209.
2. Julien P, Despres JP, Angel A. Scanning electron microscopy of very small fat cells and mature fat cells in human obesity. J Lipid Res 1989; 30:293–299.
3. Ailhaud G, Grimaldi P, Négrel R. Cellular and molecular aspects of adipose tissue development. Annu Rev Nutr 1992; 12:207–233.
4. Keller GM. In vitro differentiation of embryonic stem cells. Curr Opin Cell Biol 1995; 7:862–869.
5. Moulin K, Truel N, André M, Arnauld E, Bibbelink M, Cousin B, Dani C, Pénicaud L, Casteilla L. Emergence during development of the white-adipocyte cell phenotype is independent of the brown-adipocyte cell phenotype. Biochem J 2001; 356:659–664.
6. Hausman GJ. Identification of adipose tissue primordia in perirenal tissues of pig fetuses: utility of phosphatase histochemistry. Acta Anat 1987; 128: 236–242.
7. Poissonnet CM, Burdi AR, Garn SM. The chronology of adipose tissue appearance and disturbance in human fetus. Early Hum Dev 1984; 10:1–11.
8. Crandall DL, Hausman GJ, Kral JG. A review of the microcirculation of adipose tissue: anatomic, metabolic, and angiogenic properties. Microcirculation 1997; 4:211–232.
9. Bartness TJ, Manshad M. Innervation of mammalian white adipose tissue: implications for the regulation of total body fat. Am J Physiol 1998; 275:R1399–R1411.
10. Dobson DE, Kambe A, Block E, Dion T, Lu H, Castellt JJ Jr, Spiegelman BM. 1-Butyrylglycerol: a novel angiogenesis factor secreted by differentiating adipocytes. Cell 1990; 61:223–230.
11. Bouloumié A, Drexler HCA, Lafontan M, Busse R. Leptin, the product of Ob gene, promotes angiogenesis. Circ Res 1998; 83:1059–1066.
12. Sierra-Honigmann MR, Nath AK, Murakami C, Garcia-Cardena G, Papapetropoulos A, Sessa WC, Madge LA, Schechner JS, Schwab MB, Polverini PJ, Flores-Riveros JR. Biological action of leptin as an angiogenic factor. Science 1998; 281:1683–1686.
13. Wassermann F. The development of adipose tissue. In: Renold AE, Cahill GF, eds. Handbook of Physiology. Section 5: Adipose Tissue. Washington: American Physiological Society, 1965:87–100.
14. Poissonnet CM, Burdi AR, Bookstein FL. Growth and development of human adipose tissue during early gestation. Early Hum Dev 1983; 8:1–11.
15. Hager A, Sjöström L, Arvidsson B, Björntorp P, Smith U. Body fat and adipose tissue cellularity in infants: a longitudinal study. Metabolism 1977; 26: 607–614.
16. Sjöström L, William Olsson T. Prospective studies on adipose tissue development in man. Int J Obes 1981; 5:597–604.
17. Boulton TJC, Dunlop M, Court JM. The growth and development of fat cells in infancy. Pediatr Res 1978; 12:908–911.
18. Salans LB, Cushman SW, Weismann RE. Studies of human adipose tissue. Adipose cell size and number in nonobese and obese patients. J Clin Invest 1973; 52: 929–941.
19. Baum D, Beck RQ, Hammer LD, Brasel JA, Greenwood MRC. Adipose tissue thymidine kinase activity in man. Pediatr Res 1986; 20:118–121.
20. Hauner H, Wabitsch M, Pfeiffer EF. Proliferation and differentiation of adipose tissue derived stromal-vascular cells from children at different ages. In: Björntorp P, Rössner S, eds. Obesity in Europe 88: Proceedings of the 1st European Congress on Obesity. London: Libbey, 1989:195–200.
21. Knittle JL, Timmers K, Ginsberg-Fellner F, .Brown RE, Katz DP. The growth of adipose tissue in children and adolescents. Cross-sectional and longitudinal studies of adipose cell number and size. J Clin Invest 1979; 63:239–246.
22. Hirsch J, Batchelor B. Adipose tissue cellularity in human obesity. J Clin Endocrinol Metab 1976; 5:299–311.
23. Hauner H, Entenmann G, Wabitsch M, Gaillard D, Négrel R, Ailhaud G, Pfeiffer EF. Promoting effect of glucocorticoids on the differentiation of human adipocyte precursor cells cultured in a chemically defined medium. J Clin Invest 1989; 84: 1663–1670.
24. Entenmann G, Hauner H. Relationship between replication and differentiation in cultured human adipocyte precursor cells. Am J Physiol 1996; 270: C1011–C1016.
25. Zuk PA, Zhu M, Mizuno H, Huang J, Futrell JW, Katz AJ, Benhaim P, Lorenz HP, Hedrick MH. Multilineage cells from human adipose tissue: implications for cell-based therapies. Tissue Eng 2001; 7: 211–228.
26. Levine JA, Jensen MD, Eberhardt NL, O'Brien TO. Adipocyte macrophage colony-stimulating factor is a mediator of adipose tissue growth. J Clin Invest 1998; 101:1557–1564.
27. Levacher C, Sztalryd C, Kinebanyan MF, Picon L. Effects of thyroid hormones on adipose tissue development in Sherman and Zucker rats. Am J Physiol 1984; 246:C50–C56.
28. Hausman GJ. The influence of thyroxine on the differentiation of adipose tissue and skin during fetal development. Pediatr Res 1992; 32:1255–1261.
29. Geloen A, Collet AJ, Guay G, Bukowiecki LJ. Insulin stimulates in vivo cell proliferation in white adipose tissue. Am J Physiol 1989; 256:C190–C196.
30. Accili D, Taylor SI. Targeted inactivation of the

insulin receptor gene in mouse 3T3-L1 fibroblasts via homologous recombination. Proc Natl Acad Sci USA 1991; 88:4708–4712.
31. Chaika OV, Chaika N, Volle DJ, Wilden PA, Pirucello SJ, Lewis RE. CSF-1 receptor/insulin receptor chimera permits CSF-1-dependent differentiation of 3T3-L1 preadipocytes. J Biol Chem 1997; 272:11968–11974.
32. Amri E-Z, Grimaldi P, Négrel R, Ailhaud G. Adipose conversion of ob17 cells. Insulin acts solely as modulator in the expression of the differentiation program. Exp Cell Res 1984; 152:368–377.
33. Wiederer O, Löffler G. Hormonal regulation of the differentiation of rat adipocyte precursor cells in primary culture. J Lipid Res 1987; 28:649–658.
34. Bonnet F, Lodeweyckx MV, Eckels R, Malvaux P. Subcutaneous adipose tissue and lipids in blood in growth hormone deficiency before and after treatment with human growth hormone. Pediatr Res 1974; 8:800–805.
35. Rosenbaum M, Gertner JM, Leibel RL. Effects of systemic growth hormone (GH) administration on regional adipose tissue distribution and metabolism in GH-deficient children. J Clin Endocrinol Metab 1989; 69:1274–1281.
36. Bengtsson B-A, Eden S, Lönn L, Kvist H, Stokland A, Lindstedt G, Bosaeus I, Tölli J, Sjöström L, Isaksson OGP. Treatment of adults with growth hormone (GH) deficiency with recombinant human GH. J Clin Endocrinol Metab 1993; 76:309–317.
37. Ottosson M, Vikman-Adolfsson K, Enerbäck S, Elander A, Björntorp P, Eden S. Growth hormone inhibits lipoprotein lipase activity in human adipose tissue. J Clin Endocrinol Metab 1995; 80:936–941.
38. Harant I, Beauville M, Crampes F, Riviere D, Tauber M-T, Tauber J-P, Garrigues M. Response of fat cells to growth hormone (GH): effect of long-term treatment with recombinant human GH in GH-deficient adults. J Clin Endocrinol Metab 1994; 78: 1392–1395.
39. Gaskins HR, Kim J-W, Wright JT, Rund LA, Hausman GJ. Regulation of insulin-like growth factor-I ribonucleic acid expression, polypeptide secretion, and binding protein activity by growth hormone in porcine preadipocyte cultures. Endocrinology 1990; 126:622–630.
40. Nougues J, Reyne Y, Barenton B, Chery T, Darandel V, Soriano J. Differentiation of adipocyte precursors in a serum-free medium is influenced by glucocorticoids and endogenously produced insulin-like growth factor-I. Int J Obes 1993; 17:159–167.
41. Wabitsch M, Braun S, Hauner H, Heinze E, Ilondo M, Shymko R, De Meyts P, Teller W. Mitogenic and antiadipogenic properties of human growth hormone in human adipocyte precursor cells in primary culture. Pediatr Res 1996; 40:450–456.
42. Lönn L, Kvist H, Ernest I, Sjöström L. Changes in body composition and adipose tissue distribution after treatment of women with Cushing's syndrome. Metabolism 1994; 43:1517–1522.
43. Rebuffe-Scrive M, Krotkiewski M, Elfverson J, Björntorp P. Muscle and adipose tissue morphology and metabolism in Cushing's syndrome. J Clin Endocrinol Metab 1988; 67:1122–1128.
44. Rebuffe-Scrive M, Brönnegard M, Nilsson A, Eldh J, Gustafsson J-A, Björntorp P. Steroid hormone receptors in human adipose tissue. J Clin Endocrinol Metab 1990; 71:1215–1219.
45. Pepin MC, Pothier F, Barden N. Impaired type II glucocorticoid-receptor function in mice bearing antisense RNA transgene. Nature 1992; 355:725–728.
46. Stenzel-Poore MP, Cameron VA, Vaughan J, Sawchenko PE, Vale W. Development of Cushing's syndrome in corticotropin-releasing factore transgene mice. Endocrinology 1992; 130:3378–2286.
47. Xu X, De Pergola G, Björntorp P. The effects of androgens on the regulation of lipolysis in adipose precursor cells. Endocrinology 1990; 126:1229–1234.
48. Pedersen SB, Börglum JD, Eriksen EF, Richelsen B. Nuclear estradiol binding in rat adipocytes. Regional variations and regulatory influences of hormones. Biochim Biophys Acta 1991; 1093:80–86.
49. Pedersen SB, Brunn JM, Hube F, Kristensen K, Hauner H, Richelsen B. Demonstration of estrogen receptor subtypes α and β in human adipose tissue: influences of adipose cell differentiation and fat depot localisation. Mol Cell Endocrinol 2001; 182: 27–37.
50. O'Brien SN, Welter BH, Mantzke KA. Identification of progesterone receptors in human subcutaneous adipose tissue. J Clin Endocrinol Metab 1988; 83:509–513.
51. De Ridder CM, de Boer RW, Seidell JC, Nieuwenhoff CM, Jeneson JAL, Bakker CJG, Zonderland MI, Erich WBM. Body fat distribution in pubertal girls quantified by magnetic resonance imaging. Int J Obes 1992; 16:443–449.
52. Kissebah AH, Krakower GR. Regional adiposity and morbidity. Physiol Rev 1994; 74:761–811.
53. Haarbo J, Marslew U, Gotfredsen A, Christiansen C. Postmenopausal hormone replacement therapy prevents central distribution of body fat after menopause. Metabolism 1991; 40:1323–1326.
54. Björntorp P. The regulation of adipose distribution in humans. Int J Obes 1996; 20:291–302.
55. Marin P, Holmäng S, Jönsson L, Sjöström L, Kvist H, Holm G, Lindstedt G, Björntorp P. The effects of testosterone treatment on body composition and metabolism in middle-aged obese men. Int J Obes 1992; 16:991–997.
56. Kvist H, Hallgren P, Jönsson L, Pettersson P, Sjöberg C, Sjöström L, Björntorp P. Distribution of adipose

tissue and muscle mass in alcoholic men. Metabolism 1993; 42:569–573.
57. Amri E, Ailhaud G, Grimaldi PA. Fatty acids as signal transducing molecules: involvement in the differentiation of preadipose to adipose cells. J Lipid Res 1994; 35:930–937.
58. Levak-Frank Sradner H, Walsh AM, Stollberger R, Knipping G, Hoefler G, Sattler W, Breslow JL, Zechner R. Muscle-specific overexpression of lipoprotein lipase causes a severe myopathy characterized by proliferation of mitochondria and peroxi-somes in transgenic mice. J Clin Invest 1995; 96: 976–986.
59. Shillaber G, Lau DC. Regulation of new fat cell formation in rats: the role of dietary fats. J Lipid Res 1994; 35:592–600.
60. Cleary MP, Phillips FC, Morton AA. Genotype and diet effects in lean and obese Incker rats fed either safflower or coconut oil diets. Proc Soc Exp Biol Med 1999; 220:153–161.
61. Shepherd PR, Gnudi L, Tozzo E, Yang H, Leach F, Kahn BB. Adipose cell hyperplasia and enhanced glucose disposal in transgenic mice overexpressing GLUT4 selectively in adipose tissue. J Biol Chem 1993; 268:22243–22246.
62. Katz EB, Stenbit AE, Hatton K, DePinho R, Charron MJ. Cardiac and adipose tissue abnormalities but not diabetes in mice deficient in GLUT4. Nature 1995; 377:151–155.
63. Faust IM, Johnson PR, Hirsch J. Adipose tissue regeneration following lipectomy. Science 1977; 197:391–393.
64. Reyne Y, Nougues J, Vezinhet A. Adipose tissue regeneration in 6-month-old and adult rabbits following lipectomy. Proc Soc Exp Biol Med 1983; 174:258–264.
65. Djian O, Roncari DAK, Hollenberg CH. Influence of anatomic site and age on the replication and differentiation in rat adipocyte precursors in culture. J Clin Invest 1983; 72:1200–1208.
66. Roth J, Greenwood MRC, Johnson PR. The regenerating fascial sheath in lipectomized Osborne-Mendel rats: morphological and biochemical indices of adipocyte differentiation and proliferation. Int J Obes 1981; 5:131–143.
67. Weber RV, Buckley MC, Fried SK, Kral JG. Subcutaneous lipectomy causes a metabolic syndrome in hamsters. Am J Physiol 2000; 279:R936–R943.
68. Barzilai N, She L, Lin B-Q, Vuguin P, Cohen P, Wang I, Rossetti L. Surgical removal of visceral fat reverses hepatic insulin resistance. Diabetes 1999; 48: 94–98.
69. Leibel RL, Edens NK, Fried SK. Physiological basis for the control of body fat distribution in humans. Annu Rev Nutr 1989; 9:417–443.
70. Gregoire F, Todoroff G, Hauser N, Remacle C. The stroma-vascular fraction of rat inguinal and epididymal adipose tissue and adipoconversion of fat cell precursors in primary culture. Biol Cell 1990; 69:215–222.
71. Wang H, Kirkland JL, Hollenberg CH. Varying capacities for replication of rat adipocyte precursor clones and adipose tissue growth. J Clin Invest 1989; 83:1741–1746.
72. Crandall DL, Goldstein BM, Huggins F, Cervoni P. Adipocyte blood flow: influence of age, anatomic location, and dietary manipulation. Am J Physiol 1984; 247:R46–R51.
73. Cousin B, Casteilla L, Lafontan M, Ambid L, Langin D, Berthault M-F, Penicaud L. Local sympathetic denervation of white adipose tissue in rats induces preadipocyte proliferation without noticeable changes in metabolism. Endocrinology 1993; 133:2255–2262.
74. Krotkiewski M, Sjöström L, Björntorp P, Smith U. Regional adipose tissue cellularity in relation to metabolism in young and middle-aged women. Metabolism 1975; 24:703–710.
75. Pettersson P, Van RLR, Karlsson M, Björntorp P. Adipocyte precursor cells in obese and nonobese humans. Metabolism 1985; 34:808–812.
76. Adams M, Montague CT, Prins JB, Holder JC, Smith SA, Sanders L, Digby JE, Sewter CP, Lazar MA, Chatterjee VK, O'Rahilly S. Activators of peroxisome prolifetor–activated receptor γ have depot-specific effects on human preadipocyte differentiation. J Clin Invest 1997; 100:3149–3153.
77. van Harmelen V, Dicker A, Rydem M, Hauner H, Lönnqvist F, Näslund E, Arner P. Increased lipolysis and decreased leptin production by human omental as compared with subcutaneous preadipocytes. Diabetes 2002; 51:2029–2036.
78. Hauner H, Entenmann G. Regional variation of adipose differentiation in cultured stromal-vascular cells from the abdominal and femoral adipose tissue of obese women. Int J Obes 1991; 15:121–126.
79. Faust IM, Johnson PR, Stern JS, Hirsch J. Diet-induced adipocyte number increase in adult rats: a new model of obesity. Am J Physiol 1978; 235: E279–E286.
80. Roncari DAK, Lau DCW, Kindler S. Exaggerated replication in culture of adipocyte precursors from massively obese persons. Metabolism 1981; 30: 425–427.
81. Gregoire FM, Johnson PR, Greenwood MRC. Comparison of the adipoconversion of preadipocytes derived from lean and obese Zucker rats in serum-free cultures. Int J Obes 1995; 19:664–670.
82. Martorell R, Stein AD, Schroeder DG. Early nutrition and later adiposity. J Nutr 2001; 131:874S–880S.
83. Miller WH, Faust IM, Goldberger AC, Hirsch J. Effects of severe long-term food deprivation and refeeding on adipose tissue cells in the rat. Am J Physiol 1983; 245:E74–E80.
84. Hausberger FX. Effect of dietary and endocrine factors on adipose tissue growth. In: Renold AE,

Cahill GF, eds. Handbook of Physiology. Section 5: Adipose Tissue. Washington: American Physiological Society, 1965:519–528.
85. Geloen A, Roy PE, Bukowiecki LJ. Regression of white adipose tissue in diabetic rats. Am J Physiol 1989; 257:E547–E553.
86. Björntorp P, Carlgren G, Isaksson B, Krotkiewski M, Larsson B, Sjöström L. Effect of an energy-reduced dietary regimen in relation to adipose tissue cellularity in obese women. Am J Clin Nutr 1975; 28:445–452.
87. Knittle JL, Ginsberg-Fellner F. Effect of weight reduction on in vitro adipose tissue lipolysis and cellularity in obese adolescents and adults. Diabetes 1972; 21:764–761.
88. Näslund I, Hallgren P, Sjöström L. Fat cell weight and number before and after gastric surgery for morbid obesity in women. Int J Obes 1988; 12:191–197.
89. Lemonnier D. Effect of age, sex, and site on the cellularity of the adipose tissue in mice and rats rendered obese by a high-fat diet. J Clin Invest 1972; 51:2907–2915.
90. Herberg L, Döppen W, Major E, Gries FA. Dietary-induced hypertrophic-hyperplastic obesity in mice. J Lipid Res 1975; 15:580–585.
91. Oscai LB, Brown MM, Miller WC. Effect of dietary fat on food intake, growth and body composition in rats. Growth 1984; 48:415–424.
92. Prins JB, Walker NI, Winterford CM, Cameron DP. Apoptosis of human adipocytes in vitro. Biochem Biophys Res Commun 1994; 201:500–507.
93. Prins JB, Niesler CU, Winterford CM, Bright NA, Siddle K, O'Rahilly S, Walker NI, Cameron DP. Tumor necrosis factor-α induces apoptosis of human adipose cells. Diabetes 1997; 46:1939–1944.
94. Zhang HH, Kumar S, Barnett AH, Eggo MC. Dexamethasone inhibits tumor necrosis factor-α–induced apoptosis and interleukin-1β release in human subcutaneous adipocytes and preadipocytes. J Clin Endocrinol Metab 2001; 86:2817–2825.
95. Loftus TM, Kuhajda FP, Lane MD. Insulin depletion leads to adipose-specific cell death in obese but not lean mice. Proc Natl Acad Sci USA 1998; 95:14168–14172.
96. Tsuboyama-Kasaoka N, Takahashi M, Tanemura K, Kim H-J, Tange T, Okuyama H, Katsai M, Ikemoto S, Ezaki O. Conjugated linoleic acid supplementation reduces adipose tissue by apoptosis and develops lipodystrophy in mice. Diabetes 2000; 49: 1534–1542.
97. Prins JB, Walker NI, Winterford CM, Cameron DP. Human adipocyte apoptosis occurs in malignancy. Biochem Biophys Res Commun 1994; 205:625–630.
98. Niesler CU, Siddle K, Prins JB. Human preadipocytes display a depot-specific susceptibiliy to apoptosis. Diabetes 1998; 47:1365–1368.
99. Sorisky A, Magun R, Gagnon AM. Adipose cell apoptosis: death in the energy depot. Int J Obes 2000; 24(suppl 4):S3–S7.
100. Petruschke T, Hauner H. Tumor necrosis factor-alpha prevents the differentiation of human adipocyte precursor cells and causes delipidation of newly developed fat cells. J Clin Endocrinol Metab 1993; 76:742–747.
101. Zhou Y-T, Wang Z-W, Higa M, Newgard CB, Unger RE. Reversing adipocyte differentiation: implications for treatment of obesity. Proc Natl Acad Sci USA 1999; 96:2391–2395.
102. Dani C, Smith AG, Dessolin S, Leroy P, Staccini L, Villageois P, Darimont C, Ailhaud G. Differentiation of embryonic stem cells into adipocytes in vitro. J Cell Sci 1997; 110:1279–1285.
103. Grégoire F, Smas C, Sul HS. Understanding adipocyte differentiation. Physiol Rev 1998; 78:783–809.
104. Ji X, Chen D, Xu C, Harris SE, Mundy GR, Yoneda T. Patterns of gene expression associated with BMP-2 induced osteoblast and adipocyte differentiation of mesenchymal progenitor cell 3T3-F442A. J Bone Miner Metab 2000; 18:132–139
105. Wabitsch M, Brüderlein S, Melzner I, Braun M, Mechtersheimer G, Möller P. LiSa-2, a novel human liposarcoma cell line with a high capacity for terminal adipose differentiation. Int J Cancer 2000; 88: 889–894.
106. Aso H, Abe H, Nakajima I, Ozutsumi K, Yamaguchi T, Takamori Y, Kodama A, Hoshino FB, Takano S. A preadipocyte clonal line from bovine intramuscular adipose tissue: nonexpression of GLUT-4 protein during adipocyte differentiation. Biochem Biophys Res Commun 1995; 213:369–375.
107. Pittenger MF, Mackay AM, Beck SC, Jaiswal RK, Douglas R, Mosca JD, Moorman MA, Simonetti DW, Craig S, Marshak DR. Multilineage potential of adult human mesenchymal stem cells. Science 1999; 284:143–147.
108. Ailhaud G, Amri E, Bertrand B, Barcellini-Couget S, Bardon S, Catalioto RM, Dani C, Deslex S, Djian P, Doglio A, Pradines-Figuères A, Forest C, Gaillard D, Grimaldi P, Négrel R, Vannier C. Cellular and molecular aspects of adipose tissue growth. In: Bray G, Ricquier D, Spiegelman B, eds. Obesity: Towards a Molecular Approach. New York: Alan R. Liss, 1990; 133:219–236.
109. Wabitsch M, Brenner RE, Melzner I, Braun M, Möller P, Heinze E, Debatin KM, Hauner H. Characterization of a human preadipocyte cell strain with high capacity for adipose differentiation. Int J Obes 2001; 25:8–15.
110. Soukas A, Socci ND, Saatkamp BD, Novelli S, Friedman JM. Distinct transcriptional profiles of adipogenesis in vivo and in vitro. J Biol Chem 2001; 276:34167–34174.

111. Diascro DD Jr, Vogel RL, Johnson TE, Wihterup KM, Pitzenberger SM, Rutledge SJ, Prescott DJ, Rodan GA, Schmidt A. High fatty acid content in rabbit serum is responsible for the differentiation of osteoblasts into adipocyte-like cells. J Bone Miner Res 1998; 13:96–106.
112. Dorheim MA, Sullivan M, Vandapani V, Wu X, Hudson J, Segarini PR, Rosen DM, Aulthouse AL, Gimble JM. Osteoblastic gene expression during adipogenesis in hematopoietic supporting murine bone marrow stromal cells. J Cell Physiol 1993; 154:317–328.
113. Teboul L, Gaillard D, Staccini L, Inadera H, Amri EZ, Grimaldi P. Thiazolidinediones and fatty acids convert myogenic cells into adipose-like cells. J Biol Chem 1995; 276:28183–28187.
114. Ross SE, Hemati N, Longo AK, Bennett CN, Lucas PC, Erickson RL, MacDougald OA. Inhibition of adipogenesis by Wnt signaling. Science 2000; 289: 950–953.
115. Kirkland JL, Hollenberg CH, Gillon WS. Age, anatomic site, and the replication and differentiation of adipocyte precursors. Am J Physiol 1990; 258: C206–C210.
116. Lu Z, Pineyro MA, Kirkland IL, Li ZH, Gregerman RI. Prostaglandin-sensitive adenylyl cyclase of cultured preadipocytes and mature adipocytes of the rat: probable role of Gi in determination of stimulatory or inhibitory action. J Cell Physiol 1988; 136: 1–12.
117. Aubert J, Dessolin S, Belmonte N, Li M, McKenzie FR, Staccini L, Villageois P, Barhanin B, Vernallis A, Smith AG, Ailhaud G, Dani C. Leukemia inhibitory factor and its receptor promote adipocyte differentiation via the mitogen-activated protein cascade. J Biol Chem 1999; 274:24965–24972.
118. Vassaux G, Gaillard D, Darimont C, Ailhaud G, Négre R. Differential response of preadipocytes and adipocytes to PGI_2 and PGE_2: physiological implications. Endocrinology 1992; 131:2393–2398.
119. Börglum JD, Pedersen SB, Ailhaud G, Négrel R, Richelsen B. Differential expression of prostaglandin receptor mRNAs during adipose cell differentiation. Prostaglandins Other Lipid Mediat 1999; 57:305–317.
120. Miller CW, Casimir DA, Ntambi JM. The mechanism of inhibition of 3T3-L1 preadipotcyte differentiation by prostaglandin $PGF_{2\alpha}$. Endocrinology 1996; 137:5641–5650.
121. Börglum J, Vassaux G, Gaillard D, Darimont C, Ailhaud G, Richelsen B, Négrel R. Changes in adenosine A_1- and A_2-receptor expression during adipose cell differentiation. Mol Cell Endocrinol 1996; 117:17–25.
122. Smas CM, Chen L, Sul HS. Cleavage of membrane-associated pref-1 generates a soluble inhibitor of adipocyte differentiation. Mol Cel Biol 1997; 17: 977–988.
123. Garcés C, Ruiz-Hidalgo MJ, Bonvini E, Goldstein J, Laborda J. Adipocyte differentiation is modulated by secreted delta-like (dlk) variants and requires the expression of membrane associated dlk. Differentiation 1999; 64:103–114.
124. Pedersen SB, Fuglsig S, Sjögren P, Richelsen B. Identification of steroid receptors in human adipose tissue. Eur J Clin Invest 1996; 26:1051–1056.
125. Mizutani I, Nishikawa Y, Adachi H, Enomoto T, Ikegami H, Kurachi H, Nomura T, Miyake A. Identification of estrogen receptor in human adipose tissue and adipocytes. J Clin Endocrinol Metab 1994; 78:950–954.
126. Safonova I, Darimont C, Amri E, Grimaldi P, Ailhaud G, Reichert U, Shroot B. Retinoids are positive effectors of adipose cell differentiation. Mol Cell Endocrinol 1994; 104:201–211.
127. Flores-Delgado G, Marsh-Moreno M, Kuri-Harcuch W. Thyroid hormone stimulates adipocyte differentiation of 3T3 cells. Mol Cell Biochem 1987; 76:35–43.
128. Darimont C, Gaillard D, Ailhaud G, Négrel. Terminal differentiation of mouse preadipocyte cells: adipogenic and antimitogenic role of triiodothyronine. Mol Cell Endocrinol 1993; 98:67–73.
129. Amri EZ, Bonino F, Ailhaud G, Abumrad NA, Grimaldi PA. Cloning of a protein that mediates transcriptional effects of fatty acids in preadipocytes. Homology to peroxisome proliferator–activated receptors J Biol Chem 1995; 270:2367–2371.
130. Lemberger T, Desvergne B, Wahli W. Peroxisome proliferator-activated receptors: A nuclear receptor signaling pathway in lipid physiology. Annu Rev Dev Biol 1996; 12:335–363.
131. Liu PCC, Phillips MA, Matsumura F. Alteration by 2,3,7,8-tetrachlorodibenzo-p-dioxin of CCAAT/enhancer binding protein correlates with suppression of adipocyte differentiation in 3T3-L1 cells. Mol Pharmacol 1996; 49:989–997.
132. Alexander DL, Ganem LG, Fernandez-Salguero P, Gonzalez F, Jefcoate CR. Arylhydorcarbon receptors is an inhibitory regulator of lipid synthesis and of commiment to adipogenesis. J Cell Sci 1998; 111:3311–3322.
133. Brodie AE, Manning VA, Hu Cy. Inhibitors of preadipocyte differentiation induce COUP-TF binding to a PPAR/RXR binding sequence. Biochem Biophys Res Commun 1996; 228:655–661.
134. Shimba S, Todoroki K, Aoyagi T, Tezuka M. Depletion of arylhydrocarbon receptor during adipose differentiation in 3T3-L1 cells. Biochem Biophys Res Commun 1998; 249:131–137.
135. Reusch JEB, Colton LA, Klemm DJ. CREB activation induces adipogenesis in 3T3-L1 cells. Mol Cell Biol 2000; 20:1008–1020.

136. Wu Z, Xie Y, Bucher NLR, Farmer SR. Conditional ectopic expression of C/EBPβ in NIH-3T3 cells induces PPARγ and stimulates adipogenesis. Genes Dev 1995; 9:2350–2363.
137. Kim JB, Spiegelman BM. ADD1/SREBP1 promotes adipocyte differentiation and gene expression linked to fatty acid metabolism. Genes Dev 1996; 10: 1096–1107.
138. Mandrup S, Lane MD. Regulating adipogenesis. J Biol Chem 1997; 272:5367–5370.
139. Lane MD, Tang QQ, Jiang MS. Role of CCAAT/enhancer binding proteins (C/EBPs) inadipocyte differentiation. Biochem Biophys Res Commun 1999; 266:677–683.
140. Jiang MS, Tang QQ, McLenithan J, Geiman D, Shillinglaw W, Henzel WJ, Lane MD. Derepression of the C/EBPα gene during adipogenesis: identification of AP-2α as a repressor. Proc Natl Acad Sci USA 1998; 95:3467–3471.
141. Moldes M, Lasnier F, Fève B, Pairault J, Djian P. Id3 prevents differentiation of preadipose cells. Mol Cell Biol 1997; 17:1796–1804.
142. Moldes M, Boizard M, Lepievre X, Fève B, Dugail I, Pairault J. Functional antagonism between inhibitor of DNA binding (Id) and adipocyte determination and differentiation factor 1/sterol regulatory element-binding protein-1c (ADD1/SREBP-1c) trans-factors for the regulation of fatty acid synthase promoter in adipocytes. Biochem J 1999; 344:873–880.
143. Tong Q, Dalgin G, Xu H, Ting CN, Leiden JM, Hotamisligil GS. Function of GATA transcription factors in preadipocyte-adipocyte transition. Science 2000; 290:134–138.
144. Garcès C, Ruiz-Hidalgo MJ, Font de Moras J. Notch-1 controls the expression of fatty acid–activated transcription factors and is required for adipogenesis. J Biol Chem 1997; 272:29729–29734.
145. Smas CM, Chen L, Zhao L, Latasa MJ, Sul HS. Transcriptional repression of pref-1 by glucocorticoids promotes 3T3-L1 adipocyte differentiation. J Biol Chem 1999; 274:12632–12641.
146. Gaillard D, Wabitsch M, Pipy B, Négrel R. Control of terminal differentiation of adipose precursor cells by glucocorticoids. J Lipid Res 1991; 32:569–579.
147. Börglum J, Richelsen B, Darimont C, Pedersen SB, Négrel R. Expression of the two isoforms of prostaglandin endoperoxide synthase (PGHS-1 and PGHS-2) during adipose differentiation. Mol Cel Endocrinol 1997; 131:67–77.
148. Wu Z, Bucher NLR, Farmer SR. Induction of peroxisome proliferator-activated receptor γ during the conversion of 3T3 fibroblasts into adipocytes is mediated by C/EBPβ, C/EBPδ and glucocorticoids. Mol Cell Biol 1996; 16:4128–4136.
149. Vassaux G, Gaillard D, Ailhaud G, Négrel R. Prostacyclin is a specific effector of adipose cell differentiation: its dual role as a cAMP- and Ca^{2+}-elevating agent. J Biol Chem 1992; 267:11092–11097.
150. Yarwood SJ, Kilgour E, Anderson NG. Cyclic AMP potentiates growth hormone–dependent differentiation of 3T3-F442A preadipocytes: possible involvement of the transcription factor CREB. Mol Cell Endocrinol 1998; 138:41–50.
151. Shi H, Halvorsen YD, Ellis PN, Wilkison WO, Zemel MB. Role of intracellular calcium in human adipocyte differentiation. Physiol Genomics 2000; 3:75–82.
152. Aubert J, Saint-Marc P, Belmonte N, Dani C, Négrel R, Ailhaud G. Prostacyclin IP receptor up-regulates the early expression of C/EBPβ and C/EBPδ in preadipose cells. Mol Cell Endocrinol 2000; 160:149–156.
153. Belmonte N, Phillips B, Massiéra F, Villageois P, Nichols J, Aubert J, Saeki K, Yuo A, Narumiya S, Ailhaud G, Dani C. Activation of extracellular signal-regulated kinases and CREB/ATF-1 mediate the expression of C/EBPβ and C/EBPδ in preadipocytes. Mol Endocrinol 2001; 15:2037–2049.
154. Accili D, Taylor SI. Targeted inactivation of the insulin receptor gene in mouse 3T3-L1 fibroblasts via homologous recombination. Proc Natl Acad Sci USA 1991; 88:4708–4712
155. Benito M, Potras A, Nebreda AR, Santos E. Differentiation of 3T3-L1 fibroblasts to adipocytes induced by transfection of ras oncogenes. Science 1991; 253:565–568.
156. Klemm DJ, Leitner JW, Watson P, Nesterova A, Reusch JEB, Goalstone ML, Draznin B. Insulin-induced adipocyte differentiation: activation of CREB rescues adipogenesis from the arrest caused by inhibition of prenylation. J Biol Chem 2001; 276: 28430–28435.
157. Magun R, Burgering BMT, Coffer P, Pardasani D, Lin Y, Chabot J, Sorisky A. Expression of a constitutively activated form of protein kinase B (c-Akt) in 3T3-L1 preadipose cells causes spontaneous differentiation. Endocrinology 1996; 137:3590–3593.
158. Gagnon AM, Chen CS, Sorisky A. Activation of protein kinase B and induction of adipogenesis by insulin in 3T3-L1 preadipocytes. Contribution of phosphoinositide-3,4,5-triphosphate versus phosphoinositide-3,4-biphosphate. Diabetes 1999; 48:691–698.
159. Xia X, Serrero G. Inhibition of adipose differentiation by phosphatidylinositol 3-kinase inhibitors. J Cell Physiol 1999; 178:9–16.
160. Boney CM, Smith R, Gruppuso P. Modulation of insulin-like growth factor-1 mitogenic signaling in 3T3-L1 preadipocyte differentiation. Endocrinology 1998; 139:1638–1644.
161. Boney CM, Gruppuso P, Faris RA, Frackelton AR Jr. The critical role of Shc in insulinlike growth factor-I–mediated mitogenesis and differentiation in 3T3-L1 preadipocytes. Mol Endocrinol 2000; 14:805–813.

162. Hu E, Kim JB, Sarraf P, Spiegelman BM. Inhibition of adipogenesis through MAP kinase–mediated phosphorylation of PPARgamma. Science 1996; 274:2100–2103.
163. Reginato MJ, Krakow SL, Bailey ST, Lazar MA. Prostaglandins promote and block adipogenesis through opposing effects on peroxisome proliferator–activated receptor gamma. J Biol Chem 1998; 273:1855–1858.
164. Valet P, Pagès C, Jeanneton O, Daviaud D, Barbe P, Record M, Saulnier-Blache JS, Lafontan M. Alpha$_2$-adrenergic receptor-mediated release of lysophosphatidic acid by adipocytes. A paracrine signal for preadipocyte growth. J Clin Invest 1998; 101:1431–1438.
165. Pagès C, Rey A, Lafontan M, Valet P, Saulnier Blache JS. Ca^{2+}-independent phospholipase A2 is required for α2-adrenergic-induced preadipocyte spreading. Biochem Biophys Res Commun 1999; 265:572–576.
166. Pagès C, Daviaud D, An S, Krief S, Lafontan M, Valet P, Saulnier-Blache JS. Endothelial differentiation gene-2 receptor is involved in lysophosphatidic acid-dependent control of 3T3-F442A preadipocyte proliferation and spreading. J Biol Chem 2001; 276:11599–11605.
167. Doglio A, Dani C, Grimaldi P, Ailhaud G. Growth hormone stimulates c-fos gene expression via protein kinase C without increasing inositol lipid turnover. Proc Natl Acad Sci USA 1989; 86:1148–1152.
168. Kamai Y, Mikawa S, Endo K, Sakai H, Komano T. Regulation of insulin-like factor-I expression in mouse preadipocyte Ob1771 cells. J Biol Chem 1996; 271:9883–9886.
169. Catalioto RM, Gaillard D, Ailhaud G, Négrel R. Terminal differentiation of mouse preadipocyte cells: the mitogenic-adipogenic role of growth hormone is mediated by the protein kinase C signalling pathway. Growth Factors 1992; 6:255–264.
170. Yarwood SJ, Sale EM, Sale GJ, Houslay MD, Kilgour E, Anderson NG. Growth hormone–independent differentiation of 3T3-F442A preadipocytes requires Janus kinase/Signal transducer and activator of transcription but not mitogen-activated protein kinase or p70 S6 kinase signaling. J Biol Chem 1999; 274:8662–8668.
171. Teglund S, McKay C, Schuetz E, Van Deursen JM, Stravopodis D, Wang D, Brown M, Bodner, Grosveld G, Ihle JN. Stat5a and STAT5b proteins have essential and nonessential or redundant roles in cytokine responses. Cell 1998; 93:841–850.
172. Wabitsch M, Heinze E, Hauner H, Shymko RM, Teller WM, De Meyts P, Ilondo MM. Biological effects of human growth hormone in rat adipocyte precursor cells and newly differentiated adipocytes in primary culture. Metabolism 1996; 45:34–42.
173. Hansen LH, Madsen B, Teisner B, Nielsen JH, Billestrup N. Characterization of the inhibitory effect of growth hormone on primary preadipocyte differentiation. Mol Endocrinol 1998; 12:1140–1149.
174. Nanbu-Wakao R, Fujitani Y, Masuho Y, Muramatu M, Wakao H. Prolactin enhances CCAAT enhancer-binding protein-β (C/EBPβ) and peroxisome proliferator–activated receptor γ (PPARγ) messenger RNA expression and stimulates adipogenic conversion of NIH-3T3 cells. Mol Endocrinol 2000; 14:307–316.
175. Grimaldi P, Djian P, Négrel R, Ailhaud G. Differentiation of Ob17 preadipocytes to adipocytes: requirement of adipose conversion factor(s) for fat cell cluster formation. EMBO J 1982; 1:687–692.
176. Darimont C, Gaillard D, Ailhaud G, Négrel R. Terminal differentiation of mouse preadipocyte cells: adipogenic and antimitogenic role of triiodothyronine. Mol Cell Endocrinol 1993; 98:67–73.
177. Xue JC, Schwartz EJ, Chawla A, Lazar MA. Distinct stages in adipogenesis revealed by retinoid inhibition of differentiation after induction of PPARγ. Mol Cell Biol 1996; 16:1567–1575.
178. Amri E, Bertrand B, Ailhaud G, Grimaldi P. Regulation of adipose cell differentiation I. Fatty acids are inducers of the aP2 gene expression. J Lipid Res 1991; 32:1449–1456.
179. Gaillard D, Négrel R, Lagarde M, Ailhaud G. Requirement and role of arachidonic acid in the differentiation of preadipose cells. Biochem J 1989; 257:389–397.
180. Négrel R, Gaillard D, Ailhaud G. Prostacyclin as a potent effector of adipose cell differentiation. Biochem J 1989; 257:399–405.
181. Forman BM, Vhen J, Evans RM. Hypolipidemic drugs, polyunsaturated fatty acids, and eicosanoids are ligands for peroxisome proliferator-activated receptors α and δ. Proc Natl Acad Sci USA 1997; 94:4312–4317.
182. Négrel R, Ailhaud G. Metabolism of arachidonic acid and prostaglandin synthesis in Ob17 preadipocyte cell line. Biochem Biophys Res Commun 1981; 98: 768–777.
183. Cassis LA, Saye J, Peach M. Location and regulation of rat angiotensinogen messenger RNA. Hypertension 1988; 11:591–596.
184. Aubert J, Darimont C, Safonova I, Ailhaud G, Négrel R. Regulation by glucocorticoids of angiotensinogen gene expression and secretion in adipose cells. Biochem J 1997; 328:701–706.
185. Jones B, Standbridge MK, Moustaid N. Angiotensin II increases lipogenesis in 3T3-L1 and human adipose cells. Endocrinology 1997; 138:1512–1519.
186. Darimont C, Vassaux G, Ailhaud G, Négrel R. Differentiation of preadipose cells: paracrine role of prostacyclin upon stimulation of adipose cells by angiotensin II. Endocrinology 1994; 135:2030–2036.
187. Engeli S, Négrel R, Sharma AM. Physiology and pathophysiology of the adipose tissue renin-angiotensin system. Hypertension 2000; 35:1270–1277.

188. Massiéra F, Block-Faure M, Ceiler D, Murakami K, Fukamizu A, Gasc JM, Quignard-Boulangé A, Négrel R, Ailhaud G, Seydoux J, Meneton P, Teboul M. Adipose angiotensinogen is involved in adipose tissue growth and blood pressure regulation. FASEB J 2001. In press.
189. Selvarajan S, Lund LR, Takeuchi T, Craik CS, Werb Z. A plasma kallikrein–dependent plasminogen cascade required for adipocyte differentiation. Nat Cell Biol 2001; 3:267–275.
190. Vassaux G, Négrel R, Ailhaud G, Gaillard D. Proliferation and differentiation of rat adipose precursor cells in chemically defined medium: differential action of anti-adipogenic agents. J Cell Physiol 1994; 161:249–256.
191. Zhang B, Berger J, Hu E, Szalkowski D, White-Carrington S, Spiegelman BM, Moller DE. Negative regulation of peroxisome proliferator–activated receptor-γ gene expression contributes to the antiadipogenic effects of tumor necrosis factor-α. Mol Endocrinol 1996; 10:1457–1466.
192. Lyle RE, Richon VM, McGehee Jr RE. TNFα disrupts mitotic clonal expansion and regulation of retinoblastoma proteins p130 and p107 during 3T3-L1 adipocyte differentiation. Biochem Biophys Res Commun 1998; 274:373–378.
193. Harmon AW, Harp JB. Differential effects of flavonoids on 3T3-L1 adipogenesis and lipolysis. Am J Physiol 2001; 280:C807–C813.
194. Kawada T, Aoki N, Kamei Y, Maeshige K, Nishiu S, Sugimoto E. Comparative investigation of vitamins and their analogs on terminal differentiation, from preadipocytes to adipocytes, of 3T3-L1 cells. Comp Biochem Physiol 1990; 96:323–326.
195. Jehl-Pietri C, Bastié C, Gillot I, Luquet S, Grimaldi PA. Peroxisome proliferator–activated receptor delta mediates the effects of long-chain fatty acids on post-confluent cell proliferation. Biochem J 2000; 350: 93–98.
196. Hansen JB, Zhang H, Rasmussen TH, Petersen RK, Flindt EN, Kristiansen K. Peroxisome proliferator-activated receptor δ (PPARδ)-mediated regulation of preadipocyte proliferation and gene expression is dependent on cAMP signaling. J Biol Chem 2001; 276:3175–3182.
197. Bastié C, Holst D, Gaillard D, Jehl-Pietri C, Grimaldi P. Expression of peroxisome proliferator-activated receptor PPARs promotes induction of PPARγ and adipocyte differentiation in 3T3C2 fibroblasts. J Biol Chem 1999 274:21920–21925.
198. Bastié C, Luquet S, Holst D, Jehl-Pietri C, Grimaldi P. Alterations of peroxisome proliferator–activated receptor delta activity affect fatty acid–controlled adipose differentiation. J Biol Chem 2000; 275: 38768–38773.
199. Morrisson RF, Farmer SR. Role of PPARγ in regulating a cascade expression of cyclin-dependent kinase inhibitors, p18(INK4c) and p21(Waf1/Cip1), during adipogenesis. J Biol Chem 1999; 274:17088–17097.
200. Rosen ED, Sarraf P, Troy AE, Bradwin G, Moore K, Milstone DS, Spiegelman BM, Mortensen RM. PPARγ is required for the differentiation of adipose tissue in vivo and in vitro. Mol Cell 1999; 4:611–617.
201. Barak Y, Nelson MC, Ong ES, Jones YZ, Ruiz-Lozano P, Chien KR, Koder A, Evans RM. PPARγ is required for placental, cardiac and adipose tissue development. Mol Cell 1999; 4:585–595.
202. King FJ, Hu E, Harris DF, Sarraf P, Spiegelman BM, Roberts TM. DEF-1, a novel Src SH3 binding protein that promotes adipogenesis in fibroblastic cell lines. Mol Cell Biol 1999; 19:2330–2337.
203. Fajas L, Schoonjans K, Gelman I, Kim JB, Najib J, Martin G, Fruchart JC, Briggs M, Spiegelman BM, Auwerx J. Regulation of peroxisome proliferator–activated receptor γ expression by adipocyte differentiation and determination factor 1/sterol regulatory element binding protein 1: implications for adipocyte differentiation and metabolism. Mol Cell Biol 1999; 19:54995–5503.
204. Kim JB, Sarraf P, Wright M, Yao KM, Mueller E, Solanes G, Lowell BB, Spiegelman BM. Nutritional and insulin regulation of fatty acid synthase and leptin gene expression through ADD1/SREBP-1c. J Clin Invest 1998; 101:1–9.
205. Sorisky A. From preadipocyte to adipocyte: differentiation-directed signals of insulin from the cell surface to the nucleus. Crit Rev Clin Lab Sci 1999; 36:1–34.
206. Kubota N, Terauchi Y, Miki H, Tamemoto H, Yamauchi T, Komeda K, Satoh S, Nakano R, Ishii C, Sugiyama T, Eto K, Tsubamoto Y, Okuno A, Murakami K, Sekihara H, Hasegawa G, Naito M, Toyoshima Y, Tanaka S, Shiota K, Kitamura T, Fujita T, Ezaki O, Aizawa S, Nagai R, Tobe K, Kimura S, Kadowaki T. PPARγ mediates high-fat diet–induced adipocyte hypertrophy and insulin resistance. Mol Cell 1999; 4:597–609.
207. Ron D, Habener JF. CHOP, a novel developmentally regulated nuclear protein that dimerizes with transcription factors C/EBP and LAP and functions as a dominant-negative inhibitor of gene transcription. Genes Dev 1992; 6:439–453.
208. Tang QQ, Lane MD. Role of C/EBP homologous protein (CHOP-10) in the programmed activation of CCAAT/enhancer-binding protein-β during adipogenesis. Proc Natl Acad Sci USA 2000; 97:12446–12450.
209. Tang QQ, Jiang MS, Lane D. Repressive effect of Spl on the C/EBPα gene promoter: role in adipocyte differentiation. Mol Cell Biol 1999; 19: 4855–4865.

210. Soloveva V, Graves RA, Rasenick MM, Spiegelman BM, Ross SR. Transgenic mice overexpressing the β1-adrenergic receptor in adipose tissue are resistant to obesity. Mol Endocrinol 1997; 11:27–38.
211. Valet P, Grujic D, Wade J, Ito M, Zingaretti MC, Soloveva V, Ross SR, Graves RA, Cinti S, Lafontan M, Lowell BB. Expression of human α2-adrenergic receptors in adipose tissue of β3-adrenergic receptor–deficient mice promotes diet-induced obesity. J Biol Chem 2000; 275:34797–34802
212. Kopecky J, Clarke G, Enerbäck S, Spiegelman B, Kozak LP. Expression of the mitochondrial uncoupling protein gene from the aP2 gene promoter prevents genetic obesity. J Clin Invest 1995; 96:2914–2923.
213. Mynatt RL, Miltenberger RJ, Klebig ML, Zemel MB, Wilkinson JE, Wilkison WO, Woychik RP. Combine effects of insulin treatment and adipose tissue-specific agouti expression on the development obesity. Proc Natl Acad Sci USA 1997; 94:919–922.
214. Moitra J, Mason MM, Olive M, Krylov D, Gavrilova O, Marcus-Samuels B, Feigenbaum L, Lee E, Aoyama T, Eckhaus M, Reitman ML, Vinson C. Life without white fat: a transgenic mouse. Genes Dev 1998; 12:3168–3181.
215. Shimomura I, Hammer RE, Richardson JA, Ikemoto S, Bashmakov Y, Goldstein JL, Brown MS. Insulin resistance and diabetes mellitus in transgenic mice expressing nuclear SREBP-1c in adipose tissue: model for congenital generalized lipodystrophy. Genes Dev 1998; 12:3182–3194.
216. Cederberg A, Grönning LM, Ahrén B, Taskén K, Carlsson P, Enerbäck S. FOXC2 is a winged helix gene that counteracts obesity, hypertriglyceridemia, and diet-induced insulin resistance. Cell 2001; 106: 563–573.
217. Osuga J, Ishibashi S, Oka T, Yagyu T, Tozawa R, Fujimoto A, Shionoiri F, Yahagi N, Kraemer FB, Tsutsumi O, Yamada N. Targeted disruption of hormone-sensitive lipse results in male sterility and adipocyte hypertrophy, but not in obesity. Proc Natl Acad Sci USA 2000; 97:787–792.
218. Martinez-Botas J, Anderson JB, Tessier D, Lapillonne A, Chang BHJ, Quast MJ, Gorenstein D, Chen KH, Chan L. Absence of perilipin results in leanness and reverses obesity in Lepr db/db mice. Nat Genet 2000; 26:474–479.
219. Smith SJ, Cases S, Jensen DR, Chen HC, Sande E, Tow B, Sanan DA, Raber J, Eckel RH, Farese RV Jr. Obesity resistance and multiple mechanisms of triglyceride synthesis in mice lacking Dgat. Nat Genet 2000; 25:87–90.
220. Elchebly M, Payette P, Michaliszyn, Cromlish W, Collins S, Loy AL, Normandin D, Cheng A, Himms-Hagen J, Chan CC, Ramachandran C, Gresser MJ, Tremblay ML, Kennedy BP. Increased insulin sensitivity and obesity resistance in mice lacking the protein tyrosine phosphatase-1B gene. Science 1999; 283: 1544–1548.
221. Klaman LD, Boss O, Peroni OD, Kim JK, Martino JL, Zabolotny JM, Moghal N, Lubkin M, Kim YB, Sharpe AH, Stricker-Krongrad A, Shulman GI, Neel BG, Kahn BB. Increased energy expenditure, decreased adiposity, and tissue-specific insulin sensitivity in protein-tyrosine phosphatase 1B–deficient mice. Mol Cell Biol 2000; 20:5479–5489.
222. Abu-Elheiga L, Matzuk MM, Abo-Hashema KAH, Wakil SJ. Continuous fatty acid oxidation and reduced fat storage in mice lacking acetyl-CoA carboxylase 2. Science 2001; 291:2613–2616.
223. Beattie JH, Wood AM, Newman AM, Bremner I, Choo KHA, Michalska AE, Duncan JS, Trayhurn P. Obesity and hyperleptinemia in metallothionein (-I and -II) null mice. Proc Natl Acad Sci USA 1998; 95:358–363.
224. Stubdal H, Lynch CA, Moriarty A, Fang Q, Chickering T, Deeds JD, Fairchild-Huntress V, Charlat O, Dunmore JH, Kleyn P, Huszar D, Kapeller R. Targeted deletion of the *tub* mouse obesity gene reveals that *tubby* is a loss-of-function mutation. Mol Cell Biol 2000; 20:878–882.
225. Cummings DE, Brandon EP, Planas JV, Motamed K, Idzerda RL, McKnight GS. Genetically lean mice result from targeted disruption of the RIIβ subunit of protein kinase A. Nature 1996; 382:622–626.
226. Massiéra F, Seydoux J, Geloen A, Quignard-Boulangé A, Turban P, Saint Marc P, Fukamizu A, Négrel R, Ailhaud G, Teboul M. Angiotensinogen-deficient mice exhibit impairment of diet-induced weight gain with alteration in adipose tissue development and increased locomotor activity. Endocrinology 2001; 142:5220–5225.
227. Dong ZM, Gutierrez-Ramos JC, Coxon A, Mayadas TN, Wagner DD. A new class of obesity genes encodes leukocyte adhesion receptors. Proc Natl Acad Sci USA 1997; 94:7526–7530.
228. Freemark M, Fleenor D, Driscoll P, Binart N, Kelly PA. Body weight and fat deposition in prolactin receptor–deficient mice. Endocrinology 2001; 142:532–537.
229. Goudriaan JR, Tacken PJ, Dahlmans VE, Gijbels MJ, Van Dijk KW, Havekes LM, Jong MC. Protection from obesity in mice lacking the VLDL receptor. Arterioscler Thromb Vasc Biol 2001; 21: 1488–1493.
230. Costet P, Legendre C, Moré J, Edgard A, Galtier P, Pineau T. Peroxisome proliferator–activated receptor PPARα-isoform deficiency leads to progressive dyslipidemia with sexually dimorphic obesity and steatosis. J Biol Chem 1998; 273:29577–29585.
231. Peters JM, Lee SST, Li W, Ward JM, Gavrilova O, Everett C, Reitman ML, Hudson LD, Gonzalez FJ. Growth, adipose, brain, and skin alterations resulting

from targeted disruption of the mouse peroxisome proliferator–activated receptor β(δ). Mol Cell Biol 2000; 20:5119–5128.

232. Wang N, Finegold MJ, Bradley A, Ou CN, Abdelsayed SV, Wilde MD, Taylor LR, Wilson DR, Darlington GJ. Impaired energy homeostasis in C/EBPα knockout mice. Science 1995; 269:1108–1112.

233. Tanaka T, Yoshida N, Kishimoto T, Akira S. Defective adipocyte differentiation in mice lacking the C/EBPβ and/or C/EBPδ gene. EMBO J 1997; 24: 7432–7443.

234. Imai T, Jiang M, Chambon P, Metzger D. Impaired adipogenesis and lipolysis in the mouse upon selective ablation of the retinoid X receptor α mediated by tamoxifen-inducible chimeric Cre recombinase (Cre-ER^{T2}) in adipocytes. Proc Natl Acat Sci USA 2001; 98:224–228.

235. Anand A, Chada K. In vivo modulation of Hmgic reduces obesity. Nat Genet 2000; 24:377–380.

18

Lipolysis and Lipid Mobilization in Human Adipose Tissue

Dominique Langin and Max Lafontan

Obesity Research Unit, INSERM U586, Louis Bugnard Institute, Université Paul Sabatier-Centre Hospitalier Universitaire de Rangueil, Toulouse, France

I INTRODUCTION

Adipose tissue is the body's largest energy reservoir. Energy is stored in fat cells as triacylglycerols (TG). Factors that control the storage and mobilization of TG in adipocytes are important regulators of fat accumulation in various fat areas (1). The major source for adipocyte TG comes from chylomicrons and very low density lipoproteins (VLDL). TG in the lipoprotein particles are hydrolyzed by lipoprotein lipase (LPL) located on the capillary walls of adipose tissue so that nonesterified fatty acids (NEFA) and monoacylglycerol are formed. NEFA are probably taken up by the fat cell through passive and active transport. Indeed, specific NEFA-transporting proteins have been described (2–4). Once taken up by the fat cells, NEFA are esterified to TG. The circulating albumin-bound NEFA can also be taken up by the fat cells and esterified to TG.

Adipose tissue lipolysis, i.e., the catabolic process leading to the breakdown of triglycerides into NEFA and glycerol, is often considered as a simple and well-understood metabolic pathway. However, it is not firmly established what truly sets the rate of adipose tissue lipolysis. Newly released NEFA can be reesterified in the adipocytes. Quantitative studies are lacking in vivo. Catecholamines and insulin represent the major regulators of lipolysis. However, the physiological role of a number of other lipolytic and antilipolytic agents remains to be elucidated. During lipolysis, intracellular TG undergo hydrolysis through the action of a neutral lipase located inside the fat cell, hormone-sensitive lipase (HSL). NEFA and glycerol leave the fat cells and are transported by the bloodstream to other tissues (mainly liver for glycerol; liver, skeletal muscle, and heart for NEFA). NEFA act as signaling molecules as well as metabolic substrates.

In addition to their role in adipose tissue metabolism, they can regulate glucose utilization in muscle and are important signals to the liver and beta cells as well. Some of the NEFA that are formed during lipolysis do not, however, leave the fat cell and can be reesterified into intracellular TG. The glycerol formed during lipolysis is not reutilized to a major extent by fat cells because they contain only minimal amounts of the enzyme glycerol kinase. In normal-weight man, the mean turnover rate of TG in the total fat mass is ~100–300 g TG per day. An imbalance between hydrolysis and synthesis of TG can be important for the development of obesity. Altered lipolysis could be an element leading to obesity and interindividual variations in AT lipolysis are of importance for the rate of weight loss. Conversely, excessive lipolytic rates, in conjunction with impairment in NEFA utilization by muscle and liver, may be a major contributor to the metabolic abnormalities found in persons with android or upper-body obesity and lead to non-insulin-dependent diabetes mellitus (NIDDM).

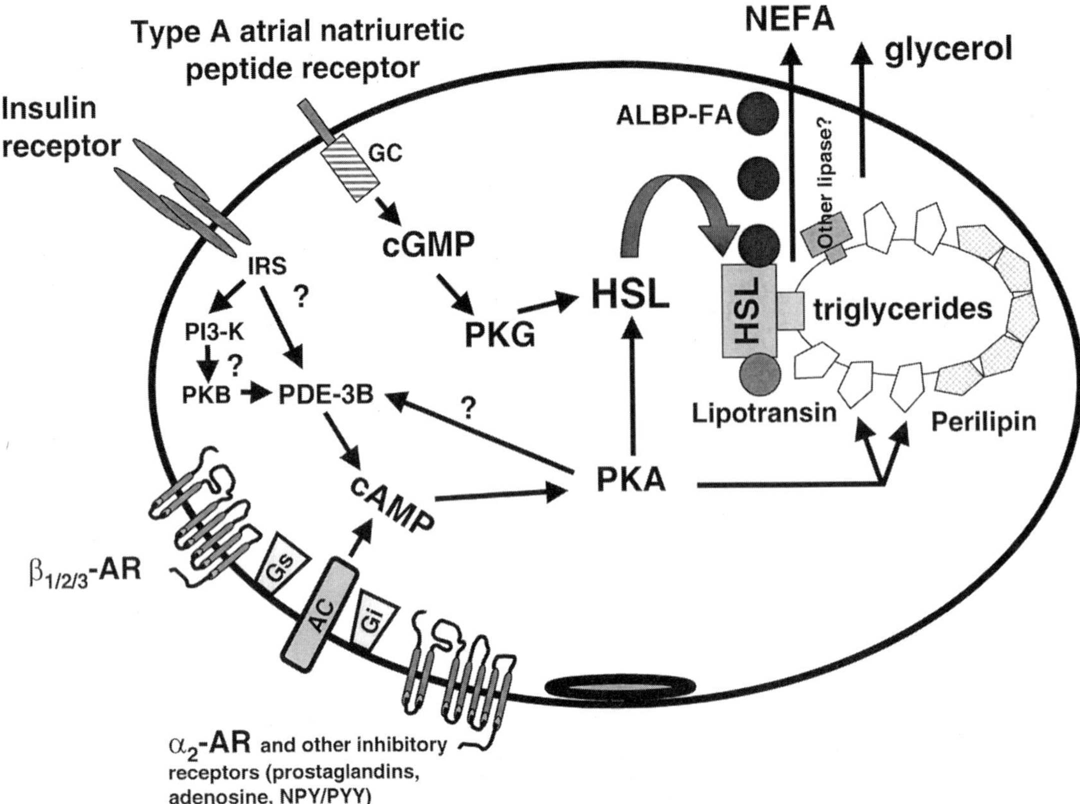

Figure 1 Control of human adipocyte lipolysis. Diagram of signal transduction pathways for catecholamines via adrenergic receptors (AR), atrial natriuretic peptide via type A receptor and insulin. Protein kinases (PKA, PKG, and PKB) are involved in target proteins phosphorylations. HSL phosphorylation promote its translocation from the cytosol to the surface of the lipid droplet. Perilipin phosphorylation induces an important physical alteration of the droplet surface that facilitates the action of HSL and lipolysis. Docking of ALBP to HSL favors the evacuation of NEFA released by the hydrolysis of triglycerides. Question marks show pathways which are still hypothetical or the relevance of which has not been fully demonstrated in human fat cells. Abbreviations: AC, adenylyl cyclase; ALBP, adipocyte lipid-binding protein; AR, adrenergic receptor; FA, fatty acid; GC, guanylyl cyclase; Gi, inhibitory GTP-binding protein; Gs, stimulatory GTP-binding protein; HSL, hormone-sensitive lipase; IRS, insulin receptor substrate; NEFA, nonesterified fatty acid; PDE-3B, phosphodiesterase 3B; P13-K, phosphatidylinositol-3-phosphale kinase; PKA, protein kinase A; PKB, protein kinase B; PKG, protein kinase G.

This chapter reviews quantitative and regulatory aspects of lipid mobilization in human adipose tissue. Several hundred articles have been published relating to adipose tissue metabolism. In light of space limitations, we will as often as possible cite reviews that cover a large number of major publications in the area. A diagram of the mechanisms involved in the control of human fat cell lipolysis is given in Figure 1.

II TRIGLYCERIDE HYDROLYSIS

A Protein-Lipid Interactions

The hydrolysis of the triglycerides stored in the fat cell lipid droplets is a complex phenomenon. One mole of triglyceride is broken in a stepwise fashion via diglyceride and monoglyceride intermediates into 3 moles of free fatty acid and 1 mole of glycerol. In vitro, HSL catalyzes the hydrolysis of triglycerides into diglycerides, and diglycerides into monoglycerides. The first step occurs at a 10-fold lower rate than the second step. The enzyme is also responsible for the hydrolysis of cholesterol and retinyl esters. Although HSL has the capacity to hydrolyze monoglycerides in vitro, monoglyceride lipase (MGL) is required to obtain complete hydrolysis of monoglycerides in vivo. It is important to note that MGL also hydrolyzes 2-monoglycerides resulting from the action of lipoprotein lipase. Unlike other known mammalian triglyceride lipases, HSL phosphorylation by protein kinase A

(PKA) leads to an activation of the enzyme. Through modulation of 0cAMP levels, catecholamines and insulin therefore control HSL activity. Three phosphorylation sites have been characterized—Ser^{563}, Ser^{659}, and Ser^{660} (5). The latter two were shown to be responsible for in vitro activation of HSL, whereas the role of Ser^{563} remains elusive. Activation of the extracellular signal-regulated kinase pathway is able to activate lipolysis by phosphorylating HSL on Ser^{660} (6). Whether this pathway is important in vivo remains to be demonstrated.

Comparison of in vitro and in vivo activation of HSL implies that a simple conformational change of phosphorylated HSL leading to a higher affinity for its substrate does not fully account for fat cell lipolysis stimulation. By analogy with other lipases, HSL may exist in two conformational states—an active, open form with exposure of a hydrophobic area that interacts with lipids to unmask the catalytic site, and an inactive, closed form (7). Phosphorylation of HSL would be required to trigger the transition from the closed to the open form. In vivo, an important step in lipolysis activation seems to be the translocation of HSL from a cytosolic compartment to the surface of the lipid droplet (8–10). In unstimulated cells, HSL is diffusively distributed throughout the cytosol. Upon stimulation with a beta-adrenergic agonist, the enzyme translocates concomitantly to the onset of lipolysis. This rapid process does not require protein synthesis and apparently does not involve cytoskeleton.

HSL is classically considered as the key enzyme catalyzing the rate-limiting step of adipose tissue lipolysis. Mice lacking HSL are not obese (11,12). Catecholamine-induced lipolysis is markedly blunted as expected, but basal (or unstimulated) lipolysis is unaltered in isolated adipocytes. Accumulation of diglyceride in AT shows that HSL is the rate-limiting enzyme for the catabolism of diglycerides but not triglycerides (13). The data therefore suggest the existence of a triglyceride lipase different from HSL. It is not known whether the high activity of the novel lipase does result from a compensatory mechanism associated with the lack of HSL.

Proper activation of lipolysis relies on proteins that are not directly involved in the catalytic process. Two proteins have recently been shown to interact with HSL: adipocyte lipid-binding protein (ALBP or aP2), and lipotransin (14,15). ALBP is an intracellular fatty acid–binding protein highly expressed in adipocytes. ALBP interacts with HSL N-terminal region and increases the lipolytic activity of HSL through its ability to bind and sequester fatty acids and via specific protein-protein interaction. Consistent with such a role for ALBP is the observation that ALBP-null mice exhibit decreased lipolytic capacity (16,17). Lipotransin is a member of the katanin family that may dock the protein to the surface of the lipid droplet. The exact contribution of lipotransin to catecholamine lipolytic and insulin antilipolytic effect awaits further studies.

Access to the lipid droplet constitutes another potential mechanism for the control of lipolysis. Perilipins are proteins covering the large lipid droplets in adipocytes (18): They shield stored triglycerides from cytosolic lipases. It has been hypothesized that, upon phosphorylation, perilipins allow access to the lipid droplet and thereby allow lipase to interact with its substrates. In two independent studies, ablation of perilipin results in mice with decreased fat mass and increased lean body mass (19,20). The mice are resistant to diet-induced obesity. Moreover, double mutant $Lepr^{db/db}$/Plin-/- mice are protected against the obesity phenotype owing to mutation in the leptin receptor. No hepatic steatosis or alteration of the lipid profile was observed, which might be due to the increased metabolic rate of the mutant animals. Basal lipolysis is increased in perilipin-deficient adipocytes, which is in line with a role of perilipin as a suppressor of lipolysis in quiescent cells.

B Selective Mobilization of Fatty Acid

The selectivity of fatty acid mobilization from rat and human adipose tissue has been reported during fasting in vivo (21,22) and during stimulated lipolysis on isolated fat cells (23,24). The composition of NEFA released by adipose tissue was compared to that of the triglycerides from which they originated. For some fatty acids, their percentage in NEFA was different from that in TAG. As a rule, the relative mobilization decreases with increasing chain length for a given unsaturation degree and increases with increasing unsaturation for a given chain length. The contribution of HSL to the selective mobilization was studied using purified HSL and stable lipid emulsions (25,26). The fatty acid specificities of HSL do not seem to be oriented toward a special demand by tissues or toward a preferential sparing of particular fatty acids. Comparison of the relative hydrolysis of fatty acids by HSL and their mobilization rates from adipocytes supports the view that the low mobilization of some fatty acids could derive from a low release of fatty acids by HSL, whereas the high mobilization of other fatty acids seems unrelated to the enzymological properties of HSL. Because HSL can explain only part of fatty acid mobilization, it is possible that ALBP and perilipin contribute to the fatty acid selectivity.

C Control of HSL Gene Expression

Factors modulating HSL gene expression have been studied in mature adipocytes using murine preadipose cell lines. cAMP and phorbol esters were shown to decrease HSL mRNA and lipase activity levels through independent mechanism, suggesting that sustained activations of protein kinase A and C pathways exert a negative control on HSL gene expression (27). In rodent and human adipocytes, glucose is a positive regulator of HSL expression. Glucose deprivation results in a decrease of HSL mRNA and lipase activity levels (28). The effect of glucose is reversible and is not due to an impairment of the differentiation program. In primary culture of rat adipocytes, prolonged treatment with glucose and insulin results in an increase of basal and stimulated lipolysis and a maintenance of HSL protein levels (29). Long-chain fatty acids do not seem to affect HSL expression.

The 775-amino-acid-long adipocyte HSL is encoded by nine exons spanning 11 kb (30). A short 5′ noncoding exon located 1.5-kb upstream of exon 1 contains the transcriptional start site (31). The proximal 5′ flanking region contains an E-box that binds upstream stimulatory factors, and two GC-boxes that bind Sp1 and Sp3 (32). The *cis*-acting elements are essential for promoter activity. The E-box also mediates the response to glucose, but the nature of the transcription factor complex responsible for glucose induction is unknown. Besides transcriptional mechanisms, alternative splicing of pre-mRNA has an important role in the regulation of gene expression. An alternatively spliced form of human HSL has been identified in AT (33). In-frame skipping of exon 6 generates a catalytically inactive but phosphorylatable protein. The short-form HSL mRNA represents ~20% of HSL transcripts.

III MECHANISMS OF THE HORMONAL CONTROL OF LIPOLYSIS

A G-protein-Coupled Receptors and Adenylyl Cyclase Regulation

Activators and inhibitors of the adenylyl cyclase system and hormones and enzymes controlling intracellular cyclic AMP levels are direct regulators of lipolysis. Intracellular cyclic AMP (cAMP) increases lipolysis while antilipolysis is associated with the lowering of cAMP levels. In vitro studies on human fat cells have established that the tuning of cAMP levels and lipolysis by hormones and paracrine agents is dependent on the balanced cross-talk between stimulatory and inhibitory pathways mediating the control of adenylyl cyclase on one hand and fat cell cyclic nucleotide phosphodiesterases (PDEs) on the other. PDEs, by hydrolyzing cAMP and cyclic GMP, are critical in terminating cyclic nucleotide signals and therefore regulate biological processes mediated by second messengers. Activation of adenylyl cyclase activity stimulates the formation of cAMP from ATP. Stimulating receptors coupled to Gs-protein activate adenylyl cyclase while activation of inhibitory receptors coupled to Gi-proteins inhibit the activity of the enzyme.

1 Gs-protein-Coupled Receptors

In human fat cells, both $beta_1$- and $beta_2$-adrenergic receptors are known to stimulate cAMP production and lipolysis in vitro (34) and in vivo (35). The physiological role of the $beta_3$-adrenergic receptor in human adipose tissue remains questionable. The receptor does not contribute to catecholamine-induced lipolysis in human subcutaneous adipocytes (36). The action of $beta_3$-agonists exerting some lipolytic activity in vitro has not been convincingly validated in vivo. Moreover, one of these agonists, CGP 12177, exerts its effect through a so-called $beta_4$-adrenergic receptor effect, which was, in fact, atypical interaction of the drug with $beta_1$-adrenergic receptors (37–40). Confirmation of the lack of $beta_3$-adrenergic effect in humans has also been provided by in vivo studies. During isoproterenol infusion at dosages < 200 ng/kg min, there was no evidence for a $beta_3$-adrenergic receptor-mediated increase in human lipolysis, energy expenditure and lipid oxidation (41).

Similar conclusions were obtained when using in situ microdialysis (35). The other hormones which are known to exert lipolytic effects in rodent fat cells through Gs-protein-coupled receptors, such as glucagon, parathyroid hormone, TSH, α-MSH, and ACTH, are either ineffective or very weak activators of lipolysis in human adipocytes.

2 Gi-protein-Coupled Receptors

In addition to lipolysis-promoting agents neuropeptides, paracrine factors, and autacoid agents (adenosine, prostaglandins and their metabolites) originating from the adipocytes themselves, preadipocytes, endothelial cells, macrophages, and sympathetic nerve terminals are known to negatively control adenylyl cyclase activity and inhibit lipolysis by their interaction with plasma membrane receptors belonging to the seven-transmembrane domain receptor family. The major antilipolytic pathways involve alpha$_2$-adrenergic receptors, A$_1$-adenosine-receptors, EP$_3$-prostaglandin E$_2$ receptors, and neuropeptide Y/peptide YY (NPY-1) receptors. Existence of inhibitory nicotinic acid-receptors is proposed to explain the well-known antilipolytic action of nicotinic acid, but as yet, the receptor protein has not been identified. Antilipolytic responses (initiated by alpha$_2$-adrenergic receptor agonists, prostaglandins, adenosine, NPY/PYY) are less easy to investigate than simulating effects in vitro, and some controversies exist in the design of the experiments and the results.

Recent studies have focused on the diversity and the abundance (number of binding sites) of lipolysis-inhibiting receptors in human fat cells. The human fat cell NPY receptor is an NPY-1 receptor subtype which, when stimulated, sustains a strong antilipolytic effect (42). Adrenaline and noradrenaline have a higher affinity for alpha$_2$- than for beta$_1$/beta$_2$-adrenergic receptors, suggesting the existence of a role for the alpha$_2$-adrenergic pathway in the control of lipolysis in humans (43). Concerning adenosine and prostaglandins, these compounds are probably metabolized very rapidly in vivo as well as in vitro (44,45). Nevertheless, substantial amounts of adenosine were found in the interstitial fluid of adipose tissue (46). Endogenous inhibitory agents may therefore have a stronger effect on TG hydrolysis than previously suspected. Giα_2 is a major transducer of the inhibitory response in adipose tissue, and provides tonic suppression of basal adenylyl cyclase activity in vivo (47). The fact that unrestrained fat cell adenylyl cyclase proceeds at increased rates suggests that a certain degree of inhibition might be necessary for fat cell adenylyl cyclase to be susceptible to stimulation. Under in vivo conditions, in the presence of the endogenous ligands, Gi-dependent inhibitory pathways may be undersustained and permanent inhibition, since the inhibitory pathways driven by prostaglandins, catecholamines, and adenosine are always activated at the low concentrations of the agents (43,48). Convincing in vivo demonstration of existence of such mechanisms in human adipose tissue is necessary.

B Tyrosine-Kinase Receptors and Signaling Pathways

Insulin and IGF-1 receptors are prototypic members of this family of receptors that are characterized by an extracellular binding domain, a single transmembrane portion, and a large intracellular catalytic domain. In parallel to their control of glucose uptake by fat cells, insulin and IGF-1 control cAMP levels and lipolysis through PDE3B-dependent degradation of cyclic AMP to 5′AMP, decrease in cyclic AMP level, inactivation of PKA, and reduced phosphorylation of HSL. Insulin and IGF-1 tyrosine-kinase receptors are coupled to phosphatidyl inositol kinase-3 (PI3-K). PI3-K is a heterodimer composed of two subunits: a p85 regulatory subunit, which contains two Src homology 2 (SH2) domains, and one Src homology 3 (SH3) domain, as well as the p110 catalytic subunit. PI3-K possesses both lipid-kinase and serine-kinase activities. The antilipolytic effect of insulin is mediated through the activation of the cGMP-inhibited phosphodiesterase3B (PDE3B).

The activation cascade is rather complex, and some points remain unclear. When insulin binds to its receptor, the receptor is activated by phosphorylation on tyrosine residues, which causes tyrosine phosphorylation on intracellular substrates such as insulin receptor substrate I, II and (IRS-I and II), and binding of the p85 subunit of PI3-K. This binding activates the lipid-kinase, which phosphorylates the phosphoinositol at the D-3 position of the inositol ring. In addition, the PI3-K serine kinase autophosphorylates both the p85 regulatory subunit and the p110 catalytic subunit. This step is followed by PKB/Akt phosphorylation/activation, PDE3B activation, and cAMP breakdown (49).

Recent studies in human adipocytes have shown that PDE3B is associated with the insulin receptor; its association does not appear to be regulated by insulin. Insulin increases binding and capacity of the PI3-K-serine kinase associated with the insulin receptor, leading to an increased phosphorylation and activation of PDE3B (50). cAMP-mediated pathways may either oppose or facilitate the actions of insulin and/or growth factors that signal via receptor tyrosine kinases (51).

C Other Lipolytic Pathways

1 Natriuretic Peptides

A new hormonal lipolytic pathway has been discovered in human fat cells (52). Atrial natriuretic peptide (ANP) and brain natriuretic peptide (BNP) stimulate human fat cell lipolysis as much as isoproterenol. The rank order of potency for stimulation of lipolysis (ANP > BNP > CNP) and the existence of an ANP-induced cyclic GMP production suggested the presence of a functional type A natriuretic peptide receptor in human fat cells. Expression of ANP receptors mRNAs and binding studies have confirmed the presence of type A and C ANP receptors. Activation or inhibition of PDE-3B and inhibition of adenylyl cyclase activity do not modify ANP-induced lipolysis (52). In vitro studies have shown that HSL could be phosphorylated by cyclic GMP-dependent protein kinase (53). Cyclic GMP–dependent activation of protein kinase G and phosphorylation of HSL occur after ANP stimulation in human adipocytes (Sengenes et al., unpublished results). In situ microdialysis experiments have confirmed the potent lipolytic effect of ANP in abdominal subcutaneous AT of healthy subjects, and intravenous administration of ANP promotes a striking rise in plasma levels of NEFA and glycerol in normal and obese subjects (54). ANP-induced lipid mobilizing effect was enhanced after a low-calorie diet in obese subjects (55). These results raise questions about the physiological and/or pathological relevance of this novel lipolytic pathway in normal subjects and obese patients.

2 Growth Hormone

Growth hormone (GH) stimulates lipolysis in human adipocytes; however, the exact mechanism of action is not fully clarified. Although GH treatments in adults reduce abdominal obesity and improve insulin sensitivity as well as blood lipid profiles, the physiological contribution of GH to the control of human adipose tissue lipid mobilization has remained elusive and is not yet entirely clear. Recent studies have assessed its role; small physiological GH pulses increase interstitial glycerol concentrations in both femoral and abdominal adipose tissue (56). Moreover, normal nocturnal rise in plasma GH concentrations also leads to site-specific regulation of lipolysis in adipose tissue (57). Of putative pharmacological interest, a small synthetic peptide sequence of human GH (AOD-9041) has been shown to increase human and rodent fat cell lipolysis in vitro. Its efficiency on lipid mobilization has been observed after chronic oral administration in rodents; mechanisms of action remain to be clarified (58).

3 Tumor Necrosis Factor-α

TNFα is a macrophage product, also released by fat cells, which has been suggested to signal the loss of body weight through the decrease in AT and muscle mass. Macrophages release cytokine(s) in response to lipopolysaccharide that stimulate lipolysis in freshly isolated rat adipocytes. TNFα can account for most of the action on adipocytes. Stimulation of lipolysis by TNFα is not direct, since it becomes apparent only after long-lasting exposure of human and rodent adipocytes to the cytokine (59). Exploration of TNFα mechanisms of action has been performed in rodent fat cells.

To demonstrate the role of the different TNFα receptors in the induction of the lipolytic effects, experiments were performed on preadipocyte cell lines established from wild-type mice (TNFR1 +/+ R2 +/+) and from mice lacking TNFR1 (TNFR1 -/-), TNFR2 (TNFR2 -/-) or both (TNFR1 -/- R2 -/-). The studies demonstrated that TNFα-induced lipolysis as well as inhibition of insulin-stimulated glucose transport are predominantly mediated by TNFR1 (60). Additional experiments have demonstrated that TNFα could regulate lipolysis, in part, by decreasing perilipin protein levels at the lipid droplet surface (61). Blunting the endogenous inhibition of lipolysis through Gi protein downregulation is another possible mechanism (62). In human fat cells, TNFα activates the three mammalian mitogen activated protein kinases (MAPK) in a distinct time- and concentration-dependent manner. TNFα-induced lipolysis is mediated by only p44/42 and Jun Kinase but not by p38 (63).

4 Miscellaneous Agents

Nitric oxide (NO) or related redox species like NO^+/INO^- have been proposed as potential regulators of lipolysis in rodent and human fat cells (64,65). A number of experiments have reported the production by cachexia-inducing tumors of a lipid-mobilizing factor (LMF) that causes immediate release of glycerol when incubated with murine adipocytes. Induction of lipolysis by LMF was associated with an increase in intracellular cAMP levels. LMF has not yet been characterized, but its activity was shown to be attenuated by eicosapentaenoic acid (66). The serum and urine of cachectic cancer patients contain LMF, the activity of which correlated with the extent of weight loss (67).

IV IN VIVO REGULATION OF LYPOLYSIS IN HUMAN ADIPOSE TISSUE

In normal subjects, regulation of lipolysis in response to feeding, fasting, and exercise is based on HSL expression/activity upon and interactions with several regulators discussed above, principally plasma insulin and sympathetic nervous system activity modulation (68). In humans, several studies have been performed to explore the relationship between HSL expression and lipolytic rate in physiological and pathological situations. In human subcutaneous adipocytes, a good correlation was found between HSL protein and mRNA levels and maximal lipolysis independently of fat cell size (69).

Concerning the various regulators, in vitro studies on human fat cells have established that the tuning of cAMP levels and lipolysis by catecholamines is dependent on the balanced cross-talk between beta- and $alpha_2$-adrenergic receptor–dependent pathways

(43,70–72). A number of in vitro studies have clearly established that the repertoire and the expression level of human adipocyte adrenergic receptors largely differ according to anatomical location of AT depots, sex, and age of the subjects and genetic determinants.

A Body Fat Distribution and Lipid Mobilization

Body fat distribution differs between normal-weight men and women. A peripheral distribution is usually found in women while a more central one is described in men. Human adipose tissue displays significant regional differences in preadipocyte capacities for replication and differentiation, adipocyte size, basal metabolic activities, and hormonal responsiveness (73). These differences appear to determine regional fat deposition. Adipose site-related differences in the regulation of lipolysis have been shown in vitro and in vivo in normal-weight subjects (43,71,74–76). Lipolytic response of isolated fat cells to catecholamines is weaker in the subcutaneous gluteal/femoral than in the subcutaneous abdominal and visceral adipose tissue. These site-related differences are more noticeable in women than in men. In vitro studies have revealed an enhanced alpha$_2$-adrenergic responsiveness associated with a concomitant decrease in beta-adrenergic responsiveness explains the lower lipolysic effect of catecholamines in gluteal/femoral fat cells of women. Conversely, visceral fat adipocytes exhibit the highest lipolytic responsiveness to catecholamines. In vitro studies have shown that concomitant variations in beta$_2$- and alpha$_2$-adrenergic sensitivity in adipocytes may be predictive of weight loss during dieting or very low calorie diets (77,78). The mechanisms explaining the regional differences have been investigated in vitro (72,79,80). Moreover, microdialysis studies have confirmed the sex-related differences revealed in in vitro assays.

Site-related differences are also found in the antilipolytic action of insulin, prostaglandins, and adenosine. In vitro studies have demonstrated that regional differences exist in the antilipolytic effects of insulin. Omental adipocytes are less sensitive to the antilipolytic effect of insulin than abdominal subcutaneous adipocytes; mechanisms have been explored (81). Regional heterogeneity of insulin-regulated NEFA release has been confirmed in vivo, indicating that visceral adipose tissue lipolysis is more resistant to insulin suppression than is leg lipolysis in humans (82). Whatever the mechanistic interest of the in vitro approaches, tissue-specific investigations, using in situ microdialysis, must be extended to delineate the physiological relevance of previous studies on antilipolytic agents.

B Aging

Aging is associated with a diminished ability to mobilize fatty acids and to use fat as a fuel (increase skeletal muscle fatty acid uptake and oxidation) during beta-adrenergic receptor stimulation (83). There is a selective decrease in the beta-adrenergic lipolytic capacity with aging, which may be caused by disturbances at the adrenergic receptor level or at the postadrenergic receptor level. These alterations are independent from the age-expected increase in total adiposity (84). The impairment in sympathetic nervous system (SNS)-mediated lipolysis and fat oxidation may be of importance in the age-related increase in adiposity and obesity.

C Stress

In diverse stressful conditions such as surgery, trauma, or severe burns, most of the studies have described incremental lipolysis which could be activated to an inappropriate level and lead to excess of plasma NEFA. Activation of lipolysis is due to an increased SNS drive and stress hormones secretion, which both facilitate lipid mobilization and reduce insulin secretion (68,85). Sustained changes in SNS activity or plasma catecholamine levels have commonly been associated with altered beta-adrenergic function in target cells leading to desensitization. Desensitization of beta-adrenergic receptor–mediated lipolysis to catecholamines exposure has extensively been studied in vitro (70). Repeated adrenaline treatment has been shown to suppress basal- and adrenaline-stimulated lipolysis in lean and obese subjects. Plasma insulin concentration increased after repeated adrenaline treatment, and could contribute to the loss of adrenaline efficacy (86). The in vivo lipolytic response of the AT to adrenaline is desensitized by prior adrenaline exposure (87). However, no cardiovascular desensitization was observed in these conditions. It remains to be established if this phenomenon is related to a noticeable beta-adrenergic receptor desensitization, to the appearance of a change in the balance between beta- and alpha$_2$-adrenergic receptor–dependent effects, or to an incremental increase in plasma insulin level.

D Exercise

Exercise represents, with fasting, the main physiological situation of increased lipolysis; sustained exercise of moderate intensity is characterized by marked increases in lipolysis (88). Much of the lipolytic response to exercise can be blocked by beta-adrenergic receptor antagonists. Possible limiting factors to exercise while taking beta-blockers include local alterations to AT blood flow and reduction of adipose tissue and intramuscular lipolysis (89). Aerobic physical training in obese male subjects, when designed to have no effect on body weight, modifies AT lipolysis through an enhancement of beta-adrenergic responses and a concomitant blunting of adipocyte antilipolytic activity (90–92). Adrenaline- and isoproterenol-stimulated lipolytic responses in vitro are higher in fat cells of trained than of sedentary women, whereas alpha$_2$-adrenergic responses are lower. Maximal lipolysis initiated by agents acting at the postreceptor level is also higher (93). Microdialysis studies have revealed a higher exercise-induced lipolysis in trained than in untrained subjects; beta-adrenergic response is largely responsible for this effect, since the alpha$_2$-adrenergic receptor–mediated antilipolytic action is not involved in the regulation of lipolysis in subcutaneous abdominal adipose tissue of the trained subjects during exercise (94).

V DYSREGULATION OF LIPOLYSIS IN OBESITY

As in normal-weight subjects, the distribution of body fat is subject to variation, with noticeable differences between sexes in obesity. Gender and obesity appear to influence these regional differences. Obese men have a tendency to develop central (abdominal) obesity, while a more peripheral form of obesity usually exists women. Epidemiological studies have suggested that visceral obesity has strong associations with metabolic and cardiovascular complications (73). An extended intra-abdominal fat depot appears to be the major factor contributing to increased endocrine and metabolic disorders. However, not all investigators attribute the metabolic complications of obesity to visceral adiposity (75,95). In vitro studies of adipocytes taken from different body fat regions suggest substantial differences in lipolysis between intra-abdominal (omental, visceral), lower-body subcutaneous, and abdominal subcutaneous regions.

In situ measurements of glycerol release from adipose tissue have provided further evidence that regional heterogeneity of lipolysis occurs in humans (76). In upper-body obesity, the regional variations in lipolysis between visceral and subcutaneous fat cells are more important than in normal-weight subjects. It is not clearly established whether NEFA reesterification is altered in obesity. Theoretically, primary defects might exist in adipose tissue of certain obese individuals. Approximately 50% of newly hydrolyzed NEFA are reesterified in subcutaneous adipose tissue of weight-stable obese individuals; during weight reduction, this proportion drops to 10% (96). The true role of NEFA reesterification remains to be clarified in normal-weight, obese, and postobese, weight-stable subjects.

A Basal Rate of Lipolysis

The basal rate of lipolysis in vitro is increased in enlarged fat cells of obese subjects. The differences existing in the basal rate of lipolysis in vitro between lean and obese subjects disappears when fat cell size is taken into account. It is known that circulating NEFA levels are increased in obese subjects and that an in vivo increase in the overall rate of lipolysis exists during fasting in obesity. Interpretation of results is more complex since when fat mass is taken in account, the increase is not observed (68). Microdialysis studies performed after an overnight fast in obese subjects have revealed that the lipolytic rate per tissue weight was normal in obesity (97). The mass effect due to the enlargement of body fat deposits might explain the increased overall rates of "basal" lipolysis in vivo, and probably explains the origin of increased plasma NEFA levels commonly found in obese subjects. The relative contribution of the various fat deposits to this increase in plasma NEFA levels represents an important factor which merit attention.

B Differences in HSL Activity

Larger fat cells, usually found in subcutaneous deposits of obese subjects, have higher lipolysis rates, HSL activity, and HSL mRNA expression levels. Lipolysis rates correlate with fat cell size regardless of the adipose tissue region (98). Comparison of two groups of young adult nonobese subjects with or without a family trait for overweight showed that adipocyte maximal lipolytic capacity and HSL expression were lower in subjects with obese relatives (99). The data suggest a defect in fat cell lipolysis caused by an impaired expression of HSL in normal-weight subjects with a family history of obesity. Impaired lipolysis could therefore constitute an early event in the development of obesity. Moreover, a defect in HSL expression linked to an impaired lipolytic capacity in subcutaneous adipocytes was observed in massively obese subjects (100).

During a 4-week very low calorie diet, an increase in HSL expression in subcutaneous AT of obese women was reported (101). This physiological adaptation might be important to allow an intense mobilization of fatty acids which are, during this type of calorie restriction, the preferred fuels in the body. In two independent weight reduction programs combining hypocaloric diet followed by stabilization at the new weight, the level of HSL after weight stabilization was lower than the HSL level before the program (102,103). These data show that variations in AT lipolysis and HSL expression differ between the hypocaloric and isocaloric phases of weight reduction programs. It is tempting to speculate that hereditary alterations in the regulation of fat cell lipolysis may contribute to the increase in fat mass in some subjects.

C Catecholamine Action

It is commonly accepted that the action of catecholamines is impaired in obesity. This defect might be an early event since it has been observed in obese adolescents (104,105). A summary of the modifications of the lipolytic responses described on human isolated fat cells in vitro or when using in situ microdialysis is given in Table 1. It is probable that this link between abnormal in vivo regulation of lipolysis and upper-body obesity is caused by regional variations of lipolysis regulation. Greater resistance to the lipolytic effect of catecholamines and the antilipolytic effect of insulin is found in subjects with abdominal than in those with peripheral obesity (71). Another important AT component, modulated by SNS activity, insulin, paracrine factors, and autacoid agents released by the adipocytes could also interfere with adipocyte function and AT physiology, which is adipose tissue blood flow (ATBF). Changes in ATBF contribute to TG clearance and facilitate the removal of NEFA and glycerol produced during lipolysis. Failure to regulate ATBF may be a feature of obesity and insulin resistance (106).

The theory on regional fat lipolysis results from a number of in vitro observations. Differences in the

Table 1 Physiological and Pathological Modifications of the Human Lipolytic Responses to Catecholamines In Vitro in Isolated Fat Cells and In Situ Using Adipose Tissue Microdialysis

Physiological and pathological situations	Lipolytic response[a]	Modulatory effects	Ref.
Neonatal period	Decreased[1]	α_2-adrenergic responsiveness ↑	142
Aging	Decreased[1]	Activation of HSL ↓	143
Sex-related differences	Variable[1]	Changes in the balance between α_2- and β-adrenergic effects	78
		HSL expression correlated positively with fat cell size	144
Anatomical differences	Variable[1]	idem	107,108
Very low calorie diet	Increased[1]	HSL expression ↑	101
Endurance training	Increased[1,2]	β-adrenergic response ↑	91
Obesity	Decreased[1]	HSL expression ↓	100
		β_2-adrenergic receptor expression ↓	145
		α_2-adrenergic receptor response ↑	107
Insulin resistance syndrome	Decreased[1]	HSL activation ↓	117
		β2-adrenergic receptor number ↓	
Catecholamine resistance in normal population	Decreased[1]	β_2-adrenergic response ↓	80
		β_2-adrenergic receptor number ↓	
Combined familial hyperlipidemia	Decreased[1]	HSL expression ↓	146
Polycystic ovary syndrome	Decreased[1]	HSL activation ↓	147
		β_2-adrenergic receptor number ↓	
Hypothyroidism	Decreased[1]	HSL activation	148
Hyperthyroidism	Increased[1]	β-adrenergic receptor number ↑	148
Cushing syndrome	Decreased[1]	Unknown	79
Phaeochromocytoma	Decreased[1]	Unknown	149
Type I diabetes	Increased[2]	β-adrenergic response ↑	150
Microgravity	Increased[2]	β-adrenergic response ↑	151
Adrenaline infusion	Decreased[2]	β-adrenergic response ↓	87

HSL, hormone-sensitive lipase.
[a] Data obtained in vitro ([1]) and situ ([2]).

lipolytic response of adipocytes to catecholamines in obese compared with lean subjects are associated with variations in the functional balance between beta- and alpha$_2$-adrenergic receptors in AT (107,108). Reduced beta$_2$-adrenergic lipolytic responsiveness has been reported in subcutaneous fat cells from obese subjects (109) or subjects with a reduced isoprenaline sensitivity (80). In addition, an increased antilipolytic responsiveness linked to alpha$_2$-adrenergic receptors stimulation has also been found in subcutaneous adipocytes of obese of both sexes (107). Conversely, in visceral fat, catecholamines action is increased owing to an increased beta-adrenergic responsiveness and decreased alpha$_2$-adrenoceptor function (110). To sum up, the lipolytic defects described in the adipose tissue of obese subjects can originate from direct HSL alterations (expression and/or function) or from multiple defects in catecholamine signal transduction pathways (beta/alpha$_2$-adrenergic receptor balance, Gs/Gi-proteins level, and function and decreased ability of cyclic AMP and PKA to stimulate HSL).

A number of in vivo studies have shown blunted catecholamine-induced lipolysis in subcutaneous fat cells of obese subjects. Studies performed in adults with long-standing obesity have shown a reduced lipolytic sensitivity to catecholamines in subcutaneous abdominal adipose tissue. Unresponsiveness of the subcutaneous adipose tissue to neurally stimulated lipolysis has been described in obese subjects (111). The lipolytic defects in obese subjects have been confirmed by different groups (104,112,113). Using in situ microdialysis, a specific impairment in the capacity of beta$_2$-adrenergic receptor agonists to promote lipolysis has been reported in the subcutaneous abdominal adipose tissue of obese adolescent girls (105). Moreover, when performing IV administration of selective beta$_1$- and beta$_2$-adrenergic receptor agonists, the increase in lipolysis and thermogenesis promoted by a selective beta$_2$-adrenergic stimulation (salbutamol) was reduced in obese subjects. Conversely, beta$_1$-adrenergic receptor-mediated (dobutamine) metabolic processes (i.e. lipolysis, thermogenesis, and lipid oxidation) were similar in obese and lean men. In conclusion, beta$_2$-adrenergic-mediated increases in thermogenesis and lipid oxidation are impaired in the obese. It is suspected that a dysfunction of the beta$_2$-adrenergic pathway or of the beta$_2$-adrenergic receptor density may play a role in the etiology or maintenance of a relatively increased fat mass and, consequently, obesity. A lipolytic defect associated with a reduced NEFA availability may be the cause of an impairment of responses in energy expenditure and lipid oxidation during beta-adrenergic receptor stimulation (114).

In vivo studies of regional NEFA release have confirmed that adipose tissue lipolysis varies between upper- and lower-body fat. Release of NEFA from lower-body adipose tissue is less than that from upper-body adipose tissue in obese men and women (76). Although women have a higher percentage of body fat than men, there are a number of studies showing that lipolysis and the proportion of energy derived from fat during exercise is higher in women than in men (115). A recent study has demonstrated that the physiological activation of antilipolytic alpha$_2$-adrenergic receptors could inhibit lipid mobilization in subcutaneous AT of exercising obese men. The physiological stimulation of adipocyte alpha$_2$-adrenergic receptors during exercise-induced SNS activation contributes to the blunted lipolysis observed in subcutaneous AT of obese men (116).

However, the alpha$_2$-adrenergic effect is weaker in the subcutaneous adipose tissue of obese women (Stich V., unpublished results). These in vivo results provide evidence of the contribution of fat cell alpha$_2$-adrenergic receptors on the physiological control of lipolysis in subcutaneous AT of obese men. In hypertrophic human fat cells which express a high level of alpha$_2$-adrenergic receptors, any reduction of the beta-adrenergic receptor–mediated lipolytic response will disturb the functional balance between alpha$_2$- and beta-adrenergic receptor–mediated effects and amplify the reduction of the lipolytic response initiated by the physiological amines. Alpha$_2$-adrenergic receptors in subcutaneous AT of obese subjects may have important physiopathological implications in men developing large subcutaneous fat deposits and in women with excessive hip and femoral fat deposits. Reduced AT lipolytic sensitivity to catecholamines occurring in subcutaneous AT deposits probably represent an adaptive process of the hypertrophied adipocyte. A rise in alpha$_2$-adrenergic receptors and alpha$_2$-adrenergic activity has beneficial effects by limiting excessive rates of lipolysis and NEFA release into the systemic circulation. Such a regulation could represent a valuable adaptative process to adjust lipolytic responsiveness to catecholamines to fat accumulation; the mechanisms leading to alpha$_2$-adrenergic receptor overexpression are not established. It is tempting to speculate that adipocyte alpha$_2$-adrenergic receptors may have a major contribution to the resistance of subcutaneous AT to fat loss during very low calorie diets and during physical training programs in obese subjects.

Taken together, these in vitro and in vivo findings suggest that catecholamine-induced lipolysis is decreased in subcutaneous fat but increased in visceral fat following SNS activation. This would promote a marked increase in portal NEFA in relation to peripheral venous NEFA. Excess in portal NEFA could be a mechanism responsible for the hepatic insulin resistance usually observed in abdominal obesity. Unfortunately, a number of these speculations are based on in vitro studies and in vivo measurements of subcutaneous adipose tissue responses. For practical and ethical reasons, it is difficult to perform a direct study of portal NEFA flux in vivo in humans; it is the major limitation of such studies.

Moreover, in addition to catecholamines, and owing to technical limitations, the contribution of other hormones and paracrine agents exerting antilipolytic actions has not been investigated so deeply in visceral obesity. It is not clear to what extent insulin action is altered in obesity. Controversial results have been published. Insulin resistance has been demonstrated in obese subjects when insulin action is studied on glucose transport and glucose uptake by adipose tissue. Data on insulin-induced antilipolysis have shown that insulin exerts a stronger antilipolytic action in subcutaneous than in visceral fat deposits; controversies persist probably owing to the difficulties existing for the investigation of the antilipolytic actions of insulin in obese subjects. Increased, decreased or normal antilipolytic actions of insulin have been described in fat cells obtained from obese subjects (79,117). Preservation or partial or tissue-dependent reduction of antilipolytic actions of insulin could be important for the maintenance or acceleration of obesity in overweight subjects. There is a generalized resistance to insulin suppression of lipolysis in type 2 diabetes compared with equally obese nondiabetic individuals (118). Modifications of other antilipolytic mechanisms may also be involved in the adipocyte of obese subjects. Decreased antilipolytic actions of prostaglandins and adenosine have been reported in subcutaneous fat cells of obese subjects in vitro. These results must be interpreted cautiously since the design of in vitro assays for in vivo demonstrations do not exist for the moment. Whatever the number of in vitro studies on isolated adipocytes and small tissue samples, it is still difficult to extrapolate a number of in vitro findings to the in vivo situation.

VI GENETICS OF FAT CELL LIPOLYSIS

Hereditary influences have repeatedly been reported in the control of catecholamine-induced lipolysis (101,119–121). Beta-adrenergic receptors are candidate genes for obesity because of their role in catcholamine-induced lipolysis and energy homeostasis. Polymorphisms in the beta$_1$-, beta$_2$-AR-, and beta$_3$-adrenergic receptors could influence adipocyte lipolysis and have an effect on the development of obesity-related metabolic disorders. Altered coupling properties of the Arg389Gly gene variant of the beta$_1$-adrenergic receptor have been reported in recombinant cells. Nevertheless, distribution of the Arg389Gly polymorphism of the beta$_1$-adrenergic receptor is similar in lean and obese subjects, and has no apparent effect on the lipolytic responsiveness (122). The rare beta$_2$-adrenergic receptor polymorphism Thr164Ile is associated with a decreased lipolytic responsiveness of subcutaneous fat cells, suggesting that the genetic variance of the beta$_2$-adrenergic receptor might be an important determinant of catecholamines responsiveness in fat cells (123). In addition, the Gln27Glu substitution in the beta$_2$-AR was found twice as common in obese as in nonobese subjects in a group of women with a large variation in body fat mass.

Homozygotes for Glu27 had an average fat mass in excess of 20 kg and ~50% larger fat cells than controls (124,125). Nevertheless, change in beta$_2$-AR lipolytic function was not observed. The frequency of the Glu27 is also higher in patients with type 2 diabetes, but this association could be secondary to obesity. The problem is complex and probably depends on sex-related determinants, since the positive association between obesity and the Glu27 variant in the beta$_2$-AR exists in females, while, conversely, in males there is a negative correlation between the Glu27 variant and obesity (126).

The Arg16Gly polymorphism was associated with altered beta$_2$-AR function with Gly16 carriers showing a fivefold increased agonist sensitivity. The frequency of Gly16 homozygotes was lower in obese than in nonobese women; women bearing the Arg16 allele had higher BMI values than Gly16Gly women. Women carriers of the Arg16Arg genotype had lower fasting plasma NEFA and greater suppression of NEFA after an oral glucose load than women bearing the Gly16 allele. Moreover, the effect of the Arg16Arg genotype on the suppression of NEFA levels was modified by physical activity level (127).

A recent population study on unselected subjects of the WHO-MONICA project in the North of France has shown that the Glyl6Arg and Gln27Glu polymorphism were in strong linkage disequilibrium, as two-thirds of the women investigated carried both Gly16 and Glu27 in a hetero- or homozygous form. The study has also shown that men bearing the Gln27Gln genotype had higher body weight, body mass index, and waist-hip ratio and increased risk of obesity. If Gln27Gln men were bearing in addition the Arg16 allele, the increase in body weight and BMI, and waist-to-hip ratio was more important (128). Physical activity counterbalanced the effect of the genetic predisposition to increase body weight, body fat, and obesity described in Gln27Gln subjects. Obese individuals with the beta$_2$-AR Gln27Gln genotype may benefit from physical activity to reduce their weight (129). These findings suggest that polymorphisms in the coding sequence in the human beta$_2$-AR gene could be of importance for obesity, energy expenditure, and beta$_2$-AR-dependent lipolytic function in AT. Since some controversies still exist (130,131), deeper investigations are required before final conclusions may be reached. Determination of putative alterations of in vitro lipolysis and whole body lipolytic sensitivity to adrenaline is needed to complete the delineation of the various phenotypes.

Missense mutation of beta$_3$-AR gene (Trp64Arg) has been reported to be associated with high BMI, abdominal obesity, increased capacity to gain weight, and resistance to insulin and early onset of type 2 diabetes. However, a number of controversial reports exist. Some studies did not reveal any phenotypic effect of the polymorphism. It is difficult to reach a consensus at the present time (132). The Trp64Arg polymorphism may have some influence on body weight and various metabolic parameters. However, the beta$_3$-AR gene cannot be considered as a major obesity gene. Polymorphism-related questions become more complex when combinations of polymorphisms are considered. A recent report has shown that common variants in the beta$_2$-(Gln27Glu)- and beta$_3$-(Trp64Arg)-adrenergic receptor genes are associated with increased fasting insulin and NEFA concentrations, and could increase susceptibility to type II diabetes. Subjects homozygous for the protective alleles (Glu27 and Trp64) had a lower prevalence of diabetes than subjects with other phenotypes combinations (133).

The HSL gene is a candidate gene in obesity and related disorders because of its pivotal role in the control of lipid metabolism. Two highly polymorphic dinucleotide repeats have been found within introns 6 and 7. The microsatellites have been used in association and family studies within the Caucasian population. Two independent studies showed an association between the polymorphisms and obesity and type 2 diabetes (134,135). Moreover, allele 5 of the intron 6 polymorphism is associated with a marked decrease in the lipolytic rate of subcutaneous fat cells (136). Linkage analysis on families with one or more morbidly obese subject(s) was negative (137). In families with type 2 diabetes, an extended transmission disequilibrium test showed distorted transmission of alleles to abdominally obese offspring (135). The data suggest that the HSL gene may participate in the polygenic background of obesity and/or may be a susceptibility gene important for obesity-related phenotypes.

Quantitative sib-pair linkage analysis was recently performed in dizygotic women twins to study the possible involvement of loci for lipases in changes of lipoprotein variables over 10 years (138). A linkage was demonstrated between the HSL locus and age-adjusted changes in plasma triglyceride levels, suggesting that variation at the locus may underlie a portion of the interindividual variations in this coronary heart disease risk factor. Several amino acid polymorphisms have been identified in the HSL gene. The Arg309Cys mutation found in the Japanese population is extremely rare in Caucasians (139). The more prevalent Glu620Asp and Ser681Ile have no impact on insulin sensitivity of lipolysis or glucose disposal in a lean, healthy population (140). The impact of these mutations in obese and diabetic subjects has not been investigated. A C to G change was found in the proximal adipocyte promoter and appeared to affect promoter activity (139). Women with the -60G allele may be protected against insulin resistance (141).

VII CONCLUSIONS AND FUTURE TRENDS

The last decade has been marked by the discovery of a number of mechanisms able to clarify the control of fat storage and mobilization. Genetic variation and altered gene expression may modify HSL and adrenergic receptor function and play a noticeable role in the development of obesity. Future studies must be devoted to the delineation of the defects affecting genes encoding the various elements of the transduction pathways and the enzymes involved in the regulation of the lipolytic and antilipolytic mechanisms as well as lipogenesis. Further work will also help to understand the complex interplay between genetic and nongenetic determinants of AT function.

Altered SNS impact on its target cells could lead to the development of obesity. Reduced efficiency of beta-adrenergic receptor–dependent lipolysis and/or enhanced alpha$_2$-AR-mediated antilipolysis could both impair lipolysis and lead to catecholamine resistance and promote the development and/or stabilization of obesity. It is the increased rate of visceral fat cell lipolysis that is commonly believed to play a pathophysiological role. The reduced lipolysis commonly reported in subcutaneous AT of obese subjects could be viewed as a physiological adaptive mechanism limiting excess rate of lipolysis. Sequestration of NEFA, in the form of TG, in hypertrophic subcutaneous fat cells may limit deleterious metabolic actions of these metabolites. Environmental factors such as sedentary life-style may worsen a hereditary defect affecting beta-adrenergic receptor-dependent lipolysis, while physical exercise may counterbalance the influence of the hereditary defect. Much information is needed about the disturbances affecting all the steps of the lipolytic cascade and the genetic factors impacting these events. There is no doubt that studies of the interactions between genetic factors and environmental conditions will be of great interest to explain why energy storage differs so widely.

REFERENCES

1. Bouchard C, Després J-P, Mauriège P. Genetic and nongenetic determinants of regional fat distribution. Endocr Rev 1993; 14:72–93.
2. Abumrad N, Harmon C, Ibrahimi A. Membrane transport of long-chain fatty acids: evidence for a facilitated process. J Lipid Res 1998; 39:2309–2318.
3. Hamilton JA, Kamp F. How are free fatty acids transported in membranes? Is it by proteins or by free diffusion through the lipids? Diabetes 1999; 48:2255–2269.
4. Frohnert BI, Bernlohr DA. Regulation of fatty acid transporters in mammalian cells. Prog Lipid Res 2000; 39:83–107.
5. Anthonsen MW, Rönnstrand L, Wernstedt C, Degerman E, Holm C. Identification of novel phosphorylation sites in hormone-sensitive lipase that are phosphorylated in response to isoproterenol and govern activation properties in vitro. J Biol Chem 1998; 273:215–221.
6. Greenberg AS, Shen WJ, Muliro K, Patel S, Souza SC, Roth RA, Kraemer FB. Stimulation of lipolysis and hormone-sensitive lipase via the extracellular signal-regulated kinase pathway. J Biol Chem 2001; 276: 45456–45461.
7. Holm C, Osterlund T, Laurell H, Contreras JA. Molecular mechanisms regulating hormone-sensitive lipase and lipolysis. Annu Rev Nutr 2000; 20:365–393.
8. Hirsch AH, Rosen OM. Lipolytic stimulation modulates the subcellular distribution of hormone-sensitive lipase in 3T3-L1 cells. J Lipid Res 1984; 25:665–677.
9. Egan JJ, Greenberg AS, Chang M-K, Wek SA, Moos J, Londos C. Mechanism of hormone-stimulated lipolysis in adipocytes: translocation of hormone-sensitive lipase to the lipid storage droplet. Proc Natl Acad Sci USA 1992; 89:8537–8541.
10. Brasaemle DL, Levin DM, Adler-Wailes DC, Londos C. The lipolytic stimulation of 3T3-L1 adipocytes promotes the translocation of hormone-sensitive lipase to the surfaces of lipid storage droplets. Biochim Biophys Acta 2000; 1483:251–262.
11. Osuga J, Ishibashi S, Oka T, Yagyu H, Tozawa R, Fujimoto A, Shionoiri F, Yahagi N, Kraemer FB, Tsutsumi O, Yamada N. Targeted disruption of hormone-sensitive lipase results in male sterility and adipocyte hypertrophy, but not in obesity. Proc Natl Acad Sci USA 2000; 97:787–792.
12. Wang SP, Laurin N, Himms-Hagen J, Rudnicki MA, Levy E, Robert M-F, Pan L, Oligny L, Mitchell GA. The adipose tissue phenotype of hormone-sensitive lipase deficiency in mice. Obesity Res 2001; 9:119–128.
13. Haemmerle G, Zimmermann R, Hayn M, Theussl C, Waeg G, Wagner E, Sattler W, Magin TM, Wagner E, Zechner R. Hormone-sensitive lipase deficiency in mice causes diglyceride accumulation in adipose tissue, muscle and testis. J Biol Chem 2002; 277:4806–4815.
14. Shen WJ, Sridhar K, Bernlohr DA, Kraemer FB. Interaction of rat hormone-sensitive lipase with adipocyte lipid-binding protein. Proc Natl Acad Sci USA 1999; 96:5528–5532.
15. Syu LJ, Saltiel AR. Lipotransin: a novel docking protein for hormone-sensitive lipase. Mol Cell 1999; 4:109–115.
16. Scheja L, Makowski L, Uysal KT, Wiesbrock SM, Shimshek DR, Meyers DS, Morgan M, Parker RA, Hotamisligil GS. Altered insulin secretion associated with reduced lipolytic efficiency in aP2-/- mice. Diabetes 1999; 48:1987–1994.
17. Coe NR, Simpson MA, Bernlohr DA. Targeted disruption of the adipocyte lipid-binding protein (aP2 protein) gene impairs fat cell lipolysis and increases cellular fatty acid levels. J Lipid Res 1999; 40:967–972.
18. Londos C, Brasaemle DL, Schultz CJ, Adler-Wailes DC, Levin DM, Kinimel AR, Rondinone CM. On the control of lipolysis in adipocytes. Ann NY Acad Sci 1999; 892:155–168.
19. Martinez-Botas J, Anderson JB, Tessier D, Lapillonne A, Chang BH, Quast MJ, Gorenstein D, Chen KH, Chan L. Absence of perilipin results in leanness and reverses obesity in Leprdb/db mice. Nat Genet 2000; 26:474–479.
20. Tansey JT, Sztalryd C, Gruia-Gray J, Roush DL, Zee JV, Gavrilova O, Reitman ML, Deng C-X, Li C, Kimmel AR, Londos C. Perilipin ablation results in a lean mouse with aberrant adipocyte lipolysis, enhanced leptin production, and resistance to diet-induced obesity. Proc Natl Acad Sci USA 2001; 98:6494–6499.
21. Raclot T, Groscolas R. Selective mobilization of adipose tissue fatty acids during energy depletion in the rat. J Lipid Res 1995; 36:2164–2173.
22. Halliwell KJ, Fielding BA, Samra JS, Humphreys SM,

Frayn KN. Release of individual fatty acids from human adipose tissue in vivo after an overnight fast. J Lipid Res 1996; 37:1842–1848.
23. Raclot T, Mioskowski E, Bach AC, Groscolas R. Selectivity of fatty acid mobilization: a general metabolic feature of adipose tissue. Am J Physiol 1995; 269:R1060–R1067.
24. Raclot T, Langin D, Lafontan M, Groscolas R. Selective release of human adipocyte fatty acids according to molecular structure. Biochem J 1997; 324: 911–915.
25. Raclot T, Holm C, Langin D. A role for hormone-sensitive lipase in the selective mobilization of adipose tissue fatty acids. Biochim Biophys Acta 2001; 1532:88–96.
26. Raclot T, Holm C, Langin D. Fatty acid specificity of hormone-sensitive lipase and its implication in the selective hydrolysis of adipose tissue triacylglycerols. J Lipid Res 2001; 42:2049–2057.
27. Plée-Gauthier E, Grober J, Duplus E, Langin D, Forest C. Inhibition of hormone-sensitive lipase gene expression by cAMP and phorbol esters in 3T3-F442A and BFC-1 adipocytes. Biochem J 1996; 318:1057–1063.
28. Raclot T, Dauzats M, Langin D. Regulation of hormone-sensitive lipase expression by glucose in 3T3-F442A adipocytes. Biochem Biophys Res Commun 1998; 245:510–513.
29. Botion LM, Green A. Long-term regulation of lipolysis and hormone-sensitive lipase by insulin and glucose. Diabetes 1999; 48:1691–1697.
30. Langin D, Laurell H, Stenson Holst L, Belfrage P, Holm C. Gene organization and primary structure of human hormone-sensitive lipase: possible significance of a sequence homology with a lipase of *Moraxella* TA144, an antarctic bacterium. Proc Natl Acad Sci USA 1993; 90:4897–4901.
31. Grober J, Laurell H, Blaise R, Fabry B, Schaak S, Holm C, Langin D. Characterization of the promoter of human adipocyte hormone-sensitive lipase. Biochem J 1997; 328:453–461.
32. Smih F, Rouet P, Lucas S, Mairal A, Sengenes C, Lafontan M, Vaulont S, Casado M, Langin D. Transcriptional regulation of adipocyte hormone-sensitive lipase by glucose. Diabetes 2002; 51:293-300.
33. Laurell H, Grober J, Vindis C, Lacombe T, Dauzats M, Holm C, Langin D. Species-specific alternative splicing generates a catalytically inactive form of human hormone-sensitive lipase. Biochem J 1997; 328: 137–143.
34. Mauriège P, Pergola GD, Berlan M, Lafontan M. Human fat cell beta-adrenergic receptors: beta agonist–dependent lipolytic responses and characterization of beta-adrenergic binding sites on human fat cell membranes with highly selective beta1-antagonists. J Lipid Res 1988; 29:587–601.
35. Barbe P, Millet L, Galitzky J, Lafontan M, Berlan M. In situ assessment of the role of the β1-, β2-, and β3-adrenoceptors in the control of lipolysis and nutritive blood flow in human subcutaneous adipose tissue. Br J Pharmacol 1996; 117:907–913.
36. Tavernier G, Barbe P, Galitzky J, Berlan M, Caput D, Lafontan M, Langin D. Expression of β3-adrenoceptors with low lipolytic action in human subcutaneous fat cells. J Lipid Res 1996; 37:87–97.
37. Arch JRS, Wilson S. Prospects for β3-adrenoceptor agonists in the treatment of obesity and diabetes. Int J Obes 1996; 20:191–199.
38. Galitzky J, Langin D, Verwaerde P, Montastruc J-L, Lafontan M, Berlan M. Lipolytic effects of conventional β3-adrenoceptor agonists and of CGP 12,177 in rat and human fat cells: preliminary pharmacological evidence for a putative β4-adrenoceptor. Br J Pharmacol 1997; 122:1244–1250.
39. Galitzky J, Langin D, Montastruc JL, Lafontan M, Berlan M. On the presence of a putative fourth beta-adrenoceptor in human adipose tissue. Trends Pharmacol Sci 1998; 19:164–166.
40. Konkar AA, Zhai Y, Granneman JG. β1-adrenergic receptors mediate β3-adrenergic-independent effects of CGP12177 in brown adipose tissue. Mol Pharmacol 2000; 57:252–258.
41. Schiffelers SLH, Blaak EE, Saris WHM, Van Baak MA. In vivo β3-adrenergic stimulation of human thermogenesis and lipid utilization. Clin Pharmacol Ther 2000; 67:558–566.
42. Serradeil–Le Gal C, Lafontan M, Raufaste D, Marchand J, Pouzet B, Casellas P, Pascal M, Maffrand J-P, Fur GL. Characterization of NPY receptors controlling lipolysis and leptin secretion in human adipocytes. FEBS Lett 2000; 475:150–156.
43. Lafontan M, Berlan M. Fat cell α2-adrenoceptors: the regulation of fat cell function and lipolysis. Endocr Rev 1995; 16:716–738.
44. Kather H. Purine accumulation in human fat cell suspensions. J Biol Chem 1988; 263:8803–8809.
45. Kather H. Pathways of purine metabolism in human adipocytes: further evidence against a role of adenosine as an endogenous regulator of human fat cell function. J Clin Invest 1990; 265:96–102.
46. Lönnroth P, Jansson P-A, Fredholm BB, Smith U. Microdialysis of intercellular adenosine concentration in subcutaneous adipose tissue in humans. Am J Physiol 1989; 256:E250–E255.
47. Moxham CM, Hod Y, Malbon CC. Gi-alpha2 mediates the inhibitory regulation of adenylyl cyclase in vivo: analysis in transgenic mice with Gi-alpha2 suppressed by inducible antisense RNA. Dev Genet 1993; 14:266–273.
48. Kather H, Simon B. Biphasic effects of prostaglandin E2 on the human fat cell adenylate cyclase. J Clin Invest 1979; 64:609–612.

49. Saltiel AR, Pessin JE. Insulin signaling pathways in time and space. Trends Cell Biol 2002; 12:65–71.
50. Rondinone CM, Carvalho E, Rahn T, Manganiello VC, Degerman E, Smith UP. Phosphorylation of PDE3B by phosphoinositol 3-kinase associated with the insulin receptor. J Biol Chem 2000; 275:10093-10098.
51. Graves LM, J C Lawrence J. Insulin, growth factors and cAMP. Antagonism in the signal transduction pathways. Trends Endocrinol Metab 1996; 7:43–50.
52. Sengenes C, Berlan M, De Glisezinski I, Lafontan M, Galitzky J. Natriuretic peptides: a new lipolytic pathway in human adipocytes. FASEB J 2000; 14:1345–1351.
53. Strålfors P, Belfrage P. Phosphorylation of hormone-sensitive lipase by cyclic GMP–dependent protein kinase. FEBS Lett 1985; 180:280–284.
54. Galitzky J, Sengenes C, Thalamas C, Marques M-A, Senard J-M, Lafontan M, Berlan M. The lipid mobilizing effect of atrial natriuretic peptide is unrelated to sympathetic nervous system activation or obesity in young men. J Lipid Res 2001; 42:536–544.
55. Sengenes C, Stich V, Berlan M, Hejnova J, Lafontan M, Pariskova Z, Galitzky J. Increased lipolysis in adipose tissue and lipid mobilization to natriuretic peptides during low-calorie diet in obese women. Int J Obes 2002; 26:24–32.
56. Gravholt CH, Schmitz O, Simonsen L, Bulow J, Christiansen JS, Moller N. Effects of a physiological GH pulse on interstitial glycerol in abdominal and femoral adipose tissue. Am J Physiol 1999; 277:E848–E854.
57. Samra JS, Clark ML, Humphreys SM, Macdonald IA, Bannister PA, Matthews DR, Frayn KN. Suppression of the nocturnal rise in growth hormone reduces subsequent lipolysis in subcutaneous adipose tissue. Eur J Clin Invest 1999; 29:1045–1052.
58. Hefferman MA, Jiang WJ, Thorburn AW, Ng FM. Effects of oral administration of a synthetic fragment of human growth hormone on lipid metabolism. Am J Physiol 2000; 279:E501–E507.
59. Hauner H, Petruschke T, Russ M, Röhrig K, Eckel J. Effects of tumor necrosis factor alpha (TNFα) on glucose transport and lipid metabolism of newly differentiated human fat cells in culture. Diabetologia 1995; 38:764–771.
60. Sethi J, Xu H, Uysal K, Wiesbrock S, Scheja L, Hotamisligil G. Characterisation of receptor-specific TNFα functions in adipocyte cell lines lacking type 1 and 2 TNF receptors. FEBS Lett 2000; 469:77–82.
61. Souza SC, De Vargas LM, Yamamoto MT, Lien P, Franciosa MD, Moss LG, Greenberg AS. Overexpression of perilipin A and B blocks the ability of tumor necrosis factor-α to increase lipolysis in 3T3-L1 adipocytes. J Biol Chem 1998; 273:24665–24669.
62. Gasic S, Tian B, Green A. Tumor necrosis factor alpha stimulates lipolysis in adipocytes by decreasing Gi protein concentrations. J Biol Chem 1999; 274: 6770–6775.
63. Ryden M, Dicker A, Harmelen VV, Hauner H, Brunnberg M, Perbeck L, Lönnqvist F, Amer P. Mapping of early signalling events in TNF-α-mediated lipolysis in human fat cells. J Biol Chem 2002; 277:1085–1091.
64. Gaudiot N, Jaubert A-M, Charbonnier E, Sabourault D, Lacasa D, Giudicelli Y, Ribière C. Modulation of white adipose tissue lipolysis by nitric oxide. J Biol Chem 1998; 273:13475–13481.
65. Andersson K, Gaudiot N, Ribière C, Elizalde M, Giudicelli Y, Arner P. A nitric oxide–mediated mechanism regulates lipolysis in human adipose tissue in vivo. Br J Pharmacol 1999; 126:1639–1645.
66. Tisdale M. Wasting in cancer. J Nutr 1999; 129 (1suppl):243S–246S.
67. Groundwater M, Bulcavage L, Barton C, Adamson C, Ferrier I, Tisdale M. Alteration of serum and urinary lipolytic activity with weight loss in cachectic cancer patients. Br J Cancer 1990; 62:816–821.
68. Coppack SW, Jensen MD, Miles JM. In vivo regulation of lipolysis in humans. J Lipid Res 1994; 35: 177–193.
69. Large V, Arner P, Reynisdottir S, Grober J, Harmelen VV, Holm C, Langin D. Hormone-sensitive lipase expression and activity in relation to lipolysis in human fat cells. J Lipid Res 1998; 39:1688–1695.
70. Lafontan M, Berlan M. Fat cell adrenergic receptors and the control of white and brown fat cell function. J Lipid Res 1993; 34:1057–1091.
71. Arner P. Catecholamine-induced lipolysis in obesity. Int J Obes 1999; 23(suppl 1):10–13.
72. Langin D, Lucas S, Lafontan M. Millenium fat-cell lipolysis reveals unsuspected novel tracks. Horm Metab Res 2000; 32:443–452.
73. Kissebah A, Krakower GR. Regional adiposity and morbidity. Physiol Rev 1994; 74:761–811.
74. Leibel R, Edens NK, Fried SK. Physiologic basis for the control of body fat distribution in humans. Annu Rev Nutr 1989; 9:417–443.
75. Abate N, Garg A. Heterogeneity in adipose tissue metabolism: causes, implications and management of regional adiposity. Prog Lipid Res 1995; 34:53–70.
76. Jensen MD. Lipolysis: contribution from regional fat. Annu Rev Nutr 1997; 17:127–139.
77. Hellström L, Rössner S, Hagström-Toft E, Reynisdottir S. Lipolytic catecholamine resistance linked to β2-adrenoceptor sensitivity—a metabolic predictor of weight loss in obese subjects. Int J Obes 1997; 21:314–320.
78. Mauriège P, Imbeault P, Langin D, Lacaille M, Alméras N, Tremblay A, Després JP. Regional and gender variations in adipose tissue lipolysis in response to weight loss. J Lipid Res 1999; 40:1559–1571.

79. Arner P. Control of lipolysis and its relevance to development of obesity in man. Diabetes Metab Rev 1988; 4:507–515.
80. Lönnqvist F, Wahrenberg H, Hellstrom L, Reynisdottir S, Arner P. Lipolytic catecholamine resistance due to decreased β2-adrenoceptor expression in fat cells. J Clin Invest 1992; 90:2175–2186.
81. Zierath J, Livingston J, Thorne A, Bolinder J, Reynisdottir S, Lonnqvist F, Arner P. Regional difference in insulin inhibition of non-esterified fatty acid release from human obese adipocytes: relation to insulin receptor phosphorylation and intracellular signalling through the insulin receptor substrate-1 pathway. Diabetologia 1998; 41:1343–1354.
82. Meek SE, Nair KS, Jensen MD. Insulin regulation of regional free fatty acid metabolism. Diabetes 1999;48: 10–14.
83. Blaak EE. Adrenergically stimulated fat utilization and ageing. Ann Med 2000; 32:380–382.
84. Imbeault P, Prud'Homme D, Tremblay A, Després J, Mauriège P. Adipose tissue metabolism in young and middle-aged men after control for total body fatness. J Clin Endocrinol Metab 2000; 85:2455–2462.
85. Wolfe R. Substrate utilization/insulin resistance in sepsis/trauma. Bailleres Clin Endocrinol Metab 1997; 11:645–657.
86. Townsend R, Klein S, Wolfe R. Changes in lipolytic sensitivity following repeated epinephrine infusion in humans. Am J Physiol 1994; 266:E155–E160.
87. Stallnecht B, Bülow J, Frandsen E, Galbo H. Desensitization of human adipose tissue to adrenaline stimulation studied by microdialysis. J Physiol 1997;500:271–282.
88. Horowitz J, Klein S. Lipid metabolism during endurance exercise. Am J Clin Nutr 2000; 72(suppl):558S–563S.
89. Head A. Exercise metabolism and β-blocker therapy. An update. Sports Med 1999; 27:81–96.
90. Stallknecht B, Simonsen L, Bülow J, Vinten J, Galbo H. Effect of training on epinephrine-stimulated lipolysis determined by microdialysis in human adipose tissue. Am J Physiol 1995; 269:E1059–E1066.
91. De Glisezinski I, Crampes F, Harant I, Berlan M, Hejnova J, Langin D, Rivière D, Stich V. Endurance training changes in lipolytic responsiveness of obese adipose tissue. Am J Physiol 1998; 275:E951–E956.
92. Stich V, De Glisezinski I, Galitzky J, Hejnova J, Crampes F, Rivière D, Berlan M. Endurance training increases the β-adrenergic lipolytic response in subcutaneous adipose tissue in obese subjects. Int J Obes 1999; 23:374–381.
93. Mauriège P, Prud'Homme D, Marcotte M, Yoshioka M, Tremblay A, Després JP. Regional differences in adipose tissue metabolism between sedentary and endurance-trained women. Am J Physiol 1997; 273:E497–E506.
94. De Glisezinski I, Marion-Latard F, Crampes F, Berlan M, Hejnova J, Cottet-Emard J-M, Stich V, Rivière D. Lack of alpha2-adrenergic antilipolytic effect during exercise in subcutaneous adipose tissue of trained men. J Appl Physiol 2001; 91:1760–1765.
95. Abate N, Garg A, Peshock RM, Stray-Gundersen J, Grundy SM. Relationships of generalized and regional adiposity to insulin sensitivity in men. J Clin Invest 1995; 96:88–98.
96. Leibel RL, Hirsch J, Berry EM, Gruen RK. Alterations in adipocyte free fatty acid re-esterification associated with obesity and weight reduction in man. Am J Clin Nutr 1985; 82:198–206.
97. Jansson P-A, Larsson A, Smith U, Lönnroth P. Glycerol production in subcutaneous adipose tissue of lean and obese humans. J Clin Invest 1992; 89: 1610–1617.
98. Reynisdottir S, Dauzats M, Thorne A, Langin D. Comparison of hormone-sensitive lipase activity in visceral and subcutaneous human adipose tissue. J Clin Endocrinol Metab 1997; 82:4162–4166.
99. Hellström L, Langin D, Reynisdottir S, Dauzats M, Arner P. Adipocyte lipolysis in normal weight subjects with obesity among first degree relatives. Diabetologia 1996; 39:921–928.
100. Large V, Reynisdottir S, Langin D, Fredby K, Klannemark M, Holm C, Arner P. Decreased expression and function of adipocyte hormone-sensitive lipase in subcutaneous fat cells of obese subjects. J Lipid Res 1999; 40:2059–2066.
101. Stich V, Harant I, De Glisezinski I, Crampes F, Berlan M, Kunesova M, Hainer V, Dauzats M, Rivière D, Garrigues M, Holm C, Lafontan M, Langin D. Adipose tissue lipolysis and hormone-sensitive lipase expression during very-low-calorie diet in obese female identical twins. J Clin Endocrinol Metab 1997; 82:739–744.
102. Reynisdottir S, Langin D, Carlström K, Holm C, Rössner S, Arner P. Effects of weight reduction on the regulation of lipolysis in adipocytes of women with upper-body obesity. Clin Sci 1995; 89:421–429.
103. Klein S, Luu K, Gasic S, Green A. Effect of weight loss on whole body and cellular lipid metabolism in severely obese humans. Am J Physiol 1996; 270:E739–E745.
104. Bougnères P, Le Stunff C, Pecqueur C, Pinglier E, Adnot P, Ricquier D. In vivo resistance of lipolysis to epinephrine. A new feature of childhood onset obesity. J Clin Invest 1997; 99:2568–2573.
105. Enoksson S, Talbot M, Rife F, Tamborlane WV, Sherwin RS, Caprio S. Impaired in vivo stimulation of lipolysis in adipose tissue by selective β2-adrenergic agonist in obese adolescent girls. Diabetes 2000; 49:2149–2153.
106. Summers LKM, Samra JS, Frayn KN. Impaired postprandial regulation of blood flow in insulin re-

sistance: a determinant of cardiovascular risk? Atherosclerosis 1999; 147:11–15.
107. Mauriège P, Després JP, Prud'homme D, Pouliot MC, Marcotte M, Tremblay A, Bouchard C. Regional variation in adipose tissue lipolysis in lean and obese men. J Lipid Res 1991; 32:1625–1633.
108. Mauriège P, Prud'homme D, Lemieux S, Tremblay A, Després J-P. Regional differences in adipose tissue lipolysis from lean and obese women: existence of postreceptor alterations. Am J Physiol 1995; 269: E341–E350.
109. Reynisdottir S, Wahrenberg H, Carlström K, Rössner S, Arner P. Catecholamine resistance in fat cells of women with upper-body obesity due to decreased expression of beta2-adrenoceptors. Diabetologia 1994; 37:428–435.
110. Lönnqvist F, Thorne A, Large V, Arner P. Sex differences in visceral fat lipolysis and metabolic complications of obesity. Arterioscler Thromb Vasc Biol 1997; 17:1472–1480.
111. Dodt C, Lonnroth P, Fehm HL, Elam M. Intraneural stimulation elicits an increase in subcutaneous interstitial glycerol levels in humans. J Physiol 1999; 521:545–552.
112. Carel JC, Stunff CL, Condamine L, Mallet E, Chaussain JL, Adnot P, Garabedian M, Bougnères P. Resistance to the lipolytic action of epinephrine: a new feature of protein Gs deficiency. J Clin Endocrinol Metab 1999; 84:4127–4131.
113. Horowitz JF, Klein S. Whole body and abdominal lipolytic sensitivity to epinephrine is suppressed in upper body obese women. Am J Physiol 2000; 278: E1144–E1152.
114. Schiffelers SLH, Saris WHM, Van Baak MA. The effects of an increased NEFA concentration on thermogenesis and substrate oxidation in obese and lean men. Int J Obes 2001; 25:33–38.
115. Blaak EE. Gender differences in fat metabolism. Curr Opin Clin Nutr Metab Care 2001; 4:499–502.
116. Stich V, De Glisezinsky I, Crampes F, Hejnova J, Cottet-Emard J-M, Galitzky J, Lafontan M, Rivière D, Berlan M. Activation of alpha2-adrenergic receptors impairs exercise-induced lipolysis in SCAT of obese subjects. Am J Physiol 2000; 279:R499–R504.
117. Reynisdottir S, Ellerfeldt K, Wahrenberg H, Lithell H, Arner P. Multiple lipolysis defects in the insulin resistance (metabolic) syndrome. J Clin Invest. 1994; 93:2590–2599.
118. Basu A, Basu R, Shah P, Vella A, Rizza RA, Jensen MJ. Systemic and regional free fatty acid metabolism in type 2 diabetes. Am J Physiol 2001; 280:E1000–E1006.
119. Mauriège P, Després J-P, Marcotte M, Tremblay A, Nadeau A, Moorjani S, Lupien P, Dussault J, Fournier G, Thèriault G, Bouchard C. Adipose tissue lipolysis after long-term overfeeding in identical twins. Int J Obes 1992; 16:219–225.
120. Hellström L, Reynisdottir S. Influence of heredity for obesity on adipocyte lipolysis in lean and obese subjects. Int J Obes 2000; 24:340–344.
121. Arner P. Genetic variance and lipolysis regulation: implications for obesity. Ann Med 2001; 33: 542–546.
122. Ryden M, Hoffstedt J, Eriksson P, Brigman S, Arner P. The Arg389 Gly β1-adrenergic receptor gene polymorphism and human fat cell lipolysis. Int J Obesity 2001; 25:1599–1603.
123. Hoffstedt J, Iliadou A, Pedersen NL, Schalling M, Arner P. The effect of the beta2-adrenoceptor gene Thr164Ile polymorphism on human adipose tissue lipolytic function. Br J Pharmacol 2001; 133:708–712.
124. Large V, Hellström L, Reynisdottir S, Lönnqvist F, Eriksson P, Lannfelt L, Arner P. Human beta2-adrenoceptor gene polymorphism are highly frequent in obesity and associated with altered adipocyte beta2-adrenoceptor function. J Clin Invest 1997; 100:3005–3013.
125. Ishiyama-Shigemoto S, Yamada K, Yuan X, Ichikawa F, Nonaka K. Association of polymorphisms in the beta2-adrenergic receptor gene with obesity, hypetriglyceridemia and diabetes mellitus. Diabetologia 1999; 42:98–101.
126. Hellström L, Large V, Reynisdottir S, Wahrenberg H, Arner P. The different effects of a Gln27Glu beta2-adrenoceptor gene polymorphism on obesity in males and females. J Intern Med 1999; 245:253–259.
127. Meirhaeghe A, Luan J, Selberg-Franks P, Hennings S, Mitchell J, Halsall D, O'Rahilly S, Wareham NJ. The effect of the Gly16Arg polymorphism of the beta2-adrenergic receptor gene on plasma free fatty acid levels is modulated by physical activity. J Clin Endocrinol Metab 2001; 86:5881–5887.
128. Meirhaeghe A, Cottel D, Helbecque N, Amouyel P. Impact of polymorphisms in the human β2-adrenoceptor gene on obesity in French population. Int J Obes 2000; 24:382–387.
129. Meirhaeghe A, Helbecque N, Cottel D, Amouyel P. β2-Adrenoceptor gene polymorphism, body weight and physical activity. Lancet 1999; 353:236.
130. Oberkofler H, Esterbauer H, Hell E, Krempler F, Patsch W. The Gln27Glu polymorphism in the beta2-adrenergic receptor gene is not associated with morbid obesity in Austrian women. Int J Obes 2000; 24:388–390.
131. Kortner B, Wolf A, Wendt D, Beisiegeel U, Evans D. Lack of association between a human beta2-adrenoceptor gene polymorphism (Gln27Glu) and morbid obesity. Int J Obes 1999; 23:1099–1100.
132. Allison DB, Heo M, Faith MS, Pietrobelli A. Meta-analysis of the association of the Trp64Arg polymorphism in the β(3-adrenergic receptor with body mass index. Int J Obes 1998; 22:559–566.
133. Carlsson M, Orho-Melander M, Hedenbro J, Groop

LC. Common variants of the beta2-(Gln27Glu) and beta3-(Trp64Arg)-adrenoceptor genes are associated with elevated serum NEFA concentrations and type II diabetes. Diabetologia 2001; 44:629–636.

134. Magré J, Laurell L, Fizames C, Antoine PJ, Dib C, Vigouroux C, Bourut C, Capeau J, Weissenbach J, Langin D. Human hormone-sensitive lipase: genetic mapping, identification of a new dinucleotide repeat and association with obesity and NIDDM. Diabetes 1998; 47:284–286.
135. Klannemark M, Orho M, Langin D, Laurell H, Holm C, Reynisdottir S, Arner P, Groop L. The putative role of the hormone-sensitive lipase gene in the pathogenesis of type II diabetes mellitus and abdominal obesity. Diabetologia 1998; 41:1516–1522.
136. Hoffstedt J, Arner P, Schalling M, Pedersen NL, Sengul S, Ahlberg S, Iliadou A, Lavebratt C. A common hormone-sensitive lipase i6 gene polymorphism is associated with decreased human adipocyte lipolytic function. Diabetes 2001; 50:2410–2413.
137. Clément K, Dina C, Basdevant A, Chastang N, Pelloux V, Lahlou N, Berlan M, Langin D, Guy-Grand B, Froguel P. A candidate gene study in French families with morbid obesity: indication for linkage with islet 1 locus on chromosome 5q. Diabetes 1999; 48(2):398–402.
138. Friedlander Y, Talmud PJ, Edwards KL, Humphries SE, Austin MA. Sib-pair linkage analysis of longitudinal changes in lipoprotein risk factors and lipase genes in women twins. J Lipid Res 2000; 41:1302–1309.
139. Talmud PJ, Palmen J, Walker M. Identification of genetic variation in the human hormone-sensitive lipase gene and 5′sequences: homology of 5′ Sequences with mouse promoter and identification of potential regulatory elements. Biochem Biophys Res Commun 1998; 252:661–668.
140. Stumvoll M, Wahl HG, Jacob S, Rettig A, Machicao F, Haring H. Two novel prevalent polymorphisms in the hormone-sensitive lipase gene have no effect on insulin sensitivity of lipolysis and glucose disposal. J Lipid Res 2001; 42:1782–1788.
141. Talmud PJ, Palmen J, Luan Ja, Flavell D, Byrne CD, Waterworth DM, Wareham NJ. Variation in the promoter of the human hormone sensitive lipase gene shows gender specific effects on insulin and lipid levels: results from the Ely study. Biochim Biophys Acta 2001; 1537:239–244.
142. Marcus C, Karpe B, Bolme P, Sonnenfeld T, Arner P. Changes in catecholamine-induced lipolysis in isolated human fat cells during the first year of life. J Clin Invest 1987; 79:1812–1818.
143. Lönngvist F, Nyberg B, Wahrenberg H, Arner P. Catecholamine-induced lipolysis in adipose tissue of the elderly. J Clin Invest 1990; 85:1614–1621.
144. Reynisdottir S, Dauzats M, Thörne A, Langin D. Comparison of hormone-sensitive lipase activity in visceral and subcutaneous adipose human adipose tissue. J Clin Endocrinol Metab 1997; 82:4162–4166.
145. Reynisdottir S, Wahrenberg H, Carlström K, Rössner S, Arner P. Catecholamine resistance in fat cells of women with upper-body obesity due to decreased expression of β2-adrenoceptors. Diabetologia 1994; 37:428–435.
146. Reynisdottir S, Eriksson M, Angelin B, Arner P. Impaired activation of adipocyte lipolysis in familial combined hyperlipidemia. J Clin Invest 1995; 95:2161–2169.
147. Ek I, Arner P, Bergqvist A, Carlstrom K, Wahrenberg H. Impaired adipocyte lipolysis in nonobese women with the polycystic ovary syndrome: a possible link to insulin resistance? J Clin Endocrinol Metab 1997; 82:1147–1153.
148. Wahrenberg H, Wennlund A, Amer P. Adrenergic regulation of lipolysis in fat cells from hyperthyroid and hypothyroid patients. J Clin Endocrinol Metab 1994; 78:898–903.
149. Wesslau C. Coupling between the beta-adrenergic receptor and the adenylate cyclase—pathophysiological implications. Acta Med Scand 1983; 672:S17–20.
150. Bolinder J, Sjöberg S, Arner P. Stimulation of adipose tissue following insulin-induced hypoglycaemia: evidence of increased beta-adrenoceptor-mediated lipolytic response in IDDM. Diabetologia 1996; 39:845–853.
151. Barbe P, Galitzky J, De Glisezinski I, Rivière D, Thalamas C, Sénard J-M, Crampes F, Lafontan M, Berlan M. Simulated microgravity increases β-adrenergic lipolysis in human adipose tissue. J Clin Endocrinol Metab 1998; 83:619–625.

19

Lipodystrophy and Lipoatrophy

Steven R. Smith

Pennington Biomedical Research Center, Louisiana State University, Baton Rouge, Louisiana, U.S.A.

I INTRODUCTION

Excess adipose tissue is associated with metabolic disturbances and disease, i.e., the metabolic syndrome (1,2). Somewhat paradoxically, inadequate adipose tissue manifests itself in a similar fashion (3,4). This observation demonstrates that adipose tissue is required for normal metabolic function. The inherited and acquired lipodystrophies constitute a heterogeneous group of disorders that share the common feature of inadequate adipose tissue stores.

Although the lipodystrophic disorders represent a variety of underlying pathophysiological states, their common sequelae are instructive, as they are likely to be similar to the metabolic complications associated with "garden-variety" obesity/metabolic syndrome X. Our understanding of the pathophysiology of these patients and parallel models of lipodystrophy in animals point toward the concept of an "optimal" adipose tissue mass that matches the energy requirements of the organism. In addition, these disorders illustrate the central role of adipose tissue to (1) sequester lipid, and (2) adipose tissue as an endocrine organ.

This chapter is divided into three main sections. First, the characterized lipodystrophies and their salient features will be briefly reviewed. Second, the common pathophysiological mechanisms will be discussed in light of the available animal models. Last, based on the mechanisms by which inadequate adipose tissue leads to disease, potential therapeutic strategies are discussed.

The following classification schema follows that of Garg (5), with reference to the schema presented by the Online Mendelian Inheritence in Man (OMIM) by McKusick (6). The reader is referred to the latter reference for a continual update of the rarer lipodystrophy syndromes and a comprehensive bibliography: http://www.ncbi.nlm.nih.gov/Entrez/.

II LIPODYSTROPHIES

A Congenital Generalized Lipodystrophy (CGL)

CGL, OMIM 269700, i.e., Berardinelli-Seip syndrome, is an autosomal-recessive disorder that manifests at birth as a complete absence of adipose tissue, hepatomegaly, and severe nonketotic insulin resistant diabetes. Additional features include acanthosis nigricans and an elevated basal metabolic rate. Mechanical fat in the hands, feet, orbit, scalp, and periarticular fat are usually preserved (3).

B Familial Partial Lipodystrophy (FPL)

FPL, OMIM 151660, familial partial lipodystrophy, an autosomal-dominant disorder, is differentiated from congenital generalized lipodystrophy, an autosomal-recessive disorder, by the timing of the onset (4). FPL manifests during or after puberty, while CGL is present from birth. The FPL syndrome occurs in both men and women, but is most apparent in women owing to the muscular appearance of the extremities and the greater amount of body fat of women in general. Patients are severely insulin resistant, have dyslipidemia with elevated triglycerides and a low HDL, and often develop overt diabetes at an early age. Three "varieties" have been described.

The ***Dunnigan variety*** (OMIM 151660) is characterized by loss of fat in the limbs and trunk, except for the vulva. Excess fat can accumulate in the neck, supraclavicular space, and face, and is sometimes confused with Cushing's syndrome. Acanthosis nigricans and polycystic ovarian syndrome are uncommon. The ***Köbberling variety*** (OMIM 151660) is characterized by loss of subcutaneous fat in the limbs; however, the face and trunk are spared. The ***mandibuloacral dysplasia variety*** (OMIM 248370) demonstrates other congenital defects such as a hypoplastic mandible, severe dental crowding, persistently wide cranial sutures, and multiple Wormian bones. Acro-osteolysis is a hallmark of this syndrome.

C Acquired Lipodystrophy

There are at least three forms of acquired lipodystrophy. ***Acquired generalized lipodystrophy*** **(AGL)** is most likely an autoimmune disease. It is characterized by a generalized progressive loss of adipose tissue, with women more commonly affected than men. Loss of fat from the soles of the feet and palms of the hands may occur. ***Acquired partial lipodystrophy*** **(APL; Barraquer-Simons)** affects the face and neck and spreads downward with sparing of the pelvic girdle and lower extremities (7). Many of these patients exhibit altered complement activation and develop glumerulonephritis with subsequent renal failure. Metabolic complications, such as insulin resistance and dyslipidemia, are uncommon. This is probably due to the sequestration of lipid in the lower extremities and the absence of increased visceral adiposity.

HIV and HIV therapy are associated with an acquired lipodystrophy (8–10). This association was recognized prior to the advent of highly active antiretroviral therapy (HAART). HIV-HAART-associated lipodystrophy was first described in individuals taking a new class of anti-HIV drugs known as the protease inhibitors, although most antiretroviral drugs have been associated with the syndrome. The first features recognized were a "buffalo hump" similar to that seen in Cushing's disease, central-visceral obesity, and loss of fat on the extremities. More recently, the syndrome is known to include elevated triglycerides, insulin resistance, a decrease in facial fat, particularly in the cheeks and temporal area, and loss of subcutaneous fat in the buttocks, arms, and legs. These latter changes have been described as "roping" of the superficial veins in the arms and a muscular appearance to the lower extremities.

III SHARED PATHOPHYSIOLOGY

Several features are shared across the lipodystrophic syndromes. Several of these features are indicative of inadequate adipose tissue to sequester adipose tissue, but may also occur as a manifestation of endocrine deficits, such as hypoleptinemia, that coincide with the decreased adipose tissue mass. A hallmark of the lipodystrophic syndromes is elevated triacylglycerol levels.

At least two anatomic sites exhibit increased lipid infiltration in lipodystrophic patients—skeletal muscle and liver. The aberrant lipid storage manifests as hepatic steatosis, hepatomegaly, and an increase in skeletal muscle lipid on NMR spectroscopy. The pancreatic beta-cell has been proposed as a third site of aberrant lipid storage, but direct evidence of this in humans is lacking. These sites are also affected in patients with the metabolic syndrome X (11–13).

The insulin-resistant state associated with the lipodystrophic syndrome is frequently severe, leading to early-onset diabetes mellitus. Indeed, large doses of insulin are often ineffective at controlling blood glucose. Recent reports suggest that cardiovascular disease is accelerated, with a greater incidence in women than men (14).

A Specific Pathophysiology/Genetics

1 Familial Partial Lipodystrophy

Simultaneous mapping efforts from several laboratories resulted in the determination that the genetic defect in FPL was located at chromosome 1q21-q22. The lamin A/C gene was identified as a positional candidate, and mutations in this gene were subsequently identified in patients with FPLD in 2000 (15,16). The lamins are structural components of the nuclear pore that are thought to be involved in the trafficking of molecules between the cytoplasm and nucleus (17). Lamins A and C differ only in their differentially spliced C-terminal domains. Curiously, FPL mutations are clustered in one portion of the molecule. Mutations in other regions are associated with Emery-Dreifuss muscular dystrophy (18), limb girdle muscular dystrophy 1B (19), or autosomal-dominant dilated cardiomyopathy and conduction system disease (20). The exact mechanism(s) by which Laminin mutations result in a partial loss of adipose tissue are not known (21).

2 PPAR-γ and Familial Partial Lipodystrophy

Recently, several pedigrees were described with severe insulin resistance, diabetes, and peripheral fat wasting (21a). The manifestation of this inherited partial lipodystrophy syndrome is quite similar to the metabolic syndrome X, with the exception that these patients do not respond to the antidiabetic thiazolidinediones (TZDs). These families were found to have mutations in the PPAR-γ nuclear transcription factor gene at the ligand-binding pocket (21b). This results in impaired activation of gene transcription by the TZDs. Newer PPAR-γ ligands with a different structural backbone may bypass this mutation in vitro. Although rare, these mutations are instructive in the sense that the metabolic sequelae are almost identical to the "garden-variety" obesity/syndrome X.

3 Congenital Generalized Lipodystrophy

Lamin does not appear to be involved in congenital generalized lipodystrophy, and the genetic mutation for CGL is unknown. Mapping studies demonstrate linkage to chromosome 9q34. The exact mutation has not been identified (22).

4 Acquired Lipodystrophy

Little is known about the immunological mechanisms that lead to the development of the acquired lipodystrophies. Many of these patients exhibit laboratory features of an autoimmune syndrome and glomerulonephritis (23).

5 HIV-HAART-Associated Lipodystrophy

The drugs used to treat HIV, i.e., highly active antiretroviral therapy, HAART, have themselves been associated with metabolic disturbances in individuals without HIV. However, lipodystrophy syndromes were present before HAART. As such, it is unclear at this time whether the HIV-HAART-associated lipodystrophy can be solely blamed on the pharmacotherapy. Several studies suggest that activation and rebound of the immune system during HAART are associated with lipodystrophy (8,9). In addition, almost all of the effective HIV drugs are associated with lipodystrophy. This is unusual for diverse chemical classes to manifest similar toxicities. Because of these paradoxes, it is possible that reconstitution of the immune system plays a role in the development of HIV-HAART associated lipodystrophy.

B Animal Models

Recent progress in our understanding of the transcriptional cascade involved in the differentiation of adipocyte precursors into mature adipocytes led to the development of transgenic models of lipodystrophy. These models came from the laboratories of Shimomura (24) and Reitman (25). The models are instructive regarding the pathophysiology of the adipose tissue deficiency and are useful in testing pharmacological interventions. A spontaneous mutation in the *lipin* gene is responsible for the ***fld lipodystrophic mouse***, a novel model of the complete lipodystrophy syndrome (26,27). Detailed studies of these animal models may reveal unexpected mechanisms by which a failure to develop adipose tissue results in diabetes and metabolic derangements (28–31).

IV THERAPY

Because of the rarity of these syndromes, little is known regarding specific therapies for lipodystrophy. There are three basic approaches based on the pathophysiology of the syndromes.

First, given that an inability to sequester lipid in adipose tissue is likely to lead to the accumulation of lipid in abnormal locations such as the liver and skeletal muscle, creating a negative fat and calorie balance is recommended. This is difficult in practice, however, and may be due to anecdotal reports of increased appetite, especially in the setting of uncontrolled diabetes. Along these same lines, the "standard" medical therapies for dyslipidemia are indicated, but for patients with hypertriglyceridemia in the face of maximal lipid and diabetes medications, plasmapheresis may be necessary. Newer therapies that target specific metabolic defects are likely to supplant this therapy.

A second approach is based on the known pathways affecting insulin sensitivity. For example, the thiazolidinediones have been used with success in the treatment of these patients (32). As a cautionary note, one of these patients developed liver complications during therapy with troglitazone, and liver enzyme testing at regular intervals may be more important than in the routine diabetic patient. Given this caveat, the newer TZDs, which are less likely to cause liver toxicity, are likely to become a first-line therapy for lipodystrophic metabolic syndromes.

A third approach is based on the observation that patients with CGL and FPL have low leptin levels. Preliminary data from the lipodystrophy groups in Dallas and Bethesda support the concept that leptin replacement is a useful therapeutic strategy. Short-term therapy with leptin resulted in a fall in triglyceride levels and a reduction in hepatomegaly in patients with lipodystrophy. This suggests that the actions of leptin to increase fat oxidation results in a decrease in tissue stores of fatty acids. This makes sense given that in in vivo systems, leptin regulates fat oxidation (33,34). As more patients are enrolled in these experimental protocols and our understanding of the pathophysiology progresses, specific therapies are likely to follow these encouraging results.

V THE FUTURE

Understanding the underlying genetic causes of the CGL syndrome is an important short-term milestone. As we understand the common mechanism by which inadequate adipose tissue stores contribute to disease, we will develop specific therapies. These therapies will consist of treatment not only for the metabolic sequelae but also for the defects in adipocyte proliferation and/or differentiation that cause these diverse syndromes. Several of these can be anticipated; i.e., drugs that increase fat oxidation, improve insulin resistance, or replace decreased hormones (e.g., leptin) are likely to occur in a shorter time span. Other therapies will not be obvious until we understand the complex mechanisms of genes such as laminin A/C or lipin and the pathophysiology of CGL.

NOTE ADDED IN PROOF

Recent genetic studies revealed mutations in the triglyceride synthetic enzyme AGPAT2 as the cause of some, but not all, cases of CGL (35). Other cases are due to mutations in Seipin (36), also known as guanine nucleotide binding protein, gamma 3. The exact mechanism(s) responsible for the lack of adipose tissue development are still unclear (37–39).

REFERENCES

1. Bjorntorp P. Visceral obesity: a civilization syndrome. Obes Res 1993; 1:206–222.
2. Bouchard C, Despres JP, Mauriege P. Genetic and nongenetic determinants of regional fat distribution. Endocr Rev 1993; 14:72–93.
3. Seip M, Trygstad O. Generalized lipodystrophy, congenital and acquired (lipoatrophy). Acta Paediatr Suppl 1996; 413:2–28.
4. Kobberling J, Dunnigan MG. Familial partial lipodystrophy: two types of an X linked dominant syndrome, lethal in the hemizygous state. J Med Genet 1986; 23:120–127.
5. Garg A. Lipodystrophies. Am J Med 2000; 108:143–152.
6. Hamosh A, Scott AF, Amberger J, Valle D, McKusick VA. Online Mendelian Inheritance in Man (OMIM). Hum Mutat 2000; 15:57–61.
7. Spranger S, Spranger M, Tasman AJ, Reith W, Voigtlander T, Voigtlander V. Barraquer-Simons syndrome (with sensorineural deafness): a contribution to the differential diagnosis of lipodystrophy syndromes. Am J Med Genet 1997; 71:397–400.
8. Ledru E, Christeff N, Patey O, De Truchis P, Melchior JC, Gougeon MI. Alteration of tumor necrosis factor-alpha T-cell homeostasis following potent antiretroviral therapy: contribution to the development of human immunodeficiency virus-associated lipodystrophy syndrome. Blood 2000; 95: 3191–3198.
9. Mynarcik DC, McNurlan MA, Steigbigel RT, Fuhrer J, Gelato MC. Association of severe insulin resistance with both loss of limb fat and elevated serum tumor necrosis factor receptor levels in HIV lipodystrophy. J AIDS 2000; 25:312–321.
10. Carr A, Samaras K, Thorisdottir A, Kaufmann GR, Chisholm DJ, Cooper DA. Diagnosis, prediction, and natural course of HIV-1 protease-inhibitor-associated lipodystrophy, hyperlipidaemia, and diabetes mellitus: a cohort study. Lancet 1999; 353:2093–2099.
11. Ryysy L, Hakkinen AM, Goto T, Vehkavaara S, Westerbacka J, Halavaara J, Yki-Jarvinen H. Hepatic fat content and insulin action on free fatty acids and glucose metabolism rather than insulin absorption are associated with insulin requirements during insulin therapy in type 2 diabetic patients. Diabetes 2000; 49:749–758.
12. Krssak M, Falk Petersen K, Dresner A, DiPietro L, Vogel SM, Rothman DL, Roden M, Shulman GI. Intramyocellular lipid concentrations are correlated with insulin sensitivity in humans: a ^{1}H NMR spectroscopy study. Diabetologia 1999; 42:113–116.
13. Shulman GI. Cellular mechanisms of insulin resistance in humans. Am J Cardiol 1999; 84:3J–10J.
14. Hegele RA. Premature atherosclerosis associated with monogenic insulin resistance. Circulation 2001; 103: 2225–2229.
15. Speckman RA, Garg A, Du F, Bennett L, Veile R, Arioglu E, Taylor SI, Lovett M, Bowcock AM. Mutational and haplotype analyses of families with familial partial lipodystrophy (Dunnigan variety) reveal recurrent missense mutations in the globular C-terminal domain of lamin A/C. Am J Hum Genet 2000; 66: 1192–1198.
16. Cao H, Hegele RA. Nuclear lamin A/C R482Q muta-

tion in Canadian kindreds with Dunnigan-type familial partial lipodystrophy. Hum Mol Genet 2000; 9:109–112.

17. Genschel J, Schmidt HH. Mutations in the LMNA gene encoding lamin A/C. Hum Mutat 2000;16:451–459.
18. Emery AE. Emery-Dreifuss muscular dystrophy—a 40 year retrospective. Neuromuscul Disord 2000; 10:228–232.
19. Kitaguchi T, Matsubara S, Sato M, Miyamoto K, Hirai S, Schwartz K, Bonne G. A missense mutation in the exon 8 of lamin A/C gene in a Japanese case of autosomal dominant limb-girdle muscular dystrophy and cardiac conduction block. Neuromuscul Disord 2001; 11:542–546.
20. Jakobs PM, Hanson EL, Crispell KA, Toy W, Keegan H, Schilling K, Icenogle TB, Litt M, Hershberger RE. Novel lamin A/C mutations in two families with dilated cardiomyopathy and conduction system disease. J Card Fail 2001; 7:249–256.
21. Nagano A, Arahata K. Nuclear envelope proteins and associated diseases. Curr Opin Neurol 2000; 13:533–539.

21a. Agarwal AK, Garg A. A novel heterozygous mutation in peroxisome proliferator-activated receptor-gamma gene in a patient with familial partial lipodystrophy. J Clin Endocrinol Metab 2002; 87:408–411.

21b. Barroso I, Gurnell M, Crowley VE, et al. Dominant negative mutations in human PPARgamma associated with severe insulin resistance, diabetes mellitus and hypertension. Nature 1999; 402:880–883.

22. Garg A, Wilson R, Barnes R, Arioglu E, Zaidi Z, Gurakan F, Kocak N, O'Rahilly S, Taylor SI, Patel SB, Bowcock AM. A gene for congenital generalized lipodystrophy maps to human chromosome 9q34. J Clin Endocrinol Metab 1999; 84:3390–3394.
23. Levy Y, George J, Yona E, Shoenfeld Y. Partial lipodystrophy, mesangiocapillary glomerulonephritis, and complement dysregulation. An autoimmune phenomenon. Immunol Res 1998; 18:55–60.
24. Shimomura I, Hammer RE, Richardson JA, Ikemoto S, Bashmakov Y, Goldstein JL, Brown MS. Insulin resistance and diabetes mellitus in transgenic mice expressing nuclear SREBP-1c in adipose tissue: model for congenital generalized lipodystrophy. Genes Dev 1998; 12:3182–3194.
25. Reitman ML, Mason MM, Moitra J, Gavrilova O, Marcus-Samuels B, Eckhaus M, Vinson C. Transgenic mice lacking white fat: models for understanding human lipoatrophic diabetes. Ann NY Acad Sci 1999; 892:289–296.
26. Peterfy M, Phan J, Xu P, Reue K. Lipodystrophy in the fld mouse results from mutation of a new gene encoding a nuclear protein, lipin. Nat Genet 2001; 27: 121–124.
27. Reue K, Xu P, Wang XP, Slavin BG. Adipose tissue deficiency, glucose intolerance, and increased atherosclerosis result from mutation in the mouse fatty liver dystrophy (fld) gene. J Lipid Res 2000; 41:1067–1076.
28. Ebihara K, Ogawa Y, Masuzaki H, Shintani M, Miyanaga F, Aizawa-Abe M, Hayashi T, Hosoda K, Inoue G, Yoshimasa Y, Gavrilova O, Reitman ML, Nakao K. Transgenic overexpression of leptin rescues insulin resistance and diabetes in a mouse model of lipoatrophic diabetes. Diabetes 2001; 50:1440–1448.
29. Yamauchi T, Kamon J, Waki H, Terauchi Y, Kubota N, Hara K, Mori Y, Ide T, Murakami K, Tsuboyama-Kasaoka N, Ezaki O, Akanuma Y, Gavrilova O, Vinson C, Reitman ML, Kagechika H, Shudo K, Yoda M, Nakano Y, Tobe K, Nagai R, Kimura S, Tomita M, Froguel P, Kadowaki T. The fat-derived hormone adiponectin reverses insulin resistance associated with both lipoatrophy and obesity. Nat Med 2001; 7:941–946.
30. Kim JK, Gavrilova O, Chen Y, Reitman ML, Shulman GI. Mechanism of insulin resistance in A-ZIP/F-1 fatless mice. J Biol Chem 2000; 275:8456–8460.
31. Gavrilova O, Marcus-Samuels B, Graham D, Kim JK, Shulman GI, Castle AL, Vinson C, Eckhaus M, Reitman ML. Surgical implantation of adipose tissue reverses diabetes in lipoatrophic mice. J Clin Invest 2000; 105:271–278.
32. Arioglu E, Duncan-Morin J, Sebring N, Rother KI, Gottlieb N, Lieberman J, Herion D, Kleiner DE, Reynolds J, Premkumar A, Sumner AE, Hoofnagle J, Reitman ML, Taylor SI. Efficacy and safety of troglitazone in the treatment of lipodystrophy syndromes. Ann Intern Med 2000; 133:263–274.
33. Muoio DM, Dohm GL, Fiedorek FT Jr, Tapscott EB, Coleman RA, Dohn GL. Leptin directly alters lipid partitioning in skeletal muscle. Diabetes 1997; 46:1360–1363.
34. Muoio DM, Dohm GL, Tapscott EB, Coleman RA. Leptin opposes insulin's effects on fatty acid partitioning in muscles isolated from obese ob/ob mice. Am J Physiol 1999; 276:E913–E921.
35. Agarwal AK, Arioglu E, De Almeida S, et al. AGPAT2 is mutated in congenital generalized lipodstrophy linked to chromosome 9q34. Nat Genet 2002; 81:21–23.
36. Magre J, Delepine M, Khallouf E, et al. Identification of the gene altered in Berardinelli-Seip congenital lipodystrophy on chromosome 11q13. Nat Genet 2001; 28:365–370.
37. Lloyd DJ, Trembath RC, Shackleton S. A novel interaction between lamin A and SREBP1: implications for partial lipodystrophy and other laminopathies. Hum Mol Genet 2002; 11:769–777.
38. Dhe-Paganon S, Werner ED, Chi YI, Shoelson SE. Structure of the globular tail of nuclear lamin. J Biol Chem 2002; 277:17381–17384.
39. Pages C, Daviaud D, An S, Krief S, Lafontan M, Valet P, Saulnier-Blache JS. Endothelial differentiation gene-2 receptor is involved in lysophosphatidic acid-dependent control of 3T3F442A preadipocyte proliferation and spreading. J Biol Chem 2001; 276:11599–11605.

20

Uncoupling Proteins

Daniel Ricquier

UPR 9078, Centre National de la Recherche Scientifique, Faculty of Medicine, Necker-Sick Children, Paris, France

Leslie P. Kozak

Pennington Biomedical Research Center, Louisiana State University, Baton Rouge, Louisiana, U.S.A.

I INTRODUCTION

The coupling of respiration to ADP phosphorylation in mitochondria represents the coupling of exergonic and endergonic processes. Actually, such a coupling is never complete and results in energy dissipation as heat. Apart from a role in thermogenesis, uncoupling of respiration limits ATP synthesis and allows NADH reoxidation. In the absence of uncoupling mechanisms, a high level of ATP would inhibit respiration and NADH reoxidation. Two types of mechanisms have been proposed to explain the molecular basis of respiration uncoupling. The first is based on a decreased efficiency of the respiratory chain or "slippage" of respiratory chains; the second one postulates the existence of proton leaks in the mitochondrial inner membrane. Analysis of thermogenic mechanisms in brown adipocytes has established that UCP1 in the inner mitochondrial membrane works as a regulatable proton leak and an uncoupler that stimulates fatty acid oxidation (see below). The recent identification of homologues of UCP1 has extended this regulatory mechanism based on the possible mitochondrial proton leaks to virtually all other tissues. Accordingly, this phenomenon of mitochondrial proton leaks represents a widespread strategy for controlling substrate utilization, and energy partitioning through changes in metabolic efficiency.

II UCP1

A UCP1 in Energy Expenditure and Body Weight Regulation

Pharmacological and genetic manipulations of experimental rodents suggest that nonshivering thermogenesis is one of the most effective strategies for reducing adiposity in obese individuals. While there are many systems of thermogenesis that are theoretically capable of increasing energy expenditure, in fact, a body of evidence confirming that a specific mechanism for increasing thermogenesis is effective in reducing adiposity is available only for mitochondrial uncoupling protein (UCP1)-dependent thermogenesis of brown adipose tissue. The previous edition of the Handbook of Obesity described the biology of brown adipose tissue, the biochemistry of UCP1, and the adrenergic signaling mechanisms that controlled the activation of nonshivering thermogenesis. Although the effectiveness of UCP1 in reducing adiposity in obese rodents is clear its relevance to obesity in humans has remained questionable because of the paucity of brown adipocytes in adult humans. Since the previous edition of the handbook was issued, important developments in mitochondrial uncoupling proteins and the regulation of brown adipocyte differentiation research suggest that a review of uncoupling proteins in body weight regulation is indicated.

The prevailing paradigm guiding obesity research for the past several decades has been the thrifty metabolism ideas originally formulated by Neel (1) and subsequently developed by Coleman (2) and others in their interpretation of not only of human obesity, but also of obesity in rodent models. Briefly, modern human beings are descended from individuals who have adapted to survive during a time when caloric deprivations were common and when high levels of daily physical activity were the norm. In this environment, human evolution selected for individuals with an efficient metabolism—i.e., a maximum level of productive work per unit of food consumed. However, this efficient metabolism in the current world of plentiful food with a high caloric density and physical inactivity has resulted in an epidemic of obesity. One solution to this problem is to develop strategies that reduce metabolic efficiency. The most direct means would be to increase energy expenditure by thermogenesis, i.e., to maximize metabolic inefficiency. As noted above, uncoupling respiration from oxidative phosphorylation is an effective mechanism for heat production, but as important as the mechanism for producing heat itself is, the mechanism for the regulation of nonshivering thermogenesis is equally important. This regulation is controlled by the hypothalamus and mediated by the sympathetic nervous system. As long as adrenergic signaling mechanisms are associated with the control of expression, it is probable that the consequences of overexpression—namely, hyperthermia—will be avoided. In this section we will describe efforts to utilize heat production by the brown fat specific UCP1 for manipulating energy expenditure and adiposity.

The underlying assumption underpinning the hypothesis that UCP1-based thermogenesis could be used to reduce excess body weight, is that this mechanism of thermogenesis functions to regulate the efficiency of energy metabolism as well as to protect the animal from cold exposure. The brown fat is therefore viewed as a pathway for dissipating excess calories by thermogenesis, thereby increasing metabolic inefficiency. This view of brown fat emerged following the landmark paper of Rothwell and Stock (3), who showed that a cafeteria diet could induce nonshivering thermogenesis in rats. The implication of this finding was that in rodents, brown fat thermogenesis was not only induced by exposure to cold, but also by dietary conditions that would lead to an increased, abnormal deposition of fat. In support of this hypothesis are much data indicating that mice and rats with single gene mutations and lesions to the hypothalamus causing hyperphagia and obesity almost invariably have reduced nonshivering thermogenesis [see review by Himms-Hagen (4)]. It suggests that in rodents a normal function of UCP1-based thermogenesis is the regulation of body weight.

However, we do not understand how this putative function of brown fat in body weight regulation is balanced and integrated with its role in regulating body temperature. Evidence that *Ucp1* expression is modulated by leptin and other orexigenic and anorexic peptides provides a biological basis for the idea that the regulation of body weight by these hormones includes the regulation of energy expenditure by UCP1. The relative balance of these functions for brown fat becomes important when attempting to extrapolate from the mouse to the human, because small body size has made brown fat much more important for the regulation of body temperature in the mouse than in the human. Does the primary and dominant role for UCP1 in maintaining body temperature in the rodent provide a secondary but important role in body weight regulation?

The possibility that agents that stimulated brown fat thermogenesis could be useful as antiobesity agents quickly led to the identification of a class of pharmacological agents that were selected on the basis of their ability to stimulate lipolysis and respiration in isolated brown adipocytes (5–7). These agonists were found to interact with atypical beta-adrenergic receptors on adipocytes (8) and were subsequently cloned and called the β3-adrenergic receptor (9). While the β3-adrenergic receptor agonists have proven to be effective agents to stimulate brown fat respiration, lipolysis, *Ucp1* expression, and thermogenesis and to reduce body fat in rodents and dogs (10,11), their effectiveness in treating human obesity has not been established.

There is strong evidence emerging that the discovery of mechanisms for stimulating brown adipocyte thermogenesis in a controlled manner could be an effective means for reducing adiposity. Because of the low levels of UCP1 and brown adipocytes in humans, the primary strategy will be to determine mechanisms that control both the regulation of the *Ucp1* gene and the proliferation and differentiation of the brown adipocyte in adult fat tissue. Molecular genetic approaches that have been used to explore these regulatory problems in the mouse and rat will be described below.

B Overexpression of *Ucp1* with Heterologous Promoters in Transgenic Mice

Treating mice, rats, and dogs with β3-adrenergic receptor agonists has increased the expression of *Ucp1* and brown adipocytes, stimulated lipolysis, and reduced both dietary and genetic obesity (10–13). These weight-reducing effects of the β3-agonists could be due to the effects of adrenergic stimulated breakdown of triglycerides in fat and subsequent oxidation of fatty acids in the muscle. However, two genetic models—one in which *Ucp1* was constitutively expressed in both white and brown fat from the aP2 gene promoter (14), and the other in which *Ucp1* was expressed in muscle from the myosin light chain promoter (MLC-*Ucp1*)—both gave very similar phenotypes (15). The aP2-*Ucp1* transgenic mice were resistant to both genetic and dietary obesity (14,16), and the MLC-*Ucp1* transgenic mice were resistant to dietary obesity, and both transgenes reduced the hyperglycemia and insulin resistance that develops in the background strains used when fed a high-fat diet.

Transgenic systems for overexpression of *Ucp1* have underscored the effectiveness of UCP1-mediated uncoupling on reduction of adipose stores and increasing insulin sensitivity. Since the levels of UCP1 in white fat and the level of UCP1 in muscle in transgenic mice hemizygous for the transgenes were both ~1% of normal brown fat levels, it indicates that very small increases in uncoupling-based thermogenesis are effective in reducing adiposity (15). They also show that it is not necessary to have expression of UCP1 in brown fat or even in white fat to be effective. However, the experiments also illustrate how important it is to control the limits of overexpression. Transgenic mice homozygous for the aP2-*Ucp1* transgene lose ~95% of their brown adipocytes owing to cytotoxicity of UCP1 at excessive levels in brown adipocytes (17), and mice homozygous for the low-expressing MLC-*Ucp1* transgenic animal have severely reduced body weights (15). Since the levels of muscle phosphocreatine and ATP were 60% of normal in mice homozygous for the MLC-*Ucp1* transgene, it suggests that excessive uncoupling by UCP1 is lethal to the cell. The inability of the muscle to maintain ATP levels in the face of excessive uncoupling suggests that normal mechanisms of controlling proton flux at the membrane level are not sufficiently effective in preventing excessive uncoupling (18). Although the transgenic mice were not hyperthermic, it is clear that controlling the level of UCP1 is very important if one is to avoid serious side effects. One problem with an approach to overexpression that is modeled after the transgenic mice described above, is that unlike the normal endogenous *Ucp1* gene, which is stringently regulated by the adrenergic nervous system, the aP2 and MCL promoters are constitutive promoters that are not known to modulate expression through the action of effectors, hormones, etc. Thus, any approach to upregulating the *Ucpl* gene must occur where tight regulatory control is maintained, optimally its own adrenergic signaling system. The value of these transgenic animals is that they have established the principle that upregulation of UCP1 can reduce both obesity and insulin resistance.

C Natural Variation in the Expression of Brown Adipocytes in White Fat Depots

An alternative approach to increasing *Ucpl* gene expression is based on increasing the number of brown adipocytes in an individual. This approach directly addresses the problem of limiting numbers of brown adipocytes in adult humans that preclude a robust response to an adrenergic agonist. It has been observed among several mammalian species that chronic sympathetic stimulation by either cold exposure or adrenergic agonists leads to an increase in brown adipocytes in traditional white fat depots as evidenced by increases in the *Ucpl* expression or by the histological appearance of adipocytes with a multilocular morphology (10,11,19,20). This inductive response may also occur in humans. For example, Finnish laborers working outdoors in the winter months are reported to have larger deposits of brown adipocytes (21), and patients carrying catecholamine-secreting pheochromocytoma develop large depots of brown fat (22). The former report suggests that the increase in brown adipocytes enhances the thermogenic capacity of the laborers; the latter report underscores the possibility that humans have the capacity to increase the number of brown adipocytes.

There is evidence that increased numbers of brown adipocytes in rats treated with β3-adrenergic agonists reduce obesity caused by either a mutation to the leptin receptor or a high-fat diet (11,13). Rats treated with the drugs lost weight and also had elevated numbers of brown adipocytes. However, it is not clear whether rats with induced levels of brown adipocytes lost weight because of increased energy expenditure derived from increased numbers of brown adipocytes or weight was lost by some other mechanism. Similarly, when inbred strains of mice that varied in the numbers of brown adipocytes were treated with a β3-agonist, those strains with more brown adipocytes lost more adipose tissue (23). The same caveat holds for this experiment, since it is possible that other biochemical differences, rather than brown adipocyte number among the strains, affected adiposity.

There has been a careful quantification of *UCP1* expression in human adipose tissue from lean and obese individuals by quantitative RTPCR (24). In this study, it was estimated that approximately one of every one to two hundred adipocytes in human fat depots is a brown adipocyte (24). This is quite a significant level of expression given the fact that expression of a *Ucp1* transgene in mouse muscle at only 1% the level detected in brown fat is able to reduce adiposity and insulin resistance (15). The data of Oberkofler et al. (24) also suggested that *Ucp1* mRNA levels were reduced in the fat depots of the obese individuals, and those researchers speculated that this reduction could reduce energy expenditure in these individuals. Further work needs to be done in both nontransgenic obese animal models and obese humans to establish whether variation in *Ucpl* expression in white adipose tissue can contribute to the level of adiposity.

With the finding that the induction of brown adipocytes in white fat depots varied among inbred strains of mice (23,25), an effort is under way to identify novel cell signaling and transcriptional pathways that can be used to induce brown adipocyte numbers in traditional white fat depots. The objective is to use quantitative genetic methods to map and clone genes that control brown adipocyte differentiation. Quantitative trait locus (QTL) analysis has defined regions on chromosomes 2, 3, 8, and 19 that control brown fat induction in mice (26). Only the QTL on chromosome 8 carries a known gene that could be involved in UCP1 expression and that gene is *Ucp1* itself. However, the genetic data cannot define with sufficient precision the location of the variant genes to any of the QTLs, including those on chromosome 8, to ascribe confidently to them a function in *Ucp1* induction. Since the QTLs on chromosomes 2, 3, and 19 do not carry genes known to be associated with either *Ucp1* expression or adipogenesis, it is highly probable that novel rate-controlling steps in the signaling or transcription of *Ucp1* expression will be discovered from these genetic studies. The evidence that complex interactions between chromosomes 8 and 19 are involved in the regulation of *Ucp1* induction suggests that epistatic gene interactions are controlling *Ucp1* expression.

These genetic studies on brown adipocyte induction are still at early stages. In addition, they have only addressed the regulation of *Ucp1* expression and have not yet investigated the regulation of mitochondrial biogenesis nor other aspects of brown adipocyte differentiation. While *Ucp1* expression and mitochondrial biogenesis will likely share some regulatory mechanisms, such as the known involvement of PGC1 in both, we expect that there will be mechanisms that are unique for each process. Considering that the brown adipocyte in the human is similar to that in other species in its dependence on adrenergic signalling, it is quite possible that the pathways that control variation in the expression of brown adipocytes in the mouse will also exist in the human. The genetic dissection of the regulation of brown fat induction in mice will hopefully identify the details of the inductive pathways and provide alternatives sites for pharmacological intervention.

D Variation in *Ucp1* Expression in Transgenic and Knockout Models

Transgenic mice have the potential to provide insight into the regulation of brown adipocyte expression. To date, the major phenotype is one in which hypertrophy of interscapular brown fat occurs because of the effects of the transgene on energy expenditure and thermogenesis. Overexpression of the cytoplasmic glycerol-3-phosphate dehydrogenase induces thermogenesis systemically, possibly by a substrate cycling mechanism, with the consequence that a large increase of the lipid droplets occurs in the brown adipocytes because of reduced lipolysis and thermogenesis as evidenced by reduced *Ucp1* expression and elevated leptin (27). Inactivation of the hormone-sensitive lipase gene causes a similar hypertrophy because of the reduced capacity of the tissue to utilize its lipid stores (28). A dramatic increase in brown fat due to accumulation of lipid occurs in mice carrying the sterol regulatory element-binding protein (29). These mice have virtually undetected levels of *Ucp1* mRNA, in brown fat, which is peculiar since the levels of leptin mRNA are also very low. Normally, if brown fat is inactive owing to reduced sympathetic input, leptin expression is increased. The phenotype of this mouse in which brown fat is enlarged, white fat is shrunken, and both leptin and *Ucp1* expressions are reduced suggests that overexpression of SREBP-1 by the aP2 promoter has caused a major disruption of the adipocyte differentiation program.

An important mechanism for both enhancing the expression of *Ucp1* in the brown fat and stimulating the conversion of brown adipocytes in white fat depots has emerged from two disparate studies. In one study, the targeted gene inactivation of the RIIβ regulatory subunit of protein kinase A resulted in animals that showed striking reductions in adiposity, especially in mice fed a high-fat diet (30). These animals had elevated levels of UCP1 in brown fat owing to an increase in protein kinase A activity that occurred when the inactivation RIIβ subunit gene was compensated by an increase in the levels of the RIα regulatory subunit. In mutant mice, the holoenzyme of protein kinase A with the RIα subunit binds cAMP with higher avidity than in wild-type mice, thereby lowering its threshold for activation and subsequent stimulation of CREB-mediated transcription. In a second study, a winged helix/forkhead transcription factor FOXC2 was overexpressed in adipose tissue of transgenic mice with the aP2 promoter (31). Similar to the RIIβ regulatory subunit targeted mice, the FOXC2 transgenic mice had increased expression of *Ucp1* in brown adipose tissue and, in addition, had an increase in the expression of the brown adipocytes in white fat depots. The increase in PGC1, PPARγ, and ADD1/SREBP in the white fat depots of transgenic mice suggests that the overexpression of FOXC2 stimulates the brown adipocyte differentiation program in the white fat depots. The mechanism by which FOXC2 induces these changes appears to be mediated by changes in the expression of the regulatory subunits of protein kinase A. FOXC2 preferentially stimulates the expression of the RIα regulatory subunit, thereby establishing a cAMP system with heightened activity. The results with FOXC2 show how the induction of both *Ucp1* expression and the brown adipocyte differentiation are exquisitely sensitive to cAMP signaling. Consistent with these models is an earlier transgenic model in which the β1-adrenergic receptor was overexpressed from the aP2 promoter and resulted in an increase in brown adipocyte expression (32). However, in a follow-up analysis of the effects of the RIIβ subunit gene inactivation on gene expression associated with lipolysis and gene expression in white fat depots, those effects that would indicate a striking increase in brown adipocyte expression in the white fat of the knockout mice were much more modest (33). Whether the differences between the RIIβ knockout and FOXC2 overexpression systems are due to background strain effects, sex, or type of fat pads analyzed need to be resolved.

In summary, alternative strategies are being discovered by which an enhancement of cAMP signalling can activate the brown adipocyte differentiation program in white fat as follows: 1.) The FOXC2 transgenic model has revealed a novel mechanism by which sensitivity of PKA signalling can be modulated by regulating expression of the PKA regulatory subunits; 2.) the genetic analysis of brown fat induction in mice has identified at least four more chromosomal regions in which reside novel genes that can also stimulate *Ucp1* expression. Accordingly, it is possible that additional strategies for upregulating brown adipocyte differentiation will be discovered. The fact that FOXC2 is abundantly expressed in human adipose tissue suggests that the machinery for inducing brown fat expression also exists in the human (31).

E UCP1 and Hormones of Feeding Behavior

Shortly after the discovery of ob/ob mice, Alonso and Maren (34) demonstrated that the total body weight of ob/ob mice pair-fed with nonmutant littermates was similar to that of controls, but the percent body fat was still similar to that of ob/ob mice fed ad libitum. Several years later, in a repeat of this experiment that included db/db mutant mice, Coleman noted that hyperphagia, although a major contributory factor to the amount of fat accretion, was not essential for the development of either obesity or diabetes (35). Rather, he concluded, the *ob* and *db* genes have major effects on the partitioning of calories. With the cloning of the *ob* gene, the effects of leptin on body composition, presumably through its action on energy expenditure, was confirmed when *ob/ob* mice treated with leptin showed normalized food intake and total body weight as well as a normal body composition (36). Several laboratories have now demonstrated that in addition to the effects of leptin on food intake, it also increases energy expenditure by stimulating *Ucp1* expression in brown fat via the sympathetic nervous system (37–40). The ability of neuropeptides of food intake to have peripheral effects on energy expenditure is not restricted to leptin, but is a property shared by other anorexic agents, including the melanocortin system.

Similar to leptin action, the melanocortin system for the regulation of food intake and body weight is a system of agonists (α-MSH) and antagonists (agouti-related protein and agouti protein) acting on the MC3R and MC4R receptors. Inactivation of the receptors by gene targeting or treatment with antagonists causes increases in food intake and the development of obesity in a manner resembling mutations to leptin or the leptin receptor (41,42). In fact, the pathway for action of leptin signaling in the hypthalamus appears to be partially mediated by MC3R and MC4R (43,44). Although the evidence is not as clear as in the experiments with ob/ob mice, mice with mutated MC3R or MC4R genes or mice treated with an antagonist have an increase in adiposity even when pair-fed to control/untreated animals (45).

An important finding in these studies is that *Ucp1* expression is upregulated when energy expenditure is increased and downregulated when energy expenditure is reduced. The emerging conclusion is that leptin and α-MSH inhibition of food intake stimulates sympathetic nervous activity to brown adipose tissue to induce *Ucp1* expression, while AGRP and NPY stimulate food intake and attenuated expression of *Ucp1* (46,47). The implication of these phenotypes is that UCP1 plays a role in determining changes in peripheral energy expenditure initiated by the action of leptin. Given that even UCP1-deficient mice are not obese (48), the relative contributions that changes in *Ucp1* expression may have in modulating energy expenditure and adiposity by anorexic and orexigenic peptides remains uncertain. Even more uncertain is the contribution that this mechanism has in modulating energy expenditure in humans.

F Regulation of the Endogenous *Ucp1* Gene

Ucp1 is activated in response to growth and development, environmental temperature, and nutrition status. Much of this regulation is coordinated centrally from the hypothalamus via the sympathetic nervous system; however, other aspects of regulation appear to proceed independent of the sympathetic nervous system, and some regulation may require both the SNS and mechanisms independent of the SNS. In parallel with these expression studies, several research groups have been characterizing the regulatory motifs, located in the 5′ flanking region of the gene, and identifying the transcription factors that interact with these motifs. The picture emerging from these studies is that a number of motifs and factors have been identified that may interact in various combinations to regulate *Ucp1* transcription under a specific set of conditions. What these combinations may be for a given function remains to be determined.

The general structure of the 5′ regulatory region of *Ucp1*, depicted in Figure 1, highlights two major domains—the proximal promoter, and a distal enhancer region. These regions are highlighted because expression studies based on transgenic mice and transient expression assays in cultured cells of the regulatory motifs from the mouse and rat genes have shown consistent results. Other motifs, principally those located between the proximal promoter and the distal enhancer, have been identified by comparative sequence analysis, but have not been clearly verified by expression studies. In addition, there is evidence for a silencer located ~1 kb from the transcription start site, but the identity of the sequences specifying this function has not been determined. Finally, strong DNase hypersensitive regions 16 kb upstream of the transcription start site of *Ucp1* have been mapped. Whether these sites are the location of *Ucp1* regulatory motifs, such as a distal locus-controlling element, is not known.

An absolute requirement for a CRE in the proximal promoter has been shown by site-direct mutagenesis of the CRE in both the mouse and the rat gene (49,50). It is probable that cJun is involved in regulation from this

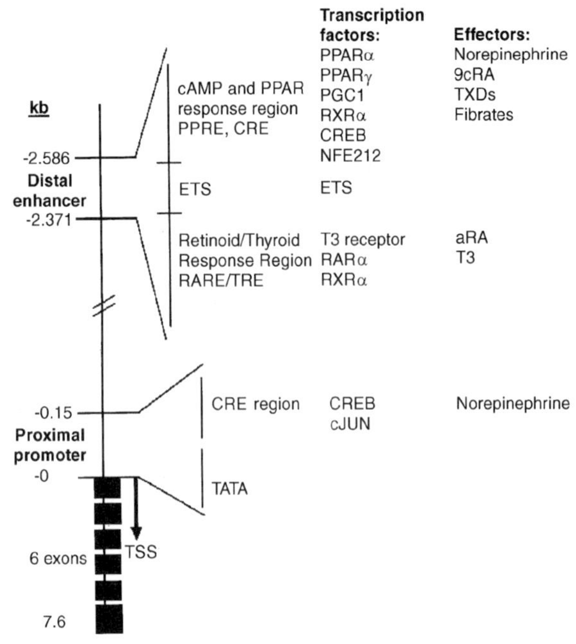

Figure 1 Schematic representation of the 5′ flanking regulatory region of the *Ucp1* gene. Known transcription factors and effectors are listed. The nucleotide positions of the enhancers and proximal promoter regions are those that have been determined for the mouse gene, but the mouse and human genes have comparable locations for these regulatory elements. The overall size and relationship of transmembrane domains to exon/intron structure is also similar among the rat, mouse, and human (173–175). Additional elements are likely to reside between the proximal promoter and distal enhancer, but these have not been well characterized at this time.

site, but it is not determining the differentiation-dependent expression of *Ucp1* (50). Whether the proxima CRE is required for retinoic acid–dependent induction of gene expression is not known. Sp1 and NF1 motifs have been identified by sequence analysis; however, there is no other evidence that these motifs have a function in the promoter (51).

The distal enhancer region is extremely complex with evidence for the involvement of 10 or more transcription factors (Fig. 1). The importance of this region was first identified in transgenic mice (52) and subsequently by deletion and mutation analysis in transient expression assays in brown adipocyte cultures (49,53). PPRE region in the distal enhancer was rigorously characterized as the PPARγ-binding site by Sears et al. (54), thereby providing the groundwork that led to the discovery of PGC1 as a coactivator of PPARγ together with RXRα (55). Corroboration of the importance of the PPRE site and its interaction with PPARγ and RXRα and its role in *Ucp1* regulation has also established by analysis of the rat *Ucp1* gene (56). Importantly, not only PPARγ, but also PPARα, has a role in the regulation of *Ucp1* (56). A second site in the distal enhancer contains motifs for regulation by retinoic acid and thyroid hormone (57–59). Mutation analysis in both the mouse and rat genes has also identified an ETS binding domain located between the PPRE/CRE region and the more proximal RARE/TRE domain (49,51).

The human *UCP1* gene also has a multipartite element in an upstream enhancer (located between -3.82 and -3.47 kb from the transcription start site) that mediates its expression. As determined in mouse cells by transient expression analysis, maximal expression depends on simultaneous addition of retinoic acid, isoproterenol and thiazolidinediones (60). Very little expression could be detected with addition of only one of these effectors independently, and only low expression was detected when one of the three effectors was absent. The requirement for thiazolidinediones occurred even though a consensus PPRE motif could not be detected. These results suggest that upregulation of the human *UCP1* will depend on transcription mechanisms similar to those that control the rodent gene.

Why does there seem to be so much redundancy built into the regulatory mechanisms? Does regulation of the *Ucp1* require all of these transcription factors all the time, or are there physiological conditions when only a subset of factors is required? It has been proposed by Villaroya and colleagues that retinoic acid, which has been shown to induce *Ucp1* expression, as well as norepinephrine, albeit with a delayed time course (57,59), could be the primary transcription mechanism controlling *Ucp1* expression during in utero development between 18 and 19 days (61). This mechanism assumes that in utero *Ucp1* is not capable of being stimulated by adrenergic signaling. Given that dopamine β-hydroxylase-deficient mice die in utero and that β-adrenergic signaling stimulates brown adipocyte proliferation and differentiation (62,63) in tissue culture, further experimentation needs to be performed to understand the effects of adrenergic signalling on *Ucp1* expression in utero. The discovery by Villarroya and colleagues that *Ucp1* is regulated by effectors of PPARα as well as PPARγ (56) suggests that while PPARγ is required for expression of *Ucp1* during BAT differentiation, PPARα upregulates *Ucp1* during active thermogenesis when PPARα also controls the expression of genes encoding enzymes for fatty acid oxidation.

G Genetic Variants in UCP1 and Susceptibility to Obesity

Whether genetic variation in *UCP1* expression could increase susceptibility to obesity in humans is a question that is still unresolved. Genetic studies evaluating this issue are inconclusive, since some studies have reported significant associations between *UCP1* polymorphisms and body weight (64–66) while others have not (67–69). Without knowledge of some functional change associated with a given polymorphism, it is difficult to interpret these association and linkage data, and there is little information on UCP1 function. Oberkofler et al. (24) found lower *UCP1* mRNA levels in the intraperitoneal fat depots, but not extraperitoneal fat depots, of morbidly obese subjects compared to lean controls. Whether this difference is indicative of lower energy expenditure in the obese individuals and is causally linked to the development of obesity is unknown.

H Perspectives on UCP1

Even a small increase in the expression of *Ucp1* has been shown to have strong effects in reducing the development of obesity and type 2 diabetes in rodent models. Much of this information has come from transgenic and gene knockout models. However, these genetic models have not only established that stimulation of UCP1 is effective as an antiobesity target, but they have also revealed novel signalling and transcription pathways that will promote the emergence of differentiated brown adipocytes in white fat tissues. As this manuscript goes to press, two studies have elegantly shown this, one on the effects of overexpression of FOXC2, a transcription factor (31), and the other on the targeted inactivation of 4E-BP1, an inhibitor of translation (70). Both mechanisms for the control of gene expression result in the same phenotype, that is, increases in brown adipocytes in traditional white fat depots and concomitant reductions in adiposity. The emergence of a multitude of targets for unregulating *Ucp1* in the mouse provides much hope that some of these will become effective targets for the unregulation of *UCP1* and brown adipocyte–derived thermogenesis in human.

III THE NOVEL UCPS

Brown fat mitochondria are characterized by an active proton pathway that can be uncoupled by an adrenergic stimulation by activation of UCP1. Data from several studies finding that the coupling of respiration to ATP synthesis in mitochondria from several tissues was less than perfect and also due to proton leaks (71). With the identification of UCP2 and UCP3, two homologs of the brown fat UCP in 1997, the hypothesis emerged that mitochondrial proton leaks in skeletal muscle or in liver or brain mitochondria were due to proteins homologous to brown fat UCP. UCP2 is widely expressed in tissues, whereas UCP3 is mainly expressed in skeletal muscle and brown adipose tissue. The high level of identity among UCP2, UCP3, and UCP1, as well as preliminary functional, physiological, and genetic studies (72–77), supported a putative role for these novel UCPs in energy expenditure and metabolic regulation. However, subsequent studies, in particular the observation that UCP2 and UCP3 gene expression was induced in skeletal muscles in humans (78) or rodents (79) during starvation and that UCP2 was present in ectothermic vertebrates (80), questioned the role for the novel UCPs in energy expenditure. In this chapter, we will not discuss the roles of other mitochondrial carriers identified in mammals, plants, or birds that are more or less related to the UCPs and are referred to as BMCP1 (81), UCP4 (82), plant UCP (83), and avian UCP (84,85). This section of the review on UCP2 and UCP3 will present data from biochemical, genetic, physiological, and pathophysiological studies in human and rodent models as well as data from the analysis of transgenic mice.

A Biochemical Studies

The questions to address are: Are the novel UCPs true uncouplers of respiration? Do they work as proton translocators? Are they regulated by fatty acids or nucleotides? Do they affect ATP level in cells?

Expression of UCP1 in yeast or reconstitution studies of UCP1 into liposomes was previously used to demonstrate its ability to uncouple respiration and translocate protons. In these systems, UCP1 uncoupling activity is increased by addition of fatty acids and is decreased in presence of nucleotides, as it is in brown adipocyte mitochondria (86–88). Similarly, expression of human or rodent UCP2 or UCP3 in yeast induces a marked uncoupling of respiration and thermogenesis (73,74,89–92). In addition, liposomes reconstituted with UCP2 or UCP3 purified from recombinant bacteria were able to catalyze an electrophoretic flux of protons (93). Using a similar approach, Echtay et al. also observed a proton transport activity in lipidic vesicles reconstituted with UCP2 or UCP3 (94). However, the physiological significance of uncoupling activity of UCP2 or UCP3 in recombinant yeast was recently criticized by Brand and colleagues who reported that physiological levels of UCP2 were unable to significantly uncouple respiration of yeast mitochondria (95). These authors claimed that the observed uncoupling of respiration might be due to damaged mitochondria from the large excess of recombinant proteins. They also draw attention to the fact that the increase of UCP3 mRNA in the skeletal muscle of starved rats was not accompanied by a change of proton conductance (96). A problem with interpretation of many of the reconstituted systems, whether from yeast or liposomes, has been the lack of careful quantification of the protein in these preparations.

In isolated yeast mitochondria, unlike UCP1, UCP2, or UCP3, activity is regulated by neither fatty acids nor nucleotides (91,92). However, a direct activation of UCP2 by retinoids was observed in yeast mitochondria (92). This effect of retinoids on UCP2 was confirmed in a reconstitution system (97). In contrast to studies in yeast, the reconstituted proton transport activity of UCP2 or UCP3 in liposomes has an obligatory requirement for fatty acids (94,98). Proton flux was also inhibited by nucleotides in liposomes, but with much lower affinity than observed with UCP1 (98). Klingenberg and coworkers have recently reported on the striking effects of coenzyme Q as an obligatory cofactor for the H^+ transport in liposomes reconstituted with UCP1, UCP2, and UCP3 (99). They also proposed that these H^+ transport activities conducted in the presence of coenzyme Q are regulated by the concentration of free ATP and ADP and by the ATP/ADP ratio (94).

The biochemical functions of UCP2 and UCP3 have been explored by overexpression of the proteins in mammalian cells and transgenic mice, and by inactivation of their genes in mice targeted by homologous recombination (the data referring to transgenic mice are reviewed below). Overexpression of UCP2 in rat pancreatic islets (100,101) or insulinoma cells (102) resulted in a severe blunting of glucose-stimulated insulin secretion and significantly reduced ATP content (101,102) and mitochondrial membrane potential (101). Consistent with these effects of overexpression, UCP2-deficient mice had higher islet ATP levels and increase of glucose-stimulated insulin secretion. These studies support a true uncoupling activity of UCP2 and a negative role for UCP2 in the control of insulin secretion. The presence of UCP2 in pancreas (73,74, 101,103–105) and the well-known control of insulin secretion by ATP/ADP ratios in β-cells also support their findings from these genetic studies. Overexpression of human UCP3 in L6 myotubes or H9C2 cardiomyoblasts stimulates glucose uptake and GLUT4 translocation to the cell surface by activating a PI3K-dependent pathway (106). Such an effect could be related to uncoupling activity of UCP3 and a subsequent requirement for substrate utilization. Another study of overexpression of human UCP3 in cultured human muscle was shown to favor fatty acid over glucose oxidation (107).

In summary, it is obvious that unphysiological levels of UCP2 or UCP3 can uncouple respiration in yeast or mammalian cell and translocate protons through a membrane, but it is not certain whether the low physiological levels of these proteins may be sufficient to induce a net uncoupling of respiration in vivo. The divergent observations of the regulation of the activities of UCP2 or UCP3 by fatty acids or nucleotides will require further studies. Interestingly, Moore et al. recently proposed that UCP2 and UCP3 could export fatty acid anion under conditions of elevated fatty acid oxidation (108). Expression studies of UCP2 in pancreatic cells agree with an uncoupling activity, but the demonstration that a concomitant decrease of ATP content directly results from respiration uncoupling should be further confirmed. Another important role for UCP2 and UCP3 may be related to the control of reactive oxygen species (this point is discussed in the section on transgenic mice).

B Genetic Studies

The *UCP2* and *UCP3* genes are adjacent genes on human chromosome 11 and mouse chromosome 7 (109–112). Sequence analysis has shown a similar distribution of the coding domain over six exons and a similar localization of exon/intron boundaries, which suggests that *UCP2* and *UCP3* have evolved by duplication from a common ancestor, as their juxtaposition on the chromosome predicts (109,112–116). In comparison with the UCP1 gene, the *UCP2* gene contains two additional exons in the 5′ side, whereas the *UCP3* gene contains one additional untranslated exon in the 5′ side. Exon 1 of *UCP2* is untranslated and exon 2 contains an open reading frame of an unknown 36–amino acid peptide (112). Actually, exon 2-ORF seems to limit UCP2 synthesis and may be important for the translational regulation of the *UCP2* gene (117). In contrast to *UCP3* promoter (116), the UCP2 promoter lacks both TATA and CAAT boxes and is GC rich (112,115). Promoter studies have identified a positive regulatory region in the proximal part of *UCP2* and *UCP3* promoters (112,114,116), and a double E-box mediating PPARγ response in *UCP2* promoter (118). The UCP3 promoter contains several MyoD-binding motifs (119), and its activity in vitro is largely dependent on MyoD (120).

The genetic linkage of the *Ucp2* locus to hyperinsulinemia in mouse (73) and the putative respiration uncoupling activity of the novel *UCPs* stimulated geneticists to investigate the contribution of these genes to metabolic physiology and pathophysiology in humans. The first genetic analysis in the human revealed a significant linkage of an anonymous marker, D11S911, lying close to the *UCP2* and *UCP3* genes, to resting metabolic rate in Caucasians (77). This first study hinted at a potential role of the novel *UCPs* in energy expenditure. A genomic scan for genes affecting body composition before and after exercise training in Caucasians identified the *UCP2/UCP3* locus as a region linked to change in percent fat (121). However, another study failed to find significant linkage between the *UCP2/UCP3* region and obesity in familial type 2 diabetes (122). In another analysis, the D11S911 marker in the *UCP2/UCP3* gene cluster was associated with anorexia nervosa in a cohort of 170 female Caucasians (123).

Two common polymorphisms were identified in human *UCP2* gene: one nucleotide substitution at codon 55 in exon 5 replacing an alanine with a valine (124–126), and a 45-bp insertion/deletion variant in the untranslated region of exon 8 (127). A rare variant resulting in an alanine/threonine substitution at position 232 was also described (128). The alanine/valine substitution polymorphism was related to metabolic efficiency, fat oxidation, and energy cost of physical exercise in a Danish population (129,130). However, this alanine/valine polymorphism was not associated with the pathogenesis of juvenile or maturity-onset obesity or insulin resistance in Caucasians (124,131) or with basal metabolic rate and susceptibility to obesity in Caucasians or Japanese (126,128). The 45-bp insertion/deletion polymorphism in exon 8 is associated with body mass index in South Indian subjects but not in obese Caucasians (132) or in morbidly diabetic obese French subjects (131). Confirming a genomic scan analysis, the insertion/deletion polymorphism in the 3′ untranslated region of exon 8 was calculated to be associated with gain in fat mass over 12 years, suggesting that *UCP2* might be associated with an increased susceptibility to gain fat with age (121). Yanovski et al. reported that this polymorphism was associated with body mass index in childhood-onset obesity (133). An association with obesity was also observed in German adults (134).

More recently, another common variant in the promoter region of human *UCP2* was described (G/A at position bp -866 relative to the transcriptional start site); this variant is associated with decreased risk of obesity in middle-aged humans in a cohort of 790 individuals (135).

The different variants identified in the human *UCP3* gene are the following: four nucleotide substitutions in the intron 3, and two silent amino acids (Tyr/Tyr at position 99 in exon 3, Tyr/tyr at position 200 in exon 5); substitution of a glycine residue for a serine residue at position 84 of amino acids in exon 3 (113); substitution of a valine for an isoleucine at position 102 in exon 3; a mutation introducing a stop codon in exon 4 (arginine residue at position 143); a terminal polymorphism in the splice donor junction of exon 6, resulting in a short form of UCP3 protein lacking the N-terminal transmembrane helix (136); substitution of a valine for a methionine at position 9 in exon 2; and substitution of an arginine for a tryptophan at position 308 in exon 7 (137). It is unlikely that variants in exons 3 and 4 of the UCP3 gene contribute to the pathogenesis of juvenile-onset obesity among Danish Caucasians (113) or obesity in French (137) or Isle of Ely Caucasians (138). In contrast with these studies, Argyropoulos et al. (136) observed that the exon 6–splice donor polymorphism correlated significantly with basal fat oxidation and respiratory quotient in morbidly diabetic obese Gullah-speaking African-Americans (but not in Caucasians). They proposed a role for UCP3 in metabolic fuel partitioning. However, these data were not confirmed in an independent population of African-Americans (139). In other respects, a GA polymorphic site in intron 6 of *UCP3* gene was calculated to be strongly associated with body mass index and body fat content in the Quebec family study (140). C-to-T substitution in the UCP3 promoter, 55 bp upstream of the transcriptional start site, has been detected; this polymorphism is associated with UCP3 mRNA levels (141,142). The C-to-T polymorphism in the 5′ sequence of the *UCP3* gene is negatively associated to body mass index (138,143). Interestingly, in the group with the C/C genotype, body mass index was negatively associated with physical activity, suggesting that the *UCP3* gene might contribute to corpulence and alter the benefit of physical activity (143). Therefore, although the *UCP2* and *UCP3* genes are not major genes for human obesity or metabolic diseases, several studies identified the *UCP2/UCP3* locus as a region possibly implicated in the control of resting metabolic rate, fat oxidation, and adiposity in humans.

C Physiological and Pathophysiological Studies

Several studies have aimed at understanding the physiological significance and regulation of UCP2 and UCP3. These studies were related to (1) effects of hormones, substrates or drugs on UCP expression, (2) status of UCPs in obese or diabetic patients, and (3) the relationship between UCP2 and UCP3 and physical exercise.

The identification of UCP homologs able to uncouple respiration in recombinant systems prompted the authors to propose that such proteins were involved in basal or regulatory thermogenesis. In agreement with this hypothesis, Barbe et al. reported that the level of *UCP2* mRNA in adipose tissue of obese humans after 25 days of hypocaloric diet correlated with resting metabolic rate adjusted for lean body mass (144). The hypothesis that the UCP homologs could stimulate thermogenesis is supported by several studies showing that they were upregulated by thyroid hormones in rodents (76,145,146). The effect of thyroid hormones was tested in humans receiving an amount of T_3 causing a 1.7-fold increase in plasma-free T3 level, a 14% increase in resting metabolic rate, a small decrease in respiratory quotient, and no change in plasma level of nonesterified fatty acids (147). In this study, T3 increased *UCP2* mRNA levels in adipose tissue as well as *UCP2* and *UCP3* mRNA levels in skeletal muscle. In addition, the direct effect of T3 on skeletal muscle and adipose tissue *UCP2* and *UCP3* mRNA was demonstrated in vitro with human primary cultures. A marked upregulation of *UCP2* mRNA was also described in adipose tissue of hyperthyroid patients (148).

Soon after the discovery of *UCP2* and *UCP3*, an upregulation of *UCP2* and *UCP3* mRNAs upon starvation was described both in humans (78) and rodents (79,149). Such data questioned the hypothetical role for the novel *UCP*s in energy expenditure in the face of depleted energy reserves; however, it was suggested that the *UCP*s could provide for the important function of maintaining body temperature that could occur during starvation. Dulloo and Samec have proposed that the function of *UCP2* and *UCP3* was rather to adapt cell metabolism to lipid utilization rather than thermogenesis (149). In agreement with this proposal, the upregulation of *UCP2* and *UCP3* mRNAs by a high-fat diet in humans is more pronounced in humans with high proportions of type IIA fibers, which are known to have a high capacity to shift from carbohydrate to fat oxidation (150).

To explain *Ucp3* induction in skeletal muscle during food restriction of rats, Weigle et al. proposed that the free fatty acids are the mediators of such a change (151). In agreement with this work, infusion of lipids for 5 hr in human volunteers induces a rise in nonesterified fatty acids and a doubling of *UCP3* mRNA level in skeletal muscles (152). Thiazolidinediones stimulate *UCP2* expression in rat or human skeletal muscle cells in culture (153,154). A positive effect of a PPARβ agonist on *UCP3* mRNA levels in rat L6 myotubes was obtained (155). Chevillotte et al. demonstrated that omega-6 polyunsaturated fatty acids, acting through PPARβ, can stimulate *UCP2* expression in primary culture of human skeletal muscle cells (154). Fatty acids have been shown to induce *UCP2* expression in adipocyte cultures of both rodents (153,156) and humans (157).

A survey of articles reporting on *UCP2* or *UCP3* mRNA levels in humans does not give a clear picture. Identical (78,158) or reduced *UCP2* gene expression was measured in skeletal muscle (159) and intraperitoneal adipose tissue (160) of human obese subjects compared to lean individuals. Although body mass index was negatively correlated with *UCP2* expression in skeletal muscle of Pima Indians (161), in two other studies it was found that *UCP3* mRNA levels in skeletal muscle did not differ between obese and lean subjects (78,162). However, a prolonged hypocaloric diet downregulated *UCP3* mRNA expression in muscle of obese patients (162). No difference in the mRNA level of *UCP2* in skeletal muscle was measured between NIDDM and control subjects; in contrast, mRNA levels of *UCP3* is significantly reduced in skeletal muscle of NIDDM patients (163).

In comparison with untrained subjects, exercise-trained subjects exhibit lower levels of *UCP3* mRNA in their skeletal muscle (141). These data led the authors to hypothesize that endurance training makes athletes more energy efficient. The status of *UCP2* and *UCP3* was also investigated in skeletal muscle of tetraplegic subjects before and after an 8-week exercise program consisting of electrically stimulated leg cycling (164). In agreement with data of able-bodied people trained to physical exercise (141), tetraplegia was shown to be associated with increased expression of *UCP2* and *UCP3* in skeletal muscle, and exercise training of tetraplegic patients normalized *UCP2* mRNA levels. Although it is difficult to understand the significance of decreased *UCP* expression during exercise and increased *UCP* expression in absence of exercise, it appears that physical activity regulates *UCP* expression in skeletal muscle. Whether expression of UCP2 and UCP3 in skeletal muscle is related to oxygen utilization remains to be investigated.

In conclusion, an unclear picture emerges from analysis of *UCP2* and *UCP3* expression in physiological or pathophysiological situations. On the one hand, the upregulation of the *UCP*s in skeletal muscle during starvation, as well as the level of mRNAs in obese individuals compared to lean individuals do not illustrate an obvious role for UCP2 or UCP3 in substrate utilization and energy partitioning. On the other hand, the positive effect of T3, a hormone known to induce mitochondrial proton leak and substrate oxidation, on expression of *UCP2* and *UCP3* in tissues, supports their possible role in energy dissipation. Analysis of *UCP2* and *UCP3* function in nonactive or activated skeletal muscle of tetraplegic patients indicates that a role for the UCPs in thermogenesis and maintenance of body temperature cannot be ruled out.

D Studies from Transgenic Mice

Mice overexpressing human *UCP3* in skeletal muscle were created (165). These mice weigh less than the wild-type littermates although they are hyperphagic. The predominant factor contributing to reduced body weight is a 50% decrease in the amount of adipose tissue in the transgenic mice. Moreover, these mice exhibit a lower insulinemia and lower fasting glycemia. Muscle temperature is increased but core temperature is not affected. The resting oxygen consumption of the transgenic mice is markedly increased. These data support a role for UCP3 in activating substrate oxidation and decreasing body fat content. A decrease in respiratory control ratio illustrated by increased state 4 respiration and decreased membrane potential in mitochondria isolated from muscle of the transgenic animals, confirms that overexpression of UCP3 induces respiration uncoupling. These data are in agreement with a respiration uncoupling activity of a high level of UCP3 and its potential role in treatment of obesity. However, a critical point seems to be the question of the amount of UCP3 necessary to induce a significant respiration uncoupling and have an effect on body weight, since Clapham et al. (165) created mice with a very high level of UCP3. Curiously, the same authors concluded that UCP3 in normal mice had no uncoupling activity since UCP3 induction in skeletal muscle of starved rats does not change the mitochondrial proton conductance (96). Moreover, it was shown that treatment of rats by T3 increases mitochondrial ATP production in oxidative muscle despite increased expression of UCP3 (166). No data corresponding to transgenic mice overexpressing UCP2 have been published yet.

Coincident with the creation of transgenic mice overexpressing UCP3, two other teams inactivated UCP3 by gene targeting (167,168). In contrast to the marked decreased in fat content of mice overexpressing UCP3 (see above), the Ucp3 -/- mice are not obese; they have a normal body temperature and no change in oxygen consumption. The absence of phenotype is surprising since analysis of the mitochondria of the Ucp3 -/- mice showed a reduced proton leak (167), a decreased state 4 respiration, and increased ROS production (168), these three changes supporting the hypothesis of respiration uncoupling activity of UCP3. Moreover, the rate of ATP synthesis, measured by NMR analysis, is strongly increased in skeletal muscle of Ucp3 -/- mice, and this increased efficiency of ATP production in mutant mice is consistent with a role for the uncoupling activity of UCP3 in skeletal muscle in vivo in controlling energy status (169). Therefore, the data obtained from mice made null for the UCP3 gene are rather contradictory, since it appears that disruption of a mitochondrial protein able to uncouple respiration does not induce phenotypic changes.

Similar to the observation with Ucp3 -/- mice, the disruption of the UCP2 gene did not induce obesity of the mice, even when they were put on an adipogenic diet (105,170). These data challenge the expected role of the novel UCPs in energy metabolism. However, analysis of the Ucp2 -/- mice identified two interesting roles of UCP2. Guided by the fact that UCP2 is expressed at high level in the immune system (73), Arsenijevic et al. found that the mutant mice were more resistant to infection by a parasite (170). In fact, disruption of the *Ucp2* gene provokes an elevation of ROS level that facilitates the killing of the pathogens. It is unknown whether such an effect results directly from a net change in respiration coupling in mitochondria or from a modification of the mitochondrial membrane potential that controls mitochondrial ROS production. Moreover, whether the increase of ROS in macrophages of Ucp2 -/- mice represents the main effect on pathogens or precedes an activation of NADPH oxidase in phagocytes remains to be studied. These data support a role for UCP2 in limiting ROS level in cells as predicted (171,172). In other respects, Zhang et al. observed that the Ucp2 -/- mice were hypoglycemic and hyperinsulinemic (105). This is due to a higher insulin secretion in response to glucose by pancreatic islets. The authors explained this higher insulin secretion as a consequence of increased ATP levels in the absence of UCP2 uncoupling activity in islets of mutant mice. The more pronounced insulin secretion by pancreatic islets of the Ucp2 -/- mice was confirmed in another study (Picard et al., unpublished data). These data are in agreement with experiments of overexpression of UCP2 in pancreatic islets (see above). Therefore, UCP2 controls negatively insulin secretion.

To summarize studies from genetically modified mice, strong overexpression of UCP3 or deletion of the UCP3 gene or the UCP2 gene tends to support an uncoupling activity of UCP3, but the in vivo uncoupling activity of UCP2 is still a matter of debate. Whereas disruption of the UCP3 gene did not clarify its physiological role, disruption of the UCP2 gene reveals its significant physiological role both in the control of ROS production and insulin secretion.

E UCP2 and UCP3, Conclusions and Perspectives

Besides UCP1, which has a well-demonstrated uncoupling activity and an essential role in maintenance of body temperature in small rodents exposed to the cold, the exact biochemical and physiological roles of UCP2 and UCP3 remain to be further identified. Certain data support a true activity of these UCPs in respiration uncoupling; other data do not agree with a role for these UCPs in controlling body weight or adiposity. Whereas the physiological role of UCP3 remains rather unknown, UCP2 and UCP3 appear to be genes limiting ROS level in cells and UCP2 as a gene controlling insulin secretion.

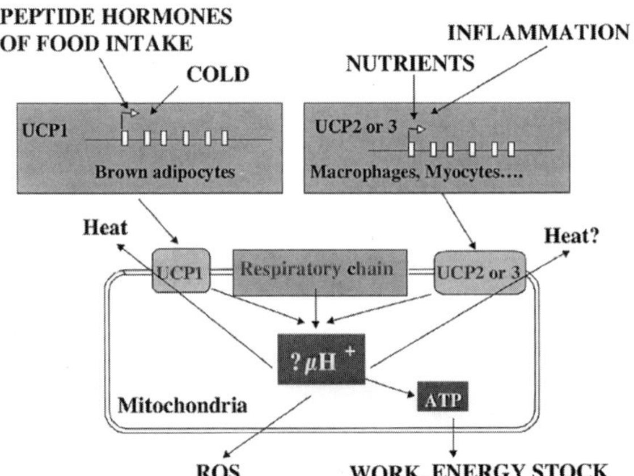

Figure 2 Models of physiological activities of UCP1, UCP2, and UCP3. The *UCP1* gene is only transcribed in brown adipocytes. The *UCP1* gene is activated following exposure of animals to the cold whereas the activity of the *UCP2* and *UCP3* genes can be modulated in response to the flux of glucidic or lipidic substrates. The activity of the *UCP2* gene can also be activated during inflammatory responses in macrophages. Activated UCPs tend to decrease the mitochondrial proton gradient. This gradient controls ATP synthesis and ROS production. Physiologically, the main effects of UCP1 are substrate oxidation and regulatory thermogenesis. The roles of UCP2 and UCP3 in cellular thermogenesis and control of ATP level require further studies. These two UCPs decrease ROS production by mitochondria.

Since UCP2 and UCP3 homologues exist in ectothermic animals, it may be hypothesized that UCP2 and UCP3 are closer to a UCP ancestor than is UCP1, which only exists in mammals. The UCPs belong to the family of the mitochondrial anion carriers. UCP1 translocates protons, whereas UCP2 and UCP3 can also transport protons. The ability of UCP2 and UCP3 to transport ions other than protons should be investigated. A depiction of the putative functions for the UCPs is provided in Figure 2.

Undoubtedly, a central question is that of the amount of UCP2 and UCP3 in tissues. Experiments of overexpression of the novel UCPS in transgenic mice or mammalian cells have shown that these proteins can uncouple respiration from ATP synthesis and therefore represent putative targets for antiobesity compounds. However, the amount of UCP2 or UCP3 normally present in vivo seems to be very low and insufficient to provoke a discernible uncoupling of respiration. It remains to be determined whether the amount (or activity?) of UCP2 or UCP3 in cells can be sufficiently elevated to uncouple respiration under selective natural or pharmacological conditions. The observation that the level of UCP2 protein can be rapidly and strongly increased in tissues in absence of variation in the amount of *UCP2* mRNA indicates that a rather high level of UCP2 can be obtained, at least in certain cells. It should not be forgotten that a very small, but prolonged, change in level of coupling of mitochondrial respiration, i.e., change in efficiency of substrate oxidation, can significantly affect body adiposity.

REFERENCES

1. Neel JV. Diabetes mellitus: A "thrifty" genotype rendered detrimental by "progress." Am J Hum Genet 1962; 14:353–362.
2. Coleman DL. Obesity genes: beneficial effects in heterozygous mice. Science 1979; 203:663–665.
3. Rothwell NJ, Stock MJ. A role for brown adipose tissue in diet-induced thermogenesis. Nature 1979; 281: 31–35.
4. Himms-Hagen J. Brown adipose tissue thermogenesis and obesity. Prog Lipid Res 1989; 28:67–115.
5. Arch JRS, Ainsworth AT, Cawthorne MA, Piercy V, Senitt MV, Thody VE, Wilson C, Wilson S. Atypical β-adrenoreceptor on brown adipocytes as targets for antiobesity drugs. Nature 1984; 309:163–165.
6. Holloway BR, Howe R, Rao BS, Stribling D, Mayers RM, Briscoe MG, Jackson JM. ICI D7114 a novel selective beta-adrenocoptor agonist selectively stimulates brown fat and increases whole body oxygen consumption. Br J Pharmacol 1991; 104:97–104.
7. Bloom JD, Dutia MD, Johnson BD, Wissner A, Burns MG, Largis EE, Dolan JA, Claus TH. Disodium (R,R)-5-[2-[(2-(3-chlorophenyl)-2-hydroxyethyl]-amino]propyl]-l,3-benzodioxole-2,2-dicarboxylate (CL 316,243). A potent beta-adrenergic agonist virtually specific for beta 3 receptors. A promising antidiabetic and antiobesity agent. J Med Chem 1992; 35:3081–3084.
8. Arch JRS. The brown adipocyte β-adrenoceptor. Proc Nutr Soc 1989; 48:215–223.
9. Emorine LJ, Marullo S, Briend-Sutren M-M, Patey G, Tate K, Delavier-Klutchko C, Strosberg AD. Molecular characterization of the human β3-adrenergic receptor. Science 1989; 245:1118–1121.
10. Champigny O, Ricquier D, Blondel O, Mayers RM, Briscoe MG, Holloway BR. Beta 3-adrenergic receptor stimulation restores message and expression of brown-fat mitochondrial uncoupling protein in adult dogs. Proc Natl Acad Sci USA 1991; 88:10774–10777.
11. Himms-Hagen J, Cui J, Danforth E Jr, Taatjes DJ, Lang SS, Waters BL, Claus TH. Effect of CL-316,243, a thermogenic beta 3-agonist, on energy balance and brown and white adipose tissues in rats. Am J Physiol 1994; 266:R1371–R1382.
12. Ghorbani M, Claus TH, Himms-Hagen J. Hypertrophy of brown adipocytes in brown and white adipose tissues and reversal of diet-induced obesity in rats treated with a β3-adrenoreceptor agonist. Biochem Pharmacol 1997; 54:121–131.
13. Ghorbani M, Himms-Hagen J. Appearance of brown adipocytes in white adipose tissue during CL 316,243-induced reversal of obesity and diabetes in Zucker *fa/fa* rats. Int J Obes 1997; 21:465–475.
14. Kopecky J, Clarke G, Enerback S, Spiegelman B, Kozak LP. Expression of the mitochondrial uncoupling protein gene from the aP2 gene promoter prevents genetic obesity. J Clin Invest 1995; 96:2914–2923.
15. Li B, Nolte LA, Ju JS, Han DH, Coleman T, Holloszy JO, Semenkovich CF. Skeletal muscle respiratory uncoupling prevents diet-induced obesity and insulin resistance in mice. Nat Med 2000; 6:1115–1120.
16. Kopecky J, Hodny Z, Rossmeisl M, Syrovy I, Kozak LP. Reduction of dietary obesity in aP2-Ucp transgenic mice: physiology and adipose tissue distribution. Am J Physiol 1996; 270:E768–E775.
17. Stefl B, Janovska A, Hodny Z, Rossmeisl M, Horakova M, Syrovy I, Bemova J, Bendlova B, Kopecky J. Brown fat is essential for cold-induced thermogenesis but not for obesity resistance in aP2-Ucp mice. Am J Physiol 1998; 274:E527–E533.
18. Matthias A, Ohlson KB, Fredriksson JM, Jacobsson A, Nedergaard J, Cannon B. Thermogenic responses in brown fat cells are fully UCP1-dependent. UCP2 or UCP3 do not substitute for UCP1 in adrenergically or

fatty acid–induced thermogenesis. J Biol Chem 2000; 275:25073–25081.
19. Young P, Arch JRS, Ashwell M. Brown adipose tissue in the parametrial fat pad of the mouse. FEBS Lett 1984; 167:10–14.
20. Loncar D, Afzelius BA, Cannon B. Epididymal white adipose tissue after cold stress in rats. II. Mitochondrial changes. J Ultrastruct Mol Struct Res 1988; 101:199–209.
21. Huttunen P, Hirvonen J, Kinnula V. The occurrence of brown adipose tissue in outdoor workers. Eur J Appl Physiol 1981; 46:339–345.
22. Ricquier D, Nechad M, Mory G. Ultrastructural and biochemical characterization of human brown adipose tissue in pheochromocytoma. J Clin Endocrinol Metab 1982; 54:803–807.
23. Guerra C, Koza RA, Yamashita H, Walsh K, Kozak LP. Emergence of brown adipocytes in white fat in mice is under genetic control. Effects on body weight and adiposity. J Clin Invest 1998; 102:412–420.
24. Oberkofler H, Dallinger G, Liu Y-M, Hell E, Krempler F, Patsch W. Uncoupling protein gene: quantification of expression levels in adipose tissues of obese and nonobese humans. J Lipid Res 1997; 38:2125–2133.
25. Collins S, Daniel KW, Petro AE, Surwit RS. Strain-specific response to beta 3-adrenergic receptor agonist treatment of diet-induced obesity in mice. Endocrinology 1997; 138:405–413.
26. Koza RA, Hohmann SM, Guerra C, Rossmeisl M, Kozak LP. Synergistic gene interactions control the induction of the mitochondrial uncoupling protein (Ucpl) gene in white fat tissue. J Biol Chem 2000; 275:34486–34487.
27. Kozak LP, Kozak UC, Clarke GT. Abnormal brown and white fat development in transgenic mice over-expressing glycerol 3-phosphate dehydrogenase. Genes Dev 1991; 5:2256–2264.
28. Osuga J, Ishibashi S, Oka T, Yagyu H, Tozawa R, Fujimoto A, Shionoiri F, Yahagi N, Kraemer FB, Tsutsumi O, Yamada N. Targeted disruption of hormone-sensitive lipase results in male sterility and adipocyte hypertrophy, but not in obesity. Proc Natl Acad Sci USA 2000; 97:787–792.
29. Shimomura I, Hammer RE, Richardson JA, Ikemoto S, Bashmakov Y, Goldstein JL, Brown MS. Insulin resistance and diabetes mellitus in transgenic mice expressing nuclear SREBP-lc in adipose tissue: model for congenital generalized lipodystrophy. Genes Dev 1998; 12:3182–3194.
30. Cummings DE, Brandon EP, Planas JV, Motamed K, Idzerda RL, McKnight GS. Genetically lean mice result from targeted disruption of the RII beta subunit of protein kinase A. Nature 1996; 382:622–626.
31. Cederberg A, Gronning LM, Ahren B, Tasken P, Carlsson P, Enerback S. *FOXC2* is a winged helix gene that counteracts obesity, hypertriglceridemia, and diet-induced insulin resistance. Cell 2001; 106:563–573.
32. Soloveva V, Graves RA, Rasenick MM, Spiegelman BM, Ross SR. Transgenic mice overexpressing the β1-adrenergic receptor in adipose tissue are resistant to obesity. Mol Endocrinol 1997; 11:27–38.
33. Planas JV, Cummings DE, Idzerda RL, McKnight GS. Mutation of the RIIbeta subunit of protein kinase A differentially affects lipolysis but not gene induction in white adipose tissue. J Biol Chem 1999; 274:36281–36287.
34. Alonso LG, Maren TH. Effect of food restriction on body composition of hereditary obese mice. Am J Physiol 1955; 183:284–290.
35. Coleman DL. Increased metabolic efficiency in obese mutant mice. Int J Obes 1985; 9(suppl 2):69–73.
36. Halaas JL, Gajiwala KS, Maffei M, Cohen SL, Chait BT, Rabinowitz D, Lallone RL, Burley SK, Friedman JM. Weight-reducing effects of the plasma protein encoded by the obese gene. Science 1995; 269:543–546.
37. Scarpace PJ, Matheny M. Leptin induction of UCP1 gene expression is dependent on sympathetic innervation. Am J Physiol 1998; 275:E259–E264.
38. Arvaniti K, Ricquier D, Champigny O, Richard D. Leptin and corticosterone have opposite effects on food intake and the expression of UCP1 mRNA in brown adipose tissue of lep(ob)/lep(ob) mice. Endocrinology 1998; 139:4000–4003.
39. Commins SP, Watson PM, Padgett MA, Dudley A, Argyropoulos G, Gettys TW. Induction of uncoupling protein expression in brown and white adipose tissue by leptin. Endocrinology 1999; 140:292–300.
40. Commins SP, Marsh DJ, Thomas SA, Watson PM, Padgett MA, Palmiter R, Gettys TW. Norepinephrine is required for leptin effects on gene expression in brown and white adipose tissue. Endocrinology 1999; 140:4772–4778.
41. Huszar D, Lynch CA, Fairchild-Huntress V, Dunmore JH, Fang Q, Berkemeier LR, Gu W, Kesterson RA, Boston BA, Cone RD, Smith FJ, Campfield LA, Burn P, Lee F. Targeted disruption of the melanocortin-4 receptor results in obesity in mice. Cell 1997; 88:131–141.
42. Chen AS, Marsh DJ, Trumbauer ME, Frazier EG, Guan XM, Yu H, Rosenblum CI, Vongs A, Feng Y, Cao L, Metzger JM, Strack AM, Camacho RE, Mellin TN, Nunes CN, Min W, Fisher J, Gopal-Truter S, MacIntyre DE, Chen HY, Van der Ploeg LH. Inactivation of the mouse melanocortin-3 receptor results in increased fat mass and reduced lean body mass. Nat Genet 2000; 26:97–102.
43. Satoh N, Ogawa Y, Katsuura G, Numata Y, Masuzaki H, Yoshimasa Y, Nakao K. Satiety effect and sympathetic activation of leptin are mediated by hypothalamic melanocortin system. Neurosci Lett 1998; 249:107–110.
44. Marsh DJ, Hollopeter G, Huszar D, Laufer R, Yagaloff KA, Fisher SL, Burn P, Palmiter RD.

Response of melanocortin-4 receptor–deficient mice to anorectic and orexigenic peptides. Nat Genet 1999; 21:119–122.
45. Ste Marie L, Miura GI, Marsh DJ, Yagaloff K, Palmiter RD. A metabolic defect promotes obesity in mice lacking melanocortin-4 receptors. Proc Natl Acad Sci USA 2000; 97:12339–12344.
46. Billington CJ, Briggs JE, Harker S, Grace M, Levine AS. Neuropeptide Y in hypothalamic paraventricular nucleus: a center coordinating energy metabolism. Am J Physiol 1994; 266:R1765–R1770.
47. Small CJ, Kim MS, Stanley SA, Mitchell JR, Murphy K, Morgan DG, Ghatei MA, Bloom SR. Effects of chronic central nervous system administration of agouti-related protein in pair-fed animals. Diabetes 2001; 50:248–254.
48. Enerback S, Jacobsson A, Simpson EM, Guerra C, Yamashita H, Harper ME, Kozak LP. Mice lacking mitochondrial uncoupling protein are cold-sensitive but not obese. Nature 1997; 387:90–94.
49. Kozak UC, Kopecky J, Teisinger J, Enerback S, Boyer B, Kozak LP. An upstream enhancer regulating brown-fat-specific expression of the mitochondrial uncoupling protein gene. Mol Cell Biol 1994; 14:59–67.
50. Yubero P, Barbera MJ, Alvarez R, Vinas O, Mampel T, Iglesias R, Villarroya F, Giralt M. Dominant negative regulation by c-Jun of transcription of the uncoupling protein-1 gene through a proximal cAMP-regulatory element: a mechanism for repressing basal and norepinephrine-induced expression of the gene before brown adipocyte differentiation. Mol Endocrinol 1998; 12:1023–1037.
51. Cassard-Doulcier AM, Larose M, Matamala JC, Champigny O, Bouillaud F, Ricquier D. In vitro interactions between nuclear proteins and uncoupling protein gene promoter reveal several putative trans-activating factors including Ets1, retinoid X receptor, thyroid hormone receptor, and a CACCC box-binding protein. J Biol Chem 1994; 269:24335–24342.
52. Boyer BB, Kozak LP. The mitochondrial uncoupling protein gene in brown fat: correlation between DNase I hypersensitivity and expression in transgenic mice. Mol Cell Biol 1991; 11:4147–4156.
53. Cassard-Doulcier AM, Gelly C, Fox N, Schrementi J, Raimbault S, Klaus S, Forest C, Bouillaud F, Ricquier D. Tissue-specific and beta-adrenergic regulation of the mitochondrial uncoupling protein gene: control by cis-acting elements in the 5′-flanking region. Mol Endocrinol 1993; 7:497–506.
54. Sears IB, MacGinnitie MA, Kovacs LG, Graves RA. Differentiation-dependent expression of the brown adipocyte uncoupling protein gene: regulation by peroxisome proliferator-activated receptor gamma. Mol Cell Biol 1996; 16:3410–3419.
55. Puigserver P, Wu Z, Park CW, Graves R, Wright M, Spiegelman BM. A cold-inducible coactivator of nuclear receptors linked to adaptive thermogenesis. Cell 1998; 92:829–839.
56. Barbera MJ, Schluter A, Pedraza N, Iglesias R, Villarroya F, Giralt M. Peroxisome proliferator–activated receptor alpha activates transcription of the brown fat uncoupling protein-1 gene. A link between regulation of the thermogenic and lipid oxidation pathways in the brown fat cell. J Biol Chem 2001; 276:1486–1493.
57. Alvarez R, De Andres J, Yubero P, Vinas O, Mampel T, Iglesias R, Giralt M, Villarroya F. A novel regulatory pathway of brown fat thermogenesis. Retinoic acid is a transcriptional activator of the mitochondrial uncoupling protein gene. J Biol Chem 1995; 270:5666–5673.
58. Rabelo R, Schifman A, Rubio A, Sheng X, Silva JE. Delineation of thyroid hormone-responsive sequences within a critical enhancer in the rat uncoupling protein gene. Endocrinology 1995; 136:1003–1013.
59. Larose M, Cassard-Doulcier AM, Fleury C, Serra F, Champigny O, Bouillaud F, Ricquier D. Essential cis-acting elements in rat uncoupling protein gene are in an enhancer containing a complex retinoic acid response domain. J Biol Chem 1996; 271:31533–31542.
60. Del Mar Gonzalez-Barroso M, Pecqueur C, Gelly C, Sanchis D, Alves-Guerra MC, Bouillaud F, Ricquier D, Cassard-Doulcier AM. Transcriptional activation of the human ucpl gene in a rodent cell line. Synergism of retinoids, isoproterenol, and thiazolidinedione is mediated by a multipartite response element. J Biol Chem 2000; 275:31722–31732.
61. Giralt M, Martin I, Iglesias R, Vinas O, Villarroya F, Mampel T. Ontogeny and perinatal modulation of gene expression in rat brown adipose tissue. Unaltered iodothyronine 5′-deiodinase activity is necessary for the response to environmental temperature at birth. Eur J Biochem 1990; 193:297–302.
62. Bronnikov G, Houstek J, Nedergaard J. β-Adrenergic, cAMP-mediated stimulation of proliferation of brown fat cells in primary culture. J Biol Chem 1992; 267:2006–2013.
63. Kozak UC, Kozak LP. Norepinephrine-dependent selection of brown adipocyte cell lines. Endocrinology 1994; 134:906–913.
64. Kogure A, Yoshida T, Sakane N, Umekawa T, Takakura Y, Kondo M. Synergic effect of polymorphisms in uncoupling protein 1 and beta3-adrenergic receptor genes on weight loss in obese Japanese. Diabetologia 1998; 41:1399.
65. Oppert J, Vohl M, Chagnon M, Dionne FT, Cassard-Doulcier A-M, Ricquier D, Pérusse L, Bouchard C. DNA polymorphism in the uncoupling protein (UCP) gene and human body fat. Int J Obes 1994; 18:526–531.
66. Fumeron F, Durack-Bown I, Betoulle D, Cassard-Doulcier AM, Tuzet S, Bouillaud F, Melchior JC,

Ricquier D, Apfelbaum M. Polymorphisms of uncoupling protein (UCP) and beta 3 adrenoreceptor genes in obese people submitted to a low calorie diet. Int J Obes Relat Metab Disord 1996; 20:1051–1054.

67. Urhammer SA, Fridberg M, Sorensen TI, Echwald SM, Andersen T, Tybjaerg-Hansen A, Clausen JO, Pedersen O. Studies of genetic variability of the uncoupling protein 1 gene in Caucasian subjects with juvenile-onset obesity. J Clin Endocrinol Metab 1997; 82:4069–4074.
68. Gagnon J, Lago F, Chagnon YC, Pérusse L, Näslund I, Lissner L, Sjöström L, Bouchard C. DNA polymorphism in the uncoupling protein 1 (UCP1) gene has no effect on obesity related phenotypes in the Swedish Obese Subjects cohorts. Int J Obes Relat Metab Disord 1998; 22:500–505.
69. Lepretre F, Vionnet N, Budhan S, Dina C, Powell KL, Genin E, Das AK, Nallam V, Passa P, Froguel P. Genetic studies of polymorphisms in ten non-insulin-dependent diabetes mellitus candidate genes in Tamil Indians from Pondichery. Diabetes Metab 1998; 24:244–250.
70. Tsukiyama-Kohara K, Poulin F, Kohara M, DeMaria CT, Cheng A, Wu Z, Gingras AC, Katsume A, Elchebly M, Spiegelman BM, Harper ME, Tremblay ML, Sonenberg N. Adipose tissue reduction in mice lacking the translational inhibitor 4E- BP1. Nat Med 2001; 7:1128–1132.
71. Stuart JA, Cadenas S, Jekabsons MB, Roussel D, Brand MD. Mitochondrial proton leak and the uncoupling protein 1 homologues. Biochim Biophys Acta 2001; 1504:144–158.
72. Boss O, Samec S, Dulloo A, Seydoux J, Muzzin P, Giacobino J-P. Tissue-dependent upregulation of rat uncoupling protein-2 expression in response to fasting or cold. FEBS Lett 1997; 412:111–114.
73. Fleury C, Neverova M, Collins S, Raimbault S, Champigny O, Levi-Meyrueis C, Bouillaud F, Seldin MF, Surwit RS, Ricquier D, Warden CH. Uncoupling protein-2: a novel gene linked to obesity and hyperinsulinemia. Nat Genet 1997; 15:269–272.
74. Gimeno RE, Dembski M, Weng X, Deng N, Shyjan AW, Gimeno CJ, Iris F, Ellis SJ, Woolf EA, Tartaglia LA. Cloning and characterization of an uncoupling protein homolog: a potential molecular mediator of human thermogenesis. Diabetes 1997; 46:900–906.
75. Vidal-Puig A, Solanes G, Grujic D, Flier JS, Lowell BB. UCP3: an uncoupling protein homologue expressed preferentially and abundantly in skeletal muscle and brown adipose tissue. Biochem Biophys Res Commun 1997; 235:79–82.
76. Gong DW, He Y, Karas M, Reitman M. Uncoupling protein-3 is a mediator of thermogenesis regulated by thyroid hormone, beta3-adrenergic agonists, and leptin. J Biol Chem 1997; 272:24129–24132.
77. Bouchard C, Perusse L, Chagnon YC, Warden C, Ricquier D. Linkage between markers in the vicinity of the uncoupling protein 2 gene and resting metabolic rate in humans. Hum Mol Genet 1997; 6:1887–1889.
78. Millet L, Vidal H, Andreelli F, Larrouy D, Riou JP, Ricquier D, Laville M, Langin D. Increased uncoupling protein-2 and -3 mRNA expression during fasting in obese and lean humans. J Clin Invest 1997; 100:2665–2670.
79. Boss O, Samec S, Kuhne F, Bijlenga P, Assimacopoulos-Jeannet F, Seydoux J, Giacobino JP, Muzzin P. Uncoupling protein-3 expression in rodent skeletal muscle is modulated by food intake but not by changes in environmental temperature. J Biol Chem 1998; 273:5–8.
80. Stuart JA, Harper JA, Brindle KM, Brand MD. Uncoupling protein 2 from carp and zebrafish, ectothermic vertebrates. Biochim Biophys Acta 1999; 1413:50–54.
81. Sanchis D, Fleury C, Chomiki N, Goubern M, Huang Q, Neverova M, Gregoire F, Easlick J, Raimbault S, Levi-Meyrueis C, Miroux B, Collins S, Seldin M, Richard D, Warden C, Bouillaud F, Ricquier D. BMCP1, a novel mitochondrial carrier with high expression in the central nervous system of humans and rodents, and respiration uncoupling activity in recombinant yeast. J Biol Chem 1998; 273:34611–34615.
82. Mao W, Yu XX, Zhong A, Li W, Brush J, Sherwood SW, Adams SH, Pan G. UCP4, a novel brain-specific mitochondrial protein that reduces membrane potential in mammalian cells [published erratum appears in FEBS Lett 1999; 449(2–3):293]. FEBS Lett 1999; 443:326–330.
83. Laloi M, Klein M, Riesmeier JW, Muller-Rober B, Fleury C, Bouillaud F, Ricquier D. A plant cold-induced uncoupling protein. Nature 1997; 389:135–136.
84. Raimbault S, Dridi S, Denjean F, Lachuer J, Couplan E, Bouillaud F, Bordas A, Duchamp C, Taouis M, Ricquier D. An uncoupling protein homologue putatively involved in facultative muscle thermogenesis in birds. Biochem J 2001; 353: 441–444.
85. Vianna CR, Hagen T, Zhang CY, Bachman E, Boss O, Gereben B, Moriscot AS, Lowell BB, Bicudo JE, Bianco AC. Cloning and functional characterization of an uncoupling protein homolog in hummingbirds. Physiol Genomics 2001; 5:137–145.
86. Rial E, Gonzalez-Barroso MM. Physiological regulation of the transport activity in the uncoupling proteins UCP1 and UCP2. Biochim Biophys Acta 2001; 1504:70–81.
87. Bouillaud F, Couplan E, Pecqueur C, Ricquier D. Homologues of the uncoupling protein from brown adipose tissue (UCP1): UCP2, UCP3, BMCP1 and UCP4. Biochim Biophys Acta 2001; 1504:107–119.
88. Klingenberg M, Echtay KS. Uncoupling proteins: the issues from a biochemist point of view. Biochim Biophys Acta 2001; 1504:128–143.

89. Paulik MA, Buckholz RG, Lancaster ME, Dallas WS, Hull-Ryde EA, Weiel JE, Lenhard JM. Development of infrared imaging to measure thermogenesis in cell culture: thermogenic effects of uncoupling protein-2, troglitazone, and beta-adrenoceptor agonists. Pharm Res 1998; 15:944–949.
90. Hinz B, Schroder H. Vitamin C attenuates nitrate tolerance independently of its antioxidant effect. FEBS Lett 1998; 428:97–99.
91. Zhang CY, Hagen T, Mootha VK, Slieker LJ, Lowell BB. Assessment of uncoupling activity of uncoupling protein 3 using a yeast heterologous expression system. FEBS Lett 1999; 449:129–134.
92. Rial E, Gonzalez-Barroso M, Fleury C, Iturrizaga S, Sanchis D, Jimenez-Jimenez J, Ricquier D, Goubern M, Bouillaud F. Retinoids activate proton transport by the uncoupling proteins UCP1 and UCP2. EMBO J 1999; 18:5827–5833.
93. Jaburek M, Yarov-Yarovoy V, Paucek P, Garlid KD. State-dependent inhibition of the mitochondrial KATP channel by glyburide and 5-hydroxydecanoate. J Biol Chem 1998; 273:13578–13582.
94. Echtay KS, Winkler E, Frischmuth K, Klingenberg M. Uncoupling proteins 2 and 3 are highly active H(+) transporters and highly nucleotide sensitive when activated by coenzyme Q (ubiquinone). Proc Natl Acad Sci USA 2001; 98:1416–1421.
95. Stuart JA, Harper JA, Brindle KM, Jekabsons MB, Brand MD. Physiological levels of mammalian uncoupling protein 2 do not uncouple yeast mitochondria. J Biol Chem 2001; 276:18633–18639.
96. Cadenas S, Buckingham JA, Samec S, Seydoux J, Din N, Dulloo AG, Brand MD. UCP2 and UCP3 rise in starved rat skeletal muscle but mitochondrial proton conductance is unchanged. FEBS Lett 1999; 462:257–260.
97. Chomiki N, Voss JC, Warden CH. Structure-function relationships in UCP1, UCP2 and chimeras: EPR analysis and retinoic acid activation of UCP2. Eur J Biochem 2001; 268:903–913.
98. Jaburek M, Vaecha M, Gimeno RE, Dembski M, Jezek P, Zhang M, Burn P, Tartaglia LA, Garlid KD. Transport function and regulation of mitochondrial uncoupling proteins 2 and 3. J Biol Chem 1999; 274:26003–26007.
99. Echtay KS, Winkler E, Klingenberg M. Coenzyme Q is an obligatory cofactor for uncoupling protein function. Nature 2000; 408:609–613.
100. Chan CB, MacDonald PE, Saleh MC, Johns DC, Marban E, Wheeler MB. Overexpression of uncoupling protein 2 inhibits glucose-stimulated insulin secretion from rat islets. Diabetes 1999; 48:1482–1486.
101. Chan CB, De Leo D, Joseph JW, McQuaid TS, Ha XF, Xu F, Tsushima RG, Pennefather PS, Salapatek AM, Wheeler MB. Increased uncoupling protein-2 levels in beta-cells are associated with impaired glucose-stimulated insulin secretion: mechanism of action. Diabetes 2001; 50:1302–1310.
102. Hong Y, Fink BD, Dillon JS, Sivitz WI. Effects of adenoviral overexpression of uncoupling protein-2 and -3 on mitochondrial respiration in insulinoma cells. Endocrinology 2001; 142:249–256.
103. Kassis N, Bernard C, Pusterla A, Casteilla L, Penicaud L, Richard D, Ricquier D, Ktorza A. Correlation between pancreatic islet uncoupling protein-2 (UCP2) mRNA concentration and insulin status in rats. Int J Exp Diabetes Res 2000; 1:185–193.
104. Lameloise N, Muzzin P, Prentki M, Assimacopoulos-Jeannet F. Uncoupling protein 2: a possible link between fatty acid excess and impaired glucose-induced insulin secretion? Diabetes 2001; 50:803–809.
105. Zhang CY, Baffy G, Perret P, Krauss S, Peroni O, Grujic D, Hagen T, Vidal-Puig AJ, Boss O, Kim YB, Zheng XX, Wheeler MB, Shulman GI, Chan CB, Lowell BB. Uncoupling protein-2 negatively regulates insulin secretion and is a major link between obesity, beta cell dysfunction, and type 2 diabetes. Cell 2001; 105:745–755.
106. Huppertz C, Fischer BM, Kim YB, Kotani K, Vidal-Puig A, Slieker LJ, Sloop KW, Lowell BB, Kahn BB. Uncoupling protein 3 (UCP3) stimulates glucose uptake in muscle cells through a phosphoinositide 3-kinase-dependent mechanism. J Biol Chem 2001; 276:12520–12529.
107. Garcia-Martinez C, Sibille B, Solanes G, Darimont C, Mace K, Villarroya F, Gomez-Foix AM. Overexpression of UCP3 in cultured human muscle lowers mitochondrial membrane potential, raises ATP/ADP ratio, and favors fatty acid vs. glucose oxidation. FASEB J 2001; 15:2033–2035.
108. Moore GB, Himms-Hagen J, Harper ME, Clapham JC. Overexpression of UCP-3 in skeletal muscle of mice results in increased expression of mitochondrial thioesterase mRNA. Biochem Biophys Res Commun 2001; 283:785–790.
109. Solanes G, Vidal-Puig A, Grujic D, Flier JS, Lowell BB. The human uncoupling protein-3 gene. Genomic structure, chromosomal localization, and genetic basis for short and long form transcripts. J Biol Chem 1997; 272:25433–25436.
110. Surwit RS, Wang S, Petro AE, Sanchis D, Raimbault S, Ricquier D, Collins S. Diet-induced changes in uncoupling proteins in obesity-prone and obesity-resistant strains of mice. Proc Natl Acad Sci USA 1998; 95:4061–4065.
111. Gong DW, He Y, Reitman ML. Genomic organization and regulation by dietary fat of the uncoupling protein 3 and 2 genes. Biochem Biophys Res Commun 1999; 256:27–32.
112. Pecqueur C, Cassard-Doulcier AM, Raimbault S, Miroux B, Fleury C, Gelly C, Bouillaud F, Ricquier D. Functional organization of the human uncoupling

protein-2 gene, and juxtaposition to the uncoupling protein-3 gene. Biochem Biophys Res Commun 1999; 255:40–46.

113. Urhammer SA, Dalgaard LT, Sorensen TI, Tybjaerg-Hansen A, Echwald SM, Clausen JO, Pedersen O. Organisation of the coding exons and mutational screening of the uncoupling protein 3 gene in subjects with juvenile-onset obesity. Diabetologia 1998; 41: 241–244.
114. Yamada M, Hashida T, Shibusawa N, Iwasaki T, Murakami M, Monden T, Satoh T, Mori M. Genomic organization and promoter function of the mouse uncoupling protein 2 (UCP2) gene. FEBS Lett 1998; 432:65–69.
115. Tu N, Chen H, Winnikes U, Reinert I, Marmann G, Pirke KM, Lentes KU. Molecular cloning and functional characterization of the promoter region of the human uncoupling protein-2 gene. Biochem Biophys Res Commun 1999; 265:326–334.
116. Tu N, Chen H, Winnikes U, Reinert I, Pirke KM, Lentes KU. Functional characterization of the 5′-flanking and the promoter region of the human UCP3 (hUCP3) gene. Life Sci 2000; 67:2267–2279.
117. Pecqueur C, Alves-Guerra MC, Gelly C, Levi-Meyrueis C, Couplan E, Collins S, Ricquier D, Bouillaud F, Miroux B. Uncoupling protein 2, in vivo distribution, induction upon oxidative stress, and evidence for translational regulation. J Biol Chem 2001; 276:8705–8712.
118. Medvedev AV, Snedden SK, Raimbault S, Ricquier D, Collins S. Transcriptional regulation of the mouse uncoupling protein-2 gene. Double E-box motif is required for peroxisome proliferator-activated receptor-gamma-dependent activation. J Biol Chem 2001; 276:10817–10823.
119. Acin A, Rodriguez M, Rique H, Canet E, Boutin JA, Galizzi JP. Cloning and characterization of the 5′ flanking region of the human uncoupling protein 3 (UCP3) gene. Biochem Biophys Res Commun 1999; 258:278–283.
120. Solanes G, Pedraza N, Iglesias R, Giralt M, Villarroya F. The human uncoupling protein-3 gene promoter requires MyoD and is induced by retinoic acid in muscle cells. FASEB J 2000; 14:2141–2143.
121. Chagnon YC, Rice T, Perusse L, Borecki IB, Ho-Kim MA, Lacaille M, Pare C, Bouchard L, Gagnon J, Leon AS, Skinner JS, Wilmore JH, Rao DC, Bouchard C. Genomic scan for genes affecting body composition before and after training in Caucasians from HERITAGE. J Appl Physiol 2001; 90:1777–1787.
122. Elbein SC, Leppert M, Hasstedt S. Uncoupling protein 2 region on chromosome 11q13 is not linked to markers of obesity in familial type 2 diabetes. Diabetes 1997; 46:2105–2107.
123. Campbell DA, Sundaramurthy D, Gordon D, Markham AF, Pieri LF. Association between a marker in the UCP-2/UCP-3 gene cluster and genetic susceptibility to anorexia nervosa. Mol Psychiatry 1999; 4:68–70.
124. Urhammer SA, Dalgaard LT, Sorensen TI, Moller AM, Andersen T, Tybjaerg-Hansen A, Hansen T, Clausen JO, Vestergaard H, Pedersen O. Mutational analysis of the coding region of the uncoupling protein 2 gene in obese NIDDM patients: impact of a common amino acid polymorphism on juvenile and maturity onset forms of obesity and insulin resistance. Diabetologia 1997; 40:1227–1230.
125. Argyropoulos G, Brown AM, Peterson R, Likes CE, Watson DK, Garvey WT. Structure and organization of the human uncoupling protein 2 gene and identification of a common biallelic variant in Caucasian and African-American subjects. Diabetes 1998; 47:685–687.
126. Klannemark M, Orho M, Groop L. No relationship between identified variants in the uncoupling protein 2 gene and energy expenditure. Eur J Endocrinol 1998; 139:217–223.
127. Walder K, Norman RA, Hanson RL, Schrauwen P, Neverova M, Jenkinson CP, Easlick J, Warden CH, Pecqueur C, Raimbault S, Ricquier D, Silver MHK, Shuldiner AR, Solanes G, Lowell BB, Chung WK, Leibel RL, Pratley R, Ravussin E. Association between uncoupling protein polymorphisms (UCP2-UCP3) and energy metabolism/obesity in Pima Indians. Hum Mol Genet 1998; 7:1431–1435.
128. Kubota T, Mori H, Tamori Y, Okazawa H, Fukuda T, Miki M, Ito C, Fleury C, Bouillaud F, Kasuga M. Molecular screening of uncoupling protein 2 gene in patients with noninsulin-dependent diabetes mellitus or obesity. J Clin Endocrinol Metab 1998; 83:2800–2804.
129. Astrup A, Toubro S, Dalgaard LT, Urhammer SA, Sorensen TI, Pedersen O. Impact of the v/v 55 polymorphism of the uncoupling protein 2 gene on 24-h energy expenditure and substrate oxidation. Int J Obes Relat Metab Disord 1999; 23:1030–1034.
130. Buemann B, Schierning B, Toubro S, Bibby B, Sorensen T, Dalgaard L, Pedersen O, Astrup A. The association between the val/ala-55 polymorphism of the uncoupling protein 2 gene and exercise efficiency. Int J Obes Relat Metab Disord 2001; 25:467–471.
131. Otabe S, Clement K, Rich N, Warden C, Pecqueur C, Neverova M, Raimbault S, Guy-Grand B, Basdevant A, Ricquier D, Froguel P, Vasseur F. Mutation screening of the human UCP 2 gene in normoglycemic and NIDDM morbidly obese patients: lack of association between new UCP 2 polymorphisms and obesity in French Caucasians. Diabetes 1998; 47:840–842.
132. Cassell PG, Neverova M, Janmohamed S, Uwakwe N, Qureshi A, McCarthy MI, Saker PJ, Albon L, Kopelman P, Noonan K, Easlick J, Ramachandran A, Snehalatha C, Pecqueur C, Ricquier D, Warden C, Hitman GA. An uncoupling protein 2 gene variant is

associated with a raised body mass index but not type II diabetes. Diabetologia 1999; 42:688–692.
133. Yanovski JA, Diament AL, Sovik KN, Nguyen TT, Li H, Sebring NG, Warden CH. Associations between uncoupling protein 2, body composition, and resting energy expenditure in lean and obese African American, white, and Asian children. Am J Clin Nutr 2000; 71:1405–1420.
134. Evans D, Minouchehr S, Hagemann G, Mann WA, Wendt D, Wolf A, Beisiegel U. Frequency of and interaction between polymorphisms in the beta3-adrenergic receptor and in uncoupling proteins 1 and 2 and obesity in Germans. Int J Obes Relat Metab Disord 2000; 24:1239–1245.
135. Esterbauer H, Schneitler C, Oberkofler H, Ebenbichler C, Paulweber B, Sandhofer F, Ladurner G, Hell E, Strosberg AD, Patsch JR, Krempler F, Patsch W. A common polymorphism in the promoter of UCP2 is associated with decreased risk of obesity in middle-aged humans. Nat Genet 2001; 28:178–183.
136. Argyropoulos G, Brown AM, Willi SM, Zhu J, He Y, Reitman M, Gevao SM, Spruill I, Garvey WT. Effects of mutations in the human uncoupling protein 3 gene on the respiratory quotient and fat oxidation in severe obesity and type 2 diabetes. J Clin Invest 1998; 102:1345–1351.
137. Otabe S, Clement K, Dubois S, Lepretre F, Pelloux V, Leibel R, Chung W, Boutin P, Guy-Grand B, Froguel P, Vasseur F. Mutation screening and association studies of the human uncoupling protein 3 gene in normoglycemic and diabetic morbidly obese patients. Diabetes 1999; 48:206–208.
138. Halsall D, Luan J, Saker P, Huxtable S, Farooqi I, Keogh J, Wareham N, O'Rahilly S. Uncoupling protein 3 genetic variants in human obesity: the c-55t promoter polymorphism is negatively correlated with body mass index in a UK Caucasian population. Int J Obes Relat Metab Disord 2001; 25:472–477.
139. Chung WK, Luke A, Cooper RS, Rotini C, Vidal-Puig A, Rosenbaum M, Chua M, Solanes G, Zheng M, Zhao L, LeDuc C, Eisberg A, Chu F, Murphy E, Schreier M, Aronne L, Caprio S, Kahle B, Gordon D, Leal SM, Goldsmith R, Andreu AL, Bruno C, DiMauro S, Leibel RL. Genetic and physiologic analysis of the role of uncoupling protein 3 in human energy homeostasis. Diabetes 1999; 48:1890–1895.
140. Lanouette CM, Giacobino JP, Perusse L, Lacaille M, Yvon C, Chagnon Y, Kuhne F, Bouchard C, Muzzin P. Association between uncoupling protein 3 gene and obesity-related phenotypes in the Quebec Family Study. Mol Med 2001; 7:433–441.
141. Schrauwen P, Troost FJ, Xia J, Ravussin E, Saris WH. Skeletal muscle UCP2 and UCP3 expression in trained and untrained male subjects. Int J Obes Relat Metab Disord 1999; 23:966–972.
142. Schrauwen P, Xia J, Walder K, Snitker S, Ravussin E. A novel polymorphism in the proximal UCP3 promoter region: effect on skeletal muscle UCP3 mRNA expression and obesity in male non-diabetic Pima Indians. Int J Obes Relat Metab Disord 1999; 23:1242–1245.
143. Otabe S, Clement K, Dina C, Pelloux V, Guy-Grand B, Froguel P, Vasseur F. A genetic variation in the 5′ flanking region of the UCP3 gene is associated with body mass index in humans in interaction with physical activity. Diabetologia 2000; 43:245–249.
144. Barbe P, Millet L, Larrouy D, Galitzky J, Berlan M, Louvet JP, Langin D. Uncoupling protein-2 messenger ribonucleic acid expression during very-low-calorie diet in obese premenopausal women. J Clin Endocrinol Metab 1998; 83:2450–2453.
145. Lanni A, Beneduce L, Lombardi A, Moreno M, Boss O, Muzzin P, Giacobino JP, Goglia F. Expression of uncoupling protein-3 and mitochondrial activity in the transition from hypothyroid to hyperthyroid state in rat skeletal muscle. FEBS Lett 1999; 444:250–254.
146. De Lange P, Lanni A, Beneduce L, Moreno M, Lombardi A, Silvestri E, Goglia F. Uncoupling protein-3 is a molecular determinant for the regulation of resting metabolic rate by thyroid hormone. Endocrinology 2001, 142:3414 3420.
147. Barbe P, Larrouy D, Boulanger C, Chevillotte E, Viguerie N, Thalamas C, Trastoy MO, Roques M, Vidal H, Langin D. Triiodothyronine-mediated upregulation of UCP2 and UCP3 mRNA expression in human skeletal muscle without coordinated induction of mitochondrial respiratory chain genes. FASEB J 2001; 15:13–15.
148. Hoffstedt J, Folkesson R, Wahrenberg H, Wennlund A, Van Harmelen V, Amer P. A marked upregulation of uncoupling protein 2 gene expression in adipose tissue of hyperthyroid subjects. Horm Metab Res 2000; 32:475–479.
149. Dulloo AG, Samec S. Uncoupling proteins: their roles in adaptive thermogenesis and substrate metabolism reconsidered. Br J Nutr 2001; 86:123–139.
150. Schrauwen P, Hoppeler H, Billeter R, Bakker A, Pendergast D. Fiber type dependent upregulation of human skeletal muscle UCP2 and UCP3 mRNA expression by high-fat diet. Int J Obes Relat Metab Disord 2001; 25:449–456.
151. Weigle DS, Selfridge LE, Schwartz MW, Seeley RJ, Cummings DE, Havel PJ, Kuijper JL, BeltrandelRio H. Elevated free fatty acids induce uncoupling protein 3 expression in muscle: a potential explanation for the effect of fasting. Diabetes 1998; 47:298–302.
152. Khalfallah Y, Fages S, Laville M, Langin D, Vidal H. Regulation of uncoupling protein-2 and uncoupling protein-3 mRNA expression during lipid infusion in human skeletal muscle and subcutaneous adipose tissue. Diabetes 2000; 49:25–31.
153. Camirand A, Marie V, Rabelo R, Silva JE. Thiazolidinediones stimulate uncoupling protein-2 expression

in cell lines representing white and brown adipose tissues and skeletal muscle. Endocrinology 1998; 139:428–431.

154. Chevillotte E, Rieusset J, Roques M, Desage M, Vidal H. The regulation of uncoupling protein-2 gene expression by omega-6 polyunsaturated fatty acids in human skeletal muscle cells involves multiple pathways, including the nuclear receptor peroxisome proliferator-activated receptor beta. J Biol Chem 2001; 276:10853–10860.

155. Nagase I, Yoshida S, Canas X, Irie Y, Kimura K, Yoshida T, Saito M. Up-regulation of uncoupling protein 3 by thyroid hormone, peroxisome proliferator–activated receptor ligands and 9-cis retinoic acid in L6 myotubes. FEBS Lett 1999; 461:319–322.

156. Aubert J, Champigny O, Saint-Marc P, Negrel R, Collins S, Ricquier D, Ailhaud G. Up-regulation of UCP-2 gene expression by PPAR agonists in preadipose and adipose cells. Biochem Biophys Res Commun 1997; 238:606–611.

157. Viguerie-Bascands N, Saulnier-Blache JS, Dandine M, Dauzats M, Daviaud D, Langin D. Increase in uncoupling protein-2 mRNA expression by BRL49653 and bromopalmitate in human adipocytes. Biochem Biophys Res Commun 1999; 256:138–141.

158. Millet L, Vidal H, Larrouy D, Andreelli F, Laville M, Langin D. mRNA expression of the long and short forms of uncoupling protein-3 in obese and lean humans. Diabetologia 1998; 41:829–832.

159. Nordfors L, Hoffstedt J, Nyberg B, Thorne A, Arner P, Schalling M, Lonnqvist F. Reduced gene expression of UCP2 but not UCP3 in skeletal muscle of human obese subjects. Diabetologia 1998; 41:935–939.

160. Oberkofler H, Liu YM, Esterbauer H, Hell E, Krempler F, Patsch W. Uncoupling protein-2 gene: reduced mRNA expression in intraperitoneal adipose tissue of obese humans. Diabetologia 1998; 41:940–946.

161. Schrauwen P, Xia J, Bogardus C, Pratley RE, Ravussin E. Skeletal muscle uncoupling protein 3 expression is a determinant of energy expenditure in Pima Indians. Diabetes 1999; 48:146–149.

162. Esterbauer H, Oberkofler H, Liu YM, Breban D, Hell E, Krempler F, Patsch W. Uncoupling protein-1 mRNA expression in obese human subjects: the role of sequence variations at the uncoupling protein-1 gene locus. J Lipid Res 1998; 39:834–844.

163. Krook A, Digby J, O'Rahilly S, Zierath JR, Wallberg-Henriksson H. Uncoupling protein 3 is reduced in skeletal muscle of NIDDM patients. Diabetes 1998; 47:1528–1531.

164. Hjeltnes N, Fernstrom M, Zierath JR, Krook A. Regulation of UCP2 and UCP3 by muscle disuse and physical activity in tetraplegic subjects. Diabetologia 1999; 42:826–830.

165. Clapham JC, Arch JR, Chapman H, Haynes A, Lister C, Moore GB, Piercy V, Carter SA, Lehner I, Smith SA, Beeley LJ, Godden RJ, Herrity N, Skehel M, Changani KK, Hockings PD, Reid DG, Squires SM, Hatcher J, Trail B, Latcham J, Rastan S, Harper AJ, Cadenas S, Buckingham JA, Brand MD. Mice overexpressing human uncoupling protein-3 in skeletal muscle are hyperphagic and lean. Nature 2000; 406:415–418.

166. Short KR, Nygren J, Barazzoni R, Levine J, Nair KS. T(3) increases mitochondrial ATP production in oxidative muscle despite increased expression of UCP2 acid -3. Am J Physiol Endocrinol Metab 2001; 280: E761–E769.

167. Gong DW, Monemdjou S, Gavrilova O, Leon LR, Marcus-Samuels B, Chou CJ, Everett C, Kozak LP, Li C, Deng C, Harper ME, Reitman ML. Lack of obesity and normal response to fasting and thyroid hormone in mice lacking uncoupling protein-3. J Biol Chem 2000.

168. Vidal-Puig Al, Grujic D, Zhang CY, Hagen T, Boss O, Ido Y, Szczepanik A, Wade J, Mootha V, Cortright R, Muoio DM, Lowell BB. Energy metabolism uncoupling protein 3 gene knockout mice. J Biol Chem 2000.

169. Cline GW, Vidal-Puig AJ, Dufour S, Cadman KS, Lowell BB, Shulman GI. In vivo effects of uncoupling protein-3 gene disruption on mitochondrial energy metabolism. J Biol Chem 2001; 276:20240–20244.

170. Arsenijevic D, Onuma H, Pecqueur C, Raimbault S, Manning BS, Miroux B, Couplan E, Alves-Guerra MC, Goubern M, Surwit R, Bouillaud F, Richard D, Collins S, Ricquier D. Disruption of the uncoupling protein-2 gene in mice reveals a role in immunity and reactive oxygen species production [in process citation]. Nat Genet 2000; 26:435–439.

171. Negre-Salvayre A, Hirtz C, Carrera G, Cazenave R, Troly M, Salvayre R, Penicaud L, Casteilla L. A role for uncoupling protein-2 as a regulator of mitochondrial hydrogen peroxide generation. Faseb J 1997; 11:809–815.

172. Diehl AM, Hoek JB. Mitochondrial uncoupling: role of uncoupling protein anion carriers and relationship to thermogenesis and weight control "the benefits of losing control." Bioenerg Biomembr 1999; 31:493–506.

173. Kozak LP, Britton JH, Kozak UC, Wells JM. The mitochondrial uncoupling protein gene. Correlation of exon structure to transmembrane domains. J Biol Chem 1988; 263:12274–12277.

174. Bouillaud F, Raimbault S, Ricquier D. The gene for rat uncoupling protein: complete sequence, structure of primary transcript and evolutionary relationship between exons. Biochem Biophys Res Commun 1988; 157:783–792.

175. Cassard AM, Bouillaud F, Mattei MG, Hentz E, Raimbault S, Thomas M, Ricquier D. Human uncoupling protein gene: structure, comparison with rat gene, and assignment to the long arm of chromosome 4. J Cell Biochem 1990; 43:255–264.

21

Peroxisome Proliferator–Activated Receptor γ and the Transcriptional Control of Adipogenesis and Metabolism

Lluis Fajas and Johan Auwerx

Institut de Génétique et de Biologie Moléculaire et Cellulaire, Illkirch, and Université Louis Pasteur, Strasbourg, France

I INTRODUCTION

The peroxisome proliferator–activated receptor gamma (PPARγ) is one of three PPARs, which together constitute a distinct subfamily of the nuclear receptor superfamily and which are all activated by naturally occurring fatty acids or fatty acid derivatives. PPARγ heterodimerizes with retinoid X receptors (RXR) and alters the transcription of numerous target genes after binding to specific response elements or PPREs, which are found in several genes involved in fat metabolism. Coordinate regulation of genes involved in fat uptake and storage by PPARγ underlies its effects on adipocyte differentiation. PPARγ's claim to fame is due to its pivotal roles in adipogenesis and its implication in insulin sensitization. A number of additional functions were attributed to PPARγ, which suggests a more pleiotropic role affecting multiple fundamental pathways in the cell with wide-ranging biomedical implications.

II THE PPARγ GENE, RNA, AND PROTEIN

The human PPARγ gene, which is mapped to a locus on chromosome 3p25, has nine exons and spans over 100 kb of genomic DNA (1). In contrast to mice, in which only two PPARγ isoforms have been described so far (2), in man, three PPARγ mRNA isoforms have been identified—PPARγ1, γ2(1), and γ3 (3). Alternate transcription start sites and alternative splicing generate these three PPARγ mRNAs, which differ at their 5′ ends. Consistent with the production of three PPARγ mRNAs, there are three PPARγ promoters, each with a specific and distinctive expression pattern, (1,3). Whereas the PPARγl and γ3 mRNAs give rise to an identical protein product, i.e., PPARγ1, the PPARγ2 mRNA encodes for the PPARγ2 protein, which in man contains 28 additional amino acids encoded by the B exon.

Little is known about the expression of PPARγ during development in mammals (4). In adult animals, PPARγ expression is relatively confined. Adipose tissue, large intestine, and hematopoietic cells express the highest levels of PPARγ; kidney, liver, and small intestine have intermediate levels; whereas PPARγ is barely detectable in muscle (1,5). Related to the subtype distribution, PPARγ2 is much less abundant in all tissues relative to PPARγl, the predominant PPARγ form. The only tissue expressing significant amounts of PPARγ2 is adipose tissue, where PPARγ2 mRNA makes up 30% of total PPARγ mRNA (5). PPARγ3 mRNA expression is restricted to macrophages and large intestine (3,6).

In man, short-term changes in food intake do not affect the expression levels of PPARγ (5), whereas hypocaloric diets for a longer period result in a downregulation of PPARγ expression (7). In rodents, PPARγ was downregulated by fasting and insulin-dependent diabetes mellitus (8), whereas its expression was induced by a high-fat diet. Most interesting, however, was the observation that in normal-weight subjects PPARγ expression is highly enriched in subcutaneous fat, whereas its expression in visceral adipose tissue is significantly higher in obese subjects (9). Insulin and glucocorticoids induce PPARγ expression in cultured human adipocytes (7,10), whereas TNFα was reported to decrease PPARγ expression (11,12).

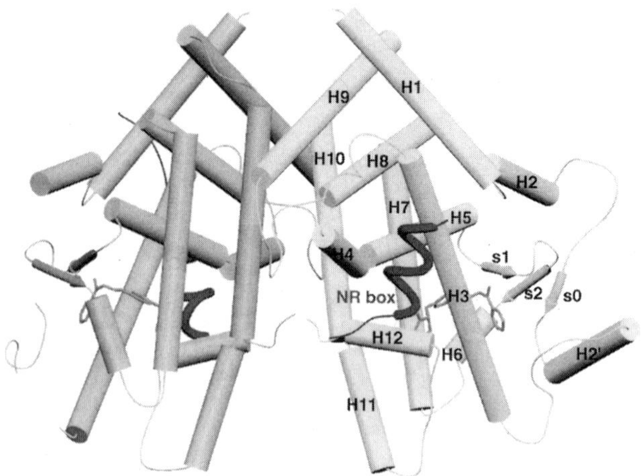

Figure 1 Crystallographic structure of the ternary complex hPPARγ LBD homodimer/rosiglitazone/coactivator peptide ((27) and PDB entry 2PRG). One LBD monomer is in green and the other one in yellow. Helices are depicted as cylinders and β-strands as arrows. In one monomer (the green one), residues 239–247 and 257–272 are not seen in the electron density map, and thus s0 and H2′ are not present. Rosiglitazone is in blue and the coactivator peptide is depicted as a red ribbon. Only the NR boxes of the coactivator peptide are seen in the electron density map; each NR box forms a helix that fits in a hydrophobic cleft on the LBD surface comprising the C-terminus of H3, loop H3-H4,H4, and H12.

III SOME STRUCTURAL ISSUES

As in all nuclear receptors (NRs), PPARγ has a modular structure composed of several domains: the NH_2 terminal A/B domain, harboring a ligand-independent transcriptional activation function (AF-1); the C domain, which contains two zinc fingers, responsible for DNA binding; the D or hinge region, which is important for cofactor docking; and the E COOH-terminal region, which among others contains the ligand-binding domain (LBD) and the ligand-dependent activation domain AF-2 (reviewed in 13). In recent years a large body of information has accumulated related to the three dimensional structures of the LBDs of multiple NRs (14). In general, the unliganded (apo) LBD of a prototypical NR is organized in 12 highly conserved α-helices which are folded into three layers to create a central hydrophobic ligand-binding pocket. The x-ray crystallographic structures of the LBD of PPARγ are similar to those reported for the other receptors (15,16).

The ligand-binding pocket of PPARγ is formed by residues from helix (H), 2′, H3, H5, H7, H11, H12, and the β-sheet (Fig. 1). In contrast to the LBDs of other NRs, the PPARγ ligand-binding pocket is exposed to the solvent between H3 and the β-sheet, and PPARγ has a more accessible ligand-binding cavity, which at ≈ 1300 Å^3 is almost twice the size of that of other receptors (≈ 600 Å^3) (15–17). The PPARγ apo-LBD (unliganded receptor) has a highly dynamic character, and agonist binding leads to a strong decrease of conformational freedom (18). In the crystal structure of the PPARγ apo-LBD homodimer (15), the activation helix H12 extends one subunit away from the LBD core, as in the RXR apo-LBD (19), while in the other subunit H12 is packed against the LBD core, sealing the pocket on one side, as in the retinoic acid receptor (RAR) bolo-LBD (liganded form) (20). This indicates that H12 is in equilibrium between at least these two conformations that are trapped by the crystal packing. In the PPARγ (16) apo-LBD monomer structure, H12 is also in a "hololike" conformation, folded against the LBD core. The structure of rosiglitazone-bound PPARγ LBD homodimer as a ternary complex with a fragment of the SRC-1 coactivator has also been reported (15). Rosiglitazone occupies ~40% of the ligand-binding pocket and is stabilized there by a combination of hydrogen bonds and Van der Waals contacts. The SRC-1 fragment contains two conserved LXXLL motifs ("NR boxes") with each LXXLL motif bound to one LBD monomer (21–23). The helix of the LXXLL peptide is positioned in a hydrophobic cleft on the LBD surface, formed by H3, the loop H3-H4, H4, and H12, through what has been called a "charge clamp." When H12 is in a hololike conformation in the PPARγ apo-LBD crystal structures, its position is slightly different from that in the agonist-bound structure. This emphasizes the crucial role of the direct or indirect contacts between the ligand and H12 in the transactivation process. The bound agonist tightens the position of H12 to provide a precise anchoring surface for the coactivator together with H3-H4. Interestingly, in the structure with the partial agonist GW0072, H12 does not seem to interact directly with the ligand and hence is found in a position more similar to the unliganded (apo) than to the liganded (holo) structure (24). Unlike full agonists, partial agonists would therefore not be able to stabilize the activation helix in the proper position, owing to the lack of a few key interactions, and such a slight malpositioning of H12 may result in an attenuated transcriptional response.

Recently, the structure of a PPARγ-RXRα LBD heterodimer was reported (25). The heterodimerization interface is topologically the same as the homodimerization interface in RXR (19), ER (26), and PPAR (15), and as the heterodimerization interface in the RARα-RXRα heterodimer (27). An interesting feature is the salt bridge between the C-terminal carboxylate of PPARγ (Tyr477, 4 residues downstream of H12) and Lys431 in H10 of RXRα. In the case of heterodimers, transcription may be regulated by the respective ligands for both receptors, such as is the case in the permissive PPAR-RXR heterodimer, whereas this is not the case for the nonpermissive RAR-RXR and TR-RXR heterodimers (28). The interaction between the C-terminus of the PPARγ LBD and H10 of RXR suggests a structural basis for such permissiveness, as it may stabilize H12 of PPARγ in the holo conformation allowing the recruitment of coactivators, even in the absence of a bound agonist (25).

IV A COORDINATOR FOR THE THRIFTY RESPONSE

Adipose tissue is mainly composed of adipocytes, which store energy in the form of triglycerides during periods of nutritional affluence and release it as free fatty acids at times of nutritional deprivation (for review see 29,30). Excessive accumulation of adipose tissue leads to obesity, whereas its absence is associated with lipodystrophic syndromes. The molecular mechanisms that control adipocyte differentiation from adipose precursor cells (adipoblasts) are complex and are affected by numerous signaling pathways. The adipocyte differentiation process starts after fibroblastic precursor cells become contact-hibited in their growth. Those cells then re-enter the cell cycle after appropriate hormonal induction, in a process termed clonal expansion. Later on, cells arrest this second proliferation phase again, undergo terminal adipocyte differentiation, and start to accumulate lipids (Fig. 2). We will discuss these two phases separately in the sections below.

A Control of the Early Phases of Adipogenesis

Whereas the terminal stages of adipocyte differentiation are well understood, the molecular mechanisms underlying the transition between cell proliferation and differentiation of preadipocytes remain elusive. Since these early phases of adipogenesis involve clonal expansion of the precursor cells, it was logical to start looking for factors that are involved in the control of the cell cycle as potential triggers for these early phases. The E2F family of transcription factors, which are major regulators of the cell cycle and which have been shown to have an important role in the regulation of other differentiation systems, were hence good candidates (31–33). E2Fs trigger the expression of PPARγ directly by binding to and transactivating the PPARγl promoter during the clonal expansion of the adipocyte differentiation process. In contrast to E2Fs, the role of the retinoblastoma (RB) protein family members, or the pocket proteins RB, p130, and p107, in adipocyte differentiation seems more complex. The negative role of pocket proteins in cell cycle progression, repressing the expression of the E2F target genes, has been demonstrated in several settings (for review see 34,35). Pocket proteins are inactivated by phosphorylation by the cyclin-dependent kinases, resulting in the activation of the E2F target genes. Consistent with an active cell cycle in the early stages of adipogenesis, pocket proteins have been found to be hyperphosphorylated following hormonal induction of preadipocytes (36). However, an apparent paradox arises from the finding that pRB inactivation by SV40 large T-antigen inhibits adipogenesis (37). Moreover, pRB-deficient fibroblasts fail to differentiate into adipocytes when properly stimulated (38,39). This apparent paradox was explained by the participation of RB in the growth arrest following clonal expansion (39a). This suggests that RB is involved in two phases of adipocyte differentiation. First, inactivation of RB enables clonal expansion, whereas growth arrest after this expansion phase requires active RB, which positively influences adipocyte differentiation. A different role, independent of the control of cell cycle, has also been attributed to RB in another aspect of the regulation of adipogenesis, i.e., the enhancement of the transactivation capability of C/EBPα and β, via direct protein-protein interaction (39). In contrast to RB, the other members of the retinoblastoma family, p130 and p107, have been

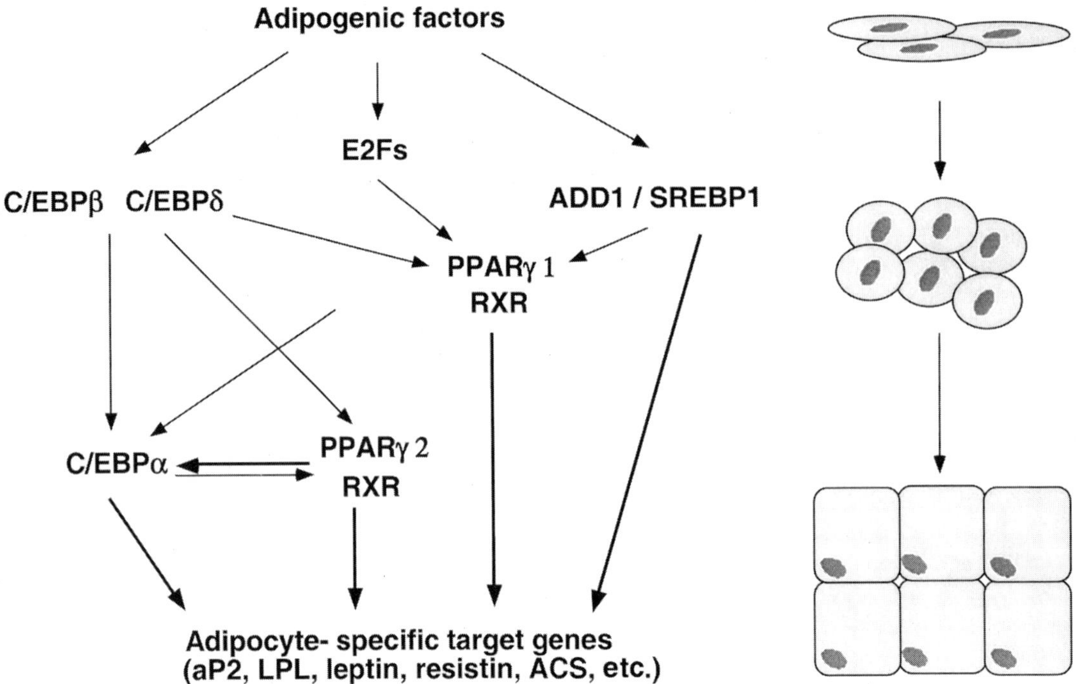

Figure 2 Coordinate regulation of adipogenesis by E2Fs, PPARγ, C/EBPs, and ADD-1/SREBP-1. Interactions among these different transcription factors determine the cascade of events during adipocyte differentiation. The right part of the figure depicts the three different cellular stages—adipocyte precursors, adipoblasts, and adipocytes. The quiescent adipocyte precursor cells undergo an obligatory phase of clonal expansion which requires reentry into the cell cycle. This phase generates adipoblasts, which upon further lipid accumulation become mature adipocytes.

reported to negatively regulate adipogenesis (36,38). Indeed, fibroblasts deficient in both p130 and p107 differentiate spontaneously into adipocytes, whereas the wild-type cells do not (38). Furthermore, reintroduction of p130 and p107 in these cells inhibits adipocyte differentiation. These effects of p107 and p130 in adipogenesis have been suggested to be mediated through downregulation of PPARγ activity.

In the context of the early phases of adipocyte differentiation, we will now discuss the transcriptional regulators that have been shown to inhibit adipogenesis. The adipocyte enhancer-binding protein 1 (AEBP-1) is a carboxypeptidase which was first described as a transcriptional repressor that inhibits the expression of the adipocyte fatty acid–binding protein aP2 (40). Expression of AEBP-1 is downregulated during the adipocyte differentiation process (40). Recently, it was shown that the γ5 subunit of the heterotrimeric G protein binds to AEBP-1 and that it attenuates its transcriptional repression activity (41). Adipogenic stimulation selectively decreased Gγ5 level and enhanced the transcriptional repression activity of AEBP-1 during the mitotic clonal expansion at the onset of adipogenesis (41). Which set of genes is inhibited by this increased AEBP-1 activity during clonal expansion phase is at present unknown, but it is tempting to speculate that some of the genes driving terminal adipocyte differentiation, such as PPARγ and the C/EBP family of transcription factors, could be AEBP-1 targets.

It has been suggested that adipogenesis is also inhibited by several transcription factors of the GATA-binding protein family (42). GATA-2 and -3 are strongly and selectively expressed in adipose tissue (42). Although these GATA factors are enriched in adipose tissue, there is good evidence that they play a negative role in adipogenesis. This is based on the observation that in four independent mouse models of obesity, including the *ob/ob*, *db/db*, and *tub/tub*, and KKA^y mice, expression of GATA-2 and GATA-3 was decreased in adipose tissue (42). Constitutive expression of GATA-2 and GATA-3 results furthermore in a decrease in PPARγ expression and a consequent inhibition of adipocyte differentiation (42). This effect is mediated by a direct inhibitory effect of these GATA factors on PPARγ transcription. Consistent with such an inhibitory effect of GATA-3 on adipocyte differentiation, it was shown that GATA-3 -/- embryonic stem cells differentiated much more efficiently into adipocytes than wild-type ES cells (42).

The retinoic acid receptor (RAR) is another transcription factor of the NR family that is capable of blocking early steps of adipocyte differentiation. In fact, downregulation of RARγ 1 expression during adipocyte differentiation correlates well with the loss of responsiveness to the inhibitory effects of retinoic acid on adipocyte differentiation (43). Along similar lines, ectopic expression of RAR extends the retinoic acid responsive period (43). One mechanism by which retinoic acid might block adipogenesis is by interfering with C/EBPβ-mediated transcription, which is only essential in the early stages of adipogenesis (44), thereby explaining why retinoic acid is less effective when added later in the adipocyte differentiation program. In addition, retinoic acid can inhibit PPARγ action by favoring the formation of the nonpermissive RAR/RXR heterodimer over the PPAR/RXR dimer (45) (see also Fig. 2). Alternatively, RA has been shown to induce the expression of the repressive orphan receptor COUP-TF (46), which also competes with PPARγ for binding to a DR-1.

Several other signaling pathways have been suggested to inhibit this early phase of adipogenesis; tumor necrosis factor alpha (TNF)-α, Pref-1, and Wnt. TNFα is a potent inhibitor of adipocyte differentiation and exposure of 3T3-L1 adipocytes or primary adipocytes to TNFα results in lipid depletion and a complete reversal of adipocyte differentiation (47). An important mechanism by which TNFα exerts its antiadipogenic action is downregulation of the expression of adipogenic factors such as C/EBPα (48,49) and PPARγ (11,47). Interestingly, several other polypeptides, such as TGFβ and bFGF, as well as PKC-activating agents and calcium ionophores, are capable of reversing adipocyte differentiation through a decreased expression of adipogenic transcription factors (11,50). How these agents mediate this decrease in expression is unclear, but further studies are required to investigate the role of NF-κB, AP1, and other transcription factors in the inhibition and reversal of adipocyte differentiation.

Pref-1 is a 45 to 60 kDa transmembrane protein with six tandem EGF-like repeats, which has some similarities to the *Drosophila* cell-fate determination proteins Notch and Delta (51). Pref-1 is expressed in preadipocytes but is absent in adipocytes (51), and its constitutive expression inhibits expression of PPARγ and C/EBPα and blocks adipocyte differentiation (52), suggesting that it functions as a negative regulator of adipogenesis. The inhibitory action of Pref-1 can be exerted either in a juxtacrine manner, as a transmembrane protein affecting adjacent cells, or in a paracrine manner, as a soluble inhibitor of adipocyte differentiation, released by cleavage of the membrane-associated form (52). There are four major forms of Pref-1 which result from alternate splicing (53). Although all four transcripts generate transmembrane Pref-1, only two of them undergo processing to a soluble form of Pref-1, corresponding to their respective complete ectodomains. The other two Pref-1 proteins have a deletion that includes the putative processing site proximal to the membrane, and therefore do not produce a soluble form (53). The mode of inhibition, i.e., juxtacrine or paracrine, therefore depends on the specific alternate Pref-1 form expressed, and underscores the importance of alternate splicing in the determination of Pref-1's range of action (53). However, the mechanism of action of Pref-l or which signaling pathway is implicated remains to be elucidated. Some pro-adipogenic hormones, such as dexamethasone, have been shown to inhibit expression of Pref-1 (54).

Finally, the Wnt family of signaling factors also negatively affects adipocyte differentiation (55). Wnts, signaling molecules that play a major role in the regulation of cell growth and development (56), have been implicated in the inhibition of adipocyte differentiation. It was recently demonstrated that forced expression of Wnt-1 in 3T3-F442A cells inhibited the formation of adipose tissue when these cells were grafted into nude mice (55). Furthermore, 3T3-L1 cells ectopically expressing a dominant negative form of TCF4, a transcriptional mediator of Wnt signaling, undergo adipogenesis without any hormonal induction (55). Repression of PPARγ and C/EBPα expression was suggested as the mechanism by which activation of the Wnt signaling inhibited adipogenesis.

B The Terminal Phases of Adipocyte Differentiation

The terminal phases of adipogenesis are relatively well understood (for review see 30,57), and it is at this stage that PPARγ is suggested to be the predominant player. This was initially based on the fact that the infection of fibroblasts with a retrovirus encoding PPARγ-induced fibroblast (58) and muscle cells (59) undergo terminal adipocyte differentiation. This adipogenic property, however, seems hardly unique, since a whole range of transcription factors affect adipogenesis. It is currently thought that full-fledged adipogenesis requires an interplay between the PPARγ/RXR heterodimer and two other groups of transcription factors: the CCAATT enhancer-binding proteins (C/EBP), and ADD-1/SREBP-1 (reviewed in 29,30) (Fig. 2). Although all of these transcription factors can independently induce adipocyte differentiation in vitro, they act synergistically in vivo.

During the initial phases of these terminal stages of adipogenesis, C/EBPβ and δ are induced in response to adipogenic hormones such as insulin or glucocorticoids (60–62). Both these C/EBPs induce the transcription of PPARγ2, via interaction with a C/EBP site in the PPARγ2 promoter (63). Ectopic expression of C/EBPβ is sufficient to induce differentiation of 3T3-L1 cells in the absence of hormonal induction, whereas overexpression of C/EBPδ accelerates adipose conversion, but only in the presence of hormonal inducers (60). Furthermore, induction of C/EBPβ levels results in the differentiation of NIH-3T3 fibroblasts, which cannot differentiate spontaneously. Additional evidence that both these C/EBPs play an important role in the control of the adipocyte differentiation process in vivo comes from the characterization of animals with mutations in the C/EBPβ and δ genes. Mice lacking either of these factors have normal white adipose tissue, although their brown adipose tissue accumulates less lipids (64). The reduced fraction of mice (15%) that survive the deletion of both C/EBPβ and δ genes have a severe decrease in both brown and white adipose tissue mass, despite normal levels of expression of PPARγ and C/EBPα (64). In contrast to the role of C/EBPβ and δ in regulating the expression of PPARγ2, expression of PPARγ1 seems to be independent of these factors. Indeed, a dominant negative C/EBPβ isoform (also termed LIP) suppresses adipogenesis and the expression of PPARγ2, whereas PPARγ1 was still expressed (65). However, addition of PPARγ agonists bypassed the block in adipogenesis imposed by LIP, suggesting that C/EBPβ might not only induce the expression of PPARγ2 (63), but also participates in the generation of PPARγ ligands during adipogenesis (65).

RXR, the obligate heterodimeric partner of PPARγ, constitutes another pivotal sensor during adipocyte differentiation (45). On DR-1 response elements, such as most PPREs, RXR is a nonpermissive inactive partner when heterodimerized with RAR, whereas it is a permissive partner in the context of the PPARγ/RXR heterodimer. The levels of RAR and PPARγ change considerably during the induction of adipocyte differentiation, with RAR expression being strongly reduced and PPARγ levels being induced (43). A change in the relative levels of RAR and PPARγ in the differentiating adipocytes will hence induce a switch for RXR from one partner to another one (43,45). This will change RXR activity from the nonpermissive state when bound to RAR to the permissive state when complexed to PPARγ. This switch in partners induces the recruitment of a distinct set of cofactors, ultimately translating in an alteration of the transcriptional activity of the downstream target genes (Fig. 3) (45). Such a switch in partners might underlie not only how PPARγ agonists but also how RXR agonists exert their effects on adipogenesis and glucose homeostasis. Proof that RXR is involved in adipose tissue homeostasis in vivo was recently provided by the spatiotemporally controlled mutagenesis of the RXRα gene in adipose tissue (66). Mice lacking RXRα in fat tissue have significantly reduced fat mass and are resistant against the induction of obesity (66). This model further points out that most likely both partners of the RXR/PPARγ heterodimer are important in inducing and maintaining adipose tissue homeostasis.

The basic helix-loop-helix (bHLH) protein ADD-1/SREBP-1c is also induced during terminal adipocyte differentiation (67,68). ADD-1/SREBP-1c accelerates

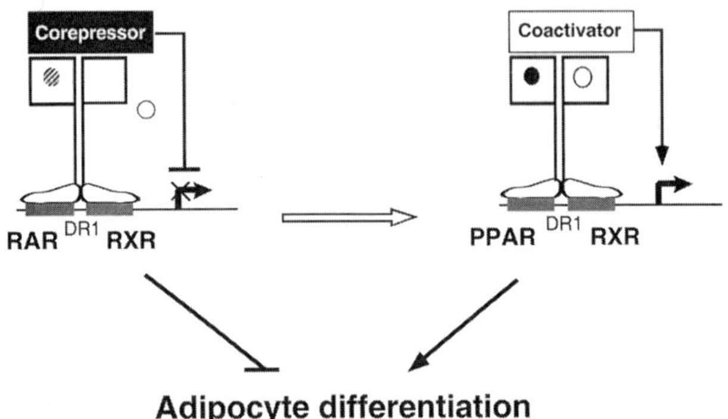

Figure 3 Switch in RXR partners stimulates adipocyte differentiation. PPAR/RXR and RAR/RXR heterodimers respectively activate and repress DR-1 containing promoters. When the RAR/RXR heterodimer is bound to a DR-1, RAR blocks the binding of ligands to RXR, keeping the heterodimer in an inactive state due to the binding of corepressors such as N-CoR or SMRT. In contrast, the PPAR/RXR heterodimer configuration permits ligand binding to RXR, allowing for activation of both partners in the PPAR/RXR heterodimer.

adipocyte differentiation when coexpressed in fibroblasts, which also contain PPARγ. ADD-1/SREBP-1 belongs to a family of transcription factors that are synthesized as membrane-bound precursors that are released by proteolysis (69). Whereas the proteolytic cleavage of SREBP-2 is regulated by cellular cholesterol levels, it is at present unknown what controls the cleavage of ADD-1/SREBP-1 (69). ADD-1/SREBP-1c induces the expression of several genes involved in lipogenesis in both adipocytes and liver. These genes include the genes encoding for fatty acid synthase (68,70,71), acetyl coenzyme A carboxylase (71,72), glycerol-3-phosphate acyltransferase (73), and the lipoprotein lipase (LPL) gene (68,71) (74). Stimulation of lipogenesis contributes to the massive cholesterol and fatty acid accumulation seen in the livers of transgenic animals expressing the mature form of SREBP-1a (71), and to the more moderate fatty acid accumulation observed upon overexpression of the weaker transactivator SREBP-1c (75). The observation that transgenic mice overexpressing SREBP-1c under the control of the adipose tissue-specific aP2 promoter are lipodystrophic (76) appears inconsistent with these adipo- and lipogenic effects (68,71,75) and suggests that SREBP-1c, under certain conditions, could also negatively influence adipogenesis. The differences between this last study (76) and previous work (68,71,75) are unclear and will require further investigation.

Finally, terminal adipocyte differentiation requires the concerted action of PPARγ and C/EBPα (58,59, 77), another C/EBP family member which appears only relatively late in the differentiation process. In contrast to the relatively early effects of C/EBPβ and δ, C/EBPα seems to play an important role in the later stages of differentiation by sustaining high levels of PPARγ expression and by maintaining the differentiated adipocyte phenotype. Several lines of evidence support an important role of C/EBPα in adipocyte differentiation. First, temporal activation of C/EBPα expression occurs immediately before the coordinate expression of a group of adipocyte-specific genes, suggesting its involvement in their regulation. Second, antisense C/EBPα RNA can inhibit adipocyte differentiation. Third, premature induction or overexpression of C/EBPα triggers adipocyte differentiation. And finally, adipocytes from C/EBPα -/- mice failed to accumulate lipids in adipose tissue (78,79). PPARγ controls not only the expression of C/EBPα, but this last factor in its turn also induces PPARγ gene expression, via interaction with C/EBP response elements present in the human (63) and mouse (2,77) PPARγ promoter. Interestingly, introduction of PPARγ in cells deficient for C/EBPα enabled adipocyte differentiation, whereas the reverse, i.e., overexpression of C/EBPα in PPARγ deficient cells, did not result in differentiation.

C Other Factors Involved in Adipogenesis

1 Signal Transducers and Activators of Transcription (STATs)

The STAT family of transcription factors is composed of six family members that are phosphorylated as a cellular response to various cytokines and peptide hormones (80,81). After phosphorylation and translocation to the nucleus, they regulate the transcription of specific target genes. Three members of the STAT family—STATs 1, 3, and 5a and b—are highly induced during adipocyte differentiation in a manner similar to C/EBPα and PPARγ (82). Furthermore, inhibition of adipogenesis by TNFα correlates with the repression of STATs in 3T3-L1 cells (82). Adipose tissue contains several receptors of the cytokine receptor superfamily, such as the growth hormone and the prolactin receptor, both of which are induced during the differentiation process (83,84) and which have been shown to control the expression of adipocyte genes, such as LPL (85,86). Interestingly, prolactin, a lactogenic hormone that triggers the STAT pathway, was shown to increase C/EBPβ and PPARγ mRNA expression and stimulate adipocyte differentiation of NIH-3T3 cells (87). Furthermore, it was shown that STAT5a transactivated the expression of the aP2 promoter in a prolactin-dependent manner. Further support for a role of STAT5a and b in adipogenesis came from the analysis of mice deficient in these transcription factors. Targeted deletion of either STAT5a or STAT5b results in animals with markedly reduced adipose tissue mass (88). In contrast to STAT5, participation of STAT3 in the adipocyte differentiation process seems to be restricted to the proliferative phases of the clonal expansion (89). Unfortunately, STAT3-deficient mice are not viable (90), and tissue-specific STAT3-deficient animals will be required to further assess the role of this member of the family in adipogenesis. Altogether, these data suggest that cytokines and peptide hormones, through their effects on STAT-mediated gene expression (and perhaps other transcription factors), could play a significant role in the development and/or maintenance of the adipose phenotype.

2 Glucocorticoid Receptor

Activated glucocorticoid receptor (GR) is thought to have multiple pro-adipogenic effects, several of them enhancing PPARγ activity. First, glucocorticoids inhibit the expression of Pref-1 (54). The transcriptional repression of Pref-1 is an early action of dexamethasone in 3T3L1 adipocyte differentiation, suggesting that downregulation of Pref-1 by glucocorticoids may be a prime mechanism for promoting adipogenesis. Second, activated GR will increase the expression of early adipogenic genes, including the C/EBPs, which in their turn will switch on PPARγ. It has also been suggested that GR might directly stimulate the expression of PPARγ, although further studies are required to elucidate whether there is a functional GR binding site in the PPARγ promoter. In addition, glucocorticoids are known to activate phospholipase A2, stimulating the production of prostanoid ligands of PPARγ (91). Another important issue to bring up at this time is the relationship between hypercorticosteroidism and insulin resistance. Corticosteroid activity is in part regulated by the activity of the enzyme 11β-hydroxysteroid dehydrogenase (11β-HSD), which converts cortisone into the active glucocorticoid cortisol. Activation of PPARγ has been shown to reduce 11β-HSD activity in adipose tissue, and the ensuing decrease in cortisol levels will contribute to the antidiabetic effects of PPARγ activators (92).

D Adipocyte Apoptosis

PPARγ is a crucial element not only in the control of adipocyte differentiation but also in the modulation of programmed cell death in the adipocytes (93) (J. Auwerx, unpublished results). Activation of PPARγ has been shown to induce adipocyte apoptosis, an event mainly restricted to large fully differentiated adipocytes, which express high amounts of PPARγ. This pro-apoptotic effect of PPARγ activation on large adipocytes,

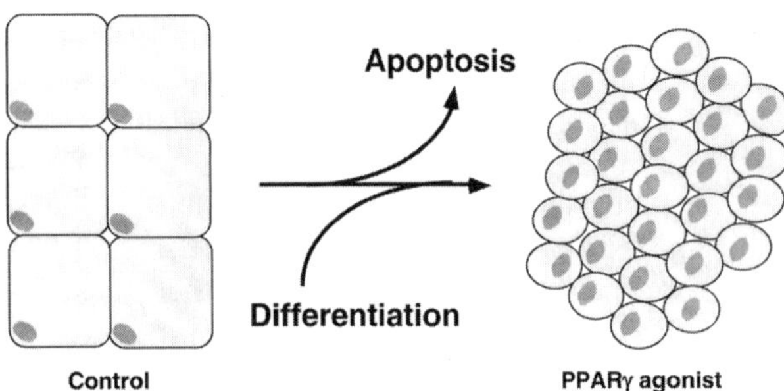

Figure 4 Remodeling of white adipose tissue by PPARγ activation. Activation of PPARγ in adipocytes will not only translate in apoptosis of the fully differentiated adipocytes, but will also induce de novo differentiation of preadipocytes. This will result in a continuous remodeling of the adipose tissue.

coupled with its capacity to enhance de novo differentiation of adipocytes, favors the formation of small adipocytes which tend to replace the large adipocytes normally constituting white adipose tissue (93,94). It is therefore tempting to speculate that PPARγ activation results in a continuous remodeling of adipose tissue (Fig. 4). The ultimate fate of these small freshly differentiated adipocytes remains unclear. It will therefore be important to determine whether over time they will store more and more energy and finally become hypertrophic leading to a state of resistance to PPARγ activation.

V PPARγ CONTROLS ADIPOCYTE-SPECIFIC GENE EXPRESSION

The enhanced adipocyte differentiation, which ensues from PPARγ activation, translates in the induction of the expression of adipocyte-specific genes. In fact, functional PPREs have been identified in several genes implicated in adipocyte differentiation, most of them involved in lipid storage and control of metabolism. Good examples are the lipid-binding protein aP2 (95), phosphoenolpyruvate carboxykinase (PEPCK) (96), acyl-CoA synthase (ACS) (97), fatty acid transport protein-1 (FATP-1) (98), and LPL (99), which are all regulated by PPARγ. PPARγ can also influence and control the generation and cellular uptake of its own ligands or activators, suggesting that PPARγ and its target genes play an interdependent role in adipocyte differentiation. This hypothesis is supported by the observation that fatty acids and fatty acid analogs induce the expression of adipocyte-specific genes, enhance adipocyte conversion, and maintain the mature adipocyte phenotype by creating a positive feedforward loop, which involves PPARγ and several of the above mentioned target genes (for review see 29,30,100). Some of these adipocyte-specific genes are also coordinately regulated by the other transcription factors discussed above (74,99), resulting in a strong and sustained expression of these genes.

In addition to these genes, which are mainly involved in adipocyte metabolism, cytokinelike signaling factors produced by the adipocytes, such as leptin, TNFα, and resistin, also appear to be functioning in this adipocyte sustaining positive regulatory loop. Leptin is an adipocyte-derived signaling factor which after interaction with specific cytokinelike receptors induces a pleiotropic response including control of body weight and energy expenditure (reviewed in 101). Leptin gene expression is regulated in an opposite fashion by PPARγ and C/EBPα, the first one reducing its expression (102–104), whereas the second induces its expression (105–107). The decrease in circulating leptin levels upon PPARγ activation is associated with an increase in food intake, which will provide substrates, subsequently to be stored in the adipocytes. A similar hypothesis can be formulated in relation to adipose tissue TNFα production. TNFα, which was originally described as cachectin, is a potent inhibitor of adipocyte differentiation, and exposure of 3T3-L1 adipocytes to TNFα results in lipid depletion and a complete reversal of adipocyte differentiation (108) (reviewed in 109). TNFα exerts this antiadipogenic action in part by the downregulation of the expression of adipogenic factors such as C/EBPα (48,49) and PPARγ (11,12,110). Interestingly, obesity characterized by increased adipose tissue mass is associated with increased TNFα expression in adipose tissue. Although the exact role of high TNFα levels in obesity is unclear, it might constitute a regulatory mechanism to limit further increase in adipose tissue mass. This increase in TNFα levels in obesity also interferes with the insulin signaling pathways (111), contributing to the insulin resistance characteristic of the obese state (112,113). Consistent with the opposing effects of PPARγ and TNFα in adipose tissue, treatment of obese animals with PPARγ agonists reduces adipose tissue expression of TNFα, contributing to weight gain (93,114). PPARγ activation furthermore blocks the inhibitory effects of TNFα on insulin signaling (110) as well as the TNFα-induced glycerol and free fatty acid release (115). PPARγ activation would not only favor adipocyte differentiation by affecting adipocyte metabolism, but in addition would trigger an adipocyte-sustaining endocrine, paracrine, or autocrine response consisting of decreased levels of two important adipocyte-derived signaling factors, leptin and TNFα. PPARγ therefore seems to be a master gene controlling a coordinated thrifty response.

Another adipose tissue protein whose expression has been shown to be decreased by PPARγ activation is resistin (116). Resistin was identified in a screen of genes downregulated by the PPARγ agonist rosiglitazone in fully differentiated adipocytes (116). Resistin is a secreted protein, and its levels in plasma are increased in several animal models of obesity. The group of Lazar et al. hypothesized that resistin is a signaling molecule, which reduces glucose utilization by insulin-sensitive tissues. To prove this point, it was shown that decreasing resistin levels by injection of resistin antibodies improves glucose homeostasis, whereas a deterioration of glucose homeostasis is observed after administration of recombinant resistin to animals (116). Two new resistinlike molecules, RELMα and RELMβ, have been described recently (117). Interestingly, the expression pattern of these two proteins is restricted to two tissues with high levels of PPARγ expression, i.e., adipose tissue and colon (117). Further studies are required to elucidate the exact function of the resistin protein family, but it is highly likely that they act as signaling molecules.

VI NATURAL AND SYNTHETIC PPARγ ACTIVATORS

PPARγ, like the other PPARs, seems to be a very promiscuous receptor when it comes to activation, which can be achieved by a wide variety of naturally occurring and synthetic compounds (118). This property could be linked to its spacious ligand-binding cavity (15,16). For some of these PPARγ agonists, it was subsequently shown that they not only activate, but also bind to, the receptor. Most attention has been paid to some of the naturally occurring arachidonic acid metabolites derived from the cyclooxygenase pathway, such as 15-deoxy-Δ12,14-prostaglandin J2 (119–121) and Δ12-prostaglandin J2 (122). Although 15-deoxy-Δ12,14-prostaglandin J2 was shown to be the most potent of the naturally occurring ligands, it is still unclear whether it is produced in sufficient quantities in vivo in cells expressing PPARγ. In contrast, Δ12-prostaglandin J2 has been demonstrated to be made in vivo. A report that estrogen induces the production of Δ12-prostaglandin J2 in duck uropygial gland was interesting in this context, since it could point to an especially interesting dialog between estrogen and peroxisome proliferator–stimulated signaling pathways (122). Other eicosanoids and unsaturated fatty acids are also reported to bind and activate PPARγ (121,123,124). This has been demonstrated for the ω-3 polyunsaturated fatty acids, α-linolenic (18:3), eicosapentaenoic (20:5;EPA), and docohexanoic acid (22:6; DHA) (121,123,124). Two eicosanoids present in oxidized low-density lipoproteins (oxLDL), 9-hydroxyoctadecadienoic and 13-hydroxyoctadecadienoic acid, are also potent PPARγ ligands (125). Finally, an oxidatively modified alkyl phospholipid, hexadecyl azelaoyl phosphatidylcholine (azPC), which is present in the oxLDL particles, has been identified as a high-affinity ligand of PPARγ.

In addition to the above-mentioned natural PPARγ ligands, several classes of synthetic PPARγ agonists have been described (Fig. 5). Most is known about the thiazolidinediones (TZDs), which are potent insulin sensitizers currently used in the treatment of type 2

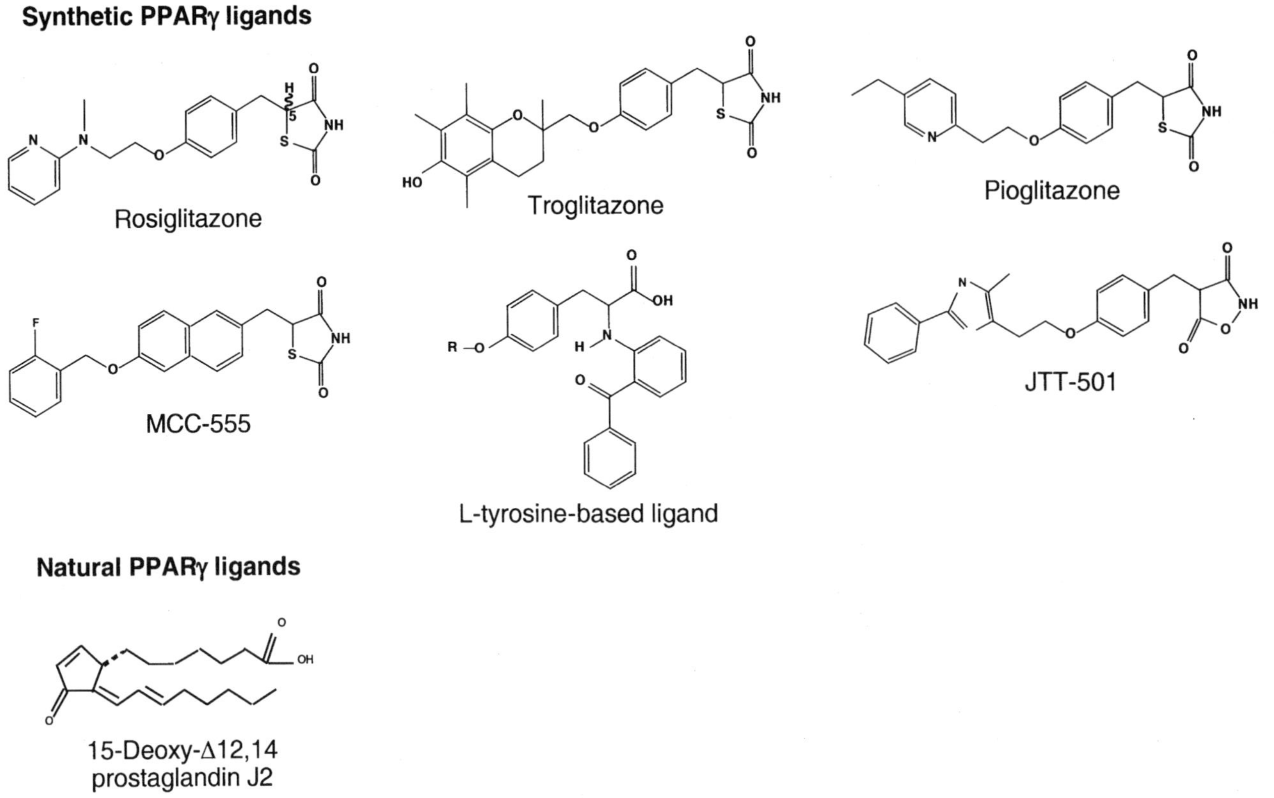

Synthetic PPARγ ligands

Rosiglitazone

Troglitazone

Pioglitazone

MCC-555

L-tyrosine-based ligand

JTT-501

Natural PPARγ ligands

15-Deoxy-Δ12,14 prostaglandin J2

Figure 5 Natural and synthetic PPARγ ligands. Rosiglitazone, troglitazone, pioglitazone, and MCC-555 are members of the thiazolidinedione family of PPARγ ligands, whereas L-tyrosine-based ligands and JTT-501 are not. Rosiglitazone, troglitazone, and pioglitazone have all received market approval, but only rosiglitazone and pioglitazone are actually on the market.

diabetes mellitus (126). L-tyrosine-based PPARγ ligands are another group of promising synthetic PPARγ agonists, which are under development (127). Finally, certain nonsteroidal anti-inflammatory drugs (NSAIDs) (128) were demonstrated to be high-affinity ligands for PPARγ. It is interesting that the relative potency of most TZDs to bind to and to activate PPARγ in vitro seems to correlate with their antidiabetic potency in vivo, suggesting that PPARγ mediates at least in part their antidiabetic effect (126,129). The involvement of PPARγ in insulin sensitization and glucose homeostasis is furthermore supported by the observation that activation of RXR, the heterodimeric partner of PPARγ, also induces a certain degree of adipocyte differentiation and improves glucose homeostasis (130). These observations argue that the active moiety involved in ameliorating glucose metabolism is the heterodimer PPARγ/RXR. Move recent work, however, clearly underscores that PPARγ and RXR activation can also have distinct biological effects (131), although a fair number of overlapping effects exists. Furthermore, the recent observation that synthetic as well as natural PPARγ ligands retain the capacity to exert some modulatory effects in PPARγ -/- macrophages (132,133), points to the fact that certain of these compounds also could have PPARγ independent effects in glucose homeostasis.

Since the current PPARγ agonists are rather weak in monotherapy and because these compounds all have some unwanted side effects (118), there is no doubt that the future will bring another dimension to the development of PPARγ modulators, which until now was focused on the development of simple agonists. First, novel ligands, such as the TZD derivative, KRP-297 and JTT-501, with activity toward both PPARα and γ are being developed, widening both their tissue-specific activity and pharmacological properties (134,135). Administration of a combination of PPARα and γ agonists (136) or a single dual-agonist (134), with effects on both liver and adipose tissue, can clearly widen the therapeutic window and enhance their efficacy in complex metabolic disturbances such as insulin resistance and type 2 diabetes. Although little is known about their pharmacological properties, ligands capable of binding and activating both PPARγ and β have recently been reported (137). These dual PPARγ and β agonists could become highly relevant compounds in the treatment of the many facets of the metabolic syndrome, since they might combine the insulin sensitizing activities of PPARγ activation with the HDL raising activities of PPARβ activation.

Second, the discovery of a novel TZD, MCC-555, with significant antidiabetic properties but only weak capacities to bind to PPARγ, makes a notable exception to the rule that PPARγ binding correlates with clinical efficacy (126,129). MCC-555 can function either as a full or partial agonist or as an antagonist pending on cell type and the sequence recognition site. This property can be explained by unique cofactor recruitment by this compound and demonstrates that it will be possible to produce tissue- and promoter-specific PPARγ modulators. Another PPARγ modulator, i.e., FMOC-L-Leucine (FMOC-L-Leu), was recently described in our laboratory (137a). FMOC-L-Leu has some similarity to the tyrosine-based PPARγ ligands but, unlike these last compounds, have a rather weak affinity for PPARγ. Interestingly, two molecules of FMOC-L-Leu bind to the ligand-binding domain of the receptor, as demonstrated by mass spectrometry of the PPARγ ligand-binding domain and FMOC-L-Leu. This unique binding to PPARγ changes the cofactor preference of PPARγ, relative to classical agonist ligands, and results in distinct biological effects characterized by strong insulin sensitization without weight gain.

VII ADIPOSE TISSUE, TRANSCRIPTION FACTORS, AND FATTY ACIDS IN INSULIN SENSITIVITY

On a whole-body level, adipose tissue is absolutely required for glucose homeostasis. Indeed, subjects with lipoatrophy (138) and transgenic animals that are engineered to lack adipose tissue (76,139) are extremely insulin resistant. This seems therefore to indicate that storage of energy in the adipocytes favors insulin sensitivity and that the important adipogenic activity of PPARγ contributes to the insulin sensitization of PPARγ agonists. Despite the fact that PPARγ seems to have its primary effects on adipose tissue, it is unclear how PPARγ agonists improve insulin sensitivity in muscle. Normally, adipose tissue and liver contribute only minimally to glucose disposal, whereas muscle is responsible for most of the glucose uptake, yet muscle expresses only trace amounts of PPARγ. This questions whether these minute quantities of PPARγ are sufficient or, alternatively, might be induced during TZD treatment, leading to an eventual direct PPARγ-mediated response of the muscle to these insulin sensitizers. Alternatively, PPARγ activators may generate an adipocyte-derived signal affecting insulin sensitivity in muscle. Both proteins and lipids have been proposed as nonmutually exclusive signaling molecules, which can affect the muscle.

The prototypical examples of protein signaling molecules are the adipocytokines (140). TNFα is the prime example of molecules belonging to this group. Increased adipose tissue TNFα production has been shown to induce systemic insulin resistance by interference with the insulin signaling cascade (111,112). TZDs have been shown to reduce TNFα expression, which may contribute to the improved insulin sensitivity (93,114). More recently, it was demonstrated that also leptin might interfere with insulin signaling in vitro (141–143), although its in vivo activity on glucose homeostasis suggests otherwise (144,145). Two other adipocytokines were recently shown to affect glucose homeostasis—resistin and adipo-Q. Resistin reduces glucose utilization and its expression is decreased by PPARγ activation (116). Although a proteolytically cleaved fragment of adipo-Q improves glucose disposal, it is unknown whether TZDs affect this pathway in vivo (146). Other adipocyte-derived proteins, such as adipsin (147), angiotensinogen (148), and plasminogen activator inhibitor I (140), could also be involved in a similar signaling process, although experimental proof of this is still missing.

A second group of important mediators that affect insulin sensitivity in both muscle and liver and that are derived from adipose tissue, consists of fatty acids. Since the original observation by Randle (149) (reviewed in 150), it has been well established that increased fatty acid concentrations in the muscle decrease glucose metabolism in that tissue (151). Perhaps the most extreme example of fatty acid and triglyceride accumulation in muscle and liver occurs when adipose tissue is completely absent, such as the case in lipoatrophy (152), a condition characterized by extreme insulin resistance (153). In the liver, fatty acids stimulate gluconeogenesis, suggesting that hormonal control of lipolysis in the adipocyte indirectly controls hepatic glucose production (154). This observation is particularly relevant in visceral adipose tissue, which is less sensitive to insulin than subcutaneous fat and which drains directly to the liver via the portal circulation.

Interestingly, treatment with PPARγ activators induces LPL, aP2, FATP-1, and ACS (all genes involved in fatty acid uptake) selectively in adipose tissue, whereas they do not seem to change the expression of these genes in muscle or hepatic tissue (reviewed in 150). This might on a whole-body level induce a "fatty acid steal" due to a specific PPARγ-mediated increase in lipid and fatty acid clearance by adipose tissue, without a concomitant increase in fatty acid delivery to the muscle and liver (155). The resulting "trapping" of fatty acids in fat tissue leads to a decreased systemic availability and a diminished fatty acid uptake by the muscle and liver, potentially improving both muscle insulin sensitivity according to the mechanisms proposed by Randle (149) and hepatic glucose output (154).

From all the above it is clear that the majority of PPARγ regulated genes are involved in fatty acid and/or lipid metabolism and seem to be linked to adipocyte differentiation. In contrast, very little is known about regulation by PPARγ of genes directly involved in glucose homeostasis and insulin signaling. The mRNAs encoding for both the glucose transporter Glut-4 (156) and the insulin receptor substrate 2 (IRS-2) (157) were reported to be induced by PPARγ agonists, although a direct regulation on the promoter activity of the above mentioned genes by PPARγ has not been studied. Similarly, it was demonstrated that the c-Cbl associated protein (CAP) was induced by activation of PPARγ (158). CAP, which is only expressed in cells that are metabolically sensitive to insulin, is involved in insulin-stimulated tyrosine phosphorylation of c-Cbl (158). Upon phosphorylation, the c-Cbl/CAP complex translocates to lipid raft domains of the cell membrane (159) and recruits additional signaling molecules to these lipid rafts, resulting in the activation of the G-protein TC10. This molecular switch provides then a second signal to the Glut-4 protein, parallel to phosphatidylinositol 3-kinase (PI-3K) (159). Also the p85α subunit of PI-3K was shown to be dose dependently induced by both PPARγ and RXR agonists in isolated human adipocytes, directly proving the implication of the RXR/PPARγ heterodimer in its induction (160). Finally, it is important to stress that other adipose tissue–independent and perhaps PPARγ-independent mechanisms also contribute to the insulin-sensitizing effects of TZDs. In fact, these PPARγ agonists retain some insulin-sensitizing activity in transgenic mice that totally lack adipose tissue (161), and furthermore these agonists have significant anti-inflammatory effects in PPARγ -/- macrophages (132,133). The exact nature of these nonadipose tissue and PPARγ-independent effects, however, is unclear at present and warrants more detailed investigation.

The extensive cross-regulation among C/EBPs, PPARγ/RXR, and ADD-1/SREBP-1 to induce and sustain adipocyte differentiation suggests that these factors also are of importance in glucose homeostasis (see discussion below). Fasting and feeding regulate ADD-1/SREBP-1c levels via insulin in both fat (162) and liver (163), indicating that ADD-1/SREBP-1c is an intermediate or a target of insulin signaling. SREBP-1c furthermore increases the expression of several genes involved in gluconeogenesis and lipogenesis (74,162–164). Interestingly, hepatic SREBP-1c levels are both increased in a mouse model of lipoatrophy, as well as in the *ob/ob* mouse, a model that reflects the relative leptin deficiency in obesity-induced diabetes (165). Administration of leptin could normalize this effect (145). This led to the suggestion that increased expression of SREBP-1c underlies the mixed insulin resistance/sensitivity, with increased and inappropriate rates of both gluconeogenesis (as a sign of insulin resistance) and lipogenesis (as a sign of insulin sensitivity) (165). A further link between SREBPs and glucose homeostasis is provided by the fact that SREBPs induce the expression of PPARγ (166), and that their lipogenic effects will stimulate the generation of fatty acids ligands for PPARγ (167).

Also the C/EBP family of transcription factors seems to play an important role in glucose homeostasis. Mice homozygous for a mutation in the C/EBPα gene have diminished glycogen stores in the liver and fail to activate gluconeogenic pathways (78,79,168). This leads to premature death of mutant C/EBPα -/- animals postpartum because of severe hypoglycemia (78,79). Defective gluconeogenesis and low glycogen synthase activity was recapitulated in animals in which the C/EBPα gene was disrupted in adult mouse liver with a temporally and spatially controlled strategy using an adenovirus to express the Cre recombinase (169). Also adult C/EBPβ -/- mice have a significant hypoglycemia after fasting, which is accompanied by lower hepatic glucose output (170). These mice have also a decrease in fasting plasma fatty acid levels (170). All this work suggests that anti-C/EBP strategies could be of value to suppress excessive gluconeogenesis. Whereas these data refer to the effects of C/EBPs on liver glucose homeostasis, there are also some recent data suggesting that C/EBPα is involved in the induction of insulin sensitivity during adipocyte differentiation. Insulin regulation of Glut4 in the adipocytes requires C/EBPα, which is involved in the stimulation of gene expression and tyrosine phosphorylation of the insulin receptor and the insulin receptor substrate-1 (IRS-1) (77). In view of the extensive cross-regulation between PPARγ and C/EBPα, C/EBPα could be an important indirect target to explain the antidiabetic effects of PPARγ agonists (77). The role of C/EBPα in muscle glucose utilization is less clear.

VIII GENETIC STUDIES SUPPORT A ROLE OF PPARγ IN ADIPOGENESIS

Approximately 70% of the variance in body mass index (BMI) is genetically determined (171). In this context, the PPARγ gene was also analyzed for mutations. A rare Pro115Gln mutation in the NH_2-terminal ligand-independent activation domain of PPARγ has been described in four very obese subjects (172). This mutation resulted in a permanently active PPARγ since it inhibited phosphorylation of the protein at Ser114 and led to increased adipocyte differentiation capacity in vitro (172). Furthermore, modification of the A/B domain by phosphorylation of this residue was reported to reduce ligand-binding affinity through interdomain communication between the A/B and the ligand-binding pocket in the DEF domain of PPARγ. Phosphorylation at Ser114 was proposed as a mechanism by which growth factors and insulin, through mitogen-activated protein kinase, decreased PPARγ activity and adipocyte differentiation (173–176).

In addition, a much more common Pro 12Ala substitution in the PPARγ2-specific exon B has been described (177–180). The PPARγ2 Ala allele, whose frequency ranges from ~0.12 among Caucasians to 0.02 in Japanese-Americans (177,178), was associated with lower BMI, improved insulin sensitivity, and higher plasma HDL cholesterol levels (178). The association with insulin sensitivity disappeared when corrected for BMI, indicating that the primary effect of this mutation was on body weight. Among Japanese-American subjects, a significantly lower frequency of the Ala allele amongst type 2 diabetics was observed relative to normals. The PPARγ Ala allele exhibited a reduced ability to transactivate responsive promoters (178). These observations were confirmed in a very large study, which independently demonstrated that this Pro12Ala mutation was associated with a reduction in BMI and significant insulin sensitization (181). Together with the observations of the Pro115Gln substitution, these results provide strong evidence of a role of PPARγ in the control of adipogenesis in vivo, such that a more active PPARγ (Pro115Gln) results in increased BMI (172), whereas the opposite is seen with a less active PPARγ (Pro12Ala)(178). Although these studies provide strong evidence for a role of PPARγ in the control of adipogenesis and insulin resistance, some smaller studies in more heterogeneous patient populations found only a weak or no association of the Pro12Ala substitution with BMI and insulin sensitivity (180,182). These apparently conflicting data indicate the importance of gene environment interactions in the determination of the phenotype.

The genetic and functional data on the Pro12Ala substitution point to the importance of the PPARγ2-specific B exon in determining the activity of PPARγ more particularly in adipocytes, the only tissue known to express significant amounts of PPARγ2. The exon B–encoded 28 NH_2-terminal residues were previously shown to be dispensable in in vitro assays of transcriptional activation and adipocyte differentiation (58). In apparent contradiction to this observation, the NH_2-terminus of PPARγ2 was shown to be 5–10 times more potent in transactivation assays than the NH_2-terminus of PPARγ1 (183). The sequence of the first 13 of these 28 residues in PPARγ2 is evolutionarily conserved between mouse, pig, cow, and human, indicating that they may be functionally important in vivo (unpublished data) (1). The function of the NH_2-terminal residues of PPARγ2 is unknown. This domain may modulate nuclear import, ligand binding, DNA binding, or transcriptional activation by inducing a conformational change, or it may endow PPARγ2 with unique capacities to interact with coactivators or corepressors that have been shown to interact with nuclear receptors. Support for the role of the NH_2-terminus of PPARγ in transcriptional activity not only comes from the presence of a ligand-independent AF-1 domain in this part of the molecule (183) but also from its allosteric effects on ligand-dependent transcriptional activity through interdomain communication (184). The identification and characterization of proteins interacting with the NH_2-terminus of PPARγ in the future will point to mechanisms by which this domain affects adipose tissue accumulation and metabolism.

In combination, these human genetic studies suggested that the major function of PPARγ was fat formation, not insulin sensitization, as was stipulated from pharmacological characterization of the receptor. Additional genetic support for a role of PPARγ in the determination of body fat comes from the fact that one of the loci with suggestive linkage to obesity (LOD = 2.0) in Pima Indians maps close to the location of *PPARG* in the 3p25-p24 region (185). Furthermore, the striking phenotype observed in mice with a mutation in the PPARγ gene confirmed the validity of the human genetic studies. Whereas homozygous PPARγ-/- mice are not viable (most likely due to the complete absence of adipose tissue) (186), heterozygous PPARγ -/+ mice are characterized by a decrease in adipose tissue mass and, contrary to general expectations, by a marked insulin sensitization (187,188). Although these knockout (KO) data appear at odds with pharmacological studies with PPARγ agonists, they are fully in line with the above-mentioned human genetic studies on the Pro12Ala and Pro115Gln. In fact, both the human and mouse genetic studies demonstrate that the prime activity of PPARγ is to stimulate adipocyte differentiation and suggest that its effect on insulin sensitivity are associated with the changes in adipose tissue mass. These studies hence also clearly demonstrate an inherent problem of currently marketed PPARγ agonists, which all stimulate PPARγ activity and induce weight gain, a highly undesirable profile in diabetic patients.

Interestingly, the above-discussed genetic studies demonstrated an association between (1) the Pro12Ala substitution in the PPARγ2 gene and (2) increased HDL cholesterol and reduced total triglycerides levels (178). The genetic association of HDL levels and PPARγ2 Ala allele suggests that adipose tissue mass has important implications on reverse cholesterol transport (196,197). In addition, these genetic data support a role of adipose tissue in the complex metabolic abnormalities associated with visceral obesity/insulin resistance syndrome, such as elevated triglyceride, small dense LDL, low HDL levels, and increased predisposition to atherosclerosis (198,199). Support for the hypothesis that PPARγ could be involved in certain aspects of the visceral obesity/insulin resistance syndrome, and more particularly in the protection against atherosclerosis, was recently provided both by in vitro (132,133) and in vivo (200,201) studies. Activation of PPARγ could in fact protect against foam cell formation in vitro (132,133), whereas administration of agonists of PPARγ (200,201) or of its heterodimeric partner RXR (201) could reduce atherosclerotic lesions in two different and validated animal models of atherosclerosis.

IX PPARγ AND THE CONTROL OF LIPID METABOLISM AND ATHEROSCLEROSIS

In addition to its role in fat storage in the adipocytes, PPARγ is also important in extracellular lipid metabolism, more particularly in that of triglyceride-rich lipoproteins (reviewed in 13,100). Steady-state triglyceride levels are determined on the one hand by their production rates in the liver and gut, a process controlled to a large extent by substrate (fatty acid) availability, and on the other hand by their clearance rate, a process under the control of LPL and apolipoprotein C-III. In fact, activation of either PPARα and/or PPARγ has pronounced triglyceride-lowering effects, but the mechanisms by which they achieve this are largely different. Whereas TZDs predominantly affect triglyceride clearance, fibrates, which are weak PPARα ligands, exert their effects both on triglyceride clearance and production rates (reviewed in 13,189). PPARα activation will reduce the production of apo C-III and triglyceride-rich lipoproteins in the liver (190,191), whereas activation of PPARγ will induce adipose tissue LPL gene expression (99,136), both resulting in a more efficient lipolysis-mediated clearance of triglycerides from the circulation. The induction of the LPL-mediated lipolysis of triglyceride-rich lipoproteins is most likely underlying the increase in LDL particles, often observed after the use of certain TZDs in animal models (such as the *db/db* mouse) or humans with elevated levels of triglyceride-rich lipoproteins (192–195).

X REGULATING PPARγ ACTIVITY THROUGH PROTEIN-PROTEIN INTERACTIONS

A new functional class of proteins, called "cofactors," was recently shown to play an important role in transcriptional control. Such cofactors also interact with nuclear receptors, and they can either repress (corepressors) or enhance (coactivators) their transcriptional activities (202). Initially, it was thought that cofactors simply bridge transcription factors with the basic transcription machinery, such as in the case of p300, which is also a component of TATA-binding protein complexes (203), or for the p300 homologous protein, CREB (cAMP-responsive binding protein)–binding protein (CBP), which has been shown to be associated with the RNA polymerase II via RNA helicase A (204). Although this bridging function is definitely important, several cofactors also have enzymatic activities, suggesting that they could control gene expression by specifically modifying DNA and chromatin structure. The discovery that several cofactors had either chromatin-remodeling or -modifying activities, which controlled the transition of chromatin from a closed to a more open conformation, and hence affected gene expression, was particularly relevant (Fig. 6).

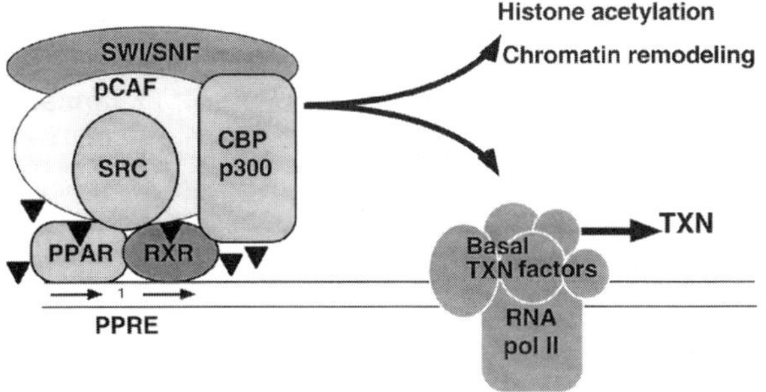

Figure 6 Schematic representation of the recruitment of cofactors to the PPARγ/RXR heterodimer. Transcriptional activation of nuclear receptors requires in general the release of corepressor complexes, which contain histone deacetylase activity (HDAC). Coactivators, such as the SRC family members, CBP/p300, pCAF, or the chromatin remodeling SWI/SNF complex, are then recruited to the receptors. These coactivators either facilitate contact of the basal transcription machinery, remodel chromatin, and/or target histone acetyl transferases (HAT) to the promoters of the target genes of the nuclear receptors. The differential docking of cofactors is facilitated by structural changes brought about by ligand binding or receptor phosphorylation.

One group of cofactors, which has ATP-dependent chromatin-remodeling activity, contains a central ATPase that has homology to yeast SWI2/SNF2. The SWI/SNF and related complexes remodel the chromatin structure and hence facilitate the binding of transcription modulators to its DNA binding sites resulting in either stimulation or inhibition of transcription (205–207). Implication of the SWI/SNF chromatin remodeling complex in the transcription mediated by hormone nuclear receptors has so far been shown only for the glucocorticoid receptor (208–210), the estrogen receptor (211), the retinoic acid receptor (212,213), where chromatin remodeling induced by the SWI/SNF complex together with histone acetylation-deacetylation contributes to NR signaling. The modification of PPARγ signaling by chromatin remodeling has not yet been described, although it will most likely be similar to that described for other nuclear receptors. Other proteins involved in the regulation of chromatin structure and function are the family of "high-mobility group" (HMG) chromosomal proteins. HMGI-C belongs to this family of architectural DNA-binding proteins that are abundant, heterogeneous, nonhistone components of chromatin (214). Although they do not have transcriptional activity by themselves, they change the conformation of DNA and may hence influence transcription. Support for the involvement of HMGI-C in adipogenesis is provided by the observation that the mouse mutant *pygmy*, characterized by its small size and disproportionally reduced body fat content, was found to be a null allele of HMGI-C (215). Further evidence comes from the finding that in certain lipomas gene rearrangements were found in which the HMGI-C DNA-binding domain was fused to either a LIM or an acidic transactivation domain (216,217). In the first case, the LIM domain of the translocation partner could recruit transcriptional activators to the DNA site, whereas in the second case, the fusion of the HMGI-C protein to an acidic transactivation domain could turn the chimeric protein into a powerful transcriptional activator. Thus, the lack or reduced expression of HMGI-C could predispose to leanness, whereas the juxtaposition of its DNA-binding motif to transcriptional regulatory domains could promote adipogenesis. Furthermore, transgenic mice carrying a truncated HMGI-C gene, which contains only the AT hook domains, develop a giant phenotype and abdominal and pelvic lipomatosis (218). In addition to its role in regulating chromatin structure during adipogenesis, it has been shown that another member of the HMG i.e., HMG-(Y), mediates adipocyte differentiation by physically interacting with C/EBPβ, enhancing its transcriptional activity (219).

Members of three groups of coactivators—the p160 steroid receptor coactivator family (SRC); CBP/p300, the p300/CBP associated factor (p/CAF)/GCN family; and the nuclear receptor coactivator ACTR—have been reported to acetylate histones (220–225) as well as other proteins of the transcription complex, such as TFIIEβ and TFIIF (226). In contrast, corepressors such as the silencing mediator for retinoid and thyroid hormone receptors (SMRT) and nuclear receptor corepressor (NCoR) occur in complexes which show histone deacetylase activity (227–229). Histone hypoacetylation is associated with transcriptionally silent and condensed nucleosomes, whereas acetylation is associated with increased transcription, suggesting that alterations of nucleosome conformation modulate accessibility of promoter regions. Regulation of the acetylation of histones and of other DNA binding proteins seems therefore to be of prime importance for transcriptional activation, which often occurs as a multistep process involving first removal of histone deacetylases (HDACs) from DNA with subsequent recruitment of histone acetyl transferases (HATs) (Fig. 5). In general, unactivated nuclear receptors are complexed with corepressors, which extinguish their transcriptional activity by the recruitment of HDACs. Activation of the receptor induces then a conformational change which results in the dissociation of corepressors and the recruitment of coactivator complexes that contain proteins with HAT activity, which facilitates target gene transcription (for review, see 230). A further issue of discussion is how the different groups of cofactors mentioned above interface in controlling the transcription of PPARγ target genes.

An important number of putative cofactors interact with PPARγ, but a firm role in the regulation of the transcriptional activity of PPARγ has not always been established. In the section below we will specifically focus on cofactors for PPARγ, which have been shown not only to bind to but also to modulate its transcriptional activity. SMRT is a corepressor that inhibits retinoic acid receptor and thyroid hormone receptor–dependent transcription in absence of their respective ligands and targets HDACs to the DNA (231,232). In presence of ligands, SMRT dissociates from these receptors allowing the recruitment of coactivators. Lavinsky et al. suggested that SMRT may also be involved in down-modulating PPARγ-mediated gene transcription (233). Indeed, EGF enhances the interaction of PPARγ and SMRT in whole-cell extracts from CV-1 cells. Furthermore, antibodies directed against SMRT can relieve the MAP kinase–dependent inhibition of the PPARγ transcriptional activity (233). Interestingly, microinjection of antibodies directed against SMRT could relieve SMRT corepression of PPAR's activity, whereas antibodies directed related NCoR were ineffective (233). However, these data seem at odds with the observation that PPARγ seems only to be capable to interact with SMRT and N-CoR in solution, but not when bound as a heterodimer with RXR to its cognate response element (45,234). Furthermore, PPARs seem to be lacking the conserved CoR box (45), previously determined to be required for binding of corepressors to the receptors. These conflicting data sets therefore leave the question open, whether unliganded PPARγ has any constitutive repressive activity on gene expression in vivo.

Members of at least two families of histone acetylases, CBP/p300 and the SRC family, are reported to interact with PPARγ. CBP and p300 are two related and widely expressed (235) cofactors that were originally identified as CREB (236) and E1A (237) interacting factors (for review see 238). CBP/p300 coactivates numerous transcription factors including several nuclear receptors (239–244), and was reported to have intrinsic HAT activity (220,223,225). We have observed that CBP/p300 interacts with PPARγ through multiple domains in each protein (245). Most notably, the NH_2-terminal region of PPARγ can dimerize with CBP/p300 in absence of ligand, and this association enhances its constitutive AF-1 transcriptional activity (245). The constitutive presence of cofactors such as CBP/p300 could hence enhance the basal ligand–independent transcriptional activity of PPARγ in vivo and could together with the absence of well-documented interactions with compressors explain the high level of basal activity of PPARγ. A last point worth noting is that CBP/p300 seems to be able to contact other cofactors, such as SRC-1 and its related family members (246). This suggests that CBP/p300 could facilitate the assembly of multiprotein complexes involved in gene activation.

The SRC family of cofactors is also of notable interest for PPARγ. SRC-1 was initially isolated as a progesterone receptor (PR) coactivator (247) but has since also been shown to interact in a yeast two-hybrid system with the PPARγ LBD (248). Like CBP/p300, SRC-1 has an intrinsic HAT activity (224) and is ubiquitously expressed (235,247). SRC-1 has a lower affinity for PPARγ than to CBP/p300 (249). SRC-1 has been shown to have two PPAR binding domains, each containing the LXXLL consensus receptor interaction motifs (23,250). However, also some residues COOH-terminal to the LXXLL motifs are involved in receptor interaction (251). The liganded PPARγ LBD has been cocrystallized with a region of SRC-1 that contains two LXXLL motifs (15). The structural data reveal that the SRC-1 fragment interacted with two PPARγ LBDs, with each of its LXXLL motifs contacting conserved residues in H12 (contains the AF-2) and H3 (15). Mutation of the AF-2 is associated with a loss in transcriptional activity and a loss of the capacity to interact with SRC-1 or CBP (249). Also other related members of the SRC family of cofactors, such as Tif2/Grip1 and ACTR/RAC3/AIB/pCIP, have been shown to interact with PPARγ in a manner similar to SRC-1. One interesting issue related to this family of cofactors, which requires further investigation, is whether these different SRC family members are recruited specifically by different PPARγ ligands and whether these different SRC family members exert distinct effects on transcription of target genes and would in consequence have different biological activity. Our comparative studies with rosiglitazone and FMOC-L-Leu, discussed above, would suggest that such a ligand-specific differential cofactor recruitment is in fact possible (137a).

Since both p300/CBP and SRC family of cofactors are not specific for PPARγ, several labs have tried to identify PPARγ-specific coactivators. Two coactivators, PPAR-binding protein (PBP) (252) and PPAR gamma coactivator-1 (PGC-1) (253), were isolated using this approach, but they turned out later not to be specific for PPARγ. In addition, and in contrast to

CBP/p300 and the SRC-1 families, it is not established whether these proteins contain any HAT activity. The first of these proteins isolated on the basis of its interaction with the LBD of PPARγ in a yeast two-hybrid screen of a mouse liver cDNA library is PBP (252). PPARγ and PBP are constitutively associated both in vitro and in vivo, but the presence of a ligand reinforces this interaction. PBP stimulates PPARγ transcriptional activity only modestly but a truncated form bearing only the receptor-binding domain acts as a dominant-negative repressor, suggesting that PBP is a genuine coactivator for PPARγ. PBP is expressed in a wide range of tissues, including several tissues where PPARγ is of physiological importance, such as adipose tissue, colon, and breast (254).

PBP has been shown to be identical to TRAP 220 (255) and DRIP 205 (256), two proteins that were isolated as part of a multiprotein complex interacting in a ligand-dependent fashion with the thyroid and vitamin D receptor, respectively. The TRAP/DRIP complexes were subsequently reported to be similar to the activator-recruited cofactor (ARC)(257) and Srb/Mediator coactivator (SMCC)(258) complexes. The TRAP/DRIP/ARC/SMCC complex lacks CBP/p300 or SRC proteins and is recruited to the AF-2 domain via a single LXXLL motif of TRAP 220/DRIP 205 (259,260). Interestingly, the TRAP/DRIP/ARC/SMCC complex is absolutely required for transcriptional activation by nuclear receptors in cell-free in vitro transcription assay (255,256) and on chromatin-organized templates (259). Evidence that this complex might also be involved in PPARγ signaling and adipogenesis came from the observation that cells derived from the PBP -/- animals had a decreased capacity for ligand dependent activation of PPARγ (261). Furthermore, the phenotype of the KO animals for TRAP 220 and PBP shared some features with the PPARγ -/- mice in that the TRAP 220 -/- animals, were small and have heart defects (262), whereas the PBP -/- animals have a defect in placenta formation (261). Further exploration as to whether adipogenesis is defective is required to unequivocally establish a role of PBP in PPARγ signaling.

The coactivator PGC-1 was isolated in a yeast two-hybrid screen of a mouse brown fat cell cDNA library (253). PGC-1 again turned out to be not specific for PPARγ, since it also interacts with other receptors such as PPARα, TR, and a set of mitochondrial transcription factors (253,263,264). Interestingly, the interaction between PGC-1 on the one hand and PPARγ and PPARα on the other hand is ligand independent both in vitro and in vivo and seems independent of the LXXLL motif. This LXXLL motif is, however, involved in the ligand-dependent interaction of PGC-1 and other nuclear receptors, such as the estrogen and glucocorticoid receptors (265,266). In addition, PGC-1 seems in its turn to interact with both SRC-1 and CBP/p300, leading to a model in which interaction of PGC-1 with PPARγ stimulates recruitment of the SRC-1 and CBP/p300 coactivators (267). PGC-1 is expressed in brown fat, heart, kidney, and brain, all tissues in which PPARγ might be of physiological importance, and its expression is induced upon cold exposure in brown fat and skeletal muscle. When PGC-1 is ectopically expressed in white adipose cells, PGC-1 activates expression of the uncoupling protein (UCP)-1, a key mitochondrial enzyme of the respiratory chain, normally restricted in expression to brown adipose tissue (253,263). PGC-1 has been shown to activate the nuclear respiratory factor 1 (NRF-1), a transcription factor that regulates genes in mitochondrial DNA replication and transcription, stimulating in this way mitochondrial biogenesis (263).

In addition, PGC-1 contributes to the induction of genes important for the oxidative phosphorylation pathway in the mitochondria, such as the genes for cytochome c oxydase subunits II and IV, and ATP synthetase in muscle and fat cells (253,263). These observations suggest that PGC-1 could play a role in linking nuclear receptors to adaptive thermogenesis and indicate that it could be involved in the initiation of brown adipose tissue formation. Recently, PGC-1 has been demonstrated to regulate also certain aspects of glucose homeostasis. In fact, PGC-1 expression restores Glut4 levels in myoblast cell liner (268). This effect is mediated in part through activation of the muscle-specific transcription factor MEF2C (268). Finally, it was recently demonstrated that PGC-1 is not only involved in transcriptional induction of gene expression, but also in posttranscriptional aspects of gene regulation such as in mRNA processing (269). This mRNA processing activity is the result of a direct association of PGC-1 with splicing factors and other components of the polymerase II elongation and mRNA processing complex.

From the above it is evident that although several cofactors interact with PPARγ, none of these cofactors seem to be specific for PPARγ. Understanding how these cofactor complexes interact and modulate receptor activity will require detailed structural studies, careful reconstitution of PPARγ transcriptional activity in purified reconstituted transcription systems, and a detailed characterization of their biological implication in vivo in animal model systems. Furthermore, several cofactors seem to be interacting as multiprotein complexes, suggesting a certain degree of redundancy. The mode of action of the receptor interacting protein 140

(RIP140) suggests that some of them are mutually exclusive when interacting with the same receptor (270), pointing to the importance of the stoichiometry of the different components in the transcription complexes. Therefore it will also be of interest in the future to better characterize the expression profiles of the various cofactors as well as to get more insight into the regulation of their respective promoters.

XI CONCLUSIONS AND PERSPECTIVES

Although PPARγ is today one of the best-characterized nuclear receptors, there are still enormous challenges ahead of us before the complex function of this transcription factor in the control of adipogenesis will be unraveled. In view of the fact that PPARγ represents an important therapeutic target for the treatment of insulin resistance and type 2 diabetes, a careful understanding of its exact role in physiology is an absolute requirement. This implies a detailed knowledge of all activities of PPARγ, which are much broader than a strict function in adipose tissue. Most important, perhaps, is our need to understand the role of PPARγ in the control of cell proliferation and differentiation. In addition, we need to identify novel ways to modulate PPARγ activity, without inducing unwanted side effects, such as the potential to enhance macrophage foam cell formation (6,125,271), stimulate colon carcinogenesis (272,273), and induce acute liver dysfunction (274). This will require thorough understanding about how this receptor interacts with cofactors and how it activates transcription. Furthermore, the restricted expression of certain PPARγ isoforms, such as the adipose-restricted PPARγ2 form, suggests the feasibility of the development of PPARγ modulators affecting only one specific tissue, such as adipose tissue. All these developments will undoubtedly facilitate the more rational design of new classes of PPARγ modulators, which might not be restricted to agonists, but might also include antagonists or inverse agonists, which could also have interesting therapeutic applications beyond the treatment of metabolic diseases.

ACKNOWLEDGMENTS

We thank Laurent Gelman and Jean-Paul Renaud for help with the cofactor and structural sections, respectively. The members of the "Auwerx" lab are acknowledged for support and discussions. Actual work in the laboratory of the authors is supported by grants of CNRS, INSERM, CHU de Strasbourg, ARC (contract 9943), the Juvenile Diabetes Foundation (1-1999-819), the European community RTD program (QLG1-CT-1999-00674), Ligue Nationale Contre le Cancer, and the Human Frontier Science Program (RG0041/1999-M). L.F. is a research associate of INSERM, and J.A. is a research director with CNRS.

REFERENCES

1. Fajas L, Auboeuf D, Raspe E, Schoonjans K, Lefebvre AM, Saladin R, Najib J, Laville M, Fruchart JC, Deeb S, Vidal-Puig A, Flier J, Briggs MR, Staels B, Vidal H. Organization, promoter analysis and expression of the human PPARγ gene. J Biol Chem 1997; 272:18779–18789.
2. Zhu Y, Qi C, Korenberg JR, Chen X-N, Noya D, Rao MS, Reddy JK. Structural organization of mouse peroxisome proliferator activated receptor γ (mPPARγ) gene: alternative promoter use and different splicing yield two mPPARγ isoforms. Proc Natl Acad Sci USA 1995; 92:7921–7925.
3. Fajas L, Fruchart JC, Auwerx J. PPARγ3 mRNA: a distinct PPARγ mRNA subtype transcribed from an independent promoter. FEBS Lett 1998; 438:55–60.
4. Dreyer C, Krey G, Keller H, Givel F, Helftenbein G, Wahli W. Control of the peroxisomal β-oxidation pathway by a novel family of nuclear hormone receptors. Cell 1992; 68:879–887.
5. Auboeuf D, Rieusset J, Fajas L, Vallier P, Frering V, Riou JP, Laville M, Staels B, Auwerx J, Vidal H. Tissue distribution and quantification of the expression of PPARs and LXRα in humans: no alterations in adipose tissue of obese and NIDDM patients. Diabetes 1997; 48:1319–1327.
6. Ricote M, Huang J, Fajas L, Li A, Welch J, Najib J, Witztum JL, Auwerx J, Palinski W, Glass CK. Expression of the peroxisome proliferator-activated receptor γ (PPARγ) in human atherosclerosis and regulation in macrophages by colony stimulating factors and oxidized low density lipoprotein. Proc Natl Acad Sci USA 1998; 95:7614–7619.
7. Vidal-Puig AJ, Considine RV, Jimenez-Linan M, Werman A, Pories WJ, Caro JF, Flier JS. Peroxisome proliferator-activated receptor gene expression in human tissues: effects of obesity, weight loss, and regulation by insulin and glucocorticoids. J Clin Invest 1997; 99:2416–2422.
8. Vidal-Puig A, Jimenez-Linan M, Lowell BB, Hamann A, Hu E, Spiegelman B, Flier JS, Moller DE. Regulation of PPARγ gene expression by nutrition and obesity in rodents. J Clin Invest 1996; 97:2553–2561.
9. Lefebvre AM, Laville M, Vega N, Riou JP, Van Gaal L, Auwerx J, Vidal H. Depot-specific differences in

adipose tissue gene expression in lean and obese subjects. Diabetes 1998; 47:98–103.
10. Rieusset J, Andreelli D, Auboeuf D, Roques P, Valier P, Riou JP, Auwerx J, Laville M, Vidal H. Insulin acutely regulates the expression of the peroxisome proliferator-activated receptor γ in human adipocytes. Diabetes 1999; 48:699–705.
11. Xing H, Northrop JP, Grove JR, Kilpatrick KE, Su JL, Ringold GM. TNFα-mediated inhibition and reversal of adipocyte differentiation is accompanied by suppressed expression of PPARγ without effects on Pref-1 expression. Endocrinology 1997; 138:2776–2783.
12. Hill M, Young M, McCurdy C, Gimble J. Decreased expression of murine PPARγ in adipose tissue during endotoxinemia. Endocrinology 1997; 138:3073–3076.
13. Schoonjans K, Staels B, Auwerx J. Role of the peroxisome proliferator activated receptor (PPAR) in mediating effects of fibrates and fatty acids on gene expression. J Lipid Res 1996; 37:907–925.
14. Moras D, Gronemeyer H. The nuclear receptor ligand-binding domain: structure and function. Curr Opin Cell Biol 1998; 10(3):384–391.
15. Nolte RT, Wisely GB, Westin S, Cobb JE, Lambert MH, Kurokawa R, Rosenfeld MG, Willson TM, Glass CK, Milburn MV. Ligand binding and co-activator assembly of the peroxisome proliferator-activated receptor γ. Nature 1998; 395:137–143.
16. Uppenberg J, Svensson C, Jaki M, Bertilsson G, Jendeberg L, Berkenstam A. Crystal structure of the ligand binding domain of the human nuclear receptor PPARγ. J Biol Chem 1998; 273:31108–31112.
17. Xu HE, Lambert MH, Montana VG, Parks DJ, Blanchard SG, Brown PJ, Sternbach DD, Lehmann JM, Wisely GB, Willson TM, Kliewer SA, Milburn MV. Molecular recognition of fatty acids by peroxisome proliferator-activated receptors. Mol Cell 1999; 3(3):397–403.
18. Johnson BA, Wilson EM, Li Y, Moller DE, Smith RG, Zhou G. Ligand-induced stabilization of PPAR-gamma monitored by NMR spectroscopy: implications for nuclear receptor activition. J Mol Biol 2000; 298(2):187–194.
19. Bourguet W, Ruff M, Chambon P, Gronemeyer H, Moras D. Crystal structure of the ligand-binding domain of the human nuclear receptor RXR-α. Nature 1995; 375:377–382.
20. Renaud JP, Rochel N, Ruff M, Vivat V, Chambon P, Gronemeyer H, Moras D. Crystal structure of the RAR-gamma ligand-binding domain bound to all-trans retinoic acid. Nature 1995; 378(6558):681–689.
21. Le Douarin B, Nielsen AL, Garnier JM, Ichinose H, Jeanmougin F, Losson R, Chambon P. A possible involvement of TIF1 alpha and TIF1 beta in the epigenetic control of transcription by nuclear receptors. EMBO J 1996; 15(23):6701–6715.
22. Torchia J, Rose DW, Inostroza J, Kamei Y, Westin S, Glass CK, Rosenfeld MG. The transcriptional co-activator p/CIP binds CBP and mediates nuclear-receptor function [see comments]. Nature 1997; 387(6634):677–684.
23. Heery DM, Kalkhoven E, Hoare S, Parker MG. A signature motif in transcriptional coactivators mediates binding to nuclear receptors. Nature 1997; 387:733–736.
24. Oberfield JL, Collins JL, Holmes CP, Goreham DM, Cooper JP, Cobb JE, Lenhard JM, Hull-Ryde EA, Mohr CP, Blanchard SG, Parks DJ, Moore LB, Lehmann JM, Plunket K, Miller AB. A peroxisome proliferator-activated receptor gamma ligand inhibits adipocyte differentiation. Proc Natl Acad Sci USA 1999; 96(11):6102–6106.
25. Gampe RTJ, Montana VG, Lambert MH, Miller AB, Bledsoe RK, Milburn MV, Kliewer SA, Willson TM, Xu HE. Asymmetry in the PPAR gamma-RXR alpha crystal structure reveals the molecular basis of heterodimerization among nuclear receptors. Mol Cell 2000; 5:545–555.
26. Brzozowski AM, Pike AC, Dauter Z, Hubbard RE, Bonn T, Engstrom O, Ohman L, Greene GL, Gustafsson JA, Carlquist M. Molecular basis of agonism and antagonism in the oestrogen receptor. Nature 1997; 389(6652):753–758.
27. Bourguet W, Vivat V, Wurtz JM, Chambon P, Gronemeyer H, Moras D. Crystal structure of a heterodimeric complex of RAR and RXR ligand-binding domains. Mol Cell 2000; 5:289–298.
28. Mangelsdorf DJ, Evans RM. The RXR heterodimers and orphan receptors. Cell 1995; 83:841–850.
29. Spiegelman BM, Flier JS. Adipogenesis and obesity: rounding out the big picture. Cell 1996; 87:377–389.
30. Fajas L, Fruchart JC, Auwerx J. Transcriptional control of adipogenesis. Curr Opin Cell Biol 1998; 10:165–173.
31. Ding Q, Wang Q, Dong Z, Evers BM. Characterization and regulation of E2F activity during Caco-2 cell differentiation. Am J Physiol Cell Physiol 2000; 278(1):C110–C117.
32. Rempel RE, Saenz-Robles MT, Storms R, Morham S, Ishida S, Engel A, Jakoi L, Melhem MF, Pipas JM, Smith C, Nevins JR. Loss of E2F4 activity leads to abnormal development of multiple cellular lineages. Mol Cell 2000; 6(2):293–306.
33. Persengiev SP, Kondova, II, Kilpatrick DL. E2F4 actively promotes the initiation and maintenance of nerve growth factor-induced cell differentiation. Mol Cell Biol 1999; 19(9):6048–6056.
34. Harbour JW, Dean DC. The Rb/E2F pathway: expanding roles and emerging paradigms. Genes Dev 2000; 14(19):2393–2409.
35. Helin K. Regulation of cell proliferation by the E2F transcription factors. Curr Opin Genet Dev 1998; 8(1):28–35.

36. Richon V, Lyle RE, McGehee REJ. Regulation and expression of retinoblastoma proteins p107 and p130 during 3T3-L1 adipocyte differentiation. J Biol Chem 1997; 272:10117–10124.
37. Higgins C, Chatterjee S, Cherington V. The block of adipocyte differentiation by a C-terminally truncated, but not by full-length, simian virus 40 large tumor antigen is dependent on an intact retinoblastoma susceptibility protein family binding domain. J Virol 1996; 70(2):745–752.
38. Classon M, Kennedy BK, Mulloy R, Harlow E. Opposing roles of pRB and p107 in adipocyte differentiation [in process citation]. Proc Natl Acad Sci USA 2000; 97(20):10826–10831.
39. Chen PL, Riley DJ, Chen Y, Lee WH. Retinoblastoma protein positively regulates terminal adipocyte differentiation through direct interaction with C/EBPs. Genes Dev 1996; 10(21):2794–2804.
39a. Fajas L, Egler V, Reiter R, Hausen J, Kristiansen K, Debril M-B, Miarol S, Auwerx J. The retinoblastoma-histone deacetylase 3 complex inhibits PPARJ and adipocyte differentiation. Developmental Cell 2002; 3:903–910.
40. He GP, Muise A, Li AW, Ro HS. A eucaryotic transcriptional repressor with carboxypeptidase activity. Nature 1995; 378:92–96.
41. Park J-G, Muise A, He G-P, Kim S-W, Ro H-S. Transcriptional regulation by the γ5 subunit of a heterotrimeric G protein during adipogenesis/. EMBO J 1999; 18:4004–4012.
42. Tong Q, Dalgin G, Xu H, Ting CN, Leiden JM, Hotamisligil GS. Function of GATA transcription factors in preadipocyte-adipocyte transition [in process citation]. Science 2000; 290(5489):134–138.
43. Xue JC, Schwarz EJ, Chawla A, Lazar MA. Distinct stages in adipogenesis revealed by retinoid inhibition of differentiation after induction of PPARγ. Mol Cell Biol 1996; 16:1567–1575.
44. Schwarz EJ, Reginato MJ, Shao D, Krakow SL, Lazar MA. Retinoic acid blocks adipogenesis by inhibiting C/EBPβ-mediated transcription. Mol Cell Biol 1997; 17(3):1552–1561.
45. DiRenzo J, Soderstrom M, Kurokawa R, Ogliastro MH, Ricote M, Ingrey S, Horlein A, Rosenfeld MG, Glass CK. Peroxisome proliferator-activated receptors and retinoic acid receptors differentially control the interactions of retinoid X receptor heterodimers with ligands, coactivators and corepressors. Mol Cell Biol 1997; 17:2166–2176.
46. Brodie AE, Manning VA, Hu CY. Inhibitors of preadipocyte differentiation induce COUP-TF binding to PPAR/RXR binding sequences. Biochem Biophys Res Commun 1996; 228:655–661.
47. Zhang B, Berger J, Hu E, Szalkowski D, White-Carrington S, Spiegelman BM, Moller DE. Negative regulation of peroxisome proliferator-activated receptor-γ gene expression contributes to the adipogenic effect of tumor necrosis factor-α. Mol Endocrinol 1996; 10:1457–1466.
48. Williams PM, Chang DJ, Danesch U, Ringold GM, Heller RA. CCAAT/enhancer binding protein expression is rapidly extinguished in TA1 adipocyte cells treated with tumor necrosis factor. Mol Endocrinol 1992; 6:1135–1141.
49. Ron D, Brasier AR, McGehee REJ, Habener JF. Tumor necrosis factor-induced reversal of adipocytic phenotype of 3T3-L1 cells is preceded by a loss of nuclear CCAAT/enhancer binding protein (C/EBP). J Clin Invest 1992; 89:223–233.
50. Ntambi JM, Takova T. Role of Ca2+ in the early stages of murine adipocyte differentiation. Differentiation 1996; 60:151–158.
51. Smas CM, Sul HS. Pref-1, a protein containing EGF-like repeats, inhibits adipocyte differentiation. Cell 1993; 73:725–734.
52. Smas CM, Chen L, Sul HS. Cleavage of membrane-associated pref-1 generates a soluble inhibitor of adipocyte differentiation. Mol Cell Biol 1997; 17:977–988.
53. Sul HS, Smas C, Mei B, Zhou L. Function of pref-1 as an inhibitor of adipocyte differentiation. Int J Obes Relat Metab Disord 2000; 24(suppl 4):S15–S19.
54. Smas CM, Chen L, Zhao L, Latasa MJ, Sul HS. Transcriptional repression of pref-1 by glucocorticoids promotes 3T3-L1 adipocyte differentiation. J Biol Chem 1999; 274(18):12632–12641.
55. Ross SE, Hemati N, Longo KA, Bennett CN, Lucas PC, Erickson RL, MacDougald OA. Inhibition of adipogenesis by Wnt signaling. Science 2000; 289(5481):950–953.
56. Cadigan KM, Nusse R. Wnt signaling: a common theme in animal development. Genes Dev 1997; 11: 3286–3305.
57. Rosen ED, Walkey CJ, Puigserver P, Spiegelman BM. Transcriptional regulation of adipogenesis. Genes Dev 2000; 14(11):1293–1307.
58. Tontonoz P, Hu E, Spiegelman BM. Stimulation of adipogenesis in fibroblasts by PPARγ2, a lipid-activated transcription factor. Cell 1994; 79:1147–1156.
59. Hu E, Tontonoz P, Spiegelman BM. Transdifferentiation of myoblasts by the adipogenic transcription factors PPARγ and C/EBPα. Proc Natl Acad Sci USA 1995; 92:9856–9860.
60. Yeh WC, Cao Z, Classon M, McKnight S. Cascade regulation of terminal adipocyte differentiation by three members of the C/EBP family of leucine zipper proteins. Genes Dev 1995; 9:168–181.
61. Wu Z, Xie Y, Bucher NLR, Farmer SR. Conditional ectopic expression of C/EBPβ in NIH-3T3 cells induces PPARγ and stimulates adipogenesis. Genes Dev 1995; 9:2350–2363.

62. Wu Z, Bucher NLR, Farmer SR. Induction of peroxisome proliferator-activated receptor γ during the conversion of 3T3 fibroblasts into adipocytes is mediated by C/EBPβ, C/EBPδ, and glucocorticoids. Mol Cell Biol 1996; 16:4128–4136.
63. Saladin R, Fajas L, Dana S, Halvorsen YD, Auwerx J, Briggs M. Differential regulation of peroxisome proliferator activated receptor γ1 (PPARγ1) and PPARγ2 mRNA expession in early stages of adipogenesis. Cell Growth Differ 1999; 10:43–48.
64. Tanaka T, Yoshida N, Kishimoto T, Akira S. Defective adipocyte differentiation in mice lacking the C/EBPbeta and/or C/EBPdelta gene. EMBO J 1997; 16(24):7432–7443.
65. Hamm JK, Park BH, Farmer SR. A role for C/EBP{beta} in regulating PPAR {gamma} activity during adipogenesis in 3T3-L1 preadipocytes. J Biol Chem 2001; 27:27.
66. Imai T, Jiang M, Chambon P, Metzger D. Impaired adipogenesis and lipolysis in the mouse upon selective ablation of the retinoid X receptor alpha mediated by a tamoxifen-inducible chimeric Cre recombinase (Cre-ERT2) in adipocytes. Proc Natl Acad Sci USA 2001; 98(1):224–228.
67. Tontonoz P, Kim JB, Graves RA, Spiegelman BM. ADD1: a novel helix-loop-helix transcription factor associated with adipocyte determination and differentiation. Mol Cell Biol 1993; 13:4753–4759.
68. Kim JB, Spiegelman BM. ADD1/SREBP1 promotes adipocyte differentiation and gene expression linked to fatty acid metabolism. Genes Dev 1996; 10:1096–1107.
69. Brown MS, Goldstein JL. The SREBP pathway: regulation of cholesterol metabolism by proteolysis of a membrane-bound transcription factor. Cell 1997; 89:331–340.
70. Bennet MK, Lopez JM, Sanchez HB, Osborne TF. Sterol regulation of fatty acid synthase promoter; coordinate feedback regulation of two major lipid pathways. J Biol Chem 1995; 270:25578–25583.
71. Shimano H, Horton JD, Hammer RE, Shimomura I, Brown MS, Goldstein JL. Overproduction of cholesterol and fatty acids causes massive liver enlargement in transgenic mice expressing truncated SREBP-1a. J Clin Invest 1996; 98:1575–1584.
72. Lopez JM, Bennett MK, Sanchez HB, Rosenfeld JM, Osborne TF. Sterol regulation of acetyl coenzyme A carboxylase: a mechanism for coordinate control of cellular lipid. Proc Natl Acad Sci USA 1996; 93:1049–1053.
73. Ericsson J, Jackson SM, Kim JB, Spiegelman BM, Edwards PA. Identification of glycerol-3-phosphate acyltransferase as an adipocyte determination and differentiation factor 1- and sterol regulatory element-binding protein-responsive gene. J Biol Chem 1997; 272:7298–7305.
74. Schoonjans K, Gelman L, Haby C, Briggs M, Auwerx J. Induction of LPL gene expression by sterols is mediated by a sterol regulatory element and is independent of the presence of multiple E boxes. J Mol Biol 2000; 304(3):323–334.
75. Shimano H, Horton JD, Shimomura I, Hammer RE, Brown MS, Goldstein JL. Isoform 1c of sterol regulatory element binding protein is less active than isoform 1a in liver of inorganic mice and in cultured cells. J Clin Invest 1997; 99:846–854.
76. Shimomura I, Hammer RE, Richardson JA, Ikemoto S, Bashmakov Y, J.L. G, Brown MS. Insulin resistance and diabetes mellitus in transgenic mice expressing nuclear SREBP-1c in adipose tissue: a model for congenital generalized lipodystrophy. Genes Dev 1998; 12:3182–3194.
77. Wu Z, Rosen ED, Brun R, Hauser S, G. A, Troy AE, McKeon C, Darlington GJ, Spiegelman BM. Cross-regulation of C/EBPα and PPARγ controls the transcriptional pathway of adipogenesis and insulin sensitivity. Mol Cell 1999; 3:143–150.
78. Wang ND, Finegold MJ, Bradley A, Ou C, Abdelsayed SV, Wilde MD, Taylor LR, Wilson DR, Darlington GJ. Impaired energy homeostasis in C/EBPα knockout mice. Science 1995; 269(5227):1108–1112.
79. Flodby P, Barlow C, Kylefjord H, Ahrlund-Richter L, Xanthopoulus KG. Increased hepatic cell proliferation and lung abnormalities in mice deficient in CCAAT/enhancer binding protein alpha. J Biol Chem 1996; 271(40):24753–24760.
80. Horvath CM, Darnell JE. The state of the STATs: recent developments in the study of signal transduction to the nucleus. Curr Opin Cell Biol 1997; 9(2):233–239.
81. Ihle JN. The Stat family in cytokine signaling. Curr Opin Cell Biol 2001; 13(2):211–217.
82. Stephens JM, Morrison RF, Pilch PF. The expression and regulation of STATs during 3T3-L1 adipocyte differentiation. J Biol Chem 1996; 271: 10441–10444.
83. McAveney KM, Gimble JM, Lee LY. Prolactin receptor expression during adipocyte differentiation of bone marrow stroma. Endocrinology 1996; 137:5723–5726.
84. Zou L, Menon RK, Sperling MA. Induction of mRNAs for the growth hormone receptor gene during 3T3-L1 preadipocyte differentiation. Metabolism 1997; 46:114–118.
85. Pradines-Figueres A, Barcellini-Couget S, Dani C, Vannier C, Ailhaud G. Transcriptional control of the expression of lipoprotein lipase gene by growth hormone in preadipocyte Ob1771 cells. J Lipid Res 1990; 31:1283–1291.
86. Francis SM, Enerback S, Moller C, Enberg B, Norstedt G. A novel in vitro model for studying

signal transduction and gene regulation via growth hormone receptor. Mol Endocrinol 1993; 7:972–978.
87. Nanbu-Wakao R, Fujitani Y, Masuho Y, Muramatu M, Wakao H. Prolactin enhances CCAAT enhancer-binding protein-beta (C/EBP beta) and peroxisome proliferator-activated receptor gamma (PPAR gamma) messenger RNA expression and stimulates adipogenic conversion of NIH-3T3 cells. Mol Endocrinol 2000; 14(2):307–316.
88. Teglund S, McKay C, Schuetz E, van Deursen JM, Stravopodis D, Wang D, Brown M, Bodner S, Grosveld G, Ihle JN. Stat5a and Stat5b proteins have essential and nonessential, or redundant, roles in cytokine responses. Cell 1998; 93(5):841–850.
89. Deng J, Hua K, Lesser SS, Harp JB. Activation of signal transducer and activator of transcription-3 during proliferative phases of 3T3-L1 adipogenesis. Endocrinology 2000; 141(7):2370–2376.
90. Takeda K, Noguchi K, Shi W, Tanaka T, Matsumoto M, Yoshida N, Kishimoto T, Akira S. Targeted disruption of the mouse Stat3 gene leads to early embryonic lethality. Proc Natl Acad Sci USA 1997; 94(8):3801–3804.
91. Negrel R, Gaillard D, Ailhaud G. Prostacyclin as a potent effector of adipose-cell differentiation. Biochem J 1989; 257:399–405.
92. Berger J, Tanen M, Elbrecht A, Hermanowski-Vosatka A, Moller DE, Wright SD, Thieringer R. PPAR{gamma} ligands inhibit adipocyte 11 {beta}-hydroxysteroid dehydrogenase type 1 expression and activity. J Biol Chem 2001; 22:22.
93. Okuno A, Tamemoto H, Tobe K, Ueki K, Mori Y, Iwamoto K, Umesono K, Akanuma Y, Fujiwara T, Horikoshi H, Yazaki Y, Kadowaki T. Troglitazone increases the number of small adipocytes without the change of white adipose tissue mass in obese Zucker rats. Journal of Clinical Investigation 1998; 101:1354–1361.
94. Hallakou S, Doare L, Foufelle F, Kergoat M, Guerre-Millo M, Berthault MF, Dugail I, Morin J, Auwerx J, Ferre P. Pioglitazone induces in vivo adipocyte differentiation in the obese Zucker fa/fa rat. Diabetes 1997; 46:1393–1399.
95. Tontonoz P, Hu E, Graves RA, Budavari AI, Spiegelman BM. mPPARγ2: tissue-specific regulator of an adipocyte enhancer. Genes Dev 1994; 8:1224–1234.
96. Tontonoz P, Hu E, Devine J, Beale EG, Spiegelman BM. PPARγ2 regulates adipose expression of the phosphoenolpyruvate carboxykinase gene. Mol Cell Biol 1995; 15:351–357.
97. Schoonjans K, Watanabe M, Suzuki H, Mahfoudi A, Krey G, Wahli W, Grimaldi P, Staels B, Yamamoto T, Auwerx J. Induction of the acyl-coenzyme A synthetase gene by fibrates and fatty acids is mediated by a peroxisome proliferator response element in the C promoter. J Biol Chem 1995; 270:19269–19276.
98. Martin G, Schoonjans K, Lefebvre A, Staels B, Auwerx J. Coordinate regulation of the expression of the fatty acid transport protein (FATP) and acyl CoA synthetase genes by PPARα and PPARγ activators. J Biol Chem 1997; 272:28210–28217.
99. Schoonjans K, Peinado-Onsurbe J, Lefebvre AM, Heyman R, Briggs M, Deeb S, Staels B, Auwerx J. PPARα and PPARγ activators direct a tissue-specific transcriptional response via a PPRE in the lipoprotein lipase gene. EMBO J 1996; 15:5336–5348.
100. Schoonjans K, Martin G, Staels B, Auwerx J. Peroxisome proliferator-activated receptors, orphans with ligands and functions. Curr Opin Lipidol 1997; 8:159–166.
101. Auwerx J, Staels B. Leptin. Lancet 1998; 351:737–742.
102. De Vos P, Lefebvre AM, Miller SG, Guerre-Millo M, Wong K, Saladin R, Hamann L, Staels B, Briggs MR, Auwerx J. Thiazolidinediones repress *ob* gene expression via activation of PPARγ. J Clin Invest 1996; 98:1004–1009.
103. Zhang B, Graziano MP, Doebber TW, Leibowitz MD, White-Carrington S, Szalkowski DM, Hey PT, Wu M, Cullinan CA, Bailey P, Lollmann B, Frederich R, Flier JS, Strader CD, Smith RG. Down-regulation of the expression of the *obese* gene by antidiabetic thiazolidinedione in Zucker diabetic fatty rats and *db*/*db* mice. J Biol Chem 1996; 271:9455–9459.
104. Kallen CB, Lazar MA. Antidiabetic thiazolidinediones inhibit leptin (ob) gene expression in 3T3-L1 adipocytes. Proc Natl Acad Sci USA 1996; 93:5793–5796.
105. Miller SG, De Vos P, Guerre-Millo M, Wong K, Hermann T, Staels B, Briggs MR, Auwerx J. The adipocyte specific transcription factor, C/EBPα modulates human ob gene expression. Proc Natl Acad Sci USA 1996; 93:5507–5511.
106. He Y, Chen H, Quon MJ, Reitman M. The mouse *obese* gene. Genomic organization, promoter activity, and activation by CCAAT/enhancer-binding protein alpha. J Biol Chem 1995; 270:28887–28891.
107. Hollenberg AN, Susulic VS, Madura JP, Zhang B, Moller DE, Tontonoz P, Sarraf P, Spiegelman BM, Lowell BB. Functional antagonism between CCAAT/enhancer binding protein-α and peroxisome proliferator-activated receptor-γ on the leptin promoter. J Biol Chem 1997; 272:5283–5290.
108. Torti FM, Dieckman B, Beutler B, Cerami A, Ringold GM. A macrophage factor inhibits adipocyte gene expression; an in vitro model for cachexia. Science 1985; 229:867–869.
109. Beutler B, Cerami A. Cachectin (tumor necrosis factor): a macrophage hormone governing cellular metabolism and inflammatory response. Endocr Rev 1988; 9:57–66.
110. Peraldi P, Xu M, Spiegelman BM. Thiazolidinediones block tumor necrosis factor-α-induced inhibition of insulin signalling. J Clin Invest 1997; 100:1863–1869.

111. Hotamisligil GS, Shargill NS, Spiegelman BM. Adipose tissue expression of tumor necrosis factor-α: direct role in obesity-linked insulin resistance. Science 1993; 259:87–91.
112. Hotamisligil GS, Peraldi P, Budavari A, Ellis R, White MF, Spiegelman BM. IRS-1-mediated inhibition of insulin receptor tyrosine kinase activity in TNF-α- and obesity-induced insulin resistance. Science 1996; 271:665–668.
113. Hotamisligil GS, Murray DL, Choy LN, Spiegelman BM. Tumor necrosis factor α inhibits signaling from the insulin receptor. Proc Natl Acad Sci USA 1994; 91:4854–4858.
114. Hofmann C, Lorenz K, Braithwaite SS, Colca JR, Palazuk BJ, Hotamisligil GS, Spiegelman BM. Altered gene expression for tumor necrosis factor-α and its receptor during drug and dietary modulation of insulin resistance. Endocrinology 1994; 134:264–270.
115. Souza SC, Yamamoto MT, Franciosa MD, Lien P, Greenberg AS. BRL 49653 blocks lipolytic actions of tumor necrosis factor-alpha: a potential new insulin-sensitizing mechanism for thiazolidinediones. Diabetes 1998; 47:691–695.
116. Steppan CM, Bailey ST, Bhat S, Brown EJ, Banerjee RR, Wright CM, Patel HR, Ahima RS, Lazar MA. The hormone resistin links obesity to diabetes. Nature 2001; 409(6818):307–312.
117. Steppan CM, Brown EJ, Wright CM, Bhat S, Banerjee RR, Dai CY, Enders GH, Silberg DG, Wen X, Wu GD, Lazar MA. A family of tissue-specific resistin-like molecules. Proc Natl Acad Sci USA 2001; 98(2):502–506.
118. Schoonjans K, Auwerx J. Thiazolidinediones: an update [In Process Citation]. Lancet 2000; 355(9208): 1008–1010.
119. Forman BM, Tontonoz P, Chen J, Brun RP, Spiegelman BM, Evans RM. 15-Deoxy-Δ12,14 prostaglandin J2 is a ligand for the adipocyte determination factor PPARγ. Cell 1995; 83:803–812.
120. Kliewer SA, Lenhard JM, Willson TM, Patel I, Morris DC, Lehman JM. A prostaglandin J2 metabolite binds peroxisome proliferator-activated receptor γ and promotes adipocyte differentiation. Cell 1995; 83:813–819.
121. Krey G, Braissant O, L'Horset F, Kalkhoven E, Peroud M, Parker MG, Wahli W. Fatty acids, eicosanoids, and hypolipidemic agents identified as ligands of peroxisome proliferator-activated receptors by co-activator-dependent receptor ligand assay. Mol Endocrinol 1997; 11:779–791.
122. Ma H, Sprecher HW, Kolattukudy PE. Estrogen-induced production of a peroxisome proliferator-activated receptor (PPAR) ligand in PPARγ-expressing tissue. J Biol Chem 1998; 273:30131–30138.
123. Kliewer SA, Sundseth SS, Jones SA, Brown PJ, Wisely GB, Koble CS, Devchand P, Wahli W, Willson TM, Lenhard JM, Lehmann JM. Fatty acids and eicosanoids regulate gene expression through direct interactions with peroxisome proliferator-activated receptors α and γ. Proc Natl Acad Sci USA 1997; 94:4318–4323.
124. Forman BM, Chen J, Evans RM. Hypolipidemic drugs, polyunsaturated fatty acids, and eicosanoids are ligands for peroxisome proliferator-activated receptors α and δ. Proc Natl Acad Sci USA 1997; 94:4312–4317.
125. Nagy L, Tontonez P, Alvarez JG, Chen H, Evans RM. Oxidized LDL regulates macrophage gene expression through ligand activation of PPARγ. Cell 1998; 93: 229–240.
126. Willson TM, Cobb JE, Cowan DJ, Wiethe RW, Correa ID, Prakash SR, Beck KD, Moore LB, Kliewer SA, Lehmann JM. The structure activity relationship between peroxisome proliferator activated receptor γ agonism and the antihyperglycemic activity of thiazolidinediones. J Med Chem 1996; 39:665–668.
127. Henke BR, Blanchard SG, Brackeen MF, Brown KK, Cobb JE, Collins JL, Harrington WW, Jr., Hashim MA, Hull-Ryde EA, Kaldor I, Kliewer SA, Lake DH, Leesnitzer LM, Lehmann JM, Lenhard JM. N-(2-benzoylphenyl)-L-tyrosine PPARgamma agonists. 1. Discovery of a novel series of potent antihyperglycemic and antihyperlipidemic agents. J Med Chem 1998; 41(25):5020–5036.
128. Lehmann JM, Lenhard JM, Oliver BB, Ringold GM, Kliewer SA. Peroxisome proliferator–activated receptors α and γ are activated by indomethacin and other non-steroidal anti-inflammatory drugs. J Biol Chem 1997; 272:3406–3410.
129. Berger J, Bailey P, Biswas C, Cullinan CA, Doebber TW, Hayes NS, Saperstein R, Smith RG, Leibowitz MD. Thiazolidinediones produce a conformational change in peroxisomal proliferator-activated receptor-γ: binding and activation correlate with antidiabetic actions in db/db mice. Endocrinology 1996; 137:4189–4195.
130. Mukherjee R, Davies PAJ, Crombie DL, Bischoff ED, Cesario RM, Jow L, Hamann LG, Boehm MF, Mondon CE, Nadzan AM, Paterniti JR, Heyman RA. Sensitization of diabetic and obese mice to insulin by retinoid X receptor agonists. Nature 1997; 386:407–410.
131. Davies PJ, Berry SA, Shipley GL, Eckel RH, Hennuyer N, Crombie DL, Ogilvie KM, Peinado-Onsurbe J, Fievet C, Leibowitz MD, Heyman RA, Auwerx J. Metabolic effects of rexinoids: tissue-specific regulation of lipoprotein lipase activity. Mol Pharmacol 2001; 59(2):170–176.
132. Chawla A, Barak Y, Nagy L, Liao D, Tontonoz P, Evans RM. PPAR-gamma dependent and independent effects on macrophage-gene expression in lipid metabolism and inflammation. Nat Med 2001; 7(1):48–52.

133. Moore KJ, Rosen ED, Fitzgerald ML, Randow F, Andersson LP, Altshuler D, Milstone DS, Mortensen RM, Spiegelman BM, Freeman MW. The role of PPAR-gamma in macrophage differentiation and cholesterol uptake. Nat Med 2001; 7(1):41–47.
134. Murakami K, Tobe K, Ide T, Mochizuki T, Ohashi M, Akanuma Y, Yazaki Y, Kadowaki K. A novel insulin sensitizer acts as a coligand for peroxisome proliferator-activated receptor α and γ. Effect of PPARα activation on normal lipid metabolism in liver of Zucker fatty rats. Diabetes 1998; 47:1841–1847.
135. Shibata T, Matsui K, Nagao K, Shinkai H, Yonemori F, Wakitani K. Pharmacological profiles of a novel oral antidiabetic agent, JTT-501, an isoxazolidininedione derivative. Eur J Pharmacol 1999; 364:211–219.
136. Lefebvre A-M, Peinado-Onsurbe J, Leitersdorf I, Briggs MR, Paterniti JR, Fruchart J-C, Fievet C, Auwerx J, Staels B. Regulation of lipoprotein metabolism by thiazolidinediones occurs through a distinct, but complementary mechanism relative to fibrates. Arterioscler Thromb Vasc Biol 1997; 17:1756–1764.
137. Berger J, Leibowitz MD, Doebber TW, Elbrecht A, Zhang B, Zhou G, Biswas C, Cullinan CA, Hayes NS, Li Y, Tanen M, Ventre J, Wu MS, Berger GD, Mosley R. Novel peroxisome proliferator activated receptor (PPAR) γ and PPARδ ligands produce distinct biological effects. J Biol Chem 1999; 274: 6718–6725.
137a. Rocchi S, Picarol F, Vamecq J, Gelman L, Potier N, Zeyer D, Dubuquoy L, Bac P, Champy M-F, Plunket KD, Leesnitzer LA, Blanchard SG, Desreumaux P, Moras D, Renaud J-P, Auwerx J. A unique PPARγ ligand with potent insulin-sensitizing yet weak adipogenic activity. Mol Cell 2001; 8:737–747.
138. Moller DE, Flier JS. Insulin resistance-mechanisms, syndromes, and implications. N Engl J Med 1991; 325:938–948.
139. Moitra J, Mason MM, Olive M, Krylov D, Gavrilova O, Marcus-Samuels B, Feigenbaum L, Lee E, Aoyama T, Eckhaus M, Reitman ML, Vinson C. Life without fat: a transgenic mouse. Genes Dev 1998; 12:3168–3181.
140. Shimomura I, Funahashi T, Takahashi M, Maeda K, Kotani K, Nakamura T, Yamashita S, Miura M, Fukuda Y, Takemura K, Tokunaga K, Matsuzawa Y. Enhanced expression of PAI-1 in visceral fat: possible contributor to vascular disease in obesity. Nat Med 1996; 2:800–803.
141. Cohen B, Novick D, Rubinstein M. Modulation of insulin activities by leptin. Science 1996; 274:1185–1188.
142. Muller G, Ertl J, Gerl M, Preibisch G. Leptin impairs metabolic actions of insulin in isolated rat adipocytes. J Biol Chem 1997; 272:10585–10593.
143. Liu YL, Emilson V, Cawthorne MA. Leptin inhibits glycogen synthesis in isolated soleus muscle of obese (ob/ob) mice. FEBS Lett 1997; 411:351–355.
144. Kamohara S, Burcelin R, Halaas JL, Friedman JM, Charron MJ. Acute stimulation of glucose metabolism in mice by leptin treatment. Nature 1997; 389:374–377.
145. Shimomura I, Hammer RE, Ikemoto S, Brown MS, Goldstein JL. Leptin reverses insulin resistance and diabetes mellitus in mice with congenital lipodystrophy. Nature 1999; 401(6748):73–76.
146. Fruebis J, Tsao TS, Javorschi S, Ebbets-Reed D, Erickson MR, Yen FT, Bihain BE, Lodish HF. Proteolytic cleavage product of 30-kDa adipocyte complement-related protein increases fatty acid oxidation in muscle and causes weight loss in mice. Proc Natl Acad Sci USA 2001; 98(4):2005–2010.
147. Rosen B, Cook KS, Yaglom J, Groves DL, Volonakis JE, Damm D, White T, Spiegelman BM. Adipsin and complement factor D activity: an immune-related defect in obesity. Science 1989; 244:1483–1487.
148. Frederich RC, Kahn BB, Peach MJ, Flier JS. Tissue-specific nutritional regulation of angiotensinogen in adipose tissue. Hypertension 1992; 19:339–344.
149. Randle PJ, Garland PB, Hales CN, Newsholme EA. The glucose-fatty acid cycle: its role in insulin sensitivity and metabolic disturbances of diabetes mellitus. Lancet 1961; i:785–789.
150. Martin G, Schoonjans K, Staels B, Auwerx J. PPARγ activators improve glucose homeostasis by stimulating fatty acid uptake in the adipocytes. Atherosclerosis 1998; 137:75–80.
151. Perseghin G, Scifo P, De Cobelli F, Pagliato E, Battezzati A, Arcelloni C, Vanzulli A, Testolin G, Pozza G, Del Maschio A, Luzi L. Intramyocellular triglyceride content is a determinant of in vivo insulin resistance in humans: a ^{1}H-^{13}C nuclear magnetic resonance spectroscopy assessment in offspring of type 2 diabetic parents. Diabetes 1999; 48(8):1600–1606.
152. Kim JK, Gavrilova O, Chen Y, Reitman ML, Shulman GI. Mechanism of insulin resistance in A-ZIP/F-1 fatless mice. J Biol Chem 2000; 275(12):8456–8460.
153. Gavrilova O, Marcus-Samuels B, Graham D, Kim JK, Shulman GI, Castle AL, Vinson C, Eckhaus M, Reitman ML. Surgical implantation of adipose tissue reverses diabetes in lipoatrophic mice. J Clin Invest 2000; 105(3):271–278.
154. Bergman RN, Ader M. Free fatty acids and pathogenesis of type 2 diabetes mellitus. Trends Endocrinol Metab 2000; 11(9):351–356.
155. Oakes ND, Camilleri S, Furler SM, Chisholm DJ, Kraegen EW. The insulin sensitizer, BRL 49653, reduces systemic fatty acid supply and utilization and tissue availability in the rat. Metabolism 1997; 46:935–942.

156. Wu Z, Xie Y, Morrison RF, Bucher NLR, Farmer SR. PPARγ induces the insulin-dependent glucose transporter GLUT4 in absence of C/EBPα during the conversion of 3T3 fibroblast into adipocytes. J Clin Invest 1998; 101:22–32.
157. Smith U, Gogg S, Johansson A, Olausson T, Rotter V, Svalstedt B. Thiazolidinediones (PPARgamma agonists) but not PPAR alpha agonists increase IRS-2 gene expression in 3T3-L1 and human adipocytes. FASEB J 2001; 15(1):215–220.
158. Ribon V, Johnson JH, Camp HS, Saltiel AR. Thiazolidinediones and insulin resistance: peroxisome proliferator–activated receptor γ activation stimulates expression of the CAP gene. Proc Natl Acad Sci USA 1998; 95:14751–14756.
159. Baumann CA, Ribon V, Kanzaki M, Thurmond DC, Mora S, Shigematsu S, Bickel PE, Pessin JE, Saltiel AR. CAP defines a second signalling pathway required for insulin-stimulated glucose transport. Nature 2000; 407(6801):202–207.
160. Rieusset J, Auwerx J, Vidal H. Regulation of gene expression by activation of the peroxisome proliferator–activated receptor gamma with rosiglitazone (BRL 49653) in human adipocytes. Biochem Biophys Res Commun 1999; 265(1):265–271.
161. Burant CF, Sreenan S, Hirano K-I, Tai T-AC, Lohmiller J, Lukens J, Davidson NO, Ross S, Graves RA. Troglitazone action is independent of adipose tissue. J Clin Invest 1997; 100:2900–2908.
162. Kim JB, Sarraf P, Wright M, Yao KM, Mueller E, Solanes G, Lowell BB, Spiegelman BM. Nutritional and insulin regulation of fatty acid synthetase and leptin gene expression through ADD1/SREBP1. J Clin Invest 1998; 101:1–9.
163. Shimomura I, Bashmakov Y, Ikemoto S, Horton JD, Brown MS, Goldstein J. Insulin selectively increases SREBP-1c mRNA in the livers of rats with streptozotocin-induced diabetes. Proc Natl Acad Sci USA 1999; 96:13656–13661.
164. Foretz M, Guichard C, Ferré P, Foufelle F. Sterol regulatory element binding protein 1c is a major mediator of insulin action on the hepatic expression of glucokinase and lipogenesis-related genes. Proc Natl Acad Sci USA 1999; 96:12737–12742.
165. Shimomura I, Matsuda M, Hammer RE, Bashmakov Y, Brown MS, Goldstein JL. Decreased IRS-2 and increased SREBP-1c lead to mixed insulin resistance and sensitivity in livers of lipodystrophic and ob/ob mice [In Process Citation]. Mol Cell 2000; 6(1):77–86.
166. Fajas L, Schoonjans K, Gelman L, Kim JB, Najib J, Martin G, Fruchart JC, Briggs M, Spiegelman BM, Auwerx J. Regulation of PPARγ expression by ADD-1/SREBP-1: implications for adipocyte differentiation and metabolism. Mol Cell Biol 1999; 19:5495–5503.
167. Kim JB, Wright HM, Wright M, Spiegelman BM. ADD1/SREBP1 activates PPARγ through the production of endogeneous ligand. Proc Natl Acad Sci USA 1998; 95:4333–4337.
168. Croniger C, Trus M, Lysek-Stupp K, Cohen H, Liu Y, Darlington GJ, Poli V, Hanson RW, Reshef L. Role of the isoforms of CCAAT/enhancer-binding protein in the initiation of phosphoenolpyruvate carboxykinase (GTP) gene transcription at birth. J Biol Chem 1997; 272(42):26306–26312.
169. Lee YH, Sauer B, Johnson PF, Gonzalez FJ. Disruption of the c/ebp alpha gene in adult mouse liver. Mol Cell Biol 1997; 17(10):6014–6022.
170. Liu S, Croniger C, Arizmendi C, Harada-Shiba M, Ren J, Poli V, Hanson RW, Friedman JE. Hypoglycemia and impaired hepatic glucose production in mice with a deletion of the C/EBPbeta gene. J Clin Invest 1999; 103(2):207–213.
171. Bouchard C, Perusse L. Genetics of obesity. Annu Rev Nutrition 1993; 13:337–354.
172. Ristow M, Muller-Wieland D, Pfeiffer A, Krone W, Kahn CR. Obesity associated with a mutation in a genetic regulator of adipocyte differentiation. N Engl J Med 1998; 339:953–959.
173. Hu E, Kim JB, Sarraf P, Spiegelman BM. Inhibition of adipogenesis through MAP-kinase mediated phosphorylation of PPARγ. Science 1996; 274: 2100–2103.
174. Adams M, Reginato MJ, Shao D, Lazar MA, Chatterjee VK. Transcriptional activation by peroxisome proliferator-activated receptor gamma is inhibited by phosphorylation at a consensus mitogen-activated protein kinase site. J Biol Chem 1997; 272:5128–5132.
175. Camp HS, Tafuri SR. Regulation of peroxisome proliferator-activated receptor gamma activity by mitogen-activated protein kinase. J Biol Chem 1997; 272:10811–10816.
176. Zhang B, Berger J, Zhou G, Elbrecht A, Biswas S, White-Carrington S, Szalkowski D, Moller DE. Insulin and mitogen-activated protein kinase-mediated phosphorylation and activation of peroxisome proliferator-activated receptor gamma. J Biol Chem 1996; 271:31771–31774.
177. Yen CJ, Beamer BA, Negri C, Silver K, Brown KA, Yarnall DP, Burns DK, Roth J, Shuldiner AR. Molecular scanning of the human peroxisome proliferator activated receptor gamma gene in diabetic Caucasians: identification of a Pro12Ala PPARgamma 2 missense mutation. Biochem Biophys Res Commun 1997; 241:270–274.
178. Deeb S, Fajas L, Nemoto M, Laakso M, Fujimoto W, Auwerx J. A Pro12Ala substitution in the human peroxisome proliferator-activated receptor gamma2 is associated with decreased receptor activity, improved insulin sensitivity, and lowered body mass index. Nat Genet 1998; 20:284–287.
179. Vigouroux C, Fajas L, Khallouf E, Meier M, Gyapay

G, Auwerx J, Weissenbach J, Capeau J, Magre J. Human peroxisome proliferator-activated receptor gamma 2: genetic mapping, identification of a variant in the coding sequence, and exclusion as the gene responsible for lipoatrophic diabetes. Diabetes 1998; 47:490–492.

180. Beamer BA, Yen CJ, Andersen RE, Muller D, Elahi D, Cheskin LJ, Andres R, Roth J, Shuldiner AR. Association of the Pro12Ala variant in peroxisome proliferator–activated receptor gamma2 gene with obesity in two Caucasian populations. Diabetes 1998; 47:1806–1808.
181. Altshuler D, Hirschhorn JN, Klannemark M, Lindgren CM, Vohl MC, Nemesh J, Lane CR, Schaffner SF, Bolk S, Brewer C, Tuomi T, Gaudet D, Hudson TJ, Daly M, Groop L. The common PPARgamma Pro12Ala polymorphism is associated with decreased risk of type 2 diabetes [In Process Citation]. Nat Genet 2000; 26(1):76–80.
182. Mori Y, Kim-Motoyama H, Katakura T, Yasuda K, Kadowaki H, Beamer BB, Shuldiner AR, Akanuma Y, Yazaki Y, Kadowaki T. Effect of the Pro12Ala variant of the human peroxisome proliferator activated receptor γ2 gene on adiposity, fat distribution, and insulin sensitivity in Japanese men. Biochem Biophys Res Commun 1998; 251:195–198.
183. Werman A, Hollenberg A, Solanes G, Bjorbaek C, Vidal-Puig A, Flier JS. Ligand-independent activation domain in the N terminus of peroxisome proliferator–activated receptor γ (PPARγ). J Biol Chem 1997; 272:20230–20235.
184. Shao D, Rangwala SM, Bailey ST, Krakow SL, Reginato MJ, Lazar MA. Interdomain communication regulating ligand binding by PPAR gamma. Nature 1998; 396(6505):377–380.
185. Norman RA, Thompson DB, Foroud T, Garvey WT, Bennett PH, Bogardus C, Ravussin E. Genomewide search for genes influencing percent body fat in Pima Indians: suggestive linkage at chromosome 11Q21 Q22. Am J Hum Genet 1997; 60:166–173.
186. Barak Y, Nelson MC, Ong ES, Jones YZ, Ruiz-Lozano P, Chien KR, Koder A, Evans RM. PPAR-gamma is required for placental, cardiac, and adipose tissue development. Mol Cell 1999; 4:585–595.
187. Kubota N, Terauchi Y, Miki H, Tamemoto H, Yamauchi T, Komeda K, Satoh S, Nakano R, Ishii C, Sugiyama T, Eto K, Tsubamoto Y, Okuno A, Murakami K, Sekihara H. PPARg mediates high-fat diet–induced adipocyte hypertrophy and insulin resistance. Mol Cell 1999; 4:597–609.
188. Miles PD, Barak Y, He W, Evans RM, Olefsky JM. Improved insulin-sensitivity in mice heterozygous for PPAR-gamma deficiency. J Clin Invest 2000; 105(3): 287–292.
189. Schoonjans K, Staels B, Auwerx J. The peroxisome proliferator–activated receptors (PPARs) and their effects on lipid metabolism and adipocyte differentiation. Biochim Biophys Acta 1996; 1302: 93–109.
190. Staels B, Vu-Dac N, Kosykh V, Saladin R, Fruchart JC, Dallongeville J, Auwerx J. Fibrates down-regulate apolipoprotein C-III expression independent of induction of peroxisomal Acyl Co-enzyme A Oxidase. J Clin Invest 1995; 95:705–712.
191. Hertz R, Bishara-Shieban J, Bar-Tana J. Mode of action of peroxisome proliferators as hypolipidemic drugs, suppression of apolipoprotein C-III. J Biol Chem 1995; 270:13470–13475.
192. Castle CK, Colca JR, Melchior GW. Lipoprotein profile characterization of the KKAy mouse, a rodent model of type II diabetes, before and after treatment with the insulin-sensitizing agent pioglitazone. Arterioscler Thromb 1993; 13:302–309.
193. Schwartz S, Raskin P, Fonseca V, Graveline JF. Effect of troglitazone in insulin-treated patients with type II diabetes. N Engl J Med 1998; 338:861–866.
194. Kumar S, Boulton AJM, Beck-Nielsen H, Berthezene F, Muggeo M, Persson B, Spinas GA, Donoghue S, Lettis S, Stewart-Long P. Troglitazone, an insulin action enhancer, improves metabolic control in NIDDM patients. Diabetologia 1996; 39:701–709.
195. Ghazzi MN, Perez JE, Antonucci TK, Driscoll JH, Huang SM, Faja BW, Whitcomb RW. Cardiac and glycemic benefits of troglitazone treatment in NIDDM. Diabetes 1997; 46:433–439.
196. Berthezene F. Non-insulin dependent diabetes and reverse cholesterol transport. Atherosclerosis 1996; 124:S39–S42.
197. Sasahara T, Yamashita T, Sviridov D, Fidge N, Nestel P. Altered properties of high density lipoprotein subfractions in obese subjects. J Lipid Res 1997; 38:600–611.
198. Vague J. The degree of masculine differentiation of obesities: a factor determining predisposition to diabetes, atherosclerosis, gout and uric calculous disease. Am J Clin Nutr 1956; 34:416–422.
199. Wajchenberg BL. Subcutaneous and visceral adipose tissue: their relation to the metabolic syndrome. Endocr Rev 2000; 21:697–738.
200. Li AC, Brown KK, Silvestre MJ, Willson TM, Palinski W, Glass CK. Peroxisome proliferator–activated receptor gamma ligands inhibit development of atherosclerosis in LDL recepto–deficient mice. J Clin Invest 2000; 106(4):523–531.
201. Claudel T, Leibowitz MD, Fievet C, Tailleux A, Wagner B, Repa JJ, Torpier G, Lobaccaro JM, Paterniti JR, Mangelsdorf DJ, Heyman RA, Auwerx J. Reduction of atherosclerosis in apolipoprotein E knockout mice by activation of the retinoid X receptor. Proc Natl Acad Sci USA 2001; 98(5):2610–2615.
202. Glass CK, Rose DW, Rosenfeld MG. Nuclear receptor coactivators. Curr Opin Cell Biol 1997; 9:222–232.

203. Abraham SE, Lobo S, Yaciuk P, Heidi HG, Moran E. p300 and p300-associated proteins, are components of the TATA-binding protein (TBP) complexes. Oncogene 1993; 8:1639–1647.
204. Nakajima T, Uchida C, Anderson S, Lee CG, Hurwitz J, Parvin JD, Montmimy M. RNA helicase A mediates association of CBP with RNA polymerase II. Cell 1997; 90:1107–1112.
205. Kingston RE, Narlikar GJ. ATP-dependent remodeling and acetylation as regulators of chromatin fluidity. Genes Dev 1999; 13(18):2339–2352.
206. Vignali M, Hassan AH, Neely KE, Workman JL. ATP-dependent chromatin-remodeling complexes. Mol Cell Biol 2000; 20(6):1899–1910.
207. Sudarsanam P, Winston F. The Swi/Snf family nucleosome-remodeling complexes and transcriptional control [In Process Citation]. Trends Genet 2000; 16(8):345–351.
208. Muchardt C, Yaniv M. A human homologue of *Saccharomyces cerevisiae SNF2/SW12* and *Drosophila brm* genes potentiates transcriptional activation by the glucocorticoid receptor. EMBO J 1993; 12(11):4279–4290.
209. Fryer CJ, Archer TK. Chromatin remodelling by the glucocorticoid receptor requires the BRGI complex. Nature 1998; 393(6680):88–91.
210. Wallberg AE, Neely KE, Hassan AH, Gustafsson JA, Workman JL, Wright AP. Recruitment of the SWI-SNF chromatin remodeling complex as a mechanism of gene activation by the glucocorticoid receptor taul activation domain. Mol Cell Biol 2000; 20(6):2004–2013.
211. Di Lorenzo D, Williams P, Ringold G. Identification of two distinct nuclear factors with DNA binding activity within the glucocorticoid regulatory region of the rat alpha-1-acid glycoprotein promoter. Biochem Biophys Res Commun 1991; 176:1326–1332.
212. Chiba H, Muramatsu M, Nomoto A, Kato H. Two human homologues of *Saccharomyces cerevisiae SWI2/SNF2* and *Drosophila brahma* are transcriptional coactivators cooperating with the oestrogen receptor and the retinoic acid receptor. Nucl Acids Res 1994; 22(10):1815–1820.
213. Dilworth FJ, Fromental-Ramain C, Yamamoto K, Chambon P. ATP-Driven chromatin remodeling activity and histone acetyltransferases act sequentially during transactivation by RAR/RXR In vitro. Mol Cell 2000; 6(5):1049–1058.
214. Lovell-Badge R. Living with bad architecture. Nature 1995; 376:725–726.
215. Zhou X, Benson KF, Ashar HR, Chada K. Mutation responsible for the mouse pygmy phenotype in the developmentally regulated factor HMGI-C. Nature 1995; 376(6543):771–774.
216. Schoenmakers EFPM, Wanschura S, Mols R, Bullerdiek J, Van den Berghe H, Van de Ven WJW. Recurrent rearrangements in the high mobility group protein gene, HMGI-C, in benign mesenchymal tumours. Nat Genet 1995; 10:436–443.
217. Ashar HR, Schoenberg Fejzo M, Tkachenko A, Zhou X, Fletcher JA, Weremowicz S, Morton CC, Chada K. Disruption of the architectural factor HMGI-C: DNA binding AT hook motifs fused in lipomas to distinct transcriptional regulatory domains. Cell 1995; 82(1):57–65.
218. Battista S, Fidanza V, Fedele M, Klein-Szanto AJ, Outwater E, Brunner H, Santoro M, Croce CM, Fusco A. The expression of a truncated HMGI-C gene induces gigantism associated with lipomatosis. Cancer Res 1999; 59(19):4793–4797.
219. Melillo RM, Pierantoni GM, Scala S, Battista S, Fedele M, Stella A, De Biasio MC, Chiappetta G, Fidanza V, Condorelli G, Santoro M, Croce CM, Viglietto G, Fusco A. Critical role of the hmgi(y) proteins in adipocytic cell growth and differentiation. Mol Cell Biol 2001; 21(7):2485–2495.
220. Bannister AJ, Kouzarides T. The CBP co-activator is a histone acyltransferase. Nature 1996; 384:641–643.
221. Chen H, Lin RJ, Louis Schiltz L, Chakravarti D, Nash A, Nagy L, Privalsky ML, Nakatani Y, Evans RM. Nuclear receptor coactivator ACTR is a novel histone acetyltransferase and forms multimeric activation complexes with P/CAF and CBP/p300. Cell 1997; 90:569–580.
222. Korzus E, Torchia J, Rose DW, Xu L, Kurokawa R, McInerney EM, Mullen TM, Glass CK, Rosenfeld MG. Transcription factor–specific requirements for coactivators and their acetyltransferase functions. Science 1998; 279:703–707.
223. Ogryzko VV, Schiltz RL, Russanova V, Howard BH, Nakatani Y. The transcriptional coactivators p300 and CBP are histone acetyltransferases. Cell 1996; 87:953–959.
224. Spencer TEJ, G., Burcin MM, Allis CD, Zhou J, Mizzen CA, McKenna NJ, Onate SA, Tsai SY, O'Malley BW. Steroid receptor coactivator-1 is a histone acetyltransferase. Nature 1997; 389:194–198.
225. Martinez-Balbas MA, Bannister AJ, Martin K, Haus-Seuffert P, Meisterernst M, Kouzarides T. The acetyltransferase activity of CBP stimulates transcription. EMBO J 1998; 17:2886–2893.
226. Imhof A, Yang XJ, Ogryzko VV, Nakatani Y, Wolffe AP, Ge H. Acetylation of general transcription factors by histone acetyltransferases. Curr Biol 1997; 7:689–692.
227. Nagy L, Kao HK, Chakravarti D, Lin RJ, Hassig CA, Ayer DE, Schreiber SL, Evans RM. Nuclear receptor repression mediated by a complex containing SMRT, mSin3A, and histone deacetylase. Cell 1997; 89:373–380.
228. Alland L, Muhle R, Hou H, Potes J, Chin L, Schreiber-Agus N, DePinho RA. Role for N-CoR

and histone deacetylase in Sin3-mediated transcriptional repression. Nature 1997; 387:49–55.

229. Heinzel T, Lavinsky RM, Mullen TM, Soderstrom M, Laherty CD, Torchia J, Yang W-M, Brard G, Davie JR, Seto E, Eisenman RN, Rose DW, Glass CK, Rosenfeld MG. A complex containing N-CoR, mSin3 and histone deacetylase mediates transcriptional repression. Nature 1997; 387:43–48.
230. Glass CK, Rosenfeld MG. The coregulator exchange in transcriptional functions of nuclear receptors. Genes Dev 2000; 14(2):121–141.
231. Chen JD, Evans RM. A transcriptional co-repressor that interacts with nuclear hormone receptors. Nature 1995; 377:454–457.
232. Chen DJ, Umesono K, Evans RM. SMRT isoforms mediate repression and anti-repression of nuclear receptor heterodimers. Proc Natl Acad Sci USA 1996; 93:7567–7571.
233. Lavinsky RM, Jepsen K, Heinzel T, Torchia J, Mullen TM, Schiff R, Del-Rio AL, Ricote M, Gemsch J, Hilsenbeck SG, Osborne CK, Glass CK, Rosenfeld M, Rose DW. Diverse signalling pathways modulate nuclear receptor recruitment of N-CoR and SMRT complexes. Proc Natl Acad Sci USA 1998; 95:2920–2925.
234. Zamir I, Zhang J, Lazar M. Stochiometric and steric principles governing repression by nuclear hormone receptors. Genes Dev 1997; 11:835–846.
235. Misiti S, Schomburg L, Yen PM, Chin WW. Expression and hormonal regulation of co-activator and co-repressor genes. Endocrinology 1998; 139:2493–2500.
236. Chrivia JC, Kwok RP, Lamb N, Hagiwara M, Montminy MR, Goodman RH. Phosphorylated CREB binds specifically to the nuclear protein CBP. Nature 1993; 365:855–859.
237. Eckner R, Ewen ME, Newsome D, Gerdes M, DeCaprio JA, Bentley Lawrence J, Livingston DM. Molecular cloning and functional analysis of the adenovirus E1A-associated 300 kD protein (p300) reveals a protein with properties of a transcriptional adaptator. Genes Dev 1994; 8:869–884.
238. Janknecht R, Hunter T. Transcriptional control: versatile molecular glue. Curr Biol 1996; 6:951–954.
239. Chakravarti D, LaMorte VJ, Nelson MC, Nakajima T, Schulman IG, Juguilon H, Montminy M, Evans RM. Role of CBP/p300 in nuclear receptor signalling. Nature 1996; 383:99–103.
240. Kamei Y, Xu L, Heinzel T, Torchia J, Kurokawa R, Gloss B, Lin S-C, Heyman RA, Rose DW, Glass CK, Rosenfeld MG. A CBP integrator complex mediates transcriptional activation and AP-1 inhibition by nuclear receptors. Cell 1996; 85:403–414.
241. Hanstein B, Eckner R, DiRenzo J, Halachmi S, Liu H, Searcy B, Kurokawa R, Brown M. p300 is a component of an estrogen receptor coactivator complex. Proc Natl Acad Sci USA 1996; 93:11540–11545.
242. Smith CL, Onate SA, Tsai MJ, O'Malley BW. CREB binding protein acts synergistically with steroid receptor coactivator-1 to enhance steroid receptor–dependent transcription. Proc Natl Acad Sci USA 1996; 93:8884–8888.
243. Kraus WL, Kadonaga JT. p300 and estrogen receptor cooperatively activate transcription via differential enhancement of initiation and reinitiation. Genes Dev 1998; 12:331–342.
244. Dowell P, Ishmael JE, Avram D, Peterson VJ, Nevrivy DJ, Leid M. p300 functions as a co-activator for the peroxisome proliferator-activated receptor α. J Biol Chem 1997; 272:33435–33433.
245. Gelman L, Zhou G, Fajas L, Raspe E, Fruchart JC, Auwerx J. p300 interacts with the N- and C-terminal part of PPARγ2 in a ligand-independent and -dependent manner respectively. J Biol Chem 1999; 274:7681–7688.
246. Yao TP, Ku G, Zhou N, Scully R, Livingston DM. The nuclear hormone receptor coactivator SRC-1 is a specific target of p300. Proc Natl Acad Sci USA 1996; 93(20):10626–10631.
247. Onate SA, Tsai SY, Tsai MJ, O'Malley BW. Sequence and characterization of a coactivator for the steroid hormone receptor superfamily. Science 1995; 270:1354–1357.
248. Zhu Y, Qi C, Calandra C, Rao MS, Reddy J. Cloning and identification of mouse steroid receptor coactivator-1 (mSRC-1), as a coactivator of peroxisome proliferator–activated receptor γ. Gene Expr 1996; 6:185–195.
249. Zhou G, Cummings R, Li Y, Mitra S, Wilkinson H, Elbrecht A, Hermes D. Schaeffer J, Smith R, Moller D. Nuclear receptors have distinct affinities for coactivators: characterization by fluorescence resonance energy transfer. Mol Endocrinol 1998; 12:1594–1604.
250. Voegel JJ, Heine MJ, Tini M, Vivat V, Chambon P, Gronemeyer H. The coactivator TIF2 contains three nuclear receptor binding motifs and mediates transactivation through CBP binding–dependent and –independent pathways. EMBO J 1998; 17:507–519.
251. McInermey E, Rose D, Flynn S, Westin S, Krones A, Inostroza J, Torchia J, Nolte R, Assa-Munt N, Milburn M, Glass C, Rosenfeld M. Determinants of coactivator LXXLL motif specificity in nuclear receptor transcriptional activation. Genes Dev 1998; 12:3357–3368.
252. Zhu Y, Qi C, Rao MS, Reddy JK. Isolation of and characterization of PBP, a protein that interacts with peroxisome proliferator activated receptor. J Biol Chem 1997; 272:25500–25506.
253. Puigserver P, Wu Z, Park CW, Graves R, Wright M, Spiegelman BM. A cold-inducible coactivator of nuclear receptors linked to adaptive thermogenesis. Cell 1998; 92:829–839.

254. Jain S, Pulikuri S, Zhu Y, Qi C, Kanwar YS, Yeldandi AV, Rao MS, Reddy JK. Differential expression of the peroxisome proliferator-activated receptor γ (PPARγ) and its coactivators steroid receptor coactivator-1 and PPAR-binding protein PBP in the brown fat, urinary bladder, colon, and breast of the mouse. Am J Pathol 1998; 153:349–354.
255. Fondell JD, Ge H, Roeder RG. Ligand induction of a transcriptionally active thyroid hormone receptor coactivator complex. Proc Natl Acad Sci USA 1996; 93(16):8329–8333.
256. Rachez C, Suldan Z, Ward J, Chang CP, Burakov D, Erdjument-Bromage H, Tempst P, Freedman LP. A novel protein complex that interacts with the vitamin D3 receptor in a ligand-dependent manner and enhances VDR transactivation in a cell-free system. Genes Dev 1998; 12(12):1787–1800.
257. Naar AM, Beaurang PA, Zhou S, Abraham S, Solomon W, Tjian R Composite co-activator ARC mediates chromatin-directed transcriptional activation. Nature 1999; 398(6730):828–832.
258. Gu W, Malik S, Ito M, Yuan CX, Fondell JD, Zhang X, Martinez E, Qin J, Roeder RG. A novel human SRB/MED-containing cofactor complex, SMCC, involved in transcription regulation. Mol Cell 1999; 3(1):97–108.
259. Rachez C, Lemon BD, Suldan Z, Bromleigh V, Gamble M, Naar AM, Erdjument-Bromage H, Tempst P, Freedman LP. Ligand-dependent transcription activation by nuclear receptors requires the DRIP complex. Nature 1999; 398(6730):824–828.
260. Yuan CX, Ito M, Fondell JD, Fu ZY, Roeder RG. The TRAP220 component of a thyroid hormone receptor–associated protein (TRAP) coactivator complex interacts directly with nuclear receptors in a ligand-dependent fashion [published erratum appears in Proc Natl Acad Sci USA 1998; 95(24):14584]. Proc Natl Acad Sci USA 1998; 95(14):7939–7944.
261. Zhu Y, Qi C, Jia Y, Nye JS, Rao MS, Reddy JK. Deletion of PBP/PPARBP, the gene for nuclear receptor coactivator peroxisome proliferator–activated receptor-binding protein, results in embryonic lethality. J Biol Chem 2000; 275(20):14779–14782.
262. Ito M, Yuan CX, Okano HJ, Darnell RB, Roeder RG. Involvement of the TRAP220 component of the TRAP/SMCC coactivator complex in embryonic development and thyroid hormone action. Mol Cell 2000; 5(4):683–693.
263. Wu Z, Puigserver P, Andersson U, Zhang C, Adelmant G, Mootha V, Troy A, Cinti S, Lowell B, Scarpulla RC, Spiegelman BM. Mechanisms controlling mitochondrial biogenesis and respiration through the thermogenic coactivator PGC-1. Cell 1999; 98(1): 115–124.
264. Vega RB, Huss JM, Kelly DP. The coactivator PGC-1 cooperates with peroxisome proliferator–activated receptor alpha in transcriptional control of nuclear genes encoding mitochondrial fatty acid oxidation enzymes. Mol Cell Biol 2000; 20(5):1868–1876.
265. Tcherepanova I, Puigserver P, Norris JD, Spiegelman BM, McDonnell DP. Modulation of estrogen receptor-alpha transcriptional activity by the coactivator PGC-1. J Biol Chem 2000; 275(21):16302–16308.
266. Knutti D, Kaul A, Kralli A. A tissue-specific coactivator of steroid receptors, identified in a functional genetic screen. Mol Cell Biol 2000; 20(7):2411–2422.
267. Puigserver P, Adelmant G, Wu Z, Fan M, Xu J, O'Malley B, Spiegelman BM. Activation of PPAR-gamma coactivator-1 through transcription factor docking. Science 1999; 286(5443):1368–1371.
268. Michael LF, Wu Z, Cheatham RB, Puigserver P, Adelmant G, Lehman JJ, Kelly DP, Spiegelman BM. Restoration of insulin-sensitive glucose transporter (GLUT4) gene expression in muscle cells by the transcriptional coactivator PGC-1. Proc Natl Acad Sci USA 2001; 98(7):3820–3825.
269. Monsalve M, Wu Z, Adelmant G, Puigserver P, Fan M, Spiegelman BM. Direct coupling of transcription and mRNA processing through the thermogenic coactivator PGC-1. Mol Cell 2000; 6(2):307–316.
270. Treuter E, Albrektsen T, Johansson L, Leers J, Gustafsson JA. A regulatory role for RIP140 in nuclear receptor activation. Mol Endocrinol 1998; 12(6):864–881.
271. Tontonoz P, Nagy L, Alvarez JG, Thomazy VA, Evans RM. PPARγ promotes monocyte/macrophage differentiation and uptake of oxidized LDL. Cell 1998; 93:241–252.
272. Lefebvre A, Chen I, Desreumaux P, Najib J, Fruchart J, Geboes K, Briggs M, Heyman R, Auwerx J. Activation of the peroxisome proliferator-activated receptor γ promotes the development of colon tumors in C57BL/6J-APC^{Min} /+ mice. Nat Med 1998; 4:1053–1057.
273. Saez E, Tontonoz P, Nelson MC, Alvarez JGA, Ming UT, Baird SM, Thomazy VA, Evans RM. Activators of the nuclear receptor PPARγ enhance colon polyp formation. Nat Med 1998; 4:1058–1061.
274. Watkins PB, Whitcomb RW. Hepatic dysfunction associated with troglitazone. N Engl J Med 1998; 338:916–917.

22

Biology of Visceral Adipose Tissue

Susan K. Fried

University of Maryland and Baltimore Veterans Administration Medical Center, Baltimore, Maryland, U.S.A.

Robert R. Ross

Queen's University, Kingston, Ontario, Canada

I INTRODUCTION

A Visceral Obesity and Health–A Brief Historical Perspective

In humans and other mammals, fat is deposited within anatomically discrete depots that are located throughout the body. In humans, while most fat is present in subcutaneous depots, up to 20% of total body fat is deposited in adipose depots within the abdominal cavity (see Table 1). The pattern of fat distribution is a main determinant of variations in body shape (1–3). Vague first noted that that an upper body (android or male-type) fat distribution is associated with development of diabetes, atherosclerosis, and gout (4,5). Kissebah et al. (6,7) and Krotkiewski et al. (6), among others, confirmed and extended Vague's hypothesis, finding evidence for correlations of upper-body obesity and enlarged abdominal subcutaneous fat cells to hypertension, insulin resistance, and hyperlipidemia in clinical studies. Epidemiological studies showed that upper-body fat distribution, measured by the ratio of waist to hip circumferences, was a significant determinant of diabetes, cardiovascular disease, and premature death in both men and women (3). These statistical associations were independent of overall obesity, as assessed by the body mass index. Thus, much research attention became focused on the phenomenon of abdominal obesity.

With the application of imaging technology to the study of fat distribution, it became possible to better define fat distribution by distinguishing the relative sizes of intra-abdominal and subcutaneous fat compartments. It was realized that increased waist circumference was a heterogeneous phenotype associated in some cases with high amounts of intra-abdominal fat, and in others with mostly subcutaneous abdominal fat. Many studies found that the size of intra-abdominal fat stores as measured by computerized tomography (CT) or magnetic resonance imaging (MRI) was most closely linked with the metabolic complications of obesity (1,7–9).

B The Portal Hypothesis

The statistical association between abdominal obesity and health risk does not prove a causal relationship (10). Thus, investigators addressed potential mechanistic links between the size of specific fat depots and alterations in systemic metabolism. As noted by Björntorp (10), there was accumulating evidence in the literature from 1960s and 1970s that fat cells from different fat depots exhibit marked differences in functional capaci-

Table 1 Major Fat Depots in Humans and Rodents

Humans
- I. Intra-abdominal or visceral[a] adipose tissue depots
  - A. Intraperitoneal
    - 1. omental—greater and lesser
    - 2. mesenteric—small intestine, colon-rectum, epiploic
    - 3. umbilical/round/falciform ligament
  - B. Extraperitoneal (including pre- or properitoneal)
    - 1. perirenal[b]
    - 2. peripancreatic[b]
    - 3. urogenital (bladder, uterus, prostate)
- II. Subcutaneous fat depots (deep and superficial compartments)
  - A. Truncal (anterior or posterior chest)
  - B. Mammary (only one compartment)
  - C. Abdominal
  - D. Lumbar
  - E. Gluteal
  - F. Femoral

Rodents
- I. Intra-abdominal
  - A. Mesenteric
  - B. Omental
  - C. Gonadal (parametrial or epididymal)
  - D. Perirenal ("retroperitoneal")
- II. Subcutaneous
  - A. Truncal
    - 1. cervical[b]
    - 2. axillary[b]
    - 3. interscapular[c]
    - 4. dorsal
  - B. Inguinal

[a] Operationally defined as "intra-abdominal" on CT or MRI images.
[b] Contains some brown adipose tissue.
[c] Mainly brown adipose tissue.

ties and responsiveness to nutritional manipulations (11). In particular, a consistent finding was that omental fat cells were more lipolytically active than subcutaneous ones (12–14). Because the omental (and mesenteric) fat depots drained their venous blood into the portal vein, it was hypothesized that these 'portal' adipose tissues would be the most metabolically dangerous by virtue of the impact of high levels of lipolytic products on hepatic metabolism. Indeed, evidence that fatty acids caused deleterious effects on hepatic metabolism, including decreased insulin degradation, impaired insulin sensitivity, and increased VLDL output, fueled acceptance of the 'portal hypothesis' of Björntorp (15). However, in part because of the difficulty of directly measuring portal concentrations of fatty acids, there is no clear evidence that the high in vitro lipolytic rates of portal adipose tissues are translated into high in vivo activity and therefore high portal fatty acid delivery in humans (16,17). Some animal data do support the possibility that an increased mass of visceral adipose tissues lead to increased portal fatty acids levels in vivo (18–20).

C Extending the Portal Hypothesis

Recent evidence that adipose tissues are also heterogeneous in their endocrine functions raises the possibility for additional mechanistic links between visceral adiposity and metabolic derangements (18,21). A growing body of literature indicates that there are marked differences in the secretory products of visceral and subcutaneous adipose tissues, including leptin, interleukin-6, plasminogen activator inhibitor-1, and adiponectin, that may contribute to the development of the metabolic syndrome (21,22).

D Goals of this Chapter

The size of intra-abdominal fat stores, as determined by CT, is strongly influenced by genetic factors, and the genes associated with intra-abdominal fatness are different from those determining overall obesity (23). Thus, visceral fat appears to represent a subset or type of adipose tissue that has distinct determinants and metabolic characteristics. The main goals of this chapter are to define 'visceral fat' from a biologic and clinical perspective and to review our knowledge of its cellular composition and its metabolic and endocrine properties, focusing mainly on data in humans. We will also discuss physiologic determinants of the size of visceral fat depots and the influence of therapeutic interventions on visceral adiposity.

II DEFINITION, ANATOMICAL DESCRIPTION, AND MEASUREMENT OF VISCERAL ADIPOSE TISSUE

It is now well established that CT and MRI are the preferred methods for measuring visceral adipose tissue (VAT) in vivo and that the two methods provide images of the abdomen that are comparable and that are characterized by good tissue contrast (for further details see the chapter by Heymsfield et al.) However, despite evidence that CT (24) and MRI (25) provide accurate estimates of VAT by comparison to cadaver sections, the best way to apply these methods to the measurement of VAT in vivo is not firmly established. Thus several issues require clarification.

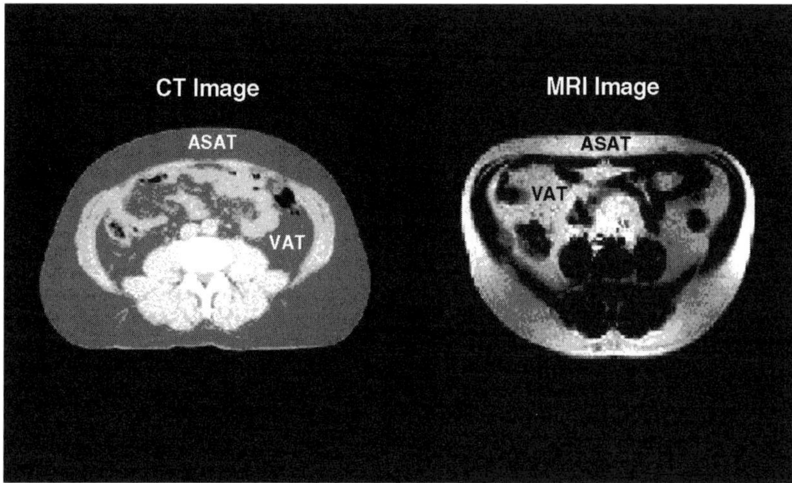

Figure 1 Axial computerized tomography (CT) and magnetic resonance imaging (MRI) images obtained in the midabdomen. Adipose tissue appears black on the CT image and white on the MRI image. VAT, visceral adipose tissue; ASAT, abdominal subcutaneous adipose tissue.

A Visceral Adipose Tissue Defined

Despite the acknowledged importance of VAT in the etiology of metabolic risk (7,26), there is no consensus as to the ideal protocol for measuring VAT in research settings. Anatomically defined VAT is that contained within the visceral peritoneum (i.e., omental and mesenteric). The visceral peritoneum is the membrane that covers, with few exceptions, the abdominal organs of the gastrointestinal tract. This definition excludes retroperitoneal adipose tissue, which, from a clinical point of view, is reasonable, given the hypothetical role of free fatty acids liberated from omental and mesenteric adipose tissue in the etiology of metabolic risk, the so-called portal theory (15). However, because the peritoneum is not visible on either CT or MRI images, separation of VAT into intraperitoneal (omental and mesenteric) and retroperitoneal (i.e., perirenal) components, has relied on arbitrary criteria (27,28). Accordingly, efforts to determine whether separation of VAT into intraperitoneal and retroperitoneal provides additional insight into the relationship between the VAT depot and metabolic risk provide equivocal results (29–33). However, at present the weighted evidence from clinical studies appears to suggest that subdivision of VAT into intraperitoneal and retroperitoneal depots is not warranted and thus, in practice, VAT on CT and MRI axial images within the abdomen region includes all visible intra-abdominal adipose tissue (Fig. 1). However, as discussed in Section IV, there is heterogeneity in the functional properties of the intraperitoneal and retroperitoneal fat depots of humans that may be relevant to understanding the relationships between so-called visceral adiposity and metabolic disease.

As illustrated in Figure 2, it is clear from a coronal perspective that VAT deposition extends throughout the abdominal region. Moreover, it is well established that the accumulation of VAT differs according the level of the abdomen at which the CT or MRI image is

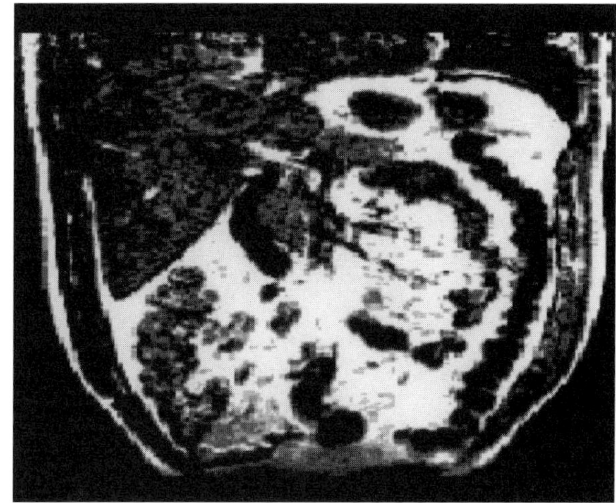

Figure 2 Visceral adipose tissue depicted by magnetic resonance imaging in the coronal plane.

obtained (34–37) (Fig. 3). However, as illustrated in Figure 3, the relative difference between those with high and low VAT is relatively homogeneous throughout the abdomen. This may partially explain why the relationship between VAT and metabolic risk factors is not influenced by the level of the abdomen at which VAT is measured (31,36). Thus, while a universally accepted definition of VAT awaits resolution, it would appear that the ability to determine individual health risk, as conveyed by the accumulation of VAT, can be determined by a single MRI or CT image of the abdomen. This is generally true for axial images acquired in a region of the abdomen bordered by S1-L5 and L1-T12 (31,34,38).

To summarize, human VAT for practical reasons includes all visible intra-abdominal adipose tissue on CT or MRI images. Although the anatomical landmarks that define VAT are not yet established, evidence suggests that the relationship between VAT and metabolic risk factors appears to be similar independent of the level of the abdomen at which VAT is measured; thus, observations from images obtained at different levels of the abdomen are comparable.

It should also be noted that subcutaneous fat can be divided into deep versus superficial subcutaneous fat layers) that are observable on CT images above and below Scarpa's fascia (fascia superficialis). The volume of the deep abdominal subcutaneous fat layer is independently associated with insulin resistance and dyslipidemia (36,39). As most studies do not distinguish subcompartments of subcutaneous fat, these findings may explain some discrepancies in the literature on the contribution of VAT to metabolic complications.

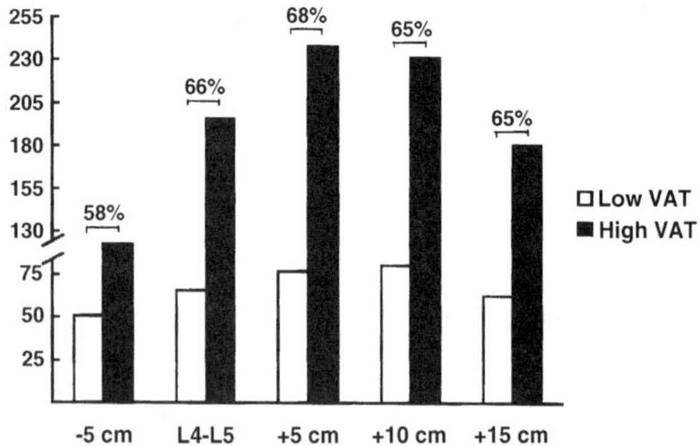

Figure 3 Visceral adipose tissue at the L4-L5 level, 5 cm below, 5 cm above, 10 cm above, and 15 cm above L4-L5 in 91 Caucasian men with low visceral adipose tissue (<125 cm^2 at L4-L5) and 110 Caucasian men with high visceral adipose tissue (>125 cm^2 at L4-L5). The numbers represent the relative difference between the high and low visceral adipose tissue groups for each of the five abdominal images.

B VAT in Rodent Models

Intra-abdominal fat depots of rats include the perirenal, retroperitoneal, gonadal, and mesenteric and omental (40) (note that in rodents, the so-called retroperitoneal fat depot is not outside the peritoneal cavity). Of these, only the mesenteric depot is associated with the digestive tract, is substantial in size, and drains portally. The omental fat depot in rodents, in contrast to that in humans, is much smaller than mesenteric and not usually dissected or studied. Thus, the mesenteric depot of rodents would probably be the best "model" of a human (visceral)portal depot. Data from Warden (41) indicate that genes that determine the size of mesenteric depot are distinct from those regulating the size of other depots, supporting the contention that this visceral fat depot is anatomically and probably metabolically distinct.

The relative distribution of fat appears to differ in humans and rats because the latter deposits relatively more total fat within intra-abdominal depots. Over 50% of the total fat mass of rats is accounted for by intraabdominal fat (42). In contrast, in humans the total intra-abdominal (including omental and mesenteric) fat mass is only ~20% of the total (most is subcutaneous). Furthermore, whereas in humans the size of subcutaneous fat cells are as large as or larger than intra-abdominal ones, in rats subcutaneous fat cells tend to be smaller than those from intra-abdominal depots such as epididymal or retroperitoneal (40,42,43). Thus, the metabolic effects of removal of intra-abdominal fat depots should not be assumed to be comparable to the removal of the "portal" adipose tissues. Caution should be used in extrapolating data about the metabolic effects of altered fat distribution in rodent models to the human (e.g., 44).

III DESCRIPTIVE CHARACTERISTICS—EFFECTS OF GENDER, RACE

A Gender

It is generally reported that, for a given BMI (38) or body fat (45), the accumulation of VAT is lower in women than in men. Lemieux et al. (45) studied a cohort of 89 men and 74 premenopausal women varying in total and visceral adiposity. In that study, the authors report that men have significantly greater quantities of VAT than women after correction for differences in total adiposity. Because VAT is a strong correlate of metabolic risk (7,26), these observations may partially explain the greater obesity-related health risk that characterize men by comparison to obesity-matched women. This notion is reinforced by Couillard et al. (46), who report that the well established gender dimorphism in postprandial triglyceride response (women less than men) is eliminated when men and women are matched for VAT accumulation.

The relative masses of deep vs. superficial subcutaneous fat also varies by gender and because this covaries with VAT volume, this may factor into metabolic risk (36,39). Men have relatively more deep than superficial SAT (36) than women. However, type 2 diabetic men have less superficial but similar amounts of deep SAT as women (47).

B Race

It is generally reported that African-American men and women have less VAT than Caucasian men and women (36,48–50). The race differences in men remain after statistical control for differences in total adiposity (36,48). However, in women the racial dimorphism between African-American women and Caucasian women disappears after control for variation in total adiposity (36,48). However, Albu found that after adjusting for total fat, black women had less VAT and VAT/SCAT for any waist-to-hip ratio (50). This racial difference in VAT accumulation is apparent in childhood as it is commonly reported that African-American children have less VAT by comparison to age-matched Caucasian-American children (51,52). This clinical or metabolic importance of VAT accumulation in children is unclear. Goran et al. (51) report that in both African-American and Caucasian children insulin sensitivity is more closely related to total body fat than to VAT. This may not be surprising given that in children the vast majority of VAT is located posterior to the peritoneum (i.e., is not portally drained). Thus, if the "portal theory" (15) is the mechanism that links VAT and metabolic risk, given the relatively small accumulation of omental and mesenteric fat (Fig. 4) in children, one would not expect VAT to be a strong marker of metabolic risk in children.

Apart from comparisons of African-American with Caucasian men and women, it has recently been reported that healthy Asian-American women have greater quantities of VAT than European-American women after adjustment for differences in total adiposity and age (53). However, no differences in VAT accumulation were observed after control for differences in age and total adiposity in Asian-American men by comparison to their European-American counterparts.

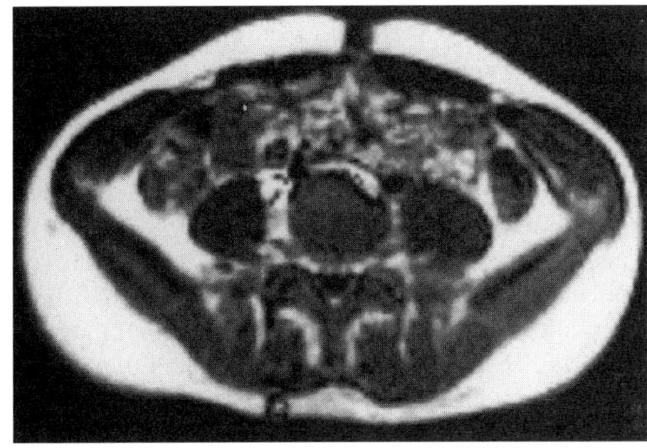

Figure 4 Magnetic resonance image obtained at the level of the umbilicus in a 12-year-old girl.

IV COMPOSITION OF VISCERAL FAT DEPOTS

A Types of Cells Within Visceral and Subcutaneous Fat Depots

All fat depots contain adipocytes, preadipocytes, endothelial cells, mast cells, and fibroblasts. There are no systematic studies that characterize and quantify the different cell types present in visceral compared to subcutaneous fat. The omental fat depot is also rich in mesothelial cells, apparently derived from the peritoneum (54–56).

There appear to be more macrophages present in omental than subcutaneous adipose tissue (57). The abundance of lymph nodes in visceral depots may also be of importance in determining the metabolic activity of surrounding adipocytes (58).

The number of preadipocytes in omental fat may be lower than in subcutaneous (59). Because nonadipose cells including preadipocytes produce many cytokines including tumor necrosis factor-α (60) and interleukin-6 (61,62) and other proteins that may influence adipocyte metabolism, it seems likely that the paracrine environment of different depots differs between visceral and subcutaneous fat, at least in part, by virtue of the different cell types present. These differences in cellular composition may underlie regional differences in adipocyte metabolism, and hence variations in the regional deposition of fat or its function.

B Size of Visceral Adipocytes

In lean men and women, omental fat cells are smaller than subcutaneous ones (63–66). In obese men, most studies indicate that omental fat cells are similar in size to subcutaneous (66–69). In obese women, however, omental fat cells are ~20-30% smaller (68–70). Variations among studies are probably due to the relatively small number of subjects studied in each (usually 10–20) and random variations in fat distribution that may add to variability. Some studies also pool small numbers of women and men. Mesenteric fat cells of severely obese individuals are reported in several studies to be larger than omental (70), most markedly in men (68,69). However, some studies (67) find no difference between omental and mesenteric adipocytes. Round ligament adipocytes tend to be larger than omental, mesenteric, or subcutaneous (71,72).

V METABOLIC CHARACTERISTICS OF VISCERAL ADIPOSE TISSUE

Increased catecholamine sensitivity and lower insulin sensitivity may contribute to higher turnover of fatty acids (FA) in visceral versus subcutaneous adipocytes. Most studies of lipolysis in visceral adipose tissue have studied omental fat cells (12). Limited data indicate that omental and mesenteric adipocytes behave similarly, with only minor, gender-specific differences detected in some studies (65,67,73). Adipocytes from the round ligament appear to be markedly different (72).

A Basal Lipolysis Is Lower in Omental Than in Subcutaneous Fat Cells

Most studies indicate that adipocytes isolated from the omental depot of lean or obese men and women exhibit lower basal lipolysis, even when the rates are corrected for cell size (surface area) (12,70,72,74). Similar results are obtained when basal lipolysis is assessed in the absence or presence of adenosine deaminase (ADA) to permit maximally disinhibited lipolysis (12,74). However, when high concentrations of fat cells were incubated in the absence of ADA, no differences in basal lipolysis were detectable (65,75). The low rates of basal lipolysis under these conditions may make it difficult to detect differences. Indeed, omental fat cells are reportedly less sensitive to adenosine inhibition of lipolysis (76). Similarly, studies of intact fragments of adipose tissue from obese subjects revealed no difference in basal lipolysis in men, but did show a clearly lower lipolytic rate in women (77). Thus, it is possible that there may be gender-specific differences in the sensitivity of omental adipocytes to paracrine regulators. Overall, available data indicate that omental adipocytes exhibit lower basal lipolytic capacity. The higher expression of the constituitively active endothelial nitric oxide synthetase (eNOS) in omental fat has been implicated in its lower basal lipolysis (78).

B Sensitivity and Responsiveness to Lipolytic Agonists Are Greater in Visceral Fat

Maximally beta-adrenergic-stimulated rates of lipolysis by a nonspecific agonist are similar in omental and subcutaneous adipose tissues (72,73). Because of the lower basal, the increment (delta) over basal is higher in omental than in subcutaneous. Mesenteric fat cells appear to also exhibit increased responsiveness to isoproterenol, particularly in men (73). Omental fat cells exhibit about twofold higher responses to physiologic catecholamines that activate both beta (stimulatory) and alpha$_2$- (inhibitory) adrenergic receptors (66). Only minor but statistically higher responses to beta$_1$-adrenergic receptors occur in omental than in subcutaneous fat cells of lean men (66). However, there are impressive differences in the sensitivity of omental fat cells to adrenergic receptor subtypes. Omental fat cells of obese men exhibit markedly increased sensitivity (ED_{50}) as well as increased responsiveness to beta-adrenergic agonists, particularly to the beta$_3$ agonist CGP 12177 and decreased responsiveness to the antilipolytic effects of alpha$_2$-adrenergic receptors (66,72,79,80). Omental fat cells of men as compared to women are markedly more sensitive to the lipolytic effects of beta-adrenergic agonist, particularly the beta$_3$ component (79).

The differences in beta-adrenergic responsiveness between omental and subcutaneous fat cells appear to derive from alterations in receptor expression rather than postreceptor events (74). No differences in Gi or Gs subtypes (76) are reported. Levels of HSL expression (protein and mRNA) are reported to be lower in omental than in subcutaneous (SC), predicting the lower maximal rates of lipolysis in omental that were in fact observed is some studies (64).

C Antilipolytic Effect of Insulin Is Lower in Omental Than in Subcutaneous Adipocytes

Studies are consistent in reporting a decreased sensitivity and responsiveness to the antilipolytic effect of insulin in omental compared to fat cells. The ED50 for insulin antilipolysis is higher in omental (71,81). Zierath et al. reported that insulin was two- to fourfold less potent in stimulating insulin receptor autophosphorylation and IRS-1 phosphorylation times in omental than in subcutaneous adipocytes. IRS1 protein expression was only half that in omental than SC. In parallel with these alterations in insulin signaling, insulin was less effective in suppressing lipolysis and increasing FA reesterification in omental adipocytes (81). These in vitro results are consistent with the reports that splanchnic lipolysis is less suppressible by insulin in vivo (82).

D Is Lipolysis in Visceral Fat Increased In Vivo?

The rate of lipolysis in vivo depends on the balance of lipolytic and antilipolytic regulators. For example, the rise in catecholamines with fasting is coupled with a lowering of circulating insulin levels. Because catecholamines sensitivity is markedly greater and insulin sensitivity is lower in omental than in subcutaneous fat, the in vitro studies would predict higher rates of lipolysis. In the fed state (high insulin, low catecholamines), determinants of "basal" lipolysis as well as insulin sensitivity likely factor into the rate of lipolysis, and it is therefore difficult to predict. In vivo studies reveal that under hyperinsulinemic conditions, the contribution of visceral (splanchnic) lipolysis to total systemic lipolysis increased from ~10% to 40%, suggesting the physiologic importance of the lower insulin sensitivity of omental adipocytes (82). Nevertheless, in vivo studies appear to indicate that non-splanchnic, upper body subcutaneous fat depots make a larger contribution to hepatic FFA delivery than visceral fat (83). Surprisingly, in subjects with NIDDM in whom visceral fat depots were enlarged, the relative contribution of visceral depots to hepatic FFA delivery is not disproportionately increased (83). In vivo studies also show an increased lipolytic responsiveness to isoproterenol and mixed adrenergic agonist (epinephrine), but this does not appear to be due to the enhanced lipolysis in visceral fat depots (84). Thus, the pathophysiologic importance of the alterations in the cellular regulation of lipolysis in visceral fat depots are debatable (16,17).

E Triacylglycerol Synthesis in Visceral Fat

1 Capacity for Glucose Uptake and Conversion to Triglyceride

If lipolysis is higher in visceral adipocytes, maintenance of the size of this depot implies that triglyceride synthesis must be increased in parallel. In vivo studies (85) demonstrated that the uptake of orally administered labelled triolein was greater in omental than in subcutaneous adipose tissues of lean to moderately obese men. Consistent with the idea that triglyceride turnover is increased in omental fat cells, glucose transport and glut4 mRNA and protein expression tended to be higher in omental than in subcutaneous (71), though one study found the opposite result with respect to glut4 mRNA (86). In vitro studies of glucose metabolism in omental and subcutaneous adipose tissue are few. One study found that in the presence of glucose and fatty acids, omental exhibited lower rates of glucose conversion to total lipids, with lower relative rates of conversion of triacylglycerol, but higher conversion of diacylglycerol (77). The physiological meaning of the apparently lower acylglyerol synthesis in omental adipose tissue is unclear. The fact that glucose transport capacity is at least as high in omental fat cells indicates that under in vivo conditions where fatty acid delivery is high, rates of triacylglycerol synthesis in vivo must be at high enough to balance the greater rate of lipolysis. In vivo factors such as regional differences in blood flow or innervation may also influence rates of triglyceride deposition and lipolysis in omental versus subcutaneous adipose tissues.

2 Acylation-Stimulating Protein

Acylation-stimulating protein (ASP), or C3a desarg, is a circulating protein that is synthesized in adipose tissue among other tissues (87,88). Serum ASP concentration, as well as adipose production, rises after a meal and stimulates triacylglycerol synthesis in an additive fashion with insulin. The binding capacity and affinity of subcutaneous fat cells exceed those of omental in both lean and obese subjects, and in both males and females (88). ASP is thought to act by stimulating diacylglyceroacyltransferase. It seems reasonable to hypothesize that its lower activity in omental may explain the relatively higher accumulation of newly synthesized diacylglycerol in this depot (77). No previous studies have examined regional differences in ASP production, although one small study showed no higher production of adipsin, the precursor of ASP, in omental adipose tissue (89). Although adipose tissue is not the sole site of ASP production in vivo, further studies of regional differences in its production appear warranted. It seems possible that local production of ASP is higher in omental, leading to a downregulation of its receptor affinity or number; thus, the net effect of ASP in omental and subcutaneous adipocytes may depend on the balance of its concentration and activity. The finding that subcutaneous adipocytes of obese women show the highest affinity for ASP suggests that this protein may promote subcutaneous fat deposition.

3 Lipoprotein Lipase

The activity of lipoprotein lipase (LPL) is responsible for local hydrolysis of circulating triacylglycerol that provide fatty acids for storage or utilization within peripheral tissues. LPL activity in omental vs subcutaneous adipose tissue is reportedly similar (in men) or slightly lower (women) (69,90). A number of studies did not find differences in LPL activity or its mRNA expression in omental versus subcutaneous adipose tissue, probably because of the small number of subjects and studies and the pooling of men and women, or expression of data on a per-gram rather than a per–fat cell basis (65,67,75,91). In vivo analysis shows that LPL provides an excess of triglyceride fatty acids to the adipocytes to be esterified in subcutaneous adipose tissue (92). Thus, it seems likely that there is sufficient LPL activity to provide ample substrate (FA) for high rates of triacylglycerol synthesis in both depots in vivo. However, there are no data comparing regional differences in omental versus subcutaneous LPL activity in the fed state (because of problems sampling the omental depot).

Differences in the activities of enzymes and proteins involved in regulating adipocyte triacylglyceride metabolism as a function of changes in nutritional status may derive from altered responsiveness to chronic effects of hormones on their expression. For example, omental adipose tissue is more responsive to glucocorticoid and less responsive to insulin. Whereas culture with dexamethasone increases LPL expression in omental adipose tissue, no effect is observed in subcutaneous adipose tissue. Conversely, culture with insulin leads to increased LPL activity in subcutaneous but not omental adipose tissue (68).

Depot differences in the expression or activity of key transcription factors such as sterol regulatory element binding protein-1c/ADD1 and peroxisome proliferator receptor-γ may be of importance determinants of depot differences in the expression of lipogenic genes, including LPL (93,94).

F Fatty Acid Transport and Metabolism

Omental adipocytes appear to have an increased intrinsic capacity to take up fatty acids. Kirkland's laboratory demonstrated that fatty acid transport was higher in newly differentiated preadipocytes derived from human omental than in subcutaneous adipose tissue (95). Depot differences in rates of fatty acid uptake and the activities of acyl CoA synthetases, and in expression of fatty acids binding proteins (adipocyte and keratinocyte are both increased), were also documented. The expression of the adipocyte fatty acid–binding protein and the ratio of the adipocyte to the keratinocyte fatty acid–binding protein were higher in omental than in Sc(96). The biochemical or physiological consequences of alterations in the expression of fatty acid–binding proteins are uncertain, as there are discrepant results in the literature on the phenotype of the adipocyte fatty acid binding protein knockout mouse (97–99).

The fatty acid composition of omental fat does not differ markedly from that of subcutaneous, suggesting no major depot differences in fatty acid metabolism, including desaturase reactions (100).

G Other Metabolic Differences

Some research attention has addressed a number of other metabolic features of omental adipose tissue. For example, this depot also expresses higher levels of uncoupling protein 2 mRNA, with no gender or obesity effect (101). Only subcutaneous, not omental, fat responded with an increase in UCP2 expression in response to a PPARγ agonist (101). The implications for adipocyte metabolism are not clear at this time.

VI PHYSIOLOGICAL DETERMINANTS OF VISCERAL ADIPOSE TISSUE FUNCTION

The major metabolic differences between omental and subcutaneous adipose tissues are summarized in Table 2. It is tempting to speculate that adipocytes of the visceral versus subcutaneous depots represent different "types" of fat, with intrinsic, genetically programmed differences in functional capacities. Such "intrinsic" differences could explain the differential growth of these two fat compartments as a function of developmental stage, age, endocrine status, genetics, and disease (1). The concomitant growth of visceral fat while subcutaneous fat depots become depleted in patients with acquired immunodeficiency syndrome provides yet another indication that these depots are functionally distinct "types" of fat. However, it is equally plausible that the local environment within these fat depots, i.e., blood flow, innervation, and paracrine influences, leads secondarily to the variations in metabolism.

Table 2 Summary of Differences Between Omental (Om) and Abdominal Subcutaneous (SC) Adipose Tissues

A. Metabolism
  1. Lipolysis
    a. Basal (Om < SC)
    b. Response to stimulatory agonist
      1. Beta-adrenergic (Om > SC)
    c. Response to inhibitory hormones
      1. alpha2-adrenergic (Om < SC)
      2. insulin (omental < SC)
      3. adenosine (omental < SC)
  2. Triglyceride deposition
    a. lipoprotein lipase activity (Om < SC in females)
    b. glucose transport (basal and insulin-stimulated, Om < SC)
    c. glucose conversion to triacylglycerol (Om < SC)
    d. glucose conversion to diacylglycerol (Om > SC)
    e. acylation stimulating protein (Om < SC)
B. Endocrine
  1. leptin (Om < SC)
  2. interleukin-6 (Om < SC)
  3. cortisone → cortisol conversion (Om > SC, stromal culture)
  4. ACRP30 (Om < SC)
C. Coagulation
  1. PAI1 (inconsistent reports)
D. Expression of transcription factors
  1. SREBP1c (SC > Om)
  2. PPARγ (SC = Om)

A Blood Flow

Blood flow to the rat mesenteric fat pad is about fivefold higher than other intra-abdominal depots (102,103). Other than casual observations that visceral adipose tissues are highly enriched in endothelial cells, suggesting high vascularization, no published information is available comparing the rate of blood flow or its regulation in these depots in humans.

B Innervation

We could find no data comparing the sympathetic innervation of human visceral versus subcutaneous adipose tissues. In the rat, mesenteric adipose may receive a richer sympathetic input than subcutaneous or other intra-abdominal depots (104,105).

C Hormonal Determinants

1 Sex Steroids

Studies in transsexuals given hormone replacement indicate that estrogen produces proportionately greater increases in subcutaneous than in visceral fat (106). Testosterone administration to female-to-male transsexuals decreased subcutaneous fat but increased visceral fat (106,107). In contrast, Marin et al. (85) found that testosterone decreased the deposition of radiolabeled triglyceride into omental and retroperitoneal fat. This result is consistent with the finding that serum testosterone is negatively correlated with visceral fat area in men (108,109). It appears that the effects of sex steroids on visceral fat deposition vary in men and women, perhaps owing to the effects of progestins (106).

The biochemical or molecular basis for the regional differences in sex steroid effects on adipose metabolism are not well elucidated. However, estrogen appears to produce a greater stimulation of preadipocyte proliferation in subcutaneous than in omental fat (110,111). Also, estrogen and testosterone influence the expression of adrenergic receptors through direct effects on the adipocyte (112–116).

2 Growth Hormone

Administration of growth hormone tends to selectively deplete visceral fat mass as analyzed by CT (117–121). Chronic growth hormone decreases lipoprotein lipase activity and increases basal lipolysis (122) in vitro. To our knowledge, there are no in vitro studies comparing the sensitivity or responsiveness to the effects of growth hormone on adipocyte metabolism in visceral versus subcutaneous adipose tissue of humans.

3 Cortisol

Cortisol excess (Cushing's syndrome) is associated with a truncal and visceral accumulation of fat, often with wasting of peripheral fat that is reversible with therapy (123). The metabolic basis of this is altered fat distribution thought to be the increased number of glucocorticoid receptors on omental versus subcutaneous fat cells (1,31,124–127). Additionally, greater responsiveness, but not sensitivity, to glucocorticoid effects has been demonstrated in omental versus abdominal subcutaneous adipose tissues of obese humans (68,128).

Cortisol can be synthesized locally within adipose tissue. HSD1 activity is higher in stromal cultures derived from omental as compared to subcutaneous fat (129,130). It has been suggested that higher local production of cortisol in omental may produce visceral obesity by promoting local hypertrophy of adipocytes, essentially "Cushing's" of the omentum (129). Further studies of regional HSD1 activity in subjects of varying degrees of visceral adiposity are needed to test this attractive hypothesis. No information is available on variations in visceral and subcutaneous HSD1 activity as a function of gender, age, fat distribution, or metabolic status.

Proof of principle that local cortisol production within adipose tissue can lead to visceral obesity was recently reported. Transgenic mice in which the aP2 promoter was used to drive expression of the gene for HSD1 in adipose tissue exhibited the preferential growth of mesenteric fat, as well as a generalized increase in fatness (20), particularly when placed on a high-fat diet. It seems likely that the increased growth of the mesenteric fat depot was due to increased glucocorticoid receptor expression (127), as supported by the observation that the expression of lipoprotein lipase was markedly increased in this depot. This new mouse model strongly supports that hypothesis that local production of cortisol within adipose tissue can drive fat deposition and that depot variations in the local production of cortisol (or responsiveness to its action) are important determinants of regional adiposity.

D Genetic Determinants of Visceral Adiposity

It appears that genes factor in the control of the size of visceral fat stores, independent of total fat mass in humans (23,131) and in a mouse model (41). A number of candidate genes and loci that modulate visceral fat deposition were identified, including several that are involved in steroid metabolism and food intake regulation (23,132). One interesting possibility is that polymorphisms in the glucocorticoid receptor gene may also exert an effect on regional fat distribution (133,134). Heterozygosity for a missense mutation in the melanocortin-4 receptor gene was associated with higher visceral adiposity and morning cortisol levels (132).

E Effect of Thiazolidinedione (TDZ) Drugs on Fat Distribution

The antidiabetic TDZs are ligands of peroxisome proliferating–activating receptor-γ (PPARγ) and thus increase adipogenesis as well as improving insulin sensitivity. TDZs appear to be less potent in stimulating preadipocyte differentiation in cultures derived from human omental versus subcutaneous fat depots despite similar levels of PPARγ. Clinical studies show that treatment of type 2 diabetics with troglitazone leads to a selective decrease in visceral adiposity and may also increase the mass of subcutaneous fat stores (135,136). This TDZ is no longer in clinical use, and there are as yet no reports of other TZD effects on human fat distribution. In rats, pioglitazone has more potent adipogenic effects on intraabdominal depots (ovarian and retroperitoneal vs. subcutaneous fat, the mesenteric was not examined) (137).

VII ENDOCRINE AND SECRETORY FUNCTIONS OF VISCERAL ADIPOCYTES AND ADIPOSE TISSUE

A Endocrine Function of Visceral Adipose Tissue

Adipose tissue is now recognized as an important endocrine organ that produces protein hormones including leptin, interleukin-6 (IL-6), adiponectin (also known as ACRP30 or adipoQ), angiotensinogen (and all components of the renin angiotensin system), and resistin (21,138). Considerable depot differences in leptin production add to the concept of the visceral adipocytes as a functionally distinct subtype of adipocytes. The lower leptin production by omental may not be an intrinsic property, however, because long-term culture with insulin plus dexamethasone abolished this depot difference (128). Thus, in vivo factors such as increased responsiveness of omental adipocytes to β-adrenergic agonists may contribute to the lower leptin expression (139). Depot differences in IL-6 production, however, persist after long-term culture (62). The majority of the tissue IL-6 derives from nonadipose (stromal) cells within adipose tissue. Differences in the cellular composition of visceral versus subcutaneous adipose tissues may therefore have pathophysiological implications, and deserve further study. The fact that the size of different fat depots is regulated by different genes in mice strongly supports the concept of different "types" of fat, although secondary effects cannot be ruled out (41).

1 Leptin Expression Is Lower in Visceral Adipose Tissue

The adipocyte hormone leptin has been studied extensively with regard to depot differences. Omental adipose tissue expressed lower levels of leptin mRNA, and produces less leptin (per cell or per gram) independent of fat cell size in lean and obese men and women (63,89,128,140,141). Thus, omental adipose tissue production of leptin is a minor determinant of systemic levels, but may be of importance via its impact on hepatic metabolism via the portal circulation.

B IL-6 Production Is Higher in Omental Than in Subcutaneous Fat

IL-6 is considered an adipose hormone because arteriovenous studies show a net release of IL-6 across the abdominal subcutaneous fat in vivo (16,142,143). Of note, in vivo and in vitro production of IL-6 in subcutaneous fat and serum IL-6 levels are increased in proportion to BMI (144,145). One study indicates that omental produces more IL-6 in severely obese subjects (men and women) (62). Further studies of omental IL-6 production in lean and moderately obese subjects are needed, because it could be playing an important paracrine as well as endocrine role. It has been suggest that IL-6 overproduction by visceral fat delivered directly to the liver via the portal vein may contribute to the development of the metabolic syndrome (62). Animal studies show that IL-6 increases VLDL production and increasing the synthesis of acute phase proteins, both features of visceral obesity. Most of the IL-6 produced derives from stromal elements, but adipocytes also appear to produce it (62). More needs to be known about cell-specific and depot-specific regulation of IL-6 synthesis and secretion. Interestingly, isoproternol administration in vivo appears to increase serum and adipose tissue IL-6 (145–147). As the omental depot is more responsive to β-adrenergic effects, this may be one factor in the increased omental production of this cytokine.

High levels of omental IL-6 and perhaps other cytokines (if they are secreted from the omentum) may also greatly impact hepatic metabolism. Both these hormones may contribute to hepatic insulin resistance, and IL-6 is a potent stimulator of hepatic VLDL production and the acute phase protein synthesis that appears to be a feature of visceral obesity (148–150).

1 Expression of Other Cytokines in Visceral Fat

Adipose tissue also synthesizes a number of cytokines (TNFα, IL-1β, IL-8, IL-10) and chemokines (146,151–156) that appear to act mainly on the paracrine level. Depot differences in cytokine production have not been extensively studied. Tumor necrosis factor-α does not appear to be released from adipose tissue (at least from the subcutaneous depot), and may therefore serve an exclusively paracrine role. Several studies have not found a depot difference in TNF expression (22,89). Other cytokines have not been examined for possible depot differences.

The expression of the cellular inhibitor of apoptosis protein 2 is higher in omental and subcutaneous preadipocytes (89,157). However, this depot difference does not persist after culture of preadipocytes derived from each depot (157), suggesting an altered pro-apoptotic environment in vivo, in omental fat.

2 Adiponectin

The adipocyte hormone adiponectin is implicated in the pathogenesis of insulin resistance (158–160). The extent of the reduction of adiponectin expression in subcutaneous fat in type 2 diabetes appears be less than in omental fat (161), but depot differences in its expression are not yet well characterized.

3 Sex Steroid Metabolism

Estrogen is produced via P450 aromatase that is expressed in the stromal compartment of adipose tissue, particularly in postmenopausal women (162). Adipose tissue also possesses enzymes involved in androgen metabolism (109). Possible depot differences in sex steroid metabolism have not yet been extensively studied. However, there appears to be evidence to depot-specific estrogen action. The estrogen receptor-α limits fat deposition (163,164). The expression of the estrogen receptor-α is poorly feedback-regulated in human omental as compared to subcutaneous fat, suggesting a mechanism for depot-specific effects of estrogen on fat distribution (165). Additionally, estrogen receptor-β is expressed in lower relative abundance in omental than subcutaneous adipose tissue of women and men (116), but the physiological implications of this observation are unclear.

4 Cortisone-Cortisol Interconversion in Visceral Versus Subcutaneous Fat: Endocrine Aspects

As discussed in Section IV.C.3, adipose tissue is also a site of conversion of cortisone (inactive) to cortisol (active). 11-Beta-hydroxysteroid dehydrogenase 1(HSD1) is expressed in both stromal and fat cells where it may serve an endocrine as well as a paracrine role (166–169). In vivo, arteriovenous difference studies show that here is a net production of cortisol across the abdominal subcutaneous fat depot (170), indicating that adipose tissue may participate in the increased cortisol turnover observed in the obese (170). Although HSD1 activity was found to be lower in cultures of stromal cells from subcutaneous vs omental fat (129), homogenates of subcutaneous adipose tissue were able to convert cortisone to cortisol, and the activity was increased in obese men (171). Because of the greater volume of subcutaneous adipose tissue, this depot may be a more important contributor to circulating cortisol levels than visceral depots.

5 Renin-Angiotensin System

All components of the renin-angiotensin system are expressed in adipose tissue, and expression is increased in obesity and response to nutritional alterations. Omental adipose tissue appears to express higher levels of angiotensinogen, particularly in the obese (22,172,173).

C Adipocyte Secretory Products Involved in Systemic Metabolism: Contribution from Visceral Versus Subcutaneous Fat

Adipose tissue also secretes proteins involved in lipid and lipoprotein metabolism [cholesterol ester transfer protein (CETP), phosholipid transfer protein (PLTP), ASP, apolipoprotein E], as discussed previously (174). CETP expression is higher in subcutaneous than omental fat, but PLTP does not differ (172); apoE expression has not yet been studied. ASP expression in omental versus subcutaneous fat was discussed in Section V.B.4.

D Omental Adiposity and Fibrinolysis

Proteins involved in fibrinolysis, including plasminogen activators and plasminogen inhibitor 1 (PAI1), are expressed in adipose tissue (175). Many authors have found that PAI1 expression is higher in omental than in subcutaneous fat (22,176–178), but others find an elevation with obesity but no regional difference (179,180). The source of the PAI1 production in samples of human adiose tissue is unclear (54), and human preadipocytes in culture derived from omental and subcutaneous fat release similar amounts of PAI1 (181). In addition, whether subcutaneous fat actually releases PAI1 to the systemic circulation has been questioned (182). The degree to which the depot-specific production of PAI1 accounts for the association of hypercoaguability with the metabolic syndrome require further in vivo and in vitro studies, but local actions within each adipose depot are also likely. For example, PAI1 may promote preadipocyte migration and cluster formation during adipogenesis (183). Furthermore, obese (obob) mice null for PAI1 showed lower TNFα expression in fat and improved insulin sensitivity, providing a potential mechanism linking adipose PAI1 expression to metabolic complications of obesity (184).

E Lipodystrophies

Depletion of subcutaneous fat stores occurs in cases of genetic and acquired lipodystrophies (185). The fat maldistribution associated with the acquired immunodeficiency syndrome (186) provides a dramatic example of differences between visceral and subcutaneous fat depots. The central adiposity in this syndrome may be exacerbated by protease inhibitors, but were reported before the use of these drugs (186). Whether the adipose tissue depots have a special role in responding to the immune challenge remains to be determined (187,188). Depot differences in responsiveness or altered sensitivity to catabolic or apoptotic effects of systemic or local cytokines may contribute to depot differences in responses to altered metabolic states.

VIII THERAPEUTIC STRATEGIES FOR REDUCTION OF VISCERAL ADIPOSITY

A Methodological Considerations

As reported above, the correlation coefficients between VAT and metabolic risk factors appears to be relatively constant independent of the level of the abdomen at which VAT is measured. Preliminary evidence also suggests that the mobilization of VAT (cm^2) in response to weight loss at different levels of the abdomen are comparable (35,189,190); that is, the relative reduction observed at the level of L4-L5 is not different from that observed at the L2-L3 level. The relatively uniform reduction in VAT remains true independent of the method of inducing weight loss (e.g., diet- or exercise-induced weight loss) (189). Although this observation is based in large measure on data from Caucasian men and women, Conway et al. (49) report that in obese African-American women the reductions in VAT at the L2-L3 level are not different from those observed at the L4-L5 level.

Illustrated in Figure 5 is the influence of weight loss on both VAT and abdominal subcutaneous adipose tissue in a large cohort of overweight and obese men and women. Inspection of Figure 5 reveals that the relative (%) reduction in VAT area (cm^2) for four MRI images obtained in the abdomen is uniform and similar to the relative reduction in VAT mass derived using the four abdominal images. These data suggest that the influence of weight loss on VAT determined using a single CT or MR image obtained in a region bordered by S1-L5 and about L2-L3 will provide similar results. In other words, the distribution of VAT does not appear to be influenced by weight loss in the order of 10% (35,189).

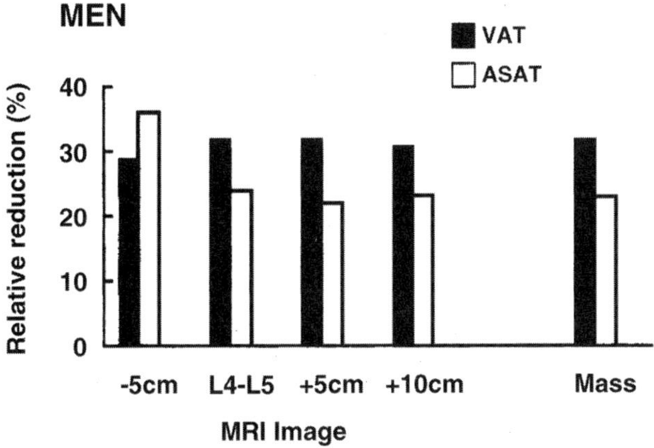

Figure 5 Relative reduction in visceral and abdominal subcutaneous adipose tissue at the L4-L5 level, 5 cm below, 5 cm above, and 10 cm above L4-L5, as well as visceral and abdominal subcutaneous adipose tissue mass derived using five abdominal images. The reductions in visceral and abdominal subcutaneous fat were observed in response to a 10% weight loss in 61 men (left) and 56 women (right). VAT, visceral adipose tissue; ASAT, abdominal subcutaneous adipose tissue.

B Lifestyle-Based Strategies

1 Exercise

The effects of exercise on abdominal adipose tissue distribution have recently been considered and the reader is referred to these citations for detailed reviews (191–193). For simplicity, we review here those studies that consider the effects of exercise with or without weight loss separately on abdominal adiposity, in particular, VAT.

2 Exercise Without Weight Loss

Ross et al. (194) observed a 16% reduction in VAT independent of any change in abdominal subcutaneous or total adipose tissue in obese men who performed daily, aerobic exercise (brisk walking, ~60 min) for 3 months. This finding confirms an earlier report wherein Mourier et al. (195) observed large reductions in both VAT (~48%) and abdominal subcutaneous adipose tissue (~18%) in response to moderate exercise performed three times per week for 8 weeks in men and women with type II diabetes. Thomas et al. (196) also examined the effects of exercise training without weight loss in 17 nonobese, healthy women. In that study, the women performed aerobic-type exercise under supervision 3 days per week for 6 months. Despite no change in total and subcutaneous adipose tissue, a 25% reduction in VAT was observed. Together these results suggest that regularly performed aerobic exercise without weight loss results in marked reductions in VAT, which are in general greater than the change in total or abdominal subcutaneous adipose tissue.

In contrast to these observations, Poehlman et al. (197) report that 6 months of either endurance or resistance exercise training did not reduce VAT or abdominal subcutaneous adipose tissue in young, premenopausal women, a finding consistent with that of DiPietro et al. (198), who report that in older men and women, 4 months of supervised aerobic exercise had no effect on abdominal subcutaneous or visceral adipose tissue. A rationale to explain the equivocal findings is unknown. However, it is noted that in the Poehlman et al. (197) study, the average VAT values pretreatment for the exercise groups approximated 40 cm^2, a value substantially below the values thought to be associated with metabolic risk (199,200). Taken together, available evidence does not permit firm conclusions regarding the effects of exercise training in the absence of weight loss on VAT distribution.

3 Exercise-Induced Weight Loss

Inspection of Table 3 reveals that few studies have examined the effects of exercise-induced weight loss on VAT distribution. Schwartz et al. (1991) report marked reduction in both abdominal subcutaneous (~20%) and visceral (~25%) adipose tissue in response to aerobic-type exercise in older men despite very modest weight loss (2.5 kg) (201). Consistent with the findings of this study, Wilmore et al. (202) report that 5 months of cycling exercise performed three times per week by 557 men and women varying widely in age, race, and adiposity resulted in significant but relatively small reductions in visceral adipose tissue (~6%) in association with a minor change in body weight and total fat (<1 kg). Bouchard et al. (203) studied seven twin pairs who exercised on a stationary bicycle 6 days a week for 3 months such that 1000 kcal was expended each day. In that study, the authors prescribed an isocaloric diet to ensure that the negative energy balance was induced by exercise alone. The exercise program resulted in a 5-kg reduction in body weight that was associated with a 35% and 27% reduction in visceral and abdominal subcutaneous adipose tissue, respectively. Unfortunately, very little is known regarding whether exercise-induced weight loss influences the visceral to abdominal subcutaneous adipose tissue ratio. In other words, whether exercise alters adipose tissue

Table 3 Influence of Exercise Training on Visceral and Abdominal Subcutaneous Adipose Tissue

Reference	Subjects	BMI (kg/m^2)	Treatment	Study duration (months)	Reduction in weight (kg)	Reduction in body fat (kg)	Reduction in VAT (cm^2) [%]	Reduction in ASAT (cm^2) [%]
Randomized, controlled trials								
Ross et al., 2000 (194)	Men	31	Control group	3	0.8	0.6	0 [0]	[3]
		33	Exercise (WL)		7.6[a]	6.1[a]	52 [28][a]	[18][a]
		32	Exercise (WWL)		0.5	0.8	32 [16][a]	[6]
Poehlman et al., 2000 (197)	Young women	22	Control group	6	+1.0	0.0	+4 [11]	NR
		22	Aerobic exercise		+2.0	+1.0	0 [0]	0
		22	Resistance exercise		0.0	−1.0	+1 [2]	1
DiPietro et al., 1998 (198)	Older men and women	27	Control group	4	0.0	NR	18 [13]	+20 [8]
		27	Aerobic exercise		1.0		10 [9]	+11 [6]
Mourier et al., 1997 (195)	Diabetic men and women	30	Control group	2	0.2	0.8	5 [3]	9 [3]
		30	Aerobic exercise		1.5	0.8	76 [48][a]	41 [18][a]
Nonrandomized trials								
Thomas et al., 2000 (196)	Young women	25	Aerobic exercise	6	0.6	1.9 L	0.4 L [25]	NR
Wilmore et al., 1999 (202)	Men	26	Aerobic exercise	5	0.4[b]	0.9[b]	6 [7][b]	10 [5][b]
	Women	25	Aerobic exercise		0.1	0.5[b]	3 [5][b]	8 [3][b]
Treuth et al., 1995 (217)	Older women	25	Resistance exercise	4	0.1	0.4	14 [10][b]	17 [6]
Bouchard et al., 1994 (203)	Young men	[82]	Aerobic exercise	3	5.0[b]	5.0[b]	29 [36][b]	67 [27][b]
Schwartz et al., 1991 (201)	Young men	26	Aerobic exercise	7	0.5	1.6	11 [17][b]	21 [10][b]
	Old men	26	Aerobic exercise		2.5[b]	2.4[b]	35 [25][b]	35 [20][b]
Després et al., 1991 (218)	Young women	34	Aerobic exercise	14	3.7[b]	4.6[b]	3 [3]	60 [11][b]

WL, weight loss; WWL, without weight loss; BMI, body mass index: VAT, visceral adipose tissue; ASAT, abdominal subcutaneous adipose tissue; NR, not reported; L, liters.

[a] Significantly different from change in control group ($P < .05$).

[b] Significant within group change ($P < .05$).

distribution by inducing a greater reduction in visceral versus subcutaneous fat is unclear (191).

4 Diet (Caloric Restriction)

Caloric restriction has been the principal means of assessing the influence of weight loss on VAT (Table 4). From the studies reviewed it is noted that the magnitude of the diet-induced weight loss ranges from 4.4 to 18.8 kg (Table 4). The corresponding reductions in VAT vary according to the weight loss; the greater the weight loss, the greater the reduction in VAT. When expressed per kilogram of body weight lost [mean absolute VAT loss (cm^2) ÷ mean weight loss (kg)], the corresponding reduction in VAT varied from 2.5 to 13.8 cm^2/kg. In relative terms (i.e., controlling for initial differences in VAT accumulation), the relative loss per kg is ~3% (4). Thus, for a 10-kg weight loss, the relative reduction in VAT is ~30%. It is important to note the large interindividual variations observed in VAT reduction (Table 4) and that the observation is generally restricted to obese Caucasian adults.

The data in Table 4 also suggest that in response to diet-induced weight loss, there is a preferential reduction in VAT. Whether the observation is based on data obtained from a single image or by comparing relative reductions in VAT and subcutaneous adipose tissue volume (liters) derived from multiple images, for a given weight loss, the relative reduction in VAT is greater than those observed for subcutaneous adipose tissue (Table 4).

5 Pharmacotherapy

The potential of pharmacotherapy for the treatment of obesity is promising. When used as an adjunct to the traditional approaches of diet- and/or exercise-induced weight loss it would appear that the addition of available pharmacological agents are useful in helping patients achieve and maintain weight loss (204). At

Table 4 Influence of Diet-Induced Weight Loss on Visceral and Abdominal Subcutaneous Adipose Tissue

Study	Subjects N	Subjects Sex	BMI (kg/m²)	Duration (weeks)	Weight loss Abs [kg] (%)	VAT loss[a] Abs [cm²] (%)	VAT loss/kg weight loss Abs [cm²] (%)	ASAT loss[a] Abs [cm²] (%)
Bosello et al., 1990 (219)	19	Young women	40	2–3	6.7 (6)	29.1 (20)	4.3 (3.0)	34.4 (6)
Fujioka et al., 1991 (220)	14	Young women	34	8–10	12.0 (14)	2.6 (38)[b]	(3.2)	3.1 (25)[b]
	26	VO SO	36		12.3 (14)	1.3 (33)[b]	(2.7)	4.0 (23)[b]
Gray et al., 1991 (221)	10	Young women	35	10	10.5 (12)	26 (27)	2.5 (2.6)	62 (13)
Stallone et al., 1991 (222)	11	Older women	37	26	18.8 (20)	52.9 (36)	2.8 (1.9)	152.8 (33)
Armellini et al., 1991 (223)	26	Women	39	2	6 (6)	24 (15)	4.0 (2.5)	6 (1)
Leenen et al., 1992 (224)	40 38	Young women, men	31 30	13	11.7 (14) 12.6 (13)	35 (30) 61 (39)	3.0 (2.6) 4.8 (3.1)	117 (30) 113 (36)
Chowdhury et al., 1993 (225)	9	Men	35	1	4.4 (4)	0.9 (10)[b]	−2.3	1.0 (6)[b]
Zamboni et al., 1993 (226)	16	Young women	38	16	16.2 (16)	73.7 (44)	4.5 (2.7)	145.3 (24)
Nicklas et al., 1997 (227)	9	Older women	74	26	9.8 (12)	26 (17)	2.7 (1.7)	65 (15)
Zamboni et al., 1997 (228)	34	Men and women	~36	2	7.0 (7)	27.3 (16)	3.9 (2.3)	35.9 (10)
Janand-Delenne et al., 1998 (229)	13	Young women	34	4	6.6 (7)	29 (22)	4.4 (3.3)	55 (15)
Goodpaster et al., 1999 (230)	17 15	Young women, men	34 34	16	12.2 (13) 17.6 (16)	44 (30) 78 (47)	3.6 (2.5) 4.4 (2.7)	118 (23) 159 (34)
Janssen and Ross, 1999 (231)	10 10	Young women, men	34 32	16	10.7 (11) 11.7 (12)	51 (37) 58 (30)	4.8 (3.5) 4.9 (2.6)	7 (18) 6 (23)
Kockx et al., 1999 (232)	25 25	Young women, men	31 30	13	11.4 (13) 12.1 (12)	32 (33) 61 (39)	2.8 (2.9) 5.0 (3.2)	122 (30) 109 (35)
Riches et al., 1999 (233)	12	Men	34	16	10.2 (9)	100 (31)[c]	9.8 (3.0)	NR
Ross et al., 1994 (38)	38	Young women	34	26	8.2 (9)	15 (19)	1.8 (2.3)	6 (21)
Doucet et al., 2000 (234)	45	Young women, men	93 103	2	7.9 (9) 10.7 (11)	27 (18) 79 (38)	3.4 (2.3) 7.4 (3.6)	56 (10) 84 (21)
Kamel et al., 2000 (235)	19 17	Young women, men	33 33	26	10.6 (12) 9.5 (9)	106 (44) 132 (37)	10.0 (4.2) 13.8 (3.9)	204 (21) 177 (24)
Ross et al., 2000 (194)	14	Men	31	12	7.4 (8)	44 (26)	5.9 (3.5)	NR

Abs = absolute reduction; % = percentage (relative) reduction; VAT = visceral adipose tissue; ASAT = abdominal subcutaneous adipose tissue; NR = not reported; VO = visceral obesity; SO = subcutaneous obesity.

[a] Image obtained at L4-L5 unless otherwise indicated.

[b] Volume (liters).

[c] L3 level.

present there is limited evidence regarding the independent influence of the two drugs currently approved for obesity treatment in North America. We are unaware of trials wherein the effects of orlistat, a pancreatic lipase inhibitor, on VAT are considered. Preliminary evidence suggests that the serotonin reuptake inhibitor sibutramine is associated with marked reduction of VAT (~22%) in response to a 6-month trial (205). However, in that trial the subjects received sibutramine in conjunction with a hypocaloric diet and were encouraged to exercise. Given the demonstrated importance of visceral obesity in the development of metabolic risk, further study to consider the independent effects of pharmacotherapy on VAT is warranted.

IX IS THE METABOLIC SYNDROME DUE TO TOO MUCH VISCERAL OR TOO LITTLE SUBCUTANEOUS FAT?

Although there is agreement in the literature that increased central obesity is associated with a metabolic syndrome that increase risk for development of type 2 diabetes and cardiovascular disease, there is considerable controversy about which fat compartment that is the main culprit. Numerous careful studies find that visceral fat volume is the strongest independent predictor of metabolic risk (insulin resistance, dyslipidemia) in men or women carefully matched for total body fat but differing in visceral fat mass (1,8,206,207). Nevertheless, not all studies assessed whether the associations were independent of total body fat (32,208).

It has been suggested that visceral adiposity was a marker of the metabolic syndrome (i.e., a secondary effect of an altered hormonal milieu that affects fat distribution *and* metabolism), rather than its primary cause (208). Indeed, Abate et al. (32) found that insulin sensitivity was best correlated with the mass of truncal subcutaneous (not visceral or retroperitoneal) fat in nondiabetic middle-aged men and in subjects with NIDDM. More recently, two groups have noted that the relative amount of deep subcutaneous adipose tissue also predicts metabolic risks associated with obesity (36,209). Addition of visceral adipose tissue volume to the equation only slightly increased the regression coefficient. In another study, the size of posterior (vs. anterior) subcutaneous fat stores was best correlated with intra-abdominal (visceral) fat, and was a better predictor of insulin resistance in nondiabetic men (210).

Very little is known about the metabolic features of the deep versus the superficial subcutaneous fat layers, or posterior versus anterior subcutaneous fat. However, a recent microdialysis study indicates that the superficial subcutaneous fat layer that is usually sampled in adipocyte metabolic studies is more responsive to the lipolytic action of epinephrine compared to deep subcutaneous or preperitoneal depots (211). Thus, deep subcutaneous may be less active than visceral adipose tissue; why its mass correlates with metabolic risk remains obscure. Nevertheless, future studies of the influence of visceral adiposity on systemic metabolic should consider potentially confounding effects of variation in deep subcutaneous fat mass.

It is also possible that the level of visceral adiposity influences the metabolic activity of subcutaneous fat cells, and that this in turn contributes to metabolic abnormalities including increased systemic fatty acid turnover. For instance, decreased sensitivity to the antilipolytic action of insulin was noted in abdominal subcutaneous adipose cells from viscerally obese women (212). In men, subcutaneous adipocytes from viscerally obese patients show higher maximal responses to alpha2-adrenergic receptor agonists, and this may be related to the greater hyperinsulinemia associated with visceral fatness (213). Thus, the influence of visceral fat stores on fatty acid metabolism is likely to be exerted through multiple mechanisms, and may extend beyond the lipolytic activity of the visceral fat cells per se.

Lipectomy of the two main intra-abdominal (but nonportal) adipose tissues of rats, the perirenal and epididymal, led to a marked improvement in hepatic insulin resistance (44). However, this experiment cannot distinguish an effect of a decrease in total body fat from a regionally specific effect. For instance, it is not known whether removal of subcutaneous fat that produced an equivalent decrease in total body fat would similarly lead to alterations in hepatic insulin action in the rat. Nevertheless, the results of this experiments indicates that nonportal abdominal adipose tissue can influence glucose-insulin homeostasis.

An alternate hypothesis to explain the association between visceral adiposity and metabolic risk is that the metabolic effects of obesity are related to "subcutaneous fat deficiency" (214,215). Indeed, subcutaneous fat lipectomy in hamsters also leads to a metabolic syndrome, despite no measurable increase in the size of the major intra-abdominal depots (214). Thus, subcutaneous fat may be a "safe" place to deposit excess triglyceride, while other tissues, e.g., liver and muscle, as well as visceral fat, may not be (214,216).

Resolution of the controversy on the importance of abdominal subcutaneous versus visceral fat will require studies in which the sizes of specific intra-abdominal and subcutaneous regions are quantified, e.g, by whole-body MRI or other methods.

X SUMMARY AND CONCLUSIONS

The relative importance of visceral and subcutaneous abdominal cells in the etiology of the metabolic syndrome is a matter of debate. Nevertheless, the biology of visceral fat remains of considerable interest, as these fat depots undoubtedly play an important, although probably not an exclusive, role in the metabolic derangements associated with abdominal obesity. Abundant evidence indicates that visceral adipose tissue, particularly the better-studied omental depot, has distinct metabolic properties from subcutaneous fat. Recent studies indicate that the influence of the visceral fat depots likely extends beyond glucose and fatty acid metabolism, and includes the regulation of blood pressure, coagulation, and perhaps immunity. Thus, further understanding of the nature of visceral fat depots has far-reaching implications.

It will be essential for our field to better define our use of the term visceral fat. From a clinical and practical perspective, the term indicates all intra-abdominal depots, but from a mechanistic perspective, it is important to distinguish those that are associated with digestive organs and drain portally (i.e., omental and mesenteric). It will also be important to discern whether the metabolic behavior of these "portal" depots is due to intrinsic (genetic) differences among truly different "types" of fat cells, or they are induced by variations in the local neural, endocrine, and paracrine environment within each fat depot.

ACKNOWLEDGMENTS

We thank Dr. John Kral for insightful discussions and his contributions to Table 1, and Dr. Colleen Russell for helpful comments on the manuscript.

REFERENCES

1. Bouchard C, Despres JP, Mauriege P. Genetic and nongenetic determinants of regional fat distribution. Endocr Rev 1993; 14(1):72–93.
2. Katzmarzyk PT, Malina RM, Perusse L, Rice T, Province MA, Rao DC, Bouchard C. Familial resemblance for physique: heritabilities for somatotype components. Ann Hum Biol 2000; 27(5):467–477.
3. Kissebah AH, Krakower GR. Regional adiposity and morbidity. Physiol Rev 1994; 74(4):761–811.
4. Vague J. The degree of masculine differentiation of obesities: a factor determining predisposition to diabetes, atherosclerosis, gout and uric calculous disease. Am J Clin Nutr 1956; 4:20–34.
5. Vague J. La différenciation sexuelle: factueur déterminant des formes del'obésité. Presse Med 1947; 55:339–340.
6. Krotkiewski M, Bjorntorp P, Sjostrom L, Smith U. Impact of obesity on metabolism in men and women. Importance of regional adipose tissue distribution. J Clin Invest 1983; 72(3):1150–1162.
7. Despres JP, Nadeau A, Tremblay A, Ferland M, Moorjani S, Lupien PJ, Theriault G, Pinault S, Bouchard C. Role of deep abdominal fat in the association between regional adipose tissue distribution and glucose tolerance in obese women. Diabetes 1989; 38(3): 304–309.
8. Despres JP, Moorjani S, Lupien PJ, Tremblay A, Nadeau A, Bouchard C. Regional distribution of body fat, plasma lipoproteins, and cardiovascular disease. Arteriosclerosis 1990; 10(4):497–511.
9. Seidell JC, Bouchard C. Abdominal adiposity and risk of heart disease. JAMA 1999; 281(24):2284–2285.
10. Björntorp P. Hazards in subgroups of human obesity. Eur J Clin Invest 1984; 14(4):239–241.
11. Krotkiewski M, Sjostrom L, Bjorntorp P, Smith U. Regional adipose tissue cellularity in relation to metabolism in young and middle-aged women. Metabolism 1975; 24(6):703–710.
12. Ostman J, Arner P, Engfeldt P, Kager L. Regional differences in the control of lipolysis in human adipose tissue. Metabolism 1979; 28(12):1198–1205.
13. Micheli H, Carlson LA, Hallberg D. Comparison of lipolysis in human subcutaneous and omental adipose tissue with regard to effects of noradrenaline, theophylline, prostaglandin E1 and age. Acta Chir Scand 1969; 135(8):663–670.
14. Carlson LA, Hallberg D, Micheli H. Quantitative studies on the lipolytic response of human subcutaneous and omental adipose tissue to noradrenaline and theophylline. Acta Med Scand 1969; 185(6):465–469.
15. Björntorp P. "Portal" adipose tissue as a generator of risk factors for cardiovascular disease and diabetes. Arteriosclerosis 1990; 10:493–496.
16. Frayn KN, Samra JS, Summers LK. Visceral fat in relation to health: is it a major culprit or simply an innocent bystander? Int J Obes Relat Metab Disord 1997; 21(12):1191–1192.
17. Jensen MD. Lipolysis: contribution from regional fat. Annu Rev Nutr 1997; 17:127–139.
18. Bergman RN, Van Citters GW, Mittelman SD, Dea MK, Hamilton-Wessler M, Kim SP, Ellmerer M. Central role of the adipocyte in the metabolic syndrome. J Inves Med 2001; 49(1):119–126.

19. Getty L, Panteleon AE, Mittelman SD, Dea MK, Bergman RN. Rapid oscillations in omental lipolysis are independent of changing insulin levels in vivo. J Clin Invest 2000; 106(3):421–430.
20. Masuzaki H, Paterson J, Shinyama H, Morton NM, Mullins JJ, Seckl JR, Flier JS. A transgenic model of viseral obesity and the metabolic syndrome. Science 2001; 294:2166–2170.
21. Montague CT, O'Rahilly S. The perils of portliness: causes and consequences of visceral adiposity. Diabetes 2000; 49(6):883–888.
22. Arner P. Regional differences in protein production by human adipose tissue. Biochem Soc Trans 2001; 29(Pt 2):72–75.
23. Perusse L, Rice T, Chagnon YC, Despres JP, Lemieux S, Roy S, Lacaille M, Ho- Kim MA, Chagnon M, Province MA, Rao DC, Bouchard C. A genome-wide scan for abdominal fat assessed by computed tomography in the Quebec Family Study. Diabetes 2001; 50(3):614–621.
24. Rossner S, Bo WJ, Hiltbrandt E, Hinson W, Karstaedt N, Santago P, Sobol WT, Crouse JR. Adipose tissue determinations in cadavers—a comparison between cross-sectional planimetry and computed tomography. Int J Obes 1990; 14(10):893–902.
25. Abate N, Burns D, Peshock RM, Garg A, Grundy SM. Estimation of adipose tissue mass by magnetic resonance imaging: validation against dissection in human cadavers. J Lipid Res 1994; 35(8):1490–1496.
26. Matsuzawa Y, Shimomura I, Nakamura T, Keno Y, Kotani K, Tokunaga K. Pathophysiology and pathogenesis of visceral fat obesity. Obes Res 1995; 3(suppl 2):187S–194S.
27. Baumgartner RN, Heymsfield SB, Roche AF, Bernardino M. Abdominal composition quantified by computed tomography. Am J Clin Nutr 1988; 48(4): 936–945.
28. Kvist H, Sjostrom L, Tylen U. Adipose tissue volume determinations in women by computed tomography: technical considerations. Int J Obes 1986; 10(1):53–67.
29. Rissanen J, Hudson R, Ross R. Visceral adiposity, androgens, and plasma lipids in obese men. Metabolism 1994; 43(10):1318–1323.
30. Ross R, Rissanen J, Pedwell H, Clifford J, Shragge P. Influence of diet and exercise on skeletal muscle and visceral adipose tissue in men. J Appl Physiol 1996; 81(6):2445–2455.
31. Ross R, Aru J, Freeman J, Hudson R, Janssen I. Abdominal adiposity and insulin resistance in obese men. Am J Physiol Endocrinol Metab 282:E657–663.
32. Abate N, Garg A, Peshock RM, Stray-Gundersen J, Grundy SM. Relationships of generalized and regional adiposity to insulin sensitivity in men. J Clin Invest 1995; 96(1):88–98.
33. Abate N, Garg A, Peshock RM, Stray-Gundersen J, Adams-Huet B, Grundy SM. Relationship of generalized and regional adiposity to insulin sensitivity in men with NIDDM. Diabetes 1996; 45(12):1684–1693.
34. Ross R, Leger L, Morris D, de Guise J, Guardo R. Quantification of adipose tissue by MRI: relationship with anthropometric variables. J Appl Physiol 1992; 72(2):787–795.
35. Ross R, Rissanen J. Mobilization of visceral and subcutaneous adipose tissue in response to energy restriction and exercise. Am J Clin Nutr 1994; 60(5): 695–703.
36. Smith SR, Lovejoy JC, Greenway F, Ryan D, deJonge L, De la Bretonne J, Volafova J, Bray GA. Contributions of total body fat, abdominal subcutaneous adipose tissue compartments, and visceral adipose tissue to the metabolic complications of obesity. Metabolism 2001; 50(4):425–435.
37. Han TS, Kelly IE, Walsh K, Greene RM, Lean ME. Relationship between volumes and areas from single transverse scans of intra-abdominal fat measured by magnetic resonance imaging. Int J Obes Relat Metab Disord 1997; 21(12):1161–1166.
38. Ross R, Shaw KD, Rissanen J, Martel Y, de Guise J, Avruch L. Sex differences in lean and adipose tissue distribution by magnetic resonance imaging: anthropometric relationships. Am J Clin Nutr 1994; 59(6): 1277–1285.
39. Kelley DE, Thaete FL, Troost F, Huwe T, Goodpaster BH. Subdivisions of subcutaneous abdominal adipose tissue and insulin resistance. Am J Physiol Endocrinol Metab 2000; 278(5):E941–E948.
40. Newby FD, Sykes MN, Digirolamo M. Regional differences in adipocyte lactate production from glucose. Am J Physiol 1988; 255(5 Pt 1):E716–E722.
41. Warden CH, Fisler JS, Shoemaker SM, Wen PZ, Svenson KL, Pace MJ, Lusis AJ. Identification of four chromosomal loci determining obesity in a multifactorial mouse model. J Clin Invest 1995; 95(4):1545–1552.
42. Digirolamo M, Fine JB, Tagra K, Rossmanith R. Qualitative regional differences in adipose tissue growth and cellularity in male Wistar rats fed ad libitum. Am J Physiol 1998; 274(5 Pt 2):R1460–R1467.
43. Fried SK, Lavau M, Pi-Sunyer FX. Variations of glucose metabolism by fat cells from three adipose depots of the rat. Metabolism 1982; 31(9):876–883.
44. Barzilai N, She L, Liu BQ, Vuguin P, Cohen P, Wang J, Rossetti L. Surgical removal of visceral fat reverses hepatic insulin resistance. Diabetes 1999; 48(1): 94–98.
45. Lemieux S, Prud'homme D, Bouchard C, Tremblay A, Despres JP. Sex differences in the relation of visceral adipose tissue accumulation to total body fatness. Am J Clin Nutr 1993; 58(4):463–467.
46. Couillard C, Bergeron N, Prud'homme D, Bergeron J, Tremblay A, Bouchard C, Mauriege P, Despres JP. Gender difference in postprandial lipemia: importance

of visceral adipose tissue accumulation. Arterioscler Thromb Vasc Biol 1999; 19(10):2448–2455.
47. Kelley DE, Williams KV, Price JC, McKolanis TM, Goodpaster BH, Thaete FL. Plasma Fatty acids, adiposity, and variance of skeletal muscle insulin resistance in type 2 diabetes mellitus. J Clin Endocrinol Metab 2001; 86(11):5412–5419.
48. Hill JO, Sidney S, Lewis CE, Tolan K, Scherzinger AL, Stamm ER. Racial differences in amounts of visceral adipose tissue in young adults: the CARDIA (Coronary Artery Risk Development in Young Adults) study. Am J Clin Nutr 1999; 69(3):381–387.
49. Conway JM, Yanovski SZ, Avila NA, Hubbard VS. Visceral adipose tissue differences in black and white women. Am J Clin Nutr 1995; 61(4):765–771.
50. Albu JB, Murphy L, Frager DH, Johnson JA, Pi-Sunyer FX. Visceral fat and race-dependent health risks in obese nondiabetic premenopausal women. Diabetes 1997; 46(3):456–462.
51. Goran MI, Bergman RN, Gower BA. Influence of total vs. visceral fat on insulin action and secretion in African American and white children. Obes Res 2001; 9(8):423–431.
52. Goran MI, Nagy TR, Treuth MS, Trowbridge C, Dezenberg C, McGloin A. Visceral fat in white and African American prepubertal children. Am J Clin Nutr 1997; 65(6):1703–1708.
53. Park YW, Allison DB, Heymsfield SB, Gallagher D. Larger amounts of visceral adipose tissue in Asian Americans. Obes Res 2001; 9(7):381–387.
54. Takahashi K, Hata J, Mukai K, Sawasaki Y. Close similarity between cultured human omental mesothelial cells and endothelial cells in cytochemical markers and plasminogen activator production. In Vitro Cell Dev Biol 1991; 27A(7):542–548.
55. Chung-Welch N, Patton WF, Shepro D, Cambria RP. Two-stage isolation procedure for obtaining homogenous populations of microvascular endothelial and mesothelial cells from human omentum. Microvasc Res 1997; 54(2):121–134.
56. Chung-Welch N, Patton WF, Shepro D, Cambria RP. Human omental microvascular endothelial and mesothelial cells: characterization of two distinct mesodermally derived epithelial cells. Microvasc Res 1997; 54(2):108–120.
57. Bornstein SR, Abu-Asab M, Glasow A, Path G, Hauner H, Tsokos M, Chrousos GP, Scherbaum WA. Immunohistochemical and ultrastructural localization of leptin and leptin receptor in human white adipose tissue and differentiating human adipose cells in primary culture. Diabetes 2000; 49(4):532–538.
58. Mattacks CA, Pond CM. Interactions of noradrenalin and tumour necrosis factor alpha, interleukin 4 and interleukin 6 in the control of lipolysis from adipocytes around lymph nodes. Cytokine 1999; 11(5): 334–346.
59. Adams M, Montague CT, Prins JB, Holder JC, Smith SA, Sanders L, Digby JE, Sewter CP, Lazar MA, Chatterjee VK, O'Rahilly S. Activators of peroxisome proliferator-activated receptor gamma have depot-specific effects on human preadipocyte differentiation. J Clin Invest 1997; 100(12):3149–3153.
60. Hube F, Lee YM, Rohrig K, Hauner H. The phosphodiesterase inhibitor IBMX suppresses TNF-alpha expression in human adipocyte precursor cells: a possible explanation for its adipogenic effect. Horm Metab Res 1999; 31(6):359–362.
61. Path G, Bornstein SR, Gurniak M, Chrousos GP, Scherbaum WA, Hauner H. Human breast adipocytes express interleukin-6 (IL-6) and its receptor system: increased IL-6 production by beta-adrenergic activation and effects of IL-6 on adipocyte function. J Clin Endocrinol Metab 2001; 86(5):2281–2288.
62. Fried SK, Bunkin DA, Greenberg AS. Omental and subcutaneous adipose tissues of obese subjects release interleukin-6: deot difference and regulation by glucocorticoid. J Clin Endocrinol Metab 1998; 83:847–850.
63. van HV, Reynisdottir S, Eriksson P, Thorne A, Hoffstedt J, Lonnqvist F, Arner P. Leptin secretion from subcutaneous and visceral adipose tissue in women. Diabetes 1998; 47(6):913–917.
64. Reynisdottir S, Dauzats M, Thorne A, Langin D. Comparison of hormone-sensitive lipase activity in visceral and subcutaneous human adipose tissue. J Clin Endocrinol Metab 1997; 82(12):4162–4166.
65. Rebuffe-Scrive M, Andersson B, Olbe L, Bjorntorp P. Metabolism of adipose tissue in intraabdominal depots of nonobese men and women. Metabolism 1989; 38:453–458.
66. Hoffstedt J, Arner P, Hellers G, Lonnqvist F. Variation in adrenergic regulation of lipolysis between omental and subcutaneous adipocytes from obese and non-obese men. J Lipid Res 1997; 38(4):795–804.
67. Rebuffe-Scrive M, Anderson B, Olbe L, Bjorntorp P. Metabolism of adipose tissue in intraabdominal depots in severely obese men and women. Metabolism 1990; 39(10):1021–1025.
68. Fried SK, Russell CD, Grauso NL, Brolin RE. Lipoprotein lipase regulation by insulin and glucocorticoid in subcutaneous and omental adipose tissues of obese women and men. J Clin Invest 1993; 92(5): 2191–2198.
69. Fried SK, Kral JG. Sex differences in regional distribution of fat cell size and lipoprotein lipase activity in morbidly obese patients. Int J Obes 1987; 11(2): 129–140.
70. van HV, Lonnqvist F, Thorne A, Wennlund A, Large V, Reynisdottir S, Arner P. Noradrenaline-induced lipolysis in isolated mesenteric, omental and subcutaneous adipocytes from obese subjects. Int J Obes Relat Metab Disord 1997; 21(11):972–979.

71. Marette A, Mauriege P, Marcotte B, Atgie C, Bouchard C, Theriault G, Bukowiecki LJ, Marceau P, Biron S, Nadeau A, Despres JP. Regional variation in adipose tissue insulin action and GLUT4 glucose transporter expression in severely obese premenopausal women. Diabetologia 1997; 40(5):590–598.
72. Mauriege P, Marette A, Atgie C, Bouchard C, Theriault G, Bukowiecki LK, Marceau P, Biron S, Nadeau A, Despres JP. Regional variation in adipose tissue metabolism of severely obese premenopausal women. J Lipid Res 1995; 36(4):672–684.
73. Fried SK, Leibel RL, Edens NK, Kral JG. Lipolysis in intraabdominal adipose tissues of obese women and men. Obes Res 1993; 1:443–448.
74. Hellmer J, Marcus C, Sonnenfeld T, Arner P. Mechanisms for differences in lipolysis between human subcutaneous and omental fat cells. J Clin Endocrinol Metab 1992; 75(1):15–20.
75. Rebuffe-Scrive M, Andersson B, Olbe L, Bjorntorp P. Metabolism of adipose tissue in intraabdominal depots of nonobese men and women. Metabolism 1989; 38(5): 453–458.
76. Vikman HL, Ranta S, Kiviluoto T, Ohisalo JJ. Different metabolic regulation by adenosine in omental and subcutaneous adipose tissue. Acta Physiol Scand 1991; 142(3):405–410.
77. Edens NK, Fried SK, Kral JG, Hirsch J, Leibel RL. In vitro lipid synthesis in human adipose tissue from three abdominal sites. Am J Physiol 1993; 265(3 Pt 1): E374–E379.
78. Ryden M, Elizalde M, Ohlund A, Hoffstedt J, Bringman S, Andersson K. Increased expression of eNOS protein in omental versus subcutaneous adipose tissue in obese human subjects. Int J Obes Relat Metab Disord 2001; 25(6):811–815.
79. Lonnqvist F, Thorne A, Large V, Arner P. Sex differences in visceral fat lipolysis and metabolic complications of obesity. Arterioscler Thromb Vasc Biol 1997; 17(7):1472–1480.
80. Mauriege P, Galitzky J, Berlan M, Lafontan M. Heterogeneous distribution of beta and alpha-2 adrenoceptor binding sites in human fat cells from various fat deposits: functional consequences. Eur J Clin Invest 1987; 17:156–165.
81. Zierath JR, Livingston JN, Thorne A, Bolinder J, Reynisdottir S, Lonnqvist F, Arner P. Regional difference in insulin inhibition of non-esterified fatty acid release from human adipocytes: relation to insulin receptor phosphorylation and intracellular signalling through the insulin receptor substrate-1 pathway. Diabetologia 1998; 41(11):1343–1354.
82. Meek SE, Nair KS, Jensen MD. Insulin regulation of regional free fatty acid metabolism. Diabetes 1999; 48(1):10–14.
83. Basu A, Basu R, Shah P, Vella A, Rizza RA, Jensen MD. Systemic and regional free fatty acid metabolism in type 2 diabetes. Am J Physiol Endocrinol Metab 2001; 280(6):E1000–E1006.
84. Guo Z, Johnson CM, Jensen MD. Regional lipolytic responses to isoproterenol in women. Am J Physiol 1997; 273(1 Pt 1):E108–E112.
85. Marin P, Lonn L, Andersson B, Oden B, Olbe L, Bengtsson BA, Bjorntorp P. Assimilation of triglycerides in subcutaneous and intraabdominal adipose tissues in vivo in men: effects of testosterone. J Clin Endocrinol Metab 1996; 81(3):1018–1022.
86. Lefebvre AM, Laville M, Vega N, Riou JP, van Gaal L, Auwerx J, Vidal H. Depot-specific differences in adipose tissue gene expression in lean and obese subjects. Diabetes 1998; 47(1):98–103.
87. Maslowska MH, Sniderman AD, Maclean LD, Cianflone K. Regional differences in triacylglycerol synthesis in adipose tissue and in cultured preadipocytes. J Lipid Res 1993; 34:219–227.
88. Saleh J, Christou N, Cianflone K. Regional specificity of ASP binding in human adipose tissue. Am J Physiol 1999; 276(5 Pt 1):E815–E821.
89. Montague CT, Prins JB, Sanders L, Zhang J, Sewter CP, Digby J, Byrne CD, O'Rahilly S. Depot-related gene expression in human subcutaneous and omental adipocytes. Diabetes 1998; 47(9):1384–1391.
90. Panarotto D, Poisson J, Devroede G, Maheux P. Lipoprotein lipase steady-state mRNA levels are lower in human omental versus subcutaneous abdominal adipose tissue. Metabolism 2000; 49(9):1224–1227.
91. Pedersen SB, Jonler M, Richelsen B. Characterization of regional and gender differences in glucocorticoid receptors and lipoprotein lipase activity in human adipose tissue. J Clin Endocrinol Metab 1994; 78(6): 1354–1359.
92. Frayn KN, Coppack SW, Fielding BA, Humphreys SM. Coordinated regulation of hormone-sensitive lipase and lipoprotein lipase in human adipose tissue in vivo: implications for the control of fat storage and fat mobilization. Adv Enzyme Regul 1995; 35:163–178.
93. Kolehmainen M, Vidal H, Alhava E, Uusitupa MI. Sterol regulatory element binding protein 1c (SREBP-1c) expression in human obesity. Obes Res 2001; 9(11): 706–712.
94. Ribot J, Rantala M, Kesaniemi YA, Palou A, Savolainen MJ. Weight loss reduces expression of SREBP1c/ADD1 and PPARgamma2 in adipose tissue of obese women. Pflugers Arch 2001; 441(4):498–505.
95. Caserta F, Tchkonia T, Civelek VN, Prentki M, Brown NF, McGarry JD. Fat depot origin affects fatty acid handling in cultured rat and human preadipocytes. Am J Physiol Endocrinol Metab 2001; 280(2): E238–E247.
96. Fisher RM, Eriksson P, Hoffstedt J, Hotamisligil GS, Thorne A, Ryden M. Fatty acid binding protein expression in different adipose tissue depots from

lean and obese individuals. Diabetologia 2001; 44(10): 1268–1273.

97. Hotamisligil GS, Johnson RS, Distel RJ, Ellis R, Papaioannou VE, Spiegelman BM. Uncoupling of obesity from insulin resistance through a targeted mutation in aP2, the adipocyte fatty acid binding protein. Science 1996; 274(5291):1377–1379.
98. Uysal KT, Scheja L, Wiesbrock SM, Bonner-Weir S, Hotamisligil GS. Improved glucose and lipid metabolism in genetically obese mice lacking aP2. Endocrinology 2000; 141(9):3388–3396.
99. Shaughnessy S, Smith ER, Kodukula S, Storch J, Fried SK. Adipocyte metabolism in adipocyte fatty acid binding protein knockout mice (aP2-/-) after short-term high-fat feeding: functional compensation by the keratinocyte fatty acid binding protein. Diabetes 2000; 49(6):904–911.
100. Schoen RE, Evans RW, Sankey SS, Weissfeld JL, Kuller L. Does visceral adipose tissue differ from subcutaneous adipose tissue in fatty acid content? Int J Obes Relat Metab Disord 1996; 20(4):346–352.
101. Digby JE, Crowley VE, Sewter CP, Whitehead JP, Prins JB, O'Rahilly S. Depot-related and thiazolidinedione-responsive expression of uncoupling protein 2 (UCP2) in human adipocytes. Int J Obes Relat Metab Disord 2000; 24(5):585–592.
102. West DB, Prinz WA, Greenwood MR. Regional changes in adipose tissue blood flow and metabolism in rats after a meal. Am J Physiol 1989; 257(4 Pt 2): R711–R716.
103. Crandall DL, Goldstein BM, Huggins F, Cervoni P. Adipocyte blood flow: influence of age, anatomic location, and dietary manipulation. Am J Physiol 1984; 247(1 Pt 2):R46–R51.
104. Bartness TJ, Bamshad M. Innervation of mammalian white adipose tissue: implications for the regulation of total body fat. Am J Physiol 1998; 275(5 Pt 2):R1399–R1411.
105. Rebuffe-Scrive M. Neuroregulation of adipose tissue: molecular and hormonal mechanims. Int J Obes Relat Metab Disord 1991; 15:83–86.
106. Elbers JM, Asscheman H, Seidell JC, Gooren LJ. Effects of sex steroid hormones on regional fat depots as assessed by magnetic resonance imaging in transsexuals. Am J Physiol 1999; 276(2 Pt 1):E317–E325.
107. Elbers JM, Asscheman H, Seidell JC, Megens JA, Gooren LJ. Long-term testosterone administration increases visceral fat in female to male transsexuals. J Clin Endocrinol Metab 1997; 82(7):2044–2047.
108. Seidell JC, Bjorntorp P, Sjostrom L, Kvist H, Sannerstedt R. Visceral fat accumulation in men is positively associated with insulin, glucose, and C-peptide levels, but negatively with testosterone levels. Metabolism 1990; 39(9):897–901.
109. Tchernof A, Labrie F, Belanger A, Prud'homme D, Bouchard C, Tremblay A, Nadeau A, Despres JP. Relationships between endogenous steroid hormone, sex hormone-binding globulin and lipoprotein levels in men: contribution of visceral obesity, insulin levels and other metabolic variables. Atherosclerosis 1997; 133(2):235–244.
110. Anderson LA, McTernan PG, Barnett AH, Kumar S. The effects of androgens and estrogens on preadipocyte proliferation in human adipose tissue: influence of gender and site. J Clin Endocrinol Metab 2001; 86(10): 5045–5051.
111. Roncari DA, Van RL. Promotion of human adipocyte precursor replication by 17beta-estradiol in culture. J Clin Invest 1978; 62(3):503–508.
112. Pecquery R, Dieudonne MN, Cloix JF, Leneveu MC, Dausse JP, Giudicelli Y. Enhancement of the expression of the alpha 2-adrenoreceptor protein and mRNA by a direct effect of androgens in white adipocytes. Biochem Biophys Res Commun 1995; 206(1): 112–118.
113. Bouloumie A, Valet P, Dauzats M, Lafontan M, Saulnier-Blache JS. In vivo upregulation of adipocyte alpha 2-adrenoceptors by androgens is consequence of direct action on fat cells. Am J Physiol 1994; 267(4 Pt 1):C926–C931.
114. Giudicelli Y, Dieudonne MN, Lacasa D, Pasquier YN, Pecquery R. Modulation by sex hormones of the membranous transducing system regulating fatty acid mobilization in adipose tissue. Prostaglandins Leukot Essent Fatty Acids 1993; 48(1):91–100.
115. Xu XF, De Pergola G, Bjorntorp P. Testosterone increases lipolysis and the number of beta-adrenoceptors in male rat adipocytes. Endocrinology 1991; 128(1): 379–382.
116. Pedersen SB, Bruun JM, Hube F, Kristensen K, Hauner H, Richelsen B. Demonstration of estrogen receptor subtypes alpha and beta in human adipose tissue: influences of adipose cell differentiation and fat depot localization. Mol Cell Endocrinol 2001; 182(1): 27–37.
117. Lo JC, Mulligan K, Noor MA, Schwarz JM, Halvorsen RA, Grunfeld C, Schambelan M. The effects of recombinant human growth hormone on body composition and glucose metabolism in HIV-infected patients with fat accumulation. J Clin Endocrinol Metab 2001; 86(8):3480–3487.
118. Roemmich JN, Huerta MG, Sundaresan SM, Rogol AD. Alterations in body composition and fat distribution in growth hormone-deficient prepubertal children during growth hormone therapy. Metabolism 2001; 50(5):537–547.
119. Brummer RJ. Effects of growth hormone treatment on visceral adipose tissue. Growth Horm IGF Res 1998; 8(suppl B):19–23.
120. Nam SY, Kim KR, Cha BS, Song YD, Lim SK, Lee HC, Huh KB. Low-dose growth hormone treatment combined with diet restriction decreases insulin re-

sistance by reducing visceral fat and increasing muscle mass in obese type 2 diabetic patients. Int J Obes Relat Metab Disord 2001; 25(8):1101–1107.
121. Johannsson G, Marin P, Lonn L, Ottosson M, Stenlof K, Bjorntorp P, Sjostrom L, Bengtsson BA. Growth hormone treatment of abdominally obese men reduces abdominal fat mass, improves glucose and lipoprotein metabolism, and reduces diastolic blood pressure. J Clin Endocrinol Metab 1997; 82(3):727–734.
122. Ottosson M, Vikman-Adolfsson K, Enerback S, Olivecrona G, Bjorntorp P. The effects of cortisol on the regulation of lipoprotein lipase activity in human adipose tissue. J Clin Endocrinol Metab 1994; 79(3): 820–825.
123. Lonn L, Kvist H, Ernest I, Sjostrom L. Changes in body composition and adipose tissue distribution after treatment of women with Cushing's syndrome. Metabolism 1994; 43(12):1517–1522.
124. Joyner JM, Hutley LJ, Cameron DP. Glucocorticoid receptors in human preadipocytes: regional and gender differences. J Endocrinol 2000; 166(1):145–152.
125. Miller LK, Kral JG, Strain GW, Zumoff B. Differential binding of dexamethasone to ammonium sulfate precipitates of human adipose tissue cytosols. Steroids 1987; 49(6):507–522.
126. Rebuffe-Scrive M, Lundholm K, Bjorntorp P. Glucocorticoid hormone binding to human adipose tissue. Eur J Clin Invest 1985; 15(5):267–271.
127. Sjogren J, Weck M, Nilsson A, Ottosson M, Bjorntorp P. Glucocorticoid hormone binding to rat adipocytes. Biochim Biophys Acta 1994; 1224(1):17–21.
128. Russell CD, Petersen RN, Rao SP, Ricci MR, Prasad A, Zhang Y, Brolin RE, Fried SK. Leptin expression in adipose tissue from obese humans: depot-specific regulation by insulin and dexamethasone. Am J Physiol 1998; 275(3 Pt 1):E507–E515.
129. Bujalska IJ, Kumar S, Stewart PM. Does central obesity reflect "Cushing's disease of the omentum"? Lancet 1997; 349(9060):1210–1213.
130. Bujalska IJ, Kumar S, Hewison M, Stewart PM. Differentiation of adipose stromal cells: the roles of glucocorticoids and 11beta-hydroxysteroid dehydrogenase. Endocrinology 1999; 140(7):3188–3196.
131. Katzmarzyk PT, Malina RM, Perusse L, Rice T, Province MA, Rao DC, Bouchard C. Familial resemblance in fatness and fat distribution. Am J Human Biol 2000; 12(3):395–404.
132. Rosmond R, Chagnon M, Bouchard C, Bjorntorp P. A missense mutation in the human melanocortin-4 receptor gene in relation to abdominal obesity and salivary cortisol. Diabetologia 2001; 44(10):1335–1338.
133. Rosmond R, Chagnon YC, Chagnon M, Perusse L, Bouchard C, Bjorntorp P. A polymorphism of the 5′-flanking region of the glucocorticoid receptor gene locus is associated with basal cortisol secretion in men. Metabolism 2000; 49(9):1197–1199.
134. Rosmond R, Bouchard C, Bjorntorp P. Tsp5091 polymorphism in exon 2 of the glucocorticoid receptor gene in relation to obesity and cortisol secretion: cohort study. BMJ 2001; 322(7287):652–653.
135. Nakamura T, Funahashi T, Yamashita S, Nishida M, Nishida Y, Takahashi M. Thiazolidinedione derivative improves fat distribution and multiple risk factors in subjects with visceral fat accumulation–double-blind placebo-controlled trial. Diabetes Res Clin Pract 2001; 54(3):181–190.
136. Kelly IE, Han TS, Walsh K, Lean ME. Effects of a thiazolidinedione compound on body fat and fat distribution of patients with type 2 diabetes. Diabetes Care 1999; 22(2):288–293.
137. De Souza CJ, Eckhardt M, Gagen K, Dong M, Chen W, Laurent D. Effects of pioglitazone on adipose tissue remodeling within the setting of obesity and insulin resistance. Diabetes 2001; 50(8):1863–1871.
138. Ahima RS, Flier JS. Adipose tissue as an endocrine organ. Trends Endocrinol Metab 2000; 11(8):327–332.
139. Ricci MR, Fried SK. Isoproterenol decreases leptin expression in adipose tissue of obese humans. Obes Res 1999; 7(3):233–240.
140. Arner P. Differences in lipolysis between human subcutaneous and omental adipose tissues. Ann Med 1995; 27(4):435–438.
141. Montague CT, Prins JB, Sanders L, Digby JE, O'Rahilly S. Depot- and sex-specific differences in human leptin mRNA expression: implications for the control of regional fat distribution. Diabetes 1997; 46(3):342–347.
142. Frayn KN. Visceral fat and insulin resistance–causative or correlative? Br J Nutr 2000; 83(suppl 1):S71–S77.
143. Mohamed-Ali V, Goodrick S, Rawesh A, Katz DR, Miles JM, Yudkin JS, Klein S, Coppack SW. Subcutaneous adipose tissue releases interleukin-6, but not tumor necrosis factor-alpha, in vivo. J Clin Endocrinol Metab 1997; 82(12):4196–4200.
144. Kern PA, Ranganathan S, Li C, Wood L, Ranganathan G. Adipose tissue tumor necrosis factor and interleukin-6 expression in human obesity and insulin resistance. Am J Physiol Endocrinol Metab 2001; 280(5):E745–E751.
145. Bastard JP, Jardel C, Bruckert E, Blondy P, Capeau J, Laville M, Vidal H, Hainque B. Elevated levels of interleukin 6 are reduced in serum and subcutaneous adipose tissue of obese women after weight loss. J Clin Endocrinol Metab 2000; 85(9):3338–3342.
146. Mohamed-Ali V, Bulmer K, Clarke D, Goodrick S, Coppack SW, Pinkney JH. Beta-adrenergic regulation of proinflammatory cytokines in humans. Int J Obes Relat Metab Disord 2000; 24(suppl 2):S154–S155.
147. Orban Z, Remaley AT, Sampson M, Trajanoski Z, Chrousos GP. The differential effect of food intake and beta-adrenergic stimulation on adipose-derived

hormones and cytokines in man. J Clin Endocrinol Metab 1999; 84(6):2126–2133.

148. McCarty MF. Interleukin-6 as a central mediator of cardiovascular risk associated with chronic inflammation, smoking, diabetes, and visceral obesity: down-regulation with essential fatty acids, ethanol and pentoxifylline. Med Hypotheses 1999; 52(5):465–477.

149. Vozarova B, Weyer C, Hanson K, Tataranni PA, Bogardus C, Pratley RE. Circulating interleukin-6 in relation to adiposity, insulin action, and insulin secretion. Obes Res 2001; 9(7):414–417.

150. Forouhi NG, Sattar N, McKeigue PM. Relation of C-reactive protein to body fat distribution and features of the metabolic syndrome in Europeans and South Asians. Int J Obes Relat Metab Disord 2001; 25(9): 1327–1331.

151. Mohamed-Ali H, Pinkney JH, Coppack SW. Adipose tissue as an endocrine and paracrine organ. Int J Obes 1998; 22(12):1145–1158.

152. Gerhardt CC, Romero IA, Cancello R, Camoin L, Strosberg AD. Chemokines control fat accumulation and leptin secretion by cultured human adipocytes. Mol Cell Endocrinol 2001; 175(1 2):81–92.

153. Coppack SW. Pro-inflammatory cytokines and adipose tissue. Proc Nutr Soc 2001; 60(3):349–356.

154. Bruun JM, Pedersen SB, Richelsen B. Interleukin-8 production in human adipose tissue. inhibitory effects of anti-diabetic compounds, the thiazolidinedione ciglitazone and the biguanide metformin. Horm Metab Res 2000; 32(11-12):537–541.

155. Bruun JM, Pedersen SB, Richelsen B. Regulation of interleukin 8 production and gene expression in human adipose tissue in vitro. J Clin Endocrinol Metab 2001; 86(3):1267–1273.

156. Zhang HH, Kumar S, Barnett AH, Eggo MC. Intrinsic site-specific differences in the expression of leptin in human adipocytes and its autocrine effects on glucose uptake. J Clin Endocrinol Metab 1999; 84(7): 2550–2556.

157. Niesler CU, Prins JB, O'Rahilly S, Siddle K, Montague CT. Adipose depot-specific expression of cIAP2 in human preadipocytes and modulation of expression by serum factors and TNFalpha. Int J Obes Relat Metab Disord 2001; 25(7):1027–1033.

158. Yamauchi T, Kamon J, Waki H, Terauchi Y, Kubota N, Hara K, Mori Y, Ide T, Murakami K, Tsuboyama-Kasaoka N, Ezaki O, Akanuma Y, Gavrilova O, Vinson C, Reitman ML, Kagechika H, Shudo K, Yoda M, Nakano Y, Tobe K, Nagai R, Kimura S, Tomita M, Froguel P, Kadowaki T. The fat-derived hormone adiponectin reverses insulin resistance associated with both lipoatrophy and obesity. Nat Med 2001; 7(8):941–946.

159. Berg AH, Combs TP, Du X, Brownlee M, Scherer PE. The adipocyte-secreted protein Acrp30 enhances hepatic insulin action. Nat Med 2001; 7(8):947–953.

160. Combs TP, Berg AH, Obici S, Scherer PE, Rossetti L. Endogenous glucose production is inhibited by the adipose-derived protein Acrp30. J Clin Invest 2001; 108(12):1875–1881.

161. Statnick MA, Beavers LS, Conner LJ, Corominola H, Johnson D, Hammond CD, Rafaeloff-Phail R, Seng T, Suter TM, Sluka JP, Ravussin E, Gadski RA, Caro JF. Decreased expression of apM1 in omental and subcutaneous adipose tissue of humans with type 2 diabetes. Int J Exp Diabetes Res 2000; 1(2): 81–88.

162. Singh A, Purohit A, Ghilchik MW, Reed MJ. The regulation of aromatase activity in breast fibroblasts: the role of interleukin-6 and prostaglandin E2. Endocr Relat Cancer 1999; 6(2):139–147.

163. Cooke PS, Heine PA, Taylor JA, Lubahn DB. The role of estrogen and estrogen receptor-alpha in male adipose tissue. Mol Cell Endocrinol 2001; 178(1-2): 147–154.

164. Heine PA, Taylor JA, Iwamoto GA, Lubahn DB, Cooke PS. Increased adipose tissue in male and female estrogen receptor-alpha knockout mice. Proc Natl Acad Sci USA 2000; 97(23):12729–12734.

165. Anwar A, McTernan PG, Anderson LA, Askaa J, Moody CG, Barnett AH, Eggo MC, Kumar S. Site-specific regulation of oestrogen receptor-alpha and -beta by oestradiol in human adipose tissue. Diabetes Obes Metab 2001; 3(5):338–349.

166. Napolitano A, Voice MW, Edwards CR, Seckl JR, Chapman KE. 11Beta-hydroxysteroid dehydrogenase 1 in adipocytes: expression is differentiation-dependent and hormonally regulated. J Steroid Biochem Mol Biol 1998; 64(5-6):251–260.

167. Ricketts ML, Verhaeg JM, Bujalska I, Howie AJ, Rainey WE, Stewart PM. Immunohistochemical localization of type 1 11beta-hydroxysteroid dehydrogenase in human tissues. J Clin Endocrinol Metab 1998; 83(4):1325–1335.

168. Tomlinson JW, Bujalska I, Stewart PM, Cooper MS. The role of 11beta-hydroxysteroid dehydrogenase in central obesity and osteoporosis. Endocr Res 2000; 26(4):711–722.

169. Tomlinson JW, Moore J, Cooper MS, Bujalska I, Shahmanesh M, Burt C, Strain A, Hewison M, Stewart PM. Regulation of expression of 11beta-hydroxysteroid dehydrogenase type 1 in adipose tissue: tissue-specific induction by cytokines. Endocrinology 2001; 142(5):1982–1989.

170. Katz JR, Mohamed-Ali V, Wood PJ, Yudkin JS, Coppack SW. An in vivo study of the cortisol-cortisone shuttle in subcutaneous abdominal adipose tissue. Clin Endocrinol (Oxf) 1999; 50(1):63–68.

171. Rask E, Olsson T, Soderberg S, Andrew R, Livingstone DEW, Johnson O, Walker BR. Tissue-specific dysregulation of cortisol metabolism in human obesity. J Clin Endocrinol Metab 2001; 86:1418–1421.

172. Dusserre E, Moulin P, Vidal H. Differences in mRNA expression of the proteins secreted by the adipocytes in human subcutaneous and visceral adipose tissues. Biochim Biophys Acta 2000; 1500(1):88–96.
173. Giacchetti G, Faloia E, Sardu C, Camilloni MA, Mariniello B, Gatti C, Garrapa GG, Guerrieri M, Mantero F. Gene expression of angiotensinogen in adipose tissue of obese patients. Int J Obes Relat Metab Disord 2000; 24(suppl 2):S142–S143.
174. Fried SK, Russell CD. Diverse roles of the adipose tissue in the regulation of systemic metabolism and energy balance. In: Bray GA, Bouchard C, James WPT eds. Handbook of Obesity. New York: Marcel Dekker, 1998:397–413.
175. Seki T, Miyasu T, Noguchi T, Hamasaki A, Sasaki R, Ozawa Y, Okukita K, Declerck PJ, Ariga T. Reciprocal regulation of tissue-type and urokinase-type plasminogen activators in the differentiation of murine preadipocyte line 3T3-L1 and the hormonal regulation of fibrinolytic factors in the mature adipocytes. J Cell Physiol 2001; 189(1):72–78.
176. Giltay EJ, Elbers JM, Gooren LJ, Emeis JJ, Kooistra T, Asscheman H. Stehouwer CD Visceral fat accumulation is an important determinant of PAI-1 levels in young, nonobese men and women: modulation by cross-sex hormone administration. Arterioscler Thromb Vasc Biol 1998; 18(11):1716–1722.
177. Gottschling-Zeller H, Birgel M, Rohrig K, Hauner H. Effect of tumor necrosis factor alpha and transforming growth factor beta 1 on plasminogen activator inhibitor-1 secretion from subcutaneous and omental human fat cells in suspension culture. Metabolism 2000; 49(5):666–671.
178. Eriksson P, van HV, Hoffstedt J, Lundquist P, Vidal H, Stemme V, Hamsten A, Arner P, Reynisdottir S. Regional variation in plasminogen activator inhibitor-1 expression in adipose tissue from obese individuals. Thromb Haemost 2000; 83(4):545–548.
179. Alessi MC, Peiretti F, Morange P, Henry M, Nalbone G, Juhan-Vague I. Production of plasminogen activator inhibitor 1 by human adipose tissue: possible link between visceral fat accumulation and vascular disease. Diabetes 1997; 46(5):860–867.
180. Polac I, Cierniewska-Cieslak A, Stachowiak G, Pertynski T, Cierniewski CS. Similar pai-1 expression in visceral and subcutaneous fat of postmenopausal women. Thromb Res 2001; 102(5):397–405.
181. Crandall DL, Quinet EM, Morgan GA, Busler DE, McHendry-Rinde B, Kral JG. Synthesis and secretion of plasminogen activator inhibitor-1 by human preadipocytes. J Clin Endocrinol Metab 1999; 84(9): 3222– 3227.
182. Yudkin JS, Coppack SW, Bulmer K, Rawesh A, Mohamed-Ali V. Lack of evidence for secretion of plasminogen activator inhibitor-1 by human subcutaneous adipose tissue in vivo. Thromb Res 1999; 96(1): 1–9.
183. Crandall DL, Busler DE, McHendry-Rinde B, Groeling TM, Kral JG. Autocrine regulation of human preadipocyte migration by plasminogen activator inhibitor-1. J Clin Endocrinol Metab 2000; 85(7):2609–2614.
184. Schafer K, Fujisawa K, Konstantinides S, Loskutoff DJ. Disruption of the plasminogen activator inhibitor 1 gene reduces the adiposity and improves the metabolic profile of genetically obese and diabetic ob/ob mice. FASEB J 2001; 15(10):1840–1842.
185. Garg A. Lipodystrophies. Am J Med 2000; 108(2): 143–152.
186. Engelson ES, Kotler DP, Tan Y, Agin D, Wang J, Pierson RN Jr, Heymsfield SB. Fat distribution in HIV-infected patients reporting truncal enlargement quantified by whole-body magnetic resonance imaging. Am J Clin Nutr 1999; 69(6):1162–1169.
187. Esterbauer H, Krempler F, Oberkofler H, Patsch W. The complement system: a pathway linking host defence and adipocyte biology. Eur J Clin Invest 1999; 29(8):653–656.
188. Choy LN, Rosen BS, Spiegelman BM. Adipsin and an endogenous pathway of complement from adipose cells. J Biol Chem 1992; 267(18):12736–12741.
189. Ross R, Fortier L, Hudson R. Separate associations between visceral and subcutaneous adipose tissue distribution, insulin and glucose levels in obese women. Diabetes Care 1996; 19(12):1404–1411.
190. Pare A, Dumont M, Lemieux I, Brochu M, Almeras N, Lemieux S, Prud'homme D, Despres JP. Is the relationship between adipose tissue and waist girth altered by weight loss in obese men? Obes Res 2001; 9(9):526–534.
191. Ross R, Janssen I. Is abdominal fat preferentially reduced in response to exercise-induced weight loss? Med Sci Sports Exerc 1999; 31(11 suppl):S568–S572.
192. Ross R, Janssen I, Stallknecht B. Influence of endurance exercise on adipose tissue distribution. In: Nicklas B,. Endurance Exercise and Adipose Tissue Boca Raton, FL: CRC Press, 2001:122–152.
193. Ross R, Janssen I. Physical activity, total and regional obesity: dose-response considerations. Med Sci Sports Exerc 2001; 33(6 suppl):S521–S527.
194. Ross R, Dagnone D, Jones PJ, Smith H, Paddags A, Hudson R, Janssen I. Reduction in obesity and related comorbid conditions after diet-induced weight loss or exercise-induced weight loss in men. A randomized, controlled trial. Ann Intern Med 2000; 133(2): 92–103.
195. Mourier A, Gautier JF, De Kerviler E, Bigard AX, Villette JM, Garnier JP, Duvallet A, Guezennec CY, Cathelineau G. Mobilization of visceral adipose tissue related to the improvement in insulin sensitivity in response to physical training in NIDDM, Effects of branched-chain amino acid supplements. Diabetes Care 1997; 20(3):385–391.

196. Thomas EL, Brynes AE, McCarthy J, Goldstone AP, Hajnal JV, Saeed N, Frost G, Bell JD. Preferential loss of visceral fat following aerobic exercise, measured by magnetic resonance imaging. Lipids 2000; 35(7):769–776.
197. Poehlman ET, Dvorak RV, DeNino WF, Brochu M, Ades PA. Effects of resistance training and endurance training on insulin sensitivity in nonobese, young women: a controlled randomized trial. J Clin Endocrinol Metab 2000; 85(7):2463–2468.
198. DiPietro L, Seeman TE, Stachenfeld NS, Katz LD, Nadel ER. Moderate-intensity aerobic training improves glucose tolerance in aging independent of abdominal adiposity. J Am Geriatr Soc 1998; 46(7): 875–879.
199. Despres JP, Lamarche B. Effects of diet and physical activity on adiposity and body fat distribution: implications for the prevention of cardiovascular disease. Nutr Res Rev 1999; 6:137–159.
200. Williams MJ, Hunter GR, Kekes-Szabo T, Trueth MS, Snyder S, Berland L, Blaudeau T. Intra-abdominal adipose tissue cut-points related to elevated cardiovascular risk in women. Int J Obes Relat Metab Disord 1996; 20(7):613–617.
201. Schwartz RS, Shuman WP, Larson V, Cain KC, Fellingham GW, Beard JC, Kahn SE, Stratton JR, Cerqueira MD, Abrass IB. The effect of intensive endurance exercise training on body fat distribution in young and older men. Metabolism 1991; 40(5):545–551.
202. Wilmore JH, Despres JP, Stanforth PR, Mandel S, Rice T, Gagnon J, Leon AS, Rao D, Skinner JS, Bouchard C. Alterations in body weight and composition consequent to 20 wk of endurance training: the HERITAGE Family Study. Am J Clin Nutr 1999; 70(3):346–352.
203. Bouchard C, Tremblay A, Despres JP. The response to exercise with constant energy intake in identical twins. Obes Res 1994; 2:400–410.
204. Glazer G. Long-term pharmacotherapy of obesity 2000: a review of efficacy and safety. Arch Intern Med 2001; 161(15):1814–1824.
205. Van Gaal LF, Wauters MA, Peiffer FW, De Leeuw IH. Sibutramine and fat distribution: is there a role for pharmacotherapy in abdominal/visceral fat reduction? Int J Obes Relat Metab Disord 1998; 22(suppl 1):S38–S40.
206. Marcus MA, Murphy L, Pi-Sunyer FX, Albu JB. Insulin sensitivity and serum triglyceride level in obese white and black women: relationship to visceral and truncal subcutaneous fat. Metabolism 1999; 48(2): 194–199.
207. Albu JB, Curi M, Shur M, Murphy L, Matthews DE, Pi-Sunyer FX. Systemic resistance to the antilipolytic effect of insulin in black and white women with visceral obesity. Am J Physiol 1999; 277(3 Pt 1):E551–E560.
208. Seidell J, Bouchard C. Visceral fat in relation to health: is it a major culprit or simply an innocent bystander? Int J Obes 1997; 21:626–631.
209. Goodpaster BH, Thaete FL, Simoneau JA, Kelley DE. Subcutaneous abdominal fat and thigh muscle composition predict insulin sensitivity independently of visceral fat. Diabetes 1997; 46(10):1579–1585.
210. Chandalia M, Abate N, Garg A, Stray-Gundersen J, Grundy SM. Relationship between generalized and upper body obesity to insulin resistance in Asian Indian men. J Clin Endocrinol Metab 1999; 84(7): 2329–2335.
211. Enevoldsen LH, Simonsen L, Stallknecht B, Galbo H, Bulow J. In vivo human lipolytic activity in preperitoneal and subdivisions of subcutaneous abdominal adipose tissue. Am J Physiol Endocrinol Metab 2001; 281(5):E1110–E1114.
212. Johnson JA, Fried SK, Pi-Sunyer FX, Albu JB. Impaired insulin action in subcutaneous adipocytes from women with visceral obesity. Am J Physiol Endocrinol Metab 2001; 280(1):E40–E49.
213. Mauriege P, Brochu M, Prud'homme D, Tremblay A, Nadeau A, Lemieux S, Despres JP. Is visceral adiposity a significant correlate of subcutaneous adipose cell lipolysis in men? J Clin Endocrinol Metab 1999; 84(2):736–742.
214. Weber RV, Buckley MC, Fried SK, Kral JG. Subcutaneous lipectomy causes a metabolic syndrome in hamsters. Am J Physiol Regul Integr Comp Physiol 2000; 279(3):R936–R943.
215. Terry RB, Stefanick ML, Haskell WL, Wood PD. Contributions of regional adipose tissue depots to plasma lipoprotein concentrations in overweight men and women: possible protective effects of thigh fat. Metabolism 1991; 40(7):733–740.
216. Reitman ML, Arioglu E, Gavrilova O, Taylor SI. Lipoatrophy revisited. Trends Endocrinol Metab 2000; 11(10):410–416.
217. Treuth MS, Hunter GR, Kekes-Szabo T, Weinsier RL, Goran MI, Berland L. Reduction in intra-abdominal adipose tissue after strength training in older women. J Appl Physiol 1995; 78(4):1425–1431.
218. Despres JP, Pouliot MC, Moorjani S, Nadeau A, Tremblay A, Lupien PJ, Theriault G, Bouchard C. Loss of abdominal fat and metabolic response to exercise training in obese women. Am J Physiol 1991; 261(2 Pt 1):E159–E167.
219. Bosello O, Zamboni M, Armellini F, Zocca I, Bergamo AI, Smacchia C, Milani MP, Cominacini L. Modifications of abdominal fat and hepatic insulin clearance during severe caloric restriction. Ann Nutr Metab 1990; 34(6):359–365.
220. Fujioka S, Matsuzawa Y, Tokunaga K, Tarui S. Contribution of intra-abdominal fat accumulation to the impairment of glucose and lipid metabolism in human obesity. Metabolism 1987; 36(1): 54–59.

221. Gray DS, Fujioka K, Colletti PM, Kim H, Devine W, Cuyegkeng T, Pappas T. Magnetic resonance imaging used for determining fat distribution in obesity and diabetes. Am J Clin Nutr 1991; 54(4):623–627.
222. Stallone DD, Stunkard AJ, Wadden TA, Foster GD, Boorstein J, Arger P. Weight loss and body fat distribution: a feasibility study using computed tomography. Int J Obes 1991; 15(11):775–780.
223. Armellini F, Zamboni M, Rigo L, Bergamo-Andreis IA, Robbi R, De Marchi M, Bosello O. Sonography detection of small intra-abdominal fat variations. Int J Obes 1991; 15(12):847–852.
224. Leenen R, Droop A, Seidell JC, Deurenberg P, Weststrate JA, Hautvast JG. Visceral fat loss measured by magnetic resonance imaging in relation to changes in serum lipid levels of obese men and women. Arterioscler Thromb 1993; 13(4):487–494.
225. Chowdhury B, Kvist H, Andersson B, Bjorntorp P, Sjostrom L. CT-determined changes in adipose tissue distribution during a small weight reduction in obese males. Int J Obes Relat Metab Disord 1993; 17(12): 685–691.
226. Zamboni M, Armellini F, Turcato E, Todesco T, Bissoli L, Bergamo-Andreis IA, Bosello O. Effect of weight loss on regional body fat distribution in premenopausal women. Am J Clin Nutr 1993; 58(1): 29–34.
227. Nicklas BJ, Rogus EM, Goldberg AP. Exercise blunts declines in lipolysis and fat oxidation after dietary-induced weight loss in obese older women. Am J Physiol 1997; 273(1 Pt 1):E149–E155.
228. Zamboni M, Facchinetti R, Armellini F, Turcato E, Bergamo AI, Bosello O. Effects of visceral fat and weight loss on lipoprotein(a) concentration in subjects with obesity. Obes Res 1997; 5(4):332–337.
229. Janand-Delenne B, Chagnaud C, Raccah D, Alessi MC, Juhan-Vague I, Vague P. Visceral fat as a main determinant of plasminogen activator inhibitor 1 level in women. Int J Obes Relat Metab Disord 1998; 22(4): 312–317.
230. Goodpaster BH, Kelley DE, Wing RR, Meier A, Thaete FL. Effects of weight loss on regional fat distribution and insulin sensitivity in obesity. Diabetes 1999; 48(4):839–847.
231. Janssen I, Ross R. Effects of sex on the change in visceral, subcutaneous adipose tissue and skeletal muscle in response to weight loss. Int J Obes Relat Metab Disord 1999; 23(10):1035–1046.
232. Kockx M, Leenen R, Seidell J, Princen HM, Kooistra T. Relationship between visceral fat and PAI-1 in overweight men and women before and after weight loss. Thromb Haemost 1999; 82(5):1490–1496.
233. Riches FM, Watts GF, Hua J, Stewart GR, Naoumova RP, Barrett PH. Reduction in visceral adipose tissue is associated with improvement in apolipoprotein B-100 metabolism in obese men. J Clin Endocrinol Metab 1999; 84(8):2854–2861.
234. Doucet E, St Pierre S, Almeras N, Mauriege P, Despres JP, Richard D, Bouchard C, Tremblay A. Fasting insulin levels influence plasma leptin levels independently from the contribution of adiposity: evidence from both a cross-sectional and an intervention study. J Clin Endocrinol Metab 1999; 85(11): 4231–4237.
235. Kamel EG, McNeill G, Van Wijk MC. Change in intra-abdominal adipose tissue volume during weight loss in obese men and women: correlation between magnetic resonance imaging and anthropometric measurements. Int J Obes Relat Metab Disord 2000; 24(5):607–613.

23

Resting Energy Expenditure, Thermic Effect of Food, and Total Energy Expenditure

Yves Schutz and Eric Jéquier

University of Lausanne, Lausanne, Switzerland

I METHODS OF MEASURING ENERGY EXPENDITURE IN HUMANS

A Introduction

Three main methods are used to measure energy expenditure in man: indirect calorimetry, direct calorimetry, and the doubly labeled water technique. These methods are based on different principles and do not measure the same type of energy.

Indirect calorimetry is the best method to measure resting energy expenditure, the thermic effect of food and the energy expended for physical activity. It has the great advantage of being relatively simple; it can be used either with a ventilated hood system (for a resting subject), or with a respiration chamber, when a 24-hr measurement is needed. A first advantage of indirect calorimetry is the immediate response of oxygen consumption (measured by the method of respiratory gas exchange) in relation with the real oxygen consumption in the tissues and organs within the body. There is no delay in measuring oxygen consumption because the body has negligible O_2 stores. A second advantage of indirect calorimetry in comparison with other methods is the possibility to assess nutrient oxidation rates, when oxygen consumption, CO_2 production, and urinary nitrogen excretion are measured.

Direct calorimetry is the method of choice for studies aiming at assessing thermoregulatory responses. The method consists in measuring heat losses, not heat production. In many circumstances, heat losses differ from heat production and there is a change in heat stored. For instance, after a meal, heat production begins to rise 20–30 min after the onset of eating, whereas heat loss increases only later on; the consequence of the different time courses of heat production and heat loss is a rise in body temperature.

The method of direct calorimetry consists in the measurement of the heat dissipated by the body by radiation, convection, conduction, and evaporation (1). Under conditions of thermal equilibrium in a subject at rest and in postabsorptive conditions, heat production, measured by indirect calorimetry, is identical to heat dissipation, measured by direct calorimetry (Fig. 1). This is an obvious confirmation of the first law of thermodynamics—that the energy released by oxidative processes is ultimately transformed into heat (and external work during exercise). In steady-state conditions, the identity between heat production and heat loss in a resting subject (Fig. 1) corroborates the validity (for the whole body) of the method of indirect calorimetry.

Doubly labeled water technique is the third method and is based on the difference in the rates of turnover of $^{2}H_2O$ and $H_2{}^{18}O$ in body water. The subject is given a single oral dose of $^{2}H_2{}^{18}O$ to label body water with both isotopes ^{2}H and ^{18}O. A rapid exchange of ^{18}O occurs between water and carbon dioxide owing to the action of carbonic anhydrase. As a result, after

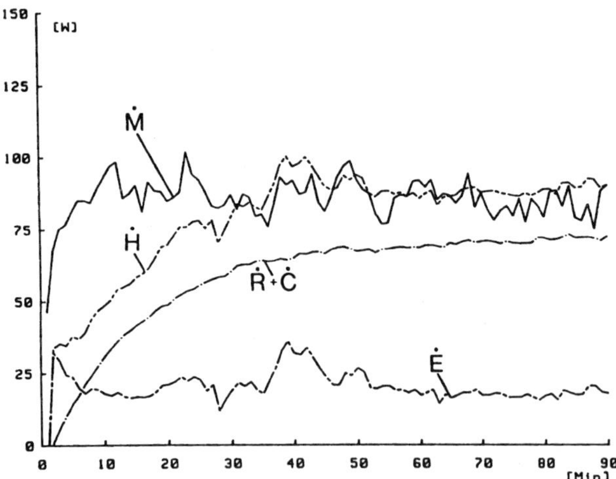

Figure 1 Metabolic rate ($\dot{M}$), total heat losses ($\dot{H}$), radiative and convective heat losses ($\dot{R} + \dot{C}$), and evaporative heat losses ($\dot{E}$) in a male subject aged 25 years, exposed at 28°C in a direct calorimeter. Note that after 30 min of temperature equilibration within the calorimeter, the values of $\dot{M}$ and $\dot{H}$ are similar, indicating that heat production is identical to heat losses.

equilibrium of $^2H_2$ ^{18}O in the water pool and equilibrium of ^{18}O with carbon dioxide, ^{18}O is lost both as $H_2{}^{18}O$ and $CO^{18}O$, whereas ^2H is lost only as $^2H_2$ O. The difference in the rate of turnover of $H_2{}^{18}O$ and ^2H_2O is an estimate of CO_2 production rate. In order to calculate the subject's energy expenditure, the mean respiratory quotient (RQ) must be known. Energy expenditure is obtained by multiplying $\dot{V}CO_2$ by the energy equivalent of CO_2 production. The latter varies from 21.0 to 27.7 kJ/L CO_2 at respiratory quotients of 1.0–0.7, respectively. The disappearance rates of the isotopes can be measured in urine, blood or saliva, for a period equivalent to two to three biologic half-lives. This corresponds to ~14 days in adult subjects. Thus, the method provides a mean value of energy expenditure for a 2-week period. It is not possible to calculate the day-to-day variation in energy expenditure with the doubly labeled water technique.

Several validation studies in both infants and adults have consistently shown a good agreement between the $\dot{V}CO_2$ determined by the doubly labeled water and that assessed by indirect calorimetry. Issues have been raised in regard to the question of two-point versus multiple points isotopic sampling, the extent of the fractionation of the isotopes, the difference between the oxygen and hydrogen dilution space, as well as the inherent precision of the analysis by mass spectrometry (2). Roberts et al. (3) have recently conducted an interlaboratory comparison of the doubly labeled water method using standards containing varying amounts of $^2H_2$ and ^{18}O as well as dose specimens. Surprisingly, there was substantial variability between laboratories in the results, and some laboratories obtained physiologically impossible energy expenditure (i.e., below the resting value). The type of calculation used had little effect on the accuracy of the technique. As a result, the average coefficient of variation for the doubly labeled water method, which is often claimed to be 5%, was not attained by a few laboratories, mostly owing to the quality of the isotopic analysis. The impact of deuterium and ^{18}O pool size determination on the calculation of total energy expenditure constitutes an important issue (4) since hydrogen tracer dilutes into a pool significantly larger than the body water pool due to the presence of labile hydrogen. This justifies the need for a correction factor for the isotope pool size. It seems that the best approach is to use a pool size based upon the average of the deuterium and ^{18}O pool space (4).

A recent study by Speakman (5) indicated that the error for $\dot{V}CO_2$ estimated by doubly labeled water was not normally distributed. Depending on the difference in the elimination rate constants of the two labels, the duration of the experiment, and the initial isotopic dose, the precision error (99% confidence interval for mean) using duplicate analysis varied enormously (between 3% and 47%). By increasing the number of replicates from two to five, the error could be substantially reduced. The issue of shifts in baseline abundance of deuterium of ^{18}O tracers is important since it may generate errors in the derivation of CO_2 and H_2O turnover rates and hence calculated energy expenditure. Jones (6) suggested that optimally the subject should first equilibrate with the new water source when a doubly labeled water study is performed. Alternatively, correction for shifting baseline can be made by measuring isotopic abundance changes in a control group of subjects who do not receive the doubly labeled water dose, but ingest the same diet as the experimental group and perform similar activities.

B Indirect Calorimetry: The Method of Choice to Measure Energy Expenditure and Nutrient Oxidation Rates

1 Measurement of Energy Expenditure

The term "indirect calorimetry" stems from the fact that the heat released by chemical processes within the body can be indirectly calculated from the rate of oxygen consumption ($\dot{V}O_2$). The main reason for the close relation between energy metabolism and $\dot{V}O_2$ is that the oxidative phosphorylation in the respiratory chain is coupled with a continuous synthesis of adenosine triphosphate (ATP). The energy expended within the body to maintain electrochemical gradients, to support biosynthetic processes, and to generate muscular contractions cannot be directly provided by nutrient oxidation. Almost all chemical processes requiring energy depend on ATP hydrolysis. It is the rate of ATP utilization that determines the overall rate of substrate oxidation and therefore $\dot{V}O_2$. With the exception of anaerobic glycolysis, ATP synthesis is coupled with substrate oxidation. Because there is a proportionality between $\dot{V}O_2$ and ATP synthesis, and because each mole of ATP synthesized is accompanied by the production of a given amount of heat, one understands the rationale of using $\dot{V}O_2$ measurement to calculate heat production within the body (7).

The study of the regulation of energy metabolism and nutrient utilization in humans has recently raised a great interest thanks to advances in the construction of open-circuit ventilated hood indirect calorimeters and comfortable respiration chambers.

With the measurement of $\dot{V}O_2$ (in liters of O_2/min) at STPD conditions [standard temperature (O°C), pressure (760 mmHg), and gas dry], metabolic rate (M), which corresponds to heat production, can be calculated (in kJ/min) as follows:

$$M = 20.3 \times \dot{V}O_2 \qquad (1)$$

The number 20.3 is a mean value (in kJ/L) of the energy equivalent for the consumption of 1 L (STPD) oxygen. The value of the energy equivalent of oxygen depends on the composition of the fuel mixture oxidized (Table 1). The error in using Eq. (1) instead of an equation that takes into account the type of fuels oxidized [Eqs. (2) and (3); see below] is not greater than ± 2%.

The heat released by the oxidation of each of the three macronutrients (carbohydrates, fats, and proteins) can be calculated from three measurements: oxygen consumption ($\dot{V}O_2$), carbon dioxide production ($\dot{V}CO_2$), and urinary nitrogen excretion (N).

Simple equations for computing metabolic rate (or energy expenditure) from these three determinations are written under the form:

$$M = a\ \dot{V}O_2 + b\ \dot{V}CO_2 - c\ N \qquad (2)$$

The factors a, b, and c depend on the respective constants for the amount of O_2 used and the amount of CO_2 produced during oxidation of the three classes of nutrients (Table 1). An example of such a formula (Brouwer's equation) is given below:

$$M = 16.18\ \dot{V}O_2 + 5.02\ \dot{V}CO_2 - 5.99\ N \qquad (3)$$

where M is in kilojoules per unit of time, $\dot{V}O_2$ and $\dot{V}CO_2$ are in liters STPD per unit of time, and N is in grams per unit of time. Slightly different factors for the amounts of O_2 used and of CO_2 produced during oxidation of the nutrients are used by other authors, and the values for the factors a, b, and c are modified accordingly. The difference in energy expenditure calculated by the various formulae is not greater than 3%. Detailed information about these calculations is given elsewhere (9,10).

Table 1 Oxygen Consumed, CO_2 Produced, and Heat Released from Oxidation of Nutrients

				Heat released (per gram)		Energy equivalent (per liter STPD) of:			
						$\dot{V}O_2$		$\dot{V}CO_2$	
Nutrients	O_2 consumed[a]	CO_2 produced[a]	RQ	kJ/g	kcal/g	kJ/L	kcal/L	kJ/L	kcal/L
Starch	0.829	0.829	1.00	17.6	4.20	21.2	5.06	21.2	5.06
Saccharose	0.786	0.786	1.00	16.6	3.96	21.1	5.04	21.1	5.04
Glucose	0.746	0.746	1.00	15.6	3.74	21.0	5.01	21.0	5.01
Lipid	2.019	1.427	0.71	39.6	9.46	19.6	4.69	27.7	6.63
Protein	1.010	0.844	0.83	19.7	4.70	19.5	4.66	23.3	5.58
Lactic acid	0.746	0.746	1.00	15.1	3.62	20.3	4.85	20.3	4.85

[a] In liters per gram of substrate oxidized.
RQ = respiratory quotient = $\dot{V}CO_2/\dot{V}O_2$; kJ = kilojoules.
Source: Ref. 8.

2 Measurement of Nutrient Oxidation Rates

As an example, let us assume that a subject is oxidizing g grams per minute of carbohydrate (as glucose), f g/ min of fat, and is excreting n g/min of urinary nitrogen. The following equations, based on Table 1, describe $\dot{V}O_2$ and $\dot{V}CO_2$:

$$\dot{V}O_2 = 0.746\ g + 2.02\,f + 6.31\ n \qquad (4)$$

$$\dot{V}CO_2 = 0.746\ g + 1.43\,f + {\sim}5.27\ n \qquad (5)$$

We can solve Eqs. (4) and (5) for the unknown g and f as follows:

$$g = 4.59\ \dot{V}CO_2 - 3.25\ \dot{V}O_2 - 3.68\ n \qquad (6)$$

$$f = 1.69\ \dot{V}O_2 - 1.69\ \dot{V}CO_2 - 1.72\ n \qquad (7)$$

Because 1 g urinary nitrogen arises from ~6.25 g protein, the protein oxidation rate (p in g/min) is given by the equation:

$$p = 6.25n \qquad (8)$$

Other metabolic processes (such as lipogenesis, gluconeogenesis, and ketogenesis) may influence the calculated oxidation rates of nutrients. However, intermediate metabolic processes do not influence the results of Eqs. (6) and (7), provided intermediate substrates do not accumulate within the body or are not excreted from the body. When there is accumulation or excretion of an intermediate or end product other than CO_2 and H_2O, this approach to compute the oxidation rates of nutrients is no longer valid, and correction factors must be applied to take into account the changes in the pool size of the intermediates or end products.

II RESTING AND BASAL METABOLIC RATES (RMR AND BMR)

A Whole-Body, Organ, and Tissue Metabolic Rates

There is an arbitrary distinction between RMR and BMR in the literature. RMR may be considered equivalent to BMR if the measurements are made in postabsorptive conditions. It seems difficult to partition RMR into various subcomponents since the metabolic rates of individual organs and tissues are difficult to assess in humans under noninvasive experimental conditions. By measuring the arteriovenous difference in concentration of O_2 across an organ or tissue, combined with the assessment of blood flow perfusing this organ or tissue, the $\dot{V}O_2$ of an organ or tissue can be estimated in vivo (based on the reverse Fick equation), but this requires invasive procedures such as arterial and venous catheterization. The error of measurement will largely increase if the rate of blood perfusion of an organ is high compared to its $\dot{V}O_2$, indicating a low arteriovenous oxygen difference.

Elia (11) has written an excellent review of the contribution of organs and tissue to the metabolic rate. The major part of the whole-body RMR stems from organs with high metabolic activity such as the liver, kidneys, brain, and heart, although these account for a small proportion of the total body weight (5%; Table 2). Per unit body weight, the kidneys and heart have a metabolic rate more than twice as high as the liver and the brain. In contrast, the metabolic rate of muscle per unit body weight is nearly 35 times lower than that of the heart and kidneys. Since the propor-

Table 2 Contribution of Different Organs and Tissues to Total Body Weight and Basal Metabolic Rate (BMR) in an Average Man of 70 kg with a BMR of 1680 kcal/day (7.03 MJ/day)

	Tissue or organ weight (kg)	Contribution of tissue or organ weight to body weight (%)	Organ metabolic rate per unit weight (kcal/kg/day)	Contribution to BMR (% total)
Liver	1.8	2.6	200	21
Brain	1.4	2.0	240	20
Heart	0.33	0.5	440	9
Kidneys	0.31	0.4	440	8
Muscle	28.0	40.0	13	22
Adipose tissue	15.0	21.4	4.5	4
Δ = miscellaneous tissues (bones, skin, intestines, lungs, etc.)	23.2	33.1	12	16
Total	70.00	100	24	100

Source: Ref. 11.

tion of muscle to nonmuscle changes with age from birth to adulthood, the RMR per unit body weight is not constant with age (12). The tissue with the lowest metabolic activity per unit body weight is adipose tissue, which accounts for only 4% of the whole-body RMR in nonobese subjects. Calculations show that this value can increase up to 10% or more in obese subjects with a large excess in body fat (Schutz et al., unpublished). The "residual" metabolic rate (16%) not explained by the tissues and organs mentioned above can be accounted for by skin and intestines (which have a relatively large protein mass and protein turnover), as well as bones and lungs.

B Body Composition: Effect of Fat-Free Mass and Fat Mass

The excess body weight of the obese is primarily constituted by fat tissue, but also a small component of associated lean tissue. Although the exact nature of extra lean tissue in obesity is largely unknown, it seems logical to expect a greater absolute RMR in obese adults (13) and children (14) characterized by an excess fat mass and a slight increase in fat-free mass (FFM). Numerous studies have demonstrated that the major factor explaining the variation in RMR between individuals is FFM (15). FFM is a heterogeneous component that can be partitioned into muscle mass and nonmuscle mass. Unfortunately, there is no simple and accurate way to assess these two subcomponents. Owing to the larger variation, between individuals, in fat mass, as compared to FFM, and because, in grossly obese women, fat mass can represent a nonnegligible component of total RMR, the prediction models for RMR that include both FFM and fat mass explain significantly more variance in RMR than FFM alone (15). In addition, age, sex, and family membership are additional factors which should be taken into account.

The effects of gender on resting metabolic rate are explained by differences in body composition. Caution should be used when comparing resting metabolic rate expressed per kilogram FFM in men and women, because the composition of FFM is influenced by gender. The muscle mass of men being larger than that of women, this fact tends to lower the value of RMR per kilogram FFM in men when compared to that of women. This is explained by a greater component of a tissue with a low metabolic rate (resting muscle) in men than in women (Table 2). According to recent data (16,17), women have a lower RMR than men (3–10%) even after adjustment for FFM, fat mass, age, and VO_2max. Various mechanisms could explain this observation such as hormonal status, differences in the composition of the FFM, muscular fiber type composition (18), and Na,K-ATPase activity (19) as well as differences in the activity of the neoglucogenic pathway, differences in the central body temperature and sympathetic nervous system activity (16).

Physiological variations in sex hormones during the phases of the menstrual cycle in women offer the opportunity to assess, in addition to the change in basal body temperature, the effect of hormonal variation on RMR. Previous studies have indicated an increase in RMR (20) and sleeping metabolic rate (21) in the luteal phase of the menstrual cycle, although recent data in Indian (22) and Dutch (23) women did not show any differences. In a study in which heat production and heat losses were measured by both direct and indirect calorimetry (24), we failed to find any significant differences in RMR (heat production) and heat losses during the luteal phase of the menstrual cycle in young women. By combining indirect calorimetry, direct calorimetry, and thermometry, skin thermal conductance and skin blood flow could be calculated. We observed a decrease in these two latter parameters during the luteal phase that indicates an increase in cutaneous thermal insulation. We concluded that during the luteal phase, the decreased thermal conductance in women exposed to a neutral environment allows the maintenance of a higher internal temperature (24).

Aging leads to a progressive decrease in RMR. Classically, this has been attributed to the reduction in muscle mass accompanying aging (25). A drop in the metabolic activity per unit tissue mass is also likely to occur if the loss of FFM does not fully account for the lower RMR (26). In a recent study, we explored the change in RMR and whole body protein turnover in healthy elderly and lean Gambian men (27). It was found that adjusted for FFM, the RMR was significantly lower (by 13%) in elderly than in young individuals. This was not explained by a decrease in protein turnover, since the protein turnover adjusted for FFM was not different between the two groups. The extent of the decline in RMR in obese male and female individuals remains to be investigated.

C Effect of Previous Dietary Intake

Postabsorptive RMR (or BMR) is typically measured 12 hr after the last meal, in order to diminish the effect of "residual" postprandial thermogenesis. Nevertheless, the relative composition of the diet eaten the previous days (i.e., the food quotient; FQ), largely influences the respiratory quotient during postabsorptive RMR (28).

Isocaloric substitution of low versus high carbohydrate diets have much more influence on the RQ than on the rate of RMR (29). The extent to which short-term overfeeding will increase both the RQ and the RMR depends on the duration of overfeeding: one single-day surfeit energy intake increases the RQ above the FQ (indicating fat storage), but the rise in RMR is very limited and most of the effect is seen on dietary-induced thermogenesis (30).

D Hormonal Factors

Many studies have demonstrated that catecholamines increase RMR (31–33). Both β_1 and β_2-adrenoceptors are involved in this sympathetically mediated thermogenesis (34). Subcutaneous or intravenous injections of epinephrine increase the RMR by about 20% with large interstudy variation and in a dose-dependent manner (31). Many different organs are involved in the epinephrine-mediated thermogenesis, but the major part of the effect seems to occur in skeletal muscles and in the heart. The mechanism by which epinephrine exerts its thermogenic action may be via a specific stimulation at the cellular level, extrasubstrate cycling (e.g., Cori cycle), and activation of skeletal muscle and cardiac activities.

It is well known that thyroid hormones increase BMR since BMR measurement was used, several decades ago, as a diagnostic tool of hyperthyroidism until hormonal concentrations could be determined. Hyperthyroid patients have an increased metabolic rate which is dependent upon the T3 plasma concentration and may reach up to 180% of the standard reference value (34). There is no general agreement about the mechanisms whereby thyroid hormones stimulate heat production; they may increase the Na,K-ATPase activity in various tissues and may stimulate the rate of protein turnover. Thyroid hormones also potentiate the effects of the sympathetic nervous system at the level of the adrenergic receptor and adenyl cyclase complex. Thyroid hormones act in a permissive manner to allow sympathetic activity to accelerate production of heat.

E Familial and Genetic Effects

Almost two decades ago, Bogardus et al. (35) observed that part of the unexplained variance in RMR could be accounted for by family membership, indicating that the level of RMR is partially genetically determined. The twins studies of Bouchard et al. (36) have shown that the RMRs of monozygotic twins have more resemblance than that of dizygotic twins after statistical adjustment for differences in body size and body composition. An excellent account of the part played by genetic factors in the etiology of human obesity as well as their metabolic implications has been published by Bouchard (37).

F Uncoupling Proteins and Energy Expenditure

Mitochondria of brown adipose tissue have an inducible proton conductance catalyzed by an uncoupling protein, UCP_1 (38). Cold exposure in rodents induces UCP_1 mRNA and protein in brown adipose tissue. The activated UCP_1 catalyzes proton leak across the mitochondrial inner membrane leading to an increased heat production which is called nonshivering thermogenesis (NST). It was then shown (39) that NST was used by rodents not only to protect against cold stress, but also to maintain energy homeostasis in response to excessive caloric intake through an efficient control of adaptive thermogenesis. In rodents, obesity can arise from impaired adaptive thermogenesis, and pharmacological stimulation of brown adipose tissue thermogenesis by β_3-adrenoreceptor agonists is an effective mechanism for reducing obesity (40). In adult humans, however, the absence of detectable brown adipose tissue depots explains why adaptive thermogenesis in response to overfeeding is lacking (41); it also accounts for the failure of β_3-adrenoreceptor agonists as potential therapeutic agents to treat human obesity (40).

The recent discovery of homologs of UCP_1, particularly the expression of high levels of UCP_2 mRNA in white adipose tissue and of UCP_3 mRNA in skeletal muscle of humans, has given hope that mechanisms unrelated to UCP_1 and to brown adipose tissue might be involved in the stimulation of energy expenditure (42,43). Several studies indicate that these UCPs also have proton transport activity across the mitochondrial inner membrane (42,43). Since UCP_2 and UCP_3 have uncoupling activity and are expressed widely, it has been proposed that they could contribute to adaptive thermogenesis. However, the observation that the expression of UCP_2 and UCP_3 messenger RNA increases with starvation, a condition known to be associated with a reduction in energy expenditure, argues against the view of a role of UCP_2 and UCP_3 in stimulating adaptive thermogenesis.

The conditions that modulate expression of UCP_2 and UCP_3 messenger RNA have been much studied over the past 2 years. Expression of UCP_2 mRNA was found to be elevated in white adipose tissue of obese animals, but discordant results were reported on UCP_2

expression in white adipose tissue of obese humans (44). Regarding stimulation of UCP_3 mRNA expression, increased circulating free fatty acids levels play a major role (45). Thus, starvation, which is characterized by elevated circulating free fatty acids, is accompanied by a stimulation of UCP_3 (and also UCP_2) expression in skeletal muscle. These UCPs have therefore no thermogenic effect (because energy expenditure is reduced by starvation), but they may play a role in the stimulation of lipid oxidation (46).

In conclusion, while it is well documented that UCP_1 increases energy dissipation in brown adipose tissue and thus plays a major role in thermoregulation of rodents and human newborns, it is not yet established whether or not UCP_2 and/or UCP_3 are involved in the regulation of energy metabolism. Recently, J.E. Silva (47) postulated that the activity, rather than the concentrations of these uncoupling proteins, could be regulated; the capacity of the cells to produce their energetic currency, ATP, is such a vital process that it must be under tight control through regulation of uncoupling protein activity. This new area of investigation needs to be addressed if we want to understand their physiological role.

G Leptin and Resting Energy Expenditure

Leptin, the product of the ob gene, is mainly synthesized in adipose tissue and released into the circulation. It represents an afferent hormonal signal to the hypothalamus where it acts on specific receptors and induces a decrease in appetite and an increase in energy expenditure in rodents. In humans, it is likely that leptin decreases appetite, but a role in the control of resting energy expenditure is not established.

Human studies investigating the relationship between serum leptin concentrations and energy expenditure have yielded inconsistent results. Several studies showed that serum leptin concentrations were not related to resting energy expenditure (48–50). By contrast, Jorgensen et al. (51) reported that in men, serum leptin levels were a strong determinant of resting metabolic rate (RMR). The body composition of the individuals studied may, however, account for an apparent effect of leptin on energy expenditure. Fat mass is strongly related to serum leptin concentrations, and, besides fat-free mass, fat mass is also a predictor of RMR. Therefore, multiple regression analysis should be carried out to adjust RMR for FFM and fat mass, before concluding that leptin stimulates RMR. In a recent study in a free-living elderly population, Neuhäuser-Berthold et al. (52) clearly showed that leptin was not a significant predictor of RMR, when the effects of FFM and fat mass on RMR are taken into account.

In conclusion, in humans, leptin is probably not involved in the regulation of RMR. In rats, leptin acting on hypothalamic receptors stimulates the CRH pathway which induces a stimulation of sympathetic activity and activates brown adipose tissue metabolism through adrenergic β_3 receptors (53). The latter tissue being virtually absent in adult humans, this may explain why leptin has no effect on resting energy expenditure.

III THERMIC EFFECT OF FOOD IN HUMANS

The energy expenditure increases significantly after a meal, which has first been attributed to the intake of protein under the term of "specific dynamic action." It was subsequently recognized that not only protein intake, but also carbohydrate and, to a lesser extent, fat intake, stimulate energy expenditure. This effect is nowadays called dietary-induced thermogenesis, or the thermic effect of food.

The thermic effect of food is mainly due to the energy cost of nutrient absorption, processing, and storage. The total thermic effect of food over 24 hr represents ~10% of the total energy expenditure in sedentary subjects.

A Techniques for Measurement of the Thermic Effect of Food

The best technique to assess the thermic effect of a meal is to measure the energy expenditure following a meal during 3–5 hr and to compare the values with a control test during the same period of time, after a zero-energy drink is given. Alternatively, one often measures resting energy expenditure in a postabsorptive subject during 1 hr to get a stable baseline. Thereafter, a meal is given to the subject and energy expenditure is continuously measured with a ventilated hood during 3–5 hr. The area under the curve over the baseline (considered a constant reference value) represents the thermic effect of the meal. It is important that the period of measurement be of sufficient duration to include the entire thermogenic response (54).

B Effect of Energy Intake and Dietary Composition on the Thermic Effect of Food

The thermic effect of nutrients mainly depends on the energy costs of processing and/or storing the nutrient.

Expressed in percent of the energy content of the nutrient, values of 8%, 2%, 20–30%, and 22% have been reported for glucose, fat, protein, and ethanol, respectively (9,55,56).

Glucose-induced thermogenesis mainly results from the cost of glycogen synthesis and substrate cycling (9). Glucose storage as glycogen requires 2 mol ATP/mol. In comparison with the 38 mol ATP produced on complete oxidation of glucose, the energy cost of glucose storage as glycogen corresponds to 5% (or 2/38) of the energy content of glucose stored. Cycling of glucose to glucose-6-phosphate and back to glucose, to fructose -1,6-diphosphate and back to glucose-6-phosphate, or to lactate and back to glucose, is occurring at variable rates and are energy-requiring processes which may increase the thermic effect of carbohydrates.

The thermic effect of dietary fat is very small; an increase of 2% of its energy content has been described during infusion of an emulsion of triglyceride (57). This slight increase in energy expenditure is explained by the ATP consumption in the process of free fatty acid reesterification to triglyceride. As a consequence, the dietary energy of fat is used very efficiently.

The thermic effect of proteins is the highest of all nutrients (20–30% of the energy content of proteins). Ingested proteins are degraded in the gut into amino acids. After absorption, amino acids are deaminated, their amino group transferred to urea, and their carbon skeleton converted to glucose. These biochemical processes require the consumption of energy amounting to ~25% of the energy content of amino acids. The second pathway of amino acid metabolism is protein synthesis. The energy expended for the synthesis of the peptide bonds also represents ~25% of the energy content of amino acids. Therefore, irrespective of their metabolic pathway, the thermogenesis induced after amino acids absorption represents ~25% of their energy content.

The thermic effect of ethanol amounts to ~22% of its energy content (56). The acute effects of ethanol ingestion include a decrease in the plasma free fatty acids level and a change in the cellular redox state in the liver cells, with an inhibition of lipid oxidation.

C Effect of Gender, Menstrual Cycle, and Age on the Thermic Effect of Food

The thermic effect of food is apparently not influenced by gender. More than a decade ago, we observed that the thermic effect of an oral load of glucose was negatively correlated with age (58). The effects of age on the thermic effect of food are entirely explained by the decrease in fat-free mass with age (59). Thus, when the thermic effect of food is corrected for the fat-free mass, both young and elderly subjects have similar values (59). A clear effect of menstrual cycle has not been observed since the thermic effect of food was found blunted during the luteal phase (60) or unchanged (61).

D Effect of Body Composition and Nutritional Status on the Thermic Effect of Food

The effect of body composition on the thermic effect of food has been much studied. The hypothesis of a "thrifty gene," a genetic propensity to increase the efficiency of energy utilization has been proposed to explain how humans have survived during periods of famine over the millions of years of evolution. According to this hypothesis, there has been a strong selective pressure to eliminate individuals with a low metabolic efficiency, whereas those with a thrifty gene have had greater chance of survival thanks to a more efficient energy metabolism. When exposed to conditions of plenty, those with a thrifty gene have an increased risk to become obese.

In support of this hypothesis, it has been reported that thermogenesis is decreased in most obese individuals (62). The reduction of postprandial thermogenesis in obesity is related to the degree of insulin resistance, which may be influenced by a low sympathetic activity (63). Thermogenesis is the energy expenditure above basal metabolic rate due to food intake, cold exposure, thermogenic agents, and psychological influences. The most important factor that stimulates thermogenesis is food intake (9). However, note that caffeine (64) and nicotine (65) are thermogenic agents that stimulate energy expenditure. Cold exposure does not play a significant role in stimulating energy expenditure under usual life conditions (66). Humans avoid cold exposure by wearing clothes and maintaining room temperature in the comfort zone. Dietary thermogenesis includes two components: the "obligatory" costs of digesting, absorbing, processing, and storing the nutrients, and a "facultative" component. The facultative component of thermogenesis depends on the sympathetic nervous system (67). Carbohydrate overfeeding induces a sustained rise of urinary norepinephrine (68), and infusions of glucose and insulin increase plasma norepinephrine levels (69). Additional evidence of the activation of the sympathetic nervous system after carbohydrate infusion is the reduction of the glucose-induced thermogenic response by β-adrenergic blockade with propranolol (70).

The possible contribution of a thermogenic defect in the etiology of obesity is controversial. The thermogenic responses to glucose or meal ingestion are either decreased (71–80) or unaltered (81–87) in obese subjects. The thermic effect of infused insulin-glucose was found to be reduced in insulin resistant and non-insulin-dependent diabetes mellitus (NIDDM) obese patients (88–90). The thermic effect of insulin-glucose was found to be proportional to the rate of glucose storage. This concept is supported by Ravussin et al. (91), who showed a similar thermic effect of glucose in lean and obese subjects when they were infused at the rate of insulin needed to obtain a predetermined glucose uptake. Obese subjects had to be infused with a larger rate of insulin infusion in order to get the same rate of glucose uptake as that of lean subjects. With a similar rate of glucose uptake, the thermogenic response was the same in lean and obese subjects. It can be concluded that obese subjects with impaired glucose tolerance and NIDDM obese patients have a decreased rate of glucose storage after a meal (or a glucose load) accompanied by a reduced rate of storage of glucose as glycogen in muscles, with an economy of energy expenditure.

It is interesting to evaluate the possible role of a thermogenic defect in the weight gain that occurs in most patients after cessation of an hypocaloric therapy. We calculated that a thermogenic defect can account for a maximal energy saving of approximately 125 kcal/d. Because the increase in body weight is accompanied by a rise in energy expenditure of ~25 kcal/d/kg weight gain, it can be calculated that a weight gain of 5 kg (i.e., a rise in energy expenditure of ~125 kcal/day) completely offsets the effect of the thermogenic defect (92). Therefore, a thermogenic defect is a factor that contributes to the weight gain after cessation of dietary therapy but it has a modest effect (92). It is likely that an abnormality in the control of food intake plays the most important role in the development of obesity or in relapse of body weight gain after an hypocaloric diet. Obese individuals, even those with a low basal metabolic rate per unit lean body mass, expend more energy than lean sedentary individuals (93). Thus, the important conclusion is that the concept of "small eaters" who remain obese with daily energy intake less than 1800 kcal/d is certainly wrong.

E Control of the Thermic Effect of Food by the Autonomic Nervous System and by Hormones

The sympathetic nervous system (SNS) plays a role in the control of energy expenditure. As already described, the thermogenic response to food ingestion includes a facultative component that depends on the activity of the SNS (70). Recent evidence shows that oral (94) or intravenous (95) glucose administration stimulates muscle sympathetic nerve activity (MSNA). Increased activity of the SNS may contribute to the thermic effect of food since β-adrenergic blockade with propranolol decreases glucose-induced thermogenesis (70,96). However, the metabolic effects of catecholamines released at sympathetic nerve endings or by the adrenal medulla remain unclear (97).

Since the parasympathetic nervous system is involved in the cephalic phase of insulin secretion at the beginning of a meal (98), a role for this system has also been investigated in the control of the thermic effect of food (99). Cholinergic blockade with atropine decreases the thermic effect of a meal (99). This effect can be explained in part by the fact that atropine slows gastric emptying and reduces intestinal motility. Thus, the thermogenic mechanisms which are dependent on the parasympathetic nervous system may be related to intestinal absorption and the subsequent rate of storage of the absorbed nutrients.

The main hormone involved in the thermic effect of a meal is insulin. There is a reduced thermogenic response to a meal in obese subjects with insulin resistance and in obese NIDDM patients. Thus, either insulin resistance or a relative defect in insulin secretion (or both) induces a reduced glucose-induced thermogenesis. The latter is due in part to an impaired rate of glucose storage as glycogen in muscles; whether a reduced activation of the SNS plays a role is still unknown.

F Familial and Genetic Effects on Thermic Effect of Food

Genetic factors may contribute to the interindividual differences observed in the components of energy expenditure. Studies on the genetic effect of energy expenditure associated with the thermic effect of food are limited. Bouchard et al. (36) measured the thermic effect of a 1000-kcal meal during 4 hr in 21 pairs of dizygotic twins and 37 pairs of monozygotic twins, as well as in 31 parent-offspring pairs. The results suggest a genetic effect of less than one-third of the total thermic effect of food. Expressed in absolute values, the standard deviation of the thermic effect of food over 4 hr reached ~20 kcal, and the 95% confidence intervals were therefore ± 40 kcal, or ± 4% of the energy intake. These data confirm that the variance of the thermic effect of food between individuals represents a relatively small proportion of the total energy turnover. By comparison, the 95% confidence intervals were ~ ± 250 kcal/day for resting energy expenditure, or ± 10% of total energy expenditure.

IV COMPONENTS OF TOTAL ENERGY EXPENDITURE IN THE LEAN AND OBESE STATES

A Absolute Versus Relative Values

It has been customary to distinguish among the following different components of total energy expenditure (TEE): basal metabolic rate, postprandial thermogenesis (or thermic effect of food), and physical activity. This partition is important since the reasons for an abnormal 24-hr energy expenditure can be ascribed to a combination of abnormal subcomponents. As defined in preceding sections, the basal metabolic rate represents the energy expended in resting conditions under fasting state and comfortable environmental conditions; the thermic effect of food represents the net increase in postabsorptive resting metabolic rate in response to the ingestion of a meal or to an increase in total food intake (diet induced thermogenesis). In addition, extra non-meal-mediated thermogenic stimuli may occur owing to cold or heat exposure, as well as psychological factors (emotion or stress) or results from the administration of hormones and drugs. However, physical activity is the most variable (and hence least predictable) component of total energy expenditure. In contrast to the other components, it can be voluntarily modified by the behavior of the subject. In absolute terms, the total energy expenditure of the obese has been shown to be greater than that of lean individuals, both in the confinement of a respiration chamber (13,62,85) and in free-living conditions (100).

The relative rate of TEE can be expressed as a multiple of some baseline values such as RMR. This approach has been used by an international expert committee for calculating the energy requirement in the so called "factorial" method (101). Since both the RMR and TEE of obese subjects are greater in absolute value, it seems of interest to calculate the ratio between the latter and the former. This provides a rough index of physical activity ("physical activity level; PAL), but the contribution of the thermic effect of foods represents a small confounding factor. Since the energy cost for a given activity is proportional to body weight, in particular for weight-bearing activities, the absolute energy expenditure during weight bearing activity will be linearly related to body weight (102). A flat (or a negative) relationship between the energy expenditure due to physical activity and the degree of obesity would indicate that the greater absolute cost of physical activity among obese subjects is largely offset by the depressed activity level. A study by Rising et al. (103) has shown that obesity was associated with lower levels of physical activity. The key question is to know whether a low level of physical activity is the *consequence* or the *cause* of obesity, or both.

Normalization of total energy expenditure in the obese appears to be difficult since the RMR is proportional to FFM (and fat mass) whereas the energy expenditure related physical activity is proportional to body weight. Although there is a statistical bias in normalizing the TEE by RMR (104), it seems to be a reasonable way (as compared to other alternatives) to express as such the free-living energy expenditure. The fact that both the absolute RMR and the energy cost for a given activity are greater in the obese explain why the TEE expressed in relative value (TEE/RMR) is not expected to be dramatically different from that observed in a nonobese subject. In this context, it seems of interest to review the magnitude of the ratio TEE/RMR in nonobese and obese adult subjects. Table 3 shows an overview of different experimental studies recently published in the literature (105–112). Globally considered, there is no strong evidence that the ratio TEE/RMR is systematically lower in obese individuals than in lean subjects, although the variations among and within studies was substantial (Table 3). This confirms our previous results in the respiration chamber (13).

Compilations of total daily energy expenditure results (using a meta-analysis approach) in individuals of various body weight and gender have been made by Schulz and Schoeller (113) and Carpenter et al. (104). In all these studies, energy expenditure was assessed by the doubly labeled water technique. In the former study (113), it was found that the increased weight of men (but not of women) was associated with a tendency for the TEE/RMR ratio to be lower, corroborating the notion that obesity tends to depress physical activity in obese men. This tendency was confirmed in a subsequent meta-analysis by Prentice et al. (109).

Because of the increase in prevalence and incidence of childhood obesity, it seems also important to study the energy metabolism in children as they grow through puberty in order to initiate early therapeutic intervention and prevent subsequent obesity in adults. Blunted physical activity due to a greater placidity and sedentary life-style are associated with low TEE (114–116). A classic study by Dietz et al. (117) has shown that the amount of time dedicated to watch television

Table 3 Total Energy Expenditure (TEE) Expressed as a Multiple of Resting Metabolic Rate (RMR) in Obese and Nonobese Subjects (Physical Activity Level; PAL)

	Authors	Ref.	TEE/RMR
Obese individuals			
American women	Lichtman et al. (1992)	105	1.68
American women	Welle et al. (1992)	106	1.73
British women	Livingstone et al. (1990)	107	1.39
Pima Indian	Ravussin et al. (1991)	108	1.56
Average overweight men (BMI 25–30)	Prentice et al. (1996)	109	1.86
Average overweight women (BMI 25–30)	Prentice et al. (1996)	109	1.73
Average moderately obese men (BMI 30–35)	Prentice et al. (1996)	109	1.82
Average moderately obese women (BMI 30–35)	Prentice et al. (1996)	109	1.73
Average obese men (BMI $\geq$ 35)	Prentice et al. (1996)	109	1.52
Average obese women (BMI $\geq$ 35)	Prentice et al. (1996)	109	1.65
Nonobese individuals			
American men	Goran et al. (1993)	110	1.70
American men	Roberts et al. (1991)	111	1.98
British men	Livingstone et al. (1990)	107	1.88
Dutch men	Westerterp et al. (1991)	112	1.64
Average men (affluent society)	Prentice et al. (1996)	109	1.80
Average women (affluent society)	Prentice et al. (1996)	109	1.67

was related to the degree of obesity in childhood. The relationship between a low level of physical activity and the accumulation of body fat in children has been the subject of a number of studies in both infants and children of Caucasian and Pima Indian origin (114, 118,119). The classic study by Roberts et al. (119) suggested that infants who were overweight at 1 year of age had a low total energy expenditure 9 months earlier (i.e., at 3 months of age) compared with a control group of children. The blunted rate of energy expenditure can be considered as one of the causal factors since at the time the infants were measured (3 months) they were not overweight.

Although the total daily energy expenditure in free-living condition in obese children is, expressed in absolute value, either greater than (120) or similar to (121) a matched group of lean children, this does not imply that the obese children have the same level of physical activity since the same type of activity will involve a greater energy cost in obese children. Taken together, these studies suggest that a reduced physical activity–related energy expenditure constitutes an important factor in the etiology of the subsequent weight gain. The study of Davies et al. (122) has shown a negative association between the level of physical activity as determined by the ratio between TEE and resting metabolic rate (physical activity level) and the percentage body fat in a sample of 77 boys and girls. A review on the available measures of physical activity indexes has just been published (123).

B Effect of Weight Loss on Energy Expenditure

When significant weight loss occurs, energy expenditure decreases, whereas weight gain leads to a rise in energy expenditure. This will depend on the respective effect of the individual factors influencing the three components of TEE: resting energy expenditure will decrease as a function of the loss of FFM; the absolute thermic effect of food will be lower as a result of the restricted dietary intake; and, for a given rate of physical activity, the absolute energy expenditure due to physical activity will drop because of the lower body size. In a prospective study of weight loss and relapse in body weight gain, we found that the rate of TEE and RMR essentially followed the change in body weight and body composition. The progressively reduced (or increased) energy expenditure accompanying weight loss (or weight gain) constitutes one of the major factors that explain the decrease in the rate of weight loss (or weight gain) with time. Another factor is the change in dietary compliance during dieting, which seems to be an individual characteristic.

Finally, it should be recalled that the compensatory energetic processes mentioned above tend to jeopardize the persistence of the altered body weight in obese individuals, accounting for the generally poor long-term efficacy of obesity treatments. (124).

REFERENCES

1. Jéquier E. Direct and indirect calorimetry in man. In: Garrow JS, Halliday D, eds. Substrate and Energy Metabolism. London: Libbey, 1985:82–92.
2. Schoeller DA, Taylor PB, Shay K. Analytic requirements for the doubly labeled water method. Obes Res 1995; 3(suppl 1):15–20.
3. Roberts SB, Dietz W, Sharp T, Dallal GE, Hill JO. Multiple laboratory comparison of the doubly labeled water technique. Obes Res 1995; 3(suppl 1):3–13.
4. Matthews DE, Gilker CD, Impact of ^{2}H and ^{18}O pool size determinations on the calculation of total energy expenditure. 1995; 3(suppl 1):21–29.
5. Speakman JR. Estimation of precision in DLW studies using the two-point methodology. Obes Res 1995; 3 (suppl 1):31–39.
6. Jones PJH. Correction approaches for doubly labeled water in situations of changing background water abundance. Obes Res 1995; 3(suppl 1):41–48.
7. Jéquier E, Acheson K, Schutz Y. Assessment of energy expenditure and fuel utilization in man. Annu Rev Nutr 1987; 7:187–208.
8. Livesey G, Elia M. Estimation of energy expenditure, net carbohydrate utilization, and net fat oxidation and synthesis by indirect calorimetry: evaluation of errors with special reference to the detailed composition of fuels. Am J Clin Nutr 1988; 47:608–628.
9. Jéquier E, Acheson K, Schutz Y. Assessment of energy expenditure and fuel utilization in man. Annu Rev Nutr 1987; 7:187–208.
10. Frayn KN. Calculation of substrate oxidation rates in vivo from gaseous exchange. J Appl Physiol 1983; 55:628–634.
11. Elia M. Organ and tissue contribution to metabolic rate. In: Kinney JM, Tucker HN, eds. Energy Metabolism. Tissue Determinants and Cellular Corollaries. New York: Raven Press, 1992:61–79.
12. Weinsier R, Schutz Y, Bracco D. Reexamination of the relationship of resting metabolic rate to fat-free mass and to the metabolically active components of fat-free mass in humans. Am J Clin Nutr 1992; 55:790–794.
13. Schutz Y, Jéquier E. Energy expenditure. Lancet 1986; 101–102.
14. Maffeis C, Schutz Y, Zoccante L, Pinelli L. Resting metabolic rate in six-to-ten-year-old obese and nonobese children. J Pediatr 1993; 122:556–562.
15. Nelson K, Weinsier RL, Long CL, Schutz Y. Prediction of resting energy expenditure from fat-free mass and fat mass. Am J Clin Nutr 1992; 56:848–856.
16. Ferraro R, Lillioja S, Fontvielle AM, Rising R, Bogardus C, Ravussin E. Lower sedentary metabolic rate in women compared to men. J Clin Invest 1992; 90:1–5.
17. Arciero PJ, Goran MI, Poehlman ET. Resting metabolic rate is lower in women than in men. J Appl Physiol 1993; 75:2514–2520.
18. Zurlo F, Larson K, Bogardus C, Ravussin E. Skeletal muscle metabolism is a major determinant of resting energy expenditure. J Clin Invest 1990; 86:1423–1427.
19. Poehlman ET, Toth MJ, Webb GD. Erythrocyte Na-K pump activity contributes to the age-related decline in resting metabolic rate. J Clin Endocrinol Metab 1993; 76:1054–1057.
20. Solomon SJ, Kurzer MS, Calloway DH. Menstrual cycle and basal metabolic rate in women. Am J Clin Nutr 1982; 36:611–616.
21. Bisdee JT, James WPT, Shaw MA. Changes in energy expenditure during the menstrual cycle. Br J Nutr 1989; 61:187–199.
22. Piers LS, Diggavi SN, Rijskamp J, van Raaij JM, Shetty PS, Hautvast JG. Resting metabolic rate and thermic effect of a meal in the follicular and luteal phases of the menstrual cycle in well-nourished Indian women. Am J Clin Nutr 1995; 61:296–302.
23. Weststrate JA. Resting metabolic rate and diet-induced thermogenesis: a methodological reappraisal. Am J Clin Nutr 1993; 58:592–601.
24. Frascarolo P, Schutz Y, Jéquier E. Decreased thermal conductance during the luteal phase of the menstrual cycle in women. J Appl Physiol 1990; 69:2029–2033.
25. Shock NW, Yiengst MJ. Age changes in basal respiratory measurements and metabolism in males. J Gerontol 1955; 10:31–40.
26. Poehlman ET, Goran MI, Gardner AW. Determinants of decline in resting metabolic rate in aging females. Am J Physiol 1993; 264:E450–E455.
27. Benedek C, Berclaz P-Y, Jéquier E, Schutz Y. Resting metabolic rate and protein turnover in apparently healthy elderly Gambian men. Am J Physiol 1995; 268:E1083–E1088.
28. Acheson KJ, Schutz Y, Bessard T, Ravussin E, Jéquier E, Flatt JP. Nutritional influences on lipogenesis and thermogenesis after a carbohydrate meal. Am J Physiol 1984; 246:E62–E70.
29. Schutz Y. Abnormalities of fuel utilization as predisposing to the development of obesity in humans. Obes Res 1995; 3(suppl 2):173S–178S.
30. Schutz Y. The adjustment of energy expenditure and oxidation to energy intake: the role of carbohydrate and fat balance. Int J Obes 1993; 17(suppl 3):S23–S27.
31. Sjöstrom L, Schutz Y, Gudinchet F, Hegnell L, Pittet PG, Jéquier E. Epinephrine sensitivity with respect to metabolic rate and other variables in women. Am J Physiol 1983; 245:E431–E442.

32. Staten MA, Matthews DE, Cryer PE, Bier M. Physiological increments in epinephrine stimulate metabolic rate in humans. Am J Physiol 1987; 253: E322–E330.
33. Mansel PI, Fellows IW, Macdonald IA. Enhanced thermogenic response to epinephrine after 48-h starvation in humans. Am J Physiol 1990; 258:R87–R93.
34. Randin J-P, Schutz Y, Scazziga B, Lemarchand-Béraud T, Felber J-P, Jéquier E. Unaltered glucose-induced thermogenesis in Graves disease. Am J Clin Nutr 1986; 43:738–744.
35. Bogardus C, Lillioja S, Ravussin E, et al. Familial dependence of the resting metabolic rate. N Engl J Med 1986; 315:96–100.
36. Bouchard C, Tremblay A, Nadeau A, et al. Genetic effect in resting and exercise metabolic rates. Metabolism 1989; 38:364–370.
37. Bouchard C. Genetics of obesity: overview and research directions. In: Bouchard C, ed. The Genetics of Obesity. Boca Raton: CRC Press, 1994:223–233.
38. Nicholls DG, Locke RM. Thermogenic mechanisms in brown fat. Physiol Rev 1984; 64:1–64.
39. Rothwell NJ, Stock MJ. A role for brown adipose tissue in diet-induced thermogenesis. Nature 1979; 281: 31–35.
40. Weyer C, Gautier JF, Danforth EJ. Development of beta3-adrenoceptor agonists for the treatment of obesity and diabetes—an update. Diabetes Metab 1999; 25:11–21.
41. Ravussin E, Schutz Y, Acheson KJ, Dusmet M, Bourquin L, Jéquier E. Short-term, mixed-diet overfeeding in man: no evidence for "Luxuskonsumption." Am J Physiol 1985; 249:E470–E477.
42. Fleury C, Neverova M, Collins S. Uncoupling protein-2: a novel gene linked to obesity and hyperinsulinemia. Nat Genet 1997; 15:269–272.
43. Boss O, Samec S, Paoloni-Giacobino A, et al. Uncoupling protein-3: a new member of the mitochondrial carrier family with tissue-specific expression. FEBS Lett 1997; 408:39–42.
44. Kozak LP, Harper ME. Mitochondrial uncoupling proteins in energy expenditure. Annu Rev Nutr 2000; 20:339–363.
45. Boss O, Bobbioni-Harsch E, Assimacopoulos-Jeannet F, et al. Uncoupling protein-3 expression in skeletal muscle and free fatty acids in obesity. Lancet 1998; 35:1933.
46. Samec S, Seydoux J, Dulloo AG. Role of UCP homologues in skeletal muscles and brown adipose tissue: mediators of thermogenesis or regulators of lipids as fuel substrate? FASEB J 1998; 12:715–724.
47. Silva JE. The physiological role of the novel uncoupling proteins: view from the chair. Int J Obes 1999; 23(suppl 6):S72–S74.
48. Roberts SB, Nicholson M, Staten M, et al. Relationship between circulating leptin and energy expenditure in adult men and women aged 18 years to 81 years. Obes Res 1997; 5:459–463.
49. Kennedy A, Gettys TW, Watson P, et al. The metabolic significance of leptin in humans: gender-based differences in relationship to adiposity, insulin sensitivity, and energy expenditure. J Clin Endocrinol Metab 1997; 82:1293–1300.
50. Campostano A, Grillo G, Bessarione D, De Grandi R, Adami GF. Relationships of serum leptin to body composition and resting energy expenditure. Horm Metab Res 1998; 30:646–647.
51. Jorgensen JO, Vahl N, Dall R, Christiansen JS. Resting metabolic rate in healthy adults: relation to growth hormone status and leptin levels. Metabolism 1998; 47:1134–1139.
52. Neuhauser-Berthold M, Herbert BM, Luhrmann PM, et al. Resting metabolic rate, body composition, and serum leptin concentrations in a free-living elderly population. Eur J Endocrinol 2000; 142:486–492.
53. Haynes WG, Morgan DA, Walsh SA, Mark AL, Sivitz WI. Receptor-mediated regional sympathetic nerve activation by leptin. J Clin Invest 1997; 100:270–278.
54. Reed GW, Hill JO. Measuring the thermic effect of food. Am J Clin Nutr 1996; 63:164–169.
55. Tappy L, Jéquier E. Fructose and dietary thermogenesis. Am J Clin Nutr 1993; 58(suppl):766S–770S.
56. Suter PM, Jéquier E, Schutz Y. Effect of ethanol on energy expenditure. Am J Physiol 1994; 266:R1204–R1212.
57. Thiébaud D, Acheson K, Schutz Y, et al. Stimulation of thermogenesis in men after combined glucose long-chain triglyceride infusion. Am J Clin Nutr 1983; 37: 603–611.
58. Golay A, Schutz Y, Broquet C, Moeri R, Felber JP, Jéquier E. Decreased thermogenic response to an oral glucose load in older subjects. J Am Geriatr Soc 1983; 31:144–148.
59. Bloesch D, Schutz Y, Breitenstein E, Jéquier E, Felber JP. Thermogenic response to an oral glucose load in man: comparison between young and elderly subjects. J Am Coll Nutr 1988; 7:471–483.
60. Tai MM, Castillo TP, Pi-Sunyer FX. Thermic effect of food during each phase of the menstrual cycle. Am J Clin Nutr 1997; 66:1110–1115.
61. Melanson KJ, Saltzman E, Russell R, Roberts SB. Postabsorptive and postprandial energy expenditure and substrate oxidation do not change during the menstrual cycle in young women. J Nutr 1996; 126: 2531–2538.
62. Jéquier E, Schutz Y. Energy expenditure in obesity and diabetes. Diabetes Metab Rev 1988; 4:583–593.
63. De Jonge L, Bray GA. The thermic effect of food and obesity: a critical review. Obes Res 1997; 5:622–631.
64. Bracco D, Ferrarra JM, Arnaud MJ, Jéquier E, Schutz Y. Effects of caffeine on energy metabolism, heart rate,

and methylxanthine metabolism in lean and obese women. Am J Physiol 1995; 269:E671–E678.
65. Hofstetter A, Schutz Y, Jéquier E, Wahren J. Increased 24-hour energy expenditure in cigarette smokers. N Engl J Med 1986; 314:79–82.
66. Jéquier E, Gygax PH, Pittet PH, Vannotti A. Increased thermal body insulation: relationship to the development of obesity. J Appl Physiol 1974; 36:674–678.
67. Welle S, Lilavivat U, Campbell RG. Thermic effect of feeding in man: increased norepinephrine levels following glucose but no protein or fat consumption. Metabolism 1981; 30:953–958.
68. Schutz Y, Acheson KJ, Jéquier E. Twenty-four-hour energy expenditure and thermogenesis: response to progressive carbohydrate overfeeding in man. Int J Obes 1985; 9:111–114.
69. Rowe JW, Young JB, Minaker KL, Stevens AL, Pallota J, Landsberg L. Effects of insulin and glucose infusions on sympathetic nervous system activity in normal man. Diabetes 1981; 30:219–225.
70. Acheson KJ, Ravussin E, Wahren J, Jéquier E. Thermic effect of glucose in man: obligatory and facultative thermogenesis. J Clin Invest 1984; 74:1572–1580.
71. Bessard T, Schutz Y, Jéquier E. Energy expenditure and postprandial thermogenesis in obese women before and after weight loss. Am J Clin Nutr 1983; 38:680–693.
72. Kaplan ML, Léveillé GA. Calorigenic response in obese ans non-obese women. Am J Clin Nutr 1976; 29:1108–1113.
73. Pittet P, Chappuis P, Acheson KJ, De Techtermann F, Jéquier E. Thermic effect of glucose in obese subjects studied by direct and indirect calorimetry. Br J Nutr 1976; 35:281–289.
74. Shetty PS, Jung RT, James WPT, Barrand MA, Callingham BA. Postprandial thermogenesis in obesity. Clin Sci 1981; 60:519–525.
75. Danforth EJ, Daniels RJ, Katzeff HL, Ravussin E, Garrow JS. Thermogenic responsiveness in Pima Indians. Clin Res 1981; 29:663.
76. Golay A, Schutz Y, Meyer HU. Glucose induced thermogenesis in nondiabetic and diabetic obese subjects. Diabetes 1982; 31:1023–1028.
77. Schwartz RS, Ravussin E, Massari M, O'Connell M, Robbins DC. The thermic effect of carbohydrate versus fat feeding in man. Metabolism 1983; 32:581–589.
78. Schutz Y, Bessard T, Jéquier E. Diet-induced thermogenesis measured over a whole day in obese and nonobese women. Am J Clin Nutr 1984; 40:542–552.
79. Swaminatham R, King RFGJ, Holmfield J, Siwek R, Baker M, Wales JK. Thermic effect of feeding carbohydrates, fat protein and mixed meal in lean and obese subjects. Am J Clin Nutr 1985; 42:177–181.
80. Segal KR, Gutin B, Pi-Sunyer FX. Thermic effect of food at rest, during exercise, and after exercise in lean and obese men of similar body weight. J Clin Invest 1985; 76:1107–1112.
81. Sharief NN, MacDonald I. Differences in dietary-induced thermogenesis with various carbohydrates in normal and overweight men. Am J Clin Nutr 1982; 35:267–272.
82. Welle SL, Campbell RG. Normal thermic effect of glucose in obese women. Am J Clin Nutr 1983; 37:87–92.
83. Felig P, Cunningham J, Levitt M, Hendler R, Nadel E. Energy expenditure in obesity in fasting and post-prandial state. Am J Physiol 1983; 244:E45–E51.
84. Segal KR, Gutin B. Thermic effect of food and exercise in lean and obese women. Metabolism 1983; 32:581–589.
85. Blaza S, Garrow JS. Thermogenic response to temperature, exercise and food stimuli in lean and obese women, studied by 24 h direct calorimetry. Br J Nutr 1983; 49:171–180.
86. Anton-Kuchly B, Laval M, Choukroun ML, Manciet G, Roger P, Varene P. Postprandial thermogenesis and hormonal release in lean and obese subjects. J Physiol (Paris) 1985; 80:321–329.
87. Vernet O, Christin L, Schutz Y, Danforth E, Jéquier E. Enteral vs parenteral nutrition: comparison of energy metabolism in lean and moderately obese women. Am J Clin Nutr 1986; 43:194–209.
88. Ravussin E, Acheson KJ, Vernet O, Danforth EJ, Jéquier E. Thermic effect of infused glucose and insulin in man. Decreased response with increased insulin resistance in obesity and noninsulin dependent diabetes mellitus. J Clin Invest 1983; 72:893–902.
89. Bogardus C, Lillioja S, Mott D, Zawadski J, Young A, Abbott W. Evidence for reduced thermic effect of insulin and glucose infusions in Pima Indians. J Clin Invest 1985; 75:1264–1269.
90. Golay A, Schutz Y, Felber JP, DeFronzo RA, Jéquier E. Lack of thermogenic response to glucose/insulin infusion in diabetic obese subjects. Int J Obes 1986; 10:107–116.
91. Ravussin E, Acheson KJ, Vernet O, Danforth EJ, Jéquier E. Evidence that insulin resistance is responsible for the decreased thermic effect of glucose in human obesity. J Clin Invest 1985; 76:1268–1273.
92. Weinsier RL, Bracco D, Schutz Y. Predicted effects of small decreases in energy expenditure on weight gain in adult women. Int J Obes 1993; 17:693–700.
93. Ravussin E, Lillioja S, Knowler WC, et al. Reduced rate of energy expenditure as a risk factor for body-weight gain. N Engl J Med 1988; 318:467–472.
94. Berne C, Fagius J, Niklasson F. Sympathetic response to oral carbohydrate administration. Evidence from microelectrode nerve recordings. J Clin Invest 1989; 84:1403–1409.
95. Vollenweider P, Tappy L, Randin D. Differential

effects of hyperinsulinemia and carbohydrate metabolism on sympathetic nerve activity and muscle blood flow in humans. J Clin Invest 1993; 92:147–154.
96. Acheson KJ, Jéquier E, Wahren J. Influence of β-adrenergic blockade on glucose-induced thermogenesis in man. J Clin Invest 1983; 72:981–986.
97. Tappy L, Girardet K, Schwaller N, et al. Metabolic effects of an increase of sympathetic activity in healthy humans. Int J Obes 1995; 19:419–422.
98. Berthoud HR, Bereiter DA, Trimble ER, Siegel EG, Jeanrenaud B. Cephalic phase, reflex insulin secretion. Neuroanatomical and physiological characterization. Diabetologia 1981; 20:393–401.
99. Nacht C, Christin L, Temler E, Chiolero R, Jéquier E, Acheson K. Thermic effect of food: possible implication of parasympathetic nervous system. Am J Physiol 1987; 253:E481–E488.
100. Prentice AM, Black AE, Coward WA, et al. High levels of energy expenditure in obese women. BMJ 1986; 292:983–987.
101. Schutz Y, Jéquier E. Energy needs: assessment and requirements. In: Shils ME, Olson JA, Shike M, eds. Modern Nutrition in Health and Disease. Philadelphia: Lea & Febiger, 1994:101–111.
102. Schutz Y. Rôle de l'activité physique dans l'étiologie de l'obésité. Rev Ther 1989; 5:281–290.
103. Rising R, Harper IT, Fontvielle AM, Ferraro RT, Spraul M, Ravussin E. Determinants of total daily energy expenditure: variability in physical activity. Am J Clin Nutr 1994; 59:800–804.
104. Carpenter WH, Poehlman ET, O'Connell M, Goran MI. Influence of body composition and resting metabolic rate on variation in total energy expenditure: a meta-analysis. Am J Clin Nutr 1995; 61:4–10.
105. Lichtman SW, Pisarska K, Raynes Berman E, et al. Discrepancy between self-reported and actual caloric intake and exercise in obese subjects. N Engl J Med 1992; 327:1893–1898.
106. Welle S, Forbes GB, Statt M, Barnard RR, Amatruda JM. Energy expenditure under free-living conditions in normal weight and overweight women. Am J Clin Nutr 1992; 55:14–21.
107. Livingstone MBE, Prentice AM, Strain JJ, et al. Accuracy of weighted dietary records in studies of diet and health. BMJ 1990; 300:708–712.
108. Ravussin E, Harper IT, Rising R, Bogardus C. Energy expenditure by doubly labeled water: validation in lean and obese subjects. Am J Physiol 1991; 261:E402–E409.
109. Prentice AM, Black AE, Coward WA, Cole TJ. Energy expenditure in overweight and obese adults in affluent societies: an analysis of 319 doubly-labelled water measurements. Eur J Clin Nutr 1996; 50:93–97.
110. Goran MI, Beer WH, Wolfe RR, Poehlman ET, Young VR. Variation in total energy expenditure in young healthy free-living men. Metabolism 1993; 42: 487–496.
111. Roberts SB, Heyman MB, Evans WJ, Fuss P, Tsay R, Young VR. Dietary energy requirements of young adult men, determined by using doubly labeled water method. Am J Clin Nutr 1991; 54:499–505.
112. Westerterp KR, Meijer GAL, Saris WHM, Soeters PB, Winants Y, Hoor FT. Physical activity and sleeping metabolic rate. Med Sci Sports Exerc 1991; 23:166–170.
113. Schulz LO, Schoeller DA. A compilation of total daily energy expenditures and body weights in healthy adults. Am J Clin Nutr 1994; 60:676–681.
114. Fontvieille AM, Harper TT, Ferraro T, Spraul M, Ravussin E. Daily energy expenditure by five year old children measured by doubly labelled water. J Pediatr 1993; 123:201–206.
115. Goran MI, Carpenter WH, Poehlman ET. Total energy expenditure in 4 to 6 year old children. Am J Physiol 1993; 264:E706–E711.
116. Davies PSW, Coward WA, Tyler H, White A. Total energy expenditure and energy intake in the pre-school child. a comparison. Br J Nutr 1994; 72:13–20.
117. Dietz WH, Gortmaker SL. Do we fatten our children at the TV set? Television viewing and obesity and adolescents. Pediatrics 1985; 75:807–812.
118. Fontvielle AM, Krisha A, Ravussin E. Decreased physical activity in Pima Indians compared with Caucasian children. Int J Obes 1993; 17:445–452.
119. Roberts SB, Savage J, Coward WA, Chew B, Lucas A. Energy expenditure and intake in infants born to lean and overweight mothers. N Engl J Med 1988; 318:461–466.
120. Maffeis C, Pinelli L, Zaffanello M, Schena F, Iacumin P, Schutz Y. Daily energy expenditure in free-living conditions in obese and non-obese children: comparison of doubly labelled water ($^2H_2$ ^{18}O) method and heart-rate monitoring. Int J Obes 1995; 19:671–677.
121. DeLany JP, Harsha DW, Kime JC, Kumler J, Melancon L, Bray GA. Energy expenditure in lean and obese prepubertal children. Obes Res 1995; 3(suppl 1):67–72.
122. Davies PS, White GA. Physical activity and body fatness in pre-school children. Int J Obes 1995; 19:6–10.
123. Schutz Y, Weinsier RL, Hunter GR. Assessment of free-living physical activity in humans: an overview of currently available and proposed new indexes. Obes Res 2001; 9:368–379.
124. Leibel RL, Rosenbaum M, Hirsch J. Changes in energy expenditure resulting from altered body weight. N Engl J Med 1995; 332:621–628.

24

Energy Expenditure in Physical Activity

James O. Hill

University of Colorado Health Sciences Center, Denver, Colorado, U.S.A.

W. H. M. Saris

University of Maastricht, Maastricht, The Netherlands

James A. Levine

Mayo Clinic, Rochester, Minnesota, U.S.A.

I ENERGY EXPENDITURE DURING PHYSICAL ACTIVITY

A Human Energy Balance

Biological entities obey physical laws, and, in this regard, humans and other mammals obey the laws of thermodynamics. Body energy stores can only increase and obesity can only occur when food intake exceeds energy expenditure (or metabolic rate). Similarly, energy stores can only be depleted when energy expenditure exceeds food intake. Thus, the balance between food intake and energy expenditure determines the body's energy stores. The quantity of energy stored by the human body is impressive; lean individuals store 2–3 months of their energy needs in adipose tissue whereas obese persons can carry a year's worth of their energy needs. The cumulative impact of energy imbalance over months and years can result in the development of obesity. The factors that regulate appetite and food intake are discussed elsewhere. In this chapter we will discuss the importance of physical activity as a component of energy expenditure.

B Components of Energy Expenditure

There are three principal components to energy expenditure in humans: basal metabolic rate, thermic effect of food, and the energy expenditure of physical activity (activity thermogenesis). Basal metabolic rate is the energy expended when an individual is lying at complete rest, in the morning, after sleep, in the postabsorptive state. In individuals with sedentary occupations basal metabolic rate accounts for ~60% of total daily energy expenditure. About 75% of the variability in basal metabolic rate is predicted by lean body mass within and across species (1,2). Resting energy expenditure, in general, is within 10% of basal metabolic rate and is measured in subjects at complete rest in the postabsorptive state. The second component of energy expenditure is the thermic effect of food (3–6). This is the increase in energy expenditure associated with the digestion, absorption, and storage of food and accounts for ~10% of total daily energy expenditure; many believe there to be facultative (adaptive) as well as fixed components. The third component of energy expenditure is the energy expenditure of physical activity, "activity thermogenesis." There are additional components of energy expenditure that may contribute to the whole, such as the energetic costs of altered temperature, medications, and emotion. Each of these components of energy expenditure is highly variable, and the sum effect of these variances determines the variability in daily energy expenditure between individuals.

It is likely that activity thermogenesis contributes substantially to the inter- and intraperson variability in energy expenditure. If three-quarters of the variance of resting energy expenditure is accounted for by variance in lean body mass, and if the thermic effect of food represents 10% of total energy expenditure, then the majority of the variance in total energy expenditure that occurs independent of body weight must be accounted for by the variance in physical activity. Evidence indeed suggests that this is so. The range of activity thermogenesis is wide, ranging from ~15% of total daily energy expenditure in very sedentary individuals to 50% or more of total daily energy expenditure in highly active individuals (7,8). Because this component of energy expenditure is the most variable component of energy expenditure, both within and between subjects (9), its potential role in body weight regulation and in the etiology of obesity deserves close examination. For example, Dauncey (8) estimates that differences in minor activity throughout the day can account for differences of 20% in 24-hr energy expenditure. Such differences, if not compensated for by changes in energy intake, can lead to significant changes in body weight and/or body composition.

Activity thermogenesis can be readily divided into that associated with purposeful exercise and that associated with nonexercise activities, such as the activities of daily living. Exercise is exertion for the specific purpose of physical fitness. Nonexercise activities include the myriad of activities of daily living that are not undertaken as purposeful exercise; they include maintaining posture, walking from the bus stop to work, tapping one's foot or hand while talking, and cleaning the house. The energy expenditure associated with each activity is the product of the time spent performing the activity and the energy cost of that activity per unit time. Thus, to assess activity thermogenesis as a whole, one needs to define each exercise and nonexercise task an individual performs, the time engaged in each activity, and the energy cost of each activity. The ability to do this accurately in free-living humans is technically demanding and is why the importance of activity thermogenesis in energy balance and obesity has been difficult to quantify and define.

In this chapter we will discuss activity thermogenesis, how it is measured, its components, and the impact of activity thermogenesis on other components of energy expenditure and energy balance as a whole.

II METHODOLOGY

Before we can begin to understand the role of activity thermogenesis in energy balance and the pathogenesis of obesity, we must first quantify the nature and duration of exercise and nonexercise activities.

A Quantifying the Nature and Duration of Exercise

A series of tools has been used and, in some cases, validated to quantifying exercise. One approach has been to employ prospective methods (10). Prospective measures include the use of diaries or other recording media (e.g., handheld tape machine) to have subjects record the nature and intensity of exercise performed over a defined time period. The disadvantages of this approach are the reliance on the subjects to record data precisely and the subjective nature of the intensity determinations. An alternative or complementary method for prospective data collection is to record physiological variables, such as pulse rate or respiration, over the period of interest (11). For example, a subject is fitted with a pulse recorder (12) that records along with a time stamp. In this fashion, objective information is gained regarding the duration over which exercise is likely to have been performed (i.e., the time periods during which pulse exceeded a predefined cutoff). The disadvantage of this approach is that no information is gained regarding the nature or intensity of exercise. Studies have repeatedly demonstrated that the magnitude of the change in pulse does not reflect the energetic cost of the exercise performed because heart rate and stroke volume do not change linearly with exercise intensity (13,14).

Retrospective approaches for quantifying exercise have been widely used. A variety of questionnaires (15–17) have been devised that ask subjects to recall their habitual levels and intensities of exercise or to recollect exercise bouts over a defined period. These assessments are often relatively straightforward to perform (many using self-administered questionnaires), rapid, and inexpensive. This approach enables large groups of subjects to be studied. The disadvantage of retrospective surveys of exercise is the inability to verify the precision of the data. On balance, the validated tools are applicable for group comparisons either in cross-sections or longitudinal studies.

B Quantifying the Nature and Duration of Nonexercise Activities

Nonexercise activities are enormously varied and include body postures, locomotion, fidgeting, talking, and brushing hair. Quantifying nonexercise activity is extremely taxing, and little information is available about the energy expended in these activities. Furthermore, the physical activities can be expressed in a variety of units; as the time period of activity (hours, minutes), as units of movements (counts), or even as a numerical score derived from responses to a questionnaire. Activity can also be defined as an overt intentional behavior (e.g., the number of social contacts).

1 Activity Recall and Time and Motion Studies

Nonspecific information about habitual and occupational activity can be obtained using questionnaires, interviews, or time-and-motion studies. Predictably, substantial errors are introduced through inaccurate recall and inadequate data recording. These approaches can be used, however, for following trends in certain activities, particularly with relation to occupational practices (18).

2 Kinematic Measurements

In kinematic measurements, a subject's movements are quantified. Some techniques are specific for confined spaces such as radar tracking and cinephotography (19,20). Other techniques have been used in free-living individuals and generally focus on pedometers and accelerometers of varying sophistication. Pedometers typically detect the displacement of a subject with each stride. However, pedometers tend to lack sensitivity because they do not quantify stride length or total body displacement and overall, therefore, become poor predictors of total activity thermogenesis (21) although potentially of value for quantifying walking (e.g., to determine compliance with a walking program). Accelerometers detect body displacement electronically with varying degrees of sensitivity—uniaxial accelerometers in one axis and triaxial accelerometers in three axes. Portable uniaxial accelerometer units have been widely used to detect physical activity (22–24). Careful evaluation demonstrates that these instruments are not sufficiently sensitive to quantify the physical activity of a given free-living subject but rather they are more valuable for comparing activity levels between groups of subjects. Greater precision has been obtained using triaxial accelerometers (25–27). In free-living subjects, data from these devices correlate well with total daily energy expenditure, measured using doubly labeled water divided by basal metabolic rate (28). The utility of motion tracking using approaches such as Global Positioning Systems has not been fully defined for human studies.

Thus, methods are available for quantifying the amounts of exercise and nonexercise activities that an individual performs. Because of the variable precision of these measures, caution is recommended in applying these techniques for measurements and when interpreting reported studies.

C Quantifying the Energy Cost of Exercise and Nonexercise Activities

The energy costs of specific exercise and nonexercise activities are readily measurable. The technique most often used is indirect calorimetry, whereby oxygen consumption, carbon dioxide production, or both of these variables are measured before and during the activity of interest. Energy expenditure is then calculated by means of established formula (29,30).

Indirect calorimeters vary in sophistication and cost (31). In the laboratory, ventilated open-circuit calorimeters are most often used. Here expired air is collected by means of a mouthpiece, a mask, or a hood or from a sealed chamber (32,33). The air is then mixed, the rate of flow is measured, and oxygen and carbon dioxide concentrations are determined. Measurements to within 1% of chemical standards can be achieved using these devices. In the field, Douglas bags or portable expiratory open circuit calorimeters are most often used. The Douglas bag (34–37) comprises a polyvinyl chloride (or other leakproof material) bag of ~100–150 L (38). After collection of the expired air, the volume of expired air in the bag is measured and a sample analyzed to determine oxygen and/or carbon dioxide concentrations. The technique is highly operator dependent and under optimal conditions the error of energy expenditure measurements undertaken with Douglas bags can be small ($< 3\%$). A variety of portable expiratory open-circuit systems have been devised (39–42). In most, expiratory flow is measured, as are expired oxygen and/or carbon dioxide concentrations. Although less precise than laboratory based instruments, their flexibility allows data to be collected on daily physical activities in the most germane setting.

The techniques for measuring the energy costs of exercise and nonexercise activities are readily defined and, when carefully executed, provide reliable and precise measurements in both the laboratory and field settings.

D Quantifying Activity Thermogenesis

Little information is available regarding the time period of measurement needed to gain a representative assessment of physical activity. We estimate that approximately 7 days of measurement are likely to provide a representative assessment of activity thermogenesis for a given 3- or 4-month block of time. Such 7-day measurements can be repeated to understand the importance of season and changing occupational roles.

There are three principal approaches to estimating activity thermogenesis. The first is to measure it directly in a chamber-style calorimeter. Although this is the only means of directly measuring activity thermogenesis, the approach is enormously limited because subjects are confined to a small (e.g., 12 m^2) room for the measurement duration and so cannot perform their normal daily activities (9,32). Measurement of activity thermogenesis in free-living individuals is more challenging. Broadly, investigators have either tried to sum the energetic equivalents for each activity a subject undertakes, termed the factoral method (39,43,44), or total daily, free-living energy expenditure is measured using doubly labeled water (45) with no attempt made to ascertain the constituents of activity thermogenesis.

Prentice et al. (46) have noted the importance of considering differences in body size when interpreting measurements of physical activity. Caution must be used when making comparisons of energy expended in physical activity between individuals who differ markedly in body size. The physical activity level (PAL) is a calculation often used to express activity thermogenesis values relative to body size. The PAL is calculated as total daily energy expenditure (TEE) divided by RMR. For sedentary subjects the PAL is ~1.5. This value can increase to around 3.5–4.5 under extreme exercise conditions. Alternatively, activity thermogenesis can be calculated from:

$$\begin{aligned}&\text{Activity thermogenesis}\\&\quad= \text{total energy expenditure}\\&\qquad- (\text{basal metabolic rate}\\&\qquad+ \text{thermic effect of food})\end{aligned}$$

Here, thermic effect of food is often not measured but assumed to equal 10% of total energy expenditure.

1 Activity Logs and the Factorial Method

This is a frequently used approach for estimating activity thermogenesis in free-living individuals. First, a subject's physical activities are logged over the time period of interest (e.g., 1 week). The energy equivalent of each of these activities is measured or estimated using a calorimeter or tables, respectively (39,43,44). The time spent in each activity is then multiplied by the energy equivalent for that activity. These values are then summed to derive an estimate of activity thermogenesis.

Errors for the factoral method may first result from inaccurate recording of activities and, secondly, from inaccurate determinations of the energy costs of the activities. To log activity, subjects are often asked to record in a diary the nature and amount of time spent performing each of their activities throughout the day (47). This has several limitations: subjects may be illiterate or anumerate, may report their activities inaccurately or incompletely, and/or may alter their normal activity patterns during periods of assessment. To limit these sources of error, one approach is to have trained enumerators follow subjects and objectively record the subject's activities (18). This is time-consuming and expensive but potentially a valuable source of accurate and objective data.

Newer image gathering technologies may be useful in the future for this purpose. To determine the energy costs of physical activities, standard tables are often used. However, these may introduce substantial (albeit systematic) errors. First, the tables may not include the precise activity the subject performed. Second, the energy cost for a given activity is highly variable between subjects even independent of gender. Third, calorimeter methods for measuring the energy costs of activities have not been standardized between investigators so that precision and accuracy of data in the activity tables cannot always be assured.

To limit these errors, the energy costs of each or most of the activities that the subjects of interest perform can be measured using calorimeters, as described above. At best, the energy costs for each subject's activities would be measured but clearly this is rarely practical except for small studies. In general, population-, gender-, age-specific group means for the majority of the studied subjects activities represents a standard that is worth achieving where optimum precision is warranted.

2 Doubly Labeled Water (DLW)

In the doubly labeled water method (45,48–52), both the hydrogen and oxygen of water are labeled or "tagged" using stable, nonradioactive isotopes (D_2O^{18}). Elimination of administered D_2O^{18} may be used to estimate carbon dioxide production and energy expenditure.

The principle of this technique is as follows. In body water, the O_2 of expired CO_2 is in equilibrium with the O_2:

$$CO_2 + H_2O \leftrightarrow H_2CO_3$$

Thus, if the O_2 in body water is tagged with the tracer O^{18}, the label will distribute not only in body water but also in circulating H_2CO_3 and in expired CO_2. Over time the concentration of the O_2 label in body water will decrease as CO_2 is expired and body water is lost in urine, perspiration, and respiration. If the H_2 in body water is tagged with the tracer D2, the label will distribute solely in the circulating H_2O and H_2CO_3. Over time, the concentration of the H_2 label will decrease, as body water is lost (some of the hydrogen can become partitioned into body protein or fat, however). Thus, if both the O_2 and H_2 in body water are tagged, with known amounts of tracers at the same time, the differences in the elimination rates of the O_2 and H_2 tracers will represent the elimination rate of CO_2.

Subjects are usually given DLW orally after baseline samples of urine, saliva, or blood have been collected. Time is allowed for complete mixing of isotopes to occur within the body water space and then samples of urine, saliva, or blood are collected over 7–21 days. These samples are used for measurements of D_2 and O^{18} enrichments using mass spectroscopy. Changes in D_2 and O^{18} concentrations in body water are then calculated over time, and CO_2 production and energy expenditure are calculated. Energy expenditure can be measured over 7–21 days using this technique with an error of ~6–8% (52). This error can be decreased to a small degree, by collecting samples repeatedly over the measurement period rather than by collecting samples only before and after the measurement period.

Doubly labeled water allows total energy expenditure to be measured to within ~6–8% of actual. Basal metabolic rate can be measured to within 1% of actual, so the cumulative error for measurements of PAL is ~7%. This is impressive considering the measurements are performed in completely free-living individuals. A major limitation of this approach is, however, that no information is gleaned regarding the components of physical activity and how these contribute relative to others. It can thus be difficult to discriminate the impact of exercise from nonexercise or to ascertain the importance of the different components of nonexercise activity thermogenesis (NEAT).

It is thereby possible to measure activity thermogenesis. No approach is ideal, but these available technologies readily enable hypotheses to be addressed regarding activity thermogenesis and its role in energy balance in free-living individuals.

III AMOUNT OF PHYSICAL ACTIVITY HUMANS PERFORM

There are several sources of data that allow information to be gleaned regarding the quantities of exercise and nonexercise activities that humans perform.

A Amount of Exercise Humans Perform

Several comprehensive surveys have provided data on exercise levels in adults in the United States, a population where obesity is epidemic: the National Health Interview Survey (53), the Behavioral Risk Factor Surveillance System (54), and the Third National Health and Nutrition Examination Survey (55). Approximately 22–29% of adults report no participation in leisure time physical activity within 2–4 weeks of the point of survey. Individuals at greater risk for undertaking no exercise are those who are female, black or Hispanic, older, less educated, and receiving lower income. About 20–24% of individuals participate in regular sustained physical activity (five or more times a week for >30 min duration per occasion). The individuals most likely to participate in regular exercise are those who were male, white, younger, more educated, and receiving greater income. The most common forms of exercise are (in descending order) walking for purposeful exercise, gardening or yardwork, stretching exercises, and bicycling. More worrisome still are U.S. survey data derived from children. A quarter of U.S. individuals aged 12–21 years report no exercise, and participation in all types of physical activity declines toward adulthood. These data are echoed by others from developed countries.

B Amount of Nonexercise Activities Humans Perform

Because, as noted above, the variety of nonexercise activity is so enormous and the ability to quantify it so poor, it is very difficult to gain a true estimate of free-living individuals' nonexercise activities. Some of the better-quality data have been derived from approaches where trained enumerators follow individuals and record their physical activities at short time intervals.

These data allow precise determination of the range and type of physical activities performed by specific populations (45,49,56). What transpires from reviewing these surveys is, not surprisingly, that an individual's cultural environment defines the vast majority of the variability in the amount of nonexercise activity performed. The two key components of this cultural environment appear to be first the individual's occupation, and second the "sedentariness" of the indigenous population.

The occupational impact on nonexercise activity can be overt—for example, when comparing nonexercise activity between physical laborers and civil servants (57–59). More subtle occupational effects on physical activity include the impact of factors such as gender. For example, in many populations where women work both in home and out of the home, their cumulative work burden exceeds that of male cohabitants by several hours per day (56).

The importance of population sedentariness is well illustrated by studies of physical activity levels for individuals moving from agricultural communities to urban environments or of the effects of industrialization. In many populations where this has occurred, urbanization been associated with decreased physical activity and increased obesity. Sedentary cues are unmistakable in developed countries often through services designed to optimize convenience and throughput at the expense of necessitating locomotion. Examples include drive-through restaurants and banks, televisions, remote controls, escalators, motorized walkways and clothes washing machines. The sedentariness of a population is likely to be affected by a variety of specific factors that include genetics, age, gender, body composition, education, and season.

1 Variation Due to Genetic Background

It is likely that genetics play some role in determining the amount of physical activity performed. Data in support of this notion was reviewed by Bouchard et al. (60). Based on twin and family studies, the heritability for physical activity level has been estimated as between 29% and 62%. Analysis of self-reports of physical activity from the Finnish Twin Registry, consisting of 1537 monozygotic and 3057 dizygotic twins, estimated a 62% heritability level for age-adjusted physical activity (61). Analyses of self-reported physical activity from the Quebec Family Study, consisting of 1610 members of 375 families, showed a heritability level of 29% for habitual physical activity (62).

2 Variation Due to Age

Many datasets consistently show a decline in physical activity with aging (63–65), with the decline occurring in both men and women. However, some data suggest that during the period 1986–1990, activity levels decreased more in elderly subjects than in young adults (65).

3 Variation Due to Gender

Adult men and women in the United States report similar levels of aerobic and moderate physical activity (65,66). In other countries, such as Canada, England, and Australia, men report 1.5–3 times more aerobic or moderate activity than women (64,67,68). Women in the United States appear to have increased their physical activity more than men during the period 1986–1990 (65,66). In children, a consistent gender difference is found, with boys being more active than girls (69). Gender may influence physical activity in more subtle ways such as through the influence of culturally defined gender occupational roles.

4 Variation Due to Body Composition

There are substantial data to suggest that overweight individuals are less active than their lean counterparts (70–72). This appears to be true across all ages, for both genders, and for all ethnic groups. We cannot, however, conclude on the basis of available evidence that a low level of physical activity contributes to development of obesity. It is equally possible that development of obesity leads to a reduction in physical activity. Reduced activity may partly be balanced by increased energy cost of weightbearing activities. In fact, moving around with a higher body mass implies a higher energy cost.

5 Variation Due to Education

Groups with more education consistently report more leisure time physical activity than groups with less education. In the United States, highly educated groups are two to three times more likely to be active than those with less education (63,65,66).

6 Seasonal Variations in Physical Activity

Limited data are available regarding differences in amount of physical activity performed during different seasons. Data from Canada suggest wide differences in time spent in physical activity due to season. Time spent in these activities was twice as high during the summer months as in the winter months (67).

IV ENERGY COST OF PHYSICAL ACTIVITIES

The other major determinant of activity thermogenesis is the efficiency with which exercise and nonexercise activities (i.e., work) are performed. Work efficiency can be defined as the amount of work performed divided by the energy expended in performing the work. While it is clear that work efficiency is not constant for all human subjects, the extent of individual differences and their importance in body weight regulation is unclear. Several studies have reported differences in work efficiency between groups of subjects, and these will be discussed below. It seems logical that differences in morphology/metabolism of skeletal muscle may play a role in determining work efficiency. Blei et al. (73), using 31P NMR spectroscopy, reported that human muscle varied nearly twofold in both energy cost per twitch (energy cost) and recovery time constants (oxidative capacity) across individuals.

A Data on the Metabolic Cost of Exercise

Since for the average adult the resting metabolic rate (RMR) is fairly close to 3.5 mL/kg min of oxygen, or 1 kcal/kg of body weight h, the energy cost of activities can be expressed as multiples of RMR and called METs (an abbreviation of "metabolic"). The use of METs is a simple approach to estimate energy expenditure, taking body weight into account. Ainsworth et al. (74) have published an extensive compendium of MET values of all type of activities. MET values provide an indication of intensity of physical activity and, when summed over time, can be used to compare level of physical activity between individuals.

The gross energy cost of exercise that can be maintained for more than a few minutes roughly varies between 2.0 METs (leisure walking) and 8.0 METs (running 5 mph). However, to expend more energy (e.g., 18 METs; running 10 mph) for a longer period of time, the aerobic fitness of an individual has to be far beyond the level that is observed in general population. An individual who has an aerobic fitness of 35 mL/kg min, which is the average for a normal weight 40-year-old female, is not able to expend more than 7 METs (corresponding to 70% of her VO_2max) for >30 min. A deterioration in aerobic fitness can thus reduce the ability to be active.

B Postexercise Energy Expenditure

Energy expenditure does not return to preexercise levels immediately upon cessation of the physical activity, and the period of increased energy expenditure following exercise is called excess postexercise energy expenditure. The factors that determine the extent to which postexercise energy expenditure occurs have not been clearly defined, leaving a controversy regarding the overall importance of postexercise energy expenditure for overall energy balance (75). Some have suggested energy expenditure can be elevated as long as 24 hr after a bout of exercise (76); others have suggested baseline energy expenditure is restored within a few minutes after exercise cessation (77). Further, it appears that the magnitude and duration of the postexercise increase in energy expenditure is related to the intensity and duration of the exercise bout, with longer, more intense exercise likely to produce a more significant post exercise increase in energy expenditure (78). Over a 12-hr period excess postexercise energy expenditure has been found to vary between 24 kcal after 120 min cycling at 100 Watt and 157 kcal after cycling 80 min at 70% VO_2max (79). Compared to the energy expenditure during exercise itself, the postexercise increase above RMR is modest and has been found to increase energy expenditure by exercise by another 3–15%.

In a review of this phenomenon, Poehlman et al. (80) concluded that, from a practical point of view, an exercise prescription for the general public that consists of low (<50% VO_2max) and moderate intensity (50–70% VO_2max) would result in an extra postexercise energy expenditure of only 9–30 kcal per bout. It is unlikely that these differences will significantly influence body weight regulation. In this regard, it is questionable whether the moderate exercise usually prescribed for moderately obese humans is sufficient to produce appreciable postexercise increase in energy expenditure.

C Data on the Metabolic Cost of Nonexercise Activities

It has long been known that even trivial movement is associated with substantial deviation in energy expenditure above resting values. For example, even mastication is associated with deviations in energy expenditure of 20% above resting (81). Very low levels of physical activity such as fidgeting can increase energy expenditure above resting levels by 20–40% (82). It is not surprising that ambulation whereby body weight is supported and translocated is associated with substantial excursions in energy expenditure (28). Even walking at 1 mph doubles energy expenditure and purposeful walking pace (2–3 mph) is associated with doubling or tripling of energy expenditure. When body translocation is logged using a triaxial accelerometer attached to the back, the output from this unit correlates with nonresting energy expenditure. This implies that ambulation is likely to have a profound influence on NEAT and most likely total energy expenditure in many individuals. The energy costs of a multitude of occupational and nonoccupational physical activities have been charted and tabulated in a series of publications (74). What is noteworthy is the manyfold variance in the energy costs of occupational related activities ranging from <1 MET (e.g., typing) to 5–10 METs (e.g., wood cutting, harvesting, or physical construction).

D Factors that Affect the Energy Costs of Physical Activities

It is recognized that several factors affect the energetic efficiency of exercise and nonexercise activities.

1 Body Weight/Body Composition

It requires more energy to move a larger body mass, and several investigators (83–85) demonstrated that energy expended in physical activity during weightbearing physical activity increased with increasing body mass. It is important to take into account the greater cost of physical activity of a larger body mass when assessing differences in physical activity between obese and non obese subjects. An obese person who is slightly less active than a lean counterpart may expend as much or more total energy in physical activity.

It is less clear whether work efficiency varies with body composition, independently of body weight. Some studies (86–89) have found no differences in work efficiency between obese and nonobese subjects, while others (90,91) have found a greater work efficiency in the obese. Most studies not finding differences in work efficiency have used cycle ergometers with a moderate workload, while those finding differences have used cycle ergometers with heavy loads or treadmills. Work efficiency may vary with type and intensity of physical activity. There are some data suggesting that oxygen consumption increases more rapidly in obese than lean individuals as workload increases (90). This would be consistent with a greater work efficiency in the obese.

2 Effects of Changes in Body Weight/Body Composition

Several studies have reported that efficiency of work is reduced following weight reduction. Foster et al. (92) measured the energy cost of walking in 11 obese women before weight loss and at 9 and 22 weeks after weight loss. They determined that the energy cost of walking (after controlling for loss of body weight) decreased substantially by 22 weeks after weight loss. They estimated that with a 20% loss of body weight, subjects would expend ~427 kJ/hr less during walking than before weight loss. Geissler et al. (93) compared energy expenditure during different physical activities and found that energy expenditure was 15% lower in the postobese than in controls across different activities. DeBoer (94) found that sleeping metabolic rate declined appropriately for the decline in fat-free mass (FFM) when obese subjects lost weight but that total energy expenditure declined more than expected for the change in FFM. Similar results were obtained by Leibel et al. (95), who speculate that an increased work efficiency may be partially responsible for weight regain following weight loss.

Alternatively, Froidevaux (96) measured the energy cost of walking in 10 moderately obese women before and after weight loss and during refeeding. Total energy expended during treadmill walking declined with weight loss, but was entirely explained by the decline in body mass. Net efficiency of walking did not change. Poole and Henson also found no change in efficiency of cycling after caloric restriction in moderately obese women (88). Weigle and Brunzell demonstrated that ~50% of the decline in energy expenditure with weight loss was eliminated when they replaced weight lost by energy restriction with external weight worn in a specially constructed vest (97). Thus, while it is clear that total energy expenditure declines with weight loss, the extent to which changes in work efficiency contribute to this decline is controversial.

3 Role of Skeletal Muscle Metabolism in Determining Work Efficiency

Differences in skeletal muscle morphology/metabolism have been suggested to play a role in differences in work efficiency. Henriksson (98) has suggested that changes in muscle morphology in response to energy restriction lead to changes in the relative proportion of type I versus type II fibers in human subjects. Some studies suggest that type II fibers have a greater fuel economy than type I fibers (99,100). Since type II fibers appear to be better preserved during starvation than type I fibers (98), overall fuel economy and work efficiency may be increased following energy restriction and loss of body mass. However, a study on muscle fiber type before and after a 10.8-kg weight loss in obese females did not show any changes in the fiber type distribution (101).

The potential contribution of skeletal muscle differences to differences in work efficiency between weight stable lean and obese subjects is more controversial. Substantial data suggest that obese subjects oxidize proportionally more carbohydrate and less fat than lean subjects in response to perturbations in energy balance (102–104) and that differences in morphology/metabolism of skeletal muscle and sympathetic nervous system activity (105) may underlie some of the whole-body differences (104,106). However, it is not clear to what extent such differences contribute to differences in work efficiency. Further, such differences may arise both from genetic and environmental causes.

4 Genetic Contributions to Work Efficiency

Very little information is available to allow estimation of the genetic contribution to differences in efficiency of work. Bouchard et al. (107) assessed the energy cost associated with common body postures (sitting, standing) and low-intensity activities (walking, stair climbing, etc.) in 22 pairs of dizygotic and 31 pairs of monozygotic twins. All subjects were classified as sedentary. A significant genetic effect for energy expenditure was found with activities from 50 to 150 watts even after correction for differences in body weight. No genetic effect was seen for activities requiring energy expenditure greater than six times resting energy expenditure.

5 Effects of Age on Work Efficiency

Work efficiency may vary with age. For example, Villagra et al. (108) demonstrated that children are ~ 10% more energy efficient during squatting exercises than adults. There is little information available to evaluate the effects of aging in adults on work efficiency. Skeletal muscle mass is often lost as a subject ages, and if the loss involves a greater proportion of type I than type II fibers, work efficiency could increase with age.

6 Effects of Exercise Training on Work Efficiency

If work efficiency varies as a function of exercise training, training induced effects in skeletal muscle could be important. Alterations in physical activity can alter the fiber type proportions of skeletal muscle as well as induce significant changes in enzyme activities. Aerobic exercise training results primarily in the transformation of type IIb into type IIa fibers, while transformation of type II fibers into type I fibers is not common unless the exercise training has been extremely intense over a long period of time. Type I fibers have a greater mitochondrial density and are more oxidative and more fatigue-resistant than type IIb fibers. Type IIb fibers are glycolytic in nature with lower mitochondrial content and are more prone to fatigue. Type IIa fibers are intermediate in their mitochondrial content and, in humans, closely resemble type I fibers in oxidative capacity. However, an overlap of oxidative capacity exists between fiber types groups. Type I and type IIa fibers are more energy efficient than type IIb fibers, and the proportions of these fiber types will vary according to the type of exercise training performed. It has been shown that even independently of fiber type alterations, the activities of important enzymes in oxidative and glycolytic pathways can be modified as a result of exercise training, and can lead to improvements in metabolic efficiency.

Sharp et al. (109) found that there was not a significant relationship between VO_2max and activity thermogenesis in a group of men and women studied in a whole-room calorimeter. Cross-sectional studies indicate that training may increase the efficiency of the activity when being trained. Elite runners and cyclists have lower energy expenditure at a certain speed than not specifically trained individuals. Differences can be accounted for 15% (running) up to 50% (swimming) (110,111). Children have a higher energy cost calculated per kg body weight for the same activity than do adults.

7 Effects of Gender on Work Efficiency

There are several reports that female athletes, unlike male athletes, are more energy efficient than their sedentary counterparts (112–114). There are reports in the literature for increased energy efficiency in female runners (112), dancers (113), and swimmers (114) as compared to sedentary females. However, most reports make conclusions regarding energetic efficiency based on indirect rather than direct measurements of energy intake and/or expenditure. For example, Mulligan et al. (112) concluded that female runners had increased energy efficiency since their self-reported energy intake was less than their estimated energy expenditure. In the few studies in which both intake and expenditure were measured directly, no evidence of increased energy efficiency was seen in female runners (115) or female cyclists (116). Thus, the question of whether female athletes show a different energy efficiency than sedentary females is controversial. If this proves to be true, the extent to which such differences might be due to differences in work efficiency is unknown.

V ACTIVITY THERMOGENESIS AND TOTAL DAILY ENERGY EXPENDITURE

Measurements of activity thermogenesis have provided insight into the energy needs of individuals and into the physiology of energy balance. In terms of understanding the energy needs of individuals, data on PAL values have provided information regarding the energy expenditure associated with different occupations and the impacts of culture, gender, and physical states such as pregnancy and lactation. This information is invaluable in terms of understanding the energy requirements of individuals. This information has also guided how statutory agencies have defined the energy needs of populations (117). What is becoming clear is that the greater the quality of data on activity thermogenesis for a given population, the better the estimates will be of that population's energy needs. With fast-advancing technologies that allow data from activity sensors to be combined with doubly labeled water, enormous advance in this arena is anticipated.

VI SUBSTRATE OXIDATION DURING PHYSICAL ACTIVITY

Body weight regulation involves balancing total energy intake and expenditure. It also involves maintaining over time a balance between intake and oxidation of protein, carbohydrate, and fat. Thus, it is useful to consider factors that influence both the amount and composition of fuel used during physical activity. When assessing factors that influence substrate oxidation, it is important to consider influences both during performance of exercise and during the postexercise recovery period.

A Characteristics of Physical Activity

Skeletal muscle tissue has the ability to convert chemical energy to mechanical energy required for physical activity using the myosin motor proteins as a lever arm to produce movement (118). The immediate source of chemical energy required for contraction is provided by the hydrolysis of adenosine triphosphate (ATP) catalyzed by myosin ATPase.

Intracellular ATP stores are small and can be depleted within seconds of maximal contraction if they are not adequately replenished. The ATP synthesis pathways include the phosphagen system and (anaerobic) glycolysis. The phosphagen system includes the breakdown of creatine phosphate (CrP) as well as the regeneration of ATP from ADP by the adenylate kinase reaction. The anaerobic glycolysis pathway allows a five to six times higher ATP synthesis, than the oxidative glycolysis of glucose. The rate by which ATP can be generated depends on the biochemical pathways that are followed as well as on the substrate source.

In Table 1, the high-energy phosphate (HEP) formation rates following the aerobic and/or anaerobic breakdown of carbohydrates and fat are given. The rate of HEP formation depends clearly on the type of oxidation (anaerobic > aerobic), locations of the fuel source (endogenous > bloodborne), as well as the fuel type (carbohydrate > fat). Based on the examples given in Table 1, it can be seen that the maximal rate of ATP synthesis from fat can provide only enough energy to sustain exercise at 55–70% of maximal oxygen intake (VO_2max) depending on the training status. However, the rate of energy generated from carbohydrate, both anaerobic and aerobic, can provide enough energy to sustain exercise up to maximal level for a short period of time.

Table 1 Maximum Rate of High-Energy Phophate (HEP) Regeneration from Carbohydrate and Lipid Substrates Compared to Utilization of HEP During Various Types of Exercise

Maximum rate of HEP regeneration

Substrate utilized	Max. rate of formation HEP Mol HEP.min-1
Endogenous glycogen (anaerobic)	2.4
Endogenous glycogen (aerobic)	1.0
Bloodborne glucose (aerobic)	0.37
Bloodborne fatty acids (aerobic)	0.40

Rate of HEP utilization

Type of exercise	Rate of utilization
Rest	0.07
Walking	0.3
100 m sprint	2.6
800 m sprint	2.0
1500 m sprint	1.7
Marathon	1.0

m, meters.
Source: Ref. 126.

During endurance moderate-intensity exercise ATP demands can be provided entirely by oxidative phosphorylation of both intramuscular and bloodborne carbohydrate and fat. Substrate oxidation during exercise is often estimated from the whole-body respiratory quotient (RQ), which provides an indication of the relative proportion of carbohydrate and fat being oxidized. In comparing RQ between exercise conditions, it is important to consider total energy expended as well as RQ. Especially at low-intensity exercise, a relatively high proportion of lipids are oxidized, mainly as a result of the preferential oxidation of free fatty acids in the type I fibers. For example, at 20% VO_2max, RQ is ~0.80, meaning that 62% of the local substrate utilization is derived from fat. At 80% VO_2max, more type II fibers are involved and RQ value is 0.9, leading to a contribution of fat oxidation of only 21%.

The relative contribution of fat and carbohydrate oxidation to total energy expenditure during exercise can vary enormously and strongly depends on exercise intensity, training status, and diet (119).

Quantifying the rates of utilization of the different substrate sources during exercise is of importance to gain more insight into the metabolic consequences of physical activity. It enables us to evaluate the effects of dietary and training interventions on a whole-body level, thereby also contributing to our understanding of the metabolic defect(s) associated with obesity and non-insulin-dependent diabetes mellitus (NIDDM), (120,121).

1 Exercise Intensity

While the intensity of exercise is the major determinant of amount of energy expenditure as well as substrate source, both the intensity and duration of exercise influence the source of fuel used for exercise (119).

Substrate utilization rates in relation to exercise intensity have been derived by Romijn et al. (122) using stable isotopes to estimate whole body oxidation rate of all endogenous substrate sources as a function of exercise intensity. In Figure 1, the endogenous substrate utilization during exercise at low (25% VO_2max), moderate (65% VO_2max), and high (85% VO_2max) intensity is depicted. The main fuel source during high-intensity exercise (>70–75% VO_2max) is carbohydrate as glycogen from the muscle. Generally, the oxidation of plasma FFA provides the majority of energy during low-intensity exercise with little or no net utilization of intramuscular triglycerides (IMTG) or lipoprotein derived TG (122–124).

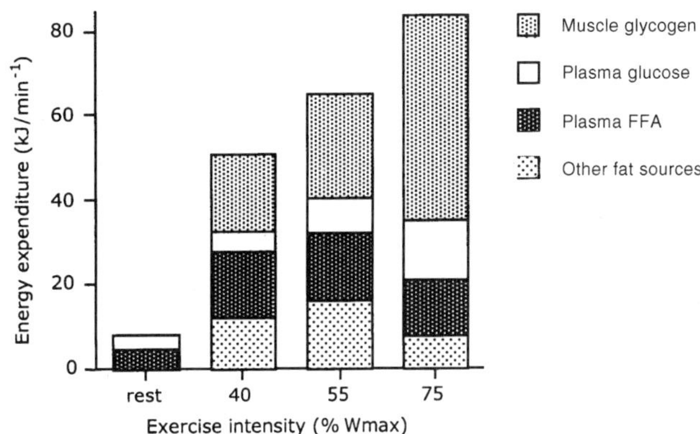

Figure 1 Endogenous substrate utilization (mol HEP per min) during exercise of various intensities. (From Ref. 122.)

During moderate-intensity exercise (40–65% VO_2 max) fat oxidation, from an absolute point of view, reaches maximal rates, with the endogenous IMTG stores (including possibly lipoprotein-derived TG) contributing ~50% of total energy expenditure (122,125).

The majority of the carbohydrates oxidized are derived from muscle glycogen stores. With increasing intensity, fat oxidation decreases substantially from a relative as well as a qualitative point of view. The precise mechanisms that explain the increase and the limitations in fat oxidation during exercise are not well understood. From rest to moderate-intensity exercise, the increase in fat oxidation is enabled by an increase in adipose tissue lipolytic rate, followed by an increase in plasma FFA availability. However, plasma FFA oxidation is limited by yet undetermined factors, which likely include FFA transport from the vascular space into the intramyocellular compartment (126). This has led to an increased interest in the contribution of IMTG as endogenous fat source during moderate-intensity exercise (122). An increase in exercise intensity will result in an increased oxidation of IMTG, enabled by an increase in intracellular FA availability and an increase in the activity of the enzymes involved in the transport of FA over the mitochondrial membrane (127,128). By contrast, protein oxidation during exercise is small (129).

2 Exercise Duration

With increased duration of exercise the intramuscular fuel sources will diminish while the contribution from the circulating fuels will increase (122,130–135). During the initial phase of exercise, carbohydrate is mainly supplied from intramuscular glycogen stores (136,137).

After ~30–40 min of exercise, the contribution of blood glucose increases (131) and remains relatively constant (122,136) until the later stages of prolonged exercise, when it declines (137). The blood glucose level is maintained through an increase in hepatic glucose production (131,137). Initially, this is mainly due to hepatic glycogenolysis, but with prolonged exercise, gluconeogenesis becomes more important (131,138–140). Optimal carbohydrate ingestion can completely suppress hepatic glucose production during exercise (141).

Also, IMTG appears to be utilized more during the initial phase of moderate exercise with an increasing contribution from circulating FFA as time progresses. Although the contribution of protein to fuel utilization during exercise is small, < 11% of total energy expended (142), this can increase with very prolonged exercise. Protein contributes to energy production directly via oxidation of branched chain amino acids (BCAA) and indirectly through the increased release of the gluconeogenic precursor alanine (129). Protein synthesis in muscle declines whereas proteolysis in other tissues can increase the circulating BCAA (129,143). This increases the amino acid pool available for oxidation. As gluconeogenesis becomes more important during exercise, alanine release also rises (144).

B Characteristics of the Exercising Individual

Both the amount of energy expended during exercise and the source of fuel for the added energy expenditure are influenced by several characteristics of the exercising individual.

1 Training Status

Christensen and Hansen (145), in their classic studies, observed that endurance training leads to an increased capacity to utilize fat as a fuel source. This training-induced change in substrate utilization has been confirmed in numerous studies (125,146–148). The contribution of fat as a fuel source during exercise has been shown to be increased in an endurance-trained state, compared at the same absolute and the same relative (and therefore higher absolute) workload (139). Saris (120) calculated that during 30 min of exercise at 60% VO_2max, trained individuals would oxidize an extra 10 g of fat as compared to sedentary individuals. The main metabolic adaptations to endurance training that are responsible for the increased fat oxidative capacity include an increase in both the size and number of mitochondria and a concomitant enhanced activity of enzymes involved in the uptake and oxidation of fatty acids, as well as enzymes involved in the TCA cycle and respiratory chain (127,149).

Increased proportions of oxidative type I fibers and decreased proportions of type IIb fibers (except in sprint athletes) result following exercise training, so skeletal muscle is more adapted to fat oxidation. Similarly, the activity of important enzymes in fat and carbohydrate oxidation is modified. Exercise training leads to an increased ability to remove FFA from the circulation (142), which will also facilitate an increase in FFA oxidation. This is most probably mediated by an increase in membrane-associated fatty acid-binding proteins (FABP) (150). In addition, some of the increased fat oxidation in trained individuals may be due to a greater reliance on IMTG as an exercise fuel source. This is suggested by a greater decline in IMTG postexercise following a period of training (147) and an inability of the increased FFA uptake to account for all the increase in total fat oxidation observed during exercise (125,151). However postexercise fat intake repletes IMTG but not faster in trained than in sedentary individuals (152). This increased lipid oxidation essentially spares both muscle glycogen and blood glucose (125,147,151). Other training adaptations relating to carbohydrate metabolism include a greater capacity for muscle glycogen storage (153) and an increased lactate clearance, which provides more gluconeogenic substrate (154).

2 Gender

There is abundant evidence that the proportion of energy derived from fat during exercise is higher in women than in men (155,156). Most studies have shown a greater fat oxidation (adjusted for energy expenditure) during submaximal exercise in women than in men (157–159). Also, a lower skeletal muscle glucose uptake (159) and attenuated muscle glycogen utilization (160) have been reported during exercise in women.

One factor of importance may be the differences in FFA availability. It has been shown that lipolysis as indicated by the rate of appearance of glycerol is higher in women than in men during exercise (159). Others, however, did not find a difference in rate of appearance of FFA (157,161). Also, a higher level of IMTG was found in women compared to men matched for lifestyle habits and insulin sensitivity (162).

This could indicate that higher IMTG oxidation may contribute to the increased fat oxidation of women during exercise as suggested before (160). Also, higher expression of FABP mRNA was found in women compared to men (163). From all these indications it becomes clear that women have a higher capacity for FA transport and storage in the muscle, leading to a higher fat oxidation rate at the same relative exercise intensity.

The stage of menstrual cycle in females may also affect the pattern of fuel oxidation. Although few adequately controlled studies have been performed in this area, there is a suggestion of increased lipid oxidation during exercise performed in the luteal versus follicular phase of the menstrual cycle (164,165). Further work is warranted to more accurately elucidate potential gender-related aspects of exercising fuel metabolism. This will also give more information about the regulatory factors influencing fat versus carbohydrate oxidation during exercise.

3 Age

It has been suggested that the ability to oxidize fat during exercise declines with age (166). If true, this could be due to changes in the morphology and metabolism of skeletal muscles, and/or to availability of lipid substrate during exercise.

4 Body Composition

In the past years new data suggest that increases in body fatness promote insulin resistance and NIDDM. The progression in insulin resistance is accompanied by increased circulating concentrations of FFA. On the one hand, these increased FFA concentrations may result from the expended adipose tissue stores in obesity and NIDDM by a mass action effect or by a diminished ability of insulin to inhibit lipolysis. Both the beta-adrenergic stimulation and exercise stimulation of lipolysis and fat oxidation are impaired in the obese and NIDDM subjects (167–169). On the other hand, the uptake of FFA is impaired in skeletal muscle of the obese and obese NIDDM subjects during exercise (167,169). An increased IMTG has been hypothesized to be a key feature in the development of skeletal muscle insulin resistance (170). This is most probably mediated by a lower ability to increase muscle lipolysis during exercise as was shown in NIDDM (171) and obese (172,173) subjects. In Figure 2, relative fat source utilization during moderate intensity exercise is depicted from selected groups of subjects using the same measurement protocol (174,169,175).

Sedentary untrained and trained as well as highly trained healthy subjects are compared with obese and obese NIDDM subjects. Although subjects are not matched for age and body fatness, the figure illustrates clearly the low contribution of other fat sources

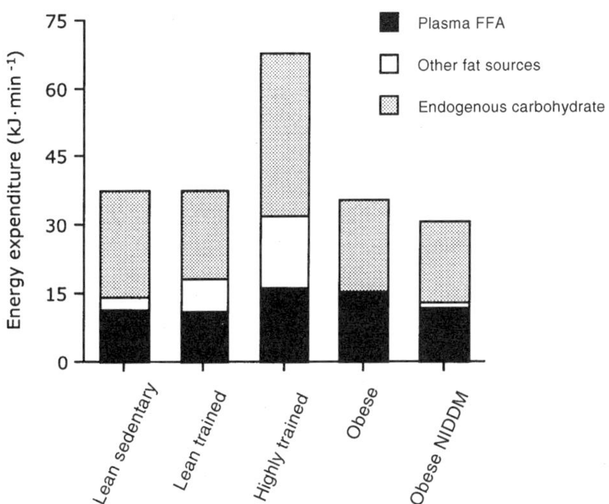

Figure 2 Relative endogenous carbohydrate and fat source utilization during moderate-intensity exercise in lean sedentary subjects before and after a 3-month training period (from Ref. 220), highly trained athletes (from Ref. 174), and obese and obese NIDDM subjects (from Ref. 169).

(IMTG and lipoprotein-derived TG) in the substrate utilization during moderate intensity exercise in the obese state. Although not measured, it is assumed based on the available literature that in the obese and NIDDM groups the IMTG is higher than in the lean sedentary and trained subjects. In highly trained athletes, high levels of IMTG are found. Despite the similar high levels of IMTG in the obese and obese NIDDM groups, trained athletes show a very large capacity to use the other fat sources, in particular the IMTG stores. This topic clearly needs further attention in future studies because it can give us more insight in the detrimental role of fat stores in obesity and NIDDM.

VII ROLE OF PHYSICAL ACTIVITY IN THE ETIOLOGY OF OBESITY

The most recent report from the National Health and Examination Survey (176) shows that the prevalence of obesity in the United States continues to increase, and was at 31%. While this is further evidence that factors in the U.S. environment are contributing to the population weight gain, it is not clear whether these environmental factors are influencing energy intake, energy expenditure, or both. Dramatic changes in the food supply and in the need for physical activity in daily life have both occurred over the past century, and each could be contributing to weight gain. Unfortunately, population-based records of food intake are not very accurate, and physical-activity data (especially lifestyle or nonleisure physical activity) have not been systematically recorded. It is interesting to note that national household surveys of several different countries show a decrease in energy intake over time. For example, in Great Britain, energy intake decreased by more than 500 kcal from 1970 to 1990 (177). During the same time, however, body mass index and average body weight increased by 1.0 BMI unit and 2.5 kg, respectively. These figures would imply that energy expenditure must have declined by even >500 kcal. The problem is, we do not have any data to show whether this might be the case other than anecdotal information on the number of automobiles and occupational mechanization. While definitive data may be lacking, in this section we will examine the available data suggesting a causal link between physical activity and obesity.

A Relationship Between Physical Activity and Body Fatness

Epidemiological studies have consistently shown a negative relationship between measures of physical activity (usually self-reports) and indices of obesity (usually body mass index) (178). This relationship is present in most datasets obtained from the general U.S. population (179,180). The relationship appears to be similar in men and women, and across all ages (181–184). Further, there is evidence for a similar relationship in African-Americans (185), Hispanics (186), and Native Americans (187). This inverse relationship between BMI and physical activity has been seen using both self-reports of amount of physical activity (180) and actual energy expended in physical activity assessed from doubly labeled water measures (188,189).

Given that there is a negative relationship between obesity and physical activity and given that obesity is increasing dramatically in the population, can we attribute some of this weight gain to reduced energy expenditure due to declines in energy expended in physical activity, and can we reduce this weight gain with efforts to promote physical activity?

B Do Low Levels of Physical Activity Increase the Risk of Obesity?

Despite the lack of randomized, controlled studies, there is substantial evidence that low levels of physical activity may be contributing to the increased prevalence of obesity in the United States population. In several cohort studies where indices of obesity over time were assessed without intervention, associations between low levels of physical activity and indices of obesity were found (190–193). In these studies, baseline measures of physical activity were inversely related to BMI. In some, low levels of physical activity predicted high weight gain over the follow-up period (191–193), and decreases in physical activity over time were associated with high weight gain (191–193).

Reduced levels of physical activity with age in the general population may play a role in the development of obesity. Reductions in physical activity could alter fiber type composition toward a greater proportion of glycolytic type IIb fibers that have a reduced capacity for fat utilization and may predispose to fat accumulation. This could lead to a vicious cycle of reduced physical activity resulting in further increased type IIb fiber proportions and decline in fat oxidation, thus promoting obesity. If a low level of physical activity contributes to weight gain, can we document a decline in overall physical activity that coincides with the increased prevalence of obesity seen over the past two decades?

C Secular Trends in Physical Activity

For our purposes, we can divide total physical activity into that activity performed intentionally during leisure time (leisure time physical activity; LTPA) or activity performed in daily living (lifestyle physical activity; LSPA). Are there clear secular trends in LTPA and LSPA?

While there are ample data indicating that the vast majority of Americans get little or no LTPA, there is little evidence that this has changed dramatically over the past two decades (194–196). It is not possible from existing data to conclude that substantial decreases in LTPA have occurred simultaneously with the onset of the obesity epidemic. It is more likely that declines in LSPA have contributed to the increased prevalence of obesity, but unfortunately it is difficult to quantify this contribution. While most obesity experts accept that technological advances have reduced the amount of LSPA required, this decline has not been documented to the extent to allow quantification of the changes. In fact, it is only in recent years that attempts have begun to measure LSPA. All indications are that work-related physical activity has declined. The only prospective data available come from Finland, where a 225 kJ/d decline in work-related physical activity has occurred over 10 years (197). Similarly, there is reason to believe that other forms of energy expended in activities of daily living have declined rapidly over the past two or three decades. One can, for example, estimate the energy savings due to proliferation of televisions and computers, remote control devices, microwave ovens and increased use of prepared foods. While each may reduce physical activity only slightly, together these energy savings accumulate and can have a significant impact on total energy expenditure. Declines in energy expended for transportation have also likely occurred in recent years. This can best be illustrated with data from the National Personal Transportation Survey (198). In the United States between 1990 and 1995, the number of annual walking trips had declined 12.4%, while the number of daily car trips had increased nearly an identical amount (12.3%).

The total amount of energy expended in physical activity may also be declining owing to an increase in attractive sedentary activities such as television watching, video games, and computer interactions. Again, we do not have good measures of sedentary activity that would allow us to examine how time spent in these activities has changed over the past few years. It is likely, however, that these highly attractive sedentary activities are successfully competing with LTPA for our leisure time.

D Does Increasing Physical Activity Prevent Weight Gain?

If declines in physical activity have contributed to weight gain, it may be possible to prevent or slow weight gain by increasing physical activity. There have been surprisingly few prospective intervention studies to examine this question, but several observational studies are relevant. DiPietro et al. (199) measured a group of adults coming to the Cooper Clinic at baseline and 7.5 years later. They found that higher levels of aerobic fitness were associated with lower weight gain in this population. However, they reported that, over time, increases in fitness were necessary for subjects to remain weight stable. Williams (200) found that even among a highly active group of runners, increasing amounts of physical activity with increasing age were needed to prevent weight gain. Ching et al. (201) found that the combination of high levels of physical activity and a low amount of time spent watching television/VCR was associated with a lower BMI at baseline and with lower weight gain over time. Sherwood et al. (202) found that a high level of physical activity was one of the factors that were protective against weight gain in the Pound study. These authors point out, however, that a number of factors seem to interact to influence weight gain over time.

In children, prospective intervention studies do suggest that increasing physical activity can prevent weight gain. Epstein et al. (203) and Robinson (204) have reported success in increasing physical activity through reduction in sedentary activities (e.g., TV, video games).

E How Much Physical Activity Is Required to Prevent Weight Gain?

There is no consensus about how much physical activity is required to prevent weight gain. The Surgeon-General recommends accumulation of at least 30 min of moderate-intensity physical activity on most days and on at least 3 days a week (205). At the time of development of these recommendations, there were few or no data relating amount of physical activity to weight gain, so the recommendations were made using data about physical-activity level and risk of cardiovascular disease and mortality rates. The question if whether the data now available are helpful in defining physical activity recommendations to prevent weight gain.

It may be helpful to consider prevention of weight gain separately from prevention of weight regain. We have more data about the amount of physical activity required to prevent weight regain in reduced-obese subjects than we have about the amount of physical activity required to prevent weight gain over time in the never-obese. It is not clear if more physical activity is required to prevent weight regain than to prevent weight gain, but this should be considered as a possibility.

F Prevention of Weight Regain

There is surprising consensus about the amount of physical activity that seems to help maintain weight loss and prevent weight regain. This amount may be 60–90 min of moderate-intensity physical activity each day—substantially more physical activity than recommended for health by the Surgeon-General. Schoeller et al. (206) found that a PAL of 1.75 ($1.75 \times$ basal metabolic rate) was protective against weight regain in a group of obese-reduced subjects. They recommended 80 min/day of moderate-intensity physical activity to prevent weight regain. Studies of the National Weight Control Registry show that subjects maintaining an average weight loss of 30 kg for an average of 5.5 years reported expending from 2545 kcal/week (women) to 3293 kcal/week (men) in physical activity (207). This would be equivalent to 60–90 min of moderate-intensity physical activity.

Jakicic et al. (208) found that reduced-obese subjects who engaged in at least 200 min/week of physical activity were less likely to regain weight than those who engaged in less physical activity. Finally, Weinsier et al. (209) studied women who maintained or gained weight over time. They found that weight maintainers were more physically active than weight gainers. They estimated that it may take as much as 80 min/day to maintain body weight (depending on diet). It should be noted, however, that the weight maintainers included some women who were previously obese and some who had never been obese.

G Prevention of Weight Gain

There are far fewer data available about how much physical activity is required to prevent the weight gain over time seen in the general population. This amount of weight gain may be on the order of 0.5–1.0 kg/year (55). Theoretically, an adult could gain 1 kg of body fat over 1 year with an energy imbalance of <50 kcal/d. This might suggest that the amount of physical activity required to prevent this weight gain could be relatively small. However, we have no prospective studies that have tested this assumption.

H What Characteristics of Physical Activity Are Important in Preventing Weight Gain?

At present there are insufficient data to recommend specific types of physical activity for prevention of weight gain. Some have suggested that more vigorous physical activity may be better, independent of total energy expended (210); others suggest that resistance training may be useful (211). It is interesting to note that subjects in the National Weight Control Registry report engaging in weightlifting to a greater extent than is seen in the general population. On the other hand, Westerterp (212) noted that the cumulative impact of low-intensity activities over greater duration is of greater energetic impact than short bursts of high-intensity physical activities in free-living individuals. Thus, not only are recommendations for exercise germane but also those to reverse sedentariness.

I How to Increase Physical Activity?

While definitive randomized controlled studies showing that increasing physical activity can prevent weight gain are lacking, substantial indirect evidence suggests that increasing physical activity is likely to be one of our most effective strategies for reducing the weight gain seen in the general population. The evidence is strong enough that we should expand the efforts toward understanding how to get the population more physically active.

Attempts to increase physical activity by increasing LTPA have not met with overwhelming success, since LTPA has not increased over the past decade (194–196), but efforts to increase LSPA may be more promising (213,214). Increasing walking could be effective in increasing physical activity sufficiently to prevent weight gain (215). A limitation in promoting LSPA has been the difficulty in measuring it, but technological advances have brought pedometers and accelerometers that allow the individual some feedback about amount of LSPA performed (216–218). These devices may prove to be very useful in population efforts to increase physical activity. It will also be necessary to consider policy strategies to promote physical activity, as was reviewed elsewhere (219).

REFERENCES

1. Dériaz O, Fournier G, Tremblay A, Despres JP, Bouchard C. Lean-body-mass composition and resting energy expenditure before and after long-term overfeeding. Am J Clin Nutr 1992; 56:840–847.
2. Ford LE. Some consequences of body size. Am J Physiol 1984; 247:H495–H507.
3. Hill JO, DiGirolamo M, Heymsfield SB. Thermic effect of food after ingested versus tube-delivered meals. Am J Physiol 1985; 248:E370–E374.
4. D'Alessio DA, Kavle EC, Mozzoli MA, Smalley KJ, Polansky M, Kendrick ZV, Owen LR. Thermic effect of food in lean and obese men. J Clin Invest 1988; 81:1781–1789.
5. Kinabo JL, Durnin JV. Thermic effect of food in man: effect of meal composition, and energy content. Br J Nutr 1990; 64:37–44.
6. Reed GW, Hill JO. Measuring the thermic effect of food. Am J Clin Nutr 1996; 63:164–169.
7. Livingstone MBE, Strain JJ, Prentice AM, Coward WA, Nevin GB, Barker ME, Hickey HJ, McKenna PG, Whitehead RG. Potential contribution of leisure activity to the energy expenditure patterns of sedentary populations. Br J Nutr 1991; 65:145–155.
8. Dauncey MJ. Activity and energy expenditure. Can J Physiol Pharmacol 1990; 68:17–27.
9. Ravussin E, Lillioja S, Anderson TE, Christin L, Bogardus C. Determinants of 24-hour energy expenditure in man: methods and results using a respiratory chamber. J Clin Invest 1986; 78:1568–1578.
10. Baranowski T, Smith M, Thompson WO, Baranowski

J, Herbert D, DeMoor C. Intraindividual variability and reliability in a 7-day exercise record. Med Sci Sports Exerc 1999; 31:1619–1622.
11. Lamonte MJ, Ainsworth BE. Quantifying energy expenditure and physical activity in the context of dose response. Med Sci Sports Exerc 2001; 33:S370–S378.
12. Baker JA, Humphrey SJ, Wolff HS. Socially acceptable monitoring instruments (SAMI). J Physiol 1967; 188:4–5P.
13. Proctor DN, Sinning WE, Bredle DL, Joyner MJ. Cardiovascular and peak VO_2 responses to supine exercise: effects of age and training status. Med Sci Sports Exerc 1996; 28:892–899.
14. Wilmore JH, Ewy GA, Freund BJ, Hartzell AA, Jilka SM, Joyner MJ, Todd CA, Kinzer SM. Cardiorespiratory alterations consequent to endurance exercise training during chronic beta-adrenergic blockade with atenolol and propranolol. Am J Cardiol 1985; 55:142D–148D.
15. Sirard JR, Pate RR. Physical activity assessment in children and adolescents. Sports Med 2001; 31:439–454.
16. Westerterp KR. Assessment of physical activity level in relation to obesity: current evidence and research issues. Med Sci Sports Exerc 1999; 31:S522–S525.
17. Melanson EL Jr, Freedson PS. Physical activity assessment: a review of methods. Crit Rev Food Sci Nutr 1996; 36:385–396.
18. University UN. Research Methods in Nutritional Anthropology 1989.
19. Schutz Y, Ravussin E, Diethelm R, Jequien E. Spontaneous physical activity measured by radar in obese and control subjects studied in a respiration chamber. Int J Obes 1982; 6:23–28.
20. Mayer J. Physical activity and anthropometric measurements of obese adolescents. Fed Proc 1966; 25:11–14.
21. Gretebeck RJ, Montoye HJ. Variability of some objective measures of physical activity. Med Sci Sports Exerc 1992; 24:1167–1172.
22. Bassett DR Jr, Ainsworth BE, Swartz AM, Strath SJ, O'Brien WL, King GA. Validity of four motion sensors in measuring moderate intensity physical activity. Med Sci Sports Exerc 2000; 32:S471–S480.
23. Melanson EL Jr, Freedson PS. Validity of the Computer Science and Applications, Inc. (CSA) activity monitor. Med Sci Sports Exerc 1995; 27:934–940.
24. Pambianco G, Wing RR, Robertson R. Accuracy and reliability of the Caltrac accelerometer for estimating energy expenditure. Med Sci Sports Exerc 1990; 22: 858–862.
25. Bouten CV, Westerterp KR, Verduin M, Janssen JD. Assessment of energy expenditure for physical activity using a triaxial accelerometer. Med Sci Sports Exerc 1994; 26:1516–1523.
26. Westerterp KR, Bouten CV. Physical activity assessment: comparison between movement registration and doubly labeled water method. Ernahrungswiss Z 1997; 36:263–267.
27. Levine JA, Baukol PA, Westerterp KR. Validation of the Tracmor triaxial accelerometer system for walking. Med Sci Sports Exerc 2001; 33:1593–1597.
28. Bouten CV, Verboeket–Van de Venne WP, Westerterp KR, Verduin M, Janssen JD. Daily physical activity assessment: comparison between movement registration and doubly labeled water. J Appl Physiol 1996; 81:1019–1026.
29. Cunningham JJ. Calculation of energy expenditure from indirect calorimetry: assessment of the Weir equation. Nutrition 1990; 6:222–223.
30. Weir JB. New methods for calculating metabolic rate with special reference to protein metabolism. Nutrition 1949; 6:213–221.
31. Jequier E, Felber JP. Indirect calorimetry. Baillieres Clin Endocrinol Metab 1987; 1:911–935.
32. Sun M, Reed GW, Hill JO. Modification of a whole room indirect calorimeter for measurement of rapid changes in energy expenditure. J Appl Physiol 1994; 76:2686–2691.
33. Levine JA, Schleusner SJ, Jensen MD. Energy expenditure of nonexercise activity. Am J Clin Nutr 2000; 72:1451–1454.
34. Lum L, Saville A, Venkataraman ST. Accuracy of physiologic deadspace measurement in intubated pediatric patients using a metabolic monitor: comparison with the Douglas bag method. Crit Care Med 1998; 26:760–764.
35. De Groot G, Schreurs AW, Van Ingen Schenau GJ. A portable lightweight Douglas bag instrument for use during various types of exercise. Int J Sports Med 1983; 4:132–134.
36. Yoshida T, Nagata A, Muro M, Takevchi N, Suda Y. The validity of anaerobic threshold determination by a Douglas bag method compared with arterial blood lactate concentration. Eur J Appl Physiol Occup Physiol 1981; 46:423–430.
37. Douglas CG. A method for determining the total respiratory exchange in man. J Physiol 1911; 42:17–18.
38. Daniels J. Portable respiratory gas collection equipment. J Appl Physiol 1971; 31:164–167.
39. Sujatha T, Shatrugna V, Venkataramana Y, Begom N. Energy expenditure on household, childcare and occupational activities of women from urban poor households. Br J Nutr 2000; 83:497–503.
40. Consolazio CF. Energy expenditure studies in military populations using Kofranyi-Michaelis respirometers. Am J Clin Nutr 1971; 24:1431–1437.
41. Rietjens GJ, Kuipers H, Kester AD, Keizer HA. Validation of a computerized metabolic measurement system (Oxycon-Pro) during low and high intensity exercise. Int J Sports Med 2001; 22:291–294.

42. McLaughlin JE, King GE, Howley ET, Bassett DR, Ainsworth BE. Validation of the COSMED K4 b2 portable metabolic system. Int J Sports Med 2001; 22:80–84.
43. Morio B, Beaufrere B, Montaurier C, Ritz P, Fellmann N, Boirie Y, Vermorel M. Gender differences in energy expended during activities and in daily energy expenditure of elderly people. Am J Physiol 1997; 273:E321–E327.
44. Banerjee B, Khew KS, Saha N. A comparative study of energy expenditure in some common daily activities of non-pregnant and pregnant Chinese, Malay and Indian women. J Obstet Gynaecol Br Commonw 1971; 78:113–116.
45. Black AE, Coward WA, Cole TJ, Prentice AM. Human energy expenditure in affluent societies: an analysis of 574 doubly-labelled water measurements. Eur J Clin Nutr 1996; 50:72–92.
46. Prentice AM, Goldberg GR, Murgatroyd PR, Cole TJ. Physical activity and obesity: problems in correcting expenditure for body size. Int J Obes 1996; 20:688–691.
47. Ferro-Luzzi A, Scaccini C, Taffese S, Aberra B, Demeke T. Seasonal energy deficiency in Ethiopian rural women. Eur J Clin Nutr 1990; 44(suppl 1):7–18.
48. Coward WA, Roberts SB, Cole TJ. Theoretical and practical considerations in the doubly-labelled water ($2H_2O^{18}$) method for the measurement of carbon dioxide production rate in man. Eur J Clin Nutr 1988; 42:207–212.
49. Coward WA. Contributions of the doubly labeled water method to studies of energy balance in the third world. Am J Clin Nutr 1998; 68:962S–969S.
50. Goran MI, Poehlman ET, Nair KS, Danforth E. Deuterium exchange in humans: effect of gender, body composition and age. Basic Life Sci 1993; 60: 79–81.
51. Kurpad AV, Borgonha S, Shetty PS. Measurement of total energy expenditure by the doubly labelled water technique in free living Indians in Bangalore city. Indian J Med Res 1997; 105:212–219.
52. Schoeller DA, Taylor PB. Precision of the doubly labelled water method using the two-point calculation. Hum Nutr Clin Nutr 1987; 41:215–223.
53. National Health Interview Survey Electronic citation. http://www.cdc.gov/nchs/nhishtm
54. Mokdad AH, Bowman BA, Ford ES, Vinicor F, Marks JS, Loplan JP. The continuing epidemic of obesity and diabetes in the United States. JAMA 2001; 286(10):1195–1200.
55. Kuczmarski RJ, Flegal KM, Campbell SM, Johnson CL. Increasing prevalence of overweight among US adults. JAMA 1994; 272:205–211.
56. Levine JA, Weisell R, Chevassus S, Martinez CD, Burlingam B, Coward WA. The work burden of women. Science 2001; 294:812.
57. Davey Smith G, Shipley MJ, Batty GD, Morris JN, Marmot M. Physical activity and cause-specific mortality in the Whitehall study. Public Health 2000; 114: 308–315.
58. Chave SP, Morris JN, Moss S, Semmence AM. Vigorous exercise in leisure time and the death rate: a study of male civil servants. J Epidemiol Commun Health 1978; 32:239–243.
59. Shetty PS, Henry CJ, Black AE, Prentice AM. Energy requirements of adults: an update on basal metabolic rates (BMRs) and physical activity levels (PALs). Eur J Clin Nutr 1996; 50(suppl 1):S11–S23.
60. Bouchard C, Dériaz O, Pérusse L, Tremblay A. Genetics of energy expenditure in humans. In: Bouchard C, ed. The Genetics of Obesity. Boca Raton: CRC Press, 1994:135–146.
61. Kaprio J, Koskenvuo M, Sarna S. Cigarette smoking, use of alcohol, and leisure-time physical activity among same sexed adult male twins. Prog Clin Biol Res 1981; 69:37–46.
62. Pérusse L, Tremblay A, Leblanc C, Bouchard C. Genetic and environmental influences on level of habitual physical activity and exercise participation. Am J Epidiol 1989; 129:1012–1022.
63. Stephens T, Caspersen CJ. The demography of physical activity. In: Bouchard C, Shephard RJ, Stephens T, eds. Physical Activity, Fitness, and Health. Champaign, IL: Human Kinetics Publishers, 1994: 203–213.
64. Activity and Health Research. Allied Dunbar National Fitness Survey: Main Findings. London: Sports Council and the Health Education Authority, 1992.
65. Caspersen CJ, Merritt RK. Trends in physical activity patterns among older adults: the behavioral risk factor surveillance system, 1986–1990. Med Sci Sports Exerc 1992; 24:S26.
66. Merritt RK, Caspersen CJ. Trends in physical activity patterns among young adults: the behavioral risk factor surveillance system, 1986–1990. Med Sci Sports Exerc 1992; 24:S26.
67. Stephens T, Craig CL. The Well-Being of Canadians: Highlights of the 1988 Campbell's Survey. Ottawa: Canadian Fitness and Lifestyle Research Institute, 1990.
68. Risk Factor Prevalence Study Management Committee Risk Factor Prevalence Study: Survey No 3 1989. Canberra: National Heart Foundation of Australia and Australian Institute of Health, 1990.
69. Saris WHM, Elvers JWH, Van't Hof M, Binkhorst RA. Changes in physical activity profiles of children aged 6 to 12 years. In: Rutenfranz J, ed. Children and Exercise XII. Champaign, Il: Human Kinetics, 1986: 121–130.
70. Matsushima M, Kriska A, Tajima N, LaPorte R. The epidemiology of physical activity and childhood obesity. Diabetes Res Clin Pract 1990; 10(suppl 1): S95–S102.

71. Pacy PJ, Webster J, Garrow JS. Exercise and obesity. Sports Med 1986; 3:89–113.
72. Thompson JK, Jarvie GJ, Lahey BB, Cureton KJ. Exercise and obesity: etiology, physiology, and intervention. Psychol Bull 1982; 91:55–79.
73. Blei ML, Conley KE, Odderson IR, Esselman PC, Kushmerick MJ. Individual variation in contractile cost and recovery in human skeletal muscle. Proc Natl Acad Sci USA 1993; 90:7396–7400.
74. Ainsworth BE, Haskell WL, Leon AS, Jacobs DR Jr, Montoye HJ, Sallis JF, Paffenbarger RS. Compendium of physical activities. Classification of energy costs of human physical activities. Med Sci Sports Exerc 1993; 25:71–80.
75. Bahr R. Excess post exercise oxygen consumption—magnitude, mechanisms, and practical implications. Acta Physiol Scand 1992; 144(suppl 605):1–70.
76. Bielinski R, Schutz Y, Jequier E. Energy metabolism during the postexercise recovery in man. Am J Clin Nutr 1985; 42:69–82.
77. Freedman-Akabas S, Colt E, Kissileff HR, Pi-Sunyer FX. Lack of sustained increase in VO_2 following exercise in fit and unfit subjects. Am J Clin Nutr 1985; 41:545–549.
78. Brehm BA, Gutin B. Recovery energy expenditure for steady state exercise in runners and nonexercisers. Med Sci Sports Exerc 1986; 18:205–210.
79. Saris WHM, Van Baak MA. Consequences of exercise on energy expenditure. In: Hill AP, Wahlqvist ML, eds. Exercise and Obesity. London: Smith Gordon, 1994: 85–101.
80. Poehlman ET. A review: exercise and its influence on resting energy metabolism in man. Med Sci Sports Exerc 1989; 21:515–525.
81. Levine JA, Baukol PA, Pavlidis Y. The energy expended chewing gum. N Engl J Med 1999; 341:2100.
82. Haymes EM, Byrnes WC. Walking and running energy expenditure estimated by Caltrac and indirect calorimetry. Med Sci Sports Exerc 1993; 25:1365–1369.
83. Miller AT, Blyth CS. Influence of body type and body fat content on the metabolic cost of work. J Appl Physiol 1955; 8:139–141.
84. Passmore R. Daily energy expenditure in man. Am J Clin Nutr 1956; 4:692–708.
85. Jéquier E, Schutz Y. The contribution of BMR and physical activity to energy expenditure. In: Cioffi LA, James WPT, Van Itallie TB, eds. The Body Weight, Regulatory System: Normal and Disturbed Mechanisms. New York: Raven Press, 1981:89–96.
86. Bray GA, Whipp BJ, Koyal SN, Wasserman K. Some respiratory and metabolic effects of exercise in moderately obese men. Metabolism 1977; 26:403–412.
87. Hanson JS. Exercise responses following production of experimental obesity. J Appl Physiol 1973; 35:587–591.
88. Poole DC, Henson LC. Effect of acute caloric restriction on work efficiency. Am J Clin Nutr 1988; 47:15–18.
89. Whipp BJ, Bray GA, Koyal SN. Exercise energetics in normal man following acute weight gain. Am J Clin Nutr 1973; 26:1284–1286.
90. Dempsey JA, Reddan W, Balke B, Rankin J. Work capacity determinants and physiologic cost of weight-supported work in obesity. J Appl Physiol 1966; 21:1815–1820.
91. Maloiy GMO, Heglund NC, Prager LM, Cavagna CA, Taylor CR. Energetic cost of carrying loads: have African women discovered an economic way? Nature 1986; 319:668–669.
92. Foster GD, Wadden TA, Kendrick ZV, Letizia KA, Lander DP, Conill AM. The energy cost of walking before and after significant weight loss. Med Sci Sports Exerc 1995; 27:888–894.
93. Geissler CA, Miller DS, Shah M. The daily metabolic rate of the post-obese and the lean. Am J Clin Nutr 1987; 45:914–920.
94. DeBoer JO, Roovers LCA, Van Raaij JM, Hautvast JG. Adaptation of energy metabolism of overweight women to low-energy intake, studied with whole-body calorimeters. Am J Clin Nutr 1986; 44:585–595.
95. Leibel RL, Rosenbaum M, Hirsch J. Changes in energy expenditure resulting from altered body weight. N Engl J Med 1995; 332:621–628.
96. Froidevaux F, Schutz Y, Christin L, Jéquier E. Energy expenditure in obese women before and during weight loss, after refeeding, and in the weight-relapse period. Am J Clin Nutr 1993; 57:35–42.
97. Weigle DS, Brunzell JD. Assessment of energy expenditure in ambulatory reduced-obese subjects by the techniques of weight stabilization and exogenous weight replacement. Int J Obes 1990; 14(suppl 1):69–81.
98. Henriksson J. The possible role of skeletal muscle in the adaptation to periods of energy deficiency. Eur J Clin Nutr 1990; 44(suppl 1):55–64.
99. Wendt IR, Gibbs CL. Energy production of rat extensor digitorum longus muscle. Am J Physiol 1973; 224:1081–1086.
100. Crow M, Kushmerick MJ. Chemical energetics of slow and fat-twitch muscles of the mouse. J Gen Physiol 1982; 79:147–166.
101. Saris WHM, Kempen KPG, Van Baak MA. Muscle fiber type, body fatness and substrate oxidation during exercise in obese females. Int J Obes 1994; 18(suppl 2):96.
102. Thomas CD, Peters JC, Reed GW, Abumrad NN, Sun M, Hill JO. Nutrient balance and energy expenditure during ad libitum feeding of high-fat and high-carbohydrate diets in humans. Am J Clin Nutr 1992; 55: 934–942.
103. Zurlo F, Lillioja S, Esposito-Del Puente A, Nyomba BL, Raz I, Saad MF, Swinburn BA, Knowler WC,

Bogardus C, Ravussin E. Low ratio of fat to carbohydrate oxidation as predictor of weight gain: study of 24-h RQ. Am J Physiol 1990; 259:E650–E657.
104. Zurlo F, Nemeth PM, Choksi RM, Sesodia S, Ravussin E. Whole-body energy metabolism and skeletal muscle biochemical characteristics. Metabolism 1994; 43:481–486.
105. Blaak EE, Van Baak MA, Kemerink GJ, Pakbiers MTW, Herdendal GAR, Saris WHM. β-Adrenergic stimulation of energy expenditure and forearm skeletal muscle metabolism in lean and obese men. Am J Physiol 1994; 267:E316–E322.
106. Chang S, Graham B, Yakubu F, Lin D, Peters JC, Hill JO. Metabolic differences between obesity-prone and obesity-resistant rats. Am J Physiol 1990; 259:R1103–R1110.
107. Bouchard C, Tremblay A, Nadeau A, Després JP, Thériault G, Boulay MR, Lortie G, Leblanc C, Fournier G. Genetic effect in resting and exercise metabolic rates. Metabolism 1989; 38:364–370.
108. Villagra F, Cooke CB, McDonagh MJN. Metabolic cost and efficiency in two forms of squatting exercise in children and adults. Eur J Appl Physiol 1993; 67:549–553.
109. Sharp TA, Reed GW, Sun M, Abumrad NN, Hill JO. Relationship between aerobic fitness level and daily energy expenditure in weight-stable humans. Am J Physiol 1992; 263:E121–E128.
110. Costill DL. Inside Running: Basics of Sport Physiology. Indianapolis: Benchmark Press, 1986.
111. Holmer I. Physiology of swimming man. Acta Physiol Scand 1974; 407:1–55.
112. Mulligan K, Butterfield GE. Discrepancies between energy intake and expenditure in physically active women. Br J Nutr 1990; 64:23–36.
113. Dahlstrom M, Jansson E, Nordevang E, Kaijser L. Discrepancy between estimated energy intake and requirements in female dancers. Clin Physiol 1990; 10: 11–25.
114. Jones PJ, Leitch CA. Validation of doubly labeled water for measurement of caloric expenditure in collegiate swimmers. J Appl Physiol 1993; 74:2909–2914.
115. Schulz LO, Alger S, Harper I, Wilmore JH, Ravussin E. Energy expenditure of elite female runners measured by respiratory chamber and doubly labeled water. J Appl Physiol 1992; 72:23–28.
116. Horton TJ, Drougas HJ, Sharp TA, Martinez LR, Reed GW, Hill JO. Energy balance in endurance-trained female cyclists and untrained controls. J Appl Physiol 1994; 76:1937–1945.
117. FAO. The State of Food Insecurity in the World 2000. Rome: Food and Agriculture Organization of the United Nations, 2000.
118. Geeves MA. Stretching the lever-arm theory. Nature 2002; 415:129–131.
119. Gollnick PD. Metabolism of substrates: energy substrate metabolism during exercise as modified by training. Fed Proc 1985; 44:353–357.
120. Saris WHM. Physical activity and body weight regulation. In: Bouchard C, Bray GA, eds. Regulation of Body Weight. Chichester, England: John Wiley & Sons, 1996:135–148.
121. Kelley DE, Mandarino LS. Fuel selection in human skeletal muscle in insulin resistance: a re-examination. Diabetes 2000; 49:677–683.
122. Romijn JA, Coyle EF, Sidossis LS, Gastaldelli A, Jorowitz JF, Endert E, Wolfe RR. Regulation of endogenous fat and carbohydrate metabolism in relation to exercise intensity and duration. Am J Physiol 1993; 265:E380–E391.
123. Holloszy JO, Kohrt WM. Regulation of carbohydrate and fat metabolism during and after exercise. Annu Rev Nutr 1996; 10:121–138.
124. Klein S, Coyle EF, Wolfe RR. Fat metabolism during low intensity exercise in endurance trained and untrained men. Am J Physiol 1994; 267:E924–E940.
125. Martin WH, Dalsky GP, Hurley BF, Matthews DE, Bier DM, Hagberg JM, Rogers MA, King DS, Holloszy JO. Effect of endurance training on plasma free fatty acid turnover and oxidation during exercise. Am J Physiol 1993; 265:E708–E714.
126. Van der Vusse GJ, Reneman RS. Lipid metabolism in muscle. In: Rowell LB, Sheperd JT, eds. Handbook of Physiology, Section 12. Exercise: Regulation and Integration of Multiple Systems. New York: Oxford University Press, 1996:952–994.
127. Hoppeler H. Skeletal muscle substrate metabolism. Int J Obes 1999; 23:S7–S10.
128. Guo Z, Burquera D, Jensen MD. Kinetics of intramuscular triglyceride fatty acids in exercising humans. J Appl Physiol 2000; 89:2057–2064.
129. Hood DA, Terjung RL. Amino acid metabolism during exercise and following endurance training. Sports Med 1990; 9:23–35.
130. Jeukendrup AE, Raben A, Gijsen A, Stegen JH, Brouns F, Saris WH, Wagenmakers AJ. Glucose kinetics, during prolonged exercise in highly trained human subjects: effect of glucose ingestion. J Physiol 1999; 515:579–589.
131. Ahlborg G, Felig P, Hagenfeldt, Hendler R, Wahren J. Substrate turnover during prolonged exercise in man Splanchnic and leg metabolism of glucose, free fatty acids, and amino acids. J Clin Invest 1974; 53:1080–1090.
132. Jansson E, Kaijser L. Effect of diet on the utilization of blood-borne and intramuscular substrates during exercise in man. Acta Physiol Scand 1982; 115:19–30.
133. Hargreaves M, Kiens B, Richter EA. Effect of increased free fatty acid concentrations on muscle metabolism in exercising men. J Appl Physiol 1991; 70: 194–201.
134. Griffiths AJ, Humphreys SM, Clark MOL, Frayn KN.

Forearm substrate utilization during exercise after a meal containing both fat and carbohydrate. Clin Sci 1994; 86:169–175.
135. Turcotte LP, Richter EA, Kiens B. Increased plasma FFA uptake and oxidation during prolonged exercise in trained vs. untrained humans. Am J Physiol 1992; 262:E791–E799.
136. Wahren J. Glucose turnover during exercise in man. Ann NY Acad Sci 1977; 301:45–55.
137. Essen B, Hagenfeldt L, Kaijser L. Utilization of blood-borne and intramuscular substrates during continuous and intermittent exercise in man. J Physiol 1977; 265: 489–506.
138. Bosch AN, Dennis SC, Noakes TD. Influence of carbohydrate ingestion on fuel substrate turnover and oxidation during prolonged exercise. J Appl Physiol 1994; 76:2364–2372.
139. Bergstrom J, Hultman E. A study of the glycogen metabolism during exercise in man. Scand J Clin Lab Invest 1967; 19:218–228.
140. Ahlborg G, Juhlin-Dannfelt A. Effect of β-receptor blockade on splanchnic and muscle metabolism during prolonged exercise in men. J Appl Physiol 1994; 76: 1037–1042.
141. Jeukendrup AE, Wagenmakers AJ, Stegen JH, Gijsen AP, Brouns F, Saris WH. Carbohydrate can completely suppress endogenous glucose production during exercise. Am J Physiol 1999; 276:E672–E683.
142. Friedman JE, Lemon PWR. Effect of chronic endurance exercise on retention of dietary protein. Int J Sports Med 1989; 10:118–123.
143. Millward DJ, Bowtell JL, Pacy P, Rennie MJ. Physical activity, protein metabolism and protein requirements. Proc Nutr Soc 1994; 53:223–240.
144. Felig P, Wahren J. Amino acid metabolism in exercising man. J Clin Invest 1971; 50:2703–2714.
145. Christensen EH, Hansen O. Respiratorischer quotient und O_2-aufnahme. Scand Arch Physiol 1929; 81:180–189.
146. Kiens B, Essen-Gustavsson B, Christensen NJ, Saltin B. Skeletal muscle substrate utilization during submaximal exercise in man: effect of endurance training. J Physiol 1993; 469:459–478.
147. Hurley BF, Nemeth PM, Martin WH, Hagberg JM, Dalsky GP, Holloszy JO. Muscle triglyceride utilization during exercise: training effect. J Appl Physiol 1986; 60:562–567.
148. Holloszy JO, Coyle EF. Adaptations of skeletal muscle to endurance exercise and their metabolic consequences. J Appl Physiol 1984; 56:831–838.
149. Gollnick PD, Saltin B. Significance of skeletal muscle oxidative enzyme enhancement with endurance training. Clin Physiol 1982; 2:1–12.
150. Kiens B, Kristiansen S, Jensen P, Richter EA, Turcotte LP. Membrane associated fatty acid binding protein (FABP) in human skeletal muscle is increased by endurance training. Biochem Biophys Res Commun 1997; 231:463–465.
151. Jansson E, Kaijser L. Substrate utilization and enzymes in skeletal muscle of extremely endurance-trained men. J Appl Physiol 1987; 62:999–1005.
152. Decombaz J, Schmitt B, Ith M, Decarli B, Biem P, Kreis R, Hoppeler H, Boesch C. Postexercise fat intake repletes intramyocellular lipids but no faster in trained than in sedentary subjects. Am J Physiol Regul Integr Comp Physiol 2001; 281:R760–R769.
153. Saltin G. Metabolic fundamentals in exercise. Med Sci Sports Exerc 1973; 5:137–146.
154. Donovan CM, Brooks GA. Endurance training affects lactate clearance not lactate production. Am J Physiol 1983; 244:E83–E92.
155. Tarnopolsky LJ, MacDougall JD, Atkinson SA, Tarnopolsky MA, Sutton JR. Gender differences in substrate for endurance exercise. J Appl Physiol 1990; 308:302–308.
156. Blaak E. Gender difference in fat metabolism. Curr Opinion Clin Nutr Med Care 2001; 4:499–502.
157. Toth MJ, Gardner AW, Arciero PJ, Calles-Escandon J, Poehlman ET. Gender differences in fat oxidation and sympathetic nervous system activity at rest and during submaximal exercise in older individuals. Clin Sci 1998; 95:59–66.
158. Horton TJ, Pagliassotti MJ, Hobbs K, Hill JO. Fuel metabolism in men and women during short and long-duration exercise. J Appl Physiol 1998; 85:1823–1832.
159. Carter SL, Rennie C, Tarnapolsky MA. Substrate utilisation during endurance exercise in men and women after endurance training. Am J Physiol 2001; 280:E898–E907.
160. Tarnapolsky MA. Gender differences in lipid metabolism during exercise and rest. In: Tarnapolsky MA, ed. Gender Differences in Metabolism Practical and Nutritional Implication. Boca Raton: CRC Press, 1999:179–199.
161. Burguera B, Proctor D, Dietz N, Guo Z, Joyner M, Jensen MD. Leg free fatty acid kinetics during exercise in men and women. Am J Physiol Endocrinol Metab 2000; 278:E113–E117.
162. Perseghin G, Scifo P, Pagliato E. Gender factors affect fatty acids induced insulin resistance in non obese humans. Effects of oral steroidal contraception. J Clin Endocrinol Metab 2001; 86:3188–3196.
163. Binnert C, Koistinen HA, Martin G, Andreelli F, Ebeling P, Koivisto VA, Laville M, Auwerx J, Vidal H. Fatty acid transport protein-1 mRNA expression in skeletal muscle and in aclipose tissue in humans. J Physiol 2000; 279:E1072–E1079.
164. Nicklas BJ, Hackney AC, Sharp RL. The menstrual cycle and exercise: performance, muscle glycogen, and substrate responses. Int J Sports Med 1989; 10:264–269.
165. Hackney AC, McCracken-Compton MA, Ainsworth

B. Substrate responses to submaximal exercise in the midfollicular and midluteal phases of the menstrual cycle. Int J Sport Nutr 1994; 4:299–308.
166. Calles-Escandón J, Arciero PJ, Gardner AW, Bauman C, Poehlman ET. Basal fat oxidation decreases with aging in women. J Appl Physiol 1995; 78:266–271.
167. Blaak EE, Van Baak MA, Kemerink GJ, Pakbiers MT, Heidendal GA, Saris WH. Beta adrenergic stimulation of whole body energy expenditure and skeletal muscle metabolism in lean and obese men. Am J Physiol 1994; 267:306–315.
168. Blaak EE, Saris WHM, Wolffenbuttel B. Substrate utilisation and thermogenic responses to beta adrenergic stimulation in obese subjects with NIDDM. Int J Obes Relat Metab Disord 1999; 2:411–418.
169. Blaak EE, Van Aggel-Leijssen DPC, Wagenmakers AJ, Saris WH, Van Baak MA. Impaired oxidation of plasma-derived fatty acids in NIDDM subjects during moderate intensity exercise. Diabetes 2000; 49:2102–2107.
170. Jacobs DR Jr, Hahn LP, Folsom AR, Hannan PJ, Sprafka JM, Burke GL. Time trends in leisure-time physical activity in the upper Midwest 1957–1987: University of Minnesota studies. Epidemiology 1991; 2:8–15.
171. Virkamaki A, Korsheninnikova E, Seppata-Lindroos A, Vehkavaara S, Goto T, Halavaara J, Yki-Jarvinen H. Intra-myocellular lipid is associated with resistance to in vivo insulin actions on glucose uptake, anti-lipolysis and early insulin signalling pathways in human skeletal muscle. Diabetes 2001; 50:2337–2343.
172. Malenfant P, Tremblay A, Doucet E, Imbeault P, Simoneau JA, Joanisse DR. Elevated intramyocellular lipid concentrations in obese subjects is not reduced after diet and exercise training. Am J Physiol Endocrinol Metab 2001; 280:E632–639.
173. Malenfant P, Joanisse DR, Theriaulb R. Fat content in individual muscle fibers of lean and obese subjects. Int J Obes Relat Metab Disord 2001; 25: 1316–1321.
174. Van Loon L, Greenhaff PL, Constantin-Teodosiu D, Saris WH, Wagenmakers AJ. The effects of increasing exercise intensity on muscle fuel utilisation in humans. J Physiol 2001; 536:295–304.
175. Schrauwen P, Van Aggel PPC, Wagenmakers AJM, Van Baak MA, Saris WHM. Low intensity exercise training increases non-plasma derived triglyceride oxidation. Int J Obes 2000; 24:S181.
176. National Center for Health Statistics. Prevalence of Overweight and Obesity Among Adults. Atlanta: National Center for Health Statistics, 1999. www.cdc.gov/nchs.
177. MAFF. Household food consumption and energy expenditure (annual reports). London: AMSO, 1940–1994.
178. DiPietro L. Physical activity, body weight and adiposity: an epidemiologic perspective. Exerc Sports Sci Rev 1995; 23:275–303.
179. Hill JO. Physical activity, body weight and body fat distribution. In Leon A, ed. In: Physical Activity and Cardiovascular Health. Champaign, IL: Human Kinetics, 1997:80–92.
180. Kuczmarski RJ, Flegal KM, Campbell SM, Johnson CL. Increasing prevalence of overweight among US adults. JAMA 1994; 272:205–211.
181. Eck LH, Hackett-Renner C, Klesges LM. Impact of diabetic status, dietary intake, physical activity, and smoking status on body mass index in NHANES II. Am J Clin Nutr 1992; 56:329–333.
182. Reaven PD, Barrett-Connor E, Edelstein S. Relation between leisure-time physical activity and blood pressure in older women. Circulation 1991; 83:559–565.
183. Obarzanek E, Schreiber GB, Crawford PB, Goldman SR, Barrier PM, Frederick MM, Lakatos E. Energy intake and physical activity in relation to indexes of body fat: the National Heart, Lung and Blood Institute Growth and Health Study. Am J Clin Nutr 1994; 60:15–22.
184. Capersen CJ, Nixon PA, Durant RH. Physical activity epidemiology applied to children and adolescents. Exerc Sport Sci Rev 1998; 26:341–404.
185. Slattery ML, McDonald A, Bild DE, Cann BJ, Hilner JE, Jacobs DR Jr, Liu K. Associations of body fat and its distribution with dietary intake, physical activity, alcohol, and smoking in blacks and whites. Am J Clin Nutr 1992; 55:943–949.
186. Mayer EJ, Burchfiel CM, Eckel RH, Marshall JA, Haskell WL, Hamman RF. The role of insulin and body fat in associations of physical activity with lipids and lipoproteins in a biethnic population: the San Luis Valley Diabetes Study. Arterioscler Thromb 1991; 11:973–984.
187. Fontvieille AM, Kriska A, Ravussin E. Decreased physical activity in Pima Indian compared with Caucasian children. Int J Obes 1993; 17:445–452.
188. Davies PSW, Gregory J, White A. Physical activity and body fatness in pre-school children. Int J Obes 1995; 19:6–10.
189. Schulz LO, Schoeller DA. A compilation of total daily energy expenditures and body weights in healthy adults. Am J Clin Nutr 1994; 60:676–681.
190. Williamson DF, Madans J, Anda RF, Kleinman JC, Kahn HS, Byers T. Recreational physical activity and ten-year weight change in a US national cohort. Int J Obes Relat Metab Disord 1993; 17:279–286.
191. Owens JF, Matthews KA, Wing RR, Kuller LH. Can physical activity mitigate the effects of aging in middle-aged women. Circulation 1992; 85:1265–1270.
192. French SA, Jeffery RW, Forster JL, McGovern PG, Kelder SH, Baxter JE. Predictors of weight change over two years among a population of working adults:

the Healthy Worker Project. Int J Obes 1994; 18:145–154.
193. Rissanen AM, Heliovaara M, Knekt P, Reonanen A, Aromaa A. Determinants of weight gain and overweight in adult Finns. Eur J Clin Nutr 1991; 45:419–430.
194. Paffenbarger RS, Wing AL, Hyde RT. Physical activity as an index of heart attack risk in college alumni. Am J Epidemiol 1978; 108:161–175.
195. Racette S, Schoeller DA, Kushner RF. Comparison of heart rate and physical activity recall with doubly labeled water in obese women. Med Sci Sports Exerc 1995; 27:126–133.
196. Crespo CJ, Keteyian SJ, Heath GW, Sempos CT. Leisure-time physical activity among US adults. Results from the Third National Health and Nutrition Examination Survey. Arch Intern Med 1996; 156: 93–98.
197. Fogelholm M, Mannisto S, Vartiainen E, Pietinen P. Determinants of energy balance and overweight in Finland 1982 and 1992. Int J Obes Relat Metab Disord 1996; 20:1097–1104.
198. Hu PS, Young JR. U.S. Personal Transportation Survey. Washington, DC: U.S. Department of Transportation, 1995.
199. DiPietro L, Kohl HW, Barlow CE, Blair SN. Improvements in cardiorespiratory fitness attenuate age-related weight gain in healthy men and women: the Aerobics Center Longitudinal Study. Int J Obes 1998; 22:55–62.
200. Williams PT. Evidence for the incompatibility of age-neutral overweight and age-neutral physical activity standards from runners. Am J Clin Nutr 1997; 65:1391–1396.
201. Ching PLYH, Willett WC, Rimm EB, Colditz GA, Gortmaker SL, Stampfer MJ. Activity level and risk of overweight in male health professionals. Am J Public Health 1996; 86:25–30.
202. Sherwood NE, Jeffery RW, French SA, Hannah PJ, Murray DM. Predictors of weight gain in the Pound of Prevention study. Int J Obes Relat Metab Disord 2000; 2:95–100.
203. Epstein LH, Paluch RA, Gordy CC, Dorn J. Decreasing sedentary behaviors in treating pediatric obesity. Arch Ped 2000; 154:220–226.
204. Robinson TN. Reducing children's television viewing to prevent obesity: a randomized controlled trial. JAMA 1999; 282:1561–1567.
205. U.S. Department of Health and Human Services Physical Activity and Health: A Report of the Surgeon General. Atlanta: U.S. Department of Health and Human Services, Centers for Disease Control and Prevention, National Center for Chronic Disease Prevention and Health Promotion, 1996.
206. Schoeller DA, Shay K, Kushner RF. How much physical activity is needed to minimize weight gain in previously obese women? Am J Clin Nutr 1997; 66:551–556.
207. Wing RR, Hill JO. Successful weight loss maintenance. Annu Rev Nutr 2001; 21:323–341.
208. Jakicic JM, Winters C, Lang W, Wing RR. Effects of intermittent exercise and use of home exercise equipment on adherence, weight loss and fitness in overweight women: a randomized trial. JAMA 1999; 282: 1554–1560.
209. Weinsier RL, Hunter GR, Desmond RA, Byrne NM, Zuckerman PA, Darnell BE. Free-living activity energy expenditure in women who are successful and unsuccessful in maintaining a normal body weight. Am J Clin Nutr 2002; 75:499–504.
210. Tremblay A, Després J-P, Leblanc C, Craig CL, Ferris B, Stephens T, Bouchard C. Effect of intensity of physical activity on body fatness and fat distribution. Am J Clin Nutr 1990; 51:153–157.
211. Broeder CE, Burrhus KA, Svanevik LS, Wilmore JH. The effects of either high-intensity resistance or endurance training on resting metabolic rate. Am J Clin Nutr 1992; 55:802–810.
212. Westerterp KR. Pattern and intensity of physical activity. Nature 2001; 410:539.
213. Dunn AL, Marcus BH, Kampert JB, Garcia ME, Kohl WH 3rd, Blair SN. Comparisons of lifestyle and structured interventions to increase physical activity and cardiorespiratory fitness. JAMA 1999; 281(2): 327–334.
214. Anderson RE, Wadden TA, Bartlett SJ, Zemel B, Verde TJ, Franckowiak SC. Effects of lifestyle activity vs structured aerobic exercise in obese women. JAMA 1999; 281:335–339.
215. Fogelholm M, Kukkonen-Harjula K, Nenonen A, Pasanen M. Effects of walking training on weight maintenance after a very-low-energy diet in premenopausal obese women. Arch Intern Med 2000; 106: 2177–2184.
216. Hendelman D, Miller K, Baggette C, Debold E, Freedson P. Validity of accelerometry for the assessment of moderate intensity physical activity in the field. Med Sci Sports Exerc 2000; 32:S442–S449.
217. Welk GJ, Differding JA, Thompson RW, Blair SN, Dziura J, Hart P. The utility of the Digi-Walker step counter to assess daily physical activity patterns. Med Sci Sports Exerc 2000; 32:S481–S488.
218. Westerterp KR. Assessment of physical activity level in relation to obesity: current evidence and research issues. Med Sci Sports Exerc 1999; S522–S525.
219. Sallis JF, Bauman A, Pratt M. Environmental and policy interventions to promote physical activity. Am J Prev Med 1998; 15:379–397.
220. Schrauwen P, Van Aggel-Leijssen DPC, Wagenmakers AJM, Van Baak AM, Saris WHM. Low intensity exercise training increases non plasma derived triglyceride oxidation. Int J Obes Relat Metab Disord 2000; 24:S181.

25

Endocrine Determinants of Obesity

Jonathan H. Pinkney

University of Liverpool, Liverpool, England

Peter G. Kopelman

Barts and the London Queen Mary's School of Medicine and Dentistry, University of London, London, England

I INTRODUCTION

Obesity is a fundamental disorder of energy balance in which excessive energy stores accumulate in the form of fat in response to sustained high energy intake and/or low expenditure. While genetic factors influence obesity through endocrine mechanisms, the majority of endocrine changes observed in obese subjects are consequences of obesity. The endocrine mechanisms giving rise to disturbances of fat distribution, and by which obesity gives rise to its principal complications—diabetes, cardiovascular disease, and female reproductive dysfunction—are becoming clear. In this chapter we consider the unusual primary endocrine causes of obesity, including recently described genetic syndromes, and then focus on the more common alterations in endocrine function that are characteristic of obesity—disturbances in insulin secretion and action, adrenocortical function, sex steroid secretion, the growth hormone insulinlike growth factor and pituitary-thyroid axes. The evidence that these changes play a role in either the determination of corpulence or the perpetuation of the obese state is considered.

II PRIMARY ENDOCRINE DISEASE AS A CAUSE OF OBESITY

Diseases in which primary endocrine disturbances are the cause of obesity are unusual in clinical practice. This group of disorders (Table 1) includes structural lesions of the hypothalamus, of which craniopharyngioma, or its treatment with surgery or radiotherapy, is the commonest. The mechanisms responsible for weight gain in this situation include hyperphagia, reduced resting metabolic rate, and autonomic imbalance leading to hyperinsulinemia (1). Treatment, which reduces insulin secretion, promotes weight loss in a subset of such patients (2). Patients with growth hormone (GH) deficiency secondary to pituitary/hypothalamic disease also have increased body fat and reduced muscle mass, and this is corrected by GH replacement (3–7). Genetic defects affecting the function of this brain region include Prader-Willi syndrome, until recently the commonest known monogenic form of obesity. Mutations in leptin, leptin receptor, pro-opiomelanocortin (POMC), and melanocortin-4 receptor (MC4R) have now been described in obese humans (8–11), but these are rare

Table 1 Primary Endocrine Causes of Obesity in Humans

Structural damage to hypothalamus
Craniopharyngioma
Pituitary macroadenoma with suprasellar extension
Other space-occupying lesions
Trauma
Infiltration
Inflammation
Surgery and radiotherapy
Other contributing factors
GH deficiency
Hypogonadism
Panhypopituitarism
Genetic syndromes of obesity with hypothalamic dysfunction
Prader-Willi syndrome
Leptin deficiency
Leptin receptor deficiency
POMC mutation
Melanocortin-4 receptor mutation

in clinical practice. Hyperphagia is the main mechanism leading to obesity. MC4R mutations, however, appear to be more common, present in possibly 4% of morbidly obese patients (12). As genome scans identify other loci linked to human obesity new genes await discovery. However, overt endocrine defects of primary significance are seldom observed in the obesity clinic, confirming that most of the observed endocrine changes are adaptations to obesity.

III INSULIN SECRETION AND ACTION IN OBESITY

A major consequence of obesity is impaired insulin action, and this leads to increased insulin secretion from islet β-cells. This abnormality is fundamental to understanding the metabolic complications of obesity (Fig. 1). Insulin resistance and hyperinsulinemia are central to the pathogenesis of ischemic heart disease (13), and, in individuals whose β-cells are unable to compensate for insulin resistance, glucose tolerance is progressively impaired and type 2 diabetes supervenes (14).

Although obesity is characterized by elevated fasting insulin and exaggerated insulin response to oral glucose (15), it is intra-abdominal fat deposition—central obesity—that is particularly associated with a decline in insulin sensitivity (16). Hepatic insulin extraction is reduced in central obesity (17), further increasing plasma insulin levels. While increased body weight moderately reduces hepatic and peripheral insulin sensitivity, central obesity causes far greater impairments. With the advent of computed tomography and magnetic resonance imaging, it has been possible to confirm that visceral, rather than overall, adipose tissue mass is primarily related to the decline in insulin sensitivity and accompanying defects (18).

Several mechanisms account for the effects of obesity on insulin action. Plasma fatty acid (FA) levels are elevated in obese subjects despite normal glucose homeostasis (19). Fatty acids impair insulin-stimulated

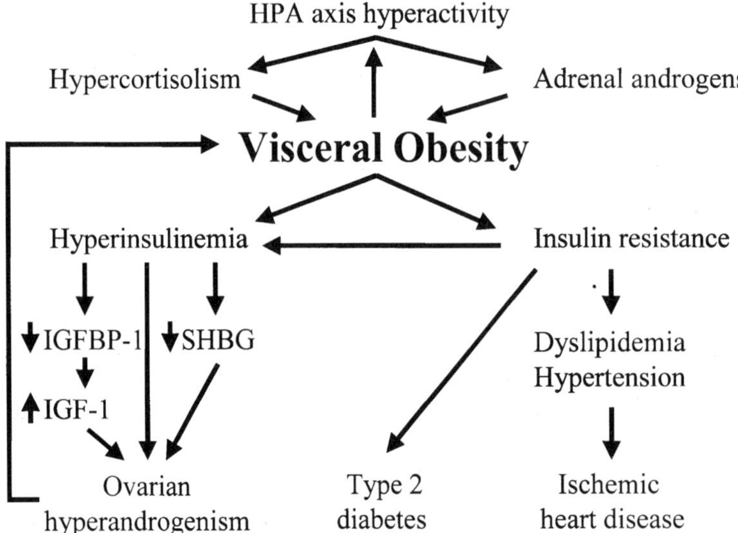

Figure 1 Endocrine relationships among visceral obesity, insulin resistance, and steroid metabolism.

glucose uptake and oxidation in muscle (20) and insulin-mediated suppression of hepatic glucose output (21). It has been suggested that FA released by visceral fat play a key role in the impairment of liver and muscle insulin sensitivity (22). Recently, it has been suggested also that FA accumulation in muscle may be a key event in the impairment of insulin sensitivity (23).

Impaired glucose transport and insulin signaling have attracted attention as possible explanations for insulin resistance. In premenopausal women, insulin-stimulated activity of the enzyme glycogen synthase in quadriceps muscle declined with increasing obesity and insulin resistance during a somatostatin-insulin-dextrose infusion (24). An inverse relationship was observed between insulin receptor numbers and a measure of upper-body obesity, waist-to-hip ratio (WHR). Obesity was also associated with depletion of adipocyte glucose transporters (GLUT4) (25). Severe insulin resistance in type 2 diabetic patients was associated with a still greater fall in GLUT4 mRNA compared to simple obesity that involved both plasma membrane and cytosolic compartments. In both patient groups, suppression of GLUT4 mRNA expression entirely accounted for impaired insulin responsiveness in adipose tissue. In contrast, no differences were seen in skeletal muscle GLUT4 content or mRNA from control subjects (26). These studies support the concept of a primary defect in GLUT4 in adipocytes but not in muscle.

More recently, it has been shown in animal models that knockout of GLUT4 in adipose tissue leads to insulin resistance in liver and muscle (27). The mechanism responsible for this remains to be determined but FA are a leading candidate. Declining muscle insulin sensitivity may also result from decreased functional activity of GLUT4 or impairment of insulin-stimulated translocation of intracellular GLUT4 to the cell surface. It has been demonstrated that chronic exposure to high concentrations of glucose and insulin reduces insulin-stimulated glucose transporter translocation (28). Thus hyperglycemia and/or hyperinsulinemia may contribute to insulin resistance.

Many other hormones and mediators are released by adipose tissue (29), some affecting insulin secretion and/or action. Leptin was found by some (30,31), but not all, investigators to inhibit insulin signaling. However, leptin also inhibits insulin secretion (32), and this may impair glucose tolerance. TNFα is also expressed in adipocytes and may cause insulin resistance in obesity (33). A comprehensive discussion of other factors is beyond the scope of this chapter. These include prostanoids, angiotensinogen, IGF-1, IL-6, adiponectin, complement components and related molecules, and resistin. It is clear that there are many potential mechanisms through which an increased adipose tissue mass can influence insulin secretion and action.

IV ADRENOCORTICAL FUNCTION IN OBESITY

Obesity is associated with complex changes in the hypothalamic-pituitary (HPA) axis (Table 2). Obese subjects have normal plasma and urinary cortisol levels but accelerated cortisol production and degradation (34,35), and the daytime variation is reduced with diminished morning peaks (36–38). A moderate elevation of plasma ACTH levels is seen in obesity (39), with the ACTH response to insulin-induced hypoglycemia positively correlating with body weight (40). Furthermore, HPA axis activation after a meal is greater in women with central than peripheral obesity or normal weight (41). Hyperreactivity of the HPA axis in obese subjects to both neuropeptides and stress is also observed (42). Elevations in stress-related salivary cortisol profiles have been associated with central obesity in men (43), which supports the concept that stress may predispose to central obesity through HPA axis activation.

There are several additional lines of evidence that demonstrate the association of increased HPA activity and central obesity. Cortisol inhibits the antilipolytic effects of insulin in adipocytes, and this may be more pronounced in visceral adipose tissue (VAT), which contains increased numbers of glucocorticoid receptors (44). Increased cortisol clearance may result from a decrease in cortisol-binding globulin, as well as increased glucocorticoid receptor binding (45), especially in visceral adipocytes with a high density of glucocorticoid receptors (46). It has been suggested that increased expression of 11-β-hydroxysteroid dehydrogenase in omental fat also may increase local cortisol production, thereby promoting central obesity (47).

Table 2 Principal Abnormalities of the HPA Axis in Obesity

Increased stress-induced ACTH secretion
Increased cortisol secretion
Decreased cortisol-binding globulin
Increased cortisol clearance
Flat diurnal cortisol profile
Reduced morning cortisol peak
Impaired dexamethasone suppression
Increased adrenal androgen production
Normal 24-hr urinary cortisol levels

The obesity-related acceleration in adrenocortical function and cortisol clearance is associated with an increased adrenal androgen production and increased urinary 17-ketosteroid excretion. (48). Increased dehydroepiandrosterone (DHEA) turnover occurs in obese women (49), and androgen clearance correlates with WHR. In premenopausal women serum DHEA correlates positively with truncal but negatively with leg fat, whereas these effects are not seen in men (50,51). In women, a shift toward central fat deposition may be an androgenic effect of DHEA. In healthy postmenopausal women, androgen levels are inversely related to fasting plasma glucose levels, and predict central obesity 15 years later (52). A positive correlation is reported between body weight and changes in DHEA and DHEA/17-hydroxyprogesterone ratio after administration of ACTH (53). In vitro studies also suggest less inhibition of 17-hydroxylase compared to 17,20-desmolase by DHEA (54), favoring further androgen production. Thus, DHEA may contribute to abdominal fat cell accumulation with resulting insulin resistance and hyperinsulinemia. The latter depresses SHBG, resulting in an increase in free testosterone levels and further visceral fat accumulation.

In conclusion, dysregulation of the HPA axis in obesity—especially central obesity—results from two distinct alterations. The first is central and characterized by altered ACTH secretory dynamics and hyperresponsiveness of the HPA axis. The other is located in the periphery, including visceral adipose tissue, and is characterized by supranormal cortisol production and tissue response.

V CUSHING'S SYNDROME AND OBESITY

There are many similarities between central obesity and Cushing's syndrome. Cushing's syndrome is characterized by insulin resistance, impaired glucose tolerance, hypertension, dyslipidemia, central obesity, and muscle weakness (55). In addition, decreased plasma SHBG and raised free testosterone levels are features of Cushing's syndrome. Furthermore, women with central obesity and women with Cushing's syndrome do not show the typical female increase in fat cell size and LPL activity in femoral versus abdominal adipocytes. Instead, LPL activity in enlarged abdominal fat cells is increased two to three times that of normal-weight women. It is likely that this results from a combined action of increased cortisol and insulin: human adipose tissue exposed in vitro to high concentrations of cortisol shows increased LPL activity in the presence of insulin (44). These findings suggest cortisol has a preferential effect on abdominal fat because no clear difference from normal is found in femoral fat. This may reflect increased glucocorticoid receptors in abdominal fat (46). Diminished lipolysis in Cushing's syndrome results in a decreased capacity of abdominal fat cells to mobilize fat, leading to adipocyte enlargement. Thus, central obesity in Cushing's syndrome may result from increased LPL activity and reduced lipolysis.

Muscle changes in central obesity and Cushing's syndrome are also similar. Subjects with central obesity show a relative decrease in type I muscle fibers, as in Cushing's syndrome (55). In women with Cushing's syndrome, vastus lateralis muscle contains normal glycogen levels but very low glycogen synthase activity, the likely consequence of reduced insulin sensitivity (55). Fiber composition in such women (and in women with central obesity who were not cushingoid) is characterized by relative abundance of type IIb and scarcity of type I fibers compared to women with gynoid obesity. Moreover, a correlation is seen between the proportion of type I fibers and insulin sensitivity, and between type IIb and insulin resistance: type I fibers show higher insulin sensitivity and bind insulin more efficiently. Thus, the muscle fiber composition in Cushing's syndrome resembles that seen in central obesity.

VI REGIONAL DISTRIBUTION OF ADIPOSE TISSUE

Fat topography can be defined at two levels: first, by individual differences in adipose tissue cell characteristics, and second, by the anatomical distribution of body fat (56,57). The factors controlling fat localization are not fully understood, but regional differences in lipolysis may play a role. Human adipose tissue is richly endowed with β_2-, β_3-, and α_2-adrenoceptors; agonists at β_2/β_3-receptors enhance lipolysis whereas α_2-agonists inhibit lipolysis. In both men and women, the lipolytic response to norepinephrine is more marked in abdominal than gluteal or femoral fat (56). Furthermore, analysis in men and women suggests that male fat distribution reflects predominence of α_2- over β-adrenergic activity in abdominal fat (58). There is considerable evidence that LPL activity influences regional fat distribution. There are significant gender and regional differences in LPL activity that parallel variations in adiposity. Premenopausal women have higher LPL activities in gluteal and femoral regions than men, but this difference disappears after the menopause (59). In addition, women have quantitatively more LPL in gluteal and femoral fat, which contains larger cells, than they do in abdominal adipocytes. These differences in fat distribution between men and women may be explained by the tendency for premenopausal women to deposit fat preferentially in subcutaneous depots. A regional difference is seen in the response of adipose tissue to catecholamine-induced lipolysis, which is probably localized at the adrenoceptor level: stimulation of protein kinase abolishes the lipolytic differences between site and gender (60). Insulin is permissive for LPL synthesis, and glucocorticoids enhance the activity of LPL when added with insulin in vitro (44). Sex steroids are strongly implicated in the regional distribution of body fat, and gender differences are seen also in LPL activity particularly during pregnancy and lactation (61). It is likely that regional variation in receptors for glucocorticoids and sex steroids plays an important role in determining regional fat distribution. Endocrine determinants of fat distribution are discussed at length elsewhere in this volume.

VII SEX STEROID SECRETION IN OBESITY

Excess fat accumulation in women is associated with ovulatory dysfunction, hyperandrogenism, and the development of hormone-sensitive carcinomas (62). Both overall adiposity and fat distribution correlate with these changes (63,64). Menarche frequently occurs at a younger age in obese girls and menstrual abnormalities are common in adulthood (65). Weight loss has a salutary effect on ovulatory function with the return of menses in previously amenorrheic obese women. Obese women exhibit distinct changes in sex steroid levels (64). Androstenedione and testosterone plasma concentrations are often elevated, sex hormone–binding globulin (SHBG) levels reduced, and the plasma ratio of estrone to estradiol increased. This is similar to the patterns found in women with polycystic ovary syndrome. Evans and colleagues (63) showed that body weight and WHR correlate inversely with SHBG levels and directly with free testosterone. Others describe a higher production rate from the adrenal cortex and ovaries and increased clearance of testosterone and dihydrotestosterone (64). The clearance of testosterone increases as SHBG decreases, the consequence of an increased fraction of unbound testosterone available for hepatic extraction and clearance (65). Fat is able to sequester steroids, including androgens, because of their lipid solubility, and most sex steroids are preferentially concentrated within adipocytes rather than plasma (66). As a result, the steroid pool is greater in obese than in lean subjects; the fat volume in obese subjects is much larger than the intravascular space, and tissue steroid levels are 2–13 times higher than in plasma. Fat serves not only as a reservoir but also as a site for steroid metabolism. Androgens are irreversibly aromatized to estrogens or reversibly converted to other androgens (67).

There are two possible explanations for the obesity-related increase in androgen production rate. The first is hypothalamic-pituitary-gonadal and adrenal compensation for increased clearance. Alternatively, the increase in ovarian and adrenal production is stimulated by factors such as insulin and, with falling SHBG production, increased bioactivity and clearance of free steroid (68). Increased androgen levels favor central fat deposition with an additional increase in steroid clearance through adipose tissue sequestration and metabolism. Unlike most hormone receptors, the number of androgen receptors in fat cells increases with exposure to testosterone. Interestingly, hypogonadism in men is associated with a significant decrease in the lipolytic response to catecholamines while treatment with testosterone normalizes this response and increases triglyceride turnover. The lipolytic effect of testosterone is mediated by an increase in β-adrenoceptor numbers and the activity of adenylate cyclase, protein kinase A, and hormone-sensitive lipase. The density of abdominal subcutaneous adipose tissue α-adrenoceptors is higher in men than in women. Thus, although the main effect of androgens is lipolytic, these hormones may also increase the number of antilipolytic adrenoceptors. Long-term treatment with testosterone of hypogonadal men leads to a marked decrease in both LPL activity and FA uptake in abdominal but not femoral subcutaneous fat. Moreover, the inhibition of lipid uptake after testosterone administration is more apparent in visceral than in abdominal subcutaneous adipose tissue. Such results are in line with studies that show androgen receptors have a higher density in visceral fat than in subcutaneous fat cells (69).

Obesity in men is characterized by reductions in total and free testosterone, and SHBG concentrations. Such men with lower free testosterone have lower lipolytic responses to catecholamines and higher LPL activity in adipose tissue. These metabolic adaptations may contribute to the lower triglyceride turnover and body fat accumulation in these subjects (70). In addition, there is a strong negative correlation between leptin and free testosterone that is independent of plasma insulin concentration. This may be the explanation for the lower serum leptin levels in men compared to women (71).

VIII ESTROGEN METABOLISM IN OBESITY

Excess body fat leads to changes in the hypothalamic-pituitary-ovarian axis and ovarian function (72). The production of estrogen and its precursors, including androstenedione and testosterone, decreases with age and after the menopause. In premenopausal women, mean 24-hr plasma estrone and estradiol levels do not differ in obese and lean women (73). However, obese women have lower SHBG levels and increased free estrogen. In postmenopausal obese women, serum estrone and estradiol correlate with fat mass (74). SHBG levels are also lower in older women, further elevating free estradiol levels. Aromatization of androstenedione to estrone occurs in adipose tissue of premenopausal and postmenopausal women and is closely related to body weight (75). Aromatization increases with age and is two to four times higher in postmenopausal women (76). Androstenedione is the major substrate for estrogen formation; although only a small amount of testosterone is aromatized, this may be of greater significance. Longcope and colleagues (77) have reported associations between body weight and the conversion of testosterone to estradiol. The interconversion of estrone to estradiol is also greater in omental than subcutaneous fat (78,79). Furthermore, adipose tissue 17-hydroxysteroid dehydrogenase activity, measured by the conversion of estrone to estradiol, is higher in premenopausal than postmenopausal women, and women have higher activity than men (78). Estrogens should not be considered as passive byproducts of obesity because they positively promote preadipocyte proliferation, preservation, and further expansion of adipose tissue (79).

IX SEX HORMONE–BINDING GLOBULIN IN OBESITY

Sex hormone–binding globulin (SHBG), produced by the liver, binds to sex steroids in high affinity but low capacity (80). Levels of SHBG are inversely related to fat mass and WHR (63), so obesity results in increased free steroid levels and clearance. Aromatization rates correlate with free rather than total androgen. The lower affinity of SHBG for estradiol relative to testosterone also results in an estrogen amplification effect on sensitive tissues (particularly the liver) with decreasing SHBG levels (80). Central obesity in women is characterized by higher total testosterone, with increased production rates, increased estradiol, and reduced SHBG compared to lower body obesity (81).

Obesity probably influences SHBG production by several mechanisms. Obesity-related hyperandrogenism may itself reduce SHBG levels, increasing clearance of testosterone and estradiol (72). However, insulin inhibits SHBG synthesis (82), and hyperinsulinemia is probably the main mechanism leading to the fall in SHBG production in central obesity. Hyperinsulinemia, in conjunction with increased free IGF-1, further increases ovarian androgen secretion, thereby contributing to a vicious circle of events (68,83).

X POLYCYSTIC OVARY SYNDROME AND OBESITY

The polycystic ovary syndrome (PCOS) (84) is the most common endocrine disorder of reproduction. Moderate degrees of excess bodyweight are frequently observed in the syndrome, fueling speculation that obesity is a causal factor. The multiple endocrine and metabolic defects associated with PCOS are summarized in Table 3.

The ovaries in PCOS show thickened cortices and increased numbers of atretic follicles. The androgen-producing stroma are usually hyperplastic. There is hyperplasia of thecal cells, and immature granulosa cells are unable to convert androgens to estrogens. Many of these features are seen in obese women with normal menstrual function, but in this circumstance the ovary is not enlarged (85). Similar morphology is seen in women with Cushing's disease and congenital adrenal hyperplasia, syndromes also associated with hyperandrogenism (86). What are the common features of PCOS and obesity, and is it possible to distinguish PCOS from obesity?

Table 3 Principal Metabolic Abnormalities Associated with Obesity and the PCOS

Insulin resistance
Hyperinsulinemia
Impaired glucose tolerance
Type 2 diabetes
Dyslipidemia
Increased adrenal androgen secretion
Increased ovarian testosterone secretion
Increased aromatization of androstenedione
Increased estrone/estradiol ratio
Decreased SHBG
Decreased IGFBP-1
Increased free steroid concentrations

In contrast to obesity, the ovaries in PCOS are the major source of androgens, with LH-dependent production (86). PCOS is characterized by increased plasma androstenedione and testosterone and a reversed estradiol:estrone ratio. SHBG is also reduced in PCOS, as in obesity (63,87). Testosterone is formed in peripheral tissues by conversion from androstenedione, DHEA, and DHEAS, while estrone is both secreted by the ovaries and derived from extragonadal aromatization. In both PCOS and obesity, aromatization rates of androstenedione to estrone by adipose tissue correlate with body weight (88). In contrast to obesity, however, PCOS is marked by increased LH secretion, reflecting increased pituitary sensitivity to gonadotropin-releasing hormone (GnRH).

The etiology of PCOS is controversial. Much evidence supports a key role for insulin resistance, and this may explain the association of PCOS with obesity. Insulin increases free testosterone levels in PCOS by increasing production of testosterone and suppressing that of SHBG (89). Women with PCOS are insulin resistant and hyperinsulinemic, and often develop impaired glucose tolerance and type 2 diabetes (90). Although the degree of hyperinsulinemia is proportional to body weight, lean women with PCOS are also insulin resistant. In PCOS, as in obesity, increasing central obesity is associated with insulin resistance and reduced hepatic insulin extraction (68). Obese women with PCOS are significantly more hyperinsulinemic than nonobese women with PCOS (91). However, suppression of gonadal steroidogenesis with a long-acting GnRH analog does not affect plasma insulin levels or insulin sensitivity (92), which argues against steroids as the cause of insulin resistance. Hyperinsulinemia may drive ovarian steroidogenesis to produce PCOS (68). Nestler and colleagues (93) observed a fall in plasma insulin and testosterone levels in obese women with PCOS given diazoxide, with no effect on gonadotropin release. Subsequent studies with the insulin-sensitizing agents metformin and thiazolidinediones (94–96) confirm the findings with diazoxide. Ovarian P450c17α-hydroxylase activity declines markedly in obese and lean women with PCOS after the reduction of serum insulin with metformin (97).

An additional mechanism by which insulin influences androgen secretion involves IGFBP-1. Lean women with PCOS show a positive correlation between plasma insulin and IGF-1 concentrations and a negative one with IGFBP-1, a pattern identical to that in obesity (98). Since IGFBP-1 acts as an inhibitor of IGF-1 action, its suppression by insulin favors increased androgen production by increasing ovarian levels of free IGF-1. IGF-1 is a potent amplifier of LH-induced androgen synthesis (99).

An alternative theory for the etiology of PCOS is the gonadotropin hypothesis, which postulates a primary role for increased LH secretion relative to FSH. Against a primary role for the hypothalamus in PCOS, however, is the fact that increased LH secretion is not a usual finding in most obese women of reproductive age, and this argues against increased gonadotropin secretion as the initial event in the obesity-PCOS relationship. Finally, the finding that weight loss improves menstrual function in obese women with PCOS (100) supports the contention that obesity is a cause of the ovarian disturbance.

XI THE GROWTH HORMONE/INSULINLIKE GROWTH FACTOR AXIS IN OBESITY

The growth hormone (GH)/insulinlike growth factor (IGF) axis is an important regulator of body composition throughout life. Multiple GH-IGF axis defects are present in obese individuals (Table 4), although these are usually maladaptive consequences, rather than primary etiological factors. However, GH hyposecretion is physiologically relevant to increasing body fatness. Subcutaneous fat is markedly increased in GH-deficient subjects (101), and abdominal rather than peripheral adiposity is closely associated with GH hyposecretion (102). In one study of GH-deficient subjects, visceral fat was decreased by 30% after 6 months' treatment with GH (103). GH deficiency is associated with impairments of lipolysis in fat and protein synthesis in muscle (104)—an unfavorable combination in the context of obesity. Several mechanisms contribute to reduced GH levels in obesity including inhibition of secretion by nutrient and neuroendocrine signals, increased binding, and clearance. GH secretion is reduced in response to both pharmacological and physiological stimuli (105). The reduction in GH secre-

Table 4 Principal Abnormalities of the GH-IGF Axis in Obesity

Decreased GH secretion
Increased GHBP secretion
Decreased IGFBP-1
Decreased IGFBP-3
Low/normal total IGF-1
Increased free IGF-1
Decreased ghrelin secretion

tion is due mainly to a reduction in pulse amplitude rather than frequency (106). The clearance of both exogenous GH and endogenous GH is increased in obesity (107,108), and the consequences of reduced GH secretion are further amplified by increased levels of GH-binding protein (GHBP) (109), particularly in central obesity (110).

Circulating FA levels are increased in obesity, and contribute to the downregulation of GH secretion. Thus, an intravenous lipid infusion impairs the GH response to GHRH in humans (111). A direct inhibitory effect of FA on pituitary GH secretion explains this phenomenon (112). The usual inhibitory effect of glucose on GH secretion is blunted in obesity, suggesting a disturbance of hypothalamic glucose sensing (113). Chronic carbohydrate overfeeding impairs GH responses without any increase in body weight (114). It is currently unclear whether this results from direct nutrient effects or neuroendocrine mechanisms. Insulin suppresses GH secretion in vitro (115), so hyperinsulinemia may contribute to GH hyposecretion in obesity. Other factors involved in the downregulation of GH secretion are IGF-1 and its binding proteins. IGF-binding protein 1 and 3 (IGFBP-1, IGFBP-3) are reduced in obesity; the decreased serum IGFBP-1 levels are inversely related to fasting insulin and WHR (116,117). Insulin stimulates synthesis of IGF-1 and suppresses that of IGFBP-1. The hyperinsulinemia of obesity, in conjunction with increased IGF-1 output from an expanded adipose tissue mass, may explain the elevated levels of free IGF-1 in obesity (118). Free IGF-1 exerts negative feedback on GH secretion in pituitary cells. Confirming this mechanism, the GH response to GHRH in obese humans is suppressed by exogenous IGF-1 (119). A final mechanism for GH hyposecretion is suggested by the recent finding of reduced plasma ghrelin levels in obesity (see below).

Evidence that GH hyposecretion contributes to the maintenance, and perhaps the pathophysiology, of the obese state, is provided by clinical trials of administering GH to obese subjects. In a 9-month study of rhGH in men with central obesity, total body and visceral fat declined by 9.2% and 18.1%, with improved glucose tolerance, lipid profile, and blood pressure (120). The mechanisms responsible for the beneficial effect on fat mass are probably multiple, including increased lipolysis (121), lean body mass, and resting metabolic rate (122). There is evidence that GH may augment plasma leptin levels in GH-deficient humans (123), which could promote negative energy balance, although GH has no effect on leptin in obese adults (122). Lastly, in preadipocytes, IGF-1 promotes and GH suppresses adipocyte differentiation (124,121), raising the interesting possibility that the high IGF-1/low GH environment of obesity favors adipocyte differentiation. Finally, the observation that weight loss reverses the defects in GH and IGF-1 secretion (125) and reduces GHBP levels (126), confirms that these abnormalities are indeed secondary to obesity.

XII GHRELIN AND OBESITY

A discussion of obesity and the GH-IGF axis would no longer be complete without mention of ghrelin. Ghrelin is a 28–amino acid GH secretagogue expressed in gut neuroendocrine cells—mainly in the gastric fundus, as well as the arcuate nucleus of the hypothalamus (127). Ghrelin is the endogenous ligand for the previously identified growth hormone secretagogue receptor (128). Whether administered to pituicytes in vitro, ICV to animals, or by peripheral injection to animals and humans, ghrelin powerfully elicits GH secretion (129). Unexpectedly, both ICV and peripheral injection of ghrelin in animals and humans also elicited strong feeding responses, and weight gain was observed in animals. Gastric ghrelin expression and secretion increase with fasting and decline in the postprandial state. In the stomach, ghrelin has a prokinetic effect, whereas circulating ghrelin appears to stimulate feeding and induce weight gain and gastric acid secretion through central effects.

The effect on weight is probably mediated through central antagonism of leptin and other anorectic cytokines through signals delivered via vagal afferents, rather than a direct bloodborne effect on the hypothalamus (130). This action is mediated through increased expression of hypothalamic neuropeptide- Y (130) and Agouti-related protein (AGRP) (131). Reduced plasma ghrelin concentrations have been reported now in human obesity (132), and may result from the higher leptin or insulin levels in obese subjects. Both leptin and interleukin-1β reduce ghrelin expression in the stomach (130). Thus, circulating ghrelin controls hypothalamic sensitivity to anorectic signals while some of the same signals regulate peripheral ghrelin release.

Although the role of ghrelin in energy homeostasis remains to be fully clarified, on the basis of these data it has been proposed that both centrally released and peripheral circulating ghrelin of gastric origin are involved in the regulation of GH secretion and feeding, and therefore that circulating ghrelin explicitly impacts central control of feeding and GH secretion. Further research should clarify the extent to which these actions are distinct or intrinsically linked. Given this apparent dual role, however, it is possible that circulating ghrelin couples activity of the GH-IGF axis to signals that induce negative energy balance such as leptin and cytokines. The defence of lean body mass in the fasting state—an important function of the GH-IGF axis—would be more efficient if concurrent anorectic and thermogenic signals could be shut down. However, while ghrelin downregulation in the stomach may be an appropriate adaptation to obesity, by potentiating the central actions of signals that induce negative energy balance, and reducing gastric acid secretion and motility, it is also possible that low ghrelin secretion might have less desirable effects including contributing to the maladaptive reduction of GH secretion characteristic of the obese state.

XIII THE PITUITARY-THYROID AXIS IN OBESITY

Although hypothyroidism can present with weight gain, the hypothalamic-pituitary-thyroid (HPT) axis is not considered to play a major role in the etiology of obesity. However, thyroid hormone is an important regulator of genes for energy homeostasis (133–137). An additional direct nongenomic effect of 3,5-di-iodothyronine on mitochondrial respiration has been suggested (138). During fasting, overfeeding, and in obesity, adaptations occur at all levels of the HPT axis. The availability of free hormone measurements and sensitive thyrotropin-stimulating hormone (TSH) assays over the past two decades has aided research in this area. Although a study in obese adults found no change in free thyroid hormone levels (139), a study of lean and obese children reported that the median TSH and thyroid hormone levels were elevated in obese subjects, although still within the reference ranges (140). Increased TSH and decreased prolactin responses to TRH are also seen in obesity (141), suggesting central upregulation. Levels of TSH also correlate with body fat and plasma leptin in obese subjects (142), consistent with central upregulation. Experimental data in humans confirm that the HPT axis is under nutritional control. Overfeeding increases total levels of thyroid hormone and reduces levels of reverse-T3, (143), whereas fasting reduces free T3 and free T4 levels in obese subjects (144). Although 5′-deiodinase activity is under nutritional control and regulates T4-T3 conversion, the fasting-induced fall in T3 is mainly due to reduced thyroid secretion (145). Therefore, the main nutritional and obesity-related changes in the HPT axis occur centrally. The mechanism for this involves the action of leptin in the arcuate nucleus on POMC and NPY-containing neurones (146,147). Thus, the HPT axis makes appropriate adaptations to fasting, defending body weight and muscle mass. As with other endocrine mechanisms, the HPT axis has little capacity for the reverse adaptation in the obese state. Thyroid hormones have attracted interest in obesity treatment, but their primary effect is to reduce lean rather than fat mass (148). This and other side effects confirm that therapeutic hyperthyroidism is not a treatment option for obesity.

XIV CONCLUSIONS

Obesity causes many endocrine adaptations and defects related to fuel metabolism, energy storage, and reproduction (Fig. 2). Overt endocrine causes of

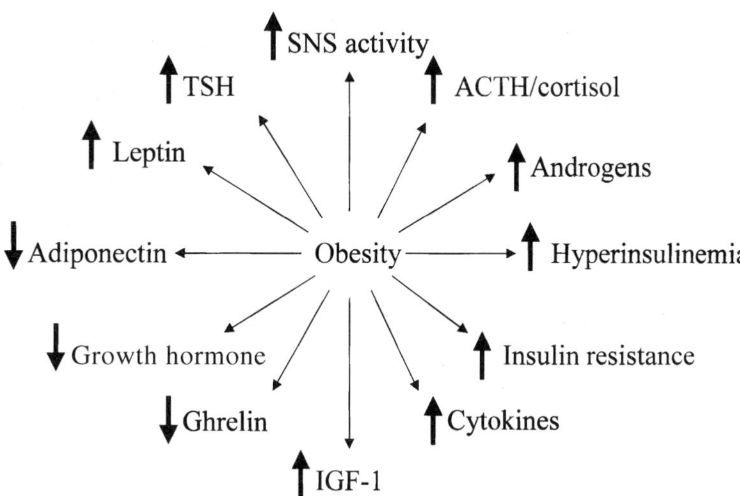

Figure 2 Endocrine consequences of obesity.

obesity are unusual, but advances in genetics are identifying a small number of genes predisposing to obesity. The endocrine adaptations to obesity, with the exception of glucocorticoids and sex steroids, and their effect on fat distribution, are not important in the causation of obesity. They may, however, contribute to the perpetuation of corpulence. Such endocrine adaptations have evolved to store fuel efficiently during times of plenty and to defend the lean body mass in times of famine. Unfortunately, they have little capacity for reverse adaptations in the face of continuous positive energy balance and consequential obesity.

REFERENCES

1. Pinkney JH, Wilding JPH, Williams G, MacFarlane I. Hypothalamic obesity in humans: What do we know and what can be done? Obesity Reviews 2002; 3:27–34.
2. Lustig RH, Rose SR, Burgben GA, et al. Hypothalamic obesity caused by cranial insult in chldren: altered glucose and insulin dynamics and reversal by a somatostatin agonist. J Pediatr 1999; 135:162–168.
3. Li Voon Chong JS, Benbow S, Foy P, Wallymahmed ME, Wile D, MacFarlane IA. Elderly people with hypothalamic-pituitary disease and growth hormone deficiency: lipid profiles, body composition and quality of life compared with control subjects. Clin Endocrinol 2001; 53:551–559.
4. Rosenfalck AM, Mahgsoudi S, Fuisker S, et al. The effect of 30 months of low dose replacement therapy with recombinant human growth hormone (rhGH) on insulin and C-peptide kinetics, insulin secretion, insulin sensitivity, glucose effectiveness, and body composition in GH-deficient adults. J Clin Endocrinol Metab 2000; 85:4173–4181.
5. Chrisoulidou A, Beshyah SA, Rutherford O, et al. Effects of 7 years of growth hormone replacement therapy in hypopituitary adults. J Clin Endocrinol Metab 2000; 85:3762–3769.
6. Biller BM, Sesmilo G, Baum HB, Hayden D, Shoenfeld D, Klibanski A. Withdrawal of long term physiological growth hormone (GH) administration: differential effects on bone density and body composition in men with adult onset GH deficiency. J Clin Endocrinol Metab 2000; 85:970–976.
7. Stouthart PJ, De Ridder CM, Rekers-Mombarg LT, Van der Wall HA. Changes in body composition during 12 months after discontinuation of growth hormone therapy in young adults with growth hormone deficiency from childhood. J Pediatr Endocrinol Metab 1999; 12:335–338.
8. Farooqi IS, Jebb SA, Langmack G. Effects of recombinant leptin therapy in a child with congenital leptin deficiency. N Engl J Med 1999; 341:879–884.
9. Clement K, Vaisse C, lahlou N, et al. A mutation in the human leptin receptor gene causes obesity and pituitary dysfunction. Nature 1998; 392:398–401.
10. Krude H, Biebermann H, Luck W, Hom R, Brabant G, Gruters A. Severe early onset obesity, adrenal insufficiency and red hair pigmentation caused by POMC mutations in humans. Nat Genet 1998; 19: 155–157.
11. Yeo GS, Farooqi IS, Aminian S, Halsall DJ, Stanhope RG, O'Rahilly S. A frameshift mutation in MC4R associated with dominantly inherited hman obesity. Nat Genet 1998; 20:111–112.
12. Vaisse C, Clement K, Durand E, Hercberg S, Guy-Grand B, Froguel P. Melanocortin-4 receptor mutations are a frequent and heterogeneous cause of morbid obesity. J Clin Invest 2000; 106:253–262.
13. Reaven GM. Role of insulin resistance in human disease. Diabetes 1988; 37:1595–1607.
14. DeFronzo RA. The triumvirate: B-cell, muscle, liver. A collusion responsible for NIDDM. Diabetes 1988; 37:667–687.
15. Kolterman OG, Insel J, Sackow M, Olefsky JM. Mechanisms of insulin resistance in human obesity. J Clin Invest 1980; 65:1272–1284.
16. Kissebah AH, Vydelingum N, Murray R, et al. Relation of body fat distribution to metabolic complications of obesity. J Clin Endocrinol Metab 1982; 54:254–260.
17. Peiris AN, Mueller RASGA. Splanchnic insulin metabolism in obesity: influence of body fat distribution. J Clin Invest 1986; 78:1648–1657.
18. Pouliot MC, Despres JP, Nadeau A, Moorjani S, Prud'homme D, Lupien PJ. Visceral obesity in men. associations of glucose tolerance, plasma insulin, and lipoprotein levels. Diabetes 1992; 41:826–834.
19. Golay A, Swislicki AL, Chen YD, Jaspan JD, Reaven GM. Effect of obesity on ambient plasma glucose, free fatty acid, insulin, growth hormone, and glucagon concentrations. J Clin Endocrinol Metab 1986; 63:481–484.
20. Randle PJ, Garland PB, Hales CN, Newsholme EA. The glucose fatty acid cycle. Its role in insulin sensitivity and the metabolic disturbance of diabetes mellitus. Lancet 1963; 785–789.
21. Boden G, Chen X, Ruiz J, White JV, Rossetti L. Mechanisms of fatty acid-induced inhibition of glucose uptake. J Clin Invest 1994; 93:2438–2446.
22. Bjorntorp P. 'Portal' adipose tissue as a generator of risk factors for cardiovascular disease and diabetes. Arteriosclerosis 1990; 10:493–496.
23. Shulman GI. Cellular mechanisms of insulin resistance. J Clin Invest 2000; 106:171–176.
24. Evans DJ, Murray R, Kissebah AH. Relationship between skeletal muscle insulin resistance, insulin-mediated glucose disposal and insulin binding effects of obesity and body fat topography. J Clin Invest 1984; 74:1515–1525.

25. Garvey WT, Maianu L, Huecksteadt TP, et al. Pretranslational suppression of a glucose transporter protein causes cellular insulin resistance in non-insulin-dependent diabetes and obesity. J Clin Invest 1991; 87: 1072–1081.
26. Garvey WT, Maianu L, Hancock JA, Golichowski AM, baron A. Gene expression of GLUT4 in skeletal muscle from insulin resistant patients with obesity, IGT, GDM and NIDDM. Diabetes 1992; 41:465–475.
27. Abel ED, Peroni O, Kim JK, et al. Adipose-selective targeting of the GLUT4 gene impairs insulin action in muscle and liver. Nature 2001; 409:729–733.
28. Garvey WT, Olefsky JM, Matthaei S, Marshall S. Glucose and insulin coregulate the glucose transport system in primary cultured adipocytes: a new mechanism of insulin resistance. J Biol Chem 1987; 262: 189–197.
29. Mohamed-Ali V, Pinkney JH, Coppack SW. Adipose tissue as an endocrine and paracrine organ. Int J Obes 1998; 22:1145–1158.
30. Muller G, Ertl J, Gerl M, Preibisch G. Leptin impairs metabolic actuions of insulin in isolated rat adipocytes. J Bio Chem 1997; 272:10585–10593.
31. Walder K, Filippis A, Clark S, Zimmet P, Collier GR. leptin inhibits insulin binding in isolated rat adipocytes. J Endocrinol 1997; 155:R5–R7.
32. Cases JA, Gabriely I, Ma XH, et al. Physiological increase in plasma leptin markedly inhibits insulin secretion in vivo. Diabetes 2001; 50:348–352.
33. Hotamisligil GS, Spiegelman BM. Tumor necrosis factor—a key component of the obesity-diabetes link. Diabetes 1994; 43:2409–2415.
34. Migeon CJ, Green OC, Eckert JP. Study of adrenocortical function in obesity. Metabolism 1963; 12:718–730.
35. Galvao-Tales A, Graves L, Burke CW, et al. Free cortisol in obesity: effect of fasting. Acta Endocrinol 1976; 81: 321–329.
36. Strain GW, Zumoff B, Strain JJ, levin J, Fukushima DK. Cortisol production in obesity. Metabolism 1980; 29:980–985.
37. Ljung T, Andersson B, Bengtsson B-A, Bjorntorp P, Marin P. Inhibition of cortisol secretion by dexamethasone in relation to body fat distribution: a dose response study. Obes Res 1996; 4:277–282.
38. Marin P, Darin N, Amemiya T, Andersson B, Jern S, Bjorntorp P. Cortisol secretion in relation to body fat distribution in obese premanopausal women. Metabolism 1992; 41:882–886.
39. Slavnov VN, Epstein EV. Somatotrophic, thyrotriphic and adenotrophic functions of the anterior pituitary in obesity. Endocrinologie 1977; 15:213–218.
40. Weaver JU, Kopelman PG, McLoughlin L, et al. Hyperactivity of the hypothalamo-pituitary-adrenal axis in obesity: a study of ACTH, AVP, b-lipotropin and cortisol responses to insulin-induced hypoglycaemia. Clin Endocrinol 1993; 39:345–350.
41. Korbonits M, Trainer PJ, Nelson MI, et al. Differential stimulation of cortisol and dehydroepiandrosterone levels by food in obese and normal subjects: relation to body fat distribution. Clin Endocrinol 1996; 45:699–706.
42. Pasquali R, Biscotti M, Spinucci G. Pulsatile rhythm of ACTH and cortisol in premenopausal women: effect of obesity and body fat distribution. Clin Endocrinol 1998; 48:603–612.
43. Rosmond R, Dallman MF, Bjorntorp P. Stress-related cortisol secretion in men: relationships with abdominal obesity and endocrine, metabolic and hemodynamic abnormalities. J Clin Endocrinol Metab 1998; 83: 1853–1859.
44. Cigolini M, Smith U. Human adipose tissue in culture. VIII. Studies on the insulin antagonist effect of glucocorticoids. Metabolism 1979; 28:502–510.
45. Rebuffe-Scrive M, Bronnegard M, Nilsson A. Steroid hormone receptors in human adipose tissues. J Clin Endocrinol Metab 1990; 71:1215–1219.
46. Bronnegard M, Arner P, Hellstrom L, et al. Gluocorticoid receptor messenger ribonucleic acid in different regions of human adipose tissue. Endocrinology 1990; 127:1689–1696.
47. Bujalska IJ, Kumar S, Stewart PM. Does central obesity reflect Cushing's disease of the omentum? Lancet 1997; 349:1210–1213.
48. Simkin V. 17-Ketosteroid and 17-ketogenic steroid excretion in obese patients. N Engl J Med 1961; 264: 974–977.
49. Kurtz BR, Givens JR, Kominder S, et al. maintenance of normal circulating levels of D-androstenedione and dehydroepiandrosterone in simple obesity despite increased metabolic clearance rates: evidence for a servo-controlled mechanism. J Clin Endocrinol Metab 1987; 64:1261–1267.
50. Williams DP, Boyden TW, Pamenter RW, et al. Relationship of body fat percentage and fat distribution with dehydroepiandrosterone sulfate in premanopausal females. J Clin Endocrinol Metab 1993; 77:80–85.
51. Usiskin KS, Butterworth S, Clore JN, et al. Lack of effect of dehydroepiandrosterone sulphate in obese men. Int J Obes 1990; 14:457–463.
52. Khaw K-T, Barret-Connor E. Fasting plasma glucose levels and endogenous androgens in non-diabetic postmenopausal women. Clin Sci 1991; 80: 199–203.
53. Brody S, Carlstrom K, Lagrelius K, et al. Adrenal steroid in postmenopausal women: relation to obesity and bone mineral content. Maturitas 1987; 9:25–32.
54. Couch RM, Muller J, Winter JSD. Regulation of the activities of 17-hydroxylase and 17,20-desmolase in the human adrenal cortex: genetic analysis and inhibition by endogenous steroids. J Clin Endocrinol Metab 1986; 63:613–618.

55. Rebuffe-Scrive M, Krotkiewski M, Elfverson J, Bjorntorp P. Muscle and adipose tissue morphology and metabolism in Cushing's syndrome. J Clin Endocrinol Metab 1988; 67:1122–1128.
56. Krotkiewski M, Bjorntorp P, Sjostrom L, Smith U. Impact of obesity on metabolism in men and women. Importance of regional adipose tissue distribution. J Clin Invest 1983; 72:1150–1162.
57. Bouchard C, Bray GA, Hubbard V. Basic and clinical aspects of regional fat distribution. Am J Clin Nutr 1990; 52:946–950.
58. La Fontan M, Dang-Tran L, Berlan M. Alpha-adrenergic antilipolytic effect of adrenaline in human fat cells of the thigh: comparison with adrenal responsiveness of different fat deposits. Eur J Clin Invest 1975; 9:261–266.
59. Rebuffe-Scrive M, Bjorntorp P. Regional adipose tissue metabolism in man. In: Vague J, Bjorntorp P, Guy-Grand B, eds. Metabolic Complications of Human Obesities. Amsterdam: Elsevier North-Holland, 1985:149–159.
60. Wahrenberg H, Lonnqvist F, Arner P. Mechanisms underlying regional differences in lipolysis in human adipose tissue. J Clin Invest 1989; 84:458–467.
61. Rebuffe-Scrive M, Enk L, Crona L, et al. Fat cell metabolism in different regions in women. Effects of menstrual cycle, pregnancy and lactation. J Clin Invest 1985; 75:1973–1976.
62. Kirschner MA, Schneider G, Ertl NH, Worton E. Obesity, androgens, oestrogens and cancer risk. Cancer Res 1982; 42:3281–3285.
63. Evans DJ, Hoffman RG, Kalkhoff R, Kissebah AH. Relationship of androgenic activity of body fat topography, fat cell morphology and metabolic aberrations in postmenpausal women. J Clin Endocrinol Metab 1983; 57:304–310.
64. Samojlik E, Kirschner MA, Silber D, et al. Elevated production and metabolic clearance rates of androgens i morbidly obese women. J Clin Endocrinol Metab 1984; 59:949–954.
65. Vermulen A, Ando S. Metabolic clearance rate and interconversion of androgens and the influence of free androgen fractions. J Clin Endocrinol Metab 1979; 48:320–326.
66. Feher T, Brodrogi L. A comparative study of steroid concentrations in human adipose tissue and peripheral circualation. Clin Chim Acta 1982; 126:135–141.
67. Longcope C, Kato T, Orton R. Conversion of blood androgens to estrogens in normal adult men and women. J Clin Invest 1969; 48:2191–2201.
68. Barbieri RL, Hornstein MD. Hyperinsulinaemia and ovarian hyperandrogenism: cause and effect. Endocrinol Metab Clin North Am 1988; 17:685–703.
69. Sjögren L, Min P. Androgen hormone binding to adipose tissue in rats. Biochim Biophys Acta 1995; 1244:117–120.
70. Marin P, Lonn L, Andersson B, et al. Assimilation of triglycerides in subcutaneous and intraabdominal adipose tisusue in vivo in men. J Clin Invest 1996; 81: 1018–1022.
71. Vettor R, De Pergola G, Pagano C, et al. Gender differences in obese people. Relationship with testosterone, body fat distribution and insulin secretion. Eur J Clin Invest 1997; 27:1016–1024.
72. Aziz R. Reproductive endocrinologic alterations in female asymptomatic obesity. Fertil Steril 1989; 52: 703–725.
73. Zhang Y-W, Stern B, Rebar RW. Endocrine comparison of obese menstruating and amenorrhoeic women. J Clin Endocrinol Metab 1984; 58:1077–1083.
74. Meldrum DR, Davidson BJ, Tatryn IV, Judd HL. Changes in circulating steroids with ageing in postmenopausal women. Obstet Gynecol 1981; 57:404–408.
75. Schinder AE, Ebert A, Friedrich E. Conversion of androstenedione to oestrone by human fat tissue. J Clin Endocrinol Metab 1972; 35:627–630.
76. Hemsell DL, Grodin JM, Brenner PF, et al. Plasma precursors of oestrogen. II. Correlation of the extent of conversion of plasma androstenedione to oestrone with age. J Clin Endocrinol Metab 1974; 38:476–479.
77. Longcope C, Baker R, Johnston CCJ. Androgen and estrogen metabolism: relationship to obesity. Metabolism 1986; 35:235–237.
78. Deslypere JP, Verdonek L, Vermulen A. Fat tissue: a steroid reservoir and site of steroid metabolism. J Clin Endocrinol Metab 1987; 61:564–570.
79. Roncari DAK, Van RLR. Promotion of human adipocyte precursor replication by 17-b-oestradiol in culture. J Clin Endocrinol Metab 1987; 61:564–570.
80. Anderson DC. Sex hormone binding globulin. J Clin Endocrinol Metab 1974; 3:69–96.
81. Kirschner MA, Samojlik M, Drejka M, et al. Androgen-oestrogen metabolism in women with upper body obesity versus lower body opbesity. J Clin Endocrinol Metab 1990; 70:479.
82. Plymate SR, Matej LA, Jones RA, Friedl KE. Inhibition of sex hormone binding globulin production in human hepatoma (HepG2) cell line by insulin and prolactin. J Clin Endocrinol Metab 1988; 67:460–464.
83. Barbieri RR, Makris A, Randall RW, et al. Insulin stimulates androgen accumulation in incubations of ovarian stroma obtained from women with hyperandrogenism. J Clin Endocrinol Metab 1986; 62:904–910.
84. Stein IF, Leventhal LM. Amenorrhoea associated with bilateral polycystic ovaries. Am J Obstet Gynecol 1935; 29:181–191.
85. Fisher ER, Gregonon R, Stephen T. Ovarian changes in women with morbid obesity. Obstet Gynecol 1974; 44:839–844.
86. Dunaif A. Polycystic ovary syndrome and obesity. In:

Bjorntorp P, Brodoff PN, eds. Obesity. Philadelphia: Lippincott, 1992:594–605.

87. Hausner H, Ditschieneit HM, Pal SB, et al. Fat distribution, endocrine and metabolic profile in obese women with and without hirsutism. Metabolism 1988; 37:281–286.
88. Edman CD, MacDonald PC. Effect of obesity on conversion of plasma androstendione to oestrone in ovulatory and anovulatory young women. Am J Obstet Gynecol 1978; 130:456–461.
89. Nestler JE, Powers LP, Matt DW, et al. A direct effect of hyperinsulinemia on serum sex hormone binding globulin levels in obese women with polycytstic ovary syndrome. J Clin Endocrinol Metab 1991; 72:83–89.
90. Oberfield SE. Metabolic lessons from the study of young adolescents with polycystic overy syndrome—is insulin, indeed, the culprit? J Clin Endocrinol Metab 2001; 85:3520–3525.
91. Franks S, Kiddy D, Sharp P, et al. Obesity and polycystic ovary syndrome. Ann NY Acad Sci 1991; 626:201–206.
92. Geffner ME, Kaplan SA, Bersch N, et al. Persistence of insulin resistance in polycystic ovary disease after inhibition of ovarian steroid secretion. Fertil Steril 1986; 45:327–333.
93. Nestler JE, Barlascini CO, Matt DW, et al. Suppression of serum insulin by diazoxide reduces serum testosterone levels in obese women with PCOS. J Clin Endocrinol Metab 1989; 68:1027–1032.
94. Velasquez EM, Mendoza S, Hamer, et al. Metformin therapy in polycystic ovary syndrome reduces hyperinsulinemia, hyperandrogenemia and systolic blood pressure while facilitating menses and pregnancy. Metabolism 1994; 43:647–654.
95. Dunaif A, Scott D, Finegood D. The insulin-sensitizing agent troglitazone improves metabolic and reproductive abnormalities in polycystic ovary syndrome. J Clin Endocrinol Metab 1996; 81:3299–3306.
96. Iuonro MJ, Nestler JE. Insulin-lowering drugs in polycystic ovary syndrome. Obstet Gynecol Clin North Am 2001; 28:153–164.
97. Nestler JE, Jakubowicz DJ. Decreases in ovarian cytochrome P450c17 alpha activity and serum free testosterone after reduction of insulin secretion in polycystic ovary syndrome. N Engl J Med 1996; 335: 617–623.
98. Conway GS, Jacobs HS, Holly JMP, Wass JAH. Effects of luteinizing hormone, insulin-like growth factor small binding protein-1 in the polycystic ovary syndrome. Clin Endocrinol 1990; 33:593–603.
99. Erickson GF, Magoffin DA, Dyer CA, Hofeditz C. The ovarian androgen producing cells: a review of structure/function relationships. Endocr Rev 2001; 6: 371–399.
100. Kiddy DS, Hamilton-Fairley D, Bush A, et al. Improvements in endocrine and ovarian function during dietary treatment of obese women. Clin Endocrinol 1992; 36:105–111.
101. Tanner JM, Whitehouse RH. The effect of human growth hormone on subcutaneous fat thickness in hyposomatrophic and hypopituitary dwarfs. J Endocrinol 1967; 39:263–275.
102. Vahl N, Jorgensen JOL, Skjaerbaek C, Veldhuis JD, Orskov H, Christiansen JS. Abdominal adiposity rather than age and sex predicts mass and regularity of GH secretion in healthy adults. Am J Physiol 1997; 272:E1108–E1116.
103. Bengtsson BA, Eden S, Lonn L, et al. Treatment of adults with growth hormone deficiency with recombinant human GH. J Clin Endocrinol Metab 1994; 78:960–967.
104. Jorgensen JO, Moller N, Wolthers T, et al. Fuel metabolism in growth hormone–deficient adults. Metabolism 1995; 44:103–107.
105. Maccario M, Grotolli S, Procopio M, et al. The GH/IGF-1 axis in obesity: influence of neuroendocrine and metabolic factors. Int J Obes 2000; 24:S96–S99.
106. Veldhuis J, Liem A, South S, et al. Differential impact of age, sex steroid hormones, and obesity on basal vs pulsatile growth hormone secretion in men as assessed in an ultrasensitivie chemiluminescence assay. J Clin Endocrinol Metab 1995; 80:3209–3222.
107. Langendonk JG, Meinders AE, Burggraaf J. Influence of obesity and body fat distribution on growth hormone kinetics in humans. Am J Physiol 1999; 277:E824–E829.
108. Veldhuis JD, Iranmanesh A, Ho KK, Waters MJ, Johnson ML, Lizarralde G. Dual defects in pulsatile growth hormone secretion and clearance subserve the hyposomatotropism of obesity in man. J Clin Endocrinol Metab 1991; 72:51–59.
109. Postel-Vinay MC, Saab C, Gourmelen M. Nutritional status and growth hormone binding protein. Horm Res 1995; 44:177–181.
110. Fisker S, Vahl N, Jorgense JO, Christiansen JS, Orskov H. Abdominal fat determines growth hormone–binding protein levels in healthy nonobese adults. J Clin Endocrinol Metab 1997; 82:123–128.
111. Maccarrio M, Arvat E, Procopio M, et al. Metabolic modulation of growth hormone–releasing activity of hexarelin in man. Metabolism 1995; 44:134–138.
112. Alvarez CV, Mallo F, Burguera B, Caciedo L, Dieguez C, Casanueva FF. Evidence for a direct pituitary inhibition by free fatty acids of in vivo growth hormone responses to growth hormone-releasing hormone in the rat. Neuroendocrinology 1991; 53:185–189.
113. Maccario M, Procopio M, Grotolli S, et al. In obesity the somatotrope response to either growth hormone–releasing hormone or arginine is inhibited by somatostatin or pirenzepine but not by glucose. J Clin Endocrinol Metab 1995; 80:3774–3778.

114. Merimee TJ, Fineberg SE. Dietary regulation of human growth hormone secretion. Metabolism 1973; 22:1491–1497.
115. Yamashita S, Melmed S. Effect of insulin on rat anterior pituitary cells. Diabetes 1986; 35:440–447.
116. Weaver JU, Kopelman PG, Holly JMP, et al. Decreased sex hormone binding globulin (SHBG) and insulin-like growth factor-1 (IGFBP-1) in extreme obesity. Clin Endocrinol 1990; 32:641–646.
117. Bang P, Brismar K, Rosenfeld RG, Hall K. Fasting affects serum insulin-like growth factors (IGFs) and IGF-binding proteins in patients with non-insulin-dependent diabetes versus healthy nonobese and obese subjects. J Clin Endocrinol Metab 1994; 78:960–967.
118. Frystyk J, Skjaerbaek E, Morgensen CE, Orskov H. Free insulin-like growth factor in human obesity. Metabolism 1995; 44:37–44.
119. Maccario M, Tassone F, Gianotti L. Effects of recombinant human insulin-like growth factor 1 administration on the growth hormone (gh) response to GH-releasing hormone in obesity. J Clin Endocrinol Metab 2001; 86:167–171.
120. Johansson G, Marin P, Lonn L. Growth hormone treatment of abdominally obese men reduces abdominal fat mas, improves glucose and lipoprotein metabolism, and reduces diastolic blood pressure. J Clin Endocrinol Metab 1997; 82:727–734.
121. Richelsen B. Action of growth hormone in adipose tissue. Horm Res 1997; 48:105–110.
122. Karlsson C, Stenlof K, Johansson G. Effects of growth hormone treatment on the leptin system and on energy expenditure in abdominally obese men. Eur J Endocrinol 1998; 138:408–414.
123. Bianda TL, Glatz Y, Boeni-Schnetzler M, Froesch ER, Schmid C. Effects of growth hormone (GH) and insulinlike growth factor-1 on serum leptin in GH-deficient adults. Diabetologia 1997; 40:363–364.
124. Smith PJ, Wise LS, Berkowitz R, Wan C, Rubin CS. Insulin-like growth factor-1 is an essential regulator of the differentiation of 3T3-L1 adipocytes. J Biol Chem 1988; 263:9402–9408.
125. Rasmussen MH, Hvidberg AJA, Main KM, Gotfredsen A, Skakkebaek NE, Hilsted J. Massive weight loss restores 24-hour growth hormone release profiles and serum insulin-like growth factor-1 levels in obese subjects. J Clin Endocrinol Metab 1995; 80:1407–1415.
126. Rasmussen MH, Ho KK, Kjems L, Hilsted J. Serum growth hormone–binding protein in obesity: effect of short term, very low calorie diet and diet-induced weight loss. J Clin Endocrinol Metab 1996; 81:1519–1524.
127. Kojima M, Hosoda H, Date Y, Nakazato M, Matsuo H, Kangawa K. Ghrelin is a growth-hormone-releasing acylated peptide from stomach. Nature 1999; 402:656–660.
128. Kojima M, Hosoda H, Matsuo H, Kangawa K. Ghrelin: discovery of the natural endogenous ligand for the growth hormone secretagogue receptor. Trends Endocrinol Metab 2001; 12:118–122.
129. Dieguez C, Casanueva FF. Ghrelin: a step forward in the understanding of somatotroph cell function and growth regulation. Eur J Endocrinol 2000; 142:413–417.
130. Shintani M, Ogawa Y, Ebihara K, et al. Ghrelin, an endogenous growth hormone secretagogue, is a novel orexigenic peptide that antagonizes leptin action through the activation of hypothalamic neuropeptide Y/Y1 receptor pathways. Diabetes 2001; 50:227–232.
131. Kamegai J, Tamura H, Shimizu T, Ishii S, Sugihara H, Wakabayashi I. Central effect of ghrelin, an endogenous growth hormone secretagogue, on hypothalamic peptide gene expression. Endocrinology 2000; 141:4797–4800.
132. Tschöp M, Weyer C, Tataranni PA, Devanarayan V, Ravussin E, Heiman ML. Circulating ghrelin leveles are decreased in human obesity. Diabetes 2001; 50:707–709.
133. Zhang J, Lazar MA. The mechanism of action of thyroid hormones. Annu Rev Physiol 2000; 62:439–466.
134. Pillar TM, Seitz HJ. Thyroid hormone and gene expression in the regulation of mitochondrial respiratory function. Eur J Endocrinol 1997; 136:231–239.
135. El Hadri K, Pairault J, Feve B. Triiodothyronine regulates beta 3-adrenoceptor expression in 3t3-F442A differentiating adipocytes. Eur J Biochem 1996; 239: 519–525.
136. Rabelo R, Reyes C, Schifman A, Silva JE. Interactions among receptors, thyroid hormone response elements, and ligands in the regulation of the rat uncoupling protein gene expression by thyroid hormone. Endocrinology 1996; 137:3478–3487.
137. Gong D-W, He Y, Karas M, Reitman M. Uncoupling protein-3 is a mediator of thermogenesis regulated by thyroid hormone and b3-adrenergic agonists and leptin. J Biol Chem 1997; 272:24129–24132.
138. Arnold S, Goglia F, Kadenbach B. 3,5-Diiodothyronine binds to subunit Va of cytochrome-c oxidase and abolishes the allosteric inhibition of ATP. Eur J Biochem 1998; 253:325–330.
139. Buscemi S, Verga S, Maneri R, Blunda G, Galluzzo A. Influences of obesity and weight loss on thyroid hormones. A 3–3.5 year follow-up study on obese subjects with surgical biliopancreatic bypass. J Endocrinol Invest 1997; 20:276–281.
140. Stichel H, l'Allemand D, Gruters A. Thyroid function and obesity in children and adolescents. Horm Res 2000; 54:14–19.
141. Scaglione R, Averna MR, Dichiara MA, et al. Thyroid function and release of thyroid-stimulating hormone and prolactin from the pituitary in human obesity. J Int Med Res 1991; 19:389–394.

142. Pinkney JH, Goodrick S, Katz J, et al. Leptin and the pituitary-thyroid axis: comparative study in lean, obese, hyperthyroid and hypothyroid subjects. Clin Endocrinol 1998; 49:583–588.
143. Davidson MB, Chopra IJ. Effect of carbohydrate and non-carbohydrate sources of calories on plasma 3,5,3-triiodothyronine concentrations in man. J Clin Endocrinol Metab 1979; 48:577–581.
144. Kvetny J. Nuclear tyroxine receptors and cellular metabolism of thyroxine in obese subjects before and after fasting. Horm Res 1995; 21:60–65.
145. Kinlaw WB, Schwartz HL, Oppenheimer JH. Decreased serum triiodothyronine in starving rats is due primarily to diminished thyroidal secretion of thyroxine. J Clin Invest 1985; 75:1238–1241.
146. Legradi G, Emerson CH, Ahima RS, Flier JS, Lechan RM. Leptin prevents fasting-induced suppression of prothyrotropin-releasing hormone messenger ribonucleic acid in neurons of the hypothalamic paraventricular nucleus. Endocrinology 1997; 138:2569–2576.
147. Fekete C, Legradi G, Mihaly E. Alpha-melanocyte-stimulating hormone is contained in nerve terminals in thyrotropin-releasing hormone–synthesising neurons in the hypothalamic paraventricular nucleus and prevents fasting-induced suppression of prothyrotropin-releasing hormone gene expression. J Neurosci 2000; 20:1550–1558.
148. Koppeschaar HP, Meinders AE, Shwarz F. Metabolic responses in grossly obese subjects treated with a very-low-calorie diet with and without triiodothyronine treatment. Int J Obes 1983; 7:133–141.

26

Endocrine Determinants of Fat Distribution

Renato Pasquali, Valentina Vicennati, and Uberto Pagotto

University of Bologna and S. Orsola-Malpighi General Hospital, Bologna, Italy

I INTRODUCTION

Obesity is a heterogeneous disorder with wide variations in risks for complicating diseases. The recognition of the marked differences between excess fat localized in different parts of the body has markedly increased the knowledge of mechanisms by which metabolic and cardiovascular risk factors and diseases aggregate to specific phenotypes of obesity. At the same time, emerging scientific interest has increased our understanding of the main metabolic and hormonal factors involved in the pathophysiology of different obesity phenotypes.

This chapter will focus on the concept of adipose tissue as an endocrine organ, the regulation of the lipolytic/lipogenetic balance, the physiology of hormone regulation of different adipose tissue depots, and the role of hormonal derangements in the pathophysiology of different obesity phenotypes, particularly the abdominal phenotype.

II ADIPOSE TISSUE AS AN ENDOCRINE ORGAN

Adipocytes are well known for their essential role as triglyceride depots, from which energy is called forth at times of need in the form of free fatty acids (FFAs) and glycerol. However, in the past few years, it has been definitively established that adipose tissue may also act as an endocrine organ. In fact, adipocytes express and secrete a number of peptidergic hormones and cytokines, which help to maintain homeostasis; vasoactive peptides, whose proteolytic products regulate vascular tone; and leptin, which plays a central role in regulating energy balance (1). Adipose tissue can also produce active steroid hormones, including estrogens and cortisol, by conversion of androgen precursors and inactive glucocorticoids, respectively. Through such secreted products, adipocytes may deeply influence local adipocyte biology, as well as systemic metabolism at sites as diverse as brain, liver, muscle, pancreatic β-cells, gonads, lymphoid organs, and systemic vasculature (2).

Adipose tissue is also tightly regulated in its differentiation process and in its metabolic functions by many hormones. Each hormone has its own peculiar effect, according to the receptor expression pattern, to gender and age, and to the different adipose tissue sites. These effects are particularly related to regulating the balance between fat accumulation (lipogenesis) and breakdown (lipolysis). There are several differences in the balance between lipogenesis and lipolysis among adipose tissues located in subcutaneous or visceral sites. These effects mainly depend on the activity of lipoprotein lipase and hormone-sensitive lipase, respectively.

III FUNCTIONS OF ADIPOSE TISSUE: LIPOGENESIS AND LIPOLYSIS

A Lipoprotein Lipase: Lipogenesis

Lipoprotein lipase (LPL) is an extrahepatic enzyme responsible for the hydrolysis of triglycerides into chylomicra and very low density lipoprotein (VLDL), and controls the rate-limiting step in the removal of FFAs from the bloodstream. LPL is mainly located at the endothelial surface, and at the level of adipose and muscular tissues as well (3). In vitro studies have shown that adipocyte precursors have no LPL activity during their growth phase in culture, whereas a high enzymatic activity, correlated with adipocyte size, is noticeable during postconfluence differentiation of the cells (3). Insulin, glucocorticoids (GCs), catecholamines, interleukin (IL)-6, IL-1, and other factors differently modulate LPL activity in the various fat depots. The regulation of LPL secretion is related to posttranslational changes in the LPL enzyme at the level of Golgi cisternae and exocytotic vesicles (4). Interestingly, this enzyme displays a specific gender difference (4), due to the different types of receptors expressed by adipocytes in both sexes. In men, LPL activity, measured by radiolabeled triglyceride uptake, is 50% higher in the omentum than in abdominal subcutaneous fat (5). On the contrary, an opposite pattern is observed in women, in whom the omental adipocytes are smaller and the activity of LPL located in abdominal fat depots is lower than that in subcutaneous fat, regardless of the presence of obesity (4).

B Hormone-Sensitive Lipase (HSL): Lipolysis

Adipose tissue releases energy in response to the body's demands (6). Lipolysis in adipose tissue has been extensively investigated in vivo and in vitro because it is easy to quantify the end products such as FFAs and glycerol induced by the lipolytic process. A specific hormone binding to plasma membrane-bound receptors initiates the lipolytic cascade. These receptors are coupled with a G-protein, which may have both stimulatory (Gs) and inhibitory (Gi) effect. Gs proteins are able to activate the intracellular catalytic moiety of adenyl-cyclase converting ATP to cyclic AMP (cAMP). cAMP binds to the regulatory subunit of protein kinase, releasing an active catalytic subunit able to phosphorylate and activate HSL, the rate-limiting enzyme of lipolysis (6). The Gi inhibits the breakdown of ATP into cAMP, thus blocking the lipolytic cascade. Only insulin and catecholamines have marked acute effects on lipolysis. Insulin inhibits lipolysis (7) whereas catecholamines have dual effects: stimulation through different β-receptors and inhibition through α2-receptors (8). HSL activity is also increased by ACTH, glucagon, TSH (3), cAMP (6), and caffeine and teophylline (3). It has been shown in vitro that HSL mRNA and activity are higher in subcutaneous than in omental fat cells. Moreover, subcutaneous adipocytes are larger in the subcutaneous than in the omental region, and the lipolysis rate is significantly correlated to fat cell size regardless of either the region of origin or gender, indicating that the regulation of HSL activity is to a large extent dependent on fat cell size (9). Antilipolytic parahormones such as adenosine and prostaglandins, which are produced locally, are also of importance for the regulation of lipolysis in humans.

IV PHYSIOLOGY OF HORMONE REGULATION OF BODY FAT DISTRIBUTION

A Insulin

The adipocyte is a highly insulin-responsive cell type. In fact, insulin is a critical regulator of virtually all the metabolic step aspects of adipocyte physiology (2). Insulin promotes adipocyte triglyceride storage by several mechanisms, including fostering the differentiation of preadipocytes to adipocytes and stimulating glucose transport and triglyceride synthesis, as well as inhibiting lipolysis in mature adipocytes. By stimulating LPL activity in adipose tissue insulin also increases the uptake of fatty acids derived from circulating lipoproteins (Table 1). Insulin's metabolic effects are mediated by rapid changes in protein phosphorylation and function, as well as by changes in target gene expression (2). Insulin and GCs represent the main physiological stimulants of the LPL activity; their association plays an important role in the regulation of body fat topography. When omental adipose tissue, resistant to insulin action, is exposed to a combination of insulin and dexamenthasone for 7 days, a large increase in mRNA LPL is observed (10). GLUT4 is the main insulin-responsive glucose transporter and is located primarily in muscle cells and adipocytes (11,12). In the presence of insulin, GLUT4 is translocated from intracellular storage to the plasma membrane, leading to a rise in the maximal velocity of glucose transport into the cell (12). The initial molecular signal for insulin action involves the activation of the insulin receptor substrates (IRSs), the activation of phosphoinositide 3′ kinase (PI3K), leading to the translocation of GLUT4 to the plasma membrane (13–15). Whereas activation of PI3K is necessary for full stimulation of glucose transport by insulin, emerging evidence suggests that the other metabolic effects of insulin might be mediated by another pathway with differential sensitivity to insulin (14). For example, the antilipolytic effect of insulin requires much lower insulin concentrations than stimulation of glucose transport. Hence, even in insulin-resistant states in which glucose transport is impaired, sensitivity to insu-

Table 1 Comparison of Lipolysis and Lipogenesis in Omental and Subcutaneous Fat in Nonobese and Obese Individuals (Insulin and Catecholamines Are the Most Important Hormones in the Regulation of Lipolysis)

Omental fat		Subcutaneous fat	
Nonobese[a]	Obese[b]	Nonobese	Obese[c]
Lipolysis		Lipolysis	
β_1: ↑	β_1: =	β_1: ↓	β_1: =
β_2: ↑	β_2: =	β_2: ↓	β_2: ↓
β_3: ↑	β_3: ↑ ↑ ↑	β_3: 0	β_3: 0
Antilipolysis		Antilipolysis	
Adenosine: =	Adenosine: =	Adenosine: =	Adenosine: =
α_2: =	α_2: ↓	α_2: =	α_2: =
Insulin: ↓	Insulin: ↓↓	Insulin: ↑	Insulin: ↓
Lipogenesis		Lipogenesis	
LPL: ↓	LPL: ↑	LPL: ↑	LPL: ↑↑
Insulin: ↓	Insulin: ↓↓	Insulin: ↑	Insulin: ↓

[a] Omental vs. subcutaneous nonobese.
[b] Omental obese vs. omental nonobese.
[c] Subcutaneous obese vs. subcutaneous nonobese.
Source: Ref. 119.

lin's antilipolytic effect is relatively preserved, resulting in maintenance or expansion of adipose stores.

Insulin also plays an important role in the regulation of leptin secretion, even though there are discordant data in the literature. In fact, it has been shown that both acute (hours) and chronic (days) administration of insulin in vivo or in vitro increases *ob* mRNA in rodents and humans (16–19). On the contrary, Sinha et al. did not find any correlation between 24-hr profiles of circulating leptin and insulin levels (20). However, this does not exclude the possibility that chronic hyperinsulinemia, which characterizes obesity, may cause and maintain an elevated leptin expression. It has been shown that the fasting condition or the diabetic state, both of which are known to decrease the circulating insulin level, causes a dramatic reduction in leptin expression, as indicated by changes in the level of the leptin message on adipose tissue (16,21). This decrease can be rapidly, i.e., within hours, reversed by refeeding or insulin administration (16,21). It is likely that insulin acts directly on the adipocyte, rather than indirectly via hormones produced by remotely located tissue, because leptin mRNA level is markedly increased by insulin in epididymal fat explants and adipocyte cell lines (22). Insulin has a favoring role on cortisol-induced LPL activation. These combined actions might, at least in part, explain the different LPL activity in visceral than subcutaneous fat depots, considering that abdominal fat shows a higher glucocorticoid receptor density (23).

B Catecholamines

Catecholamines may specifically activate four adrenergic receptors: β1, β2, β3, and α2, all members of the super family of G-protein-coupled receptors (24). There are significant species differences in adrenergic receptors, and significant differences in affinity of each receptor for the ligand. The order of affinity of the adrenergic receptors is $\alpha2 > \beta1 \geq \beta2 > \beta3$ for norepinephrine (25), and $\alpha2 > \beta2 > \beta1 > \beta3$ for epinephrine (24). The biological significance of the presence of three different β-receptors in adipocytes is unclear but it has been suggested that each receptor subtype might display a different signaling role (26). All three β-receptors are Gs coupled and all may activate adenylyl cyclase. Only β3-receptors have been shown to also interact with Gi in adipocyte membranes, suggesting a different crosstalk of these receptors with inhibitory receptors (26). β1-receptors, which are more sensitive to catecholamines and desensitize rapidly, may mediate acute effects of low level catecholamine stimulation. On the other hand, β3-receptors, which require higher levels of catecholamines to be activated and are more resistant to desensitization, deliver a more sustained signal (27, 28). The presence of the inhibitory α2-receptor provides the cell with the opportunity of dual regulation of cyclase activity. It has been demonstrated that gluteal adipocytes isolated from females have more α2-receptors than adipocytes from males (29). Microdialysis experiments suggest that the α2-adrenoreceptors may regulate lipolysis in the resting phase, while the β-receptors regulate lipolysis during exercise (30). Males have a larger visceral fat cell volume, which seems to be associated with a decrease in α2-receptors and an increase in the β3-adrenoreceptor function (31). These differences may account for gender-specific differences observed in the balance between lipolysis and lipogenesis. In vitro studies have shown a different regional sensitivity to both sympathetic nervous system (SNS) and insulin action. In both genders, the subcutaneous abdominal adipocytes have higher β1- and β2-adrenoreceptor density and sensitivity and a reduced α2-receptor affinity and number than the femoral and gluteal adipocytes (7). Thus, femoral and gluteal depots show a lower lipolytic response to catecholamines than subcutaneous depots (30). On the other hand, visceral adipocytes are equally sensitive to both catecholamine-induced stimulation and inhibition of lipolysis, but they are less sensitive to the antilipolytic effect of insulin when compared to the subcutaneous abdominal or femoral adipose tissue (31,32). Thus in visceral adipose tissue there is a higher turnover of lipids than in the other fat depots, with greater sensitivity to catecholamine-induced lipolysis and decreased sensitivity to insulin antilipolysis (7) (Table 1).

C Glucocorticoids

Glucocorticoid receptors (GCRs), located at intracellular level, function as transcription factors by inducing and/or repressing the expression of a host of target genes. The GCRs are members of the steroid-thyroid intracellular receptor superfamily. The ligand binding to receptors is modulated by "prereceptor" metabolism (33). Recently, it has been demonstrated that pre-receptor metabolism of GCs is an important determinant of tissue-specific responses. There is strong evidence for such a role for 11β-hydroxysteroid-dehydrogenase (11βHSD) enzymes. In adipose tissue, 11βHSD isoform type 1 is involved in the conversion of cortisone to cortisol. In human adipocyte culture, 11βHSD1 activity is higher in the omental than in the subcutaneous fat (23) and GCRs show a regional difference in density, being higher in visceral fat depots (23). In vitro studies have shown that cortisol induces the LPL activity in human adipose tissue (34) and that RU486, a glucocorticoid receptor antagonist, induces an efficient inhibition of cortisol-induced LPL expression (35,36). The cortisol effects on LPL in human adipose tissue are dependent on insulin. LPL is efficiently expressed in a dose-dependent manner, and is apparently a combined effect of transcription of the LPL gene and a stabilization of enzyme activity (35,36). Abdominal adipose tissue shows a higher expression of cortisol-induced LPL. Visceral adipose tissue has not yet been examined with respect to LPL activity and expression, but the high density of the GCRs (35,36) in visceral adipose tissue strongly suggests the possibility that the expression of LPL by cortisol is higher in visceral than in subcutaneous adipose tissue. Cortisol is also involved in the regulation of lipolysis. In the presence of insulin, when LPL activity is efficiently expressed, catecholamine-induced lipolysis is inhibited by cortisol (34). Finally, it has been demonstrated both in animal and human adipose cell lines that GCs are involved in the regulation of leptin secretion (17). In fact, glucocorticoids stimulate ob gene expression both in cultured explants of human adipose tissue (37) and in humans (38). Treatment of normal rats with different types of GCs at catabolic doses rapidly induces leptin expression in adipose tissue followed by a concordant decrease in body weight gain and food intake (39). Exposure of isolated rat adipocytes to dexamethasone was reported to increase leptin mRNA four- to eightfold within hours as well as leptin secretion (40).

D Androgens

Male sex steroid hormones play an important role in the determination of body fat distribution and pattern of obesity. It is well known that androgens bind specific intracellular receptors. Androgen receptors (ARs) have been shown to be present in a very low level in hamster and human adipocytes (41). On the contrary, high levels of ARs have been described in male rat and human preadipocytes (42). Moreover, the number of ARs is more abundant in preadipocytes derived from abdominal than from subcutaneous fat deposits (43). These site-related differences in AR distribution between different fat depots constitute the rationale to explain divergent differentiation processes and metabolic responses observed between intra-abdominal and subcutaneous adipose tissues. Importantly, stimulation with androgens seems to upregulate the expression of their own receptor (42). Androgens stimulate lipolysis in adipose tissue. In primary culture of rat preadipocytes, chronic stimulation with androgens induced an antiadipogenic effect (43). In males, administration of testosterone (T) was followed by a reduction in LPL and FFA uptake in abdominal but not in subcutaneous adipose tissue (44). It is worth mentioning that growth hormone (GH) presence largely contributes to developing the full androgen action at the level of fat depots. In conclusion, the final effect of androgens is a mobilization of lipids which induces a reduction of visceral fat.

E Progesterone and Estrogens

Little is known about the effect of progesterone on fat distribution (45,46). Both isoforms of progesterone receptors (PR-A and PR-B) have been detected more in the stromal-vascular cells than in the adipocytes (45), being strikingly different from estrogen receptors which are mainly localized in the adipocytes (47). This different cellular distribution, recalling that reported at the level of the uterus endometrium (48), points to a complex interaction between estrogen and progesterone in modulating adipose tissue differentiation and function.

Estrogens bind with similar affinity to two different types of receptors, named estrogen receptor (ERs) ERα and ERβ. However, as observed in many organs, the activation of each receptor is supposed to mediate different transactivating properties (49). ERs in adipose tissue have only recently been documented, early studies being unable to detect ER (33,50,51). The development of more sensitive assays has made it possible to detect ERα mRNA, protein as well as specific estrogen binding sites in human subcutaneous adipose tissue (51,52). More recently, also ERβ mRNA has been found in human subcutaneous tissue (52). Altogether these findings clearly indicate that adipose cells are targets for estrogen actions. These data have been reinforced by functional studies in animal models. In rats, ovariectomy leads to an increase in body fat mass, which is reversible after estradiol (E_2) administration (53). The definite proof that the effects mentioned above must be attributed to the ER activation is provided by the studies on mice in which ERs have been knocked out by genetic disruption. After sexual maturation, female mice having homozygous either ER-α or both subtypes deletion showed an increase in total body fat and enhanced serum leptin levels, demonstrating that ERα is responsible for the obese phenotype (54). Importantly, a second paper adopting the same molecular strategy and similar animal models detected the same phenotype also in male mice, indicative of the importance of ERα for normal development and function of adipose tissue in both genders (55). Estrogen replacement in ovarietomized animals resulted in decreased LPL enzyme activity (56).

In women, studies of the effects of hormone replacement therapy on LPL activity levels have been somewhat contradictory. Rebuffé-Scrive et al. (57) showed that the oral administration of sequential combination of estradiol valerate and levonorgesterol to postmenopausal women significantly increased the adipose tissue LPL activity, but data about the effect of estrogens alone were missing from that study. In contrast, Iverius et al. (58) showed an inverse correlation between serum E_2 levels and adipose tissue LPL levels in obese women. Adipose tissue is one of the main sites of E_2 interconversion into estrone, particularly the gluteofemoral region. Price et al. (59) showed that the effect of female sex steroids is different depending on the menopause status. In fact, in premenopausal women progesterone is responsible for the stimulation of LPL activity, with deposition of adipose tissue in the gluteofemoral area rather than the abdominal region. On the contrary, in postmenopausal women progesterone production declined, and localized production of estrone predominates, with a decrease in LPL activity. Because estrone production is higher in the gluteofemoral region, LPL activity decreases in this area to a greater extent than does activity in the abdominal region. Thus, this change in activity is associated with abdominal deposition of body fat. After all, the effects of estrogens partly depend on those of androgens. However, to date, there is very little information on the mechanisms by which androgens and estrogens act separately and which cellular and molecular mechanisms are involved in the differentiation of adipose tissue morphology and function between the sexes.

F Thyroid Hormones

Thyroid hormones have multiple catabolic effects on adipocytes by interacting with the adrenergic receptor signal transduction system (8). Increased concentrations and appearance rates of plasma nonesterified fatty acids (NEFA) and glycerol reflect this action (60). The mechanisms of thyroid hormone action on lipolysis in vitro is unclear. The increased lipolytic rate produced by thyroid hormones in vivo might be related to the increased subcutaneous blood-flow (60) or to a modification of the lipolytic action of catecholamines; it is known that in the hyperthyroid state there is an increase in the total number of β-adrenoreceptors (β1 and β2), unaltered function of the α2-receptors and enhancement of the lipolytic response to catecholamines in gluteal fat (61,62). However, recovery from hyperthyroidism affects visceral and subcutaneous fat differently, since Lonn et al. (63) showed that during the first 3 months of therapy there was an increase of visceral fat, whereas only after 12 months of therapy has an increase of subcutaneous adipose tissue been described (63). On the other hand, there are data showing that in the hyperthyroidism state, muscle LPL activity is increased whereas adipose tissue LPL is unchanged (64). These apparent discrepancies clearly indicate the need for further studies on this topic. Additional studies are also needed to investigate the role of the hyperthyroid state on human body fat regulation and fat distribution.

G GH

It is known that GH exerts its action mainly by inducing insulinlike growth factor (IGF-I) release from the liver; this growth factor is consequently believed to mediate the physiological effect of GH on the different target organs. However, GH is also able to directly affect some distinct target tissues such as adipose tissue. It has been known for many years that both rodent and human adipocytes express GH receptors (65). It is worth mentioning that human adipose tissue also expresses the splice variant (1–279) of the GH receptor at a high level (66), encoding for an isoform having intact extracellular and transmembrane domains but lacking more than 90% of the intracellular domain. This variant has no signaling capacity, but can inhibit GH action mediated by wild-type receptor in a dominant negative manner. However, the significance of this finding is at present still unclear. In rodent and human adipose tissue, GH exerts a lipolytic action either directly, by stimulating basal lipolysis (67), or indirectly, by influencing the ability of fat cells to respond to lypolitic hormones such as catecholamines (68).

At molecular level, GH is thought to increase lipolysis by increasing HSL expression and phosphorylation (69), by upregulating β3-adrenergic receptor level (70), by inhibiting Gi protein (71), and/or by preventing insulin-induced antilipolysis. Recently, new analogs of GH have been provided and tested in animals. These compounds have specific and discrete functional domains of GH. Therefore, there is now evidence supporting the concept that some discrete structural domains within GH might be responsible for the different metabolic functions of the intact GH. Importantly, one of these compounds (AOD-9401) is composed of the carboxy-terminal fragment of the GH molecule and it appears to mainly regulate the lipid metabolism without being associated with alterations of the glucose metabolism as the whole peptide is. In rodents, this compound was able to reduce body weight and when assessed in adipose tissue in culture AOD-9401 significantly reduced lipogenic activity and increased lipolytic activity (72). Further in vivo studies are needed to definitively prove the mode of action of this compound; however, this preliminary report may open new avenues for the full comprehension of GH interaction in adipose tissue. Even more interesting information, at present lacking, will be provided in the future by the use of the recently developed drug pegvisomant, which disables the functional dimerization of the two GH receptors involved in the signal transduction pathway (73).

H Synthetic GH Secretagogues and Ghrelin

Growth hormone secretagogues (GHSs) are compounds able to stimulate GH release by parallel routes to those used by GHRH (74). In 1996, a specific receptor for these peptides was cloned and localized in different central and peripheral organs (75), and a few years later ghrelin, an endogenous ligand for this receptor, was discovered (76). The most important source of production of ghrelin is the stomach, suggesting that this peptide may act as an endocrine signal from gut to hypothalamus. Recently, ghrelin has been shown to play an important role in the development of obesity (77). Interestingly, these data were anticipated by data in which also GHSs were shown to enhance lean body mass and bone mass (78). However, it was difficult to discern whether the stimulatory effect of GHSs on food intake or that on GH secretion prevailed in determining changes in body composition. In fact, chronic stimulation of food intake by GHSs may result in increased body fat, whereas chronic stimulation of GH may result in reduction of body fat, GH being a lipolytic hormone. Recently, the usage of ghrelin in GH-deficient mice (lit/lit), has clearly confirmed that ghrelin displays a GH-independent effect on body weight increasing the fat mass (78). This adipogenic effect is brilliantly mirrored by the simultaneous increased level of circulating leptin, whereas it is well known that GH itself downregulates leptin levels. The precise mechanisms by which ghrelin or GHSs induces adiposity are still unclear, although it has been suggested that reduced levels of ghrelin may represent a physiological adaptation to the positive energy balance associated with obesity (79).

I Leptin

Leptin, a 16-kDa protein, is the well-known product of the ob gene, mainly synthesized by adipose cells and secreted into the bloodstream (80). Leptin was discovered in genetically obese rodents (*ob*/*ob* mice), which are unable to produce an anorexic factor. Correction of leptin deficiency in these animals causes a marked reduction in food intake and a normalization of the obesity syndrome (81). The role of leptin is to control food intake and energy metabolism. Leptin presents structural similarities to the cytokine family (82). Leptin receptors (OB-Rs) have been found at the level of hypothalamus, the brain center responsible for satiety (83). However, OB-R are not confined to the brain but exhibit a widespread distribution, including liver, heart, kidneys, lungs, small intestine, spleen, pancreas, and adipose tissue (83). The OB-Rs belong to the class I cytokine receptor family (84). The receptors have an extracellular domain, a transmembrane domain, and a variable intracellular domain characteristic for each of the five isoforms. OB-Rs act through Janus kinases (JAK) and signal transducers and activators of transcription (STAT). JAK proteins are phosphorylated, thus activating the translocation to the nucleus and stimulation of transcription (84). It has been shown that omental adipocytes have a lower leptin mRNA expression than the subcutaneous fat (85). There is evidence of a direct autocrine/paracrine effect of leptin on the lipolytic activity of isolated adipocytes (85). In addition, leptin has been shown to repress acetyl-CoA carboxylase gene expression, fatty acid synthesis, and lipid synthesis, biochemical reactions that contribute to lipid accumulation without the participation of centrally mediated pathways. Thus, leptin appears to be involved in the direct regulation of adipose tissue metabolism by both inhibiting lipogenesis and stimulating lipolysis (85).

J IL-6

Similarly to leptin, IL-6 binds class I cytokine receptors, and in this way activates JAK and STATs. The IL-6 receptor expression pattern in the different fat depots localization is still unknown. IL-6 circulating levels are positively correlated with body mass index (86); this finding supports that notion that adipose tissue has to be considered a main reservoir of this cytokine. It has in fact been proposed that one-third of circulating IL-6 derives from fat cells (87). IL-6 is released from subcutaneous adipose tissue and threefold more from visceral depots (87,88). However, cells other than adipocytes, such as fibroblasts, immune cells, and vascular cells composing the whole architecture of adipose tissue, constitute the main source of IL-6 (88), making it possible to speculate a mixed autocrine and paracrine role of this cytokine. However, since the liver is the direct target of the venous drainage from omental fat depots, the metabolic impact of IL-6 produced by omental adipose tissue might be of pathophysiological relevance for alterations in lipid synthesis and metabolism. IL-6 has been shown to increase triglyceride secretion in rat liver (89), so IL-6 secreted by omental depots may contribute to maintain hypertriglyceridemia associated with abdominal obesity. IL-6 decreases adipose LPL activity (90) and increases lipolysis (91). These effects have been correlated with the fat depletion occurring during cachectic states characterized by high circulating IL-6 levels (90). IL-6 production from adipose tissue can be stimulated by TNFα (92) and catecholamines (93), whereas GCs downregulate its production (93). The hyperactivation of hypothalamic-pituitary-adrenal (HPA) axis and the increased cortisol turnover are features of the visceral obese state (see below). IL-6 is capable of directly activating this axis at all three levels (94), so IL-6 produced by the adipose tissue may act as a feedforward regulator of this axis, playing an important role in contributing to modulate the differential fat distribution that occurs in patients displaying HPA hyperactivation.

K TNFα

TNFα is involved in the induction of insulin resistance (95) and in the loss of body fat occurring in wasting disorders (96). In humans, TNFα binds p60 and p80 receptors (97). Some authors found an increase in the expression of both receptors in obese subjects (98), whereas others detected only an increase of the p80 receptor (99). Activation of p80 stimulates differentiation in human preadipocytes, whereas p60 seems to induce the opposite effect (100). Soluble circulating TNFα receptor subtypes, which have been detected in the bloodstream, are supposed to inhibit TNFα action. Increased levels of both these soluble subtypes have been recently described in obese patients (98), whereas another report showed an in vivo release of soluble type 1 by human adipose subcutaneous tissue (101). TNFα is produced in greater amounts by subcutaneous than visceral fat (95,102). However, a positive correlation has recently been shown in female subjects between circulating TNFα levels and visceral obesity, which has been attributed to the higher lipolytic action occurring in this adipose tissue district (103). TNFα expression and/or secretion positively correlates with hyperinsulinemia (100). By suppressing LPL, TNFα exerts a prominent catabolic effect on the adipose tissue (100). Moreover, TNFα is supposed to activate HSL, leading to lipid mobilization and an increased delivery of FFA to the liver (104). TNFα is also able to inhibit leptin synthesis (105), confirming that a close interaction seems to occur between the network of cytokines produced in adipose tissue and leptin.

L Resistin

A new peptide named resistin has recently been identified in adipose tissue after a screening for genes induced during adipocyte differentiation. Resistin is specifically expressed in white adipose tissue, circulates in the serum, and can be downregulated by thiazolidinediones. Increased resistin circulating levels have been shown in mouse genetic and diet-induced forms of obesity. Insulin-stimulated glucose uptake in adipocytes was increased by using neutralizing resistin antiserum and resistin administration in mice was shown to reduce glucose tolerance and to decrease the sensitivity to the effects of insulin (106). Resistin is a member of tissue-specific resistin-like molecules (RELMs), and other components such as RELMα, which is a secreted protein abundant in white adipose tissue, or RELMβ, which is expressed in the gastrointestinal tract, have recently been described (107). Isoproterenol treatment was shown to reduce resistin expression in 3T3-L1 adipocytes via β-receptor activation (108). Thus, one may speculate that catecholamines may influence resistin expression more in visceral adipose tissue in which the concentrations of receptors are higher compared to subcutaneous adipose depots. Rather surprisingly,

Table 2 Hormones and Other Factors Involved in the Regulation of Body Fat Distribution and Their Mechanisms of Action

Hormones and factors	Biological functions and mechanisms of action
Insulin	Synergism with GC in increasing LPL activity. Reduced sensitivity of the visceral adipocytes on antilipolytic activity. Stimulation of leptin mRNA expression.
Glucocorticoids (GC)	GC receptors highly expressed, particularly in the visceral adipose tissue. 11β-HSD highly expressed in the visceral adipose tissue. Increased LPL activity (synergism with insulin). In the presence of insulin when LPL if efficiently expressed, catecholamine-induced lipolysis is inhibited by cortisol. Stimulation of leptin mRNA expression.
Androgens (testosterone)	Receptors highly expressed in the visceral adipose tissue. Stimulation of lipolysis and reduced LPL activity in males. These effects are counteracted by estrogens in females. Regulation of leptin mRNA expression.
Estrogens	Estrogen receptors (ERs) highly expressed in the subcutaneous gluteofemoral adipocytes. Inhibition of LPL activity, particularly in the subcutaneous fat. Gluteofemoral adipocytes preferentially transform estradiol to estrone (the most important estrogen after menopause in women).
Progesterone	Receptors found in the stromal-vascular cells. Increase of LPL activity.
GH and related peptides	Stimulation of basal and catecholamine-induced lipolysis. Increase of HSL activity. Variants may be involved in reducing lipogenesis and increasing lipolysis. Ghrelin seems to favor fat gain.
Iodothyronines	Stimulation of lipolysis (increased blood flow or synergism with catecholamines?). Increase of β1- and β2- and reduction of α2-receptors.
Catecholamines	Lipolysis in the visceral adipose tissue highly stimulated (*see Table 1 for different receptor functions in visceral and subcutaneous fat*). Stimulation of IL-6 release from adipose tissue (differences between visceral and subcutaneous?).
Leptin	Omental adipocytes have lower leptin mRNA expression than subcutaneous fat. Paracrine effects on lipolysis (stimulation) and lipogenesis (inhibition).
IL-6	Released by the stromal-vascular cells in the visceral fat more than in subcutaneous fat. Decreased LPL activity and increased lipolysis. Downregulated by GC but exerts stimulation of the HPH axis (therefore it may regulate GB effects on the visceral fat).
TNFα	Stimulation of IL-6 production from the adipose tissue P80 receptors involved in adipocytes differentiation. Production in different adipose tissue depots controversial (visceral < subcutaneous?). Inhibition of leptin synthesis. Activation of HSL (?) and release of FFA to the liver favored.
Resistin	Expressed in the adipose tissue. Regulation by catecholamines more in the visceral than subcutaneous fat (?)

a recent report was not able to confirm the original data from Lazar's study (107) showing that resistin was severely decreased in the white adipose tissue of genetic obese mice and in animals with diet-induced obesity. Moreover, the same group showed that different PPARγ agonists stimulate resistin expression in two rodent models of type 2 diabetes (109). In conclusion, further studies are needed to fully clarify the potential implications of resistin and RELMs in the regulation of adipose tissue function and distribution. Table 2 summarizes all main hormonal actions and functions involved in the regulation of fat distribution in humans.

V BODY FAT DISTRIBUTION IN ENDOCRINE DISORDERS CHARACTERIZED BY HORMONE EXCESS AND DEFICIENCY

A Cushing's Syndrome

Cushing's syndrome is characterized by a redistribution of adipose tissue from peripheral to central sites of the body, mainly in the truncal region and visceral depots. This may occur as a result of the dual effect of GCs which on the one hand downregulate HPL and increase lipolysis, and on the other hand favor preadipocyte differentiation and stimulate substrates to gluconeogenesis and FFA to central fat. Centralization of visceral fat depots tends to be markedly reduced in patients with Cushing's syndrome after eradication of causes of cortisol excess, and this process can be successfully completed within 1–2 years after interventional surgical treatment at pituitary or adrenal level.

B Male Hypogonadism

Hypogonadic males are characterized by increased amounts of visceral fat in both childhood and adult age, and these effects can be completely reversed after T replacement (110). Mechanisms by which T deficiency increases visceral fat depend on the lipogenetic/lipolytic balance in the visceral adipose tissue, due to a different receptor density compared to the subcutaneous tissue (see Sec. IV.D above). The same phenotype can be observed in elderly men, when an increase and redistribution of body fat occurs, with a specific tendency to a greater increase of the abdominal/visceral fat areas. The decline of T production and of circulating levels in elderly individuals plays a dominant role in this context. This is further supported by the decrease in fat mass, particularly in the visceral depots, after long-term treatment with T, provided that physiological levels are achieved and maintained over time.

C Hyperandrogenism in Women

More than 50% of women with the polycystic ovary syndrome (PCOS), the most common cause of hyperandrogenism in females, are overweight or obese. Moreover, most of them are characterized by abdominal fat distribution, particularly if they are obese. Obesity and the abdominal phenotype make it possible to distinguish a large cohort of PCOS women in which the metabolic syndrome is also frequently associated, even though this latter syndrome may also occur in normal-weight PCOS. Insulin resistance and hyperinsulinemia play a key role in the pathogenesis of hyperandrogenism. Mechanisms responsible for the great persistence of the abdominal phenotype in PCOS women largely depend on the coordinate effects of hyperinsulinemia and hyperandrogenism on fat balance. In addition, an excess of androgens may directly produce insulin insensitivity in the muscles by stimulating type II fibers, which are less sensitive to insulin and to increasing FFA efflux (36). Indirect evidence of the role of androgens in determining enlarged visceral fat in women is further supported by the fact that androgen administration in postmenopausal women increases visceral fat depots (111) and tends to reduce whole-body insulin sensitivity.

D GH Deficiency

The profound lipolytic effect of GH have been clearly confirmed by in vivo studies in which GH replacement has been proposed in either children or adult GH-deficient subjects. In fact, several groups have demonstrated a redistribution of adiposity from the subcutaneous trunk to more peripheral regions after GH therapy (112) and a stimulation of FFA release (112). In general, fat redistribution after therapy has been associated with GH-induced reduction of the antilipolytic effect of insulin, which varies according to the fat depot localization.

E Acromegaly

Pathological and inappropriate GH circulating levels characterize acromegaly. In patients affected by this disease there is a reduction in visceral adipose tissue, with an increase in lean body mass (113). The short-term reduction in GH level obtained by octreotide treatment has been shown to reduce lean body mass (114).

VI PATHOPHYSIOLOGY OF DIFFERENT OBESITY PHENOTYPES: THE ROLE OF HORMONES

A Sex Hormones in Women

It is well known that an increase in body weight and fat tissue is associated with several abnormalities of sex steroid balance in premenopausal women. Such alterations involve both androgens and estrogens and overall their carrier protein, sex hormone binding globulin (SHBG), which binds T and dihydrotestosterone (DHT) with high affinity and estrogens with lower affinity. Changes in SHBG concentrations lead to an alteration of androgen and estrogen delivery to target tissues. SHBG plasmatic levels are regulated by a complex of factors, including estrogens, iodothyronines, and GH as stimulating agents, and androgens and insulin as inhibiting factors (115). The net balance of this regulation is probably responsible for the SHBG concentration decrease in obesity, which is inversely related to the increase in body weight (115). Body fat distribution has been demonstrated to substantially affect SHBG concentrations in obese women. In fact, female subjects with central obesity usually have lower SHBG concentrations in comparison to their age- and weight-matched counterparts with peripheral obesity (116). This seems to be dependent on higher circulating insulin in abdominally obese women and on the inhibiting capacity of insulin on SHBG liver synthesis. Reduction of circulating SHBG determines an increase in the metabolic clearance rate of circulating SHBG-bound steroids, specifically T, DHT, and androstenediol (A-diol), which is the principal active metabolite of DHT (116). However, this effect is compensated for by a consequent elevation of production rates. Obesity also affects the metabolism of the androgens not bound to SHBG. In fact, both production rates and metabolic clearance rates of dehydroepiandrostenedione (DHEA) and androstenedione (A) are equally increased in obesity (117,123).

The pattern of body fat distribution can regulate androgen production and metabolism to a significant extent. In fact premenopausal women with central obesity have higher T production rates than those with peripheral obesity (119). Accordingly, metabolic clearance rates of T and DHT are significantly higher in women with central than with peripheral obesity. The maintenance of normal circulating levels of these hormones in obesity may tend to predict the presence of a sophisticated regulation, which can adjust both the production rate and the metabolic clearance rate of these hormones to body size. Owing to the greater reduction of SHBG concentrations, percentage free T fraction tends to be higher in women with central obesity than in those with peripheral obesity (116). An inverse correlation exists between waist to hip ratio (WHR) (or other indices of body fat distribution) and T or SHBG concentrations, regardless of body mass index (BMI) values (116). Therefore, a condition of "relative functional hyperandrogenism" appears to be associated with the central obesity phenotype in women. Androgens play an important role in determining body fat distribution in the female sex. Mechanisms of action have been previously discussed (see Sec. IV.D). This can explain the significant positive association between the abdominal phenotype and hyperandrogenism, as occurs particularly in women with PCOS (120). The observation that visceral fat accumulation occurs only in female-to-male transsexuals after oophorectomy suggests that the remaining estrogen production before surgery was in fact protective (121). Direct evidence of the action of androgens in women is also provided by a controlled study showing that exogenous androgen administration in obese postmenopausal women has been shown to cause a significant gain in visceral fat (as measured by CT scan) and a relatively greater loss of subcutaneous fat in comparison with placebo (111). Mechanisms leading to "functional hyperandrogenism" in obese women are depicted in Figure 1.

Obesity can also be considered a condition of increased estrogen production, since the estrogen production rate significantly correlates with body weight and the amount of body fat (118). Reduced SHBG concentrations may in turn lead to an increased exposure of target tissues to free estrogens. In addition, obesity is associated with a decreased formation of inactive 17β-E_2 metabolites, such as 2-hydroxyestrogens, which are virtually devoid of peripheral estrogen activity, and a higher production of estrone sulfate, an important reservoir of active estrogens. Altogether, these alterations lead to an increased ratio of active to inactive estrogens as a final result. However, in spite of these alterations, blood estrogen concentrations are usually normal or only slightly elevated in both premenopausal and postmenopausal obese women (118). This finding may be attributed to the ability of an enlarged body fat to act as storage for excess formed estrogen, contributing in this way to maintain normal levels of circulating hormone. In addition, there are no systematic differences in the estrogen blood concentrations in women

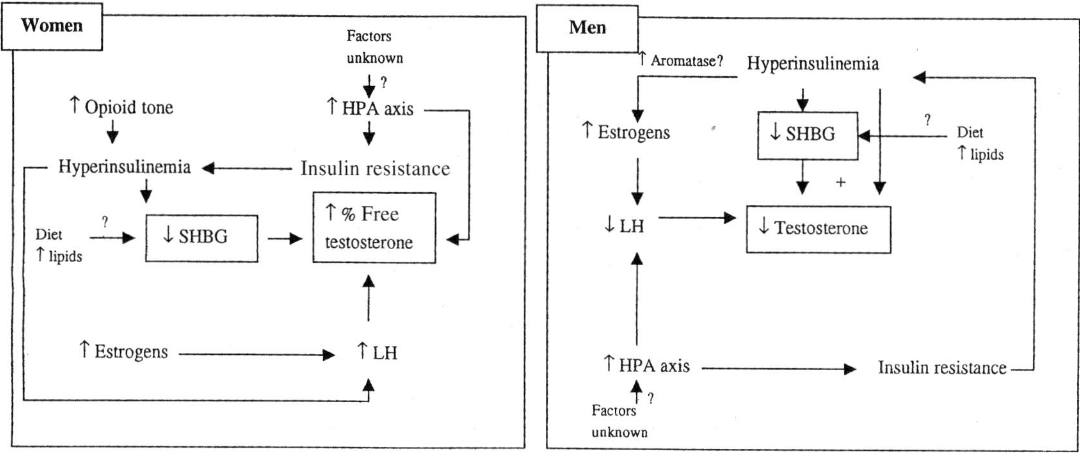

Figure 1 Schematic representation of sex hormone alterations in obese women (left panel) and men (right panel).

with different obesity phenotypes (122), although estrogen production rates have been found to be particularly increased in women with peripheral obesity. Together with the aforementioned protective effects of estrogens on visceral fat development, there is, however, evidence that they play a key role in the regulation of subcutaneous adipocytes, particularly during pregnancy and lactation (58). After menopause, a sudden decrease of estrogens occurs, due to the physiological ovarian failure. Whether the occurrence of menopause alters body weight and fat distribution remains controversial. In fact, while many women claim an increase in body weight during the transition period toward menopause and after menopause, most but not all studies (123) have shown that although the weight of postmenopausal women is greater than before menopause, this difference tends to disappear after adjusting for age values, thus suggesting that age and not the menopausal status per se is probably responsible for weight increase.

Some discrepancies have also been found with regard to the effects of menopause on fat distribution, since there are studies reporting that postmenopausal women had higher WHR values than premenopausal women, whereas others did not observe any effect (123). On the other hand, as discussed in a previous paragraph (see Sec. IV.E above), it should be taken into account that the androgen/estrogen balance differently regulates the adipose tissue morphology and function in the subcutaneous and visceral sites after menopause, thereby potentially favoring some change in the phenotype pattern. The lack of detailed studies investigating the specific role of each class of hormones could therefore explain the aforementioned discrepancies of the effects of hormone replacement therapy in postmenopausal years.

Weight loss is associated with an increase of SHBG levels and the free androgen fraction in women with obesity (121). Moreover, in those with PCOS it not only improves insulin resistance but also the hyperandrogenic state, thereby restoring normal menses and improving fertility rate in a large part of them. Administration of insulin sensitizers such as metformin, added to a hypocaloric diet, further extends these effects and, additionally, seems to favor a greater reduction of the visceral adipose tissue depots (124). These beneficial effects appear to be dependent on the coordinated action of reduced androgen and insulin concentrations and improved insulin sensitivity.

Similar effects have been obtained by using thiazolidinediones, which are selective ligands for peroxisome proliferation–activated receptor (PPAR)γ, a member of the nuclear receptor superfamily of ligand-activated transcription factor (125). Although their mechanisms of action are not yet fully elucidated, they markedly improved insulin-mediated glucose disposal (126) and, at high doses, may suppress basal hepatic glucose production. Studies performed in PCOS women using troglitazone (127) have demonstrated its capability to significantly improve insulin sensitivity, decrease fasting and stimulated insulin levels, reduce the degree of hyperandrogenism, and in several cases, improve spontaneous ovulation. On the other hand, there are studies suggesting that long-term treatment with thiazolidinediones may weakly but significantly increase body weight (128). This may not be surprising, since cell culture studies have demonstrated that after activation of PPARγ, these compounds promote differentiation of pluripotent stem cells and preadipocytes into mature adipocytes (125). Whether changes in body fat occur in the same extent in both subcutaneous and visceral depots has not been clarified. This critical issue needs therefore to be defined by further long-term studies in both diabetic and non diabetic individuals.

Other agents, such as diazoxide, have been proved to selectively reduce hyperinsulinemia and hyperandrogenism in short-term studies performed in obese PCOS women (129). In the unique double-blind placebo-controlled trial performed so far, Alemzadeh and coworkers found that in a group of hyperinsulinemic obese patients, 8-week treatment with diazoxide (2 mg/kg BW) associated with a low-calorie diet reduced insulin levels, body weight, and body fat significantly more than placebo, without altering glucose tolerance (130). However, larger, long-term studies seem justified to evaluate the therapeutic effect of diazoxide, particularly in abdominal obesity.

In obese women with PCOS a weak but significant improvement of insulin resistance and hyperinsulinemia can also be achieved by antiandrogen administration. These effects have been observed regardless of the type of antiandrogen used (131). Preliminary data from our group, obtained in a 6-month study on a group of obese PCOS women, seem to be consistent with the possibility that a potent antiandrogen flutamide, when added to hypocaloric dieting and metformin, may further and selectively reduce visceral body fat by ~50%, these effects being associated with a normalization of androgen levels (unpublished data). These findings further support the concept that androgens are an important determinant of the abdominal obesity phenotype in women.

B Sex Hormones in Males

In contrast to what has been observed in obese women, in the obese male total and free T blood concentration levels progressively decrease with increasing body weight, as clearly exemplified in subjects affected by Klinefelter syndrome (132). Moreover, such a reduction is associated with a progressive decrease of SHBG concentrations (133). Spermatogenesis and fertility are not impaired in the majority of obese men. However, these parameters have been described to be reduced in subjects with massive obesity (132). Androstenedione and DHT circulating levels are usually normal or slightly reduced in obese patients (134). However, other C19 steroids can also be reduced in obesity (134). Similarly to what has been reported for women, in male obesity, estrogen production rates are increased in proportion to body weight, and blood concentrations of all major estrogens, particularly estrone, have been described as normal (132) or only slightly elevated (115). Aromatase activity of the adipose tissue, responsible for active conversion of androgens into estrogens, may explain the altered estrogen metabolism in obesity. Alterations in gonadotropin secretion have also been described in male obesity. Obese men show a reduction of total luteinizing hormone (LH) secretion, probably due to impaired secretion of the gonadotropin releasing hormone at the hypothalamic level, producing a reduced LH secretory mass per secretory burst without any change in burst number (135). The absence of clinical signs of hypogonadism can be explained by the fact that the T freefraction represents only 2% of total T, and that obesity predominantly affects circulating bound T, owing to the concurrent decrease of SHBG production. Although T levels are inversely related to obesity, it is still under debate whether T correlates with fat distribution in male obesity. Some studies (136) found an association between T and WHR values, whereas others, using anthropometry or magnetic resonance, showed no correlation (137,138). This suggests that the relationship between sex steroids to WHR may be the result of the shared covariance of WHR and total adiposity, rather than a direct relationship. This reflects the evidence that obesity in males is invariably associated with a parallel increase in abdominal and visceral fat, meaning that the central distribution of body fat in males depends on the actual presence of obesity.

Other studies have confirmed that the reduction of C19 steroid precursors are predominantly associated with body fatness rather than with excess visceral fat accumulation (134). Glucuronic acid is able to conjugate steroids influencing their biological activity. Notably 3-androstenediol glucuronide (3A-Diol-G) levels were found to be significantly higher in obese men having a visceral phenotype (134). This association between 3A-Diol-G and visceral fatness suggests that an increased visceral adipose tissue corresponds to a state in which the steroid metabolism is altered. Glucuronide conjugates must therefore be considered a more appropriate marker of peripheral androgen metabolism than circulating free steroids.

Both SHBG and T are negatively correlated with insulin levels, even after adjusting for BMI and WHR values (137). Such an inverse relationship is due to the ability of insulin to inhibit hepatic SHBG synthesis in the liver (139). However, as has been demonstrated in women, particularly in those with PCOS (131), there are data consistent with a stimulatory role of insulin on T production even in men (139). Therefore, reduced T levels in obese males appear to result from several complementary factors, including lower gonadotropin secretion and the balanced effects of insulin on SHBG (inhibition) and T (stimulation). Mechanisms leading to reduced T levels in obese men are depicted in Figure 1.

Weight reduction by both dietary intervention or surgical procedures can increase T and SHBG concentrations, provided substantial weight loss is achieved (115). When massively obese men restore a near-normal BMI, SHBG concentrations fall within the reference values for normal-weight individuals. Although there are no kinetic data on estrogen production following weight loss in obese men, it is presumable that estrogen metabolism and peripheral production improve as weight loss increases. Interestingly, the correction of the hypotestosteronemia by exogenous T replacement has been found to provide a beneficial effect not only by reducing body fat, particularly visceral fat, but also on all major parameters of the metabolic syndrome, by reducing hyperlipidemia and improving peripheral insulin sensitivity (140).

C The GH/IGF-I Axis

Growth hormone is substantially reduced in obesity, mainly owing to a significant reduction of GH secretory burst mass in the pituitary (141). The entity of this alteration appears to be inversely proportional to the increase in body fat (132). Blunted GH secretion to all stimuli of GH release, including GHRH, insulin-induced hypoglycemia, L-dopa, arginine, glucagon, exercise, opioid peptides, clonidine, nicotinic acid, or states such as deep sleep, is a common feature in obese subjects (132). The mechanisms responsible for reduced GH levels in obesity are multiple and not yet fully clarified. It is known that GH metabolic clearance rate is increased in proportion to body weight, as demonstrated in monkeys (142) and humans (120). Moreover, an enhanced somatostatinergic tone may further contribute to the reduced levels of GH in obese patients (143). However, as mentioned above, other still unknown central factors may be hypothesized to be involved in the impaired GH secretion in obesity. Peripheral factors have also been implicated in contributing to reduce GH levels. The increase of FFA production characterizing obesity may inhibit basal GH secretion, by mechanisms independent of effects on somatostatinergic tone (132). Sex steroids, specifically T and E_2, have positive effects on GH secretion, probably by influencing the pulsatile mode of GH release (139). Basal GH secretory bursts, which are reduced in obesity, are positively correlated with E_2 and T concentrations (139), further indicating a close relationship between sex steroid imbalance and GH secretory dynamics in the obese state.

The role of IGF-I in obesity is still under debate. The normal growth of obese children, in spite of the fact that they have lower GH levels in basal conditions and after stimulatory testing, seems to suggest that IGF-I action in the target tissues for growth is indeed adequate for growth and development before, during, and after puberty (132). However, the finding that free IGF-I levels are elevated in obese subjects (144) makes it possible to speculate that, via an inhibitory feedback on GH secretion at pituitary level, IGF-I may take part in the decline in obesity-associated GH levels. Importantly, subjects with visceral obesity have reduced circulating IGF-I levels (132). Since insulin regulates IGF-I metabolism, stimulating the synthesis of IGF binding protein (IGFBP)-I, alterations in circulating levels of IGF-I in visceral obesity may reflect a prevailing hyperinsulinemia in the blood circulation.

The potent lipolytic activity attributed to GH levels may be of relevance taking into account the reduced GH levels in obesity. Therefore, an unbalanced lipogenetic condition might be responsible for the perpetuation of the obese state once established. In fact, obese subjects have elevated insulin levels as a consequence of the insulin resistance state with respect to carbohydrate metabolism, but the adipose tissue remains sensitive to the antilipolytic effects of insulin. Evidence from animal and human studies supports the hypothesis that GH administration in obesity may stimulate lipolytic pathways and can provide a valuable adjunct to diet in inducing weight loss. In GH-deficient children, many of whom are obese, GH administration reduces body fat (145). The same occurs in subjects with adult GH deficiency (146) and in elderly subjects who have undergone therapy with GH to increase lean body mass and improve fitness (32). Exogenous GH administration also reduces fat stores, particularly in the visceral deposits, in GH-deficient adult subjects (147). These effects can be additive to those dependent on diet restriction, but they may also occur in conditions of eucaloric intake (148). One limitation of GH administration is related to the possibility that long-term GH treatment worsens glucose tolerance and insulin resistance, although the contrary has been reported by some studies (147). Perhaps the administration of GH in a manner that stimulates normal physiological secretion rather than pharmacological doses would circumvent or lessen its effects on carbohydrate metabolism in the long term.

D Glucocorticoids and the HPA Axis

Cortisol excess may have a key role in the development of enlarged abdominal or visceral fat in obese individuals of both sexes. This derives from the combination of the effects produced by hyperinsulinemia, from the GH reduction and from the decreased (in male obesity) or increased (in female obesity) free androgen availability in peripheral tissues, which are the above-mentioned features of abdominal phenotype of obesity (149). Most studies found normal ACTH and cortisol levels in visceral obesity, although slightly reduced morning cortisol levels have been described by some authors (150). Visceral obese women had higher ACTH pulse frequency and lower ACTH pulse amplitude, particularly in the morning, despite similar mean ACTH basal concentrations, than women with peripheral obesity and normal weight controls (151). However, the dysregulation of the system in abdominal obesity has been more convincingly demonstrated by many dynamic studies, which showed high secretions of cortisol after laboratory stress test, elevated ACTH and cortisol secretion after administration of CRF alone or combined with arginine-vasopressin (AVP), and elevated cortisol concentrations after challenges with maximal or low-dose ACTH (152) in abdominal obese patients. This might indicate sensitized and/or hyperresponsive hypothalamic centers, pituitary as well as adrenal regulatory mechanisms, that result in slightly but inappropriately elevated net cortisol production, either continuous or episodic, in individuals with abdominal obesity.

Among the dynamics, dexamethasone suppression test has been proposed as the gold standard to discriminate between a normal and a pathological activation of the HPA axis. However, maximal suppression with dexamethasone cannot provide adequate information on the feedback sensitivity at both pituitary and suprapituitary levels. At variance, it has been suggested that the utilization of lower dexamethasone doses may give good insight into the individual feedback sensitivity of the HPA axis. Preliminary studies from Ljiung et al. (153), performed in a group of men with different obesity phenotypes, found a blunted inhibition of cortisol secretion by submaximal (0.50 mg overnight) dexamethasone administration, thus suggesting a reduced sensitivity to inhibition by dexamethasone via down-regulation of central glucocorticoid receptors. We recently performed an extensive study in a large cohort of obese and normalweight individuals by using different doses (0.0035 mg, 0.0070 mg, and 0.015 mg/kg BW) of dexamethasone administered orally at midnight. The results of this study showed that obesity had no effects on cortisol and ACTH concentrations following each test, whereas sex and dexamethasone blood levels represented the main factors influencing the HPA axis suppressibility in both obese and normal weight individuals (154).

It has been speculated that alterations of the HPA axis activity may derive from a dysruption of the regulatory mechanisms at central nervous system level. In this context, we have proposed that abnormal catecholaminergic regulation may take part in the hyperactivation of HPA axis. Catecholamines modulate CRH and ACTH secretion, particularly during acute and chronic stress challenges by activation of α1- and α2-adrenoreceptor subtypes. In particular, by inhibiting ACTH release in experimental animals and in humans (155), α2-adrenoreceptors may provide negative feedback mechanisms preventing an excess of glucocorticoid response to stressor stimuli. We found that yohimbine, an α2-adrenoreceptor antagonist, slightly but significantly reduced ACTH response to combined CRH + AVP challenge in normal weight controls, in comparison with that observed during the control test, whereas in obese women, particularly the abdominal phenotype, the response of ACTH was significantly increased (156). These different effects after α2-adrenoreceptor inhibition in the two groups suggest that obese women with abdominal body fat distribution may escape physiological α2-adrenoreceptor control, thus favoring inappropriate HPA axis excitation following appropriate neuropeptide stimulation.

Increased cortisol clearance (157), higher cortisol turnover, and altered cortisol metabolism in adipose tissue represent the main peripheral alterations of cortisol production and metabolism in obese patients (23,33). Many studies have shown that daily urine free cortisol excretion rate was significantly increased in subjects, particularly women, with abdominal body fat distribution (158). At variance, we recently found that nondepressed women with abdominal obesity were characterized by lower urinary free cortisol excretion rates, which is consistent with increased metabolic rates of cortisol. Theoretically, this could be due to multiple factors, including subtle abnormalities of cortisol transport, function, and metabolism. The concentrations of the corticosteroid-binding globulin, which carries cortisol into the bloodstream, may be reduced in the abdominal phenotype (150). Moreover, as stated above, visceral adipocytes show a higher number of GCRs than do subcutaneous adipocytes; the resulting increase of intracellular cortisol could therefore enhance cortisol metabolic clearance (158). In addition, alterations of enzymes such as 11βHSD1 and 5α-reductase type 1 are

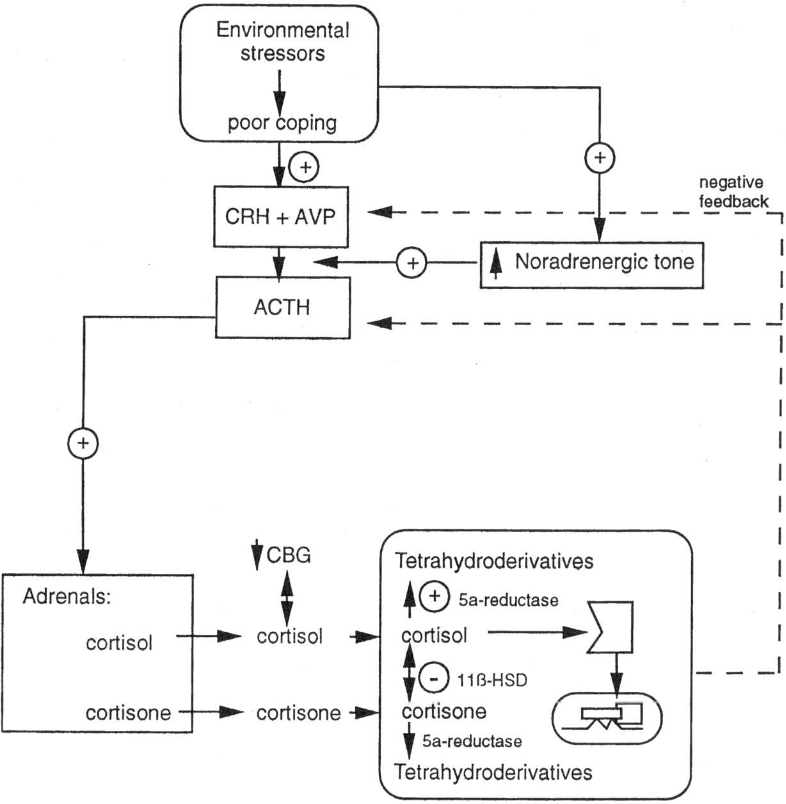

Figure 2 Schematic representation of the HPA axis–noradrenergic system alterations in the pathophysiology of abdominal obesity and the metabolic syndrome. Exaggerated response to chronic stress factors and alterations in cortisol metabolism (whose causative mechanisms are still unknown), with compensatory neuroendocrine activation, may cooperate in determining HPA hyperactivation and cortisol hypersensitivity. Also shown is a schematic target cell, in which interconversion of cortisol and cortisone by 11β-HSD dictates access of GCs to receptors and subsequent regulation of target genes, encoding those responsible for negative feedback. Cortisol and cortisone circulate in similar free concentrations, although free cortisol is in equilibrium with a pool of cortisol bound to CBG and albumin. Symbols in circles indicate increased or decreased activity. (From Refs. 68,150.)

supposed to play a role in the alteration of HPA axis. Recent studies have provided evidence for an inhibition of 11βHSD1 in patients with increased central adiposity (158), similar to what was previously observed in patients with PCOS (159). The association between reduced 11βHSD1 activity and abdominal obesity should not, however, be surprising, since high doses of insulin inhibit this enzyme's expression (160). In addition, increased 5α-reductase type 1 activity, as indicated by an increased urinary excretion rate of 5α-tetrahydrocortisol (161), has also been reported in abdominal obesity. This may further contribute to increased catabolism of cortisol in extra-adrenal tissues. At present, no studies have investigated the effects of pharmacological or behavioral manipulations in order to normalize HPA responsiveness and/or derangements in cortisol metabolism in patients with the abdominal obesity phenotype of both sexes. Both central and peripheral mechanisms responsible for altered HPA axis activity in the abdominal obesity phenotype are represented in Figure 2.

VII SUMMARY AND CONCLUSIONS

The recognition that adipose tissue has endocrine properties and represents a main target for hormone effects has reinforced research in this direction, and over the years new findings have enormously increased our knowledge on the main mechanisms of regulation of some functions of the human body, including energy balance and body composition, in both the physiological state and in diseases. Mechanisms of regulation of the differentiation and the lipogenetic/lipolytic balance in the different adipose tissue depots involve a list of hormones, cytokines, and neuropeptides not yet completely defined, acting via endocrine, paracrine, and autocrine pathways (Table 2). Among the hormones, alterations of the hypothalamic-pituitary-gonadal axis, the GH/IGF-I axis, and the HPA axis, acting in concert and with the modulatory role of insulin and the noradrenergic system, appear to play a dominant role in the pathophysiology of the abdominal obesity phenotypes in both females and males. Moreover, the endocrine axis appears to be strictly interconnected with leptin regulation and function, both in the adipose tissue and at neuroendocrine sites. An exciting area of investigation is further represented by the crosstalk between other locally acting cytokines, particularly TNFα and IL-6. The recognition of endocrine and metabolic derangements in different obesity phenotypes may be of importance in the definition and categorization of patients and in defining the pathophysiology of associated comorbodities, particularly type 2 diabetes, cardiovascular diseases, and hormone-dependent cancers. In addition, these findings pave the way for more sophisticated potential applications of hormone replacement therapy, particularly with regard to the treatment of the visceral phenotype of obesity.

REFERENCES

1. Flier JS. Leptin expression and action: new experimental paradigms. Proc Natl Acad Sci USA 1997; 94: 4242–4245.
2. Kahn BB, Flier JS. Obesity and insulin resistance. J Clin Invest 2000; 106:473–481.
3. Cryer A. Tissue lipoprotein lipase activity and its action in lipoprotein metabolism. J Biochem 1981; 13: 525–541.
4. Ailhaud G. L'adipocyte, cellule sécrétrice et endocrine. Medecine/Sciences 1998; 14:858–864.
5. Kern PA, High adipose tissue lipoprotein lipase activity plays a causal role in the etiology of obesity. In: Angel A, Anderson H, Bouchard C, Lau D, Leiter L, Mendelson R, eds. Progress in Obesity Research: Proceedings of the Seventh International Congress on Obesity (Toronto, 1994). London: John Libbey & Company, 7:89–94.
6. Carey GB. Mechanisms regulating adipocyte lipolysis. In: Richter J, ed. Skeletal Muscle Metabolism in Exercise and Diabetes New York: Plenum Press, 1998.
7. Bonadonna R, Bonora E. Glucose and free fatty acid metabolism in human obesity. Relationships to insulin resistance. Diabetes Rev 1997; 5:21–51.
8. Lafontan M, Berlan M. Fat cell adrenergic receptors and the control of white and brown fat cell function. J Lipid Res 1993; 34:1057–1091.
9. Reynisdottir S, Dauzats M, Thorne A, Langin D. Comparison of hormone-sensitive lipase activity in visceral and subcutaneous human adipose tissue. J Clin Endocrinol Metab 1997; 82:4162–4166.
10. Fried SK, Russell CD, Grauso NL, Brolin RE. Lipoprotein lipase regulation by insulin and glucocorticoids in subcutaneous and omental adipose tissues of obese women and men. J Clin Invest 1993; 92:2191–2198.
11. Shepherd PR, Kahn BB. Glucose transporters and insulin action: implications for insulin resistance and diabetes mellitus. N Engl J Med 1999; 341:248–257.
12. Gould GW, Holman GD. The glucose transporter family: structure, function, and tissue-specific expression. Biochem J 1993; 295:329–341.
13. White MF. The IRS-signaling system: a network of docking proteins that mediate insulin and cytokines action. Recent Prog Horm Res 1998; 53:119–138.
14. Czech MP, Corvera S. Signaling mechanisms that regulate glucose transport. J Biol Chem 1999; 274: 1865–1868.
15. Frevert EU, Kahn BB. Differential effects of constitutively active phosphatidylinositol 3-kinase on glucose transport, glycogen synthase activity and DNA synthesis in 3T3-L1 adipocytes. Mol Cell Biol 1997; 17:190–198.
16. Saladin R, De Vos P, Guerre-Millo M. Transient increase in obese gene expression after food intake or insulin administration. Nature 1995; 377:527–529.
17. Wabitsh M, Jensen PB, Blum WF. Insulin and cortisol promote leptin production in cultured human fat cells. Diabetes 1996; 45:1435–1438.
18. Considine RV, Sinha MK, Heiman ML, Kriauciunas A, Stephens TW, Nyce MR. Serum immunoreactive leptin concentrations in normal-weight and obese humans. N Engl J Med 1996; 334:292–295.
19. Hathout EH, Sharkey J, Racine M, Ahn D, Mace JW, Saad MF. Changes in plasma leptin during the treatment of diabetic ketoacidosis. J Clin Endocrinol Metab 1999; 84:4545–4548.
20. Sinha MK, Ohannesian JP, Heiman ML, Kriauciunas A, Stephens TW, Magosin S, Marco C, Caro JF. Nocturnal rise of leptin in lean, obese, and non-insulin-dependent diabetes mellitus subjects. J Clin Invest 1996; 97:1344–1347.
21. Becker DJ, Ongemba LN, Brichard V, Henquin JC, Brichard SM. Diet- and diabetes-induced changes in ob gene expression in rat adipose tissue. FEBS Lett 1995; 371:324–328.
22. Leroy P, Dessolin S, Villageois P, Moon BC, Friedman JM. Expression of ob gene in adipose cell. J Biol Chem 1996; 271:2365–2368.
23. Bujalska IJ, Kumar S, Stewart PM. Does central obe-

sity reflect "Cushing's disease of the omentum"? Lancet 1997; 349:1210–1213.

24. Lafontan M, Bousquet-Melou A, Galitzky J, Barbe P, Carpene C, Langin D. Adrenergic receptors and fat cells: differential recruitment by physiological amines and homologous regulation. Obes Res 1995; 3:S507–S514.
25. Sollevi A, Fredholm BB. The antilipolytic effect of endogenous and exogenous adenosine in canine adipose tissue in situ. Acta Physiol Scand 1981; 113:53–60.
26. Granneman JG. Why do adipocytes make the β3 adrenergic receptor? Cell Signal 1995; 7:9–15.
27. Richelsen B. Increased alpha-2- but similar beta-adrenergic receptor activities in subcutaneous gluteal adipocytes from females compared with males. Eur J Clin Invest 1986; 1:302–309.
28. Arner P, Kriegholm E, Engfeldt P, Bolinder J. Adrenergic regulation of lipolysis in situ at rest and during exercise. J Clin Invest 1990; 85:893–898.
29. Lonnqvist F, Thorne A, Large V, Arner P. Sex differences in visceral fat lipolysis and metabolic complications of obesity. Arterioscler Thromb Vasc Biol 1997; 17:1472–1480.
30. Mauriège P, Marette A, Atgié C, Bouchard C, Thériault G, Bukowiecki LK. Regional variation in adipose tissue metabolism of severely obese premenopausal women. J Lipid Res 1995; 36:672–684.
31. Hellmer J, Marcus C, Sonnenfeld T, Arner P. Mechanisms for differences in lipolysis between human subcutaneous and omenatl fat cells. J Clin Endocrinol Metab 1992; 75:15–20.
32. Arner P, Hellstrom L, Wahrenberg H, Bronnengard M. α-Adrenoreceptor expression in human fat cells from different regions. J Clin Invest 1992; 86:1595–1600.
33. Rebuffé-Scrive M, Bronnegard M, Nilsson N, Eldh J, Gustafsson JA, Bjorntorp P. Steroid hormone receptors in human adipose tissue. J Clin Endocrinol Metab 1990; 71:1215–1219.
34. Bjorntorp P. The regulation of adipose tissue distribution in humans. Int J Obes 1996; 20:291–302.
35. Rebuffé-Scrive M, Lundholm K, Bjorntorp P. Glucocorticoid hormone binding to human adipose tissue. Eur J Clin Invest 1985; 15:267–271.
36. Ottosson M, Marin P, Karason K, Elander A, Bjorntorp P. Blockade of the glucocorticoid receptor with RU 486: effects in vitro and in vivo on human adipose tissue lipoprotein lipase activity. Obes Res 1995; 3:233–240.
37. Lonnqvist F, Arner P, Nordfors L, Schalling M. Overexpression of the obese (ob) gene in adipose tissue of human obese subjects. Nat Med 1995; 1:950–956.
38. Masuzaki H, Ogawa Y, Hosoda K, et al. Glucocorticoid regulation of leptin synthesis and secretion in humans: elevated plasma leptin levels in Cushing's syndrome. J Clin Endocrinol Metab 1997; 82:2542–2547.
39. Marin P, Darin N, Amemya T, Andersson B, Jern S, Bjorntorp P. Cortisol secretion in relation to body fat distribution in obese premenopausal women. Metabolism 1992; 41:882–886.
40. Masuzaki H, Ogawa Y, Isse N, Satoh N, Okazaki T, Shigemoto M, Kawda T, Nakao K. Human obese gene expression. Adipocyte-specific expression and regional differences in the adipose tissue. Diabetes 1996; 44:855–858.
41. Miller LK, Kral JG, Strain GW, Zumoff B. Androgen binding to ammonium sulfate precipitates of human adipose tissue cytosols. Steroids 1990; 55:410–415.
42. De Pergola G, Xu XF, Yang SM, Giorgino R, Bjorntorp P. Up-regulation of androgen receptor binding in male rat fat pad adipose precursor cells exposed to testosterone: study in a whole cell assay system. J Steroid Biochem Mol Biol 1990; 37:553–558.
43. Dieudonne MN, Pecquery R, Boumediene A, Leneveu MC, Giudicelli Y. Androgen receptors in human preadipocytes and adipocytes: regional specificities and regulation by sex steroids. Am J Physiol 1998; 274: C1645–C1652.
44. Marin P, Oden B, Bjorntorp P. Assimilation and mobilization of triglycerides in subcutaneous abdominal and femoral adipose tissue in vivo in men: effects of androgens. J Clin Endocrinol Metab 1995; 80:239–243.
45. Gray JM, Wade GN. Cytoplasmic progestin binding in rat adipose tissues. Endocrinology 1979; 104:1377–1382.
46. O'Brien SN, Welter BH, Mantzke KA, Price TM. Identification of progesterone receptor in human subcutaneous adipose tissue. J Clin Endocrinol Metab 1998; 83:509–513.
47. Price TM, O'Brien SN. Determination of estrogen receptor messenger ribonucleic acid (mRNA) and cytochrome P450 aromatase mRNA levels in adipocytes and adipose stromal cells by competitive polymerase chain reaction amplification. J Clin Endocrinol Metab 1993; 77:1041–1045.
48. Zaino RJ, Clarke CL, Feil PD, Satyaswaroop PG. Differential distribution of estrogen and progesterone receptors in rabbit uterus detected by dual immunofluorescence. Endocrinology 1989; 125:2728–2734.
49. Ciocca DR, Roig LM. Estrogen receptors in human nontarget tissues: biological and clinical implications. Endocr Rev 1995; 16:35–62.
50. Bronnegard M, Ottosson M, Boos J, Marcus C, Bjorntorp P. Lack of evidence for estrogen and progesterone receptors in human adipose tissue. J Steroid Biochem Mol Biol 1994; 51:275–281.
51. Mizutani T, Nishikawa Y, Adachi H, Enomoto T, Ikegami H, Kurachi H, Nomura T, Miyake A. Iden-

tification of estrogen receptor in human adipose tissue and adipocytes. J Clin Endocrinol Metab 1994; 78: 950–954.

52. Crandall DL, Busler DE, Novak TJ, Weber RV, Kral JG. Identification of estrogen receptor beta RNA in human breast and abdominal subcutaneous adipose tissue. Biochem Biophys Res Commun 1998; 248:523–526.
53. Wade GN. Sex steroids and energy balance: sites and mechanisms of action. Ann NY Acad Sci 1986; 474: 389–399.
54. Ohlsson C, Hellberg N, Parini P, Vidal O, Bohlooly M, Rudling M, Lindberg MK, Warner M, Angelin B, Gustafsson JA. Obesity and disturbed lipoprotein profile in estrogen receptor-alpha-deficient male mice. Biochem Biophys Res Commun 2000; 278: 640–645.
55. Heine PA, Taylor JA, Iwamoto GA, Lubahn DB, Cooke PS. Increased adipose tissue in male and female estrogen receptor-alpha knockout mice. Proc Natl Acad Sci USA 2000; 97:12729–12734.
56. Hamosh M, Hamosh P. The effect of estrogen on the lipoprotein lipase activity of rat adipose tissue. J Clin Invest 1975; 55:1132–1135.
57. Rebuffe-Scrive M, Basdevant A, Guy-Grand B. Effect of local application of progesterone on human adipose tissue lipoprotein lipase. Horm Metab Res 1983; 15:566.
58. Iverius PH, Brunzell JD. Relationship between lipoprotein lipase activity and plasma sex steroid level in obese women. J Clin Invest 1988; 82:1106–1112.
59. Price TM, O'Brien SN, Welter BH, George R, Anandjiwala J, Kilgore M. Estrogen regulation of adipose tissue lipoprotein lipase—possible mechanism of body fat distribution. Am J Obstet Gynecol 1998; 178:101–107.
60. Pucci E, Chiovato L, Pinchera A. Thyroid and lipid metabolism. Int J Obes 2000; 24:S109–S112.
61. Wahrenberg H, Wennlund A, Arner P. Adrenergic regulation of lipolysis in fat cells from hyperthyroid and hypothyroid patients. J Clin Endocrinol Metab 1994; 78:898–903.
62. Richelsen B, Sorensen NS. α2- and β-adrenergic receptor binding and action in gluteal adipocytes from patients with hypothyroidism and hyperthyroidism. Metabolism 1987; 36:1031–1039.
63. Lonn L, Stenlof K, Ottosson M, Lindroos AK, Nystrom E, Sjostrom L. Body weight and body composition changes after treatment of hyperthyroidism. J Clin Endocrinol Metab 1998; 83:4273–4296.
64. Lithell H, Vessby B, Dahlberg PA. High muscle lipoprotein lipase activity in thyrotoxic patients. Acta Endocrinol 1985; 109:227–231.
65. Vikman K, Carlsson B, Billig H, Eden S. Expression and regulation of growth hormone (GH) receptor messenger ribonucleic acid (mRNA) in rat adipose tissue, adipocytes, and adipocyte precursor cells: GH regulation of GH receptor mRNA. Endocrinology 1991; 129:1155–1161.
66. Ballesteros M, Leung KC, Ross RJ, Iismaa TP, Ho KK. Distribution and abundance of messenger ribonucleic acid for growth hormone receptor isoforms in human tissues. J Clin Endocrinol Metab 2000; 85: 2865–2871.
67. Harant I, Beauville M, Crampes F, Riviere D, Tauber MT, Tauber JP, Garrigues M. Response of fat cells to growth hormone (GH): effect of long term treatment with recombinant human GH in GH-deficient adults. J Clin Endocrinol Metab 1994; 78:1392–1395.
68. Beauville M, Harant I, Crampes F, Riviere D, Tauber MT, Tauber JP, Garrigues M. Effect of long-term rhGH administration in GH-deficient adults on fat cell epinephrine response. Am J Physiol 1992; 263:E467–E472.
69. Dietz J, Schwartz J. Growth hormone alters lipolysis and hormone-sensitive lipase activity in 3T3-F442A adipocytes. Metabolism 1991; 40:800–806.
70. Thorburn AW, Gumbiner B, Brechtel G, Henry RR. Effect of hyperinsulinemia and hyperglycemia on intracellular glucose and fat metabolism in healthy subjects. Diabetes 1990; 39:22–30.
71. Doris R, Vernon RG, Houslay MD, Kilgour E. Growth hormone decreases the response to anti-lipolytic agonists and decreases the levels of Gi2 in rat adipocytes. Biochem J 1994; 297:41–45.
72. Heffernan MA, Jiang WJ, Thorburn AW, Ng FM. Effects of oral administration of a synthetic fragment of human growth hormone on lipid metabolism. Am J Physiol Endocrinol Metab 2000; 279:E501–E507.
73. Thorner MO, Strasburger CJ, Wu Z, Straume M, Bidlingmaier M, Pezzoli SS, Zib K, Scarlett JC, Bennett WF. Growth hormone (GH) receptor blockade with a PEG-modified GH (B2036-PEG) lowers serum insulin-like growth factor-I but does not acutely stimulate serum GH. J Clin Endocrinol Metab 1999; 84:2098–2103.
74. Bowers CY, Momany FA, Reynolds GA, Hong A. On the in vitro and in vivo activity of a new synthetic hexapeptide that acts on the pituitary to specifically release growth hormone. Endocrinology 1984; 114: 1537–1545.
75. Howard AD, Feighner SD, Cully DF, Arena JP, Liberator PA, Rosenblum CI. A receptor in pituitary and hypothalamus that functions in growth hormone release. Science 1996; 273:974–977.
76. Kojima M, Hosoda H, Date Y, Nakazato M, Matsuo H, Kangawa K. Ghrelin is a growth-hormone-releasing acylated peptide from stomach. Nature 1999; 402: 656–660.
77. Tschoep M, Smiley DL, Heiman ML. Ghrelin induces adiposity in rodents. Nature 2000; 407:908–913.
78. Locke W, Kirgis HD, Bowers CY, Abdoh AA. Intracerebroventricular growth-hormone-releasing pep-

tide-6 stimulates eating without affecting plasma growth hormone responses in rats. Life Sci 1995; 56: 1347–1352.

79. Tschoep M, Weyer C, Tataranni PA, Devanarayan V, Ravussin E, Heiman ML. Circulating ghrelin levels are decreased in human obesity. Diabetes 2001; 50:707–709.
80. Zhang Y, Proenca R, Maffei M, Barone M, Leopold L, Friedman JM. Positional cloning of the mouse obese gene and its human homologue. Nature 1994; 372:425–432.
81. Campfield LA, Smith FJ, Guisez Y, Devos R, Burn P. Recombinant mouse OB protein: evidence for a peripheral signal linking adiposity and central networks. Science 1995; 269:546–549.
82. Madej T, Bogusky MS, Bryant SH. Threading analysis suggests that the obese gene product may be a helical cytokine. FEBS Lett 1995; 373:13–18.
83. Tartaglia LA, Dembsky M, Weng X. Identification and expression cloning of a leptin receptor, OB-R. Cell 1995; 83:1263–1271.
84. Baumann H, Morella KK, White DW. The full-length leptin receptor has signaling capabilities of interleukin 6-type cytokine receptors. Proc Natl Acad Sci USA 1996; 93:8374–8378.
85. Fruhbek G, Jebb SA, Prentice AM. Leptin: physiology and pathophysiology. Clin Physiol 1998; 18:399–419.
86. Vgontzas AN, Papanicolaou DA, Bixler EO, Kales A, Tyson K, Chrousos GP. Elevation of plasma cytokines in disorders of excessive daytime sleepiness: role of sleep disturbance and obesity. J Clin Endocrinol Metab 1997; 82:1313–1316.
87. Mohamed-Ali V, Goodrick S, Rawesh A, Katz DR, Miles JM, Yudkin JS, Klein S, Coppack SW. Subcutaneous adipose tissue releases interleukin-6, but not tumor necrosis factor-alpha, in vivo. J Clin Endocrinol Metab 1997; 82:4196–4200.
88. Fried SK, Bunkin DA, Greenberg AS. Omental and subcutaneous adipose tissues of obese subjects release interleukin-6: depot difference and regulation by glucocorticoid. J Clin Endocrinol Metab 1998; 83:847–850.
89. Nonogaki K, Fuller GM, Fuentes NL, Moser AH, Staprans I, Grunfeld C, Feingold KR. Interleukin-6 stimulates hepatic triglyceride secretion in rats. Endocrinology 1995; 136:2143–2149.
90. Greenberg AS, Nordan RP, McIntosh J, Calvo JC, Scow RO, Jablons D. Interleukin 6 reduces lipoprotein lipase activity in adipose tissue of mice in vivo and in 3T3-L1 adipocytes: a possible role for interleukin 6 in cancer cachexia. Cancer Res 1992; 52:4113–4116.
91. Feingold KR, Grunfeld C. Role of cytokines in inducing hyperlipidemia. Diabetes 1992; 2:97–101.
92. Stephens JM, Butts MD, Pekala PH. Regulation of transcription factor mRNA accumulation during 3T3-L1 preadipocyte differentiation by tumour necrosis factor-alpha. J Mol Endocrinol 1992; 9:61–72.
93. Papanicolaou DA, Petrides JS, Tsigos C, Bina S, Kalogeras KT, Wilder R, Gold PW, Deuster PA, Chrousos GP. Exercise stimulates interleukin-6 secretion: inhibition by glucocorticoids and correlation with catecholamines. Am J Physiol 1996; 271:E601–E605.
94. Arzt E, Pereda MP, Castro CP, Pagotto U, Renner U, Stalla GK. Pathophysiological role of the cytokine network in the anterior pituitary gland. Front Neuroendocrinol 1999; 20:71–95.
95. Hotamisligil GS, Shargill NS, Spiegelman BM. Adipose expression of tumor necrosis factor-alpha: direct role in obesity-linked insulin resistance. Science 1993; 259:87–91.
96. Torti FM, Dieckmann B, Beutler B, Cerami A, Ringold GM. A macrophage factor inhibits adipocyte gene expression: an in vitro model of cachexia. Science 1985; 229:867–869.
97. Grell M. Tumor necrosis factor (TNF) receptors in cellular signaling of soluble and membrane-expressed TNF. J Inflamm 1995–96; 47:8–17.
98. Hube F, Birgel M, Lee YM, Hauner H. Expression pattern of tumour necrosis factor receptors in subcutaneous and omental human adipose tissue: role of obesity and non-insulin-dependent diabetes mellitus. Eur J Clin Invest 1999; 29:672–678.
99. Hotamisligil GS, Arner P, Atkinson RL, Spiegelman BM. Differential regulation of the p80 tumor necrosis factor receptor in human obesity and insulin resistance. Diabetes 1997; 46:451–455.
100. Hube F, Hauner H. The role of TNF-alpha in human adipose tissue: prevention of weight gain at the expense of insulin resistance? Horm Metab Res 1999; 31:626–631.
101. Mohamed-Ali V, Goodrick S, Bulmer K, Holly JM, Yudkin JS, Coppack SW. Production of soluble tumor necrosis factor receptors by human subcutaneous adipose tissue in vivo. Am J Physiol 1999; 277:E971–E975.
102. Hotamisligil GS, Arner P, Caro JF, Atkinson RL, Spiegelman BM. Increased adipose tissue expression of tumor necrosis factor-alpha in human obesity and insulin resistance. J Clin Invest 1995; 95:2409–2415.
103. Garaulet M, Perex-Llamas F, Fuente T, Zamora S, Tebar FJ. Anthropometric, computed tomography and fat cell data in an obese population: relationship with insulin, leptin, tumor necrosis factor-alpha, sex hormone-binding globulin and sex hormones. Eur J Endocrinol 2000; 143:657–666.
104. Feingold KR, Grunfeld C. Role of cytokines in inducing hyperlipidemia. Diabetes 1992; 2:97–101.
105. Yamaguchi M, Murakami T, Tomimatsu T, Nishio Y, Mitsuda N, Kanzaki T, Kurachi H, Shima K, Aono T, Murata Y. Autocrine inhibition of leptin production by tumor necrosis factor-alpha (TNF-alpha) through

TNF-alpha type-I receptor in vitro. Biochem Biophys Res Commun 1998; 244:30–34.
106. Steppan CM, Bailey ST, Bhat S, Brown EJ, Banerjee RR, Wright CM, Patel HR, Ahima SR, Lazar MA. The hormone resistin links obesity to diabetes. Nature 2001; 409:307–312.
107. Steppan CM, Brown EJ, Wright CM, Bhat S, Banerjee RR, Dai CY, Enders GH, Silberg DG, Weu X, Wu GD, Lazar MA. A family of tissue-specific resistin-like molecules. Proc Natl Acad Sci USA 2001; 98:502–506.
108. Fasshauer M, Klein J, Neumann S, Eszlinger M, Paschke R. Isoproterenol inhibits resistin gene expression through a G(S)-protein-coupled pathway in 3T3-L1 adipocytes. FEBS Lett 2001; 500:60–63.
109. Way JM, Gorgun CZ, Tong Q, Uysal KT, Brown KK, Harrington WW, Oliver WR Jr, Wilson TM, Kliever SA, Hotamisligil GS. Adipose tissue resistin expression is severely suppressed in obesity and stimulated by peroxisome proliferator-activated receptor gamma agonists. J Biol Chem 2001; 276:25651–25653.
110. Pasquali R, Vicennati V. Obesity and hormonal abnormalities. In: Bjorntorp P, ed. International Textbook of Obesity Chichester: John Wiley & Sons, 2001:225–239.
111. Lovejoy JC, Bray GA, Bourgeois MO, Macchiavelli R, Rood JC, Greeson C, Partington C. Exogenous androgens influence body composition and regional body fat distribution in obese postmenopausal women—a clinical research center study. J Clin Endocrinol Metab 1996; 81:2198–2203.
112. Bengtsson BA, Eden S, Lonn L, Kvist H, Stokland A, Lindstedt G, Bosaeus I, Tolli J, Sjostrom L, Isaksson OG. Treatment of adults with growth hormone (GH) deficiency with recombinant human GH. J Clin Endocrinol Metab 1993; 76:309–317.
113. O'Sullivan AJ, Kelly JJ, Hoffman DM, Freund J, Ho KK, Brummer RJ. Body composition and energy expenditure in acromegaly. J Clin Endocrinol Metab 1994; 78:381–386.
114. Hansen TB, Gram J, Bjerre P, Hagen C, Bollerslev J. Body composition in active acromegaly during treatment with octreotide: a double-blind, placebo-controlled cross-over study. Clin Endocrinol (Oxf) 1994; 41:323–329.
115. Von Shoultz B, Carlstrom K. On the regulation of sex-hormone-binding globulin. A challenge of old dogma and outlines of an alternative mechanism. J Steroid Biochem 1989; 32:327–334.
116. Pasquali R, Casimirri F, Platè L, Capelli M. Characterization of obese women with reduced sex hormone-binding globulin concentrations. Horm Metab Res 1990; 22:303–306.
117. Samojlik E, Kirschner MA, Silber D, Schneider G, Ertel NH. Elevated production and metabolic clearance rates of androgens in morbidly obese women. J Clin Endocrinol Metab 1984; 59:949–954.
118. Kirschner MA, Samojlik E, Drejka M, Szmal E, Schneider G, Ertel N. Androgen-estrogen metabolism in women with upper body versus lower body obesity. J Clin Endocrinol Metab 1990; 70:473–479.
119. Evans DJ, Hoffmann RG, Kalkhoff RK, Kissebah AH. Relationship of androgenic activity to body fat topography, fat cell morphology and metabolic aberrations in premenopausal women. J Clin Endocrinol Metab 1983; 57:304–310.
120. Pasquali R, Casimirri F. The impact of obesity on hyperandrogenism and polycystic ovary in premenopausal women. Clin Endocrinol (Oxf) 1993; 39:1–16.
121. Wajchenberg BL. Subcutaneous and visceral adipose tissue: their relation to the metabolic syndrome. Endocr Rev 2000; 21:697–738.
122. Pasquali R, Casimirri F, Cantobelli S, Morselli-Labate AM, Venturoli S, Paradisi R, Zannarini L. Insulin and androgen relationship with abdominal body fat distribution in women with and without hyperandrogenism. Horm Res 1993; 39:179–187.
123. Pasquali R, Vicennati V, Ceroni L, Cota D, Critical weight gain periods through life. In: Guy-Grand B, ed. Nutrition and Women's Health Cerin Symposium, Paris, 2001:163–173.
124. Pasquali R, Gambineri A, Biscotti D, Vicennati V, Gagliardi L, Colitta D, Fiorini S, Cognini GE, Filicori M, Morselli-Labate AM. Effect of long-term treatment with metformin added to hypocaloric diet on body composition, fat distribution, and androgen and insulin levels in abdominally obese women with and without the polycystic ovary syndrome. J Clin Endocrinol Metab 2000; 85:2767–2774.
125. Lehmann JM, Moore LB, Smith-Oliver TA, et al. An antidiabetic thiazolidinedione is a high affinity ligand for peroxisome proliferation-activated receptor g (PPARg). J Biol Chem 1995; 270:12953–12956.
126. Nolan JJ, Ludvik B, Beerdsen P. Improvement in glucose tolerance and insulin resistance in obese subjects treated with troglitazone. N Engl J Med 1994; 331:1188–1193.
127. Murphy E, Nolan JJ. Insulin sensitizers drugs. Exp Opin Invest Drugs 2000; 9:1347–1361.
128. Matthaei S, Stumvoll M, Kellerer M, Haring HU. Pathophysiology and pharmacological treatment of insulin resistance. Endocr Rev 2000; 21:585–618.
129. Nestler JE, Barlascini CO, Matt DW, Steingold KA, Plymate SR, Clore JN, Blackard WG. Suppression of serum insulin by diazoxide reduces serum testosterone levels in obese women with polycystic ovary syndrome. J Clin Endocrinol Metab 1989; 68:1027–1032.
130. Alemzadeh R, Langley G, Upchurch L, Smith P, Slonim AE. Beneficial effect of diazoxide in obese hyperinsulinemic adults. J Clin Endocrinol Metab 1998; 83:1911–1915.
131. Poretsky L, Cataldo NA, Rosenwaks Z, Giudice LC. The insulin-related ovarian regulatory system in health and disease. Endocr Rev 1999; 20:535–582.

132. Smith SR. The endocrinology of obesity. Endocr Metab Clin North Am 1996; 25:921–942.
133. Zumoff B, Strain G, Miller LK, Rosner W, Senie R, Seres D, Rosenfield RS. Plasma free and non-sex-hormone-binding-globulin-bound testosterone are decreased in obese men in proportion to their degree of obesity. J Clin Endocrinol Metab 1990; 71:929–931.
134. Tchernoff A, Després J-P, Bélanger A, Dupont A, Prud'homme D, Moorjani S, Lupien PJ, Labrie F. Reduced testosterone and adrenal C19 steroid levels in obese women. Metabolism 1995; 44:513–519.
135. Vermeulen A, Kaufman JM, Deslypere JP, Thomas G. Attenuated luteinizing hormone (LH) pulse amplitude but normal LH pulse frequency, and its relation to plasma androgens in hypogonadism of obese men. J Clin Endocrinol Metab 1993; 76:1140–1146.
136. Khaw KT, Barret-Connor E. Lower endogenous androgens predict central adiposity in men. Ann Epidemiol 1992; 2:675–682.
137. Pasquali R, Casimirri F, Cantobelli S, Melchionda N, Morselli Labate AM, Fabbri R, Capelli M, Bortoluzzi L. Effect of obesity and body fat distribution on sex hormones and insulin in men. Metabolism 1991; 40:101–104.
138. Leenen R, Van der Koy K, Seidell JC, Deurenberg P, Kopperschaar HPF. Visceral fat accumulation in relation to sex hormones in obese men and women undergoing weight loss therapy. J Clin Endocrinol Metab 1994; 78:1515–1520.
139. Pasquali R, Casimirri F, De Iasio R, Mesini P, Boschi S, Chierici R, Flamia R, Biscotti M, Vicennati V. Insulin regulates testosterone and sex hormone-binding globulin concentrations in adult normal weight and obese men. J Clin Endocrinol Metab 1995; 80:654–658.
140. Marin P, Holmang S, Jonsson L, Sjostrom L, Kvist H, Holm G, Lindstedt G, Bjorntorp P. The effects of testosterone treatment on body composition and metabolism in middle-aged obese men. Int J Obes 1992; 16:991–997.
141. Veldhuis JD, Liem AY, South S, Weltman J, Weltman J, Clemmons DA, Abbott R, Mullingan T, Johnson ML, Pincus S, Strume M, Iranmanesh A. Differential impact of age, sex steroid hormones, and obesity on basal versus pulsatile growth hormone secretion in men as assessed in an ultrasensitive chemiluminescence assay. J Clin Endocrinol Metab. 1995; 80:3209–3222.
142. Dubey AK, Hanukoglu A, Hamsen BC, Kowarski AA. Metabolic clearance rates of synthetic human growth hormone in lean and obese male rhesus monkeys. J Clin Endocrinol Metab 1988; 67:1064–1067.
143. Cordido F, Penalva A, Dieguez C, Casanueva FF. Massive growth hormone (GH) discharge in obese subjects after combined administration of GH-releasing hormone and GHRP-6: evidence for a marked somatotroph secretory capability in obesity. J Clin Endocrinol Metab 1993; 76:819–823.
144. Frystyk J, Vestbo E, Skjaerbaek C, Mogensen CE, Ørskov H. Free insulin-like growth factors in human obesity. Metabolism 1995; 44(suppl):37–44.
145. Rosembaum M, Gertner JM, Leibel R. Effects of systemic growth hormone (GH) administration on regional adipose tissue distribution and metabolism in GH-deficient children. J Clin Endocrinol Metab 1989; 69:1274–1281.
146. Solomon F, Cenco RC, Herp R, Sonksen PH. The effects of treatment with recombinant human GH on body composition and metabolism in adults with GH deficiency. N Engl J Med 1989; 321:1797–1803.
147. Hwu CM, Kwok CF, Lai TY, Shih KC, Lee TS, Hsiao LC, Lee SH, Fang VS, Ho LT. Growth hormone (GH) replacement reduces total body fat and normalize insulin sensitivity in GH-deficient adults: a report of one-year clinical experience. J Clin Endocrinol Metab 1997; 82:3285–3292.
148. Skaggs SR, Crist DM. Exogenous human growth hormone reduce body fat in obese women. Horm Res 1991; 35:19–24.
149. Bjorntorp P. Visceral obesity: "a civilization syndrome." Obes Res 1993; 1:206–222.
150. Chalew S, Nagel H, Shore S. The hypothalamic-pituitary-adrenal axis in obesity. Obes Res 1995; 3: 371–382.
151. Pasquali R, Biscotti D, Spinucci G, Vicennati V, Genazzani AD, Sgarbi L, Casimirri F. Pulsatile secretion of ACTH and cortisol in premenopausal women: effect of obesity and body fat distribution. Clin Endocrinol (Oxf) 1998; 48:603–612.
152. Pasquali R, Vicennati V. The abdominal obesity phenotype and insulin resistance are associated with abnormalities of the hypothalamic-pituitary-adrenal axis in humans. Horm Metab Res 2000; 32:521–525.
153. Ljiung T, Andersoson B, Bengtsson BA, Bjorntorp P, Marin P. Inhibition of cortisol secretion by dexamethasone in relation to body fat distribution: a dose-response study. Obes Res 1996; 4:277–282.
154. Pasquali R, Ambrosi B, Armanini D, Cavagnini F, Degli Uberti E, Del Rio G, De Pergola G, Maccario M, Mantero F, Marugo M, Rotella CM, Vettor R, on the behalf of the Study Group on Obesity of the Italian Society of Endocrinology. Cortisol and ACTH response to oral dexamethasone in obesity and effects of sex, body fat distribution and dexamethasone concentrations: a dose-response study. J Clin Endocrinol Metab 2002; 87:166–175.
155. Al-Damluji S. Adrenergic control of the secretion of anterior pituitary hormones. Baillieres Clin Endocrinol Metab 1993; 7:355–392.
156. Pasquali R, Vicennati V, Calzoni F, Gnudi U, Gambineri A, Ceroni L, Cortelli P, Menozzi R, Sinisi

R, Del Rio G. α2-Adrenoreceptor regulation of the hypothalamic-pituitary-adrenocortical axis in obesity. Clin Endocrinol (Oxf) 2000; 52:413–421.

157. Strain GW, Zumoff B, Kream J, Stain JJ, Levin J, Fukushima D. Sex differences in the influence of obesity on the 24 hr mean plasma concentration of cortisol. Metabolism 1982; 31:209–212.

158. Stewart PM, Boulton A, Kunar S, Clarck PMS. Shackleton CHL Cortisol metabolism in human obesity: impaired cortisone-cortisol conversion in subjects with central adiposity. J Clin Endocrinol Metab 1999; 84:1022–1027.

159. Rodin A, Thakkar H, Taylor N, Clayton R. Hyperandrogenism in polycystic ovary syndrome: evidence for a dysregulation of 11β-hydroxysteroid dehydrogenase. N Engl J Med 1994; 330:460–465.

160. Jamieson P, Chapman KE, Edwards CRW, Seckl JR. 11β-Hydroxysteroid dehydrogenase is an exclusive 11β-reductase in primary cultures of rat hepatocytes: effect of physicochemical and hormonal manipulations. Endocrinology 1995; 136:4754–4761.

161. Andrew R, Phillips DIW, Walker BR. Obesity and gender influence cortisol secretion and metabolism in man. J Clin Endocrinol Metab 1998; 83:1806–1809.

27

Sympathoadrenal System and Metabolism

Eric Ravussin

Pennington Biomedical Research Center, Louisiana State University, Baton Rouge, Louisiana, U.S.A.

Ian Andrew Macdonald

University of Nottingham Medical School, Nottingham, England

I INTRODUCTION

The sympathetic nervous system (SNS) is an important component of the autonomic nervous system, and thus plays a major role in the maintenance of body homeostasis. The SNS is of particular importance in the control of the cardiovascular system and of a number of metabolic processes including energy homeostasis. Alterations in SNS effects on metabolism have been implicated in the development and maintenance of obesity, and the SNS is a potential therapeutic target in the treatment of obesity. This short review provides an overview of the anatomical and physiological aspects of the SNS, before considering the evidence showing a role for the SNS in the development or treatment of obesity.

II ORGANIZATION AND STRUCTURE OF THE SNS

The autonomic nervous system consists of the sympathetic nervous system, parasympathetic nervous system (PNS), and adrenal medulla. A number of anatomical differences distinguish the SNS and the parasympathetic nervous system, which are reviewed in detail by Astrup and Macdonald (1). The important structural aspects of the SNS are that the preganglionic nerves arise from thoracic and lumbar regions of the spinal cord, and that the ganglia are close to the spinal cord. Thus, the SNS has long postganglionic nerves, which innervate almost all of the vital organs and tissues of the body. While most of these vital organs and tissues are also innervated by the parasympathetic nervous system, major exceptions are the blood vessels, sweat glands, and adipose tissue, which have only a sympathetic nerve supply. The adrenal medulla is effectively a sympathetic ganglion, but it releases hormones directly into the bloodstream instead of having a postganglionic nerve. There are many physiological and clinical situations in which activation of the SNS and adrenal medulla are dissociated, and it is more appropriate to consider them as the sympathoadrenal system than to include the adrenal medulla in the SNS. The other distinctive anatomical feature of sympathetic nerves is that they have varicosities along the length of nerve within the tissue that is innervated. Thus, each nerve releases neurotransmitters at a number of sites.

The SNS and PNS nerves, which arise from the spinal cord and supply the vital organs and tissues, represent the efferent part of the autonomic nervous system. Activation of these nerves usually occurs as part of reflex mechanisms that involve afferent signals and some processing in the central nervous system. Many of the afferent signals involved in these reflexes travel to the brain in afferent nerve fibers located in the sympathetic and parasympathetic nerve trunks. The most important structure for the integration of these afferent signals is the hypothalamus, which also receives inputs from higher brain centers. Thus, the hypothalamus is the major regulator of SNS activity, and is undoubtedly of major importance in the control of metabolism and energy homeostasis. As shown schematically in Figure 1, it is now well established that stimulation of the parasympathetic nervous system is associated with an anabolic effect (stimulation of food intake and inhibition of energy expenditure), whereas stimulation of the SNS is associated with a catabolic state in which food intake is decreased and energy expenditure is increased.

A large number of neurotransmitters and neuromodulators are involved in the central nervous control of the autonomic nervous system (2). The neuromodulators are normally peptides, coreleased with the classical neurotransmitters, and have a variety of effects to alter the response to the neurotransmitter. While the detail of such central control of autonomic (including SNS) efferent activity is beyond the scope of this review, it should be recognized that effects on the central nervous system may affect peripheral functions controlled by the SNS. The principal peripheral neurotransmitters in the autonomic nerves are acetylcholine and noradrenaline

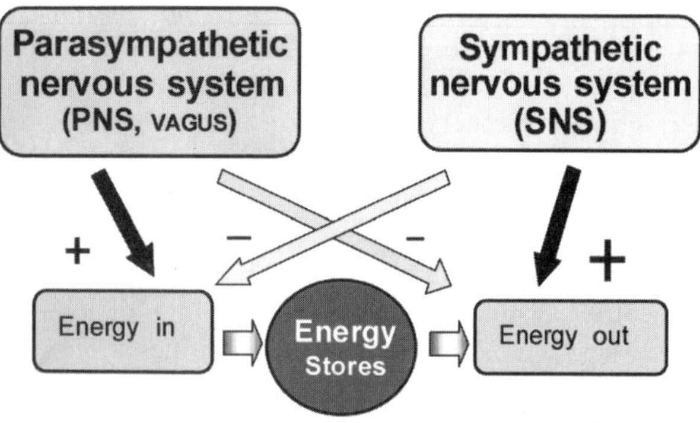

Figure 1 Schematic representation of the autonomic control of energy balance. Overall, an enhanced activity of the SNS tends to decrease the energy stores by decreasing energy intake and increasing energy expenditure, whereas an impaired activity is associated with increased energy stores and possibly obesity. On the contrary, an enhanced activity of the PNS is associated with obesity, whereas an impaired activity may be associated with leanness.

(norepinephrine). In the ganglia (both sympathetic and parasympathetic), the major neurotransmitter is acetylcholine, but a number of neuromodulatory neuropeptides are also present (3). The major postganglionic neurotransmitter in the SNS is noradrenaline (norepinephrine), while parasympathetic nerves almost exclusively release acetylcholine (and some peptides) from the nerve terminals. Some sympathetic nerves (such as those innervating the sweat glands) release acetylcholine rather than noradrenaline, and most sympathetic nerves also release a number of neuropeptides.

The predominant receptors of interest in the postganglionic sympathetic nerves are also those that mediate the effects of noradrenaline, or other catecholamines such as adrenaline (epinephrine). These catecholamine receptors are known as adrenoceptors, which are grouped into α and β subtypes. There are at least two types of α-adrenoceptor and three types of β-adrenoceptor. α-Adrenoceptors are particularly common in blood vessels, with vasoconstriction occurring when the receptors are stimulated by noradrenaline. By contrast, stimulation of β-adrenoceptors usually causes relaxation of vascular or bronchial smooth muscle. A major distinction between α- and β-adrenoceptors is in their second-messenger mechanisms. Cyclic AMP generation is a key second messenger for most if not all β-adrenoceptor-mediated responses, although the detailed mechanisms are rather complex, and vary between tissues and receptor types, involving G-proteins and other membrane components. α-Adrenoceptor activation produces different second messengers, mainly through the generation of phosphatidylinositol and diacylglycerol, causing an increase in intracellular calcium and often a decrease in cAMP.

III PHYSIOLOGICAL ROLE OF THE SNS

The aspects of SNS function that are of specific interest in relation to metabolism and obesity concern the regulation of the cardiovascular system, gastrointestinal function, pancreatic hormone secretion, and adipose tissue lipolysis. The single most important role of the SNS is the maintenance of an adequate blood pressure to maintain functioning of the vital organs. This is achieved principally by the sympathetic control of cardiac output and blood vessels, although it should be recognized that the parasympathetic innervation of the heart has a part to play. In most tissues or organs, stimulation of the sympathetic nerves produces vasoconstriction, reducing blood flow and potentially raising blood pressure. However, in some tissues (e.g., adipose tissue, skeletal muscle, and some skin areas) sympathetic activation can produce vasodilatation, increasing blood flow. Nevertheless, in most cases when tissue blood flow increases, it does so either because of effects of local metabolites or because of a reduction in sympathetic vasoconstriction. The importance of the SNS in the control of the cardiovascular system should not be overlooked, as any nonspecific stimulation or antagonism of the SNS intended to produce metabolic effects will also have significant cardiovascular effects that could be undesirable.

SNS activation has a general inhibitory effect on gastrointestinal function, reducing intestinal motility and gastric emptying. This contrasts with its general stimulatory effect on many other physiological processes. The SNS has a major role in the control of lipolysis in adipose tissue, both directly and due to the effects on pancreatic hormone secretion (1,4). The major metabolic effects of the SNS and plasma adrenaline are summarized in Figure 2.

In most physiological situations, the SNS is activated in a discrete manner, with stimulation of some tissues and no effect on others. This was clearly identified by Muntzel et al. (5), who showed that intracerebroventricular (ICV) administration of insulin to rats activated sympathetic outflow to the hind limbs (mainly skeletal muscle) but not to other areas. It is only in extreme circumstances, e.g., profound hypotension or the "fight or flight" response, that a generalized sympathetic activation may occur. In metabolic situations such as overfeeding, fasting, or hypoglycemia in rats, there is selective activation or inhibition of sympathetic activity in some organs, with no change in others (6). Thus, any

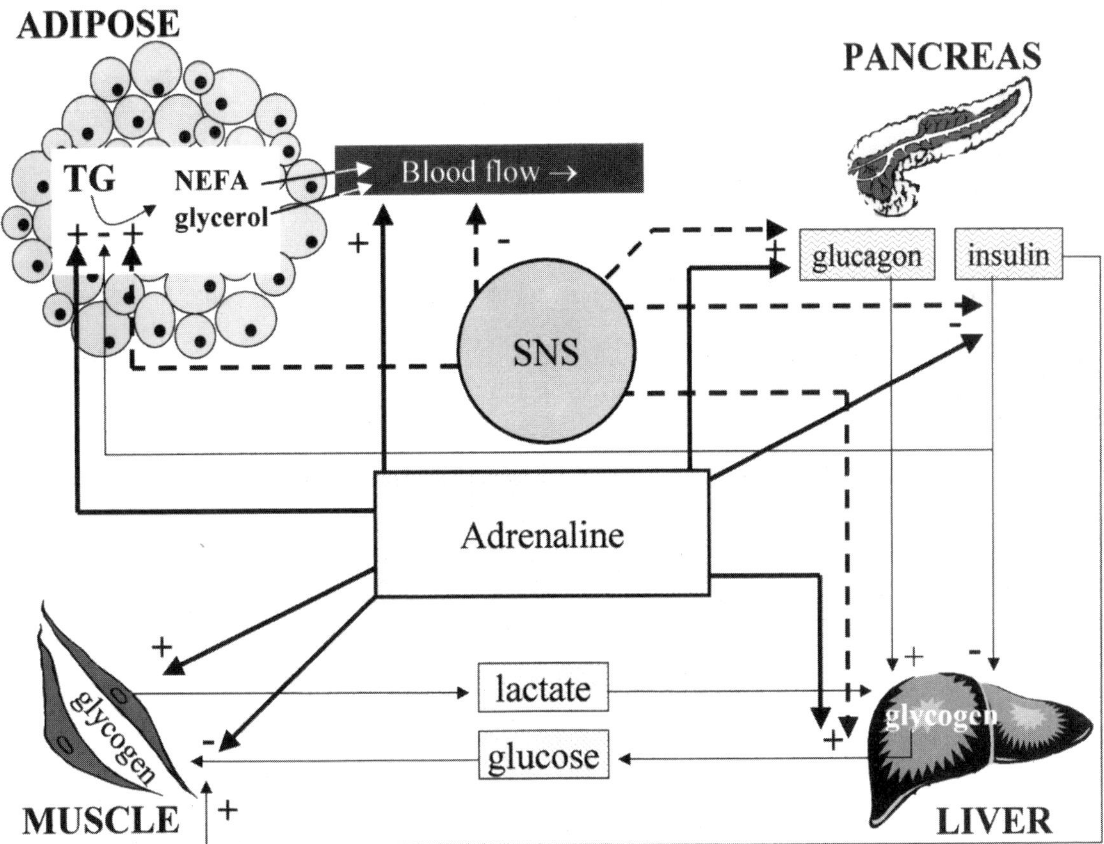

Figure 2 Summary of the metabolic effect of the sympathetic nervous system (SNS) and plasma adrenaline. Shaded boxes represent plasma compartments for hormones or substrates, solid lines represent effect of adrenaline from the adrenal medulla, and dashed lines represent activities mediated by sympathetic nerves. Other thin lines represent exchanges through the bloodstream.

consideration of the role of altered SNS or adrenal medullary activity in relation to obesity must take account of the discrete manner in which these systems are involved in physiological regulation.

IV METHODS FOR ASSESSING SNS ACTIVITY

A number of techniques are routinely used to assess SNS activity, but none of them are able to provide reliable information under all conditions. When assessing SNS activity, three important components must be recognized: the neural reflex arc, the end-organ responsiveness, and the existence of compensatory systems (7). Thus, just to obtain an index of efferent nerve activity, without some assessment of the functional consequences of any change recorded, can be misleading. Moreover, when possible, one should use more than one technique to assess SNS activity in order to obtain a more reliable assessment.

A Nerve Activity

The activity of the efferent sympathetic nerves can be determined by direct nerve recording (microneurography). The use of microneurography to assess SNS activity was pioneered by Wallin and colleagues (8). The technique involves the insertion of a fine tungsten microelectrode into a nerve, and is thus restricted to peripheral nerves such as the peroneal nerve in the leg. This technique can only provide information on SNS activity in the skin and skeletal muscle, and measurements can only be made with a subject resting quietly to avoid displacement of the electrode. The technique has been used to investigate the control of the cardiovascular system, and it is now clear that muscle sympathetic nerve activity (MSNA) is mainly related to the control of blood pressure, and that an increase in nerve firing rate is usually associated with vasoconstriction in skeletal muscle. However, this is not always the case, as there are a number of situations in which vasodilatation occurs despite an increase in muscle sympathetic nerve activity (1).

Thus, assessing peripheral sympathetic nerve firing rate in humans provides an index of the SNS supplying skeletal muscle, but in some circumstances this may not reflect overall sympathetic activity in the whole body. This is illustrated by the studies of sympathetic activity in obesity, where the measurement of plasma or urinary catecholamines in obese and non-obese subjects shows no clear consensus as to whether the obese have altered sympathetic activity. However, the few studies of muscle sympathetic nerve activity in lean and obese subjects consistently report increased activity in the obese. Thus, depending on how sympathetic activity is assessed, one would conclude the obese have either normal or elevated SNS activity (9).

B Neurotransmitter Release

It is very difficult to determine the rate of release of neurotransmitters from efferent sympathetic nerves, as the released molecules can undergo a number of different metabolic fates, including reuptake into the neuron, metabolism in the synaptic cleft, uptake into surrounding tissues, or spillover into the plasma. This last has been used as an index of SNS activity and can be obtained from radioactive tracer-based measurements of noradrenaline (10) or of urinary noradrenaline excretion (11). The use of arterial blood samples in the spillover technique allows an assessment of whole-body SNS activity, while regional venous blood sampling will allow SNS activity to be determined in a variety of tissues (12). By contrast, urinary excretion of noradrenaline provides information on the whole body, integrated over the period of the urine collection. The use of either the spillover technique or urinary noradrenaline excretion to assess the SNS relies on a constant relationship between release, spillover, and metabolism of noradrenaline. Any condition, or drug, that alters this relationship (e.g., a neuronal noradrenaline re-uptake inhibitor) could invalidate the index of SNS activity.

Plasma noradrenaline concentration per se provides limited information on SNS activity, as noradrenaline in the plasma arises from spillover from sympathetic nerves and release from the adrenal medulla. Thus, alteration in plasma noradrenaline could be the result of changes in adrenal medullary activity, although in most situations changes in SNS activity are responsible for alterations in plasma noradrenaline. If plasma noradrenaline is to be used to assess whole body SNS activity, it is more appropriate to use arterial [reviewed by Hjemdahl (13)] or arterialized venous blood samples (14) to avoid the errors produced by uptake and release of noradrenaline by forearm tissues.

In principle, the use of plasma adrenaline concentrations to assess adrenal medullary activity is more straightforward, although changes in clearance of the catecholamine from plasma can produce errors. For example, the nonselective β-adrenoceptor antagonist propranolol reduces the clearance of catecholamines from plasma and produces higher plasma concentrations of noradrenaline and adrenaline for a given rate of release or spillover (15).

V FACTORS AFFECTING SNS ACTIVITY OR RESPONSIVENESS

A variety of metabolic factors can alter the activity of the SNS or change the response to adrenoceptor activation. The classical studies of Landsberg and Young (6) showed that underfeeding of rodents led to a decrease in SNS activity, especially to the heart and brown adipose tissue, whereas overfeeding had the opposite effect. While similar effects of underfeeding on the SNS may occur in humans, starvation for up to 4 days does not reduce the lipolytic and thermogenic responses to infused catecholamines [reviewed by Macdonald and Webber (16)]. It has been argued that this reduced SNS activity during underfeeding is of survival value in reducing resting energy expenditure and thus prolonging survival. Such a mechanism would then explain possible links between reduced SNS activity and the development or maintenance of obesity discussed below.

As mentioned earlier, administration of insulin into the brain in rats increases muscle SNS activity (4), and similar effects are seen in humans when insulin is infused intravenously (i.e., muscle sympathetic nerve activity and plasma noradrenaline both increase) (17). It has long been established in clinical situations that there is a synergy between catecholamine and thyroid hormone effects on the cardiovascular system and metabolism. In situations of less severe disturbances of thyroid function, mild hyperthyroidism can increase metabolic rate and cardiac responses to administered catecholamines (18), while mild hypothyroidism reduces baseline heart rate and metabolic rate but does not affect the response to catecholamines (19).

There has been major interest in recent years in the possibility that receptor polymorphisms may be associated with altered function and have an etiological role in the development of disease. In the area of obesity, attention has been focused on the association of adrenoceptor (in particular the β_2 and β_3 adrenoceptors) or uncoupling protein (UCP1) polymorphisms, and the obese state. Most studies have failed to show convincing associations between obesity and receptor polymorphisms, although Large et al. (20) did show that a sevenfold increased relative risk of obesity was associated with a β_2-adrenoceptor polymorphism (Glu27 homozygosity). Interestingly, this polymorphism was not associated with any altered function of the β_2-adrenoceptor, while a different receptor polymorphism (Arg16Gly) was accompanied by increased receptor sensitivity in adipose tissue. More recently, Valve et al. (21) showed that combined polymorphisms of the β_3-adrenoceptor and UCP1 were associated with a low resting metabolic rate in obese Finns. However, many genetic association studies have failed to reproduce this finding (22). Taken together, these studies indicate a need to consider alterations in responsiveness to SNS activation or adrenal medullary hormone secretion as possible contributory factors to the development of obesity in humans.

VI ROLE OF LOW ENERGY EXPENDITURE IN THE PATHOGENESIS OF OBESITY

The daily energy expenditure (EE) of an individual can be divided into its components as illustrated in Figure 3. The resting metabolic rate (RMR) comprises 50–80% of the total daily EE and varies greatly among individuals. About 70–80% of this variance can be accounted for by differences in fat-free mass, fat mass, age, and gender (23). After accounting for these variables, studies in Pima Indians have indicated that an additional 7–11% of the variance in RMR is accounted for by family membership, strongly suggesting that RMR is influenced by genetic factors (24). Several studies support the idea that a low RMR is associated with weight gain. A low metabolic rate has been shown to precede body weight gain in infants (25), children (26), and adults (27). Based on the assumption that formerly obese, weight-reduced subjects exhibit the metabolic characteristics that predisposed them to obesity, several studies have compared metabolic rates in formerly obese subjects to those of weight-matched controls who have never been obese. A meta-analysis of 12 such studies corroborates the prospective data by demonstrating a 3–5% lower mean RMR in the formerly obese subjects (28). Moreover, these data indicate that a low RMR is more frequent among formerly obese subjects than among "never-obese" control subjects.

The thermic effect of food (TEF) is commonly defined as the increase in EE in response to food intake. Although TEF accounts for only ~10% of daily EE, many researchers believe that a low TEF plays a role in the development of obesity. Some data supporting this view have been presented, but the issue is still debated (29,30). Importantly, in the only prospective study to date, a low TEF was not associated with weight gain (31).

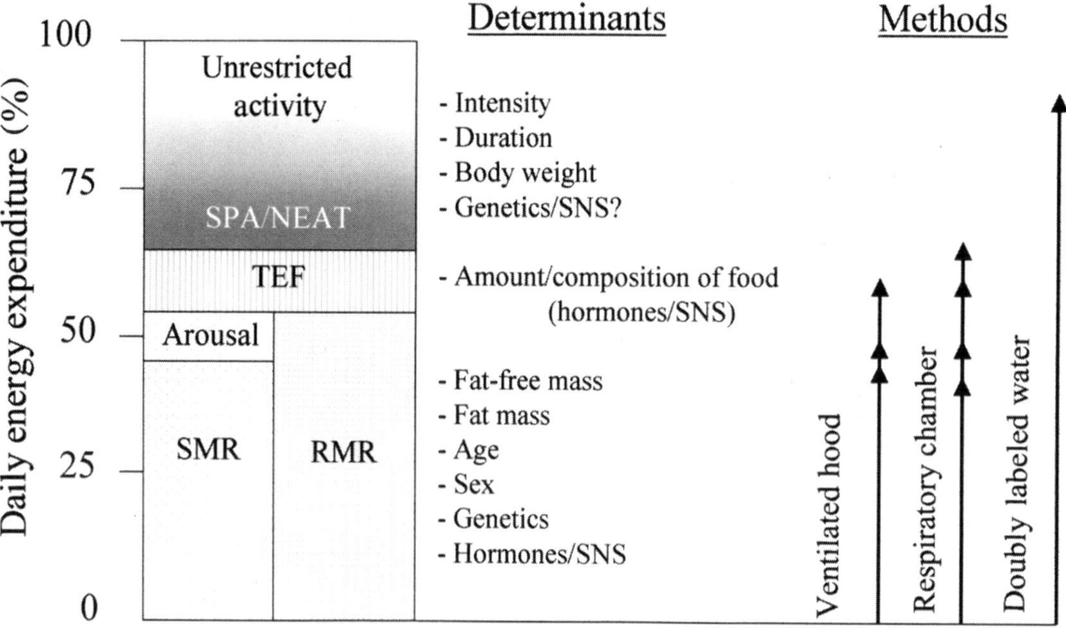

Figure 3 Components of daily energy expenditure, their major determinants and the methods by which they can be measured. SPA, spontaneous physical activity; NEAT, nonexercise activity thermogenesis; SMR, sleeping metabolic rate; RMR, resting metabolic rate; SNS, sympathetic nervous system.

When confined to a respiratory chamber, individuals differ as to how much they move around spontaneously, change position, and fidget. This *spontaneous physical activity* can be measured (23), and a low spontaneous physical activity is a risk factor for body weight gain in men (32). Recently, Levine et al. (33) showed that subjects who did unconsciously increase their spontaneous physical activity in response to overfeeding were resistant to weight gain compared to those who did not. They coined the term NEAT, for this "Non-Exercise Activity Thermogenesis" component of energy expenditure.

During indirect calorimetry measurements, the contributions of carbohydrate, lipid, and protein to total EE can be determined. The respiratory quotient (RQ) is calculated as the molar amount of CO_2 produced, divided by the amount of O_2 consumed, with a value of 1.0 indicating that glucose is the sole metabolic substrate, whereas a value of 0.71 indicates that fat is the fuel source. A high RQ (i.e., closer to 1.0 than 0.71) indicates a high oxidation of carbohydrate relative to lipid. Evidence that a high RQ predisposes to weight gain has been obtained in prospective studies (34,35) as well as in studies in formerly obese subjects (36–39). Therefore, both impaired energy expenditure and impaired fat oxidation can predispose individuals to weight gain. We here briefly discuss how the sympathetic nervous system can influence the different metabolic predictors of weight gain.

VII CONTRIBUTION OF THE SNS TO EE AND ITS COMPONENTS

A Energy Expenditure (24-hr EE and RMR)

Observations in rats indicate that the SNS stimulates thermogenesis and that dietary manipulation influences noradrenaline turnover. These findings have promoted interest in the role of the SNS in body weight regulation in humans. During short-term studies, sympathomimetic agents clearly increase EE (40). In a long-term, crossover study in seven white males, 24-hr EE tended to be lower during administration of the β-antagonist propranolol than placebo or the β_2-adrenergic agonist terbutaline (41). However, lipid oxidation was increased by terbutaline (41). In another study (42), 24-hr EE measured in a respiratory chamber was positively correlated with urinary noradrenaline excretion. Furthermore, administration of the β-antagonist propranolol caused a 4% decrease in RMR in white people but, interestingly, not in Pima

Indians (42), suggesting a dissociation of SNS and RMR in Pima Indians, a population with one of the highest prevalence rates of obesity in the world. In yet another study (43), adjusted 24-hr EE, sleeping metabolic rate, and RMR were correlated with MSNA in white people, but again, there was no relationship in Pima Indians. Noradrenaline turnover studies have shown that most of the variability in RMR unexplained by body size and composition is related to differences in SNS activity (44,45). Taken together, the above studies suggest that SNS activity does modulate RMR, the largest component of daily EE.

B Thermic Effect of Food

Studies in which β-blockade is used have demonstrated a facultative, β-adrenergically mediated component of glucose-induced thermogenesis. Furthermore, it has been shown, by measurement of plasma noradrenaline turnover (46,47), that the increased SNS activity in response to a meal accounts for at least part of the meal-induced TEF. The major drive for the increase in SNS activity in response to a meal seems to be insulin (48). Despite the clear impact of SNS activity on TEF, the contribution of TEF to total EE may be too small to have an impact on body weight gain, as suggested by prospective data (31).

C Spontaneous Physical Activity or NEAT

The relationship between spontaneous physical activity and noradrenaline appearance rate (49) is consistent with the idea that SNS activity is a determinant of how much subjects move around, change position, and fidget, all of which contribute to total EE. In other words, "fidgeters" seem to have higher activity of the SNS. It remains to be determined, however, whether the increased SNS activity in those who fidgets is a contributing factor to the fidgeting, or secondary to the increased activity associated with fidgeting. The mechanisms underlying the variability in the induction of NEAT in response to overfeeding are unknown, and it will be interesting to test the impact of the activity of the autonomic system on this variability. Recent data from the NIH group in Phoenix showed that spontaneous physical activity measured in a respiratory chamber is related to the level of physical activity in free-living conditions (50). Taken together, the results suggest that a higher sympathetic tone may drive an increase in both spontaneous physical activity and habitual physical activity, therefore protecting individuals against body weight gain.

D Substrate Oxidation

The effects of the SNS on metabolism appear to influence the relative amounts of substrate oxidized (41). Accordingly, an inverse relationship was demonstrated in white people between 24-hr RQ (measured in a respiratory chamber) and basal muscle sympathetic nerve activity (measured immediately after the stay in the respiratory chamber) (51). The relationship between RQ and SNS activity was independent of the percentage of body fat and clearly indicates an association between a low SNS activity and a low lipid oxidation. A possible explanation for this observation is the stimulatory effect of noradrenaline on intracellular lipolysis and on free fatty acids uptake in the muscle, which seem impaired in previously obese subjects (52).

E Responsiveness to Sympathetic Stimuli

Decreased *responsiveness* to sympathetic stimuli may be as equally important as decreased *activity* of the SNS for the development of obesity. Defects of catecholamine-induced lipolysis have been observed in a number of obese subjects, but polymorphisms of the β_2-(20) and β_3-receptors (53) were proposed as explanations for the impaired lipolysis. Using an in vivo model for studies of neural control of adipose tissue lipolysis (intraneural electrical stimulation of the lateral cutaneous femoral nerve), Dodt et al. (54) showed that human obesity is characterized by a profound unresponsiveness of the subcutaneous adipose tissue to lipolysis. Decreased responsiveness could possibly be caused by polymorphisms in the genes encoding the various types of adrenoceptors, but may also be due to a reduced number of those receptors in the obese. A variant in the gene encoding for the β_3-adrenoceptor, resulting in the substitution of tryptophan with arginine in position 64 (trp64arg) of the receptor protein, has been associated with obesity and diabetes in some studies (55), and exhibits impaired signaling when expressed in Chinese hamster ovary (CHO) cells under certain, but not all, experimental conditions (56,57). A number of genetic polymorphisms in the β_2-adrenoceptor have also been reported (20), some of which are associated with functional abnormalities, and some of which are associated with obesity, but none of which are associated with both (20). At the intracellular level, cAMP released owing to SNS stimulation may affect the expression and the thermogenic function of the uncoupling proteins (UCPs). Lately, attention has been focused on UCP3, which is mostly expressed in muscle. UCP3 mRNA expression increases in response to overfeeding and fasting (probably through increased availability of NEFAs) and in response to adrenergic stimulation. The UCP3 and UCP2 genes are located adjacent to each other in a region implicated in linkage studies as contributing to obesity (58), and a polymorphism in the gene encoding for UCP3 has been associated with reduced fat oxidation (59). However, the potential uncoupling activity of UCP2 and UCP3 is still debated (60) despite the fact that massive overexpression of human UCP3 in mice was associated with increased metabolic rate (61).

VIII LOW SNS ACTIVITY IS ASSOCIATED WITH WEIGHT GAIN

In rodents, administration of the adipocyte hormone leptin promotes negative energy balance, the latter partly mediated by increased SNS outflow to a number of organs including brown adipose tissue. Accordingly, animals with defective leptin biosynthesis or receptor function (e.g., the *ob/ob* mouse, the *db/db* mouse, or the *fa/fa* rat) have markedly reduced SNS activity and become obese. Rodents made obese by lesions of the ventromedial hypothalamus have a reduced firing rate of sympathetic nerves to the brown adipose tissue in the basal state and in response to dietary and environmental stimuli. This reduced SNS activity is associated with low metabolic rate and hyperphagia (62). Studies in humans in whom SNS activity or adrenal medullary function is compared between lean and obese subjects have yielded very conflicting results, as reviewed (63), probably because comparisons of lean and obese subjects provide only very limited information about the role of the SNS in the etiology of obesity as they do not discern between causes and consequences of weight gain. A better approach is to establish the relationship between SNS activity and subsequent weight gain. The only such report we are aware of (64) demonstrates a relationship between low urinary noradrenaline excretion and weight gain, and a relationship between low urinary adrenaline excretion and the development of central obesity. These results strongly suggest that a low SNS activity is also a risk factor for weight gain in humans. SNS activity increases in response to weight gain, thereby attenuating the original impairment. It is of interest to note that basal MSNA for a given percentage of body fat is lower in Pima Indians compared to white people (41,43), possibly contributing to the propensity to obesity in the Pima Indians.

IX SNS ACTIVITY AS A PREDICTOR OF WEIGHT LOSS DURING TREATMENT OF OBESITY

Because sympathetic activity is an important determinant of EE and plays a role in the propensity to weight gain in some individuals, it is likely that constitutional differences in SNS activity may contribute to explain the large variability in weight loss among obese individuals on dietary treatment programs. Sympathetic activation has also been associated with enhanced meal-induced satiety (65), which suggests that the SNS exerts a dual effect, i.e., working on both sides of the energy balance equation. Pharmacological blockade of the SNS is difficult to achieve, but a certain functional inhibition occurs during chronic treatment with a number of agents, such as β-adrenergic antagonists (1). Treatment of hypertensive or other patients with β-antagonist produces an average of 2- to 5-kg weight increase, which can be entirely accounted for by fat gain (66). Even if other unknown regulatory mechanisms may counteract further weight gain (67), it is interesting that some individuals experience a rather large weight gain during inhibition of their SNS.

The habitual SNS activity may also play a role in variability in weight loss during the treatment of obese patients. Three studies have assessed the relationship between pretreatment SNS activity of obese subjects and weight loss outcome during hypoenergetic dieting. In a study of obese females who underwent 36 weeks of 4.2-MJ d^{-1} diet, pretreatment levels of postprandial plasma noradrenaline were positively associated with the maximum achieved weight loss, and a low plasma noradrenaline level was found to be a risk factor for a small weight loss (68). Similarly, pretreatment levels of both plasma noradrenaline and adrenaline were found to be positively associated with fat loss in 63 obese patients undergoing an 8-week, very low energy diet (2.8 MJ d^{-1}) (69). In a third study, Hellström et al. (70) found that plasma noradrenaline and α_2-adrenoceptor sensitivity was associated with fat loss during 4 weeks on a 1.6-MJ d^{-1} diet. These studies suggest that obese patients with low SNS activity are less responsive to diet-induced weight loss programs and that plasma noradrenaline can be used as a prognostic marker of weight loss.

X DIETARY STIMULATION OF SNS

It is not entirely clear from the literature if basal metabolic rate (BMR) and 24hr EE can be influenced by the dietary macronutrient composition. However, there are some studies indicating that the carbohydrate content of the diet may slightly increase EE. Toth and Poehlman (45) studied the diet composition and RMR of vegetarians and nonvegetarians. Vegetarians reported a greater intake of carbohydrates than nonvegetarians (62% vs. 51%), whereas no difference was found in body composition or aerobic capacity. Vegetarians had an 11% higher RMR, which could be explained by their higher SNS activity due to the higher carbohydrate intake (45). Some, but not all, intervention studies also support that a high-carbohydrate diet increases EE. One group found that, despite a weight loss during 20 weeks on an ad libitum low-fat, high-carbohydrate diet, energy intake was 19% higher than a control group consuming a high-fat diet (71). An analysis of physical activity level could not identify any change in daily activity level, which suggests that other components of EE were affected (72). Strictly controlled dietary intervention studies have demonstrated that EE is increased only by high-carbohydrate diets with high contents of simple sugars. Vasilaras et al. (73) compared the impact of high-sucrose versus high-starch diet on 24-hr EE and SNS activity. After 14 days on the sucrose diet, 24-hr EE, as well as postprandial plasma adrenaline and noradrenaline concentrations, was significantly higher than on the high-starch diet and on a high-fat control diet. The results have been confirmed by the European multicenter randomized trial CARMEN, in which about 300 overweight and obese subjects completed 6 months ad libitum intake of low-fat diets, rich in either simple or complex carbohydrates (74). Only the diet rich in simple carbohydrates increased EE, whereas no effect was seen with the complex carbohydrates. The reason for the differences between the carbohydrates is probably to be found in the effect of fructose on EE and SNS activity. Several studies have found that fructose and sucrose increase EE after intake, compared with glucose and starch (74,75). However, this advantage of simple over complex carbohydrates should be balanced against the reverse effects on satiety and energy intake.

REFERENCES

1. Astrup A, Macdonald IA. Sympathoadrenal system and metabolism. In: Bray GA, Bouchard C, James WPT, eds. Handbook of Obesity. New York: Marcel Dekker, 1998:491–511.
2. Bennaroch EE. Central neurotransmitters and neuromodulators in cardiovascular regulation. In: Bannister R, Mathias CJ, eds. Autonomic Failure. Oxford: Oxford University Press, 1992:36–53.
3. Matthews MR. Autonomic ganglia in multiple system atrophy and pure autonomic failure. In: Bannister R, Mathias CJ, eds. Autonomic Failure. Oxford: Oxford University Press, 1992:593–621.
4. Webber J, Macdonald IA. Metabolic actions of catecholamines in man. Baillieres Clin Endocrinol Metab 1993; 7:393–413.
5. Muntzel MS, Morgan DA, Mark AL, Johnson AK. Intracerebroventricular insulin produces nonuniform regional increases in sympathetic nerve activity. Am J Physiol 1994; 267:R1350–R1355.
6. Landsberg L, Young JB. The influence of diet on the sympathetic nervous system. Neuroendocr Perspect 1985; 4:191–218.
7. Mathias CJ, Bannister R. Investigation of autonomic disorders. In: Bannister R, Mathias CJ, eds. Autonomic Failure. Oxford: Oxford University Press, 1992:225–290.
8. Wallin BG, Sundlof G, Lindblad LE. Baroreflex mechanisms controlling sympathetic outflow to the muscles in man. In: Sleight P, ed. Arterial Baroreceptors and Hypertension. Oxford: Oxford University Press, 1980:101–108.
9. Macdonald IA. Advances in our understanding of the role of the sympathetic nervous system in obesity. Int J Obes Relat Metab Disord 1995; 19(suppl 7):S2-S7.
10. Esler M, Jennings G, Lambert G, Meredith I, Horne M, Eisenhofer G. Overflow of catecholamine neurotransmitters to the circulation: source, fate, and functions. Physiol Rev 1990; 70:963–985.
11. Kopp U, Bradley T, Hjemdahl P. Renal venous outflow and urinary excretion of norepinephrine, epinephrine, and dopamine during graded renal nerve stimulation. Am J Physiol 1983;244: E52–E60.
12. Cox HS, Kaye DM, Thompson JM, Turner AG, Jennings GL, Itsiopoulos C, Esler MD. Regional sympathetic nervous activation after a large meal in humans. Clin Sci (Colch) 1995; 89:145–154.
13. Hjemdahl P. Plasma catecholamines—analytical challenges and physiological limitations. Baillieres Clin Endocrinol Metab 1993; 7:307–353.
14. Liu D, Andreasson K, Lins PE, Adamson UC, Macdonald IA. Adrenaline and noradrenaline responses during insulin-induced hypoglycaemia in man: should the hormone levels be measured in arterialized venous blood? Acta Endocrinol (Copenh) 1993; 128:95–98.
15. Cryer PE, Rizza RA, Haymond MW, Gerich JE. Epinephrine and norepinephrine are cleared through beta-adrenergic, but not alpha-adrenergic, mechanisms in man. Metabolism 1980; 29:1114–1118.
16. Macdonald IA, Webber J. Feeding, fasting and starvation: factors affecting fuel utilization. Proc Nutr Soc 1995; 54:267–274.
17. Berne C, Fagius J, Pollare T, Hjemdahl P. The sympathetic response to euglycaemic hyperinsulinaemia. Evidence from microelectrode nerve recordings in healthy subjects. Diabetologia 1992; 35:873–879.

18. Gelfand RA, Hutchinson-Williams KA, Bonde AA, Castellino P, Sherwin RS. Catabolic effects of thyroid hormone excess: the contribution of adrenergic activity to hypermetabolism and protein breakdown. Metabolism 1987; 36:562–569.
19. Johnson AB, Webber J, Allison SP, Gallen IW, Mansell PI, Macdonald IA. Effects of hypothyroidism on the physiological responses to infused adrenaline. Endocrinol Metab 1995; 43:747–751.
20. Large V, Hellstrom L, Reynisdottir S, Lonnqvist F, Eriksson P, Lannfelt L, Arner P. Human beta-2 adrenoceptor gene polymorphisms are highly frequent in obesity and associated with altered adipocyte beta-2 adrenoceptor function. J Clin Invest 1997; 100:3005–3013.
21. Valve R, Heikkinen S, Rissanen A, Laakso M, Uusitupa M. Synergistic effect of polymorphisms in uncoupling protein 1 and beta3-adrenergic receptor genes on basal metabolic rate in obese Finns. Diabetologia 1998; 41:357–361.
22. Allison DB, Heo M, Faith MS, Pietrobelli A. Meta-analysis of the association of the Trp64Arg polymorphism in the beta3 adrenergic receptor with body mass index. Int J Obes Relat Metab Disord 1998; 22:559–566.
23. Ravussin E, Lillioja S, Anderson TE, Christin L, Bogardus C. Determinants of 24-hour energy expenditure in man. Methods and results using a respiratory chamber. J Clin Invest 1986; 78:1568–1578.
24. Bogardus C, Lillioja S, Ravussin E, Abbott W, Zawadzki JK, Young A, Knowler WC, Jacobowitz R, Moll PP. Familial dependence of the resting metabolic rate. N Engl J Med 1986; 315:96–100.
25. Roberts SB, Savage J, Coward WA, Chew B, Lucas A. Energy expenditure and intake in infants born to lean and overweight mothers. N Engl J Med 1988; 318:461–466.
26. Griffiths M, Payne PR, Stunkard AJ, Rivers JP, Cox M. Metabolic rate and physical development in children at risk of obesity. Lancet 1990; 336:76–78.
27. Ravussin E, Lillioja S, Knowler WC, Christin L, Freymond D, Abbott WG, Boyce V, Howard BV, Bogardus C. Reduced rate of energy expenditure as a risk factor for body-weight gain. N Engl J Med 1988; 318:467–472.
28. Astrup A, Gotzsche PC, Van de Werken K, Ranneries C, Toubro S, Raben A, Buemann B. Meta-analysis of resting metabolic rate in formerly obese subjects. Am J Clin Nutr 1999; 69:1117–1122.
29. Ravussin E, Swinburn BA. Energy metabolism. In: Stunkard AJ, Wadden TA, eds. Obesity: Theory and Therapy. New York: Raven Press, 1993:97–123.
30. De Jonge L, Bray GA. The thermic effect of food and obesity: a critical review. Obes Res 1997; 5:622–631.
31. Tataranni PA, Larson DE, Snitker S, Ravussin E. Thermic effect of food in humans: methods and results from use of a respiratory chamber. Am J Clin Nutr 1995; 61:1013–1019.
32. Zurlo F, Ferraro RT, Fontvielle AM, Rising R, Bogardus C, Ravussin E. Spontaneous physical activity and obesity: cross-sectional and longitudinal studies in Pima Indians. Am J Physiol 1992; 263:E296–E300.
33. Levine JA, Eberhardt NL, Jensen MD. Role of nonexercise activity thermogenesis in resistance to fat gain in humans. Science 1999; 283:212–214.
34. Zurlo F, Lillioja S, Esposito-Del Puente A, Nyomba BL, Raz I, Saad MF, Swinburn BA, Knowler WC, Bogardus C, Ravussin E. Low ratio of fat to carbohydrate oxidation as predictor of weight gain: study of 24-h RQ. Am J Physiol 1990; 259:E650–E657.
35. Seidell JC, Muller DC, Sorkin JD, Andres R. Fasting respiratory exchange ratio and resting metabolic rate as predictors of weight gain: the Baltimore Longitudinal Study on Aging. Int J Obes Relat Metab Disord 1992; 16:667–674.
36. Larson DE, Ferraro RT, Robertson DS, Ravussin E. Energy metabolism in weight-stable post obese individuals. Am J Clin Nutr 1995; 62:735–739.
37. Filozof CM, Murua C, Sanchez MP, Brailovsky C, Perman M, Gonzalez CD, Ravussin E. Low plasma leptin concentration and low rates of fat oxidation in weight-stable post-obese subjects. Obes Res 2000; 8: 205–210.
38. Kelley DE, Goodpaster B, Wing RR, Simoneau JA. Skeletal muscle fatty acid metabolism in association with insulin resistance, obesity, and weight loss. Am J Physiol 1999; 277:E1130–E1141.
39. Ballor DL, Harvey-Berino JR, Ades PA, Cryan J, Calles-Escandon J. Decrease in fat oxidation following a meal in weight-reduced individuals: a possible mechanism for weight recidivism. Metabolism 1996; 45:174–178.
40. Schiffelers SL, Blaak EE, Saris WH, Van Baak MA. In vivo beta3-adrenergic stimulation of human thermogenesis and lipid use. Clin Pharmacol Ther 2000; 67: 558–566.
41. Acheson KJ, Ravussin E, Schoeller DA, Christin L, Bourquin L, Baertschi P, Danforth E Jr, Jequier E. Two-week stimulation or blockade of the sympathetic nervous system in man: influence on body weight, body composition, and twenty four-hour energy expenditure. Metabolism 1988; 37:91–98.
42. Saad MF, Alger SA, Zurlo F, Young JB, Bogardus C, Ravussin E. Ethnic differences in sympathetic nervous system–mediated energy expenditure. Am J Physiol 1991; 261:E789–E794.
43. Spraul M, Ravussin E, Fontvieille AM, Rising R, Larson DE, Anderson EA. Reduced sympathetic nervous activity. A potential mechanism predisposing to body weight gain. J Clin Invest 1993; 92:1730–1735.
44. Poehlman ET, Arciero PJ, Goran MI. Endurance exercise in aging humans: effects on energy metabolism. Exerc Sport Sci Rev 1994; 22:251–284.

45. Toth MJ, Poehlman ET. Sympathetic nervous system activity and resting metabolic rate in vegetarians. Metabolism 1994; 43:621–625.
46. Schwartz RS, Jaeger LF, Silberstein S, Veith RC. Sympathetic nervous system activity and the thermic effect of feeding in man. Int J Obes 1987; 11:141–149.
47. Schwartz RS, Jaeger LF, Veith RC. The thermic effect of feeding in older men: the importance of the sympathetic nervous system. Metabolism 1990; 39:733–737.
48. Anderson EA, Hoffman RP, Balon TW, Sinkey CA, Mark AL. Hyperinsulinemia produces both sympathetic neural activation and vasodilation in normal humans. J Clin Invest 1991; 87:2246–2252.
49. Christin L, O'Connell M, Bogardus C, Danforth E Jr, Ravussin E. Norepinephrine turnover and energy expenditure in Pima Indian and white men. Metabolism 1993; 42:723–729.
50. Snitker S, Tataranni PA, Ravussin E. Spontaneous physical activity in a respiratory chamber is correlated to habitual physical activity. Int J Obes 2001; 25:1481–1486.
51. Snitker S, Tataranni PA, Ravussin E. Respiratory quotient is inversely associated with muscle sympathetic nerve activity. J Clin Endocrinol Metab 1998; 83:3977–3979.
52. Blaak EE, Van Baak MA, Kemerink GJ, Pakbiers MT, Heidendal GA, Saris WH. Beta-adrenergic stimulation of skeletal muscle metabolism in relation to weight reduction in obese men. Am J Physiol 1994; 267:E316–E322.
53. Clement K, Vaisse C, Manning BS, Basdevant A, Guy-Grand B, Ruiz J, Silver KD, Shuldiner AR, Froguel P, Strosberg AD. Genetic variation in the beta3-adrenergic receptor and an increased capacity to gain weight in patients with morbid obesity. N Engl J Med 1995; 333:352–354.
54. Dodt C, Lonnroth P, Fehm HL, Elam M. The subcutaneous lipolytic response to regional neural stimulation is reduced in obese women. Diabetes 2000; 49:1875–1879.
55. Fujisawa T, Ikegami H, Kawaguchi Y, Ogihara T. Meta-analysis of the association of Trp64Arg polymorphism of beta3-adrenergic receptor gene with body mass index. J Clin Endocrinol Metab 1998; 83:2441–2444.
56. Pietri-Rouxel F, St John Manning B, Gros J, Strosberg AD. The biochemical effect of the naturally occurring Trp64→Arg mutation on human beta3-adrenoceptor activity. Eur J Biochem 1997; 247:1174–1179.
57. Candelore MR, Deng L, Tota LM, Kelly LJ, Cascieri MA, Strader CD. Pharmacological characterization of a recently described human beta3-adrenergic receptor mutant. Endocrinology 1996; 137:2638–2641.
58. Bouchard C, Perusse L, Chagnon YC, Warden C, Riquier D. Linkage between markers in the vicinity of the uncoupling protein 2 gene and resting metabolic rate in humans. Hum Mol Gen 1997; 11:1887–1889.
59. Argyropoulos G, Brown AM, Willi SM, Zhu J, He Y, Reitman M, Gevao SM, Spruill I, Garvey WT. Effects of mutations in the human uncoupling protein 3 gene on the respiratory quotient and fat oxidation in severe obesity and type 2 diabetes. J Clin Invest 1998; 102: 1345–1351.
60. Stuart JA, Harper JA, Brindle KM, Jekabsons MB, Brand MD. Physiological levels of mammalian uncoupling protein 2 do not uncouple yeast mitochondria. J Biol Chem 2001; 276:18633–18639.
61. Clapham JC, Arch JR, Chapman H, Haynes A, Lister C, Moore GB, Piercy V, Carter SA, Lehner I, Smith SA, Beeley LJ, Godden RJ, Herrity N, Skehel M, Changani KK, Hockings PD, Reid DG, Squires SM, Hatcher J, Trail B, Latcham J, Rastan S, Harper AJ, Cadenas S, Buckingham JA, Brand MD, Abuin A. Mice overexpressing human uncoupling protein-3 in skeletal muscle are hyperphagic and lean. Nature 2000; 406:415–418.
62. Bray GA. Reciprocal relation of food intake and sympathetic activity: experimental observations and clinical implications. Int J Obes Relat Metab Disord 2000; 24(suppl 2):S8–S17.
63. Young JB, Macdonald IA. Sympathoadrenal activity in human obesity: heterogeneity of findings since 1980. Int J Obes Relat Metab Disord 1992; 16:959–967.
64. Tataranni PA, Young JB, Bogardus C, Ravussin E. A low sympathoadrenal activity is associated with body weight gain and development of central adiposity in Pima Indian men. Obes Res 1997; 5:341–347.
65. Raben A, Holst JJ, Christensen NJ, Astrup A. Determinants of postprandial appetite sensations: macronutrient intake and glucose metabolism. Int J Obes Relat Metab Disord 1996; 20:161–169.
66. Astrup AV, Christensen NJ, Simonsen L, Bulow J. Effects of nutrient intake on sympathoadrenal activity and thermogenic mechanisms. J Neurosci Methods 1990; 34:187–192.
67. Leibel RL, Rosenbaum M, Hirsch J. Changes in energy expenditure resulting from altered body weight. N Engl J Med 1995; 332:621–628.
68. Astrup A, Buemann B, Gluud C, Bennett P, Tjur T, Christensen N. Prognostic markers for diet-induced weight loss in obese women. Int J Obes Relat Metab Disord 1995; 19:275–278.
69. Kempen KPG. Predictors of fat loss during very-low calorie diet in obese females. Maastricht, Holland: University of Maastricht, 1996.
70. Hellstrom L, Rossner S, Hagstrom-Troft E, Reynisdottir S. Lipolytic catecholamine resistance linked to alpha2-adrenoceptor sensitivity—a metabolic predictor of weight loss in obese subjects. Int J Obes 1995; 21:314–320.
71. Astrup A, Toubro S, Raben A, Skov AR. The role of low-fat diets and fat substitutes in body weight

management: what have we learned from clinical studies? J Am Diet Assoc 1997; 97:S82–S87.
72. Raben A, Macdonald I, Astrup A. Replacement of dietary fat by sucrose or starch: effects on 14 d ad libitum energy intake, energy expenditure and body weight in formerly obese and never-obese subjects. Int J Obes Relat Metab Disord 1997; 21:846–859.
73. Vasilaras TH, Raben A, Astrup A. Six months intake of simple carbohydrates increases energy expenditure obese subjects. Int J Obes 1998; 22:S256.
74. Tappy L, Randin JP, Felber JP, Chiolero R, Simonson DC, Jequier E, DeFronzo RA. Comparison of thermogenic effect of fructose and glucose in normal humans. Am J Physiol 1986; 250:E718–E724.
75. Raben A, Kiens B, Richter EA. Differences in glycaemia, hormonal response and energy expenditure after a meal rich in mono- and disaccharides compared to a meal rich in polysaccharides in physically fit and sedentary subjects. Clin Physiol 1994; 14:267–280.

28

Energy Expenditure and Substrate Oxidation

Jean-Pierre Flatt

University of Massachusetts Medical School, Worcester, Massachusetts, U.S.A.

Angelo Tremblay

Laval University, Sainte-Foy, Quebec, Canada

I FACTORS DETERMINING TOTAL SUBSTRATE OXIDATION

The rate of substrate oxidation varies considerably during the day, being dictated by the body's need to regenerate the adenosine triphosphate (ATP) used in carrying out its metabolic functions, in digesting and storing nutrients, in moving, and in performing physical tasks. The amount of heat generated is generally sufficient to allow maintenance of body temperature by regulation of heat dissipation, aided when necessary by measures seeking to maintain comfort through appropriate clothing and control of environmental temperatures. Situations where substrate oxidation is activated for the sake of thermogenesis are avoided as much as possible.

The energy expended in the resting state depends primarily on the size of the lean body mass, plus the metabolic costs for processing ingested nutrients. The energy expended for specific physical activities is highly reproducible and in many cases roughly proportional to body weight (1). Overall energy expenditure for weight maintaining adults is thus determined primarily by body size and by the intensity and duration of the physical activities undertaken. In sedentary individuals total daily energy expenditure (TEE) varies typically between 1.3 and 1.5 times the rate of resting energy expenditure (REE) extrapolated to 24 hr.

A Efficiency of Oxidative Phosphorylation and P:O Ratio

It is difficult to assess the efficiency of oxidative phosphorylation and the P:O ratio in intact cells, because the ATP turnover due to the cell's metabolic activities is not readily measurable. Pahud et al. (2) were nevertheless able to assess the efficiency of oxidative phosphorylation in man by combining direct and indirect calorimetry measurements in young men pedaling on a bicycle ergometer at different levels of work output. During sustained aerobic work, the mechanical work performed was equivalent to 27% of the energy contained in the increment in substrate oxidation elicited by pedaling. During the first minutes of pedaling against a suddenly increased resistance, the mechanical work produced (measured electrically with the bicycle ergometer) plus the energy appearing in the form of heat (measured by direct calorimetry and from the increase in the subjects' body temperature) exceeded the energy liberated by substrate oxidation (determined by indirect calorimetry). This implies that preformed high-energy bonds (ATP and creatine-phosphate) were utilized to accomplish part of the mechanical work during this phase of the test. The characteristics of this latter process allowed them to determine that the *coupling coefficient*, which describes the efficiency with which chemical energy can be converted into work in muscles, is 41%. The difference in the two observed efficiencies is due to the fact that a fraction only of the energy liberated by the oxidation of metabolic fuels is recovered in the form of ATP. The ratio 27%/41% = 0.66 thus provides an estimate of the efficiency with which the energy liberated by substrate oxidation is recovered in the form of ATP in human muscles.

During the complete oxidation of 1 mol of glucose, ~689 (ΔG, kcal/mol) × 0.66 = 450 kcal of free energy is therefore recovered in the form of high-energy bonds. Since the ΔG for ATP hydrolysis in muscle is ~ −14.3 kcal/mol and oxidative phosphorylation operates at near equilibrium conditions, one would expect 450/14.3 = 31.5 mol ATP to be formed, which corresponds to a P:O ratio of 31.3/12 = 2.6 (3). This is in reasonably good agreement with other evaluations of the P:O ratio in intact cells (3). In reality, such experiments provide evaluations of the increments in ATP generation divided by the increments in oxygen consumption, i.e., a "ΔP:ΔO ratio." This is higher than the P:O ratio prevailing in resting cells, in which the P:O ratio is lower due to a certain rate of proton leakage through the mitochondrial membrane (4), which may account for 20% of resting energy expenditure (5). While ATP turnover based on estimates of the ΔP:ΔO ratio will thus be overestimated, this uncertainty is of lesser importance when increments in ATP turnover are to be assessed. Considering the number of assumptions and sources of possible errors inherent in these estimates, a value of 2.6 still seems to be compatible with the "traditional" values of three and two high-energy bonds regenerated per mitochondrial NADH and per $FADH_2$ or cytoplasmic NADH reoxidized, respectively. In order to maintain consistency with common practices, these values were used in computing the amounts of ATP yielded by the oxidation of metabolic fuels (Table 1) (6,7) and in the assessment of the metabolic costs of processes based on their ATP-related stoichiometries (Fig. 1) (6).

Extramitochondrial reactions with oxygen are catalyzed by peroxidases, and for diverse hydroxylations catalyzed by oxygenases (where the ultimate reaction

Table 1 Stoichiometry of Substrate Oxidation and High-Energy Bond Production

Substrate	RQ	Products
$C_6H_{12}O_6$ + 6 O_2 Glucose	RQ = 1.00 (4.99 kcal/L O_2)	6 CO_2 + 6 H_2O + 670 kcal[a] [+38 − 2 = +36~][b]
$C_6H_{10}O_5$ + 6 O_2 Glucosyl-	RQ = 1.00 (5.05 kcal/L O_2)	6 CO_2 + 6 H_2O + 678 kcal[a] [+38 − 1 = + 37~]
[c]4.5 $C_6H_{12}O_6$ + 4 O_2 Glucose	RQ = 2.75 (7.06 kcal/L O_2)	$C_{16}H_{32}O_2$ + 11 CO_2 + 11 H_2O + 630 kcal Palmitate [+40 − 34 = 6~]
$C_{16}H_{32}O_2$ + 23 O_2 Palmitate	RQ = 0.696 (4.68 kcal/L O_2)	16 CO_2 + 16 H_2O + 2398 kcal [+131 − 2 = + 129~]
[d]$C_{57}H_{107}O_6$ + 78 O_2 [e]Triglyceride	[d]RQ = 0.71 [a](4.69 kcal/L O_2)	57 CO_2 + 52 H_2O + 8139 kcal [+459 − 7 = + 452~]
[f]$C_{4.6}H_{8.4}O_{1.8}N_{1.25}$ + 1.5 O_2 0.2 H_2O	(RQ = 0.40) (*liver*)	0.6 Urea + 0.6 CO_2 + 0.35 Gluc + 0.3 KB [+8.2 − 4.6 = + 3.6~]
[f]Protein 0.35 Gluc + 0.3 KB + 3.3 O_2	(RQ = 1.0) (*periphery*)	3.3 CO_2 + 3.1 H_2O [+20.6 − 1 = + 19.6~]
$C_{4.6}H_{8.4}O_{1.8}N_{1.25}$ + 4.8 O_2 [g]Protein	[e]RQ = .835 [e](4.66kcal/L O_2)	0.6 Urea + 4.0 CO_2 + 2.9 H_2O + 520 kcal [g][+28.8 − 5.6 = +23.2~]

KB, Ketone bodies.
[a] Handbook of Chemistry and Physics, 57th ed, 1970 (13).
[b] The number of high-energy bonds (~) produced, minus those utilized, as well as the overall ~ yield is shown in square brackets.
[c] Based on stoichiometry reported for lipogenesis in rat adipose tissue (7).
[d] Palmityl-stearyl-oleyl triglyceride, which is representative of the usual fatty acid pattern in human adipose fat.
[e] Coefficients given by Livesey and Elia (15).
[f] Approximate composition of a protein mixture containing 1000 mmol of amino-acyl residues in 110 g, to have 16% of its weight as N and 50% as C, to be oxidized with an RQ of 0.835 and to generate 3.6 g glucose per g N.
[g] ATP stoichiometry is based on McGilvery (16).
Source: Ref. 6.

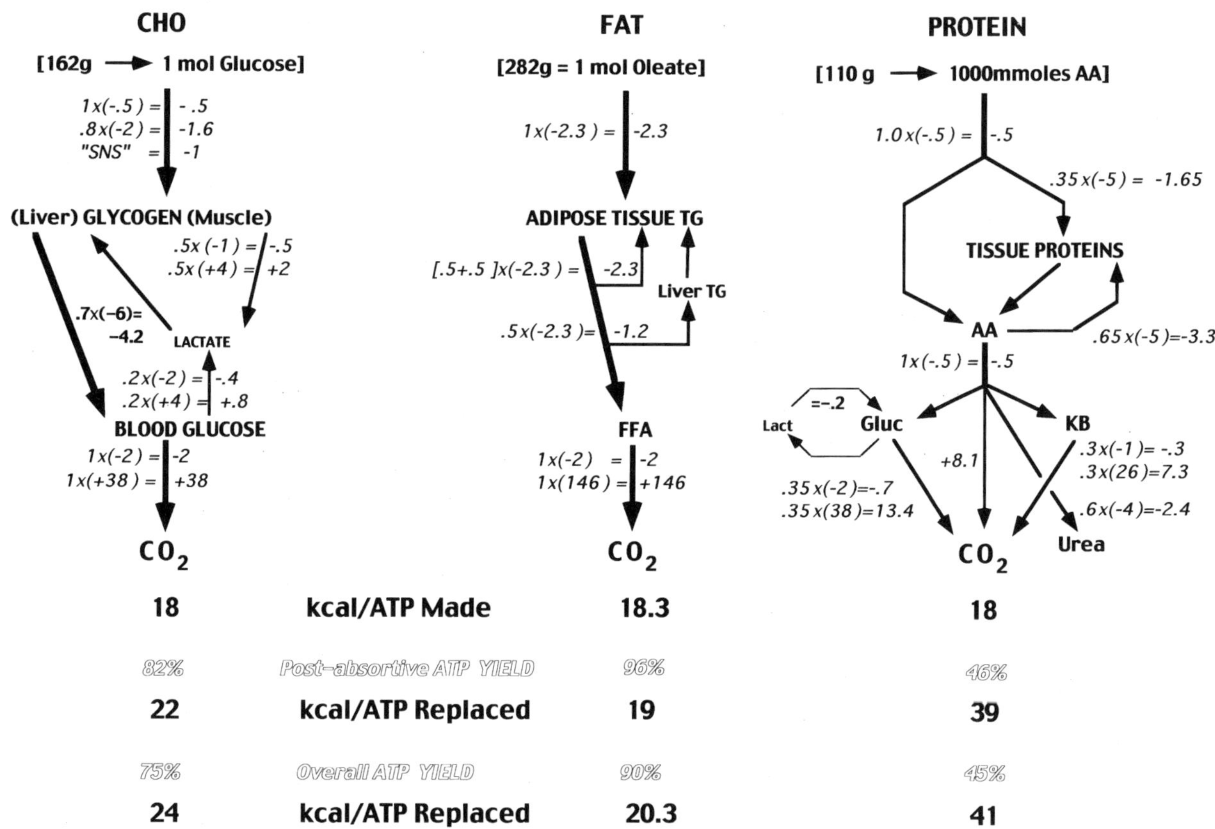

Figure 1 ATP yields during oxidation of carbohydrate, fat, and protein. The numbers printed in brackets show moles of substrate flowing through various metabolic pathways, and, in parenthesis, the moles of ATP produced and expended per mole substrate metabolized, assuming a P:O ratio of 3 for the reoxidation of mitochondrial NADH. (From Ref. 6.)

with oxygen is often catalyzed by the cytoplasmic cytochrome P450), but they account for only 10% of resting O_2 consumption (5). Reactions of the H generated during substrate degradation with oxygen are primarily mediated by cytochrome oxidase, the ultimate enzyme in the mitochondrial respiratory chain, which carries out oxidative phosphorylation. This explains why substrate oxidation in vivo is closely controlled by the rate of ADP formation (i.e., the rate of ATP utilization) under most circumstances, except in brown adipose tissue (BAT). BAT mitochondria contain an uncoupling protein (UCP). In the presence of fatty acids produced by catecholamine-stimulated lipolysis (8) this protein creates a proton-conducting pathway which allows NADH reoxidation to occur at rates much higher than those determined when proton reentry is coupled to ATP regeneration. This permits rapid substrate oxidation and heat production, important for the maintenance of body temperature in small animals exposed to cold, as well as in raising body temperature during arousal from hibernation. Activation of this proton conductance pathway during overfeeding can play an important role in enhancing energy dissipation, thereby limiting fat accumulation during overfeeding in small animals (9,10). This mechanism for energy dissipation does not appear to operate to a significant extent in man (8,11).

B Costs Associated with ATP Generation

The number of mol of ATP formed per mol glucose, fatty acid, and amino acid oxidized are shown in Table 1, as well as the number of ATP required to initiate their degradation (negative numbers), and in the case of amino acid oxidation to carry out gluconeogenesis and ureagenesis. In order to evaluate the costs of ATP expenditures associated with these and other metabolic processes, the amount of substrate which needs to be oxidized to regenerate a given amount of ATP must be assessed. Such evaluations depend therefore not only on the P:O ratio, but also on the amounts of ATP expended for the transport, activation, and handling of the metabolic fuels whose oxidation provides the energy for ATP regeneration.

1 Substrate Handling and Storage Costs

In the case of glucose, 38 ATPs are produced during the oxidation of one glucose molecule, but two are used for its activation to glucose-6-P and fructose-di-P, so that the ATP yield is 36/38 = 95%. If one allows for the fact that some 15–25% of the glucose released by the liver is recycled via the *Cori cycle* and the *glucose-alanine cycle* (at a net cost of 4 ATP/glucose recycled), only some 90% of the ATP generated by oxidation of glucose derived from liver glycogen are available to replace ATPs used in peripheral tissues. Significant portions of the carbohydrates supplied by the diet are initially stored in the form of muscle glycogen (12), so that a substantial part of the glucose released by the liver is in fact regenerated from lactate released by breakdown of muscle glycogen. The cost of gluconeogenesis would then consume additional ATP. Assuming that this applies to half of the glucose released by the liver, the net ATP yield during glycogen oxidation is reduced to ~82% (Fig. 1). The heat of combustion (ΔH) for glucose is 670 kcal/mol (13). Note that the ΔH is very similar to the ΔG for this process, i.e., −689 kcal/mol, which is generally the case when complete oxidation of biological substrates are considered. The ΔH for fructose-1,6-di-P oxidation may be estimated at 685 kcal/mol. The release of 685 kcal, then reflects the turnover of 38 mol of ATP or 685/38 = 18 kcal/mol ATP when glucose is the metabolic fuel oxidized. However, since 18% of the ATP generated merely replaces the ATP spent for substrate handling, an amount of glucose containing 18/0.82 = 22 kcal must be oxidized to replace 1 mol of ATP consumed by a given metabolic process.

To evaluate the energy expended in regenerating ATP by oxidation of fat, one has to consider that some of the free fatty acids (FFA) produced by triglyceride hydrolysis in adipose tissue are reesterified before leaving adipose tissue, at a cost of 7 ATP/triglyceride reconstituted. Some of the FFA released into the circulation are removed and reesterified by the liver, to be reexported in the form of lipoproteins, requiring twice 2.33 ATP/FFA (Fig. 1) (6). The extent to which the lipolytic rate exceeds the rate of fatty acid oxidation appears to be rather variable (14). If one assumes that lipolysis proceeds at twice the rate of fat oxidation and that half of the fatty acids that escape oxidation are reesterified in adipose tissue while the other half are returned to adipose tissue via lipoproteins secreted by the liver, 3.5 ATP is expended per mol fatty acid oxidized.

Oleate is the most common fatty acid in human triglycerides. During its oxidation 146 ATP/mol are generated, while 2 ATP are expended for its activation to oleyl-CoA. The ATP yield for fat oxidation is thus ~140.5/146 = 96%. In view of the large amount of ATP generated per mol fatty acid oxidized, some variations in the relative rate of FFA reesterification will not greatly modify this yield. The ΔH for oleate oxidation is 2657 kcal/mol (13), and that for oleyl-CoA can be estimated at 2670 kcal/mol, so that 2670/146 = 18.3 kcal are released per mole ATP turned over. The energy expenditure per mole of ATP utilized and replaced by fatty acid oxidation thus comes to 18.3/096 = 19 kcal/mol ATP (as compared to 22 kcal/mol ATP during glycogen oxidation) (Fig. 1).

By taking into account the known heats of combustion and the amino acid content of various proteins, Livesey and Elia (15) concluded that the RQ during protein oxidation is 0.835, and that 4.7 kcal is released per gram protein metabolized to CO_2, water, and urea, rather than 0.80 and 4.32, respectively, which were generally used (15). With protein, 110 g represents an assembly of 1000 mmol of various amino acids (Table 1). In the course of the oxidation of 1 mol of protein, 110 g × 4.70 kcal/g = 517 kcal and 28.8 mol of ATP are generated (16), or 517/28.8 = 18 kcal/mol ATP. (With the old coefficients, the corresponding value would be 16.5 kcal/mol ATP generated, which is not consistent with the values of 18.0 to 18.3 kcal/mol ATP generated during carbohydrate and fat oxidation.) Since the costs of gluconeogenesis and ureagenesis consume 5.5 mol ATP/1000 mmol mixed AA oxidized, or ~20% of the amount generated (Table 1), the oxidation of 18/0.8 = 22 kcal of protein is required to generate 1 mol of ATP.

Only some of the amino acids produced by protein breakdown are oxidized (possibly about 1/3) (17), so oxidation of amino acids derived from endogenous protein turnover is always accompanied by protein resynthesis, a process requiring ~5 ATP/amino acid reincorporated into protein (i.e., four for the synthesis of the peptide bond plus an estimated 1 additional mol for amino acid transport, mRNA synthesis, etc.). This would consume 10 ATP in addition to the 5.5 utilized for glucose and urea synthesis per mol amino acid oxidized. The net ATP yield associated with the oxidation of amino acids derived from the turnover of endogenous proteins would accordingly be in the order of (28.8–15.5)/28.8 = 46%. When amino acids contribute either 15% or 20% of the fuel mix oxidized, assuming commensurate differences in protein turnover rates would predict a 3% difference in metabolic rates. Part of the variability in basal metabolic rates is indeed explained by differences in protein turnover (18). Furthermore it is well known that elevations in urinary nitrogen excretion and in resting metabolic rates run a parallel course following trauma or during sepsis (19).

The ATP yielded by different nutrients is further decreased when one takes into account the costs incurred for their initial transport and storage after ingestion. Assuming that in addition to the 2 ATP used for the synthesis of glycogen, 0.5 ATP is expended for active transport and intestinal enzyme synthesis and motility, this would entail an energy expenditure equivalent to 2.5 × (22.5 kcal per mol ATP replaced at a postprandial RQ of 0.89) = 56 kcal, or 56/670 = 8% for the storage of dietary carbohydrate as glycogen. That some of the ingested glucose is used without prior conversion into glycogen (assumed to be 20% in Fig. 1) is approximately offset by the stimulation of the sympathetic nervous system induced by carbohydrate intake (20). In studies in which the amount of glycogen synthesis could be calculated from indirect calorimetry data, the predicted energy expended for glucose storage amounted to 4–6% of the glucose energy infused, and accounted for about two-thirds of the observed increase in energy expenditure above the fasting rate, the remainder being attributable primarily to increased catecholamine secretion (20).

When the catecholamine effect is curtailed by administration of adrenergic blocking agents, the thermic effect observed is consistent with the predicted metabolic expense for glucose storage. Taking into account the energy dissipated during the postprandial phase, the net ATP yield from dietary carbohydrate comes to ~0.92 × 82% (the net ATP yield for glycogen oxidation) = 75%. In the case of fat, the predictable cost for the initial deposition of dietary fat comes to about 3% of the energy provided by dietary fat, though addition of fat generally appears to raise postprandial energy expenditure by 5–10% of the energy provided by the added fat (21). The net ATP yield from dietary fat would thus be reduced to about 0.93% × 96% (the yield from endogenous fat), or some 90%. These considerations suggest that the oxidation of 18/0.75 = 24 kcal of dietary carbohydrate, or the oxidation of 18.3/0.90 = 20.3 kcal of dietary fat is needed to replace 1 mol of ATP, or that some 15–20% more energy may be required to sustain metabolism with dietary carbohydrate than with dietary fat, even in the absence of lipogenesis.

2 Diet Composition and Energy Expenditure

In animal studies, Donato and Hegsted (22) reported that 35% of the energy consumed in excess of maintenance requirements was retained when the excess was provided in the form of fat, as compared to 28% when the excess was carbohydrate. In mice whose 24-hr energy expenditure was measured individually for many consecutive days, the use of carbohydrate as a fuel, as compared to fat, was accompanied by 9–12% higher rates of energy expenditure (6). Hurni et al. (23) found sleeping metabolic rates, basal metabolic rates (BMRs), and 24-hr energy expenditure to be 5–8% higher in a group of volunteers when they were consuming a high-carbohydrate diet (80% of energy as CHO, 5% as fat), as compared to a mixed diet (55% CHO, 30% fat). On the other hand, Abbott et al. (24) could find no difference in 24-hr expenditure among obese Pima Indians adapted to diets providing 42% fat and 43% carbohydrate, or 20% fat and 65% carbohydrate. However, in many studies in which total daily energy expenditure was measured while the proportions of CHO and fat in the diet differed substantially, slightly higher energy expenditures on high-carbohydrate than on high-fat diets have been observed, though the differences were not statiscally significant (25,26,27). Since a 15% difference in net ATP yields, applied to the proportion of carbohydrate exchanged for fat, would only lead to a relatively minor difference in overall expenditure, this effect remains uncertain, though it can be concluded that its practical impact is negligible.

The increase in resting energy expenditure, i.e., the *thermic effect of food* (TEF) (cf. Chap. 25), elicited by protein consumption varies between 20% and 30% (28,29). The ATP required to absorb and transport dietary amino acids into cells, and then to convert them into protein, may be estimated at ~5.5 mol ATP/mol mixed amino acids. If the amino acids are oxidized instead, the ATP expenditure for transport, ureagenesis, and gluconeogenesis also comes to ~5.5 mol ATP (16,30). The TEF of protein is therefore essentially the same when either (or any combination) of these two processes is involved: (5.5 × 22.5 kcal/ATP replaced)/(110 g × 4.70 kcal/g) = 25% (31). However, depending on the proportion of amino acids initially converted into protein, subsequent costs for protein turnover will vary, until an amount of amino acids equivalent to that initially incorporated into protein has in turn been degraded and converted into glucose and urea. Protein intake can thus be expected to influence energy expenditure beyond the postprandial phase. For instance, in patients receiving fixed amounts of energy by intravenous infusion, but in whom 0.31 g of dextrose/kg body weight (BW)/d was replaced by an equicaloric amount of amino acids (to provide 364 instead of 180 mg of amino acid nitrogen/kg BW/d), an increase in energy expenditure of 2.2 kcal/kg/d was observed (32). This is equivalent to 40% of the energy content of the additional dose of amino acids. Considering that the amino acids were provided intravenously, and that there was a concomitant decrease in metabolic costs for handling glucose, one would expect dietary protein to raise the metabolic rate by an amount approaching half of its energy content.

Based on the "best guesses" described above, the ATP expended for substrate handling (transport, storage, recycling, and activation) dissipates ~10%, 25%, or 45% of the ATP produced in the metabolic degradation of dietary fat, carbohydrate and protein, respectively. The *net ATP yields* are thus estimated to decline from 90% with fat, to 75% with carbohydrate, to 45% with protein. On this basis, a change in protein intake from 75 to 100 g/d would be expected to increase energy expenditure by ~50 kcal/d. Depending on the composition of the diet consumed and the time elapsed after food intake, the cost for replacing one mol of ATP would be expected to vary between 20 and 22 kcal. This is some 10–20% more than the 18 kcal released per mol ATP turned over.

3 Cost for Glucose Conversion to Fat

Several reactions in the fatty acid–synthesizing pathway require ATP, so conversion of glucose into fat requires a substantial energy investment. If the costs for prior conversion of glucose into glycogen, as well as for the transport of fatty acid synthesized in the liver to adipose tissue are also included, the cost for conversion of dietary carbohydrate into fat may be assessed at ~25% (7,33). In subjects consuming a Western diet, fatty acid synthesis from glucose appears to be of minor quantitative significance (34,35), as even the ingestion of an unusually large carbohydrate load of 500 g is accommodated by expansion of the glycogen reserves, without increases in body fat (36). Contrary to still commonly held expectations, dissipation of dietary energy by conversion of glucose into fat is therefore not a reason that could explain why high-carbohydrate diets are less conducive to obesity than high-fat diets.

4 Costs for Maintaining Energy Reserves

The costs for nutrient storage include not only the ATP expenditure required for their initial incorporation into the body's stores, but also those involved in maintaining and moving the tissues which contain these reserves. The resting metabolic rate increases by ~7–10 kcal/d/kg additional body weight in adult women and men (37). However, owing to the cost of moving the additional weight, this causes a greater increase in daily energy expenditure ranging from 10–15 in sedentary to 20–30 kcal/d/kg additional body weight in moderately active to very active individuals. Typically it takes ~1 year for these costs to be equal to the initial energy investment. The degree of physical activity is thus another factor affecting the cost of energy storage, even though it does not imply any change in the efficiency with which metabolic processes or ATP turnover occur. Furthermore, the self-correcting effect which changes in body weight exert in compensating for deviations from the energy balance is greater in physically active and in "fidgety" subjects (38) than in sedentary individuals, a phenomenon that totally escapes detection when resting metabolic rates are compared.

5 Futile Cycles

Interconversion of intracellular substrates can cause ATP dissipation if they involve ATP-consuming reactions (e.g., fructose-1,6-diphosphate hydrolysis by fructose diphosphatase and resynthesis by phosphofructokinase). Such *substrate cycles*, which cause no net change in the organism but dissipate ATP, have sometimes been referred to as *futile cycles*. Elaborate mechanisms have evolved to regulate the activity of enzymes involved in catalyzing opposite transformation so as to prevent high rates of wasteful substrate interconversions. Complete suppression of these interconversions is not always achieved, however, as it may not be compatible with the quick responses needed to allow for rapid changes in ATP production when needed (39). Other intracellular substrate cycles include interconversions of glucose and glucose-6-P, or synthesis and breakdown of phosphoenolpyruvate by enzymes involved in the gluconeogenic pathway. When fatty acids are produced by triglyceride hydrolysis in adipose tissue, some are reesterified on the spot. In spite of this, free fatty acids are released from adipose tissue in amounts greater than used for energy production; the excess is reesterified in the liver, to be reexported to adipose tissue in the form of lipoproteins (14). This also causes ATP dissipation without net change in the system, but the fact that lipolysis proceeds at higher-than-minimal rates helps to ensure an adequate supply of circulating FFA and promotes fat oxidation, since fat oxidation is enhanced by high circulating FFA levels (40).

It has been difficult to design tracer studies capable of providing accurate estimates of some of these substrate cycling rates, but the available information suggests that they account for only a small percentage of total energy expenditure (41). The increase in peripheral substrate mobilization caused by higher catecholamine levels during overfeeding, and the increased release of various mobilizing hormones during periods of stress cause an increase in substrate traffic, which may account for about one-fourth of the rise in resting metabolic rates under these conditions (42).

There has also been interest in examining the possibility that transfer of reducing equivalents from mitochondrial to cytoplasmic NADH, through a set of reactions involving glycerol-3-phosphate dehydrogenase (GPDH), may alter metabolic efficiency, since only two instead of three high-energy bonds can be generated from cytoplasmic NADH (43). Overexpression of GPDH in transgenic mice considerably reduces their body fat content (44), but the extent to which this enzyme affects the turnover of reducing equivalent is unknown. Its influence would be reflected in the resting metabolic rates, as are the effects of futile cycles.

The activity of substrate cycles tends to be enhanced by thyroid hormones (45) and their potential role in energy dissipation have therefore been of some interest. However, their impact on energy expenditure is far less than that of the ATP-dependent sodium extrusion constantly carried out by the cell membranes' sodium-potassium ATPase, which may account for ~20% of basal energy expenditure, though data to establish this with some certainty are not available (5,46). Proton leakage through the mitochondrial membrane also demands a certain rate of substrate oxidation at rest to maintain a proton gradient sufficient to drive ATP resynthesis, which may account for 20% of energy expenditure (5). Even though these two phenomena do not result in changes in the system, maintenance of K^+ gradients across cell membrane and of H^+ gradients across mitochondrial membranes cannot really be considered to be futile, since these gradients are essential in maintaining membrane potentials and cell integrity. Increases in sodium-potassium ATPase activity induced by thyroxine suggest that enhanced Na^+ pumping may account for increases in energy expenditure caused by elevation of thyroxine levels, though a higher number of ATPase molecules does not by itself cause or prove that Na^+ fluxes are increased. Thyroid status also appears to affect the rate of proton leakage through the mitochondrial membrance (47).

C Metabolic Efficiency

When compared to daily energy turnover, the amount of energy retained during growth and during the development of obesity is rather small, amounting to a difference of only a few percent between intake and expenditure. Because a positive energy balance can, in principle, be attributed to excessive intake or to reduced expenditure, there has been considerable interest in the possible significance of even small differences in *metabolic efficiency* for the development, or the prevention of obesity.

Metabolic efficiency can be defined in many ways. The most readily applied approach is to relate physical work output to energy expenditure. During low-intensity exertion, the efficiency of the process appears to be low, because most of the energy expended serves to regenerate the ATP dissipated for maintenance metabolism. The intensity of the workload, relative to resting energy expenditure, is thus the major variable determining the apparent *overall metabolic efficiency*. To obtain a better measure of metabolic efficiency, it is important to relate the amount of work produced to the change in metabolic rate it causes. Typical values for the *net efficiency* of aerobic work range from 25% to 27% in man and animals (2,28). Relating energy deposited in the carcass to total amount of food energy consumed is an important practical consideration in judging *feed efficiency* in the production of meat. As in the case of increasing workloads, overall or *gross nutrient efficiency* rises markedly as the amount of excess energy consumed becomes larger relative to maintenance energy expenditure (Fig. 2). In a situation characterized by rather small changes in body size over time, gross nutrient efficiency is close to zero, which in terms of characterizing potential metabolic differences between lean and obese is essentially meaningless. In trying to assess the efficiency with which food energy is processed, it is therefore important to assess energy retention relative to the amount consumed in excess of maintenance requirements. The accuracy of such an approach is limited, particularly in man, because the maintenance energy requirements account for a rather large fraction of the energy consumed, and because these requirements keep changing as body weight and physical activities vary during the weeks needed to produce measurable changes in body composition. Thus, even small errors in estimating maintenance requirements have a considerable impact on the net efficiency value obtained

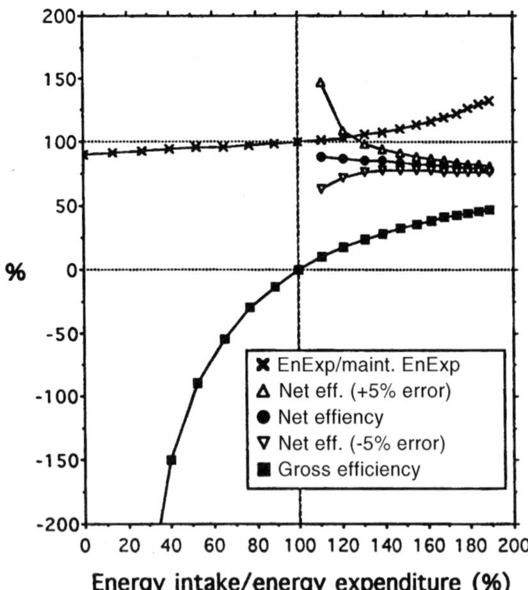

Figure 2 Effect of level of energy intake on "gross" and "net" nutrient efficiencies. Energy expenditure (x) is considered to increase during overfeeding (dissipating 20% of the energy consumed above maintenance requirements), and to decline during underfeeding (attenuating the energy deficit) by 5%). "Gross nutrient efficiency" describes the % of energy retained relative to energy consumed (■). It is determined primarily by the level of energy intake. "Net nutrient efficiency" (●) describes the fraction of the energy consumed above maintenance levels that is retained. It is greatly affected by minor errors (i.e., a 5% overestimate △, or a 5% underestimate ▽), particularly in the range of modest excess intakes.

(Fig. 2), and the reliability of such evaluations in characterizing potential differences in metabolic efficiencies is questionable.

Differences in ATP dissipation through ion pumping, futile cycles, and protein turnover are all included in the measured resting metabolic rates. These are closely correlated with the size of the fat-free mass and the fat mass, and resting energy expenditures are thus higher in obese than in lean subjects of the same heights (48), though a certain degree of variability among individuals remains. The importance often attributed to such differences appears to be founded on the presumption that changes in energy expenditure will not be offset by changes in energy intake. Under conditions where energy intake could be "clamped" at some particular level, a 5% difference in resting energy expenditure would be offset by a difference in body weight of 5–8 kg in a sedentary individual, or less in a physically active individual. When access to food is not restricted, energy balance is determined overwhelmingly by the factors influencing food intake, and by the adjustments in food intake that serve to compensate for recent substrate imbalances, rather than by the overall rate of energy turnover (49). Pregnancy, for instance, leads to the deposition of a few kg of additional fat in spite of an increase in resting energy expenditure (50). Arguments about the possible role of minor differences in resting metabolic rates in promoting or preventing obesity and in playing a role in body weight maintenance are therefore hollow if they are not linked to considerations of the factors controlling energy intake; if they fail to do so, they may end up creating a conceptual trap.

D Cold Exposure

Exposure to low environmental temperatures raises energy expenditure and can modify the composition of the fuel mix oxidized. Thus the RQ of ad libitum–fed rats was 0.92 at thermal neutrality, 0.87 during acute cold exposure (acclimation to 25°C and test at 15°C), and 0.77 at chronic cold (acclimation and test at 15°C) (51). This is consistent with other data showing a preferential contribution of lipid to nonshivering thermogenesis in cold-exposed animals (52,53).

The impact of cold exposure has also been studied in man. Acute exposure to a temperature of 5°C causes resting O_2 consumption to nearly double after 2 hr (54). Under these conditions changes in the respiratory exchange ratio over the 2 hr of cold exposure were not significant at rest and during exercise. Spending a day in a respiratory chamber at 16°C was perceived to be uncomfortably cool, and rectal temperatures in the morning were 0.11°C lower than when the ambient temperature was 24°C. Yet this elicited only a 2% increase in 24-hr energy expenditure, covered by increased glucose oxidation (55). When one considers that individuals generally adjust clothing when exposed to cold, the changes in resting energy expenditure induced by a cold environment are not likely to be substantial. Since a wide range of cold exposures can be survived, the use of glucose obviously can adjust itself to carbohydrate intake, regardless of the stimuli that may cause changes in the RQ at the onset of cold exposure. However, one may keep in mind some incidental observations, whose validity remains to be established. For instance, cold exposure may elicit vigorous movements reflecting efforts to restore blood flow and to raise body temperature, or on the contrary, it may inhibit motion.

There also seems to be a prevailing perception of increased hunger when subjects are exposed to a cold environment, and of a tendency to gain fat during the cold season.

II MEASUREMENT OF SUBSTRATE OXIDATION AND ENERGY EXPENDITURE

Changes in the body's substrate content due to metabolism can be calculated from CO_2 production, O_2 consumption, and urinary nitrogen excretion data. This experimental approach has provided a wealth of data on human energy expenditure (28,29,56,57). The results of this "indirect calorimetry" are consistent with data obtained by direct measurement of heat production, i.e., "direct calorimetry" but the former has the advantage of providing information on the relative amounts of carbohydrate, fat, and protein used. Attention must be given to careful calibrations to permit accurate determinations of the respiratory quotient and hence of the relative proportions of carbohydrate and fat oxidized. When combined with precise assessment of the amounts of nutrients consumed, indirect calorimetry can establish substrate or nutrient balances over periods of 1 day or several days, which are far too small to be established by body composition measurements (27). In recent years, indirect calorimetry has been complemented by the application of the doubly labeled water (DLW) technique, which has allowed to determine energy expenditure (but not substrate balances) in free-living subjects (48).

A 24-Hr Energy Expenditure by Indirect Calorimetry Using Metabolic Chambers

Modern gas analyzers and online data processing have stimulated the construction of respiratory chambers in which subjects can be studied over 24-hr periods or for several consecutive days with reasonable comfort. In such a confining environment, sedentary behavior can be modified by prescribed amounts of exercise on a treadmill or equivalent device (56,58). Reproducible measurements of daily energy expenditure can be achieved that are accurate within a few percent. Under the best conditions, errors in carbohydrate and fat balances can be reduced to ± 20 and ± 10 g/d, respectively (59). Numerous studies have been performed to quantify daily energy expenditure and substrate balances, notably to compare differences in energy expenditure in lean and obese subjects and the effects of overfeeding. Among other things, they indicated that a high 24-hr RQ is a risk factor for long-term body weight gain (60,61). Twenty-four-hour indirect calorimetry also provides the means to study the adjustment of the fuel mix oxidized to changes in the diet's composition (26,27,62). Other important results relate to the role of sympathetic nervous system activity on daily macronutrient utilization (63) and to the measurement of net lipogenesis induced by deliberate and sustained overconsumption of carbohydrates (33).

B 24-Hr Energy Expenditure Based on Heart Rate Measurements

Continuous heart rate monitoring offers a possibility to measure energy expenditure around the clock, but it requires that the relationship between heart rate and oxygen consumption be established individually. The approach has been validated by concomitant indirect calorimetry and DLW measurements (64,65). This "heart rate O_2 method" has been successfully used in trained and untrained individuals to measure daily energy expenditure and compensations in non-prescribed daily activities (66).

C Energy Turnover in Free-Living Subjects

The lack of means to assess energy expenditure and substrate oxidation under free-living conditions has long been a major barrier for obesity research. This problem was finally resolved thanks to a method conceived by Lifson et al. in the 1950s (67) to assess energy expenditure in small animals. It is based on the administration of an initial dose of $^2H_2{}^{18}O$. The difference in the rate of ^{18}O elimination, which is lost in water and CO_2, relative to the rate of deuterium (^2H) elimination, lost as water only, allows assessment of the CO_2 production rate, which correlates closely with oxygen consumption and energy expenditure (68). It took nearly three decades before the first paper describing the application of this DLW technique in humans was published (69). A number of methodological problems and potential pitfalls were encountered, leading on occasions to physiologically impossible results. Comparison of results obtained by several groups of investigators have confirmed the validity of the method, and the conditions and calculations for its successful applications have been defined with increasing detail (70).

Measurements of energy turnover by the DLW method in sedentary subjects led to downward revisions of common assumptions about minimum maintenance requirements (71). Other studies (72) led to a reduction of the additional energy allowances during pregnancy from 500 to 300 kcal/d (50). The long-held belief about the low maintenance energy requirements in overweight "small eaters" was shown to be attributable to underreporting of habitual food intake (48,73,74). It also became possible to assess energy expenditure under conditions of extreme physical demand, demonstrating energy turnovers reaching 5000–8000 kcal/d in bicycle racers (75). According to Goran and Poehlman (76), the technique can be used to evaluate compensations in energy expenditure in response to exercise training.

D Diet-Induced Thermogenesis

Diet-induced thermogenesis (DIT) includes all increases in resting energy expenditure induced by food consumption, which comprise the TEF during the postprandial periods (see Chap. 25), as well as increases in resting energy expenditure between meals induced by excessive food consumption. In man, most of these increments in resting energy expenditure are explained by "obligatory" factors such as digestion, metabolism, and storage of macronutrients including the cost for the synthesis of the constituents of newly formed tissues, and the physiological processes essential for their maintenance (31). "Nonobligatory" or "facultative" components contributing to DIT are catecholamine-mediated increases in energy expenditure elicited by carbohydrate consumption during the TEF, and the stimulation of substrate oxidation in BAT through activation of a protein-conducting pathway elicited by SNS innervation, which has the effect of uncoupling substrate oxidation from oxidation phosphorylation (8,9). The quantitative importance of facultative thermogenesis can be substantial in animals, and suppression of BAT thermogenesis greatly enhances the development of obesity in animals (10).

Investigations into the physiological role of BAT in humans has not yielded comparable results. Although the presence of BAT has been demonstrated in humans (77), experimental evidence suggests that skeletal muscle is the main site of cold-influenced thermogenesis (78). A number of overfeeding studies have been performed to evaluate the potential role of DIT in human studies in which energy expenditure was directly measured either by indirect calorimetry or by the DLW method, but dissipation of excess dietary energy through *Luxuskonsumption* (a term sometimes used to describe elevated DIT during overfeeding) could not be detected. Most of the increase in 24-hr energy expenditure found during overfeeding could be explained by the cost of substrate handling, tissue accretion, and maintenance of an enlarged body (79–82).

E Physical Activity

The metabolic changes observed during and for many hours after exercise can substantially modify macronutrient utilization and energy expenditure. As depicted in Figure 3, RQ increases during exercise, indicating that initially carbohydrate is the main substrate contributing to the increase in energy production. The figure also illustrates that the RQ during exercise is influenced by numerous factors such as the intensity and duration of exercise. It is well established that RQ is increased to a greater extent by high than low to moderate intensity exercise (83) and that the RQ progressively declines with increasing exercise duration. Exercise RQ also tends to belower in trained than in nontrained individuals (84).

Resting RQ can be reduced for 15–20 hr after prolonged vigorous exercise (85,86). However, no data are available to establish how long and how much the resting RQ is decreased after exercise. Since high intensity exertion is as effective in inducing fat loss as aerobic work (87), one can infer that high-intensity exercise must have a substantial effect in enhancing postexercise lipid oxidation. This may be due to the glycogen depletion which it induces, but another important observation is that high-intensity training increases the potential of skeletal muscle to oxidize lipid to a greater extent than aerobic exercise of moderate intensity, at least as judged by the rise in muscle β-hydroxy-acyl-CoA dehydrogenase (HADH) activity (87).

Since exercise permits weight maintenance at lower degrees of adiposity, it substitutes for an expansion of

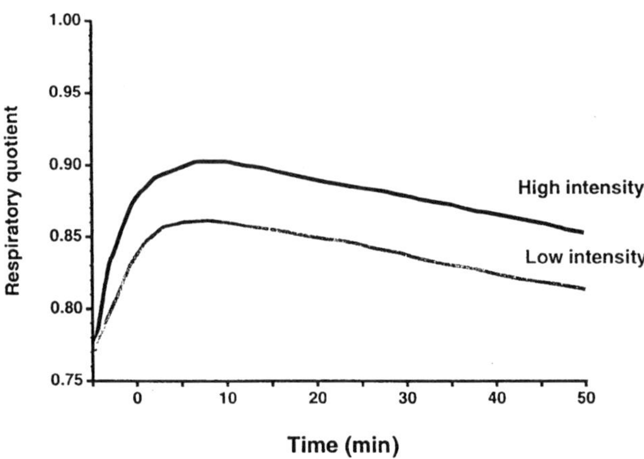

Figure 3 Variations in respiratory quotient during a low- and a high-intensity exercise. (From Ref. 83.)

the fat mass in bringing about rates of fat oxidation commensurate with fat intake. The overall effect of exercise is therefore to increase fat oxidation more than glucose oxidation (88). Human subjects who are high fat oxidizers during exercise consumed less food when they subsequently could eat at will, and they were more likely to be in negative energy and lipid balance compared to low fat oxidizers (89,90). Of particular interest is the hypothesis that exercise is likely to induce greater fat losses in obese individuals who have a high capacity to oxidize fat during and after exercise. The potential link between exercise-induced changes in substrate oxidation and postexercise energy intake and balance needs to be investigated.

F Variability of Daily Energy Expenditures, Intakes, and Balances

Daily energy expenditures of subjects confined to a respiratory chamber are substantially lower than in free-living subjects (91,92), and the spontaneous variations in physical activity associated with free-living conditions cannot manifest themselves. On the other hand, DLW measurements, which provide assessment of overall energy expenditure over periods of 7–10 days, do not allow to define variations in energy expenditure from day to day. Future methodological developments may permit us to assess substrate oxidation under free-living conditions, a potential suggested by recent animal studies (93). These variations must be evaluated on the basis of estimates calculated from activity logs. Many more data are available on daily food intakes. The coefficients of variations for intraindividual daily food intake are large, averaging ±22% among adults (94), and ranging from ±15 to ±33% in children (95). It seems to be generally held that variations in food intake are substantially greater than variations in energy expenditure. Deviations from the energy balance are thus probably comparable in size to the variability in intakes. The extent of daily variations in food intake and energy expenditure, and the size of daily deviations from energy balance potentially influence body weight maintenance, inasmuch as changes in food intake in response to positive or negative energy balances may not occur with the same accuracy (96,97).

III FACTORS DETERMINING SUBSTRATE OXIDATION RATES

Overall energy expenditure is determined by an individual's size and physical activity, and it is only modestly affected by nutrient intake. Amino acid oxidation rates vary only moderately, increasing somewhat after protein ingestion (17) and during vigorous exertion (98), but declining when protein intakes are reduced. By contrast, the organism is able to rapidly and powerfully alter the relative contributions made by glucose and FFAs to the fuel mix oxidized. Such great flexibility in fuel utilization is made possible by the ability of most cells to interchangeably use metabolic intermediates derived from carbohydrates, fats, and proteins to regenerate ATP. It allows adaptation to food supplies varying widely in their macronutrient distribution (provided that proteins provide at least some 10%, and essential fatty acids at least 1–2% of total energy) (50).

A Substrate Oxidation by Different Tissues

The contribution made by various tissues to the body's oxygen consumption, or in effect to overall energy turnover, is described in Table 2 (16), whereas their contribution to overall fuel utilization also depends on their metabolic functions (99). The central nervous system's rate of energy expenditure is particularly high for its size (2% of body weight), as it accounts for nearly 20% of resting energy expenditure in adults (100). Since it cannot use FFA, it is critically dependent on an adequate supply of glucose (~80 mg/min). However, after adaptation to starvation, ketone bodies can provide about two-thirds of the brain's energy needs (101). Red blood cells also depend on glucose, as they lack mitochondria and must generate ATP by substrate-level phosphorylation during glucose degradation to lactate. They use ~1 g of glucose per hour (100,102), but this has very little impact on the body's fuel economy, since 98% is converted to lactate (102), which can be reconverted into glucose by the liver.

Table 2 Relative Oxygen Consumption of Different Tissues

	At rest	Light work	Heavy work
Brain	0.20	0.20	0.20
Abdominal organs	0.25	0.24	0.24
Kidneys	0.07	0.06	0.07
Skin	0.02	0.06	0.08
Heart	0.11	0.23	0.40
Skeletal muscles	0.30	2.05	6.95
Other	0.05	0.06	0.06
Total	1.00	3.00	8.00

(whole body at rest = 1.00; actual value near 3.8 mL O_2 min^{-1} kg^{-1})
Source: Ref. 16.

About one-quarter of resting energy expenditure occurs in the splanchnic bed (103). It has become evident that the gut derives a substantial part of its energy by partial degradation of glutamine, its glucogenic moiety reaching the liver (30). Conversion of the glucogenic moieties of the amino acids is a feature of amino acid degradation even under fed conditions (30). One can therefore presume that conversion of pyruvate to acetyl-CoA in the liver is effectively inhibited during most of the day, a conclusion which is consistent with the lack of hepatic fatty acid synthesis under habitual living conditions (34).

The heart accounts for ~10% of resting energy expenditure. Its constant and critical requirement for fuel is aptly matched by its ability to utilize all types of substrates that may be available, including notably some of the lactate produced by working skeletal muscles (104). Although skeletal muscles make up three-quarters of the body cell mass, the muscle accounts for only 20–30% of energy expenditure at rest (5,100). During exertion substrate oxidation in the muscle mass can increase 20-fold (Table 2) (16), with the increase being even greater in particular muscle groups. In the postabsorptive state, fatty acids are the main oxidized fuel in muscle (99,105), whereas during exertion, great demands are initially placed on the muscles' own glycogen reserve, with a subsequent shift toward increasingly greater use of fatty acids, mobilized from muscle fat stores as well as from adipose tissue (Fig. 3). Since muscle is ready to oxidize fatty acids as well as glucose (40,106), exercise enhances the body's ability to adjust the use of glucose and fatty acids to the dietary supply (Fig. 4). This may explain why fat oxidation can more readily keep up with fat intake in physically active adults and in most children and adolescents as they are naturally more physically active than adults.

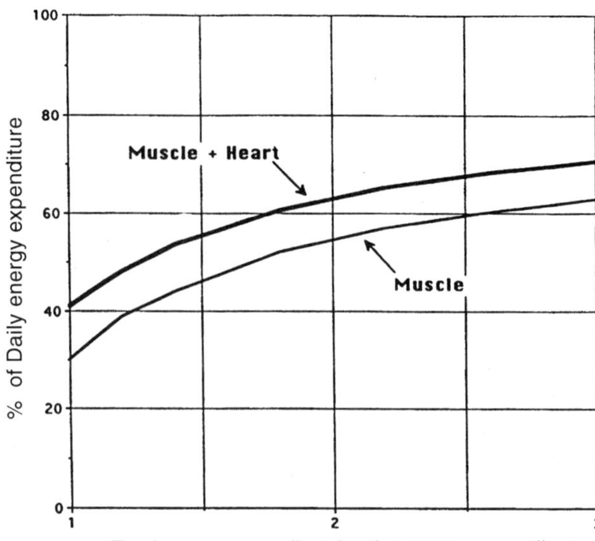

Figure 4 Impact of physical activity (described as the ratio of total to resting energy expenditure) on the contribution of skeletal and heart muscle metabolism to total energy turnover. (Calculated from the information provided in Table 3, assuming that half of the exercise-induced increase in energy expenditure is due to work of light and half to work of heavy intensity.)

B Glucose Turnover and Glucose Oxidation

Some of the glucose utilized by various tissues is converted to lactate (*Cori cycle*) or to alanine (*glucose-alanine cycle*), which are readily reconverted into glucose by the liver. Glucose turnover is thus substantially greater than the rate of glucose oxidation. Carbohydrate oxidation determined by indirect calorimetry describes the change in the body's carbohydrate content. It should be noted at this point that the energy content of glycogen (4.18 kcal/g) and of glucose (3.7 kcal/g) differ by 10% (because 1 mol of water is removed when glucose is incorporated into the glycogen or starch). It is thus important to be consistent and to specify which of the two is being considered. During the degradation of amino acid mixtures, 55–60 g of glucose is generated by gluconeogenesis from 100 g of protein, and this occurs even in the fed state when plenty of glucose is available (30). In indirect calorimetry calculations, the oxidation of the glucose formed by gluconeogenesis from amino acids is included in the coefficients describing CO_2 production and oxygen consumption from protein. Glucose oxidation determined with the help of tracers is thus measurably greater than carbohydrate disappearance established by indirect calorimetry. Similarly, the glycerol liberated during the oxidation of triglycerides (about 10 g/100 g triglycerides, or 5% of the triglyceride energy) is converted into glucose before being oxidized, the CO_2 produced and the oxygen consumed being again included in the coefficients for fat oxidation. This is why the RQ for triglyceride oxidation (0.71) is slightly higher than that for fatty acid oxidation (0.70) (15).

C Starvation Ketosis

The body's glycogen reserves are limited to a few hundred grams (107), and during periods of starvation or marked carbohydrate deprivation they can provide enough glucose to the brain for a few days only (101,108). Survival during starvation is made possible by the induction of ketogenesis in the liver, when insulin levels become very low and FFA levels concomitantly rise (109). Acetoacetate plus β-hydroxybutyrate production reaches 100–120 g/day by the third day of total starvation. Circulating ketone body levels rise only progressively, as some are used by skeletal muscle during the initial days of starvation, since muscle is ready to use ketone bodies whenever they are produced—e.g., during prolonged physical efforts. When starvation ketosis is fully developed, ketone body levels reach a plateau of 5–6 mM. At this level, they provide about two thirds of the brain's fuel needs, but 5–15 g of β-hydroxybutyrate and acetoacetate is lost in the urine per day. The urinary loss of limited amounts of these anions can be offset by excretion of N in the form of ammonium instead of urea. This provides the cations needed, thereby preventing the development of metabolic acidosis (101). In the total absence of insulin, ketone levels rise to far higher levels, in part because the overabundance of circulating fuels decreases peripheral ketone body utilization. Urinary losses then become far greater, leading to metabolic acidosis.

D Regulation of Substrate Oxidation

In view of the critical need to maintain high ATP levels, of the functional importance of proteins, and of the need to ensure a sufficient supply of glucose for the brain, the main goals for metabolic fuel regulation are to assure the distribution of substrates in amounts sufficient to support oxidative phosphorylation at the required rates, to maintain homeostasis, and to bring about the use of metabolic fuels in such proportions as to minimize changes in protein content and to maintain glycogen levels within a desirable range. This is detrimental to the body's ability to regulate the fat balance (110), which is not a problem in the short term, since such gains or losses of fat are very small in comparison to the body's large fat stores (50,000–200,000 kcal in adults and even more in obese subjects). However, if the fat balance is not accurately regulated, neither is the overall energy balance.

1 Hormonal Regulation of Substrate Availability

The composition of the fuel mix oxidized is mainly controlled by adjustment of circulating substrate and hormone levels. These levels are markedly influenced by nutrient intake. The impact of changes in substrate levels on their rates of utilization during the postprandial phase is enhanced by the release of insulin, which promotes transport and storage of glucose, amino acids, and fats while inhibiting the release of glucose from the liver and of fatty acids from adipose tissue. The decline in circulating FFA levels, brought about by the antilipolytic action of insulin complemented by the direct and indirect effects of insulin in activating pyruvate dehydrogenase (PDH) (111) lead to an increase in glucose oxidation and to a commensurate decrease in fatty acid oxidation. The decline in insulin secretion when glucose absorption from the gut is completed, complemented by the release of catecholamines and glucagon, activates the mobilization of the body's glycogen and fat reserves to assure an adequate supply of glucose and FFA in the circulation (112,113). These effects are greatly enhanced when the demand for metabolic fuels is magnified by physical efforts.

2 Body Composition and Fuel Composition

Between meals and efforts, the composition of the fuel mix oxidized is influenced by the size of the body's protein pools, the degree of repletion of its glycogen reserves, and the size and distribution of the adipose tissue depots. This is the simple consequence of the fact that the influence of hormones on substrate fluxes is determined by the intensity of the endocrine signals and by the size of the targets they influence, and that hormone secretion is itself influenced by prevailing substrate levels.

The gains or losses that occur when the oxidation of glucose, FFA, and amino acids do not match their intakes lead to changes in body composition until the impacts of these changes on the composition of the fuel mixture oxidized complement the body's endocrine and enzymatic regulatory mechanisms such that the fuel mix oxidized matches, on average, the macronutrient distribution in the diet (114). As evidenced by the commonly observed stability of body composition, the effect of these changes in bringing about the adjustment of fuel composition to nutrient intake is universal and remarkably effective, but the body composition for which this adjustment is achieved can vary greatly between individuals, depending on interactions between inherited and circumstantial factors (113).

3 Adjustment of Amino Acid Oxidation to Protein Intake

The ability to quantify changes in the body's protein content by monitoring the N balance has led to the early recognition of the organism's tendency to maintain a stable protein content, or to allow for an appropriate rate of protein accretion during growth or recovery from disease or undernutrition. This occurs regardless of differences in the carbohydrate-to-fat ratio of the diet. Detailed metabolic studies during starvation have revealed how the organism is able to minimize protein losses during food deprivation (112). Its regulatory features also enable it to avoid needless and costly buildup of its protein content when high-protein diets are consumed, but the mechanisms accounting for this are not well understood. Daily protein intakes, generally between 50 and 100 g in adults, are small compared to the body's total protein content, of which about half (~6 kg) is intracellular and engaged in active turnover. When changing from situations of high to low protein intake, or vice versa, a few days are required before N balance is again achieved. The small gains or losses of proteins which are thereby incurred appear to be prerequisites for the reestablishment of N balance, demonstrating that relatively minor changes in protein content play a significant role in the adjustment of amino acid oxidation rates to protein intake. Small gains or losses of protein thus appear able to influence amino acid oxidation and to bring about the corrective responses needed to compensate for the small deviations from even N balance which occur from day to day.

4 Adjustment of Glucose Oxidation to Carbohydrate Intake: Influence of Glycogen Stores

The body's glycogen stores (200–500 g in adults) (107) are not much larger than the amount of carbohydrate usually consumed in one day. In view of the importance of the hepatic glycogen stores in maintaining stable blood glucose levels and of muscle glycogen availability in permitting appropriate muscular responses to sudden demands, biological evolution led to regulatory mechanisms (including endocrine signals) that give high priority to the adjustment of carbohydrate oxidation to carbohydrate availability (114,115). Glucose oxidation thus declines rapidly when ingestion of food fails to replenish the glycogen reserves in a timely fashion. On the other hand, the body's metabolism quickly shifts to the predominant use of glucose after carbohydrate ingestion. This manifests itself by a prompt postprandial rise in the RQ to an extent and for periods determined by the amounts and the types of carbohydrates consumed. This response is important since inappropriate curtailment of fat oxidation when carbohydrates provide the bulk of food energy would lead to a negative fat balance, or require substantial de novo fat synthesis (at substantial metabolic cost) during part of the day.

After large carbohydrate intakes, high rates of carbohydrate oxidation persist for many hours, allowing dissipation of the built-up glycogen reserves (36). If massive consumption of carbohydrates is deliberately kept up for several days, glycogen stores become saturated and further accumulation is prevented by conversion of glucose into fat, which may drive the overall RQ to values > 1.0 (33). However, the regulation of appetite is such that glycogen levels are spontaneously maintained far below the range at which de novo lipogenesis is induced, and loss of carbohydrate by conversion into fat is quantitatively insignificant (< 5 g/d) in adults consuming mixed diets (34,35).

The degree of repletion of the body's glycogen stores thus greatly influences the contribution made by glucose to the fuel mix oxidized. Gains or losses of glycogen are therefore effective in bringing about changes in glucose oxidation when the influx of carbohydrate varies (26,116) or when physical exertion has caused unusual glycogen depletion. As in the case of protein, this is in part a simple mass effect, since insulin is less effective in curtailing glucose release from the liver when the hepatic glycogen reserves have been built up (117).

5 Adjustment of Fat Oxidation to Fat Intake: Influence of Adipose Tissue Mass and Distribution

Because amino acid and glucose oxidation rates adjust themselves to the amounts of protein and carbohydrate consumed, fat oxidation is determined primarily by the gap between total energy expenditure and the amounts of energy ingested in the form of carbohydrates and proteins (49). Fat oxidation rates are thus set primarily by parameters unrelated to the body's fat economy, rather than by the amounts of fat consumed. Furthermore, short-term gains or losses of fat are so small in comparison to the body's large fat stores that they are unlikely to elicit changes in food intake or in fat oxidation. Given the lack of direct regulatory mechanisms serving to adjust fat oxidation to fat intake (118), one may wonder why body fat contents should nevertheless tend to remain fairly constant, even when diets differing widely in fat content are consumed.

Various factors contribute to this adjustment. For instance, if fat replaces carbohydrate in meals, the postprandial inhibition of fat oxidation is lessened, since the postprandial rise in RQ is related primarily to the amount of carbohydrate consumed. The presence of fat in a meal delays its absorption, and this will also attenuate the post-prandial rise in the RQ. When meals containing very large amounts of fat are consumed (e.g., 80 g) (119), some of the fatty acids liberated from chylomicrons by lipoprotein lipase escape capture by adipose cells and enter the pool of circulating free fatty acids, promoting fat oxidation, though only modestly (e.g., 10 g in 6 hr) (119). Finally, glycogen levels may tend to be maintained in a lower range when the proportion of carbohydrate in the diet is reduced, resulting in lower insulin levels and hence higher rates of FFA release and oxidation between meals (26). However, this cannot be expected to produce an exact compensation, since FFA levels and oxidation rates are controlled by insulin whose secretion is determined primarily by the need to maintain appropriate blood glucose levels.

While short-term errors in the fat balance are too small to affect the size of the body's fat stores, circulating FFA levels, fat oxidation, or food intake, the cumulative effects of repeated imbalances between fat intake and fat oxidation can in time lead to substantial changes in the size of the adipose tissue mass. Expansion of the fat mass leads to higher FFA levels and turnover (120). The role that change in the adipose tissue mass plays in the establishment of the steady state of weight maintenance can be inferred by considering the changes in substrate balances induced by a period of food restriction. After a few days on reduced intake, or after the first few days during a subsequent period of weight regain, further losses or gains of protein and glycogen are minimal and account for only a minor part of the energy imbalance. Owing to the contribution made by endogenous fat to the fuel mix oxidized during caloric deprivation, the average RQ is lower than usual during the period of weight loss. During weight regain, on the other hand, the 24-hr RQ is greater than usual, reflecting the oxidation of a fuel mix containing a higher proportion of glucose than the diet, as part of the fat consumed is stored. At some point, the situation is encountered for which the two conditions necessary for weight maintenance are again satisfied; i.e., food intake is commensurate with energy expenditure and the average RQ matches the diet's "food quotient" (FQ), which describes the ratio of CO_2 produced to O_2 consumed during the biological oxidation of a representative sample of the diet (31,114). What one would like to know in this regard is whether this should be attributed to the increase in energy expenditure associated with weight gain, or whether some other phenomenon is involved.

This issue could be precisely examined in mice (Fig. 5) (113). The unusually elevated rate of food consumption following a period of food restriction abated when the fat mass had regained its initial size. The balance between energy expenditure and food intake was not achieved by an increase in energy expenditure due to weight gain, but by a decrease in food consumption, as the degree of adiposity was approached, for which the RQ became again equal to the FQ. Enlargement

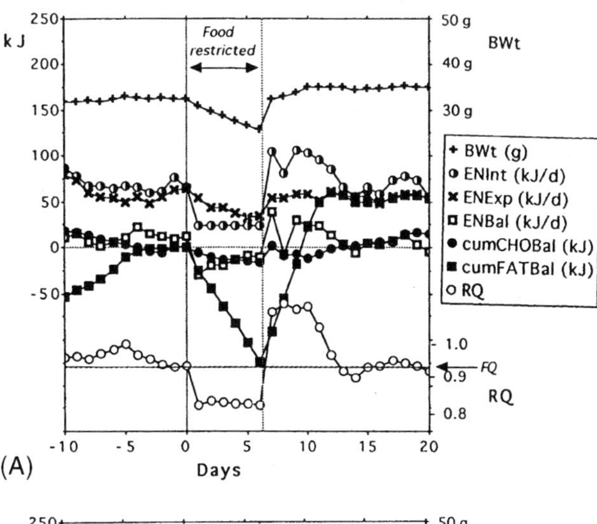

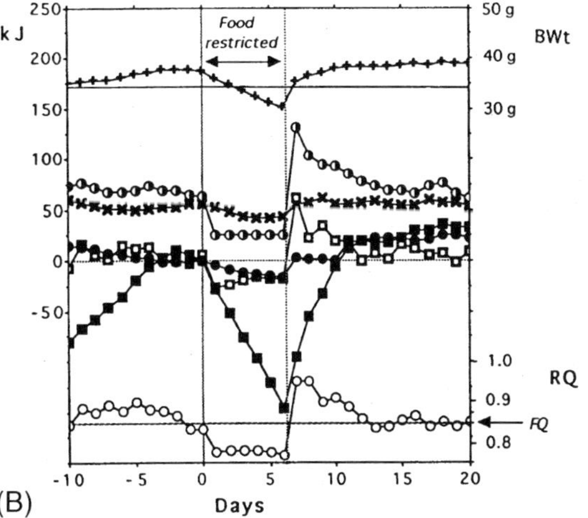

Figure 5 Effect of temporary food restriction on body fat and glycogen content in mice. The figure shows average body weights, cumulative carbohydrate and fat balances, and daily energy expenditures, intakes, and balances in two groups of five fed female CD1 mice, during a 6-day period of food restriction to 40% of average ad libitum intake, and during the preceding and following days of ad libitum intake. One group was maintained on a diet containing 13% (panel A), the other on a diet containing 41% (panel B) of dietary energy as fat, 19% as casein and the balance as corn starch plus sucrose (1:1). (From Ref. 113.)

of the fat depots thus promotes fat oxidation, just as well as filled glycogen stores promote glucose oxidation (27,117), but the increase in fat oxidation brought about by expansion of the adipose tissue mass is *chronic*, rather than related to recent food consumption. This chronic effect can be enhanced by a type of insulin resistance typically induced by excessive fat accumulation, whose effect is to promote fatty acid, but to inhibit glucose oxidation (49,61,121). The influence of the adipose tissue mass on the composition of the fuel mix oxidized explains why the particular body composition will in time be reached (or approached) for which the fat oxidation is commensurate with fat intake.

6 Alcohol Intake and Oxidation

Alcohol is not generally considered to contribute greatly to dietary energy intake, but alcohol sales data indicate that alcohol provides ~5% of overall energy intake in the United States. In the Quebec Family Study, alcohol energy represented 17% and 11% of daily energy intake of adult males and females, respectively, in the upper quartile for alcohol intake (122).

Many epidemiological studies have investigated the association between alcohol consumption and the intake of macronutrients. Some reported a negative association between alcohol and carbohydrate intake (122,123); others found reduced protein, fat, and carbohydrate intake in moderate alcohol drinkers (124). However, other studies showed that energy and macronutrient intakes were not altered by alcohol intake, suggesting that alcohol energy often represents just an additional source of dietary energy (125–129). Studies on the impact of alcohol intake on energy expenditure show that the thermic effect of alcohol is slightly higher than that of carbohydrate, but lower than that of protein (130). Alcohol drives its oxidation, regardless of the level of other fuels, but only up to a rate that covers a minor fraction of total energy turnover. The maximal rate of alcohol oxidation varies among individuals, being generally higher in men than in women, and enhanced in habitual alcohol consumers (131). In examining the impact of alcohol oxidation on the use of other fuels, one sees that its main effect is to reduce fat oxidation (129,132). The inhibitory effect of alcohol on fat oxidation means that alcohol intake is equivalent to fat intake in influencing the fat and energy balances. Alcohol consumption was indeed found to raise total energy intake, particularly when a high-fat diet was consumed (Fig. 6) (122), in a manner that could not be explained by the high energy density of the items consumed (133). Inactive individuals reporting a high fat and alcohol intake are characterized by increased subcutaneous adiposity, particularly in the trunk area (122).

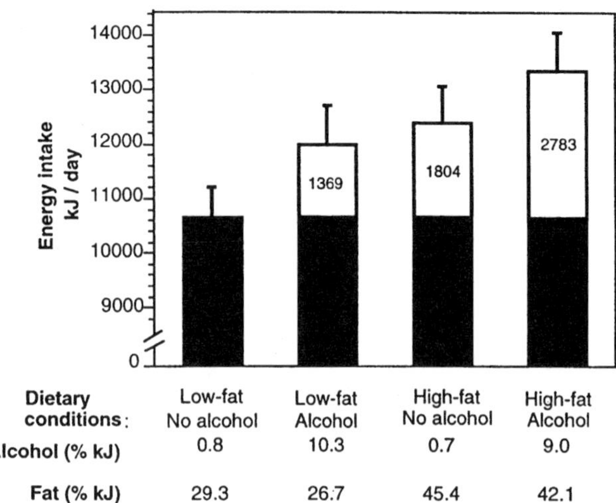

Figure 6 Effect of dietary fat content and alcohol on daily energy intake (means ± SE). (From Ref. 122.)

IV SUBSTRATE BALANCES AND WEIGHT MAINTENANCE

When the steady state of weight maintenance has become established, the concept of "nutrient partitioning" is rather meaningless, since over a period of a few days all the nutrients consumed are oxidized, whereas the type of nutrient retained preferentially varies from day to day to compensate for short-term deviations from equilibrated substrate balances. It is the nature of these compensatory responses that needs to be examined to understand what brings about body weight stability.

A Fuel Composition and Energy Balance

Because of the organism's tendency to adjust glucose oxidation to carbohydrate intake and to maintain stable glycogen stores, the fuel mix oxidized on days during which excess food is consumed is enriched in carbohydrate. This manifests itself by an elevated 24-hr RQ that reveals that fat oxidation is inhibited on such days in spite of increased intake (114). Excess energy will therefore be retained primarily in the form of fat. When food consumption is insufficient to cover energy expenditure, the substrates obtained from food have to be supplemented by drawing on the body's energy reserves, primarily from endogenous fat, in order to prevent excessive glycogen losses. The addition of endogenous fat to the fuel mix oxidized causes the 24-hr RQ to be lower than on days during which energy balance is achieved. There is thus a strong positive correlation between the RQ and the energy balance (114,134,135). Figure 7 (left panel) shows that the relationship between energy balance and RQ depends on the carbohydrate content of the diet. Solid lines show the correlations for diets providing 25%, 40%, or 55% of dietary energy as fat, assuming that carbohydrate balance is exactly preserved. The slope of these correlations is attenuated when part of the imbalance in the energy balance is absorbed by gains or losses of glycogen, as shown by the dotted lines, which are based on the assumption that 20% of the energy imbalance is absorbed by changes in the glycogen stores.

B RQ/FQ Concept and Energy Balance

To avoid ambiguity about the implications which a particular RQ value may have in judging whether the fuel mix oxidized contains more or less fat than the diet, it is convenient to compare the RQ to the FQ. The relationship between RQ and energy balance can be normalized by considering the RQ/FQ ratio in relation to the ratio of energy intake divided by energy expenditure (right panel of Fig. 7). That the slopes of the lines are slightly different for different diets does not deter the fact that RQ/FQ ratios >1.0 imply positive energy balances, whereas RQ/FQ ratios <1.0 indicate negative energy balances. Weight maintenance, which depends on protein, carbohydrate, and fat balances being all close to zero, corresponds to the situation where the respiratory quotient is equal, on average, to the diet's FQ (114).

The need to satisfy the RQ = FQ condition creates constraints in the system, as it shows that a balance must be reached between the influences which the body's glycogen stores and the size of the adipose tissue exert on the relative proportions of glucose and FFA being oxidized (113,114). This creates a reason for a particular degree of fatness to become established as long as an individual's diet and lifestyle, as well as habitual glycogen levels, are constant (cf. Fig. 5). It is therefore not necessary to postulate the existence of some mysterious set-point to explain body weight stability.

C Importance of Food Intake Regulation and Variations in Energy Expenditure in Bringing About Weight Maintenance

Numerous factors capable of influencing food intake have been recognized and studied, but their relative importance and contributions to weight maintenance have been difficult to establish in man, in whom non-

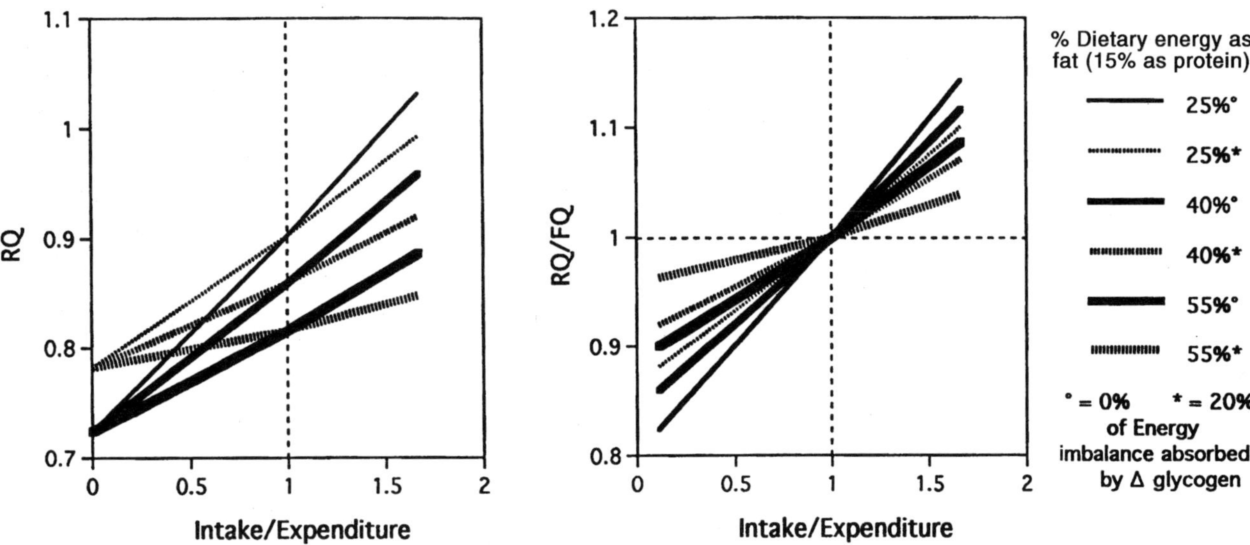

Figure 7 Relationships among the RQ, the RQ/FQ ratio, and energy balance, assuming that carbohydrate balances are equilibrated (solid lines) or that 20% of the energy imbalances are absorbed by gains or losses of glycogen (dotted lines). (From Ref. 135.)

physiological factors contribute to stabilize or to alter food consumption. Whatever the mechanisms may be, the drive to eat provides for the maintenance of glycogen levels adequate for carrying out habitual workloads and sufficient to prevent hypoglycemia. On the other hand, spontaneous restraint of appetite keeps glycogen levels well below the range for which appreciable rates of de novo lipogenensis would be induced, even when there is free access to a large variety of appetizing food (33,36). Regulation of food intake also prevents overloading the digestive system (136), but this does not prevent the occurrence of substantial day-to-day deviations from energy and substrate balances, or the existence of individual weekly patterns of food intake (137). In spite of considerable short-term deviations from energy balance, most individuals maintain stable body fat contents during prolonged periods of their lives. Since changes in energy expenditure can only modestly attenuate the impact of excessive or insufficient food intakes, it is evident that weight stability is achieved through corrective changes in food consumption and that these adjustments are effective in compensating the daily energy imbalances which occur in free-living individuals (113).

D Body Composition for Which Substrate Oxidation Matches Nutrient Intake

1 Impact of Dietary Fat Content

One of the most significant changes in dietary habits during the 20th century was a marked increase in the fat content of the diet, generally believed to have contributed significantly to the increased incidence of obesity in affluent societies (89,138,139), although other factors (113), notably a reduced level of physical activity, are important contributory factors (140). The overfeeding associated with the consumption of mixed diets providing substantial amounts of fat can be attributed in part to the high energy density of high fat foods (141), to the inability of fat intake to promote fat oxidation (118,142), and to *passive overconsumption* due to the failure of dietary lipid to promote an adequate level of satiety, as suggested by the fact that fat preloads suppress subsequent energy intake less than carbohydrate preloads (143,144). Animal studies show that the steady state of weight maintenance under ad libitum feeding conditions becomes established for higher body fat contents as the fat content of the diet increases, apparently because expansion of the fat mass is required to raise fat oxidation (113,114). This supports the concept that obesity represents an adaptation to high fat diets (145). A certain predilection for fat in the foods consumed has often been noted in overweight subjects, and epidemiological data show correlations between dietary fat consumption and adiposity (89,138, 146,147).

2 Impact of Physical Activity

Vigorous physical activity is known to influence body weight and fat stores, and it has been repeatedly observed that obese individuals tend to be less physically active than lean subjects. The Canada Fitness Survey demonstrated that individuals reporting regular practice of vigorous activities were leaner than those not performing such activities (148). In addition, obese individuals who had managed to lose weight and maintained an exercise routine regained less weight than those who did not (149). The negative association between activity level and body fatness is shown by relating body fat content to the ratio of total to resting energy expenditure (TEE/REE), a commonly used index of physical activity (150).

Intervention studies in which exercise was prescribed show that the weight loss achieved depends on the amount of exercise performed (151). Exercise is more likely to induce negative energy balance in subjects with a high capacity to oxidize fat (90) and when postexercise consumption of high-fat food is avoided (152,153). When the effect of a high-intensity intermittent training program was compared to that of an aerobic training program of moderate intensity (which raised energy expenditure more than twice as much), the former was found to cause a ninefold greater subcutaneous fat loss when expressed per MJ expended in training. In addition, the high intensity program induced a greater increase in the potential of skeletal muscle to oxidize fatty acids, as judged by muscle β-hydroxy-acylCoA dehydrogenase activity (87).

When fat loss becomes sufficient to decrease fat mobilization and oxidation (88,154), the ability of exercise to induce negative fat and energy balances declines. The effect of exercise in promoting fat oxidation is then offset by the decline of the fat mass, and a new steady state, at a lower degree of adiposity, is approached.

3 Synergestic Effect of High-Fat Diet and Sedentary Lifestyle

Situations in which low physical activity is associated with the consumption of diets with a high fat content appear to be particularly conducive to the development of obesity. Indeed, these two conditions must prevail simultaneously for the prevalence of obesity to reach epidemic proportions. The reasons for this may be that oxidizing fat at the rate at which it is consumed is problematic, when the contribution of muscle, the largest compartment in the body able to rapidly oxidize fatty acids, is low (Fig. 4). Indeed, the impact of running activity on the energy balance among ad libitum–fed mice is greater on mixed than on low-fat diets (88). Recent indirect calorimetry studies in men also reveal the significance of this linkage, not only because adjustment of fat oxidation to higher fat intake is prompter in physically active than in sedentary subjects (155), but also because this adjustment appears to be facilitated by concurrent physical activity (58).

4 Impact of Hormones

Hormones can influence substrate oxidation by altering overall energy expenditure and the relative proportions of amino acids, glucose, and fatty acids being oxidized. The impact on body weight most clearly attributable to hormone-induced changes in energy expenditure occurs in cases of frank hypothyroidism or hyperthyroidism, whereas the effect of other hormones on adiposity is elicited primarily through their influence on the control of food intake and/or substrate metabolism.

In the case of amino acids and glucose, the effect of altered hormone levels or of altered responsiveness to their action can be offset by changes in the size of the protein and amino acid pools, and in glycogen stores and blood glucose levels, without affecting body composition in a readily detectable manner. Hormones that reduce fat oxidation, by inhibiting fat mobilization or by enhancing glucose oxidation, tend to raise the amount of body fat needed for fat oxidation to become commensurate with fat intake, and this can lead to changes in body composition and body weight that are clearly perceived and quantifiable.

Insulin is the main hormone curtailing fat oxidation, whereas growth hormone and catecholamines have the opposite effect. An important site for the expression of the antagonistic effects of these hormones is on the regulation of PDH, the enzyme catalyzing the irreversible step in the oxidation of carbohydrate. Thus, insulin promotes the activation of PDH, whereas increases in FFA and acetyl-CoA levels, elicited by catecholamines and growth hormone or by expansion of the adipose tissue mass, inhibit PDH (111). Interestingly, insulin and FFA levels are both elevated in obesity. The balance between the effects of elevated insulin and FFA levels on PDH activity would appear to have some importance, since body weight gain over several years tends to be less in obese subjects exhibiting insulin resistance (121).

The effect of β-adrenergic agonists tends to be more pronounced on lipid oxidation than on thermogenesis, whereas administration of β-blockers such as propranolol over a 2-week period resulted in a decrease in daily lipid oxidation three times greater than the decrease in energy expenditure, while carbohydrate oxidation was increased (63). Acute stimulation of sympathetic activity by exposing the lower body to negative pressure was found to induce a substantial increase in lipid oxidation, whereas energy expenditure was not altered (156). According to the RQ/FQ concept (114), a decrease in the use of fat relative to glucose is likely to increase food consumption, and a high RQ has indeed been a predictor for weight gain (60,61).

The situation is in reality much more complex than it appears by considering only the effects of hormones on peripheral fuel metabolism, notably because the neurosystems involved in the regulation of food intake are also influenced by insulin (157). Furthermore, hyperinsulinemia increases plasma noradrenaline (158) and muscle sympathetic nerve activity (159,160). Increases in sympathetic activity decrease energy intake and stimulate thermogenesis (8,9,161). However, since muscle sympathetic nerve activity represents only one component of sympathetic nervous system activity, it is not yet possible to generalize from this peripheral effect. In addition, high insulin levels in the central nervous system inhibit food intake (162), in part by inhibiting the fasting-related increase in the synthesis and release of neuropeptide Y (163), which is known to increase energy intake and to reduce thermogenesis (164). The hyperinsulinemia brought about by enlargement of the fat stores thus tends to restrain further weight gain through central effects (157). Conversely, the normalization of insulinemia achieved by weight reduction (165,166) may explain increasing resistance to further weight loss. Glucocorticoid hormones promote fat deposition, and they are in fact essential for the development of obesity in many genetically obese animals (167). As in the case of insulin, their action appears to be mediated by central nervous system as well as by peripheral effects (161). Growth hormone exerts the opposite influence; among other effects, it promotes fat oxidation relative to glucose oxidation (168). The balance of these various endocrine effects ultimately has to be judged by the impact they have on the size of the fat mass at which weight maintenance tends to occur.

5 Impact of Drugs

Considerable efforts have been made to develop drugs that induce body weight loss, either by increasing energy expenditure or by curtailing food intake. At present, most of the commonly used weight-reducing drugs act through their anorectic effects. When food intake is not restricted, the effectiveness of thermogenic stimuli for weight reduction depends on food intake not increasing enough to compensate for the drug-induced increase in energy expenditure. The phenomena regulating food intake thus remain an essential component in any rationale by which the impact of increases in energy expenditure in eliciting weight reduction is to be explained. The ultimate issue in explaining the weight-reducing influences of drugs (as well as of exercise) is why food intake regulation did not elicit an increase in food intake commensurate with the increase in energy expenditure. Since the RQ must on average be below the FQ to achieve weight reduction (49), weight-reducing drugs could be selected for their ability to help in achieving this condition, rather than merely for increasing energy expenditure.

E Daily Substrate Oxidation Patterns in Lean and Obese Individuals

Fat oxidation after an overnight fast is higher in obese than in lean subjects, in part owing to higher BMR and in part to lower RQ (154). The negative correlation between RQ and adiposity reflects the influence of the adipose tissue mass in raising FFA levels and in promoting fat relative to glucose oxidation. However, one should also allow for the fact that obese subjects often tend to consume diets with a higher fat content (89, 146,147) which could contribute to their relatively low postabsorptive RQ. Whatever the case may be, the average 24-hr RQ is equal to the diet's FQ in weight-stable subjects, be they lean or obese. If one assumes that the lower postabsorptive RQ observed in obese individuals is not imputable to a difference in the macronutrient composition of their diet, one would have to predict that the RQ would be higher in obese than in normal subjects during some periods of the day. This issue remains to be explored.

F Substrate Oxidation and Predisposition to Obesity

Most individuals reach a state of approximate weight maintenance in which the average composition of the fuels mix they oxidize matches the nutrient distribution in their diets. A rate of fat accumulation resulting in a gain of 1 kg of adipose tissue in a year represents a retention of only ~1% of the energy consumed, making it difficult to detect differences in fuel oxidation under normal conditions. Nevertheless, under rigorously standardized conditions, it was found that subjects tending to have high 24-hr RQ, i.e., those tending to burn more glucose but less fat, were at a higher risk of gaining weight during subsequent years (60,61). The view that difficulty in burning as much fat as is consumed is an important factor in promoting obesity is further supported by the fact that adjustment of fat oxidation to increased fat intake occurs more slowly in obese than in lean subjects (25), placing them at greater risk for weight gain. Furthermore it was found that a low skeletal muscle oxidative capacity is associated with increased adiposity (169) and that skeletal muscle fatty acid utilization was reduced in women displaying visceral obesity (170).

Since adjustment of fuel oxidation to intake is achieved in lean and in obese subjects, once the fat mass has reached the size needed for fat oxidation to be commensurate with fat intake, it is necessary to compare postobese individuals to lean controls to identify possible differences in metabolic regulation. Such studies show daily fat oxidation measured by indirect calorimetry to be lower in the postobese subjects (55,171, 172). Furthermore, fat oxidation rises more slowly in postobese subjects than in lean individuals in response to an increase in dietary fat content (173,174). It thus appears that individuals predisposed to obesity are characterized by a reduced fat oxidation when they are tested in a postobese state. In formerly obese long-distance runners tested after a 39.5-kg weight loss, epinephrine stimulated adipose tissue lipolysis was much less than in runners who had never experienced problems with body weight control (175).

G Interactions Between Genetic and Environmental Factors

The powerful role of inheritance on obesity has long been recognized (176). However, the great increase in the prevalence of obesity in industrialized countries (177), in populations whose gene pool has been relatively constant, shows that environmental factors also assume considerable importance. These facts can be reconciled by recognizing that some genotypes are more affected than others when exposed to environmental factors that influence substrate oxidation and balances. The genotype-environment interactions have been investigated by subjecting monozygotic twins to well-defined nutritional and exercise conditions, and by comparing within-pair to between-pair responses. Such studies suggest that heredity is a significant determinant of changes in body weight, energy expenditure, and body fatness induced by training (178,179) or overfeeding (180–182). The observation that weight gain was greatest in subjects predisposed to obesity (because at least one of their parents was overweight) and consuming diets with a relatively high fat content (183) supports the view that genetic traits affecting the regulation of glucose versus fat oxidation influence the risk for developing obesity.

V CONCLUSIONS

When access to foods is unrestricted, stability of body weight is achieved in spite of differences in energy expenditure, whether these are due to differences in resting metabolic rates, in metabolic efficiency, or in physical activity. Since energy expenditure is not markedly affected by variations in food intake in man, maintenance of energy balance is overwhelmingly determined by the factors controlling food intake. Adjustment of the composition of the substrate mix oxidized to the macronutrient distribution in the diet is crucial in enabling control of food intake to occur in a manner bringing about short-term corrections in food consumption that sustain long-term weight stability. In individuals in whom fat oxidation tends to be low relative to glucose oxidation, substantial expansion of the adipose tissue mass is often necessary before this weight stability is reached.

REFERENCES

1. Astrand P-O, Rodahl K. Textbook of Work Physiology, 2nd ed. New York: McGraw-Hill, 1977.
2. Pahud P, Ravussin E, Jéquier E. Energy expended during oxygen deficit period of submaximal exercise in man. J Appl Physiol 1980; 48:770–775.
3. Flatt JP, Pahud P, Ravussin E, Jéquier E. An estimate of the P:O ratio in man. TIBS 1984; 9:251–255.
4. Brand MD, Couture P, Else PL, Withers KW, Hulbert AJ. Evolution of energy metabolism. Proton permeability of the inner membrane of liver mitochondria is greater in a mammal than in a reptile. Biochem J 1991; 275:81–86.
5. Rolfe DFS, Brown GC. Cellular energy utilization and molecular origen of standard metabolic rate in mammals. Physiol Rev 1997; 77(3):731–758.
6. Flatt JP. Energy costs of ATP synthesis. In: Kinney JH, Tucker H, eds. Energy Metabolism: Tissue Determinants and Cellular Corollaries. New York: Raven Press, 1992:319–342.
7. Flatt JP. Conversion of carbohydrate to fat in adipose tissue: an energy-yielding and, therefore, self-limiting process. J Lipid Res 1970; 11:131–143.
8. Himms-Hagen J. Thermogenesis in brown adipose tissue as an energy buffer: implications for obesity. N Engl J Med 1984; 311:1549–1558.
9. Rothwell NJ, Stock MJ. Regulation of energy balance. Annu Rev Nutr 1981; 1:235–256.
10. Lowell BB, S-Susulic V, Hamann A, Lawitts JA, Himms-Hagen J, Boyer BB, Kozak LP, Flier JS. Development of obesity in transgenic mice after genetic ablation of brown adipose tissue. Nature 1993; 366: 740–742.
11. Schrauwen P, Walder K, Ravussin E. Human uncoupling proteins and obesity. Obes Res 1998; 7(1):97–105.
12. DeFronzo RA, Ferrannini E. Regulation of hepatic glucose metabolism in humans. Diabetes/Metab Rev 1987; 3:415–459.
13. Weast RC. Handbook of Chemistry and Physics, 57th ed. Cleveland: CRC Press, 1976.
14. Elia M, Zed C, Neale G. Livesey G. The energy cost of triglyceride-fatty acid recycling in non-obese subjects after an overnight fast and four days of starvation. Metabolism 1987; 36:251–255.
15. Livesey G, Elia M. Estimation of energy expenditure, net carbohydrate utilization, and net fat oxidation and synthesis by indirect calorimetry: evaluation of errors with special reference to the detailed composition of fuels. Am J Clin Nutr 1988; 47:608–623.
16. McGilvery RW, Goldstein G. Biochemistry. A Functional Approach. Philadelphia: W.B. Saunders, 1979.
17. Garlick PJ, Clugston GA, Swick RW, Waterlow JC. Diurnal pattern of protein and energy metabolism in man. Am J Clin Nutr 1980; 33:1983–1986.
18. Welle S, Nair KS. Relationship of resting metabolic rate to body composition and protein turnover. Am J Physiol 1990; 258:E990–E998.
19. Kinney JM, Elwyn DH. Protein metabolism and injury. Annu Rev Nutr 1983; 3:433–466.
20. Acheson KJ, Ravussin E, Wahren J, Jéquier E. Thermic effect of glucose in man, obligatory and facultative thermogenesis. J Clin Invest 1984; 74:1572–1580.
21. Dallosso HM, James WPT. Whole-body calorimetry studies in adult men 1. The effect of fat over-feeding on 24 h energy expenditure. Br J Nutr 1984; 52:49–64.
22. Donato KA, Hegsted DM. Efficiency of utilization of various energy sources for growth. Proc Natl Acad Sci USA 1985; 82:4866–4870.
23. Hurni M, Burnand B, Pittet PH, Jéquier E. Metabolic effects of a mixed and a high-carbohydrate low-fat diet in man, measured over 24 h in a respiration chamber. Br J Nutr 1982; 47:33–43.
24. Abbott WGH, Howard BV, Ruotolo G, Ravussin E. Energy expenditure in humans: effects of dietary fat and carbohydrate. Am J Physiol 1990; 258:E347–E351.

25. Thomas CD, Peters JC, Reed GW, Abumrad NN, Sun M, Hill JO. Nutrient balance and energy expenditure during ad libitum feeding of high fat and high carbohydrate diets in humans. Am J Clin Nutr 1992; 55:934–942.
26. Shetty PS, Prentice AM, Goldberg GR, Murgatroyd PR, McKenna APM, Stubbs RJ, Volschenk PA. Alterations in fuel selection and voluntary food intake in response to isoenergetic manipulation of glycogen stores in humans. Am J Clin Nutr 1994; 60:534–543.
27. Stubbs RJ, Harbron CG, Murgatroyd PR, Prentice AM. Covert manipulation of dietary fat and energy density: effect on substrate flux and food intake in men eating ad libitum. Am J Clin Nutr 1995; 62:316–329.
28. Kleiber M. The Fire of Life and Introduction to Animal Energetics. New York: Robert E. Krieger, 1975.
29. Lusk G. The Elements of the Science of Nutrition, 4th ed. Philadelphia: W.B. Saunders, 1928.
30. Jungas RL, Halperin ML, Brosnan JT. Quantitative analysis of amino acid oxidation and related gluconeogenesis in humans. Physiol Rev 1992; 72:419–448.
31. Flat JP. The biochemistry of energy expenditure. Rec Adv Obes Res 1978; 2:211–228.
32. Shaw SN, Elwyn DH, Askanazi J, Iles M, Schwarz Y, Kinney JM. Effects of increasing nitrogen intake on nitrogen balance and energy expenditure in nutritionally depleted adult patients receiving parenteral nutrition. Am J Clin Nutr 1983; 37:930–940.
33. Acheson KJ, Schutz, Y, Bessard T, Anantharaman K, Flatt JP, Jéquier E. Glycogen storage capacity and de novo lipogenesis during massive carbohydrate overfeeding in man. Am J Clin Nutr 1988; 48:240–247.
34. Hellerstein MK, Christiansen M, Kaempfer S, Kletke C, Wu K, Reid JS, Mulligan K, Hellerstein NS, Shackleton CHL. Measurement of de novo hepatic lipogenesis in humans using stable isotopes. J Clin Invest 1991; 87:1841–1852.
35. Guo ZK, Cella LK, Baum C, E R, Schoeller DA. De novo lipogenesis in adipose tissue of lean and obese women: application of deuterated water and isotope ratio mass spectrometry. Int J Obes 2000; 24:932–937.
36. Acheson KJ, Schutz Y, Bessard T, Ravussin E, Jéquier E, Flatt JP. Nutritional influences on lipogenesis and thermogenesis after a carbohydrate meal. Am J Physiol 1984; 246:E62–E70.
37. Owen OE, Holup JL, D'Alessio DA, Craig ES, Polansky M, Smalley KJ, Kavle EC, Bushman MC, Owen LR, Mozzoli MA, Kendrick ZV, Boden GH. A reappraisal of the caloric requirements of men. Am J Clin Nutr 1987; 46:875–885.
38. Ravussin E, Lillioja S, Anderson TE, Christin L, Bogardus C. Determinants of 24-h energy expenditure in man. J Clin Invest 1986; 78:1568–1578.
39. Newsholme EA, Leech AR. Biochemistry for the Medical Sciences. Chichester: Wiley & Sons, 1983.
40. Randle PJ, Hales CN, Garland PB, Newsholme EA. The glucose fatty-acid cycle: its role in insulin sensitivity and the metabolic disturbances of diabetes mellitus. Lancet 1963; i:785–789.
41. Wolfe RR. The role of triglyceride–fatty acid cycling and glucose cycling in thermogenesis and amplification of net substrate flux in human subjects. In: Müller MJ, Danforth E, Burger AG, eds. Hormones and Nutrition in Obesity and Cachexia. New York: Springer, 1990.
42. Wolfe RR, Herndon DN, Jahoor F, Miyoshi H, Wolfe M. Effect of severe burn injury on substrate cycling by glucose and fatty acids. N Engl J Med 1987; 317:403–408.
43. Lardy H, Su CY, Kneer N, Wielgus S. Dehydroepiandrosterone induces enzymes that permit thermogenesis and decrease metabolic efficiency. In: Lardy H, Stratman F, eds. Hormones, Thermogenesis, and Obesity. New York: Elsevier, 1989:415–426.
44. Kozak LP, Kozak UC, Clarke GT. Abnormal brown and white fat development in transgenic mice overexpressing glycerol 3-phosphate dehydrogenase. Genes Dev 1991; 5:2256–2264.
45. Shulman GI, Ladenson PW, Wolfe MH, Ridgway EC, Wolfe RR. Substrate cycling between gluconeogenesis and glycolysis in euthyroid, hypothyroid, and hyperthyroid in man. J Clin Invest 1985; 76:757–764.
46. Clausen T, Van Hardeveld C, Everts ME. Significance of cation transport in control on energy metabolism and thermogenesis. Physiol Rev 1991; 71:733–774.
47. Brand MD, Steverding D, Kadenbach B, Stevenson PM, Hafner RP. The mechanism of the increase in mitochondrial proton permeability induced by thyroid hormones. Eur J Biochem 1992; 206:775–781.
48. Schoeller DA, Field CR. Human energy metabolism: what we have learned from the doubly labeled water method. Annu Rev Nutr 1991; 11:355–373.
49. Flatt JP. Importance of nutrient balance in body weight regulation. Diabetes/Metab Rev 1988; 4:571–581.
50. Recommended Dietary Allowances, 10th ed. Washington: National Academy Press, 1989.
51. Refinetti R. Effect of ambient temperature on respiratory quotient of lean and obese Zucker rats. Am J Physiol 1989; 256:R236–R239.
52. Pagé E, Chénier L. Effects of diets and cold environment on the respiratory quotient of the white rat. Rev Can Biol 1953; 12:530–541.
53. Wilson S, Thurlby PL, Arch JRS. Substrate supply for thermogenesis induced by the B-adrenoceptor agonist BRL 26830A. Can J Physiol Pharm 1987; 65: 113–119.
54. Graham TE, Sathasivam P, MacNaughton KW. Influence of cold, exercise, and caffeine on catechol-

amine and metabolism in men. J Appl Physiol 1991; 70:2052–2058.
55. Buemann B, Astrup A, Christensen N, Madsen J. Effect of moderate cold exposure on 24 h energy expenditure: similar response in postobese and nonobese women. Am J Physiol 1992; 263:E1040–E1045.
56. Jéquier E, Acheson K, Schutz Y. Assessment of energy expenditure and fuel utilization in man. Annu Rev Nutr 1987; 7:187–208.
57. McLean JA. Animal and Human Calorimetry. Cambridge: Cambridge University Press, 1987.
58. Smith SR, De Jonge L, Zachwieja JJ, Heli R, Nguyen T, Rood JC, Windhauser MM, Volaufova J, Bray GA. Concurrent physical activity increases fat oxidation during the shift to a high-fat diet. Am J Clin Nutr 2000; 72:131–138.
59. Murgatroyd PR, Shetty PS, Prentice AM. Techniques for the measurement of human energy expenditure: a practical guide. Int J Obes 1993; 17:549–568.
60. Zurlo F, Lillioja S, Esposito-Del Puente A, Nyomba BL, Raz I, Saad MF, Swinburn BA, Knowler WC, Bogardus C, Ravussin E. Low ratio of fat to carbohydrate oxidation as predictor of weight gain: study of 24h RQ. Am J Physiol 1990; 259:E650 E657.
61. Seidell JC, Muller DC, Sorkin JD, Andres R. Fasting respiratory exchange ratio and resting metabolic rate as predictors of weight gain: the Baltimore Longitudinal Study on Aging. Int J Obes 1992; 16:667–674.
62. Hill JO, Peters JC, Reed GW, Schlundt DG, Sharp T, Greene HL. Nutrient balance in humans: effects of diet composition. Am J Clin Nutr 1991; 54:10–17.
63. Acheson KJ, Ravussin E, Schoeller DA, Christin L, Bourquin L, Baertschi P, Danforth E, Jéquier E. Two-week stimulation or blockade of the sympathetic nervous system in man: influence on body weight, body composition, and twenty four-hour energy expenditure. Metabolism 1988; 37:91–98.
64. Spurr GB, Prentice AM, Murgatroyd PR, Goldberg GR, Reina JC, Christman NT. Energy expenditure from minute-by-minute heart-rate recording: comparison to indirect calorimetry. Am J Clin Nutr 1988; 48: 552–559.
65. Livingstone MBE, Prentice AM, Coward WA, Ceesay SM, Strain JJ, McKenna PG, Nevin GB, Baker ME, Hickey RJ. Simultaneous free-living energy expenditure by the doubly labeled water method and the heart-rate monitoring. Am J Clin Nutr 1990; 52:59–65.
66. Alméras N, Mimeault N, Serresse O, Boulay MR, Tremblay A. Non-exercise daily energy expenditure and physical activity pattern in male endurance athletes. Eur J Appl Physiol 1991; 63:184–187.
67. Lifson N, Gordon GB, Mc Clintock R. Measurement of total carbon dioxide production by means of $D_2{}^{18}O$. J Appl Physiol 1955; 7:704–710.
68. Elia M. Energy equivalents of CO_2 and their importance in assessing energy expenditure when using tracer techniques. Am J Physiol 1991; 260:E75–E88.
69. Schoeller DA, Van Santen E. Measurement of energy expenditure in humans by doubly labeled water method. J Appl Physiol 1982; 53:955–959.
70. Roberts SB, Dietz W, Sharp T, Dallal GE, Hill JO. Multiple laboratory comparison of the doubly labeled water technique. Obes Res 1995; 3:S3–S13.
71. Prentice AM, Coward WA, Davies HL, Murgatroyd PR, Black AE, Goldberg GR, Ashford J, Sawyer M, Whitehead RG. Unexpectedly low levels of energy expenditure in health women. Lancet 1985; i:1419–1422.
72. Heini A, Schutz Y, Diaz E, Prentice AM, Whitehead RG, Jequier E. Free-living energy expenditure measured by two independent techniques in pregnant and nonpregnant Gambian women. Am J Physiol 1991; 261:E9–E17.
73. Tremblay A, Seale J, Alméras N, Conway J, Moe P. Energy requirements of a postobese man reporting a low intake at weight maintenance. Am J Clin Nutr 1991; 54:1–3.
74. Prentice AM, Black AE, Coward WA, Cole TJ. Energy expenditure in overweight and obese adults in affluent societies: an analysis of 319 doubly-labelled water measurements. Eur J Clin Nutr 1996; 50:93–97.
75. Westerterp KR, Saris WHM, Van Es M, Ten Hoor F. Use of the doubly labelled water technique in humans during heavy sustained exercise. J Appl Physiol 1986; 61:2162–2167.
76. Goran MI, Poehlman ET. Endurance training does not enhance total energy expenditure in healthy elderly persons. Am J Physiol 1992; 263:E950–E957.
77. Heaton JM. The distribution of brown adipose tissue in the human. J Anat 1972; 112:35–39.
78. Astrup A, Bülow J, Madsen J, Christensen NJ. Contribution of brown adipose tissue and skletal muscle to thermogenesis induced by ephedrine in man. Am J Physiol 1985; 248:E507–E515.
79. Norgan NG, Durnin JVGA. The effect of 6 weeks of overfeeding on the body weight, body composition, and energy metabolism of young men. Am J Clin Nutr 1980; 33:978–988.
80. Ravussin E, Schutz Y, Acheson KJ, Dusmet M, Bourquin L, Jéquier E. Short-term, mixed-diet overfeeding in man: no evidence for "Luxuskonsumption." Am J Physiol 1985; 249:E470–E477.
81. Diaz EO, Prentice AM, Goldberg GR, Murgatroyd PR, Coward WA. Metabolic response to experimental overfeeding in lean and overweight healthy volunteers. Am J Clin Nutr 1992; 56:641–655.
82. Tremblay A, Després JP, Thériault G, Fournier G, Bouchard C. Overfeeding and energy expenditure in humans. Am J Clin Nutr 1992; 56:857–862.

83. Wasserman K, Hansen EJ, Sue DY, Whipp BJ. Principles of Exercise Testing and Interpretation. Philadelphia: Lea and Febiger, 1987:274.
84. Coggan AR, Kohrt MW, Spina RJ, Bier DM, Holloszy JO. Endurance training decreases plasma glucose turnover and oxidation during moderate-intensity exercise in men. J Appl Physiol 1990; 68: 990–996.
85. Tremblay A, Fontaine E, Nadeau A. Contribution of postexercise increment in glucose storage to variations in glucose-induced thermogenesis in endurance athletes. Can J Physiol Pharm 1985; 63:1165–1169.
86. Bielinski R, Schutz Y, Jéquier E. Energy metabolism during the post-exercise recovery in man. Am J Clin Nutr 1985; 42:69–82.
87. Tremblay A, Simoneau J-A, Bouchard C. Impact of exercise intensity on body fatness and skeletal muscle metabolism. Metabolism 1994; 43:814–818.
88. Flatt JP. Integration of the overall effects of exercise. Int J Obes 1995; 19:S31–S40.
89. Tremblay A, Plourde G, Després JP, Bouchard C. Impact of dietary fat content and fat oxidation on energy intake in humans. Am J Clin Nutr 1989; 49: 799–805.
90. Alméras N, Lavallée N, Després J-P, Bouchard C, Tremblay A. Exercise and energy intake: effect of substrate oxidation. Physiol Behav 1995; 57:995–1000.
91. Ravussin E, Lillioja S, Knowler WC, Christin L, Freymond D, Abbott WGH, Boyce V, Howard BV, Bogardus C. Reduced rate of energy expenditure as a risk factor for body-weight gain. N Engl J Med 1988; 318:467–472.
92. Stubbs JR, Ritz P, Coward WA, Prentice AM. Covert manipulation of the ratio of dietary fat to carbohydrate and energy density: effect on food intake and energy balance in free-living men eating ad libitum. Am J Clin Nutr 1995; 62:330–337.
93. Speakman JR, Racey PA. The equilibrium concentration of oxygen-18 in body water: implications for the accuracy of the doubly-labelled water technique and a potential new method of measuring RQ in free-living animals. J Theor Biol 1987; 127:79–95.
94. Bingham SA, Gill C, Welch A, Day K, Cassidy A, Khaw KT, Sneyd MJ, Key TJA, Roe L, Day NE. Comparison of dietary assessment methods in nutritional epidemiology: weighed records v. 24h recalls, food-frequency questionnaires and estimated-diet records. Br J Nutr 1994; 72:619–643.
95. Birch LL, Johnson SL, Andresen G, Peters JC, Schulte MC. The variability of young children's energy intake. N Engl J Med 1991; 324:232–235.
96. Mattes RD, Pierce CB, Friedman MI. Daily caloric intake of normal weight adults: response to changes in dietary energy density of a luncheon meal. Am J Clin Nutr 1988; 48:214–219.
97. Ramirez I, Tordoff MG, Friedman MI. Dietary hyperphagia and obesity: what causes them? Physiol Behav 1989; 45:163–168.
98. Romjin JA, Coyle EF, Sidossis LS, Gastaldelli A, Horowitz JF, Endert E, Wolfe RR. Regulation of endogenous fat and carbohydrate metabolism in relation to exercise intensity and duration. Am J Physiol 1993; 265:E380–E391.
99. Elia M. General integration and regulation of metabolism at the organ level. Proc Nutr Soc 1995; 54:213–232.
100. Geigy. Scientific Tables, 7th ed. Ardsley, NY: Geigy Pharmaceuticals, 1970.
101. Cahill GF. Starvation in man. N Engl J Med 1970; 282(12):668–675.
102. Murphy JR. Erythrocyte metabolism. II. Glucose metabolism and pathways. J Lab Clin Med 1960; 55: 286–302.
103. Müller MJ. Hepatic fuel selection. Proc Nutr Soc 1995; 54:139–150.
104. Brooks GA, Mercier J. Balance of carbohydrate and lipid utilization during exercise: the "crossover" concept. J Appl Physiol 1994; 76(6):2253–2261.
105. Coppack SW, Frayn KN, Humphreys SM, Whyte PL, Hockaday TDR. Arteriovenous differences across human adipose and forearm tissues after overnight fast. Metabolism 1990; 39(4):384–390.
106. Nuutila P, Koivisto VA, Knuuti J, Ruotsalainen U, Teras M, Haaparanta M, Bergman J, Solin O, Voipio-Pulkki LM, Wegelius U, Yki-Jarvinen H. Glucose-free fatty acid cycle operates in human heart and skeletal muscle in vivo. J Clin Invest 1992; 89:1767–1744.
107. Björntorp P, Sjöström L. Carbohydrate storage in man: speculations and some quantitative considerations. Metabolism 1978; 27:1853–1865.
108. Klein S, Wolfe RR. Carbohydrate restriction regulates the adaptive response to fasting. Am J Physio 1992; 262: 631–636.
109. Keller U, Lustenberger J, Müller-Brand J, Gerber PPG, Stauffacher W. Human ketone body production and utilization studied using tracer techniques: regulation by free fatty acids, insulin, catecholamines, and thyroid hormones. Diabetes/Metab Rev 1989; 5:285–298.
110. Abbott WGH, Howard BV, Christin L, Fremond D, Lilloja S, Boyce VL, Anderson TE, Bogardus C, Ravussin E. Short-term energy balance: relationship with protein, carbohydrate, and fat balances. Am J Physiol 1988; 255:E332–E337.
111. Randle PJ, Priestman DA, Mistry SC, Halsall A. Glucose fatty acid interactions and the regulation of glucose disposal. J Cell Biochem 1994; 55S:1–11.
112. Cahill GF Jr. Physiology of insulin in man. Diabetes 1971; 20:785–799.
113. Flatt JP. McCollum Award Lecture, 1995. Diet, lifestyle and weight maintenance. Am J Clin Nutr 1995; 62:820–836.
114. Flatt JP. Dietary fat, carbohydrate balance, and weight

maintenance: effects of exercise. Am J Clin Nutr 1987; 45:296–306.
115. Mayer J, Thomas DW. Regulation of food intake and obesity. Science 1967; 156:328–337.
116. Stubbs RJ, Murgatroyd PR, Goldberg GR, Prentice AM. Carbohydrate balance and the regulation of day-to-day food intake in humans. Am J Clin Nutr 1993; 57:897–903.
117. Clore JN, Helm ST, Blackard WG. Loss of hepatic autoregulation after carbohydrate overfeeding in normal man. J Clin Invest 1995; 96:1967–1972.
118. Flatt JP, Ravussin E, Acheson KJ, Jéquier E. Effects of dietary fat on postprandial substrate oxidation and on carbohydrate and fat balances. J Clin Invest 1985; 76:1019–1024.
119. Griffiths AJ, Humphreys SM, Clark ML, Fielding BA, Frayn KN. Immediate metabolic availability of dietary fat in combination with carbohydrate. Am J Clin Nutr 1994; 59:53–59.
120. Björntorp P, Bergman H, Varnauskas E, Lindholm B. Lipid mobilization in relation to body composition in man. Metabolism 1969; 18:840–851.
121. Swinburn BA, Nyomba BL, Saad MF, Zurlo F, Raz I, Knowler WC, Lillioya S, Bogardus C, Ravussin E. Insulin resistance associated with lower rates of weight gain in Pima Indians. J Clin Invest 1991; 88:168–173.
122. Tremblay A, Wouters E, Wenker M, St.-Pierre S, Bouchard C, Després J-P. Alcohol and a high-fat diet: a combination favoring overfeeding. Am J Clin Nutr 1995; 62:639–644.
123. Colditz GA, Giovannucci E, Rimm ER, Stampfer MJ, Rosner B, Speizer YE, Gordis E, Walter CW. Alcohol intake in relation to diet and obesity in women and men. Am J Clin Nutr 1991; 54:49–55.
124. Jones BR, Barrett-Connor E, Criqui MH, Holbrook MJ. A community study of calorie and nutrient intake in drinkers and nondrinkers of alcohol. Am J Clin Nutr 1982; 35:135–139.
125. Bebb HT, Houser HB, Witschi JC, Litell AS, Fuller RK. Calorie and nutrient contribution of alcoholic beverages to the usual diets of 155 adults. Am J Clin Nutr 1971; 24:1042–1052.
126. Gruchow HW, Sobocinski KA, Barboriak JJ, Scheller JG. Alcohol consumption, nutrient intake and relative body weight among US adults. Am J Coll Nutr 1985; 42:289–295.
127. De Castro JM, Orozco S. Moderate alcohol intake and spontaneous eating patterns of humans: evidence of unregulated supplementation. Am J Clin Nutr 1990; 52:246–253.
128. Veenstra J, Schenkel JAA, Van Erp-Baart AMJ, Brants HAM, Hulshof KFAM, Kistemaker C, Schaafsma G, Ockhuizen T. Alcohol consumption in relation to food intake and smoking habits in the Dutch National Food Consumption Survey. Eur J Clin Nutr 1993; 47:482–489.
129. Prentice AM. Alcohol and obesity. Int J Obes 1995; 19:S44–S50.
130. Suter PM, Jéquier E, Schutz Y. Effect of ethanol on energy expenditure. Am J Physiol 1994; 266:R1204–R1212.
131. Lieber CS. Herman Award Lecture, 1993. A personal perspective on alcohol, nutrition, and liver. Am J Clin Nutr 1993; 58:430–442.
132. Suter PM, Schutz Y, Jéquier E. The effect of ethanol on fat storage in healthy subjects. N Engl J Med 1992; 326:983–987.
133. Tremblay A, St-Pierre S. The hyperphagic effect of high-fat and alcohol persists after control for energy density. Am J Clin Nutr 1996; 63:479–482.
134. Jéquier E. Calorie balance versus nutrient balance. In: Kinney JH, Tucker H, eds. Enery Metabolism: Tissue Determinants and Cellular Corollaries. New York: Raven Press, 1992:123–134.
135. Flatt JP. The RQ/FQ concept and weight maintenance. In: Angel A, Anderson H, Bouchard C, eds. Progress in Obesity Research 7. London: Libbey, 1996: 49–66.
136. Russek M. Current status of the hepatostatic theory of food intake control. Appetite 1981; 2:137–143.
137. Tarasuk V, Beaton GH. The nature and individuality of within subject variation in energy intake. Am J Clin Nutr 1991; 54:464–470.
138. Lissner L, Heitmann BL. Dietary fat and obesity: evidence from epidemiology. Eur J Clin Nutr 1995; 49: 79–90.
139. Bray GA, Popkin BM. Dietary fat intake does affect obesity! Am J Clin Nutr 1998; 68:1157–1173.
140. Prentice AM, Jebb SA. Obesity in Britain: gluttony or sloth? BMJ 1995; 311:437–439.
141. Porikos KP, Booth G, Van Italie TB. Effect of covert nutritive dilution on the spontaneous food intake of obese individuals: a pilot study. Am J Clin Nutr 1977; 30:1638–1644.
142. Schutz Y, Flatt JP, Jéquier E. Failure of dietary fat intake to promote fat oxidation: a factor favoring the development of obesity. Am J Clin Nutr 1989; 50:307–314.
143. Rolls BJ, Kim-Harris S, Fischman MW, Foltin RW, Moran TH, Stoner SA. Satiety after preloads with different amounts of fat and carbohydrate: implications for obesity. Am J Clin Nutr 1994; 60:476–487.
144. Blundell JE, Cotton JR, Delargy H, Green S, Greenough A, King NA, Lawton CL. The fat paradox: fat-induced satiety signals versus high fat overconsumption. Int J Obes 1995; 19:832–835.
145. Astrup A, Buemann B, Western P, Toubro S, Raben A, Christensen NJ. Obesity as an adaptation to a high fat diet: evidence from a cross-sectional study. Am J Clin Nutr 1994; 59:350–355.
146. Dreon DM, Frey-Hewitt B, Ellsworth N, Williams PT,

Terry RB, Wood PD. Dietary fat: carbohydrate ratio and obesity in middle aged men. Am J Clin Nutr 1988; 47:995–1000.
147. Romieu I, Willett WC, Stampfer MJ, Colditz GA, Sampson L, Rosner B, Hennekens CH, Speizer FE. Energy intake and other determinants of relative weight. Am J Clin Nutr 1988; 47:406–412.
148. Tremblay A, Després J-P, Leblanc C, Craig CL, Ferris B, Stephens T, Bouchard C. Effect of intensity of physical activity on body fatness and fat distribution. Am J Clin Nutr 1990; 51:153–157.
149. Ewbank PP, Darga LL, Lucas CP. Physical activity as a predictor of weight maintenance in previously obese subjects. Obes Res 1995; 3:257–264.
150. Rising R, Harper IT, Fontvielle AM, Ferraro RT, Spraul M. Determinants of total daily energy expenditure: variability in physical activity. Am J Clin Nutr 1994; 59:800–804.
151. Ballor DL, Keesey RE. A meta-analysis of the factors affecting exercise-induced changes in body mass, fat mass, and fat-free mass in males and females. Int J Obes 1991; 15:717–726.
152. Tremblay A, Alméras N, Boer J, Kranenbarg EK, Després JP. Diet composition and postexercise energy balance. Am J Clin Nutr 1994; 59:975–979.
153. King NA, Blundell JE. High-fat foods overcome the energy expenditure induced by high-intensity cycling or running. Eur J Clin Nutr 1995; 49:114–123.
154. Schutz Y, Tremblay A, Weinsier RL, Nelson KM. Role of fat oxidation in the long term stabilization of body weight in obese women. Am J Clin Nutr 1992; 55:670–674.
155. Smith SR, De Jonge L, Zachwieja JJ, Heli R, Nguyen T, Rood JC, Windhauser MM, Bray GA. Fat and carbohydrate balances during adaptation to a high-fat diet. Am J Clin Nutr 2000; 71:450–457.
156. Tappy L, Girardet K, Shwaller N, Vollenweider L, Jéquier E, Nicod P, Scherrer U. Metabolic effects of an increase of sympathetic activity in healthy humans. Int J Obes 1995; 19:419–422.
157. Woods SC, Figlewicz Latteman DP, Schwartz MW, Porte D. A re-assessment of the regulation of adiposity and appetite by the brain insulin system. Int J Obes 1990; 14:69–76.
158. Rowe JW, Young JB, Minaker KL, Steven AL, Pallotta J, Lansberg L. Effect of insulin and glucose infusions on sympathetic nervous system activity in normal man. Diabetes 1981; 30:219–225.
159. Berne C, Fagius J, Pollare T, Hemjdahl P. The sympathetic response to euglycaemic hyperinsulinemia. Diabetologia 1992; 35:873–879.
160. Vollenweider P, Randin D, Tappy L, Jéquier E, Nicod P, Scherrer U. Impaired insulin-induced sympathetic neural activation and vasodilation in skeletal muscle in obese humans. J Clin Invest 1994; 93:2365–2371.
161. Bray GA. Obesity—a state of reduced sympathetic activity and normal or high adrenal activity (the autonomic and adrenal hypothesis revisited). Int J Obes 1990; 14:77–92.
162. Kaiyala KJ, Woods SC, Schwartz MW. New model for the regulation of energy balance and adiposity by the central nervous system. Am J Clin Nutr 1995; 62: 1123S–1134S.
163. Schwartz MJ, Marks J, Sipols AJ, Baskin DG, Wood SC, Kahn SE, Porte D. Central insulin administration reduces neuropeptide Y mRNA expression in the arcuate nucleus of food-deprived lean (Fa/Fa) but not obese (fa/fa) Zucker rats. Endocrinology 1991; 128: 2645–2647.
164. Williams G, McKibbin PE, McCarthy HD. Hypothalamic regulatory peptides and the regulation of food intake and energy balance: signals or noise? Proc Nutr Soc 1991; 50:527–544.
165. Tremblay A, Sauvé L, Després JP, Nadeau A, Thériault G, Bouchard C. Metabolic characteristics of postobese individuals. Int J Obes 1989; 13: 357–366.
166. Tremblay A, Després J-P, Maheux J, Pouliot MC, Nadeau A, Moorjani PJ, Lupien PJ, Bouchard C. Normalization of the metabolic profile in obese women by exercise and a low fat diet. Med Sci Sports Exerc 1991; 23(12):1326–1331.
167. Saito M, Bray GA. Adrenalectomy and food restriction in the genetically obese (ob/ob) mouse. Am J Physiol 1984; 246:R20–R25.
168. Salomon F, Cuneo RC, Hesp R, Sönksen PH. The effects of treatment with recombinant human growth hormone on body composition and metabolism in adults with growth hormone deficiency. N Engl J Med 1989; 321:797–803.
169. Simoneau JA, Bouchard C. Skeletal muscle metabolism and body fat content in men and women. Obes Res 1995; 3:23–29.
170. Colberg S, Simoneau J, Thaete F, Kelley D. Skeletal muscle utilization of free fatty acids in women with visceral obesity. J Clin Invest 1995; 95:1846–1853.
171. Lean MEJ, James WPT. Metabolic effects of isoenergetic nutrient exchange over 24 hours in relation to obesity in women. Int J Obes 1988; 8:641–648.
172. Buemann B, Astrup A, Madsen J, Christensen NJ. A 24-h energy expenditure study on reduced-obese and nonobese women: effect of β-blockade. Am J Clin Nutr 1992; 56:662–670.
173. Astrup A, Buemann B, Christensen NJ, Toubro S. Failure to increase lipid oxidation in response to increasing dietary fat content in formerly obese women. Am J Physiol 1994; 266:E592–E599.
174. Raben A, Anderson HB, Christensen NJ, Madsen J, Holst JJ, Astrup A. Evidence for an abnormal postprandial response to a high fat meal in women predisposed to obesity. Am J Physiol 1994; 267:E549–E559.

175. Tremblay A, Després JP, Bouchard C. Adipose tissue characteristics of ex-obese long-distance runners. Int J Obes 1984; 8:641–648.
176. Bouchard C, Pérusse L. Heredity and body fat. Annu Rev Nutr 1988; 8:259–277.
177. Kuczmarksi RJ, Flegal KM, Campbell SM, Johnson CL. Increasing prevalence of overweight among US adults. JAMA 1994; 272:205–211.
178. Poehlman ET, Tremblay A, Nadeau A, Dussault J, Thériault G, Bouchard C. Heredity and changes in hormones and metabolic rates with short-term training. Am J Physiol 1986; 250:E711–E717.
179. Bouchard C, Tremblay A, Després JP, Thériault G, Nadeau A, Lupien PJ, Moorjani S, Prudhomme D, Fournier G. The response to exercise with constant energy intake in identical twins. Obes Res 1994; 2:400–410.
180. Poehlman ET, Tremblay, Fontaine E, Després JP, Nadeau A, Bouchard C. Genotype dependency of dietary induced thermogenesis: its relation with hormonal changes following overfeeding. Metabolism 1986; 35: 30–36.
181. Poehlman ET, Tremblay A, Després JP, Fontaine E, Pérusse L, Thériault G, Bouchard C. Genotype-controlled changes in body composition and morphology following overfeeding in twins. Am J Clin Nutr 1986; 43:723–731.
182. Bouchard C, Tremblay A, Despres JP, Nadeau A, Lupien PJ, Thériault G, Dussault J, Moorjani S, Pinault S, Fournier G. The response to long term overfeeding in identical twins. N Engl J Med 1990; 322: 1477–1482.
183. Heitman BL, Lissner L, Sørensen TIA, Bengtsson C. Dietary fat intake and weight gain in women genetically predisposed for obesity. Am J Clin Nutr 1995; 61: 1213–1217.

29

Skeletal Muscle and Obesity

David E. Kelley

University of Pittsburgh, Pittsburgh, Pennsylvania, U.S.A.

Len Storlien

University of Wollongong, Wollongong, New South Wales, Australia, and AstraZeneca, Mölndal, Sweden

I INTRODUCTION

In obesity, there is increased nonadipose tissue as well as increased adiposity. The increase of nonadipose tissue entails an increase in skeletal muscle mass. Recent data indicate that obesity affects not only the quantity, but also the "quality" of skeletal muscle, and this will be one area of focus for this chapter. One manifestation of a change in the composition of skeletal muscle in obesity is an increased lipid content within and around muscle fibers. How this occurs is an important question. Altered composition of skeletal muscle may arise only as a consequence of having become obese, reflecting the general increase in adiposity in multiple organs. Yet, there are data that strongly suggest that changes in the physiology and biochemistry of skeletal muscle in obesity dispose to an accumulation of lipid within muscle. Indeed, these changes in muscle in fuel partitioning of lipid, between oxidation and storage of fat calories, may contribute to the pathogenesis of obesity and precede its development. This hypothesis could be of central importance to our understanding of this chronic disease and therefore will be carefully considered in this chapter.

A related theme of the chapter will be that skeletal muscle insulin resistance, a well-recognized metabolic complication of obesity, entails perturbations not only of glucose but also in fatty acid metabolism. In metabolic health, skeletal muscle physiology is characterized by the capacity to utilize either lipid or carbohydrate fuels, and to effectively transition between these fuels. We will review recent findings that indicate that in obesity, skeletal muscle manifests a loss of the capacity for transition between lipid and carbohydrate fuels. This inflexibility in fuel selection by skeletal muscle, as well as differences in fuel partitioning, is a key pathophysiological characteristic that contributes to an altered composition of muscle in obesity and to the insulin resistance of muscle.

II NONINVASIVE STUDIES OF SKELETAL MUSCLE COMPOSITION IN OBESITY

A Skeletal Muscle Quantity

Adipose tissue mass is certainly increased in obesity, and contributes substantially to increased weight. However, body composition analyses also suggest that there is an increased amount of nonadipose tissue components in obesity, including increased skeletal muscle mass. Two-compartment methods for estimating body composition, such as dual-energy x-ray absorptiometry (DXA) or underwater weighing, indicate that fat-free mass is increased in obesity. Part of the increase in fat-free mass in obesity is represented by greater muscle mass than is present in lean individuals, otherwise paired for age and sex. Using DEXA in a region-specific manner, an increase of skeletal muscle can be shown in the extremities (1). Equally, Landin et al. (2) examined lean and obese middle-aged men and women using a method to detect total body potassium, a classic method of body composition that determines tissue mass apart from adipose tissue, due to the low potassium content of fat cells. Total body potassium, calculated from the natural isotope K^{40} determined in a whole-body counter, was higher in obese men and obese women than in their lean counterparts, indicative of increased skeletal muscle mass. In general, obese individuals with a body mass index (BMI) ranging from 35 to 40 kg/m^2 and weighing ~ 100 kg have ~ 5 kg more fat-free mass than do lean subjects with a BMI of 25 and weighing ~ 70 kg. In addition, Ross et al. (3) compared total and regional lean tissue distribution in obese men and women using magnetic resonance imaging. It was found, not unexpectedly, that obese women have significantly less total lean tissue than obese men. This difference was observed regardless of which body segment (head and arms, abdomen and torso, hip and pelvic region, and legs) was evaluated.

B Skeletal Muscle Quality—Imaging of Fat and Lean Compartments

While quantitative muscle mass may be higher in obesity, a considerable body of literature has accumulated that shows that qualitatively this muscle mass is quite different in obesity with one of the features being different levels and localization of fats. Both computed tomography and magnetic resonance imaging are appropriate and sensitive tools for investigations of such issues (4).

1 Computed Tomography

Computed tomography (CT) is a powerful in vivo imaging technique of growing sophistication [see (5) for a recent review of the technique]. CT is particularly effective at distinguishing between water and lipid and this is because the attenuation values measured by CT reflect the chemical composition of tissue. Using water as a reference value [set to 0 Hounsfield units (HU)], adipose tissue imaged by CT has a strongly negative attenuation value, generally ranging from −200 to −1 Hounsfield units. Thus, for example, a finding of lower attenuation in skeletal muscle in obesity is indicative of increased fat deposition within muscle, and recent chemical phantom studies by Goodpaster et al. (5) have confirmed the relationship between lipid content and CT attenuation values.

During the past decade, a substantial body of data has emerged that indicate that the tissue composition of skeletal muscle differs between obese and nonobese individuals. Moreover, in obese individuals who undergo weight loss, the tissue composition of muscle can change. The differences in skeletal muscle composition between lean and obese individuals can be demonstrated both at the whole-organ level, using novel regional methods for body composition that have emerged in the past decade, and at the cellular level, using methods of microscopy and biochemistry. What is perhaps the most compelling finding is that skeletal muscle composition is a strong determinant of insulin resistance in obesity.

One of the earlier studies in this area was from the Kelley laboratory using CT of the thigh for regional analysis of skeletal muscle composition (6). In that study, and as later reaffirmed by Simoneau (7) and then Goodpaster et al. (1), in obesity there is increased cross-sectional area of skeletal muscle compared to lean individuals. These studies also reaffirmed the concept that women have less muscle mass than men, even when matched for degree of obesity. However, the more novel finding from these studies was that the "quality" of skeletal muscle is altered in obesity. In obesity, the CT attenuation value (expressed as Hounsfield units) of skeletal muscle is lower than in lean individuals, as shown in Figure 1. It is of interest that following weight loss the density of skeletal muscle increases and approaches the range of values found in lean individuals (8). This change in muscle reflects the fact that not only the quantity of muscle mass, but also its composition, is altered during periods of weight gain and weight loss. Reduced attenuation values for skeletal muscle are associated with aging and with gender, with lower values in older individuals and among women (9). The questions that arise therefore are what is being revealed by the reduced attenuation value of skeletal muscle, and why is this related to insulin resistance. As discussed below, muscle lipid content is a strong determinant of the CT attenuation values, and likely accounts for the association between CT attenuation values and insulin sensitivity and aspects of physical performance.

In situ imaging of skeletal muscle, as obtained by CT imaging, provides data concerning the impact of obesity on muscle structure that is not readily revealed by more classic two-compartment models, such as underwater weighing or DXA. To employ a two-compartment analysis, these approaches need to assume a constant density

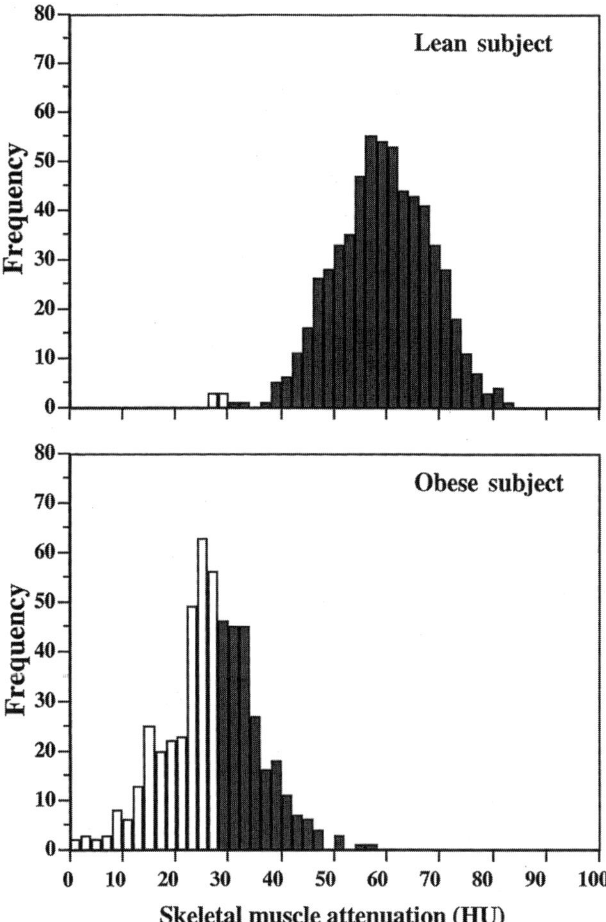

Figure 1 Shown in the upper and lower panels are histograms of the distributions of skeletal muscle attenuation values, in Hounsfield units, measured by computed tomography imaging of the midthigh skeletal muscle. The dark shaded bars for muscle from a lean subject represent the normal distribution (95% confidence levels established in a group of lean, healthy volunteers). In muscle from the obese subject, the distribution of attenuation values is shifted to the left, and just approximately half of the pixels are within the normal range.

for fat-free mass. In situ imaging modalities have revealed some of the limitations of this assumption with respect to obesity.

There is an important physiological significance to the altered composition of skeletal muscle as revealed by CT imaging. Across several studies it has been found that the altered composition of skeletal muscle in obesity, as reflected in the lower CT attenuation values, is a correlate of the severity of insulin resistance (1,7,10). This association between muscle density and insulin sensitivity is at least partially independent of the adverse effect of visceral adiposity to aggravate insulin resistance, a point to which we will return. Also, muscle attenuation values correlate to maximal aerobic capacity in young and middle-aged adults and with muscle performance in older individuals. In the Health ABC Study, a longitudinal study of the effects of aging on body composition and functional status, muscle strength and fatigue was correlated with muscle density, as revealed by CT attenuation values, after adjusting for the amount of muscle area (9).

2 Magnetic Resonance Imaging of Skeletal Muscle Lipid Content

A limitation of the computed tomography method is that the spatial resolution is not sufficient to fully distinguish between lipid contained within, and that present outside, myocytes. Areas of adipose tissue that are large enough to form a CT pixel can be identified as adipose tissue based on a negative attenuation value whereas a smaller deposit, not filling an entire pixel, might not meet attenuation characteristics to be imaged as adipose tissue. Another imaging approach, one that does seem to have a capability for distinguishing between intramyocyte and extramyocyte lipid, is magnetic resonance spectroscopy (MRS). Using MRS, and more specifically, using MRS to exploit fairly subtle chemical shift differences in these two lipid depots, it is possible to identify peaks that correspond to the methylene carbon of triglyceride from intra- and extramyocyte triglyceride (11). The extramyocyte triglyceride is contained within adipocytes within muscle, while the intramyocyte triglyceride is located within muscle fibers. Intramyocyte triglyceride is increased in obesity and is correlated with the severity of insulin resistance (12). Increases of intramyocyte triglyceride have been found in nonobese, first-degree relatives of individuals with type 2 diabetes mellitus and to relate to insulin resistance in this condition (13). The data suggest that the regional deposition of fat within skeletal muscle may be an early body composition abnormality in relation to insulin resistance, obesity, and type 2 diabetes rather than arising only as a late complication of excess adiposity.

The biochemical mechanisms that might contribute to the increased partitioning of fatty acids into muscle triglyceride are discussed later in this chapter. The fact that lipid accumulation can be seen relatively early in the development of insulin resistance adds to the concept that perturbed lipid metabolism by skeletal muscle may have a pivotal role in the development of obesity and its comorbidities.

C Regional Adipose Tissue Distribution Adjacent to Skeletal Muscle

There is another aspect of muscle composition, from the whole-organ perspective, that has been learned from the application of regional CT imaging, and this concerns the distribution of adipose tissue outside skeletal muscle. There can be substantial subcutaneous adipose tissue located near muscle, and this is especially true with respect to the lower extremities. In general, and as opposed to depots such as visceral adipose tissue, adipose tissue located in the extremities has been regarded as relatively benign with respect to insulin resistance. However, recent studies suggest that this perspective needs to be modified to account for adipose tissue distribution, or sublocations. In the lower extremities, the majority of adipose tissue is in a subcutaneous location, above the muscle fascia. In CT imaging of the midthigh, the fascial plane formed by the *fascia lata* can be discerned and it has been found that adipose tissue located beneath the *fascia lata* is significantly correlated with insulin sensitivity (negatively). In contrast, the much greater depot located above this fascia is not significantly related to insulin sensitivity in either men or women (14).

The mechanisms that account for the association of subfascial AT but not subcutaneous AT with IR are not well understood. At this juncture, only speculations can be made. Potential factors might be related to effects of fatty acids released by adipocytes adjacent to muscle, or it is also possible that in a paracrine manner, there are secreted products of this depot of adipocytes (e.g., cytokines) that influence insulin action within the adjacent skeletal muscle.

III MICROSCOPIC STUDIES OF SKELETAL MUSCLE FIBERS IN OBESITY

A Lipid Content in Muscle Fibers

Another approach to the study of lipid content within skeletal muscle is to directly examine tissue obtained by muscle biopsy. A number of studies have used muscle obtained by percutaneous biopsy of the vastus lateralis. Pan et al. (15) used this method and extracted lipid from the biopsy samples. Triglyceride was greater in skeletal muscle in obesity and was related to the severity of insulin resistance. However, even with careful removal of visibly identifiable adipose tissue, a potential limitation of performing lipid extraction from muscle biopsy samples is that the respective contributions of intra- and extramyocyte triglyceride cannot be determined. Direct visualization of muscle fibers using microscopy can circumvent this issue (16).

In situ staining of neutral lipid with Oil Red O has been used to not only to ascertain that lipid droplets are contained within muscle fibers, but by the use of contemporary computer-assisted image analyses, this method can be used to obtain quantitative assessments. Several ultrastructural investigations of human skeletal muscle have shown that lipid droplets account for ~1% of cell volume within muscle cells in lean, healthy individuals. For instance, the volume percentage occupied by lipid in skeletal muscle of women represents values ranging from 0.5% to 0.7% depending on the fiber type investigated (17). Goodpaster et al. (18) observed that the volume of lipid droplets in skeletal muscle is increased in obesity and type 2 diabetes mellitus. In that study, the approximate volume within myocytes occupied by lipid droplets was 1.5% in lean volunteers, 3–4% in obesity, and slightly greater yet in type 2 diabetes mellitus. Also, following weight loss, the microscopic analysis of muscle tissue revealed less triglyceride, as would be consistent with the data from CT imaging of skeletal muscle.

In another study using light microscopy and the Oil Red O method method, it was noted that not only the volume, but also the cellular distribution, of lipid droplets may differ in muscle from obese compared to lean individuals (19). In muscle from obese volunteers, the size of the lipid droplets did not appear to differ from those observed in muscle from nonobese individuals; simply, the muscle from obese individuals had more lipid droplets. However, in muscle from obese individuals, a higher proportion of lipid droplets appeared to be located more centrally within the muscle fiber (19). Additional research with higher resolution microscopy (e.g., electron microscopy) might be useful to further address the relation between lipid droplets and mitochondria and whether this is perturbed in muscle from obese individuals. It might be speculated that a more central location of lipid droplets within myocytes sequesters lipid, rendering it less likely to be utilized for energy. Certainly trained athletes have higher levels of intramyocellular triglyceride (20). That they are not insulin resistant may reflect both the increased mitochondrial density and possibly the distribution and relationship of the lipid droplets to those mitochondria (i.e., increased ability to utilize the fats).

B Interaction of Muscle Fiber Type and Lipid Content in Obesity

One of the striking features that can be noted when examining the Oil Red O staining patterns in skeletal muscle, especially human skeletal muscle, is that there is considerable heterogeneity between muscle fibers in the amount of lipid staining. This heterogeneity is related to muscle fiber type. It is well known, based on prior work with rat skeletal muscle, that muscle fiber types differ in their respective content of lipid (21–23). In general, type 1, or slow-twitch, oxidative (endurance) fibers contain greater lipid than type 2 fibers, and within the type 2 fibers, fast-twitch oxidative (sprint) fibers contain more lipid than do fast-twitch glycolytic (intermediate) fibers. Therefore, the question arises whether the increase in muscle triglyceride content in human obesity reflects an interdependence upon difference in muscle fiber type that might occur with obesity. To address this issue, He et al. (24) performed single-fiber analyses, in which serial sections of a muscle biopsy sample were stained for muscle lipid content (Oil Red O staining), muscle fiber type, muscle oxidative enzyme activity, and muscle glycolytic enzyme activity, as shown in Figure 2.

By serially measuring these characteristics for each muscle fiber, an overall profile for each fiber type could be ascertained. In the study by He et al. (24), vastus lateralis muscle from lean, obese, and obese type 2 diabetic men and women were examined. Lipid content was noted to be highest in type 1 fibers and lowest in type 2b fibers, with an intermediate value in type 2a fibers. This pattern was observed in all three groups of subjects, but skeletal muscle from obese and type 2 diabetic individuals was found to have increased lipid content regardless of fiber type. In each fiber type, muscle from obese individuals had greater lipid content than lean individuals, and this was also found for individuals with type 2 diabetes mellitus.

An additional and equally important finding from the study by He et al. (24) was that skeletal muscle from obese individuals and from those with type 2 diabetes mellitus had a reduced oxidative enzyme activity, as determined by standard histochemical methods. As would be expected, type 1 fibers had the highest oxidative enzyme activity, followed in order by types 2a and 2b. Within each fiber type, oxidative enzyme activity was lower in individuals with obesity and with type 2 diabetes mellitus. The ratio of oxidative enzyme activity to lipid content was also examined. In lean individuals, this ratio was relatively consistent across fiber types, despite substantial differences between fiber types in content of lipid and oxidative enzyme activities. In muscle from obese or type 2 diabetic individuals, the ratio of lipid content to oxidative capacity was also relatively consistent across fiber types, but this ratio differed markedly from that found in lean individuals. The physiological meaning of this proportionality is

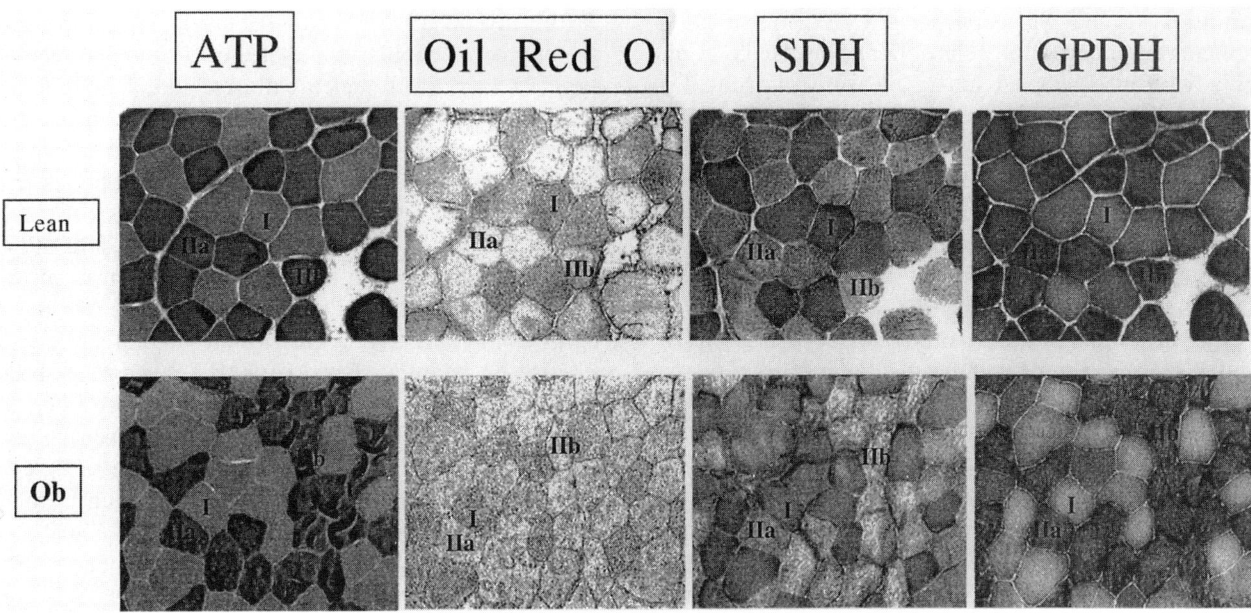

Figure 2 Skeletal muscle, biopsied from vastus lateralis muscle, is shown stained for fiber type (ATPase), lipid content (Oil Red O), oxidative enzyme capacity (SDH), and glycolytic enzyme activity (GPDH). A biopsy from a lean volunteer and one from an obese volunteer are shown. The cryosections from muscle are stained in serial order so that these respective characteristics can be assessed within single fibers.

uncertain, though it might be speculated that a homeostatic balance between fuel stores and capacity for oxidative metabolism is present in lean individuals. If this is so, then the pattern in the muscle of individuals with obesity and type 2 diabetes mellitus suggests that lipid storage is increased out of proportion to the capacity of these myocytes for substrate oxidation.

C Relation of Obesity to Muscle Fiber Type Distribution, Size, and Capillary Density

There have been several important studies that address whether the patterns of fiber type distribution differ in obesity and whether this is related to the pathogenesis of insulin resistance. It is commonly thought that type I muscle fibers in humans are better endowed for substrate oxidation than type II fibers. Reflecting this concept, it has been proposed that fiber type composition of skeletal muscle, in which type II fibers predominate, would be a determinant of obesity due to the lower substrate oxidation potential of this fiber type. In the testing of this hypothesis, conflicting results have been obtained.

A number of studies have reported that individuals with a high percentage of total body fat exhibit a low percentage of type 1 fibers in the vastus lateralis muscle (25–27). Wade et al. (26), on the basis of a rather small group of men ($N=11$), suggested that at least 40% ($r=-.65$) of the variability in fatness was related to variation in fiber type 1 proportion of vastus lateralis muscle. Similar results were obtained by Helge et al. (27), who also showed that a measure of trunk fat (central adiposity), obtained by DXA, was well related to % type 1 fibers ($r=-.58$, $P<.01$, $n=21$). A more modest correlation coefficient ($r=-.32$; $P<.01$) was reported between the fiber type 1 proportion of vastus lateralis muscle and percent body fat in the study of Lillioja et al. (25) that involved 23 Caucasians and 41 Pima Indian nondiabetic men.

On the other hand, Krotkiewski et al. (28) have shown an absence of significant relationship between the proportion of type 1 fibers and obesity. It is possible that the significant relationships previously found could have been confounded by physical fitness of the subjects, which was not controlled.

The true relation between muscle fiber type and obesity should then be determined when level of fitness is controlled. Even here, however, the results are not entirely consistent. Simoneau and Bouchard (29) did not find a significant relationship between the proportion of type 1 muscle fibers and the amount of subcutaneous fat. That study examined a large cohort of women and of men with substantial differences in subcutaneous fat content, but who were paired (within gender) on the basis of VO_2 max expressed per kg body weight. In that study, there was a lack of difference in the proportion of type 1 muscle fibers between lean and obese individuals. In contrast, Segal et al. (30) found a significantly higher proportion of type 2b fibers in vastus lateralis muscle of obese individuals (29% vs. 17%) among lean and obese subjects paired on the basis of fat-free mass and VO_2 max (30). Since it is the type 2b fibers that are glycolytic and have such limited capacity to utilize lipid for energy, it may be that this elevation as a percentage of total fibers is the critical factor. However, as we will come to below, fiber proportionality may be less relevant than oxidative capacity.

On another relevant aspect of muscle morphology, two studies from Krotkiewski et al. (28,31) have reported significant and positive correlation (with an r of $\sim .4$) between total body fat and type 1 or type 2 muscle fiber areas. These results also indicate larger muscle fibers in obesity, and thus fit nicely with the results described previously indicating elevated fat-free mass in obese subjects.

The number of capillaries surrounding muscle fibers may also play an important role in substrate and hormone delivery, and therefore in determining insulin resistance. A reduced capillary density of muscle has been described in obesity. Krotkiewski et al. (31) have reported significant and negative correlations between fasting insulin level (indicative of insulin resistance) and the number of capillaries per area of type 1 ($r=-.80$) or type 2a ($r=-.62$) skeletal muscle fibers in human. Lillioja et al. (25) confirmed that observation using a direct measure of insulin action (the hyperinsulinemic, euglycemic clamp), although the relationship was less striking. As reviewed by Björntorp (32), if a reduced capillarity of skeletal muscle is a common phenotype of obesity, then a limited transfer of insulin from the capillaries to interstitial space and the surface of myocytes could affect the kinetics of insulin action in obesity. Substantial support for this concept has been obtained. The kinetics of insulin action in skeletal muscle is slower in obesity, and this has been largely attributed to slower transcapillary diffusion of insulin more than to a reduced rate of postbinding cellular signaling.

Finally, muscle's capacity for oxidative metabolism, and particularly to utilize fat, may decline with age. While the weight of evidence suggests no major change in proportion between type 1 and type 2 fibers with age (see, e.g., 33), there is one report in an Australian population of an age-related increase in type 2b ($r=.45$,

$P = .01$) at the expense of type 2a fibers (34). In that study, both BMI and waist circumference were positively related to the percentage of type 2b fibers ($r = .44$ and .49, respectively, both $P = .01$). Interestingly, infants of age <2 years were found to have extremely low levels of type 2b fibers (~6% vs. 20+% in adults). In contrast, a comparison with a young adult population of obesity-prone Pima Indians showed this latter group to have a much higher (approximately double) percentage of type 2b fibers than would have been predicted from the regression line of age versus % type 2b for the Australian subjects. From these studies, it seems clear that fiber type changes over the life span to forms with less oxidative capacity and less able to burn fat for fuel. In addition, there may be genetic predisposition either to higher proportions of type 2b fibers at birth, or to an increased rate of transition to type 2b fibers, with age. It is not clear whether an active or sedentary lifestyle contributes to the rate of change with aging, but certainly a relatively intense exercise program can shift the proportion of type 2b toward type 2a fiber (20). This may suggest that habitual exercise will help to maintain skeletal muscle capacity for fat utilization across the life span, a suggestion that has recently received experimental support (35).

IV BIOCHEMISTRY AND MOLECULAR BIOLOGY OF SKELETAL MUSCLE IN OBESITY

A Oxidative and Glycolytic Enzyme Profiles

Though the concept that fiber type distribution per se denotes metabolic capacity of skeletal muscle for insulin sensitivity and substrate oxidation has been a useful perspective, it is not entirely sufficient. Previous studies involving microphotometric determinations (36), ultrastructural investigations (37), or microbiochemical activity determinations in dissected single fibers (38) have shown that large variation exists in the metabolic profile within each fiber type of human skeletal muscle. Although the studies do report higher average mitochondrial enzyme activities or volume density in type 1 than in type 2a or type 2b fibers, > 50% of type 1 fibers have aerobic-oxidative enzyme activities that are similar to type 2 fibers (36,37). Accordingly, it is important to distinguish between muscle enzyme capacities for substrate oxidation and muscle fiber type per se. Skeletal muscles with given enzyme activity levels may exhibit large differences in fiber type distribution, or vice versa (39). Rather than solely examining fiber type proportions, another, arguably better description of the metabolic potential of skeletal muscle would be to directly determine muscle enzyme activities.

One strategy for determining the activity of muscle enzymes is to select key marker enzymes, chosen because they regulate diverse metabolic pathways and catalyze rate-controlling reactions for distinct, critical pathways of substrate utilization. Simoneau's laboratory carried out a number of such studies by assaying a panel of key enzymes. These included key regulatory enzymes of glycolysis (PFK, HK), glycogenolysis (PHOS), aerobic oxidative metabolism (CS), oxidative phosphorylation (COX), fatty acid oxidation (CPT, HADH), and anaerobic regeneration of ATP (CK). The rationale for assaying maximal activity of regulatory enzymes, as previously justified (40), is based on conventional Michaelis-Menten kinetics. The biochemical methodology most commonly used has been to determine maximal activity (Vmax) of each enzyme chosen for the metabolic profile. The activities of enzymes catalyzing nonequilibrium reactions (i.e., regulatory enzymes) provide a semiquantitative index of both maximal metabolic flux and fuel utilization. Activities of enzymes catalyzing reactions close to equilibrium provide only qualitative information about the importance of particular metabolic pathways and the principal fuels supporting activity (41). Importantly, and what is most pertinent to a consideration of substrate metabolism in obesity, is that the influence of maximal enzyme activity may be greatest at substrate concentrations below the K_m of the enzyme (40), and these are the conditions which prevail during daily living.

In these studies, Simoneau and Kelley and others found that the activities of several marker enzymes of oxidative and glycolytic capacity were altered in obesity. Citrate synthase (CS), an enzyme of the TCA cycle activity and a strong marker of oxidative capacity, was shown to be negatively correlated with visceral obesity ($r = -.51$, $P < .05$) (42). This was confirmed in an entirely different population (Pima Indians) both for central adiposity and for % total body fat ($r = -43$, $P < .01$) (43). Conversely, CS activity was positively correlated with rates of lipid oxidation across the leg during fasting conditions and positively correlated with both whole-body insulin action and rates of glucose uptake during insulin stimulated conditions (7,44). These data indicate that oxidative capacity, as exemplified by CS activity, influences both postabsorptive utilization of FFA and insulin sensitivity. Conversely, glycolytic potential of muscle, as reflected by activity of phosphofructokinase (PFK), a regulatory enzyme in the glycolytic pathway, is increased in individuals with visceral obesity. In particular, the ratio of PFK/CS activity is a strong marker of insulin resistance. Also, creatine kinase (CK), a cytosolic enzyme that catalyzes a key step in anaerobic regeneration of ATP, is increased in proportion to obesity and insulin resistance. Taken together, this pattern of enzyme activity indicates that insulin-resistant muscle is disposed toward anaerobic and glycolytic generation of energy. Our interpretation of the enzyme and metabolic data is that obesity adversely affects substrate metabolism by skeletal muscle during both basal and insulin-stimulated conditions.

In a recently published study, Sun et al. (45) examined whether the glycolytic and oxidative enzyme characteristics of vastus lateralis skeletal muscle and fiber type proportions in this muscle predicted the response to a 100-day supervised overeating protocol carried out in identical twins. The proportion of type 1 fibers correlated inversely with the overfeeding (1000 kcal/d, 6 days per week) induced weight gain, while the proportion of type 2a fibers correlated in a positive manner with the induced change in weight (45). This would suggest that muscle with a higher capacity for fat oxidation (type 1 compared to type 2a) might protect against weight gain in the setting of sustained positive energy balance. In further support, these investigators found the ratio between oxidative to glycolytic enzyme activities was an equally strong correlate. These data suggest the key role that skeletal muscle oxidative enzyme capacity might have in protecting against, or, conversely, increasing, the risk for obesity in an environment of access to high energy intake and reduced physical activity, as prevails in modern society, and stresses the need for future research of longer periods of observation.

B Capacity for Fatty Acid Oxidation

Several clinical investigations suggest that the capacity for lipid oxidation is reduced in human skeletal muscle. Ferraro et al. (46) found that skeletal muscle lipoprotein lipase activity was decreased in obesity and that this was related to a decreased reliance on fat oxidation, as measured in a whole-body calorimetry chamber. Zurlo et al. (47), using a similar approach, found that marker enzymes of the beta-oxidation pathway are reduced in obesity. Simoneau (48) found reduced activity of CPT in skeletal muscle in obesity. The reduction in skeletal muscle CPT activity was of approximately the same proportion as the decrease in activity of other marker enzymes of mitochondria, such as citrate synthase for the TCA cycle and cytochrome C oxidase of the electron transport chain. This suggests a decrease in mitochondria number or function, or both. Interestingly, following weight loss the subjects in the study by Simoneau (48) did not have improvement in the capacity for fat oxidation as measured by activities of CPT, CS, and cytochrome C oxidase. In that same study, an increased content of cytosolic fatty acid binding protein was found in obesity, with an additional gender-related effect of higher concentrations in women. However, other groups have found diminished content of cytosolic fatty acid–binding protein in skeletal muscle in obese individuals with type 2 diabetes (49).

Another line of investigation into the capacity of skeletal muscle for lipid oxidation concerns malonyl CoA. Although skeletal muscle has a relatively limited capacity for de novo lipogenesis, it does synthesize malonyl CoA. Ruderman and colleagues (50) have found that muscle content of malonyl CoA in rodents increases in response to insulin and glucose, and can be increased in insulin resistance and following denervation. Similar studies by Winder and colleagues (51) indicate that increased muscle glucose metabolism in skeletal muscle of the rat leads to an increased malonyl CoA concentration. This is potentially germane to the capacity for lipid oxidation because an increase in malonyl CoA can inhibit CPT I, the muscle isoform of which is particularly sensitive to inhibition by malonyl CoA (52). Several groups have studied the regulation of acetyl CoA carboxylase (ACC), the enzyme responsible for synthesizing malonyl CoA from carbohydrate (53,54). The thrust of this line of investigation is that conditions may prevail in obesity and glucose intolerance, as well as inactivity, for accumulation of malonyl CoA in skeletal muscle and thus lead to allosteric inhibition of CPT I and, consequently, an inhibition of lipid oxidation. Certainly, prolonged inhibition of CPT1 has been shown to increase intramyocellular triglyceride in studies on rodents (55). Then, excess triglyceride or FFA in muscle might lead to increased long chain acyl-CoA concentrations (56–58), which in turn might lead to further insulin resistance. We will return to this issue.

Still another line of inquiry concerns uncoupling proteins. Uncoupling proteins are postulated to influence thermogenesis, as is well supported by the role of UCP 1 in brown adipose tissue and suggested for homologs UCP 2 and 3. These findings have potential implications for the pathogenesis of obesity. Nordfors et al. (59) reported decreased expression of UCP 2 in skeletal muscle of human obese subjects. However, Simoneau et al. (60) found increased protein content UCP 2 in human skeletal muscle from obese individuals, and examined the potential relation to energy expenditure and substrate oxidation, as well as to insulin resistance, which is common in obesity. Skeletal muscle UCP 2 content was significantly higher in obesity and was positively correlated with %FM ($r = .60$; $P < .05$). However, UCP 2 content in muscle was not correlated with basal energy expenditure ($r = .03$; $P = .93$), nor with insulin stimulated rates of glucose metabolism Rd ($r = -.21$; $P = .47$) (60). There was a significant correlation between muscle UCP 2 and patterns of macronutrient substrate oxidation within skeletal muscle, such increased UCP 2 was associated with higher fasting values of leg RQ ($r = .57$; $P < .05$), suggesting that UCP 2 may help to regulate nutrient partitioning within muscle and favor carbohydrate oxidation. Several lines of evidence suggest that UCP 3 expression is related to fatty acid availability (61).

C Structural and Storage Lipid Subtypes and Lipid Signaling in Obesity

Lipids play a role in muscle metabolism not only as an energy source. As with all tissues of the body they are the major structural components of plasma and organelle membranes and act as potent metabolic intermediates in cellular signaling with their actions strongly dependent on the fatty acid subtypes involved. The fatty acid composition of structural and storage lipid in skeletal muscle is influenced both by genetic predisposition and by environment (particularly dietary fatty acid profile).

There is now considerable evidence linking obesity and skeletal muscle insulin resistance to the fatty acid composition of both phospholipid, the major membrane structural lipid (15,62,63) and myocellular storage triglyceride (64). These studies show that an increased proportion of saturated fatty acids in both lipid compartments relate directly and positively to impaired insulin action and to various measures of regional and total increased adiposity. A number of mechanisms have been postulated. Increased saturation of membrane lipids should decrease membrane fluidity, leakiness to ions and protons and hence decrease metabolic rate (see 65). Interestingly, increased membrane unsaturation improves intrinsic activity of ion transporters thus providing the conditions, in concert, to allow maintenance of ion homeostasis (66). Equally, it has been demonstrated that beta-adrenergic receptor affinity is decreased with dietary treatment emphasizing saturated fat intake (67), which is also consistent with decreased metabolic rate.

The indirect effects on energy balance via modulation of insulin action by lipid intermediates is likely to involve a complex series of cellular metabolic interactions which, pleasingly, the data are now beginning to clarify. Briefly, saturated fatty acids like palmitate specifically inhibit PKB/Akt activation and, concomitantly, insulin-stimulated glucose uptake in primary myocyte cultures (68). Equally, PKB activation has been shown to inhibit insulin stimulation of glycogen synthase kinase-3, thus impairing cellular capacity for glycogen synthesis (69,70). Both of these observations are likely to involve ceramide production; ceramide is a sphingolipid derivative of palmitate, being the condensation product of serine and palmitoylCoA. Ceramides are on the synthetic pathway for, and are also formed from the breakdown of, sphingomyelins. Sphingomyelin concentrations in adipose tissue and plasma have been shown to be positively related to obesity (71,72). Cytokines like tumor necrosis factor-alpha (TNF-α) increase breakdown of sphingomyelins. Interestingly, salicylates (aspirin is acetylsalicylate) inhibit sphingomyelin-generated ceramide production and high doses have been shown to reduce obesity and improve insulin action (73,74) although other mechanisms are also likely to be important in explaining this observation.

Additional mechanisms of fatty acid modulation of muscle lipid metabolism are likely to come via influences on the sterol regulatory element–binding proteins (SREBPs). Activation particularly of SREBP1c induces a number of enzymes in the pathways of de novo fatty acid synthesis and through to triglyceride formation (see 75). It has recently been shown that while palmitate slightly induces SREBP1 expression in cell systems, more unsaturated fatty acids are powerfully inhibitory (76). Equally, it has been shown that diacylglycerol (DAG) accumulation, from an increase in fatty acyl-CoA availability, specifically from palmitate impairs insulin-stimulated glucose uptake in primary myocyte cultures (68). DAGs activate a number of isoforms of protein kinase C (PKC), and it is likely that a mechanism linking DAG accumulation from palmitate to impaired insulin action involves the known PKC inhibition of glucose transporter translocation. Palmitate is the major end product of endogenous lipogenesis via the fatty acid synthase cascade. In this regard it is interesting that mice with absent or reduced fatty acid synthase activity (knockout or cerulenin-treated) are lean and resistant to high-fat feeding-induced obesity (77). While the contribution of endogenous lipogenesis to the total fatty acid pool in humans is a matter of controversy, it is now clear that saturated fatty acids play both a direct and indirect role in a range of skeletal muscle metabolic processes that will combine to predispose obesity.

V CLINICAL INVESTIGATIONS OF FATTY ACID METABOLISM BY SKELETAL MUSCLE IN OBESITY

A Postabsorptive Patterns of Fatty Acid Use by Skeletal Muscle

Skeletal muscle can oxidize either lipid or carbohydrate to yield energy. During postabsorptive conditions, as occur after an overnight fast, skeletal muscle predominately relies on lipid oxidation. This is reflected in a respiratory quotient (RQ) across the forearm in lean individuals of approximately 0.71 to 0.82 (78–80). There is also a high rate of extraction of plasma FFA by skeletal muscle during fasting conditions, of ~40% (79). Oxidation of plasma FFA taken up by muscle, if these were to be completely oxidized, would account for nearly 80% of resting oxygen consumption by muscle. Thus, it is clear that skeletal muscle can have an important role in systemic patterns of fatty acid utilization, especially during postabsorptive metabolism.

In obesity, skeletal muscle has an increased content of triglyceride, as was emphasized in the preceding section. Accordingly, it is important to inquire as to the mechanisms that could account for increased skeletal muscle lipid deposition in obesity. Rates of de novo lipogenesis are low within skeletal muscle (81). Accordingly, skeletal muscle accretion of triglyceride in obesity would seem to arise as a consequence of an imbalance between the "importation" of plasma fatty acids and rates of fatty acid oxidation. Such a putative imbalance might result from increased fatty acid uptake, perhaps driven by increased plasma concentrations of fatty acids. Recent work from Boden and coworkers (82) has provided strong support for this possibility. In healthy young volunteers, they increased FFA levels by a combination of intralipid and heparin during a prolonged hyperinsulinemic, euglycemic clamp. They then measured both insulin action and accumulation of intramyocellular triglyceride by NMR spectroscopy. Even within 3–4 hr there was significant accumulation of intramyocellular triglyceride which related significantly to both the magnitude of elevation of the plasma FFA levels and, importantly, to the FFA-induced insulin resistance (82). Alternatively (or additionally), the excess accumulation of skeletal muscle triglyceride in obesity might arise from diminished rates of fat oxidation. Given the normal high reliance of skeletal muscle on lipid oxidation during postabsorptive conditions, it would seem logical to inquire whether any defect in lipid oxidation in obesity is evident in this physiological context.

During the past decade and more, a number of studies have begun to address whether patterns of lipid utilization by skeletal muscle differ in obese compared to nonobese individuals. Ravussin and colleagues found that obesity is associated with an impaired capacity for oxidation of fat calories (46,83). These studies included data which suggest that higher values for RQ predict weight gain over several subsequent years (83). Two of the principal areas of investigation of the Kelley laboratory, especially in those studies carried out in collaboration with the late Jean-Aime Simoneau, have been to examine whether skeletal muscle capacity for lipid oxidation is reduced in obesity and whether there is a link between fasting patterns of muscle FFA utilization and insulin resistance.

An initial study in these directions, by Colberg et al. (44) was carried out in healthy young women who had a range of body mass index from 19 to 39 kg/m^2. A key finding was that postabsorptive rates of FFA utilization by muscle were diminished in relation to visceral obesity. Women with increased visceral fat had neither lower plasma FFA nor lower rates for systemic appearance of FFA, yet manifested a reduced rate of plasma FFA uptake across the leg. The study also provided initial data that defects of lipid utilization by skeletal muscle and defects of insulin-stimulated glucose utilization might occur together. This was suggested by the correlation between fasting rates of lipid oxidation in muscle and insulin-stimulated rates of glucose storage in muscle ($r = .61$, $P < .05$).

B Metabolic Inflexibility of Substrate Utilization by Skeletal Muscle in Obesity

Based on the findings from that initial study by Colberg (44) and similar data from other investigators (84), Kelley and Simoneau undertook a larger clinical investigation involving both men and women, and involving a weight loss intervention among the obese individuals (10). The first objective was to examine fasting patterns of lipid metabolism in order to test the hypothesis that reliance on lipid oxidation is reduced in obesity. The second objective was to determine whether fasting patterns of lipid metabolism were associated with the phenotype of insulin resistance in obesity. A close corollary to this was to assess how fasting patterns of lipid metabolism related to lipid metabolism during insulin-stimulated conditions. A third goal was to assess the impact of weight loss. The effects of weight loss are described in the subsequent section.

Volunteers for this study were approximately 60 healthy young adults. One-third of the group was lean. The rest were overweight or obese with BMIs >25 kg/m^2 and ranging to an upper limit of 40. Leg balance measurements (product of arteriovenous differences and blood flow) for glucose and FFA uptake (based on the fractional extraction of [9, 10 ^{3}H] oleate) were carried out during fasting and insulin-stimulated conditions. Also, indirect calorimetry across the leg was performed to estimate substrate oxidation during fasting and insulin-stimulated conditions. The constant infusion of labeled oleate permitted measurement of uptake of plasma FFA across the leg despite the negative net balance of plasma FFA that occurs during postabsorptive conditions. Muscle tissue was obtained by percutaneous biopsy of the *vastus lateralis* muscle. Following baseline studies, the obese volunteers entered a weight loss intervention.

During fasting conditions, there was robust fractional extraction (FEX) of labeled FFA across the leg, of ~40%, indicative of the uptake of plasma FFA by leg tissues. The FEX was similar in lean and obese subjects and was approximately 10- to 15-fold higher during fasting conditions than corresponding FEX for glucose. Rates of FFA uptake across the leg were similar in lean and obese subjects. However, despite similar rates of FFA uptake across the leg, rates of fat oxidation across the leg during fasting conditions were less in obese compared to lean subjects ($P<.01$). During fasting conditions, obese subjects had an elevated leg RQ (0.90 ± 0.01 vs. 0.83 ± 0.02 in lean controls; $P<.01$). The RQ values across the leg in obesity denoted a reduced reliance on lipid oxidation, such that only a third of energy production was accounted for by fat oxidation while nearly twice that proportion was found in muscle of lean volunteers. In both lean and obese volunteers, the fasting rates of fatty acid uptake across the leg were greater than the fasting rates of lipid oxidation, indicating a modest net surplus of fatty acid uptake, as has been well described in animal studies (22,23). These rates of "net storage" of fatty acids were greater in obesity. Thus, a paradigm suggested by these findings is that in obesity, skeletal muscle accrues triglyceride owing to a reduced rate of lipid oxidation in the face of rates of fatty acid uptake that are equivalent to those of lean individuals.

A further key objective of the study of Kelley et al. (10) was to address the potential relation between insulin-resistant glucose metabolism and patterns of fatty acid uptake and oxidation during both fasting and insulin-stimulated conditions. Considering all subjects, lean and obese, a decreased reliance on lipid oxidation during fasting conditions was associated with resistance to insulin stimulation of glucose metabolism, as shown in Figure 3. Fasting values for leg RQ were negatively correlated with insulin sensitivity ($r = -.57$, $P<.001$). Thus, in addition to group differences in fasting leg RQ, there was significant correlation between the individual variation in the severity of obesity-related insulin resistance and fasting patterns of glucose and lipid oxidation in leg tissues. This observation extends our perceptions of what constitutes the phenotype of skeletal muscle insulin resistance since it reveals metabolic defects beyond those of insulin-stimulated metabolism. Thus, the phenotype of skeletal muscle insulin resistance in obesity appears to entail a broader concept of a organ system poorly performing its homeostatic function of substrate utilization. This concept may be central to understanding the role of skeletal muscle in the pathogenesis of obesity and obesity-related comorbid conditions, such as type 2 diabetes mellitus.

The hypothesis that insulin resistance is associated with decreased fasting fatty acid oxidation is a novel reformulation of the concept that perturbed skeletal muscle fatty acid metabolism may contribute to skeletal

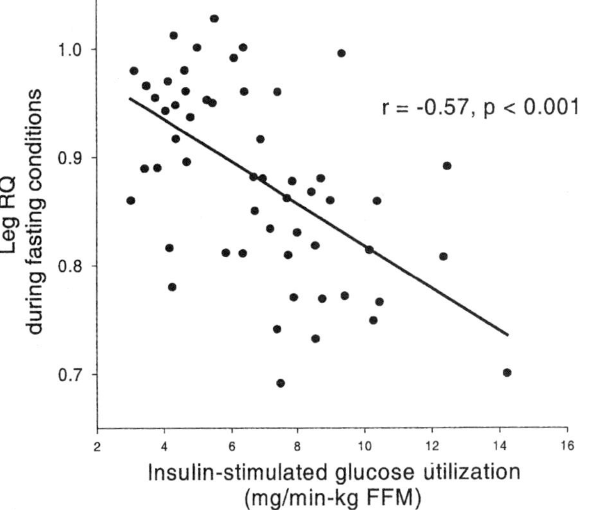

Figure 3 Values for the respiratory quotient across the leg, during fasting conditions, measured by arteriovenous differences for oxygen and carbon dioxide in lean and obese volunteers are plotted against the respective values for insulin-stimulated rates of glucose utilization, measured using the glucose clamp method. There was a significant negative correlation between these variables. Individuals with a low value for leg RQ during fasting conditions, signifying a greater reliance on fat oxidation during fasting conditions, had a higher value for insulin sensitivity than did those individuals with a lower reliance on fat oxidation (as signified by the higher values for leg RQ) during fasting conditions.

muscle insulin resistance. The more classic concept of substrate competition in relation to insulin resistance is that "excessive" lipid oxidation reduces glucose utilization by skeletal muscle. It is appropriate to ask whether the finding that reduced fat oxidation during fasting conditions is related to insulin resistance of obesity is a contradiction to the "classic" Randle hypothesis of substrate competition and insulin resistance. Several recent studies indicate that glucose inhibits fat oxidation (85,86), a so-called reverse Randle cycle, which could be pertinent to the observation that insulin-resistant skeletal muscle in animal models of obesity has increased malonyl CoA (50) and that inhibition of ACC2 which decreases malonyl CoA results both in lower body fatness and improved glucose tolerance in mice (87).

In the study by Kelley et al. (10) insulin-stimulated conditions were examined, and therefore the role of fat oxidation during this physiological context was assessed in obesity and in relation to insulin-stimulated glucose metabolism. Under the stimulation of insulin, utilization of fatty acids by skeletal muscle is normally suppressed (88), though this can be disturbed by increased availability of plasma fatty acids (89,90). In lean subjects in these studies (10), infusion of insulin stimulated a significant increase in leg RQ ($P < .001$), as shown in Figure 4, whereas in obese subjects, the insulin-stimulated values for leg RQ did not differ from fasting values of leg RQ. In lean subjects, infusion of insulin also stimulated a significant increase in rates of energy expenditure across the leg ($P < .01$), whereas in obese subjects, rates of energy expenditure across the leg were unchanged compared to fasting conditions. Insulin-stimulated values for leg RQ were significantly greater in lean compared to obese subjects (0.99 ± 0.03 vs. 0.91 ± 0.02; $P < .01$). Thus, during insulin-stimulated conditions, obese subjects manifested a failure to suppress lipid oxidation and rates of lipid oxidation were unchanged from fasting conditions.

During insulin infusions, rates of leg lipid oxidation were negatively correlated to insulin sensitivity ($r = -.45$, $P < .001$); that is, greater lipid oxidation during insulin-stimulated conditions predicted insulin-resistant glucose metabolism, whereas during postabsorptive conditions, lower rates of lipid oxidation predicted insulin-resistant glucose metabolism. These findings are not disparate, but instead are interconnected pieces of the puzzle of how insulin resistance is manifest within skeletal muscle in obesity. The concept that links these two findings is one of metabolic flexibility as a component of insulin sensitivity in lean individuals and metabolic inflexibility as a component of insulin resistance in obesity. Obese subjects had less change in leg RQ in response to insulin infusion than did lean subjects.

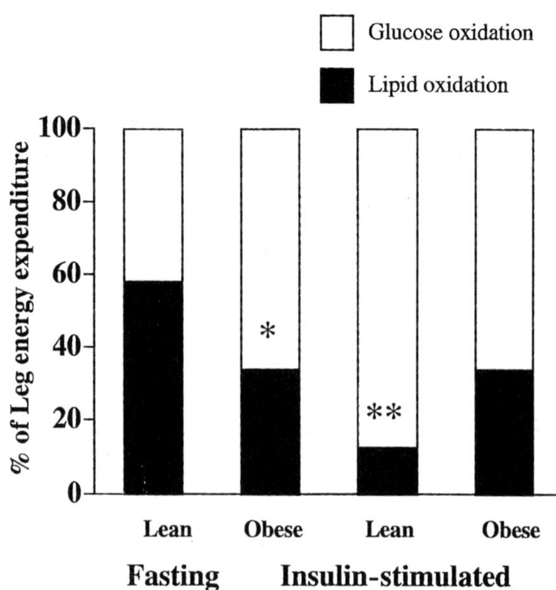

Figure 4 The contrast between a metabolic flexibility in the transition seen in lean subjects from a predominant oxidation of fat during fasting condition to predominant oxidation of carbohydrate during insulin-stimulated conditions is contrasted to a metabolic inflexibility in skeletal muscle in obese subjects, in whom there is little change in the relative proportions of carbohydrate and fat oxidation in the transitions from fasting to insulin-stimulated conditions, or vice versa.

Across the entire cohort, the amplitude of insulin-stimulated change in leg RQ (Δ leg RQ: insulin-stimulated leg RQ $-$ fasting leg RQ) correlated significantly with insulin-stimulated increases in glucose metabolism ($r = .66$, $P < .001$). This indicates responsiveness to insulin in modulation of leg RQ is related to capacity to respond to insulin stimulation of glucose uptake.

In obesity, the effect of insulin to suppress lipid oxidation was blunted, as has been previously reported (91, 92), and this clearly fits with the classic concept of fatty acid induced insulin resistance (93). Not only was incomplete suppression of lipid oxidation during insulin stimulation observed among the obese volunteers in this study, but rates of muscle lipid oxidation during insulin infusion were correlated with the severity of insulin-resistant glucose metabolism.

In summary, these observations do not indicate that fatty acid oxidation within insulin-resistant muscle is persistently "increased." While insulin infusion did not suppress muscle lipid oxidation in obesity (compared to strong suppression in lean individuals), these rates of fat oxidation were unchanged from fasting conditions. During fasting conditions, rates of fat oxidation in skeletal muscle were lower in obese than in lean individuals.

Thus, in regard to the nature of substrate competition, muscle in obesity manifested a severe inflexibility in the modulation of fatty acid oxidation, with neither suppression by insulin infusion nor an appropriate enhancement in response to an overnight fast.

C Effects of Weight Loss on Skeletal Muscle Lipid Metabolism

A critical issue is that of etiology, that is, whether impairments within the pathways of fatty acid utilization in skeletal muscle in obesity are primary defects or arise secondarily, after an individual has become obese. This is difficult to effectively address by cross-sectional comparisons of lean and obese subjects. A prospective clinical study has indicated that a decreased reliance on lipid oxidation is a risk factor for weight gain (83) and collateral analyses of skeletal muscle enzyme activities have implicated skeletal muscle in impaired lipid oxidation (46,47). A reduced reliance on lipid oxidation has also been identified as a risk factor for weight regain following weight loss (84,94,95). These data raise the possibility that a potential impairment in capacity for lipid oxidation might be a primary defect in obesity. Equally, weight loss can substantially improve insulin-resistant glucose metabolism in skeletal muscle (96) and at least aspects of muscle fat transport (97). This would seem to indicate that there may be also an acquired or secondary component of obesity-related insulin resistant glucose metabolism.

The third objective of the study by Kelley and colleagues (10), described earlier, was therefore to assess whether weight loss, undertaken by dietary restriction, could modulate patterns of skeletal muscle metabolism of fatty acids and how this would compare with the effect on glucose metabolism. Weight loss was achieved through restricted calorie intake and without changes in physical activity patterns or maximal aerobic capacity. A substantial weight loss was achieved (14.0 ± 0.9 kg, of which 10.3 ± 0.8 kg was loss of fat mass) and then followed by a 1-month period of careful weight stabilization prior to re-assessments of metabolism. Fasting plasma insulin decreased (117 ± 5 vs. 62 ± 5 pmol/L; $P < .01$), as did plasma leptin (from 39 ± 2 to 21 ± 2 ng/mL in women and from 16 ± 3 to 6 ± 2 ng/mL in men). There were reductions in fasting plasma triglycerides, apoB, and total cholesterol. Systemic insulin-stimulated glucose metabolism increased following weight loss (5.9 ± 0.4 vs. 7.5 ± 0.5 mg/kg FFM; $P < .001$), and there was a twofold increase in arteriovenous differences for glucose following weight loss ($P < .001$).

With respect to fasting patterns of skeletal muscle fatty acid metabolism, the effect of loss of weight was relatively modest. Skeletal muscle oxidative enzyme activity was slightly diminished, and activity of CPT was unchanged (and remained lower than in lean subjects). Not unexpectedly (98,99), rates of resting energy expenditure measured by limb balance were lower following weight loss, and rates of fatty acid uptake were slightly reduced. Yet, the leg RQ was unchanged from pre–weight loss values; thus, reliance of skeletal muscle on fat oxidation during fasting conditions was not improved. The observation that weight loss had a lesser effect on fatty acid metabolism than on glucose metabolism raises the provocative question as to whether abnormal fatty acid metabolism by muscle is a primary rather than an acquired metabolic impairment in obesity or obesity-prone individuals. Persistent impairment of fatty acid metabolism has been previously reported following weight loss (84,94,95,100). These data would suggest that these defects could be primary impairments, leading to obesity rather than merely resulting from obesity. Furthermore, it is interesting to speculate on what might have happened had the intervention included aerobic exercise. In lean sedentary subjects, aerobic exercise training promotes an increase in oxidative enzyme capacity and this is accompanied by an increased rate of fatty acid oxidation during exercise conditions (40,101).

Two changes that did occur in muscle fatty acid metabolism following weight loss were that insulin infusion stimulated a significant rise in leg RQ (compared to fasting values) and a significant suppression of fat oxidation, and there was an overall increase in muscle attenuation values on CT imaging (indicating a loss of muscle fat). Furthermore, following weight loss, rates of fatty acid uptake during insulin-stimulated conditions were nearly equivalent to rates of fat oxidation, whereas the rate of fat oxidation had exceeded fatty acid uptake during insulin infusions prior to weight loss. This change in insulin-stimulated patterns of muscle fatty acid metabolism is indicative of more complete suppression of lipolysis of muscle triglyceride.

VI INSULIN-RESISTANT GLUCOSE METABOLISM OF OBESITY

While the perspective of this chapter has been to give emphasis to the emerging concepts of altered fatty acid metabolism in skeletal muscle, it is also important to review the substantial body of data concerning insulin resistant glucose metabolism in obesity. In obesity, skeletal muscle typically manifests insulin resistance. This observation derived from seminal clinical investigations, conducted nearly three decades ago (102,103).

The insulin resistance of obesity seems to affect the pathway of glucose storage more severely than that of glucose oxidation (91,104,105). Recognition of this metabolic pattern in the insulin resistance of obesity has spurred a thorough examination of the insulin regulation of the glycogen synthesis pathway, with particular focus on the enzyme glycogen synthase, which is generally regarded as a rate-limiting step in glycogen synthesis (41). Obesity is associated with impairment in insulin activation, via dephosphorylation, of glycogen synthase (104), and the magnitude of this defect is correlated to the defect in nonoxidative glucose metabolism and overall systemic insulin resistance. Thus, these findings affirm the importance of impaired glycogen formation within muscle as a key process in the pathophysiology of insulin resistance in obesity.

In the past decade, several novel methods for studying proximal steps of glucose metabolism (i.e., glucose transport and phosphorylation) within skeletal muscle have been developed for clinical investigations and again NMR is important for imaging substrate concentrations within tissue. In addition, positron emission tomography (PET) is a region-specific imaging method that provides spatial mapping of metabolism. Both of these methods have been applied to the study of skeletal muscle insulin resistance. In a series of elegant studies, Shulman and colleagues (106–108) have used NMR to investigate skeletal muscle metabolism. By combining NMR with infusion of ^{13}C glucose, these investigators have been able to quantify rates of insulin-stimulated glycogen formation in skeletal muscle, and have found that this metabolic pathway is profoundly disturbed in the insulin resistance of type 2 diabetes mellitus, and with the insulin resistance of obesity. This group has also used phosphorous NMR to study accretion of glucose-6-phosphate during insulin-stimulated conditions, as a means to study insulin regulation of glucose transport and phosphorylation. These studies indicate that in obesity, there is impairment of these proximal steps of glucose metabolism. A similar overall conclusion has been achieved using a limb balance approach combined with isotope tracers to separately study glucose transport and phosphorylation (109,110), though this method has not been used in obesity per se, but only in obesity complicated by type 2 diabetes mellitus. Dynamic PET imaging, combined with mathematical modeling of the tissue activity curves of the uptake of the tracer ^{18}F-deoxy-glucose has revealed that in obesity there are potentially separate impediments of insulin activation of both glucose transport and phosphorylation (111,112). These findings from NMR, PET, and the forearm triple-tracer method indicate that glucose transport and phophorylation are rate-controlling sites of insulin action in skeletal muscle.

Among overweight individuals, the severity of insulin resistance is correlated with the degree of obesity, though in a nonlinear manner (113). In males, beyond a body fat content of $\sim 30\%$, the impairment of insulin sensitivity is not further aggravated by greater adiposity. Also in men, and to an even more pronounced extent in women, the relationship between obesity and insulin resistance is influenced by body fat distribution and is greater in proportion to upper body fat distribution (114).

The issue of body fat distribution as it relates to insulin-resistant glucose metabolism in skeletal muscle is a particularly interesting topic and can be extended beyond consideration of upper- versus lower-body fat distribution. As cited previously, fat deposition within muscle is a powerful marker of insulin resistance, and this component of fat distribution contributes to insulin resistance independently from overall adiposity (42). These results were paralleled by those of Pan et al. (15), who showed that skeletal muscle triglyceride concentrations and a measure of central adiposity were both strong, independent influences on whole-body insulin action in a nondiabetic group of adult Pima Indians. The negative effects of obesity to cause insulin resistance can be modulated by physical activity and training (as reviewed in 115) such that insulin resistance tends to be less severe among obese individuals with higher indices of aerobic power (116).

In the diet intervention study in obese men and women described earlier (10), an additional purpose was to examine whether the amount of weight loss or the amount of change within a specific aspect of regional fat determined the extent of improvement in insulin-resistant glucose metabolism in skeletal muscle. The average weight loss was 15% of baseline weight, and there were substantial and significant losses of fat mass, visceral adipose tissue (measured by cross-sectional CT imaging), and abdominal subcutaneous adiposity, as well as thigh subcutaneous adiposity (8). There was of course, individual variation in the amount of weight loss and of weight loss associated changes in the various components of regional adiposity, and as well, in the amount of change in insulin sensitivity of muscle glucose uptake. The amount of weight loss, or loss of fat mass (absolute or as a percentage), did not significantly correlate with the amount of improvement in insulin resistance. However, the percentage change in visceral adiposity did significantly correlate with the improvement in insulin resistance (8). This was the first clinical investigation to demonstrate a specific link between changes in insulin sensitivity and changes in visceral adiposity, though earlier studies had shown a correlation with improved glucose tolerance. These findings add additional credence to the concept that the amount of visceral fat, although a relatively small proportion of total body adipose tissue mass, is nevertheless of special significance for muscle metabolism.

In recent studies carried out in 23 men and women with type 2 diabetes mellitus, using PET imaging to measure muscle insulin sensitivity of glucose metabolism, the level of insulin-suppressed fatty acids was found to be a strong determinant ($r = -.81, P < .001$), and in turn, the level of insulin-suppressed fatty acids was found to be correlated with visceral adiposity but not with other depots of adipose tissue or fat mass. Thus, it will be crucial to continue to examine the link between muscle insulin resistance and visceral adiposity in order to advance our understanding of the metabolic complications of obesity.

VII SUMMARY AND CONCLUSIONS

In summary, the composition and biochemistry of skeletal muscle are altered in obese as compared to nonobese individuals. These alterations dispose to a reduction in the role of skeletal muscle in oxidation of lipid calories and to a pattern of macronutrient partitioning that increases lipid storage within skeletal muscle and systemically. Such a key role for skeletal muscle in the pathogenesis of obesity is certainly consistent with the capacity which skeletal muscle has to utilize both carbohydrate and lipid fuels and with the major role which skeletal muscle can have in overall fuel balance. An important morphological characteristic of skeletal muscle in obesity is increased content of fat, particularly the intramyocellular component. Accretion of fat within muscle tissues appears to strongly correlate with insulin resistance. This fat accretion within muscle of obese individuals may not be simply a passive process, paralleling fat storage in other tissues. Instead, and of particular metabolic interest, is the emerging concept that biochemical characteristics of skeletal muscle in obese individuals dispose to fat accumulation in muscle and may contribute substantially to the development and maintenance of the obese state. These biochemical characteristics of muscle in obese individuals have long been recognized to include insulin resistance in pathways of glucose metabolism, and more recent studies indicate as well a reduced capacity for the utilization of fat calories. Again, it must be emphasized that a key feature of skeletal muscle in obesity is a marked inflexibility in modulation of fat utilization.

Further research is needed to define the stages at which these patterns emerge. Whether these factors exist prior to the onset of increased rates of weight gain and obesity or whether they occur in response to these changes has not been clearly delineated. An important area of investigation is to assess skeletal muscle characteristics in longitudinal studies, relating skeletal muscle characteristics (oxidative enzyme levels, fiber proportions, etc.) to subsequent development of obesity and stratified for levels of physical activity. Such studies should be possible on cohorts of individuals studied one to two decades ago and would increase enormously our understanding of the role of muscle morphology in the etiology of obesity.

The task at present is to more precisely define the nature of the defects within the pathways of fat metabolism, to discern the contribution of environmental and genetic influences, and to utilize these insights to develop effective treatment strategies. An effort to modify skeletal muscle of obese individuals so that its capacity for substrate utilization (and in particular, fat oxidation) is improved should be among the goals of treatment for obesity. Whether capacity for fat oxidation by muscle can be enhanced by pharmacological treatment is largely unknown, and though it is clear that nutritional and exercise interventions can improve insulin sensitivity of skeletal muscle in obese individuals, there remains much to be learned about optimal behavioral methods to attain this goal.

ACKNOWLEDGMENTS

The authors would like foremost to acknowledge and remember the valuable contributions of Dr. Jean-Aimé Simoneau, who passed away in 1999. Dr. Simoneau was an insightful investigator of obesity and the role of skeletal muscle in the pathogenesis of obesity. This chapter is dedicated to his memory. We would also like to acknowledge the helpful comments of many colleagues, and the cooperation of the many research volunteers, without whom this knowledge could not have been gained.

REFERENCES

1. Goodpaster BH, Thaete FL, Simoneau J-A, Kelley DE. Subcutaneous abdominal fat and thigh muscle composition predict insulin sensitivity independently of visceral fat. Diabetes 1997; 46:1579–1585.
2. Landin K, Lindgärde F, Saltin B, Wilhelmsen L. Decreased skeletal muscle potassium in obesity. Acta Med Scand 1988; 223:507–513.

3. Ross R, Shaw KD, Rissanen J, Martel Y, De Guise J, Avruch L. Sex differences in lean and adipose tissue distribution by magnetic resonance imaging: anthropometric relationships. Am J Clin Nutr 1994; 59:1277–1285.
4. Mitsiopoulos N, Baumgartner RN, Heymsfield SB, Lyons W, Gallagher D, Ross R. Cadaver validation of skeletal muscle measurement by magnetic resonance imaging and computerized tomography. J Appl Physiol 1998; 85:115–122.
5. Goodpaster BH, Kelley DE, Thaete FL, He J, Ross R. Skeletal muscle attenuation determined by computed tomography is associated with skeletal muscle lipid content. J App Physiol 2000; 89:104–110.
6. Kelley DE, Slasky S, Janosky J. Effects of obesity and non-insulin dependent diabetes mellitus. Am J Clin Nutr 1991; 54:509–515.
7. Simoneau J-A, Kelley DE. Altered glycolytic and oxidative capacities of skeletal muscle contribute to insulin resistance in NIDDM. J Appl Physiol 1997; 83:166–171.
8. Goodpaster BH, Kelley DE, Wing RR, Meier A, Thaete FL. Effects of weight loss on insulin sensitivity in obesity: Influence of regional adiposity. Diabetes 1999; 48:839–847.
9. Goodpaster BH, Carlson CL, Visser M, Kelley DE, Scherzinger A, Harris TB, Stamm E, Newman AB. Attenuation of skeletal muscle and strength in the elderly: The Health ABC Study. J Appl Physiol 2001; 90:2157–2165.
10. Kelley DE, Goodpaster BH, Wing RR, Simoneau J-A. Skeletal muscle fatty acid metabolism in association with insulin resistance, obesity and weight loss. Am J Physiol Endocrinol Metab 1999; 40(277):E1130–E1141.
11. Boesch C, Slotboom J, Hoppeler H, Kreis R. In vivo determination of intra-myocellular lipids in human muscle by means of localized 1H-MR-spectroscopy. Magn Reson Med 1997; 37:484–493.
12. Szcepaniak LS, Babcock EE, Schick F, Dobbins RL, Garg A, Burns DK, McGarry JD, Stein DT. Measurement of intracellular triglyceride stores by H spectroscopy: validation in vivo. Am J Physiol Endocrinol Metab 1999; 276:E977–E989.
13. Perseghin G, Scifo P, De Cobelli F, Pagliato E, Battezzati A, Arcelloni C, Vanzulli A, Testolin G, Pozza G, Del Maschio A, Luzi L. Intramyocellular triglyceride content is a determinant of in vivo insulin resistance in humans: a ^{1}H-^{13}C nuclear magnetic resonance spectroscopy assessment in offspring of type 2 diabetic parents. Diabetes 1999; 48:1600–1606.
14. Goodpaster BH, Thaete FL, Kelley DE. Thigh adipose tissue distribution is associated with insulin resistance in obesity and in type 2 diabetes mellitus. Am J Clin Nutr 2000; 71:885–892.
15. Pan DA, Lillioja S, Milner MR, Kriketos AD, Baur LA, Bogardus C, Storlien LH. Skeletal muscle membrane lipid composition is related to adiposity and insulin action. J Clin Invest 1995; 96:2802–2808.
16. Phillips DW, Caddy S, Llic V, Frayn KN, Borthwick AC, Taylor R. Intramuscular triglycerides and muscle insulin sensitivity: evidence for a relationship in nondiabetic subjects. Metabolism 1996; 45:947–950.
17. Wang N, Hikida RS, Staron RS, Simoneau JA. Muscle fiber types of women after resistance training—quantitative ultrastructure and enzyme activity. Pflugers Arch 1993; 424:494–502.
18. Goodpaster BH, Theriault R, Watkins SC, Kelley DE. Intramuscular lipid content is increased in obesity and decreased by weight loss. Metabolism 1999; 49:467–472.
19. Malenfant P, Theriault R, Goodpaster BH, Kelley DE, Simoneau J-A. Fat content in individual muscle fibers of lean and obese subjects. Int J Obes Relat Metab Disord 2001; 25:1316–1321.
20. Hoppeler H, Howald H, Conley K, Lindstedt SL, Claasen H, Vock P, Weibel ER. Endurance training in humans: aerobic capacity and structure of skeletal muscle. J Appl Physiol 1985; 59:320–327.
21. Bonen A, Luiken JJ, Liu S, Dyck DJ, Kiens B, Kristiansen S, Turdotte LP, Van der Vusse GJ, Glatz JFC. Palmitate transport and fatty acid transporters in red and white muscles. Am J Physiol Endocrinol Metab 1998; 275:E471–E478.
22. Budohoski L, Gorski J, Nazar K, Kaciuba-Uscilko H, Terjung RL. Triacylglycerol synthesis in the different skeletal muscle fiber sections of the rat. Am J Physiol Endocrinol Metab 1996; 271:E574–E581.
23. Dyck DJ, Peters SJ, Glatz J, Gorski J, Keizer H, Kiens B, Liu S, Richter EA, Spriet LL, Van der Vusse GJ, Bonen A. Functional differences in lipid metabolism in resting skeletal muscle of various fiber types. Am J Physiol Endocrinol Metab 1997; 272:E340–E351.
24. He J, Watkins S, Kelley DE. Skeletal muscle lipid content and oxidative enzyme activity in relation to muscle fiber type in type 2 diabetes and obesity. Diabetes 2001; 50:817–823.
25. Lillioja S, Young A, Culter C, Ivy J, Abbot W, Zawadzki J, Yki-Järvinen H, Christin L, Secomb T, Bogardus C. Skeletal muscle capillary density and fiber type are possible determinants of in vivo insulin resistance in man. J Clin Invest 1987; 80:415–424.
26. Wade A, Marbut M, Round J. Muscle fiber type and aetiology of obesity. Lancet 1990; 335:805–808.
27. Helge JW, Fraser AM, Kriketos AD, Jenkins AB, Calvert GD, Ayre KJ, Storlien LH. Interrelationships between muscle fibre type, substrate oxidation and body fat. Int J Obes Relat Metab Disord 1999; 23:986–991.
28. Krotkiewski M, Seidell JC, Björntorp P. Glucose tolerance and hyperinsulinaemia in obese women: role of adipose tissue distribution, muscle fibre characteristics and androgens. J Int Med 1990; 228:385–392.
29. Simoneau JA, Bouchard C. Skeletal muscle metabolism

and body fat content in men and women. Obes Res 1995; 3:23–29.

30. Segal K, Chatr-Aryamontri B, Rosenbaum M, Simoneau JA. Effects of hypertension and obesity on postprandial thermogenesis in men. Am J Clin Nutr 1995; 61:895.
31. Krotkiewski M, Bylund-Fallenius AC, Holm J, Björntorp P, Grimby G, Mandroukas K. Relationship between muscle morphology and metabolism in obese women: the effects of long-term physical training. Eur J Clin Invest 1983; 13:5–12.
32. Björntorp P. Insulin resistance: the consequence of a neuroendocrine disturbance? Int J Obes 1995; 1:S6–S10.
33. Grimby G, Aniansson A, Zetterberg C, Saltin B. Is there a change in relative muscle fibre composition with age? Clin Physiol 1984; 4:189–194.
34. Kriketos AD, Baur LA, O'Conner JO, Carey D, King S, Caterson ID, Storlien LH. Muscle fibre type composition in infant and adult populations and relations with obesity. Int J Obes Relat Metab Disord 1997; 21:796–801.
35. Morio B, Hocquette J-F, Moontaurier C, Boirie Y, Bouteloup-Demange C, McCormack C, Fellman N, Beaufrere B, Ritz P. Muscle fatty acid oxidative capacity is a determinant of whole body fat oxidation in elderly people. Am J Physiol Endocrinol Metab 2001; 280:E143–E149.
36. Reichmann H, Pette D. A comparative microphotometric study of succinate dehydrogenase activity levels in type I, IIA and IIB fibres of mammalian and human muscles. Histochemistry 1982; 74:27–41.
37. Hoppeler H. The range of mitochondrial adaptation in muscle fibers. In: Pette D, ed. The Dynamic State of Muscle Fibers. Berlin: Walter de Gruyter, 1990:567–586.
38. Lowry CV, Kimmey JS, Felder S, Chi MM, Kaiser KK, Passonneau PN, Kirk KA, Lowry OH. Enzyme patterns in single human muscle fibers. J Biol Chem 1978; 253:8269–8277.
39. Simoneau J-A, Lortie G, Boulay MR, Thibalt MC, Theriault G, Bouchard C. Skeletal muscle histochemical and biochemical characteristics in sedentary male and female subjects. Can J Physiol Pharmacol 1985; 63:30–35.
40. Gollnick PD, Saltin B. Significance of skeletal muscle oxidative enzyme enhancement with endurance training. Clin Physiol 1982; 2:1–12.
41. Newsholme EA, Leech AR. Biochemistry for the Medical Sciences. Chicester: John Wiley and Sons, 1983.
42. Simoneau JA, Colberg SR, Thaete FL, Kelley DE. Skeletal muscle glycolytic and oxidative enzyme capacities are determinants of insulin sensitivity and muscle composition in obese women. FASEB J 1995; 9:273–278.
43. Kriketos AD, Pan DA, Lillioja S, Cooney GJ, Baur LA, Milner MR, Sutton JR, Jenkins AB, Bogardus C, Storlien LH. Interrelationships between muscle morphology, insulin action, and adiposity. Am J Physiol Endocrinol Metab 1996; 270:R1332–R1339.
44. Colberg SR, Simoneau J-A, Thaete LF, Kelley DE. Skeletal muscle utilization of free fatty acids in women with visceral obesity. J Clin Invest 1995; 95:1846–1853.
45. Sun G, Ukkola O, Rankinen T, Joanisse D, Bouchard C. Skeletal muscle characteristics predict body fat gain in response to overfeeding in never-obese young men. Metabolism 2002; 51:451–456.
46. Ferraro R, Eckel R, Larson E, Fontvielle A, Rising R, Jesnen D, Ravussin E. Relationship between skeletal muscle lipoprotein lipase activity and 24-hour macronutrient oxidation. J Clin Invest 1993; 92:441–445.
47. Zurlo F, Nemeth PM, Choski RM, Sesodia S, Ravussin E. Whole body energy metabolism and skeletal muscle biochemical characteristics. Metabolism 1994; 43:481–486.
48. Simoneau J-A, Veerkamp JH, Turcotte LP, Kelley DE. Markers of capacity to utilize fatty acids in human skeletal muscle: relation to insulin resistance and obesity and effects of weight loss. FASEB J 1999; 13:2051–2060.
49. Blaak EE, Wagenmakers AJM, Glatz JFC, Wolffenbuttel BHR, Kemerink GJ, Langenberg CJM, Heidendal GAK, Saris WHM. Plasma FFA utilization and fatty acid–binding protein content are diminished in type 2 diabetic muscle. Am J Physiol Endocrinol Metab 2000; 279:146–154.
50. Ruderman NB, Saha AK, Vavvas D, Witters LA. Malonyl-CoA, fuel sensing, and insulin resistance. Am J Physiol Endocrinol Metab 1999; 276:E1–E18.
51. Winder WW, Arogyasami J, Elayan IM, Cartmill D. Time course of exercise-induced decline in malonyl-CoA in different muscle types. Am J Physiol Endocrinol Metab 1990; 259:E266–E271.
52. McGarry JD, Brown NF. The mitochondrial carnitine palmitoyltransferase system: from concept to molecular analysis. Eur J Biochem 1997; 224:1–14.
53. Winder WW, MacLean PS, Lucas JC, Fernley JE, Trumble GE. Effect of fasting and refeeding on acetyl-CoA carboxylase in rat hindlimb muscle. J Appl Physiol 1995; 78:578–582.
54. Witters LA, Watts TD, Daniels DL, Evans JL. Insulin stimulates the dephosphorylation and activation of acetyl-CoA carboxylase. Proc Natl Acad Sci USA 1988; 85:5473–5477.
55. Dobbins RL, Szczepaniak LS, Bentley B, Esser V, Myhill J, McGarry JD. Prolonged inhibition of muscle carnitine palmitoyltransferase-1 promotes intramyocellular lipid accumulation and insulin resistance in rats. Diabetes 2001; 50:123–130.
56. Ellis BA, Poynten A, Lowy AJ, Furler SM, Chisholm DJ, Kraegen EW, Cooney GJ. Long-chain acyl-CoA

esters as indicators of lipid metabolism and insulin sensitivity in rat and human muscle. Am J Physiol Endocrinol Metab 2000; 279:E554–E560.

57. Oakes ND, Bell KS, Furler SM, Camilleri S, Saha AK, Ruderman NB, Chisholm DJ, Kraegen EW. Diet-induced muscle insulin resistance in rats is ameliorated by acute dietary lipid withdrawal or a single bout of exercise: parallel relationship between insulin stimulation of glucose uptake and suppression of long-chain fatty acyl-CoA. Diabetes 1997; 46:2022–2028.
58. Faergman NJ, Knudsen J. Role of long-chain fatty acyl-CoA esters in the regulation of metabolism and cell signaling. Biochem J 1997; 323:1–12.
59. Nordfors L, Hoffstedt J, Nyberg B, Thorne A, Arner P, Schalling M, Lonnqvist F. Reduced gene expression of UCP2 but not UCP3 in skeletal muscle of human obese subjects. Diabetologia 1998; 41:935–939.
60. Simoneau J-A, Kelley DE, Neverova M, Wardin CH. Overexpression of muscle uncoupling protein-2 content in human obesity associates with reduced skeletal muscle lipid utilization. FASEB J 1998; 12:1739–1745.
61. Boss O, Bobbioni-Harsch E, Assimacopooulos-Jeannet F, Muzzin P, Murger R, Giacobino J-P, Golay A. Uncoupling protein-3 expression in skeletal muscle and free fatty acids in obesity. Lancet 1998; 351:1933.
62. Borkman M, Storlien LH, Pan DA, Jenkins AB, Chisholm DJ, Campbell LV. The relationship between insulin sensitivity and the fatty acid composition of phospholipids of skeletal muscle. N Engl J Med 1993; 328:238–244.
63. Vessby B, Tengblad S, Lithell H. Insulin sensitivity is related to the fatty acid composition of serum lipids and skeletal muscle phospholipids in 70-year-old men. Diabetologia 1994; 37:1044–1050.
64. Manco M, Mingrone G, Greco AV, Capristo E, Gniuli D, De Gaetano A, Gasbarrini G. Insulin resistance directly correlates with increased saturated fatty acids in skeletal muscle triglycerides. Metabolism 2000; 49:220–224.
65. Storlien LH, Hulbert AJ, Else PL. Polyunsaturated fatty acids, membrane function and diseases such as diabetes and obesity. Curr Opin Clin Nutr Metab Care 1998; 1:559–563.
66. Else PL, Wu BJ. What role for membranes in determining the higher sodium pump molecular activity of mammals compared to ectotherms? J Comp Physiol B 1999; 169:296–302.
67. Matsuo T, Sumida H, Suzuki M. Beef tallow diet decreases beta-adrenergic receptor binding and lipolytic activities in different adipose tissues of rat. Metabolism 1995; 44:1271–1277.
68. Storz P, Doppler H, Wernig A, Pfizenmaier K, Muller G. Cross-talk mechanisms in the development of insulin resistance of skeletal muscle cells palmitate rather than tumour necrosis factor inhibits insulin-dependent protein kinase B (PKB)/Akt stimulation and glucose uptake. Eur J Biochem 1999; 266:17–25.
69. Hajduch E, Balendran A, Batty IH, Litherland GJ, Blair AS, Downes CP, Hundal HS. Ceramide impairs the insulin-dependent membrane recruitment of protein kinase B leading to a loss in downstream signalling in L6 skeletal muscle cells. Diabetologia 2001; 44:173–183.
70. Hajduch E, Litherland GJ, Hundal HS. Protein kinase B (PKB/Akt): a key regulator of glucose transport? FEBS Lett 2001; 492:199–203.
71. Zeghari N, Vidal H, Younsi M, Ziegler O, Drouin P, Donner M. Adipocyte membrane phospholipids and PPAR-γ expression in obese women: relationship to hyperinsulinemia. Am J Physiol Endocrinol Metab 2000; 279:E736–E743.
72. Zeghari N, Younsi M, Meyer L, Donner M, Drouin P, Ziegler O. Adipocyte and erythrocyte plasma membrane phospholipid composition and hyperinsulinemia: a study in nondiabetic and diabetic obese women. Int J Obes Relat Metab Disord 2000; 24:1600–1607.
73. Kim JK, Kim Y-J, Fillmore JJ, Chen Y, Moore I, Lee J, Yuan M, Li ZW, Karin M, Perret P, Shoelson SE, Shulman GI. Prevention of fat-induced insulin resistance by salicylate. J Clin Invest 2001; 108:437–446.
74. Yuan M, Konstantopoulos N, Lee J, Hansen L, Li ZW, Karin M, Shoelson SE. Reversal of obesity- and diet-induced insulin resistance with salicylates or targeted disruption of IKKB. Science 2001; 293:1673–1677.
75. Horton JD, Shimomusa I. Sterol regulatory element-binding proteins: activators of cholesterol and fatty acid biosynthesis. Curr Opin Lipidol 1999; 10:143–150.
76. Hannah VC, Ou J, Luong A, Goldstein JL, Brown MS. Unsaturated fatty acids down-regulate SREBP isoforms 1a and 1c by two mechanisms in HEK-293 cells. J Biol Chem 2001; 276:4365–4372.
77. Loftus TM, Jaworsky DE, Frehywot GL, Townsend CA, Ronnett GV, Lane MD, Kuhajada FP. Reduced food intake and body weight in mice treated with fatty acid synthase inhibitors. Science 2000; 288:2379–2381.
78. Andres R, Cader G, Zierler K. The quantitatively minor role of carbohydrate in oxidative metabolism by skeletal muscle in intact man in the basal state. Measurement of oxygen and glucose uptake and carbon dioxide and lactate production in the forearm. J Clin Invest 1956; 35:671–682.
79. Dagenais G, Tancredi R, Zierler K. Free fatty acid oxidation by forearm muscle at rest, and evidence for an intramuscular lipid pool in the human forearm. J Clin Invest 1976; 58:421–431.
80. Baltzan M, Andres R, Cader G, Zierler K. Heterogeneity of forearm metabolism with special reference to free fatty acids. J Clin Invest 1962; 41:116–125.
81. Schwarz J, Schwarz JM, Neese RA, Turner S, Dare D, Hellerstein MK. Short-term alterations in carbohydrate energy intake in humans. Striking effects on hepatic glucose production, de novo lipogenesis, lipolysis, and whole-body fuel selection. J Clin Invest 1995; 96:2735–2743.

82. Boden G, Lebed B, Schatz M, Homko C, Lemieux S. Effects of acute changes of plasma free fatty acids on intramyocellular fat content and insulin resistance in healthy subjects. Diabetes 2001; 50:1612–1617.
83. Zurlo F, Lillioja S, Esposito-DelPuente A, Nyomba BL, Raz I, Saad MF, Swiunburn WC, Knowler WC, Bogardus C, Ravussin E. Low ratio of fat to carbohydrate oxidation as a predictor of weight gain: a study of 24-h RQ. Am J Physiol Endocrinol Metabol 1990; 259:E650–E657.
84. Blaak EE, Van Baak MA, Kemerink GJ, Pakbiers MT, Heidendal GA, Saris WH. Beta-adrenergic stimulation of skeletal muscle metabolism in relation to weight reduction in obese men. Am J Physiol Endocrinol Metabol 1994; 267:E316–E322.
85. Mandarino LJ, Consoli A, Jain A, Kelley DE. Interaction of carbohydrate and fat fuels in human skeletal muscle: impact of obesity and NIDDM. Am J Physiol Endocrinol Metab 1996; 33:E463–E470.
86. Sidossis LS, Stuart CA, Shulman GI, Lopaschuk GD, Wolfe RR. Glucose plus insulin regulate fat oxidation by controlling the rate of fatty acid entry into the mitochondria. J Clin Invest 1996; 98:2244–2250.
87. Abu-Elheiga L, Matzuk MM, Abo-Hashema KA, Wakil SJ. Continuous fatty acid oxidation and reduced fat storage in mice lacking acetyl-CoA carboxylase 2. Science2001; 2613–2616.
88. Kelley DE, Reilly J, Veneman T, Mandarino LJ. The influence of physiologic hyperinsulinemia on skeletal muscle glucose storage, oxidation and glycolysis in man. Am J Physiol 1990; 258:E923–E929.
89. Kelley DE, Mokan M, Simoneau J-A, Mandarino LJ. Interaction between glucose and free fatty acid metabolism in human skeletal muscle. J Clin Invest 1993; 92:93–98.
90. Boden G, Jadali F, White J, Liang Y, Mozzoli M, Chen X, Coleman E, Smith C. Effect of fat on insulin-stimulated carbohydrate metabolism in normal men. J Clin Invest 1991; 88:960–966.
91. Felber JP, Ferrannini E, Golay A, Meyer H, Thiebaud D, Curchod B, Maeder E, Jéquier E, DeFronzo R. Role of lipid oxidation in the pathogenesis of insulin resistance of obesity and type II diabetes. Diabetes 1987; 36:1341–1350.
92. Lillioja S, Bogardus C, Mott D, Kennedy A, Knowler W, Howard B. Relationship between insulin-mediated glucose disposal and lipid metabolism in man. J Clin Invest 1985; 75:1106–1115.
93. Randle PJ, Garland PB, Hales CN, Newsholme EA. 1 The glucose fatty acid cycle: its role in insulin insensitivity and the metabolic disturbances of diabetes mellitus. Lancet 1963; i:785–789.
94. Bryson JM, King SE, Burns CM, Baur LA, Swaraj S, Caterson ID. Changes in glucose and lipid metabolism following weight loss produced by a very low calorie diet in obese subjects. Int J Obes 1996; 20:338–345.
95. Valtuena S, Salas-Salvado J, Lorda PG. The respiratory quotient as a prognostic factor in weight-loss rebound. Int J Obes 1997; 21:811–817.
96. Friedman JE, Dohm L, Leggett-Frazier N, Elton CW, Tapscott EB, Pories WP, Caro JF. Restoration of insulin responsiveness in skeletal muscle of morbidly obese patients after weight loss. J Clin Invest 1992; 89:701–705.
97. Kempen KPG, Saris WHM, Kuipers H, Glatz JFC, Van der Vusse GJ. Skeletal muscle metabolic characteristics before and after energy restriction in human obesity: fibre type, enzymatic β-oxidative capacity and fatty acid bind protein content. Eur J Clin Invest 1998; 28:1030–1037.
98. Amatruda JM, Statt MC, Welle SL. Total and resting energy expenditure in obese women reduced to ideal body weight. J Clin Invest 1993; 92:1236–1242.
99. Leibel RL, Rosenbaum M, Hirsch J. Changes in energy expenditure resulting from altered body weight. N Engl J Med 1995; 332:621–628.
100. Ranneries C, Bulow J, Buemann B, Christensen NJ, Madsen J, Astrup A. Fat metabolism in formerly obese women. Am J Physiol 1998; 274:E155–E161.
101. Turcotte LP, Richter EA, Kiens B. Increased plasma FFA uptake and oxidation during prolonged exercise in trained versus untrained humans. Am J Physiol 1992; 262:E791–E799.
102. Olefsky JM, Farquhar JW, Reaven G. Relationship between fasting plasma insulin level and resistance to insulin-mediated glucose uptake in normal and diabetic subjects. Diabetes 1973; 22:507–513.
103. Olefsky JM. Decreased insulin binding to adipocytes and monocytes from obese subjects. J Clin Invest 1976; 57:1165–1172.
104. Bogardus C, Lillioja S, Stone K, Mott D. Correlation between muscle glycogen synthase activity and in vivo insulin action in man. J Clin Invest 1984; 73:1185–1190.
105. Yki-Järvinen H, Mott D, Young AA, Stone K, Bogardus C. Regulation of glycogen synthase and phosphorylase activities by glucose and insulin in human skeletal muscle. J Clin Invest 1987; 80:95–100.
106. Rothman DL, Shulman RG, Shulman GI. ^{31}P nuclear magnetic resonance measurements of muscle glucose-6-phosphate: evidence for reduced insulin-dependent muscle glucose transport or phosphorylation activity in non-insulin-dependent diabetes mellitus. J Clin Invest 1992; 89:1069–1075.
107. Roden M, Price TB, Perseghin G, Petersen KF, Rothman DL, Cline GW, Shulman GI. Mechanism of free fatty acid-induced insulin resistance in humans. J Clin Invest 1996; 97:2859–2865.
108. Shulman GI, Rothman D, Jue T, Stein P, DeFronzo R, Shulman R. Quantitation of muscle glycogen synthesis in normal subjects and subjects with non-insulin-dependent diabetes by ^{13}C nuclear magnetic resonance spectroscopy. N Engl J Med 1990; 322:223–228.
109. Saccomani MP, Bier DM, DeFronzo RA, Cobelli C. A

model to measure insulin effects on glucose transport and phosphorylation in muscle: a three-tracer study. Am J Physiol 1996; 270:E170–E185.

110. Bonadonna RC, Bonora E, Saccomani MP, Gulli G, Natali A, Frascerra S, Pecori N, Ferrannini E, Bier D, Cobelli C, DeFronzo RA. Roles of glucose transport and glucose phosphorylation in muscle insulin resistance of NIDDM. Diabetes 1996; 45:915–925.

111. Kelley DE, Mintun MA, Watkins SC, Simoneau JA, Jadali F, Fredrickson A, Beattie J, Theriault R. The effect of non-insulin-dependent diabetes mellitus and obesity on glucose transport and phosphorylation in skeletal muscle. J Clin Invest 1996; 97:2705–2713.

112. Kelley DE, William KV, Price JC. Insulin regulation of glucose transport and phosphorylation in skeletal muscle assessed by positron emission tomography. Am J Physiol Endocrinol Metab 1999; 277:E361–E369.

113. Bogardus C, Lillijoa S, Mott D, Hollenbeck C, Reaven G. Relationship between degree of obesity and in vivo insulin action in man. Am J Physiol Endocrinol Metab 1985; 248:E286–E291.

114. Evan DJ, Murray R, Kissebah AH. Relationship between skeletal muscle insulin resistance, insulin-mediated glucose disposal, and insulin binding: effects of obesity and body fat topography. J Clin Invest 1984; 74:1515–1525.

115. Kelley DE, Goodpaster BH. Effects of physical activity on insulin action and glucose tolerance in obesity. Med Sci Sports Exerc 1999; 31:S619–S623.

116. Yki-Järvinen H, Koivisto VA. Effects of body composition on insulin sensitivity. Diabetes 1983; 32:765–969.

30

Nutrient Partitioning

Samyah Shadid and Michael D. Jensen

Mayo Clinic, Rochester, Minnesota, U.S.A.

I INTRODUCTION

A General Considerations on Nutrient Partitioning

Nutrient partitioning can be defined as the process by which the organism selects fuels for storage (including protein synthesis) or oxidation. Understanding the regulation of energy balance and nutrient partitioning can potentially facilitate the treatment of obesity. Although the factors that lead to an imbalance between energy/fat intake and energy expenditure, and thus the development of obesity, remain incompletely understood, nutrient partitioning may be especially relevant to the development of obesity as it relates to the hypothesis of Flatt (1). The latter suggests that total food intake increases to meet carbohydrate needs. According to this theory, food intake is regulated, at least in part, to assure an adequate amount of carbohydrate. Consumption of a high-fat diet would require the intake of excess fat in order to satisfy carbohydrate needs and therefore lead to obesity under this scenario. The concept of a diet "relatively" deficient in carbohydrate becomes important in that dysregulation of substrate partitioning could potentially affect the body's sense of what constitutes adequate carbohydrate intake. For example, if fat were preferentially shunted toward storage, more carbohydrate would be required to meet oxidative needs, thereby preventing sufficient repletion of glycogen stores. This process is proposed to generate signals that stimulate appetite. Other examples where nutrient partitioning relates to obesity and body fat content include the stimulation of lean tissue synthesis at the expense of fat calories by androgens and growth hormone, and (presumably) the reverse of this process by deficiencies of these hormones.

A variety of physiological and cellular events play key roles in determining nutrient partitioning. After a general overview of these major determinants, the regulation of the major pathways of nutrient partitioning will be reviewed, followed by specific hormonal influences on each pathway. The net effects of the major nutrient partitioning hormones (insulin, growth hormone, testosterone and cortisol) on lipid, protein, and carbohydrate metabolism are summarized in Figures 1–3.

B Nutrient Partitioning and Exercise

When energy intake exceeds energy expenditure, the excess calories must be stored. Excess energy intake in sedentary, hormonally stable adults almost inevitably results in the expansion of adipose tissue triglyceride stores. Circumstances that promote lean tissue accretion, however, can allow excess energy to be stored as muscle and/or visceral proteins. The most common circumstance resulting in net lean tissue accretion with excess food intake is increased physical activity, usually in the form of resistance exercise training. The initiation of endurance exercise training in a previously sedentary

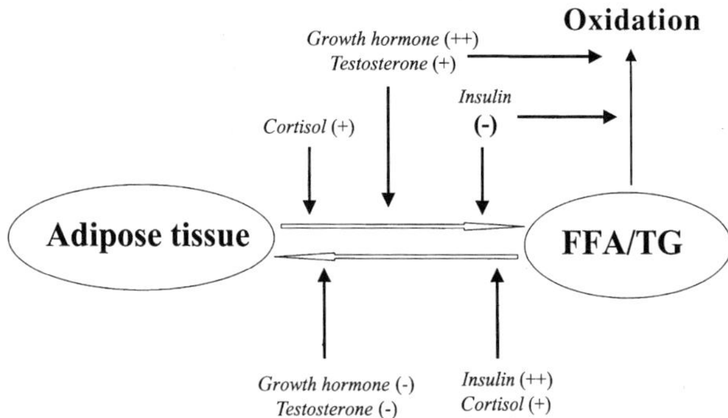

Figure 1 Endocrine control of lipid metabolism. Only direct and noncontroversial effects are depicted.

individual can have similar, albeit less pronounced, effects on lean body mass. Finally, during the recovery from catabolic illness, repletion of lost body proteins is an important fate of excess energy.

Alterations in nutrient partitioning can also occur at a relatively stable weight. For example, the reduction in protein synthesis and increased fat accumulation with aging can be considered a form of nutrient partitioning. Whether the changes are driven solely by lesser physical activity or are aggravated by other (e.g., hormonal) factors is not clear. In summary, ingested nutrients can be directed towards increasing body protein, increasing body fat, or, to a much lesser degree, expanding carbohydrate stores.

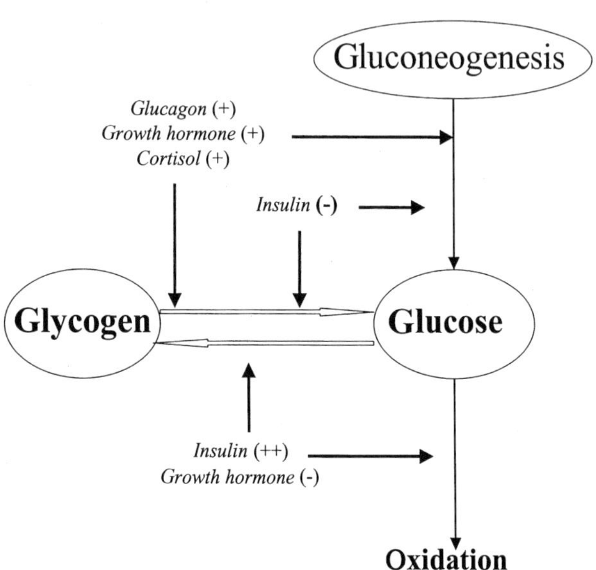

Figure 2 Endocrine control of glucose metabolism. Only direct and noncontroversial effects are depicted. Cortisol and growth hormone have additional effects to increase plasma glucose concentrations by inducing insulin resistance.

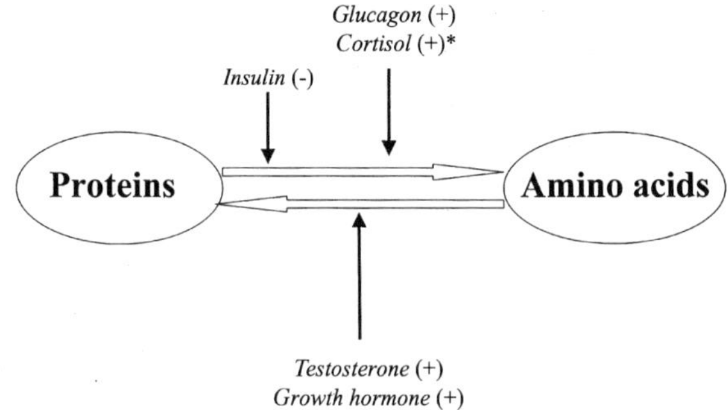

Figure 3 Endocrine control of protein metabolism. Only direct and noncontroversial effects are depicted. The enhancement of protein synthesis by insulin is controversial. *Proteolysis increases in acute hypercortisolemia, which, in chronic steroid excess, is controversial.

C Endocrine Influences on Nutrient Partitioning

Endocrine disturbances have long been associated with either the development of obesity and/or the result of obesity. Examples include Cushing's syndrome, thyroid disorders, insulin resistance, and polycystic ovarian syndrome. In some cases, endocrine influences may alter fat content and body composition by altering nutrient management without markedly changing either energy intake or expenditure.

Another point of interest is body fat distribution, a determinant of obesity-induced morbidity that is as important as the absolute amount of body fat. Upper-body obesity, which usually connotes visceral obesity, is more strongly associated with insulin resistance, hypertension, coagulation abnormalities, dyslipidemia, and cardiovascular death than obesity per se. Lower-body obesity, in which fat preferentially accumulates in the gluteofemoral region, is less strongly associated with these health hazards.

D Energy Expenditure and Metabolism

Nutrient partitioning could be accompanied or exaggerated by changes in energy expenditure. Human energy expenditure is usually broken down into three components: basal metabolic rate (BMR), the thermic effect of food, and physical activity. Basal metabolic rate is determined primarily by lean body mass, and thus hormonal effects that increase lean tissue will increase BMR. The thermic effect of food is determined primarily by the amount of carbohydrate and protein ingested, but may be reduced in insulin-resistant states. Physical activity thermogenesis is a product of the mass of the body moved and the amount of movement. Hormonal effects on energy expenditure and substrate oxidation could theoretically influence either the amount of energy expended in one of these components or the mix of fuels oxidized. To the extent that hormones influence either energy expenditure or substrate oxidation these issues will be covered.

II PROCESSING OF FUEL

The main sources of dietary energy are carbohydrates (4 kcal/g), proteins (4 kcal/g), fat (9 kcal/g), and alcohol (7 kcal/g). Alcohol will not be discussed. Fat, carbohydrates, and protein can serve functions in addition to fuel provision and the ultimate fate of these molecules depends on a variety of factors, among which hormonal influences are of importance.

A Lipid Metabolism

Dietary triglycerides are transported in chylomicrons for storage or oxidation. Effective utilization of triglycerides requires the action of lipoprotein lipase (LPL), which is present on the capillary endothelium of many tissues. Adipose tissue and muscle are the major tissues responsible for triglyceride clearance by LPL-mediated fatty acid uptake. Very low density lipoprotein (VLDL), secreted by the liver, is the other major form of circulating triglyceride. The fatty acids in these triglycerides derive largely from plasma free fatty acids (FFA), as described below.

Fat stored in adipocytes is mobilized by the action of hormone-sensitive lipase (HSL), which hydrolyzes the triglyceride, resulting in the release of glycerol and FFA. Free fatty acids circulate bound to albumin, are present at relatively low concentrations (300–600 μmol/L in the postabsorptive state) and turn over rapidly in the circulation (half-life of ~4 min). Uptake of FFA can be for use as an oxidative substrate (heart, muscle, etc.) or for reesterification (e.g., in liver) and subsequent transport in VLDL particles. At rest, FFA release and uptake rates generally exceed fatty acid oxidation rates. Hepatic reesterification of FFA and secretion as VLDL triglyceride can account for a portion of the FFA that are released in excess of fatty acid oxidation. It is thought that substantial portions of VLDL triglyceride fatty acids are re-stored in adipose tissue.

Under conditions of grossly excessive carbohydrate intake, glucose can be converted to fatty acids. This process is referred to as de novo lipogenesis, and is thought to take place primarily in the liver. It is energetically inefficient and accounts for a very small fraction of the fatty acids present in VLDL triglyceride under usual conditions.

The availability of FFA in the circulation drives fatty acid oxidation to a significant extent, as shown by the coordinate changes in fatty acid oxidation resulting from artificial elevation and lowering of plasma FFA concentrations. Some of the hormones that influence substrate partitioning may do so by in large part by altering FFA release from adipose tissue. For example, growth hormone stimulates lipolysis whereas insulin inhibits lipolysis, which in turn promotes and inhibits fatty acid oxidation. Fatty acid oxidation can also be regulated at other steps, however. It is possible for hormones to inhibit or stimulate fatty acid oxidation over and above their affects on FFA availability, thus sparing carbohydrate as an oxidative fuel. Altering the portion of fatty acids that enter reesterification pathways or altering fatty acid transport into mitochondria could modify fatty acid (and thus glucose) oxidation independent of circulating FFA availability.

1 Regulation of Lipolysis

Because of the importance of FFA availability in determining substrate oxidation, a brief overview of adipose tissue lipolysis will be provided. Under overnight postabsorptive conditions, adipose tissue lipolysis is restrained by the prevailing insulinemia; pharmacological inhibition of insulin secretion using somatostatin results in an approximate doubling of FFA release rates. Physiological hyperinsulinemia is capable of suppressing FFA release rates by 80–90% from basal levels, and FFA concentrations by >90%. Insulin-resistant obese individuals display greater maximal release of FFA during insulin withdrawal and lesser suppression of FFA during hyperinsulinemia. Catecholamines are also potent regulators of adipose tissue lipolysis. Epinephrine infusions can increase FFA release by three- to fourfold. This is similar to the stimulation of lipolysis that occurs during exercise. Catecholamines act through the stimulation of β-adrenergic receptors via a classic Gs-protein/cylic AMP mechanism that activates HSL (2). Other hormonal regulators of lipolysis include growth hormone and cortisol, although these are generally considered to be much less potent than insulin and catecholamines.

B Carbohydrate Metabolism

Most dietary carbohydrate is converted into glucose before storage or oxidation. The liver is the only organ that stores carbohydrate as glycogen for eventual export as glucose. The regulation of hepatic glucose export is under exquisite control by a variety of hormones, although insulin and glucagon are considered the most potent acute regulators of glucose availability.

There is a limited capacity for glucose storage as glycogen, such that increasing carbohydrate intake beyond usual needs quickly leads to increased carbohydrate oxidation, with an attendant reduction in fat oxidation. Increasing carbohydrate intake in the face of unchanging fat intake will result in increased fat storage as glucose replaces fat as an oxidative fuel. Massive increases in carbohydrate intake can stimulate de novo lipogenesis, although the capacity for this appears quite limited in humans (see Sec. II.A).

Reductions in carbohydrate intake are accompanied by some degree of glycogen depletion and by shifts toward greater fat oxidation. If energy intake is less than energy expenditure, fatty acids from preexisting stores are oxidized, resulting in relatively good preservation of protein stores. The shifts in carbohydrate and fatty acid oxidation that take place with changes in carbohydrate intake appear to be primarily regulated by the changes in insulin secretion that accompany the dietary changes.

C Protein Metabolism

Proteins include structural proteins, enzymes, nucleoproteins, oxygen-transporting proteins, contractile proteins, etc. The amino acids in these proteins are part of an interchangeable pool. The daily turnover of amino acids is substantially greater than the amount ingested as dietary protein; only a minor fraction of amino acids are oxidized or converted to glucose or fat.

Mechanical stimuli enhance skeletal muscle contractile protein synthesis, whereas hormonal and other factors determine the synthesis rates of many types of proteins. Given the tremendous variety of proteins in the body, many of which have specific regulatory pathways, this chapter will make only general reference to hormonal or metabolic regulation of protein metabolism.

III ENDOCRINE CONTROL OF NUTRIENT PARTITIONING

A Endocrine Control of Lipid Metabolism

1 Insulin and Lipid Metabolism

Insulin is an anabolic hormone, which promotes glucose as the preferred substrate for oxidation, sparing amino acids and fatty acids for protein and triglyceride accretion. Fat sparing is achieved via both the suppression of lipolysis and the facilitation of adipose triglyceride uptake, likely by enhancing the synthesis of adipose tissue lipoprotein lipase. It is unclear whether insulin has independent effects on FFA transport into cells. An insulin-mediated decrease in plasma FFA concentrations directly affects nutrient partitioning and substrate utilization. It is of great quantitative importance to insulin's effects on peripheral glucose uptake and oxidation: the lack of FFA supply forces peripheral tissues to intensify their use of glucose as oxidative fuel (Sec. III.B.1). In the pathological event of ineffective suppression of lipolysis following meal ingestion, such as in insulin resistance states, more fat and less glucose will be oxidized. This is proposed to be a mechanism by which the insulin resistance of obesity increases fat oxidation, thereby allowing the individual to eventually balance fat oxidation and fat intake. This will be further discussed below.

Insulin regulation of adipose tissue lipolysis displays a regional variation. Leg adipose tissue lipolysis is readily suppressed by insulin (3), with upper-body subcutaneous and visceral adipose tissue FFA release being less well inhibited (3). This is true in both lean and obese humans (3,4). If regional adipose tissue fatty acid storage were equal in all adipose tissue beds, one would expect gradual expansion of lower body fat stores. Studies of leg and abdominal subcutaneous, and of visceral adipose tissue indicate that regional variations in fatty acid uptake are in the same direction as regional variations as FFA release (5). Thus, whether regional differences in insulin action contribute to differences in body fat distribution is unknown.

2 Growth Hormone and Lipid Metabolism

The effects of GH on fuel partitioning are directed toward the use of fat as the preferred oxidative substrate. One of its main effects is, therefore, to increase FFA availability to peripheral tissues. However, its metabolic effects are biphasic: in the first ~90 min after secretion, a transient insulinlike effect is observed, characterized by accelerated glucose uptake and oxidation (6). Only after this effect has dissipated, GH adopts lipolytic and diabetogenic effects.

Regulation of fat metabolism is IGF-1 independent (7). GH stimulates fat mobilization, but in addition inhibits its uptake via the inhibition of adipose tissue LPL (8). This is reported to take place at a posttranslational level (8,9); an influence on LPL gene expression has not been consistently observed in vivo or in vitro (8,10). Whether GH affects skeletal muscle LPL is controversial (8,10,11).

Fatty acids are mobilized from adipose tissue via GH induced stimulation of HSL, of which the action, but not the production, is promoted (12). This is suggested to be mediated via increased adipocyte responsiveness to catecholamines (11,13); however, whether this is entirely responsible for the increased lipolysis is unclear.

In addition to increasing FA availability, GH directly enhances fat oxidation, at least in part, by stimulating the conversion of fatty acids to long chain acyl-CoA within responsive cells (14). This saturates the cells with fuel and thus decreases uptake of glucose (see Section II.B.2).

In clinical practice, the lipo-oxidative effect of GH is reflected in the increased and reduced fat mass in GH deficient and acromegalic patients, respectively. This can be reversed back to normal after treatment (7,15–17).

3 Testosterone and Lipid Metabolism

Testosterone has a major influence on fat metabolism. It affects fat distribution, fatty acid uptake and oxidation, and perhaps also lipolysis. This last may be related to synergistic effects with GH. These aspects have primarily been studied using testosterone supplementation in hypogonadal men and adolescents with delayed puberty, as well as by the artificial induction of testosterone deficiency in lean, healthy young men (18–20). The latter, achieved via the administration of a GnRH analog, diminishes rates of lipid oxidation and resting energy expenditure, but increases body fat mass. This suggests that testosterone-induced increases in fatty acid oxidation are not entirely due to the greater muscle mass. However, it is not clear to what extent these changes in fat oxidation result from direct effects on intracellular fatty acid trafficking versus from changes in FFA availability. Although testosterone increases adipocyte lipolytic responsiveness to catecholamines (norepinephrine, isoprotenerol and forskolin), in both in vitro and some in vivo studies, basal lipolytic rates are influenced in neither (18,21,22). Fat deposition is greatly influenced by testosterone, among others via its inhibition of LPL (22).

4 Estrogens and Lipid Metabolism

The effects of estrogens on fuel partitioning are most noticeable in the quantity and distribution of body fat. During female puberty, the latter is redistributed toward gluteofemoral deposition, which is thought to be estrogen mediated. Despite maintaining substantially more body fat (average of 30% in nonobese women compared to 15% in nonobese men), women have less visceral fat, greater amounts of lower-body fat, and lower cardiac risk factors (e.g., serum lipids) than men do. This gender difference persists throughout the adult reproductive life but begins to reverse after menopause.

However, the direct effects of estrogens on adipose tissue dynamics have been incompletely studied. Whereas a possible effect of estrogens on triglyceride uptake does not appear to have been investigated, adipose tissue fuel export has, but with conflicting results. Estrogens have been reported to increase, to decrease, or not to change lipolysis, in both animal and human studies (2,23). The only direct intervention studies, however, show that transdermal estrogen decreases adipose tissue FFA release in postmenopausal women (24) and lowers plasma FFA concentrations in ovariectomized women (25).

Equally conflicting are the data concerning the influence of estrogen on the partitioning of fat and glucose toward oxidation. One group reported that combined estrogen/progesterone supplementation of postmenopausal women did not alter basal substrate oxidation (26) but that, after a mixed meal, carbohydrate oxidation increased at the expense of lipid oxidation. This change occurred only at 30–60 min after meal ingestion, and only in the group of women given oral estrogens. Transdermal estrogen administration resulted in an opposite, but nonsignificant, effect. Another study failed to find effects of transdermal estrogen treatment on substrate oxidation under basal, insulin clamp, or adrenergic stimulation conditions (24). In contrast, inhibition of estrogen synthesis in men with an aromatase inhibitor tended ($P = .09$) to reduce basal lipid oxidation (27).

In summary, estrogens seem to alter body fat distribution and dynamics, but their exact influence remains unclear. Data on fat uptake are absent, and data on lipolysis are controversial. Nevertheless, estrogens seem to stimulate FFA release from adipose tissue and to increase lipid oxidation.

5 Glucocorticoids and Lipid Metabolism

The regulation of fat, glucose, and protein metabolism by glucocorticoids is characterized by a system that sophisticatedly redistributes nutrients over the body, according to their biological priority in stress situations (see Section II.C.4). In fat metabolism this is reflected in a net whole body lipolytic effect, which occurs simultaneously with (perhaps localized) stimulation of LPL as long as small amounts of insulin are present (28–30). The net result is an increase in FFA concentrations and fat oxidation (31,32). However, the lipolytic effect of acute hypercortisolemia, which is a facilitating effect on catecholamine-induced lipolysis, is counteracted by concomitant insulin overproduction, so that FFA release remains very limited in vivo. It has been suggested that regional stimulation of LPL might contribute to redistribution of fat by cortisol, analogous to its role in protein metabolism. Fat may be broken down in one region but stored in another under conditions of excess glucocorticoid availability: while lipolysis supplies increased amounts of FFA to peripheral tissue, circulating triglycerides (VLDL and chylomicrons), derived from increased food intake, may be preferentially stored in truncal fat (see below).

The increased FFA supply stimulates fatty acid oxidation, as shown by both indirect calorimetric measurements (decrease in RQ) (28) and appearance of ketone bodies (33). Whether cortisol also increases fat oxidation via direct intracellular effects is unclear.

In chronic hypercortisolemia, there is a net increase in fat mass and body weight despite greater fat mobilization (34). It is not completely understood why this increased fat mass is also redistributed in the centripetal pattern, typical of Cushing's syndrome. However, there is evidence that the synthesis of enzymes responsible for adipocyte fatty acid uptake is differentially regulated by cortisol, possibly mediated by regional differences in expression and/or sensitivity of cortisol receptors.

B Endocrine Control of Carbohydrate Metabolism

1 Influence of Insulin on Glucose Metabolism

Insulin largely controls glucose uptake into most cells, and stimulates both glucose oxidation and glycogen storage; skeletal muscle is the predominant site of postprandial glucose disposal. Insulin also suppresses endogenous glucose production by inhibiting hepatic glycogenolysis and gluconeogenesis. Thus, insulin largely orchestrates the disposal of meal carbohydrate by simultaneously inhibiting endogenous glucose production and stimulating the uptake and oxidation/storage of blood glucose.

The concept that failure to suppress fatty acid concentrations in the face of hyperinsulinemia will impair glucose disposal and oxidation has been confirmed. If the fall in FFA concentrations in response to hyperinsulinemia is prevented by infusing a lipid emulsion and heparin, glucose disposal and oxidation are not stimulated to the expected degree. In addition, normalizing the suppression of FFA in volunteers with type 2 diabetes (whose lipolysis is normally quite resistant to insulin) by administering acipimox, a drug with antilipolytic properties, markedly enhances insulin action with respect to glucose metabolism (35).

Insulin also promotes glucose oxidation and storage independent of its effects on substrate availability via direct action on intracellular events. Evidence for these effects has been provided by in vivo studies in which FFA concentrations have been maintained (via an intravenous lipid and heparin infusion) during hyperinsulinemic, euglycemic conditions. In these experiments, glucose uptake, storage, and oxidation increase above basal levels in response to insulin, although the rates do not equal those seen when FFA concentrations are allowed to fall normally (36). This response is clearly evident in skeletal muscle (36), but not in liver (37). These direct intracellular effects of insulin are mediated by a complex signaling cascade that regulates glucose transporter availability at the cell membrane, as well as the activity and synthesis of numerous enzymes. The details of this process are beyond the scope of this chapter.

2 Influence of Growth Hormone on Glucose Metabolism

Although GH stimulates the use of fat as the preferred oxidative substrate, it also causes plasma glucose concentrations to rise, which cannot always be compensated for by increased insulin release (7,38). This is achieved in various ways. First, the stimulation of FFA availability and the direct stimulation of fat oxidation saturate the cell with energy molecules and thus decrease cellular uptake and oxidation of glucose (7); glucose that enters the cell is deposited as glycogen. In some tissues, GH directly inhibits glucose uptake independent of FFA concentrations (39). In addition, GH stimulates hepatic glucose production (7). As a result, in situations of both acute and prolonged excess, GH has a diabetogenic effect.

3 Influence of Testosterone on Glucose Metabolism

The induction of hypogonadism in healthy men with GnRh analogs does not lead to evident changes in serum glucose levels or glucose availability. Insulin concentrations do tend to increase. Of interest, testosterone treatment in adolescents with delayed puberty causes insulin stimulated oxidative and nonoxidative glucose disposal rates to decline (18). These effects could well be temporary, as is the insulin resistance of puberty, and may be related to increased competition from greater fatty acid oxidation. In obese men, who are known to have lower plasma testosterone levels, testosterone administration increases insulin-stimulated glucose disposal rates (40). Whether this is a direct or an indirect effect, perhaps relating to changes in fat distribution or adipose tissue function, is not clear.

4 Influence of Estrogens on Glucose Metabolism

Estrogens have not been shown to influence glucose production or insulin-mediated glucose disposal in humans. Contrary to the decrease in glucose disposal found in ovariectomized rats and mice (41), insulin sensitivity in postmenopausal women is reported to be unchanged or even increased (41,42). Longitudinal studies of women going through menopause found unchanged glucose tolerance (43) and unchanged fasting glucose, but increased fasting plasma insulin concentrations (44). However, changes in fasting insulin in the perimenopausal time period are confounded by the changes in body fat and body fat distribution that commonly occur at this time of life (44). We conclude that the impact of estrogen on glucose metabolism in humans is too subtle to be clinically significant, if present at all.

5 Influence of Glucocorticoids on Glucose Metabolism

During both acute and chronic hypercortisolemia, glucose levels are almost invariably reported to increase, which is only partially attenuated by simultaneously increasing insulin levels (28,45). This is a combined effect of a decrease in insulin stimulated glucose uptake and of glucose overproduction (14,28,33). The former might be due to the increased circulating FFA, and, in chronic corticosteroid exposure, perhaps also to changes in muscle fiber types (see below). As expected, whole-body glucose oxidation diminishes (28,29). Glucose overproduction can be in part attributed to increased gluconeogenesis, which is induced by the increased supply of amino acids (especially alanine) and glycerol, derived from protein and fat mobilization (14,45,46).

It is likely that the combination of increased circulating glucose and peripheral insulin resistance, again, is a reflection of fuel redistribution: peripheral organs are forced to derive their energy from fat, saving glucose for usage in the brain. As the latter is unable to derive its energy from fat, its glucose uptake is practically insulin independent and can continue even during stress situations, during which energy use intensifies. Prolonged and/or extreme corticosteroid excess, however, can induce diabetes. The relative insulin deficiency of the diabetic state will further aggravate the protein catabolic effects of hypercortisolemia. Thus, the combination of corticosteroid excess and uncontrolled diabetes is particularly disadvantageous with respect to nutrient partitioning (47).

C Endocrine Control of Protein Metabolism

1 Insulin: Control of Protein Metabolism

The net lean tissue maintaining effect of insulin is achieved by the inhibition of proteolysis, and perhaps also by stimulating protein synthesis; the latter is somewhat controversial and is thought to occur via a direct stimulation of amino acid transport into cells, which should facilitate protein synthesis. The suppression of proteolysis reduces the release of amino acids from tissues into the circulation. In the context of a mixed meal (i.e., one providing protein as well as carbohydrate), the plasma amino acid concentrations increase as a consequence of gut delivery of amino acid into the circulation. Increased amino acid availability plays a role in stimulating protein synthesis. If insulin concentrations increase from the ingestion of pure carbohydrate or during intravenous glucose and insulin infusions, plasma amino acid concentrations and protein synthesis rates fall. Thus, the nutrient partitioning effects of insulin with respect to protein metabolism are strongly influenced by the nutrient content of the challenge.

Inherent regional and tissue differences in insulin action can potentially regulate regional nutrient partitioning. Skeletal muscle protein metabolism is affected differently by insulin than is splanchnic protein metabolism. Under overnight, postabsorptive conditions, when plasma insulin concentrations are at basal levels, skeletal muscle is a net exporter of amino acids (i.e., protein breakdown exceeds protein synthesis) whereas protein synthesis exceeds protein breakdown in the splanchnic bed (48). Increasing the plasma insulin concentration results in suppression of muscle protein breakdown without stimulating protein synthesis, but suppresses protein synthesis in the splanchnic bed without altering protein breakdown (48). The reduction in splanchnic protein synthesis in response to insulin may have been related to the fall in plasma amino acid concentrations resulting from isolated hyperinsulinemia. Thus, partitioning of amino acids between skeletal muscle and nonskeletal muscle sources is at least partially regulated by insulin.

2 Growth Hormone: Control of Protein Metabolism

GH minimizes the use of amino acids for fuel but increases their utilization for protein synthesis. GH enhances the latter by increasing cellular amino acid uptake in synergism with insulin (14,49) and modulating DNA and RNA transcription. Synergistic effects with testosterone make this more pronounced in males than in females. GH influences on protein metabolism occur via IGF-1 (7,14), although the presence of both hormones together has a greater effect than each one separately (49). Whether GH additionally inhibits proteolysis is controversial. Although many studies show no effect of GH on proteolysis (50), 6-hr GH infusions in healthy volunteers showed GH to suppress net forearm alanine, phenylalanine, and leucine release (51,52). It is unknown whether this merely reflects a decreased amino acid efflux, secondary to their increased extraction from the circulation (52), or a true suppression of proteolysis. IGF-1 has been demonstrated to induce proteolysis in animal and human studies (49). GH decreases amino acid oxidation by ~20%, as shown by GH administration to GH deficient adults (52,53) and children (7).

3 Testosterone: Control of Protein Metabolism

Acute testosterone deficiency, induced by GnRH analogs, has been shown to decrease whole-body protein synthesis and proteolysis, resulting in a decrease in fat-free mass and muscle strength (19). Testosterone supplementation studies have confirmed these conclusions, except for the effects on proteolysis, which was found to decline under the influence of testosterone.

These studies consistently reported that testosterone administration or deficiency did not change amino acid oxidation rates or plasma amino acid concentrations. This suggests that testosterone amplifies muscle mass by enhancing intracellular partitioning of amino acids toward protein synthesis (especially in muscle) rather than by increasing amino acid uptake. The latter has been confirmed in amino acid tracer studies of testosterone administration in healthy young men (54). It should be noted, however, that these studies are conducted in fasted states and that, under physiological conditions, cellular amino acid availability and uptake are expected to increase due to postprandial fluctuations in other hormones such as insulin and GH.

4 Estrogens: Control of Protein Metabolism

The influence of estrogens on protein metabolism is controversial. Although there is no question that estrogen modulates the synthesis of selected hepatic, endometrial, and other proteins in humans (55), whole-body protein pools seem to be unaffected, which has been observed in studies administrating estrogen to hypogonadal girls (55) and estrogen inhibitors (anastrozole) to young men (27). In both studies, amino acid turnover rates and amino acid oxidation were unchanged.

Apparently, estrogen affects selected protein pools without changing whole-body protein kinetics, perhaps because the tissues strongly affected account for a relatively minor fraction of total protein synthetic activity. Circulating amino acid availability does not seem to be affected by estrogens.

Of note, the estrogen inhibition in the Mauras et al. study (27) increased testosterone concentrations and decreased IGF by 18%, despite unchanged GH and IGFBP-3 concentrations. This contrasting effect on two strongly anabolic hormones, which is consistently confirmed in other studies, might blur direct measurable effects of estrogens in in vivo studies and creates yet another difficulty in the investigation of the fuel partitioning effects of estrogens. This is further complicated by the observation that GH production is stimulated by orally, but not transdermally, administered estrogens (26,56). Although the reason for this difference is not completely understood, it might influence the apparent effects of estrogen on several aspects of fuel partitioning.

5 Glucocorticoids: Control of Protein Metabolism

The well-established protein catabolic qualities of cortisol are far from random. Protein (but also fat and carbohydrate) supplies are mobilized, re-stored, and redirected according to their biological priority in stress situations. Acute hypercortisolemia increases whole-body proteolysis (28,33,45) and concomitantly decreases whole-body protein synthesis (49). However, the production of some proteins, such as some hepatic proteins and some lymphocyte proteins, is selectively stimulated (57). Overall amino acid oxidation increases (28,58).

With chronic hypercortisolemia, whole-body protein synthesis has also been shown to decrease, whereas the effects on proteolysis are controversial (47,49). In addition, with prolonged hypercortisolemia, protein catabolism progressively outpaces protein synthesis (28,57), leading to the evident protein wasting in the skeletal muscle and skin in Cushing's syndrome, which accentuates the characteristic centripetal fat redistribution.

Furthermore, over time structural changes can be observed in muscle. In addition to the above-mentioned atrophy, one study found that muscles in Cushing's syndrome may contain more type II_b (32% vs. 12%) than type I fibers (30% vs. 55%) compared to control subjects (59). Type II_b fibers have a lower glycogen synthase activity and fewer mitochondria and are therefore thought to be more insulin resistant. Interestingly, upper-body obese women display characteristics similar to those of women with Cushing's syndrome.

IV NUTRIENT PARTITIONING IN OBESITY

A General Considerations

Although the general principles of fuel partitioning are similar in obese and lean individuals, several changes in baseline endocrine physiology occur in obesity, particularly the visceral type. Although the insulin resistance is best known and studied, low GH concentrations, high or low testosterone concentrations (depending on the gender of the individual; see below), and a hyperactive hypothalamic-pituitary-adrenal axis have been observed in obesity.

None of the mechanisms has been elucidated. The many hypotheses formulated on these matters have been challenged by conflicting in vitro and in vivo observations. However, they seem likely to reflect adaptations of the body to a new environment of energy surplus, and one could well argue that the observed changes are part of a protective mechanism. Insulin resistance has been proposed as a way to limit weight gain (60), whereas the decline in GH is suggested to subdue the tendency for high FFA concentrations in central obesity, which might prevent further worsening of insulin resistance. These issues will be discussed in the following sections. The clinical relevance of this knowledge lies in a correct interpretation of lab findings in obese patients and in keeping otherwise abnormal results in perspective. Treatment aspects will not be covered.

1 Insulin and Nutrient Partitioning in Obesity

Insulin resistance with respect to glucose and fatty acid metabolism is an exceedingly common feature of obesity, being more severe and more prevalent in upper-body/visceral obesity. As noted above, this insulin resistance with respect to adipose tissue (less stimulation of LPL synthesis, less suppression of lipolysis) would theoretically act to make more lipid fuel available, thus displacing glucose as an oxidative substrate. If there is a sensing mechanism whereby the internal stimuli for energy intake are modulated by the availability of glucose, the reduced carbohydrate oxidation resulting from insulin resistance could serve to limit excess energy intake. In this regard, insulin resistance has been proposed as a mechanism to limit weight gain (60).

The development of type 2 diabetes in obese adults results in a host of nutrient partitioning changes. The relative insulin deficiency allows further excess mobilization of FFA from adipose tissue, which in theory would further depress glucose uptake and oxidation. The hyperglycemia itself, however, facilitates glucose uptake and oxidation independent of insulin, thereby limiting the extent to which fatty acid oxidation can increase. The loss of the restraining effect of insulin on skeletal muscle protein breakdown results in substantial losses of muscle in uncontrolled diabetes. In addition, glycosuria results in the nonoxidative loss of carbohydrate. This catabolic state with regard to adipose, muscle, and carbohydrate can be reversed with insulin administration or insulin secretagogues at the expense of weight gain. This weight gain could well be muscle tissue and repletion of glycogen (with its attendant water), with limited adipose accumulation. Thus, the energy deposition that occurs when uncontrolled diabetes is treated is an excellent example of nutrient partitioning into lean tissue.

In summary, insulin is involved to a major extent in virtually every aspect of nutrient partitioning. The primary issue that will face clinicians with respect to this hormone and obesity is the weight gain that attends insulin or insulin secretagogue therapy for uncontrolled type II diabetes.

2 Growth Hormone and Nutrient Partitioning in Obesity

The role of GH in obesity is complex and somewhat controversial. Although primary growth hormone deficiency leads to centripetal adiposity, visceral obesity per se results in a secondary reduction in serum GH concentrations (61). However, we view this as an adaptation to the state of energy surplus.

The differences in the pathophysiology of the two conditions are exemplified by the different IGF-1 concentrations. IGF-1 is very low in primary GH deficiency, but may be normal, high, or somewhat reduced in obesity. In the last case, IGF-1 concentrations are usually only slightly lowered from normal. Moreover, a simultaneous change in the production of IGF-binding proteins in central obesity (decreased IGFBP 1 and 2 vs. increased IGFBP 3) may result in high free, biologically active IGF-1 fractions, exceeding those in lean subjects (61). Therefore, IGF-dependent functions of GH, such as the growth ability of children, remain unchanged in obesity (61).

One could reasonably argue that reduced GH may dampen the tendency for high FFA concentrations in central obesity, thereby preventing further worsening of insulin resistance. Indeed, treatment of centrally obese adults with GH, while resulting in body fat loss, is almost uniformly associated with further increases in FFA and worsening glucose intolerance/insulin resistance.

The mechanisms behind this hyposomatotropinism in obesity have yet to be clarified. Reductions in spontaneous GH secretion (as much as 6% for each unit increase in BMI) and in the half-life of circulating GH have been reported (61). Moreover, the GH response to pharmacological (GHRH, L-dopa) and physiological stimuli, such as sleep, physical exercise, insulin-induced hypoglycemia, and corticosteroids, is impaired in adiposity (61).

Several theories have postulated explanations for the decreased GH concentrations, focusing on IGF-1, FFA, peripheral hormones, and the central nervous system. Increased plasma concentrations of FFA, IGF-1 and insulin are observed in obesity, all of which are known to provide negative feedback control on GH secretion and thus might contribute to the development of hyposomatotropinism. However, the quantitative importance of either of these feedback loops in mediating the alterations in GH dynamics in obesity is unknown. In addition, conflicting in vitro and in vivo evidence has challenged these and other theories, concentrating on leptin and the central nervous system (61).

3 Testosterone and Nutrient Partitioning in Obesity

Testosterone deficiency leads to visceral fat accumulation; however, analogously to GH, visceral obesity as a primary entity is also associated with lower free testosterone levels in men (62). As noted above, however, in women visceral obesity is associated with increased free testosterone (63). A satisfactory explanation for this paradox has yet to be found; in neither case is it clear whether this is based on a cause-and-effect relationship, or if so, whether the central fat accumulation leads to changed testosterone levels or vice versa. In both sexes, weight loss has been consistently found to reverse the abnormalities in testosterone levels (64–67). Several theories have postulated hormones such as leptin and GH to mediate the observed changes. However, neither is compatible with the changes in testosterone levels in women (68,69), and each theory is met with many other counterarguments.

In conclusion, upper-body obesity is associated with reversible high testosterone levels in women but low levels in men. Though the latter relationship has been intensively investigated, insight in the mechanism remains poor, theories varying from direct cause-and-effect relationships to indirect effects involving leptin and GH.

4 Glucocorticoids and Nutrient Partitioning in Obesity

Visceral obesity shares many characteristics with Cushing's syndrome. Both conditions are associated with large abdominal subcutaneous fat cells with high lipolytic qualities, insulin resistance, hypertension, and even buccal fat accumulation (70,71). In addition, the changes in muscle fibers described in women with Cushing's syndrome were also found in upper-body obesity (59).

As neither of these is typical of lower-body obesity, it has been suggested that visceral adiposity might be associated with changes in the hypothalamus-pituitary-adrenal (HPA) axis or cortisol receptors. Indeed, one glucocorticoid receptor polymorphism is associated with visceral obesity (72), although it is unclear how common or physiologically relevant these types of gene polymorphisms are in upper body adiposity. The fact that the HPA axis, on the other hand, is closely intertwined with food intake, makes a role in the development or sustaining of visceral obesity more plausible. CRH is a potent anorexic peptide; the increased appetite, found in most types of hypercortisolemia, is thought to be mediated by feedback inhibition of corticosteriods on CRH release. In rodent models, CRH administration reduces the body weight threshold for food hoarding behavior (73).

Therefore, obesity has been proposed to be a CRH-deficient state. However, the changes in HPA axis found in obesity, especially the abdominal type (74), are more suggestive of a hyperactive HPA axis. Secretory rates of cortisol are elevated in most, but not all, studies, even when corrected for body surface area. Plasma cortisol concentrations, however, remain normal or slightly lowered (74,75), which is thought to be a result of increased plasma cortisol clearance. Indeed, many, but not all, human studies report increased urinary cortisol excretion rates in obesity (71). In addition, the urinary excretion of 5α-reductase cortisol metabolites is positively correlated with waist circumference in nonobese men and postmenopausal women, suggesting that fat accumulation in the upper body is associated with increased cortisol turnover (76). Thus, some, but not all investigators believe cortisol production is increased in upper-body obesity. Other indications of a hyperactive HPA axis include increased adrenal sensitivity to ACTH, increased responsiveness of ACTH and cortisol to CRH, and increased postprandial HPA activation (71). However, all these parameters have also been reported to be normal by other investigators, and most studies show comparable ACTH levels in obese and lean individuals (71). The concept that obesity is a CRH-deficient state, although substantiated by rat and molecular experiments, has further been contradicted by the finding of normal to only slightly lowered cerebrospinal CRH levels in obese humans (71).

In summary, it remains difficult to unequivocally relate obesity to consistent changes in the HPA axis. It seems likely that this axis is characterized by adaptations to the state of energy excess, analogously to the other hormonal axis involved in nutrient partitioning. However, the study of the role of the HPA axis in visceral obesity is complicated by several obstacles, which might partly account for the inconsistent findings. Early investigations studied different obesity phenotypes as one entity. This may have confounded the results considerably as regards cortisol, because central obesity with its cushingoid fat distribution might be associated with different dynamics of the HPA axis than lower-body obesity.

Another important factor is the influence of the many heterogeneous and often uncontrollable variables on the HPA axis. These complicate standardization for research purposes and subsequently interpretation of the results. The most significant confounder might well be the intertwined relationship among food intake, energy balance, and the HPA axis. Changes in body weight trigger counterregulatory mechanisms aiming to maintain the steady state, which are thought to be mediated by the HPA axis. Thus, compensatory mechanisms blur the effect of weight change, which is reflected in the fact that both overfeeding and starvation experiments have been found to amplify cortisol production (74).

In summary, an intertwined and complex relationship exists among energy balance, food intake, and several components of the HPA axis. In visceral (and, to a much lesser extent, in gluteofemoral) obesity, increased cortisol secretion and clearance rates result in normal or decreased plasma concentrations. There is no evidence of an increased exposure of cells and tissues to cortisol in visceral obesity, despite its similarities with Cushing's syndrome. Whether changes on intracellular or receptor level are involved is unknown.

REFERENCES

1. Flatt JP. Carbohydrate balance and food intake regulation. Am J Clin Nutr 1995; 62(1):155–157.
2. Lafontan M, Berlan M. Fat cell α_2-adrenoceptors: the regulation of fat cell function and lipolysis. Endocr Rev 1995; 16(6):716–738.
3. Meek S, Nair KS, Jensen MD. Insulin regulation of regional free fatty acid metabolism. Diabetes 1999; 48: 10–14.
4. Guo ZK, Hensrud DD, Johnson CM, Jensen MD. Regional postprandial fatty acid metabolism in different obesity phenotypes. Diabetes 1999; 48:1586–1592.
5. Romanski SA, Nelson R, Jensen MD. Meal fatty acid uptake in adipose tissue: gender effects in non-obese humans. Am J Physiol Endocrinol Metab 2000; 279:E455–E462.
6. Bengtsson B-A, Brummer R-JM, Edén S, Sjöström L. Effects of growth hormone on fat mass and fat distribution. Acta Paediatr 1992; 383:62–65.
7. Mauras N, O'Brien KO, Welch S, Rini A, Helgeson K, Vieira NE, Yergey AL. Insulin-like growth factor I and growth hormone (GH) treatment in GH-deficient humans: differential effects on protein, glucose, lipid, and calcium metabolism. J Clin Endocrinol Metab 2000; 85(4):1686–1694.
8. Richelsen B, Pedersen SB, Kristensen K, Borglum JD, Norrelund H, Christiansen JS, Jorgensen JO. Regulation of lipoprotein lipase and hormone-sensitive lipase activity and gene expression in adipose and muscle tissue by growth hormone treatment during weight loss in obese patients. Metabolism 2000; 49(7):906–911.
9. Ottosson M, Vikman-Adolfsson K, Enerback S, Elander A, Björntorp P, Eden S. Growth hormone inhibits lipoprotein lipase activity in human adipose tissue. J Clin Endocrinol Metab 1995; 80(3):936–941.
10. Richelsen B. Effect of growth hormone on adipose tissue and skeletal muscle lipoprotein lipase activity in humans. J Endocrinol Invest 1999; 22(5 suppl):10–15.
11. Oscarsson J, Ottosson M, Vikman-Adolfsson K, Frick F, Enerback S, Lithell H, Eden S. GH but not IGF-I or insulin increases lipoprotein lipase activity in muscle tissues of hypophysectomised rats. J Endocrinol 1999; 160(2):247–255.
12. Slavin BG, Ong JM, Kern PA. Hormonal regulation of hormone-sensitive lipase activity and mRNA levels in isolated rat adipocytes. J Lipid Res 1994; 35(9):1535–1541.
13. Bjorgell P, Rosberg S, Isaksson O, Belfrage P. The antilipolytic, insulin-like effect of growth hormone is caused by a net decrease of hormone-sensitive lipase phosphorylation. Endocrinology 1984; 115(3):1151–1156.

14. Guyton AC, Hall JE. Textbook of Medical Physiology. 10th ed. Philadelphia: Saunders, 2000.
15. Biller BM, Sesmilo G, Baum HB, Hayden D, Schoenfeld D, Klibanski A. Withdrawal of long-term physiological growth hormone (GH) administration: differential effects on bone density and body composition in men with adult-onset GH deficiency. J Clin Endocrinol Metab 2000; 85(3):970–976.
16. Russell-Jones DL, Bowes SB, Rees SE, Jackson NC, Weissberger AJ, Hovorka R, Sonksen PH, Umpleby AM. Effect of growth hormone treatment on postprandial protein metabolism in growth hormone-deficient adults. Am J Physiol 1998; 274(6 Pt 1):E1050–E1056.
17. O'Sullivan AJ, Kelly JJ, Hoffman DM, Freund J, Ho KKY. Body composition and energy expenditure in acromegaly. J Clin Endocrinol Metab 1994; 78(2):381–386.
18. Arslanian S, Suprasongsin C. Testosterone treatment in adolescents with delayed puberty: changes in body composition, protein, fat, and glucose metabolism. J Clin Endocrinol Metab 1997; 82(10):3213–3220.
19. Mauras N, Hayes V, Welch S, Rini A, Helgeson K, Dokler M, Veldhuis JD, Urban RJ. Testosterone deficiency in young men: marked alterations in whole body protein kinetics, strength, and adiposity. J Clin Endocrinol Metab 1998; 83(6):1886–1892.
20. Buchter D, Behre HM, Kliesch S, Chirazi A, Nieschlag E, Assmann G, Von Eckardstein A. Effects of testosterone suppression in young men by the gonadotropin releasing hormone antagonist cetrorelix on plasma lipids, lipolytic enzymes, lipid transfer proteins, insulin, and leptin. Exp Clin Endocrinol Diabetes 1999; 107(8):522–529.
21. Xu X, De Pergola G, Bjorntorp P. The effects of androgens on the regulation of lipolysis in adipose precursor cells. Endocrinology 1990; 126:1229–1234.
22. Rebuffe-Scrive M, Marin P, Bjorntorp P. Effect of testosterone on abdominal adipose tissue in men. Int J Obes 1991; 15:791–795.
23. Mauriege P, Imbeault P, Prud'Homme D, Tremblay A, Nadeau A, Despres JP. Subcutaneous adipose tissue metabolism at menopause: importance of body fatness and regional fat distribution. J Clin Endocrinol Metab 2000; 85(7):2446–2454.
24. Jensen MD, Martin ML, Cryer PE, Roust LR. Effects of estrogen on free fatty acid metabolism in humans. Am J Physiol 1994; 266:E914–E920.
25. Pansini F, Bonaccorsi G, Genovesi F, Folegatti MR, Bagni B, Bergamini CM, Mollica G. Influence of estrogens on serum free fatty acid levels in women. J Clin Endocrinol Metab 1990; 71(5):1387–1389.
26. O'Sullivan AJ, Crampton LJ, Freund J, Ho KKY. The route of estrogen replacement therapy confers divergent effects on substrate oxidation and body composition in postmenopausal women. J Clin Invest 1998; 102:1035–1040.
27. Mauras N, O'Brien KO, Klein KO, Hayes V. Estrogen suppression in males: metabolic effects. J Clin Endocrinol Metab 2000; 85(7):2370–2377.
28. Brillon DJ, Zheng B, Campbell RG, Matthews DE. Effect of cortisol on energy expenditure and amino acid metabolism in humans. Am J Physiol Endocrinol Metab 1995; 268(31):E501–E513.
29. Stoner HB, Little RA, Frayn KN, Elebute AE, Tresadern J, Gross E. The effect of sepsis on the oxidation of carbohydrate and fat. Br J Surg 1983; 70(1):32–35.
30. Ottosson M, Vikman-Adolfsson K, Enerbäck S, Olivecrona G, Björntorp P.. The effects of cortisol on the regulation of lipoprotein lipase activity in human adipose tissue. J Clin Endocrinol Metab 1994; 79:820–825.
31. Ottosson M, Lönnroth P, Björntorp P, Edén S. Effects of cortisol and growth hormone on lipolysis in human adipose tissue. J Clin Endocrinol Metab 2000; 85(2):799–803.
32. Slavin BG, Ong JM, Kern PA. Hormonal regulation of hormone-sensitive lipase activity and mRNA levels in isolated rat adipocytes. J Lipid Res 1994; 35(9):1535–1541.
33. Shamoon H, Soman V, Sherwin RS. The influence of acute physiological increments of cortisol on fuel metabolism and insulin binding to monocytes in normal humans. J Clin Endocrinol Metab 1980; 50(3):495–501.
34. Lönn L, Kvist H, Sjostrom L. Changes in body composition and adipose tissue distribution after treatment of women with Cushing's syndrome. Metabolism 1994; 43(12):1517–1522.
35. Saloranta C, Franssila-Kallunki A, Ekstrand A, Taskinen MR, Groop L. Modulation of hepatic glucose production by non-esterified fatty acids in type 2 (non-insulin-dependent) diabetes mellitus. Diabetologia 1991; 34:409–415.
36. Kelley DE, Mokan M, Simoneau JA, Mandarino LJ. Interaction between glucose and free fatty acid metabolism in human skeletal muscle. J Clin Invest 1993; 92:91–98.
37. Rigalleau V, Binnert C, Minehira K, Stefanoni N, Schneiter P, Henchoz E, Matzinger O, Cayeux C, Jéquier E, Tappy L. In normal men, free fatty acids reduce peripheral but not splanchnic glucose uptake. Diabetes 2001; 50:727–732.
38. Seng G, Galgoti C, Louisy P, Toussain P, Drouin P, Debry G. Metabolic effects of a single administration of growth hormone on lipid and carbohydrate metabolism in normal-weight and obese subjects. Am J Clin Nutr 1989; 50(6):1348–1354.
39. Goodman HM. Effects of growth hormone on glucose utilization in diaphragm muscle in the absence of increased lipolysis. Endocrinology 1967; 81(5):1099–1103.
40. Marin P, Holmang S, Jonsson L, Sjostrom L, Kvist H, Holm G, Lindstedt G, Bjorntorp P. The effects of testosterone treatment on body composition and metabo-

lism in middle-aged obese men. Int J Obes 1992; 16:991–997.
41. Toth MJ, Sites CK, Eltabbakh GH, Poehlman ET. Effect of menopausal status on insulin-stimulated glucose disposal: comparison of middle-aged premenopausal and early postmenopausal women. Diabetes Care 2000; 23(6):801–806.
42. Walton C, Godsland IF, Proudler AJ, Wynn V, Stevenson JC. The effects of the menopause on insulin sensitivity, secretion and elimination in non-obese, healthy women. Eur J Clin Invest 1993; 23(8):466–473.
43. Tchernof A, Calles-Escandon J, Sites CK, Poehlman ET. Menopause, central body fatness, and insulin resistance: effects of hormone-replacement therapy. Coron Artery Dis 1998; 9:503–511.
44. Poehlman ET, Toth MJ, Gardner AW. Changes in energy balance and body composition at menopause: A controlled longitudinal study. Ann Intern Med 1995; 123(9):673–675.
45. Horber FF, Haymond MW. Human growth hormone prevents the protein catabolic side effects of prednisone in humans. J Clin Invest 1990; 86:265–272.
46. Gelfand RA, Matthews DE, Bier DM, Sherwin RS. Role of counterregulatory hormones in the catabolic response to stress. J Clin Invest 1984; 74:2238–2248.
47. De Feo P. Hormonal regulation of human protein metabolism. Eur J Endocrinol 1996; 135(1):7–18.
48. Meek S, Persson M, Ford GC, Nair KS. Differential regulation of amino acid exchange and protein dynamics across splanchnic and skeletal muscle beds by insulin in healthy human subjects. Diabetes 1998; 47(12):1824–1835.
49. Umpleby AM, Russell-Jones DL. The hormonal control of protein metabolism. Baillieres Clin Endocrinol Metab 1996; 10(4):551–570.
50. Garlick PJ, McNurlan MA, Bark T, Lang CH, Gelato MC. Hormonal regulation of protein metabolism in relation to nutrition and disease. J Nutr 1998; 128(2 suppl):356S–359S.
51. Moller N, Jorgensen JO, Alberti KG, Flyvbjerg A, Schmitz O. Short-term effects of growth hormone of fuel oxidation and regional substrate metabolism in normal man. J Clin Endocrinol Metab 1990; 70(4):1179–1186.
52. Fryburg DA, Barrett EJ. Growth hormone acutely stimulates skeletal muscle but not whole-body protein synthesis in humans. Metabolism 1993; 42(9):1223–1227.
53. Lucidi P, Lauteri M, Laureti S, Celleno R, Santoni S, Volpi E, Angeletti G, Santeusanio F, De Feo P. A dose-response study of growth hormone (GH) replacement on whole body protein and lipid kinetics in GH-deficient adults. J Clin Endocrinol Metab 1998; 83(2):353–357.
54. Ferrando AA, Tipton KD, Doyle D, Phillips SM, Cortiella J, Wolfe RR. Testosterone injection stimulates net protein synthesis but not tissue amino acid transport. Am J Physiol Endocrinol Metab 1998; 275(5):E864–E871.
55. Mauras N. Estrogens do not affect whole-body protein metabolism in the prepubertal female. J Clin Endocrinol Metab 1995; 80(10):2842–2845.
56. O'Sullivan AJ, Ho KK. A comparison of the effects of oral and transdermal estrogen replacement on insulin sensitivity in postmenopausal women. J Clin Endocrinol Metab 1995; 80(6):1783–1788.
57. Putignano P, Kaltsas GA, Korbonits M, Jenkins PJ, Monson JP, Besser GM, Grossman AB. Alterations in serum protein levels in patients with Cushing's syndrome before and after successful treatment. J Clin Endocrinol Metab 2000; 85:3309–3312.
58. Haymond MW, Horber FF. The effects of human growth hormone and prednisone on whole body estimates of protein metabolism. Horm Res 1992; 38(suppl 2):44–46.
59. Rebuffe-Scrive M, Krotkiewski M, Elfverson J, Björntorp P. Muscle and adipose tissue morphology and metabolism in Cushing's syndrome. J Clin Endocrinol Metab 1988; 67:1122–1128.
60. Eckel RH. Insulin resistance: an adaptation for weight maintenance. Lancet 1992; 340(8833):1452–1453.
61. Scacchi M, Pincelli AI, Cavagnini F. Growth hormone in obesity. Int J Obes Relat Metab Disord 1999; 23(3):260–271.
62. Couillard C, Gagnon J, Bergeron J, Leon AS, Rao DC, Skinner JS, Wilmore JH, Despres JP, Bouchard C. Contribution of body fatness and adipose tissue distribution to the age variation in plasma steroid hormone concentrations in men: the HERITAGE Family Study. J Clin Endocrinol Metab 2000; 85(3):1026–1031.
63. Jensen MD. Androgen effect on body composition and fat metabolism. Mayo Clin Proc 2000; 75:S65–S69.
64. Lima N, Cavaliere H, Knobel M, Halpern A, Medeiros-Neto G. Decreased androgen levels in massively obese men may be associated with impaired function of the gonadostat. Int J Obes Relat Metab Disord 2000; 24(11):1433–1437.
65. Kraemer WJ, Volek JS, Clark KL, Gordon SE, Puhl SM, Koziris LP, McBride JM, Triplett-McBride NT, Putukian M, Newton RU, Hakkinen K, Bush JA, Sebastianelli WJ. Influence of exercise training on physiological and performance changes with weight loss in men. Med Sci Sports Exerc 1999; 31(9):1320–1329.
66. Turcato E, Zamboni M, De Pergola G, Armellini F, Zivelonghi A, Bergamo-Andreis IA, Giorgino R, Bosello O. Interrelationships between weight loss, body fat distribution and sex hormones in pre- and postmenopausal obese women. J Intern Med 1997; 241(5):363–372.
67. Wabitsch M, Hauner H, Heinze E, Bockmann A, Benz R, Mayer H, Teller W. Body fat distribution and steroid hormone concentrations in obese adolescent girls before and after weight reduction. J Clin Endocrinol Metab 1995; 80(12):3469–3475.
68. Isidori AM, Caprio M, Strollo F, Moretti C, Frajese G, Isidori A, Fabbri A. Leptin and androgens in male obe-

sity: evidence for leptin contribution to reduced androgen levels. J Clin Endocrinol Metab 1999; 84(10):3673–3680.
69. Vermeulen A, Goemaere S, Kaufman JM. Testosterone, body composition and aging. J Endocrinol Invest 1999; 22(5 suppl):110–116.
70. Levine JA. Relation between chubby cheeks and visceral fat. N Engl J Med 1998; 339(26):1946–1947.
71. Pasquali R, Vicennati V. Activity of the hypothalamic-pituitary-adrenal axis in different obesity phenotypes. Int J Obes Relat Metab Disord 2000; 24(suppl 2):S47–S49.
72. Buemann B, Vohl MC, Chagnon M, Chagnon YC, Gagnon J, Perusse L, Dionne F, Despres JP, Tremblay A, Nadeau A, Bouchard C. Abdominal visceral fat is associated with a BclI restriction fragment length polymorphism at the glucocorticoid receptor gene locus. Obes Res 1997; 5(3):186–192.
73. Richard D, Huang Q, Timofeeva E. The corticotropin-releasing hormone system in the regulation of energy balance in obesity. Int J Obes Relat Metab Disord 2000; 24(suppl 2):S36–S39.
74. Björntorp P, Rosmond R. Obesity and cortisol. Nutrition 2000; 16(10):924–936.
75. Björntorp P, Rosmond R. Neuroendocrine abnormalities in visceral obesity. Int J Obes Relat Metab Disord 2000; 24(suppl 2):S80–S85.
76. Andrew R, Phillips DI, Walker BR. Influence of gender and body composition on glucocorticoid metabolism in middle-aged humans. Int J Obes Relat Metab Disord 2000; 24(suppl 2):S144–S145.

31

Obesity and Mortality Rates

Kevin R. Fontaine

Johns Hopkins University, Baltimore, Maryland, U.S.A.

David B. Allison

The University of Alabama at Birmingham, Birmingham, Alabama, U.S.A.

I INTRODUCTION

> "A certain amount of overweight has been looked upon with favor, our tendency being to consider a certain degree of hyper-nutrition to be desirable."
>
> —O. H. Rogers (1901)

> "A sudden palpitation excited in the heart of a fat man has often proved as fatal as a bullet through the thorax."
>
> —W. Wadd (1829)

Since at least the mid-19th century there has been considerable interest and debate with regard to whether and how obesity is associated with mortality. Although a common view a century ago was that weights we would consider excessive today were innocuous and perhaps even desirable, case reports coupled with data from the life insurance industry suggested that excess weight and the central distribution of this weight were associated with shortened life expectancy (1).

Over the past several decades, the question of the effect of variations in body weight on mortality has become increasingly important. This is in part because both relative body weight and rates of obesity have been dramatically and steadily increasing in the United States and most of the Western world (2–4). As agricultural and industrial technologies spread into the non-Western world, both the relative body weights and rates of obesity are increasing in those populations as well (5). Given this, it is not surprising that body weight is of considerable interest to the scientific community. Indeed, the "problem" of obesity has become the subject of governmental policies, public education campaigns, and insurance policies, and has become a major target of the food and pharmaceutical industries.

Despite efforts to address the rising rates of obesity, the effect of variations in body weight on mortality remains a controversial topic (6–9). Some studies (10–12) suggest that the relationship between measures of relative body weight (e.g., body mass index [BMI]: kg/m^2) and longevity is decreasing, indicating essentially that one can never be too thin. On the other hand, some studies suggest that BMI has little important impact on longevity (13–15). Between these two extremes are studies that suggest that the relationship between BMI and mortality is U-shaped or J-shaped, indicating higher mortalities at the extremes of the BMI distribution (16–19). To complicate matters further, studies suggest that the BMI/mortality relationship may vary considerably as a function of demographic characteristics such as age, sex, and race (20–22).

In this chapter, we review briefly the literature pertaining to the association between BMI and mortality in humans. We also examine what is known about the effects of potential confounders of this association, most notably smoking, preexisting disease, and physical inactivity. We also review briefly studies that have investigated the potential moderating effect of variables such as age and race, as well as the effect of weight loss on mortality. Finally, we summarize the literature and provide recommendations for future research.

II OVERVIEW OF THE EPIDEMIOLOGIC DATA

A Methodologic Issues

There are a number of important methodologic issues pertaining to investigations of the association between obesity and mortality. At the core of these issues are certain assumptions, largely untested, pertaining to how best to analyze data from prospective cohort studies to estimate the effect of BMI on mortality (7,8,23,24). A detailed explication of these methodologic issues is beyond the scope of this chapter (see 25). However, we will consider four of the major methodologic issues because they speak directly to the validity of the conclusions that can be drawn from the literature: the effect of smoking, the effect of preexisting disease and weight fluctuation, the effect of physical inactivity, and the use of BMI as a proxy for measures of adiposity.

B Effect of Smoking

Because smoking strongly increases mortality rate and also tends to be inversely associated with BMI (7), it is thought to contribute, artifactually, to the elevated mortality rate typically observed at the low end of the BMI continuum. If this were so, then failure to control for the effects of smoking might account for the overall J- or U-shaped BMI/mortality association commonly observed. If it is established that smoking consistently confounds this association, studies that have not controlled for the effects of smoking would have systematically underestimated the deleterious effect of high BMIs and overestimated the deleterious effect of low BMIs on mortality. Table 1 summarizes recent studies (12,17,26–36) that investigated whether smoking confounds the BMI/mortality association. As can be seen, with few exceptions (12,36), the vast majority of studies have found that the increased mortality among thin subjects (i.e., the J- or U-shaped association) persisted, though was often attenuated slightly, after smoking was controlled for.

The minimal influence of smoking on the excess mortality among thin individuals is also supported by two comprehensive analyses. Troiano et al. (18) performed a quantitative synthesis of 19 prospective cohort studies and found a U-shaped relation between BMI and mortality regardless of whether smoking was controlled for statistically or if smokers were eliminated from the analysis. The BMI in the Diverse Populations Collaborative Group (37) analyzed pooled data from 15 separate epidemiologic studies involving over 200,000 subjects and found that the BMI/mortality association remained essentially unchanged (i.e., U-shaped) irrespective of whether or how smoking was treated in the analyses. Collectively, these quantitative syntheses suggest that smoking does not appear to be a major cause of the elevated mortality observed among the thin.

C Effect of Preexisting Disease and Weight Fluctuation

In prospective studies of the BMI/mortality association it has become standard to analyze data excluding those cohort members who have died early (e.g., within the first 5 years of follow-up) as a means of controlling for confounding from preexisting diseases. The rationale for this is that many serious illnesses lead to both weight loss and an increased risk of death; thus, preexisting occult disease could confound the BMI/mortality relation and lead spuriously to the observed increase in the rate of mortality among persons with low BMIs. Thus, many reports (7,21,38) have advocated eliminating these "confounding deaths" by disregarding those persons who die early in the follow-up and analyzing only those deaths that seem less likely to have resulted from preexisting morbidities. This analytic approach seemed to become standard practice despite the absence of evidence pertaining to its effectiveness in reducing confounding due to preexisting disease.

To evaluate the effectiveness of excluding early deaths, Allison et al. (39) conducted three separate studies using analytic methods, Monte Carlo simulations, and meta-analysis. They showed that the use of "k-years exclusion" (i.e., excluding subjects who die during the first k years of follow-up) does not necessarily lead to a reduction in bias in the estimated effect of a risk factor on mortality when this relation is confounded by the presence of occult disease. Indeed, they demonstrated that such exclusion could actually increase the bias in some situations. Allison and colleagues (40) then conducted computer simulations using the

Table 1 Effect of Smoking on BMI/Mortality Association

Authors	Sample	Follow-up (years)	Deaths	Covariates	Results
Fontaine et al., 1998 (17)	1355 American women ≥50 from the Panel Study of Income Dynamics	4.5	110	Age, BMI, smoking, education, 4 health status variables	U-shaped relation with and without smoking in the model
Sempos et al., 1998 (26)	5209 Men and women from the Framingham Heart Study (28–62 yrs at baseline)	30	> 1900	Age, illness, education, smoking	J-shaped relation; similar BMI at minimum risk of death for smokers and nonsmokers
Brenner et al., 1997 (27)	Cohort of 7812 male German construction workers (25–64 yrs at baseline)	Mean 4.5	167	Age, nationality, alcohol, occupation, smoking	Excess mortality in lowest BMI category reduced but not eliminated by control of smoking
Dorn et al., 1997 (28)	1308 Men and women from the Buffalo Health Study (20–96 yrs at baseline)	29	576	Age, education, smoking	U-shaped quadratic relation
Chyou et al., 1997 (29)	8006 Japanese-American men living in Hawaii (45–68 yrs at baseline)	22	2667	Age, alcohol consumption, smoking	J-shaped relation
Seidell et al., 1996 (30)	48,287 Men & women (30–54 yrs at baseline)	Mean 12	818	Age, cholesterol, hypertension, diabetes, smoking	In men, excess mortality in lowest BMI category reduced but not eliminated by control of smoking; no relation for women
Manson et al., 1995 (12)	115,195 Women (30–55 yrs at baseline) from the Nurses' Health Study	16	4726	Age, contraception, hormone use, family history of MI, menopausal status, smoking	Apparent excess risk associated with leanness eliminated when smoking was accounted for
Wienpahl et al., 1990 (31)	5184 Black men and women (40–79 yrs at baseline) from the Kaiser Foundation Health Plan	15	676	Age, antecedent illness, education, alcohol use, smoking	J-shaped curve for men after controlling for smoking; flat association for women
Landi et al., 2000 (32)	18,316 Patients admitted to 79 Italian clinical centers	2–3	548	Comorbidities, smoking, alcohol use, cognitive impairment	U-shaped BMI/mortality association
Visscher et al., 2000 (19)	7985 European men (40–59 yrs at baseline)	15–30	3807	Age, study center	U-shaped association; underweight among all smoking categories was a predictor of mortality
Yuan et al., 1998 (33)	18,244 Chinese men (45–64 yrs at baseline)	9	1198	Age, education, alcohol consumption	U-shaped association between BMI and total mortality among lifelong nonsmokers
Rissanen et al., 1989 (34)	22,995 (age > 25 years) Finnish men	Median 12		Age, smoking, cholesterol, blood pressure	U-shaped high mortality in lean men "not entirely attributable to smoking"
Wannamethee and Shaper 1989 (35)	7735 (40–59 yrs at baseline) British men	Mean 9	660	Age, preexisting disease, smoking	Increased mortality in lean men seen only in current smokers
Garrison et al., 1983 (36)	5209 (28–62 yrs at baseline) respondents from the Framingham Heart Study	26	679	Age, smoking	BMI/mortality relation in lean subjects confounded by smoking

Source: Ref. 25.

actual BMI distribution and overall death rates from large databases representative of the U.S. population. These results were consistent with the analytical study in that removal of persons dying early in the study did not necessarily reduce bias in the estimated BMI/mortality curve due to confounding. While this simulation does not speak to whether or not the true relationship between BMI and mortality is U-shaped, it does indicate that exclusion of subjects who die early is not very effective at reducing bias, assuming such bias exists.

Finally, to investigate the effect of early death exclusion in actual data, Allison et al. (41) conducted a meta-analysis on 29 studies with almost 2 million subjects. This quantitative synthesis indicated that the difference in results when early deaths were included versus excluded was statistically significant but extremely small, and the shape of the curve did not change appreciably upon excluding early deaths. This suggests that the effects of exclusion of early deaths from the analysis are very small and not clinically significant (42).

These three lines of evidence suggest that excluding early deaths from analyses of BMI and mortality is not statistically sound. Thus, either the higher rates of mortality at lower BMIs are not simply artifacts from persons suffering from occult diseases, or such confounding does exist but eliminating early deaths is not effective in reducing this bias. To evaluate adequately the potential confounding effect of occult disease, we will need to develop more precise data collection methods to control for its influence. This will be a formidable challenge, however, since occult disease is, by definition, difficult, if not impossible, to identify.

Recently, excluding subjects who have lost more than some minimal amount of weight and/or have had more than some minimal degree of weight fluctuation has also become a popular analytic approach to address the BMI/mortality question (12,21,38,43). Like excluding early deaths, however, this practice has been used despite the absence of mathematical proofs, computer simulations, or detailed statistical discussions of its merits. Thus, before the practice of eliminating subjects with weight loss or weight fluctuation is promoted further, advocates of this technique should publish rigorous analyses and discussions of its merits.

D Effect of Physical Inactivity

It has also been suggested that the higher mortalities observed at high BMI levels could occur because many obese persons are sedentary and/or have poor cardiorespiratory fitness (44). In other words, because physical activity is an important correlate of both body weight and general health, it is possible that physical inactivity and its byproduct, low fitness, not BMI, drives the association between obesity and mortality. It is also thought that physical inactivity/low fitness may help explain the J- or U-shaped BMI/mortality curve because a sedentary lifestyle, even among the thin, may be responsible for the increased mortality often observed in the low-BMI range (45).

Support for this so-called fitness-versus-fatness hypothesis comes primarily from prospective observational data from the Aerobics Center Longitudinal Study (ACLS). In a recent representative study from these data, Wei and colleagues (46) quantified the influence of cardiorespiratory fitness on cardiovascular disease (CVD) and all-cause mortality among 25,714 men classified as normal-weight, overweight, and obese men, and compared low fitness with other established mortality predictors (e.g., hypertension, current smoking). They found that low cardiorespiratory fitness was an independent predictor of mortality in all BMI-defined groups, even after adjustment for other mortality predictors. Roughly 50% of the obese men in the sample had low fitness, which produced a population-attributable risk of 39% for CVD mortality and 44% for all-cause mortality, suggesting that low fitness is a strong and independent predictor of mortality.

Consistent with this, Blair et al. (47) report that weight loss does not appear to be as important in reducing mortality rates as does an increase in cardiorespiratory fitness. Specifically, they found that, compared with unfit men who remained unfit, unfit men who improved their fitness level experienced a 44% reduction in all-cause mortality rate, independent of changes in weight during an average follow-up time of 5 years.

Data from the ACLS cohort also indicate that the apparent effect of fitness on reducing all-cause mortality rate increases linearly with increasing BMI, suggesting that the heaviest men may benefit most from improving their fitness (44). Similar results have been obtained in the Harvard Alumni Study in that a 23% reduction in all-cause mortality rate, independent of changes in BMI, was observed in men who began to engage in moderate to vigorous sports activity (48). Collectively, these studies suggest that low fitness adds to overweight and obesity in influencing mortality adversely.

Several methodological limitations, however, may limit the conclusions that can be drawn from these studies. First, most studies were conducted with middle-aged men of mild to moderate obesity who were in the middle- to upper-socioeconomic strata. Thus, it is unclear whether these findings will generalize to, for example, severely obese persons, women, the elderly, and minority groups. Second, many studies investigating the relation among obesity and health and mortality have used relatively crude measures of self-reported physical activity as proxies for fitness. Thus, the effects of low fitness on the obesity/mortality association cannot be convincingly demonstrated with the current epidemiologic data. Third, it is important to distinguish between physical activity and physical fitness; that is, increasing physical activity may not confer the health benefits that appear to come with a quantifiable increase in aerobic fitness. Indeed, a recent meta-analysis (49) of 23 cohorts indicates that fitness and physical activity have significantly different relationships to combined CVD and coronary heart disease (CHD). Specifically, reductions in relative risk were nearly twice as great for fitness than for physical activity, suggesting that it is important to distinguish between physical fitness and physical activity, at least with regard to heart disease. Finally, because fitness, physical activity, BMI, and body composition are likely to be highly correlated, it is difficult to tease out the independent effect of these variables on mortality and morbidity.

In a recent randomized controlled clinical trial to evaluate the effects of weight loss and aerobic exercise on risk factors for coronary artery disease (CAD), Katzel et al. (50) randomized 170 healthy obese men to either (1) a 9-month weight loss (WL) intervention, (2) a 9-month aerobic exercise (AER) intervention, or (3) a weight maintenance control group. The WL group lost an average of 9.5 kg but did not change on VO_{2max}, whereas the AER group remained weight stable, but increased their VO_{2max} by 17%. The WL group has significant improvements in a variety of risk factors for CAD. Specifically, WL reduced fasting glucose concentrations by 2%, insulin by 18%, and glucose and insulin areas during oral glucose tolerance test (OGTT) by 8% and 26%, respectively. In contrast, AER did not improve fasting glucose or insulin concentrations or glucose responses during OGTT but did decrease insulin areas by 17%. Moreover, WL but not AER increased high-density lipoprotein cholesterol levels (13%) and decreased blood pressure compared with the control group. These findings indicate that weight loss improves CAD risk factors to a greater extent than does aerobic exercise training in healthy middle-aged and older obese men.

A recent published abstract (51), also from the Cooper Aerobics Fitness Center, describes the results of an analysis to investigate the association of BMI to mortality after adjusting for cardiorespiratory fitness. Using data from over 11,000 men (aged 20–89 at baseline) with at least 10 years of follow-up (10–24 years), it was found that, after adjusting for age and cardiorespiratory fitness, obesity (BMI $\geq$ 30 kg/m^2) was associated with a 1.95-fold increase in CVD mortality and a 1.46-fold increase in all-cause mortality. The association between obesity with both CVD and all-cause mortality remained strong (1.75 and 1.36, respectively) even when adjusting for, in addition to age and cardiorespiratory fitness, conventional risk factors such as smoking status, high blood pressure, diabetes, and parental CVD. This suggests, again, that obesity appears to have a potent effect on mortality, independent of cardiorespiratory fitness.

This is consistent with an analysis of data from the Buffalo Health Study (28) indicating that increased physical activity reduced the risk of all-cause (relative risk [RR] = 0.59) and coronary heart disease (CHD) (RR = 0.39) mortality among nonobese men, but not among obese men. Among women, increased physical activity reduced the risk of CHD death (RR = 0.26), but only among women aged < 60. By the same token, in an analysis of data from 631 sedentary adults from the HERITAGE Family Study (52) both body fat percentage and aerobic fitness were equally good predictors of future CHD (estimated using the revised Framingham Heart Study algorithm). However, in statistical models containing both body fat percentage and fitness (i.e., VO_{2max}), the removal of fitness from the model did not materially alter the fit of the model. In contrast, the removal of body fat percentage from the model containing only fitness changed significantly.

In sum, although some analyses of epidemiologic data demonstrate that physical inactivity and/or low cardiorespiratory fitness in overweight and obese adults are important predictors of mortality, recent randomized controlled clinical trials that have attempted to tease out the independent effects of weight loss and improved aerobic fitness suggest that weight loss may be more critical than fitness, at least with regard to improving CVD risk factors. However, a recent small-scale trial (53) suggests that, among men, exercise-induced weight loss reduces fat (particularly abdominal fat) and improves fitness significantly more than does diet-induced weight loss (see also 54). Moreover, reductions in insulin resistance, abdominal obesity, and visceral fat were similar in carefully matched subjects in the weight loss induced by diet and exercise groups. This implies that exercise alone (i.e., without dietary restriction) can be an effective strategy for reducing obesity and related comorbidities. Obviously, before definitive conclusions can be made, additional randomized clinical trials should be conducted to assess the independent and interactive effects of physical activity, fitness, and body composition on health, function, and mortality.

In any event, conceptually speaking, as with obesity-related comorbidities such as hypertension and diabetes, it is unclear whether these are best considered potential confounders of the obesity/mortality association, as mediators along the causal pathway from obesity to mortality, or as independent influence.

Using path model notation as described by Bentler (55), we present five hypothetical causal models between obesity (O), low fitness (LF), and mortality rate (MR) (see Fig. 1). In model A, O is hypothesized to cause LF, and LF increases MR. In this hypothetical situation, it is true that LF should be a stronger predictor of MR than is obesity and, after controlling for low fitness, obesity should have no independent effect on MR. However, in this case, LF is a mediating variable, not a confounder. Therefore, controlling for LF is inappropriate if one wants to ask what the total effect of O on MR is (7). In this situation, stating that O is not associated with MR after controlling for LF is akin to saying that having one's throat slit is not a risk factor for dying if one controls for blood loss. It is a true statement, but not very

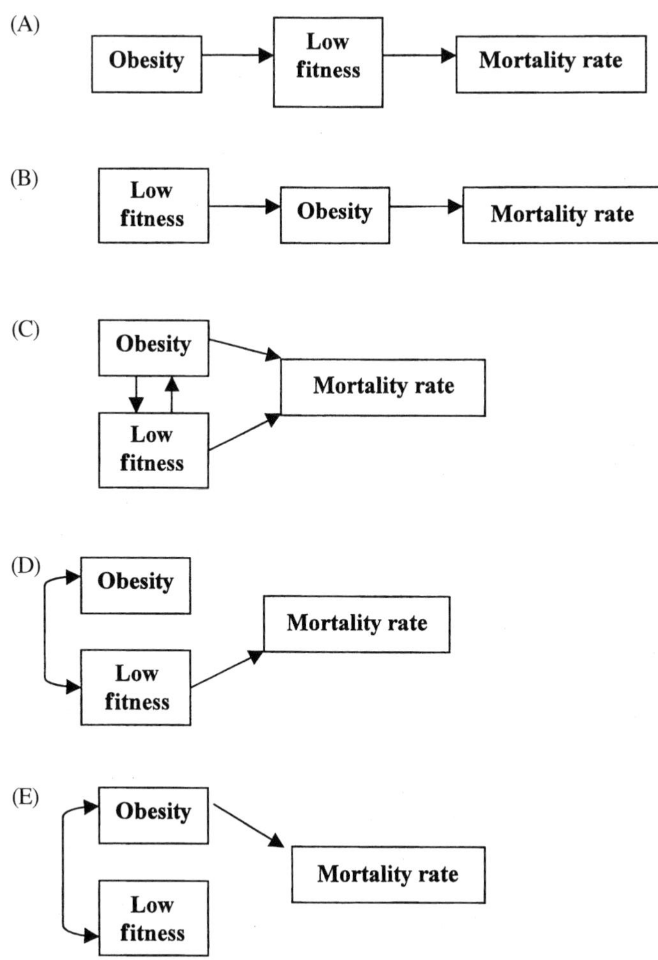

Figure 1 (A) Obesity causes low fitness and low fitness increases mortality rate. (B) Low fitness causes obesity and obesity increases mortality rate. (C) Obesity and low fitness reciprocally cause each other and collectively they increase mortality rate. (D) Obesity and low fitness are correlated but only low fitness increases mortality rate. (E) Obesity and low fitness are correlated but only obesity increases mortality rate.

informative, because it is hard to have one's throat slit and not lose blood.

In model B, LF causes O, and O increases MR. This hypothetical situation is the reverse of model A. In this instance, O should be a stronger predictor of MR than is LF and, after controlling for O, LF should have no independent effect on MR. Here, O is the mediating variable (not the confounder), and controlling for LF will not reduce the expected value of the apparent effect of O on MR. However, in finite samples, LF and O may be highly covariate and, therefore, controlling for LF may increase the variance of the estimated effect of O and cause it to be nonsignificant and/or lower even though it may have a real effect.

In model C, O and LF are strongly associated in that O is a cause of LF and LF is a cause of O and both increase MR. Controlling for O should attenuate the estimated effect of LF on MR, while controlling for LF should attenuate the estimated effect of O on MR. Due to the high correlation between O and LF, it will be difficult to "tease out" the independent effect of either O or LF on MR in such situations, and any model that includes one but not the other must be considered "misspecified" in the traditional statistical sense (56).

In model D, O and LF are correlated, perhaps due to some unspecified third factor. However, LF is the only factor that produces variation in MR. Model E is the reverse of model D in that O and LF are correlated with each other, but only O causes variation in MR. Models D and E are classic models of confounding and, under such circumstances, any model that includes one but not the other must again be considered misspecified and will lead to biased estimates of causal effects.

As models A to E illustrate, whether and how we control for O or LF when estimating the effects of either on MR depends, in part, on what we are prepared to believe about their causal relations. Moreover, each of the (nonexhaustive) possible sets of causal relations has very different biological and public health importance.

E Body Mass Index as a Proxy for Adiposity Measures

Since BMI is highly correlated (~0.70–0.80) to the percent of body weight as fat (57) and is easy to collect, it has been often used as the sole measure of relative adiposity in epidemiologic studies. However, the major difficulty in using BMI as a proxy for adiposity is that BMI is composed of two components, fat mass (FM), and fat-free mass (FFM). Thus, the use of BMI as a proxy for adiposity may mask any differential health consequences associated with both FM and FFM.

The majority of studies have shown that the rate of mortality associated with BMI is generally higher for both lower and higher BMI values and lower for moderate levels of BMI. As noted, the most common explanations for these J- or U-shaped curves are that persons with low BMI may smoke and/or suffer from preexisting diseases that increase their risk for mortality, independent of BMI. Another important hypothesis to consider, however, is that BMI, as a reflection of both adiposity and leanness, is not capable of capturing adequately the true relationship between body composition and mortality. Several studies have reported a positive health outcome for increased FFM and negative for increased FM (58). Thus, persons with low BMI may suffer from early mortality not because of BMI per se, but because inadequate levels of FFM increase their mortality rate. In other words, it may be that the risk of death increases with increasing FM and decreases with increasing FFM.

Allison and colleagues (59) investigated possible relationships between body composition and mortality using body composition measurements obtained on 1136 healthy subjects. Hypothetical mortality models were generated (using the real body composition data) in which mortality rate increased monotonically with FM and decreased monotonically with FFM. Using this model they showed that a U-shaped association between BMI and mortality could occur even when (1) mortality rate increased monotonically with FM, (2) mortality rate decreased monotonically with FFM, and (3) percent body fat increased monotonically, nearly linearly, with BMI. Thus, BMI may not capture adequately the effect of adiposity on mortality rate despite its high correlation with adiposity. This suggests that there is a need to conduct longitudinal studies that use precise body composition techniques to study the relationship between mortality rate and FM and FFM. Table 2 summarizes the few studies (60–68) that have evaluated the effects of FM and FFM (or imperfect proxies thereof) on mortality rate.

Folsom et al. (61) followed 41,837 women from the Iowa Women's Health Study Cohort for 5 years, testing the independent effects of BMI and waist-to-hip circumference ratio (WHR) on mortality rate. They found a U-shaped association between BMI and mortality rate. In contrast, WHR was strongly and positively associated with mortality in a dose-dependent manner. These findings were not altered substantially when controlling for potentially important covariates such as smoking, marital status, estrogen use, and alcohol use.

Keys et al. (60) examined 20-year coronary heart disease (CHD) incidence among 279 middle-aged Min-

Table 2 Studies Evaluating the Effects of Fat Mass (FM) and Fat-Free Mass (FFM) on Mortality Rate

Authors	Sample	Measures of FM and FFM	Effect on Mortality Rate
Keys, 1989 (60)	284 Middle-aged men from the Twin Cities Prospective Study	Hydrodensitometry	FM had greater effect on mortality rate than did BMI
Folsom et al., 1993 (61)	41,837 Women from the Iowa Women's Health Study	Anthropometry	Waist-to-hip ratio positively associated with mortality in dose-response manner
Menotti et al., 1993 (62)	9550 Adults from Seven Countries Study	Anthropometry	Among women, trend toward increased mortality with increased adiposity
Charles et al., 2000 (63)	7608 Men from the Paris Prospective Study	Anthropometry	FFM appeared protective
Baik et al., 2000 (64)	39,756 Men from the Health Professional Follow-up Study	Anthropometry	Waist circumference positively associated with CVD mortality among men $\geq$ 65 years
Heitmann et al., 2000 (65)	787 Men from Göteborg, Sweden, born in 1913	Anthropometry	FM monotonically increasing mortality rate; FFM monotonically decreasing mortality rate
Lahmann et al., 2000 (66)	28,098 Adults from the Malmo Diet and Cancer Prospective Cohort Study	Bioimpedance	% FM increased mortality rate in men but not women; FFM unrelated to mortality rate
Allison et al. (submitted) (67)	25,318 Adults from NHANES I and NHANES II follow-ups	Anthropometry	Among men: FM monotonically increasing mortality rate; FFM monotonically decreasing mortality rate
Zhu et al. (submitted) (68)			Among women: FM U-shaped association; FFM monotonically decreasing mortality rate

nesota men. Measures were taken of subjects' BMI, skinfolds, and body density by underwater weighing at baseline. Twenty-year incidence rates were then evaluated as a function of these variables. Results tended to be slightly stronger for measures of adiposity than for weight.

In a 10-year prospective study Menotti et al. (62) examined the association of BMI and skinfold measurements with mortality rate among 9550 adults. The results showed a consistent and clear U-shaped association between BMI and mortality. The analysis of skinfold data among men, however, was equivocal. Analyses of skinfold data among women, on the other hand, suggested a positive trend toward increasing mortality with increasing levels of adiposity. Notably, among women, the greatest risk was observed among those with low BMI and high skinfolds, a pattern suggestive of low FFM.

In sum, although the data are sparse (see Table 2), and the measures of adiposity are not as precise as we would like, the possibility exists that the elevated risks associated with excessively high BMIs are driven by adiposity rather than relative body weight per se.

III POTENTIAL MODERATORS

A Age

Among older adults, studies indicate weak effects of obesity on mortality rate and/or very high nadirs (i.e., BMIs associated with lowest mortality) for the BMI/mortality curves (16,17,22,28,69,70). Using data from the Build Study on 4.2 million insurance policies issued between 1950 and 1971, Andres and colleagues found that the relation between BMI and mortality was U-shaped, and that the BMI associated with minimal mortality increased consistently with age (71). In a Norwegian study (72), plots of the log of the mortality rate against BMI categories also revealed a U-shaped association. Although it was less clear whether the BMI associated with minimal mortality increased with age, the overall curves did flatten with age.

In a Finnish cohort of 17,000 women followed for 12 years, there was a U-shaped BMI-all-cause mortality relation among nonsmokers 25–64 years of age. Among women aged 65 or greater, mortality varied little according to BMI (73). Among white women from the Seventh Day Adventist cohort who never smoked, the RR of death associated with elevated BMI was lower among 55-to-74-year-olds than for 30-to-54-year-olds. For these older women, the minimal mortality was in the group with BMIs from 23 to 24.8 (74). Although the nadirs of the curves were much deeper, a recent study by Seccareccia et al. (75) of over 60,000 Italian subjects again showed the increase in the nadir with age.

Stevens et al. (21) investigated mortality over 12 years as a function of BMI across six age groups (30–44 years, 45–54, 55–64, 65–74, 75–84, and $\geq$ 85) among 324,135 never-smokers with no apparent preexisting disease from the American Cancer Society's Cancer Prevention Study I. Results indicated that, although greater BMI was associated with higher all-cause and CVD mortality, the RR associated with greater BMI declined somewhat with age (e.g., for men the RR of CVD mortality with an increment of 1.0 BMI unit was 1.10 for 30-to-44-year-olds and 1.03 for 65-to-74-year-olds).

Bender and colleagues (76) examined the effect of age on excess mortality associated with obesity among 6193 obese persons enrolled in the Dusseldorf Obesity Mortality Study (DOMS). When divided into four groups based on approximate quartiles of age and BMI, it was found that the overall risk of death increased with increased body weight, but that obesity-related excess mortality declined with age at all levels of BMI.

On the whole, these studies suggest that the relative increase in rate of death associated with increased BMI is somewhat lower for older adults than for younger adults, and that the BMI associated with minimum mortality rate increases with age. It is important to note, however, that BMI may not be a valid indicator of total fatness or fat patterning in older adults (i.e., > 65 years old). This is because older adults tend to have less muscle mass versus fat mass and more abdominal fat than younger adults at a given BMI (22). Finally, as Stevens et al. (77) point out, the absolute increase in rate of death can be higher in an older than in a younger person even when the relative increase is less.

B Race

The majority of research on the effects of BMI on mortality has been conducted on samples of European-Americans (78). While it is clear that obesity in African-Americans, most notably women, is associated with a number of risk factors (79,80), the relation between obesity and mortality among African-Americans is not as clear as it is in Caucasian individuals.

In a cohort of 2731 African-American women members of the Kaiser Foundation Health Plan who were followed for 15 years, Wienpahl et al. (31) found an essentially flat BMI/mortality association across the entire range of BMI. However, although the U-shaped relation between BMI and all-cause mortality was not significant, Stevens et al. (81) found that, among African-American men, obesity was associated with increased risk of mortality from ischemic heart disease (IHD). More recently, Stevens et al. (82) examined the association of BMI to all-cause and CVD mortality among 100,000 Caucasian and 8142 African-American women from the American Cancer Society Prevention Study I. At the 12-year follow-up, a significant interaction was observed between ethnicity and BMI for both all-cause and CVD mortality. Specifically, among white women, BMI was associated with all-cause mortality in all four groups (defined by smoking status and educational attainment). In African-American women with less than a high school education, there was no significant association between BMI and all-cause mortality. However, there was a significant association among high school–educated African-American women. Models using the lowest BMI as the reference group among never-smoking women with at least a high school education indicated a 40% higher risk of all-cause mortality at a BMI of 35.9 in the African-American women versus 27.3 in the white women. Stevens et al. (82) concluded that, although educational attainment appears to modify the impact of BMI on mortality, BMI was a less potent risk factor in the African-American women than in the Caucasian women.

Two more recent relatively large and high-quality studies have emerged with samples of African-Americans (83,84). These studies show that there clearly is a deleterious effect of obesity on mortality rate among African-Americans, though the BMIs associated with minimum mortality rate may be slightly higher among African-Americans (85). Other investigators (43,86–89) have obtained similar results, suggesting that the effect of a given BMI increase on mortality rate may be less deleterious among African-Americans than among Caucasians.

With regard to the BMI/mortality association among persons of other ethnic origins, data are sparse. In a sample of Micronesian Nauruans and Melanesian and Indian Fijians, obesity was not significantly associated with an elevated mortality rate (90). Among a sample of 8006 Japanese-American men living in Hawaii who were followed for 22 years, a significant quadratic (J-shaped) relation was found between BMI and mortality independent of the effects of smoking and alcohol consumption (29). Similarly, among a cohort of over 2000 Japanese adults over age 40, there was a U-shaped relation between BMI and mortality rate, with a nadir in the range of 23–25. However, in a cohort comprising 2,546 East Indian and Melanesian Fijians followed for 11 years, the association of BMI to all-cause and CVD mortality was generally inconsistent (91). Despite the known associations between body weight and diabetes and other obesity-related diseases found among Mexican-Americans, data have revealed lower-than-expected rates of mortality, based on known body weights (92).

Data on the BMI/mortality association among other ethnic groups (e.g., Native Americans, Alaska Natives) are limited. Hanson et al. (93) found that, among a cohort of 814 diabetic and 1814 nondiabetic Pima Indians, a U-shaped relationship between BMI and mortality was found in men but not in women. It was reported that excess mortality among lighter individuals was present in those persons who were losing weight. Thus, they concluded that preexisting illness might only partially explain the high mortality among lighter persons.

C Family History/Individualization of Optimal BMI Target

Thus far, we have primarily considered "demographic" variables as potential moderators of the BMI/mortality association. However, one important set of variables that, to our knowledge, has yet to be investigated in this regard, involves family history and genetic information. We can envision family history/genetic information entering into models for the effect of obesity on mortality rate in several ways. In turn, this may allow the use of family history/genetic information in helping individuals determine the body weights likely to be associated with minimal mortality for themselves on a case-by-case basis.

First, it is well documented that susceptibility to many, if not most, diseases is, in part, genetically determined (94). This includes several diseases for which obesity increases the risk, including heart disease (95), and at least one disease for which obesity decreases the risk, osteoporosis (96). Therefore, to the extent that individuals had a strong family history of heart disease and other diseases that are both heritable and made more likely by obesity and simultaneously had family histories of a lack of osteoporosis, lower-than-average body weights might be associated with minimal mortality for these individuals. Conversely, individuals with a strong family history of osteoporosis (or any other diseases protected against by obesity) and no family history of heart disease or other diseases made more likely by obesity, higher-than-usual BMIs might be most likely to confer the minimal rate of mortality for such individuals. Obviously, this conjecture warrants rigorous empirical evaluation before it can be accepted. Therefore, research involving related individuals in large longitudinal studies would be extremely useful. If this hypothesis is borne out, it might then be possible to use family disease history to help individuals optimize their own decisions about desired BMI levels.

Second, not only are obesity and certain obesity-related diseases partially heritable, it is possible that the propensities to suffer from ill effects of obesity are themselves partially heritable. For example, almost everyone knows some very obese person who died very early, plausibly as the result of his or her obesity. At the same time, almost everyone knows some very obese individual who lived a very long and healthy life. What factors influence these differential susceptibilities to the ill effects of obesity? To the extent that these factors are genetic, estimates of an individual's genetic susceptibility to the ill effects of obesity would be an important moderator of the BMI/mortality association. Moreover, family history might offer a potential way of providing such estimates; that is, if extensive family history about both BMIs and life spans could be obtained for individuals, one might be able to examine how much obesity did or did not confer added risk or protection within an individual family. Such information could be combined with baseline populationwide estimates of the increased or decreased risk conferred by obesity to come up with individual specific estimates. Certain random effects statistical models and empirical Bayes methods might be especially well suited to such analytic approaches.

Finally, as molecular genetic information continues to accumulate, we may eventually be able to identify specific genetic polymorphisms that are associated with the tendency for obesity to have a deleterious effect on

Table 3 Recent Weight Loss and Mortality Studies

Source	Sample	Deaths	Follow-up (years)	Results
Williamson et al. (1995) (100)	43,457 White overweight nonsmoking women	4199	12	In those with obesity-related comorbidities intentional weight loss was associated with 20% reduction in mortality rate. No association between intentional weight loss and mortality rate in women without obesity-related comorbidities. Recent intentional weight loss of >20 lbs associated with increased mortality rate.
French et al. (1999) (102)	33,017 Women from Iowa Women's Health Study	1048	3	Intentional weight loss of ≥20 lbs not associated with higher CVD mortality risk. Unintentional weight loss of ≥20 lbs associated with 26–57% higher total mortality risk and 51–114% higher CVD mortality risk.
Williamson et al. (1999) (103)	49,337 White men aged 40–64	9360	12–13	Among those with no reported health problems, intentional weight loss not associated with total, CVD, or cancer mortality rate. Among men with health problems, intentional weight loss was not associated with total or CVD mortality but with increased cancer mortality risk.
Pamuk et al. (1993) (104)	5192 Adults from NHANES I Epidemiologic Follow-Up Study	533	12–16	Weight loss of >5% maximum lifetime body weight associated with increased death rates even after excluding deaths within first 5–8 years after baseline.
Wee et al. (2000) (105)	18,494 Respondents of the 1989 National Health Interview Survey	1282	5.5 mean	Intentional weight loss of 5–10 lbs associated with lower hazard of death compared to reference group. Greater than 10-lb weight loss did not significantly increase longevity.
Lee and Paffenbarger, 1992 (106)	11,703 Men in the Harvard Alumni Study	1441	12	Both weight loss and weight gain of > 5 kg significantly increased all-cause and CHD mortality.
Blair et al., 1993 (107)	10,529 Men from the Multiple Risk Factor Intervention Trial	380	6–7	Weight loss associated with increased risk of death (range of relative risk = 1.04–3.42). Lowest mortality in weight stable.
Williamson et al., 2000 (101)	4970 Overweight adults with diabetes	1325	12	After adjusting for initial BMI, sociodemographic factors, health status, and physical activity, intentional weight loss was associated with 25% reduction in total mortality and 28% reduction in CVD and diabetes mortality.
Higgins et al., 1993 (108)	2500 Adults from the Framingham Heart Study	Not specified	20	Among men, weight loss associated with higher 20-year all-cause, cardiovascular, and CHD mortality compared with weight-stable group.
Diehr et al., 1998 (70)	4317 Nonsmoking adults from the Cardiovascular Health Study	539	5	Among overweight (BMIs 26.2–27.3) older adults (aged 65–100) a > 10-lb weight loss in the year preceding the study had 5-yr mortality rates that were similar to those who were weight stable in the year prior to the study.

longevity. If such polymorphisms could be detected and had large individual effects, then it might be possible to use such genetic information in gene by environment (or, more aptly, gene by phenotype) interaction analyses. Again, such polymorphisms could be examined for individuals to help them determine the best BMI for themselves.

Clearly, the ideas put forward in this section are concepts for which we do not currently have supporting data. Nevertheless, they are all quite consistent with existing knowledge, and we think it only a matter of time before such more complex and individualized statements about optimal BMIs with respect to longevity can be made.

D Weight Loss and Mortality

Dramatic effects of obesity on mortality rate have been demonstrated in studies of laboratory rodents (97). Specifically, when obese animals are compared to nonobese animals, the nonobese outlive the obese. These findings are consistent with the life-prolonging effects achieved by caloric restriction (CR). CR should not be confused with lower body weight or lower body fat. However, CR clearly results in lower body weight and is the most common method by which humans achieve lower body weight. Therefore, it is worth noting that CR achieved by various means and resulting in weight loss has been demonstrated to result in increased longevity in a variety of animal species (98).

Obesity, at least when severe, is clearly associated with an increased mortality rate, and weight loss is associated strongly with reductions in many risk factors (99). Therefore, it seems reasonable to conjecture that weight loss among the obese will increase life span. Indeed, some studies suggest that intentional weight loss reduces mortality rate in persons with obesity-related comorbidities such as hypertension (100) and diabetes (101). Among apparently healthy overweight and obese adults, however, the majority of studies (71,102–108) suggest that intentional weight loss is associated with an increase in mortality rate (see Table 3) (20,109). Findings such as these prompted Andres et al. (20) to conclude that no matter what population is studied, or how the data are "cleaned," treated, and analyzed, "Evidence suggests that the highest mortality rates occur in adults who either have lost weight or have gained excessive weight. The lowest mortality rates are generally associated with modest weight gain" (p 737).

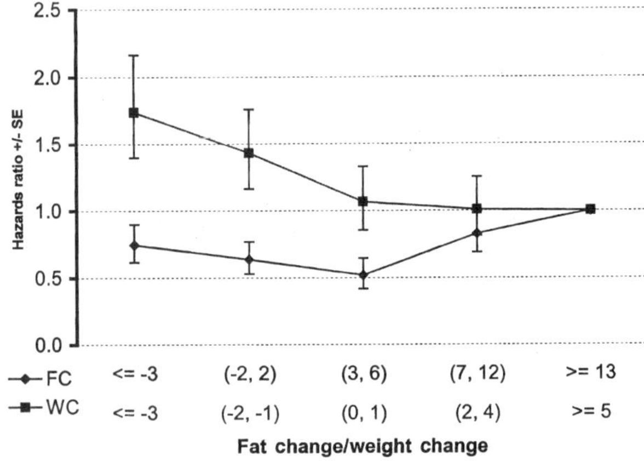

Figure 2 Estimated hazards ratios (to the last category) of individuals in the corresponding categories of weight changes in kg (WC) and fat change (FC; change in skinfolds thickness in mm), and their standard errors (SE) from the Tecumseh Community Health Study. The numbers in parentheses represent the minimum and maximum values for the corresponding quintile-defined categories. For both WC and FC, the positive and negative values represent gains and losses, respectively. (From Ref. 60.)

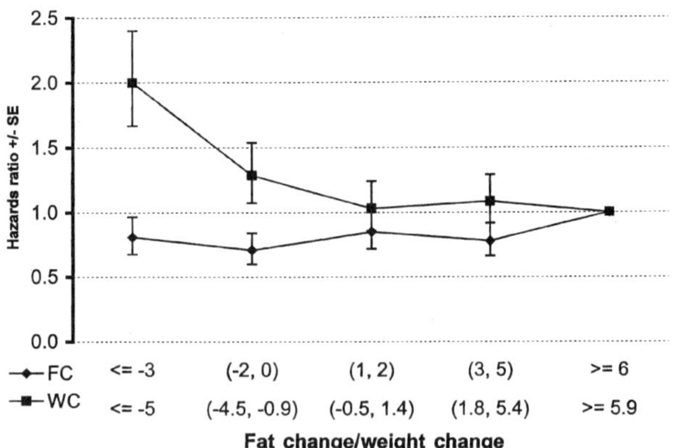

Figure 3 Estimated hazards ratios (to the last category) of individuals in the corresponding categories of weight changes in kg (WC) and fat change (FC; change in skinfolds thickness in mm), and their standard errors (SE) from the Framingham Heart Study. The numbers in parentheses represent the minimum and maximum values for the corresponding quintile-defined categories. For both WC and FC, the positive and negative values represent gains and losses, respectively. (From Ref. 60.)

This puzzling finding is the subject of considerable inquiry (110). Among the important research challenges associated with investigating the effects of weight change on mortality with current epidemiologic data are: (1) the appropriateness of basing estimates of the benefits or risks of weight loss on self-reported intentionality; (2) the potential confounding effects of smoking and preexisting disease; (3) the difficulty of assessing and accurately taking account of weight regain after weight loss; (4) assessing dietary changes during follow-up; and (5) the use of body mass index (BMI: kg/m^2) as a proxy for both fat mass and fat-free mass.

Another important issue to consider is the unknown efficacy and safety of many weight loss practices. Methods for intentionally inducing weight loss include fad diets, herbal supplements of untested safety (111), bulimia, and other potentially unsafe dietary practices. Hence, it appears ill advised to estimate the effects of weight loss achieved by medically recommended methods by studying weight loss that is merely reported to be "intentional." What is needed are studies of weight loss produced among obese humans by modern methods that are accepted by mainstream medicine.

As discussed previously, studies that have used BMI as a proxy for adiposity may not provide the best estimate of the impact of obesity or weight change on mortality. In this regard, Allison et al. (60) investigated change in weight and fat (via skinfolds), across two time points, and mortality in two epidemiologic studies—the Tecumseh Community Health Study and the Framingham Heart Study. In both studies, weight loss was associated with an increased mortality rate, while fat loss was associated with a reduced mortality rate. Specifically, each standard deviation of weight loss (~ 5.5 kg across both studies) was estimated to increase the hazard of mortality by $\sim 35\%$. In contrast, each standard deviation of fat loss (10.0 mm in Tecumseh and 4.8 mm in Framingham) reduced the hazard of mortality by $\sim 16\%$ (see Figs. 2,3). Thus, among individuals that are not severely obese, weight loss is associated with increased mortality rate, and fat loss with decreased mortality rate. If confirmed, these results suggest that weight loss should be recommended only under conditions where a sufficient proportion of the weight lost would be fat. Unfortunately, the conditions required to produce such a weight loss remain unknown, as is the exact proportion that is "sufficient."

IV SUMMARY AND RECOMMENDATIONS

A Overall Findings

The aforementioned methodological issues, most notably the use of BMI as a proxy for adiposity measures, suggest strongly that the current epidemiologic data may not provide us with the best estimates of the obesity/mortality association. Nonetheless, describing what the available data show is relatively simple. When the overall body of literature is reviewed, the data clearly show that the association between BMI and mortality is U- or J-shaped. Among nonelderly white males and females, the nadirs of the curve tend to be around the mid to high 20s for BMI. Though isolated studies may occasionally show other results, these conclusions are clearly supported by the overall body of data (18).

The relationship between BMI and mortality, however, appears to vary substantially by age and race, and it is likely that other variables, not yet identified or fully explored, may also moderate this relationship. It seems ill advised, therefore, to generalize from studies in one population (e.g., white middle-aged females) to other populations (e.g., elderly Asian females). Thus, one should refrain from making broad statements about the overall "average" relationship between BMI and mortality for the U.S. population unless such a statement is based on data that are representative of the U.S. population.

B Effect of Potential Confounders

While smoking is a plausible confounder of the BMI/mortality relationship, in practice, adjusting for smoking or excluding smokers from the analysis has very little effect on the results. This does not imply that one should not control for smoking, only that smoking does not appear to account for the U- and J-shaped relationships frequently observed in BMI/mortality studies. Nonetheless, some have argued (38) that smoking may still account for the high mortality at the lower BMI range since statistical adjustment for smoking may not address the nuances involved in smoking such as depth of inhalation and genetic susceptibility. Of course this does not explain why the J- and U-shaped association is still typically observed when "ever-smokers" are omitted from the analysis.

Excluding early deaths is not a reliable way of controlling for confounding due to occult disease. In the presence of such confounding, exclusions can either increase or decrease the bias, although in practice such exclusions appear to make little difference (39). However, because exclusions can actually increase the bias under some circumstances and result in a reduction of sample size, we do not recommend that subjects dying during the first few years be excluded from analyses. The same can be said for the practice advocated recently of excluding individuals with recent weight loss or weight fluctuation (until and unless evidence is brought to bear that shows otherwise).

A number of studies have demonstrated that low cardiorespiratory fitness increases mortality rate, suggesting that the BMI/mortality association may be confounded by fitness. It is important to note, however, that the majority of these observational studies were conducted in middle-aged white men. It is unclear, therefore, whether these results generalize to women, the elderly, and minority groups. Moreover, most studies that have investigated the relationship between obesity and health/mortality have tended to rely on self-reports of physical activity rather than fitness per se. Thus, although a physically active lifestyle may promote fitness and thus attenuate the increased rate of morbidity and mortality observed among obese persons, more sophisticated research designs and assessment techniques are required to tease out the independent effects of obesity and fitness on mortality. Indeed, recent randomized controlled clinical trials suggest that weight loss appears to have a greater effect on CVD risk factors than does improving cardiorespiratory fitness, implying that obesity may play a more central role in morbidity and mortality than fitness. Nonetheless, further research is required to disentangle the independent effects of obesity, a sedentary lifestyle, and poor fitness on health, morbidity, and mortality.

C Effects of Weight Loss

Intentional weight loss among persons with obesity-related comorbidities such as diabetes appears to reduce mortality rate. However, among apparently healthy overweight/obese adults, intentional weight loss seems to neither decrease nor increase mortality rate. Given that these findings were derived from observational studies that relied on self-reported intentionality of the weight loss, they should be interpreted with caution (110). Nonetheless, the current data suggest that remaining weight stable or increasing body weight slightly associates with lower mortality.

D BMI Versus Body Composition Measures

Though highly correlated with adiposity, BMI is not a true measure of adiposity and we cannot therefore assume that BMI will have the same relationship with mortality as will a more precise measure of body composition. Indeed, studies that have used other body composition measures suggest that distinguishing fat mass from fat-free mass may be required to determine the "true" effect of obesity on mortality, as well as the effect of intentional weight loss on mortality.

Given the quality of the data and the methodological issues outlined throughout this chapter, many of the conclusions drawn from the literature are, at best, tentative. Consistent with most clinical and basic laboratory research, however, it is clear that high levels of BMI (i.e., BMIs $>$ 30) are associated with increased mortality rate. In contrast, over the range of BMI from about 28 on down, the picture is not clear. The data suggest that lower BMIs are associated with increased mortality. However, this is inconsistent with the clinical evidence suggesting that intentional weight loss generally associates with a reduction in morbidities (99). Moreover, these data run counter to the results of animal research indicating that caloric restriction is capable of producing substantial increases in longevity (98).

E Explaining the J- or U-Shaped Association

The reasons that persons with lower levels of BMI are at greater mortality risk than those with midrange BMIs are not known. However, as we have shown, smoking is probably not a sufficient explanation for this phenomenon. A possibility that has not been considered seriously is that being in the mid-BMI range may actually cause one to be at lower risk of death from certain causes. For example, relative to thinness, it is clear that being in the mid-BMI range is protective against osteoporosis (112,113). Moreover, there is a clear biological mechanism because thinness is a significant risk factor for hip fracture (114), and these fractures, in turn, increase mortality rate (112,115).

It is also possible that lifestyle factors may explain some of the excess mortality associated with thinness. It has been demonstrated in data from the 1990 Behavioral Risk Factor Surveillance Survey that thin men and women were more likely to be sedentary and to consume high-fat diets than normal-weight adults (116). Moreover, data from the ACLS indicates that thin men and women with low aerobic fitness had the highest mortality rates (117). Thus, for at least some persons with low BMI, unhealthy lifestyles may contribute to a higher mortality rate and may help account for the J- or U-shaped BMI/mortality association.

Though more speculative, it is also possible that, relative to being in the mid-BMI range, people in the low BMI range are more potently affected by or more susceptible to certain forms of infection, injury, or disease (e.g., cancers). Finally, given that most Americans, as well as people of many other countries, do not consume adequate amounts of fruits, vegetables, fiber, and many micronutrients (e.g., 118), it may be that thin people, simply by virtue of eating less total food, are at increased risk of nutrient deficiencies despite sufficient caloric intake to remain weight stable. That is, just as laboratory animals live longer under conditions of CR, provided they have adequate micronutrient intake (119, 120), thinness in humans may be deleterious only because, for some people, it may be associated with inadequate intake of certain nutrients.

Since it is possible that thinness causes increased mortality rate, we believe potential explanations, like those we have proposed, should be investigated, and that further research is required to understand rather than simply to "explain away" the counterintuitive observation of elevated mortality rate among the thin.

V CONCLUSIONS AND FUTURE DIRECTIONS

Even if viable biological mechanisms to explain the apparent elevated mortality in the lower range of BMI were established, it is clear that the current literature has been derived from suboptimal epidemiologic data; that is, BMI, the measured independent variable, is only a proxy for adiposity, the "true" independent variable. Moreover, occult disease, the most plausible confounding factor, is not measured but inferred.

In our view, investigators have tried to compensate for the suboptimal data by using sophisticated statistical approaches. We believe, however, that no statistical technique, no matter how elegant, can produce valid conclusions from data that are unable to address directly the obesity/mortality association. We contend that valid conclusions pertaining to the obesity/mortality association are most likely to come if we use better measurements and study designs. In our view, the optimal study would be a long-term large scale randomized controlled clinical trial (121) that included: (1) a sample of persons along a broad range of BMI (mildly overweight to severely obese); (2) serial measures of body composition; (3) thorough and ongoing clinical evaluations of health status; and (4) in addition to mortality as an endpoint, the use of clinically relevant markers of subclinical disease as outcomes.

In the interim, we must rely on thoughtful and careful epidemiologic investigations using the available observational data. However, as the design and measurement techniques used in observational studies become more sophisticated and more widely used, we will be in a better position to draw valid conclusions regarding the obesity/mortality association.

ACKNOWLEDGMENT

This work was supported in part by National Institutes of Health grants RO1DK51716, P30DK56336, and R21AG17166.

REFERENCES

1. Kahn HS, Williamson DF. Abdominal obesity and mortality risk among men in nineteenth-century North America. Int J Obes Rel Metab Disord 1994; 18:686–691.
2. Kuczmarski RJ, Flegal KM, Campbell SM, Johnson CL. Increasing prevalence of overweight among US adults. The National Health and Nutrition Examination Survey, 1960–1991. JAMA 1994; 27:205–211.
3. Mokdad AH, Serdula MK, Dietz WH, Bowman BA, Marks JS, Koplan JP. The spread of the obesity epidemic in the United States, 1991–1998. JAMA 1999; 282:1519–1522.
4. Popkin BM, Doak CM. The obesity epidemic is a worldwide phenomenon. Nutr Rev 1998; 56:106–114.
5. WHO. Obesity. Preventing and Managing the Global Epidemic. Geneva: World Health Organization, 1998.
6. Simopoulos AP, Van Itallie TB. Body weight, health, and longevity. Ann Intern Med 1984; 100:285–295.
7. Manson JE, Stampfer MJ, Hennekens CH, Willett WC. Body weight and longevity: a reassessment. JAMA 1987; 257:353–358.
8. Samaras TT, Storms LH. Impact of height and weight on life span. Bull WHO 1992; 70:259–267.
9. Allison DB, Faith MS, Heo M, Kotler DP. Hypothesis concerning the U-shaped relation between body mass index and mortality. Am J Epidemiol 1997; 146:339–349.
10. Hubert HB, Feinleib M, McNamara PM, Castell WP. Obesity as an independent risk factor for cardiovascular disease: a 26-year follow-up of participants in the Framingham Heart Study. Circulation 1983; 67: 968–977.
11. Lee IM, Manson JE, Hennekens CH, Paffenbarger RS. Body weight and mortality: a 27-year follow-up of middle-aged men. JAMA 1993; 270:2823–2828.
12. Manson JE, Willett WC, Stampfer MJ, Colditz GA, Hunter DJ, Hankinson SE, Hennekens CH, Speizer FE. Body weight and mortality among women. N Engl J Med 1995; 333:677–685.
13. Carmelli D, Halpern J, Swan GE. 27-Year mortality in Western Collaborative Group Study: construction of risk groups by recursive partitioning. J Clin Epidemiol 1991; 44:1341–1351.
14. Keil JE, Sutherland SE, Knapp RG, Lackland DT, Gazes PC, Tyroler HA. Mortality rates and risk factors for coronary disease in black as compared to white men and women. N Engl J Med 1993; 329:73–78.
15. Menotti A, Descovich GC, Lanti M. Indexes of obesity and all-causes mortality in Italian epidemiological data. Prev Med 1993; 22:293–303.
16. Allison DB, Gallagher D, Heo M, Pi-Sunyer FX, Heymsfield SB. Body mass index and all-cause mortality among people age 70 and over: the Longitudinal Study of Aging. Int J Obes Relat Metab Disord 1997; 21:424–431.
17. Fontaine KR, Heo M, Cheskin LJ, Allison DB. Body mass index, smoking, and mortality among older American women. J Womens Health 1998; 7:1257–1261.

18. Troiano RP, Frongillo EA Jr, Sobal J, Levitsky DA. The relationship of body weight and mortality: a quantitative analysis of combined information from existing studies. Int J Obes Rel Metab Disord 1996; 20:63–75.
19. Visscher TLS, Seidell JC, Menotti A, Blackburn H, Nissinen A, Feskens EJM, Kromhout D. Underweight and overweight in relation to mortality among men aged 40–59 and 50–69 years: The Seven Countries Study. Am J Epidemiol 2000; 151:660–666.
20. Andres R, Muller DC, Sorkin JD. Long-term effects of change in body weight on all-cause mortality. A review. Ann Intern Med 1993; 110:737–743.
21. Stevens J, Cai J, Pamuk ER, Williamson DF, Thun MJ, Wood JL. The effect of age on the association between body-mass index and mortality. N Engl J Med 1998; 338:1–7.
22. Stevens J. Impact of age on associations between weight and mortality. Nutr Rev 2000; 58:129–137.
23. Kushner RF. Body weight and mortality. Nutr Rev 1993; 51:127–136.
24. Michels KB, Greenland S, Rosner BA. Does body mass index adequately capture the relation of body composition and body size to health outcomes? Am J Epidemiol 1998; 147:167–172.
25. Allison DB, Heo M, Fontaine KR, Hoffman DJ. Body weight, body composition, and longevity. In: Bjorntorp P, ed. International Textbook of Obesity Sussex: John Wiley & Sons, 2001:31–48.
26. Sempos CT, Durazo-Arvizu R, McGee DL, Cooper RS, Prewitt TE. The influence of cigarette smoking on the association between body weight and mortality: the Framingham Heart Study revisited. Ann Epidemiol 1998; 8:289–300.
27. Brenner H, Arndt V, Rothenbacher D, Schuberth S, Fraisse E, Fliedner TM. Body weight, pre-existing disease, and all-cause mortality in a cohort of male employees in the German construction industry. J Clin Epidemiol 1997; 50:1099–1106.
28. Dorn JM, Schisterman EF, Winkelstein W Jr, Trevisan M. Body mass index and mortality in a general population sample of men and women. The Buffalo Health Study. Am J Epidemiol 1997; 146:919–931.
29. Chyou PH, Burchfiel CM, Yano K, Sharp DS, Rodriguez BL, Curb JD, Nomura AM. Obesity, alcohol consumption, smoking, and mortality. Ann Epidemiol 1997; 7:311–317.
30. Seidell JC, Verschuren WM, Van Leer EM, Kromhout D. Overweight, underweight, and mortality: a prospective study of 48,287 men and women. Arch Intern Med 1996; 156:958–963.
31. Wienpahl J, Ragland DR, Sidney S. Body mass index and 15-year mortality in a cohort of black men and women. J Clin Epidemiol 1990; 43:949–960.
32. Landi F, Onder G, Gambassi G, Pedone C, Carbonin P, Bernabei R. Body mass index and mortality among hospitalized patients. Ann Intern Med 2000; 160:2641–2644.
33. Yuan J-M, Ross RK, Gao Y-T, Yu MC. Body weight and mortality: a prospective evaluation in a cohort of middle-aged men in Shanghai, China. Int J Epidemiol 1998; 27:824–832.
34. Rissanen A, Heliovaara M, Knekt P, Aromaa A, Reunanen A, Maatela J. Weight and mortality in Finnish men. J Clin Epidemiol 1989; 42:781–789.
35. Wannamethee G, Shaper AG. Body weight and mortality in middle aged British men: impact of smoking. Lancet 1989; 299:1497–1502.
36. Garrison RJ, Feinleib M, Castelli WP. Cigarette smoking as a contributor of the relationship between relative weight and long-term mortality: the Framingham Heart Study. JAMA 1983; 249:2199–2203.
37. BMI in Diverse Populations Collaborative Group. Effect of smoking on the body mass index-mortality relation: empirical evidence from 15 studies. Am J Epidemiol 1999; 150:1297–1308.
38. Willet WC, Dietz WH, Colditz GA. Guidelines for healthy weight. N Engl J Med 1999; 341:427–434.
39. Allison DB, Heo M, Flanders DW, Faith MS, Williamson DF. Examination of "early mortality exclusion" as an approach to control for confounding by occult disease in epidemiologic studies of mortality risk factors. Am J Epidemiol 1997; 146:672–680.
40. Allison DB, Heo M, Flanders DW, Faith MS, Carpenter KM, Williamson DF. Simulation studies of the effects of excluding early deaths on risk-factor mortality analyses in the presence of confounding due to occult disease: the example of body mass index. Ann Epidemiol 1999; 9:132–142.
41. Allison DB, Faith MS, Heo M, Townsend-Butterworth D, Williamson DF. Meta-analysis of the effect of excluding early deaths on the estimated relationship between body mass index and mortality. Obes Res 1999; 7:342–354.
42. Andres R. Beautiful hypotheses and ugly facts: the BMI-mortality association. Obes Res 1999; 7:417–419.
43. Calle EE, Thun MJ, Petreli JM, Rodriguez C, Heath CW. Body-mass index and mortality in a prospective cohort of U.S. adults. N Engl J Med 1999; 341:1097–1105.
44. Barlow CE, Kohl HW, Gibbons LW, Blair SN. Physical fitness, mortality, and obesity. Int J Obes Relat Metab Disord 1995; 19:S41–S44.
45. Gaesser GA. Thinness and weight loss: beneficial or detrimental to longevity? Med Sci Sports Exer 1999; 31:1118–1128.
46. Wei M, Kampert JB, Barlow CE, Nichaman MZ, Gibbons LW, Paffenbarger RS, Blair SN. Relationship between low cardiorespiratory fitness and mortality in normal-weight, overweight, and obese men. JAMA 1999; 282:1547–1553.
47. Blair SN, Kohl HW III, Barlow CE, Paffenbarger RS,

Gibbons LW, Macera CA. Changes in physical fitness and all-cause mortality: a prospective study of healthy men and women. JAMA 1995; 273:1093–1098.

48. Paffenbarger RS Jr, Hyde RT, Wing AL, Lee IM, Jung DL, Kampert JB. The association of changes in physical-activity level and other lifestyle characteristics with mortality among men. N Engl J Med 1993; 328:574–576.
49. Williams PT. Physical fitness and activity as separate heart disease risk factors: a meta-analysis. Med Sci Sports Exerc 2001; 33:754–761.
50. Katzel LE, Bleecker ER, Colman EG, Rogus EM, Sorkin JD, Goldberg AP. Effects of weight loss vs aerobic exercise training on risk factors for coronary disease in healthy, obese, middle-aged and older men. JAMA 1995; 274:1915–1921.
51. Wei M, Wallance J. Body mass index (BMI) as a predictor of mortality after adjustment for cardiorespiratory fitness in men with more than 10 years of follow-up. Obes Res 2000; 8(suppl 1):39S.
52. Katzmarzyk PT, Gagnon J, Leon AS, Skinner JS, Wilmore JH, Rao DC, Bouchard C. Fitness, fatness, and estimated coronary heart disease risk: the HERITAGE Family Study. Med Sci Sports Exerc 2001; 33:585–590.
53. Ross R, Dagnone D, Jones PJH, Smith H, Paddags A, Hudson R, Janssen I. Reduction in obesity and related comorbid conditions after diet-induced weight loss or exercise-induced weight loss in men: a randomized, controlled trial. Ann Intern Med 2000; 133:92–103.
54. Ross R, Freeman JA, Janssen I. Exercise alone is an effective strategy for reducing obesity and related comorbidities. Exerc Sport Sci Rev 2000; 28:165–170.
55. Bentler PM. Causal modeling via structural equation systems. In: Nesselroade JR, Cattell RB, eds. Handbook of Multivariate Experimental Psychology. 2d ed. New York: Plenum Press, 1988:317–335.
56. Berry WD. Understanding Regression Assumptions. Newbury Park: Sage, 1993.
57. Roche AF, Siervogel RM, Chumlea WC, Webb P. Grading body fatness from limited anthropometric data. Am J Clin Nutr 1981; 34:2831–2838.
58. Segal KR, Dunaif A, Gutin B, Albu J, Nyman A, Pi-Sunyer FX. Body composition, not body weight, is related to cardiovascular disease risk factors and sex hormone levels in men. J Clin Invest 1987; 80:1050–1055.
59. Allison DB, Zanolli R, Faith MS, Heo M, Pietrobelli A, VanItallie TB, Pi-Sunyer FX, Heymsfield SB. Weight loss increases and fat loss decreases all-cause mortality rate: results from two independent cohort studies. Int J Obes Relat Metab Disord 1999; 23:603–611.
60. Keys A. Longevity of men: relative weight and fatness in middle age. Ann Med 1989; 21:163–168.
61. Folsom AR, Kaye SA, Sellers TA. Body fat distribution and 5-year risk of death in older women. JAMA 1993; 142:483–487.
62. Menotti A, Keys A, Kromhout D. Inter-cohort differences in CHD mortality in the 25-year follow-up of the Seven Countries Study. Eur J Epidemiol 1993; 9:527–536.
63. Charles MA, Oppert J-M, Thibult N, Guy-Grand B, Ducimetiere P. Muscle mass, fat mass, and mortality: 15-year follow-up of the Paris Prospective Study. Obes Res 2000; 7(suppl 1):59S.
64. Baik I, Ascherio A, Rimm EB, Giovannucci E, Spiegelman D, Stampfer MJ, Willett WC. Adiposity and mortality in men. Am J Epidemiol 2000; 152:264–271.
65. Heitmann BL, Erikson H, Ellsinger B-M, Mikkelson KL, Larsson B. Mortality associated with body fat, fat-free mass and body mass index among 60-year-old Swedish men—a 22-year follow-up. Int J Obes Relat Metab Disord 2000; 24:33–37.
66. Lahmann PH, Lissner L, Gullberg B, Berglund G. All-cause mortality in relation to body fatness and central adiposity. Int J Obes Relat Metab Disord 2000; 24: S25.
67. Allison DB, Zhu S, Plankey M, Faith MS, Heo M. Differential associations of body mass index and adiposity with all-cause mortality among men in the first and second National Health and Nutrition Examination Surveys (NHANES I & NHANES II) follow-up studies. Int J Obes Relat Metab Disord 2002; 26:410–416.
68. Zhu S, Heo M, Plankey M, Faith MS, Allison DB. Associations of body mass index and anthropometric indicators of fat mass and fat free mass with all-cause mortality among women in the first and second National Health and Nutrition Examination Surveys (NHANES I & NHANES II) follow-up studies. Ann Epidemiol 2003; 13:286–293.
69. Brill PA, Giles WH, Keenan NL, Croft JB, Davis DR, Jackson KL, Macera CA. Effect of body mass index on activity limitation and mortality among older women. The National Health Interview Survery, 1986–1990. J Womens Health 1997; 6:435–440.
70. Diehr P, Bild DE, Harris TB, Duxbury A, Siscovick D, Rossi M. Body mass index and mortality in non-smoking older adults: the Cardiovascular Health Study. Am J Pub Health 1998; 88:623–629.
71. Andres R, Elahi D, Tobin J, Muller DC, Brandt L. Impact of age on weight goals. Ann Intern Med 1985; 103:1030–1033.
72. Waaler HT. Height, weight, and mortality: the Norwegian experience. Acta Med Scand Suppl 1984; 679:1–56.
73. Rissanen A, Knekt P, Heliovaara M, Aromaa A, Reunanen A, Maatela J. Weight and mortality in Finnish women. J Clin Epidemiol 1991; 44:787–795.
74. Lindsted KD, Singh PN. Body mass and 26-year risk of mortality among women who never smoked: find-

ings for the Adventist Mortality Study. Am J Epidemiol 1997; 146:1–11.

75. Seccareccia F, Lanti M, Menotti A, Scanga M. Role of body mass index in the prediction of all cause mortality in over 62,000 men and women. The Italian RIFLE Pooling Project. Risk factor and life expectancy. J Epidemiol Commun Health 1998; 52:20–26.
76. Bender R, Jockel KH, Trautner C, Spraul M, Berger M. Effect of age on excess mortality in obesity. JAMA 1999; 281:1498–1504.
77. Stevens J, Cai J, Juhaeri, Thun MJ, Williamson DF, Wood JL. Consequences of the use of different measures of effect to determine the impact of age on the association between obesity and mortality. Am J Epidemiol 1999; 150:399–407.
78. Van Itallie TB, Lew EA. In search of optimal weights for US man and women. In: Pi-Sunyer FX, Allison DB, eds. Obesity Treatment: Establishing Goals, Improving Outcomes, and Reviewing the Research Agenda. New York: Plenum, 1995:1–20.
79. Allison DB, Edlen-Nezin L, Clay-Williams G. Obesity among African American women: prevalence, consequences, causes, and developing research. Womens Health 1997; 3:243–274.
80. Nabulsi AA, Folsom AR, Heiss G, Weir SS, Chambless LE, Watson RL, Eckfeldt HH. Fasting hyperinsulinemia and cardiovascular disease risk factors in nondiabetic adults: stronger associations in lean versus obese subjects. Metabolism 1995; 44:914–922.
81. Stevens J, Keil JE, Rus PF, Tyroler HA, Davis CE, Gazes PC. Body mass index and body girths as predictors of mortality in black and white women. Arch Intern Med 1992; 152:1257–1262.
82. Stevens J. Studies of the impact of age on optimal body weight. J Nutr Biochem 1998; 9:501–510.
83. Durazo-Arvizu R, McGee D, Li Z, Cooper R. Establishing the nadir of the body mass index–mortality relationship: a case study. J Am Stat Assoc 1997; 92:1312–1319.
84. Durazo-Arvizu R, Cooper RS, Luke A, Prewitt TE, Liao Y, McGee DL. Relative weight and mortality in U.S. blacks and whites: findings from representative national population samples. Ann Epidemiol 1997; 7:383–395.
85. Sanchez AM, Reed DR, Price RA. Reduced mortality associated with body mass index in African-Americans relative to Caucasians. Ethnicity Dis 2000; 10:24–30.
86. Cornoni-Huntley JC, Harris TB, Everett DF, Albanes D, Micozzi MS, Miles TP, Feldman JJ. An overview of body weight of older persons, including the impact on morality. J Clin Epidemiol 1991; 44:743–753.
87. Johnson JL, Heineman EF, Heiss G, Hames CG, Tyroler HA. Cardiovascular disease risk factors and mortality among black women and white women aged 40–64 years in Evans County, Georgia. Am J Epidemiol 1986; 123:209–220.
88. Sorkin JD, Zonderman AB, Costa PT Jr, Andres RA. Twenty-year follow-up of the NHANES I cohort: test of methodological hypotheses. Obes Res 1996; 4:S12.
89. Stevens J, Plankey MW, Willaimson DF, Thun MJ, Rust PF, Palesch Y, O'Neil PM. The body mass index–mortality relationship in white and African American women. Obes Res 1998; 6:268–277.
90. Hodge AM, Dowse GK, Collins VR, Zimmet PZ. Mortality in Micronesian Nauruans and Melanesian and Indian Fijians is not associated with obesity. Am J Epidemiol 1997; 143:442–455.
91. Collins VR, Dowse GK, Cabealawa S, Ram P, Zimmet PZ. High mortality from cardiovascular disease and analysis of risk factors in Indian and Melanesian Fijians. Int J Epidemiol 1996; 25:59–69.
92. Stern MP, Patterson JK, Mitchell BD, Haffner SM, Hazuda HP. Overweight and mortality in Mexican Americans. Int J Obes Rel Metab Disord 1990; 14:623–629.
93. Hanson RL, McCance DR, Jacobsson LT, Narayan KM, Nelson RG, Pettitt DJ, Bennett PH, Knowler WC. The U-shaped association between body-mass index and mortality-relationship with weight-gain in a Native-American population. J Clin Epidemiol 1995; 48:903–915.
94. Collins FS. Medical and societal consequences of the human genome project. N Engl J Med 1999; 341:28–37.
95. Moatti D, Faure S, Fumeron F, Amara ME, Seknadji P, McDermott DH, Debre P, Aumont MC, Murphy PM, De Prost D, Combadiere C. Polymorphism in the fractalkine receptor CX3CR1 as a genetic risk factor for coronary heart disease. Blood 2001; 97:1925–1928.
96. Rizzoli R, Bonjour JP, Ferrari SL. Osteoporosis, genetics and hormones. J Mol Endocrinol 2001; 26:79–94.
97. Smith BA, Edwards MS, Ballachey BE, Cramer DA, Sutherland TM. Body weight and longevity in genetically obese and non-obese mice fed fat-modified diets. Growth Dev Aging 1991; 55:81–89.
98. Walford RL, Harris SB, Weindruch R. Dietary restriction and aging: historical phases, mechanisms and current discussion. J Nutr 1987; 117:1650–1654.
99. National Task Force on the Prevention and Treatment of Obesity. Overweight, obesity, and health risk. Arch Intern Med 2000; 160:898–904.
100. Williamson DF, Pamuk E, Thun M, Flanders D, Byers T, Heath C. Prospective study of intentional weight loss and mortality in never-smoking overweight US white women aged 40–64 years. Am J Epidemiol 1995; 141:1128–1141.
101. Williamson DF, Thompson TJ, Thun M, Flanders D, Pamuk E, Byers T. Intentional weight loss and mortality among overweight individuals with diabetes. Diabetes Care 2000; 23:1499–1504.
102. French SA, Folsom AR, Jeffery RW, Williamson DF.

Prospective study of intentionaity of weight loss and mortality in older women: the Iowa Women's Health Study. Am J Epidemiol 1999; 149:504–514.

103. Williamson DF, Pamuk E, Thun M, Flanders D, Byers T, Heath C. Prospective study of intentional weight loss and mortality in overweight white men aged 40–64 years. Am J Epidemiol 1999; 149:491–503.
104. Pamuk ER, Williamson DF, Serdula MK, Madans J, Byers TE. Weight loss and subsequent death in a cohort of U.S. adults. Ann Intern Med 1993; 119:744–748.
105. Wee CC, David RB, Phillips RS. The relationship between intentional weight loss and all-cause mortality. Obes Res 2000; 8(suppl 1):97S.
106. Lee IM, Paffenbarger RS. Change in body weight and longevity. JAMA 1992; 268:2045–2049.
107. Blair SN, Shaten NJ, Brownell K, Collins G, Lissner L. Body weight change, all-cause mortality, and cause-specific mortality in the Multiple Risk Factor Intervention Trial. Ann Intern Med 1993; 119:749–757.
108. Higgins M, D'Agostino R, Kannel W, Cobb J, Pinsky J. Benefits and adverse effects of weight loss: observations from the Framingham Study. Ann Intern Med 1993; 119:758–763.
109. Lee IM, Paffenbarger RS. Is weight loss hazardous? Nutr Rev 1996; 54:S116–S124.
110. Williamson DF. Intentional weight loss: patterns in the general populations and its association with morbidity and mortality. Int J Obes Relat Metab Disord 1997; 21(suppl 1):S14–S19.
111. Allison DB, Fontaine KR, Heshka S, Mentore JL, Heymsfield SB. Alternative treatments for weight loss: a critical review. Crit Rev Food Sci Nutr 2001; 41:1–40.
112. Cummings SR, Nevitt MC, Browner WS, Stone K, Fox KM, Ensrud KE, Cauley J, Black D, Vogt TM. Risk factors for hip fracture in white women. N Engl J Med 1995; 332:767–773.
113. Ensrud KE, Cauley J, Lipschutz R, Cummings SR. Weight change and fractures in older women. Study of Osteoporotic Fractures Research Group. Arch Intern Med 1997; 157:857–863.
114. Slemenda C. Protection of hip fractures: risk factor modification. Am J Med 1997; 103:65S–71S.
115. Huuskonen J, Kroger H, Arnala I, Alhava E. Characteristics of male hip fracture patients. Ann Chir Gynaecol 1999; 88:48–53.
116. Simoes EJ, Byers T, Coates RJ, Serdula MK, Mokdad AA, Heath GW. The association between leisure time physical activity and dietary fat in American adults. Am J Pub Health 1995; 85:240–244.
117. Blair SN, Kohl HW III, Barlow CE, Paffenbarger RS, Gibbons LW, Macera CA. Physical fitness and all-cause mortality: a prospective study of healthy men and women. JAMA 1989; 262:2395–2401.
118. Peterson S, Sigman-Grant M, Eissenstat B, Kris-Etherton P. Impact of adopting lower-fat food choices on energy and nutrient intakes of American adults. J Am Diet Assoc 1999; 99:177–183.
119. Frame LT, Hart RW, Leakey JE. Caloric restriction as a mechanism mediating resistance to environmental disease. Environ Health Perspect 1998; 106(suppl 1):313–324.
120. McCarter RJ. Role of caloric restriction in the prolongation of life. Clin Geriatr Med 1995; 11:553–565.
121. Stern MP. The case for randomized clinical trials on the treatment of obesity. Obes Res 1995; 3(suppl 2):299s–306s.

32

Etiology of the Metabolic Syndrome

Per Björntorp

University of Göteborg, Göteborg, Sweden

I INTRODUCTION

One significant and rapidly developing area of obesity research is the etiology of the metabolic syndrome and its prevention and treatment. The syndrome exhibits the central, visceral subtype of obesity, which is an integral part of the syndrome and bears the most serious somatic hazards of obesity, while the peripheral, subcutaneous subtype is associated mainly with mechanical problems arising from the increased body weight.

Historically, the clustering of the symptoms now called the metabolic syndrome has been observed and documented since the beginning of the 20th century. There is little consensus on the definition, although many different proposals have been advanced, particularly after addition of new components to the core of the syndrome. Most authors agree on the inclusion of insulin resistance, abdominal obesity, dyslipidemia, and hypertension, since these established risk factors for cardiovascular disease, type 2 diabetes mellitus and stroke are the reason the metabolic syndrome is of major importance.

Techniques for evaluation of the major components of the syndrome have changed little since the previous edition of the Handbook of Obesity (1998) (1), probably because the methodology continues to be adequate. However, questions exist about certain simple anthropometric measurements; for example, the waist/hip circumference ratio (WHR). It is a poor measurement of intra-abdominal, visceral fat mass, a major statistical determinant of most of the comorbidities, yet its statistical power is surprising. Possibly this measurement contains unrecognized information beyond intra-abdominal fat mass, such as a muscle component included in the hip circumference measurement. These issues are an area for more research.

At the time of the first edition, research on endocrine perturbations focused on the disturbances of regulation of the hypothalamic-pituitary-adrenal (HPA) axis and its interference with the central gonadal and growth hormone axes. Major advances have occurred with the development of new techniques, which are sensitive and discriminating enough to reveal minor regulatory errors of daily life (2–4). Research has previously addressed the peripheral consequences of the endocrine perturbations (accumulation of intra-abdominal fat and insulin resistance) (5,6), perturbations in the capillary system and in the synthesis of myosins (1). Much progress has been made in these areas and in genetics since the previous edition. The original Handbook examined the period up to 1996–1997, so this chapter will focus on the following years, including generally integrated and specific aspects of these developments covered in several recent reviews (2–9).

II DEFINITION OF THE METABOLIC SYNDROME

A syndrome is a collection of symptoms typically occurring together. Such syndromes often originate from errors not in a single organ or tissue, such as in myocardial infarction, liver cirrhosis, or brain tumors, but from overriding systemic control of the function of several organs. Multiple consequences can result, causing difficulty in diagnosis. Such syndromes often begin as basic symptomatic description, but if the basic etiology becomes clearer, treatment shifts from symptomatic to causal.

The metabolic syndrome is usually considered to include two major symptoms, insulin resistance and visceral obesity, with the addition of hypertension and dyslipidemia in the form of elevated circulating concentrations of triglycerides and triglyceride-rich very low density lipoprotein (VLDL) particles and low concentrations of high-density lipoprotein (HDL) particles. The major question is whether these apparently divergent symptoms can be collected under one common etiological mechanism.

The metabolic syndrome may arise from a component of the syndrome, acting alone or in combination with other factors. The list includes insulin resistance, visceral fat, endocrine dysregulation (cortisol, androgens, insulin, growth hormone), obesity, and/or genetics. Let us first consider the possibility that a single symptom causes the other components of the metabolic syndrome.

A Insulin Resistance as a Primary Pathogenic Factor

Reaven (10) examines whether insulin resistance could be the primary factor, resulting in dyslipidemia and hypertension. The relationship between insulin and dyslipidemia seems to be well established; however, a recent review (9) casts doubt on the concept that hypertension results from hyperinsulinemia alone. Reaven's cluster of common risk factors is the first synopsis of variables for what he terms "Syndrome X" and is supported by evidence, much from Reaven's own excellent research. Syndrome X may, however, be considered to be part of a larger syndrome, commonly called the metabolic syndrome, which also contains visceral obesity as a major component. While reasonable due to the well-documented close connection between visceral obesity and insulin resistance (11), it is difficult to imagine how insulin resistance with compensatory hyperinsulinemia might increase visceral fat mass. Therefore, other etiological primary events for the metabolic syndrome must be considered.

B Visceral Fat as a Primary Pathogenic Factor

Could the other major component of the metabolic syndrome, visceral fat accumulation, be the primary factor? One hypothesis is that free fatty acids (FFA), from the enlarged, lipolytically very active visceral fat stores delivered to the hepatic portal vein, would generate risk factors by hepatic mechanisms (12). This is an attractive hypothesis for generation of dyslipidemia in the metabolic syndrome because both insulin and delivery of FFA limit the rate of synthesis of lipoproteins in the liver. Peripheral systemic hyperinsulinemia might result from diminished hepatic clearance of portal insulin, and cause peripheral insulin resistance by a secondary downregulation of insulin receptor density. Possibly large enough concentrations of portal FFA can leak out into systemic circulation (even with 50% liver reabsorption) to cause muscular insulin resistance (13).

There are a few concerns with this hypothesis, however. First, these are theoretical considerations, lacking direct information because of the difficulty of examining the flow of FFA and insulin in the portal vein in humans. But there is indirect support (12,13) as well as recent data suggesting that hepatic exposure to FFA might well be elevated, provided FFA release from not only the portal but also the systemic circulation is included (14). Another problem is that the hypertension of the metabolic syndrome does not fit well unless hyperinsulinemia is the primary factor, which is not always the case, as discussed below. Furthermore, and most importantly, this hypothesis does not explain the apparently selective accumulation of depot fat in the visceral, "portal" adipose tissues. This is not a simple consequence of obesity in general where fat is normally harmoniously deposited in several depots, including subcutaneous regions. In summary, although this hypothesis has some merit and may apply to some symptoms of the metabolic syndrome, it does not seem to fully explain the etiology.

The remaining core symptoms of the metabolic syndrome, hypertension and dyslipidemia, are difficult to visualize as primary etiological factors for visceral obesity and insulin resistance. In principle, factors other than the cluster of symptoms in the metabolic syndrome could be involved as primary pathogenic factors.

C Hormones as a Primary Pathogenic Factor

Hormones are the major regulators of metabolic events. Could the metabolic syndrome be a consequence of endocrine dysregulation? The similarities between Cushing's syndrome and the metabolic syndrome are quite apparent, not only for distribution of fat depots but also for insulin resistance, dyslipidemia, hypertension, and certain diseases associated with these symptoms. Could the metabolic syndrome be a hypercortisolemic condition? It is a difficult question. Cortisol's effects can be hidden because it is difficult in vivo to measure, yet in general they support the hypothesis, and numerous studies show a connection.

Measurements of cortisol secretion and its regulation via the hypothalamic-pituitary-adrenal (HPA) axis are complicated, even in conditions of clearly elevated secretion, such as Cushing's syndrome. HPA axis regulation is easily disturbed by external environmental factors (15). Therefore, noninvasive sampling in ordinary circumstances is probably required to reveal minor, putative abnormalities as seen in obesity and the metabolic syndrome.

Another factor causing difficulty is the complex regulatory machinery of the HPA axis, with stimulating, amplifying and feedback inhibitory stations that result in a specific, diurnal rhythm with discrete peaks of varying magnitude and duration. This drowns single measurements of cortisol. Evidence now indicates that the kinetics of the diurnal curve might provide information different from that of total cortisol secretion (2,3); i.e., although urinary excretion of free cortisol might be measurable if the organism has been exposed to elevated circulating cortisol, a low excretion of cortisol does not necessarily equal a normal regulation of the HPA axis. Furthermore, the status of the HPA axis regulation is probably best examined by stimulatory or inhibitory tests.

III ASSOCIATION OF THE METABOLIC SYNDROME AND ELEVATED CORTISOL LEVELS

Recent studies (16,17) have shown a link between stress, salivary cortisol levels, and the metabolic syndrome, using relevant population samples (2,3) (See Fig. 1.) About two-thirds of a group of middle-aged Swedish men and women exhibited an apparently normal diurnal saliva cortisol curve, measured under ordinary life conditions and examined with low dose dexamethasone. However, ~25% of the men reported stress during the day of measurements (curve labeled "stress" in Fig. 1). In these men, the daytime saliva cortisol levels differed dramatically. Rather than a peak upon awakening followed by a sharp drop in the morning, the stress pattern peaked at lunch, and decreased drastically in the afternoon/evening hours. This resulted in an elevated total cortisol secretion over the day. Although varying effects of dexamethasone may have flawed some of these cases, indicating a need for stronger methodology (3), other studies have shown similar values (18). The immediate wake-up peak appears to be significant. Subjects in a stressful milieu have lower saliva cortisol values upon awakening which then do not "unwind" normally (19). The delayed downwinding of morning cortisol is echoed in controlled animal experiments (20), where stress exposure precedes hypersensitivity of the HPA axis at peak activity (night in rodents, early morning in humans). The tentative conclusion from this information is that ~25% of the populations examined may have an HPA axis regulation linked to stress experiences that cause elevated cortisol levels. This conclusion is significant when coupled with another finding of the Swedish study (16,17).

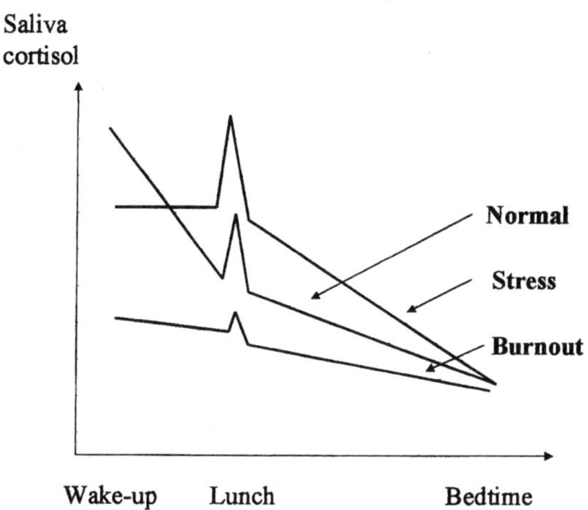

Figure 1 Saliva cortisol in men. (From Refs. 2,16.)

In the men who reported stress during the day of measurements and who had elevated total cortisol, constituting ~25% of the total population (See curve labeled "stress" in Fig. 1), there were direct associations between cortisol measurements and several features of the metabolic syndrome (16,21). Cortisol measurements, particularly those relating to perceived stress and after food intake, correlated directly with measurements of visceral obesity, insulin resistance, dyslipidemia, and blood pressure. These findings suggest a quantitative connection between cortisol secretion and the metabolic syndrome. The associations are clearer after HPA axis challenges (stress and food intake) than with baseline cortisol values in steady state (16,21). Similar observations with elevated basal and/or stimulated cortisol secretion in central, visceral obesity (22–29) and other cardiovascular risk factors (30–35) have now been made by several other laboratories.

A Effects of Cortisol

Cortisol is well known to cause peripheral insulin resistance, and the mechanisms have been clarified (36).

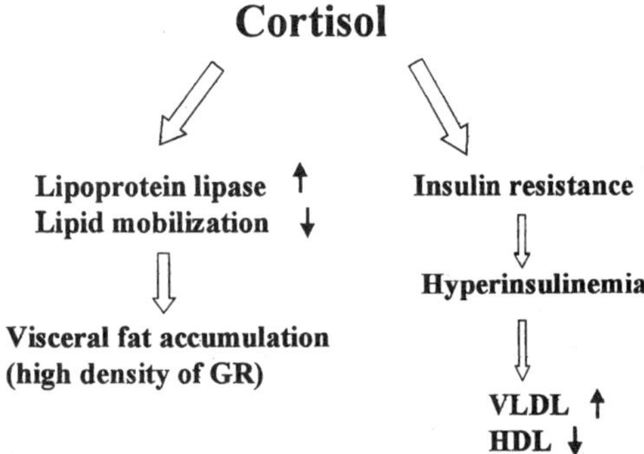

Figure 2 Cortisol, in the presence of insulin, induces visceral fat accumulation by expression of lipoprotein lipase and inhibition of lipid mobilization. Cortisol also induces insulin resistance, followed by compensatory hyperinsulinemia which is responsible for increased levels of triglyceride-rich VLDL and low levels of HDL.

Furthermore, cortisol is known to direct the storage of fat to visceral depots, as seen most typically in Cushing's syndrome, and the mechanisms have been defined at the cellular and molecular levels as reviewed previously (5). In brief, in the presence of insulin, cortisol stimulates pathways for lipid accumulation (lipoprotein lipase) while inhibiting lipid mobilization. This is mediated via the glucocorticoid receptor, with particularly high density in visceral fat. The dyslipidemia of the metabolic syndrome (high triglycerides; triglyceride-rich, low-density lipoproteins; and low high-density lipoproteins) can be derived from the insulin resistance and subsequent hyperinsulinemia via a combination of hepatic events, combined with a diminished removal of triglyceride-rich particles in the periphery (10). The remaining symptom, elevated blood pressure probably results from parallel activation of the HPA axis and sympathetic nervous system. High insulin levels might facilitate this stimulation. This is summarized in Figure 2.

In summary, cortisol elevation clearly seems to be able to induce the metabolic syndrome through known mechanisms. This is also seen in Cushing's syndrome and in patients treated with glucocorticoids, where abnormalities vanish when cortisol excess is removed (37). It may then be concluded that human subjects who show an increased cortisol secretion or who are treated with glucocorticoids will be likely to develop the metabolic syndrome as a consequence (see Fig. 2).

B Nature of Dysregulation of the HPA Axis in the Metabolic Syndrome

Cortisol secretion is innately vulnerable to regulatory errors, or dysregulation of the HPA axis, which would explain the elevated cortisol secretion in the metabolic syndrome. Factors causing regulatory errors of the HPA axis include sensitization (facilitation) of activating mechanisms, deficient feedback control, or a combination of the two. Genetic susceptibility at several levels can affect all these factors. Briefly, the pathway involves corticotropin-releasing hormone (CRH) and adrenocorticotropin hormone (ACTH), which mediate central facilitating mechanisms to regulate cortisol secretion, as does a feedback mechanism of glucocorticoid receptors found in several places, including the hippocampus (Fig. 3).

There are data supporting the hypothesis of an inefficient feedback control, although the results are not conclusive. However, the most probable point for significant regulatory errors appears to be facilitation of central regulatory mechanisms, resulting in hypersensitivity of the HPA axis and reflecting an association between long-term stress and abnormal HPA axis regulation (18–20).

That facilitation of the central regulatory mechanisms occurs is suggested by elevated cortisol secretion in the morning, during the most active phase of diurnal regulation, as seen in animal studies (20). Facilitation can result from frequent activation of the HPA axis and subsequent downregulation of the density of the central glucocorticoid receptors (38). The stress sensitivity during the examination period may arise from such facilitating factors, and has also been observed in other studies (26,27,39).

Further support is found in statistical associations with HPA axis activation. These include factors that tend to create a stressful surrounding socioeconomic and psychosocial handicaps with resulting frequent activation of the HPA axis, or depression and anxiety

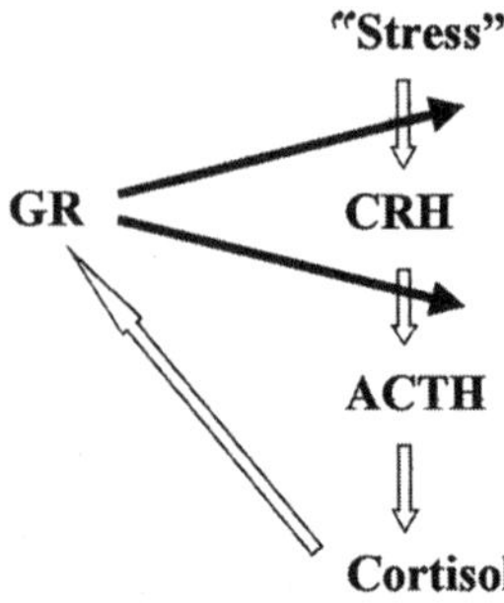

Figure 3 Regulation of the hypothalamic-pituitary-adrenal axis. Facilitating factors ("stress") induce the secretion of CRH, ACTH, and cortisol. Cortisol binds to glucocorticoid receptors in the central nervous system, which control the activity by a feedback mechanism.

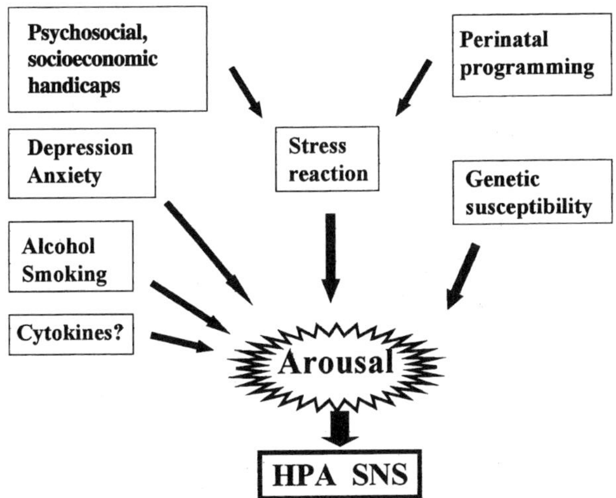

Figure 4 Arousal of the HPA and the central SNS is induced by perceived stress from psychosocial and socioeconomic handicaps. These reactions might be sensitized by perinatal programming. Depression, anxiety, alcohol use, smoking, and, possibly, cytokines cause direct activation. Genetic susceptibility predisposes for these reactions.

traits, alcohol, and smoking, which activate the HPA axis directly (39–43). Thus, in brief, environmental factors, psychological traits, and stimulants, as well as certain physiological elements, appear to negatively affect the regulation of the HPA axis, resulting in excess cortisol and consequent metabolic syndrome (Fig. 4).

IV CAUSES OF HPA AXIS DYSREGULATION IN THE METABOLIC SYNDROME

A number of factors that are known to stimulate the stress centers indirectly or directly in the metabolic syndrome in cause-effect relationships are shown in Figure 4. They can be classified as environmental stressors, stimulant usage, and physiological events.

A Environmental Stressors

Stress, both psychosocial and socioeconomic, can affect the HPA axis. Several cross-sectional studies show correlations between various psychosocial handicaps and components of the metabolic syndrome (2–4,39,40,43). Nonhuman primates, when subjected to controlled psychosocial stress, develop a submissive, depressive type of reaction. Adrenals become enlarged as a sign of increased secretory activity, and the suppressibility of cortisol secretion becomes diminished. Furthermore, sex steroid hormone secretions are diminished, a known consequence of long-term HPA axis activation (45). This is followed by insulin resistance, impaired glucose tolerance, dyslipidemia, elevated blood pressure, early coronary atherosclerosis, and visceral fat accumulation (46,47). This mirrors the metabolic syndrome effects seen in our studies with humans subjected to psychosocial stress.

Cross-sectional evidence indicates association between socioeconomic stress and the metabolic syndrome (2,3,18,39). In the Whitehall studies, a socioeconomic gradient is inversely associated with central obesity and signs of the metabolic syndrome (48). In the men of our studies, a similar socioeconomic-education gradient shows the same associations and, in addition, signs of increased stress-related cortisol secretion and a poor dexamethasone suppression. Furthermore, these endocrine and somatic risk factor phenomena are proportional to time of exposure of socioeconomic handicaps (49). These observations might be considered as prospective intervention studies and suggest that long-term socioeconomic handicaps are followed by stress reactions along the HPA axis with subsequent generation of the metabolic syndrome, which amplifies the risk for coronary artery disease and diabetes. This might be the pathway via which social inequality leads to disease.

B Psychological Traits

Mental depression classically elevates activity of the HPA axis and the sympathetic nervous system, and anxiety with panic symptoms behaves similarly (50). Depression is followed by an increased risk of developing myocardial infarction and type 2 diabetes mellitus in randomized, prospective population studies (51,52). The risk at least equals that of elevated plasma lipids, hypertension, or insulin resistance. An increased visceral fat mass has recently been demonstrated in melancholic depression (53). The metabolic syndrome is associated with minor, subclinical depressive symptoms (1,2,7,41,42). Mental depression may increase the risk for serious somatic disease via the increased cortisol secretion creating the metabolic syndrome. Depressive symptoms in the population (41,42,54) may have the same consequences. This area has recently been reviewed (7).

C Stimulant Usage

Alcohol is known to activate the HPA axis above blood concentration of ~0.1%, which is reached after about two drinks. Alcohol overconsumption without nutritional deficiencies is followed by enlargement of visceral fat depots (55). In severe cases of alcohol abuse, the so-called pseudo-Cushing syndrome may develop, which mimics the effects of the true Cushing's syndrome, and is improved or cured by alcohol abstinence (56). Alcohol consumption at moderately elevated levels has been found to be associated with signs of the metabolic syndrome (39). Alcohol may consequently be an additional factor in the generation of the metabolic syndrome through HPA activation.

Tobacco smoking is frequently found in metabolic syndrome patients (11) and is known to be followed by increased cortisol secretion (57). Smokers have an increased visceral fat mass, diminishing with smoking abstinence (58). Smoking also induces insulin resistance (59) and consequently the major factors of the metabolic syndrome.

In summary, psychosocial and socioeconomic handicaps, depression and anxiety, alcohol, and smoking are statistically associated with increased diurnal cortisol secretion. These factors have been shown in separate experiments to be followed by HPA axis activation, increased cortisol secretion, and the metabolic syndrome. Several of these studies have an intervention component, the results of which strengthen the argument for a cause-effect relationship. This suggests that the statistical association of these factors with the metabolic syndrome is caused by an elevated HPA axis activity and cortisol secretion (See Fig. 4).

It is not possible to state which of these factors is the most powerful in the individual case. It seems likely that they are mixed and interrelated. One may, for example, visualize a chain of events starting out with psychosocial or socioeconomic misfortunes, followed by abuse of stimulants and depressive symptoms. This chain might, however, start with any of the separate factors as the initial trigger.

V PHYSIOLOGICAL ELEMENTS

Certain physiological events also correlate to the metabolic syndrome, including aging, cytokine exposure, and the small-baby syndrome.

A Aging

Aging may be another stimulating factor. The changes in regulation of the HPA axis after repeated stress resemble those of aging. In aging rats, the unwinding of cortisol after a challenge is delayed, probably owing to a diminished efficacy of the controlling feedback (60). Aging humans show similar effects, but the effects cannot be separated from those of the unavoidable stressful events of a long life (61,62).

B Cytokines

Recently several studies have shown that elevations of C-reactive protein and cytokines are associated with the metabolic syndrome and risk for cardiovascular disease (63,64). Cytokines, particularly interleukin-6, are powerful stimulators of the HPA axis, probably explaining the elevated cortisol secretion during infections (65,66). It therefore seems possible that chronic infections activate the HPA axis via cytokines, inducing the same cascade of events as described above with generation of conventional risk factors (see Fig. 4). This problem is under study.

C Small-Baby Syndrome

Children born small for gestational age have been shown, with strong statistical correlations in several studies, to develop the metabolic syndrome with increased risk for cardiovascular disease and type 2 diabetes mellitus at adult age (67). Results of recent studies suggest that such subjects also show signs of an increased cortisol secretion and a sensitive HPA axis (34,35). The question, then, is, why do children small for gestational age develop a sensitive HPA axis?

Recent experimental studies in rats now provide likely explanations. Prenatal immune challenges, such as exposure to lipopolysaccharides, cytokines, or glucocorticoids, result at adulthood in apparently permanent changes in the sensitivity of the HPA axis. One common denominator for several of these agents might be a stimulation of secretion of endogenous glucocorticoids which may interfere with the sensitive development of neuroendocrine regulations. The locus of impact seems to vary with time of exposure and power of the intervention agent, and is localized to the mechanisms facilitating central HPA axis stimulation or to the feedback control by downregulation of the density of central glucocorticoid receptors responsible for the feedback signals (68–70). The consequences effect body fat mass, insulin sensitivity, and sex steroid hormones. Fetal cytokine exposure during the first 8–12 days of pregnancy produces in adulthood a condition like the metabolic syndrome in terms of stress sensitivity, sex steroid abnormalities, elevated body fat accumulation, and insulin resistance (69).

Postnatal impacts are also important for adult outcomes. For example, one injection of testosterone to newborn female rats results in metabolic syndrome–like symptoms at adulthood (71), while excess corticosterone exposure during this period results in lean adult rats (72).

These results demonstrate clearly that the perinatal period is very sensitive to various impacts which can result in permanent neuroendocrine, metabolic and body composition changes. Apparently numerous factors mediate such impacts, several of which are of potential interest for the human situation. Lipopolysaccharides and cytokines produced during maternal infections might inflict stress on the preborn baby. The original Barker (67) publications suggested that intrauterine underfeeding might be involved, inducing oversecretion of glucocorticoids as active agents in an HPA axis programming.

The Dutch Famine studies provide additional clues. Mothers subjected to the famine during early pregnancy had children who developed obesity and risk for cardiovascular disease, while children of mothers exposed late in pregnancy were small and developed hypertension and diabetes (73). It seems likely that this apparent difference in adult outcome was due to the impact of central regulatory systems at different sensitive periods.

We have recently started to examine the birth records of the subjects in our populations. Preliminarily, it appears that the HPA axis abnormalities at adulthood are found in men born small for gestational age, which agrees with the recent reports by Phillips (34,35). One aim of these studies was to estimate how often the metabolic syndrome in adulthood can be traced to birth factors. Not all birth records have been located. However, data from subjects with missing birth records do not differ from those whose birth records have been found, suggesting that selection bias is not a problem. Estimations from the prevalence of children currently born small for gestational age (< 5%) suggest that this pathway to the metabolic syndrome might not be of major importance today, whereas the prevalence of a sensitive HPA axis in middle-aged adults seems to be in the order of 25% (16). Fetal undernutrition might have been more important in the U.K. 70–80 years ago, when the subjects examined by Barker (67) were born. There may, however, be other active factors than fetal undernutrition with perinatal exposure leading to sensitization of the HPA axis, such as alcohol, tobacco smoking, and infections, which might be more important today. This is an area of major importance for observations and advice during pregnancy.

In summary, the small-baby syndrome appears to be a pathway leading to metabolic syndrome at adulthood. The mechanism might be a permanent sensitizing of the HPA axis to challenges during adult life. The pathogenic mechanism therefore probably resembles that described in the studies in adult populations (see Fig. 4). Accumulating evidence suggests that the mechanism involves interference with normal central regulations during sensitive periods of brain development. This might be compared with the long-term development of a "thrifty genotype," but is in contrast a "thrifty phenotype," developing from the impact of factors during pregnancy. The quantitative role of this pathway into the current adult prevalence of the metabolic syndrome cannot be estimated with any certainty, but the input by the condition of low birth weight appears from indirect estimations to be relatively small. This area of research has clearly demonstrated the power of perinatal factors to influence adult health.

VI OTHER VARIATIONS OF HPA AXIS DYSREGULATION

A Cortisol and Burnout

In addition to the stress pattern of cortisol secretion, another pattern is shown in Figure 1—the burnout curve, representing < 10% of the men. In that group, there was a very low morning value and low cortisol all over the day. Dexamethasone suppression seemed to be blunted, with strong associations to anthropometric, metabolic, and hemodynamic risk factors. These men also showed low values of testosterone and IGF I (16), a surrogate measurement of growth hormone secretion. In this group, cortisol by itself is unlikely to be generating the risk factor, but it seems possible that low testosterone and growth hormone secretions might be responsible. Both these hormones, when low, are followed by insulin resistance and visceral fat accumulation (5,6). When testosterone or growth hormone is added, insulin sensitivity is regained and fat is mobilized. These mechanisms are essentially known (5,6). These are opposite effects to those of cortisol, and it seems likely that the outcome in terms of the components of the metabolic syndrome is in fact dependent on the balance between cortisol on the one hand and sex steroid and growth hormone on the other. In fact, the metabolic syndrome is also seen after isolated growth hormone or testosterone deficiency (74–76) (see Fig. 5). The markedly elevated blood pressure and heart rate suggest an increased activity of the sympathetic nervous system, a known consequence of a failing HPA axis, perhaps a compensatory mechanism (77). This might amplify insulin resistance by excess mobilization of free fatty

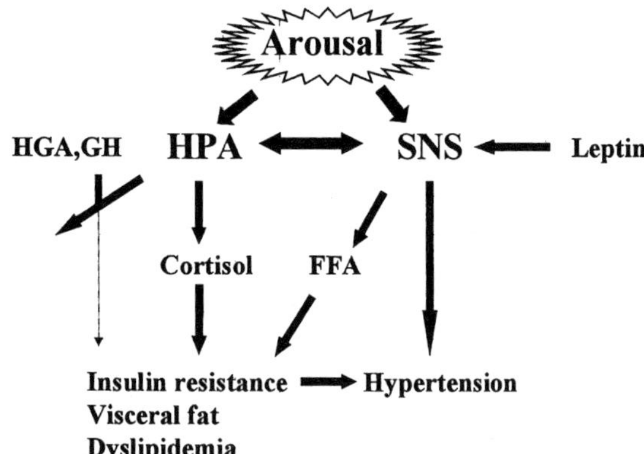

Figure 5 Arousal of the HPA is followed by elevated cortisol secretion and inhibition of the HGA and GH axes, resulting in insulin resistance, visceral fat accumulation, and dyslipidemia (the metabolic syndrome). Concomitant activation of the central SNS is followed by elevated mobilization of FFA, amplifying insulin resistance, and induces hypertension, facilitated by insulin and leptin.

acids, which are elevated in the metabolic syndrome (78) (see Fig. 5).

The reason for the pronounced derangement of the HPA axis regulation in these rather few men is not fully understood. Over time and under continuous stress, the HPA axis first reacts normally but eventually does not unwind in a normal pace after the stress challenge stops. After further development, total cortisol secretion goes down, resulting in a rigid, flat diurnal curve. This has been considered to be the case when the HPA axis is "burned out" and might, over a sufficiently long time, become irreversible and end up with actual substance loss in areas of the brain where glucocorticoid density is high, such as the hippocampus (79). These changes have been seen in "vital exhaustion," after severe "life events," in war veterans, Holocaust victims, repeated melancholic depression, and Cushing's syndrome, all conditions with prolonged elevated cortisol secretion (79). Elevated cortisol itself may have such damaging effects, which appear to be amplified by various toxins, including alcohol (38,60).

The men with a flat "burned-out" cortisol secretion also report psychosocial and socioeconomic handicaps, anxiodepressive traits, smoking, and alcohol consumption, which are slightly higher than those of the other subjects. Alcohol reporting is, however, notoriously unreliable and overuse might be a hidden factor. A time factor may also be involved, the men in question having been exposed to damaging factors longer than the others.

B Follow-up Studies of the Male Subjects

The cortisol secretory pattern of the men has been subjected to further analyses. As seen in Figure 1, three subgroups can be separated as follows. The normal group has high morning values, and lower prelunch values. The stressed men have lower morning cortisols, which are unchanged before lunch. The "burned-out" men have still lower morning values, which remain low. This means that morning and prelunch cortisols contain most of the information of interest for evaluation of the basal cortisol secretion pattern. Using only these values and the testosterone values for categorization of the neuroendocrine status of these men, essentially similar associations to risk factors remain as in the more detailed statistical analyses utilizing all measurements (16,21).

The men in this population have now been followed up after 5 years. The simplified categorization outlined above shows in preliminary analyses that the development of any new event of hypertension, diabetes mellitus, angina pectoris, or myocardial infarction can be predicted by the cortisol-testosterone measurements of 5 years ago. Consequently there are proportionally fewer events in the normal group, more in the stressed group, and the highest incidence is in the "burned-out" group (Wallerius et al., to be published).

If these observations hold true in further calculations, they strongly support the interpretation of the chain of events suggested in this overview, summarized in Figures 4 and 5, which is, as far as we know, the first longitudinal observation of the relationship between neuroendocrine stress reactions and disease. The power of this new risk factor seems impressive, providing information on development of disease or disease symptoms during such a short period of time in a comparably small cohort. These simple measurements may prove to be useful in screening for risk for development of serious somatic disease in a stressful environment.

VII WOMEN AND HYPERANDROGENICITY

The endocrine, anthropometric, and metabolic findings reported above are generally applicable to both men and women. The results in women, however, show several interesting differences (17). A major difference is the involvement of androgens in women. We were particularly interested in this phenomenon, having shown previously that a relative hyperandrogenicity (HA) is associated with a powerful risk of developing type 2 diabetes mellitus, cardiovascular disease, hypertension,

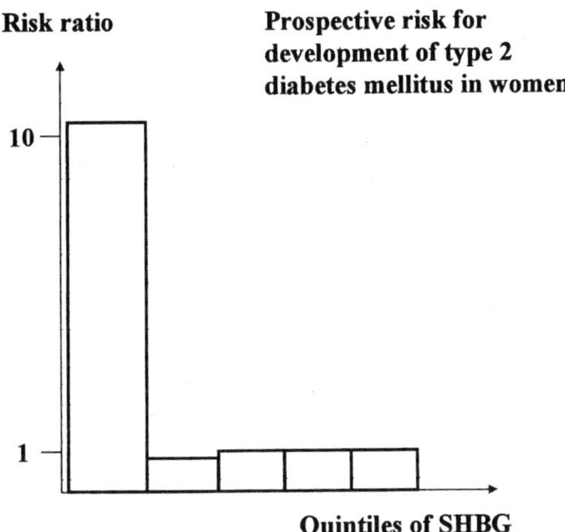

Figure 6 The risk ratio for development of type 2 diabetes mellitus in women in relation to sex hormone binding (SHBG) quintiles. (From Ref. 80.)

and endometrial cancer, followed by premature mortality (11). In fact, the risk of developing diabetes increased 10- to 20-fold among the women with HA, irrespective of menopausal state (80) (see Fig. 6). Calculations of population attributable risk indicate that HA may explain no less than 50–67% of all development of type 2 diabetes in women. HA may thus be one of the most powerful risk factors for serious disease in women. The risk seems to affect the highest quartile of testosterone values in women (17) and may therefore be considered to be a common risk factor in the general population of women. This risk factor has attracted surprisingly little attention. Androgens showed consistent, strong statistical associations to anthropometric, metabolic, and hemodynamic risk factors in women. This was particularly pronounced for free, active testosterone (T) but was also seen for cortisol, androstenedione, and dihydroepiandrosterone sulfate (DHEAS), which are secreted mainly or exclusively from the adrenals.

Values for 17β-estradiol were low. The associations to cortisol measurements were not as strong as in men, and certainly not as strong as to androgens in the women. Concentrations of the stronger androgens (T and free T) correlated closely not only with weaker androgens (androstenedione and 17-OH progesterone) but also with hormones directly associated with the activity of the HPA axis (ACTH, DHEAS, and cortisol measurements) (17). It therefore seems likely that the more powerful androgens are also at least partly of adrenal origin.

As expected, measurements of abdominal obesity also showed strong associations to the metabolic risk factors and blood pressure. Androgens and abdominal obesity were mutually dependent. Partial correlations or stepwise regression analyses performed on their associations to risk factors showed that the two contributed independently (17). It is therefore apparent that androgens and abdominal obesity both contribute to the development of disease risk in women (Fig. 7).

T administration to women is followed by accumulation of visceral fat, where estrogens might have a protective effect (81,82). T administration to women or female rats is also followed by systemic insulin resistance, localized to the glucose transporter and glycogen synthase systems in muscle (83–85). It is thus clear that androgens in women are directly associated with the metabolic syndrome, and the effect is likely to be causal. However, the generation of risk factors is in part apparently due to factors other than androgens involved in central fat distribution and obesity, which then in turn amplifies the risk factor generation (17).

Again, as in the men, the question comes up as to whether there are factors that would be suspected or known to activate the HPA axis. Indeed, approximately the same factors as in men are associated with HA, including psychosocial and socioeconomic handicaps, depression and anxiety, smoking, and alcohol (17). We believe that these factors activate the HPA axis in the same way as in the men, resulting in hypersecretions from the adrenals, where, in women, androgens seem to be more powerful in their damaging effects than cortisol, while the opposite seems true in men. It seems highly likely, although not measured, that the men with evi-

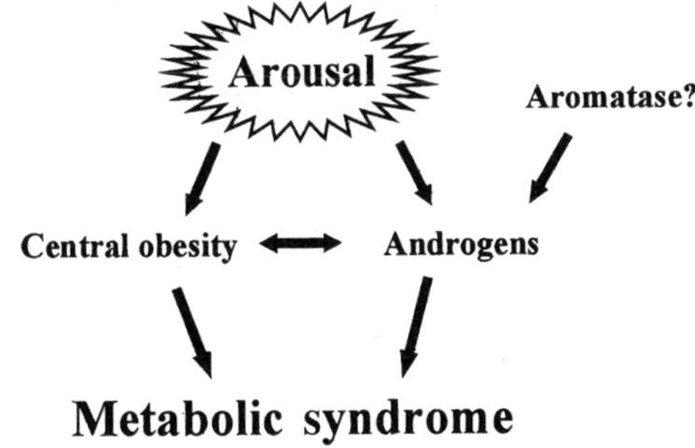

Figure 7 In women, central arousal is followed by central obesity and elevated androgens, probably at least partly of adrenal origin, which are mutually dependent and are followed by the metabolic syndrome. Aromatase might be malfunctioning, amplifying the effects of arousal of the hypothalamic-pituitary-adrenal axis. (From Ref. 17.)

dence of elevated activity of the HPA axis also secrete excess adrenal androgens, but this small increase in total androgen production in men is probably insignificant for peripheral effects, and is hidden in the much larger gonadal production. However, in the women, we cannot overlook HA generation from the ovaries.

The explanation of HA effects in the women is then likely to be at least partly due to activation of the HPA axis with androgens oversecreted from the adrenals. Androgens in circulation are converted to estrogens via the enzyme CYP-450 aromatase. Interestingly, women with HA have a polymorphism in the aromatase gene, localized to the microsatellite of the fifth intron. This microsatellite, consisting of the tetranucleotide repeat TTTA, is shorter than average in the HA women (17). The low estrogen/androgen ratio in these women is compatible with a deficient function of the aromatase, although direct measurements of enzyme activity have not yet been performed. Such a short microsatellite has previously been reported in women with an elevated risk to develop breast cancer or osteoporosis (86,87), and is therefore an association of major interest for development of serious disease in women.

It also turns out that nonsmoking women in this population, who at age 42 have managed to keep their body weight constant since the age of 21, have high estrogens and low androgens, resulting in a high estrogen/androgen ratio, compatible with an excellent function of the aromatase enzyme. Their microsatellite in the aromatase gene is longer than average, and there is no overlap between the number of tetranucleotides in the groups of abdominally obese, hyperandrogenic women, described above, and the lean women with low androgens (88) (Fig. 8). Thus, we have two groups of women who are different not only phylogenetically but are totally opposite in the obesity and risk factor pattern, in the sex steroid hormones, and in microsatellite repeat sequences in the aromatase gene.

Recently it has been shown that a knockout of the aromatase gene is followed by not only elevated androgens in female mice, but also by abdominal obesity (89). We therefore speculate that the aromatase function is a regulator not only of androgen levels in women, but also of the tendency to develop visceral obesity and the metabolic syndrome. Women with a deficient function based on an aberrant allele in the aromatase gene might be particularly susceptible to the metabolic syndrome with abdominal obesity when exposed to a stressful environment. There is a clear possibility that the short allele in the aromatase microsatellite indicates a poor function of the enzyme, followed by abdominal obesity and the metabolic syndrome.

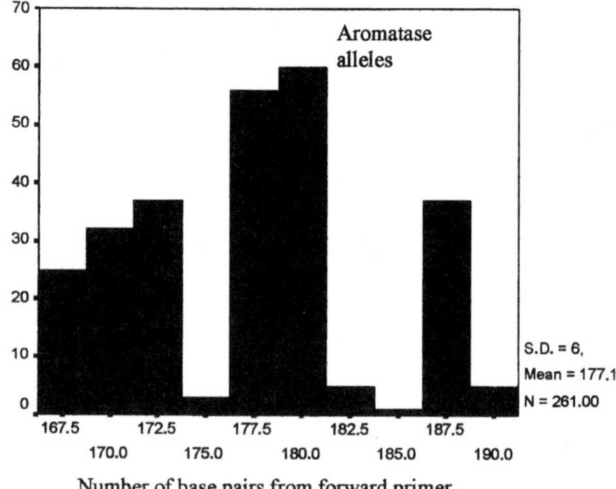

Figure 8 Distribution of tetranucleotide repeats in the microsatellite of the fifth intron of the CYP 450 aromatase gene in women in the population. Obese, hyperandrogenic women have a stretch of the tetranucleotide repeats corresponding to 168–171 bp's and lean, healthy women an average stretch of 187 bp's. (From Refs. 17,88.)

Abdominal obesity in women is closely associated with HA and increased risk to develop endometrial and mammary carcinomas (11). These are hormone-dependent cancers, and one might consider the hypothetical possibility that HA might be involved in the pathogenesis.

VIII HYPERTENSION IN THE METABOLIC SYNDROME

The relationship among blood pressure, obesity, and insulin is much debated, with controversial results (Fig. 5, right part). Numerous studies show a relationship among blood pressure, insulin resistance, and hyperinsulinemia; several others find none; still others show a mixture of results in subgroups. This was summarized in an excellent comprehensive review by Rocchini in the previous edition of the Handbook (90). Correlation studies therefore do not give much promise for this direction of research. Rocchini suggests that insulin affects blood pressure regulating mechanisms selectively, which might explain the controversies in correlative findings.

Such mechanisms include enhanced sodium retention but the picture is unclear. There is considerable evidence that insulin causes sodium retention in acute experiments, but the presumed long-term consequence—volume expansion with elevated blood pressure—does not seem to have been conclusively shown (90). Such a consequence seems rather unlikely, because volume-regulating mechanisms should prevent it (91). Furthermore, the concept of salt-induced pathogenesis of primary hypertension has in general been received with considerable doubt, at least within a normal range of salt intake variation, although a possibility exists of subgroups with genetically salt-sensitive individuals (91). Thus, the argument for an insulin-mediated retention of salt in obesity and hypertension is weak.

Another mechanistic hypothesis is that insulin may act via stimulation of the central sympathetic nervous system (92). This hypothesis is hard to prove in humans because of the difficulties in measuring activity of the sympathetic nervous system. For example, plasma concentrations or urinary outflow of catecholamines are measurements of the activity of the total sympathetic nervous system, but a concentration sufficient to regulate blood pressure might be too small to be detected.

Direct measurements of activity in sympathetic nerves in relation to insulin levels during hyperinsulinemic clamp procedures do not provide long-term information (93). Patients with insulinoma and chronically elevated insulin levels do not become hypertensive, and successful surgery is not followed by changes in blood pressure (94). A major difficulty with this entire approach to the problem is, however, that primary hypertension in humans develops through several stages; increased sympathetic nervous system activity is present only in the early stages and is absent later (91). Meaningful studies therefore need to define the stages of development of hypertension. Most studies seem to have been performed in established hypertension, where increased sympathetic nervous system activity would not have been expected to be present.

Primary hypertension develops through an initial phase of hyperkinetic circulation, due to frequent activation of the sympathetic nervous system (95). Long-term follow-up studies indicate that this transitions into a stage, which is dominated by a peripheral circulatory resistance developed through adaptive processes (96). The evidence for such a stage and the involvement of the central sympathetic nervous system in early phases are considerable, and this pathogenic pathway of hypertension seems to have reached a consensus in the field of hypertension research (97). These observations are based on subjects with or without obesity, with varying degrees of insulin resistance and hyperinsulinemia. There is evidence that insulin activates the central sympathetic nervous system (92). It may therefore be presumed that a development towards hypertension would be more likely to occur or to be more pronounced, if insulin amplifies sympathetic nervous system activity in hyperinsulinemic conditions such as in the metabolic syndrome.

There is, however, convincing evidence for other primary events. Already Brod (98) in the 1950s could show an increased stress sensitivity in early stages of hypertension. Such observations are corroborated by striking epidemiological observations. Nuns in a secluded cloister in northern Italy have been followed through decades and do not see increased blood pressure with age, unlike women of similar ages living outside the calm environmental conditions of the cloister. The difference is apparent also after adjustments for obesity, diet, alcohol intake, and childbirth (99). The difference in blood pressure development seems to be best explained by the psychosocial environment.

Another similar example comes from the Kuna Indian tribe, where individuals who moved into a large, boisterous city developed hypertension, while those remaining in their ordinary habitat, or moving to a calm environment outside the same city, remained normotensive. Salt intake does not appear to have played a role because the salt intake is rather high in this tribe and similar irrespective of habitat (100). Again these observations support the detrimental influence of a stressful environment for the development of hypertension.

Direct prospective evidence is provided by studies in the United States, where increase in blood pressure with time, carefully measured continuously during ordinary life conditions, is proportional to environmental stress (101). Taken together, this evidence strongly suggests influence by environmental stress factors as an important pathogenic feature of primary hypertension. When the metabolic syndrome with insulin resistance and hyperinsulinemia is added, it seems likely that insulin might amplify blood pressure elevation with insulin as an active component (see Fig. 5).

These results allow a consideration of another important factor. As reviewed above, the metabolic syndrome seems to have a background of HPA axis activation, due to environmental factors, where perceived stress from psychosocial and socioeconomic problems are important ingredients. In animals, there is a profile of different stress reactions depending on the perception of a threatening challenge. With apparent possibilities to cope with the challenge, the sympathetic nervous system is activated with elevated blood pressure—the fight-flight reaction. When the threat seems overwhelming, a depressive, defeat reaction occurs with activation of the HPA axis and a secondary inhibition of growth and gonadal axes. This activation may shift from one to the other depending on the situation of danger or pressure, and is often mixed (102). In humans, these profiles are less apparent. It is in fact difficult in humans to activate one of these centers without affecting the other. This is probably because the central regulation of the HPA axis and the sympathetic nervous system are tightly interconnected at several levels (45).

The primary pathogenic triggers for the metabolic syndrome seem to be central factors activating the HPA axis. The data from the hypertension research field indicate a similar origin for primary hypertension. The parallel origin opens up the possibility that primary hypertension and the metabolic syndrome might have a common central origin through parallel activation of both stress centers in the lower part of the brain, the HPA axis, and the sympathetic nervous system.

A remaining question, then, is which is the dominant factor in activation of the central sympathetic nervous system, environmental stress factors or insulin? When blood pressure is the dependent variable in partial correlation analyses correcting for several components of the metabolic syndrome, including abdominal obesity and insulin, only measurements of the HPA axis remain as a determinant of blood pressure (103). This illustrates the connection between the HPA axis and blood pressure in the men from the Swedish population sample, where the majority does not have an established hypertensive condition, which probably means that secondary regulatory factors of blood pressure such as in established hypertension are not involved. Furthermore, insulin has apparently less importance for the determination of blood pressure than HPA axis activity. More detailed studies of this problem in a smaller group of men show associations between measurements of the HPA axis against blood pressure response to laboratory stress, feeding, and corticotropin-releasing hormone administration and excretion of catecholamine metabolites (104), again indicating the close connection between the HPA axis and blood pressure regulation.

With this background it seems reasonable to suggest that the hypertension of the metabolic syndrome is actually due to a parallel activation of both stress axes, the HPA axis and the central sympathetic nervous system. The statistical associations between insulin and blood pressure, frequently reported in the literature, might therefore be due primarily to the HPA axis being responsible for the insulin elevation, with a parallel activation of the blood pressure regulating part of the central sympathetic nervous system (Fig. 5).

Another recent development of interest for the pathogenesis of hypertension in the metabolic syndrome is the connection between the leptin and the sympathetic nervous systems. Leptin is produced mainly in adipose tissue and is elevated in both obese animal models and obese humans, in proportion to adipose tissue mass (105). Although it was found early that leptin not only induces satiety via a hypothalamic receptor and stimulation of thermogenesis, recent studies have indicated that leptin also activates the part of the sympathetic nervous system that regulates blood pressure. Most obese animal models have both elevated leptin levels and elevated blood pressure. When leptin is infused systemically or intrathecally, blood pressure rises, and animals genetically engineered to overproduce excess leptin become hypertensive (106). Exceptions are the Zucker rat and the db/db mouse, which have a mutation in the leptin receptor (106). These observations indicate that leptin is responsible for the hypertension seen in obese animal models, and that this is mediated through the leptin receptor.

In human studies, polymorphisms in the leptin receptor gene locus are associated with lower blood pressure. These polymorphisms include Lys109Arg in exon 4, Gln223Arg in exon 8, and Lys656Asn in exon 14. This is particularly clear in obese subjects where the differences between subjects with normal and variant alleles are important not only statistically but clinically and are in the order of 15/10 mm Hg systolic/diastolic blood pressure. Furthermore, when hypertensive men ($>$ 140/90 mm Hg) were examined separately, they were overweight or obese and had elevated leptin levels. Only one out of 64 of these hypertensive men had normal alleles in the leptin receptor gene (107). Although not showing cause-effect relationships, these results suggest that the leptin system might also be of importance for blood pressure regulation in humans, and might show why not all obese people are hypertensive. The metabolic syndrome is often combined with obesity, so this mechanism might be of importance for blood pressure regulation in this syndrome, particularly since the central sympathetic nervous system clearly seems to be involved, as reviewed above (Fig. 5).

In summary, there are thus three major explanations of hypertension in the metabolic syndrome, namely, elevations in sympathetic nervous system activity, insulin, and leptin arising from accompanying obesity. The triggering factor in the early stages of primary hypertension is probably frequently elevated sympathetic nervous system activity. The high prevalence of hypertension in the metabolic syndrome with obesity is likely to be caused by additional effects of elevated leptin and insulin, stimulating sympathetic nervous system centers (Fig. 5).

IX ROLE OF OBESITY IN THE METABOLIC SYNDROME

Visceral fat accumulation is part of the metabolic syndrome. This is, however, not the same as obesity, which is defined as an increased body fat mass, irrespective of localization. The question, then, is whether or not obesity is part of or associated with the metabolic syndrome.

Obesity of the gluteofemoral or peripheral type may occur without the metabolic syndrome (108). Furthermore, elevated visceral fat accumulation may occur without increase of total body fat such, as with aging or smoking (11). These examples show that visceral fat and obesity are two different entities. Nevertheless, obesity and proportionally increased visceral fat accumulation frequently occur simultaneously (11). In fact, in the statistical calculations of the Swedish population samples (16,17), estimations of central waist circumference (WHR), visceral fat accumulation (abdominal sagittal diameter), and estimations of total body fat (BMI) are not only closely statistically related to each other but also to the components of the metabolic syndrome, suggesting that obesity is indeed a part of this syndrome.

Obesity is caused by a positive energy balance, by either an increased energy intake or a diminished energy output, or both. Both of these factors are regulated by a large number of complicated mechanisms. With the neuroendocrine-endocrine background of the metabolic syndrome, with the HPA axis and cortisol in a central position, one may also ask if the associated obesity might depend on similar factors.

Clinicians know that patients treated with glucocorticoids often become obese with a central localization of excess fat. Such patients often report voracious hunger, which can be objectively observed in clinical wards. Direct experimental measurements in humans show that with administration of glucocorticoids, leptin levels increase (109,110), which would be expected to decrease food intake by induction of satiety. Nevertheless, food intake clearly increases after exposure to elevated glucocorticoid levels, shown recently in fully controlled experiments with a food dispenser (111) or with automatic recording food-monitoring equipment (112).

Animal work shows that after adrenalectomy, food intake is low, such as in the clinical entity of Addisons's disease, and leptin sensitivity is elevated. With graded replacement of corticosterone, leptin sensitivity decreases and food intake increases. With doses of corticosterone, resulting in oversubstitution, food consumption rises, resulting in obesity even with high leptin levels (113). These results show that glucocorticoids can induce leptin resistance, which is characteristic of common human obesity (105). The mechanism for the action of glucocorticoids is apparently not localized to the leptin receptor (114), but may be found in the distal cascade of events after receptor binding.

These results clearly point to the possibility that the HPA axis may also regulate food intake via similar pathways. In addition, recent reports suggest that glucocorticoids might be involved in the stimulation of neuropeptide Y (NPY) secretion (115,116), shifting the NPY-leptin balance toward the former. This information is, however, not consistent and needs amplification.

Taken together (Fig. 9), evidence suggests the possibility that cortisol secretion may in fact be involved not only in the distribution of body fat to central depots, but also may increase total body fat mass by elevated food intake. This area is of considerable interest and should attract further attention. Particularly, long-term studies are needed.

Cortisol is oversecreted after stress challenges. That cortisol may increase food intake raises the question of the existence of the phenomenon of "stress eating." Some people report anecdotally that they eat more when they are stressed, and feel comfort from this, while others report that they lose their appetite. Individuals

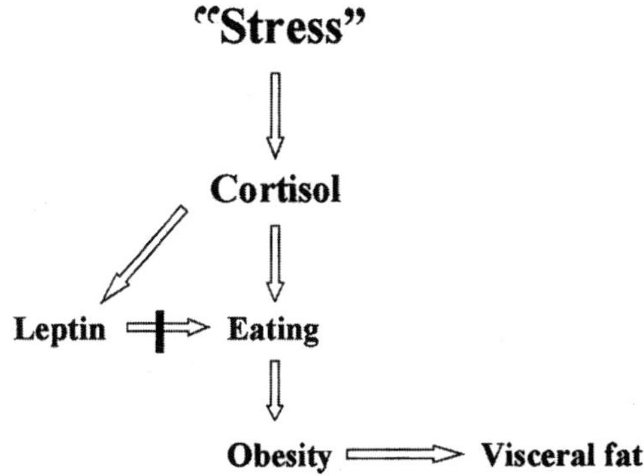

Figure 9 "Stress eating," a hypothesis. Stress induces cortisol secretion, which is followed by increased energy intake in spite of elevated leptin secretion. This results in obesity with an enlarged fraction of body fat in visceral depots (visceral obesity).

subjected to the stress of an impending operation do not increase food intake (117), while schoolgirls seem to do so before examinations (118). Other reports, including animal work, also show mixed results (119,120), and the information in this area is not conclusive. A frequent problem with this research is that the results have relied on subjective reports of both stress and food intake.

A recent report (121) seems to have resolved these problems in an ingenious way. A group of subjects were subjected to standardized laboratory stress tests, and saliva cortisol was measured. Thereafter they were allowed to eat snacks, unaware that the consumption was registered. It then turned out that those who showed elevated cortisol during the stress test also ate more afterward. This study indicates that only when stress results in neuroendocrine reactions is food intake increased, which might explain previous mixed results.

There is thus a good possibility that "stress eating" is indeed a reality and that subjects who show neuroendocrine reactions to stress normally overeat. With time and repeated stress challenges, this would be expected to result in the development of obesity. (Fig. 9). One might therefore consider that the current obesity epidemic is due not only to unlimited availability to energy-dense food and limited need for physical activity but also to current stressful life conditions. The latter may also be involved in eating under time pressure, not allowing time for the perception of satiety signals.

Other hormonal abnormalities in the metabolic syndrome might also be involved in food intake regulation. Low concentrations of sex steroid hormones are known to be followed by obesity (122), and castration is well known to increase fat contents in meat products. This might be a consequence of both increased food intake and a lower physical activity.

Physical inactivity is most likely an important part of the metabolic syndrome (123) and probably contributes to the associated obesity. This may in fact be an important factor for the pathogenesis of the entire syndrome, because physical activity has profound effects on components of the syndrome other than obesity such as insulin resistance, elevated blood pressure and depression (124–126). The direct effects of physical inactivity on the regulation of the HPA axis does not seem to have been studied. Nevertheless, physical inactivity would probably amplify the metabolic syndrome because physical activity counteracts its development and is in fact currently the only globally efficient therapeutic alternative.

In summary, the metabolic syndrome with increase of the visceral fat depots is often combined with generalized obesity. There is a possibility that this is due to concomitant interference with energy intake regulation by the neuroendocrine disturbance of the syndrome. Physical inactivity is probably an important part of this, because physical activity is an efficient treatment of the syndrome.

X GENETICS

Genetic susceptibility to develop the metabolic syndrome might be localized to a large number of genes. Since it has been considered unlikely that the components of the syndrome—visceral obesity, insulin resistance, dyslipidemia, and hypertension—can explain the pathogenesis of the entire syndrome, genetic aberrations directly associated with these components will not be discussed. Instead, since it appears that the origin of the metabolic syndrome is found in central regulatory errors, emphasis will be placed on genes involved in such pathways.

A Aromatase

The aromatase gene may be an important locus for the regulation not only of hyperandrogenicity but also of abdominal obesity with associated metabolic syndrome. In fact, alleles of the microsatellite of the fifth intron of this gene may be important for both the presence of or protection from such symptoms, via short and long alleles respectively. The long, apparently protective allele is found among ~5% of the women in the population we have examined (88). The short allele has previously been reported to be associated with an increased risk for mammary carcinoma and osteoporosis (86,87) and now also with HA (17), which predicts type 2 diabetes, cardiovascular disease, and endometrial carcinoma (11). This, then, is apparently an allele that is associated with a number of serious diseases in women. The androgen receptor gene also seems to be involved with a short microsatellite in the transactivating domain in women with hyperandrogenicity (Baghaei et al., unpublished). Since sex steroid hormones exert powerful effects on central regulation of energy balance (122), these effects may act via central regulatory events. The central regulation of energy balance and HPA axis regulation is very complex. The regulatory events involve, among several additional mechanisms, propiomelanocortin (POMC), corticotropin-releasing hormone, leptin, NPY, the serotoninergic, dopaminergic, and adrenergic systems, and insulin, as well as their connections with hormones, neuropeptides, transmitters, and receptors. The relevance for the human situation is not clear for all these factors. In our first attempts, we have directed attention primarily to the regulation of the HPA axis, the POMC system, leptin, and the neural transmitter systems.

B Leptin

As discussed above, several polymorphisms in the leptin receptor gene seem to protect against hypertension in obesity (107). A remarkable, unexpected finding in these studies is that these polymorphisms are associated with lower BMI in comparisons with subjects without these polymorphisms (107). With a poorly signaling receptor, one would have expected an elevated BMI. These findings suggest separate pathways for the regulation by leptin of blood pressure and energy intake suppression. In fact, these polymorphisms thus appear to protect against obesity. They are found in 10–25% of the population of men studied (107).

C The POMC System

The POMC gene produces several hormones, including ACTH, melanocortin, and β-endorphin, all involved in HPA axis and/or energy balance regulation (Fig. 10). A major quantitative trait locus regulating fat mass and leptin production is localized near the POMC gene locus on chromosome 2 (127). Although POMC gene knockout produces obesity (128), only two obese subjects out of many examined have been identified with a genetic defect in the POMC gene locus (129). A trinucleotide repeat in exon 3, found in 8% of Swedish men, was associated with elevated leptin levels, but without change in obesity measurements (130). This rather infrequent genetic variant then seems to protect against obesity because it is followed by elevated levels of the satiety hormone leptin.

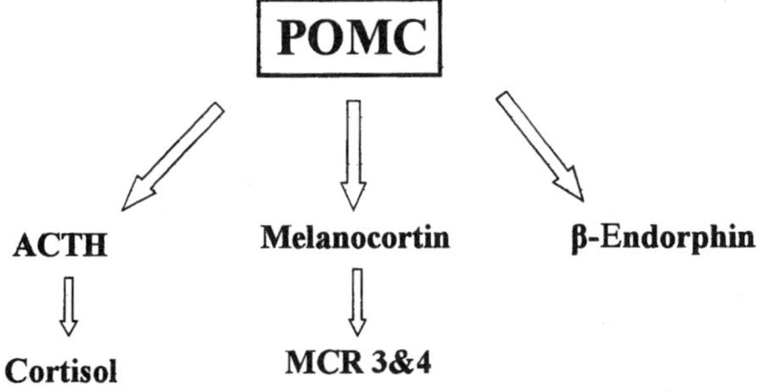

Figure 10 Factors regulating food intake. Pro-opiomelanocortin (POMC) induces ACTH and cortisol secretion, regulates the secretion of melanocortin, active via melanocortin receptors (MCR 3 and 4), and β-endorphin.

Alpha-melanocyte stimulating hormone controls energy intake via melanocortin receptors (MCR) 3 and 4 (131,132). Although early studies found only a few associations between polymorphisms in the MCR 4 and obesity (133,134), more recent studies indicate that this is a relatively frequently mutated gene in human morbid obesity (135,136), resembling the phenotype of MCR4 knockout mice (137). A G-to-A substitution in codon 103 (Val103Ile) was found in 3% of Swedish men, and there were 5% G/A heterozygotes but no A/A homozygotes (138). The G/A heterozygotes had lower measurements of abdominal obesity. Saliva cortisol measurements indicated normal kinetics of HPA axis regulation. These findings suggest that the infrequent genetic variant of a G-to-A substitution protects against abdominal obesity.

D The Serotoninergic System

Serotonin (5-hydroxytryptamine, 5HT) exerts major effects on the regulation of both the HPA axis and energy intake and is also involved in mental depression (139). Agents enhancing 5HT availability are used as efficient drugs for the treatment of depression, and have been used as antiobesity agents. Several receptors are identified with different functions (140,141). Serotonin is formed from tryptophan through hydroxylation by the rate limiting enzyme tryptophan hydroxylase. The concentration of 5HT in synapses depends on the rates of formation and reuptake, the latter regulated by the serotonin transporter. The final concentration then acts via several 5HT receptors (5HTR).

Since the 5HT system is involved in both the HPA axis regulation, depression, and energy balance, we considered it of particular interest to study this system in the metabolic syndrome, where all these variables are involved as components or potential etiological factors (2). Several of the observations mentioned in the following are preliminary and result from studies performed in women only (Baghaei et al., unpublished) with the exception of the 5HTR 2A, which has only been examined in men (Rosmond et al., unpublished).

Homozygotes for a short allele in the promoter domain of the tryptophan hydroxylase gene locus show associations to a well functioning HPA axis regulation, but not to obesity variables and their associated metabolic risk factors (unpublished). This variant has a frequency of 37.4%. Homozygotes for a short allele in the promoter domain of the gene locus for the serotonin transporter gene show elevated values of ACTH, free testosterone, and perturbations in diurnal cortisol secretion, suggesting a hyperactivity of the HPA axis. In addition, elevated abdominal sagittal diameter is an indicator of increased visceral fat mass. This genetic variant is also associated with behavioral characteristics (Baghaei et al., unpublished). It may be speculated that this genetic variation is of importance for the contents of serotonin in nerve synapses, and that the short allele therefore produces the combined effects of both a hyperactive HPA axis and visceral accumulation of body fat. The homozygotes for the short-allele variant have a frequency of ~17%, while homozygotes for the long allele are found in ~33% of cases.

Further results of studies of the serotonin system show in men associations to a genetic variant in the 5HTR 2A with a substitution of G to A at a position in the promoter (−1438). A/A homozygotes have a lower BMI, WHR, and abdominal sagittal diameter, while the G/A genotype shows a diminished suppressibility of cortisol by dexamethasone. The frequencies of the A/A and G/G homozygotes are 33% and 12% (142). It may be speculated that this genetic variation is associated with a product that promotes (G variant) or protects from (A variant) the development of abdominal obesity via serotonin influence on the HPA axis.

Similar studies of the 5HTR 2C in women so far have not revealed any associations of interest (unpublished).

E The HPA Axis

Finally, along the HPA axis, the gene for corticotropin-releasing hormone (CRH) and the GR gene have been examined. Nothing of interest seems to be present in the CRH gene (Rosmond et al., unpublished), while the GR gene shows several polymorphisms of potential interest. A microsatellite in the first coding exon, containing trinucleotide repeats (CAG), seems preliminary to be of normal length in subjects with the metabolic syndrome (143). A long allele (4.5 kb), obtained by the restriction enzyme Bcl I, cleaving the gene in the first intron, was found to be associated with abdominal obesity, insulin resistance, and hypertension (144–146). We confirmed this and found in addition a poor control of stimulated cortisol secretion (147), suggesting more directly that this polymorphism might be of functional importance for the regulation of the HPA axis. Thirteen percent of Swedish men are homozygotes for this allele, and heterozygotes (45.1%) show similar associations although less powerful. Another polymorphism in the promoter domain was found to be associated with basal cortisol secretion (148). A recent report indicated that a Tsp 5091 polymorphism in the first coding exon is strongly associated with obesity (149), which, however, we could not confirm (150).

These polymorphisms in the 5′ domain of the GR gene are of interest, although their potential functional importance is not known. It might be speculated that genetic variations in the promoter area or in the first intron might be aberrant, with consequences for the function of the GR gene transcript. If this is so, then one has to postulate that there are regional tissue differences in such polymorphisms. If the central GR is affected, then the regulatory feedback control of cortisol secretion would be expected to be inefficient, resulting in exposure of the organism to elevated cortisol levels and the metabolic syndrome. The findings suggest that this might be the correct interpretation because of the apparent association between these polymorphisms and HPA axis regulation (147). If, on the other hand, the peripheral GRs are not functionally optimal, this would presumably protect from excess cortisol effects. Tissue-specific differences in the promoter are known to be present in the GR gene (151). It may also be considered that a deficient function of the central GR, resulting in poor feedback control, may be a secondary effect due to downregulation of receptor density by elevated cortisol secretion (38).

A recent study has shown that the genetic variation in the GR gene, revealed by the Bcl I restriction enzyme, is also associated with the response to overfeeding. Subjects with the 2.3/2.3 kb gene variant were more susceptible to body weight increase as well as elevation of visceral fat mass, plasma lipids, and blood pressure than subjects with the 4.5/2.3 kb genotype (152). This is in apparent contrast to the findings in cross-sectional studies mentioned above, where the 4.5-kb allele was associated with abdominal obesity and other disease risk factors. One might consider that forced overfeeding, in contradiction to spontaneously occurring increase in fat mass, might induce pathological events in a normally regulated system.

The results of these studies are summarized in Table 1. It is apparent that there are a number of polymorphisms in these genes that are associated with the metabolic syndrome and its presumed etiological background in the central neuroendocrine pathways. The data give the impression that the frequency of protective genotypes is rather low in these population studies, at least in the aromatase, POMC, and MCR genes, suggesting that the genes promoting development toward obesity are more prevalent than the gene variants that protect. This might mean that in the general population the genes promoting obesity are more frequent than those that are protective. The

Table 1 Frequency of Genetic Variants in Central Regulatory Genes Promoting or Protecting from Obesity and the Metabolic Syndrome in Swedish Populations of Middle-Aged Men and Women

Gene locus	Protecting allele	Promoting allele	% Protecting allele
Aromatase	Long microsatellite	Short microsatellite	5
Leptin receptor	Several polymorphisms	Normal	10–25
POMC	Trinucleotide repeat	No repeat	8
MCR 4	G→A	G/G	3
TPH	Short/short	Long/long	37
SERT	Long/long	Short/short	33
5-HTR 2A	A/A	G/G	33
GR	2.3 kb	4.5 kb	39

POMC, Pro-opiomelanocortin; MCR 4, melanocortin receptor 4; TPH, tryptophan hydroxylase; SERT, serotonin transporter; 5HTR 2A, 5-hydroxytryptamine receptor 2A; GR, glucocorticoid receptor.
For explanation of alleles, see text.

situation might be different in selected cases of morbid obesity where genetic aberrations have been found in relatively small numbers in the leptin, leptin receptor, and MCR 4 genes.

Moderate obesity and overweight are now very frequent conditions (153). In fact, in several populations, those remaining lean are in the minority, as exemplified by findings in the population of middle-aged women, referred to above, where fewer than one-third have managed to keep their body weight since youth (88). The low prevalence of being lean might be due to selective mechanisms during periods of starvation in prehistoric and historical times, where those with a "thrifty" genotype survived. Such subjects may now constitute a majority of populations, and become obese in the current environment of excess food of high energy density. The minority who are able to remain lean are either restrained eaters or have a genetic predisposition protecting them from obesity. The findings in the population of a low frequency of genes protecting from obesity, as reported above, might therefore be considered to be due to evolutionary selection (154).

XI SUMMARY, SYNTHESIS, AND CONCLUSIONS

Substantial progress has been made since the previous edition of this chapter in the Handbook of Obesity. The metabolic syndrome is defined in this overview as a clustering of the symptoms insulin resistance, visceral fat accumulation, dyslipidemia, and hypertension. The metabolic syndrome might be considered to originate from a component of the syndrome, particularly when the insulin resistance and the increased visceral fat mass have been considered. It seems, however, that none of the components can explain the pathogenesis of the entire syndrome. It is difficult to visualize a pathway whereby insulin resistance may explain the accumulation of visceral fat. Visceral fat mass may, via portal free fatty acids, generate at least dyslipidemia and hepatic insulin resistance, but it is hard to understand how hypertension and systemic insulin resistance might be created through this pathway. Furthermore, this reasoning does not explain why depot fat is preferentially accumulated in the "portal" depots in the first place. It may be possible that portal free fatty acids amplify the full expression of the syndrome, but it seems unlikely that this is the primary event in the etiology of the metabolic syndrome.

This opens the possibilities of other primary pathogenic factors. We have since long entertained the possibility that this is a syndrome of central neuroendocrine dysregulations (155), resulting in multiple peripheral endocrine perturbations. The idea originated from the similarities between the metabolic syndrome and Cushing's syndrome. The major difficulty with this interpretation has been that identification of a functional hyperactivity of the HPA axis is elusive because of technical difficulties in measuring this delicate regulation. These problems are further amplified by the apparent development of different phases in the regulatory error with a first phase of increased cortisol secretion, which then appears to diminish to lower than normal values. In fact, the kinetics of the regulation of the HPA axis seems as important for the associated central and peripheral consequences as total cortisol secretion. This might explain why urinary cortisol secretion seems to be of limited help in disclosing the perturbations. Secondary inhibitions of gonadal and growth hormone axes contribute to the peripheral perturbations. The mechanisms for the peripheral effects of these endocrine and autonomic perturbations at the tissue, cellular, and molecular levels have been established. It seems somewhat surprising that these pathways have not been studied more extensively to disclose the pathogenesis of risk factors for cardiovascular disease and type 2 diabetes mellitus.

Recent findings are the powerful effects of moderate androgen elevations in women, probably at least partly originating from the adrenals. This might be amplified by a malfunction of the aromatase on a genetic basis. The view on the associations between the anthropometric and metabolic parts of the metabolic syndrome (visceral obesity, insulin resistance, and dyslipidemia) with the hemodynamic part (hypertension) is another new development. First, there is a statistical association between symptoms of the neuroendocrine perturbations and those of the sympathetic nervous system, suggesting that both stress centers are activated in parallel. This is independent of insulin, suggesting that insulin is not involved primarily. The concomitant activation of the HPA axis and the sympathetic nervous system is a well-known phenomenon from stress research. A central activation of the sympathetic nervous system is now an established view on the pathogenesis of primary hypertension. The elevated prevalence of hypertension in the metabolic syndrome might be due to the apparent dependence on leptin signals for blood pressure elevation. Insulin may well also be amplifying the central activity of the sympathetic nervous system.

Our current view on the pathogenesis of hypertension in the metabolic syndrome is therefore that a central activation of the sympathetic nervous system occurs parallel to the activation of the HPA axis, generating respectively elevated blood pressure and metabolic perturbations. The high prevalence of hypertension in the metabolic syndrome is probably due to the additional, amplifying effects of leptin and insulin. This view is strongly supported by similarities in environmental factors activating the HPA axis and the central sympathetic nervous system and thus inducing a frequent or chronic central arousal. With these considerations, the name "metabolic syndrome" may not fit as well, because it consists not only of metabolic symptoms, but also of anthropometric symptoms (visceral obesity) and hemodynamic symptoms (hypertension). It might therefore be time to consider changing the name of this cluster of symptoms to the "central arousal syndrome."

We have long been impressed by the statistical associations of the neuroendocrine, autonomic, and endocrine symptoms and their peripheral consequences to psychosocial, socioeconomic, depressive and anxiety symptoms, alcohol consumption, and smoking. The latter phenomena are all known to activate the HPA axis and the central sympathetic nervous system, either via perceived stress reactions or directly, and might therefore be primary etiological factors. These are, however, only statistical associations and need support from intervention studies. Such evidence is now accumulating. First, the Whitehall studies show a close parallelism between a decreasing socioeconomic gradient and the metabolic syndrome, which in our studies can be coupled to HPA axis perturbations and to a time axis of exposure. Furthermore, in prospective studies of the development of hypertension, similar factors are followed by elevated blood pressure. In fully controlled studies in primates, psychosocial stress is followed by all components of the metabolic syndrome, including elevated blood pressure. In addition, depression is connected to the metabolic syndrome in several ways: it can be found in the syndrome in mild, subclinical forms; it is characterized by the same neuroendocrine and autonomic perturbations; and its appearance is followed by the metabolic syndrome, which vanishes when the primary disease is cured.

A most interesting recent development is the apparent overlap in the metabolic syndrome and the small-baby syndrome. Both are characterized by the same neuroendocrine and autonomic perturbations. These seem to develop in the small-baby syndrome by sensitization of central neuroendocrine and autonomic axis due to events during the sensitive periods of brain development in the perinatal period. Originally thought to be due to intrauterine malnutrition, recent developments mainly from experimental animal work have now opened up the possibility that several other factors might be involved, including immune challenges and infections via endotoxins and cytokines. It is too early to state the extent to which perinatal factors are involved in the adult expressions of the metabolic syndrome, although the prevalence of low birth weight in relation to gestational age is currently considerably lower than the prevalence of the metabolic syndrome. This is also the case with the prevalence of HPA axis perturbations in men with low birth weight in relation to such abnormalities found in the adult population. Perinatal factors other than intrauterine malnutrition are most likely involved and need urgently to be defined (Fig. 4).

Recent developments have now opened up the possibility that obesity, defined as increased total body fat mass, is also a consequence of similar events, including HPA axis involvement. This may result in increased food intake in spite of elevated leptin levels, a condition of "leptin-resistant" obesity, typical for the prevalent human type of obesity. Elevated cortisol seems to have this ability both in controlled animal work and in humans. This increases the credibility of the phenomenon of "stress eating" in certain individuals, and might well contribute to the current epidemic of obesity.

Much of the observed phenomena associated with the metabolic syndrome may disappear with weight reduction, suggesting that obesity is the primary factor, and the neuroendocrine and autonomic phenomena secondary. Intervention studies are useful for interpretation of cause-effect relationships. There are several factors in prospective studies leading to the metabolic syndrome, such as the exposure to different stressful conditions, exposure to exogenous glucocorticoids, and, in women, to androgens, which argue in favor of the interpretation offered in this overview. Furthermore, interventions with testosterone in men or growth hormone in subjects with low secretions are followed by global improvements without necessarily affecting total body fat mass. A critical intervention here would be to normalize the HPA axis regulation, but this has so far not been possible in humans owing to the complex situation. The complications of Cushing's syndrome and glucocorticoid treatment disappear, however, after excluding excess glucocorticoid exposure. This is also the case in animal models exhibiting obesity and the metabolic syndrome.

If obesity is the primary factor, it is difficult to understand why the metabolic syndrome would appear only with visceral obesity and not with peripheral obesity. Furthermore, the associations to environmental factors with handicaps and other phenomena listed above would be difficult to understand, unless they would not also be secondary to obesity. The explanation of the effects on weight decrease on the expressions of the metabolic syndrome is probably that a weight decrease from an obese or nonobese starting point is followed by disruptions of homeostasis in several neuroendocrine and autonomic pathways, which tend to preserve energy. These phenomena appear with or without the presence of obesity or the metabolic syndrome and are probably not involved in the etiology of these conditions. If these counterregulatory mechanisms were known, the obesity treatment would be much more successful.

The elucidation of the phylogenetic expression along the pathways summarized above has made possible molecular genetic studies along these central etiological ways. Associations have been found with several steps in the POMC-MCR-HPA chain of events as well as in the serotoninergic pathway. Several of these findings seem to suggest that a genetic setup preventing obesity is rather uncommon.

Taken together, our original hypothesis, that the metabolic syndrome has its origin in central functional dysregulatory events based on environmental and genetic factors, has been considerably strengthened by continued work in our and other laboratories. The exploration of the function of the HPA axis by the development of new technology has been particularly helpful. The inclusion of the concomitant activation of the central sympathetic nervous system, resulting in hypertension, with the apparent similarities in established background factors, is another important supporting piece of information. Furthermore, independent work showing similarities in the etiology of the metabolic syndrome coming from prospective studies of psychosocially stressed nonhuman primates, socioeconomically stressed humans, mental depression, and the small-baby syndrome all provide support to the hypothesis that the metabolic syndrome has a central origin. Prospective observations indicate that perturbations in HPA axis regulation precede adverse health events. This provides additional strong support for the interpretations of available information as summarized in this overview.

The picture emerging seems to be that the current environment, be it stressful events in a competitive society, exposure to excessive energy-dense food, or physical inactivity, affects mental and bodily systems which are not adapted to such pressures. Outdated survival mechanisms and evolutionary selections are therefore now probably allowed full expression, resulting in the metabolic syndrome in combination with obesity.

REFERENCES

1. Björntorp P. Etiology of the metabolic syndrome. In: Bray GA, Bouchard C, James WPT, eds. Handbook of Obesity. New York: Marcel Dekker, 1998:573–600.
2. Björntorp P. Hypothalamic origin of prevalent human disease. In: Pfaff D, Arnold A, Etgen A, Fahrbach S, Rubin R, eds. Hormones, Brain and Behavior. San Diego: Academic Press, 2001:573–600.
3. Björntorp P, Rosmond R. Obesity and cortisol. Nutrition 2000; 16:924–936.
4. Björntorp P, Holm G, Rosmond R. Hypothalamic arousal, insulin resistance and type 2 diabetes mellitus. Diabetic Med 1999; 16:373–401.
5. Björntorp P. The regulation of adipose tissue distribution in humans. Int J Obes 1996; 20:291–302.
6. Björntorp P. Neuroendocrine perturbations as a cause

of insulin resistance. Diab/Metab Res Rev 1999; 15: 427–441.
7. Björntorp P. Epidemiology of the relationship between depression and physical illness. In: Thakore JH, ed. Depression a Stress-Related Disorder: Physical Consequences and Potential Treatment Implications. Bristol, PA: Wrightson Biomed, 2001: 427–441.
8. Björntorp P. Do stress reactions cause abdominal obesity and comorbidities? Obes Rev 2001; 2:73–86.
9. Björntorp P, Holm G, Rosmond R, Folkow B. Primary hypertension and the metabolic syndrome: closely related central origin? Blood Press 2000; 9:71–82.
10. Reaven GM. Role of insulin in human disease. Diabetes 1988; 37:1595–1607.
11. Björntorp P. Visceral obesity: A "civilization syndrome". Obes Res 1993; 1:216–222.
12. Björntorp P. "Portal" adipose tissue as a generator of risk factors for cardiovascular disease and diabetes. Arteriosclerosis 1990; 10:493–496.
13. Björntorp P. Fatty acids, hyperinsulinemia, and insulin resistance: which comes first? Curr Opin Lipid 1994; 5:166–174.
14. Martin ML, Jensen MD. Effects of body fat distribution on regional lipolysis in obesity. J Clin Invest 1991; 88:609–613.
15. Smyth J, Ockenfels MC, Porter L, Kirschbaum C, Hellhammer DH, Stone AA. Stressors and mood measured on a momentary basis are associated with salivary cortisol secretion. Psychoneuroendocrinology 1998; 23:353–371.
16. Rosmond R, Dallman MF, Björntorp P. Stress-related cortisol secretion in men: relationships with abdominal obesity and endocrine, metabolic and hemodynamic abnormalities. J Clin Endocrinol Metab 1998; 83:1853–1859.
17. Baghaei F, Rosmond R, Westberg L, Hellstrand M, Eriksson E, Holm G, Björntorp P. The CYP 19 gene and associations with androgens and abdominal obesity in premenopausal women. Obes Res 2003; 11:578–585.
18. Kristenson M, Orth-Gomér K, Kucinskiene Z, Bergdahl B, Calkausas H, Balinkyiene AG. Attenuated cortisol response to a standardised stress test in Lithuanian vs. Swedish men: the LiVicordia study. Int J Behav Med 2001; 8:23–31.
19. Wust S, Federenko I, Hellhammer DH, Kirschbaum C. Genetic factors perceived chronic stress, and the free cortisol response to awakening. Psychoneuroendocrinology 2000; 25:707–720.
20. Dallman MF, Akana SF, Scribner KA, Bradbury MJ, Walker C-D, Strack AM, Cascio CS. Stress, feedback and facilitation in the hypothalamo-pituitary-adrenal axis. J Neuroendocrinol 1992; 4:517–526.
21. Rosmond R, Holm G, Björntorp P. Food-induced cortisol secretion in relation to anthropometric, metabolic and hemodynamic variables in men. Int J Obes Relat Metabol Disord 2000; 24:416–422.
22. Pasquali R, Cantobelli S, Casimirri F. The hypothalamic-pituitary-adrenal axis in obese women with different patterns of body fat distribution. J Clin Endocrinol Metab 1993; 77:341–349.
23. Pasquali R, Anconetani B, Cattat R. Hypothalamic-pituitary-adrenal axis acticity and its relationship to the autonomic nervous system in women with visceral and subcutaneous obesity: effects of corticotropin-releasing factor/arginin-vasopressin test and of stress. Metabolism 1996; 45:531–536.
24. Hautanen A, Adlercreutz H. Altered adrenocorticotropin and cortisol secretion in abdominal obesity: implications for the insulin resistance syndrome. J Intern Med 1993; 234:461–469.
25. Pasquali R, Gagliardi L, Vicennati V. ACTH and cortisol response to combined corticotropin releasing hormone-arginine vasopressin stimulation in obese males and its relationship to body weight, fat distribution and parameters of the metabolic syndrome. Int J Obes Relat Metab Disord 1999; 23:419–423.
26. Moyer A, Rodin J, Grilo C, Rebuffé-Scrive M. Stress-induced cortisol response and fat distribution in women. Obes Res 1994; 2:255–259.
27. Epel EE, Moyer AE, Martin CD, Rebuffé-Scrive M. Stress-induced cortisol, mood, and fat distribution in men. Obes Res 1999; 7:9–12.
28. Korbonitz M, Trainer PJ, Nelson ML. Differential stimulation of cortisol and dehydroepiandrosterone levels by food in obese and normal subjects: relation to body fat distribution. Clin Endocrinol 1996; 45:699–708.
29. Liu JH, Kazer RR, Rusnussen DD. Characterization of the twenty-four hour secretion patterns of adrenocorticotropin and cortisol in normal women and patients with Cushing's disease. J Clin Endocrinol Metab 1987; 64:1027–1034.
30. Buffington CK, Givens JR, Kitabchi AE. Enhanced adrenocortical activity as a contributing factor to diabetes in hyperandrogenic women. Metabolism 1994; 43: 584–590.
31. Filipovsky J, Ducimetiere P, Eschwege E, Richard JL, Rosselin G, Claude P. The relationship of blood pressure with glucose, insulin, heart rate, fatty acids and plasma cortisol levels according to degree of obesity in middle-aged men. J Hypertens 1996; 14:229–235.
32. Stolk RP, Lamberts SWJ, De Jong FH, Pols HAP, Grobbee DE. Gender differences in the associations between cortisol and insulin sensitivity in healthy subjects. J Endocrinol 1996; 149:313–318.
33. Fraser R, Ingram MC, Anderson NH, Morrison C, Davies E, Connell J. Cortisol effects on body mass, blood pressure, and cholesterol in the general population. Hypertension 1999; 3:1374–1378.
34. Phillips DIW, Barker DJP, Fall CHD, Seckl JR, Whorwood CB, Wood PJ, Walker BR. Elevated cortisol concentrations: a link between low birth weight and the insulin resistance syndrome? J Clin Endocrinol Metab 1998; 83:757–760.

35. Phillips DIW, Walker BR, Reynolds RM, Flanagan DEH, Wood PJ, Osmond C, Barker DJP, Whorwood B. Low birth weight predicts elevated cortisol concentrations in adults from three populations. Hypertension 2001. In press.
36. McMahon M, Gerich J, Rizza R. Effects of glucocorticoids on carbohydrate metabolism. Diab Metab Rev 1988; 4:17–30.
37. Jacobs U, Klein B, Miersch WD. Dilemma: maintenance therapy enhances sclerogenic risk profile. Transplant Proc 1996; 26:3227–3230.
38. Sapolsky RM, Krey LC, McEwen BS. Stress downregulates corticosterone receptors in a site-specific manner. Endocrinology 1984; 114:287–292.
39. Rosmond R, Lapidus L, Björntorp P. The influence of occupational status and social factors on obesity and body fat distribution in middle-aged men. Int J Obes Relat Metab Disord 1996; 20:599–607.
40. Björntorp P, Rosmond R. Hypothalamic origin of the metabolic syndrome X. Ann NY Acad Sci 1999; 892:297–307.
41. Rosmond R, Björntorp P. Psychiatric ill-health of women and its relationship to obesity and body fat distribution. Obes Res 1998; 6:338–345.
42. Rosmond R, Björntorp P. Endocrine and metabolic aberrations in men with abdominal obesity in relation to anxio-depressive infirmity. Metabolism 1998; 47: 1187–1193.
43. Wing RR, Matthews KA, Kuller KH, Meilahn EN, Plantinga P. Waist to hip ratio in middle-aged women. Associations with behavioral and psychosocial factors and with changes in cardiovascular risk factors. Arterioscler Thromb 1991; 11:1250–1257.
45. Chrousos GP, Gold PW. The concept of stress and stress system disorders. Overview of physical and behavioral homeostasis. JAMA 1992; 267:1244–1252.
46. Shively CA, Laber-Laird K, Anton RF. Behavior and physiology of social stress and depression in female cynomolgus monkeys. Biol Psychiatry 1997; 41:871–882.
47. Jayo JM, Shively CA, Kaplan JR, Manuck SB. Effects of exercise and stress on body fat distribution in male *Cynomolgus* monkeys. Int J Obes 1993; 17:587–604.
48. Brunner E, Marmot MG, Nanchatal K, Shipley MJ, Stansfield SA, Juneja M. Social inequality in coronary risk: central obesity and the metabolic syndrome. Evidence from the Whitehall II study. Diabetologia 1997; 40:1341–1349.
49. Rosmond R, Björntorp P. Occupational status, cortisol secretory pattern and visceral obesity in middle-aged men. Obes Res 2000; 8:445–450.
50. Roy-Byrne PP, Uhde TW, Post RM, Gallucci W, Chrousos GP, Gold PW. The corticotropin-releasing hormone stimulation test in patients with panic disorder. Am J Psychiatry 1986; 143:896–899.
51. Pratt LA, Ford DE, Crum RM, Armenian HK, Gallo JJ, Eaton WW. Depression, psychotropic medication and risk for myocardial infarction. Prospective data from the Baltimore ECA follow-up. Circulation 1996; 94: 3123–3129.
52. Eaton WW, Armenian H, Gallo J, Pratt L, Ford DE. Depression and risk for onset of type II diabetes. A prospective population-based study. Diabetes Care 1996; 19:1097–1102.
53. Thakore JH, Richards PJ, Reznek RH, Martin A, Dinan T. Increased intra-abdominal fat deposition in patients with major depressive illness as measured by computed tomography. Biol Psychiatry 1997; 41:1140–1142.
54. Ahlberg C, Ljung T, Rosmond R, McEwen B, Holm G, Björntorp P, Åkesson HO. Depression and anxiety symptoms in relation to anthropometry and metabolism in men. Psychiatr Res 2001; 112:101–110.
55. Pettersson P, Ellsinger B-M, Sjöberg C, Björntorp P. Fat distribution and steroid hormones in women with alcohol abuse. J Intern Med 1990; 228:311–316.
56. Smals AG, Kloppenborg PW, Njo KT. Alcohol induced cushingoid syndrome. Br Med J 1976; 2: 1928.
57. Gossain VV, Sherma NK, Srivastava L, Michelakis AM, Rovner RV. Hormonal effects of smoking. II. Effects on plasma cortisol, growth hormone, and prolactin. Am J Med Sci 1986; 291:325–327.
58. Shimokata H, Tobin HJD, Muller DC, Elahi D, Coon PJ, Andres R. Studies in the distribution of body fat. I. Effects of age, sex and obesity. J Gerontol 1989; 44: M66–M73.
59. Reaven GM. Pathophysiology of insulin resistance in human disease. Physiol Rev 1995; 75:473–486.
60. Sapolsky R, Krey L, McEwen B. The neuroendocrinology of stress and aging: the glucocorticoid cascade hypothesis. Endocr Rev 1986; 7:289–301.
61. Seeman TE, Robbins RJ. Aging and the hypothalamic-pituitary-adrenal response to challenge in humans. Endocr Rev 1994; 15:233–260.
62. Björntorp P. Alterations in the ageing corticotropic stress-response axis. In: Weldhuis J, ed. The Endocrinology of Ageing. London: Wellcome Trust, 2001: 46–65.
63. Gabay C, Kushner I. Acute-phase proteins and other systemic responses to inflammation. N Engl J Med 1999; 340:448–454.
64. Rohde LEP, Hennekens CH, Ridker PM. Survey of C-reactive protein and cardiovascular risk factors in apparently healthy men. Am J Cardiol 1999; 84: 1018–1022.
65. Tsigos C, Papanicolaou DA, Defensor R, Mitsiadis CS, Kyrou I, Chrousos GP. Dose effects or recombinant human interleukin-6 on pituitary hormone secretion and energy expenditure. Neuroendocrinology 1997; 66:54–62.
66. Bornstein SR, Chrousos GP. Adrenocorticotropin (ACTH)- and non-ACTH-mediated regulation of the adrenal cortex: neural and immune inputs. J Clin Endocrinol Metab 1999; 84:1729–1736.

67. Barker DJP, Hales CN, Fall CHD, Osmond C, Phipps K, Clark PMS. Type 2 (non-insulin-dependent) diabetes mellitus, hypertension and hyperlipidemia (syndrome X): relation to fetal growth. Diabetologia 1993; 35:62–67.
68. Reul JMHM, Stec I, Wiegers GJ, Labeur MS, Linthorst ACE, Arzt E, Holsboer F. Prenatal immune challenge alters the hypothalamic-pituitary-adrenocortical axis in adult rats. J Clin Invest 1994; 93:2600–2607.
69. Dahlgren J, Nilsson C, Jennische E, Ho H-P, Eriksson E, Niklasson A, Björntorp P, Albertsson K, Wikland A, Holmäng A. Prenatal cytokine exposure results in obesity and gender-specific programming. Am J Physiol Endocrinol Metab 2001; 281:E326–E334.
70. Seckl J. Glucocorticoids, feto-placental 11 β-hydroxysteroid dehydrogenase type 2, and early life origins of adults disease. Steroids 1997; 62:89–94.
71. Nilsson C, Niklasson M, Eriksson E, Björntorp P, Holmäng A. Imprinting of female offspring with testosterone results in insulin resistance and changes in body fat distribution at adult age in rats. J Clin Invest 1998; 101:74–77.
72. Nilsson C, Larsson B-M, Jennische E, Eriksson E, Björntorp P, York DA, Holmäng A. Maternal endotoxemia results in obesity and insulin resistance in adult male offspring. Endocrinology 2001; 142:2622–2630.
73. Ravelli AC, Van der Meulen JH, Osmond C, Barker DJ, Bleker OP. Obesity at the age of 50 y in men and women exposed to famine prenatally. Am J Clin Nutr 1999; 70:811–816.
74. Johannsson G, Mårin P, Lönn L, Ottosson M, Stenlöf K, Björntorp P, Sjöström L, Bengtsson BÅ. Growth hormone treatment of abdominally obese men reduces abdominal fat mass, improves glucose and lipoprotein metabolism, and reduces diastolic blood pressure. J Clin Endocrinol Metab 1997; 82:727–734.
75. Seidell JC, Björntorp P, Sjöström L, Kvist H, Sannerstedt R. Visceral fat accumulation in men is positively associated with insulin, glucose and c-peptide levels, but negatively with testosterone levels. Metabolism 1990; 39:897–901.
76. Rosmond R, Björntorp P. The interactions between hypothalamic-pituitary-adrenal axis activity, testosterone and insulin-like growth factor I and abdominal obesity with metabolism in men. In J Obes Relat Metab Disord 1998; 22:1184–1196.
77. Plotsky PM, Cunningham ETJr, Widmaier EP. Catecholaminergic modulation of corticotrophin-releasing factor and adrenocorticotropin secretion. Endocr Rev 1989; 10:437–458.
78. Kissebah AH, Krakower GR, Sonnenberg G, Hennes MMI. Clinical manifestations of the metabolic syndrome. In: Bray GA, Bouchard C, James PCT, eds. Handbook of Obesity. New York: Marcel Dekker, 1998:601–636.
79. McEwen BS. Protective and damaging effects of stress mediators. N Engl J Med 1998; 338:171–179.
80. Lindstedt G, Lundberg PA, Lapidus L, Lundgren H, Bengtsson C, Björntorp P. Low sex-hormone-binding globuline concentration as independent risk factor for development of NIDDM: 12-yr follow-up of population study of women in Gothenburg, Sweden. Diabetes 1991; 40:123–128.
81. Lovejoy JC, Bray GA, Bourgeois MO, Macchiavelli R, Rood JC, Greeson C, Partington C. Exogenous androgens influence on body composition and regional fat distribution in obese menopausal women. A clinical research center study. J Clin Endocrinol Metab 1996; 81:189–203.
82. Elbers JM, Asscheman H, Seidell JC, Gooren LJ. Effects of sex steroid hormones on regional fat deposits as assessed by magnetic resonance imaging in transsexuals. Am J Physiol 1999; 276:E317–E325.
83. Polderman KH, Gooren LJG, Aschermann H. Induction of insulin resistance by androgens and estrogens. J Clin Endocrinol Metab 1994; 79:265–271.
84. Holmäng A, Svedberg J, Jennische E, Björntorp P. Effects of testosterone on muscle insulin sensitivity and morphology in female rats. Am J Physiol 1990; 258: E555–E560.
85. Rincon J, Holmäng A, Odegaard-Wahlström E, Lönnroth P, Björntorp P, Zierath JR, Wallberg-Henriksson H. Mechanisms behind insulin resistance in rat skeletal muscle after oophorectomy and additional testosterone treatment. Diabetes 1996; 45:615–621.
86. Riggins GJ, Lokey LK, Chastain JL, Leiner HA, Sherman SL, Wilkinson KD, Warren ST. Human genes containing polymorphic trinucleotide repeats. Nat Gene 1992; 2:186–191.
87. Comings DE. Polygenic inheritance and micro/minisatellites. Mol Psychiatry 1998; 3:21–31.
88. Baghaei F, Rosmond R, Westberg L, Hellstrand M, Landén M, Eriksson E, Holm G, Björntorp P. The lean woman. Obes Res 2002; 10:115–121.
89. Jones MEE, Thorburn AW, Britt KL, Hewitt KN, Wreford NG, Proietto J, Os OK, Leury BJ, Robertson KM, Yao S, Simpson ER. Aromatase-deficient (ArKO) mice have a phenotype of increased adiposity. Proc Natl Acad Sci USA 2000; 97:12735–12740.
90. Rocchini AP. Obesity and blood pressure regulation. In: Bray GA, Bouchard C, James WPT, eds. Handbook of Obesity. New York: Marcel Dekker, 1998:677–696.
91. Folkow B. Physiological aspects of primary hypertension. Physiol Rev 1982; 62:384–504.
92. Landsberg L, Young JB. Insulin-mediated glucose metabolism in the relation between dietary intake and sympathetic nervous system activity. Int J Obes 1985; 9:63–68.
93. Anderson EA, Hoffman RB, Baron TW, Sinkey CA, Mark AL. Hyperinsulinemia produces both sympa-

thetic neural activation and vasodilation in normal humans. J Clin Invest 1991; 87:2246–2252.
94. Tsutsu N, Nunoi K, Koama T, Nomiyama R, Iwase M, Fujishima M. Lack of association between blood pressure and insulin in patients with insulinoma. J Hypertens 1990; 8:479–482.
95. Julius S, Esler M. Autonomic nervous cardiovascular regulation in borderline hypertension. Am J Cardiol 1975; 36:685–696.
96. Lund-Johansen P. Hemodynamics of essential hypertension. In: Swales JD, ed. Textbook of Hypertension. Oxford: Blackwell Science, 1994:61–76.
97. Folkow B. Psychosocial and central nervous influences in primary hypertension. Circulation 1987; 76(suppl 1):110–119.
98. Brod J, Fencl V, Hejl Z, Jirka J, Ulrych M. General and regional hemodynamic pattern underlying essential hypertension. Clin Sci 1962; 23:339–349.
99. Timio M, Lippi G, Venanzi S. Blood pressure trend and cardiovascular events in nuns in a secluded order: a 30-year follow-up study. Blood Press 1997; 6:81–87.
100. Hollenberg NK, Martinez G, McCullough M. Aging, acculturation, salt intake, and hypertension in the Kuna of Panama. Hypertension 1997; 29:171–176.
101. Schnall PL, Schwartz JE, Landsbergis PA, Warrer K, Pickering TG. A longitudinal study of job strain and ambulatory blood pressure: results from a three-year follow-up. Psychosom Med 1988; 60:697–706.
102. Henry JP, Stephens PM. Stress, Health and the Psychosocial Environment: A Sociobiological Approach to Medicine. New York: Springer-Verlag, 1977.
103. Rosmond R, Björntorp P. Blood pressure in relation to obesity, insulin and the hypothalamic-pituitary-adrenal axis in Swedish men. J Hypertens 1998; 16: 1721–1726.
104. Ljung T, Holm G, Friberg P, Andersson B, Bengtsson B-Å, Svensson J, Dallman MF, McEwen B, Björntorp P. The activity of the hypothalamic-pituitary-adrenal axis and the sympathetic nervous system in relation to waist/hip circumference in men. Obes Res 2000; 8:1–9.
105. Considine RV, Sinha MK, Heiman ML, Kriauciunas A, Stephens TW, Nyce MR, Ohannesian JP, Marco CC, McKee LJ, Bauer TL, Caro JF. Serum immunoreactive leptin concentrations in normal-weight and obese humans. N Engl J Med 1996; 334:292–295.
106. Haynes WG, Morgan DA, Walsh SA, Mark AL, Sivitz WI. Receptor mediated regional sympathetic nerve activation by leptin. J Clin Invest 1997; 100:270–278.
107. Rosmond R, Chagnon YC, Holm G, Chagnon M, Pérusse L, Lindell K, Carlsson B, Bouchard C, Björntorp P. Hypertension in obesity and the leptin receptor gene locus. J Clin Endocrinol Metab 2000; 85:3126–3131.
108. Despres JP, Nadeau A, Tremblay A. Role of deep abdominal fat in the association between regional adipose tissue distribution and glucose tolerance in obese women. Diabetes 1989; 38:304–309.
109. Newcomer JW, Selke G, Melson AK, Gross J, Vogler GKP, Dagogo-Jack S. Dose-dependent cortisol-induced increases in plasma leptin concentration in healthy humans. Arch Gen Psychiatry 1998; 55:995–1000.
110. Dagogo-Jack S, Selke G, Melson AK, Newcomer JW. Robust leptin secretory response to dexamethasone in obese subjects. J Clin Endocrinol Metab 1997; 82:3230–3233.
111. Tataranni PA, Larson DE, Snitker S, Young JB, Flatt JP, Ravussin E. Effects of glucocorticoids on energy metabolism and food intake in humans. Am J Physiol 1996; 271:E317–E325.
112. Uddén J, Björntorp P, Arner P, Barkeling B, Meurling L, Hill M, Rössner S. Effects of glucocorticoids on leptin levels and eating behavior in women. Int Med 2003; 253:225–231.
113. Zakrzewska KE, Cusin I, Sainsbury A, Rohner-Jeanrenaud F, Jeanrenaud B. Glucocorticoids as counterregulatory hormones of leptin. Toward an understanding of leptin resistance. Diabetes 1997; 46: 717–719.
114. Uotani S, Björbaek C, Tornö J, Flier JS. Functional properties of leptin receptor isoforms. Internalization and degradation of leptin and ligand-induced receptor down-regulation. Diabetes 1999; 48:279–286.
115. Morgan CA III, Wang S, Soutwick SM, Rasmusson A, Hazlett G, Hauger RL, Charney DS. Plasma neuropeptide-Y concentrations in humans exposed to military survival training. Biol Psychiatry 2000; 47: 902–909.
116. Guidi L, Tricerri A, Vangeli M, Frasca D, Riccardo Errani A, DiGiovanni A, Antico L, Menini E, Sciamanna V, Magnavita N, Doria G, Bartoloni C. Neuropeptide Y plasma levels and immunological changes during academic stress. Neuropsychobiology 1999; 40:188–195.
117. Bellisle F, Louis-Sylvestre J, Linet N, Rocaboy B, Dalle B, Cheneau F, L'Hinoret D, Guyot L. Anxiety and food intake in men. Psychosom Med 1990; 52:452–457.
118. Michaut C, Kahn JP, Musse N, Burlet C, Nicolas JP, Mejean L. Relationships between a critical life event and eating behaviour in high-school students. Stress Med 1990; 6:57–64.
119. Grenoo CG, Wing RR. Stress-induced eating. Psychol Bull 1994; 115:444–464.
120. Allison DB, Heshka S. Emotion and eating in obesity? A critical analysis. Int J Eating Disord 1993; 13:289–295.
121. Epel E, Lapidus R, McEwen B, Brownell K. Stress may add bite to appetite in women: a laboratory study of stress-induced cortisol and eating behavior. Psychoneuroendocrinology 2001; 26:37–49.
122. Zumoff B, Strain GW. A perspective on the hormonal abnormalities of obesity: are they cause or effect? Obes Res 1994; 2:56–67.

123. Seidell J, Björntorp P, Sjöström L, Sannerstedt R, Krotkiewski M, Kvist H. Regional distribution of muscle and fat mass in men—new insight into the risk of abdominal obesity using computed tomography. Int J Obes 1989; 13:289–303.
124. Björntorp P, De Jounge K, Sjöström L, Sullivan L. The effect of physical training on insulin production in obesity. Metabolism 1970; 19:631–638.
125. Krotkiewski M, Mandroukas K, Sjöström L, Sullivan L, Wetterqvist H, Björntorp P. Effects of long-term physical training on body fat, metabolism and blood pressure in obesity. Metabolism 1979; 28:650–658.
126. Lawlor DA, Hopker SW. The effectiveness of exercise as an intervention in the management of depression: systematic review and meta-regression analysis of randomised controlled trials. BMJ 2001; 322:763–767.
127. Comuzzi AG, Hixson JE, Almasy L. A major quantitative trait locus determining serum leptin levels and fat mass is located on human chromosome 2. Nat Genet 1997; 15:273–276.
128. Yaswen L, Diehl N, Brennan MB, Hochgeschwender U. Obesity in the mouse model of pro-opiomelanocortin deficiency responds to peripheral melanocortin. Nat Med 1999; 5:1066–1070.
129. Krude H, Biebermann H, Luck W, Horn R, Brabant G, Gruters A. Severe early-onset obesity, adrenal insufficience and red hair pigmentation caused by POMC mutations in humans. Nat Genet 1998; 19:155–157.
130. Rosmond R, Ukkola O, Bouchard C, Björntorp P. Polymorphisms in exon 3 of the proopiomelanocortin gene (POMC) in relation to serum leptin, salivary cortisol and obesity in Swedish men. Metabolism 2002; 51:642–644.
131. Gantz I, Miwa H, Konda Y, Shimoto Tashiro Y, Watson SJ, DelValle J, Yamada T. Molecular cloning, expression, and gene localization of a fourth melanocortin receptor. J Biol Chem 1993; 268:15147–15179.
132. Mountjoy KG, Mortrud MT, Low MJ, Simerly RB, Cone Rd. Localization of the melanocortin-4 receptor (MC-4R) in neuroendocrine and autonomic control circuits in the brain. Mol Endocrinol 1994; 8:1298–1308.
133. Hinney A, Becker I, Heibult O, Nottebom K, Schmidt A, Ziegler A, Mayer H, Siegfried W, Blum WF, Remschmidt H, Hebebrand J. Systemic mutation screening of the proopiomelanocortin gene: identification of several genetic variants including three different insertions, one nonsense and two missense point mutations in probands of different weight extremes. J Clin Endocrinol Metab 1998; 83: 3737–3741.
134. Sina M, Hinney A, Ziegler A, Neupert T, Mayer H, Siegfried W, Blum WF, Remschmidt H, Hedebrand J. Phenotypes in three pedigrees with autosomal dominant obesity caused by haploinsufficience mutations in the melanocortin-4 receptor gene. Am J Hum Genet 1999; 65:1501–1507.
135. Faroqi IS, Yeo GS, Keogh JM, Aminian S, Jebb SA, Cheetham T, O'Rahilly S. Dominant and recessive inheritance of morbid obesity associated with melanocortin 4 receptor deficiency. J Clin Invest 2000; 106:271–279.
136. Vaisse C, Clement K, Durand E, Hercberg S, Guy-Grand B, Froguel P. Melanocortin-4 receptor mutations are a frequent and heterogenous cause of morbid obesity. J Clin Invest 2000; 106:253–262.
137. Huszar D, Lynch CA, Fairchild-Huntress V, Dunmore JH, Fang Q, Berkemeier LR, Gu W, Kesterson RA, Bostaon BA, Cone RD, Smith FJ, Campfield LA, Burn P, Lee F. Targeted disruption of the melanocortin-4 receptor results in obesity in mice. Cell 1997; 88:131–141.
138. Rosmond R, Chagnon M, Bouchard C, Björntorp P. A missense mutation in the human melanocortin-4 receptor gene in relation to abdominal obesity and salivary cortisol. Diabetologia 2002; 44:1335–1338.
139. Leibowitz SF, Alexander JT. Hypothalamic serotonin in control of eating behavior, meal size, and body weight. Biol Psychiatry 1998; 44:851–864.
140. Nonogaki K, Strack AM, Dallman MF, Tecott LH. Leptin-independent hyperphagia and type 2 diabetes in mice with a mutated serotonin 5-HT2C receptor gene. Nat Med 1998; 4:1152–1156.
141. Barnes NM, Sharp T. A review of central 5-HT receptors and their function. Neuropharmacology 1999; 38:1038–1152.
142. Rosmond R, Bouchard C, Björntorp P. 5-HT2A receptor gene promoter polymorphism in relation to abdominal obesity and cortisol. Obes Res 2002; 10:585–589.
143. Ljung T, Ottosson M, Ahlberg A-C, Edén S, Odén B, Okret S, Brönnegård M, Stierna P, Björntorp P. Central and peripheral glucocorticoid receptor function in abdominal obesity. Endocr Invest 2002; 25:229–235.
144. Weaver JU, Hitman G, Kopelman PG. An association between a Bcl I restriction fragment length polymorphism of the glucocorticoid receptor locus and hyperinsulinemia in obese women. J Mol Endocrinol 1992; 9:295–300.
145. Watt GCM, Harrap SB, Foy CJW, Holton DW, Edwards HV, Davidson HR. Abnormalities of glucocorticoid metabolism and the renin-angiotensin system: a four corners approach to identification of genetic determinants of blood pressure. J Hypertens 1992; 10:473–482.
146. Buemann B, Vohl MC, Chagnon M, Chagnon YC, Gagnon J, Pérusse L, Dionne F, Despres JP, Tremblay A, Nadeau A, Bouchard C. Abdominal visceral fat is associated with a Bcl I restriction fragment length polymorphism at the glucocorticoid receptor gene locus. Obes Res 1997; 5:186–192.
147. Rosmond R, Chagnon YC, Holm G, Chagnon M, Pérusse L, Lindell K, Carlsson B, Bouchard C, Björntorp P. A glucocorticoid receptor gene marker is

associated with abdominal obesity, leptin and dysregulation of the hypothalamic-pituitary-adrenal axis. Obes Res 2000; 8:211–218.

148. Rosmond R, Chagnon YC, Chagnon M, Pérusse L, Bouchard C, Björntorp P. A polymorphism in the 5′-flanking region of the glucocorticoid receptor gene locus is associated with basal cortisol secretion in men. Metabolism 2000; 49:1197–1199.
149. Lin RC, Wang W, Morris BJ. High penetrance, overweight, and glucocorticoid receptor variant: a case-control study. BMJ 1999; 319:1337–1338.
150. Rosmond R, Bouchard C, Björntorp P. Tsp5091 polymorphism in exon 2 of the glucocorticoid receptor gene in relation to obesity and cortisol secretion: a cohort study. BMJ 2001; 322:652–653.
151. Andrews RC, Walker BR. Glucocorticoids and insulin resistance: old hormones, new targets. Clin Sci 1999; 96:513–518.
152. Ukkola O, Rosmond R, Tremblay A, Bouchard C. Glucocorticoid receptor Bcl I variant is associated with an increased atherogenic profile in response to long-term overfeeding. Atherosclerosis 2001; 157:221–224.
153. World Health Organization. Obesity. Preventing and Managing the Global Epidemic. Report of a WHO Consultation on Obesity. WHO/NUT/NCD/981. Geneva: WHO, 1998.
154. Björntorp P. Genes in human obesity. Are we chasing ghosts? Lancet 2001; 358:1006–1008.
155. Björntorp P. Hazards in subgroups of human obesity. Eur J Clin Invest 1984; 14:239–241.

33

Obesity as a Risk Factor for Major Health Outcomes

JoAnn E. Manson

Harvard Medical School and Brigham & Women's Hospital, Boston, Massachusetts, U.S.A.

Patrick J. Skerrett

Brigham & Women's Hospital and Harvard Health Publications, Harvard Medical School, Boston, Massachusetts, U.S.A.

Walter C. Willett

Harvard School of Public Health, Boston, Massachusetts, U.S.A.

I INTRODUCTION

Until recently, excess weight was generally overlooked as a major risk factor for chronic disease. Now a rapidly expanding body of data is defining the impact of overweight and obesity on premature mortality, cardiovascular disease, type 2 diabetes mellitus, osteoarthritis, gallbladder disease, some types of cancer, and other conditions (Fig. 1) (1,2). Models using data from the Third National Health and Nutrition Examination Survey (NHANES III), the Framingham Heart Study, and other sources have demonstrated a direct, dose-dependent relationship between increasing body mass index (BMI) and lifetime risk of various conditions (Table 1) (3–5). Data from the U.S. Behavioral Risk Factor Surveillance System indicate that obesity is associated with greater morbidity and poorer health-related quality of life than smoking or problem drinking (6), and a recent conservative estimate, derived from five long-term prospective cohort studies, suggests that overweight and obesity account for >280,000 deaths each year in the United States (7). The substantial morbidity and mortality associated with excess weight underscore the pressing need to improve the education of health professionals and the public about the hazards of overweight and obesity and to remove the barriers to healthy eating and increased physical activity.

II MORTALITY

While the precise shape of the body weight/mortality curve remains controversial, there is little question that substantial excess adiposity increases mortality. A reanalysis of 12-year follow-up data of the American Cancer Society's Cancer Prevention Study I cohort that excluded smokers and those with a history of cancer or cardiovascular disease at baseline (8), as well as a new analysis of a second Cancer Prevention cohort of more than 1 million adults with 14 years of follow-up (9), showed a clear pattern of increasing mortality with increasing weight (Fig. 2). Among healthy people who had never smoked, optimal mortality was found at a BMI of 23.5–24.9 for men and 22.0–23.4 for women. These data confirm similar observations from a 27-year

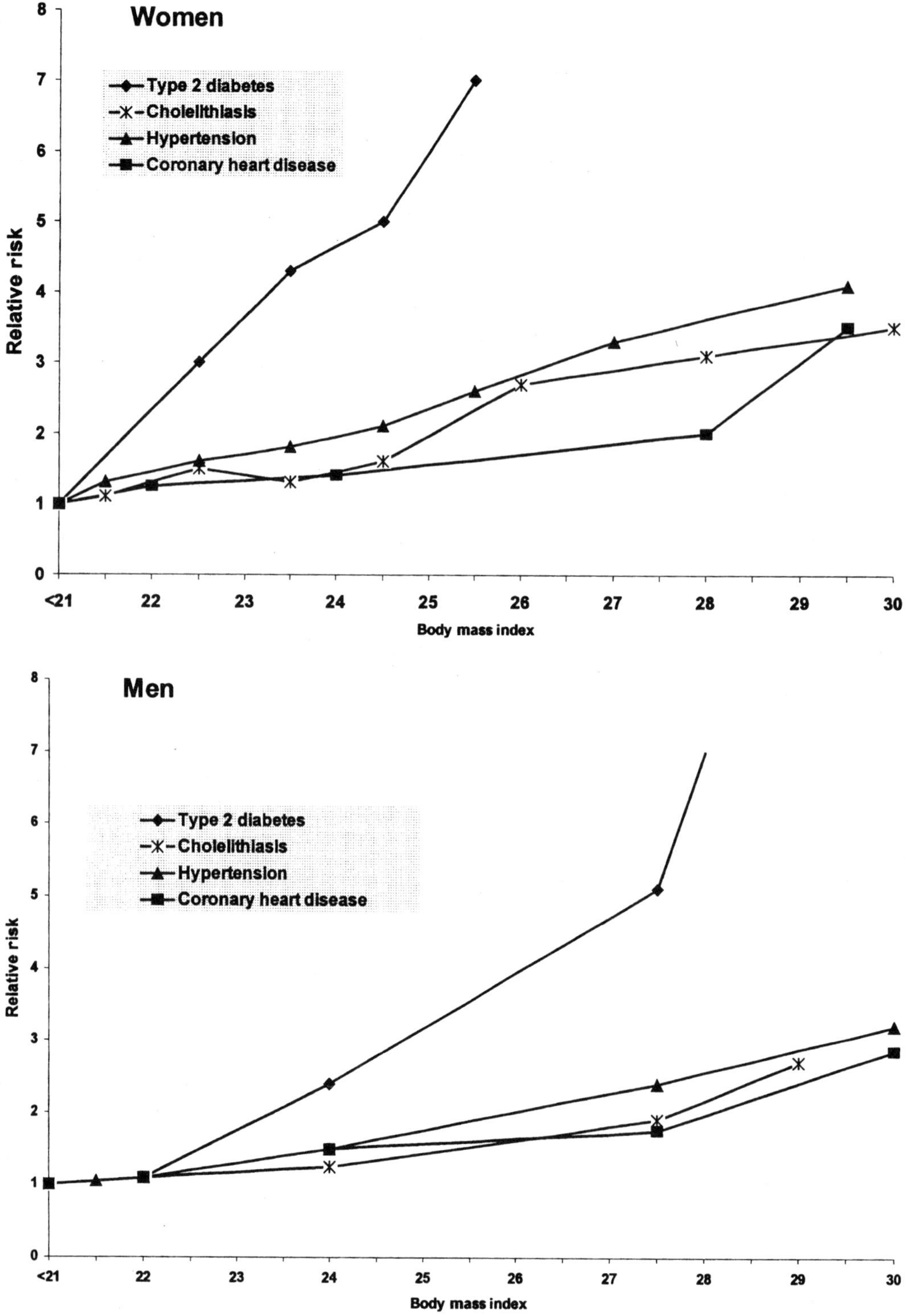

Figure 1 Relation between body mass index up to 30 and the relative risks of type 2 diabetes, cholelithiasis, hypertension, and coronary heart disease in the Nurses' Health Study and the Health Professionals Follow-up Study. (From Ref. 13.)

Table 1 Prevalence Ratios and Relative Risks of Several Weight-Related Diseases in the Third National Health and Nutrition Evaluation Survey (NHANES III),[a] the Nurses' Health Study (NHS),[b] and the Health Professionals Follow-up Study (HPFS)[c]

	Overweight (BMI 25.0–29.9 kg/m^2)	Obese (BMI 30.0–34.9 kg/m^2)	Very obese (BMI ≥35.0 kg/m^2)
Coronary heart disease			
NHANES III	1.0–1.3	1.1–1.7	2.2–3.0
NHS	1.4	1.5	1.5
HPFS	1.5	2.0	2.2
Hypertension			
NHANES III	1.1–1.6	1.2–3.2	1.4–5.5
NHS	1.7	2.1	2.3
HPFS	1.7	2.7	3.0
Hypercholesterolemia			
NHANES III	1.2–1.9	1.1–1.7	0.9–1.7
NHS	1.1	0.9	0.7
HPFS	1.3	1.2	1.3
Type 2 diabetes			
NHANES III	1.8–3.8	2.5–10.1	3.5–18.1
NHS	4.6	10.0	17.0
HPFS	3.5	11.2	23.4
Gallbladder disease			
NHANES III	1.3 1.9	1.8–4.1	2.5–21
NHS	1.9	2.5	3.0
HPFS	1.4	2.3	2.9

[a] Values are prevalence ratios for men and women aged <55 years and ≥55 years compared with individuals with BMIs of 18.0–24.9 kg/m^2.
[b] Values are relative risks compared with women with BMIs <25 kg/m^2.
[c] Values are relative risks compared with men with BMIs <25 kg/m^2.
Sources: Refs. 5, 51.

follow-up of more than 19,000 middle-aged men in the Harvard Alumni Study (10), a 16-year follow-up of 115,000 middle-aged female nurses (11), and a 12-year follow-up of nonsmoking Seventh-Day Adventists (12). Using data from five long-term prospective cohort studies, Allison and colleagues estimated the annual number of adult deaths in the United States attributable to obesity at 280,000 per year (7), making obesity second only to tobacco as a cause of preventable death in the United States.

Although some investigators have argued that the optimal weight increases with age, this observation is probably an artifact of the increasing prevalence of weight loss secondary to chronic disease and comorbidity among older individuals, the cumulative effects of cigarette smoking, and the reduced reliability of BMI as a measure of adiposity with advancing age (13). Reports from the Framingham Heart Study (14), the Adventist Health Study (15), and the American Cancer Society (8) cohorts indicate that, although the strength of the association between body weight and mortality decreases with age, being overweight remains predictive of excess mortality and that at least up to age 75, a BMI <25 kg/m^2 is associated with reduced total mortality.

III CARDIOVASCULAR DISEASE

Although obesity has been linked with cardiovascular disease for centuries, it was only formally recognized as a major modifiable coronary risk factor in 1998 (16). As described below, and in greater detail in subsequent chapters, obesity is associated with increased risks of coronary heart disease, stroke, venous thromboembolism, congestive heart failure, and cardiomyopathy. Obesity increases these risks partly through its effects on established coronary risk factors such as hypertension, dyslipidemia, and insulin resistance, as well as its effects on novel risk factors such as thrombotic and inflammatory markers. For example, in the Marks and Spencer Cardiovascular Risk Factor Study of 14,077 middle-aged women, highly significant age-adjusted

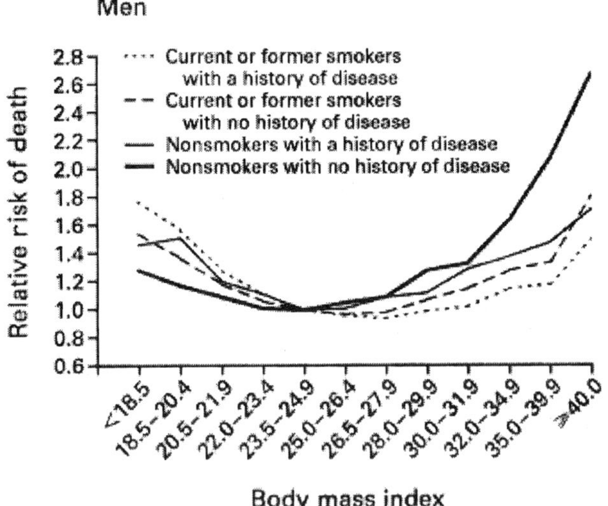

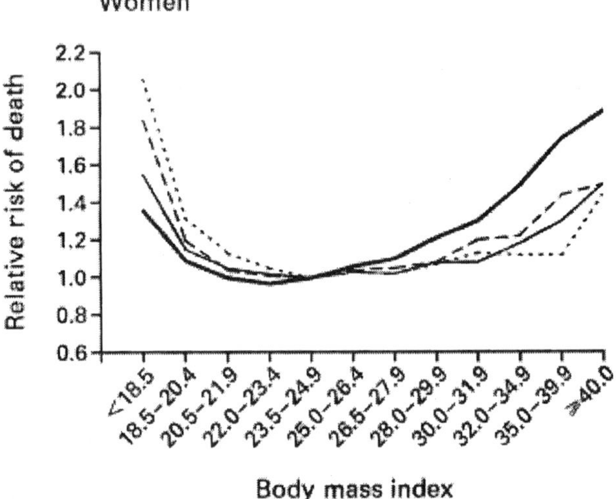

Figure 2 Multivariate relative risk of death from all causes among men and women according to body mass index, smoking status, and disease status, using subjects with a body mass index of 23.5–24.9 kg/m^2 as the referent. (From Ref. 9.)

changes were observed across seven categories of BMI (<20 to ≥ 30 kg/m^2) for systolic and diastolic blood pressure, serum total cholesterol, high-density lipoprotein (HDL) cholesterol, low-density lipoprotein (LDL) cholesterol, triglycerides, and fasting blood glucose (17). Excess weight is also associated with increases in thrombotic markers such as fibrinogen and plasminogen activator inhibitor-1, as well as increases in inflammatory markers such as C-reactive protein, that have been associated with increased risk of cardiovascular disease and diabetes (18–20). Consistent with the excess risk of coronary heart disease even among individuals with average weights, the Framingham Heart Study has demonstrated that many individuals with BMIs between 23 and 25 kg/m^2 have abnormalities in serum lipids, glucose tolerance, and blood pressure compared to those with BMIs <23 kg/m^2, and most individuals with BMIs >25 kg/m^2 have such abnormalities. In addition to its effect on these cardiovascular risk factors, obesity appears to have an independent effect on cardiovascular risk, suggesting the existence of additional mechanisms.

Limited data are available regarding the long-term benefits of intentional weight loss on cardiovascular risk. However, a number of mostly small clinical trials of varying design demonstrate benefits of weight loss among overweight and obese individuals on specific cardiovascular risk factors, including blood pressure, glucose tolerance, and lipoprotein profile, that would be expected to lower cardiovascular risk (21).

A Coronary Heart Disease

Numerous observational studies, including many long-term prospective cohort studies (22–32), have demonstrated a direct association between excess weight and coronary heart disease, the most common cause of death in the United States. The relationship appears to be linear, and even individuals of average weight (i.e., those with BMIs of 24–26 kg/m^2) at midlife are at increased risk compared with leaner individuals. In the Nurses' Health Study, for example, even after controlling for age, smoking, menopausal status, use of postmenopausal hormones, and parental history of myocardial infarction, the relative risk of coronary heart disease was 1.2 (95% CI, 0.97–1.44) for women with BMIs of 21–22.9 kg/m^2, 1.46 (95% CI 1.20–1.77) for BMIs of 23–24.9 kg/m^2, 2.06 (95% CI, 1.72–2.48) for BMIs of 25–28.9 kg/m^2, and 3.56 (95% CI, 2.96–4.29) for BMIs of 29 kg/m^2 or more, compared with women whose BMIs were <21 kg/m^2 (33). Weight gain after age 18 was also associated in a dose-dependent fashion with increased risk of coronary heart disease. When women who had lost or gained less than 5 kg were used as the referent, the risk of coronary heart disease was 1.65 (95% CI, 1.33–2.05) among those who gained 8–10.9 kg, 1.92 (95% CI, 1.61–2.29) among those who gained 11–19 kg, and 2.65 (95% CI, 2.17–3.22) among those who gained ≥ 20 kg (33). A 26-year follow-up of more than 5000 men and women in the Framingham Heart Study showed that relative weight at baseline was positively associated with coronary heart disease, coronary mortality, and congestive heart failure independent of age, cholesterol level, systolic blood pressure, smoking, and other cardiovascular risk factors (34). As in the Nurses' Health Study, weight gain after young adulthood was associated with increased risk of cardiovascular disease in both men and women.

In addition to the amount of fat, the pattern of fat deposition may also influence cardiovascular health. Adipose tissue in the waist, abdomen, and upper body is more metabolically active than that in the hip, thigh, or buttocks (35), and abdominal fat accumulation appears to be an important predictor of dyslipidemia, hypertension, and coronary heart disease, as well as of type 2 diabetes. The increased sensitivity of abdominal fat cells to lipolytic stimuli and the subsequent direct delivery of fatty acids and glycerol to the liver, thus inducing insulin resistance, are possible pathophysiologic explanations for these observed associations. Abdominal adiposity can be estimated using waist circumference or waist-to-hip ratio. A waist-to-hip ratio >0.80 in women or >0.95 in men is predictive of a substantially increased risk of cardiovascular disease (36,37). Similarly, a waist circumference of ≥35 inches in women or ≥40 inches in men is associated with increased vascular risk.

B Stroke

The clear weight-related increases in blood pressure, lipids, and blood glucose described above should be expected to translate into an increased risk of stroke. However, data regarding this association are less consistent than they are for coronary heart disease. Among male health professionals, abdominal adiposity but not BMI was related to stroke risk (38), while among female nurses, BMI and weight gain were strongly associated with increased risk of total and ischemic stroke, but not hemorrhagic stroke (39). Among Japanese men, subscapular skinfold thickness but not BMI or abdominal adiposity was related to stroke risk (40). And a recent report from the Physicians' Health Study found that increasing BMI increased the risks of total, ischemic, and hemorrhagic stroke (41). To date, there are no data from prospective studies regarding reduction in stroke risk with weight loss.

C Venous Thromboembolism

Studies of the risk factors for venous thromboembolism, which have largely been conducted among populations of hospitalized patients, have generally demonstrated an association between excess weight and deep-vein thrombosis or pulmonary embolism (42). Two prospective studies support this association. Among female nurses, the relative risk of developing primary pulmonary embolism over 14 years of follow-up was 2.9 (95% CI, 1-5–5.4) among those with BMIs of 29 kg/m^2 or greater compared with those whose BMIs were <21 kg/m^2 (43). In the Swedish study of men born in 1913, among participants in the highest decile of waist circumference (≥100 cm) the adjusted relative risk of experiencing a deep-vein thrombosis or pulmonary embolism over 26 years of follow-up was 3.92 (95% CI, 2.10–7.29) compared with men with a waist circumference <100 cm (44).

IV TYPE 2 DIABETES MELLITUS

Excess weight plays a critically important role in the etiology of type 2 diabetes mellitus (see Chap. 39). Obesity, especially central obesity, causes insulin resistance and compensatory hyperinsulinemia, which are involved in the development of type 2 diabetes (45). Data from NHANES III show a direct association between BMI and prevalence of type 2 diabetes among adults (Fig. 3) (2).

Associations between BMI and risk of type 2 diabetes have been observed in diverse populations, including female nurses (46), male health professionals (47), Mexican-Americans (48), Pima Indians (49), and Japanese railway employees (50). In the Health Professionals Follow-up Study, which included more than 50,000 middle-aged men, the relative risk of developing type 2 diabetes over 5 years of follow-up was 42 times higher in men with BMIs of 35 kg/m^2 or higher than among those with BMIs <23 kg/m^2 (47); when men with BMIs <25.0 kg/m^2 were used as the referent, the relative risk was 3.5 (95% CI, 2.9–4.1) for those with BMIs of 25.0–29.9 kg/m^2, 11.2 (95% CI, 9.3–13.6) for those with BMIs of 30.0–34.9 kg/m^2, and 23.4 (95% CI, 19.4–33.2) for those with BMIs of 35.0 kg/m^2 or greater (51). In the Nurses' Health Study, the relative risk of developing type 2 diabetes over 10 years of follow-up was 4.6-fold higher among women with BMIs of 25.0–29.9 kg/m^2 than among those with BMIs <25.0 kg/m^2, 10-fold higher among those with BMIs of 30.0–34.9 kg/m^2, and 17-fold higher among those with BMIs of 35.0 kg/m^2 or greater (51). In both of these studies, weight gain during adulthood was strongly associated with increases in risk of developing type 2 diabetes.

Given the widespread prevalence of diabetes—more than 15 million cases in the United States and 154 million cases worldwide (52)—even small reductions

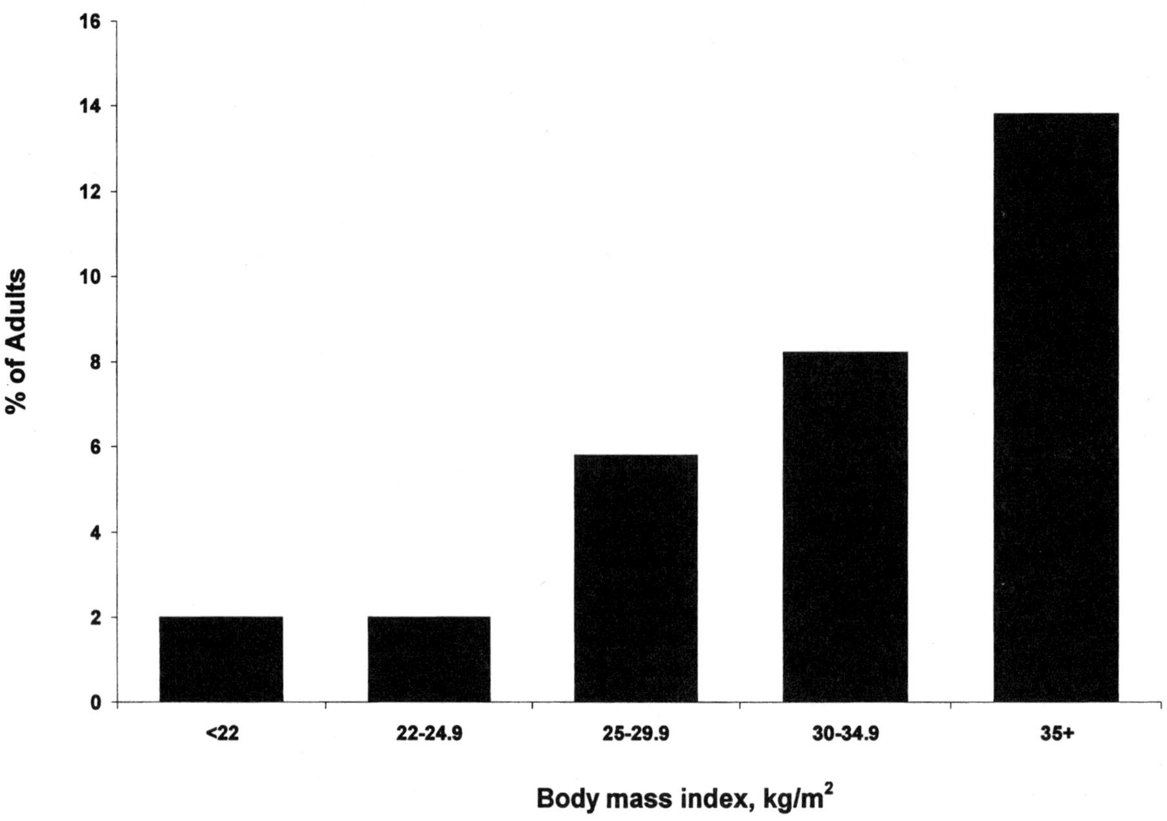

Figure 3 Prevalence of type 2 diabetes in the Third National Health and Nutrition Examination Survey by BMI categories. (From Ref. 2.)

in risk could have important effects on the global burden of this disease. Several recent studies suggest that weight loss, either alone or combined with physical activity, improves glucose levels and insulin action among individuals with type 2 diabetes (53) and lowers the risk of diabetes among overweight individuals (54). In the randomized Finnish Diabetes Prevention Study, conducted among 522 middle-aged, overweight men and women with impaired glucose tolerance, the risk of developing diabetes over 3.2 years of follow-up decreased 58% among those assigned to intervention (weight loss, improved nutrition, and increased physical activity) compared to the control group assigned to usual care (55). Bariatric surgery also appears to provide long-term control of type 2 diabetes among morbidly obese patients (56). A randomized trial funded by the National Institute of Diabetes and Digestive and Kidney Diseases, the Look AHEAD (Action for Health in Diabetes) trial, is under way to examine the effects of a lifestyle intervention designed to achieve and maintain weight loss over the long term through decreased caloric intake and increased exercise among 5000 obese individuals with type 2 diabetes (57). Results from this trial should also offer important insights into the potential beneficial effects of weight loss on risk of cardiovascular disease and other chronic conditions.

V CANCER

Ever since the landmark American Cancer Society cohort study of 750,000 U.S. adults found a highly significant age- and smoking-adjusted 33% increased risk of cancer death among obese men and a 55% increase among obese women (58), hundreds of other studies have examined the association between weight and cancer in greater detail. Most, but not all, of these studies suggest that excess weight is associated with increased risks of endometrial (59), postmenopausal breast (59), kidney (60), gallbladder (61), and colon (62) cancers. A recent meta-analysis of overweight and cancer in Europe suggests that excess weight accounts for 3.4% of cancers in men and 6.4% in women, or a total of

72,000 cases of cancer in Europe (63). By cancer site, the population attributable risk for excess weight was 39% for endometrial cancers, 25% for kidney cancers, 24% for gallbladder cancers, and 11% for colon cancers.

VI LIVER AND GALLBLADDER DISEASE

Obesity is commonly associated with morphological and functional changes in the liver. In one autopsy study, nonalcoholic steatohepatitis, a pathological condition characterized by fatty infiltration, inflammation, and fibrosis, was observed in 18.5% of markedly obese patients and 2.7% of lean patients; severe fibrosis was found in 13.8% of markedly obese patients and 6.6% of lean patients (64). Other series suggest that 70% or more of patients with nonalcoholic steatohepatitis are overweight (65). Although nonalcoholic steatohepatitis is generally a benign disease, patients with this condition occasionally develop cirrhosis, portal hypertension, and hepatic failure.

The risk of developing gallstones also increases with increasing weight, with a four-to-fivefold higher prevalence among those with BMIs of 40 kg/m^2 or higher compared with individuals with BMIs between 18.0 and 24.9 kg/m^2 (5). Among female nurses, the adjusted relative risk of cholecystectomy or new-onset gallstones was 6.0 (95% CI, 4.0–9.0) for obese women with BMIs of 32 kg/m^2 or greater and 1.7 (95% CI, 1.1–2.7) for women with BMIs of 24.0–24.9 kg/m^2, compared with women whose BMIs were <20 kg/m^2 (66). When women with BMIs of <25.0 kg/m^2 were used as the referent, the relative risks were 1.9 (95% CI, 1.7–2.0) for women with BMIs of 25.0–29.9 kg/m^2, 2.5 (95% CI, 2.3–2.7) for those with BMIs of 30.0–34.9 kg/m^2, and 3.0 (95% CI, 2.7–3.3) for those with BMIs of 35.0 kg/m^2 or greater (51). An analysis from the same cohort suggested that weight cycling was also highly associated with risk of cholecystectomy, independent of BMI (67).

VII OSTEOARTHRITIS

Arthritis is one of the leading causes of disability among U.S. adults over age 15 (68). Osteoarthritis of the knee, hip, and hand account for much of this disability among older individuals. Data from NHANES III indicate that the prevalence of osteoarthritis among women increases with increasing body weight, from 52/1000 women with BMIs between 18.0 and 24.9 kg/m^2 to 172/1000 for those with BMIs >40 kg/m^2 (Fig. 4) (5). Data for men show a similar trend. This association is most likely due predominantly to mechanical stresses on weight-bearing joints (see Chap. 42).

In the Framingham Osteoarthritis Study, among 1420 participants who had radiographs of the knee taken during a routine biennial follow-up, 468 had evidence of osteoarthritis. The relative risk of osteoarthritis was twofold higher among obese women and 1.5-fold higher among obese men than among lighter individuals (69). A similar increased risk of osteoarthritis of the knee has been observed in other cohort (70–73), twin (74), and national survey (75,76) studies. The association between obesity and osteoarthritis of the hip is less strong, with some studies showing a positive association (77–79) and others showing no association (70,73).

A recent pilot trial of exercise and weight loss among 24 elderly obese men and women showed significant improvements in pain, performance, and disability (80). Weight loss alone, achieved through diet (81), pharmacotherapy (82), or surgery (83), has also been associated with reductions in osteoarthritis-related symptoms.

VIII SLEEP APNEA

Excessive fat in the pharyngeal area, chest wall, and abdomen can profoundly alter pulmonary function via adverse effects on respiratory mechanics; respiratory muscle function, lung volume, and upper-airway narrowing (see Chap. 41).

Sleep apnea, defined as a cessation of air flow for 10 sec or longer during sleep, is a common consequence of obesity, particularly among men. More than half of men and one-third of women in the Swedish Obese Subjects Study reported snoring and apnea (84), compared with 4% of men and 2% of women in general populations (85). In the Wisconsin Sleep Cohort Study, increasing weight was a significant risk factor for sleep apnea, with a 10% increase in weight associated with a sixfold increase in the risk of developing moderate to severe sleep-disordered breathing (86).

Many patients with sleep apnea have excessive daytime sleepiness. In addition, recent epidemiologic studies have demonstrated that sleep apnea is a risk factor for hypertension (87) and may lead to the development of cardiovascular disease. In the Sleep Heart Health Study, for example, sleep-disordered breathing was significantly associated with increased risks of heart failure, stroke, and coronary heart disease (88). Weight loss significantly alleviates sleep apnea and improves nighttime breathing (86,89).

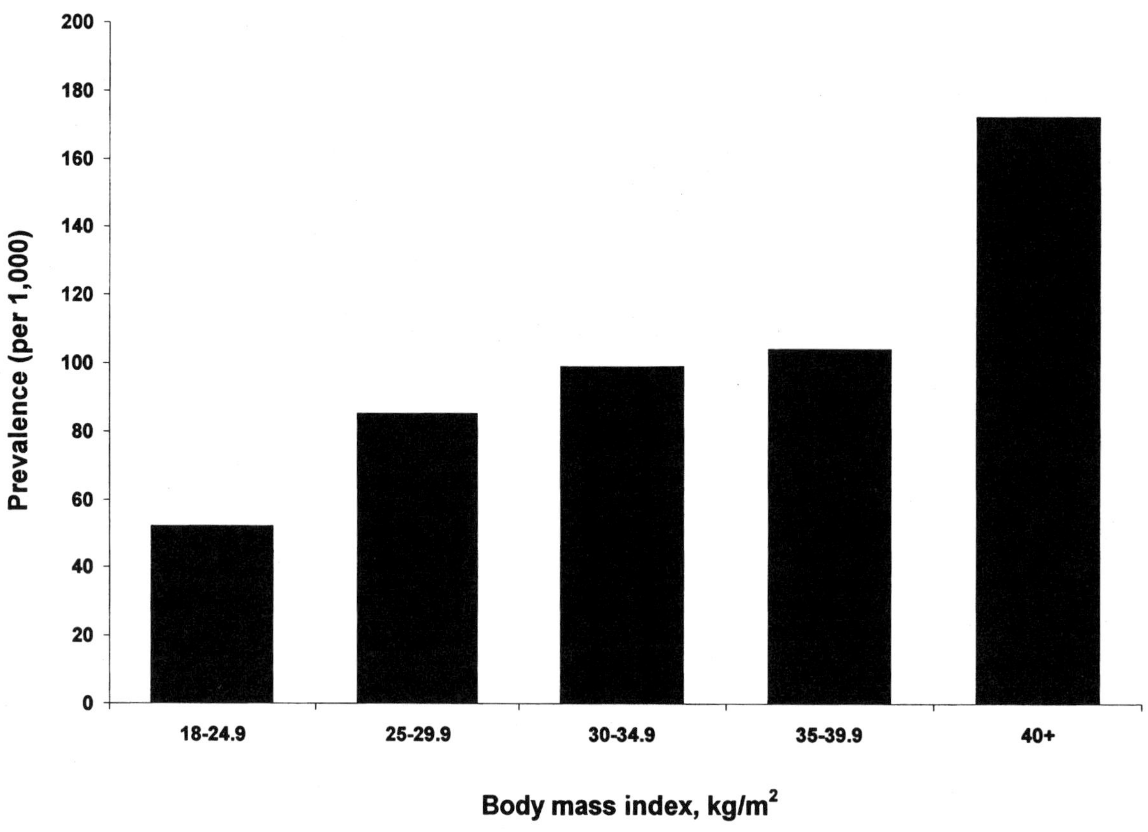

Figure 4 Prevalence of osteoarthritis among women in the Third National Health and Nutrition Examination Survey by BMI categories. (From Ref. 5.)

IX REPRODUCTIVE HEALTH

Obesity during pregnancy is related to increased morbidity for both mother and child (see Chap. 43). Maternal obesity is associated with a 10-fold increased risk of hypertension and a threefold increased risk of gestational diabetes (90,91), and is also strongly associated with the risk of pre-eclampsia (92,93). Women who are overweight or obese are also more likely to have other complications of pregnancy than women in the healthy weight range. In an analysis of more than 96,000 births in Washington state, for example, overweight and obese women were significantly more likely to have preterm deliveries, to deliver babies heavier than 4000 g, or to require caesarean section, and infants born to obese women had a twofold increased risk of death within the first year of life (94). Obesity also increases the risks associated with anesthesia, possibly due to the technical difficulties in administration (95). Excess weight may also interfere with the ability to become pregnant. Among female nurses, BMI at age 18 was strongly associated with subsequent risk of ovulatory infertility in women with and without a diagnosis of polycystic ovary syndrome, ranging from a relative risk of 1.3 among women with BMIs of 24–25.9 kg/m^2 to 2.7 among women with BMIs of 32 kg/m^2 or greater, compared with those with BMIs of 20–21.9 kg/m^2 (96).

Obesity-related risks may be borne by the developing fetus as well, with studies suggesting associations between maternal obesity and increased risk of neural tube defects (97) and other congenital malformations (98).

X QUALITY OF LIFE

Another measure of the cumulative burden of weight-related disorders is quality of life. In analyses from the Nurses' Health Study, both higher BMI and substantial weight gain during adulthood were strongly associated with reduced daily physical functioning and vitality, a greater burden of physical pain, and diminished feelings of well-being. The average decline in physical function experienced by a woman under age 65 years who gained 9 kg or more over a 4-year period was approximately three times the magnitude of that associated with cigarette smoking over the same period (99,100). In NHANES III, the proportion of participants reporting excellent health decreased in a linear fashion with increasing BMI among whites, blacks, and Hispanics, even in the absence of chronic disease conditions (101).

XI CONCLUSION

In the United States and other developed countries, the prevalence of many cardiovascular risk factors is declining. Smoking rates, average cholesterol levels, and the prevalence of hypertension in the United States have fallen significantly since the 1960s (102). At the same time, however, the prevalence of overweight and obesity continues to rise and is reaching epidemic proportions in both developed and developing countries. Given the strong associations between obesity and cardiovascular disease, type 2 diabetes, and other chronic diseases, this trend portends an enormous global burden of obesity-related morbidity and mortality in the century ahead.

Public health approaches such as those used to educate the public about the dangers of smoking, high cholesterol, and high blood pressure must be adapted for the prevention and control of overweight and obesity. In addition, health professionals must play a more active role in counseling overweight and obese patients about the health hazards of excess weight and in prescribing and encouraging sustained changes in behavior that can lead to a healthier weight. Guidelines developed by the National Heart, Lung and Blood Institute in conjunction with the North American Association for the Study of Obesity offer concrete advice for clinicians regarding the evaluation and treatment of obesity (1). Given the prevalence of overweight, helping even a small percentage of overweight or obese patients achieve a healthy weight would have a substantial impact on public health, as would helping those already in the healthy weight range maintain their weight.

REFERENCES

1. National Institutes of Health; National Heart, Lung and Blood Institute; Obesity Education Initiative. Clinical guidelines on the identification, evaluation, and treatment of overweight and obesity in adults. <http://www.nhlbi.nih.gov/guidelines/obesity/ob_gdlns.htm> Accessed on 24 July 2001.
2. National Task Force on the Prevention and Treatment of Obesity. Overweight, obesity, and health risk. Arch Intern Med 2000; 160:898–904.
3. Thompson D, Edelsberg J, Colditz GA, Bird AP, Oster G. Lifetime health and economic consequences of obesity. Arch Intern Med 1999; 159:2177–2183.
4. Oster G, Thompson D, Edelsberg J, Bird AP, Colditz GA. Lifetime health and economic benefits of weight loss among obese persons. Am J Public Health 1999; 89:1536–1542.
5. Must A, Spadano J, Coakley EH, Field AE, Colditz G, Dietz WH. The disease burden associated with overweight and obesity. JAMA 1999; 282:1523–1529.
6. Sturm R, Wells KB. Does obesity contribute as much to morbidity as poverty or smoking? Public Health 2001; 115:229–235.
7. Allison DB, Fontaine KR, Manson JE, Stevens J, Van Itallie TB. Annual deaths attributable to obesity in the United States. JAMA 1999; 282:1530–1538.
8. Stevens J, Cai J, Pamuk ER, Williamson DF, Thun MJ, Wood JL. The effect of age on the association between body-mass index and mortality. N Engl J Med 1998; 338:1–7.
9. Calle EE, Thun MJ, Petrelli JM, Rodriguez C, Heath CW Jr. Body-mass index and mortality in a prospective cohort of U.S. adults. N Engl J Med 1999; 341:1097–1105.
10. Lee IM, Manson JE, Hennekens CH, Paffenbarger RS Jr. Body weight and mortality. A 27-year follow-up of middle-aged men. JAMA 1993; 270:2823–2828.
11. Manson JE, Willett WC, Stampfer MJ, Colditz GA, Hunter DJ, Hankinson SE, Hennekens CH, Speizer FE. Body weight and mortality among women. N Engl J Med 1995; 333:677–685.
12. Singh PN, Lindsted KD, Fraser GE. Body weight and mortality among adults who never smoked. Am J Epidemiol 1999; 150:1152–1164.
13. Willett WC, Dietz WH, Colditz GA. Guidelines for healthy weight. N Engl J Med 1999; 341:427–434.
14. Garrison RJ, Kannel WB. A new approach for estimating healthy body weights. Int J Obes Relat Metab Disord 1993; 17:417–423.
15. Lindsted K, Tonstad S, Kuzma JW. Body mass index and patterns of mortality among Seventh-Day Adventist men. Int J Obes 1991; 15:397–406.
16. Eckel RH, Krauss RM. American Heart Association call to action: obesity as a major risk factor for coronary heart disease. AHA Nutrition Committee. Circulation 1998; 97:2099–2100.
17. Ashton WD, Nanchahal K, Wood DA. Body mass index and metabolic risk factors for coronary heart disease in women. Eur Heart J 2001; 22:46–55.
18. Ford ES, Galuska DA, Gillespie C, Will JC, Giles WH, Dietz WH. C-reactive protein and body mass index in children: findings from the Third National Health and Nutrition Examination Survey, 1988–1994. J Pediatr 2001; 138:486–492.

19. Duncan BB, Schmidt MI, Chambless LE, Folsom AR, Carpenter M, Heiss G. Fibrinogen, other putative markers of inflammation, and weight gain in middle-aged adults—the ARIC study. Atherosclerosis Risk in Communities. Obes Res 2000; 8:279–286.
20. Visser M, Bouter LM, McQuillan GM, Wener MH, Harris TB. Elevated C-reactive protein levels in overweight and obese adults. JAMA 1999; 282:2131–2135.
21. Stefanick ML. Exercise and weight loss. In: Hennekens CH, ed. Clinical Trials in Cardiovascular Disease: A Companion Guide to Braunwald's Heart Disease. Philadelphia: W.B. Saunders, 1999:375–391.
22. Larsson B, Svardsudd K, Welin L, Wilhelmsen L, Bjorntorp P, Tibblin G. Abdominal adipose tissue distribution, obesity, and risk of cardiovascular disease and death: 13 year follow up of participants in the study of men born in 1913. Br Med J (Clin Res Ed) 1984; 288:1401–1404.
23. Tuomilehto J, Salonen JT, Marti B, Jalkanen L, Puska P, Nissinen A, Wolf E. Body weight and risk of myocardial infarction and death in the adult population of eastern Finland. Br Med J (Clin Res Ed) 1987; 295:623–627.
24. Fitzgerald AP, Jarrett RJ. Body weight and coronary heart disease mortality: an analysis in relation to age and smoking habit. 15 years follow-up data from the Whitehall Study. Int J Obes Relat Metab Disord 1992; 16:119–123.
25. Must A, Jacques PF, Dallal GE, Bajema CJ, Dietz WH. Long-term morbidity and mortality of overweight adolescents. A follow-up of the Harvard Growth Study of 1922 to 1935. N Engl J Med 1992; 327:1350–1355.
26. Harris TB, Launer LJ, Madans J, Feldman JJ. Cohort study of effect of being overweight and change in weight on risk of coronary heart disease in old age. BMJ 1997; 314:1791–1794.
27. Huang B, Rodreiguez BL, Burchfiel CM, Chyou PH, Curb JD, Sharp DS. Association of adiposity with prevalent coronary heart disease among elderly men: the Honolulu Heart Program. Int J Obes Relat Metab Disord 1997; 21:340–348.
28. Lamarche B, Lemieux S, Dagenais GR, Despres JP. Visceral obesity and the risk of ischaemic heart disease: insights from the Quebec Cardiovascular Study. Growth Horm IGF Res 1998; 8(suppl B):1–8.
29. Folsom AR, Stevens J, Schreiner PJ, McGovern PG. Body mass index, waist/hip ratio, and coronary heart disease incidence in African Americans and whites. Atherosclerosis Risk in Communities study investigators. Am J Epidemiol 1998; 148:1187–1194.
30. Rosengren A, Wedel H, Wilhelmsen L. Body weight and weight gain during adult life in men in relation to coronary heart disease and mortality. A prospective population study. Eur Heart J 1999; 20:269–277.
31. Gray RS, Fabsitz RR, Cowan LD, Lee ET, Welty TK, Jablonski KA, Howard BV. Relation of generalized and central obesity to cardiovascular risk factors and prevalent coronary heart disease in a sample of American Indians: the Strong Heart Study. Int J Obes Relat Metab Disord 2000; 24:849–860.
32. Folsom AR, Kushi LH, Anderson KE, Mink PJ, Olson JE, Hong CP, Sellers TA, Lazovich D, Prineas RJ. Associations of general and abdominal obesity with multiple health outcomes in older women: the Iowa Women's Health Study. Arch Intern Med 2000; 160:2117–2128.
33. Willett WC, Manson JE, Stampfer MJ, Colditz GA, Rosner B, Speizer FE, Hennekens CH. Weight, weight change, and coronary heart disease in women. Risk within the 'normal' weight range. JAMA 1995; 273:461–465.
34. Hubert HB, Feinleib M, McNamara PM, Castelli WP. Obesity as an independent risk factor for cardiovascular disease: a 26-year follow-up of participants in the Framingham Heart Study. Circulation 1983; 67:968–977.
35. Carey DG. Abdominal obesity. Curr Opin Lipidol 1998; 9:35–40.
36. Rexrode KM, Carey VJ, Hennekens CH, Walters EE, Colditz GA, Stampfer MJ, Willett WC, Manson JE. Abdominal adiposity and coronary heart disease in women. JAMA 1998; 280:1843–1848.
37. Rexrode KM, Buring JE, Manson JE. Abdominal and total adiposity and risk of coronary heart disease in men. Int J Obes Relat Metab Disord 2001; 25:1047–1056.
38. Walker SP, Rimm EB, Ascherio A, Kawachi I, Stampfer MJ, Willett WC. Body size and fat distribution as predictors of stroke among US men. Am J Epidemiol 1996; 144:1143–1150.
39. Rexrode KM, Hennekens CH, Willett WC, Colditz GA, Stampfer MJ, Rich-Edwards JW, Speizer FE, Manson JE. A prospective study of body mass index, weight change, and risk of stroke in women. JAMA 1997; 277:1539–1545.
40. Curb JD, Marcus EB. Body fat, coronary heart disease, and stroke in Japanese men. Am J Clin Nutr 1991; 53:1612S–1615S.
41. Kurth T, Gaziano JM, Berger K, Kase CS, Manson JE. Body mass index and the risk of stroke in men. Neurology 2001; 56(8):A227.
42. Kearon C, Salzman EW, Hirsh J. Epidemiology, pathogenesis, and natural history of venous thrombosis. In: Colman RW, Hirsh J, Marder VJ, Clowes AW, George JN, eds. Hemostasis and Thrombosis: Basic Principles and Clinical Practice. 4th ed. Philadelphia: Lippincott Williams & Wilkins, 2001:1153–1177.
43. Goldhaber SZ, Grodstein F, Stampfer MJ, Manson JE, Colditz GA, Speizer FE, Willett WC, Hennekens CH. A prospective study of risk factors for pulmonary embolism in women. JAMA 1997; 277:642–645.
44. Hansson PO, Eriksson H, Welin L, Svardsudd K, Wilhelmsen L. Smoking and abdominal obesity: risk factors for venous thromboembolism among middle-aged

men: "the study of men born in 1913." Arch Intern Med 1999; 159:1886–1890.
45. Fujimoto WY. The importance of insulin resistance in the pathogenesis of type 2 diabetes mellitus. Am J Med 2000; 108(suppl 6a):9S–14S.
46. Colditz GA, Willett WC, Stampfer MJ, Manson JE, Hennekens CH, Arky RA, Speizer FE. Weight as a risk factor for clinical diabetes in women. Am J Epidemiol 1990; 132:501–513.
47. Chan JM, Rimm EB, Colditz GA, Stampfer MJ, Willett WC. Obesity, fat distribution, and weight gain as risk factors for clinical diabetes in men. Diabetes Care 1994; 17:961–969.
48. Wei M, Gaskill SP, Haffner SM, Stern MP. Waist circumference as the best predictor of noninsulin dependent diabetes mellitus (NIDDM) compared to body mass index, waist/hip ratio and other anthropometric measurements in Mexican Americans—a 7-year prospective study. Obes Res 1997; 5:16–23.
49. Knowler WC, Pettitt DJ, Saad MF, Charles MA, Nelson RG, Howard BV, Bogardus C, Bennett PH. Obesity in the Pima Indians: its magnitude and relationship with diabetes. Am J Clin Nutr 1991; 53:1543S–1551S.
50. Sakurai Y, Teruya K, Shimada N, Umeda T, Tanaka H, Muto T, Kondo T, Nakamura K, Yoshizawa N. Association between duration of obesity and risk of non-insulin-dependent diabetes mellitus. The Sotetsu Study. Am J Epidemiol 1999; 149:256–260.
51. Field AE, Coakley EH, Must A, Spadano JL, Laird N, Dietz WH, Rimm E, Colditz GA. Impact of overweight on the risk of developing common chronic diseases during a 10-year period. Arch Intern Med 2001; 161:1581–1586.
52. King H, Aubert RE, Herman WH. Global burden of diabetes, 1995–2025: prevalence, numerical estimates, and projections. Diabetes Care 1998; 21:1414–1431.
53. Williams KV, Kelley DE. Metabolic consequences of weight loss on glucose metabolism and insulin action in type 2 diabetes. Diabetes Obes Metab 2000; 2:121–129.
54. Resnick HE, Valsania P, Halter JB, Lin X. Relation of weight gain and weight loss on subsequent diabetes risk in overweight adults. J Epidemiol Community Health 2000; 54:596–602.
55. Tuomilehto J, Lindstrom J, Eriksson JG, Valle TT, Hamalainen H, Ilanne-Parikka P, Keinanen-Kiukaanniemi S, Laakso M, Louheranta A, Rastas M, Salminen V, Uusitupa M. Prevention of type 2 diabetes mellitus by changes in lifestyle among subjects with impaired glucose tolerance. N Engl J Med 2001; 344:1343–1350.
56. Pories WJ, Swanson MS, MacDonald KG, Long SB, Morris PG, Brown BM, Barakat HA, deRamon RA, Israel G, Dolezal JM. Who would have thought it? An operation proves to be the most effective therapy for adult-onset diabetes mellitus. Ann Surg 1995; 222:339–350.
57. National Institute of Diabetes and Digestive and Kidney Diseases. Look AHEAD: Action for Health in Diabetes. <http://www.niddk.nih.gov/patient/SHOW/lookahead.htm> Accessed on 24 July 2001.
58. Lew EA, Garfinkel L. Variations in mortality by weight among 750,000 men and women. J Chronic Dis 1979; 32:563–576.
59. Schindler AE. Obesity and cancer risk in women. Arch Gynecol Obstet 1997; 261:21–24.
60. Chow WH, Gridley G, Fraumeni JF Jr, Jarvholm B. Obesity, hypertension, and the risk of kidney cancer in men. N Engl J Med 2000; 343:1305–1311.
61. Lowenfels AB, Maisonneuve P, Boyle P, Zatonski WA. Epidemiology of gallbladder cancer. Hepatogastroenterology 1999; 46:1529–1532.
62. Tomeo CA, Colditz GA, Willett WC, Giovannucci E, Platz E, Rockhill B, Dart H, Hunter DJ. Harvard Report on Cancer Prevention. Volume 3: prevention of colon cancer in the United States. Cancer Causes Control 1999; 10:167–180.
63. Bergstrom A, Pisani P, Tenet V, Wolk A, Adami HO. Overweight as an avoidable cause of cancer in Europe. Int J Cancer 2001; 91:421–430.
64. Wanless IR, Lentz JS. Fatty liver hepatitis (steatohepatitis) and obesity: an autopsy study with analysis of risk factors. Hepatology 1990; 12:1106–1110.
65. Sheth SG, Gordon FD, Chopra S. Nonalcoholic steatohepatitis. Ann Intern Med 1997; 126:137–145.
66. Maclure KM, Hayes KC, Colditz GA, Stampfer MJ, Speizer FE, Willett WC. Weight, diet, and the risk of symptomatic gallstones in middle-aged women. N Engl J Med 1989; 321:563–569.
67. Syngal S, Coakley EH, Willett WC, Byers T, Williamson DF, Colditz GA. Long-term weight patterns and risk for cholecystectomy in women. Ann Intern Med 1999; 130:471–477.
68. Prevalence of disabilities and associated health conditions among adults—United States, 1999. MMWR 2001; 50:120–125.
69. Felson DT, Anderson JJ, Naimark A, Walker AM, Meenan RF. Obesity and knee osteoarthritis. The Framingham Study. Ann Intern Med 1988; 109:18–24.
70. Hart DJ, Spector TD. The relationship of obesity, fat distribution and osteoarthritis in women in the general population: the Chingford Study. J Rheumatol 1993; 20:331–335.
71. Hochberg MC, Lethbridge-Cejku M, Scott WW Jr, Reichle R, Plato CC, Tobin JD. The association of body weight, body fatness and body fat distribution with osteoarthritis of the knee: data from the Baltimore Longitudinal Study of Aging. J Rheumatol 1995; 22:488–493.
72. Sandmark H, Hogstedt C, Lewold S, Vingard E. Osteoarthrosis of the knee in men and women in association with overweight, smoking, and hormone therapy. Ann Rheum Dis 1999; 58:151–155.
73. Sturmer T, Gunther KP, Brenner H. Obesity, over-

weight and patterns of osteoarthritis: the Ulm Osteoarthritis Study. J Clin Epidemiol 2000; 53:307–313.
74. Cicuttini FM, Baker JR, Spector TD. The association of obesity with osteoarthritis of the hand and knee in women: a twin study. J Rheumatol 1996; 23:1221–1226.
75. Sahyoun NR, Hochberg MC, Helmick CG, Harris T, Pamuk ER. Body mass index, weight change, and incidence of self-reported physician-diagnosed arthritis among women. Am J Public Health 1999; 89:391–394.
76. Heliovaara M, Makela M, Impivaara O, Knekt P, Aromaa A, Sievers K. Association of overweight, trauma and workload with coxarthrosis. A health survey of 7,217 persons. Acta Orthop Scand 1993; 64:513–518.
77. Tepper S, Hochberg MC. Factors associated with hip osteoarthritis: data from the First National Health and Nutrition Examination Survey (NHANES-I). Am J Epidemiol 1993; 137:1081–1088.
78. Cooper C, Inskip H, Croft P, Campbell L, Smith G, McLaren M, Coggon D. Individual risk factors for hip osteoarthritis: obesity, hip injury, and physical activity. Am J Epidemiol 1998; 147:516–522.
79. Oliveria SA, Felson DT, Cirillo PA, Reed JI, Walker AM. Body weight, body mass index, and incident symptomatic osteoarthritis of the hand, hip, and knee. Epidemiology 1999; 10:161–166.
80. Messier SP, Loeser RF, Mitchell MN, Valle G, Morgan TP, Rejeski WJ, Ettinger WH. Exercise and weight loss in obese older adults with knee osteoarthritis: a preliminary study. J Am Geriatr Soc 2000; 48:1062–1072.
81. Felson DT, Zhang Y, Anthony JM, Naimark A, Anderson JJ. Weight loss reduces the risk for symptomatic knee osteoarthritis in women. The Framingham Study. Ann Intern Med 1992; 116:535–539.
82. Williams RA, Foulsham BM. Weight reduction in osteoarthritis using phentermine. Practitioner 1981; 225: 231–232.
83. McGoey BV, Deitel M, Saplys RJ, Kliman ME. Effect of weight loss on musculoskeletal pain in the morbidly obese. J Bone Joint Surg Br 1990; 72:322–323.
84. Grunstein R. Obstructive sleep apnoea as a risk factor for hypertension. J Sleep Res 1995; 4:166–170.
85. Strollo PJ Jr, Rogers RM. Obstructive sleep apnea. N Engl J Med 1996; 334:99–104.
86. Peppard PE, Young T, Palta M, Dempsey J, Skatrud J. Longitudinal study of moderate weight change and sleep-disordered breathing. JAMA 2000; 284:3015–3021.
87. Roux F, D'Ambrosio C, Mohsenin V. Sleep-related breathing disorders and cardiovascular disease. Am J Med 2000; 108:396–402.
88. Shahar E, Whitney CW, Redline S, Lee ET, Newman AB, Javier Nieto F, O'Connor GT, Boland LL, Schwartz JE, Samet JM. Sleep-disordered breathing and cardiovascular disease: cross-sectional results of the Sleep Heart Health Study. Am J Respir Crit Care Med 2001; 163:19–25.
89. Karason K, Lindroos AK, Stenlof K, Sjostrom L. Relief of cardiorespiratory symptoms and increased physical activity after surgically induced weight loss: results from the Swedish Obese Subjects study. Arch Intern Med 2000; 160:1797–1802.
90. Kumari AS. Pregnancy outcome in women with morbid obesity. Int J Gynaecol Obstet 2001; 73:101–107.
91. Michlin R, Oettinger M, Odeh M, Khoury S, Ophir E, Barak M, Wolfson M, Strulov A. Maternal obesity and pregnancy outcome. Isr Med Assoc J 2000; 2:10–13.
92. Eskenazi B, Fenster L, Sidney S. A multivariate analysis of risk factors for preeclampsia. JAMA 1991; 266: 237–241.
93. Sibai BM, Gordon T, Thom E, Caritis SN, Klebanoff M, McNellis D, Paul RH. Risk factors for preeclampsia in healthy nulliparous women: a prospective multicenter study. The National Institute of Child Health and Human Development Network of Maternal-Fetal Medicine Units. Am J Obstet Gynecol 1995; 172:642–648.
94. Baeten JM, Bukusi EA, Lambe M. Pregnancy complications and outcomes among overweight and obese nulliparous women. Am J Public Health 2001; 91:436–440.
95. Rocke DA, Murray WB, Rout CC, Gouws E. Relative risk analysis of factors associated with difficult intubation in obstetric anesthesia. Anesthesiology 1992; 77:67–73.
96. Rich-Edwards JW, Goldman MB, Willett WC, Hunter DJ, Stampfer MJ, Colditz GA, Manson JE. Adolescent body mass index and infertility caused by ovulatory disorder. Am J Obstet Gynecol 1994; 171:171–177.
97. Shaw GM, Velie EM, Schaffer D. Risk of neural tube defect-affected pregnancies among obese women. JAMA 1996; 275:1093–1096.
98. Moore LL, Singer MR, Bradlee ML, Rothman KJ, Milunsky A. A prospective study of the risk of congenital defects associated with maternal obesity and diabetes mellitus. Epidemiology 2000; 11:689–694.
99. Fine JT, Colditz GA, Coakley EH, Moseley G, Manson JE, Willett WC, Kawachi I. A prospective study of weight change and health-related quality of life in women. JAMA 1999; 282:2136–2142.
100. Coakley EH, Kawachi I, Manson JE, Speizer FE, Willet WC, Colditz GA. Lower levels of physical functioning are associated with higher body weight among middle-aged and older women. Int J Obes Relat Metab Disord 1998; 22:958–965.
101. Okosun IS, Choi S, Matamoros T, Dever GE. Obesity is associated with reduced self-rated general health status: evidence from a representative sample of white, black, and Hispanic Americans. Prev Med 2001; 32:429–436.
102. MacKay AP, Fingerhut LA, Duran CR. Health, United States, 2000. Hyattsville, MD: National Center for Health Statistics, 2000. DHHS Pub No. 2000-1232.

34

Effects of Obesity on the Cardiovascular System

Edward Saltzman

Jean Mayer USDA Human Nutrition Research Center on Aging at Tufts University and Tufts–New England Medical Center, Boston, Massachusetts, U.S.A.

Peter N. Benotti

Valley Hospital, Ridgewood, New Jersey, U.S.A.

I INTRODUCTION

Cardiovascular disease is the leading cause of death in industrialized countries, and in the United States, cardiovascular disease accounts for ~50% of all deaths (1). Obesity increases risk for coronary heart disease (CHD), congestive heart failure (CHF), arrhythmia, sudden death, and several other cardiovascular diseases (Table 1). Obesity promotes several traditional risk factors for cardiovascular disease, and in addition considerable attention has been devoted to defining the pathogenic role of excess weight that is independent of traditional risk factors. Obesity has recently been found to be associated with several nontraditional risk factors, such as disturbances in fibrinolysis, impaired endothelial function, and chronic low-grade inflammation. Regardless of the mechanism, it is clear that obesity is associated with deleterious effects on the heart and circulatory system.

In the sections below, the increased demands imposed by obesity on the heart and circulation and the resultant cardiovascular adaptation are reviewed. This is followed by discussion of the contribution of obesity to pathologic conditions such as CHF, arrhythmia, CHD, and other cardiovascular syndromes. The beneficial effects of weight loss on specific conditions and overall cardiovascular mortality is also discussed where evidence exists. Finally, the association between weight loss medications and cardiac valve disease, as well as cardiovascular effects of other appetite suppressants, is presented.

II EFFECTS OF OBESITY ON CARDIAC STRUCTURE AND FUNCTION

Obesity is characterized by expansion of fat mass, as well as expansion of skeletal muscle, viscera, and skin, all of which increase oxygen consumption (2,3). Although metabolically active, adipose tissue oxygen consumption is lower than for lean tissue, hence total body oxygen consumption expressed per kilogram of body weight in the obese is lower than in leaner persons (3–5). Obesity is also accompanied by expansion of extracellular volume, which comprises the intravascular and interstitial fluid spaces. Total blood volume and plasma volume generally increase in proportion to the degree of overweight (4,6–8). For example, in comparison to lean control groups (BMI 22 kg/m^2), nonhypertensive obese subjects (BMI ~36 kg/m^2) had 20–25% expansion of total blood volume, while the ratio of central to total blood volumes was comparatively unchanged (7,8). Expansion of blood volume leads to increased left ventricular filling, which in turn results in

Table 1 Cardiovascular Diseases Associated with Obesity

Coronary heart disease
Stroke
Hypertension
Left ventricular hypertrophy
Congestive heart failure
Sudden death
Arrhythmia
Deep-vein thrombosis
Pulmonary embolus
Venous insufficiency

increased stroke volume (6,9–11). The increase in cardiac output is generally in proportion to excess weight, reflecting the interrelationships among weight, blood volume, stroke volume, and cardiac output (4,6,7,9,12). Heart rate, the other determinant of cardiac output, remains essentially unchanged and does not significantly contribute to increased cardiac output in obesity (4,6,7, 10,11). While cardiac output is increased in absolute terms, when normalized to body surface area, values remain in the normal range (4,7). Arteriovenous oxygen extraction, another mechanism that could increase oxygen delivery, is unchanged or only slightly increased in obesity (5,9).

Reduced systemic vascular resistance accompanies elevations in cardiac output that occur in nonhypertensive obesity (4,5,7). This reduction in peripheral resistance in part explains why hypertension is not observed in all obese individuals who have elevated intravascular volume and cardiac output. A limitation to this adaptive mechanism clearly exists, however, since hypertension is commonly associated with obesity.

The initial response to increased metabolic demand and total blood volume is increased left ventricular filling, leading to chamber dilatation and increased cardiac output. However, longer-term structural changes accompany this hemodynamic adaptation. Left ventricular dilatation increases myocardial wall stress, which, over time, stimulates left ventricular myocardial growth and leads to elevated mass. In turn, wall stress is normalized, diminishing (at least in part) the stimulus for further hypertrophy. In cross-sectional observations, ventricular mass has been increased in proportion to BMI, degree of overweight or fat mass (11,13–17). In a recent trial, left ventricular mass was associated with fat mass, but was more strongly associated with fat-free mass (18), perhaps reflecting the greater relative contribution of fat-free mass than fat mass to oxygen consumption. In addition to degree of obesity, duration of obesity also appears to be predictive of left ventricular mass (15). Left ventricular mass has been directly associated with measures of central obesity, but the strengths of these associations have varied considerably between studies (11,14,18,19). Wikstrand et al. (11) have proposed that central obesity does not have an independent effect on ventricular mass, but may promote adverse loading conditions or elevated blood pressure. Metabolic factors associated with central obesity, such as insulin resistance and hyperinsulinemia (20), have also been proposed to contribute to left ventricular hypertrophy. Right ventricular dilatation and hypertrophy also have been observed in extreme obesity (21), and the presence of obstructive sleep apnea or obesity hypoventilation syndrome appears to increase risk for right as well as left ventricular hypertrophy (22).

When left ventricular dilatation and hypertrophy occur together, the usual relationship between left ventricular cavity radius and wall thickness is preserved and eccentric hypertrophy results (Fig. 1). Hypertension also promotes hypertrophy, reflecting the increased wall stress associated with elevations in systemic vascular resistance. Essential hypertension in lean patients is, in contrast to obese patients, typically characterized by

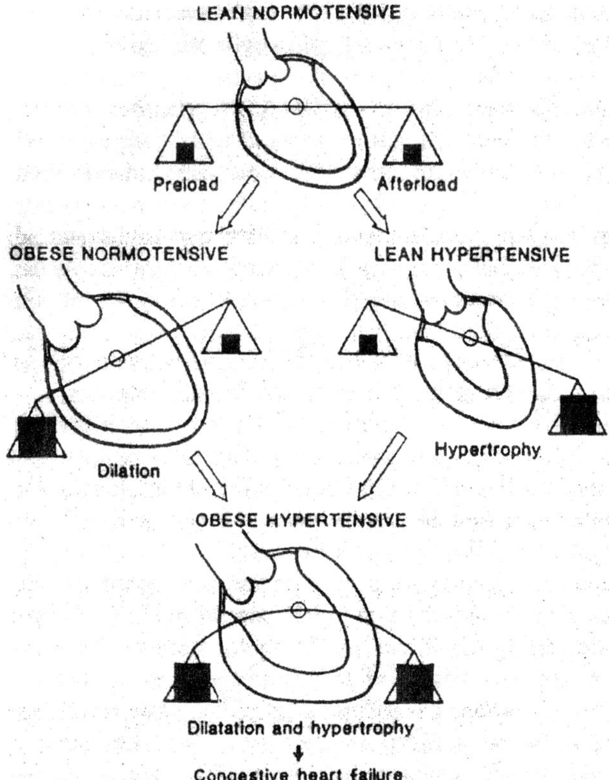

Figure 1 Effect of obesity and hypertension on cardiac structure. (Adapted from Ref. 238.)

intravascular volume contraction and elevated systemic vascular resistance (4,7,23). In obese hypertensives, the effects on blood volume expansion and systemic vascular resistance reflect either a balance of the two stimuli or favor the predominant process (7,8). In obese hypertensives, effects on ventricular mass and dimensions are independent and additive, and left ventricular mass is greater in obese hypertensives than in obese normotensives (16,17,24,25). Since intravascular volume is contracted, ventricular wall thickness due to hypertrophy is increased disproportionately to the chamber radius, resulting in a decreased ratio of chamber radius to wall thickness, or concentric hypertrophy. The separate and combined effects of obesity and hypertension on the left ventricle are depicted in Figure 1.

Autopsy studies assessing cardiac structure and pathology have been mostly limited to those who were extremely obese, which is in contrast to the studies above which assessed subjects representing a wider spectrum of leanness to obesity and employed echocardiography or other noninvasive methods. Early autopsy study by Smith and Willius (26) in 135 obese patients who died of congestive heart failure revealed a direct relationship between body weight and heart weight. Fatty infiltration of the heart (extension of epicardial fat into the myocardium and perivascular region) was also noted, leading to speculation that increased heart weight and pathology were due to fatty infiltration. Carpenter (27) subsequently observed fatty infiltration in ~3% of obese subjects at autopsy. Fatty infiltration occurs in several other disease states, including malnutrition, and despite its presence in obesity, is no longer believed to underlie most cardiac pathology in obesity (9,12). In another autopsy study, Amad et al. (28) examined the relationship between body weight and heart weight in 12 severely obese subjects without hypertension or coronary artery disease. Heart weight was far in excess of that predicted for ideal body weight, gross ventricular hypertrophy was present, and on microscopic examination the cause was noted to be myocardial hypertrophy. Other autopsy studies have noted increased left ventricular chamber size and mass associated with obesity, confirming that eccentric hypertrophy is the primary cause of increased heart weight (9).

III LEFT VENTRICULAR HYPERTROPHY AND CONGESTIVE HEART FAILURE

A Left Ventricular Hypertrophy

Left ventricular hypertrophy is an adaptive but not an entirely benign response. Left ventricular hypertrophy has been associated with greater risk of cardiovascular morbidity and all-cause mortality, CHD, congestive heart failure, arrhythmia, and sudden death (29–35). Such effects appear to be independent of traditional risk factors for cardiovascular disease such as hypertension, blood lipids, and existing CHD (29–34). In a minority of trials, effects of eccentric hypertrophy have been differentiated from those of concentric hypertrophy. Koren et al. (29) assessed mortality and cardiovascular events in 253 hypertensive patients (mean age 47 years) who had been evaluated by echocardiogram an average of 10 years previously. Patients were classified as having normal left ventricular mass, or concentric ($n = 29$) or eccentric ($n = 40$) left ventricular hypertrophy, but no information regarding obesity within each group was provided. For the whole population, left ventricular mass index (left ventricular mass/body surface area) predicted cardiovascular events or death better than several traditional risk factors. Those with baseline concentric hypertrophy experienced the greatest number of cardiovascular deaths and events (21% and 31%), while eccentric hypertrophy was intermediate (10% and 23%), and absence of hypertrophy demonstrated the lowest frequencies (0% and 11%). Gardin et al. (35) followed 5888 men and women (mean age 73 years) for 6–7 years and found that left ventricular mass at baseline was significantly higher in those with incident CHD, CHF, stroke (women only), and all-cause mortality (men only). A significant trend for incident CHD and CHF was observed across quartiles of left ventricular mass, and in those with eccentric hypertrophy the hazards ratio for incident CHD and CHF were 2.05 (95% CI 1.16–3.32) and 2.95 (95% CI 1.56–5.57). Thus, left ventricular hypertrophy is clearly associated with increased cardiovascular disease, although the specific relationships between left ventricular hypertrophy and geometry and cardiovascular outcomes in obese patients require further definition.

B Congestive Heart Failure

When the hypertrophic response is commensurate to left ventricular dilatation, filling pressures and wall stress are normalized by increased ventricular mass, and systolic function is maintained (12). Even when systolic function is maintained, however, left ventricular diastolic dysfunction may occur (15,36–38). Diminished ventricular compliance results in impaired accommodation of volume during diastole, resulting in diastolic dysfunction (15,36–38). Factors associated with diastolic dysfunction include degree and duration of overweight, degree of volume expansion, and adverse loading conditions imposed by volume overload or hypertension (15,25,36). Diastolic dysfunction may be evident on the resting echocardiogram, but may not become clinically evident until provoked by volume overload or exercise. Frank congestive heart failure due to diastolic dysfunction does occur but is most often observed in extreme obesity, and echocardiography or angiography may be needed to differentiate between underlying diastolic and systolic dysfunction (9).

When left ventricular filling exceeds favorable loading conditions and hypertrophy does not keep pace to normalize resultant wall stress, ventricular contractility is impaired and systolic dysfunction ensues (12). This is illustrated on echocardiogram as an increase in the ratio of the left ventricular cavity radius relative to wall thickness (9,12). Further evidence of systolic dysfunction was provided by two trials that demonstrated that left ventricular ejection fraction decreased inversely with BMI as well as duration of overweight (6,15). Systolic dysfunction does not occur universally in obesity, but appears to be a function of the degree and duration of overweight as well as adverse loading conditions (5,6,15,39). These and other factors that potentially contribute to the progression from physiologic adaptation and compensation, to diastolic and systolic dysfunction, and to frank decompensation, are illustrated in Figure 2.

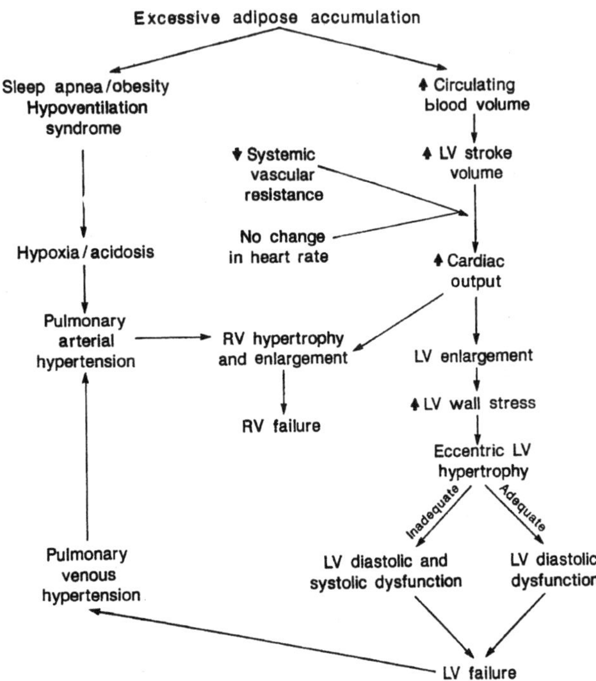

Figure 2 Pathophysiology of adaptation and congestive heart failure in obesity. (Adapted from Ref. 12.)

Evidence for an association of obesity with CHF is found in observational, clinical, and clinicopathologic trials. Body weight, independent of several traditional risk factors, was directly related to development of congestive heart failure in the Framingham Heart Study (40). In that study, incidence of congestive heart failure in those >130% of Metropolitan Relative Weight was almost twice that of subjects <110%. In the National Health and Nutrition Examination I follow-up study, overweight was associated with a modestly increased risk of developing congestive heart failure (RR 1.35, 95% CI 1.17–1.55, $P < .001$), which was only slightly weakened and remained significant when included in a multivariate model with CHD, diabetes, smoking, hypertension, and diabetes (41). In extremely obese patients, Alpert et al. (42) found that duration of obesity was strongly related to the presence of CHF. In a recent assessment of 159 consecutive patients referred for echocardiogram for congestive heart failure, 109 had preserved systolic function, and 40 of these 109 had a BMI ≥ 30 kg/m^2 (43). Kasper and colleagues (44) performed endocardial biopsy on lean and overweight patients with clinically evident dilated cardiomyopathy to assess the etiology of heart failure. Specific pathologic diagnoses were evident in 64% of the patients with BMI < 30 kg/m^2, while in those patients with BMI > 35 kg/m^2 no specific tissue diagnosis could be made in 77%, suggesting that obesity may have been the primary etiologic factor.

C Effects of Weight Loss on Cardiac Structure and Function

Weight loss is accompanied by decreases in oxygen requirements, blood volume, and cardiac output (45–47). Reductions in blood pressure occur early in weight loss and with modest amounts of lost weight (45,48–50), while greater degrees of weight loss have resulted in amelioration or resolution of severe hypertension (51–53). Given trends toward normalization of blood volume and blood pressure, parallel changes in cardiac function and structure might be expected. In mildly to moderately obese persons, weight loss in the range of 4–10 kg has only inconsistently been associated with decreased left ventricular dimension, loading conditions, and systolic function (54–60). Despite the lack of consistency in hemodynamic and functional parameters, reductions in left ventricular mass or wall thickness were observed in all but one (59) of these trials and appeared to occur independent of reductions in blood pressure (56,57). To differentiate between the effects of lost weight and reductions in blood pressure in overweight hypertensive subjects, MacMahon et al. (57) compared effects of weight loss or metoprolol treatment on left ventricular mass and blood pressure. An average weight loss of 8.3 kg resulted in a reduction in left ventricular mass/body surface area of 16%, and independent effects of weight loss and blood pressure reduction were observed.

In contrast to patients with moderate obesity, extremely obese patients who lost substantial weight following bariatric surgery showed more consistent decreases in left ventricular mass and left ventricular filling, as well as improved systolic and diastolic function (21,61–65). Improvements in structural and hemodynamic parameters appear to correlate with factors at baseline such as duration (65) and degree of obesity (62), degree of impaired loading (21), left ventricular mass (62), and degree of systolic dysfunction (63); following surgery, improvements have been correlated with percent of excess weight loss (62). Thus, improvements would be expected in those who are most obese, have the greatest baseline impairment and hypertrophy, and who lose more weight.

IV ELECTROCARDIOGRAM, ARRHYTHMIAS, AND SUDDEN DEATH

A Effects on the Electrocardiogram

Considering that obesity is associated with hemodynamic and structural changes of the heart, as well as with increased risk for sudden death, electrocardiographic (ECG) changes would not be unanticipated. Frank et al. (66) examined ECG findings in 1029 obese subjects, which were then correlated with degree of obesity, age, gender, and blood pressure. As obesity increased, there was increased leftward QRS axis, increased QRS voltage, and low QRS voltage was found in 4%. The QT interval corrected for heart rate (QTc) was abnormally prolonged in 28% and QTc prolongation correlated with degree of obesity. In trials where the ECG in obese subjects has been compared to lean controls, obese patients have had more leftward QRS axis (although pathologic left axis deviation was rare), lower QRS voltage, and more frequent T-wave flattening in the inferior and lateral leads (66–68). Alpert (67) contrasted the ECGs of 100 obese subjects (BMI 48 ± 2 kg/m^2) with 100 lean controls and found that 11/100 obese patients had low QRS voltage. None of these 11 subjects had elevated left ventricular mass/height index, although in the entire population, left ventricular mass index was elevated in 64/100. Alpert has proposed that low QRS voltage results from electrical insulation by subcutaneous or epicardial fat, and furthermore, that the relatively low prevalence of low voltage may reflect a balance between obesity-related left ventricular hypertrophy and electrical insulation by fat. This is consistent with the limited ability of the ECG to detect left ventricular hypertrophy in obese patients, as estimates of sensitivity range from 18–76% (69,70); the wide variation also reflects differing methods of indexing LV mass and criteria for hypertrophy.

Prolongation of the QT interval has been an inconsistent finding in healthy obese subjects, and among trials the prevalence of prolonged QTc has ranged from 0% to 47% (66,67,71–73). Despite inconsistencies between investigations in frank QTc prolongation, Frank et al. (66), and more recently el-Gamal et al. (71) and Carella et al. (73) observed that QTc increased directly in proportion to degree of obesity or body fat. Factors that possibly explain the variability in QT findings include inclusion of subjects who were dieting or who had subclinical electrolyte abnormalities, or failure to control for timing of meal consumption in relation to testing (since food consumption transiently prolongs the QT interval) (74).

Disturbances in heart rhythm in lean and obese subjects were assessed on standard 12-lead ECG by Alpert (67), who found no significant differences between groups in sinus bradycardia or tachycardia. Frank (66) observed bradycardia (<60 bpm) in 19% of obese subjects, in contrast to tachycardia (>100 bpm) in 0.5%. To assess the relationship between obesity and ventricular ectopy, several trials have employed longer-term ECG or Holter monitoring. In lean and obese (with and without eccentric left ventricular hypertrophy) hypertensive patients who underwent 24-hr Holter monitoring and echocardiograms, Messerli et al. (75) found that ventricular ectopy occurred 10 times more frequently in the obese and 30 times more frequently in the obese with left ventricular hypertrophy. Both left ventricular mass and diastolic diameter correlated with complexity of ectopy, and the three subjects who experienced arrhythmia had the greatest left ventricular mass and diastolic diameter. In patients without known heart disease awaiting bariatric surgery, a nonsignificant increase in ectopy was observed during 24-hr holter monitoring in comparison to lean subjects (76). In a small number of moderately obese patients referred for suspicion of arrhythmia, frequency of ventricular ectopy correlated with BMI as well as with left ventricular mass index, but in a multivariate model including age and hyperinsulinemia, both BMI and left ventricular mass became nonsignificant (77).

B Arrhythmia

Obesity promotes several risk factors for arrhythmia, including left ventricular hypertrophy, CHD, autonomic imbalance, and sleep apnea. While these factors may contribute to arrhythmia risk, documentation of malignant arrhythmias in obese patients with these risk factors has been scarce (75,77,78). Proposed mechanisms linking structural changes to arrhythmia include altered myocyte electrophysiology, fatty infiltration of the myocardium, myocardial fibrosis, myocardial ischemia resulting from diminished perfusion from dilatation and hypertrophy in combination with increased myocardial demand or work, and physical disruption of the conducting system by myocardial hypertrophy or fatty infiltration (78,79). Ventricular ectopy on 24-hr monitoring in obese patients has also been observed in association with hyperinsulinemia and with erythrocyte magnesium content in nondieting patients, possibly indicating defects in transmembrane cation exchange or abnormal intracellular concentration (77).

Abnormal heart rate variability, an index of autonomic balance reflecting sympathetic and parasympathetic contributions, is associated with risk for arrhythmia, congestive heart failure, and CHD (80,81). Reduced heart rate variability has been observed in obesity due to withdrawal of vagal activity and sympathetic predominance (76,81–84). Of interest, weight loss in the range of 9–32 kg has resulted in normalization of parasympathetic activity and heart rate variability (76,83–85). Whether weight loss–induced normalization of autonomic balance is associated with reduced cardiovascular morbidity, however, remains to be demonstrated.

Obstructive sleep apnea, a condition largely attributable to obesity, is associated with multiple rhythm disturbances including bradytachycardia (bradycardia followed by tachycardia), bradycardia, premature supraventricular and ventricular depolarizations, supraventricular tachycardia, and ventricular tachycardia (86). In 239 patients with obstructive sleep apnea, bradycardia was positively associated with BMI and severity of sleep apnea, but was observed in only 7% (87). Valencia-Flores et al. (88) conducted polysomnography in 52 consecutive patients with an average BMI of ~ 50 kg/m^2 who presented for outpatient obesity treatment. In this study, 98% had evidence of sleep-disordered breathing and 33% had severe sleep apnea. Cardiac rhythm disturbances were observed in 41% with severe apnea and in 27% of those with less severe sleep apnea. The type of rhythm disturbances noted included sinus arrhythmia (16%), premature ventricular complexes (16%), premature atrial complexes (10%), ventricular tachycardia (6%), and supraventricular tachycardia (4%). In addition, changes suggestive of cardiac ischemia during sleep occurred in 10% of subjects.

C Sudden Death

The first observation of increased risk of sudden death in obesity is attributed to Hippocrates, who over two millennia ago noted, "Sudden death is more common in those who are naturally fat than in the lean" (89). In the Framingham Heart Study, degree of overweight was highly predictive of sudden death in men (the small number of deaths observed in women precluded significance), and risk for sudden death was independent of traditional CHD risk factors (40). In the same population, a fivefold increased risk of sudden death was observed in those with congestive heart failure as compared to the general population; although the degree of obesity in those with congestive failure was unreported, there is a plausible link among obesity, congestive heart failure, and sudden death (90). In a retrospective survey by U.S. bariatric surgeons, a total of 60 sudden deaths were noted (91). In these patients, eight died awaiting gastric surgery for obesity, 14 died within 10 days following surgery, and the remainder died 12 days to 4 years after surgery. In those patients with available ECGs, 29/38 demonstrated prolonged QTc, indicating increased risk for arrhythmia. Despite the apparent increased risk for sudden death, there has been difficulty in documenting death due to malignant arrhythmia (a final lethal event in ~ 50% of patients dying of cardiovascular disease) (92).

Autopsy results from obese sudden-death patients suggest that ventricular hypertrophy or dilated cardiomyopathy is the most common finding, whereas other causes to which death could be attributed were variable. In seven young (6–32 years old) obese persons with sudden death, Bharati and Lev (79) found ventricular hypertrophy in 6/7 and greater-than-expected rates of fatty and fibrotic infiltration of the cardiac conduction system. In a study of 22 older (mean age 35 years) sudden death patients with a mean BMI of 57 kg/m^2, dilated cardiomyopathy was found in 10, hypertrophy without dilatation in four, coronary atherosclerosis in six, and pulmonary embolus in one.

In the late 1970s, 58 cases of death were reported in patients consuming very low calorie diets (93–97). Analysis of a subset of 17 of these patients revealed that death occurred during dieting in 10/17, while the remainder died during refeeding (96). Based on available ECGs, 75% had either prolonged QTc or low QRS voltage, or both. In all 11 patients who died under monitored conditions, ventricular arrhythmias were observed. Fisler (98) compiled trials reporting sudden death or ECG abnormalities in obese dieting patients prior to 1992, and several subsequent reports have now been published (72,99–102). It appears that starvation lasting more than several weeks, very low calorie diets with poor-quality protein, and surgical weight loss without nutritional monitoring were associated with QTc prolongation, low QRS voltage, and sporadic arrhythmias (93–98,103). In contrast, very low calorie diets containing sufficient quantities of good quality protein and supplemented with micronutrients (72,98–101,104–107), and starvation of brief (10 days) duration (102) have not been associated with abnormalities of cardiac conduction, voltage, or rhythm.

Sudden death is now rarely reported in patients undergoing surgical weight loss, suggesting that diet quality, preoperative assessment, and postoperative monitoring have improved. While no definitive underlying mechanism was found for sudden death during prolonged starvation or very low calorie diets, a number of factors have been proposed. Dietary factors include consumption of inadequate or poor-quality protein, electrolyte deficiencies, and copper deficiency (possibly secondary to use of collagen, a protein source low in copper) (93,98,108–110). Other proposed factors include myocardial protein depletion and increased sensitivity to the sympathetic stimulation associated with refeeding (93,98). Another proposed factor contributing to sudden death is that there is a critical threshold for loss of body weight or fat free mass. In a reanalysis in the original 58 patients, Van Itallie and Yang (93) found a direct relationship between initial BMI and months of survival on a very low calorie diet. The authors suggest that initially high levels of fat-free mass and fat might confer a survival advantage by delaying loss to a critical level of fat-free mass or myocardium.

V ATHEROEMBOLIC DISEASE: CORONARY HEART DISEASE AND STROKE

A Coronary Heart Disease

Obesity is associated with increased risk for CHD, reflecting increased risk for both atherosclerosis of the coronary arteries and ischemic events. Accordingly, the American Heart Association recently classified obesity as a major risk factor for CHD independent of traditional CHD risk factors (111). The development of atherosclerotic disease represents a progression from plaque formation to plaque rupture and thrombus formation, and finally to fibrosis (112). Obesity and central body fat distribution have been demonstrated to promote processes contributing to each of these stages (Table 2). Traditional CHD risk factors, such as diabetes, hypertension, and dyslipidemia, are discussed elsewhere in this volume. Several emerging nontraditional risk factors for CHD are associated with obesity, including the role of chronic inflammation, endothelial dysfunction, and alterations in hemostasis and coagulation.

Coronary heart disease has recently been associated with a state of chronic low-level inflammation, a state that may indicate underlying CHD, but also may contribute to pathogenesis (113–115). Several circulating markers of inflammation, such as C-reactive protein (CRP) and fibrinogen, have been identified as predictors of CHD incidence and prognosis. CRP is an acute phase protein that is elevated in response to inflammation or infection. CRP has been found to correlate directly with degree of overweight, body fat, and central fat distribution; in addition, CRP has been associated with insulin resistance, activation of coagulation, and subclinical atherosclerosis (113,114,116–121). In several trials, CRP was a significant predictor of new CHD events and prognosis after CHD events, and use of CRP has improved prediction of CHD events when combined with blood lipids (119,122,123). CRP is produced in the liver primarily under the control of interleukin-6 (IL-6), a pro-inflammatory cytokine produced in macrophages, lymphocytes, and fat cells (124). IL-6 itself has been associated with CHD (125), and also increases hepatic

Table 2 Risk Factors for CHD Associated with Obesity

Metabolic
Diabetes
Insulin resistance and hyperinsulinemia
Dyslipidemia
Androgen excess
Cardiovascular
Hypertension
Left ventricular hypertrophy
Endothelial dysfunction
Hematologic
Hyperviscosity
Pro-coagulant state
Impaired fibrinolysis
Chronic inflammation
Hyperuricemia
Obstructive sleep apnea

production of fibrinogen, induces insulin resistance, stimulates lipolysis, increases endothelial release of adhesion molecules, and increases platelet aggregation (124). Yudkin (124) has proposed a central role for IL-6 in the link between obesity and CHD, since IL-6 production and circulating levels increase in proportion to body fat. Accordingly, increased levels of circulating IL-6 may stimulate a pro-thrombotic state and endothelial dysfunction, while CRP serves as marker of inflammation. However, this model remains speculative, and the exact mechanisms relating inflammation and pro-inflammatory cytokines to obesity and CHD require further elucidation.

Obesity also appears to induce a state of hemostatic imbalance favoring coagulation. Positive relationships have been observed between BMI or body fat and fibrinogen, Von Willebrand factor, factor VII, factor VIII, and plasminogen activator inhibitor 1 (PAI-1), the primary inhibitor of fibrinolysis (126–129). In prospective epidemiologic trials, fibrinogen, Von Willebrand factor, factor VII, and PAI-1 levels have been associated with incident CHD, CHD events, or long-term survival in those with stable CHD (34,126,128,130,131).

Impaired endothelial vasodilatory responses have been proposed to increase risk for CHD, either acutely due to ischemia, or as markers of early dysregulation (vasodilatory, thrombogenic, and mitogenic functions) predisposing to CHD (132). In obese patients, endothelial nitric oxide–dependent responses to insulin, ischemia, or acetylcholine have been abnormal in peripheral (133–137) and coronary (138) arteries, while vasodilatation not dependent on endothelial nitric oxide appears largely unaffected. Abnormal nitric oxide–dependent endothelial relaxation has been observed in obese subjects in relation to degree of obesity and central fat distribution, which has been independent of traditional risk factors.

Many, but not all, epidemiologic studies have shown significant relationships between excess body weight and CHD incidence, events, or mortality (139–160). Increased risk of CHD mortality was also observed in those who were obese as adolescents, regardless of adult weight (161), and in those who gain weight in adulthood (156). The lack of consistent relationship between obesity and CHD has been attributed to a number of methodologic issues, which include misclassification bias introduced by use of anthropometric surrogates of body fat, failure to control for smoking status and body fat distribution, and use of inappropriate control populations (151,162). The most consistent relationship observed between obesity and coronary artery disease is a univariate one, without control for other CHD risk factors (163). In the Framingham Heart Study (40,164), the 26-year incidence of CHD increased proportionately to excess weight. In that population, obesity was associated with increased CHD incidence of 2.4-fold in women and twofold in men under the age of 50 years. In a prospective study of BMI and mortality, Calle et al. (165) found that CHD mortality risk in women significantly increased when BMI exceeded 25 kg/m^2, and an approximately twofold risk of CHD mortality was observed in women with BMI >35 kg/m^2. In men, CHD mortality risk increased significantly at BMI >26.5 kg/m^2, and risk of mortality was 2.9-fold with a BMI of 35 kg/m^2 (165).

A consistent relationship between CHD and body fat distribution has been observed, and increased abdominal adiposity appears to increase CHD at all levels of body weight (140,152,160,166–168). In some populations, central adiposity has been more predictive of events or mortality than degree of overweight (128, 140,152,156,158,168,169).

In multivariate models that included traditional CHD risk factors in addition to obesity, independent effects of obesity on CHD have been observed with less consistency. However, several studies have demonstrated a persistent, but diminished, contribution of body weight to CHD and myocardial infarction risk when factors such as blood pressure, blood lipids, diabetes, smoking, and age were included in multivariate models (40,139,142,156,170,171). In the Nurses' Health Study, the magnitude of elevated relative risk of coronary disease between highest and lowest BMI quintiles was diminished, but not eliminated, by adjustment for several known risk factors (RR 3.4 vs. 1.9, unadjusted vs. adjusted for other risk factors) (156).

Associations between body weight and coronary artery disease among nonwhite groups have been observed less frequently than in primarily white populations. An inconsistent relationship has been found for blacks (141,160,172,173), although two recent trials have found that obesity confers risk of CHD similar to white controls (158) or white populations. Hispanics have a disproportionate amount of obesity, central obesity, diabetes, and hypertension in comparison to non-Hispanic whites, yet in middle-aged and older Hispanics, mortality from cardiovascular disease has been less than or equal to that in non-Hispanic whites (146,174). In the Strong Heart Study (147,175), three geographically diverse subgroups of American Indians were assessed for rates of coronary heart disease and associated risk factors, revealing that obesity was a significant predictor of coronary heart disease independent of other traditional risk factors, although the overall occurrence of coronary heart disease was less than that reported in other populations.

While obesity may promote risk for CHD, diagnosis is complicated by limitations due to weight or body habitus. Accuracy of myocardial perfusion imaging may be significantly reduced when BMI exceeds 30 kg/ m^2 (176). Many exercise treadmills and angiographic tables cannot accommodate weights over 300 lb. Thus, in extreme obesity, greater reliance must be placed upon clinical factors and the electrocardiogram. In addition to difficulties in diagnosis, treatment of CHD may also be adversely influenced by obesity. In obese patients undergoing coronary artery bypass grafting, there have been increased rates of sternal wound infection (177), saphenous vein site infection (178), postoperative respiratory complications (179,180), prolonged hospital stay (181), and readmission after discharge (182).

B Stroke and Peripheral Vascular Disease

Obesity and central body fat distribution increase the risk for ischemic stroke and accelerated atherosclerotic disease of the carotid artery, but do not appear to increase the risk for hemorrhagic stroke (166,167,183–188). Effects of obesity on stroke or carotid atherosclerotic disease independent of traditional risk factors have been only inconsistently reported (166,186,189–192). In regard to peripheral vascular disease, a small number of investigators have assessed the role of obesity and have found little contribution of obesity to clinical disease (193–195). Further, noninvasive measures of carotid and femoral intima-media thickness (a measure of preclinical atherosclerosis) suggest that excess body fat is associated with thickening of only the carotid arteries (196–198).

C Effects of Weight Loss on CHD and Atherosclerosis

Weight loss in overweight, moderately obese, and extremely obese subjects has been demonstrated to improve CHD risk factors such as blood pressure (49,186, 199,200), blood glucose and insulin concentrations (201,202), and blood lipids (186,199,203). Hemostatic imbalance appears to be normalized by weight loss, as subjects who lost 8–14 kg demonstrated marked decreases in PAI-1, factor VIIc, and fibrinogen (186,203, 204). However, those who regain weight again revert toward a pro-thrombotic state. Vasodilatory function response to ischemia-induced forearm blood flow, an indicator of endothelial vasodilatory function, was significantly improved with weight losses of 5–7 kg (134). CRP was also reduced by 26% in association with an average weight loss of 8 kg in moderately obese women (205). The effects of weight loss on early atherosclerosis were assessed in two trials by pre– and post–weight loss measurement of carotid intima-media thickness. In one trial, intima-media thickness was reduced, which was independent of changes in LDL cholesterol and PAI-1 (186). In the second trial, the progression rate of intima-media thickness was slowed to that of lean controls (188).

The promising effects of weight loss on risk factors and subclinical atherosclerosis have not previously been reflected in observational trials relating CHD morbidity and mortality with weight loss, in part due to lack of differentiation between voluntary and involuntary weight loss as well as the small numbers of those who maintain lost weight over years (206). However, more recent trials limited to those reporting volitional weight loss have been more encouraging (207,208). In 4970 overweight diabetic patients, intentional weight loss over a 12-year period was associated with a 28% reduction in cardiovascular mortality (208). However, further prospective trials specifically designed to address this issue are needed to confirm effects on mortality (209).

VI CARDIOVASCULAR EFFECTS OF APPETITE SUPPRESSANTS

In July 1997, 24 cases of valvular heart disease were reported in patients taking dl-fenfluramine or dexfenfluramine, prompting the U.S. Food and Drug Administration (FDA) to issue a public health advisory. A month later descriptions of these cases, as well as an additional 29 cases, were published (210–212). Regurgitation was observed in both left- and right-sided valves, but mitral and aortic valves were more frequently involved. On gross examination and on echocardiogram, affected valves were described as having a glistening appearance on echocardiogram (210). Initial histopathology revealed changes identical to those in valvulopathy associated with carcinoid syndrome or with ergotamine use (210). Five preliminary surveys in patients taking fenfluramine alone, or in combination with phentermine, suggested that valvulopathy occurred in 33% (213), leading to withdrawal of dl-fenfluramine and dexfenfluramine from the U.S market in September 1997. These early surveys were criticized, however, for failure to employ FDA criteria for valvular disease and because they were uncontrolled. Subsequent surveys have generally used FDA criteria, and reflect a variety of methodologies. In contrast to initial estimates of valvulopathy in 33% of fenfluramine users, subsequent trials have reported a lower prevalence of valvulopathy, with estimates of fenfluramine-related valvulopathy of 0% (214,215), 4.3% (216), 6.9% (217), 7.6% (218), 8% (219), 8.8% (220), 16% (221), 16.5% (222), 23% (223), 26% (224), and 31% (225,226). Likelihood of valvulopathy was increased with duration of treatment (220–222,225–227), dosage (228), or when fenfluramine was taken in combination with phentermine (217,220,229). In patients with valvulopathy who have been reexamined by echocardiogram ~ 1 year after initial examination, there appears to be little evidence for progression of valvular dysfunction, and trends toward resolution have been observed (224,230,231). Mast et al. (231) found improvement in 17/38 patients with baseline valvulopathy, while no change was noted in 19/38 and worsening occurred in two. In another study of five patients with valvulopathy, improvement was noted in 5/5 patients with resolution in 3/5 (224).

Valvular heart disease has not been observed to occur more frequently owing to obesity itself (61,232). There also has been no valve disease associated with sibutramine, a serotonin and norepinephrine reuptake inhibitor antiobesity medication (233). Use of the serotonergic reuptake inhibitor fluoxetene in combination with phentermine has not been associated with valvulopathy in one study (234), but confirmatory trials are needed.

Use of certain over-the-counter or herbal weight loss aids has also been associated with cardiovascular morbidity and mortality. Increased risk for hemorrhagic stroke in women has been associated with use of the over-the-counter weight loss drug phenylpropanolamine, leading to its withdrawal from the U.S. market (235). Use of ephedra, an herbal preparation containing variable amounts of ephedrine alkaloids, has been associated with a number of cardiovascular side effects, including hypertension, tachycardia, myocardial infarction, and stroke (236). Further, chronic use of sympathomimetics such as ephedra may increase risk for hemodynamic instability during anesthesia secondary to catecholamine depletion (237).

VII CONCLUSION

Obesity is associated with substantial risk for cardiovascular morbidity and mortality. The obese state is characterized by hemodynamic and structural adaptation, and promotes cardiovascular disease through traditional, newly described, or as yet undefined risk factors. The salutary effects of weight loss on risk factors and cardiovascular disease itself provides encouragement that weight losses that are currently achievable will have longer-term benefit. Emerging factors linking obesity and CHD, such as chronic inflammation, not only help elucidate pathogenesis, but provide specific targets for intervention.

ACKNOWLEDGMENTS

Supported in part by the U.S. Department of Agriculture, Agricultural Research Service, under contract 53-3K06-5-10. Contents of this publication do not necessarily reflect the views or policies of the U.S. Department of Agriculture.

REFERENCES

1. American Heart Association. 2001 Heart and Stroke Statistical Update. Dallas: AHA, 2000:1–32.
2. Ravussin E. Energy expenditure and body weight. In: Brownell K, Fairburn C, eds. Eating Disorders and Obesity. New York: Guilford Press, 1995:32–37.
3. Frayn KN. Studies of human adipose tissue in vivo. In: Kinney JM, Tucker HN, eds. Energy Metabolism: Tissue Determinants and Cellular Corollaries. New York: Raven Press, 1992:267–291.
4. Messerli FH, Ventura HO, Reisin E, Dreslinski GR, Dunn FG, MacPhee AA, Frohlich ED. Borderline hypertension and obesity: two prehypertensive states with elevated cardiac output. Circulation 1982; 66:55–60.
5. De Divitiis O, Fazio S, Petitto M, Maddalena G, Contaldo F, Mancini M. Obesity and cardiac function. Circulation 1981; 64:477–482.
6. Licata G, Scaglione R, Barbagallo M, Parrinello G, Capuana G, Lipari R, Merlino G, Ganguzza A. Effect of obesity on left ventricular function studied by radionuclide angiocardiography. Int J Obes 1991; 15:295–302.
7. Messerli FH, Sundgaard-Riise K, Reisin E, Dreslinski G, Dunn FG, Frohlich E. Disparate cardiovascular effects of obesity and arterial hypertension. Am J Med 1983; 74:808–812.
8. Oren S, Grossman E, Frohlich ED. Arterial and venous compliance in obese and nonobese subjects. Am J Cardiol 1996; 77:665–667.
9. Alexander JK. The cardiomyopathy of obesity. Prog Cardiovasc Dis 1985; 27:325–334.
10. Carabello BA, Gittens L. Cardiac mechanics and function in obese normotensive persons with normal coronary arteries. Am J Cardiol 1987; 59:469–473.

11. Wikstrand J, Petterson P, Bjorntorp P. Body fat distribution and left ventricular morphology and function in obese females. J Hypertens 1993; 11:1259–1266.
12. Alpert MA. Obesity cardiomyopathy: pathophysiology and evolution of the clinical syndrome. Am J Med Sci 2001; 321:225–236.
13. Lauer MS, Anderson KM, Kannel WB, Levy D. The impact of obesity on left ventricular mass and geometry. JAMA 1991; 266:231–236.
14. Rasooly R, Sasson Z, Gupta R. Relation between body fat distribution and left ventricular mass in men without structural heart disease or systemic hypertension. Am J Cardiol 1993; 71:1477–1479.
15. Alpert MA, Lambert CR, Terry BE, Cohen MV, Mukerji V, Massey CV, Hashimi MW, Panayiotou H. Interrelationship of left ventricular mass, systolic function and diastolic filling in normotensive morbidly obese patients. Int J Obes 1995; 19:550–557.
16. Gottdiener JS, Reda DJ, Materson BJ, Massie BM, Notargiacomo A, Hamburger RJ, Williams DW, Henderson WG. Importance of obesity, race and age to the cardiac structural and functional effects of hypertension. J Am Coll Cardiol 1994; 24:1492–1498.
17. De Simone G, Devereux RB, Roman MJ, Alderman MH, Laragh JH. Relation of obesity and gender to left ventricular hypertrophy in normotensive and hypertensive adults. Hypertension 1994; 23:600–606.
18. Bella JN, Devereux RB, Roman MJ, O'Grady MJ, Welty TK, Lee ET, Fabsitz RR, Howard BV. Relations of left ventricular mass to fat-free and adipose body mass: the strong heart study. The Strong Heart Study Investigators. Circulation 1998; 98:2538–2544.
19. Urbina EM, Gidding SS, Bao W, Elkasabany A, Berenson GS. Association of fasting blood sugar level, insulin level, and obesity with left ventricular mass in healthy children and adolescents: the Bogalusa Heart Study. Am Heart J 1999; 138:122–127.
20. Sasson Z, Rasooly Y, Bhensania T, Rasooly I. Insulin resistance is an important determinant of left ventricular mass in the obese. Circulation 1993; 88:1431–1436.
21. Alpert MA, Terry BE, Kelly DL. Effect of weight loss on cardiac chamber size, wall thickness and left ventricular function in morbid obesity. Am J Cardiol 1985; 55:783–786.
22. Noda A, Okada T, Yasuma F, Nakashima N, Yokota M. Cardiac hypertrophy in obstructive sleep apnea syndrome. Chest 1995; 107:1538–1544.
23. Lavie CJ, Messerli FH. Cardiovascular adaptation to obesity and hypertension. Chest 1986; 90:275–279.
24. De la Maza M, Estevez A, Bunout D, Klenner C, Oyonarte M, Hirsch S. Ventricular mass in hypertensive and normotensive obese subjects. Int J Obes 1994; 18:193–197.
25. Lavie CJ, Amodeo C, Ventura HO, Messerli FH. Left atrial abnormalities indicating diastolic ventricular dysfunction in cardiopathy of obesity. Chest 1987; 92:1042–1046.
26. Smith HL, Willius FA. Adiposity of the heart: a clinical and pathologic study of one hundred and thirty-six obese patients. Ann Intern Med 1933; 52:930–931.
27. Carpenter HM. Myocardial fat infiltration. Am Heart J 1962; 63:491–496.
28. Amad KH, Brennan JC, Alexander JK. The cardiac pathology of chronic exogenous obesity. Circulation 1965; 32:740–745.
29. Koren MJ, Devereux RB, Casale PN, Savage DD, Laragh JH. Relation of left ventricular mass and geometry to morbidity and mortality in uncomplicated essential hypertension. Ann Intern Med 1991; 114:345–352.
30. Levy D, Garrison RJ, Savage DD, Kannel WB, Castelli WP. Left ventricular mass and incidence of coronary heart disease in an elderly cohort. Ann Intern Med 1989; 110:101–107.
31. Liao Y, Cooper RS, McGee DL, Mensah GA, Ghali JK. The relative effects of left ventricular hypertrophy, coronary artery disease, and ventricular dysfunction on survival among black adults. JAMA 1995; 273:1592–1597.
32. Ghali JK, Liao Y, Simmons B, Castaner A, Cao G, Cooper RS. The prognostic role of left ventricular hypertrophy in patients with or without coronary artery disease. Ann Intern Med 1992; 117:831–836.
33. Casale PN, Devereux RB, Milner M, Zullo G, Harshfield GA. Value of echocardiographic measurement of left ventricular mass in predicting cardiovascular morbid events in hypertensive men. Ann Intern Med 1986; 105:173–178.
34. Harjai KJ. Potential new cardiovascular risk factors: left ventricular hypertrophy, homocysteine, lipoprotein(a), triglycerides, oxidative stress, and fibrinogen. Ann Intern Med 1999; 131:376–386.
35. Gardin JM, McClelland R, Kitzman D, Lima JA, Bommer W, Klopfenstein HS, Wong ND, Smith VE, Gottdiener J. M-mode echocardiographic predictors of six- to seven-year incidence of coronary heart disease, stroke, congestive heart failure, and mortality in an elderly cohort (the Cardiovascular Health Study). Am J Cardiol 2001; 87:1051–1057.
36. Chakko S, Mayor M, Allison MD, Kessler KM, Materson BJ, Myerburg RJ. Abnormal left ventricular diastolic filling in eccentric left ventricular hypertrophy of obesity. Am J Cardiol 1991; 68:95–98.
37. Ku CS, Lin SL, Wang DJ, Chang SK, Lee WJ. Left ventricular filling in young normotensive obese adults. Am J Cardiol 1994; 73:613–615.
38. Crisostomo LL, Araujo LM, Camara E, Carvalho C, Silva FA, Vieira M, Rabelo A Jr. Comparison of left ventricular mass and function in obese versus nonobese women <40 years of age. Am J Cardiol 1999;84:1127–1129, A1111.

39. Garavaglia GE, Messerli FH, Nunez BD, Schmieder RE, Grossman E. Myocardial contractility and left ventricular function in obese patients with essential hypertension. Am J Cardiol 1988; 62:594–597.
40. Hubert HB, Feinleib M, McNamara PM, Castelli WP. Obesity as an independent risk factor for cardiovascular disease: a 26-year follow-up of participants in the Framingham Heart Study. Circulation 1983; 67:968–977.
41. He J, Ogden LG, Bazzano LA, Vupputuri S, Loria C, Whelton PK. Risk factors for congestive heart failure in US men and women: NHANES I epidemiologic follow-up study. Arch Intern Med 2001; 161:996–1002.
42. Alpert MA, Terry BE, Mulekar M, Cohen MV, Massey CV, Fan TM, Panayiotou H, Mukerji V. Cardiac morphology and left ventricular function in normotensive morbidly obese patients with and without congestive heart failure, and effect of weight loss. Am J Cardiol 1997; 80:736–740.
43. Caruana L, Petrie MC, Davie AP, McMurray JJ. Do patients with suspected heart failure and preserved left ventricular systolic function suffer from "diastolic heart failure" or from misdiagnosis? A prospective descriptive study. BMJ 2000; 321:215–218.
44. Kasper EK, Hruban RH, Baughman KL. Cardiomyopathy of obesity: a clinicopathologic evaluation of 43 obese patients with heart failure. Am J Cardiol 1992; 70:921–924.
45. Reisin E, Frohlich ED, Messerli FH, Dreslinski GR, Dunn FG, Jones MM, Batson HM Jr. Cardiovascular changes after weight reduction in obesity hypertension. Ann Intern Med 1983; 98:315–319.
46. Beretta-Piccoli C. Blood volume changes after weight reduction. Ann Intern Med 1983; 99:568–569.
47. Alpert MA. Management of obesity cardiomyopathy. Am J Med Sci 2001; 321:237–241.
48. Stevens VJ, Corrigan SA, Obarzenek E. Weight loss intervention in phase 1 of the trials of hypertension prevention. Arch Intern Med 1993; 153:849–858.
49. Blumenthal JA, Sherwood A, Gullette EC, Babyak M, Waugh R, Georgiades A, Craighead LW, Tweedy D, Feinglos M, Appelbaum M, Hayano J, Hinderliter A. Exercise and weight loss reduce blood pressure in men and women with mild hypertension: effects on cardiovascular, metabolic, and hemodynamic functioning. Arch Intern Med 2000; 160:1947–1958.
50. Minami J, Kawano Y, Ishimitsu T, Matsuoka H, Takishita S. Acute and chronic effects of a hypocaloric diet on 24-hour blood pressure, heart rate and heart-rate variability in mildly-to-moderately obese patients with essential hypertension. Clin Exp Hypertens 1999; 21:1413–1427.
51. Benotti PN, Bistrian B, Benotti JR, Blackburn G, Forse RA. Heart disease and hypertension in severe obesity: the benefits of weight reduction. Am J Clin Nutr 1992; 55:586S–590S.
52. Foley E, Benotti P, Borlase B, et al. Impact of gastric restrictive surgery on hypertension in the morbidly obese. Am J Surg 1992; 186:294–297.
53. Carson JL, Ruddy ME, Duff AE, et al. The effect of gastric bypass surgery on hypertension in morbidly obese patients. Arch Intern Med 1994; 154:193–200.
54. Wirth A, Kroger H. Improvement of left ventricular morphology and function in obese subjects following a diet and exercise program. Int J Obes 1995; 19:61–66.
55. Jordan J, Messerli F, Lavie C, Aepfelbacher F, Soria F. Reduction of weight and left ventricular mass with serotonin uptake inhibition in obese patients with systemic hypertension. Am J Cardiol 1995; 75:743–744.
56. Himeno E, Nishino K, Nakashima Y, Kuroiwa A, Ikeda M. Weight reduction regresses left ventricular mass regardless of blood pressure level in obese subjects. Am Heart J 1996; 131:313–319.
57. MacMahon SW, Wilcken DE, Macdonald GJ. The effect of weight reduction on left ventricular mass. A randomized controlled trial in young, overweight hypertensive patients. N Engl J Med 1986; 314:334–339.
58. Sido Z, Jako P, Pavlik G. The effect of moderate weight loss on echocardiographic parameters in obese female patients. Acta Physiol Hung 2000; 87:241–251.
59. Reid CM, Dart AM, Dewar EM, Jennings GL. Interactions between the effects of exercise and weight loss on risk factors, cardiovascular haemodynamics and left ventricular structure in overweight subjects. J Hypertens 1994; 12:291–301.
60. DasGupta P, Ramhanmdany E, Brigden G, Lahiri A, Baird IM, Raftery EB. Improvement in left ventricular function after rapid weight loss in obesity. Eur Heart J 1992; 13:1060–1066.
61. Karason K, Wallentin I, Larsson B, Sjostrom L. Effects of obesity and weight loss on cardiac function and valvular performance. Obes Res 1998; 6:422–429.
62. Alpert MA, Lambert CR, Terry BE, Kelly DL, Panayiotou H, Mukerji V, Massey CV, Cohen MV. Effect of weight loss on left ventricular mass in nonhypertensive morbidly obese patients. Am J Cardiol 1994; 73:918–921.
63. Alpert MA, Terry BE, Lambert CR, Kelly DL, Panayiotou H, Mukerji V, Massey CV, Cohen MV. Factors influencing left ventricular systolic function in nonhypertensive morbidly obese patients, and effect of weight loss induced by gastroplasty. Am J Cardiol 1993; 71:733–737.
64. Alpert MA, Lambert CR, Terry BE, Cohen MV, Mulekar M, Massey CV, Hashimi MW, Panayiotou H, Mukerji V. Effect of weight loss on left ventricular diastolic filling in morbid obesity. Am J Cardiol 1995; 76:1198–1201.
65. Alpert MA, Lambert CR, Panayiotou H, Terry BE, Cohen MV, Massey CV, Hashimi MW, Mukerji V. Relation of duration of morbid obesity to left ventricular mass, systolic function, and diastolic filling, and effect of weight loss. Am J Cardiol 1995; 76:1194–1197.
66. Frank S, Colliver JA, Frank A. The electrocardiogram

in obesity: statistical analysis of 1,029 patients. J Am Coll Cardiol 1986; 7:295–299.
67. Alpert MA, Terry BE, Cohen MV, Fan TM, Painter JA, Massey CV. The electrocardiogram in morbid obesity. Am J Cardiol 2000; 85:908–910, A910.
68. Alpert MA, Terry BE, Hamm CR, Fan TM, Cohen MV, Massey CV, Painter JA. Effect of weight loss on the ECG of normotensive morbidly obese patients. Chest 2001; 119:507–510.
69. Okin PM, Roman MJ, Devereux RB, Kligfield P. Electrocardiographic identification of left ventricular hypertrophy: test performance in relation to definition of hypertrophy and presence of obesity. J Am Coll Cardiol 1996; 27:124–131.
70. Okin PM, Roman MJ, Devereux RB, Kligfield P. ECG identification of left ventricular hypertrophy. Relationship of test performance to body habitus. J Electrocardiol 1996; 29:256–261.
71. el-Gamal A, Gallagher D, Nawras A, Gandhi P, Gomez J, Allison DB, Steinberg JS, Shumacher D, Blank R, Heymsfield SB. Effects of obesity on QT, RR, and QTc intervals. Am J Cardiol 1995; 75:956–959.
72. Mshui ME, Saikawa T, Ito K, Hara M, Sakata T. QT interval and QT dispersion before and after diet therapy in patients with simple obesity. Exp Biol Med 1999; 220:133–138.
73. Carella MJ, Mantz SL, Rovner DR, Willis PW III, Gossain VV, Bouknight RR, Ferenchick GS. Obesity, adiposity, and lengthening of the QT interval: improvement after weight loss. Int J Obes 1996; 20:938–942.
74. Nagy D, DeMeersman R, Gallagher D, Pietrobelli A, Zion AS, Daly D, Heymsfield SB. QTc interval (cardiac repolarization): lengthening after meals. Obes Res 1997; 5:531–537.
75. Messerli FH, Nunez BD, Ventura HO, Snyder DW. Overweight and sudden death: increased ventricular ectopy in cardiopathy of obesity. Arch Intern Med 1987; 147:1725–1728.
76. Karason K, Molgaard H, Wikstrand J, Sjostrom L. Heart rate variability in obesity and the effect of weight loss. Am J Cardiol 1999; 83:1242–1247.
77. Zemva A, Zemva Z. Ventricular ectopic activity, left ventricular mass, hyperinsulinemia, and intracellular magnesium in normotensive patients with obesity. Angiology 2000; 51:101–106.
78. Messerli F, Soria F. Ventricular dysrhythmias, left ventricular hypertrophy, and sudden death. Cardiovasc Drugs Ther 1994; 8:557–563.
79. Bharati S, Lev M. Cardiac conduction system involvement in sudden death of obese young people. Am Heart J 1995; 129:273–281.
80. Van Ravenswaaij-Arts CMA, Kollee LAA, Hopman JCW, Stoelinga GBA, Van Geijn HP. Heart rate variability. Ann Intern Med 1993; 118:436–447.
81. Colhoun HM, Francis DP, Rubens MB, Underwood SR, Fuller JH. The association of heart-rate variability with cardiovascular risk factors and coronary artery calcification: a study in type 1 diabetic patients and the general population. Diabetes Care 2001; 24:1108–1114.
82. Zahorska-Markiewicz B, Kuagowska E, Kucio C, Klin M. Heart rate variability in obesity. Int J Obes 1993; 17:21–23.
83. Emdin M, Gastaldelli A, Muscelli E, Macerata A, Natali A, Camastra S, Ferrannini E. Hyperinsulinemia and autonomic nervous system dysfunction in obesity: effects of weight loss. Circulation 2001; 103:513–519.
84. Rissanen PF-KARA. Cardiac parasympathetic activity is increased by weight loss in healthy obese women. Obes Res 2001; 9:637–643.
85. Hirsch J, Leibel RL, Mackintosh R, Aguirre A. Heart rate variability as a measure of autonomic function during weight change in humans. Am J Physiol 1991; 261:R1418–R1423.
86. Koenig SM. Pulmonary complications of obesity. Am J Med Sci 2001; 321:249–279.
87. Koehler U, Becker HF, Grimm W, Heitmann J, Peter JH, Schafer H. Relations among hypoxemia, sleep stage, and bradyarrhythmia during obstructive sleep apnea. Am Heart J 2000; 139:142–148.
88. Valencia-Flores M, Orea A, Castano VA, Resendiz M, Rosales M, Rebollar V, Santiago V, Gallegos J, Campos RM, Gonzalez J, Oseguera J, Garcia-Ramos G, Bliwise DL. Prevalence of sleep apnea and electrocardiographic disturbances in morbidly obese patients. Obes Res 2000; 8:262–269.
89. Chadwick J, Mann WN. The Medical Works of Hippocrates. Oxford: Blackwell Scientific, 1950.
90. Kannel WB, Plehn JF, Cupples LA. Cardiac failure and sudden death in the Framingham Study. Am Heart J 1988; 115:869–875.
91. Drenick EJ, Fisler JS. Sudden cardiac arrest in morbidly obese surgical patients unexplained after autopsy. Am J Surg 1988; 155:720–726.
92. Spooner PM, Albert C, Benjamin EJ, Boineau R, Elston RC, George AL Jr, Jouven X, Kuller LH, MacCluer JW, Marban E, Muller JE, Schwartz PJ, Siscovick DS, Tracy RP, Zareba W, Zipes DP. Sudden cardiac death, genes, and arrhythmogenesis: consideration of new population and mechanistic approaches from a National Heart, Lung, and Blood Institute workshop, part I. Circulation 2001; 103:2361–2364.
93. Van Itallie TB, Yang MU. Cardiac dysfunction in obese dieters: a potentially lethal complication of rapid, massive weight loss. Am J Clin Nutr 1984; 39:695–702.
94. Brown JM, Yetter JF, Spicer MJ, Jones JD. Cardiac complications of protein-sparing modified fasting. JAMA 1978; 240:120–122.
95. Singh BN, Gaarder TD, Kanegae T, Goldstein M, Montgomerie JZ, Mills H. Liquid protein diets and torsade de pointes. JAMA 1978; 240:115–119.
96. Sours HE, Frattali VP, Brand CD, Feldman RA, Forbes AL, Swanson RC, Paris AL. Sudden death associated with very low calorie weight reduction regimens. Am J Clin Nutr 1981; 34:453–461.

97. Isner JM, Sours HE, Paris AL, Ferrans VJ, Roberts WC. Sudden, unexpected death in avid dieters using the liquid-protein-modified-fast diet. Observations in 17 patients and the role of the prolonged QT interval. Circulation 1979; 60:1401–1412.
98. Fisler JS. Cardiac effects of starvation and semi-starvation diets: safety and mechanisms of action. Am J Clin Nutr 1992; 56:230S–234S.
99. Seim HC, Mitchell JE, Pomeroy C, de Zwaan M. Electrocardiographic findings associated with very low calorie dieting. Int J Obes 1995; 19:817–819.
100. Doherty JU, Wadden TA, Zuk L, Letizia KA, Foster GD, Day SC. Long-term evaluation of cardiac function in obese patients treated with a very-low-calorie diet: a controlled clinical study of patients without underlying cardiac disease. Am J Clin Nutr 1991; 53:854–858.
101. Pietrobelli A, Rothacker D, Gallagher D, Heymsfield SB. Electrocardiographic QTC interval: short-term weight loss effects. Int J Obes 1997; 21:110–114.
102. Zuckerman E, Yeshurun D, Goldhammer E, Shiran A. 24 h electrocardiographic monitoring in morbidly obese patients during short-term zero calorie diet. Int J Obes 1993; 17:359–361.
103. Pringle T, Scobie T, Murray R, Kesson C, Maccuish A. Prolongation of the QT interval during therapeutic starvation: a substrate for malignant arrhythmias. Int J Obes 1983; 7:253–261.
104. Weigle DS, Callahan DB, Fellows CL, Greene HL. Preliminary assessment of very low calorie diets by conventional and signal-averaged electrocardiography. Int J Obes 1989; 13:691–697.
105. Moyer CL, Holly RG, Amsterdam EA, Atkinson RL. Effects of cardiac stress during a very-low-calorie diet and exercise program in obese women. Am J Clin Nutr 1989; 50:1324–1327.
106. Linet OI, Butler D, Caswell K, Metzler C, Reele SB. Absence of cardiac arrhythmias during a very-low-calorie diet with high biological quality protein. Int J Obes 1983; 7:313–320.
107. Phinney SD, Bistrian BR, Kosinski E, Chan DP, Hoffer LJ, Rolla A, Schachtel B, Blackburn GL. Normal cardiac rhythm during hypocaloric diets of varying carbohydrate content. Arch Intern Med 1983; 143:2258–2261.
108. Lantigua RA, Amatruda JM, Biddle TL, Forbes GB, Lockwood DH. Cardiac arrhythmias associated with a liquid protein diet for the treatment of obesity. N Engl J Med 1980; 303:735–738.
109. Amatruda JM, Biddle TL, Patton ML, Lockwood DH. Vigorous supplementation of a hypocaloric diet prevents cardiac arrhythmias and mineral depletion. Am J Med 1983; 74:1016–1022.
110. Lowy SL, Fisler JS, Drenick EJ. Zinc and copper nutriture in obese men receiving very low calorie diets of soy or collagen protein. Am J Clin Nutr 1986; 43:272–287.
111. Eckel RH. Obesity and heart disease: a statement for healthcare professionals from the Nutrition Committee, American Heart Association. Circulation 1997; 96:3248–3250.
112. Rauch U, Osende JI, Fuster V, Badimon JJ, Fayad Z, Chesebro JH. Thrombus formation on atherosclerotic plaques: pathogenesis and clinical consequences. Ann Intern Med 2001; 134:224–238.
113. Tracy RP. Is visceral adiposity the "enemy within"? Arterioscler Thromb Vasc Biol 2001; 21:881–883.
114. Tracy RP. Inflammation in cardiovascular disease: cart, horse, or both? Circulation 1998; 97:2000–2002.
115. Ross R. Mechanisms of disease: atherosclerosis—an inflammatory disease. N Engl J Med 1999; 340:115–126.
116. Festa A, D'Agostino R, Williams K, Karter AJ, Mayer-Davis EJ, Tracy RP, Haffner SM. The relation of body fat mass and distribution to markers of chronic inflammation. Int J Obes 2001; 25:1407–1415.
117. Lemieux I, Pascot A, Prud'homme D, Almeras N, Bogaty P, Nadeau A, Bergeron J, Despres JP. Elevated C-reactive protein: another component of the atherothrombotic profile of abdominal obesity. Arterioscler Thromb Vasc Biol 2001; 21:961–967.
118. Mendall MA, Patel P, Ballam L, Strachan D, Northfield TC. C reactive protein and its relation to cardiovascular risk factors: a population based cross sectional study. BMJ 1996; 312:1061–1065.
119. Koenig W, Sund M, Frohlich M, Fischer HG, Lowel H, Doring A, Hutchinson WL, Pepys MB. C-reactive protein, a sensitive marker of inflammation, predicts future risk of coronary heart disease in initially healthy middle-aged men: results from the MONICA (Monitoring Trends and Determinants in Cardiovascular Disease) Augsburg Cohort Study, 1984 to 1992. Circulation 1999; 99:237–242.
120. Yudkin JS, Stehouwer CD, Emeis JJ, Coppack SW. C-reactive protein in healthy subjects: associations with obesity, insulin resistance, and endothelial dysfunction: a potential role for cytokines originating from adipose tissue? Arterioscler Thromb Vasc Biol 1999; 19:972–978.
121. Tracy RP, Psaty BM, Macy E, Bovill EG, Cushman M, Cornell ES, Kuller LH. Lifetime smoking exposure affects the association of C-reactive protein with cardiovascular disease risk factors and subclinical disease in healthy elderly subjects. Arterioscler Thromb Vasc Biol 1997; 17:2167–2176.
122. Ridker PM, Stampfer MJ, Rifai N. Novel risk factors for systemic atherosclerosis: a comparison of C-reactive protein, fibrinogen, homocysteine, lipoprotein(a), and standard cholesterol screening as predictors of peripheral arterial disease. JAMA 2001; 285:2481–2485.
123. Rifai N, Ridker PM. High-sensitivity C-reactive protein: a novel and promising marker of coronary heart disease. Clin Chem 2001; 47:403–411.

124. Yudkin JS, Kumari M, Humphries SE, Mohamed-Ali V. Inflammation, obesity, stress and coronary heart disease: is interleukin-6 the link? Atherosclerosis 2000; 148:209–214.
125. Ridker PM, Rifai N, Stampfer MJ, Hennekens CH. Plasma concentration of interleukin-6 and the risk of future myocardial infarction among apparently healthy men. Circulation 2000; 101:1767–1772.
126. Marckmann P. Dietary treatment of thrombogenic disorders related to the metabolic syndrome. Br J Nutr 2000; 83:S121–S126.
127. De Lorenzo F, Mukherjee M, Kadziola Z, Suleiman S, Kakkar VV. Association of overall adiposity rather than body mass index with lipids and procoagulant factors. Thromb Haemost 1998; 80:603–606.
128. Saito I, Folsom AR, Brancati FL, Duncan BB, Chambless LE, McGovern PG. Nontraditional risk factors for coronary heart disease incidence among persons with diabetes: the Atherosclerosis Risk in Communities (ARIC) Study. Ann Intern Med 2000; 133:81–91.
129. Vambergue A, Rugeri L, Gaveriaux V, Devos P, Martin A, Fermon C, Fontaine P, Jude B. Factor VII, tissue factor pathway inhibitor, and monocyte tissue factor in diabetes mellitus: influence of type of diabetes, obesity index, and age. Thromb Res 2001; 101:367–375.
130. Scarabin PY, Aillaud MF, Amouyel P, Evans A, Luc G, Ferrieres J, Arveiler D, Juhan-Vague I. Associations of fibrinogen, factor VII and PAI-1 with baseline findings among 10,500 male participants in a prospective study of myocardial infarction—the PRIME Study. Prospective Epidemiological Study of Myocardial Infarction. Thromb Haemost 1998; 80:749–756.
131. Benchimol D, Dubroca B, Bernard V, Lavie J, Paviot B, Benchimol H, Couffinhal T, Pillois X, Dartigues J, Bonnet J. Short- and long-term risk factors for sudden death in patients with stable angina. Int J Cardiol 2000; 76:147–156.
132. Rubanyi GM. The role of endothelium in cardiovascular homeostasis and diseases. J Cardiovasc Pharmacol 1993; 22:S1–S14.
133. Tack CJ, Ong MK, Lutterman JA, Smits P. Insulin-induced vasodilatation and endothelial function in obesity/insulin resistance. Effects of troglitazone. Diabetologia 1998; 41:569–576.
134. Watts GF, Herrmann S, Riches FM. Effects of diet and serotonergic agonist on hepatic apolipoprotein B-100 secretion and endothelial function in obese men. Q J Med 2000; 93:153–161.
135. Steinberg HO, Chaker H, Leaming R, Johnson A, Brechtel G, Baron AD. Obesity/insulin resistance is associated with endothelial dysfunction. Implications for the syndrome of insulin resistance. J Clin Invest 1996; 97:2601–2610.
136. Steinberg HO, Paradisi G, Cronin J, Crowde K, Hempfling A, Hook G, Baron AD. Type II diabetes abrogates sex differences in endothelial function in premenopausal women. Circulation 2000; 101:2040–2046.
137. Abdu TA, Elhadd T, Pfeifer M, Clayton RN. Endothelial dysfunction in endocrine disease. Trends Endocrinol Metab 2001; 12:257–265.
138. Al Suwaidi J, Higano ST, Holmes DR Jr, Lennon R, Lerman A. Obesity is independently associated with coronary endothelial dysfunction in patients with normal or mildly diseased coronary arteries. J Am Coll Cardiol 2001; 37:1523–1528.
139. Reed D, Yano K. Predictors of arteriographically defined coronary stenosis in the Honolulu Heart Program. Am J Epidemiol 1991; 134:111–122.
140. Rimm EB, Stampfer MJ, Giovannucci E, Ascherio A, Spiegelman D, Colditz GA, Willett WC. Body size and fat distribution as predictors of coronary heart disease among middle-aged and older US men. Am J Epidemiol 1995; 141:1117–1127.
141. Adams-Campbell LL, Peniston RL, Kim KS, Mensah E. Body mass index and coronary artery disease in African-Americans. Obes Res 1995; 3:215–219.
142. Fitzgerald A, Jarrett R. Body weight and coronary heart disease mortality: an analysis in relation to age and smoking habit. 15 years follow-up data from the Whitehall Study. Int J Obes Relat Metab Disord 1992; 16(2):119.
143. Kuhn FE, Rackley CE. Coronary artery disease in women. Arch Intern Med 1993; 153:2626–2636.
144. Keys A, Aravanis C, Blackburn H, Van Buchem F, Buzina R, Djordjevic B, Fidanza F, Karvonen M, Menotti A, Puddu V, Taylor H. Coronary heart disease: overweight and obesity as risk factors. Ann Intern Med 1972; 77:15–27.
145. Clark LT, Emerole O. Coronary heart disease in African Americans: primary and secondary prevention. Cleve Clin J Med 1995; 62:285–292.
146. Caralis PV. Coronary heart disease in Hispanic Americans: how does ethnic background affect risk factors and mortality rates? Postgrad Med 1992; 91:179–188.
147. Howard BV, Lee ET, Cowan LD, Fabsitz RR, Howard WJ, Oopik AJ, Robbins DC, Savage PJ, Yeh JL, Welty TK. Coronary heart disease prevalence and its relation to risk factors in American Indians: the Strong Heart Study. Am J Epidemiol 1995; 142:254–268.
148. Robertson TL, Kato H, Rhoads GG. Epidemiologic studies of coronary heart disease and stroke in Japanese men living in Japan, Hawaii and California: incidence of myocardial infarction and death from coronary heart disease. Am J Cardiol 1977; 39:239–243.
149. Wilson PWF. Established risk factors and coronary artery disease: the Framingham Study. Am J Hypertens 1994; 7:7S–12S.
150. Keil JE, Sutherland SE, Knapp RG, Lackland DT, Gazes PC, Tyroler H. Mortality rates and risk factors

for coronary disease in black as compared with white men and women. N Engl J Med 193; 329:73–78.
151. Barrett-Connor E. Obesity, atherosclerosis, and coronary artery disease. Ann Intern Med 1985; 103:1010–1019.
152. Clark L, Karve M, Rones K, Chang-DeMoranville B, Atluri S, Feldman J. Obesity, distribution of body fat and coronary artery disease in black women. Am J Cardiol 1994; 73:895–896.
153. Kannel WB, Neaton JD, Wentworth D, Thomas HE, Stamler J, Hulley SB, Kjelsberg MO. Overall and coronary heart disease mortality rates in relation to major risk factors in 325,348 men screened for the MRFIT. Am Heart J 1986; 112:825–836.
154. Harris TB, Ballard-Barbasch R, Madans J, Makuc DM, Feldman JJ. Overweight, weight loss, and risk of coronary heart disease in older women. Am J Epidemiol 1993; 137:1318–1327.
155. Manson JE, Colditz GA, Stampfer MJ, Willett WC, Rosner B, Monson RR, Speizer FE, Hennekens CH. A prospective study of obesity and risk of coronary heart disease in women. N Engl J Med 1990; 322:882–889.
156. Manson JE, Willett WC, Stampfer MI, Colditz GA, Hunter DI, Hankanson SE, Henneken CE, Speizer FE. Body weight and mortality among women. N Engl J Med 1995; 333:667–685.
157. Conway G, Agrawal R, Betteridge D, Jacobs H. Risk factors for coronary artery disease in lean and obese women with the polycystic ovary syndrome. Clin Endocrinol 1992; 37:119–125.
158. Folsom AR, Stevens J, Schreiner PJ, McGovern PG. Body mass index, waist/hip ratio, and coronary heart disease incidence in African Americans and whites. Atherosclerosis Risk in Communities study investigators. Am J Epidemiol 1998; 148:1187–1194.
159. Morricone L, Ferrari M, Enrini R, Inglese L, Giardini D, Garancini P, Caviezel F. The role of central fat distribution in coronary artery disease in obesity: comparison of nondiabetic obese, diabetic obese, and normal weight subjects. Int J Obes 1999; 23:1129–1135.
160. Freedman DS, Williamson DF, Croft JB, Ballew C, Byers T. Relation of body fat distribution to ischemic disease: the National Health and Nutrition Examination Survey I (NHANES I) epidemiologic follow-up study. Am J Epidemiol 1995; 142:53–63.
161. Must A, Jaques PF, Dallal GE, Bajema CJ, Dietz WH. Long-term mobidity and mortality of overweight adolescents. A follow-up of the Harvard Growth Study of 1922 to 1935. N Engl J Med 1992; 327:1350–1355.
162. Pearson TA, Derby CA. Invited commentary: should arteriographic case-control studies be used to identify causes of atherosclerotic coronary artery disease?. Am J Epidemiol 1991; 134:123–128.
163. Stern M. Epidemiology of obesity and its link to heart disease. Metabolism 1995; 44:1–3.
164. Kannel W, D'Agostino R, Cobb J. Effect of weight on cardiovascular disease. Am J Clin Nutr 1996; 63(suppl): 419S–422S.
165. Calle EE, Thun MJ, Petrelli JM, Rodriguez C, Heath CW Jr. Body-mass index and mortality in a prospective cohort of U.S. adults. N Engl J Med 1999; 341:1097–1105.
166. Lapidus L, Bengtsson C, Larson B, Pennert B, Rybo E, Sjostrom L. Distribution of adipose tissue and risk of cardiovascular disease and death: a 12 year follow up of participants in the populations study of women in Gothenburg, Sweden. BMJ 1984; 289:1257–1260.
167. Terry RB, Page WF, Haskell WL. Waist/hip ratio, body mass index and premature cardiovascular disease mortality in US Army veterans during a twenty-three year follow-up study. Int J Obes 1992; 16:417–423.
168. Rexrode KM, Carey VJ, Hennekens CH, Walters EE, Colditz GA, Stampfer MJ, Willett WC, Manson JE. Abdominal adiposity and coronary heart disease in women. JAMA 1998; 280:1843–1848.
169. Folsom AR, Kushi LH, Anderson KE, Mink PJ, Olson JE, Hong CP, Sellers TA, Lazovich D, Prineas RJ. Associations of general and abdominal obesity with multiple health outcomes in older women: the Iowa Women's Health Study. Arch Intern Med 2000; 160:2117–2128.
170. Coleman MP, Key TJA, Wang DY, Hermon C, Fentiman IS, Allen DS, Jarvis M, Pike MC, Sanders TAB. A prospective study of obesity, lipids, apolipoproteins and ischaemic disease in women. Atherosclerosis 1992; 92:177–185.
171. Rabkin SW, Mathewson FA, Hsu PH. Relation of body weight to development of ischemic heart disease in a cohort of young North American men after a 26 year observation period: the Manitoba Study. Am J Cardiol 1977; 39:452–458.
172. Kumanyika S. Searching for the association of obesity with coronary artery disease. Obes Res 1995; 3:273–275.
173. Kumanyika SK. Special issues regarding obesity in minority populations. Ann Intern Med 1993; 119:650–654.
174. Stern M, Patterson J, Mitchell B, Haffner S, Hazuda H. Overweight and mortality in Mexican-Americans. Int J Obes 1990; 14:623–629.
175. Welty TK, Lee ET, Yeh J, Cowan LD, Go O, Fabsitz RR, Le NA, Oopik AJ, Robbins DC, Howard BV. Cardiovascular disease risk factors among American Indians: the Strong Heart Study. Am J Epidemiol 1995; 142:269–287.
176. Hansen C, Woodhouse S, Kramer M. Effect of patient obesity on the accuracy of thallium-201 myocardial perfusion imaging. Am J Cardiol 2000; 85:749–754.
177. Schwann TA, Habib RH, Zacharias A, Parenteau GL, Riordan CJ, Durham SJ, Engoren M. Effects of body size on operative, intermediate, and long-term outcomes after coronary artery bypass operation. Ann Thorac Surg 2001; 71:521–530.

178. Allen KB, Heimansohn DA, Robison RJ, Schier JJ, Griffith GL, Fitzgerald EB, Isch JH, Abraham S, Shaar CJ. Risk factors for leg wound complications following endoscopic versus traditional saphenous vein harvesting. Heart Surg Forum 2000; 3:325–330.
179. Weiss YG, Merin G, Koganov E, Ribo A, Oppenheim-Eden A, Medalion B, Peruanski M, Reider E, Bar-Ziv J, Hanson WC, Pizov R. Postcardiopulmonary bypass hypoxemia: a prospective study on incidence, risk factors, and clinical significance. J Cardiovasc Vasc Anesth 2000; 14:506–513.
180. Yamagishi T, Ishikawa S, Ohtaki A, Takahashi T, Ohki S, Morishita Y. Obesity and postoperative oxygenation after coronary artery bypass grafting. Jpn J Thorac Cardiovasc Surg 2000; 48:632–636.
181. Kurki TS, Kataja M. Preoperative prediction of postoperative morbidity in coronary artery bypass grafting. Ann Thorac Surg 1996; 61:1740–1745.
182. Sabourin CB, Funk M. Readmission of patients after coronary artery bypass graft surgery. Heart Lung 1999; 28:243–250.
183. Rexrode KM, Hennekens CH, Willett WC, Colditz GA, Stampfer MJ, Rich-Edwards JW, Speizer FE, Manson JE. A prospective study of body mass index, weight change, and risk of stroke in women. JAMA 1997; 277:1539–1545.
184. Bronner LL, Kanter DS, Manson JE. Primary prevention of stroke. N Engl J Med 1995; 333:1392–1400.
185. Welin L, Svardsudd K, Wilhelmsen L, Larsson B, Tibblin G. Analysis of risk factors for stroke in a cohort of men born in 1913. N Engl J Med 1987; 317:521–526.
186. Mavri A, Stegnar M, Sentocnik JT, Videcnik V. Impact of weight reduction on early carotid atherosclerosis in obese premenopausal women. Obes Res 2001; 9:511–516.
187. Lakka TA, Lakka HM, Salonen R, Kaplan GA, Salonen JT. Abdominal obesity is associated with accelerated progression of carotid atherosclerosis in men. Atherosclerosis 2001; 154:497–504.
188. Karason K, Wikstrand J, Sjostrom L, Wendelhag I. Weight loss and progression of early atherosclerosis in the carotid artery: a four-year controlled study of obese subjects. Int J Obes 1999; 23:948–956.
189. Gillum RF. Risk factors for stroke in blacks: a critical review. Am J Epidemiol 1999; 150:1266–1274.
190. Pyorala M, Miettinen H, Laakso M, Pyorala K. Hyperinsulinemia and the risk of stroke in healthy middle-aged men: the 22-year follow-up results of the Helsinki Policemen Study. Stroke 1998; 29:1860–1866.
191. Du X, McNamee R, Cruickshank K. Stroke risk from multiple risk factors combined with hypertension: a primary care based case-control study in a defined population of northwest England. Ann Epidemiol 2000; 10:380–388.
192. Temelkova-Kurktschiev T, Koehler C, Schaper F, Henkel E, Hahnefeld A, Fuecker K, Siegert G, Hanefeld M. Relationship between fasting plasma glucose, atherosclerosis risk factors and carotid intima media thickness in non-diabetic individuals. Diabetologia 1998; 41:706–712.
193. Mainard F, Auget JL, Vest P, Madec Y. Comparative study of risk factors in patients undergoing coronary or femoropopliteal artery bypass grafting. Br Heart J 1994; 72:542–547.
194. Gofin R, Kark JD, Friedlander Y, Lewis BS, Witt H, Stein Y, Gotsman MS. Peripheral vascular disease in a middle-aged population sample. The Jerusalem Lipid Research Clinic Prevalence Study. Isr J Med Sci 1987; 23:157–167.
195. Ness J, Aronow WS, Ahn C. Risk factors for symptomatic peripheral arterial disease in older persons in an academic hospital-based geriatrics practice. J Am Geriatr Soc 2000; 48:312–314.
196. Giltay EJ, Lambert J, Elbers JM, Gooren LJ, Asscheman H, Stehouwer CD. Arterial compliance and distensibility are modulated by body composition in both men and women but by insulin sensitivity only in women. Diabetologia 1999; 42:214–221.
197. Gariepy J, Salomon J, Denarie N, Laskri F, Megnien JL, Levenson J, Simon A. Sex and topographic differences in associations between large-artery wall thickness and coronary risk profile in a French working cohort: the AXA Study. Arterioscler Thromb Vasc Biol 1998; 18:584–590.
198. Plavnik FL, Ajzen S, Kohlmann O Jr, Tavares A, Zanella MT, Ribeiro AB, Ramos OL. Intima-media thickness evaluation by B-mode ultrasound. Correlation with blood pressure levels and cardiac structures. Brazil J Med Biol Res 2000; 33:55–64.
199. MacMahon SW, Macdonald GJ, Bernstein L, Andrews G, Blacket RB. A randomized controlled trial of weight reduction and metoprolol in the treatment of hypertension in young overweight patients. Clin Exp Pharmacol Physiol 1985; 12:267–271.
200. Stevens VJ, Obarzanek E, Cook NR, Lee IM, Appel LJ, Smith West D, Milas NC, Mattfeldt-Beman M, Belden L, Bragg C, Millstone M, Raczynski J, Brewer A, Singh B, Cohen J. Long-term weight loss and changes in blood pressure: results of the Trials of Hypertension Prevention, phase II. Ann Intern Med 2001; 134:1–11.
201. Kelley D. Effects of weight loss on glucose homeostasis in NIDDM. Diabetes Rev 1995; 3:366–377.
202. Letiexhe MR, Scheen AJ, Gerard PL, Desaive C, Lefebvre PJ. Insulin secretion, clearance and action before and after gastroplasty in severely obese subjects. Int J Obes 1994; 18:295–300.
203. Marckmann P, Toubro S, Astrup A. Sustained improvement in blood lipids, coagulation, and fibrinolysis after major weight loss in obese subjects. Eur J Clin Nutr 1998; 52:329–333.
204. Rissanen P. Weight change and blood coagulability and

fibrinolysis in healthy obese women. Int J Obes 2001; 25:212–218.
205. Heilbronn LK, Noakes M, Clifton PM. Energy restriction and weight loss on very-low-fat diets reduce C-reactive protein concentrations in obese, healthy women. Arterioscler Thromb Vasc Biol 2001; 21:968–970.
206. Williamson DF, Pamuk ER. The association between weight loss and increased longevity. A review of the evidence. Ann Intern Med 1993; 119:731–736.
207. French SA, Folsom AR, Jeffery RW, Williamson DF. Prospective study of intentionality of weight loss and mortality in older women: the Iowa Women's Health Study. Am J Epidemiol 1999; 149:504–514.
208. Williamson DF, Thompson TJ, Thun M, Flanders D, Pamuk E, Byers T. Intentional weight loss and mortality among overweight individuals with diabetes. Diabetes Care 2000; 23:1499–1504.
209. Kuller LH. Invited commentary on "Prospective study of intentionality of weight loss and mortality in older women: the Iowa Women's Health Study" and "Prospective study of intentional weight loss and mortality in overweight white men aged 40–64 years". Am J Epidemiol 1999; 149:515–516.
210. Connolly HM, Crary JL, McGoon D, Hensrud DD, Edwards BS, Schaff HV. Valvular heart disease associated with fenfluramine-phentermine. N Engl J Med 1997; 337:581–588.
211. Graham DJ, Green L. Further cases of valvular heart disease associated with fenfluramine-phentermine. N Engl J Med 1997; 337:635.
212. Cannistra LB, Davis SM, Bauman AG. Valvular heart disease associated with dexfenfluramine. N Engl J Med 1997; 337:636.
213. Cardiac valvulopathy associated with exposure to fenfluramine or dexfenfluramine: U.S. Department of Health and Human Services interim public health recommendations, November 1997. MMWR 1997; 46: 1061–1066.
214. Weissman NJ, Tighe JF Jr, Gottdiener JS, Gwynne JT. An assessment of heart-valve abnormalities in obese patients taking dexfenfluramine, sustained-release dexfenfluramine, or placebo. Sustained-Release Dexfenfluramine Study Group. N Engl J Med 1998; 339:725–732.
215. Davidoff R, McTiernan A, Constantine G, Davis KD, Balady GJ, Mendes LA, Rudolph RE, Bowen DJ. Echocardiographic examination of women previously treated with fenfluramine: long-term follow-up of a randomized, double-blind, placebo-controlled trial. Arch Intern Med 2001; 161:1429–1436.
216. Wee CC, Phillips RS, Aurigemma G, Erban S, Kriegel G, Riley M, Douglas PS. Risk for valvular heart disease among users of fenfluramine and dexfenfluramine who underwent echocardiography before use of medication. Ann Intern Med 1998; 129:870–874.
217. Gardin JM, Schumacher D, Constantine G, Davis KD, Leung C, Reid CL. Valvular abnormalities and cardiovascular status following exposure to dexfenfluramine or phentermine/fenfluramine. JAMA 2000; 283:1703–1709.
218. Shively BK, Roldan CA, Gill EA, Najarian T, Loar SB. Prevalence and determinants of valvulopathy in patients treated with dexfenfluramine. Circulation 1999; 100:2161–2167.
219. Burger AJ, Sherman HB, Charlamb MJ, Kim J, Asinas LA, Flickner SR, Blackburn GL. Low prevalence of valvular heart disease in 226 phentermine-fenfluramine protocol subjects prospectively followed for up to 30 months. J Am Coll Cardiol 1999; 34:1153–1158.
220. Jollis JG, Landolfo CK, Kisslo J, Constantine GD, Davis KD, Ryan T. Fenfluramine and phentermine and cardiovascular findings: effect of treatment duration on prevalence of valve abnormalities. Circulation 2000; 101:2071–2077.
221. Kancherla MK, Salti HI, Mulderink TA, Parker M, Bonow RO, Mehlman DJ. Echocardiographic prevalence of mitral and/or aortic regurgitation in patients exposed to either fenfluramine-phentermine combination or to dexfenfluramine. Am J Cardiol 1999; 84:1335–1338.
222. Ryan DH, Bray GA, Helmcke F, Sander G, Volaufova J, Greenway F, Subramaniam P, Glancy DL. Serial echocardiographic and clinical evaluation of valvular regurgitation before, during, and after treatment with fenfluramine or dexfenfluramine and mazindol or phentermine. Obes Res 1999; 7:313–322.
223. Ristow M, Muller-Wieland D, Pfeiffer A, Krone W, Kahn R. Obesity associated with a mutation in a genetic regulator of adipocyte differentiation. N Engl J Med 1998; 339:953–959.
224. Hensrud DD, Connolly HM, Grogan M, Miller FA, Bailey KR, Jensen MD. Echocardiographic improvement over time after cessation of use of fenfluramine and phentermine. Mayo Clin Proc 1999; 74:1191–1197.
225. Lepor NE, Gross SB, Daley WL, Samuels BA, Rizzo MJ, Luko SP, Hickey A, Buchbinder NA, Naqvi TZ. Dose and duration of fenfluramine-phentermine therapy impacts the risk of significant valvular heart disease. Am J Cardiol 2000; 86:107–110.
226. Teramae CY, Connolly HM, Grogan M, Miller FA Jr. Diet drug-related cardiac valve disease: the Mayo Clinic echocardiographic laboratory experience. Mayo Clin Proc 2000; 75:456–461.
227. Jick H, Vasilakis C, Weinrauch LA, Meier CR, Jick SS, Derby LE. A population-based study of appetite-suppressant drugs and the risk of cardiac-valve regurgitation. N Engl J Med 1998; 339:719–724.
228. Li R, Serdula MK, Williamson DF, Bowman BA, Graham DJ, Green L. Dose-effect of fenfluramine use on the severity of valvular heart disease among fen-phen patients with valvulopathy. Int J Obes 1999; 23:926–928.

229. Khan MA, Herzog CA, St Peter JV, Hartley GG, Madlon-Kay R, Dick CD, Asinger RW, Vessey JT. The prevalence of cardiac valvular insufficiency assessed by transthoracic echocardiography in obese patients treated with appetite-suppressant drugs. N Engl J Med 1998; 339:713–718.
230. Weissman NJ, Panza JA, Tighe JF, Gwynne JT. Natural history of valvular regurgitation 1 year after discontinuation of dexfenfluramine therapy. A randomized, double-blind, placebo-controlled trial. Ann Intern Med 2001; 134:267–273.
231. Mast ST, Jollis JG, Ryan T, Anstrom KJ, Crary JL. The progression of fenfluramine-associated valvular heart disease assessed by echocardiography. Ann Intern Med 2001; 134:261–266.
232. Raeini-Sarjaz M, Vanstone CA, Papamandjaris AA, Wykes LJ, Jones PJ. Comparison of the effect of dietary fat restriction with that of energy restriction on human lipid metabolism. Am J Clin Nutr 2001; 73:262–267.
233. Bach DS, Rissanen AM, Mendel CM, Shepherd G, Weinstein SP, Kelly F, Seaton TB, Patel B, Pekkarinen TA, Armstrong WF. Absence of cardiac valve dysfunction in obese patients treated with sibutramine. Obes Res 1999; 7:363–369.
234. Griffen L, Anchors M. The "phen-pro" diet drug combination is not associated with valvular heart disease. Arch Intern Med 1998; 158:1278–1279.
235. Kernan WN, Viscoli CM, Brass LM, Broderick JP, Brott T, Feldmann E, Morgenstern LB, Wilterdink JL, Horwitz RI. Phenylpropanolamine and the risk of hemorrhagic stroke. N Engl J Med 2000; 343:1826–1832.
236. Haller CA, Benowitz NL. Adverse cardiovascular and central nervous system events associated with dietary supplements containing ephedra alkaloids. N Engl J Med 2000; 343:1833–1838.
237. Ang-Lee MK, Moss J, Yuan CS. Herbal medicines and perioperative care. JAMA 2001; 286:208–216.
238. Messerli FH. Cardiovascular effects of obesity. Lancet 1982; 1:1165–1168.

35

Obesity and Lipoprotein Metabolism

Jean-Pierre Després

Quebec Heart Institute, Laval Hospital Research Center, Laval University, Sainte-Foy, Quebec, Canada

Ronald M. Krauss

Children's Hospital Oakland Research Institute, Oakland, Lawrence Berkeley National Laboratory, and University of California, Berkeley, Berkeley, California, U.S.A.

I DYSLIPIDEMIC PHENOTYPES IN CORONARY HEART DISEASE: BEYOND CHOLESTEROL

The measurement of plasma lipid levels is now commonly used to assess the risk of coronary heart disease (CHD). Several epidemiological studies have shown that there is a significant positive relationship between blood cholesterol levels and deaths associated with CHD (1–3). In the Multiple Risk Factor Intervention Trial (MRFIT), Stamler et al. (4) showed that in a sample of 356,222 male subjects, increased blood cholesterol levels were associated with a progressive increase in CHD mortality. However, despite the fact that numerous studies have shown this relationship, Genest et al. (5) have reported that nearly 50% of patients having ischemic heart disease (IHD) have plasma cholesterol levels equal to or even lower than those of healthy subjects.

Accordingly, Sniderman and Silberberg (6) emphasized that although the mean blood cholesterol concentration in CHD patients is generally significantly higher than that of healthy subjects, there is a considerable overlap between CHD patients and healthy subjects. Thus, the clinical value of total cholesterol measurement alone is of limited use in distinguishing CHD patients from healthy subjects. It was therefore suggested that additional determinations of blood lipid variables were needed to more accurately assess risk.

Plasma cholesterol is a hydrophobic compound and is transported in the blood by lipoproteins. Lipoproteins vary in size, composition, and density, and four main families can be identified: chylomicrons, very low-density lipoproteins (VLDL), low-density lipoproteins (LDL), and high-density lipoproteins (HDL) (Fig. 1). Chylomicrons are large particles found after a meal which are responsible for the transport of alimentary lipids. They are generally absent from the fasting plasma of healthy subjects. Triglyceride (TG) and cholesterol molecules of hepatic origin are secreted in VLDL particles which are converted to LDL following hydrolysis by the enzyme lipoprotein lipase (LPL). During the hydrolysis of chylomicrons and VLDL, excess surface component aggregates to form nascent HDL particles. Additional newly formed and immature HDL particles originate from the intestine and the liver.

A LDL Cholesterol: A Major Culprit in CHD

Numerous prospective studies that have measured cholesterol in the lipoprotein fractions (VLDL, LDL, and HDL) have reported highly significant associations

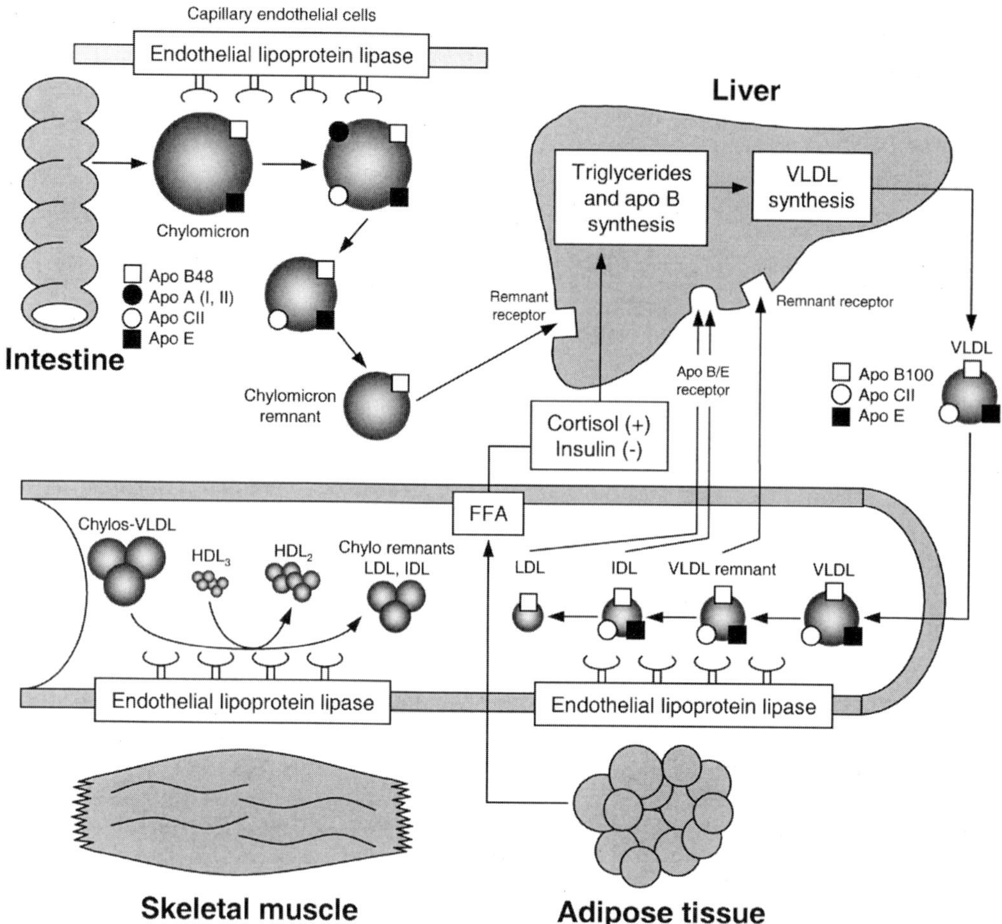

Figure 1 Simplified overview of lipoprotein metabolism. After hydrolysis of dietary triglycerides by intestinal lipase and their secretion in the lymph as chylomicrons (containing dietary cholesterol, triglycerides, phospholipids, apolipoprotein [apo] B48, and apo AI, AII, and AIV), these nascent particles acquire apo C and E in the circulation. The chylomicron binds to the enzyme lipoprotein lipase located on the surface of the endothelial cells of several tissues, including adipose tissue and skeletal muscle. This process allows the transfer of excess surface components (apo AI, AII, and AIV, of the C apolipoproteins and of phospholipids) to HDL. The chylomicron remnant particle is then cleared from the circulation via the hepatic apo E (remnant) receptor. The first step of chylomicron catabolism which involves hydrolysis by endothelial lipoprotein lipase appears to be modulated by numerous hormonal and metabolic factors. The second step, which involves the clearance of chylomicron remnants by hepatocytes, does not seem to be under close hormonal or metabolic control. Endogenous lipids are secreted by the liver as VLDL particles. Availability of lipids appears to determine the fate of constitutively synthesized apo B100 and will protect apo B against its degradation. Insulin and cortisol also seem to be important modulators of VLDL secretion via indirect (substrate availability) and direct (apo B synthesis) effects. Apo B is synthesized on ribosomes of the rough endoplasmic reticulum and associates with lipids in its smooth surface end. The nascent VLDL particle is then transported to the Golgi. Particles are packed in secretion vesicles and then secreted. VLDL particles will acquire additional apolipoproteins in the circulation. With the action of endothelial lipoprotein lipase, VLDL will be hydrolyzed into VLDL remnants, intermediate-density lipoproteins (IDL) and finally, into LDL. About 50% of the particles will be cleared as IDL by the apo B/E receptor; the others will be eliminated by extrahepatic and hepatic apo B/E receptors as LDL particles. Nascent HDL particles have multiple origins (gut, liver, plasma). However, considerable evidence suggests that hydrolysis of triglyceride-rich lipoproteins (chylomicrons and VLDL) is a major process by which excess surface components are transferred from triglyceride-rich lipoproteins to nascent HDL particles. Thus, the more efficient the hydrolysis of triglyceride-rich lipoproteins, the higher the lipoprotein lipase activity in the postheparin plasma and the higher the plasma HDL concentrations, especially the HDL_2 subfraction.

between plasma LDL cholesterol levels and the risk of CHD (4,7–10). Furthermore, with the development of HMG-CoA reductase inhibitors (statins), clinicians now have access to powerful tools to significantly lower LDL cholesterol concentrations with associated clinical benefits. Primary and secondary prevention trials have shown that LDL cholesterol lowering can reduce the risk of a first or recurrent CHD event by ~30% (11–16). Thus, the development of statins has been a remarkable breakthrough allowing clinicians to better manage CHD risk. However, these findings are of little help for the remaining 70% of statin-treated patients who remained at risk for CHD despite being treated with a LDL cholesterol–lowering drug. Furthermore, as for total cholesterol, prospective and cross-sectional studies have shown that there is a considerable overlap in the distribution of LDL cholesterol levels between CHD patients and asymptomatic individuals (5,17,18). Thus, other variables (established risk factors and other metabolic markers of CHD risk) need to be considered to refine our assessment of CHD risk.

Among those additional risk factors, several prospective studies have shown that when low HDL cholesterol is reduced, there is an increased risk of CHD and of related mortality (17,19–21). In both men and women, plasma HDL cholesterol has been inversely related to the incidence of CHD, and this relationship has been reported to be largely independent of other parameters of the lipid profile (22). These data support the notion that low HDL cholesterol levels increase CHD risk. It thus seems reasonable to assume that an intervention resulting in an increase in HDL cholesterol levels could decrease the incidence of IHD.

This hypothesis was recently tested in the Veterans Affairs High-Density Lipoprotein Intervention Trial (VA-HIT), which examined the effect of a HDL cholesterol–raising therapy using a fibrate (gemfibrozil) in a sample of middle-aged men with documented CHD who were recruited on the basis of their low HDL cholesterol levels (23). Over 5 years, fibrate therapy reduced the risk of a recurrent CHD event by 22% in the absence of any LDL cholesterol–lowering effect of gemfibrozil (23). These results confirmed that HDL cholesterol raising with fibrate therapy was relevant for the secondary prevention of CHD in patients with low HDL cholesterol levels. These results are also consistent with results from transgenic animal models which have shown that the overexpression of genes modulating HDL levels (AI, AII, etc.) resulted in a slower progression of atherosclerosis (24).

In this regard, it is also important to emphasize that patients who have low HDL cholesterol levels also frequently have elevated TG concentrations. Results of some, but not all, prospective epidemiological studies have indicated that an elevated TG concentration did not constitute an independent risk factor for CHD when statistical corrections were made for other lipoprotein or lipid variables such as HDL cholesterol (25). However, results of the PROCAM (Prospective Cardiovascular Munster) study (8), the Helsinki Heart Study (26), and the Copenhagen Male Study (27) have all shown that the presence of low HDL cholesterol levels accompanied by hypertriglyceridemia was predictive of the highest risk of CHD. Consequently, a low plasma HDL cholesterol concentration must be given special attention by the clinician, particularly when it is accompanied by elevated TG levels.

Mechanisms have been proposed in order to explain the protective effect of HDL in CHD. HDL cholesterol has been suggested to be involved in the reverse cholesterol transport, a concept introduced by Glomset (28) in the late 1960s and considerably expanded upon since the identification of the ABC-1 (adenosise triphosphate-binding cassette transporter-1) and of the SR-B1/CLA receptors (Fig. 2), which have allowed a better understanding of how free cholesterol may leave cells such as macrophages through the ABC-1 receptor, be transported by HDL, and be transferred back to the liver through the interaction of HDL with a docking receptor SR-B1/CLA-1 (29,30). There is also evidence that HDL particles can have anti-inflammatory and antioxidative properties that may contribute to atherosclerosis protection (31).

Another model suggests that the presence of high plasma HDL cholesterol levels could be indicative of effective catabolism of TG-rich lipoproteins. As shown in Figure 3, the rapid breakdown of chylomicrons and VLDL by the action of the enzyme LPL could lead to an increase in the production of HDL, more specifically, the HDL_2 subfraction, which seems to be particularly abundant when LPL activity is high. Consequently, the role of LPL in the breakdown of TG-rich lipoproteins and the production of HDL could contribute to explain the well-established inverse relationship existing between plasma TG and HDL cholesterol concentrations.

Moreover, lipid transfer proteins found in plasma allow the exchange of lipids between different lipoprotein fractions. In fact, one of these transfer proteins, cholesteryl ester transfer protein (CETP), favors the exchange of the TGs found in TG-rich lipoproteins for HDL cholesteryl esters, resulting in the depletion of cholesterol in HDL particles. In addition, and as mentioned previously, a low LPL activity contributes

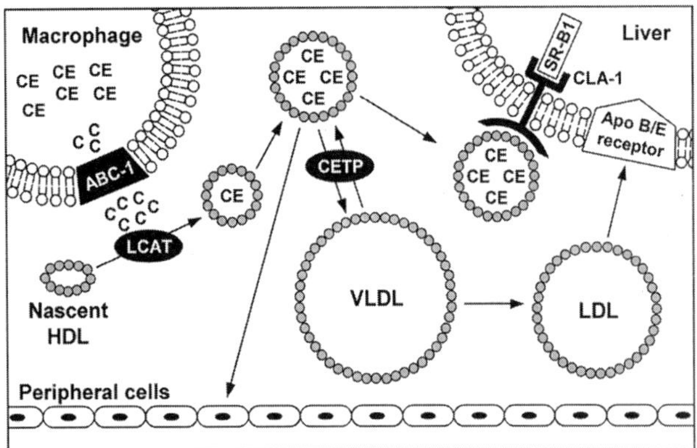

Figure 2 The role of adenosine triphosphate-binding cassette transporter (ABC-1) and of CLA-1 docking protein in cellular cholesterol efflux and of the scavenger receptor class B type 1 (SR-B1) in reverse cholesterol transport. Free cholesterol (C) may be eliminated from cells such as macrophages through a process mediated by the ABC-1 receptor. After esterification of this free cholesterol by the enzyme lecithin-cholesterol acyl transferase (LCAT), this esterified cholesterol (CE) contained in maturing HDL particles will be transported back to the liver and selectively taken up by hepatocytes through the interaction with a docking receptor SR-B1/CLA-1. Apo: apolipoprotein; CETP: cholesteryl ester transfer protein.

to a decreased production of HDL precursors originating from the aggregation of an excessive number of surface components released by the hydrolysis of VLDL and chylomicrons. In this regard, we further examined the metabolic heterogeneity underlying low HDL cholesterol levels (32). We found that individuals with low HDL cholesterol but normal TG levels did not show elevated plasma insulin levels either in the fasting state or in response to an oral glucose challenge. We also found that isolated hypertriglyceridemia was not associated with increased plasma insulin levels. However, the combination of low HDL cholesterol and of moderately elevated TG concentrations was associated with a considerable and significant increase in plasma insulin concentrations measured in the fasting state and in response to the oral glucose load, suggesting that this specific dyslipidemic state was particularly related to hyperinsulinemia stemming from resistance of tissues to insulin.

In the PROCAM Study conducted in Munster, Germany (27), and in the Helsinki Heart Study (26) the combination of high TG and low HDL cholesterol levels was associated with a significant increase in the risk of CHD and a high percentage of coronary events were specifically related to this dyslipidemia. For instance, among individuals of the PROCAM study whose TG and HDL cholesterol levels were >200 mg/dL and <35 mg/dL, respectively, the incidence of coronary events observed over a 6-year period was 5.3-fold higher (128 cases/1000 people) than among subjects with a normal lipid profile (24 cases/1000 people) (27). Consequently, this dyslipidemic profile (including hypertriglyceridemia and hypoalphalipoproteinemia) associated with hyperinsulinemia secondary to insulin resistance significantly increases the risk of CHD among individuals with this cluster of metabolic abnormalities.

Dr. Gerald Reaven (33) was the first to suggest the term "insulin resistance syndrome" to describe a cluster of metabolic abnormalities that includes hypoalphalipoproteinemia, hypertriglyceridemia, hyperinsulinemia, and increased blood pressure. To measure the sensitivity to insulin, Dr. Reaven used the euglycemic-hyperinsulinemic clamp in about 100 normal subjects as well as in glucose intolerant and type 2 diabetic patients (33). In this technique, a certain amount of insulin is

1. Increased lipid exchange due to CETP

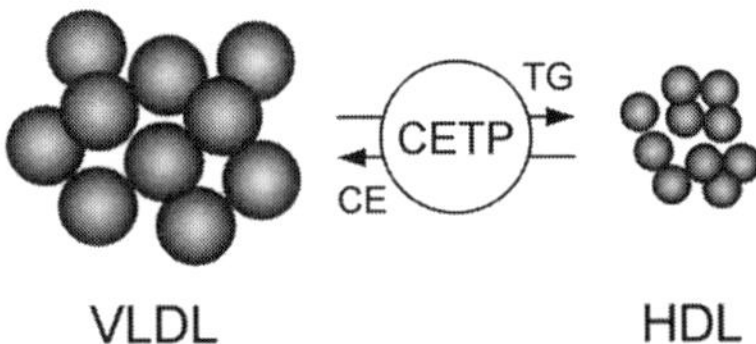

2. Low LPL activity

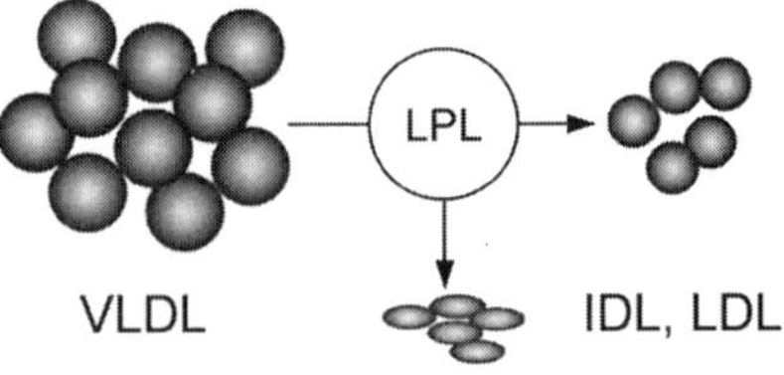

Figure 3 (1) Lipid transfer proteins contribute to the exchange of lipids between the various lipoproteins. In this case, cholesteryl ester transfer protein (CETP) allows the exchange of triglyceride (TG) from TG-rich lipoproteins for cholesteryl esters of the HDL fractions, which ultimately leads to a reduced cholesterol content of HDL particles. (2) A low lipoprotein lipase (LPL) activity contributes to a reduced production of nascent HDL particles originating from excess surface components following the hydrolysis of VLDL particles.

infused in order to induce hyperinsulinemia to a predetermined level. Obviously, the rate at which blood sugar levels drop varies if there is no simultaneous infusion of glucose. The greater the sensitivity to insulin, the faster the blood glucose levels fall, and the higher the quantity of glucose needed to maintain euglycemia. Consequently, the sensitivity to insulin, or the M value, corresponds to the amount of glucose required to maintain a normal blood glucose level under a standardized hyperinsulinemic state and this value is expressed in milligrams of glucose infused per kilogram body weigh per minute.

Reaven and colleagues (33) next subdivided the group of 100 nondiabetic subjects according to fasting insulin concentrations. The first quartile comprised individuals with the highest blood insulin levels; the fourth, individuals with the lowest. Within these four groups, considerable differences were observed in terms of in vivo sensitivity to insulin. Subjects of the lowest insulin quartile were very sensitive to insulin (M value >300), whereas subjects of the highest insulin quartile were clearly insulin resistant (M value barely above 100). Two critically important observations were made. Firstly, considerable differences in terms of sensitivity to insulin were found even among individuals with normal glucose tolerance. Furthermore, in 25% of normal individuals, the magnitude of the insulin resistant state was similar to that found among glucose-intolerant individuals or type 2 diabetic patients. Consequently, Reaven concluded that insulin resistance is prevalent in our population since 25% of nondiabetic subjects seem to have this characteristic.

There is considerable evidence indicating that insulin resistance is associated with a pro-atherogenic dyslipidemic state (34,35). Considering the recently confirmed high prevalence of insulin resistance for which the cluster of metabolic abnormalities has been defined as the "metabolic syndrome" in the recent National Cholesterol Education Program Adult Treatment Panel III (NCEP-ATP III) guidelines (36), this condition is likely to represent the most common cause of dyslipidemic states found in CHD patients (37,38).

B "Normal" LDL Cholesterol Levels in Patients with Metabolic Syndrome: Potentially Misleading Information?

Plasma LDL cholesterol levels are frequently within the normal range in patients with high TG and low HDL cholesterol concentrations and showing the features of the metabolic syndrome (17,33). However, other techniques have made it possible to conclude that this form of dyslipidemia related to insulin resistance is frequently associated with high levels of apo B (the apolipoprotein of LDL) in the presence of a relatively normal LDL cholesterol value, suggesting the presence of a greater number of LDL particles relatively depleted in cholesteryl esters. Additional analytical techniques that have used gradient gel electrophoresis to separate LDL on the basis of size have helped confirm the fact that the high TG/low HDL cholesterol dyslipidemia is associated with an increased proportion of small, dense LDL particles (39–41).

In this regard, Austin et al. (41) suggested that more than 80% of individuals characterized by a low proportion of dense LDL (phenotype A), have TG levels <92 mg/dL (1.05 mM). Consequently, it could be possible, on the basis of fasting TG concentrations, to identify a fairly large percentage of individuals with an increased proportion of dense LDL particles (phenotype B). Furthermore, >50% of patients with elevated apo B levels could also be characterized by an atherogenic phenotype that would include hypertriglyceridemia, hypoalphalipoproteinemia, and an increased proportion of smaller and denser LDL particles (41). It is appropriate to emphasize that this atherogenic phenotype is frequently observed in CHD patients with nearly normal plasma cholesterol or LDL cholesterol concentrations (37,41).

From a clinical perspective, it is interesting to note that the atherogenic B phenotype is found in ~ 20–30% of the population (25,41). This figure is similar to the estimated (33)/reported (42) prevalence of the insulin resistance syndrome (also now frequently referred to as the metabolic syndrome because of its definition in the recent NCEP-ATP III) (~25–30%) (33). Thus, the hypothesis has been put forward that a high proportion of patients characterized by hyperapobetalipoproteinemia and the atherogenic phenotype B may have a common metabolic disorder: insulin resistance.

The Québec Cardiovascular Study has published 5-year prospective data, which provided findings relevant to the present discussion (9). In this study, 2103 healthy men aged in their late 50s and initially free from clinical manifestations of IHD were followed for a period of 5 years for incidence of a first IHD event. Although plasma cholesterol concentrations were higher (7%) in men who developed IHD than in men who remained healthy, the most substantial differences were noted for the total cholesterol/HDL cholesterol ratio (16%) and apo B levels (12%) (9). We then used a simple algorithm to quantify the prevalence of dyslipidemic phenotypes in this population (9). While we found that type II dyslipidemia (hypercholesterolemia) was more prevalent among IHD men than in healthy men, hyperapo B (with or without hypertriglyceridemia) was the most prevalent abnormality among men who developed IHD. Stepwise logistic regression analyses revealed that apo B concentration analysed as a continuous variable was the best lipoprotein component predictive of IHD (43).

However, in a model excluding apo B, the total cholesterol/HDL cholesterol ratio came out as the best variable of the lipoprotein profile to predict IHD risk (43). It is important to point out that both apo B and the total cholesterol/HDL cholesterol ratio are increased in an insulin resistant state, which provides further support that insulin resistance substantially increases the risk of IHD. In this regard, no prospective study has reported data on the risk of IHD associated with an impaired in vivo insulin action. A few prospective studies, however, have measured fasting plasma insulin concentrations as a crude index of insulin sensitivity. These studies reported that hyperinsulinemia was associated with an increased risk of IHD in men (44–47). As hyperinsulinemia resulting from in vivo insulin resistance is associated with a dyslipidemic state which includes hypertriglyceridemia, elevated apo B levels, and reduced HDL cholesterol concentrations, it was still unclear whether the hyperinsulinemia-IHD relation is independent from the concomitant alterations in plasma lipoprotein levels. Results from the Paris and Caerphilly prospective studies had suggested that the risk associated with hyperinsulinemia was no longer significant after control for plasma TG levels (47–49).

C Impact of the Features of the Insulin Resistance/Metabolic Syndrome on CHD Risk: Evidence from the Québec Cardiovascular Study

The 5-year follow-up results of the Québec Cardiovascular Study provided data supporting the concept that the cluster of metabolic abnormalities which accompanies hyperinsulinemia (as a crude marker of insulin resistance) was predictive of a substantially increased risk of IHD (50). First, the 114 men who developed IHD during the 5-year follow-up period were matched for age, body mass index (BMI), smoking, and alcohol consumption with 114 men who remained healthy. We then excluded diabetic and IHD patients who could not be matched with controls because of extreme smoking habits, and we were able to match 91 nondiabetic cases and 105 controls (50). Fasting insulin concentrations were initially 18% higher in men who then developed IHD than in those who remained healthy. Furthermore, logistic regression analyses revealed that insulin levels remained associated with IHD after adjustment for concomitant variation in plasma lipoproteins including apo B concentrations (50). Two other markers of the metabolic syndrome were found to be predictive of an increased IHD risk in the Québec Cardiovascular Study: apo B concentration and small LDL particles (51,52).

As the above features of the metabolic syndrome (hyperinsulinemia, elevated apo B, and small LDL particles) are simultaneously observed, we were also interested in quantifying the IHD risk associated with this triad of metabolic abnormalities (53). We found that the presence of this atherogenic metabolic triad was predictive of a 20-fold increase in the risk of IHD in middle-aged men of the Québec Cardiovascular Study (53). Thus, the clinician dealing with type 2 diabetic patients or with nondiabetic but insulin-resistant individuals should not only focus on plasma cholesterol or LDL cholesterol levels as the simultaneous presence of hyperinsulinemia, elevated apo B, and increased proportion of small LDL, which is clearly predictive of a substantially increased IHD risk. The prevalence of this cluster of metabolic abnormalities is such that it probably represents the main cause of CHD in our population. It should also be further emphasized that this insulin resistance/metabolic syndrome will frequently be found among subjects with "normal" cholesterol and LDL cholesterol levels (37).

II OBESITY, BODY FAT DISTRIBUTION, AND DYSLIPIDEMIAS

Obesity is generally considered to be detrimental to cardiovascular health (3,54) and has long been associated with the presence of dyslipidemic states and CHD (54–56). Although some prospective studies have shown that obesity is a significant risk factor for CVD and related mortality in univariate analyses, it should be recognized that this association has generally been found to be rather weak, the relative risk ratio barely reaching 1.5 in overweight subjects in comparison with nonobese individuals (3,57–59). Multivariate analyses conducted in some studies failed to identify obesity as an independent risk factor for CVD (60,61).Thus, whether or not obesity per se is an independent predictor of CVD-related mortality has remained controversial, and this issue is still a matter of some debate in the scientific community.

In this regard, three possibilities have been raised to explain the weak association between obesity and mortality (62). First, most epidemiological studies have used anthropometric correlates of total body fat, which only provide a crude assessment of total body fatness. In addition, in order to observe the detrimental effects of disturbances in carbohydrate and lipid metabolism on clinical manifestations of CVD, it is likely that a prolonged follow-up may be necessary. Prospective studies that have reported positive associations between relative weight and mortality had follow-up periods of 10–15 years and even more (63). Finally, and most importantly, there is a body of data indicating that the health hazards of obesity are more closely related to the localization of excess body fat rather than to an elevated body weight per se. For instance, although obesity is a highly prevalent condition among patients showing metabolic aberrations, the magnitude of the associations reported has been quite variable, and clinicians have often been confronted with the metabolic heterogeneity of obesity. Therefore, it is important to adequately define obesity as a health hazard in order to develop measures aimed at the prevention and treatment of its complications (64).

Body weight expressed as a function of height has been used for a long time to obtain a crude measurement of body fatness. More than a century ago, Quetelet (65) noted that body weight (kg) was proportional to height squared (m^2). Later on, Keys and colleagues (66) redefined the Quetelet index as the BMI which also divides the body weight (kg) by height squared (m^2). This measure is now commonly used as a valuable index of relative weight and obesity (67). Some studies that have used the BMI to evaluate body composition have reported significant associations with morbidity and mortality (54,58,63,68). Although very useful to estimate overall obesity, the BMI has limitations. Individuals who do not have a large excess of body fat such as those with large muscle masses would be misclassified as having a high-risk body weight. Furthermore, the BMI does not provide information on the localization of body fat, and additional anthropometric measurements, such as the waist and hip circumferences and subcutaneous skinfolds, have been commonly used to estimate regional adipose tissue distribution (68).

Anthropometric estimates such as the waist-to-hip ratio (WHR) and skinfold measurements have generated considerable evidence to support the notion that the localization of adipose tissue rather than the accumulation of total body fat is a critical correlate of metabolic disturbances that are significant risk factors for CVD (54,55,59,69–71). Therefore, several epidemiological and metabolic studies published over the last two decades have indicated that the regional distribution of body fat was indeed the main factor involved in the relation of obesity to dyslipoproteinemias and CVD (37,38,54–56,69–90).

In this regard, Professor Jean Vague, from the University of Marseille, first proposed more than 50 years ago that body fat topography was a better correlate of the complications of obesity (diabetes, hypertension, CVD) than excess fatness per se (73). Vague defined the male type of fat distribution as "android obesity", mostly characterized by an accumulation of adipose tissue over the trunk, whereas he referred to the common fat pattern of women as "gynoid obesity," where adipose tissue accumulates mostly around the hips and thighs, this type of obesity being seldom associated with the common complications of excess fatness (73). However, it took more than four decades before these pioneering observations became widely accepted by the scientific community. During this period, the concept of adipose tissue distribution did not receive much attention, and only a few studies published in the 1960s examined this issue. In 1964, Albrink and Meigs (74) reported stronger correlations between plasma TG levels and trunk skinfolds than any other skinfold considered. Allard and Goulet (75) reached similar conclusions in the late 1960s. Although these studies showed associations between excess trunk fat and plasma TG levels, the concept of regional adipose tissue distribution only received serious consideration when prospective studies published in the 1980s indicated that excess abdominal fat was associated with an increased mortality rate in a manner which was independent of concomitant variation in total fatness as estimated by the BMI (72,76–78). These studies have shown that regional fat distribution, assessed by WHR or skinfolds, was associated with a higher incidence of diabetes and CVD, and with an increased mortality rate (76–78).

The related dyslipidemic state was an obvious possibility to explain the increased CVD risk associated with abdominal obesity, and several studies have examined the potential associations between abdominal fat accumulation and dyslipidemias. More specifically, it has been demonstrated that subjects characterized by a high accumulation of abdominal fat have elevated fasting plasma TG levels (80,82) and reduced plasma HDL cholesterol concentrations (69,80,83–85).

Studies for which HDL subfractions were measured revealed that the reduction in HDL cholesterol observed with excess abdominal fat was mainly attributed to a decrease in the concentration of plasma HDL_2 cholesterol concentrations (83–87). In addition, it has been shown that in abdominal obesity, plasma HDL cholesterol levels were reduced to a greater extent than plasma HDL-apo A1 levels and that HDL were TG enriched (88). The presence of small HDL particles is another common feature of the dyslipidemic state of abdominal obesity (91,92).

Additional work has revealed that LDL particle concentration, composition and density are altered among subjects with a high WHR (85,93). Indeed, abdominal obesity has been associated with an increased proportion of small, dense, cholesteryl ester-depleted LDL particles (39,85,93). As discussed above, the small, dense LDL phenotype is also accompanied by higher concentrations of TG and lower levels of HDL cholesterol (39), alterations that are often found in CHD patients (89).

Abdominal obesity has also been reported to relate to alterations in indices of plasma glucose-insulin homeostasis. Indeed, prospective studies have shown that an excess of abdominal fat is associated with an increased risk of diabetes (79). Although the mechanisms linking abdominal obesity to type 2 diabetes are not fully understood, it appears that a preferential accumulation of adipose tissue in the abdominal region is associated with glucose intolerance, hyperinsulinemia, and insulin resistance which are metabolic conditions predictive of an increased risk of type 2 diabetes (70,71).

Using anthropometric measurements, several studies reported that upper body obesity is more prevalent in diabetic patients than in control subjects (90). Moreover, alterations in indices of plasma glucose-insulin homeostasis are frequently observed in abdominally obese patients (71,73,81,82). More specifically, the preferential accumulation of abdominal fat has been shown to be related to hyperinsulinemia in the fasting state as well as following a glucose load (70,71). Increased insulin secretion, insulin resistance, and decreased hepatic insulin extraction are common metabolic disturbances in abdominal obesity (71,94–96). These important metabolic events may explain the resulting hyperinsulinemia found in patients with an excess of abdominal fat. Furthermore, glucose intolerance or at least an increased plasma glucose response to a glucose load are frequently found in abdominally obese patients despite the presence of hyperinsulinemia confirming the presence of insulin resistance (70,71). These alterations in lipoprotein-lipid and insulin-glucose metabolism found in abdominally obese patients contribute to explain the high prevalence of CVD and type 2 diabetes in these subjects (97).

III BODY FAT DISTRIBUTION AND DYSLIPIDEMIAS: IMPORTANCE OF VISCERAL ADIPOSE TISSUE

A Measurement of Visceral Adipose Tissue

The development in the 1980s of imaging techniques such as computed tomography (CT) has allowed the precise assessment of adipose tissue distribution (98–100). Using CT, one can easily distinguish adipose from lean tissues. Indeed, the attenuation scores generated by CT vary from -1000 (air) to +1000 (bone), depending on the level of absorption of emitted x-ray beams (100, 101). Studies that have examined the attenuation of tissues have established that the range of attenuation values (Hounsfield units, HU) for adipose tissue varies between −190 and −30 HU (100,101).

Computed tomography is also quite useful to assess precisely the amount of abdominal adipose tissue and is particularly helpful to distinguish the adipose tissue located in the abdominal cavity (the so-called intra-abdominal or visceral adipose tissue) from subcutaneous abdominal fat. When this procedure is performed, the subject is examined in the supine position with both arms stretched above the head (100,101). To measure subcutaneous and visceral abdominal adipose tissue areas, CT scans are usually performed between L4 and L5 vertebrae. Total adipose tissue areas are calculated by delineating the abdominal area with a graph pen and then computing total adipose tissue surface with an attenuation range of −190 to −30 HU (100,101). To measure the area of visceral adipose tissue, a line is drawn by passing through the muscle wall delineating the abdominal cavity (Fig. 4).

B Metabolic Disturbances Associated with Excess Visceral Adipose Tissue

Studies that have used this technique have reported that the amount of visceral adipose tissue is a critical correlate of the common metabolic complications found in obese patients. Fujioka and colleagues (102) have studied a heterogeneous group of obese patients and assessed cross-sectional areas of adipose tissue located subcutaneously or in the abdominal cavity (visceral adipose tissue). They reported that individuals with a preferential accumulation of abdominal visceral fat showed higher plasma glucose responses following an oral glucose challenge and higher fasting plasma TG levels than individuals with similar BMI values but characterized by an excess of subcutaneous abdominal fat (102–104). Several cross-sectional studies have

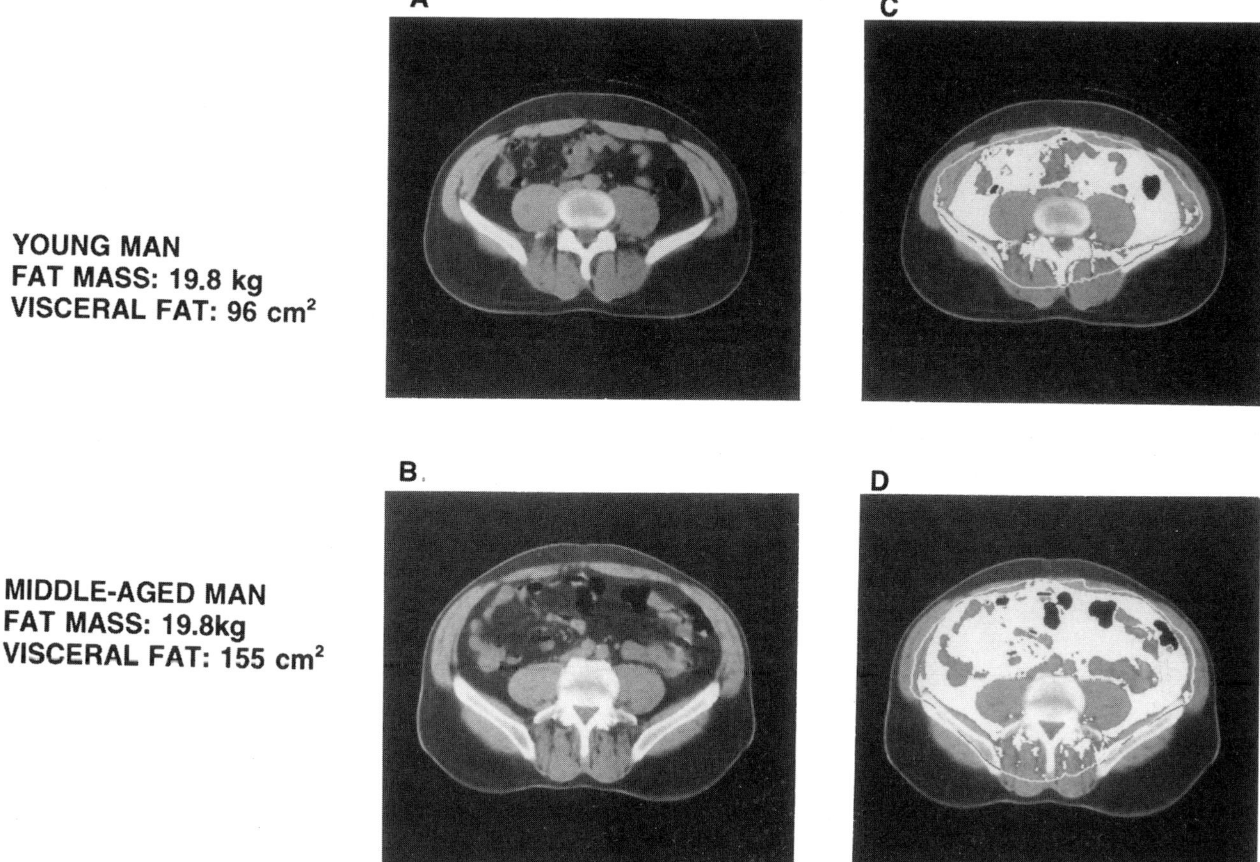

Figure 4 Cross-sectional abdominal adipose tissue areas measured by CT at L4-L5 in a middle-aged man (B,D) and a young man (A,C) with similar total body fat mass values. The visceral adipose tissue, delineated by drawing a line within the muscle wall surrounding the abdominal cavity, is highlighted (C,D).

also consistently found that an excess of abdominal visceral adipose tissue was associated with substantial alterations in indices of plasma glucose-insulin homeostasis and in plasma lipoprotein-lipid levels (86,87, 105–108).

We have examined the potential relationships between visceral adipose tissue accumulation and plasma lipoprotein levels in obese premenopausal women (86) and found that the level of visceral adipose tissue was the best correlate of lipoprotein variables that are commonly used to predict the risk of CHD. Excess visceral adipose tissue was associated with increased apo B concentrations and low plasma HDL cholesterol levels (86). We have also quantified the independent contributions of obesity versus visceral adipose tissue accumulation by comparing obese individuals with either low or high levels of visceral adipose tissue to a group of lean subjects (Fig. 5). As shown in Figure 5, the only significant difference noted between the obese subjects with low levels of visceral fat and lean individuals was a moderate increase in plasma TG levels in the obese group, whereas obese individuals with high levels of visceral fat showed important alterations in their plasma lipoprotein profile compared to lean controls. Consequently, obese individuals with a high level of visceral adipose tissue may represent the subgroup of obese individuals potentially at highest risk for CHD (69,108).

We have also compared indices of plasma glucose-insulin homeostasis among these three groups of subjects (107–109) and found that obese subjects with high levels of visceral adipose tissue had a higher glycemic response to a glucose challenge in the presence of hyperinsulinemia, reflecting an insulin resistant state (Fig. 6). In contrast, obese subjects with a low accumulation of visceral adipose tissue showed normal glucose

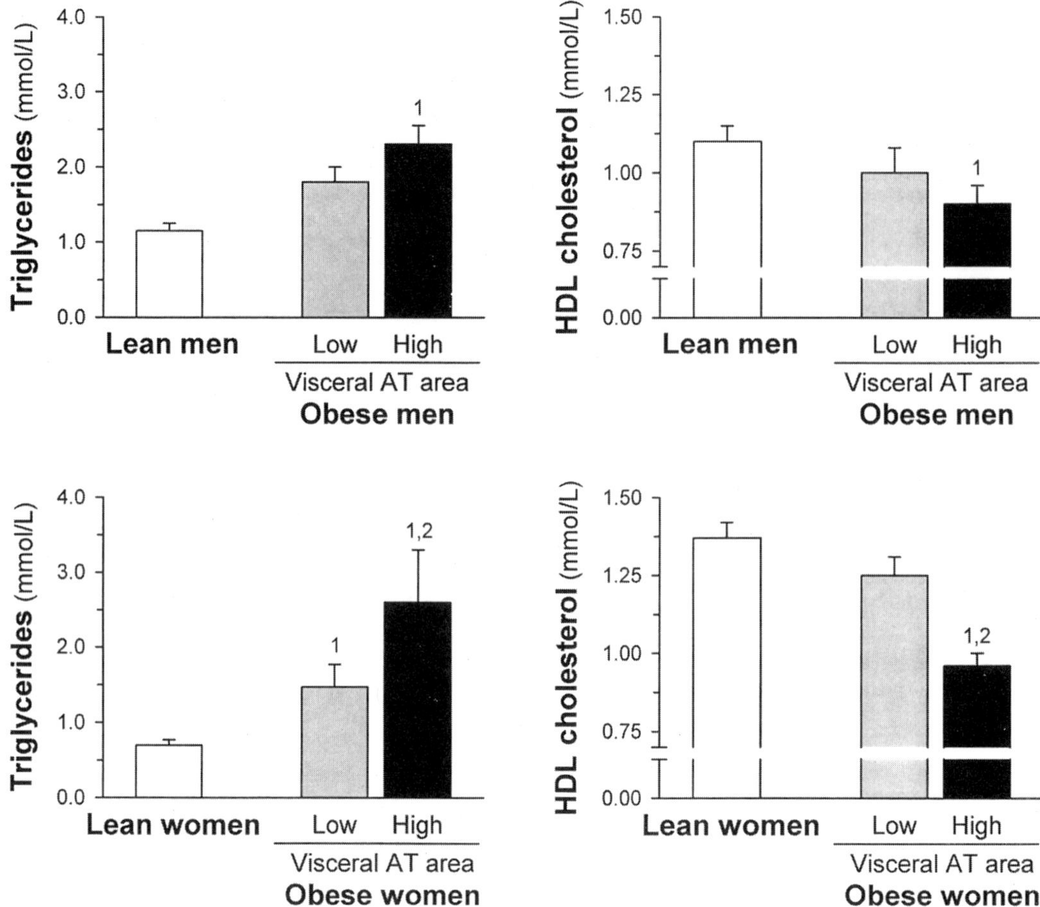

Figure 5 Plasma triglyceride and HDL cholesterol concentrations in nonobese subjects and in subgroups of obese subjects matched for body composition but having either low or high levels of visceral adipose tissue (AT) determined by computed tomography. [1]Significantly different from nonobese subjects, $P < .05$. [2]Significantly different from obese subjects with low levels of visceral adipose tissue, $P < .05$. (Adapted from Ref. 179.)

tolerance and only a slight elevation in plasma insulin levels. These analyses and group comparisons were performed in both men and women, and similar conclusions were reached (107–109). Thus, these results indicate that obesity per se is associated with moderate metabolic alterations whereas excess visceral adipose tissue accumulation is related to substantial disturbances in indices of plasma glucose-insulin homeostasis which are predictive of an increased risk of type 2 diabetes.

Using CT, it has been reported that marked gender differences exist regarding visceral adipose tissue accumulation. For instance, we found that men have almost twice the amount of abdominal visceral adipose tissue for a given body fat mass as premenopausal women (Fig. 7) (110). Furthermore, we have studied the potential contribution of gender differences in visceral adipose tissue accumulation to the sex dimorphism found in CVD risk variables (111). After control for the gender dimorphism in visceral adipose tissue accumulation, it was found that most of the differences observed in indices of plasma glucose-insulin homeostasis and in plasma lipoprotein-lipid profile were no longer significantly different between men and women (111), suggesting that the greater CVD risk noted in men compared to premenopausal women may be partly due to the preferential accumulation of visceral adipose tissue in male subjects.

Finally, in an attempt to examine whether there could be a threshold of visceral adipose tissue accumu-

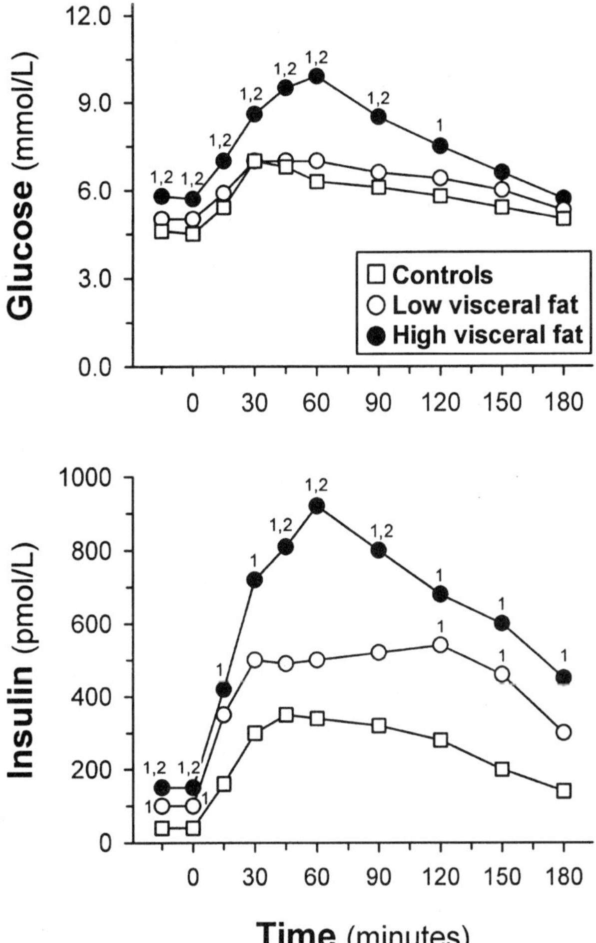

Figure 6 Plasma glucose and insulin concentrations in fasting state (−15 and 0 min) and during oral glucose tolerance test in obese women with high (●) or low (○) levels of visceral adipose tissue (n = 10 subjects/group) and in a sample of lean women (□) (n = 25). [1]Significantly different from (□). [2]Significantly different from (○), $P < .05$. (Adapted from Ref. 109.)

lation above which complications may be found, several variables predictive of CVD and type 2 diabetes were compared among samples of young adults and premenopausal women who were divided into quintiles formed on the basis of their cross-sectional visceral adipose tissue area measured by CT. Figure 8 shows that in both men and women, a value <100 cm^2 was associated with a rather favorable risk profile (112). However, a cross-sectional visceral adipose tissue area of 130 cm^2 and above was associated with a substantial deterioration in the cardiovascular risk profile (112).

C Postprandial Hyperlipidemia: Another Feature of Visceral Obesity

Analysis of lipid and lipoprotein metabolism has long been limited to the fasting state, i.e., when TG metabolism is reduced and lipid transport is presumably at equilibrium. However, considering meal frequency in Western populations, humans spend most of the day under postprandial conditions and thus, dietary fat tolerance should receive greater attention. Interest for the study of postprandial lipoprotein metabolism has been renewed since Zilversmit (113) hypothesized that chylomicron remnants, following enrichment in cholesteryl esters, could be involved in the development of atherosclerosis. This theory has been given further support, and many factors have already been reported to modulate postprandial TG-rich lipoprotein metabolism. For instance, age (114,115), male gender (114, 116,117), a high-fat diet (118), alcohol consumption (119–121), and lack of exercise (122–125) have all been associated with an exaggerated and prolonged postprandial lipemia.

Obesity is associated with numerous metabolic disturbances that have been extensively described earlier in this chapter. In addition to alterations in lipoprotein-lipid metabolism in the fasting state, obese individuals have been characterized by a greater plasma TG response following ingestion of a fatty meal (126).

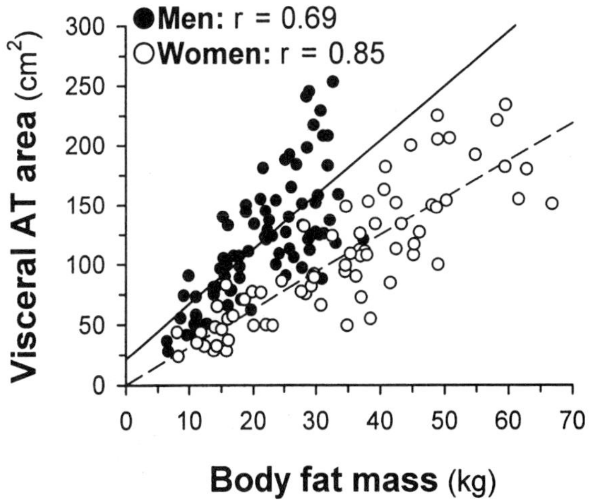

Figure 7 Relation of total body fat mass to abdominal visceral adipose tissue (AT) area measured by computed tomography in 89 men and 75 premenopausal women. Both correlations were significant at $P < .0001$. (Adapted from Ref. 110.)

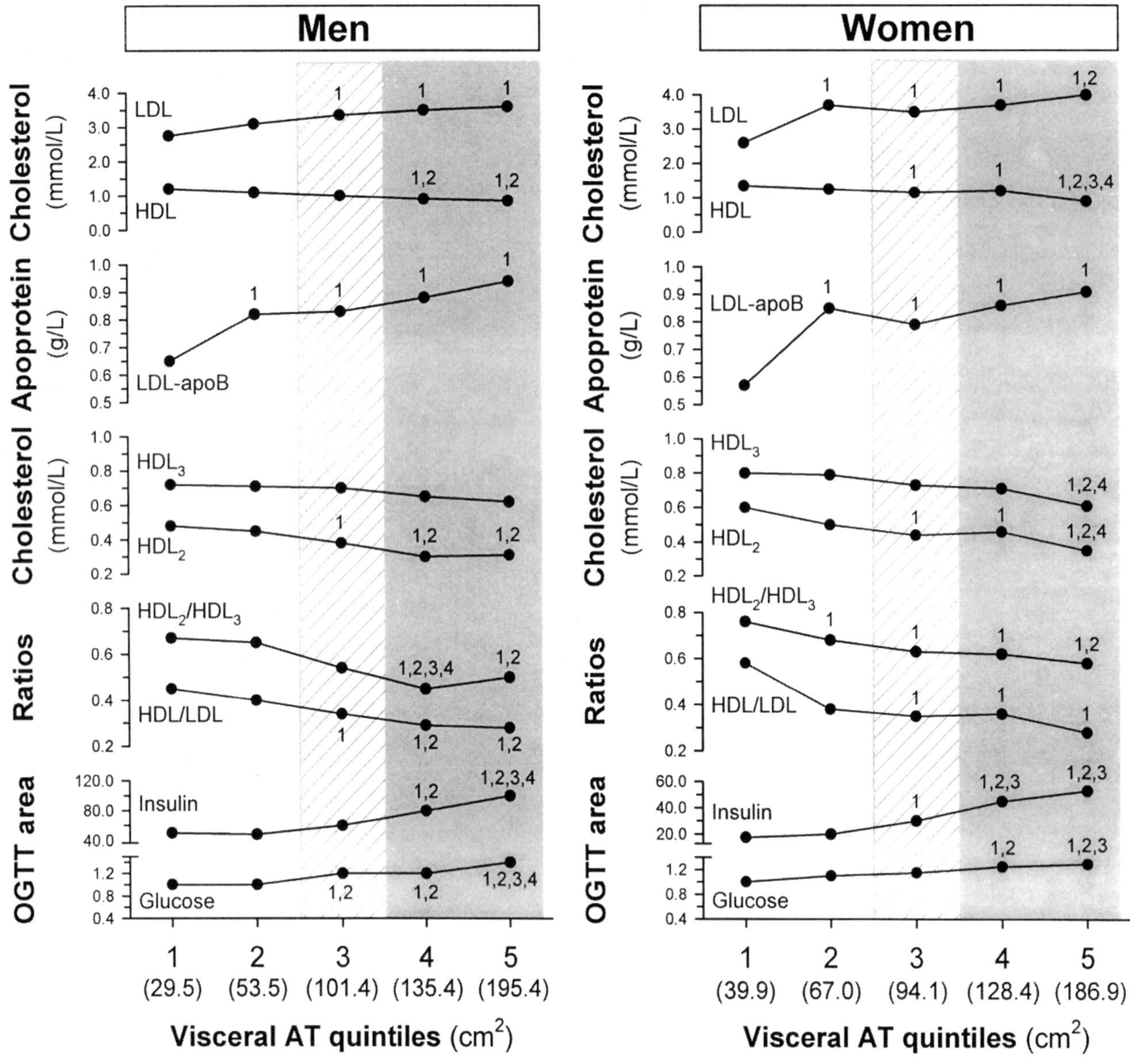

Figure 8 Relations of quintiles of abdominal visceral adipose tissue (AT) area to variables predictive of type 2 diabetes and CVD risk in samples of 115 men and 72 women, respectively. This figure shows that visceral AT areas >100 cm^2 are associated with moderate but significant metabolic changes, whereas visceral AT areas >135 cm^2 in men and 128 cm^2 in women are clearly associated with further metabolic deteriorations that suggest an increased risk of type 2 diabetes and CVD. 1, 2, 3, or 4 significantly different from quintiles 1, 2, 3, and 4, respectively ($P < .05$). Apo: apolipoprotein; OGTT: oral glucose tolerance test. (From Ref. 112.)

Although this postprandial hypertriglyceridemic state has been suggested to result from delayed clearance and/or catabolism of newly synthesized intestinal TG-rich lipoproteins, namely chylomicrons and their remnants (126), the fact that the postprandial increase of retinyl ester, a marker of TG-rich lipoproteins produced by the intestine, was of lesser magnitude compared to the TG response also suggested that a significant proportion of the postprandial TG response was due to endogenous hepatic VLDL production. In recent years, the role of abdominal fat accumulation in this metabolic alteration has been underlined. For instance, a preferential accumulation of fat in the abdominal region has been shown to be a better correlate of the impairment of postprandial TG-rich lipoprotein metabolism than excess fatness per se (127–130). In addition, we have shown that the intra-abdominal component of abdominal fat deposition was probably responsible for this deterioration (130). The importance of both intestinally and hepatically derived TG-rich lipoproteins in this postprandial hypertriglyceridemic state of abdominally obese individuals has also been underlined (129–131). Furthermore, the detrimental impact of visceral obesity was recently documented to explain the greater postprandial TG levels found in men compared to women (116). For instance, we have shown that when matched for visceral adipose tissue accumulation, men and women show comparable postprandial lipemic responses (116). Thus, and as shown in Figure 9, viscerally obese patients are not only characterized by a fasting dyslipidemic state, but they also display an exaggerated postprandial TG response and a prolonged postprandial hyperlipidemic state compared to nonobese normolipidemic subjects.

(A)

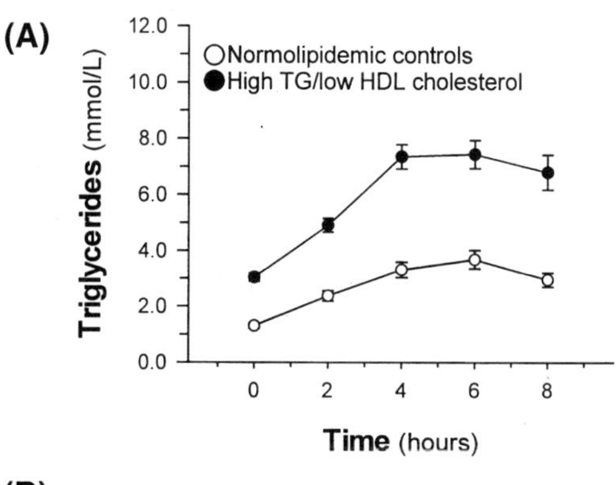

(B)

Fasting	Normolipidemic controls	High TG/ Low HDL cholesterol
Triglycerides (mmol/L)	1.31 ± 0.44	3.17 ± 0.58 *
HDL cholesterol (mmol/L)	1.10 ± 0.19	0.72 ± 0.06 *

Figure 9 Plasma triglyceride (TG) levels measured for 8 hours following the consumption of a standardized breakfast with a high lipid content (60 g dietary fat/m^2 of body surface area) in a sample of lean normolipidemic subjects as well as in a sample of viscerally obese patients with the fasting high TG/low HDL cholesterol dyslipidemia. *Significantly different from normolipidemic controls, $P < .0001$. (Adapted from Ref. 131.)

D Atherogenic Metabolic Profile of Visceral Obesity: Beyond Insulin Resistance and Related Dyslipidemias

Although it has become clear that visceral obesity is associated with diabetogenic and atherogenic metabolic alterations, studies have shown that additional metabolic disorders could explain the increased risk of CHD in these individuals. For instance, visceral obesity has been found to be associated with an impaired fibrinolysis and with an increased concentration of prothrombotic molecules such as plasminogen activator inhibitor-1 (PAI-1) (132). Recent results have also indicated that visceral obesity is characterized by a state of chronic inflammation as revealed by increased plasma levels of C-reactive protein (CRP) (133–135) likely to result from the greater cytokine production (interleukin (IL)-6, tumor necrosis factor (TNF)-α) of the expanded visceral adipose depot (133,135). Thus, visceral obesity is associated with insulin resistance and with a dyslipidemic, prothrombotic, and inflammatory profile that can contribute substantially to increase the risk of an acute coronary event (136).

IV DOES THE ATHEROGENIC DYSLIPIDEMIA OF VISCERAL OBESITY REFLECT A CAUSE-EFFECT RELATIONSHIP?

It has been suggested that enlarged omental adipocytes, which have been shown to display a high lipolytic activity, poorly inhbited by insulin (54,70,71,137), contribute to a greater flux of free fatty acids (FFA) toward the liver through the portal circulation. As shown in Figure 10, high portal FFA levels are associated with reduced hepatic insulin extraction (138,139) and lead to an increased VLDL synthesis and apo B production (55,137). Moreover, it has been suggested that increased lipid oxidation is associated with impaired glycolysis (140,141) and with a decrease in glycogen synthase activity (142). Furthermore, this elevated lipid oxidation provides precursors for gluconeogenesis (143). Thus, the evidence available suggests that insulin action is impaired in subjects displaying high FFA levels and that compensatory hyperinsulinemia is thus required to regulate plasma glucose levels in insulin resistant subjects (33).

Lipoprotein lipase is an enzyme responsible for the catabolism of TG-rich lipoproteins, and its activity has been found to be correlated with metabolic alterations

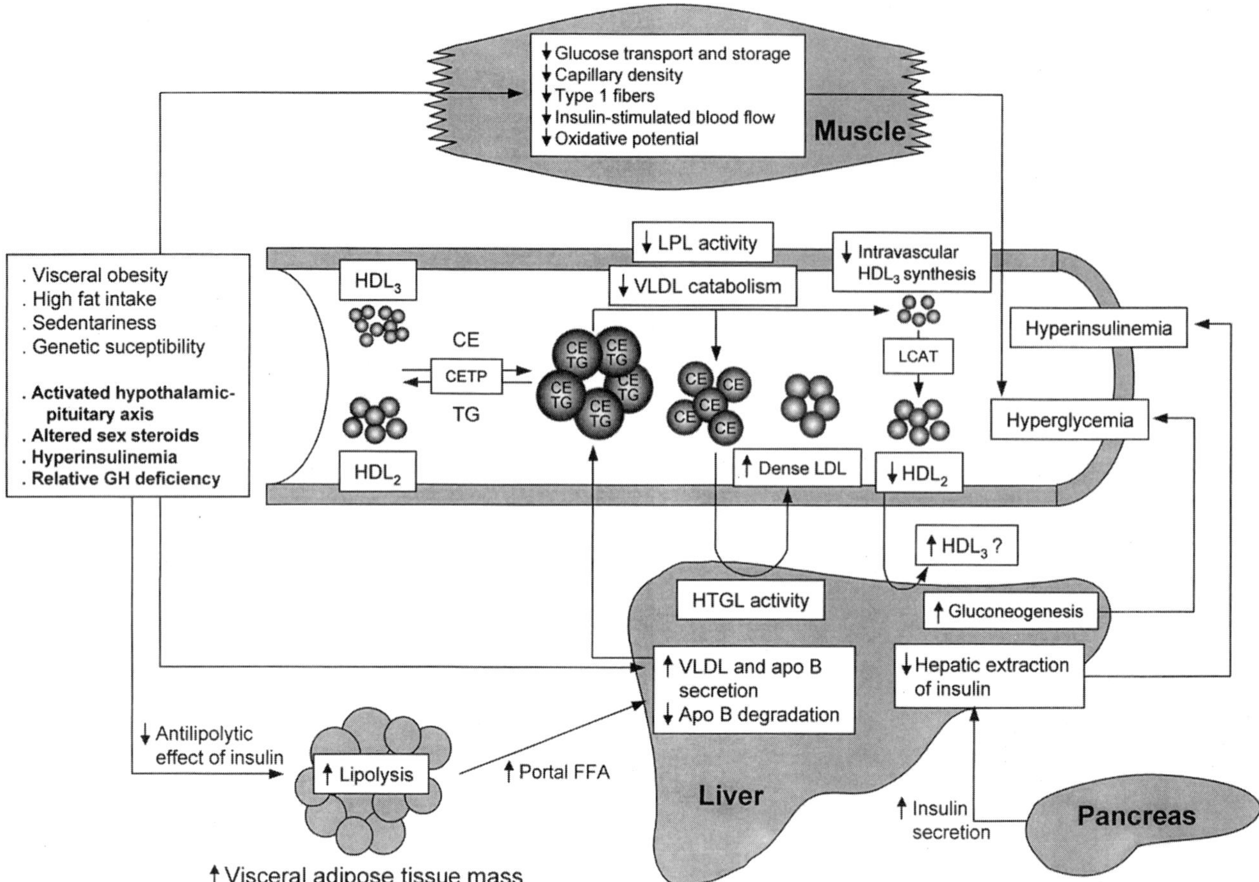

Figure 10 Complex metabolic interactions that presumably occur with the insulin resistance/dyslipidemic phenotype. In this case, insulin resistance is frequently accompanied by excess intra-abdominal (visceral) adipose tissue. The liver, via the portal circulation, becomes exposed to high levels of free fatty acids (FFA) as the compensatory hyperinsulinemia poorly inhibits the lipolysis of intra-abdominal fat cells. This phenomenon stimulates gluconeogenesis as well as VLDL synthesis and secretion. Moreover, the catabolism of TG-rich lipoproteins appears to be slow, this being attributable to the fact that LPL activity is reduced and the postprandial adipose tissue LPL response is inadequate. Impaired LPL activity may explain, at least to some degree, the low HDL cholesterol levels of insulin-resistant individuals characterized by visceral obesity. The high activity of another enzyme, hepatic lipase (HTGL), is a contributing factor in the further decrease of HDL cholesterol level. The high TG levels resulting from the increased production and slower catabolism of VLDL promotes the transfer of TG to LDL and HDL in exchange for their cholesteryl esters (CE). This phenomenon leads to an increase in VLDL CE, a process considered as atherogenic. Moreover, the TG-enriched LDL and HDL fractions represent the substrate of choice for HTGL, this process favoring the formation of dense LDL, the concentration of which is higher in coronary artery disease patients. These complex metabolic interactions increase not only the risk of diabetes but also the risk of coronary heart disease in insulin resistant individuals. CETP: cholesteryl ester transfer protein. GH: growth hormone; LCAT: lecithin-cholesterol acyl transferase; LPL, lipoprotein lipase. (Adapted from Ref. 38.)

associated with visceral obesity. Indeed, visceral obesity has been shown to be associated with decreased LPL and with increased hepatic TG lipase (HTGL) activities (87). Such a decrease in LPL activity contributes to reduce the catabolic rate of TG-rich lipoproteins (69,144), whereas higher HTGL might enhance the degradation of HDL_2 particles or lead to an increase in their conversion to HDL_3 (69,87,144). Pollare et al. (145) have reported a reduced skeletal muscle LPL activity in insulin resistant subjects and that in vivo insulin sensitivity was positively correlated with skeletal muscle LPL activity.

The higher concentrations of TG-rich lipoproteins resulting from an increased hepatic VLDL production and decreased degradation (through reduced LPL activity) are associated with an increased transfer of TG from VLDL to LDL or HDL particles (87,88) in exchange of LDL and HDL cholesteryl esters, leading to the TG enrichment of LDL and HDL. Such TG enrichment is associated with a reduced cholesterol content of HDL. Furthermore, TG-rich LDL and HDL particles represent good substrates for the enzyme HTGL, ultimately generating an atherogenic dyslipidemic phenotype including small, dense LDL and HDL particles (55,92). Thus, reciprocal changes in LPL and HTGL activities are important correlates of dyslipidemias found in an insulin resistant state associated with visceral obesity.

The mechanisms leading to in vivo insulin resistance are not fully understood, and it is also known that impaired insulin action can be present in both obese and nonobese subjects (33). These observations suggest that insulin resistance is a heterogeneous condition and provide further evidence that some genetic factors are likely to be involved. Studies conducted among insulin-resistant or type 2 diabetic subjects have shown that the presence of a familial history of diabetes may alter the relationship of abdominal fat accumulation to indices of plasma glucose-insulin homeostasis (146,147). We have previously reported that in subjects with a similar level of deterioration in plasma glucose-insulin homeostasis, those who displayed a positive familial history of diabetes had lower levels of abdominal fat than subjects without a familial history of diabetes (147). These results suggest that the presence of genetic susceptibility reduces the threshold of abdominal fat above which metabolic alterations predictive of an increased type 2 diabetes risk are observed. Thus, in abdominally viscerally obese patients, high FFA concentrations (increased lipolysis of the visceral depot), decreased LPL activity and reduced insulin sensitivity may lead to metabolic changes that are ultimately involved in the development of insulin resistance, glucose intolerance, hyperinsulinemia, dyslipoproteinemia, type 2 diabetes, and CVD.

In addition to the impaired FFA metabolism hypothesis briefly reviewed above, it has been suggested that abdominal obesity is associated with altered sex steroid levels. Results that have crudely assessed body fat distribution by the WHR have reported low levels of sex hormone binding globulin (SHBG) concentrations and high levels of free testosterone in women with excess abdominal fat (70,148–151). Moreover, the altered sex steroid concentrations observed in abdominally obese women have also been associated with variations of in vivo insulin sensitivity (70,150). Studies have also shown that the hyperinsulinemic state of abdominal obesity was partly attributed to a reduction in the hepatic extraction of insulin (148), the latter phenomenon being associated with lower SHBG concentrations. Furthermore, a reduced hepatic insulin extraction has also been related to high free testosterone levels in women (148). Thus, the associations of steroid levels with metabolic disturbances have been shown to be partly independent of the concomitant variation in adipose tissue distribution. It has also been suggested that although there is clearly an independent association between visceral fat accumulation and metabolic alterations, the dyslipidemic state observed in abdominally obese women could also partially be due to the concomitant alterations in the sex steroid profile (70).

In men, however, the associations among sex steroids, visceral obesity, and the metabolic profile are quite different from those noted in women. As opposed to abdominally obese women, visceral obesity in men is rather associated with a reduction of plasma testosterone levels (151,152). It is also not well established whether reduced levels of androgenic steroids are independently associated with an excess abdominal visceral fat accumulation after control for the concomitant variation in the amount of total body fat (152). Furthermore, the alterations found in steroid hormone levels have been found to be significantly correlated with glucose intolerance (153) and with the dyslipidemic state observed in visceral obesity (154,155). It is also relevant to note that, after controlling for variations in testosterone, the relationship between the amount of visceral adipose tissue to insulin resistance and to dyslipidemia remained significant (153,156).

In addition, the potential role of glucocorticoids on the regulation of lipid metabolism in visceral obesity must be considered (157–159). It has been proposed that the insulin-resistant state observed in subjects with excess visceral adipose tissue is partly the consequence of altered glucocorticoid levels (157–159). In this regard, environmental stress can induce an activation of the hypothalamic-pituitary-adrenal axis thereby increasing cortisol production (160). Visceral adipose cells have been reported to have the highest density of glucocorticoid receptors (161,162) in comparison to adipocytes from other fat depots, and this could explain the greater sensitivity of visceral adipose tissue to stressor agents. Furthermore, the metabolic effects of glucocorticoids (157) are in accordance with the alterations observed in visceral obesity (55,69,157). Indeed, glucocorticoids stimulate VLDL and apo B production, reduce the activity of LDL receptors, and induce insulin resistance (157).

Recently, studies have suggested that patients with growth hormone (GH) deficiencies also show the features of the metabolic syndrome including an increased visceral adipose tissue accumulation (163–166). In this regard, some intervention studies have suggested that GH replacement in relatively deficient GH patients could improve the features of the metabolic syndrome including changes in body fat distribution and visceral adipose tissue loss (163,165–167). This promising area represents a fertile area of investigation that will require further studies.

Finally, it has also been shown that adipose tissue was a remarkable endocrine organ beyond its lipid storage/mobilization functions. For instance, the expanded visceral adipose depot is a site of synthesis of pro-thrombotic molecules such as PAI-1 and of cytokines (leptin, IL-6, TNF-α). Resulting elevations in plasma IL-6 and TNF-α concentrations stimulate CRP synthesis by the liver and these cytokines therefore contribute to the inflammatory profile recently reported in viscerally obese patients (133,135). Thus, we have suggested that in addition to the model linking the expanded visceral adipose depot to an atherogenic dyslipidemic state, the pro-thrombotic and inflammatory profile of viscerally obese patients could also be linked to the intrinsic and peculiar activity of the visceral adipocytes (Fig. 11). In summary, the dyslipidemic state of visceral obesity results from complex metabolic and hormonal interactions that lead to insulin resistance and to an increased CVD risk (Fig. 10).

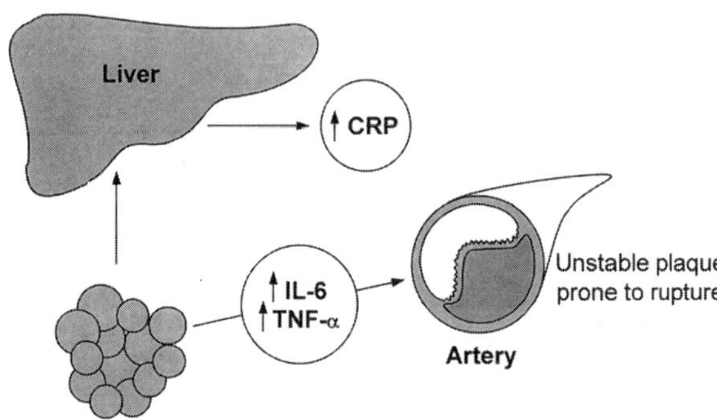

Figure 11 Model linking the expanded visceral adipose depot as an endocrine organ releasing cytokines contributing to the inflammatory component of coronary artery disease by the production of an unstable plaque with a thin fibrous cap and prone to rupture. Under this model the viscerally obese patient is at markedly elevated risk for an acute coronary syndrome as predicted by the increased levels of inflammation markers. CRP: C-reactive protein; IL-6: interleukin-6; TNF-α: tumor necrosis factor-α.

V VISCERAL OBESITY, DYSLIPIDEMIAS, AND CHD: CLINICAL IMPLICATIONS

From the evidence reviewed, the detection of the subgroup of obese patients at risk for complications associated with excess visceral adipose tissue is clinically important. Thus, an adequate estimation of visceral adipose tissue accumulation is of great relevance to better quantify the patient's risk of CVD. Although CT is very accurate and reliable, it is not accessible to most clinicians, and it was relevant to develop approaches in order to offer simple tools for the detection, prevention, and treatment of visceral obesity.

A Is Anthropometry an Appropriate Alternative to CT?

Numerous studies have examined the correlations between anthropometric measurements and cross-sectional visceral adipose tissue areas measured by CT (168,169,171). Until recently, the WHR had generally been considered as the most relevant variable in the assessment of visceral obesity (76–85), this ratio being often used in prospective and metabolic studies. Although the use of WHR has contributed to highlight the importance of body fat distribution, we have reported that visceral adipose tissue accumulation showed better correlations with the waist circumference alone than with the WHR (172). Figure 12 shows that the relation of visceral adipose tissue area to the waist girth was stronger than for the WHR, especially in women. Furthermore, the relationship between waist circumference and visceral adipose tissue was found to be similar in men and women. Moreover, waist circumference also appears to be a good correlate of total body fatness and therefore provides a better index of abdominal obesity than the WHR alone, which is a weak correlate of total adiposity (172).

For example, a nonobese woman with small hips may have a WHR value which could be similar to an obese woman with a large accumulation of abdominal fat but with also a substantial deposition of fat at the hip level (Fig. 12). Thus, despite similar WHR values in these two subjects, the obese women would have a much greater accumulation of visceral adipose tissue than the nonobese women despite the fact that their WHR are simi-

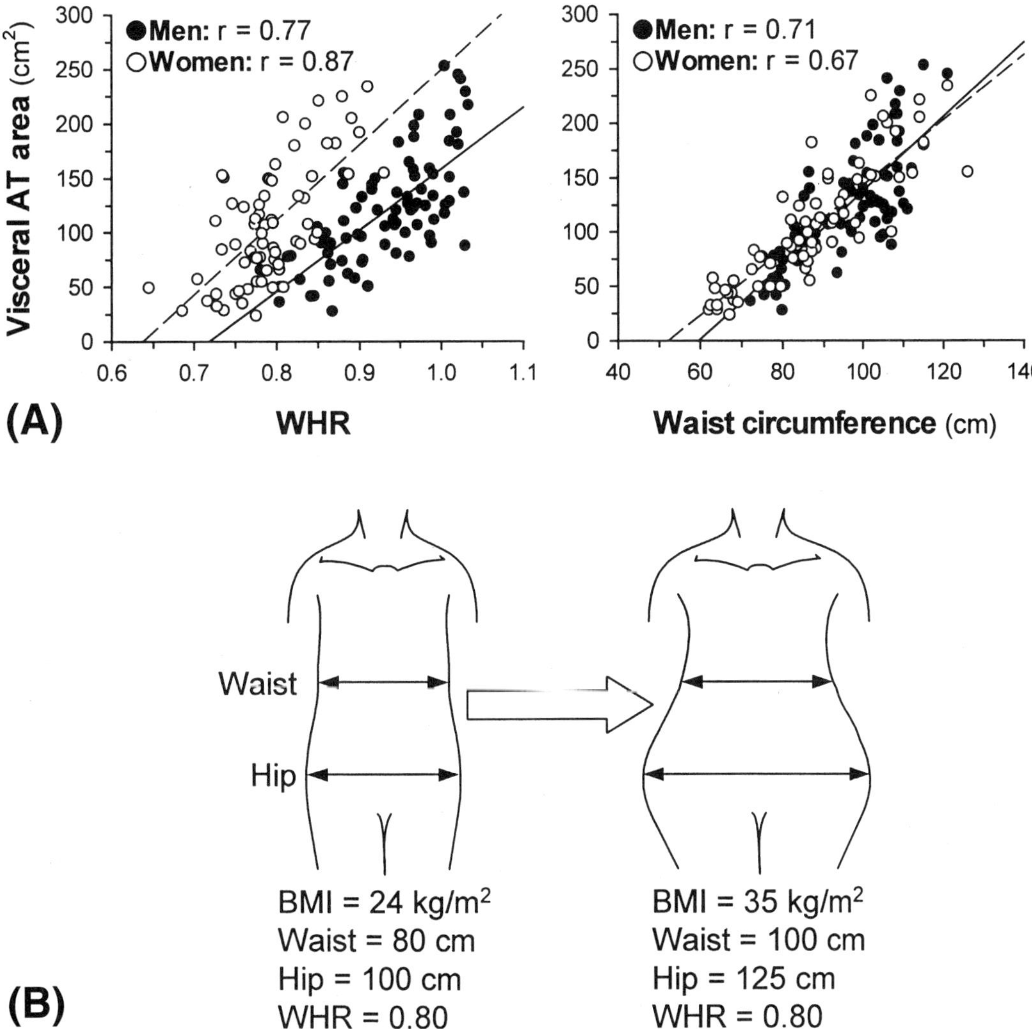

Figure 12 (A) Relation of waist-to-hip ratio (WHR) or waist circumference to abdominal visceral adipose tissue (AT) areas measured by computed tomography in men and women. (B) Misleading evaluation provided by the WHR in two women with markedly differing levels of total body fat and of visceral AT. This example illustrates the notion that the WHR is an index of the relative accumulation of abdominal fat whereas waist circumference provides a better index of the absolute amount of abdominal adipose tissue. BMI: body mass index. (Adapted from Refs. 172,178.)

lar. Consequently, the use of WHR alone can be quite misleading, whereas a high waist girth obviously indicates that excess abdominal fat and obesity are simultaneously present. Indeed, the waist circumference is positively correlated with both an accumulation of total body fat and an elevated deposition of visceral adipose tissue (172). In this context, we have proposed that the waist circumference provides a valuable index of the absolute amount of abdominal fat compared to the WHR, which rather reflects relative abdominal adipose tissue deposition (172). On that basis, the waist circumference has now been recognized as an index of abdominal fat in the NCEP-ATP III guidelines (36).

B Hypertriglyceridemic Waist: A New Phenotype Defining the High-Risk Abdominally Obese Patient

Despite the fact that waist circumference is a better predictor of visceral adipose tissue accumulation (especially over time) than BMI, abdominally obese individuals remain a heterogeneous group of patients. We were interested in the development of a simple screening approach to help physicians and health professionals identify high-risk abdominally obese patients with the features of the insulin resistance/metabolic syndrome. In a recent study, we reported that waist circumference was the simplest and best correlate of plasma insulin and apo B levels, whereas another simple parameter, fasting TG concentration, was the best predictor of LDL size (40). Sensitivity and specificity analyses revealed that the best discrimination of carriers/noncarriers of this atherogenic metabolic triad (elevated insulin and apo B levels as well as small, dense LDL particles) was obtained when using cutoff points of 90 cm for waist circumference and 2.0 mmol/L for TG in a sample of middle-aged men (Fig. 13). For instance, middle-aged men with a waist <90 cm and fasting TG levels <2.0 mmol/L had a low chance (10%) of being carriers of the triad. However, >80% of men with a waist girth ≥90 cm and TG levels ≥2.0 mmol/L had all features of the metabolic triad (40). Thus, we believe that health professionals have access to a simple and inexpensive screening test to identify a high-risk form of abdominal obesity. As there are no prospective data available in women to quantify the CHD risk associated with the metabolic triad, there is an urgent need to validate this approach in women. It should also be emphasized that there are differences in susceptibility to develop visceral obesity and related complications (diabetes, hypertension, and CHD) among ethnic groups, and our approach should only be considered as valid for Caucasian men. Specific cutoffs are likely to be obtained for instance for our Native American population as well as for the African-American and South Asian populations.

Waist circumference	+	Fasting triglycerides	Prevalence of metabolic syndrome
< 90 cm	+	< 2.0 mmol/L	~ 10%
≥ 90 cm	+	≥ 2.0 mmol/L	~ 80%

Figure 13 Description of two phenotypes predictive of either a very low or a high risk of being characterized by the atherothrombotic, inflammatory profile of the metabolic syndrome.

VI CONCLUSION. ASSESSMENT AND MANAGEMENT OF ATHEROGENIC DYSLIPIDEMIAS IN OBESE PATIENTS: WAIST GIRTH AS A VITAL SIGN

From the epidemiological and metabolic evidence available, there is no doubt that abdominal obesity is an important risk factor for the development of dyslipidemias and CVD. Several prospective studies have shown that abdominal obesity is associated with an increased mortality rate related to CVD (72,76–78,173–175). However, it is also important to acknowledge the notion that no intervention study has shown that reducing obesity and the amount of abdominal fat would lead to a reduction in the incidence of CVD and related mortality. To the best of our knowledge, the only ongoing project on this issue is the study of Swedish Obese Subjects (SOS study) (176), but these results will only apply to the question of weight loss resulting from the surgical treatment of very obese patients. However, it must be recognized that there is a considerable amount of literature that has indicated that reducing body weight and lowering the amount of abdominal fat is associated with major improvements in the CVD risk profile including reduction in blood pressure, improvement in plasma lipoprotein-lipid levels, and an increase in insulin sensitivity leading to a reduction in plasma insulin levels and to an improvement of glucose tolerance (112).

As obesity is often associated with metabolic complications causing prejudice to health, it has been suggested that obesity should be considered as a disease. However, because obesity is defined on the basis of the BMI, some healthy individuals with BMI values ≥30 are then classified as high-risk subjects (with a disease) despite the presence of a normal metabolic risk profile. This problem may explain the generally unimpressive findings reported with the pharmacotherapy of obesity, as these studies have largely included low-risk, normolipidemic obese women with a normal metabolic risk factor profile (177). Nevertheless, on the basis of the substantial metabolic improvements that can be generated by a 5–10% weight loss (56,112), the importance of targeting weight loss in high-risk viscerally obese patients with an atherogenic dyslipidemic state and identified by the hypertriglyceridemic waist phenotype rather than by the BMI should be emphasized in clinical practice (178). In this high-risk obesity phenotype, the benefits of pharmacotherapy may outweigh the potential hazards of drug therapy—a possibility that needs to be urgently tested in randomized weight loss trials.

Therefore, as for the treatment of numerous additional complications of obesity, the assessment and management of CVD risk in obese patients needs to go beyond considering only body weight as a therapeutic target. Regarding the treatment of obese dyslipidemic patients, randomized trials using lipid-lowering drugs have all shown the benefits of the pharmacotherapy irrespective of the initial patient characteristics (11–16). As most of these studies have also included overweight/obese patients, it is likely that the obese dyslipidemic patient will benefit from the pharmacotherapy of his/her dyslipidemic state either with a statin (if LDL cholesterol concentrations are elevated) or with a fibrate (in the event that HDL cholesterol levels are low). Therefore, it is important to treat the consequences of abdominal obesity in a high-risk dyslipidemic patient with CHD, as the treatment of the complications will generate clinical benefits. However, the risk of a first or recurrent CHD event associated with the management of atherogenic dyslipidemic states has been reported to be reduced by ~30%, which indicates that a substantial proportion of patients on pharmacotherapy for their dyslipidemic

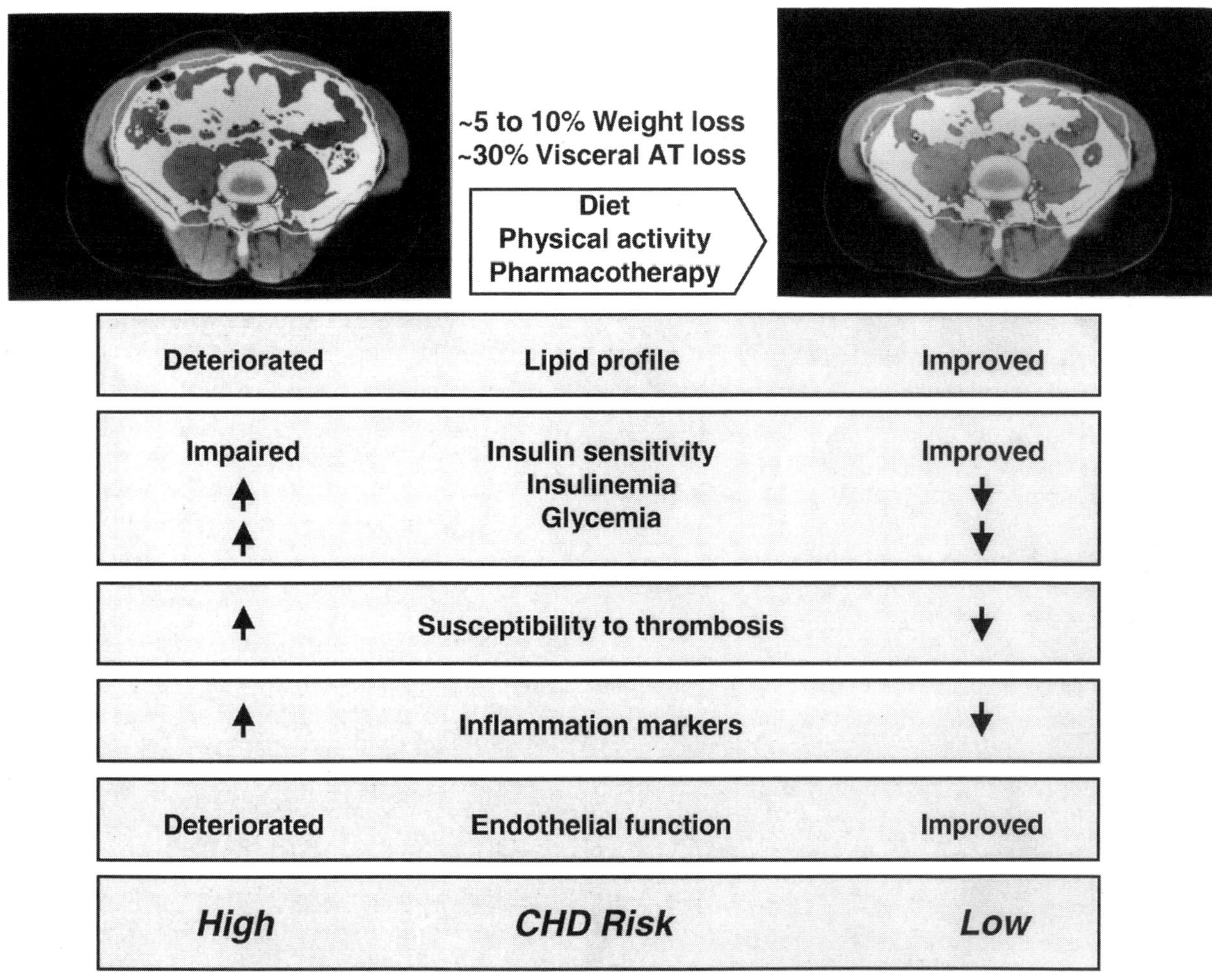

Figure 14 Potential benefits of moderate (5–10%) weight loss in a high-risk patient with the cluster of atherothrombotic, inflammatory metabolic abnormalities associated with hypertriglyceridemic waist. Weight loss in abdominally obese patients is associated with selective mobilization of diabetogenic and atherogenic visceral adipose tissue. Even a 5–10% weight loss is associated with preferential mobilization of visceral adipose tissue, leading to simultaneous improvement in all metabolic markers of coronary heart disease (CHD) risk. Thus, simultaneous metabolic improvements associated with mobilization of visceral adipose tissue may contribute to substantially reducing the risk of an acute coronary event in high-risk patients. (Adapted from Ref. 178.)

state remain nevertheless at high risk for CHD. In this context, it is proposed that CHD risk in the obese dyslipidemic patient will not be optimally managed until abdominal fat accumulation and waist reduction are considered as therapeutic targets (178). On that basis, we have proposed that waist circumference should be considered as a vital sign and incorporated in the assessment algorithm of all patients. Such recommendation has now been endorsed by the NCEP-ATP III guidelines, which recognize waist circumference as a key feature of the metabolic syndrome (36).

Finally, and as shown on the concluding last figure (Fig. 14), we believe that the reported preferential mobilization of visceral adipose tissue observed with a moderate weight loss of 5–10% (56,112) is likely to explain the greater impact of such moderate weight loss on the atherothrombotic, inflammatory profile of abdominally obese dyslipidemic patients. Again, randomized trials are needed to quantify the true impact of a selective loss of abdominal fat on the absolute and relative risk of coronary heart disease in this high-risk but prevalent subpopulation of abdominally obese dyslipidemic patients.

ACKNOWLEDGMENTS

The work of the authors reviewed in this chapter has been supported by the Canadian Institutes of Health Research and by the Canadian Diabetes Association. Jean-Pierre Després is chair professor of human nutrition, lipidology and prevention of cardiovascular diseases, which is supported by Pfizer, Provigo, and the Foundation of the Québec Heart Institute.

This work was supported by the National Institutes of Health Program Project grant HL18574 from the National Heart, Lung and Blood Institute, a grant from the National Dairy Promotion and Research Board, and administered in cooperation with the National Dairy Council, and was conducted at the Ernest Orlando Lawrence Berkeley National Laboratory.

REFERENCES

1. Keys A. Coronary heart disease in seven countries. Circulation 1970; 41(suppl I):I1–I211.
2. WHO Expert Committee on the Prevention of Coronary Heart Disease. World Health Organization Technical Reports Series 678. Geneva: World Health Organization, 1982.
3. NIH Consensus Conference. Lowering blood cholesterol to prevent heart disease. JAMA 1985; 253:2080–2086.
4. Stamler J, Wentworth D, Neaton JD. Is relationship between serum cholesterol and risk of premature death from coronary heart disease continuous or graded? Findings in 356,222 primary screenees of the Multiple Risk Factor Intervention Trial (MRFIT). JAMA 1986; 256:2823–2828.
5. Genest JJ, McNamara JR, Salem DN, Schaefer EJ. Prevalence of risk factors in men with premature coronary heart disease. Am J Cardiol 1991; 67:1185–1189.
6. Sniderman AD, Silberberg J. Is it time to measure apolipoprotein B? Arteriosclerosis 1990; 10(5):665–667.
7. Sharrett AR, Ballantyne CM, Coady SA, Heiss G, Sorlie PD, Catellier D, Patsch W. Coronary heart disease prediction from lipoprotein cholesterol levels, triglycerides, lipoprotein(a), apolipoproteins A-I and B, and HDL density subfractions: the Atherosclerosis Risk in Communities (ARIC) study. Circulation 2001; 104(10):1108–1113.
8. Assmann G, Schulte H. Relation of high-density lipoprotein cholesterol and triglycerides to incidence of atherosclerotic coronary artery disease (the PROCAM Experience). Am J Cardiol 1992; 70:733–737.
9. Lamarche B, Després JP, Moorjani S, Cantin B, Dagenais G, Lupien PJ. Prevalence of dyslipidemic phenotypes in ischemic heart disease—prospective results from the Québec Cardiovascular Study. Am J Cardiol 1995; 75:1189–1195.
10. Castelli WP. Epidemiology of coronary heart disease: the Framingham Study. Am J Med 1984; 76:4–12.
11. Downs JR, Clearfield M, Weis S, Whitney E, Shapiro DR, Beere PA, Langendorfer A, Stein EA, Kruyer W, Gotto AM Jr. Primary prevention of acute coronary events with lovastatin in men and women with average cholesterol levels: results of AFCAPS/TexCAPS, Air Force/Texas Coronary Atherosclerosis Prevention Study. JAMA 1998; 279(20):1615–1622.
12. Shepherd J, Cobbe SM, Ford I, Isles CG, Lorimer AR, MacFarlane PW, McKillop JH, Packard CJ. Prevention of coronary heart disease with pravastatin in men with hypercholesterolemia. West of Scotland Coronary Prevention Study Group. N Engl J Med 1995; 333(20):1301–1307.
13. Scandinavian Simvastatin Survival Study Group. Randomized trial of cholesterol lowering in 4444 patients with coronary heart disease: the Scandinavian Simvastatin Survival Study (4S). Lancet 1994; 344:1383–1389.
14. Sacks FM, Pfeffer MA, Moye LA, Rouleau JL, Rutherford JD, Cole TG, Brown L, Warnica JW, Arnold JMO, Wun CC, Davis BR, Braunwald E. The effect of pravastatin on coronary events after myocardial infarction in patients with average cholesterol levels. N Engl J Med 1996; 335:1001–1009.
15. Prevention of cardiovascular events and death with pravastatin in patients with coronary heart disease and

a broad range of initial cholesterol levels. The Long-Term Intervention with Pravastatin in Ischaemic Disease (LIPID) Study Group. N Engl J Med 1998; 339(19):1349–1357.

16. MRC/BHF Heart Protection Study of cholesterol lowering with simvastatin in 20,536 high-risk individuals: a randomised placebo-controlled trial. Lancet 2002; 360: 7–22.
17. Després JP, Lemieux I, Dagenais GR, Cantin B, Lamarche B. HDL-cholesterol as a marker of coronary heart disease risk: the Quebec cardiovascular study. Atherosclerosis 2000; 153(2):263–272.
18. Superko HR. Beyond LDL cholesterol reduction. Circulation 1996; 94(10):2351–2354.
19. Gordon T, Castelli WP, Hjortland MC, Kannel WB, Dawber TR. High density lipoprotein as a protective factor against coronary heart disease: the Framingham Study. Am J Med 1977; 62:707–714.
20. Miller NE, Forde OH, Thelle DS, Mjos OD. The Tromso Heart Study: high-density lipoprotein as a protective factor against coronary heart disease: a prospective case-control study. Lancet 1977; 1:965–967.
21. Castelli WP, Doyles JT, Gordon T. HDL-cholesterol and other lipids in coronary heart disease: the cooperative lipoprotein phenotyping study. Circulation 1977; 55:767–772.
22. Franceschini G. Epidemiologic evidence for high-density lipoprotein cholesterol as a risk factor for coronary artery disease. Am J Cardiol 2001; 88(12A): 9N–13N.
23. Rubins HB, Robins SJ, Collins D, Fye CL, Anderson JW, Elam MB, Faas FH, Linares E, Schaefer EJ, Schectman G, Wilt TJ, Wittes J. Gemfibrozil for the secondary prevention of coronary heart disease in men with low levels of high-density lipoprotein cholesterol. Veterans Affairs High-Density Lipoprotein Cholesterol Intervention Trial Study Group. N Engl J Med 1999; 341(6):410–418.
24. Rubin EM, Krauss RM, Spangler E, Verstuyft S, Clift S. Inhibition of early atherogenesis in transgenic mice by human apolipoprotein A-I. Nature 1991; 353:265–267.
25. Austin MA. Plasma triglyceride and coronary heart disease. Arterioscler Thromb 1991; 11:1–14.
26. Manninen V, Tenkanen L, Koskinen P, Huttunen JK, Mäntärri M, Heinonen OP, Frick MH. Joint effects of serum triglyceride and LDL-cholesterol and HDL-cholesterol concentrations on coronary heart disease risk in the Helsinki Heart Study. Implications for treatment. Circulation 1992; 85:37–45.
27. Jeppesen J, Hein HO, Suadicani P, Gyntelberg F. Relation of high TG-low HDL cholesterol and LDL cholesterol to the incidence of ischemic heart disease. An 8-year follow-up in the Copenhagen Male Study. Arterioscler Thromb Vasc Biol 1997; 17(6): 1114–1120.
28. Glomset JA. The plasma lecithin: cholesterol acyltransferase reaction. J Lipid Res 1968; 9:155–167.
29. Trigatti B, Rigotti A, Krieger M. The role of the high-density lipoprotein receptor SR-BI in cholesterol metabolism. Curr Opin Lipidol 2000; 11(2):123–131.
30. Oram JF, Vaughan AM. ABCA1-mediated transport of cellular cholesterol and phospholipids to HDL apolipoproteins. Curr Opin Lipidol 2000; 11(3):253–260.
31. Van Lenten BJ, Navab M, Shih D, Fogelman AM, Lusis AJ. The role of high-density lipoproteins in oxidation and inflammation. Trends Cardiovasc Med 2001; 11(3–4):155–161.
32. Lamarche B, Després JP, Pouliot MC, Prud'homme D, Moorjani S, Lupien PJ, Nadeau A, Tremblay A, Bouchard C. Metabolic heterogeneity associated with high plasma triglyceride or low HDL cholesterol levels in men. Arterioscler Thromb 1993; 13(1):33–40.
33. Reaven GM. Role of insulin resistance in human disease. Diabetes 1988; 37:1595–1607.
34. Laakso M, Sarlund H, Mykkänen L. Insulin resistance is associated with lipid and lipoprotein abnormalities in subjects with varying degrees of glucose tolerance. Arteriosclerosis 1990; 10:223–231.
35. Reaven GM, Ida-Chen YD, Jeppesen J, Maheux P, Krauss RM. Insulin resistance and hyperinsulinemia in individuals with small, dense, low density lipoprotein particles. J Clin Invest 1993; 92:141–146.
36. Executive Summary of the Third Report of the National Cholesterol Education Program (NCEP) Expert Panel on Detection, Evaluation, and Treatment of High Blood Cholesterol in Adults (Adult Treatment Panel III). JAMA 2001; 285(19):2486–2497.
37. Després JP. Visceral obesity: a component of the insulin resistance-dyslipidemic syndrome. Can J Cardiol 1994; 10:17B–22B.
38. Després JP, Marette A. Relation of components of insulin resistance syndrome to coronary disease risk. Curr Opin Lipidol 1994; 5:274–289.
39. Tchernof A, Lamarche B, Prud'homme D, Nadeau A, Moorjani S, Labrie F, Lupien PJ, Després JP. The dense LDL phenotype. Association with plasma lipoprotein levels, visceral obesity, and hyperinsulinemia in men. Diabetes Care 1996; 19(6):629–637.
40. Lemieux I, Pascot A, Couillard C, Lamarche B, Tchernof A, Alméras N, Bergeron J, Gaudet D, Tremblay G, Prud'homme D, Nadeau A, Després JP. Hypertriglyceridemic waist: a marker of the atherogenic metabolic triad (hyperinsulinemia; hyperapolipoprotein B; small, dense LDL) in men? Circulation 2000; 102(2):179–184.
41. Austin MA, King MC, Vranizan KM, Krauss RM. Atherogenic lipoprotein phenotype: a proposed genetic marker for coronary heart disease. Circulation 1990; 82:495–506.
42. Ford ES, Giles WH, Dietz WH. Prevalence of the metabolic syndrome among US adults: findings from

the third National Health and Nutrition Examination Survey. JAMA 2002; 287(3):356–359.
43. Lamarche B, Moorjani S, Lupien PJ, Cantin B, Bernard PM, Dagenais G, Després JP. Apolipoprotein A-I and B levels and the risk of ischemic heart disease during a five-year follow-up of men in the Québec Cardiovascular Study. Circulation 1996; 94(3):273–278.
44. Pyörälä K. Relationship of glucose tolerance and plasma insulin to the incidence of coronary heart disease: results from the two population studies in Finland. Diabetes Care 1979; 2:131–141.
45. Welborn TA, Wearne K. Coronary heart disease incidence and cardiovascular mortality in Busselton with reference to glucose and insulin concentrations. Diabetes Care 1979; 2:154–160.
46. Eschwège E, Richard JL, Thibult N, Ducimetière P, Warnet JM, Rosselin G. Coronary heart disease mortality in relation with diabetes, blood glucose and plasma insulin levels: the Paris Prospective Study, ten years later. Horm Metab Res 1985; 15(suppl):41–46.
47. Yarmell JWG, Sweetnam PM, Marks V, Teale JD, Bolton CH. Insulin in ischemic heart disease: are associations explained by triglyceride concentrations? The Caerphilly Prospective Study. Br Heart J 1994; 171: 293–296.
48. Fontbonne A, Eschwège E, Cambien F, Richard JL, Ducimetière P, Thibult N, Warnet JM, Claude JR. Hypertriglyceridemia as a risk factor of coronary heart disease mortality in subjects with impaired glucose tolerance or diabetes: results from the 11-year follow-up of the Paris Prospective Study. Diabetologia 1989; 32:300–304.
49. Fontbonne A, Charles MA, Thibult N, Richard JL, Claude JM, Warnet JM, Rosselin GE, Eschwège E. Hyperinsulinemia as a predictor of coronary heart disease mortality in a healthy population: the Paris Prospective Study. 15-year follow-up. Diabetologia 1991; 34:356–361.
50. Després JP, Lamarche B, Mauriège P, Cantin B, Dagenais GR, Moorjani S, Lupien PJ. Hyperinsulinemia as an independent risk factor for ischemic heart disease. N Engl J Med 1996; 334:952–957.
51. Lamarche B, Tchernof A, Moorjani S, Cantin B, Dagenais GR, Lupien PJ, Després JP. Small, dense low-density lipoprotein particles as a predictor of the risk of ischemic heart disease in men. Prospective results from the Québec Cardiovascular Study. Circulation 1997; 95:69–75.
52. St-Pierre AC, Ruel IL, Cantin B, Dagenais GR, Bernard PM, Després JP, Lamarche B. Comparison of various electrophoretic characteristics of LDL particles and their relationship to the risk of ischemic heart disease. Circulation 2001; 104(19):2295–2299.
53. Lamarche B, Tchernof A, Mauriège P, Cantin B, Dagenais GR, Lupien PJ, Després JP. Fasting insulin and apolipoprotein B levels and low-density lipoprotein particle size as risk factors for ischemic heart disease. JAMA 1998; 279:1955–1961.
54. Kissebah AH, Freedman DS, Peiris AN. Health risks of obesity. Med Clin North Am 1989; 73:111–138.
55. Després JP. Obesity and lipid metabolism: relevance of body fat distribution. Curr Opin Lipidol 1991; 2:5–15.
56. Després JP. Dyslipidemia and obesity. Bailleres Clin Endocrinol Metab 1994; 8:629–660.
57. Barrett-Connor E. Obesity, atherosclerosis, and coronary artery disease. Ann Intern Med 1985; 103:1010–1019.
58. Manson JE, Willett WC, Stampfer MJ, Colditz GA, Hunter DJ, Hankinson SE, Hennekens CH, Speizer FE. Body weight and mortality among women. N Engl J Med 1995; 333:677–685.
59. Bouchard C, Després JP. Variation in fat distribution with age and health implications. In: Eckert HM, Spirduso W, eds. Physical Activity and Aging. Champaign, IL: American Academy of Physical Education, 1989:78–106.
60. Bray GA, Davidson MB, Drenick EJ. Obesity: a serious symptom. An Intern Med 1972; 77:779–795.
61. Pooling Project Research Group. Relationship of blood pressure, serum cholesterol, smoking habit, relative weight and ECG abnormalities to incidence of major coronary events: final report of the Pooling Project. J Chron Dis 1978; 31:201.
62. Björntorp P. Hazards in subgroups of human obesity. Eur J Clin Invest 1984; 14:239–241.
63. Harrison GH. Height-weight tables. Ann Intern Med 1985; 103:989–994.
64. Després JP. Assessing obesity: beyond the BMI. NIN Rev 1992; 7(suppl):1–4.
65. Quetelet LAJ. Sur l'homme et le dévéloppement de ses facultés, ou essai d'une physique sociale Paris: Bachelier, 1835.
66. Keys A, Fidanza F, Karvonen MJ, Kimura N, Taylor HL. Indices of relative weight and obesity. J Chron Dis 1972; 25:329–334.
67. Garrow J, Summerbell C. Meta-analysis on the effect of exercise on the composition of weight loss. Int J Obes 1994; 18:516–517.
68. Bray GA, Gray DS. Treatment of obesity: an overview. Diabetes Metab Rev 1988; 4:653–679.
69. Després JP, Moorjani S, Lupien PJ, Tremblay A, Nadeau A, Bouchard C. Regional distribution of body fat, plasma lipoproteins, and cardiovascular disease. Arteriosclerosis 1990; 10:487–511.
70. Kissebah AH, Peiris AN. Biology of regional body fat distribution: Relationship to non-insulin-dependent diabetes mellitus. Diabetes Metab Rev 1989; 5:83–109.
71. Björntorp P. Abdominal obesity and the development of non-insulin-dependent diabetes mellitus. Diabetes Metab Rev 1988; 4:615–622.

72. Donahue RP, Abbott RD, Bloom E, Reed DM, Yano K. Central obesity and coronary heart disease in men. Lancet 1987; 1:821–824.
73. Vague J. La différenciation sexuelle, facteur déterminant des formes de l'obésité. Presse Med 1947; 30:339–340.
74. Albrink MJ, Meigs JW. Interrelationship between skinfold thickness, serum lipids and blood sugar in normal men. Am J Clin Nutr 1964; 15:255–261.
75. Allard C, Goulet C. Serum lipids: an epidemiological study of an active Montreal population. Can Med Assoc J 1968; 98:627–637.
76. Lapidus L, Bengtsson C, Larsson B, Pennert K, Rybo E, Sjöström L. Distribution of adipose tissue and risk of cardiovascular disease and death: a 12 year follow-up of participants in the population study of women in Gothenburg, Sweden. BMJ 1984; 289:1261–1263.
77. Larsson B, Svardsudd K, Welin L, Wilhemsen L, Björntorp P, Tibblin G. Abdominal adipose tissue distribution, obesity and risk of cardiovascular disease and death: 13 year follow-up of participants in the study of men born in 1913. BMJ 1984; 288:1401–1404.
78. Ducimetière P, Richard J, Cambien F. The pattern of subcutaneous fat distribution in middle-aged men and the risk of coronary heart disease: the Paris Prospective Study. Int J Obes 1986; 10:229–240.
79. Ohlsson LO, Larsson B, Svärdsudd K, Welin L, Eriksson H, Wilhelmsen L, Björntorp P, Tibblin G. The influence of body fat distribution on the incidence of diabetes mellitus—13.5 years of follow-up of the participants in the study of men born in 1913. Diabetes 1985; 34:1055–1058.
80. Anderson AJ, Sobocinski KA, Freedman DS, Barboriak JJ, Rimm AA, Gruchow HW. Body fat distribution, plasma lipids and lipoproteins. Arteriosclerosis 1988; 8:88–94.
81. Kissebah AH, Vydelingum N, Murray R, Evans DJ, Hartz AJ, Kalkhoff RK, Adams PW. Relation of body fat distribution to metabolic complications of obesity. J Clin Endocrinol Metab 1982; 54:254–260.
82. Krotkiewski M, Björntorp P, Sjöström L, Smith U. Impact of obesity on metabolism in men and women. Importance of regional adipose tissue distribution. J Clin Invest 1983; 72:1150–1162.
83. Albrink MJ, Krauss RM, Lindgren FT, Von der Groeben J, Pam S, Wood PD. Intercorrelations among plasma high density lipoprotein, obesity and triglycerides in a normal population. Lipids 1980; 15:668–676.
84. Ostlund RE, Staten M, Kohrt WM, Schultz J, Malley M. The ratio of waist-to-hip circumferences, plasma insulin level, and glucose intolerance as independent predictors of the HDL2-cholesterol level in older adults. N Engl J Med 1990; 322:229–234.
85. Terry RB, Wood PD, Haskell WL, Stefanick ML, Krauss RM. Regional adiposity pattern in relation to lipids, lipoprotein cholesterol, and lipoprotein subfraction mass in men. J Clin Endocrinol Metab 1989; 68: 191–199.
86. Després JP, Moorjani S, Ferland M, Tremblay A, Lupien PJ, Nadeau A, Pinault S, Thériault G, Bouchard C. Adipose tissue distribution and plasma lipoprotein levels in obese women: importance of intra-abdominal fat. Arteriosclerosis 1989; 9:203–210.
87. Després JP, Ferland M, Moorjani S, Tremblay A, Lupien PJ, Thériault G, Bouchard C. Role of hepatic-triglyceride lipase activity in the association between intra-abdominal fat and plasma HDL-cholesterol in obese women. Arteriosclerosis 1989; 9:485–492.
88. Després JP, Moorjani S, Tremblay A, Ferland M, Lupien PJ, Nadeau A, Bouchard C. Relation of high plasma triglyceride levels associated with obesity and regional adipose tissue distribution to plasma lipoprotein-lipid composition in premenopausal women. Clin Invest Med 1989; 12:374–380.
89. Austin MA, Breslow JL, Hennekens CH, Buring JE, Willet WC, Krauss RM. Low density lipoprotein subclass patterns and risk of myocardial infarction. JAMA 1988; 260:1917–1921.
90. Hartz AJ, Rupley DC, Kalkhoff RD, Rimm AA. Relationship of obesity to diabetes: Influence of obesity and body fat distribution. Prevent Med 1983; 12:351–357.
91. Williams PT, Haskell WL, Vranizan KM, Krauss RM. The associations of high-density lipoprotein subclasses with insulin and glucose levels, physical activity, resting heart rate, and regional adiposity in men with coronary artery disease: the Stanford Coronary Risk Intervention Project baseline survey. Metabolism 1995; 44(1): 106–114.
92. Pascot A, Lemieux I, Prud'homme D, Tremblay A, Nadeau A, Couillard C, Bergeron J, Lamarche B, Després JP. Reduced HDL particle size as an additional feature of the atherogenic dyslipidemia of abdominal obesity. J Lipid Res 2001; 42(12):2007–2014.
93. Katzel LI, Krauss RM, Goldberg AP. Relation of plasma TG and HDL-C concentrations to body composition and plasma insulin levels are altered in men with small LDL particles. Arterioscler Thromb 1994; 14:1121–1128.
94. Landin K, Lonnroth P, Krotkiewski G, Smith U. Increased insulin resistance and fat cell lipolysis in obese but not lean women with a high waist/hip ratio. Eur J Clin Invest 1990; 20:530–535.
95. Haffner SM, Stern MP, Mitchell BD, Hazuda HP, Patterson JK. Incidence of type II diabetes mellitus in Mexican Americans predicted by fasting insulin and glucose levels, obesity and body fat distribution. Diabetes 1990; 39:283–289.
96. Peiris AN, Struve MF, Kissebah AH. Relationship of body fat distribution to the metabolic clearance of insulin in premenopausal women. Int J Obes 1987; 11: 581–589.

97. Kannel WB, Gordon T, Castelli WP. Obesity, lipids and glucose intolerance. The Framingham Study. Am J Clin Nutr 1979; 32:1238–1245.
98. Borkan GA, Gerzof SG, Robbins AH, Hults DE, Silbert CK, Silbert JE. Assessment of abdominal fat content by computed tomography. Am J Clin Nutr 1982; 36:172–177.
99. Tokunaga K, Matsuzawa Y, Ishikawa K, Tarui S. A novel technique for the determination of body fat by computed tomography. Int J Obes 1983; 7:437–445.
100. Sjöström L, Kvist H, Cederblad A, Tylen U, Sjöström L, Kvist H, Cederblad A, Tylen U. Determination of total adipose tissue and body fat in women by computed tomography, 40K, and tritium. Am J Physiol 1986; 250:E736–E745.
101. Kvist H, Chowdhury B, Grangard U, Tylén U, Sjöström L. Total and visceral adipose tissue volumes derived from measurements with computed tomography in adult men and women: predictive equations. Am J Clin Nutr 1988; 48:1351–1361.
102. Fujioka S, Matsuzawa Y, Tokunaga K, Tarui S. Contribution of intra-abdominal fat accumulation to the impairment of glucose and lipid metabolism in human obesity. Metabolism 1987; 36:54–59.
103. Fujioka S, Matsuzawa Y, Tokunaga K, Kano Y, Kobatake T, Tarui S. Treatment of visceral obesity. Int J Obes 1991; 15:59–65.
104. Fujioka S, Matsuzawa Y, Tokunaga K, Kawamoto T, Kobatake T, Keno Y, Kotani K, Yoshida S, Tarui S. Improvement of glucose and lipid metabolism associated with selective reduction of intra-abdominal visceral fat in premenopausal women with visceral fat obesity. Int J Obes 1991; 15:853–859.
105. Sparrow D, Borkan GA, Gerzof SG, Wisniewski CK. Relationship of body fat distribution to glucose tolerance. Results of computed tomography in male participants of the normative aging study. Diabetes 1986; 35:411–415.
106. Peiris AN, Sothmann MS, Hennes MI, Lee MB, Wilson CR, Gustafson AB, Kissebah AH. Relative contribution of obesity and body fat distribution to alterations in glucose insulin homeostasis: predictive values of selected indices in premenopausal women. Am J Clin Nutr 1989; 49:758–764.
107. Després JP, Nadeau A, Tremblay A, Ferland M, Lupien PJ. Role of deep abdominal fat in the association between regional adipose tissue distribution and glucose tolerance in obese women. Diabetes 1989; 38: 304–309.
108. Pouliot MC, Després JP, Nadeau A, Moorjani S, Prud'homme D, Lupien PJ, Tremblay A, Bouchard C. Visceral obesity in men. Associations with glucose tolerance, plasma insulin, and lipoprotein levels. Diabetes 1992; 41:826–834.
109. Després JP. Visceral obesity, insulin resistance, and related dyslipoproteinemias. In: Rifkin H, Colwell JA, Taylor SI, eds. Diabetes 1991. Amsterdam: Elsevier Science, 1991:95–99.
110. Lemieux S, Prud'homme D, Bouchard C, Tremblay A, Després JP. Sex differences in the relation of visceral adipose tissue accumulation to total body fatness. Am J Clin Nutr 1993; 58:463–467.
111. Lemieux S, Després JP, Moorjani S, Nadeau A, Thériault G, Prud'homme D, Tremblay A, Bouchard C, Lupien PJ. Are gender differences in cardiovascular disease risk factors explained by the level of visceral adipose tissue? Diabetologia 1994; 37:757–764.
112. Després JP, Lamarche B. Effects of diet and physical activity on adiposity and body fat distribution: implications for the prevention of cardiovascular disease. Nutr Res Rev 1993; 6:137–159.
113. Zilversmit DB. Atherogenesis: a postprandial phenomenon. Circulation 1979; 60:473–485.
114. Cohn JS, McNamara JR, Cohn SD, Ordovas JM, Schaefer EJ. Postprandial plasma lipoprotein changes in human subjects of different ages. J Lipid Res 1988; 29:469–479.
115. Krasinski SD, Cohn JS, Schaefer EJ, Russell RM. Postprandial plasma retinyl ester response is greater in older subjects compared with younger subjects. Evidence for a delayed plasma clearance of intestinal lipoproteins. J Clin Invest 1990; 85:883–892.
116. Couillard C, Bergeron N, Prud'homme D, Bergeron J, Tremblay A, Bouchard C, Mauriège P, Després JP. Gender difference in postprandial lipemia—importance of visceral adipose tissue accumulation. Arterioscler Thromb Vasc Biol 1999; 19(10):2448–2455.
117. Georgopoulos A, Rosengard AM. Abnormalities in the metabolism of postprandial and fasting triglyceride-rich lipoprotein subfractions in normal and insulin-dependent diabetic subjects: effects of sex. Metabolism 1989; 38:781–789.
118. Bergeron N, Havel RJ. Assessment of postprandial lipemia: nutritional influences. Curr Opin Lipidol 1997; 8:43–52.
119. Hartung GH, Lawrence SJ, Reeves RS, Foreyt JP. Effect of alcohol and exercise on postprandial lipemia and triglyceride clearance in men. Atherosclerosis 1993; 100:33–40.
120. Frase AG, Rosalki SB, Gamble GD, Pounder RE. Inter-individual and intra-individual variability of ethanol concentration-time profiles: comparison of ethanol ingestion before or after an evening meal. Br J Clin Pharmacol 1995; 40:387–392.
121. Pownall HJ. Dietary ethanol is associated with reduced lipolysis of intestinally derived lipoproteins. J Lipid Res 1994; 35:2105–2113.
122. Weintraub MS, Rosen Y, Otto R, Eisenberg S, Breslow JL. Physical exercise conditioning in the absence of weight loss reduces fasting and postprandial triglyceride-rich lipoprotein levels. Circulation 1989; 79:1007–1014.

123. Ziogas GG, Thomas TR, Harris WS. Exercise training, postprandial hypertriglyceridemia and LDL subfraction distribution. Med Sci Sports Exerc 1997; 29:986–991.
124. Aldred HE, Perry IC, Hardman AE. The effect of a single bout of brisk walking on postprandial lipemia in normolipidemic young adults. Metabolism 1994; 43: 836–841.
125. Aldred HE, Hardman AE, Taylor S. Influence of 12 weeks of training by brisk walking on postprandial lipemia and insulinemia in sedentary middle-aged women. Metabolism 1995; 44:390–397.
126. Lewis GF, O'Meara NM, Soltys PA, Blackman JD, Iverius PH, Druetzler AF, Getz GS, Polonsky KS. Postprandial lipoprotein metabolism in normal and obese subjects: comparison after the vitamin A fat-loading test. J Clin Endocrinol Metab 1990; 71:1041–1050.
127. Wideman L, Kaminsky LA, Whaley MH. Postprandial lipemia in obese men with abdominal fat patterning. J Sports Med Phys Fitness 1996; 36:204–210.
128. Ryu JE, Craven TE, MacArthur RD, Hinson WH, Bond MG, Hagaman AP, Crouse JR. Relationship of intraabdominal fat as measured by magnetic resonance imaging to postprandial lipemia in middle-aged subjects. Am J Clin Nutr 1994; 60:586–591.
129. Mekki N, Christofilis MA, Charbonnier M, Atlan-Gepner C, Defoort C, Juhel C, Borel P, Portugal H, Pauli AM, Vialettes B, Lairon D. Influence of obesity and body fat distribution on postprandial lipemia and triglyceride-rich lipoproteins in adult women. J Clin Endocrinol Metab 1999; 84(1):184–191.
130. Couillard C, Bergeron N, Prud'homme D, Bergeron J, Tremblay A, Bouchard C, Mauriège P, Després JP. Postprandial triglyceride response in visceral obesity in men. Diabetes 1998; 47(6):953–960.
131. Couillard C, Bergeron N, Bergeron J, Pascot A, Mauriège P, Tremblay A, Prud'homme D, Bouchard C, Després JP. Metabolic heterogeneity underlying postprandial lipemia among men with low fasting high density lipoprotein cholesterol concentrations. J Clin Endocrinol Metab 2000; 85:4575–4582.
132. Juhan-Vague I, Alessi MC. PAI-1, obesity, insulin resistance and risk of cardiovascular events. Thromb Haemost 1997; 78(1):656–660.
133. Yudkin JS, Stehouwer CD, Emeis JJ, Coppack SW. C-reactive protein in healthy subjects: associations with obesity, insulin resistance, and endothelial dysfunction: a potential role for cytokines originating from adipose tissue? Aterioscler Thromb Vasc Biol 1999; 19: 972–978.
134. Lemieux I, Pascot A, Prud'homme D, Alméras N, Bogaty P, Nadeau A, Bergeron J, Després JP. Elevated C-reactive protein: another component of the atherothrombotic profile of abdominal obesity. Arterioscler Thromb Vasc Biol 2001; 21(6):961–967.
135. Tracy RP. Is visceral adiposity the "enemy within"? Arterioscler Thromb Vasc Biol 2001; 21(6):881–883.
136. Després JP. Health consequences of visceral obesity. Ann Med 2001; 33(8):534–541.
137. Björntorp P. "Portal" adipose tissue as a generator of risk factors for cardiovascular disease and diabetes. Arteriosclerosis 1990; 10:493–496.
138. Hennes M, Shrago E, Kissebah AH. Receptor and post receptor effects of FFA on hepatocyte insulin dynamics. Int J Obes 1990; 14:831–841.
139. Svedberg J, Björntorp P, Smith V, Lönnroth P. FFA inhibition of insulin binding, degradation, and action in isolated rat hepatocytes. Diabetes 1990; 39:570–574.
140. Randle PJ, Garland PB, Hales CN, Newsholme EA. The glucose fatty-acid cycle; its role in insulin sensitivity and the metabolic disturbances of diabetes mellitus. Lancet 1963; 1:785–789.
141. Taylor SI, Mukherjee C, Jungas RL. Regulation of pyruvate dehydrogenase in isolated rat liver mitochondria. J Biol Chem 1975; 250:2028–2035.
142. Felber JP. From obesity to diabetes. Pathophysiological considerations. Int J Obes 1972; 16:937–952.
143. Jahoor F, Klein S, Wolfe R. Mechanism of regulation of glucose production by lipolysis in humans. Am J Physiol 1992; 262:E353–E358.
144. Jackson RL, McLean LR, Demel RA. Mechanism of action of lipoprotein lipase and hepatic triglyceride lipase. Am Heart J 1987; 113:551–554.
145. Pollare T, Vessby B, Lithell H. Lipoprotein lipase activity in skeletal muscle is related to insulin sensitivity. Arterioscler Thromb 1991; 11:1192–1203.
146. Fujimoto WY, Leonetti DL, Newell-Morris L, Shuman WP, Wahl PW. Relationship of absence or presence of a family history of diabetes to body weight and body fat distribution in type 2 diabetes. Int J Obes 1990; 15:111–120.
147. Lemieux S, Després JP, Nadeau A, Prud'homme D, Tremblay A, Bouchard C. Heterogeneous glycaemic and insulinaemic responses to oral glucose in non-diabetic men: interactions between duration of obesity, body fat distribution and family history of diabetes mellitus. Diabetologia 1992; 35:653–659.
148. Peiris AN, Mueller RA, Struve MF, Smith GA, Kissebah AH. Relationship of androgenic activity to splanchnic insulin metabolism and peripheral glucose utilization in premenopausal women. J Clin Endocrinol Metab 1987; 64:162–169.
149. Evans DJ, Hoffmann RG, Kalkhoff RK, Kissebah AH. Relationship of androgenic activity to body fat topography, fat cell morphology, and metabolic aberrations in premenopausal women. J Clin Endocrinol Metab 1983; 57:304–310.
150. Kissebah AH, Evans DJ, Peiris A, Wilson CR. Endocrine characteristics in regional obesities: role of sex steroids. In: Vague J, Björntorp P, Guy-Grand B, eds.

Metabolic Complications of Human Obesities Amsterdam: Elsevier Science, 1985:115–130.

151. Seidell JC, Björntorp P, Sjöström L, Kvist H, Sannerstedt R. Visceral fat accumulation is positively associated with insulin, glucose and C-peptide levels, but negatively with testosterone levels. Metabolism 1990; 39:897–901.

152. Tchernof A, Després JP, Bélanger A, Dupont A, Prud'homme D, Moorjani S, Lupien PJ, Labrie F. Reduced testosterone and adrenal C19 steroid levels in obese men. Metabolism 1994; 4:513–519.

153. Tchernof A, Després JP, Dupont A, Bélanger A, Nadeau A, Prud'homme D, Moorjani S, Lupien PJ, Labrie F. Importance of body fatness and adipose tissue distribution in the relation of steroid hormones to glucose tolerance and plasma insulin levels in men. Diabetes Care 1995; 18:292–299.

154. Tchernof A, Després JP. Sex steroid hormones, sex hormone-binding globulin, and obesity in men and women. Horm Metab Res 2000; 32(11–12):526–536.

155. Tchernof A, Labrie F, Bélanger A, Prud'homme D, Bouchard C, Tremblay A, Nadeau A, Després JP. Relationships between endogenous steroid hormone, sex hormone-binding globulin and lipoprotein levels in men: contribution of visceral obesity, insulin levels and other metabolic variables. Atherosclerosis 1997; 133(2): 235–244.

156. Tchernof A, Labrie F, Bélanger A, Després JP. Obesity and metabolic complications: contribution of dehydroepiandrosterone and other steroid hormones. J Endocrinol 1996; 150(suppl):S155–S164.

157. Brindley DN, Rolland Y. Possible connections between stress, diabetes, obesity, hypertension, and altered metabolism that may result in atherosclerosis. Clin Sci 1989; 77:453–461.

158. Brindley DN. Metabolic approaches to atherosclerosis: effect of gliclazide. Metabolism 1992; 41(suppl 1):20–24.

159. Brindley DN. Neuroendocrine regulation and obesity. Int J Obes 1992; 16:S73–S79.

160. Björntorp P. Visceral fat accumulation: the missing link between psychosocial factors and cardiovascular disease? J Intern Med 1991; 230:195–201.

161. Rebuffé-Scrive M, Lundholm K, Björntorp P. Glucocorticoid binding of human adipose tissue. Eur J Clin Invest 1985; 15:267–271.

162. Pedersen SB, Jonler M, Richelsen B. Characterization of regional and gender differences in glucocorticoid receptors and lipoprotein lipase activity in human adipose tissue. J Clin Endocrinol Metab 1994; 78:1354–1359.

163. Bengtsson BA, Eden S, Lonn L, Kvist H, Stokland A, Lindstedt G, Bosaeus I, Tolli J, Sjostrom L, Isaksson OG. Treatment of adults with growth hormone (GH) deficiency with recombinant human GH. J Clin Endocrinol Metab 1993; 76(2):309–317.

164. Beshyah SA, Johnston DG. Cardiovascular disease and risk factors in adults with hypopituitarism. Clin Endocrinol (Oxf) 1999; 50(1):1–15.

165. Snel YE, Brummer RJ, Doerga ME, Zelissen PM, Bakker CJ, Hendriks MJ, Koppeschaar HP. Adipose tissue assessed by magnetic resonance imaging in growth hormone-deficient adults: the effect of growth hormone replacement and a comparison with control subjects. Am J Clin Nutr 1995; 61(6):1290–1294.

166. Rosen T, Johannsson G, Johansson JO, Bengtsson BA. Consequences of growth hormone deficiency in adults and the benefits and risks of recombinant human growth hormone treatment. A review paper. Horm Res 1995; 43(1–3):93–99.

167. Sesmilo G, Biller BM, Llevadot J, Hayden D, Hanson G, Rifai N, Klibanski A. Effects of growth hormone administration on inflammatory and other cardiovascular risk markers in men with growth hormone deficiency. A randomized, controlled clinical trial. Ann Intern Med 2000; 133(2):111–122.

168. Seidell JC, Oosterlee A, Thijssen MAO, Burema J, Deurenberg P, Hautvast JGAJ, Ruijs JHJ. Assessment of intra-abdominal and subcutaneous abdominal fat: relation between anthropometry and computed tomography. Am J Clin Nutr 1987; 45:7–13.

169. Seidell JC, Oosterlee A, Deurenberg P, Hautvast JGAJ, Ruijs JHJ. Abdominal fat depots measured with computed tomography: effects of degree of obesity, sex and age. Eur J Clin Nutr 1988; 42:805–815.

170. Ferland M, Després JP, Tremblay A, Pinault S, Nadeau A, Moorjani S, Lupien PJ, Thériault G, Bouchard C. Assessment of adipose tissue distribution by computed axial tomography in obese women: association with body density and anthropometric measurements. Brit J Nutr 1989; 61:139–148.

171. Després JP, Prud'homme D, Pouliot MC, Tremblay A, Bouchard C. Estimation of deep abdominal fat accumulation from simple anthropometric measurements in men. Am J Clin Nutr 1991; 54:471–477.

172. Pouliot MC, Després JP, Lemieux S, Moorjani S, Bouchard C, Tremblay A, Nadeau A, Lupien PJ. Waist circumference and abdominal sagittal diameter: best simple anthropometric indexes of abdominal visceral adipose tissue accumulation and related cardiovascular risk in men and women. Am J Cardiol 1994; 73:460–468.

173. Folsom AR, Kaye SA, Sellers TA, Hong CP, Cerhan JR, Potter JD, Prineas RJ. Body fat distribution and 5-year risk of death in older women. JAMA 1993; 269: 483–487.

174. Stokes J, Garrison RJ, Kannel WB. The independent contributions of various indices of obesity to the 22-year incidence of coronary heart disease: the Framingham Heart Study. In: Vague J, Björntorp P, Guy-Grand B, eds. Metabolic Complications of Human Obesities. Amsterdam: Elsevier Science, 1985:49–57.

175. Terry RB, Page WF, Haskell WL. Waist/hip ratio,

body mass index and premature cardiovascular disease mortality in US army veteran during a twenty-three year follow-up study. Int J Obes 1992; 16:417–423.

176. Sjöström L, Larsson B, Backman L, Bengtsson C, Bouchard C, Dahlgren S, Hallgren P, Jonsson E, Karls son J, Lapidus L. Swedish Obese Subjects (SOS). Recruitment for an intervention study and a selected description of the obese state. Int J Obes 1992; 16:465–479.

177. Després JP. Drug treatment for obesity. We need more studies in men at higher risk of coronary events. BMJ 2001; 322(7299):1379–1380.

178. Després JP, Lemieux I, Prud'homme D. Treatment of obesity: need to focus on high risk abdominally obese patients. BMJ 2001; 322(7288):716–720.

179. Després JP, Lemieux S, Lamarche B, Prud'homme D, Moorjani S, Brun LD, Gagné C, Lupien PJ. The insulin-resistance syndrome: contribution of visceral obesity and therapeutic implications. Int J Obes 1995; 19(suppl):S76–S86.

36

Obesity and Blood Pressure Regulation

Albert P. Rocchini

University of Michigan, Ann Arbor, Michigan, U.S.A.

I INTRODUCTION

Obesity is an independent risk factor for the development of both hypertension and cardiovascular disease. This chapter will summarize: techniques for measuring blood pressure in obese individuals and the effect of obesity on these measurements; the evidence that substantiates that obesity is an independent risk factor for the development of hypertension; an explanation of how obesity may result in the development of hypertension; a brief summary of other cardiovascular abnormalities associated with obesity; and finally a brief summary of how to manage the hypertensive obese individual.

II MEASUREMENT OF BLOOD PRESSURE IN OBESE INDIVIDUALS

For years, physicians believed that the high blood pressure observed in many obese individuals was related to a measurement error. The indirect method of measuring blood pressure usually results in an overestimation of both systolic and diastolic blood pressure. The overestimation of blood pressure is due, in part, to the fact that pressure measured by the cuff and sphygmomanometer is not just the force required to occlude the brachial artery but also includes the force required to compress the soft tissues of the arm. In the case of obesity, the increased subcutaneous fat present in the upper arm imposes a greater resistance to compression and therefore a higher cuff inflation pressure. Most of the effects of obesity on the indirect measurement of blood pressure can be corrected by using and appropriate size blood pressure cuff. Although, compared with intra-arterial measurements of blood pressure, the indirect method is less precise, nevertheless, when properly measured, elevated indirect blood pressure readings are a reliable method for diagnosing hypertension. The major errors encountered in the measurement of blood pressure include cuff size, type of instrumentation for measuring blood pressure, and observer errors.

A Cuff Size

The selection of an appropriate-size compression cuff is critical to obtaining accurate reading. The cuff consists of an inflatable bladder with a cloth cover. The dimensions of the inner bladder, not the size of the cover, determine cuff size (Fig. 1). The bladder must be the correct width for the circumference at the mid point of the upper arm (Table 1). A bladder that is too small will cause a falsely high pressure. The bladder should be wide enough to cover ~75% of the upper arm between the top of the shoulder and the olecranon. The length of the bladder also influences the accuracy of measurements. A bladder length that is roughly twice the width is ideal and should result in the cuff nearly encircling the arm. If a question arises as to which of two cuffs is appropriate, a cuff that is slightly wider and longer than

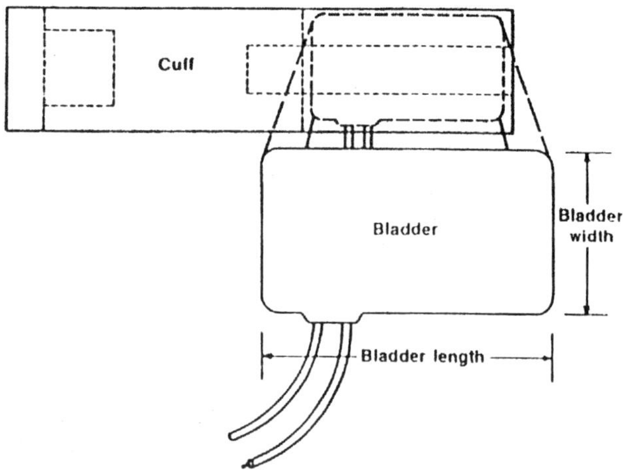

Figure 1 Schematic representation of a blood pressure cuff.

needed should be chosen. It is unlikely that slightly too large a cuff will mask hypertension, but a cuff that is too small will lead to an overestimate of blood pressure.

B Types of Equipment for Indirect Measurement of Blood Pressure

Physicians have taken reliable blood pressure measurements for nearly 90 years with a compression cuff, sphygmomanometer, and stethoscope. The major errors associated with the use sphygmomanometer and stethoscope relate to calibration of the manometer, position of the arm (if the arm is below "heart level," due to hydrostatic pressure, a falsely elevated blood pressure will be recorded), and the experience and training of the observer.

In order to eliminate observer errors automated blood pressure devices were developed. Most of these devices use the oscillometric technique. The oscillometric technique involves analysis of arterial "flutter," the lower-frequency oscillations that occur, with each heartbeat, under an occluding cuff between the systolic and diastolic pressures. A sensitive transducer attached to the cuff detects the flutter by selectively amplifying the oscillations and rejecting most artifacts. In general, these devices more reliable predict systolic than diastolic blood pressure.

C Observer Errors

An observer may record the blood pressure inaccurately because of hearing impairments, inattention, carelessness, or subconscious bias. An example of such bias is "digit preference," a well-documented phenomenon resulting in recording pressures ending with zero of five (i.e. 120 or 125 systolic or 80 or 85 diastolic) more often than expected by chance. The observer should be taught that systolic pressure is the point at which initial Korotkoff sounds are audible for two consecutive heart beats (phase I). Diastolic blood pressure should be measured at the pressure at which Korotkoff sounds disappear (phase V). With appropriate training observer errors can be greatly reduced.

D Summary

Although the indirect method of blood pressure measurement may be imprecise in the obese individual, if appropriate care is taken to use a trained observer, a large enough blood pressure cuff, and a calibrated measurement device, reliable measurements of blood pressure can be made even in extremely obese individuals.

III RELATIONSHIP BETWEEN OBESITY AND HIGH BLOOD PRESSURE

A Epidemiological Studies Linking Obesity to Hypertension

The association between obesity and hypertension has been recognized since the early 1900s. Several large epidemiological studies documented the association

Table 1 Recommended Bladder Dimensions for Blood Pressure Cuffs

Circumference of arm at midpoint[a] (cm)	Name of cuff	Bladder width (cm)	Bladder length (cm)
13–20	Child	8	13
17–26	Small adult	11	17
24–32	Adult	13	24
32–42	Large adult	17	32
42–50	Thigh	20	42

[a] Midpoint of arm is defined as half the distance from the acromion to the olecranon.

between increasing body weight and an increase in blood pressure (1–12). Symonds (2) analyzed 150,419 policyholders in the Mutual Life Insurance Corporation and documented that systolic and diastolic blood pressure increased with both age and weight. In 1925, the Actuarial Society of America also documented a similar relationship in over 500,000 men (1). The Framingham Study (4) documented that the prevalence of hypertension in obese individuals was twice that of those individuals who were normal weight. This relationship held up in all age groups of both women and men. In the National Heart Association of Australia Risk Factor Prevalence Study (12), body mass index was independently associated with blood pressure level in both men and women. In that study, obesity was felt be the cause of the hypertension in > 30% of the individuals. Stamler (2) found in a study of 1 million North Americans that the odds ratio of hypertension were significantly increased in obese compared to nonobese individuals (comparing obese with nonobese subjects the odd ratio for hypertension in subjects age 20–39 years was 2.42:1, and 1.54:1 in subjects age 40–64 years). Thus, a large number of population-based studies have documented a strong association between obesity and hypertension in both sexes, in all age groups, and for virtually every geographical and ethnic group.

B Relationship of Weight Gain to Blood Pressure Level

There have been no studies in humans that have looked at the effect of weight gain on blood pressure. However, in the dog, it has been shown that weight gain is directly related to an increase in blood pressure. Cash and Wood in 1938 (13) demonstrated that weight gain caused dogs with renal vascular hypertension to further increase their blood pressure. More recently Rocchini et al. (14,15) found that normal mongrel dogs fed a high-fat diet gained weight and developed hypertension (Fig. 2). In these dogs the hypertension was associated with sodium retention, hyperinsulinemia, and activation of the sympathetic nervous system. Hall et al. (16) have also observed that weight gain in the dog is directly associated with an increase in arterial blood pressure.

C Effect of Weight Loss on Blood Pressure Level

Weight loss is associated with a lowering of blood pressure. Haynes (17) reviewed the literature up to the mid-1980s on the relationship of weight loss to reductions in arterial pressure. He used strict criteria to examine only well-done studies and noted that there

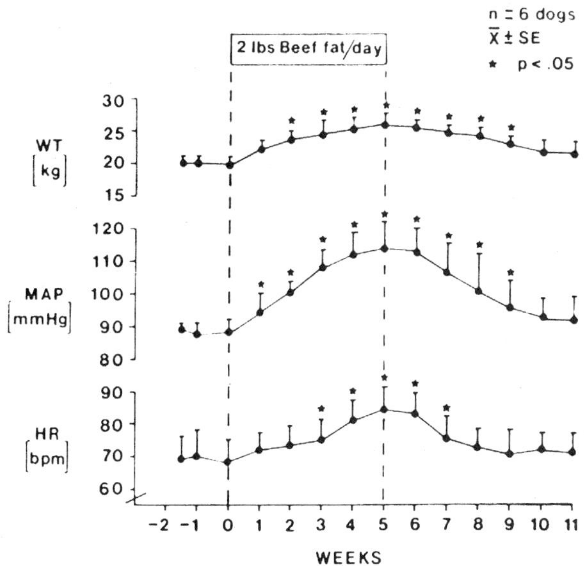

Figure 2 Weight, mean arterial pressure, and heart rate for six dogs fed a high-fat diet. With weight gain there is a significant increase in heart rate and blood pressure, and this is reversed with weight loss. (Adapted from Ref. 14.)

were only six studies available. Three of the six studies that met Haynes criteria demonstrated a clear effect of weight loss on lowering arterial pressure. Overall, many clinical trials that have been published since the late 1970s have clearly documented the blood pressure lowering effect of weight loss (17–31). However, one of the controversial aspects of these studies is whether the weight loss alone, independent of alterations in dietary sodium, was responsible for the observed reductions in blood pressure. Dahl (27) concluded that the reduced salt intake inherent in hypocaloric diets, rather than weight loss, was responsible for the lowering of blood pressure. Similarly, Fagerberg et al. (21) noted no decrease in blood pressure in individuals after weight loss using a 1230-calorie, unrestricted sodium diet; however, in another group of individuals, similar caloric restriction combined with a low-sodium diet resulted in a significant blood pressure reduction. Reisen et al. (25) reported that hypertensive individuals placed on diets designed to cause weight loss, but without sodium restriction, resulted in a substantial reduction in blood pressure. Tuck et al. (28) reported that weight loss decreased blood pressure in individual who received either a 40 mmol/d sodium diet or a 120 mmol/d sodium diet. Maxwell et al. (22) reported that in obese subjects, weight loss resulted in the same blood pressure reduction whether sodium intake was restricted to 40 mmol/d of sodium or maintained at 240 mmol/d. Gillum and coworkers (23) found that weight loss without significantly altered sodium intake resulted in blood pressure decreases. Rocchini et al. (29) demonstrated that prior to weight loss, the blood pressure of a group of obese adolescents was very sensitive to dietary sodium intake; however, after weight loss, the obese adolescents lost their blood pressure sensitivity to sodium. Finally, several large clinical trials have also documented that weight loss independent of sodium restriction results in blood pressure lowering. The Hypertension Prevention Trial (19) documented that in individuals with borderline elevations in blood pressure a mean weight loss of 5 kg was associates with as much as a 5/3 mm Hg decrease in blood pressure. The TAIM study (18) also found a significant blood pressure lowering effect of weight loss.

A limitation with the use of studies documenting that weight loss is associated with a reduction in blood pressure is that most studies do not address the long-term effect of weight change on blood pressure in subjects who are again placed on unrestricted diets. Dornfield and coworkers (30) have clearly documented that the long-term changes in blood pressure correlate with changes in body weight. In obese subjects whose blood pressure fell during a very low calorie, protein-supplemented fast, when weight loss stopped and body weight was maintained for 1 month, blood pressure did not increase. In compliant patients who regained <15 lb, 6 months after discontinuation of the very low calorie protein-supplemented fast, blood pressure increased minimally. Similarly, in another group of individuals, who were studied 21 months after being on unrestricted calorie and sodium intake but at a different body weight, Dornfield and associates also documented that differences in blood pressure correlated with differences in body weight. Reisen and Frohlich (31) reported that blood pressure remained reduced in individuals who maintained weight loss for 12–18 months. Finally, Davis et al. (20) reported that weight loss is an effective long-term therapy for maintaining blood pressure in the normal range when it is used as monotherapy or in combination with either thiazide diuretics or β-blockers. Thus, based on all of these weight loss studies, calorie restriction and weight loss are associated with a reduction in blood pressure. In addition, it is clear that even modest weight loss (i.e., 10% of body weight) improves blood pressure, and many individuals achieve normal blood pressure levels without attaining their calculated ideal weight.

However, recent data suggest that long-term weight loss does not reduce the incidence of hypertension. Sjostrom et al. (32) compared the incidence of hypertension and diabetes in 346 patients undergoing gastric surgery with 346 obese control subjects who were matched on 18 variables. After 8 years, the surgical group had maintained a 16% weight loss, whereas the control subjects had a 1% weight gain. These investigators demonstrated that the weight reduction in the surgical group had a dramatic effect on the 8-year incidence of diabetes, but had no effect on the 8-year incidence of hypertension. They (33) and others (34) previously documented that surgical weight loss positively affected blood pressure at 2 and 4 years of follow-up, but that this effect on blood pressure is lost after 8 years of follow-up. These authors have speculated that the "remaining obesity in the surgically treated patients could have induced a reappearance of hypertension during the course of the study independent on ongoing weight increase." Therefore, Sjostrom's study suggests that the relapse of blood pressure after surgically induced weight loss is more related to aging and recent small weight increase than to either initial weight or initial weight losses (35).

D Effect of Body Fat Distribution on Blood Pressure

The definition of obesity also contributes to the controversy regarding the independence of obesity as an etiological determinant of hypertension. Obesity is defined not just as an increase in body weight but rather as an increase in adipose tissue mass. Adipose tissue mass can be estimated by multiple techniques such as: skinfold thickness, body mass index ([weight in kg]/[height in meters]^2), hydrostatic weighing, bioelectrical impedance, and water dilution methods. In most clinical studies, body mass index is usually used as the index of adiposity. Obesity is generally defined as a body mass index >30 kg/m^2. In 1956, Jean Vague (36) reported that the cardiovascular and metabolic consequences of obesity were greatest in individuals whose fat distribution pattern favored the upper-body segments. Since that observation, several population-based studies have demonstrated that upper-body obesity is a more important cardiovascular risk factor than body mass index alone (37–43). The Normative Aging Study (37) has demonstrated that there is a significant relationship between abdominal circumference and diastolic blood pressure. In fact, the risk of developing hypertension was better predicted by upper body fat distribution than by either body weight or body mass index (Fig. 3). In the Bogalusa Heart Study (38), blood pressure correlated strongly with upper-body fat pattern, but not with measures of global obesity. Many investigators have

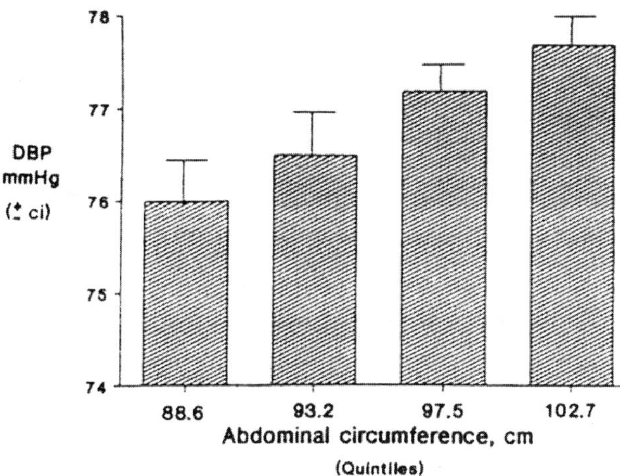

Figure 3 Relationship between diastolic blood pressure (DBP) and abdominal circumference by quintile. With increasing abdominal girth, diastolic blood pressure increases. DBP is shown with 95% confidence intervals for 1972 subjects in the Normative Aging Study. (Adapted from Ref. 37.)

demonstrated that the association of obesity to increased cardiovascular risk is primarily related to upper-body adiposity (44,45). Therefore, since most published studies investigating the role of obesity in hypertension have used total body weight or body mass index, the true role of adiposity in blood pressure regulation may have been obscured.

E Prevalence of Hypertension in Different Obese Populations

The final proof that obesity is an independent risk factor for hypertension, rather than a chance coexistence of two common clinical disorders, is that the prevalence of hypertension in obese individuals is much higher than in the general population. This increased prevalence of hypertension in obese individuals is even observed in populations with both a high (African-Americans) (2) and low (Mexican-Americans) (46) incidence of hypertension.

IV MECHANISM WHEREBY OBESITY MIGHT CAUSE HYPERTENSION

The exact mechanism whereby obesity causes hypertension is still unknown. Obesity hypertension is complex and multifactorial. It appears to involve insulin resistance, activation of the sympathetic nervous system, activation of the renin angiotensin system, abnormal renal sodium handling, possible leptin resistance, altered vascular reactivity, and alterations in the hypothalamic-pituitary-adrenal axis.

A Insulin Resistance

For years it has been recognized that hypertension is common in both obese and diabetic individuals. Glucose intolerance, independent of obesity is also associated with hypertension (47). Analysis of data from the San Antonio Heart Study has demonstrated an impressive pattern of overlap among hypertension, diabetes, and obesity. It has been estimated that by the fifth decade of life 85% of diabetic individuals are hypertensive and obese, 80% of obese subjects have abnormal glucose tolerance and are hypertensive, and 67% of hypertensive subjects are both diabetic and obese (7,46). In 1985, Modan et al. (47) demonstrated in a large epidemiological study that a strong association exists among obesity, glucose intolerance, and hypertension. There have been a number of studies in both obese and nonobese humans that demonstrate a strong relationship between insulin resistance and blood pressure (17,47–58). The relationship between insulin resistance and blood pressure has been observed in most populations (55–58). Preliminary results from the Insulin Resistance Atherosclerosis Study (59,60) suggest that after multivariate analysis, insulin resistance and body mass index, but not insulin level, predict hypertension. Therefore, insulin resistance has been suggested by many investigators to be the metabolic link that connects obesity to hypertension.

In support of the hypothesis that hyperinsulinemia may be causally linked to obesity hypertension, it has been demonstrated that in hypertensive obese subjects a 10-hr somatostatin infusion, a hormone that suppress pancreatic insulin release, causes a reduction in both plasma insulin and arterial pressure (61). Somatostatin has also been demonstrated to improve the hyperinsulinemia, hypertension, and dyslipemia associated with fructose-induced hypertension in the rat (62).

Factors known to improve insulin resistance are also associated with reductions in blood pressure. Weight loss has been documented to be associated with both a decrease in blood pressure and an improvement in insulin sensitivity (49,50). The decline in blood pressure associated with exercise training programs seems to be limited to individuals who are initially hyperinsulinemic and have the greatest fall in plasma insulin level as a result of the training program (50,63).

In addition to human data linking insulin and blood pressure, there are also animal data that suggest that insulin is an important regulator of blood pressure. Rocchini et al. (14,15) demonstrated that the weight gain associated with feeding dogs cooked beef fat is directly associated with an increase in blood pressure and insulin. Reaven and coworkers (64–67) demonstrated that normal Sprague-Dawley rats feed a fructose-enriched diet develop insulin resistance and hypertension. They have shown that the hypertension can be eliminated or attenuated by correcting the insulin resistance either with exercise training or the administration of somatostatin. Kurtz et al. (68) has shown that the genetically obese, insulin-resistant Zucker rat has an increased blood pressure compared to the genetically lean, non-insulin-resistant Zucker rat or Lewis rat. Several investigators have demonstrated that insulin resistance and hyperinsulinemia are also seen in spontaneously hypertensive rats (69–71). In addition, insulin-stimulated glucose uptake is lower in adipocytes isolated from these animals (70). Finally, Brands et al. (72) and Meehan et al. (73) have demonstrated that the infusion of insulin into normal rats results in the development of hypertension. In both studies, a rise in arterial pressure occurred within 2 days of starting the insulin infusion.

Finally, there is evidence to suggest that in normal-weight individuals, hyperinsulinemia and insulin resistance precede the development of hypertension. Young black males with borderline high blood pressure have been reported to have higher insulin levels and more insulin resistance that normotensive black men (55,56). In the Tecumseh Study (74), individuals with borderline hypertension had higher plasma insulin levels and greater weight than normotensive individuals. Normotensive children with a family history of hypertension have higher insulin levels and more insulin resistance than children with no family history of hypertension (75).

However, in contrast to these and other reports (7,47–58), linking hyperinsulinemia to hypertension, there have been studies that have been unable to establish a relationship between hyperinsulinemia and high blood pressure. There is at least one study in a group of hypertensive obese individuals (76) that did not find a correlation between hyperinsulinemia and hypertension. In normal dogs, a chronic infusion of insulin, with or without an infusion of norepinephrine, failed to increase blood pressure (21,77). In addition, even in those reports that have documented a relationship between insulin and blood pressure, there is significant overlap in insulin resistance between those individuals who are hypertensive and those who are normotensive. For example, Pollare and coworkers (49) demonstrated a significant linear relationship between insulin resistance, measured during a euglycemic insulin clamp study, and blood pressure in a group of 143 hypertensive and 51 normotensive subjects; however, ~50% of the hypertensive subjects had insulin-mediated glucose uptake values that were within 1 standard deviation of the normotensive group (that is, at least one half of the hypertensive subject were not insulin resistant). No correlation has been found between blood pressure and plasma insulin or insulin sensitivity in Pima Indians (78) or obese Mexican-American women (44). Thus, from all of these studies it is clear that not all hypertensive subjects are insulin resistant and that not all insulin-resistant subjects are hypertensive.

Based on available data in the literature, it appears that selective insulin resistance, not just hyperinsulinemia, is more likely the metabolic link that is responsible for the observed epidemiological relationship between obesity and hypertension. The term selective insulin resistance implies that although an individual or animal may have an impaired ability of insulin to cause whole body glucose uptake, some of the other physiological actions of insulin may be preserved. With respect to hypertension, one of the potentially important actions of insulin is the ability to induce renal sodium retention. Obese adolescents have selective insulin resistance in that they are resistant with respect to insulin's ability to stimulate glucose uptake yet are still sensitive to the renal sodium-retaining effects of insulin (79) (Fig. 4). The spontaneously hypertensive rat has also been documented to have impaired insulin mediated whole-rat glucose uptake yet normal insulin sensitivity to induce renal sodium retention (71). In nonobese essential hypertensives, insulin resistance has been demonstrated to involve glucose metabolism but not lipid or potassium metabolism, and is limited to the nonoxidative pathways of intracellular glucose disposal (48,80).

Thus there is evidence to indicate that in obese hypertensive subjects, insulin resistance is *selective* (mostly involving glucose metabolism), *tissue specific* (predominantly effecting skeletal muscle), and *pathway specific* (insofar as only glycogen synthesis is usually affected). Therefore, in any individual or animal the degree to which insulin resistance is tissue and/or pathway specificity may determine whether hypertension will develop. In addition to sodium retention, selective insulin resistance may modulate the development of hypertension through changes in vascular structure and function, alterations in cation flux, activation of the renin angiotensin aldosterone system, and activation of the sympathetic nervous system.

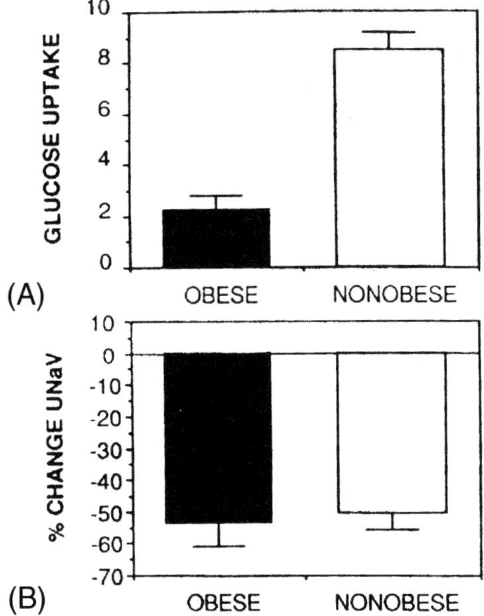

Figure 4 Panel A depicts the change in glucose uptake (M) (mg/kg/min) during euglycemic hyperinsulinemia in seven obese and five nonobese subjects. Compared to the nonobese individuals, a 40 munit/m^2/min infusion of insulin resulted in a significant depression in whole-body glucose uptake in the obese subjects ($P < .001$). The plasma insulin response to the insulin infusion was not significantly different between obese and nonobese subjects. Panel B depicts the percent change in urinary sodium excretion (% change UNaV) that occurred in the same seven obese and five nonobese subjects during water diuresis and euglycemic hyperinsulinemia. Insulin infusion resulted in a significant (~50%) decrease in urinary sodium excretion in both the obese and nonobese subjects. There was no significant difference in the response of urinary sodium excretion to hyperinsulinemia observed between the two groups. (From Ref. 79.)

B Enhanced Sodium Retention

There are ample human and animal data linking obesity hypertension to fluid retention. Rocchini et al. (29) demonstrated that when compared to nonobese adolescents, the obese adolescents have a renal-function relation (plot of urinary sodium excretion as a function of arterial pressure) that has shallower slope. The renal-function relationship is also normalized by weight loss (Fig. 5). The relationship between urinary sodium excretion and mean arterial pressure can be altered by intrinsic and extrinsic factors that are known to affect the ability of the kidney to excrete sodium. Factors that produce alterations in the renal-function curves are constriction of the renal arteries and arterioles, changes in glomerular filtration coefficients, changes in the rate of tubular reabsorption, reduced renal mass, and changing levels of renin-angiotensin activation, aldosterone, vasopressin, insulin, sympathetic nervous system activation, and atrial natriuretic hormone.

Insulin resistance and/or hyperinsulinemia can result in chronic sodium retention. Insulin can enhance renal sodium retention both directly, through its effects on renal tubules (79,81,82), and indirectly, through stimulation of the sympathetic nervous system and augmenting angiotensin II mediated aldosterone secretion (83,84). There are data to suggest that insulin resistance is directly related to sodium sensitivity in both obese and nonobese subjects. Rocchini et al. (29) have also shown in obese adolescents that insulin resistance and sodium sensitivity of blood pressure are directly related. They demonstrated that the blood pressure of obese adolescents is more dependent on dietary sodium intake than the blood pressure of nonobese adolescents and that hyperinsulinemia and increased sympathetic nervous system activity appear to be responsible for the observed sodium sensitivity and hypertension. Finta et al. (85) demonstrated that the endogenous hyperinsulinemia that occurs in obese subjects following a glucose meal

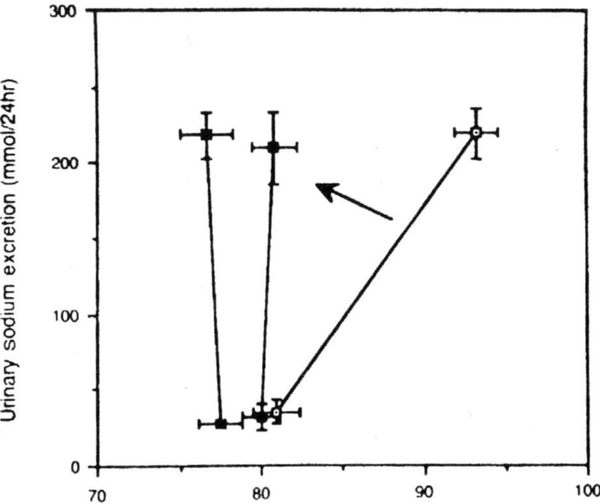

Figure 5 Renal-function relations for 18 nonobese (X), 60 obese adolescents before a weight loss program (open square) and the 36 obese adolescents who lost weight during a 20-week weight loss program (closed square). In comparison with the nonobese adolescents' renal-function relation, the obese adolescents' renal-function relation has a shallow slope ($P < .001$). In those who lost weight, the slope increased (arrow). This increase was due to a decrease in the mean arterial pressure during the two weeks of the high salt diet. (From Ref. 29.)

can result in urinary sodium retention. In that study, the investigators also demonstrated that the obese adolescents who were the most sodium sensitive had significantly higher fasting insulin concentrations, higher glucose-stimulated insulin levels, and greater urine sodium retention in response to the oral glucose load. Finally, in nonobese subjects with (82) or without (86) essential hypertension there is a direct relationship between sodium sensitivity and insulin resistance.

There are also animal data that suggest that insulin resistance may be in partly responsible for the sodium retention associated with obesity hypertension. In a dog model of obesity induced hypertension, Rocchini et al. (14,15) demonstrated that during the first week of the high-fat diet, the increase in sodium retention appeared to best relate to an increase in plasma norepinephrine activity, whereas during the latter weeks of the high-fat diet, an increase in plasma insulin appeared to be the best predictor of sodium retention. Finally, Rocchini et al. (86) demonstrated that the hypertension associated with weight gain in the dog occurs only if adequate salt is present in the diet.

In non-insulin-resistant subjects, both a concomitant decrease in proximal tubular sodium reabsorption and an increase in glomerular filtration oppose the direct effect of insulin to increase distal sodium retention (87). Hall and coworkers (88) have demonstrated that obesity-induced hypertension in the dog is associated with increased renal tubular sodium reabsorption since marked sodium retention occurred despite large increases in glomerular filtration and renal plasma flow. Ter Maaten et al. (89) have demonstrated that insulin-mediated glucose uptake was positively correlated with changes in glomerular filtration but not with changes in either proximal tubular sodium reabsorption or overall fractional sodium excretion. They speculated that insulin could only cause abnormal sodium retention if an additional antinatriuretic stimulus is present, such as through stimulation of the sympathetic activity, augmenting angiotensin II–mediated aldosterone production, and others.

Another mechanism that may link insulin and insulin resistance to salt-sensitive hypertension is alterations in insulin receptor structure or function. We characterized the change in insulin-mediated glucose uptake that occurs with feeding dogs a high-fat diet by measuring insulin-mediated glucose uptake dose response curves in dogs before and after 1, 3, and 6 weeks of the high-fat diet (90) (Fig. 6). After 1 week of the high-fat diet there was a significant increase in the amount of insulin that was required to produce a half-maximal response in glucose uptake (insulin ED_{50} dose) and little change in

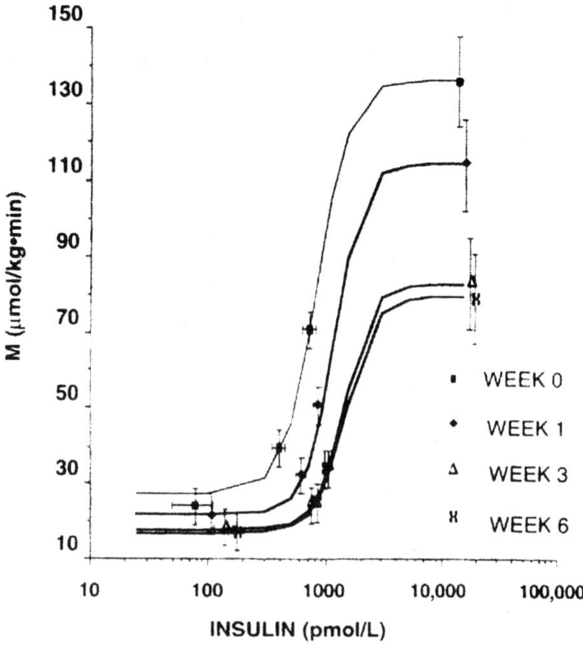

Figure 6 Rates of whole-body glucose uptake (M) determined during euglycemic clamp studies over a wide range of steady-state insulin concentrations serially in four dogs fed a high-fat diet. Weight gain resulted in a shift to right and a decrease in maximal rate of M. $P < .001$. (From Ref. 90.)

the maximal glucose uptake response. However, by 3 weeks of the high-fat diet there was a further increase in the insulin ED_{50} dose and a significant reduction in the maximal insulin-induced glucose uptake. Laasko et al. (91) reported, in obese humans, similar changes in the insulin mediated glucose uptake dose response relationship. Kolterman et al. (92) suggested that insulin resistance in obesity is due to target tissue defects (i.e., reduced sensitivity to insulin, reduced responsiveness to insulin, or a combined defect). Reduced sensitivity to insulin is believed to be due to a prereceptor or receptor defect. In this type of resistance, high concentrations of insulin overcome the defect and evoke a maximum insulin stimulation of the tissue. Alternatively, reduced responsiveness to insulin is associated with a reduced maximum insulin stimulation of the tissue, and is believed to be due to a defect that is distal to the insulin-receptor complex. Since weight gain is associated with both a reduced maximum insulin-stimulated glucose uptake and a shift of the dose response curve to the right (i.e., a significantly reduced insulin ED_{50} dose), using Kolterman's terminology, weight gain in the dog results in both a reduced sensitivity and responsiveness to insulin. We also observed that > 77% of the variance in the weekly change in blood pressure and sodium retention caused by feeding dogs a high-fat diet could be explained by the weekly insulin-stimulated glucose uptake insulin ED_{50} doses. Therefore, insulin resistance appears to be important in producing the salt-sensitive hypertension observed in obese humans and dogs. Sechi (93) reported that dietary salt content can alter insulin receptor function in the SHR rat and the fructose-fed rat. An increase in dietary salt content decreases insulin receptor number and mRNA levels only in the kidney of WKY but not SHR. Similarly, Sechi reported that when control Sprague-Dawley rats are fed a high-salt diet, renal insulin receptor number and mRNA levels decrease. However, when fructose is added to the high-salt diet, renal insulin receptor number and mRNA levels did not decrease. Therefore, Sechi has speculated that in both SHR and fructose-fed rats, the sensitivity to insulin of the kidney is unresponsive to manipulations of dietary sodium. He believes that this abnormality might contribute to sodium retention and hypertension.

Finally, there are structural changes in the kidneys of obese individuals that can cause fluid retention. The kidneys from obese animals and humans are tightly encapsulated with fat tissue. Some of the fat penetrates the renal hilum into the sinuses surrounding the renal medulla (94). The interstitial fluid hydrostatic pressure is elevated to 19 mm Hg in obese dogs, compared with on 9–10 mm Hg in lean dogs. The elevated interstitial pressure reduces medullary blood flow and causes tubular compression, thus slowing tubular flow rate and increasing fraction tubular reabsorption. Therefore, obesity, either from hormonal changes or due to physical changes in the kidney, causes fluid retention.

C Alterations in Vascular Structure and Function

Another way that obesity can cause hypertension is through alterations in vascular structure and function. Cellular metabolism of cations and other molecules may be altered in obesity and lead to changes in vascular responsiveness. Since insulin and insulinlike growth factors are mitogens capable of stimulating smooth muscle proliferation (95), hyperinsulinemia could result in vascular smooth muscle hypertrophy, narrowing of the lumen of resistance vessels, and ultimately the development of hypertension (96). Vascular abnormalities are also known to exist in obese individuals. In normal nonobese volunteers, insulin induces peripheral arterial vasodilation (97). In obese adolescents, Rocchini et al. (98) demonstrated that ischemic exercise results in a decreased maximal forearm blood flow and an increased minimum vascular resistance. These investigators demonstrated that the abnormal vascular responses to ischemic exercise directly correlate with fasting insulin and whole-body glucose uptake, and that the vascular and metabolic abnormalities improve with weight loss.

In the dog, euglycemic hyperinsulinemia increases cardiac output in a dose-dependent fashion (90). However, feeding the high-fat diet resulted in right shift of insulin's effect to increase cardiac output. Compared to the control fed dogs, the half-maximal response in the insulin-induced increase in cardiac output (insulin ED_{50} dose) was 72% ($P < .05$) higher at 1 week and 180% ($P < .01$) higher at 6 weeks. Similarly, weight gain in the dog blunts the vasodilator response to insulin in the femoral artery. Steinberg et al. (99) demonstrated that insulin enhances the release of endothelium-derived nitric oxide. Baron et al. (100) demonstrated that insulin-resistant individuals exhibit blunted insulin-mediated vasodilatation and impaired endothelium-dependent vasodilatation. Others have also demonstrated that salt-sensitive and insulin-resistant hypertensive patients manifest impaired endothelium-dependent relaxation mediated by nitric oxide (101,102).

In addition to insulin resistance possibly being associated with the development of vascular changes, there also are data that suggest that abnormalities in skeletal muscle vascular regulation may be a cause of insulin resistance. In both the dog (97) and man (97) euglycemic hyperinsulinemia has been documented to result in vasodilatation, not vasoconstriction. Even though the exact mechanism how insulin induces vasodilatation in non-insulin-resistant individuals is unknown, some investigators believe that this vasodilator response is in part due to stimulation of endothelial-dependent relaxing factor (103,104). Type 2, but not type 1, diabetic subjects respond abnormally to acetylcholine, which induces vasodilatation by stimulation of endothelial-dependent relaxing factor (105).

Insulin-mediated glucose uptake is determined both by insulin's ability to stimulate glucose extraction at the level of tissues/cells and by the rate of glucose and insulin delivery (blood flow). Thus, the relative contributions of tissue and blood flow actions of insulin will determine the overall rate of glucose uptake (i.e., degree of insulin resistance). In obese individuals with insulin resistance, an attenuated limb vasodilator reponses to hyperinsulinemia has been reported (106,107) (Fig. 7). The lack of insulin's ability to produce vasodilatation has led Baron (108) to speculate that abnormalities of skeletal muscle vascular regulation may be a cause, not a result, of insulin resistance. This hypothesis is also

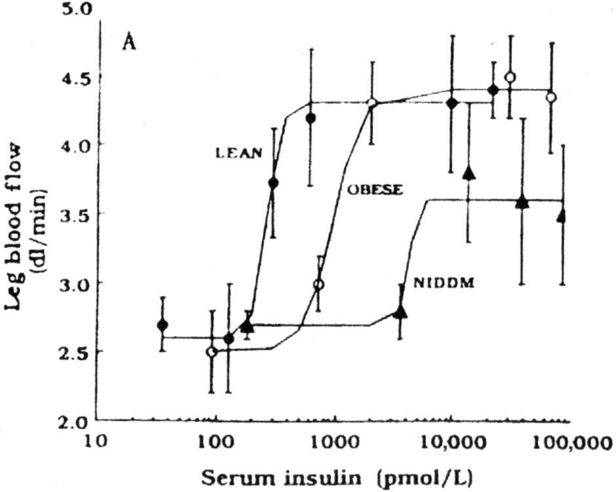

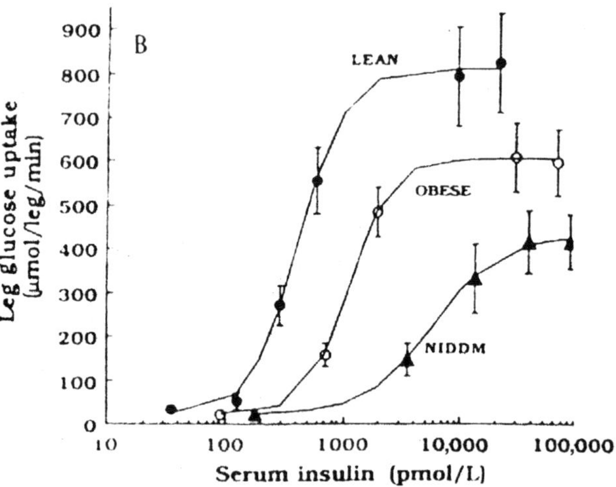

Figure 7 Rates of leg blood flow (A) and rates of leg glucose uptake (B) determined during euglycemic clamp studies over a wide range of steady-state serum insulin concentrations in lean (closed circles) and obese nondiabetic subjects (open circles) and patients with NIDDM (close triangles). Note the log scale on the abscissa. To convert the insulin concentrations from pmol/L divide by 7.175. (Adapted from Ref. 90.)

supported by the fact that antihypertensive drugs that are vasodilators (i.e., captopril, calcium channel blockers, and prazosin) tend to improve insulin resistance, whereas other antihypertensive drugs such as diuretic or beta-blockers do not (109–111).

Skeletal muscle characteristics are altered in obesity (112–115) and hypertension (116–119), and these alterations may be involved in the etiology of these two diseases. Human muscle has three categories of fiber: types I, IIa, and IIb (120). Type I fibers have high aerobic capabilities and increase capillarization. Type II fibers tend to be better suited for anaerobic metabolism. Type IIa fibers have the same capillary supply as type I fibers, whereas type IIb fibers have a reduced capillary supply. Lithell et al. (113) reported that muscle fiber diameter and capillary density correlate with fasting insulin levels. These investigators also demonstrated that obese men have an increased fiber diameter with no increase in the number of capillaries per fiber (i.e., a reduced capillary density). Lillioja et al. (112) reported similar results in a group of Pima Indians. Wade et al. (105) and Staron et al. (114) reported a significant inverse correlation between the presence of type I fibers and body fatness. However, Simoneau and Bouchard (121) found no relationship between percent body fat and the percentage of type I fibers in a group of 126 women and 213 men. The only significant correlation between body fatness and fiber type observed in this study was that obese men appeared to have an increase percentage of type IIb fibers with low aerobic enzyme activities. Krotkiewski and Bjorntrop (122) observed that upper-body obesity, increased waist-to-hip ratio, was associated with an increased percentage of type II fibers. Based on these observations, it has been speculated that the hypertension and insulin resistance observed in some obese individuals, especially those with upper-body obesity, may be due to the high percentage of type IIb muscle fibers that have low capillary density and reduced aerobic enzyme activities. In support of this theory is the observation that endurance training in obese and nonobese individuals improves insulin resistance by increasing muscle oxidative capacity and increasing capillary density (123,124).

D Alterations in Ion Transport

The fourth method by which obesity could cause hypertension is through alterations in cation transport. Insulin has been shown to affect sodium and calcium transport, although controversy still exists regarding the molecular mechanism of this effect. A direct effect of insulin on sodium/hydrogen exchange has been demonstrated in vitro (125). Insulin has been reported to both increase and decrease Na-K-ATPase activity (126). Insulin has been linked to both Na-Li countertransport and Na-K cotransport (126). In a study of leukocyte sodium content and sodium pump activity in overweight and lean hypertensive subjects, it was observed that overweight hypertensive subjects accumulated intracellular sodium probable through abnormalities of sodium pump activity (127). In obese hypertensive men, the renin-angiotensin system and sympathetic nervous system activity are reported to influence the regulation of erythrocyte sodium turnover during sodium and energy restriction (128). Thus, alteration in intracellular sodium concentration could lead to an increased intracellular calcium, an increase in vascular smooth muscle tone, and hypertension. Insulin alone has also been demonstrated to elevate cytosolic free calcium levels in adipocytes of normal subjects (129). In addition, weight loss is obese individuals is reported to be accompanied by a significant decrease in platelet-free calcium levels (130).

Insulin-mediated glucose transport is dependent on an intracellular calcium concentration of between 40 and 375 nm/L (131). Thus, increased intracellular calcium concentration might lead to insulin resistance, increased vascular resistance, and hypertension (50). In hypertensive type II diabetics a decrease in calcium adenosine-triphosphate activity is associated with increased intracellular calcium concentration (132). Insulin has also been shown to stimulate plasma membrane calcium adenosine-triphosphate activity (105) and sodium-potassium adenosine-triphosphate activity (126). Insulin resistance may blunt these pump functions and could lead to chronic increases in intracellular calcium, increased peripheral vascular resistance, and hypertension. Finally, reduced intracellular levels of magnesium are also associated with increased vascular resistance and insulin resistance (133). With the use of magnetic resonance imaging to evaluate the aorta of normal and hypertensive subjects. Resnick et al. (134) found that increased abdominal visceral fat, decreased intracellular magnesium, and advanced age were closely associated with reduced aortic distensibility vessels. Therefore, in obesity, alterations in either intracellular calcium and/or magnesium could result in the development of both hypertension and insulin resistance.

E Stimulation of the Renin-Angiotensin-Aldosterone System

A fifth way by which obesity could cause hypertension is through alterations in the renin-angiotensin-aldosterone system. The renin-angiotensin-aldosterone system is an important determinant of efferent glomerular arteriolar tone and tubular sodium reabsorption. Its activity is modulated by both dietary salt ingestion and blood pressure. Therefore alterations in the renin-angiotensin aldosterone system could be expected to alter pressure natriuresis. Enhanced activity of the renin-angiotensin system has been reported in obese humans and dogs (28,84,135–140). Tuck et al. (28) demonstrated in obese hypertensives that with weight loss plasma renin activity decreases and that the decrease in plasma renin activity was statistically correlated with the weight loss–associated decrease in mean arterial pressure. Granger and coworkers (140) reported that plasma renin activity is 170% higher in obese dogs than in control dogs. However, Hall et al. (88) demonstrated that weight-related changes in blood pressure can occur in dogs independent of changes in angiotensin II.

Obesity is also associated with abnormalities in the angiotensin-aldosterone system. In the dog, Rocchini et al. (14,15) demonstrated that the increase in blood pressure associated with weight gain is directly related to sodium retention and that this sodium retention is in part accompanied by an increase in plasma norepinephrine, insulin, and aldosterone concentrations. Tuck and associates (28) demonstrated in obese adults that weight loss lowered both plasma renin activity and aldosterone concentration. Hiramatsu et al. (136) documented in obese hypertensives that with increasing body weight, there is a progressive increase in the ratio of plasma aldosterone to plasma renin activity. Scavo et al. (137,138) reported that although obese adults have a normal plasma renin activity, they have an increased plasma aldosterone concentration and an increased aldosterone secretion rate. Sparks and coworkers (139) reported that in obese patients during the early stages of fasting there is a dissociation between plasma renin activity and aldosterone. Rocchini et al. (135) measured supine and 2-hr upright plasma renin activity and aldosterone in 10 nonobese and 30 obese adolescents before and after a 20-week weight loss program. The obese adolescents had significantly higher supine and 2-hr upright aldosterone concentrations. Although plasma renin activity was not significantly different in the two groups of adolescents, they observed that a given increment in plasma renin activity produced a greater increment in aldosterone in the obese adolescents. Compared with an obese control group, weight loss resulted in a significant decrease in plasma aldosterone. After weight loss there was also a significant decrease in the slope of the posture-induced relation between plasma renin activity and aldosterone. In addition, after weight loss there was a significant correlation between the change in plasma aldosterone and the change in mean blood pressure. The authors speculated that increased plasma aldosterone concentration in some obese subjects is caused by increased adrenal sensitivity to angiotensin II.

Insulin has been shown to influence the renin-angiotensin aldosterone system in both normal subjects (83,141) and in patients with diabetes (142). Since hyperinsulinemia is a characteristic feature of obesity, Rocchini et al. (84) hypothesized that increased aldosterone levels observed in obese individuals are caused by hyperinsulinemia and insulin's ability to augment angiotensin II–mediated aldosterone production. Rocchini et al. (84) measured the increase in plasma aldosterone after intravenous angiotensin II (5, 10, and 20 ng/kg/min for 15 min each) before and after euglycemic hyperinsulinemia in seven chronically instrumented dogs. Euglycemic hyperinsulinemia (at insulin doses of 2, 4, or 8 mU/kg/min) resulted in a significantly greater ($P < .01$) change in the angiotensin II–stimulated increments of plasma aldosterone than was observed when angiotensin II was administered alone. However, there was no dose dependence of insulin's effect on angiotensin II–stimulated aldosterone. The effect of weight gain on the angiotensin II response was also evaluated in five dogs. Weight gain significantly increased angiotensin II–stimulated aldosterone; however, with hyperinsulinemia, the response was not significantly different than that observed in the dogs prior to weight gain. The authors speculated that possible mechanisms whereby insulin could increase angiotensin II–stimulated aldosterone production include increased intracellular potassium, reduced plasma free fatty acids, and a direct action of insulin to induce increased adrenal steroidogenesis.

Hollenberg and Williams (143,144) have described a group of subjects with essential hypertension that they have called nonmodulators. These normal renin subjects appear to have a defect in their sodium-modulated tissue responsiveness to angiotensin II. Ferri et al. (145) have shown that nonmodulating hypertensives are insulin resistant. Similarly, Trevisan et al. (146) has demonstrated that IDDM patients have both an enhanced renal response to angiotensin II and insulin resistance.

F Increased Activation of the Sympathetic Nervous System

The sixth way by which obesity could cause hypertension is through stimulation of the sympathetic nervous system. For over 20 years it has been recognized that diet affects the sympathetic nervous system. Fasting suppresses sympathetic nervous system activity, whereas overfeeding with either a high-carbohydrate or high-fat diet simulates the sympathetic nervous system (147–150). Insulin is believed to be the signal that networks dietary intake and nutritional status to sympathetic activity. Glucose and insulin sensitive neurons in the ventromedial portion of the hypothalamus have been demonstrated to alter the activity of inhibitory pathways between the hypothalamus and brainstem (151). It is believed that the physiological role of the link between dietary intake and sympathetic nervous system activity is to regulate energy expenditure in a hope to maintain weight homeostasis. Landsberg and Krieger (152) have suggested that in obese individuals the sympathetic nervous system is chronically activated in an attempt to prevent further weight gain and that hypertension is a byproduct of the overactive sympathetic nervous system. They and their associates, as have others, have clearly documented that euglycemic hyperinsulinemia in both normal and obese humans and animals causes activation of the sympathetic nervous system as documented by increases in heart rate, blood pressure, and plasma norepinephrine (26,84,152–155).

More recently it has been shown that hyperinsulinemia in normal humans is associated not only with an increase in circulating catecholamines but also with an increase in sympathetic nerve activity (97). Fisher rats fed a high-fat diet develop obesity, hypertension, and insulin resistance. When euglycemic insulin infusions are performed, increases in systolic blood pressure are observed in the fat-feed animals but not in controls. The blood pressure increase is reversible by combined α-blockade and β-blockade, thus suggesting a role for increased sympathetic activity (156). Hall et al. (157) have preliminary studies suggesting that combined alpha and beta adrenergic blockade for 7 days reduced arterial pressure to a much greater extent in obese than in normal dogs. These investigators have also demonstrated that renal denervation prevents both the hypertension and sodium retention associated with obesity in the dog (158).

Although many studies in obese individuals have demonstrated increased sympathetic nervous system activity, this has not been a universal finding (159). Part of the controversy regarding the role of the sympathetic nervous system in obesity relates to relying on plasma levels of catecholamines as the index of sympathetic activity. Recent data from the Normative Aging Study (37) strongly suggest that obesity is associated with increased sympathetic nervous system activity. This study demonstrated that sympathetic activity, assessed by measuring 24-hr urinary norepinephrine excretion, is directly related to abdominal girth, waist-to-hip ratio, and body mass index. In addition, norepinephrine excretion is directly correlated with both glucose level and fasting insulin concentration (37,160). Other recent studies using the appearance rate of norepinephrine in the circulation (161) and the effects of somatostatin-induced suppression of insulin on plasma norepinephrine levels (162) provide additional corroborative data for an increase in sympathetic activity linked to obesity and driven by insulin. Sondergaard et al. (163) demonstrated that measurements of resting and 24-hr sympathoadrenal activity may differ in obese individuals. They demonstrated that sympathic activity at rest as evaluated by forearm venous plasma norepinephrine levels was increased in obese subjects. However, thrombocyte norepinephrine and epinephrine levels, which likely reflect 24-hr plasma catecholamine concentrates, were reduced in obese subjects with a body fat percentage above 40%. They speculate that the reduced thrombocyte catecholamine levels are probable due to a reduced physical activity in these subjects.

Finally, there are also ethnic differences in sympathetic tone. Weyer et al. (164) examined the relation among heart rate, blood pressure, percent body fat, fasting insulin, and muscle sympathetic nerve activity in male normotensive whites and Pima Indians. These investigators demonstrated that in both ethnic groups, heart rate and blood pressure positively related to percent body fat and muscle sympathetic nerve activity, and both were independent determinants of heart rate and blood pressure. However, muscle sympathetic nerve activity was positively related to percent body fat and fasting insulin concentration in whites but not in Pima Indians. This study emphasizes that the roles of hyperinsulinemia and increase sympathetic nervous system activity as medicator for the relation between obesity and hypertension can differ between among ethnic groups. Weyer's study (164) may explain why the Pima Indians have a low prevalence of hypertension in this population despite their high incidence of obesity and insulin resistance.

Abnormalities in the sympathetic nervous system may also play role in the actual pathogenesis of some forms of obesity. The recent identification and cloning of the β_3-adrenergic receptor have spurred great interest in the potential role of this receptor in the regulation of energy expenditure and ultimately in the development of obesity. The β_3-adrenergic receptor is predominantly expressed in omental fat tissue and gallbladder, at low levels in ileum and colon, and absent in muscle, heart, liver, lung, kidney, thyroid, and lymphocytes (165). Mutations in the β_3-adrenergic receptor gene have been detected in Pima Indians and Mexican-Americans, two populations with a high incidence of obesity and diabetes (166). Finally, preliminary studies in obese humans have demonstrated that the administration of an agent with high specificity for the β_3-adrenergic receptor results in increased energy expenditure that is accompanied by a marked improvement in insulin sensitivity and glucose tolerance (167).

Finally, there is evidence suggesting that alterations in sympathetic activity can cause insulin resistance. The acute administration of catecholamines is known to decrease insulin action (168). Diebert et al. (169) demonstrated that epinephrine, acting primarily through a beta-adrenergic receptor, markedly impairs both peripheral and hepatic resistance to the action of insulin. Jamerson et al. (170) demonstrated that a reflex increase in sympathetic tone in normotensive individuals can lead to acute insulin resistance in the forearm. These investigators speculated that reflex activation of the sympathetic nervous system caused a decrease in forearm glucose uptake that was mediated through a reduction in blood flow to the forearm. Rosen et al. (171) demonstrated that central activation of imidazoline receptors by moxonidine can prevent both the hypertension and insulin resistance associated with feeding rats a high fructose diet. Similarly, Ernsberger et al. (172) demonstrated that moxonidine completely reversed abnormal glucose tolerance and insulin resistance in obese spontaneously hypertensive rats. Finally, Rocchini et al. (173) have shown that clonidine can prevent the hypertension, sodium retention, and insulin resistance associated with feeding dogs a high-fat diet (Fig. 8). Therefore, it is possible that altered sympathetic function could be the metabolic abnormality that is responsible for obesity hypertension, salt sensitivity, and insulin resistance.

G Natriuretic Peptides

Natriuretic peptides are important regulators of volume and pressure. There are at least three natriuretic peptides that have been identified: atrial natriuretic peptide, brain natriuretic peptide, and C-type peptide. Few studies have examined the role of natriuretic peptides in obesity. Licata and coworkers (174) demonstrated that following a sodium load, obese subjects have delayed urinary sodium excretion and a blunted rise in atrial natriuretic peptide levels. Maoz and coworkers (175) demonstrated that weight loss was associated with a significant diuresis and natriuresis together with an early increase in plasma atrial natriuretic peptide levels. Finally, Dessi-Fulgheri et al. (176) reported that after caloric restriction in obese hypertensive subjects atrial natriuretic peptide infusion caused a more pronounced diuresis, natriuresis, fall in blood pressure, and an elevation in plasma cGMP levels than was observed in these subjects prior to caloric restriction. These authors suggested that relative over expression of inactive receptor Npr-C in adipose tissue might trap and clear more atrial natriuretic peptide from the circulation and thereby reduce its biologic effects on the kidney.

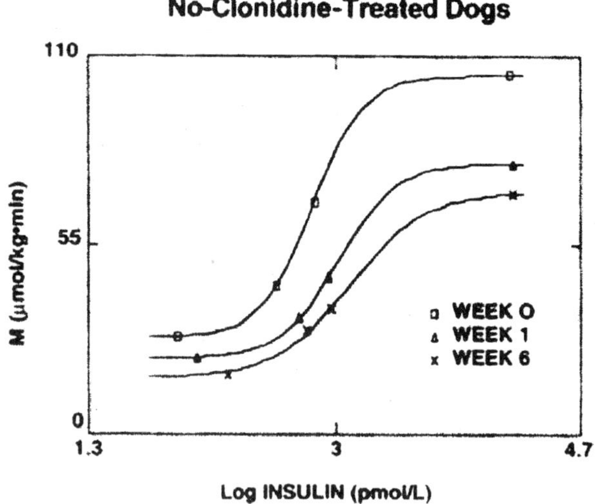

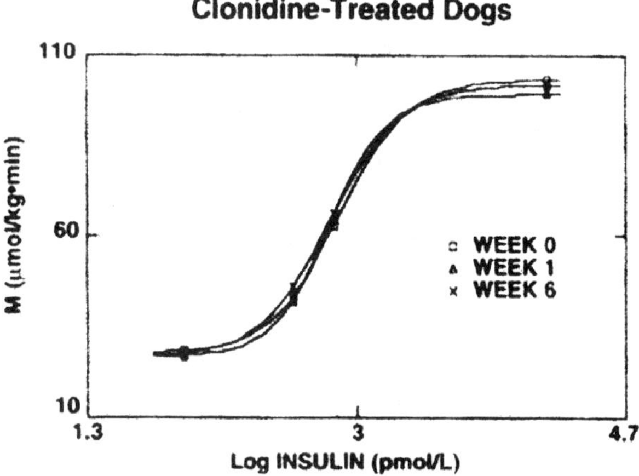

Figure 8 Rates of whole-body insulin-mediated glucose uptake (M) determined during euglycemic clamp studies over a wide range of steady-state insulin concentrations (□, week 0; Δ, week 1 of fat diet; ×, week 6 of fat diet) in dogs fed a high-fat diet with and without clonidine treatment. Weight gain resulted in a shift to the right and a decrease in the maximal rate of M ($P < .001$) in dogs not treated with clonidine; however, if the dogs were treated with clonidine, weight gain did not alter the dose-response relation. (From Ref. 173.)

H Leptin

Leptin is a 167–amino acid hormone that is secreted exclusively by adipocytes. By binding to the leptin receptor in the hypothalamus and by activating multiple neuropeptide pathways, leptin decreases appetite and increases energy expenditure, thereby decreasing adipose tissue mass and body weight. Serum leptin level is low in lean individuals and is elevated in most obese subjects (177). Since there is a strong relation between serum leptin levels and body fat mass, some authors have concluded that obesity may be associated with leptin resistance (178).

Leptin has been shown to have significant cardiovascular effects. Leptin-treated animals have a higher metabolic rate and core temperature. This may be because leptin increases sympathetic outflow and norepinephrine turnover in adipose tissue (179). Despite the increase in sympathetic outflow associated with leptin administration, no blood pressure elevation has been reported with the acute infusion of leptin (180). However, the chronic administration of leptin is associated with an increase in blood pressure, heart rate, and renal vascular resistance despite a decrease in food intake (181). Transgenic mice that overexpress leptin also are hypertensive. In these mice the elevated blood pressure can be prevented by an α-receptor blocker (182). Leptin has also been found to increase insulin sensitivity and inhibit glucose-mediated insulin secretion (183).

I Hypothalamic Origins of Obesity Hypertension

The similarities between Cushing's syndrome and the metabolic abnormalities associated with obesity hypertension has lead Bjorntrop to speculate that hypercortisolemia is involved with in the pathogenesis of obesity hypertension (184). Cortisol secretion has been measured repeatedly in obesity, but there have been conflicting results. There is evidence of increased secretion and turnover, resulting in normal or even lower than normal circulating concentration (185). Measuring salivary cortisol, investigators have been able to demonstrate that normally regulated cortisol secretion is associated with "healthy" anthropometric, metabolic, and hemodynamic variables. However, upon perceived stress cortisol secretion is increased and followed by insulin resistance, abdominal obesity, elevated blood pressure, and hyperlipidemia (186,187). In a small portion of the population a defect, "burned-out" cortisol secretion occurs. This "burnout" also is associated with decreased sex steroid and growth hormone secretions and is strongly associated with visceral adiposity, insulin resistance, and hypertension. Rosmond and Bjorntrop (188) have demonstrated that diminished dexamethasone suppression is directly associated with obesity and elevation of leptin levels. These authors suggest that a poor control of the hypothalamic-pituitary axis may be associated with obesity and inefficient leptin signals. Zahrezewska et al. (189) demonstrated in rats that glucocorticoids diminish leptin signals.

Bjorntorp and Rosmond (184) speculate that the two ways that elevated activity of the hypothalamic-pituitary adrenal axis could occur are an elevated stimulation and/or a diminished feedback control. Elevated stimulation of the HPA axis can occur owing to psychosocial and socioeconomic handicaps such as living alone, divorce, poor education, low social class, unemployment, and problems at work when employed, or even excess food intake. (190) With respect to causes of diminished feedback control of the HPA axis, Bjorntorp and others (191–193) have demonstrated that a restriction fragment length polymorphism of the glucocorticoid receptor gene is associated with poorly controlled HPA axis function, as well as abdominal obesity, insulin resistance, and hypertension. Therefore Bjorntorp has suggested that many of the cardiovascular and physiologic consequences found in obese individuals could be due to "a discretely elevated cortisol secretion, discoverable during reactions to perceived stress in everyday life" (194).

J Summary

In summary, there are conclusive data to suggest the obesity, especially upper-body fat distribution, is an independent risk factor for the development of hypertension. Calorie restriction and weight loss are associated with a reduction in blood pressure. In addition, it is clear that even modest weight loss (i.e., 10% of body weight) improves blood pressure, and many individuals achieve normal blood pressure levels without attaining their calculated ideal weight. Although controversy exists as to the role that insulin resistance and hyperinsulinemia play in the pathogenesis of obesity hypertension, there are ample data suggesting that selective insulin resistance and hypertension are related. Other hormonal systems (leptin, renin-angiotensin-aldosterone, sympathetic nervous system, and hypothalamic-pituitary-adrenal axis) have also been identified to relate to obesity, hypertension, and insulin resistance. Further studies will be necessary not only to clarify the origin of defects in insulin action that are responsible for the development of insulin resistance, but also to more precisely define the exact role that insulin resistance and the regulatory abnormalities in these other hormone systems play in blood pressure homeostasis.

V OBESITY AS A CARDIOVASCULAR RISK FACTOR

The Framingham Heart Study (4) identified obesity and hypertension as independent risk factors for the development of cardiovascular disease. Obese normotensive and hypertensive men have a higher rate of coronary heart disease (43). Manson et al. (195) also reported that, in women, the relative risk of fatal and nonfatal coronary heart disease increased from the lowest to the highest quartiles of obesity. However, other large studies (196,197) have reported an attenuated risk of cardiovascular mortality and morbidity among individuals who have both hypertension and obesity. Long-standing obesity is associated with preclinical and clinical left ventricular dilation (198) and impaired systolic function (199,200), with heart failure frequently being the ultimate cause of death in markedly overweight individuals (201).

A physiological change that may contribute to the association of obesity with left ventricular dilation is sodium retention with a concomitant increase in blood volume and cardiac output. Although many investigators (202) have reported that obesity is associated with an increased cardiac output and blood volume, when cardiac output and blood volume are indexed for body surface area, the differences between lean and fat disappear. Since obese and nonobese hypertensive subjects do not differ in their hemodynamic and volume characteristics when normalized for surface area, some investigators (203) have concluded that obesity does not result in a unique alteration in the vascular system that would produce hypertension. However, normalization for surface area may not be appropriate in the obese subject. Since the increment in cardiac output associated with obesity cannot be explained by an increase in adipose tissue perfusion alone, some have suggested that blood flow to the nonadipose mass must also be increased in obese subjects (204,205). Thus, obesity is characterized by a relative volume expansion in the presence of restricted vascular capacity.

Regional changes in organ blood flow and resistance have been studied in the dog (206). After 6 weeks of the high-fat diet, regional flows significantly increased in all measured organ beds, whereas in the control fed dogs, regional flows remained unchanged from baseline values. Weight gain was not associated with a change in vascular resistance in the heart, kidney, or brain but was associated with a significant decrease in gastrointestinal tract resistance. In addition to these data in the dog, there are also human data to suggest that regional hemodynamic abnormalities are present in obesity. Both renal and splanchnic blood flow (204) have been reported to be increased in obese subjects. In the obese adolescent, regional forearm blood flow, measured by venous occlusion plethysmography, is increased, and forearm vascular resistance is decreased (98). Both of these abnormalities are reversed with weight loss. Finally, Schmieder and Messerli (207) assessed systemic and renal hemodynamics and left ventricular function and structure in a group of 207 individuals. They noted that obese hypertensives had lower total peripheral resistance, a significantly higher stroke volume-pulse pressure index, and an elevated renal vascular resistance. They also noted that the degree of left ventricular hypertrophy was greater in the hypertensive than in the normotensive individuals, and it progressively increased with obesity.

Since obesity is associated with an increased preload to the left ventricle, dilatation and eccentric left ventricular hypertrophy (198,204,208) evolve. Hypertension increases afterload, and as a consequence the left ventricle adapts with an increase in wall thickness. The combination of obesity and hypertension therefore creates a double burden on the heart, ultimately leading to the development of impaired ventricular function (199–201,209,210).

MacMahon et al. (198) reported that 50% of individuals who are > 50% overweight have left ventricular hypertrophy. As with blood pressure, weight loss can result in a regression in the left ventricular hypertrophy (198,208,211). Unlike the universal finding of the left ventricular hypertrophy in obese individuals, not all studies have demonstrated an impairment in left ventricular function. Schmeider and Messerli (207) reported that obese hypertensive individuals have normal global left ventricular systolic function as measured by left ventricular fractional shortening and velocity of circumferential fiber shorting. However, since both of these indices of left ventricular systolic function are dependent on ventricular preload and afterload, the results of Schmeider's study do not document that left ventricular contractility is normal. In fact, Blake and coworkers (208) demonstrated that despite a normal left ventricular ejection fraction at rest, obese individuals have an impaired left ventricular ejection fraction in response to dynamic exercise. Guilermo et al. (209) reported that the end-systolic wall stress to end-systolic volume index, a load independent index of left ventricular function, is also abnormal in even mildly or moderately obese individuals. These investigators also documented a significant inverse relationship between the index of end-systolic wall stress to end-systolic volume and body mass index, diastolic diameter, and left ventricular mass index.

Abnormalities in left ventricular filling have also been reported to occur in obese individuals, i.e., decreased peak filling rate, duration of peak filling and left atrial emptying index (211), an increased isovolumic relaxation time, and an abnormal mitral valve Doppler filling pattern (210). The left ventricular hypertrophy, depressed myocardial contractility, and diastolic dysfunction can predispose individuals to excessive ventricular ectopy. Messerli et al. (212) reported that the prevalence of premature ventricular contractions was 30 times higher in obese individuals with eccentric left ventricular hypertrophy than in lean individuals.

The cardiovascular response to stress is thought to relate to cardiovascular risk. Rockstroh and associates (213) demonstrated that obese hypertensive individuals respond abnormally to stress. In their study, they evaluated the hemodynamic responses to mental and isometric stress in obese and nonobese hypertensive individuals. They observed that obese hypertensive individuals responded to mental stress with vasoconstriction and to isometric stress with an exaggerated increase in arterial pressure.

Finally, as with hypertension, insulin resistance may be related to both the cardiac hypertrophy and abnormal cardiac function that is observed in many obese individuals. Nakajima et al. (214) reported that there is a direct relationship between intraabdominal fat accumulation and the cardiac abnormalities associated with obesity. Since increased upper-body and intra-abdominal fat accumulation relates to the presence of insulin resistance even without significant overall obesity, these investigators speculated that the cardiac dysfunction observed in obese individuals may be related to insulin resistance.

A Summary

Obesity is recognized as an independent risk factor for the development of cardiovascular disease. Obesity is also is associated with the development of cardiac dysfunction. Obese individuals have an increased risk for developing left ventricular dilatation, impaired systolic and diastolic dysfunction, and the development of left ventricular hypertrophy.

VI MANAGEMENT OF THE OBESE INDIVIDUAL WITH HYPERTENSION

Weight loss is the cornerstone of hypertensive management in the obese individual. Weight loss in both adolescents and adults improves all of the cardiovascular abnormalities associated with obesity, including hypertension, dyslipemia, sodium retention, structural abnormalities in resistant vessels, and left ventricular hypertrophy and dysfunction. It is also important to realize that the method by which weight loss is accomplished is important. Although weight loss in general results in a drop in resting systolic/diastolic blood pressure and heart rate, when the weight loss is incorporated with physical conditioning, the greatest decrease in resting systolic blood pressure, peak exercise diastolic pressure, and heart rate can be achieved (26). Similarly, a weight loss program that incorporates exercise along with caloric restriction produces the most favorable effects on insulin resistance (26,63), dyslipidemia (63,215), and vascular reactivity (26,98). Endurance training in obese and nonobese individuals improves insulin resistance in part by increasing muscle oxidative capacity and increasing capillary density (123,124). Most investigators believe the additive effect of exercise to weight loss is related to the fact that exercise improves insulin resistance independently of weight loss.

Although weight loss and exercise are the cornerstones of blood pressure management in obese hypertensive individuals, most obese individuals are either unable or unwilling to lose weight or are unable to keep from regaining lost weight. Therefore, pharmacological therapy is frequently required in the hypertensive obese individual. When choosing an antihypertensive agent, it is important to remember that, depending on the antihypertensive agents used, insulin resistance has been reported to improve, worsen, or remain unchanged. In general, thiazide diuretics (54,109,216) and β-blockers (54,109) are known to impair insulin sensitivity and glucose tolerance; calcium blockers do not seem to adversely effect carbohydrate metabolism (217–219); indapaminde and potassium-sparing diuretics do not influence glucose homeostasis (220); and finally, angiotensin-converting enzyme inhibitors (109) and α_1-blockers (110,221) may even improve glucose metabolism and insulin resistance. Rocchini et al. (171) have recently demonstrated that clonidine, a centrally acting sympathetic agent, not only improved the hypertension associated with obesity but also improved the insulin resistance. Guigliano et al. (222) demonstrated that transdermal clonidine was effective in reducing blood pressure and improving insulin resistance in hypertensive individuals with non-insulin-dependent diabetes mellitus. Based on these two preliminary studies, it would appear that clonidine or other, like drugs have a favorable profile for obese individuals with hypertension.

In addition to their unfavorable effect on insulin resistance, thiazide diuretics impair pancreatic insulin secretion (223,224) and increase LDL cholesterol and total cholesterol (109,225). β-Blockers are associated with a two- to threefold incidence of inducing diabetes mellitus (226) and are associated with a significant lowering of HDL cholesterol (227,228). However, despite the different pharmacologic profiles of the antihypertensive drugs, there exists no clear recommendation for obese hypertensive individuals. Although β-blockers adversely effect the dyslipemia of obesity, Schmeider et al. (229) reported that in obese hypertensive individuals the β-blocker metroprolol decreased diastolic blood pressure to a greater extent than in those individuals receiving calcium channel blocker isradipine. Conversely, these investigators found that isradipine was more effective than metoprolol in reducing blood pressure in lean hypertensives. Frohlich (230) randomly assigned obese and lean hypertensive subjects to receive either a β-blocker or a calcium channel blocker. This study clearly suggested that that the probability of excellent blood pressure control was greater when metoprolol was given to obese individuals and isradipine to nonobese subjects. Thus, when deciding on the use of an antihypertensive in an obese individual, one must also take into account the lipid profile of the patient and the presence or risk of developing diabetes mellitus.

Finally, there are increasing data that confirm that angiotensin-converting enzyme inhibitors have specific benefit in individuals with diabetes, atherosclerosis, left ventricular dysfunction, and renal insufficiency (231). There are two other classes of agents, biguandines (metformin) and thiazolidinediones (pioglitazone, rosiglitazone, and troglitazone), that also appear to reverse insulin resistance, hypertension, and dyslipemia (232,233). However, troglitazone recently has been associated with significant liver toxicity (234). It is too early to know the role that these or similar agents will have in the treatment of obesity hypertension.

VII SUMMARY

Although weight loss is the cornerstone of hypertensive management in the obese individual, many individuals will also require pharmacologic therapy. When choosing an antihypertensive medication it is important to individualize the agent to the patient. Some agents such as thiazide diuretics and β-blockers can impair glucose tolerance and adversely alter plasma lipid levels, whereas angiotensin-converting enzyme inhibitors and centrally acting sympathetic agents improve both the hypertension and insulin resistance associated with obesity. Finally, angiotensin-converting enzyme inhibitors are also effective in reducing the development of congestive heart failure and reducing cardiovascular mortality.

ACKNOWLEDGMENTS

Supported in part by grants 1RO1 HL 52205, HL-1857-5, 2RO1-HL-35743, 2P60 AM 20572, and 2P01HL18575-24 from the National Institutes of Health.

REFERENCES

1. Dublin LI. Report of the Joint Committee on Mortality of the Association of Life Insurance Medical Directors. New York: Actuarial Society of America, 1925.
2. Stamler R, Stamler J, Riedlinger WF, Algera G, Roberts R. Weight and blood pressure: findings in hypertension screening of 1 million Americans. JAMA 1978; 240:1607–1609.
3. Symonds B. Blood pressure of healthy men and women. JAMA 1923; 8:232.
4. Hubert HB, Feinleib M, McNamara PM, Castelli WP. Obesity as an independent risk factor for cardiovascular disease: a 26-year follow-up of participants in the Framingham Heart Study. Circulation 1983; 67:968–977.
5. McMahon SW, Blacket RB, McDonald GJ, Hall W. Obesity, alcohol consumption and blood pressure in Australian men and women: National Heart Foundation of Australia Risk Factor Prevalence Study. J Hypertens 1984; 2:85–91.
6. Bloom E, Swayne R, Yano K, MacLean C. Does obesity protect hypertensives against cardiovascular disease? JAMA 1986; 256:2972–2975.
7. Ferannini E, Haffner SM, Stern MP. Essential hypertension: an insulin-resistance state. J Cardiovasc Pharmacol 1990; 15(suppl 5):S18–S25.
8. Manolio TA, Savage PJ, Burke GL, Liu KA, Wagenknecht LE, Sidney S, Jacobs DR Jr, Roseman JM, Donahue RP, Oberman A. Association of fasting insulin with blood pressure and lipids in young adults. The CARDIA Study Atherosclerosis 1990; 10:430–436.
9. Larimore JW. A study of blood pressure in relation to type of bodily habitus. Arch Intern Med 1923; 31:567.
10. Levy RL, Troud WD, White PD. Transient hypertension: its significance in terms of later development of sustained hypertension and cardiovascular-renal diseases. JAMA 1944; 126:82.
11. Hypertension Detection and Follow-Up Program Cooperative Group. Race, education and prevalence of hypertension. Am J Epidemol 1977; 106:351–361.
12. Kannel W, Brand N, Skinner J, et al. The relation of adiposity to blood pressure and development of hypertension. The Framingham Study. Ann Intern Med 1967; 67:48.
13. Cash JR, Wood JR. Observations upon the blood pressure of dogs following changes in body weight. South Med 1938; 31:270–282.
14. Rocchini AP, Moorehead C, Wentz E, Deremer S. Obesity-induced hypertension in the dog. Hypertension 1987; 9(suppl III):III64–III68.
15. Rocchini AP, Moorehead CP, DeRemer S, Bondie D. Pathogenesis of weight-related changes in blood pressure in dogs. Hypertension 1989; 13:922–928.
16. Hall JE, Brands MW, Dixon WN, et al. Obesity-induced hypertension. Renal function and systemic hemodynamics. Hypertension 1993; 22:292–299.
17. Haynes R. Is weight loss an effective treatment for hypertension? Can J Physiol Pharmacol 1985; 64:825.
18. Langford H, Davis B, Blaufox D, et al. Effect of drug and diet treatment of mild hypertension on diastolic blood pressure. Hypertension 1991; 17:210.
19. Hypertension Prevention Treatment Group. The Hypertension Trial: three-year effects of dietary changes on blood pressure. Arch Intern Med 1990; 150:153.
20. Davis BR, Blaufox D, Oberman A, Wassertheil-Smoller S, Zimbaldi N, Cutler JA, Kirchner K, Langford HG. Reduction in long-term antihypertensive medication requirements: effects of weight reduction by dietary intervention in overweight persons with mild hypertension. Arch Intern Med 1993; 153:1773–1782.
21. Fagerberg B, Andersson O, Isaksson B, et al. Blood pressure control during weight reduction in obese hypertensive men: separate effects of sodium and energy restriction. BMJ 1984; 288:11.
22. Maxwell M, Kushiro T, Dornfeld L, et al. BP changes in obese hypertensive subjects during rapid weight loss. Comparison of restricted v unchanged salt intake. Arch Intern Med 1984; 144:1581.
23. Gillum R, Prineas R, Jeffrey R, et al. Nonpharmacological therapy of hypertension: the independent effects of weight reduction and sodium restriction in overweight borderline hypertensive patients. Am Heart J 1983; 105:128.
24. Reisen E. Weight reduction in the management of hypertension: epidemiologic and mechanistic evidence. Can J Physiol Pharmacol 1985; 64:818.
25. Reisen E, Abel R, Modan M, et al. Effect of weight loss without salt restriction on the reduction of blood pressure in overweight hypertensive patients. N Engl J Med 1978; 298:1.
26. Rocchini AP, Katch V, Anderson J, Hinderliter J, Becque D, Martin M, Marks C. Blood pressure and obese adolescents: effect of weight loss. Pediatrics 1988; 82:116–123.
27. Dahl LK, Silver L, Christie RW. The role of salt in the fall of blood pressure accompanying reduction in obesity. N Engl J Med 1958; 258:1186–1192.
28. Tuck MI, Sowers J, Dornfield L, Kledzik G, Maxwell M. The effect of weight reduction on blood pressure plasma renin activity and plasma aldosterone level in obese patients. N Engl J Med 1981; 304:930–933.
29. Rocchini AP, Key J, Bondie D, Chico R, Moorehead C, Katch V, Martin M. The effect of weight loss on the

sensitivity of blood pressure to sodium in obese adolescents. N Engl J Med 1989; 321:580–585.
30. Dornfield TP, Maxwell MH, Waks AU, Schroth P, Tuck MI. Obesity and hypertension: long-term effects of weight reduction on blood pressure. Int J Obes 1985; 9:381–389.
31. Reisen E, Frohlich ED. Effects of weight reduction on arterial pressure. J Chron Dis 1982; 33:887–891.
32. Sjöström CD, Peltonen M, Wedel H, Sjöström L. Differential long-term effects of intentional weight loss on diabetes and hypertension. Hypertension 2000; 36: 20–25.
33. Sjöström CD, Lissner L, Wedel H, Sjöström L. Reduction in incidence of diabetes, hypertension, and lipid disturbances after intentional weight loss induced by bariatric surgery: the SOS Intervention Study. Obes Res 1999; 7:477–484.
34. Carson JL, Ruddy ME, Duff AE, Holems NJ, Cody RP, Brolin RE. The effect of gastric bypass surgery on hypertension in morbidly obese patients. Arch Intern Med 1994; 154:193–200.
35. Sjöström CD, Peltonen M, Sjöström L. Blood pressure and pulse pressure during long-term weight loss in the obese: the Swedish Obese Subjects (SOS) Intervention Study. Obes Res 2001; 9:188–195.
36. Vague J. The degree of masculine differentiation of obesities: a factor determining predisposition to diabetes, atherosclerosis, gout, and uric calculous disease. Am J Clin Nutr 1956; 4:20–34.
37. Landsberg L. Obesity and hypertension: experimental data. J Hypertens 1992; 10:S195–S201.
38. Shear CL, Freedman DS, Burke GL, Harsha DW, Berenson GS. Body fat patterning and blood pressure in children and young adults: the Bogalusa Heart Study. Hypertension 1987; 9:236–244.
39. Van Itallie V. Health implications of overweight and obesity in the United States. Ann Intern Med 1985; 103:983.
40. Kalkoff R, Hartz A, Rupley D, et al. Relationship of body fat distribution to blood pressure, carbohydrate tolerance, and plasma lipids in healthy obese women. J Lab Clin Med 1983; 102:621.
41. Kissebah A, Vydelingum N, Murray R, et al. Relation of body fat distribution to metabolic complications of obesity. J Clin Endocrinol Metab 1982; 54:254.
42. Peiris A, Sothmann M, Hoffmann R, et al. Adiposity, fat distribution, and cardiovascular risk. Ann Intern Med 1989; 110:867.
43. Donahue RP, Abbot RD, Bloom E, Reed DM, Yano K. Central obesity and coronary heart disease in men. Lancet 1987; 1:882–884.
44. Lapidus L, Bengtsson C, Lissner L. Distribution of adipose tissue in relation to cardiovascular and total mortality as observed during 20 years in a prospective population study of women in Gothenburg, Sweden. Diabetes Res Clin Pract 1990; 10(suppl 1):S185–S189.
45. Bjorntorp P. Portal adipose tissue as a generator of risk factors for cardiovascular disease and diabetes. Atheriosclerosis 1990; 289:333–345.
46. Haffner SM, Ferrannini E, Hazuda HP, et al. Clustering of cardiovascular risk factors in confirmed prehypertensive individuals: the San Antonio heart study. Diabetes 1992; 41:715–722.
47. Modan M, Halkin H, Almog S, et al. Hyperinsulinemia: a link between hypertension, obesity and glucose intolerance. J Clin Invest 1985; 75:809–817.
48. Ferrannini E, Buzzigoli G, Bonadonna R, et al. Insulin resistance in essential hypertension. N Engl J Med 1987; 317:350–357.
49. Pollare T, Lithell H, Berne C. Insulin resistance is a characteristic feature of primary hypertension independent of obesity. Metabolism 1990; 39:167–174.
50. Rocchini AP, Katch V, Schork A, Kelch RP. Insulin's role in blood pressure regulation during weight loss in obese adolescents. Hypertension 1987; 10:267–273.
51. Welborn TA, Breckneridge A, Rubinstein HT, Dollery CT, Russel-Fraser T. Serum insulin in essential hypertension and in peripheral vascular disease. Lancet 1966; II:1336–1337.
52. Lucas CP, Estigarribia JA, Daraga LL, Reaven GM. Insulin and blood pressure in obesity. Hypertension 1985; 7:702–706.
53. Sowers JR. Insulin resistance, hyperinsulinemia, dyslipidemia, hypertension, and accelerated atherosclerosis. J Clin Pharmacol 1992; 32:535–539.
54. Swislocki ALM, Hoffman BB, Reaven GM. Insulin resistance, glucose intolerance, and hyperinsulinemia in patients with hypertension. Am J Hypertens 1989; 2:419–423.
55. Falkner B. Differences in blacks and whites with essential hypertension: biochemistry and endocrine. Hypertension 1990; 15:681–686.
56. Falkner B, Hulman S, Tannenbaum, et al. Insulin resistance and blood pressure in young black males. Hypertension 1988; 12:352–358.
57. Shen D-C, Shieh S-M, Fuh MM-T, et al. Resistance to insulin-stimulated glucose uptake in patients with hypertension. J Clin Endocrinol Metab 1988; 66:580–583.
58. Darwin CH, Alpizar M, Buchanan TA, et al. Insulin resistance does not correlate with hypertension in Mexican American women. In 75th Annual Meeting Abstracts. Bethesda, MD: Endocrine Society Press, 1989, p. 233.
59. Hsueh WA, Buchanan TA. Obesity hypertension endocrinology and metabolism. Clin North Am 1994; 23: 405–427.
60. Meehan WP, Darwin CH, Maalouf NB, Buchanan TA, Saad MF. Insulin and hypertension: are they related? Steroids 1993; 58(12):621–634.
61. Carretta R, Fabris B, Fischetti F, Costantini M, De-Biasi F, Muiesan S, Bardelli M, Vran F, Campanacci L. Reduction of blood pressure in obese hyperinsulinemic

hypertensive patients during somatostatin infusion. J Hypertens 1989; 7(suppl 6):S196–S197.
62. Reaven GM, Ho H, Hoffman BB. Somatostatin inhibition of fructose-induced hypertension. Hypertension 1989; 14:117–120.
63. Krotkorwski M, Mandroukas K, Sjostrom L, Sullivan L, Wetterquist H, Bjorntrop P. Effect of long-term physical training on body fat, metabolism and blood pressure in obesity. Metabolism 1979; 28:650–658.
64. Zavaroni I, Sander S, Scott S, Reaven GM. Effect of fructose feeding of insulin secretion and insulin action in the rat. Metabolism 1980; 29:970–973.
65. Hwang IS, Ho H, Hoffman BB, Reaven GM. Fructose-induced insulin and hypertension in rats. Hypertension 1987; 10:512–516.
66. Reaven GM, Ho H, Hoffman BB. Attenuation of fructose-induces hypertension in rats by exercise drainage. Hypertension 1988; 12:129–132.
67. Reaven GM, Ho H, Hoffman BB. Somatostatin inhibition of fructose-induced hypertension. Hypertension 1989; 14:117–120.
68. Kurtz TW, Morris RC, Pershadsingh HA. The Zucker fatty rat as a genetic model of obesity and hypertension. Hypertension 1989; 13(6 pt 2):896–901.
69. Mondon CE, Reaven GM. Evidence of abnormalities of insulin-stimulated glucose uptake in adipocytes isolates from spontaneously hypertensive rats with spontaneous hypertension. Metabolism 1988; 37:303–305.
70. Reaven GM, Chang H, Hoffman BB, Azhar S. Resistance to insulin-stimulated glucose uptake in adipocytes isolates from spontaneously hypertensive rats. Diabetes 1989; 38:1155–1160.
71. Finch D, Davis G, Bower J, Kirchner K. Effect of insulin on renal sodium handling in hypertensive rats. Hypertension 1990; 15:514–518.
72. Brands MW, Hildebrandt DA, Mizell HL, et al. Sustained hyperinsulinemia increases arterial pressure in conscious rats. Am J Physiol 1991; 260:R764–R768.
73. Meehan WP, Buchanan TA, Hsueh WA. Chronic insulin administration elevates blood pressure in rats. Hypertension 1994; 23(pt 2):1012–1017.
74. Julius S, Jamerson K, Media A, et al. The association of borderline hypertension with target organ changes and higher coronary risk. Tecumseh Blood Pressure Study. JAMA 1990; 264:354–358.
75. Ferrari P, Weidmann P, Shaw S, et al. Altered insulin sensitivity, hyperinsulinemia, and dyslipidemia in individuals with a hypertensive parent. Am J Med 1991; 91:589–596.
76. Grugni G, Ardizzi A, Dubini A, Guzzaloni G, Sartorio A, Morabito F. No correlation between insulin levels and high blood pressure in obese subjects. Horm Metab Res 1990; 22(2):124–125.
77. Hall JE, Brands MW, Kivlighn SD, Mizelle HL, Hidebrandt DA, Gaillard CA. Chronic hyperinsulinemia and blood pressure: interaction with catecholamines? Hypertension 1990; 15:519–527.
78. Brechtold P, Jorgens V, Finke C, et al. Epidemiology and hypertension. Int J Obes 1981; 5(suppl 1):1–7.
79. Rocchini AP, Katch V, Kveselis D, Moorehead C, Martin M, Lampman R, Gregory M. Insulin and renal retention in obese adolescents. Hypertension 1989; 14:367–374.
80. DeFronzo RA, Tobin JD, Andres R. Glucose clamp technique: a method for quantifying insulin secretion and resistance. Am J Physiol 1979; D214–D223; 237: 839.
81. DeFronzo RA, Cooke CR, Andres R, Fabona GR, Davis PJ. The effect of insulin on renal handling of sodium, potassium, calcium and phosphate in man. J Clin Invest 1975; 55:845–855.
82. Baum M. Insulin stimulates volume absorption in the proximal convoluted tubule. J Clin Invest 1987; 79: 1104–1109.
83. Vierhapper H, Waldhausl W, Nowontny P. The effect of insulin on the rise in blood pressure and plasma aldosterone after angiotensin II in normal man. Clin Sci 1983; 64:383–386.
84. Rocchini AP, Moorehead C, DeRemer S, Goodfriend TL, Ball DL. Hyperinsulinemia and the aldosterone and pressor responses to angiotensin II. Hypertension 1990; 15:861–866.
85. Finta KM, Rocchini AP, Moorehead C, Key J, Katch V. Sodium retention in response to an oral glucose tolerance test in obese and nonobese adolescents. Pediatrics 1992; 90:442–446.
86. Rocchini AP. Insulin resistance, obesity, and hypertension. J Nutr 1995; 125(suppl 6):1718S–1724S.
87. Sharma AM, Spies KP, Ruland K, Distler A. Hyperinsulinemia response to oral glucose in normotensive salt-sensitive subjects. Am J Hypertens 1991; 4:13A.
88. Hall JE, Granger JP, Hester RL, Montani JP. Mechanisms of sodium balance in hypertension: role of pressure natriuresis. J Hypertens 1986; 4(suppl 4): S57–S65.
89. Ter Maaten JC, Bakker SJ, Serne EH, Ter Wee PM, Donker AJ, Gans RO. Insulin's acute effects on glomerular filtration rate correlate with insulin sensitivity whereas insulin's acute effects on proximal tubular sodium reabsorption correlate with salt sensitivity in normal subjects. Nephrol Dial Transplant 1999; 14:2357–2363.
90. Rocchini A, Marker P, Cervenka T. Time course of insulin resistance associated with weight gain in the dog: relationship to the development of hypertension. Am J Physiol 1996; 272:E147–E154.
91. Laakso M, Edelman SV, Brechtel G, Baron AD. Impaired insulin-mediated skeletal muscle blood flow in patients with NIDDM. Diabetes 1992; 41:1076–1083.
92. Kolterman O, Insel J, Saekow M, Olefsky J. Mechanisms of insulin resistance in human obesity: evidence

for receptor and post-receptor defects. J Clin Invest 1980; 65:1272–1284.
93. Sechi LA. Mechanisms of insulin resistance in rat models of hypertension and their relationships with salt sensitivity. J Hypertens 1999; 17:1229–1237.
94. Hall JE, Brands MW, Henegar JR, Shek EW. Abnormal kidney function as a cause and a consequence of obesity hypertension. Clin Exp Pharmacol Physiol 1998; 25:58–64.
95. King GL, Goodman D, Buzney S, Moses A, Kahn CR. Receptors and growth promoting effects of insulin and insulin like growth factors on cells from bovine retinal capillaries and aorta. J Clin Invest 1985; 75:1028–1036.
96. Folkow B. Cardiovascular structural adaptation: its role in the inhibition and maintenance of primary hypertension: Volhard lectures. Clin Sci 1978; 55:3s–22s.
97. Anderson EA, Hoffman RP, Balon TW, Sinkey CA, Mark AL. Hyperinsulinemia produces both sympathetic neural activation and vasolidation in normal humans. J Clin Invest 1991; 87:2246–2252.
98. Rocchini AP, Moorehead C, Katch V, Key J, Finta KM. Forearm resistance vessel abnormalities and insulin resistance in obese adolescents. Hypertension 1992; 19:615–620.
99. Steinberg HO, Brechtel G, Johnson A. Insulin mediated skeletal muscle vasodilation is nitric oxide dependent. A novel action of insulin to increase nitric oxide release. J Clin Invest 1994; 94:1172–1179.
100. Baron AD, Steinberg HO, Chaker H. Insulin mediated skeletal muscle vasodilation contributed to both insulin sensitivity and responsiveness in lean humans. J Clin Invest 1995; 96:786–792.
101. Miyoshi A, Suzuki H, Fujiwara M. Impairment of endothelial function in salt-sensitive hypertension in humans. Am J Hypertens 1997; 10:1083–1090.
102. Facchini FS, DoNascimento C, Reaven GM, Yip JW, Ni XP, Humphrey MH. Blood pressure, sodium intake, insulin resistance, and urinary nitrate excretion. Hypertension 1999; 33:1008–1012.
103. Wu HY, Jeng YY, Yue CJ, et al. Endothelial-dependent vascular effects of insulin and insulin-like growth factor-I in the rat perfused mesenteric artery and aortic rings. Diabetes 1994; 43(8):1027–1032.
104. Yagi S, Takata S, Kiyokawa H, et al. Effects of insulin on vasoconstrictive responses to norepinephrine and angiotensin II in rabbit femoral artery and vein. Diabetes 1988; 37:1064–1067.
105. Zemel MB, Sowers JR, Shehin S, et al. Impaired calcium metabolism associated with hypertension in Zucker obese rats. Metabolism 1990; 39:704–708.
106. Natali A, Buzzigoli G, Taddei S, Santoro D, Cerri M, Perdrinelli R, Ferrannini E. Effects of insulin on hemodynamics and metabolism in human forearm. Diabetes 1990; 39:490–500.
107. Laakso M, Edelman SV, Brechtel G, Baron AD. Decreased effect of insulin to stimulate skeletal muscle blood flow in obese man. J Clin Invest 1990; 85:1844–1952.
108. Baron AD, Laasko M, Brechtel G, Edelman SV. Mechanism of insulin resistance in insulin-dependent diabetes mellitus: a major role for reduced skeletal muscle blood flow. J Clin Endocrinol Metab 1991; 73: 637–643.
109. Pollare T, Lithell H, Berne C. A comparison of the effects of hydrochlorothiazide and captopril on glucose and lipid metabolism in patients with hypertension. N Engl J Med 1989; 321:868–873.
110. Swislocki AL, Hoffman BB, Sheu WH, Chen YD, Reaven GM. Effect of prazosin treatment on carbohydrate and lipoprotein metabolism in patients with hypertension. Am J Med 1989; 86:14–18.
111. Pollare T, Lithell H, Morlin C, Prantare H, Hvarfner A, Ljunghall S. Metabolic effects of diltiazem and atenolol: results from a randomized, double-blind study with parallel groups. J Hypertens 1989; 7:551–559.
112. Lillioja S, Young AA, Culter CL, et al. Skeletal muscle capillary density and fiber type are possible determinants of *in vivo* insulin resistance in man. J Clin Invest 1987; 80:415–424.
113. Lithel H, Lindgarde F, Hellsin K, Lundqvist G, Nygaard E, Vesby B, Saltin B. Body weight, skeletal muscle morphology, and enzyme activities in relation to fasting serum insulin concentration and glucose tolerance in 48-year-old-men. Diabetes 1981; 30:19–25.
114. Staron RS, Hikida RS, Hagerman FC, Dudlty GA, Murray TF. Human muscle fibre type adaptability to various workloads. J Histochem Cytochem 1984; 32: 146–152.
115. Wage AJ, Marbut MM, Round JM. Muscle fibre type and etiology of obesity. Lancet 1990; 335:805–808.
116. Juhlin-Dannfelt A, Frisk-Holmberg M, Karlsson J, Tesch P. Central and peripheral circulation in relation to muscle fibre composition in normo- and hypertensive man. Clin Sci 1979; 56:335–340.
117. Julius S, Gudbrandsson T, Jamerson K, Shahab ST, Andersson O. The hemodynamic link between insulin resistance and hypertension. J Hypertens 1991; 9:983–986.
118. Julius S, Gudbrandsson T, Jamerson K, Andersson O. The interconnection between sympathetics, microcirculation, and insulin resistance in hypertension. Blood Pressure 1992; 1:9–19.
119. Frisk-Holmberg M, Essen B, Fredrikson M, Strom G, Wibell L. Muscle fibre composition in relation to blood pressure response to isometric exercise in normotensive and hypertensive subjects. Acta Med Scand 1983; 213:21–26.
120. Bergstrom J. Muscle electrolytes in man. Scan J Clin Lab Med 1962; 14:511–513.
121. Simoneau JA, Bouchard C. Skeletal muscle metabolism in normal weight and obese men and women. Int J Obes 1993; 17(suppl 2):31.

122. Krotkiewski M, Bjorntorp P. Muscle tissue in obesity with different distribution of adipose tissue: effects of physical training. Int J Obes 1986; 10:331–341.
123. Anderson P, Henriksson J. Capillary supply of the quadriceps femoris muscle of man: adaptive response to exercise. J Physiol 1977; 270:677–690.
124. Chi MMY, Hintz CS, Henriksson J. Chronic stimulation of mammalian muscle: enzyme changes in individual fibers. Am J Physiol 1986; 251:c633–c642.
125. Lagadie-Grossman D, Chesnais JM, Fewray D. Intracellular pH regulation in papillary muscle cells from streptozotocin diabetic rats: an ion-sensitive microelectrode study. Pflugers Arch 1988; 412:613–617.
126. Tedde R, Sechi LA, Marigliano A, Scano L, Pala A. In vitro action of insulin on erythrocyte sodium transport mechanisms: its possible role in the pathogenesis of arterial hypertension. Clin Exp Hypertens 1988; 10: 545–559.
127. Ng LL, Harker M, Abel ED. Leucocyte sodium content and sodium pump activity in overweight and lean hypertensives. Clin Endocrinol (Oxf) 1989; 30(2): 191–200.
128. Herlitz H, Fagerberg B, Jonsson O, Hedner T, Andersson OK, Aurell M. Effects of sodium restriction and energy reduction on erythrocyte sodium transport in obese hypertensive men. Ann Clin Res 1988; 20 (suppl 48):61–65.
129. Draznin B, Kao M, Sussman KE. Insulin and glyburide increase in cytosolic free calcium concentration in isolated rat adipocytes. Diabetes 1987; 36:174–178.
130. Jacobs DD, Sowers JR, Hmeidan A, Niyogi T, Simpson L, Standley PR. Effects of weight reduction on cellular cation metabolism and vascular resistance. Hypertension 1993; 21:308–314.
131. Dranzin B, Sussman K, Koa M, et al. The existence of an optimal range of cystolic free calcium for insulin-stimulated glucose transport in rat adipocytes. J Biol Chem 1987; 262:1485–1488.
132. Shaefer W, Prieben J, Mannhold R, et al. Ca^{2+}-Mg^{2+}-ATPase activity of human red blood cells in healthy and diabetic volunteers. Klin Wochenschr 1987; 65: 17–21.
133. Resnick LM, Gupta RK, Gruenspan H, et al. Intracellular free magnesium in hypertension: relation to peripheral insulin resistance. J Hypertens 1988; 6: S199–S201.
134. Resnick LM, Militianu D, Cummings AJ, Pipe JG, Evelhoch JL, Soulen RL. Direct magnetic resonance determination of aortic distensibility in essential hypertension, relation to age, abdominal visceral fat, and in situ intracellular free magnesium. Hypertension 1997; 30:654–659.
135. Rocchini AP, Katch VL, Grekin R, Moorehead C, Anderson J. Role for aldosterone in blood pressure regulation of obese adolescents. Am J Cardiol 1986; 57:613–618.
136. Hiramatsu K, Yamada T, Ichikawak T, Izumiyama T, Nagata H. Changes in endocrine activity to obesity in patients with essential hypertension. J Am Geriatr Soc 1981; 29:25–30.
137. Scavo D, Borgia C, Iacobelli A. Aspetti di funzione corticosurrenalica nell'obesita'. Nota VI. Il comportamento della secrezione di aldosterone e della escrezione dei suoi metabolite nel corso di alcune prove dinamiche. Folia Endocrinol 1968; 21:591–602.
138. Scavo D, Iacobelli A, Borgia C. Aspetti fi funzione corticosurrenalica nell'obesita'. Nota V. La secrezonia giornlieia di aldosterone. Folia Endocrinol 1968; 21: 577–590.
139. Spark RF, Arky RA, Boulter RP, Saudek CD, Obrian JT. Renin, aldosterone and glucagon in the natriureses of fasting. N Engl J Med 1975; 292:1335–1340.
140. Granger JP, West D, Scott J. Abnormal pressure natriuresis in the dog model of obesity-induced hypertension. Hypertension 1994; 23(suppl I):I8–I11.
141. Trovati M, Massucco P, Anfossi G, Caralot F, Mularoni E, Mattiello L, Rocca G, Emaneulli G. Insulin influences the renin-angiotensin-aldosterone system in humans. Metabolism 1989; 38:501–503.
142. Farfel Z, Iania A, Eliahou HE. Presence of insulin-renin-aldosterone-potassium interrelationship in normal subjects, disrupted in chronic hemodialysis patients. Clin Endrocrinol Metab 1978; 47:9–17.
143. Shoback DM, Williams GH, Moore TJ, Dluhy RG, Podolsky S, Hollenberg NK. Defect in the sodium-modulated tissue responsiveness to angiotensin II in essential hypertension. J Clin Endocrinol Metab 1983; 57:764–770.
144. Hollenberg NK, Moore TJ, Shoback D, Redgrave J, Rabinowe S, Williams GH. Abnormal renal sodium handling in essential hypertension: relation to failure of renal and adrenal modulation of responses to angiotensin II. Am J Med 1986; 81:412–418.
145. Ferri C, Bellini C, Desideri G, Valenti M, De Mattia G, Santucci A, Hollenberg NK, Williams GH. Relationship between insulin resistance and nonmodulating hypertension: linkage of metabolic abnormalities and cardiovascular risk. Diabetes 1999; 48:1623–1630.
146. Trevisan R, Bruttomesso D, Vedovato M, Brocco S, Pianta A, Cinza GC, Jori E, Semplicini A, Tiengo A, Del Prato S. Enhanced responsiveness of blood pressure to sodium intake and to angiotensin II is associated with insulin resistance in IDDM patients with microalbuminuria. Diabetes 1998; 47:1347–1353.
147. Young JB, Landsberg L. Suppression of sympathetic nervous system during fasting. Science 1977; 196: 1473–1475.
148. Young JB, Landsberg L. Stimulation of the sympathetic nervous system during sucrose feeding. Nature 1977; 269:615–617.
149. Landsberg L, Young JB. Fasting, feeding and reg-

ulation of the sympathetic nervous system. N Engl J Med 1978; 298:1295–1301.

150. Young JB, Saville ME, Rothwell NJ, Stock MJ, Landsberg L. Effect of diet and cold exposure on norepinephrine turnover in brown adipose tissue in the rat. J Clin Invest 1982; 69:1061–1071.

151. Landsberg L, Young JB. Insulin-mediated glucose metabolism in the relationship between dietary intake and sympathetic nervous system activity. Int J Obes 1985; 9:63–68.

152. Landsberg L, Krieger DR. Obesity, metabolism and the sympathetic nervous system. Am J Hypertens 1989; 2:125s–132s.

153. Young JB, Kaufman LN, Saville ME, Landsberg L. Increased sympathetic nervous system activity in rats fed a low protein diet: evidence against a role for dietary tyrosine. Am J Physiol 1985; 248:r627–r637.

154. Rowe JW, Young BY, Minaker KL, Stevens AL, Pallatta J, Landsberg L. Effect of insulin and glucose infusions on sympathetic nervous system activity in normal human man. Diabetes 1981; 30:219–225.

155. O'Hare JA, Minaker K, Young JB, Rowe JW, Pallotta JA, Landsberg L. Insulin increases plasma norepinephrine (NE) and lowers plasma potassium equally in lean and obese men [abstract]. Clin Res 1985; 33:441a.

156. Assy W, Wan JM, Coyle S, Blackburn GL, Bistrain BR, Istfan NW. Fasting increases the sensitivity of blood pressure response to insulin in obese rats. Clin Res 1991; 39:a34.

157. Hall JE, Van Vliet BN, Garrity CA, Connell RD, Brands MW. Role of increased adrenergic activity in obesity-induced hypertension. Circulation 1992; 86(suppl I):I-541.

158. Kassab S, Kato T, Wilkins FC, Chen R, Hall JE, Granger JP. Renal denervation attenuates the sodium retention and hypertension associated with obesity. Hypertension 1995; 25(p2):893–897.

159. Young JB, Macdonald IA. Sympathoadrenal activity in human obesity: heterogeneity of findings since 1980. Int J Obes 1992; 16:959–967.

160. Landsberg L, Troisi R, Parker D, Young JB, Weiss St. Obesity, blood pressure and the sympathetic nervous system. Ann Epidemiol 1991; 1:295–303.

161. Elahi D, Sclater A, Waksmonski C, et al. Insulin resistance, sympathetic activity and cardiovascular function in obesity [abstract]. Clin Res 1991; 39:355a.

162. Elahi D, Krieger DR, Young JB, Landsberg L. Effects of somatostatin infusion on plasma or norepinephrine (NE) and cardiovascular function in men [abstract]. Clin Res 1991; 39:385a.

163. Sondergaard SB, Verdich C, Astrup A, Bratholm P, Christensen NJ. Obese male subjects show increased resting forearm venous plasma noradrenaline concentration but decreased 24-hour sympathetic activity as evaluated by thrombocyte noradrenaline measurements. Int J Obes Relat Metab Disord 1999; 23:810–815.

164. Weyer C, Pratley RE, Snitker S, Spraul M, Ravussin E, Tataranni A. Ethnic differences in insulinemia and sympathetic tone as links between obesity and blood pressure. Hypertension 2000; 36:531–542.

165. Krief S, Lonnquest F, Raimbault S. Tissue distribution of B_3-adrenergic receptor RNA in man. J Clin Invest 1993; 91:344–349.

166. Walston J, Silver K, Bogardus C, Knowler WC, Celi FS, Austin S, Manning B, Strosberg AD, Stern MP, Raben N. Time of onset of non-insulin-dependent diabetes mellitus and genetic variation in the beta 3-adrenergic-receptor gene. N Engl J Med 1995; 333(6): 343–347.

167. Wheeldon NM, McDevett DG, McFarlene LC, Lipworth BJ. B-adrenoceptor subtypes me dietary the metabolic effects of BRL 35135 in man. Clin Sci 1994; 86:331–337.

168. Lager I, Attrall S, Eriksson BM. Studies on the insulin-antagonistic effect of catecholamines in normal man: evidence for the importance of b2-receptor. Diabetologia 1986; 29:409–416.

169. Diebert DC, DeFronzo RA. Epinephrine-induced insulin resistance in man. J Clin Invest 1980; 65:717–721.

170. Jamerson K, Julius S, Gudbrandsson T, Andersson O, Brant D. Reflex sympathetic activation induces acute insulin resistance in the human forearm. Hypertension 1993; 21:618–623.

171. Rosen P, Ohly P, Gleochman. Experimental benefit of moxonidine on glucose metabolism and insulin secretion in the fructose-fed rat. J Hypertens 1997; 15(suppl I):S31–S38.

172. Ernsberger P, Friedman JE, Kooletsky RJ. The 11-imidazoline receptor: from binding site to therapeutic target in cardiovascular disease. J Hypertens 1997; 15(suppl I):S9–S23.

173. Rocchini AP, Mao HZ, Babu K, Marker P, Rocchini AJ. Clonidine prevents insulin resistance and hypertension in obese dogs. Hypertension 1999; 33(pt II): 548–553.

174. Licata G, Volpe M, Scanglione R, Rubattu S. Salt-regulating hormones in your normotensive obese subjects. Effect of saline load. Hypertension 1994; 3(suppl I):120–124.

175. Maoz E, Shamiss A, Peleg E, Salzberg M, Rosenthal T. The role of atrial natriuretic peptide in the natriuresis of fasting. J Hypertens 1992; 10:1041–1044.

176. Dessi-Fulgheri P, Sarzani R, Tamburrini P, Moraca A, Espinosa E, Cola G, Giantomassi L, Rappelle A. Plasma atrial natriuretic peptide and natriuretic peptide receptor gene expression in adipose tissue of normotensive and hypertensive obese patients. J Hypertens 1997; 15:1695–1699.

177. Golden P, MacCagnan TJ, Pardridge WM. Human

blood brain barrier leptin receptor binding and endocytosis in isolated human brain microvessels. J Clin Invest 1997; 99:14–18.
178. Considine RV, Sinha MK, Heiman ML, Kriauciunas A, Stephens TW. Serum immunoreactive leptin concentrations in normal-weight and obese humans. N Engl J Med 1996; 334:292–295.
179. Collins S, Kuhn CM, Petro AE, Swick AG, Chrunyk BA, Surwit RS. Role of leptin in fat regulation. Nature 1996; 380:667.
180. Haynes WG, Morgan DA, Walsh SA, Mark AL, Sivitz WI. Receptor mediated regional sympathetic nerve activation by leptin. J Clin Invest 1997; 100:270–278.
181. Shek EW, Brands MW, Hall JE. Chronic leptin infusion increases arterial pressure. Hypertension 1998; 31:409–414.
182. Ogawa Y, Masuzaki H, Aizawa M, Yura S, Satoh N, Iwai H, Hosada K, Nakao K. Blood pressure elevation in transgenic mice over-expressing leptin, the obe gene product. J Hypertens (abstract) 1989; 16:S7.
183. Haynes WG, Morgan DA, Walsh SA, Sivitz W, Mark AL. Cardiovascular consequences of obesity: role of leptin. Clin Exp Pharmacol Physiol 1998; 2565–2569.
184. Bjorntorp P, Rosmond R. Neuroendocrine abnormalities in visceral obesity. Int J Obes Relat Metab Disord 2000; 24(suppl 2):S80–S85.
185. Strain GW, Zumoff B, Strain JL. Cortisol production in obesity. Metabolism 1980; 29:980–985.
186. Rosmond R, Dallman MF, Bjorntorp P. Stress-related cortisol secretion in men: relationships with abdominal obesity and endocrine, metabolic and hemodynamic abnormalities. J Clin Endocrinol Metab 1998; 83: 1853–1859.
187. Kvist H, Chowdhury B, Grangard U, Tylen U, Sjostrom. Total and visceral adipose tissue volumes derived from measurements with computed tomography in adult men and women: predicative equations. Am J Clin Nutr 1988; 48:1351–1361.
188. Rosmond R, Bjorntorp P. The interactions between hypothalamic-pituitary-adrenal axis activity, testosterone, insulin-like growth factor I and abdominal obesity with metabolism and blood pressure in man. Int J Obes Relat Metab Disord 1998; 22:1184–1196.
189. Zahrezewska KE, Cusin J, Sainbury A, Pohner F, Jeanrenaud FR, Jeanrenaud B. Glucocorticoids are counterregulatory hormones to leptin. Towards an understanding of leptin resistance. Diabetes 1997; 46:717–719.
190. Rosmond R, Holm G, Bjorntorp P. Food-induced cortisol secretion relation to anthropometric, metabolic and hemodynamic variables in men. Int J Obes Relat Metab Disord 2000; 24:95–105.
191. Rosmond R, Chagnon YC, Holm G, Changon M, Perusse L, Lindell K, Carlsson B, Bouchard C, Bjorntorp P. A glucocorticoid receptor gene marker is associated with abdominal obesity, leptin, and dysregulation of the hypothalamic-pituitary-adrenal axis. Obes Res 2000; 8:211–218.
192. Weaver J, Hitman GA, Kopelaman PG. An association between a Bc/I restriction fragment length polymorphism of the glucocorticoid receptor gene locus and hyperinsulinemia in obese women. J Mol Endocrinol 1992; 9:295–300.
193. Buemann B, Vohl MC, Chagnon M, Chagnon YC, Gagnon J, Perusse L, Dionne F, Despres JP, Tremblay A, Nadeau A, Bouchard C. Abdominal visceral fat is associated with a Bc/I restriction fragment length polymorphism at the glucocorticoid receptor gene locus. Obes Res 1997; 5:186–189.
194. Bjorntorp P, Rosmond R. Hypothalamic origin of the metabolic syndrome X. Ann NY Acad Sci 1999; 892: 308–311.
195. Manson JE, Colditz GA, Stampfer MJ, Willnet WC, Rosner B, Monson RR, Speizer FE, Hennekens CH. A prospective study of obesity and risk of coronary heart disease in women. N Engl J Med 1990; 322:882–889.
196. Marrett-Connor E, Khaw KT. Is Hypertension more benign when associated with obesity? Circulation 1985; 72:53–60.
197. Chambien F, Chreitien JM, Docimetiere P, Guize L, Richard JL. Is the relationship between blood pressure and cardiovascular risk dependent on body mass index? Am J Epidemiol 1985; 122:434–442.
198. MacMahon SW, Wicken DEL, MacDonald GJ. Effect of weight loss on left ventricular mass: a randomized controlled trail in young overweight hypertensive patients. N Engl J Med 1985; 314:334–339.
199. Alpert MA, Singh A, Terry BE, Kelly DL, Villarreal D, Mukerji V. Effect of exercise on left ventricular systolic function and reserve in morbid obesity. Am J Cardiol 1989; 63:1478–1482.
200. De Divittis O, Fazio S, Petitto M, Maddalena G, Contaldo F, Mancini M. Obesity and cardiac function. Circulation 1981; 64:477–482.
201. Alexander JK, Pettigrove JR. Obesity and congestive heart failure. Geriatrics 1967; 22:101–108.
202. Raison HJ, Achimastos A, Bouthier J, London G, Safar M. Intravascular volume, extracellular fluid volume, and total body water in obese and non-obese hypertensive patients. Am J Cardiol 1983; 51:165–170.
203. Dustin HP, Tarazi RC, Mujais S. A comparison of hemodynamic and volume characteristics of obese and non-obese hypertensive patients. Int J Obes 1981; 5(suppl 1):19–25.
204. Reisin E, Frohlich ED, Messerli FH, Dreslinski GR, Dunn FG, Jones MM, Batson HM. Cardiovascular changes after weight reduction in obesity hypertension. Ann Intern Med 1983; 98:315–319.
205. Lesser GT, Deutsch S. Measurement of adipose tissue blood flow and perfusion in man by uptake of 85-Kr. J Appl Physiol 1967; 23:621–631.

206. Rocchini AP. Cardiovascular regulation in obesity-induced hypertension. Hypertension 1992; 19:156–159.
207. Schmeider RE, Messerli FH. Does obesity influence early target organ damage in hypertensive patients? Circulation 1993; 87:1482–1488.
208. Blake J, Devereaux RB, Borer JS, Szulc M, Pappas TW, Laragh JH. Relation of obesity, high sodium intake, and eccentric left ventricular hypertrophy to left ventricular exercise dysfunction in essential hypertension. Am J Med 1990; 88:477–485.
209. Guillermo E, Garavaglia E, Messerli FH, Nunez BD, Schmieder RE, Grossman E. Myocardial contractility and left ventricular function in obese patients with essential hypertension. Am J Cardiol 1988; 62:594–597.
210. Stoddard MF, Tseuda K, Thomas M, Dillon S, Kupersmith J. The influence of obesity on left ventricular filing and systolic function. Am Heart J 1992; 124:694.
211. Grossman E, Orren S, Messerli FH. Left ventricular filling in the systematic hypertension of obesity. Am J Cardiol 1991; 60:57–60.
212. Messerli FH, Nunez BD, Ventura HO, Snyder DW. Overweight and sudden death: increased ventricular ectopy in cardiopathy in obesity. Arch Intern Med 1987; 147:1725–1728.
213. Rockstroph JK, Schmieder RE, Schachinger H, Messerli FH. Stress response pattern in obesity and systematic hypertension. Am J Cardiol 1992; 70:1035–1039.
214. Nakajima T, Fugiola S, Tokunaga K, Matsuzawa Y, Tami S. Correlation of intraabdominal fat accumulation and left ventricular performance in obesity. Am J Cardiol 1989; 64:369–373.
215. Becque MD, Katch VL, Rocchini AP, Marks CR, Moorehead C. Coronary risk incidence of obese adolescents: reductions of exercise plus diet intervention. Pediatrics 1988; 81:605–612.
216. Beardwood DM, Alden JS, Graham CA, et al. Evidence for a peripheral action of chlorothiazide in normal man. Metabolism 1966; 15:88–93.
217. Gill JS, Al-Hussary N, Anderson DC. Effect of nifedipine on glucose tolerance, serum insulin, and serum fructosamine in diabetic patients. Clin Ther 1987; 9: 304–310.
218. Klauser R, Ptager R, Gaube S, et al. Metabolic effects on isradipine versus hydrochlorothiazide in diabetes mellitus. Hypertension 1991; 17:15–21.
219. Pollare T, Lithell H, Morlin C, et al. Metabolic effects of diltiazem and atenolol: results from a randomized, double blind study with parallel groups. J Hypertens 1989; 7:551–555.
220. Grunfeld CM, Chappell DA. Prevention of glucose intolerance of thiazide diuretics by maintenance of body potassium. Diabetes 1983; 32:106–111.
221. Pollare T, Lithell H, Selinus I, et al. Application of prazosin is associated with an increase of insulin sensitivity in obese patients with hypertension. Diabetologia 1988; 31:415–420.
222. Giugliano D, Acampora R, Marfella R, La Marca C, Marfella M, Nappo F, D'Onofrio F. Hemodynamic and metabolic effects of transdermal clonidine in patients with hypertension and non-insulin dependent diabetes mellitus. Am J Hyertens 1998; 11:184–189.
223. Fajans SS, Floyd JC, Knopf RF, et al. Benthiadiazine suppression of insulin release from normal and abnormal islet cell tissue of a man. J Clin Invest 1966; 45:481–493.
224. Amery A, Birkenhager W, Brixxo P. Glucose intolerance during diuretic therapy in elderly hypertensive patients. Med J 1986; 62:919–925.
225. Morgan TO. Metabolic effects of various antihypertensive agents. J Cardiovasc Pharmacol 1990; 15(suppl 5):s39–s45.
226. Bergtsson C, Blhme T, Lapidus D. Do antihypertensive drugs precipitate diabetes? BMJ 1984; 289:1495–1497.
227. Greenberg G, Brennan PJ, Miall WE. Effects of diuretic and β-blocker therapy in the MRC trial. Am J Med 1984; 76:45–51.
228. Gemma G, Mantanari G, Suppe G, et al. Plasma lipid and lipoprotein changes in hypertensive patients treated with propranolol and prazosin. J Cardiovasc Pharmacol 1982; 4(suppl 2):s233–s237.
229. Schmieder RE, Gatzka C, Schachinger H, Schobel H, Ruddel H. Obesity as a determinant for the response to antihypertensive treatment. BMJ 1993; 307:537–540.
230. Frohlich ED. Obesity hypertension: converting enzyme inhibitors and calcium antagonists. Hypertension 1992; 19(suppl 1):I119–I123.
231. Ferdinand KC. Update in pharmacologic treatment of hypertension. Cardiol Clin 2001; 19(2):279–294.
232. Kobayashi M, Iwanishi M, Egawa K, et al. Pioglitazone increases insulin sensitivity by activation insulin receptor kinase. Diabetes 1992; 41:476–483.
233. King AB. A comparison in a clinical setting of the efficacy and side effects of three thiazolidinediones. Diabetes Care 2000; 23:557–558.
234. Wagenaar LJ, Kuck EM, Hoekstra JB. Troglitazone: is it all over? Neth J Med 1999; 55(1):4–12.

37

Obesity and Diabetes

Jeanine Albu and F. Xavier Pi-Sunyer

Columbia University College of Physicians and Surgeons and St. Luke's-Roosevelt Hospital Center, New York, New York, U.S.A.

I ASSOCIATION BETWEEN OBESITY AND DIABETES

Obesity is rare in insulin-dependent type 1 diabetes mellitus, but is common in type 2, non-insulin-dependent, diabetes mellitus (DM). About 85% of diabetics can be classified as type 2, and of these an average of 70% are overweight, ranging from a low of 50% to a high of 90%, depending on age, gender, and race (1).

An initial observation that obesity and diabetes mellitus are associated was made by John (2) in 1929. Also, early on, it was observed that weight loss improves glucose control (3). West and Kalbfleisch (4), in the 1960s, in a series of population studies including many geographical areas, races, and cultures, noted a strong association between the prevalence of diabetes and overweight. They proposed that the largest environmental influence on the prevalence of diabetes in a population group was the degree of obesity present in that community (5). In some of these populations, diabetes was found to be as much as threefold higher in females than in males. Controlling for adiposity abolished these sex differences. In the Bedford diabetes survey of 1962, Fowler et al. (6) found that whereas in individuals <40 years of age there was no relation of weight to the prevalence of diabetes, in the 40-to-70-year-old age range the persons with diabetes were fatter. Baird et al. (7) investigated siblings of diabetic patients and siblings of nondiabetic matched controls and found that siblings of diabetics had a threefold higher prevalence of diabetes, but those with the highest prevalence were the obese siblings of nonobese diabetic propositi. More recently, Knowler et al. (8) have shown that in the Pima Indian population, the likelihood of developing diabetes rises steeply with increasing fatness (Fig. 1).

Finally, the seriousness of the present status in the United States, with regard to the increase in prevalence of type 2 diabetes mellitus, is reflected in the data from the NHANES (National Health Examination Survey) III data (1988–1994). Type 2 diabetes mellitus showed a strong increase in prevalence with increasing degree of overweight among both younger and older subjects. The prevalence was a staggering five times higher for men and 8.3 times higher for women in the most obese group compared to normal-weight individuals. As opposed to earlier studies, the prevalence ratio associated with elevated weight was three- to fourfold greater among younger overweight men and women (Fig. 2) (5–9).

There have been prospective studies in a number of countries, including the United States (10), Norway (11), Sweden (12), and Israel (13) which have shown that increasing weight increases the risk of diabetes. In the Nurses' Health Study, which has followed 114,824 women for 14 years, it has also been found that the risk of developing diabetes increases as body mass index (BMI) increases (14,15). Weight gain of even 7.0–10.9 kg after the age of 18 years was associated with a twofold increase in the risk for diabetes. It is important

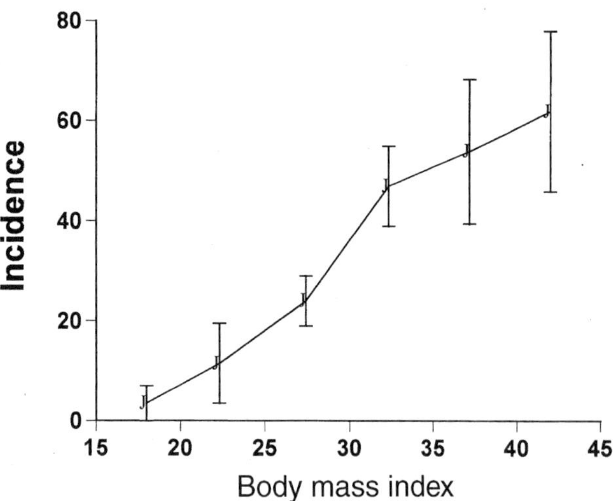

Figure 1 Age- and sex-adjusted incidence of diabetes by body mass index with 95% confidence intervals. The data are adjusted by age and sex using the 1980 U.S. white population as a standard to give average incidence rates according to body mass index. (From Ref. 8.)

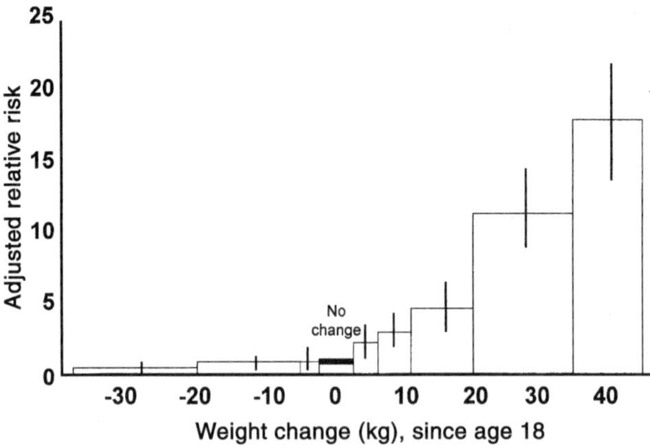

Figure 2 Age-adjusted relative risk for diabetes mellitus during 14 years of follow-up and weight change between age 18 years and 1976. (From Ref. 14.)

to note that this rise begins at levels of BMI of 22, considered generally to be a rather lean weight. These investigators observed that weight gain after the age of 18 years could be correlated to the increased incidence of diabetes, with a greater risk as the baseline of weight from which an individual started increased and also with a greater risk as weight gain increased (Fig. 3) (14,15). Other studies have found a similar risk for diabetes with increasing weight gain (16) and duration of overweight (17,18).

It is important to note that, recently, investigators analyzing results of 16 years of follow-up in the Nurses' Health Study found that lack of exercise, a poor diet, and current smoking were significantly associated with increased risk of diabetes, even after adjustment for BMI (19).

II OBESITY AS ONE OF THE MAIN FACTORS IN THE TYPE 2 GLOBAL DIABETES EPIDEMIC

The recent global type 2 diabetes epidemic has been most pronounced in non-Europid populations. This was evident in studies from Native American and Canadian communities, Pacific and Indian Ocean island populations (20), groups in India (21), and Australian Aboriginal communities (22). Zimmet et al. recently summarized the magnitude and the potential reasons for this epidemic (23). In the Pacific Island of Nauru, diabetes is present in ~40% of adults while it was virtually unknown 50 years ago (24). The highest yet reported prevalence in people of Chinese extraction comes from Mauritius. In addition, Asian Indians and Creoles experienced high rates of diabetes and a notable secular increase between 1987 and 1998 (25). Prevalence of type 2 diabetes doubled between 1984 and 1992 in Singaporean Chinese (26) and is very high in Taiwan (27). The potential for increases in the number of cases of diabetes is greatest in Asia (28). According to one estimate the number of individuals with type 2 diabetes in China will increase from 8 million in 1996 to 32 million by 2010 (23).

The current view on the reasons for this epidemic is that, apart from heightened genetic susceptibility of

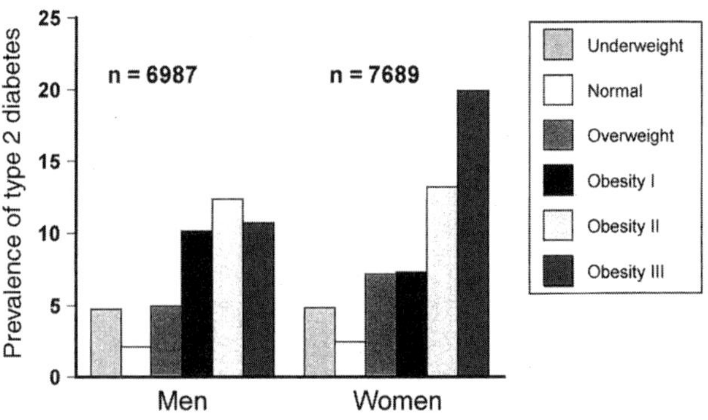

Figure 3 Prevalence of type 2 diabetes mellitus by obesity class, in men and women. Data from the Third National Health and Nutrition Examination Survey (NHANES III). (From Ref. 9.)

certain ethnic groups, environmental and behavioral factors such as sedentary lifestyle, poor nutrition, and obesity play an important role (23,29). One of the major debates in diabetes etiology is the issue of "thrifty genotype versus thrifty phenotype."

The thrifty genotype hypothesis provides an explanation for the very high prevalence of obesity and type 2 diabetes in the American Pima Indians, Australian Aborigines, and Pacific Islanders. Susceptibility for disease could result from an evolutionarily advantageous thrifty genotype that promoted fat deposition and storage of calories in times of plenty for use in times of scarcity. The present plentiful supply of a diet rich in simple carbohydrates and saturated fats and the reduction of occupational and leisure-based physical activity cause the previously favorable metabolic profile seen in "survivors" to result in obesity and type 2 diabetes. The thrifty phenotype hypothesis is based on the epidemiological observations linking low birth weight with the risk of adult disease (obesity, diabetes, and hypertension). A combination of the two may also be possible and more research is needed to clarify this problem (23).

III INFLUENCE OF THE DISTRIBUTION OF BODY FAT

The possibility of a relationship between the distribution of body fat and diabetes was first raised by Jean Vague (30), who clinically observed and reported in 1947 the occurrence of two kinds of "obesities": the android, "apple" shape or predominantly upper-body distribution of the adipose tissue, and the gynoid, "pear" shape or predominantly lower-body distribution of the adipose tissue. Subsequent cross-sectional and prospective studies have linked diabetes mellitus, dyslipidemia, and other cardiovascular risk factors to the distribution of body fat.

Feldman et al. (31), studying a group of more than 7000 people at multiple sites, found that those with diabetes were fatter and also had a more central distribution of their fat. They suggested that in diabetes there is an abnormality in hormone balance that causes women to be more like men in central fat distribution and exaggerates this effect in men. A study of more than 15,000 American women showed that clinical diabetes was related directly not only to increasing obesity but also to increasing central obesity. Women with both upper-body fat predominance and severe obesity had a relative risk of diabetes 10.3 times as great as nonobese subjects with lower-body fat predominance (32).

Distribution of body fat has been measured anthropometrically by four methods: (1) the ratio of the waist circumference to the hip circumference (WHR):(2) the "centrality index," i.e., the adipose tissue of the trunk versus that of the limbs expressed as the subscapular versus the triceps skinfold ratio (SSF/TSF): (3) the waist versus the thigh circumference ratio; or (4) the waist circumference in absolute terms.

The first reports in large population samples prospectively linking fat distribution to diabetes came from Sweden. Ohlson et al. (33) reported that WHR was an independent risk factor for the development of diabetes in men followed for 13.5 years in Göteborg, Sweden, and Lundgren et al. (34) reported that diabetes mellitus and an increase in fasting blood glucose were independently predicted by the WHR measured 13 years prior in women from Götenborg.

In the United States, the influence of body fat distribution on the incidence and prevalence of type 2 DM was studied in Mexican-Americans. This population has the second highest incidence of diabetes in the United States after the Pima Indians. Mexican-Americans with type 2 DM were found to have a history of faster adult weight gain after the age of 18, to attain a higher weight at an earlier age, and to have more trunk fat as measured by subscapular skinfold (SSF) and less leg fat than nondiabetics (35). In the San Antonio Heart Study, the WHR was better associated with type 2 DM than was the SSF/TSF overall in the Mexican-American population; however, in women, both the WHR and the SSF/TSF were associated with increased prevalence of type 2 DM (36). Prospectively, in the San Antonio Heart Study, men and women with an upper-body fat distribution measured by the highest tertile of the ratio of the SSF/TSF were more likely to get diabetes (37,38) than the other subjects. The relationship of the centrality index to conversion to diabetes was probably mediated by the relationship with insulin resistance since, in multivariate analysis, it no longer remained associated once fasting insulin and glucose were taken into account.

Results of Caucasian population studies in the United States, such as the non-Hispanic white cohort of the San Antonio Heart Study, are also consistent with a relationship between the WHR and the incidence of type 2 DM (36). In another study, of a population of 41,837 women aged 55–69 years of age, followed over 2-year period in Iowa, body fat distribution determined by self-measurement of the WHR was significantly and independently predictive of type 2 DM development (39).

Although the effect that WHR has on the development of diabetes over and above the impact of BMI is undisputed, the magnitude of this effect is controversial, with some groups reporting only a marginal effect, confined to the top 10% of the WHR distribution

(15). This may be due to the complex relationship between WHR and the development of diabetes, with insulin resistance and abdominal fat amount and metabolism both playing an important role. Waist circumference may better reflect the overall degree of insulin resistance and abdominal adiposity than WHR. Waist circumference has been found to be a better marker of abdominal fat content than WHR (40,41), across gender and BMI range (42), and across ethnic groups (43). Whether WHR imparts any independent information about disease risk beyond waist circumference is uncertain, but between the two, the waist circumference appears to carry greater prognostic significance (44,45).

IV INSULIN RESISTANCE

The reason for the relationship of obesity to diabetes mellitus is not totally clear, but two facts are incontrovertible. The accretion of excess body fat is associated with increasing insulin resistance (46), and insulin resistance is a predisposing factor for diabetes (47).

The phenomenon of excessive blood insulin level in obesity, both basal and postprandially, is one evidence of the fact that an insulin resistance or insensitivity is present. Studies of intra-arterial insulin infusions in the forearm have revealed insulin resistance in both adipose tissue and muscle (48). Also, the insulin insensitivity of muscle in obesity extends to amino acid metabolism. The amino acids usually most sensitive to the action of insulin are elevated in the blood, despite the hyperinsulinism (49).

There is experimental evidence that the liver in obese subjects also manifests insulin resistance. Obese subjects, when compared to lean subjects, have a higher splanchnic uptake of glucose precursors, have a smaller inhibition in splanchnic glucose output with equivalent insulin increases, and, if glucose is infused at rates causing comparable inhibition in splanchnic glucose output, have a greater increase in insulin (50). This is manifest in the liver by increased hepatic glucose output and in the periphery by a decreased glucose uptake by peripheral tissues, primarily muscle and adipose tissue. This is caused by both receptor and postreceptor defects in insulin action. Whether an individual with insulin resistance develops impaired glucose tolerance or frank diabetes depends on the ability of the beta cells of the pancreas to compensate for the insulin resistance by secreting more insulin. That individual whose beta cells can keep up remains euglycemic though hyperinsulinemic, while that individual whose beta cells begin to exhaust develops hyperglycemia (51).

V INSULIN RECEPTORS

Insulin signaling at the cellular level is mediated by the binding of insulin to a specific receptor. Insulin binding stimulates autophosphorylation of the intracellular region of the receptor β-subunit (52). Studies have shown that obesity is a major contributory factor for the development of reduced insulin receptor activity (53,54). In obese persons, there is a decrease in the number of insulin receptors on the cell membranes of insulin-sensitive target cells, such as adipocytes (55). This downregulation of the number of insulin receptors is thought to occur as a result of the increased circulating insulin levels (55), although it might be a primary defect. It is likely that this occurs by increased receptor internalization (56). Insulin receptor binding is thus decreased.

VI POSTRECEPTOR EFFECTS

After insulin binds to its receptor, the autophosphorylation results in activation of the tyrosine kinase activity causing a conformational change that allows ATP and receptor substrates to reach the catalytic site (57,58). The activated insulin receptor kinase results in phosphorylated IRS proteins (insulin receptor substrate proteins) on tyrosine residues. These phosphorylated IRS proteins serve as docking sites for downstream effectors (postreceptor events). Such an effector is phosphatidyl inositol 3-kinase (PI 3-kinase). This mediates most metabolic responses to insulin, i.e., protein and glycogen synthesis, antilipolysis, and antiapoptosis, as well as glucose transport, which leads to the utilization of glucose, both oxidation and storage (58,59).

While the insulin receptor is downregulated in human obesity, there is no further decrease in its activity in liver and muscle of patients with type 2 diabetes, suggesting that the more severe insulin resistance in these patients, when present, is primarily of postreceptor nature (53,60). Insulin receptor phosphorylation, IRS-1 phosphorylation, and PI 3-kinase activity are decreased in intact skeletal muscle strips from obese subjects (61). Some investigators have shown that, overall, the muscle is as equally and severely resistant to the action of insulin in those obese patients without diabetes as in those with diabetes (60). Others have shown that the PI 3-kinase is more severely reduced in patients with type 2 diabetes (61). Furthermore, adipose tissue is more insulin resistant in type 2 DM than it is in obesity (60), primarily owing to decreased insulin receptor tyrosine kinase activity in the tissue of patients with type 2 diabetes (62). Present working hypotheses for obesity-linked kinase activity inhibition are elevation in tyrosine phosphatase activity or enhanced Ser/Thr phosphorylation of the receptor that impairs its tyrosine kinase activity (58,59).

Glucose transport in insulin-sensitive cells is greatly enhanced by insulin. This occurs by translocation of glucose transporters from the intracellular pool to the plasma membrane (63). A PI 3-kinase–dependent pathway facilitates the translocation of the insulin-dependent glucose transporter 4 (Glut 4) (59). In obesity and diabetes, glucose transporters in adipose tissue are decreased due to pretranslational suppression of Glut 4 transporter gene (64). However, in muscle tissue there is impaired Glut 4 function and/or translocation to the cell membrane surface and not transporter depletion (65).

Glucose disposal is impaired in obese persons (55, 66). Use of indirect calorimetry during insulin clamp studies has allowed measurement of glucose uptake in human subjects. The difference between glucose oxidation and glucose disposal, that is, the nonoxidative glucose disposal, is used to measure glucose storage as glycogen (66,67), since there is little net glucose conversion to lipid and little of the glucose that is taken up by muscle is released as lactate. Both glucose oxidation and glucose storage are impaired in obesity, and more so in diabetes. However, the major defect of glucose metabolism is in glucose storage, since oxidation is less impaired (68). This is shown in Figure 4 taken from one of our studies (69).

Defects in glycogen synthase activity (70,71), hexokinase II (72,73), and glucose transport (72,74,75) have all

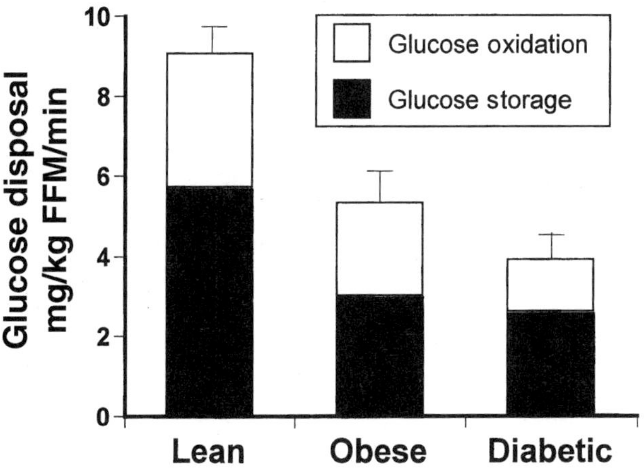

Figure 4 Total glucose disposal during euglycemic hyperinsulinemic clamp. Values are means ± SE partitioned into glucose oxidation (determined by indirect calorimetry) and nonoxidative glucose disposal (storage). $P < .001$ for glucose oxidation, glucose storage, and total glucose disposal: lean > obese > diabetic men. (From Ref. 69.)

been implicated in the loss of muscle glycogen synthesis in obesity and type 2 diabetes. Strong evidence pointing to glucose transport as the primary defect has been recently brought forth. In a series of elegant studies, Shulman et al. (76) showed that impaired glucose transport is the rate-controlling step for impaired insulin-stimulated muscle glycogen synthesis in patients with type DM and their lean nondiabetic offspring (77,78).

VII FREE FATTY ACIDS

As a rule, patients with obesity, and particularly as they develop diabetes, have elevated levels of free fatty acids (FFA) (47). The concept that elevated FFA play a key role in the development of insulin resistance in obesity and type 2 diabetes was first proposed by Randle (79). The theory stated that increased availability of FFA will increase fat oxidation, resulting in decreased glucose oxidation as well as impairment of glucose uptake. Recent studies by Boden et al. (80) and Shulman et al. (76) have clarified the sequence of these events, confirming nevertheless that elevated FFA play an important role in the impaired glucose utilization observed in obesity and type 2 diabetes.

Specifically, studies by Boden et al. suggest that chronic elevation of FFA will produce impaired glucose uptake by inhibition of glucose transport and phosphorylation, which will be followed by a decrease in the ability to store and oxidize glucose (81–83). Shulman et al. further demonstrated that the rate-controlling step for fatty acid–induced insulin resistance is glucose transport (84–86). They hypothesized that this could be a result of either a direct effect of increased intracellular FFA (or an FFA metabolite) on glucose transporters, or indirectly, from alterations in upstream signaling events such as reduced PI-3-kinase or other serine/kinase activities (87).

Other deleterious effects of high levels of FFA in obesity may be stimulation of the liver to increase gluconeogenesis, thereby enhancing hepatic glucose output (88,89). The net effect of these two phenomena is to increase circulating glucose levels and stress the beta-cell insulin secretory system (80).

VIII UPPER BODY FAT DISTRIBUTION AND VISCERAL ADIPOSITY

The large population studies on fat distribution described earlier raise the question of the mechanisms linking body fat distribution to type 2 diabetes. While a few of these mechanisms have been clarified, others are still unclear and are being studied.

Kissebah and associates published several papers relating WHR to a decreased insulin action at the muscle (90), liver (91), and adipose tissue level (92) in obese nondiabetic women. They also found an association between increased WHR and hyperinsulinemia, due to both increased insulin production and decreased hepatic insulin extraction (93). Evans et al. (90) showed that insulin binding in muscle and the sensitivity of the muscle to insulin action, as measured by the activity of glycogen synthase in muscle, decreased independently with obesity and with an increase in WHR. This can contribute to decreased glucose storage and, if plasma insulin secretory response cannot increase appropriately, development of diabetes.

Björntorp postulated that the unfavorable effects of upper body fat distribution, as measured by the WHR, are due to the accumulation of visceral adipose tissue (VAT), increased FFA flux to the liver, and subsequent hyperinsulinemia and insulin resistance in liver, muscle, and subcutaneous adipose tissue (94–96). VAT accumulation measured by CT scan as well as the visceral to the subcutaneous adipose tissue ratio (VAT/SAT) at the abdominal level were indeed found to be independently associated with glucose intolerance in males participating in the Normative Aging Study in the United States (97). VAT accumulation was found to be associated with glucose intolerance in premenopausal women (40) and in men in Canada (98) and with glucose intolerance in Japanese men and women (99). These associations were independent of the overall degree of obesity. In addition, in a cohort of Japanese-Americans, increased VAT was shown to predict the development of type 2 diabetes after 30 months of follow-up. This association was no longer significant after adjusting for the initial C-peptide level (hyperinsulinemia) (100).

The pathogenesis of the relationship of VAT with type 2 diabetes is not entirely clear. VAT has been associated with insulin resistance in women (43,101, 102) and men (103); however, this association is not always independent of the overall fat mass accumulation (43,104). On the other hand, the associations of VAT with hyperinsulinemia has been consistently independent of the degree of overall fatness (43,105).

Some researchers have postulated that the role of VAT in the associations between abdominal obesity and the insulin resistance syndrome is not as important as the role of the abdominal subcutaneous adipose tissue (SAT). Associations between the amount of abdominal subcutaneous fat (SAT) and insulin resistance have been recently reported (104,106,107), independent of the amount of VAT. Specifically, it appears that deep subcutaneous fat (107,108) and fat closer to muscle fascia as well as fat accumulated inside the myocytes may have an even closer association with insulin resistance (107,108). These findings are also consistent with results of in vivo lipolysis studies in women with upper-body and visceral obesity (109,110) which have shown that the source of excess FFA in abdominal obesity is the subcutaneous adipose tissue.

Work that we and others have published recently may bring some light to the controversial role of VAT vs. SAT in the development of insulin resistance and type 2 diabetes in obese individuals. Specifically, lipolysis in SAT was increased in women with visceral obesity independently of the overall degree of obesity, both during insulin suppression (110,111) and epinephrine stimulation (112,113). Thus we, and others (114), have postulated that the relationship between VAT and insulin resistance may be explained by their common correlate: the upper-body subcutaneous fat.

IX ROLE OF TUMOR NECROSIS FACTOR (TNF)-α AND OTHER CYTOKINES AND ADIPOSE TISSUE SECRETORY PRODUCTS IN THE PATHOGENESIS OF OBESITY-ASSOCIATED INSULIN RESISTANCE

Recently, TNFα has emerged as possibly playing a key role in the insulin resistance of obesity and type 2 DM (115,116). TNFα is a powerful inhibitor of insulin action in cultured cells, increasing the Ser phosphorylation of IRS-1 and IRS-2 and reducing the ability of these molecules to dock with the insulin receptor and interact with downstream pathways such as the PI 3-kinase (58,117,118). TNFα expression and secretion are elevated in adipose tissue of multiple experimental models of obesity and in abdominal fat and muscle tissue of obese individuals where they correlate with the degree of obesity, the levels of plasma insulin, and the degree of insulin insensitivity, and decrease with weight loss (116,119,120). Circulating levels of TNFα are increased in obesity and decrease with weight reduction (121). However, they do not correlate with the individual degree of insulin sensitivity (122). The current hypothesis is that TNFα acts in a paracrine fashion in adipose tissue and muscle (58,122) either directly on the insulin signaling cascade (123), or indirectly via stimulation of secretion of FFA or other cytokines such as leptin and/or interleukin (IL)-6 (122).

While the presence of a relationship between plasma leptin levels and/or leptin production in adipose tissue and insulin sensitivity is still controversial (59), Kern et al. have recently demonstrated that plasma IL-6 is related with the degree of insulin insensitivity to insulin action in vivo (122). They hypothesize that perhaps IL-6 represents a hormonal factor that induces muscle insulin resistance.

Other adipose secretory products identified recently and implicated in obesity-associated insulin resistance are adiponectin and resistin. Adiponectin is a novel adipose-specific protein with putative antiatherogenic and anti-inflammatory effects. Its plasma concentration was found to be decreased in individuals with obesity and type 2 DM, and was more closely associated with the degree of insulin resistance and hyperinsulinemia than with the degree of adiposity or glucose intolerance (124,125). Resistin is a newly described circulating hormone expressed primarily in adipocytes and shown to antagonize insulin action in mice (126). However, resistin gene expression in human adipocytes or muscle is very low or absent and, when present, does not appear to relate with the degree of insulin resistance (127,128).

X INSULIN SECRETION

It is generally believed that increased production of insulin by the beta cells of the pancreas is a response to the insulin resistance of obesity. In most studies, obese persons are found to be hyperinsulinemic (129,130). In general, the fatter an individual, the higher the basal or fasting insulin (131). This basal insulin is correlated to adiposity and the degree of overweight, and is related to the increasing insulin resistance that occurs with increasing adiposity (132). The degree of insulin response to glucose or other stimuli is related to basal insulin secretory levels and therefore can be correlated closely with the degree of obesity (133). This correlation between insulin response and obesity disappears if the response is expressed as a percentage of the basal value; i.e., the insulin response as a percentage of the basal value does not rise higher in the obese than in lean subjects.

In 1200 nondiabetic, normotensive European individuals the relationship between insulin resistance and insulin secretion was nonlinear (132); as insulin sensitivity declined, insulin secretion increased more than proportionally to compensate for the insulin resistance. Obesity shifted the curve upward. The relationship between insulin resistance or insulin secretion and BMI in this study was linear. The prevalence of insulin resistance and hypersecretion were quantitated in this study by defining resistance as the bottom 10% for insulin resistance and hypersecretion as the top 10% for insulin secretion. It became apparent that the prevalence of insulin hypersecretion was greater than the prevalence of insulin resistance in each category of BMI (Fig. 5) (132). In Pima Indians, there is an upper limit to this relation between adiposity and insulin secretory response. There is increasing insulin resistance as the percent of fat in the body increases up to about 35–40%; after that, insulin resistance does not increase further and insulin levels no longer rise (134).

The documented aberrations in insulin secretion in obese individuals, coupled with other hormonal abnormalities such as poor response to growth hormone and glucagon stimulation, made it unclear whether the hormonal defects seen in obesity were primary or a consequence of the obesity. The hormonal abnormalities are thought to be a consequence of the obesity since they revert to normal with effective weight loss and are found to appear after prolonged overfeeding of normal volunteers to an obese state (135). However, it is not known whether insulin hypersecretion is an earlier event at the very origin of weight gain, reflecting perhaps a central nervous system derangement. For example, hyperinsulinism may be a result, at least in part, of dietary factors rather than exclusively a consequence of insulin antagonism. Excess calories (136) and excess carbohydrate (137) may enhance insulin secretory response.

In those obese individuals who begin to develop abnormal glucose metabolism, the postprandial increase of insulin over basal values is actually decreased in comparison to normal subjects. This impairment is first observed as patients move from normal to impaired

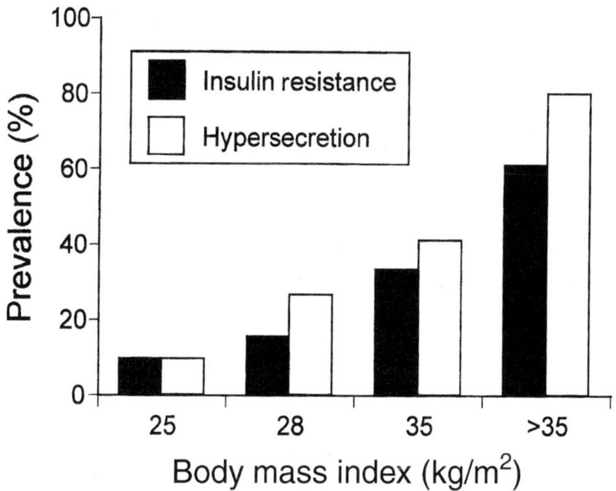

Figure 5 Prevalence of insulin resistance and insulin hypersecretion as a function of body mass index in nondiabetic, normotensive Caucasian subjects. (From Ref. 132.)

glucose tolerance to frank diabetes. Initially there is a reduction in overall insulin response (138). Subsequently, when fasting glucose begins to rise, the early phase of insulin response is lost (139), and as carbohydrate tolerance continues to deteriorate, all of the insulin response is further reduced. Most experimental data suggest that the first phase of insulin response is initially affected (140). However, there have been some studies suggesting an impairment of the second phase response, or of both (141). Even though an obese diabetic may be secreting a greater amount of insulin than a lean diabetic person, it will not be enough to maintain normal glucose tolerance, and the insulin response will be less than that of an obese person with equal adiposity who has normal glucose tolerance.

At some point, when certain individuals cannot keep up with the required increased insulin levels and become relatively hypoinsulinemic, hyperglycemia and frank diabetes supervene. The onset of hyperglycemia is not predictable in a particular individual, and seems to be determined by genetic predisposition. However, studies have suggested that the duration of obesity rather than the degree of obesity can best be correlated with carbohydrate intolerance in both obese adults and obese children (142). The genetic abnormality is likely to be an intrinsic defect in the beta cell (51,143). In fact, there is probably a heterogeneity of defects. For example, the abnormality in maturity-onset diabetes of the young is in the glucokinase gene, leading to impaired insulin release (144).

Weyer et al. (145) have recently reported on the importance of maintaining insulin secretory response in the development of type 2 DM in obese Pima Indians followed over a period of 4–7 years. All subjects followed who gained weight had a worsening of their systemic insulin-stimulated glucose disposal. However, those who also had a worsening of their insulin secretory response became glucose intolerant (IGT). Those who developed type 2 diabetes had a further increase in weight gain and worsening of both insulin-stimulated glucose disposal and an increase in the basal endogenous glucose production (145).

XI EFFECT OF EXERCISE

Obese individuals tend to lead a sedentary existence, and recent epidemiological evidence has reported that a sedentary lifestyle is a risk factor for the development of diabetes. The prevalence of both impaired glucose tolerance and type 2 DM is higher in inactive than active persons (146). In a prospective study of University of Pennsylvania male alumni, followed over 14 years, the age-adjusted incidence rates of diabetes decreased as the reported activity increased (147). This was also found in the Nurses' Health Study (148). Physical activity is inversely associated with obesity and central fat distribution, and physical training can reduce both of these conditions (149,150). In a prospective study of diabetes prevention in persons with impaired glucose tolerance, a 5-year program of diet and exercise showed that those individuals taking part in the diet-and-exercise program had less than half the progression rate to diabetes than the controls for whom no intervention was planned (151). The data are thus very suggestive of a relationship between activity and the prevention or delay of onset of type 2 DM. For this to be adequately confirmed, a randomized control trial would need to be done. So far, randomized interventional studies of lifestyle changes (both regarding diet and an increase in physical activity) in high-risk overweight patients have shown that weight reduction significantly reduces the incidence of type 2 diabetes (152,153).

The relationship between inactivity and risk for diabetes is likely to be at least partially attributed to decreased insulin sensitivity. Insulin sensitivity could be improved by exercise independently from weight reduction and changes in body composition. The muscle, liver, and fat contribute to the improvement of insulin sensitivity induced by physical exercise (154–156).

XII MACROVASCULAR DISEASE RISK

Once diabetes manifests itself, the nature of the disease can be similar to that in nonobese individuals, and all types of complications can ensue. Obesity, even independent of diabetes, is a risk factor for hypertension (157) and cardiovascular disease (158,159). When it is combined with diabetes, the risk of acquiring these illnesses is therefore greater, leading to a significantly increased morbidity and mortality (10).

The hyperinsulinemia, which occurs in obesity and in type 2 DM, is likely to abet the hypertension. Insulin has been found to be abnormally high in patients with essential hypertension, many of who manifest a degree of insulin resistance (160,161). Hypertension and glucose intolerance show a highly significant association from the mildest levels of both conditions (162). The hormone exerts a powerful effect on the kidney, increasing sodium reabsorption and thus expanding plasma volume (163).

The high levels of LDL cholesterol and triglycerides and the low levels of HDL cholesterol that are common in diabetic patients are likely to play a role in the pathogenesis of accelerated macrovascular disease (164). These abnormalities in circulating lipids are already present in obese individuals before the development of type 2 DM. In addition, as mentioned above, obese patients tend to run higher levels of FFA (47). This is particularly true of those obese individuals with central obesity (165). The enhanced FFA flux, along with the hyperinsulinemia and the ready availability of glycerol phosphate, greatly enhances the production of triglycerides in the liver. The triglycerides are packaged in the liver primarily as very low density lipoproteins (VLDL) and released into the circulation. Lipoprotein lipase released from endothelial cells in capillaries of the adipose depot helps to hydrolyze the VLDL, clear them from the circulation, and store them in the adipose tissue (166). In obesity and type 2 DM, lipoprotein lipase activity is impaired and the clearance of VLDL is delayed (167). Furthermore, in the normal process of HDL production, mature HDL is made from nascent HDL interaction with triglyceride-rich lipoprotein and lipoprotein lipase. This is defective in obese, insulin-resistant persons (168).

The final abnormality in lipids in this group of patients is the tendency to have an increased amount of small, dense LDL particles (169,170). The influence of modifiers such as hepatic lipase and cholesteryl ester transfer proteins on VLDL and HDL metabolism in patients with insulin resistance and central obesity leads to increased levels of circulating small, dense LDL cholesterol particles (171). These lipoprotein modifications are associated with atherosclerotic cardiovascular disease (ASCVD) (172). Recently it was proposed that, in the general population, this phenotype (low levels of HDL cholesterol and small dense LDL) may not be at increased risk for ASCVD unless associated with insulin resistance and an increased production of apolipoprotein B (172,173).

In type 2 diabetes, the LDL cholesterol may be oxidized and/or glycated, enhancing its atherogenicity (174). These glycated or oxidized particles are more atherogenic than larger particles and may be very important in the pathogenesis of the atherosclerosis that accompanies type 2 DM. Correction of the insulin resistance of obesity and type 2 DM with vigorous dietary and pharmacological means improves blood lipids and also hyperglycemia (175). Moreover, the current recommendations are that all patients with diabetes have reductions in LDL cholesterol to < 100 mg/dL.

Macrovascular disease is the leading cause of death in obese individuals with type 2 DM. The improvement of glucose control may, in itself, seem to have a small effect in improving the morbidity and mortality from coronary artery disease (CAD). The proof that more and/or near-optimal control of glycemia results in a reduction of macrovascular disease remains to be established (171).

It has been suggested by numerous investigators that the prevailing elevated insulin levels in these people may predispose them to CAD. A study comparing cardiovascular risk factor in normoinsulinemic and hyperinsulinemic individuals found that the hyperinsulinemic persons manifest higher triglycerides, lower HDL cholesterol, higher total cholesterols, and higher mean blood pressure (176). In addition, there have been three large epidemiological studies that have shown an association with either fasting or stimulated insulin and CAD (177–179). Monitoring risk factors in a longitudinal design, all three found an independent effect of insulin on coronary heart disease. Stout (180) has discussed the potential mechanism by which insulin may enhance the atherosclerotic process. These include increased growth factor activity leading to enhanced smooth muscle proliferation and connective tissue growth, formation of lipid plaques, and enhancing cholesterol uptake by plaque tissue. The current belief, however, is that this relationship is not cause and effect, but association (171).

Other factors that can enhance the progression of CAD in obese patients, which is abetted if they are diabetic also, are enhanced platelet aggregability, prolonged platelet survival time, and abnormal levels of plasminogen activator and plasminogen activator inhibitor 1 (181,182). These all enhance the risk of clotting in atherosclerotic blood vessels. Also, at present, much attention is being given to the relationship between endothelial dysfunction and macrovascular disease in patients with type 2 diabetes (171).

XIII MANAGEMENT OF THE OBESE DIABETIC PATIENT

As previously mentioned, obesity is present in the great majority of patients with type 2 DM. When present, obesity complicates the management of diabetes (183,184). Two issues arise in the management of the obese, insulin-resistant diabetic patient: first, glycemic control should be achieved but not at the expense of adipose tissue accumulation, especially in the visceral adipose depot with associated hyperinsulinemia and consequently, in the long run, more insulin resistance; and second, weight control must be achieved without losing sight of the need for tight glycemic control.

In the obese diabetic patient, as in any other diabetic patient, microvascular disease is primarily related to the presence of hyperglycemia (185). Uncontrolled glycemia is also responsible for an unfavorable lipoprotein pattern, an increase in glycosylation end products in all tissues, and an increased risk of thrombotic events (186). In the obese diabetic patients, tight glycemic control is thus warranted. The majority of the patients with type 2 DM are treated with oral hypoglycemic agents, which increase insulin sensitivity and enhance the beta-cell response to glucose (187). Exogenous insulin is usually necessary to control blood glucose in the obese diabetic patient when other therapeutic measures have failed to normalize blood glucose (187). Edelman et al. reviewed the use of insulin for the treatment of the type 2 diabetes (188). They concluded that obese diabetic patients could and should be evaluated for intensive insulin therapy. The candidates should be motivated and compliant and should be able to do home glucose monitoring and insulin administration. Combination therapy with insulin and oral agents can be a tool to normalize glycemia if oral agents fail. The adverse effects and potential risks of intensive insulin treatment include weight gain, which is directly associated with increased hyperinsulinemia (184,189–191). Hyperinsulinemia, as mentioned previously, has been associated with atherosclerotic risk factors, although a cause-and-effect relationship has not been proven (192). Weight control must therefore be an important part of diabetes management. It should be initiated early in the management of diabetes and it should continue throughout the duration of the treatment in the obese diabetic patient (193).

Caloric restriction and consequent weight loss in obese diabetic patients greatly improves their metabolic control because it results in improved insulin action in both liver and muscle, and frequently also results in improved beta-cell response to insulin secretory stimuli (193). In addition, weight control favorably changes cardiovascular disease risk factors such as hypertension and dyslipidemia (193). Weight control can and must be achieved through a medically supervised, moderately restricted-calorie diet and an exercise program with long-term maintenance goals (194). Recently, studies have shown that even moderate weight loss, when sustained, significantly improves the patient's metabolic profile and prolongs life expectancy (195–197). Patients with type 2 DM who underwent a 16-week lifestyle modification program and lost at least 5–10% of their initial body weight had significant improvement in HgbA1c that was still present at a 1-year follow-up. These patients also had significant reductions in their need for diabetic medications (198).

One has to be careful of the effectiveness of weight-reducing programs for obese patients with type 2 diabetes treated with large doses of insulin. In such instances, the danger of hypoglycemia must be recognized, and there is a need for close monitoring of blood glucose with frequent decreases in insulin as necessary. Some of the postulated reasons for weight gain with insulin therapy are decreased thermogenesis (199,200) and increased appetite (201); thus, it may be impossible to achieve weight loss with caloric restriction unless insulin (or oral agents that increase insulin levels) are being adequately adjusted to the lower-calorie diet prescribed.

Various classes of hypoglycemic agents, including metformin and acarbose, have been identified that, when used to normalize blood glucose, do not produce weight gain, hypoglycemia, or hyperinsulinemia (202–204). In the United Kingdom Prospective Diabetes Study (UKPDS), a randomized, controlled trial comparing sulfonylurea, insulin, and metformin therapy in patients with newly diagnosed type 2 DM that could not be controlled with diet therapy, intensive blood glucose control with insulin or sulfonylurea therapy significantly decreased progression of microvascular disease. Patients allocated to insulin gained more weight and had more hypoglycemic events than did patients allocated to sulfonylurea. Obese patients allocated to metformin gained least weight and had the fewest hypoglycemic attacks (203,204).

A new class of antidiabetic agents, the thiazolidinediones (glitazones), reduce hepatic output of glucose and increase peripheral uptake of glucose, thus enhancing insulin sensitivity and reducing the amount of exogenous insulin needed (205,206). In studies comparing insulin-glitazone treatment with insulin alone, the combination therapy resulted in better glycemic control but was associated with greater weight gain. The significance of weight gain from glitazones is difficult to assess. Despite the weight gain, the glitazones may be beneficial in that they redistribute fat from visceral to subcutaneous areas. In addition, some of the weight gain is due to peripheral edema and to an increase in extracellular fluid (207).

It is our opinion that hypoglycemic agents that are not likely to produce weight gain should be used in the obese diabetic patient whenever possible—that is, when endogenous insulin secretion is adequate. If insulin secretagogues or exogenous insulin need to be used, it would be very beneficial to combine them with an insulin-sensitizing agent like metformin to minimize weight gain and the amount of insulin needed to achieve glycemic control.

For those obese diabetic patients who require insulin, the novel recombinant insulin glargine may be preferable to NPH. It has been shown that long acting basal insulin glargine given once daily at bedtime is as effective in achieving glycemic control as NPH. The advantage of insulin glargine is that it produces less weight gain (208). The lesser weight gain seen with insulin glargine is attributed to the less frequent hypoglycemia, and thus the decreased need to increase caloric supplementation (209). Use of insulin glargine compared with NPH is also associated with lower postdinner glucose levels.

Most obese patients are unable to maintain a modest long-term reduction in their weight. Obese patients with type 2 diabetes are even more resistant to weight loss because antidiabetic drugs such as insulin and sulfonylureas often promote weight gain. These patients would likely benefit from the addition of weight management drugs as adjunctive therapy to the traditional interventions of low-calorie diet, physical activity, and behavior management (210). Two drugs in particular have been recently developed—sibutramine and orlistat. Sibutramine is a selective serotonin and noradrenaline reuptake inhibitor. Blocking of serotonin reuptake produces the satiety enhancing effect of the drug. Inhibition of noradrenaline uptake increases thermogenesis via β-3-adrenoreceptors. This results in increased energy expenditure (211,212). Orlistat, a specific inhibitor of gastrointestinal lipases, decreases the absorption of dietary triglycerides from the GI tract in a dose-dependent manner. At the maximum effective dose of 120 mg TID, orlistat reduces the absorption of dietary fat by 30% (213).

Clinical trials have shown that the use of either agent as part of an integrated program of diet, exercise, and behavior management can help nearly one-third of patients with type 2 diabetes achieve a weight loss of up to 10% of initial body weight after 1 year. As a result of the weight loss, these patients also exhibited decreased HgbA1c, decreased blood pressure, and improved lipid profiles (210–212,214). Furthermore, studies on patients with impaired glucose tolerance have shown that orlistat improves glucose tolerance and decreases the risk of progression to type 2 diabetes (215).

Other agents presently studied for weight loss may prove to be beneficial in type 2 DM. β-3-Adrenoreceptor agonists were first tried in weight reduction more than a decade ago. Animal studies had shown that selective β-3-agonists can induce weight loss and produce a weight-independent improvement in insulin resistance and glucose intolerance. Currently new β-3-agonists are being developed that have a higher selectivity for humans (210). Leptin, an adipocyte-derived hormone that is released into the bloodstream and acts as a satiety signal in the brain, has been shown to produce weight loss. In the first clinical study in humans, subcutaneous administration of a biosynthetic leptin was shown to reduce body fat and thus decrease weight in a dose-dependent manner (210). Thus, leptin is another potential weight-reducing agent for obese diabetic patients. Further studies on the safety and efficacy of leptin are needed before it can become an acceptable treatment for weight reduction (210).

Glucagonlike peptide (GLP-1), an insulinotropic gut hormone released into the bloodstream after eating, is being investigated as a promising new treatment for the obese patient with type 2 diabetes. Abnormalities in GLP-1 function are thought to contribute to the inappropriate insulin secretion seen in type 2 diabetes. This is supported by the fact that patients with type 2 diabetes have a reduced late intact GLP-1 response (216, 217). In patients with type 2 diabetes, administration of exogenous GLP-1 enhances the glucose responsiveness of pancreatic β-cells, resulting in increased insulin secretion and decreased plasma glucose (218,219). The stimulation of insulin secretion by GLP-1 is glucose dependent. Therefore, the risk of hypoglycemia with GLP-1 is low. GLP-1 has also been shown to improve glycemic control by decreasing the desire for food, delaying gastric emptying, reducing glucagon levels, and enhancing insulin sensitivity (220–222). GLP-1 also acts on the central nervous system to produce a satiating effect. Intracerebral injection of GLP-1 in normal and obese rats significantly reduces food intake and body weight (223). In patients with type 2 diabetes, GLP-1 infusion significantly enhances satiety and fullness, and reduces energy intake by 27% (224). In addition, stimulation of GLP-1 receptors in certain areas of the brain elicit strong taste aversions (225).

In a randomized, double-blind, placebo-controlled trial, 40 patients with type 2 diabetes were randomized to receive infusions of either placebo or GLP-1 at a rate of 4 ng/kg/min or 8 ng/kg/min for either 16 hr/d or 24 hr/d for a total of 7 days (226). All patients who received GLP-1 had significantly better average glucose and glucagons levels than the placebo group. The GLP-1 infusion at 8 ng/kg/min for 24 hr/d was the most efficacious dose. Those who received GLP-1 for only 16 hr/d had significantly higher nocturnal and fasting plasma glucose levels compared to those who were continuously infused for 24 hr every day. GLP-1 was well tolerated in these patients. GLP-1 and exendin-4, a more potent and longer-acting analog of GLP-1 that originates in the saliva of the Gila monster, has been shown to induce satiety and weight loss in rats (227). These agents are being investigated as potential treatments for diabetes and obesity.

Obesity surgery has become a successful method of treating obesity, especially in the diabetic patient. Studies done in the United States and in Sweden have shown that most patients with type 2 diabetes who undergo bariatric gastric surgery develop normal glucose tolerance with n 5–6 years of the surgery. This was attributed to the substantial amount of weight lost after the surgery (195,228). In one study, laparoscopic adjustable gastric banding was compared to nonsurgical treatment for obesity in patients with BMI > 35. Only the surgical patients had decreased BMI and HgbA1c. These patients also had more loss of visceral than subcutaneous adipose tissue (229).

In conclusion, the goal of the treatment for the obese diabetic patient is to achieve glycemic control, minimize weight gain, and minimize the amount of insulin required to achieve glycemic control. These goals can be achieved through effective lifestyle changes, use of antiobesity drugs such as orlistat and sibutramine, and, in particularly resistant cases of obesity, bariatric gastric surgery.

REFERENCES

1. Diabetes in America, 2d ed. Washington: National Institutes of Health; National Institute of Diabetes and Digestive Kidney Diseases, 1995. NIH Publication No. 95–1468.
2. John HJ. Summary of findings in 1100 glucose tolerance estimations. Endocrinology 1929; 13:388–392.
3. Newburgh LH. Control of hyperglycemia of obese "diabetics" by weight reduction. Ann Intern Med 1942; 17:935–942.
4. West KM, Kalbfleisch JM. Glucose tolerance, nutrition and diabetes in Uruguay, Venezuela, Malaya, and East Pakistan. Diabetes 1966; 15:9–18.
5. West KM, Kalbfleish JM. Influence of nutritional factors on prevalence of diabetes. Diabetes 1971; 20:99–108.
6. Fowler G, Butterfield WJ, Acheson RM. Physique, glycosuria and blood glucose levels in Bedford. Guy's Hosp Rep 1970; 119(4):297–314.
7. Baird JD. Diabetes mellitus and obesity. Proc Nutr Soc 1973; 32(3):199–203.
8. Knowler WC, Pettit PJ, Savage PJ, Bennett PH. Diabetes incidence in Pima Indians: contributions of obesity and parental diabetes. Am J Epidemiol 1981; 113: 144–156.
9. Must A, Spadano J, Coakley EH, Field AE, Colditz G, Dietz WH. The disease burden associated with overweight and obesity. JAMA 1999; 282:1523–1529.
10. Lew EA, Garfinkel L. Variations in mortality by weight among 750,000 men and women. J Chron Dis 1979; 32:563–576.
11. Westlund K, Nicolaysen R. Ten-year mortality and morbidity related to serum cholesterol. Scand J Clin Lab Invest 1972; 30(127):1–24.
12. Larsson B, Björntorp P, Tibblin G. The health consequences of moderate obesity. Int J Ob 1981; 5:97–116.
13. Medalie JH, Herman JB, Goldbourt U, et al. Variations in the incidence of diabetes among 10,000 adult Israeli males and factors related to their development. In: Levine R, Luft R, eds. Advances in Metabolic Disorders , New York: Academic Press, 1978:Vol 9:78.
14. Colditz GA, Willet WC, Stampfer MJ, Manson JE, Hennekens CH, Arky RA, Speizer FE. Weight as a risk factor for clinical diabetes in women. Am J Epidemiol 1990; 132:501–513.
15. Colditz GA, Willet WC, Rotnitzky A, Manson JE. Weight gain as a risk factor for clinical diabetes mellitus in women. Ann Intern Med 1995; 122:481–486.
16. Holbrook TL, Barrett-Connor E, Wingard DL. The association of lifetime weight and weight control patterns with diabetes among men and women in an adult community. Int J Obes 1989; 13:723–729.
17. Ford ES, Williamson DF, Liu S. Weight change and diabetes incidence: findings from a national cohort of US adults. Am J Epidemiol 1997; 146:214–222.
18. Wannamethee SG, Shaper AG. Weight change and duration of overweight and obesity in the incidence of type 2 diabetes. Diabetes Care 1999; 22:1266–1272.
19. Hu FB, Manson JE, Stampfer MJ, Colditz G, Liu S, Solomon CG, Willet WC. Diet, lifestyle, and the risk of type 2 diabetes mellitus in women. N Engl J Med 2001; 345:790–797.
20. De Courten M, Bennett PH, Tuomilehto J, Zimmet P. In: Alberti KGMM, Zimmet P, DeFronzo RA, Keen H, eds. International Textbook of Diabetes Mellitus, 2d ed. Chichester: Wiley, 1997:143–170.
21. Ramachandran A, Snehalatha C, Latha E, Vijay V, Viswanathan M. Rising prevalence of NIDDM in an urban population in India. Diabetologia 1997; 40:232–237.
22. O'Dea K. Westernisation, insulin resistance and diabetes in Australian Aborigines. Med J Aust 1991; 155: 258–264.
23. Zimmet P, Alberti KGMM, Shaw J. Global and societal implications of the diabetes epidemic. Nature 2001; 414:782–787.
24. Zimmet P, Dowse G, Finch C, Serjeantson S, King H. The epidemiology and natural history of NIDDM—lessons from the South Pacific. Diabetes/Metabol Rev 1990; 6:91–124.
25. Zimmet P. Diabetes epidemiology as a trigger to diabetes research. Diabetologia 1999; 42:499–518.
26. Tan C, Emmanuel S, Tan B-Y, Jacob E. Prevalence of

diabetes and ethnic differences in cardiovascular risk factors. Diabetes Care 1999; 22:241–247.
27. Chou P, Chen H, Hsiao K. Community-based epidemiological study on diabetes in Pu-Li, Taiwan. Diabetes Care 1992; 15:81–89.
28. Amos A, McCarty D, Zimmet P. The rising global burden of diabetes and its complications: estimates and projections to the year 2010. Diabetic Med 1997; 14:S1–S85.
29. Zimmet P. Kelly West Lecture 1991. Challenges in diabetes epidemiology—from West to the rest. Diabetes Care 1992; 15:232–252.
30. Vague J. Les obésités: études biométriques. Presse Med 1947; 30:339.
31. Feldman R, Sender AJ, Siegelaub AB. Difference in diabetic and non-diabetic fat distribution patterns by skinfold measurements. Diabetes 1969; 18:478–486.
32. Hartz AJ, Rupley DC Jr, Kalkhoff RD, Rimm AA. Relationship of obesity to diabetes: influence of obesity level and body fat distribution. Prev Med 1983; 12:351–357.
33. Ohlson LO, Larsson B, Svardsudd K, et al. The influence of body fat distribution on the incidence of diabetes mellitus. Diabetes 1985; 34:1055–1058.
34. Lundgren H, Bengtsson C, Biohme G, Lapidus L, Sjöström L. Adiposity and adipose tissue distribution in relation to incidence of diabetes in women: results from a prospective population study in Gothenburg, Sweden. Int J Obes 1989; 13:413–423.
35. Joos SK, Mueller WH. Diabetes alert study: weight history and upper body obesity in diabetic and non-diabetic Mexican American adults. Ann Hum Biol 1984; 2(11):167–171.
36. Haffner SM, Stern MP, Hazuda HP, Pugh J, Patterson JK. Do upper-body and centralized adiposity measure different aspects of regional body-fat distribution? Diabetes 1987; 36:43–51.
37. Haffner SM, Stern MP, Braxton DM, Hazuda HP, Patterson JK. Incidence of type II diabetes in Mexican Americans predicted by fasting insulin and glucose levels, obesity, and body-fat distribution. Diabetes 1990; 39:283–288.
38. Haffner SM, Braxton MD, Hazuda HP, Stern MP. Greater influence of central distribution of adipose tissue in women than men. Am J Clin Nutr 1991; 53:1312–1317.
39. Kaye SA, Folsom AR, Sprafka JM, Prineas RJ, Wallace RB. Increased incidence of diabetes mellitus in relation to abdominal adiposity in older women. J Clin Epidemol 1991; 44:329–334.
40. Després JP, Nadeau A, Tremblay A, Ferland M, Moorjani S, Lupien PJ, Theriault G, Pinault S, Bouchard C. Role of deep abdominal fat in the association between regional adipose tissue distribution and glucose tolerance in obese women. Diabetes 1988; 38:304–309.
41. Lean ME, Han TS, Morrison CE. Waist circumference as a measure for indicating need for weight management. BMJ 1995; 311:158–161.
42. Lemieux S, Prud'homme D, Bouchard C, Tremblay A, Després J. A single threshold value of waist girth identifies normal-weight and overweight subjects with excess visceral adipose tissue. Am J Clin Nutr 1996; 64:685–693.
43. Albu JB, Murphy I, Frager DH, Johnson JA, Pi-Sunyer FX. Visceral fat and race-dependent health risks in obese non-diabetic premenopausal women. Diabetes 1997; 46:456–462.
44. Chan JM, Rimm EB, Colditz GA, Stampfer MJ, Willet WC. Obesity, fat distribution, and weight gain as risk factors for clinical diabetes in men. Diabetes Care 1992; 41:235–240.
45. Fujimoto WY, Newell-Morris LL, Grote M, Borgstrom RW, Shuman WP. Visceral fat obesity and morbidity. Int J Obes 1991; 15(suppl 2):41–44.
46. Olefsky JM. Insulin resistance and insulin action: an in vitro and in vivo perspective. Diabetes 1981; 30:148–162.
47. Reaven GM. Role of insulin resistance in human disease. Diabetes 1988; 37:1595–1607.
48. Rabinowitz D, Zierler KL. Forearm metabolism in obesity and its response to intra-arterial insulin. Characterization of insulin resistance and evidence for adaptive hyperinsulinism. J Clin Invest 1962; 41:2173–2181.
49. Felig P, Marliss E, Cahill GF Jr. Plasma amino acid levels and insulin secretion in obesity. N Engl J Med 1969; 281:811–816.
50. Felig P, Wahren J, Hendler R, Brundin J. Splanchnic glucose and amino acid metabolism in obesity. J Clin Invest 1974; 53:582–590.
51. DeFronzo RA. The triumvirate; B cell, muscle, liver: a collusion responsible for NIDDM. Diabetes 1988; 37:644–667.
52. Kasuga M, Karisson FA, Kahn CR. Insulin stimulates the phosphorylation of the 95,000-dalton subunit of its own receptor. Science 1982; 215:185–187.
53. Caro JF, Sinha MK, Raju SM, Ittoop O, Pories WJ, Flickinger EG, Meelheim D, Dohm GL. IR kinase in human skeletal muscle from obese subjects with and without non-insulin-dependent diabetes. J Clin Invest 1987; 79:1330–1337.
54. Freidenberg GR, Reichart D, Olefsky JM, Henry RR. Reversibility of defective adipocyte insulin receptor kinase activity in non-insulin-dependent diabetes mellitus. Effect of weight loss. J Clin Invest 1988; 82:398–1406.
55. Kolterman OG, Insel J, Saekow M, Olefsky JM. Mechanisms of insulin resistance in human obesity: evidence for receptor and postreceptor defects. J Clin Invest 1980; 65:1272–1284.
56. Marshall S, Olefsky JM. Characterization of insulin-

induced receptor loss and evidence of internalization of the insulin receptor. Diabetes 1981; 30:746–753.

57. Saltiel AR. Second messengers of insulin action. Diabetes Care 1990; 13:244–253.
58. Roith DL, Zick Y. Recent advances in our understanding of insulin action and insulin resistance. Diabetes Care 2001; 24:588–593.
59. Matthaei S, Stumvoll M, Kellerer, Haring HU. Pathology and pharmacological treatment of insulin resistance. Endocr Rev 2000; 21:585–618.
60. Caro JF, Dohm LG, Pories WJ, Sinha MK. Cellular alteration in liver, skeletal muscle, and adipose tissue responsible for insulin resistance in obesity and type II diabetes. Diabetes/Metab Rev 1989; 5:665–689.
61. Goodyear LJ, Giorgino F, Sherman LA, Carey J, Smith RJ, Dohm GL. Insulin receptor phosphorylation, insulin receptor substrate - 1 phosphorylation, and phosphatidylinositol 3-kinase activity are decreased in intact skeletal muscle strips from obese subjects. J Clin Invest 1995; 95:2195–2204.
62. Thies RS, Molina JM, Ciaraldi TP, Freidenberg GR, Olefsky JM. Insulin-receptor autophosphorylation and endogenous substrate phosphorylation in human adipocytes from control, obese, and NIDDM subjects. Diabetes 1990; 39:250–259.
63. Garvey WT, Huecksteadt TP, Bimbaum MJ. Pretranslational supression of an insulin-responsive glucose transporter in rats with diabetes mellitus. Science 1989; 245:60–68.
64. Garvey WT, Maianu L, Huecksteadt TP, Birnbaum M, Molina JM, Ciaraldi TP. Pretranslational suppression of a glucose transporter protein causes insulin resistance in adipocytes from patients with non-insulin-dependent diabetes mellitus and obesity. J Clin Invest 1991; 87:1072–1081.
65. Garvey WT, Maianu L, Hancock JA, Golichowski AM, Baron A. Gene Expression of GLUT 4 in skeletal muscle from insulin-resistant patients with obesity, IGT, GDM, and NIDDM. Diabetes 1992; 41:465–475.
66. DeFronzo RA, Jacot E, Jequier E, Maeder E, Wahren J, Felber JP. The effect of insulin on the disposal of intravenous glucose. Diabetes 1981; 30:1000–1007.
67. Bogardus C, Thuillez P, Ravussin E, Vasquez B, Narimiga M, Azhar S. Effect of muscle glycogen depletion on in vivo insulin action in man. J Clin Invest 1983; 72:1605–1610.
68. Bogardus C, Lillioja S, Howard BV, Reaven G, Mott D. Relationships between insulin secretion, insulin action, and fasting glucose concentration in non-diabetic and non-insulin-dependent subjects. J Clin Invest 1984; 74:1238–1246.
69. Segal KR, Edano A, Abalos A, Albu A, Blando L, Tomas MB, Pi-Sunyer FX. Effect of exercise training on insulin sensitivity and glucose metabolism in lean, obese, and diabetic men. J Appl Physiol 1991; 71:2402–2411.
70. Bogardus C, Lillioja S, Stone K, et al. Correlation between muscle glycogen depletion and glycogen synthase activation on in vivo insulin action in man. J Clin Invest 1984; 73:1185–1190.
71. Eriksson J, Frassila-Kallunki A, Ekstrand A, Saloranta C, Widen E, Schalin C, Groop L. Early metabolic defects in persons at increased risk for non-insulin-dependent diabetes mellitus. N Engl J Med 1989; 321: 337–343.
72. Rothman DL, Shulman RG, Shulman GI. ^{31}P nuclear magnetic resonance measurements of muscle glucose-6-phosphate. Evidence for reduced insulin-dependent muscle glucose transport or phosphorylation activity in non-insulin-dependent diabetes mellitus. J Clin Invest 1992; 89:1069–1075.
73. Kelley DE, Mintun MA, Watkins SC, Simoneau JA, Jadali F, Fredrickson A, Beattie J, Theriault R. The effect of non-insulin-dependent diabetes mellitus and obesity on glucose transport and phosphorylation in skeletal muscle. J Clin Invest 1996; 97:2705–2713.
74. Bonadonna RC, Del Prato S, Bonora E, Saccomani MP, Giovanni G, Natali, Frascerra S, Pecori N, Ferrannini E, Bier D, Cobelli C, DeFronzo R. Roles of glucose transport and glucose phosphorylation in muscle insulin resistance of NIDDM. Diabetes 1996; 45:915–925.
75. Zierath JR et al. Insulin action on glucose transport and plasma membrane GLUT4 content in skeletal muscle from patients with NIDDM. Diabetologia 1996; 39:1180–1189.
76. Shulman GI. Cellular mechanism of insulin resistance. J Clin Invest 2000; 106:171–176.
77. Rothman DL, et al. Decreased muscle glucose transport/phosphorylation is an early defect in the pathogenesis on non-insulin-dependent diabetes mellitus. Proc Natl Acd Sci USA 1995; 92:983–987.
78. Cline GW, Petersen KF, Krssak M, Shen J, Hundal RS, Trajanoski Z, Inzucchi S, Dresnder A, Rothman DL, Shulman GI. Impaired glucose transport as a cause of decreased insulin-stimulated muscle glycogen synthesis in type 2 diabetes. N Engl J Med 1999; 341: 240–246.
79. Randle PJ, Garland PB, Hales CN, Newsholme EA. The glucose fatty-acid cycle. Its role in insulin sensitivity and the metabolic disturbances of diabetes mellitus. Lancet 1963; 1:785–789.
80. Boden G. Role of fatty acids in the pathogenesis of insulin resistance and NIDDM. Diabetes 1997; 46:3–10.
81. Boden G, Chen X, Ruiz J, White JV, Rosetti L. Mechanism of fatty acid induced inhibition of glucose uptake. J Clin Invest 1994; 93:2438–2446.
82. Boden G, Chen X. Effects of fat on glucose uptake and utilization in patients with non-insulin-dependent diabetes. J Clin Invest 1995; 96:1261–1268.
83. Boden G, Chen X, Rosner J, Barton M. Effects of a

48-h fat infusion on insulin secretion and glucose utilization. Diabetes 1995; 44:1239–1242.
84. Roden M, Price TB, Perseghin G, Petersen KF, Rothman DL, Cline GW, Shulman GI. Mechanism of fatty acid-induced insulin resistance in humans. J Clin Invest 1996; 97:2859–2865.
85. Dresner A, Laurent D, Marucci M, Griffin ME, Dufour S, Cline GW, Slezak LA, Andersen DK, Hundal RS, Rothman DL, Petersen KF, Shulman GI. Effects of free fatty acids on glucose transport and IRS-1 associated phosphatidylinositol 3-kinase activity. J Clin Invest 1999; 103:253–259.
86. Petersen KF, et al. $^{13}C/^{31}$ NMR studies on the mechanism of insulin resistance in obesity. Diabetes 1998; 47:381–386.
87. Griffin ME, Marcucci MJ, Cline GW, Bell K, Barucci N, Lee D, Goodyear L, Kraegen EW, White MF, Shulman GI. Free fatty acid–induced insulin resistance is associated with activation of protein kinase C θ and alterations in the insulin signaling cascade. Diabetes 1999; 48:1270–1274.
88. Ferrannini E, Barrett EJ, Bevilacqua S, De Fronzo RA. Effect of fatty acids on glucose production and utilization in man. J Clin Invest 1983; 72:1737 1747.
89. Rebrin K, Steil GM, Getty L, Bergman RN. Free fatty acid as a link in the regulation of hepatic glucose output by peripheral insulin. Diabetes 1995; 44:1038–1045.
90. Evans DJ, Hoffmann RG, Kalkhoff RN, Kissebah AH. Relationship of body fat topography to insulin sensitivity and metabolic profiles in premenopausal women. Metabolism 1984; 3:68–75.
91. Peiris AN, Struve MF, Mueller RA, Lee MB, Kissebah AH. Glucose metabolism in obesity: influence of body fat distribution. J Clin Endocrinol Metab 1988; 67:760–767.
92. Kissebah AH, Vydelingum N, Murray R, Evans DJ, Hartz AJ, Kalkhoff RK, Adams PW. Relation of body fat distribution to metabolic complications of obesity. J Clin Endocrinol Metab 1982; 54:254–260.
93. Peiris AN, Mueller RA, Smith GA, Struve MF, Kissebah AH. Splanchnic insulin metabolism in obesity. Influence of body fat. J Clin Invest 1986; 78:1648–1657.
94. Björntorp P. Visceral obesity: a "civilization syndrome". Obes Res 1993; 1:206–222.
95. Vague J, Björntorp P, Guy-Grand B, et al. Metabolic Complications of Human Obesities. Amsterdam: Elsevier, 1985.
96. Björntorp P, Smith U, Lönnroth P. Health Implications of Regional Obesity. Stockholm: Almqvist & Wiksell, 1988.
97. Sparrow D, Borkan GA, Gerzof SG, Wisniewski C, Silbert CK. Relationship of fat distribution to glucose tolerance. Diabetes 1986; 35:411–415.
98. Pouliot MC, Després JP, Ndeau A, Moorjani S, Prud'homme D, Lupien PJ, Tremblay A, Bouchard C. Visceral obesity in men. Diabetes 1992; 41:826–834.
99. Fujioka S, Matsuzawa Y, Tokunaga K, Tarui S. Contribution of intra-abdominal fat accumulation to the impairment of glucose and lipid metabolism in human obesity. Metabolism 1987; 36:54–59.
100. Bergstrom RW, Newell-Morris LL, Leonetti DL, Shuman WP, Wahl PW, Fujimoto WY. Association of elevated fasting c-peptide level and increased intra-abdominal fat distribution with development of NIDDM in Japanese-American men. Diabetes 1990; 39:104–111.
101. Bonora E, Del Prato S, Bonadonna RC, Gulli G, Solini A, Shank ML, Ghiatas AA, Lancaster JL, Kilcoyne RF, Alyassin AM, De Fronzo RA. Total body fat content and fat topography are associated differently with in vivo glucose metabolism in nonobese and obese nondiabetic women. Diabetes 1992; 41:1151–1159.
102. Carey DG, Jenkins AB, Campbell LV, Freund J, Chisholm DJ. Abdominal fat and insulin in normal and overweight women. Diabetes 1996; 45:633–638.
103. Banerji MA, Chaiken RL, Gordon D, et al. Does intra-abdominal adipose tissue in black men determine whether NIDDM is insulin-resistant or insulin-sensitive? Diabetes 1995; 44:141–146.
104. Marcus MA, Murphy L, Pi-Sunyer FX, et al. Insulin sensitivity and serum triglyceride level in obese white and black women: relationship to visceral and truncal subcutaneous fat. Metabolism 1999; 48:194–199.
105. Ross R, Fortier L, Hudson R. Separate associations between visceral and subcutaneous adipose tissue distribution, insulin and glucose levels in obese women. Diabetes Care 1996; 19:1404–1411.
106. Abate N, Garg A, Peshock RM, Stray-Gundersen J, Grundy SM. Relationships of generalized and regional adiposity to insulin sensitivity in men. J Clin Invest 1995; 96:88–89.
107. Goodpaster BH, Thaete FL, Simoneau J-A, Kelley DE. Subcutaneous abdominal fat and thigh muscle composition predict insulin sensitivity independently of visceral fat. Diabetes 1997; 46:1579–1585.
108. Kelley DE, Thaete FL, Troost F, Huwe T, Goodpaster BH. Subdivisions of subcutaneous abdominal adipose tissue and insulin resistance. Am J Physiol 2000; 278:E941–E948.
109. Guo Z, Hensrud DD, Johnson CM, Jensen MD. Regional postprandial fatty acid metabolism in different obesity phenotypes. Diabetes 1999; 48:1586–1592.
110. Albu JB, Shur M, Curi M, Murphy L, Matthews DE, Pi-Sunyer FX. Systemic resistance to the antilipolytic effect of insulin in black and white women with visceral obesity. Am J Physiol 1999; 277:E551–E560.
111. Johnson JA, Fried SK, Pi-Sunyer FX, Albu JB. Impaired insulin action in subcutaneous adipocytes from women with visceral obesity. Am J Physiol 2001; 280: E259–E264.

112. Nicklas BJ, Rogus EM, Colman EG, Goldberg AP. Visceral adiposity, increased adipocyte lipolysis, and metabolic dysfunction in obese postmenopausal women. Am J Physiol 1996; 270:E72–E78.
113. Albu JB, Johnson JA, Fried SK, Kovera AJ, Pi-Sunyer FX. Visceral adiposity and regional variation in lipolysis in obese nondiabetic women. Diabetes 2001; 50(suppl 2):A88.
114. Frayn KN. Visceral fat and insulin resistance—causative or correlative? Br J Nutr 2000; 83:S71–S77.
115. Hotamisligil GS, Spiegelman BM. Tumor necrosis factor-α: a key component of the obesity-diabetes link. Diabetes 1994; 43:1271–1278.
116. Hotamisligil GS, Arner P, Caro JF, Atkinson RL, Spiegelman BM. Increased adipose tissue expression of tumor necrosis factor-α in human obesity and insulin resistance. J Clin Invest 1995; 95:2409–2415.
117. Hofmann C, Lorenz K, Braithwaite SS, Colca JR. Altered gene expression for tumor necrosis factor-α and its receptors during drug and dietary modulation of insulin resistance. Endocrinology 1994; 134:264–270.
118. Peraldi P, Spiegelman B. TNF-α and insulin resistance: summary and future prospects. Mol Cell Biochem 1998; 182:169–175.
119. Saghizadeh M, Ong JM, Garvey WT, Henry RR, Kern PA. The expression of TNF-α by human muscle: relationship to insulin resistance. J Clin Invest 1996; 97:1111–1116.
120. Kern PA, Saghizadeh M, Ong JM, Bosch RJ, Deem R, Simsolo RB. The expression of tumor necrosis factor in human adipose tissue. Regulation by obesity, weight loss, and relationship to lipoprotein lipase. J Clin Invest 1995; 95:2111–2119.
121. Dandona P, Weinstock R, Thusu K, Abdel-Rahman E, Aljada A, Wadden T. Tumor necrosis factor-alpha in sera of obese patients: fall with weight loss. J Clin Endocrinol Metab 1998; 83:2907–2910.
122. Kern PA, Ranganathan S, Li C, Wood L, Rnaganathan G. Adipose tissue tumor necrosis factor and interleukin-6 expression in human obesity and insulin resistance. Am J Physiol 2001; 280:E745–E751.
123. Hotamisligil GS, Budavari A, Murray DL, Spiegelman BM. TNF-α inhibits signaling from insullin receptor. Proc Natl Acad Sci USA 1994; 91:4854–4858.
124. Weyer C, Funahashi T, Tanaka S, Hotta K, Matsuzawa Y, Pratley RE, Tataranni PA. Hypoadiponectinemia in obesity and type 2 diabetes: close association with insulin resistance and hyperinsulinemia. J Clin Endocrinol Metab 2001; 86:1930–1935.
125. Hotta K, Funahashi T, Bodkin NL, Ortmeyer HK, Arita Y, Hansen BC, Matsuzawa Y. Circulating concentrations of the adipocyte protein adiponectin are decreased in parallel with reduced insulin sensitivity during the progression to type 2 diabetes in rhesus monkeys. Diabetes 2001; 50:1126–1133.
126. Steppan CM, Bailey ST, Bhat S, Brown EJ, Banerjee RR, Wright CM, Patel HR, Ahima RS, Lazar MA. The hormone resistin links obesity to diabetes. Nature 2001; 409:292–293.
127. Nagaev I, Smith U. Insulin Resistance and type 2 diabetes are not related to resistin expression in human fat cells or skeletal muscle. Biochem Biophys Res Commun 2001; 285:561–564.
128. Janke J, Engeli S, Gorzelniak K, Sharma AM. Resistin gene expression in human adipocytes is not related to insulin resistance. Obes Res 2002; 10:1–5.
129. Karam JH, Grodsky GM, Forsham PH. Excessive insulin response to glucose in obese subjects as measured by immunochemical assay. Diabetes 1963; 12: 197–204.
130. Kreisberg RA, Boshell BR, DiPlacido J, Roddam RF. Insulin secretion in obesity. N Engl J Med 1967; 276: 314–319.
131. Bagdade JD, Bierman EL, Porte D Jr. Significance of basal insulin levels in the evaluation of the insulin response to glucose in diabetic and nondiabetic subjects. J Clin Invest 1967; 46:1549.
132. Ferrannini E, Camastra S. Relationship between impaired glucose tolerance, non-insulin-dependent diabetes mellitus and obesity. Eur J Clin Invest 1998; 28: 3–7.
133. Kreisberg RA, Boshell BR, DiPlacido J, Roddam RF. Insulin secretion in obesity. N Engl J Med 1967; 276: 314–319.
134. Lillioja S, Bogardus C. Obesity and insulin resistance: lessons learned from the Pima Indians. Diabetes Metab Rev 1988; 4:517–540.
135. Sims EAH, Goldman RF, Gluck CM, Horton ES, Kelleher PC, Rowe DW. Experimental obesity in man. Trans Assoc Am Physicians 1968; 81:153–170.
136. Jimenez J, Zuniga-Guarjardo S, Zinman B, Angel A. Effects of weight loss in massive obesity on insulin and C-peptide dynamics: sequential changes in insulin production, clearance, and sensitivity. J Clin Endocrinol Metab 1987; 64:661–668.
137. Ogilvie RF. Sugar tolerance in obese subjects. Q J Med 1935; 4:345.
138. Lillioja S, Mott DM, Howard BV, Bennett PH, Yki-Jarvinen H, et al. Impaired glucose tolerance as a disorder of insulin action: longitudinal and cross-sectional studies in Pima Indians. N Engl J Med 1988; 318:1217–1225.
139. Efendic S, Grill V, Luft R, Wajngot A. Low insulin response: a marker of prediabetes. Adv Exp Med Biol 1988; 246:167–174.
140. Simpson R, Benedetti A, Grodsky G, Karam J, Forsham P. Early phase of insulin release. Diabetes 1968; 17:684–692.
141. Hoker J, Rudenski A, Burnett M, Matthews D. Similar reduction of first- and second-phase B-cell responses at three different glucose levels in type II diabetes and the effect of gliclazide therapy. Metabolism 1989; 38:707–772.

142. Martin MM, Martin ALA. Obesity, hyperinsulinism, and diabetes mellitus in childhood. Pediatrics 1973; 82:192–201.
143. Pimenta W, Korytkowski M, Mitrakou A, Jenssen T. Pancreatic beta-cell dysfunction as the primary genetic lesion in NIDDM. JAMA 1995; 273:1855–1861.
144. Erikkson J, Franssila-Kallunki A, Ekstrand A, et al. Early metabolic defects in persons at increased risk for non-insulin-dependent diabetes mellitus. N Engl J Med 1989; 321:337–344.
145. Weyer C, Bogardus C, Mott DM, Pratley RE. The natural history on insulin secreatory dysfunction and insulin resistance in the pathogenesis of type 2 diabetes mellitus. J Clin Invest 1999; 104:787–794.
146. Dowse GK, Gareeboo H, Simmet PZ, Alberti KGGM, Tuomilehto J. Abdominal obesity and physical inactivity are risk factors for NIDDM and impaired glucose tolerance in Indian, Creole, and Chinese Mauritians. Diabetes Care 1991; 14:271–282.
147. Helmrich SP, Ragland DR, Leung RW, Paffenbarger RS. Physical activity and reduced occurrence of non-insulin-dependent diabetes mellitus. N Engl J Med 1991; 325:147–152.
148. Manson JE, Rimm EB, Stampfer MJ, Colditz GA, Willett WC. Physical activity and incidence of non-insulin-dependent diabetes mellitus in women. Lancet 1991; 338:774–778.
149. Després JP, Tremblay A, Nadeau A, Bouchard C. Physical training and changes in regional adipose tissue distribution. Acta Med Scand 1988; 723(suppl):205–212.
150. Krotkiewski M. Can body fat patterning be changed? Acta Med Scand 1988; 723:(suppl)213–223.
151. Eriksson KF, Lindgarde F. Prevention of type 2 (non-insulin-dependent) diabetes mellitus by diet and physical exercise. Diabetologia 1991; 34:891–898.
152. Tuomilehto J, Lindström J, Eriksson JG, et al. Prevention of type 2 diabetes mellitus by changes in lifestyle among subjects with impaired glucose tolerance. N Engl J Med 2001; 344:1343–1350.
153. Wing RR, Venditti E, Jakicic JM, Polley BA, Lang W. Lifestyle intervention in overweight individuals with a family history of diabetes. Diabetes Care 1998; 21:350–359.
154. Goodyear LJ, Kahn BB. Exercise, glucose transport, and insulin sensitivity. Annu Rev Med 1998; 49:235–261.
155. De Fronzo RA, Sherwin RS, Kraemer N. Effect of physical training on insulin action in obesity. Diabetes 1987; 36:1379–1385.
156. Koivisto VA, Yki-Jorvinen H. Effect of exercise on insulin binding and glucose transport in adipocytes of normal humans. J Appl Physiol 1987; 63:1319–1323.
157. Stamler R, Stamler J, Riedlinger WF, et al. Weight and blood pressure, findings in hypertension screening of 1 million Americans. JAMA 1978; 240:1607–1610.
158. Hubert HB, Feinleib M, McNamara PM, Castelli WP. Obesity as an independent risk factor for cardiovascular disease: a 26-year follow-up of participants in the Framingham Heart Study. Circulation 1983; 67:968–977.
159. Willett WC, Manson JE, Stampfer MJ, Colditz GA, Rosner B, Speizer FE, Hennekens CH. Weight, weight change, and coronary heart disease in women. JAMA 1995; 273(6):461–465.
160. Ferannini E, Buzzigoli G, Bonadonna R, et al. Insulin resistance in essential hypertension. N Engl J Med 1987; 317:350–357.
161. Welbom TA, Breckinridge A, Rubinstein AH, Dollery CT, Fraser TR. Serum-insulin in essential hypertension and in peripheral vascular disease. Lancet 1966; 1:1336–1337.
162. Modan M, Halkin H, Almog S, et al. Hyperinsulinemia, a link between hypertension, obesity and glucose intolerance. J Clin Invest 1985; 75:809–817.
163. De Fronzo RA, Cooke CR, Andres R, Faloona GR, Davis PJ. The effect of insulin on renal handling of sodium potassium, calcium, and phosphate in man. J Clin Invest 1975; 55:845–855.
164. Eaton RP. Lipids and diabetes: the case for treatment of macrovascular disease. Diabetes Care 1979; 2:46–50.
165. Jensen MD, Haymond MW, Rizza RA, Cryer PE, Miles JM. Influence of body fat distribution on free fatty acid metabolism in obesity. J Clin Invest 1989; 83:1168–1173.
166. Eckel RH, Yost TJ. Weight reduction increases adipose tissue lipoprotein lipase responsiveness in obese women. J Clin Invest 1987; 80:992–997.
167. Eckel RH. Lipoprotein lipase: a multifunctional enzyme relevant to common metabolic diseases. N Engl J Med 1989; 320:1060–1068.
168. Howard B. Lipoprotein metabolism I diabetes mellitus. J Lipid Res 1987; 28:613–628.
169. Austin MA, Breslow JL, Hennekens CH, Buring JE, Willett WC, Krauss RM. Low density lipoprotein subclass patterns and risk of myocardial infarction. JAMA 1988; 260:1917–1921.
170. Trible DL, Hull LG, Wood PD, Krauss RM. Variations in oxidative susceptibility among six low density lipoprotein subfractions of different density and particle size. Atherosclerosis 1992; 93:189–1942.
171. Eckel RH. Natural history of macrovascular disease and classic risk factors for atherosclerosis. Diabetes Care 1999; 22(S3):C21–C24.
172. Lamarche B, Tchemoff A, Mauriege P, Cantin B, Dagenais GR, Lupien PJ, Despres J-P. Fasting insulin and apolipoprotein B levels and low-density lipoprotein particle size as risk factors for ischemic heart disease. JAMA 1998; 279:1955–1961.
173. Després J-P, Lamarche B, Mauriege P, Cantin B, Dagenais GR, Moorjani S, Lupien PJ. Hyperinsuli-

nemia as an independent risk factor for ischemic heart disease. N Engl J Med 1996; 334:952–957.
174. Steinberg D, Parthasarathy S, Carew TE, Khoo JC, Witztum JL. Beyond cholesterol. Modifications of low density lipoprotein that increase its atherogenicity. N Engl J Med 1989; 320:915–924.
175. UKPDS Group. U.K. Prospective Diabetes Study 7 response of fasting plasma glucose to diet therapy in newly presenting type II diabetic patients. Metabolism 1990; 146:1749–1753.
176. Zavaroni I, Bonora E, Pagliara M, et al. Risk factors for coronary artery disease in healthy persons with hyperinsulinemia and normal glucose tolerance. N Engl J Med 1989; 320:702–706.
177. Pyorala K, Savolainen E, Kaukola S, Haapakoski J. Plasma insulin as coronary heart disease risk factor; relationship to other risk factors and predictive value during 9-year follow-up of the Helsinki Policemen Study population. Acta Med Scand 1985; 701:(suppl) 38–52.
178. Fontbonne AM, Eschwege EM. Insulin and cardiovascular disease: Paris Prospective Study. Diabetes Care 1991; 14:461–469.
179. Welbom TA, Wearne K. Coronary heart disease incidence and cardiovascular disease mortality in Busselton with reference to glucose and insulin concentrations. Diabetes Care 1979; 2:154–160.
180. Stout RW. Insulin and atheroma: a 20-yr perspective. Diabetes Care 1990; 13:631–654.
181. Vague P, Juhan-Vague I, Aillaud MF, et al. Correlation between blood fibrinolytic activity, plasminogen activator inhibitor level, plasma insulin level, and relative body weight in normal and obese subjects. Metabolism 1986; 2:250–253.
182. Vague P, Juhan-Vague I, Chabert V, Alessi MC, Atlan C. Fat distribution and plasminogen activator inhibitor activity in nondiabetic obese women. Metabolism 1989; 38:913–915.
183. Galloway JA. Treatment of NIDDM with insulin agonists or substitutes. Diabetes Care 1990; 13:1209–1239.
184. Genuth JF. Insulin use in NIDDM. Diabetes Care 1990; 13:1240–1246.
185. Diabetes Control and Complications Trial Research Group. The effect of intensive treatment of diabetes on the development and progression of long-term complications in insulin-dependent diabetes mellitus. N Engl J Med 1993; 329:977–986.
186. Brownlee M. Glycation products and the pathogenesis of diabetic complications. Diabetes Care 1992; 15: 1835–1843.
187. American Diabetes Association. Clinical practice recommendations, American Diabetes Association 1992–1993. Diabetes Care 1993; 16(suppl 2):1–118.
188. Edelman SV, Henry RR. Insulin therapy for normalizing glycosylated hemoglobin in type II diabetes. Application, benefits and risks. Diabetes Rev 1995; 3:308–334.
189. Henry RR, Gumbiner B, Ditzler T, Wallace P, Lyon R, Glauber HS. Intensive conventional insulin therapy for type II diabetes: metabolic effects during a 6-month outpatient trial. Diabetes Care 1993; 16:21–31.
190. Yki-Jarvinen H, Kauppila M, Kujansuu E, Lahti J, Marjanen T, Niskanen L, Rajala S, Leena R, Salo S, Seppala P, Tulokas T, Viikari J, Karjalainen J, Taskinen M-R. Comparison of insulin regimens in patients with non-insulin-dependent diabetes mellitus. N Engl J Med 1992; 327:1426–1433.
191. Kudlacek S, Schernthaner O. The effect of insulin treatment on HbA1c, body weight and lipids in type 2 diabetic patients with secondary failure to sulfonylureas: a five year follow up study. Horm Metab Res 1992; 24:478–483.
192. Stolar MW. Atherosclerosis in diabetes: the role of hyperinsulinemia. Metabolism 1988; 37(suppl 1):1–9.
193. Albu J, Konnarides C, Pi-Sunyer FX. Weight control Metabolic and cardiovascular effects. Diabetes Rev 1995; 3:335–347.
194. Beebe CA, Pastors JG, Powers MA, Wylie-Rosett J. Nutrition management for individuals with non-insulin-dependent diabetes mellitus in the 90's: a review by the Diabetes Care and Education Dietetic Practice Group. J Am Diet Assoc 1991; 91:196–207.
195. Williams G. Obesity and type 2 diabetes: a conflict of interests? Int J Obes 1999; 23(suppl 7):S2–S4.
196. Williamson DF, Thompson TJ, Thun M, et al. Intentional weight loss and mortality among overweight individuals with diabetes. Diabetes Care 2000; 23:1499–1504.
197. Leibson CL, Williamson DF, Melton LJ III, et al. Temporal trends in BMI among adults with diabetes. Diabetes Care 2001; 24:1584–1589.
198. Williams KV, Mullen ML, Kelley DE, Wing RR. The effect of short periods of caloric restriction on weight loss and glycemic control in type 2 diabetes. Diabetes Care 1998; 21:2–8.
199. Bray GA. Drug treatment of obesity. Am J Clin Nutr 1992; 55:538S–544S.
200. Bray GA. Basic mechanisms and very low calorie diets. In: Blackburn GL, Bray GA, eds. Management of Obesity by Severe Caloric Restriction Littleton, MA: PSG, 1985:129–169.
201. Flier JS. Obesity and lipoprotein disorders. In: Khan RC, Weir GC, eds. Joslin's Diabetes Mellitus. Philadelphia: Lea & Febiger, 1994:351–356.
202. Bressler R, Johnson D. New pharmacological approaches to therapy of NIDDM. Diabetes Care 1992; 15:792–805.
203. United Kingdom Prospective Diabetes Study Group. Effect of intensive blood-glucose control with metformin on complications in overweight patients with type 2 diabetes (UKPDS 34). Lancet 1998; 352:854–865.

204. United Kingdom Prospective Diabetes Study Group. UKPDS 24: a 6-year, randomized, controlled trial comparing sulfonylurea, insulin, and metformin therapy in patients with newly diagnosed type 2 diabetes that could not be controlled with diet therapy. Ann Intern Med 1998; 128:165–175.
205. Gale EAM. Lessons from the glitazones: a story of drug development. Lancet 2001; 357:1870–1875.
206. Miyazaki Y, Mahankali A, Matsuda M, et al. Improved glycemic control and enhanced insulin sensitivity in type 2 diabetic subjects treated with pioglitazone. Diabetes Care 2001; 24:710–719.
207. Yki-Järvinen H. Combination therapies with insulin in type 2 diabetes. Diabetes Care 2001; 24:758–767.
208. Rosenstock J, Schwartz SL, Clark CM Jr, et al. Basal insulin therapy in type 2 diabetes. Diabetes Care 2001; 24:631–636.
209. Yki-Järvinen H, Dressler A, Ziemen M, et al. Less nocturnal hypoglycemia and better post-dinner glucose control with bedtime insulin glargine compared with bedtime NPH insulin during insulin combination therapy in type 2 diabetes. Diabetes Care 2000; 23:1130–1136.
210. Hauner H. The impact of pharmacotherapy on weight management in type 2 diabetes. Int J Obes 1999; 23 (suppl 7):S12–S17.
211. Finer N, Bloom SR, Frost GS, Banks LM, Griffiths J. Sibutramine is effective for weight loss and diabetic control in obesity with type 2 diabetes: a randomized, double-blind, placebo-controlled study. Diabetes Obes Metab 2000; 2(2):105–112.
212. Fujioka K, Seaton TB, Rowe E, Jelinek CA, Raskin P, Lebovitz HE, Weinstein SB. Weight loss with sibutramine improves glycaemic control and other metabolic parameters in obese patients with type 2 diabetes mellitus. Diabetes Obes Metab 2000; 2(3):175–187.
213. Guerciolini R. Mode of action of orlistat. Int J Obes 1997; 21(suppl 3):S12–S23.
214. Hollander PA, Elbein SC, Hirsch IB, et al. Role of orlistat in the treatment of obese patients with type 2 diabetes. Diabetes Care 1998; 21:1288–1294.
215. Heymsfield SB, Segal KR, Hauptman J, et al. Effects of weight loss with orlistat on glucose tolerance and progression to type 2 diabetes in obese adults. Arch Intern Med 2000; 160(9):1321–1326.
216. Villsbøll T, Krarup T, Deacon CF, Madsbad S, Holst JJ. Reduced postprandial concentrations of intact biologically active glucagon-like peptide 1 in type 2 diabetic patients. Diabetes 2001; 50:609–613.
217. Mannucci E, Ognibene A, Cremasco F, et al. Glucagon-like peptide (GLP)-1 and leptin concentrations in obese patients with type 2 diabetes mellitus. Diabetic Med 2000; 17:713–719.
218. Ritzel R, Schulte M, Pørksen N, et al. Glucagon-like peptide 1 increases secretory burst mass of pulsatile insulin secretion in patients with type 2 diabetes and impaired glucose tolerance. Diabetes 2001; 50:776–784.
219. Toft-Nielsen MB, Madsbad S, Holst JJ. Determinants of the effectiveness of glucagon-like peptide-1 in type 2 diabetes. J Clin Endocrinol Metab 2001; 86:3853–386.
220. Gutzwiller JP, Drewe J, Goke B, et al. Glucagon-like peptide-1 promotes satiety and reduces food intake in patients with diabetes mellitus type 2. Am J Physiol 1999; 276:R1541–R1544.
221. Naslund E, Gutniak M, Skogar S, Rossner S, Hellstrom PM. Glucagon-like peptide 1 increases the period of postprandial satiety and slows gastric emptying in obese men. Am J Clin Nutr 1998; 68:525–530.
222. Flint A, Raben A, Rehfeld JF, Holst JJ, Astrup A. The effect of glucagon-like peptide-1 on energy expenditure and substrate metabolism in humans. Int J Obes Relat Metab Disord 2000; 24:288–298.
223. Davis HR Jr, Mullins DE, Pines JM, et al. Effect of chronic central administration of glucagon-like peptide-1 (7–36) amide on food consumption and body weight in normal and obese rats. Obes Res 1998; 6:147–156.
224. Van Dijk G, Thiele TE. Glucagon-like-peptide-1 (7–36) amide: a central regulator of satiety and interoceptive stress. Neuropeptides 1999; 33:406–414.
225. Drucker DJ. Minireview: the glucagon-like peptides. Endocrinology 2001; 142:521–527.
226. Larsen J, Hylleberg B, Ng K, Damsbo P. Glucagon-like peptide-1 infusion must be maintained for 24h/day to obtain acceptable glycemia in type 2 diabetic patients who are poorly controlled on sulfonylurea treatment. Diabetes Care 2001; 24:1416–1421.
227. Doyle ME, Egan JM. Glucagon-like-peptide-1. Rec Prog Horm Res 2001; 56:377–399.
228. Balsiger BM, Murr MM, Poggio JL, Sarr MG. Bariatric surgery. Surgery for weight control in patients with morbid obesity. Med Clin North Am 2000; 84: 477–489.
229. Bloomgarden ZT. European Association for the Study of Diabetes Annual Meeting, 2000. Diabetes Care 2001; 24:1115–1119.

38

Obesity and Gallbladder Disease

Cynthia W. Ko and Sum P. Lee

University of Washington, Seattle, Washington, U.S.A.

I INTRODUCTION

Gallstones are a common problem in the general population, and have an even higher prevalence in the obese and in those losing weight. Complications of gallstones include biliary colic, acute and chronic cholecystitis, and pancreatitis. Three conditions are necessary for cholesterol gallstone formation: supersaturation of bile with cholesterol, nucleation of cholesterol crystals, and gallbladder stasis. In obese subjects, these pathogenetic mechanisms may be modified, leading to a predisposition to gallstone formation. This chapter will review the pathogenesis of cholesterol gallstones, and the effects of obesity and weight loss on gallbladder disease.

II PATHOGENESIS OF CHOLESTEROL GALLSTONES

Bile is a complex substance composed of lipids, proteins, electrolytes, and water. There are three principal biliary lipids: cholesterol, bile acids, and phospholipids (primarily phosphatidylcholine). Many species of proteins are present, and they are derived from serum proteins as well as hepatocyte, bile duct, and gallbladder epithelial secretion. Gallstone formation is determined by the physical-chemical interactions of all of these components present in bile (1).

A Synthesis and Secretion of Biliary Lipids

1 Cholesterol

The liver is the site of primary site of cholesterol synthesis and lipoprotein metabolism in the body. Free cholesterol is synthesized in the hepatocyte endoplasmic reticulum. The rate-limiting enzyme in cholesterol synthesis is HMG-CoA reductase (2). Each day, several grams of cholesterol derived from lipoproteins are taken up by the liver. Cholesterol enters the liver in esterified form, is transported to the lysosomes, and is then converted into its free form. It is then transported to the endoplasmic reticulum and reesterified for storage. Cholesterol esters in the endoplasmic reticulum are continually undergoing hydrolysis, providing a constant supply of free cholesterol. This free cholesterol is the substrate pool for bile acid and lipoprotein synthesis and for secretion into bile. The rate of biliary excretion from this pool varies with the rate of bile salt and lipoprotein synthesis. Biliary cholesterol secretion is quantitatively correlated with bile salt secretion (2). However, the ratio of cholesterol to bile salts secreted increases as bile salt secretion decreases, in part explaining the finding of more saturated bile (higher cholesterol-to-bile salt ratio) at low bile flow rates. Cholesterol is believed to be secreted from the liver in the form of phospholipid-cholesterol vesicles (3). Leptin levels influence the amount of cholesterol secreted into bile in animal models (4), and gallstone prevalence is correlated with serum leptin levels in humans, even after controlling for body mass index (5).

2 Bile Acids

Bile acids are synthesized from cholesterol through the rate-limiting enzyme cholesterol 7α-hydroxylase, a microsomal enzyme. Bile acids, which are amphiphilic, solubilize and transport cholesterol. Two primary bile acids, chenodeoxycholic acid (3α, 7α) (CDCA) and cholic acid (3α, 7α, 12α) (CA), are synthesized in vivo. The relative proportions of these are regulated by the activity of the enzyme 12α-hydroxylase, which converts CDCA into CA. The cholesterol-carrying capacity of bile is influenced by the relative proportions of these two bile acids, since CA can solubilize less cholesterol than CDCA. 12α-Hydroxylase can be induced by estrogens, resulting in higher proportions of CA and more lithogenic bile (1,2).

After synthesis, bile acids bind to carrier proteins for transport through the hepatocyte. Here, bile acids are conjugated with glycine and taurine, increasing their water solubility. They are then actively secreted by bile acid transporters located in the biliary canalicular surface of the hepatocyte. Bile acids are initially excreted as individual molecules. However, at the critical micellar concentration, they will aggregate to form micelles that are capable of solubilizing cholesterol and phospholipids (1,2,6). After secretion, bile acids enter the intestine, where they are metabolized by intestinal bacteria, deconjugated, and dehydroxylated. In this process, CA is converted to deoxycholic acid, and CDCA to lithocholic acid. Bile acids are reabsorbed in the terminal ileum and circulate via the portal vein to the liver. Here, they are reabsorbed, reconjugated, and resecreted into bile via the enterohepatic circulation.

3 Phospholipids

Phospholipids in bile are believed to be derived from membranous structures within the hepatocyte, such as the endoplasmic reticulum or lysosomes, or from the hepatocyte canalicular membrane. Over 95% of the phospholipids are phosphatidylcholines. Phospholipids are amphiphilic molecules and, similarly to bile acids, can solubilize and transport cholesterol. It is believed that phospholipid is translocated across the canalicular lipid bilayer by a protein similar to the multidrug resistance gene protein (7,8). Cholesterol and phospholipids then aggregate and are secreted into bile as vesicles. The secretory pathway of phospholipid and cholesterol is independent of that of the bile acid transporter pathway. However, vesicular secretion is quantitatively driven by bile acid secretion (1,2).

4 Proteins

Protein composes $<5\%$ of biliary solids. Proteins in bile are derived from plasma, the hepatocyte, and biliary ductular epithelium. Most biliary proteins, such as albumin, α_2-macroglobulin, and IgG, are derived from plasma, but are present in bile in much lower concentrations. These proteins may enter bile by simple diffusion from the plasma compartment through hepatocyte tight junctions or through the epithelium of periductular capillaries. Other proteins, such as apolipoproteins, secretory IgA, or the hemoglobin-haptoglobin complex, are actively secreted into bile following nonspecific or receptor-mediated vesicular transport though the hepatocyte. The gallbladder adds to biliary proteins by secreting mucin, immunoglobulins, and other glycoproteins, which may have an important role in promoting gallstone formation (6,9).

B Physical Chemistry of Biliary Lipids

Cholesterol is a hydrophobic molecule. To be transported in an aqueous environment such as bile, it must be solubilized by amphiphilic molecules such as bile acids or phospholipids. Cholesterol is transported in two forms, micellar and nonmicellar (vesicular), in bile (8,10). The thermodynamic stability of these two forms of transport differs. Since only a limited amount of cholesterol can be solubilized by bile acids and phospholipids, the relative concentrations of cholesterol, phospholipid, and bile acids determine in part the gallstone-forming capability, or lithogenicity, of bile. Lithogenicity is expressed as the cholesterol saturation index (11,12). Bile with a cholesterol saturation index greater than one is, by definition, supersaturated. Bile supersaturation is a prerequisite for cholesterol gallstone formation.

1 Nonmicellar Cholesterol Transport

Biliary cholesterol transport can be transported in unilamellar vesicles, which are 40–70 nm in diameter and consist of a bilayer of phospholipids interdigitated with cholesterol (3,13–17). Vesicles contain very little or no bile acids. In bile with a higher concentration of bile acids, such as gallbladder bile, these vesicles may fuse and form larger, multilamellar vesicles up to 500–1000 nm in diameter (15–17). Vesicles are believed to be less thermodynamically stable than mixed micelles, and cholesterol in these vesicles may coalesce to form a metastable state (3,13,18–20). Cholesterol in vesicles is felt to be more prone to nucleate and precipitate (20–23), and gallstone patients may have a larger proportion of cholesterol transported in this form (22).

2 Micellar Cholesterol Transport

Cholesterol is also transported in mixed micelles, which have diameters of 4–8 nm (1). Cholesterol can undergo dynamic exchange between the nonmicellar and micellar forms of transport (24,25), but only the micellar form is considered thermodynamically stable. Cholesterol equilibration between nonmicellar and micellar forms starts immediately after secretion. Transfer of both cholesterol and phospholipids from the nonmicellar to the micellar fraction is facilitated by increasing bile acid concentrations, as may occur with gallbladder stasis.

During this phase of "micellation," more phospholipid than cholesterol is transferred to the forming micelle (1). The residual vesicles are thus less stable due to higher cholesterol-to-phospholipid ratio. However, with lower rates of bile acid secretion, the relative concentration of bile acids is too low to solubilize all biliary cholesterol, and therefore most cholesterol is transported in vesicular, less stable form (21). Under these circumstances, cholesterol crystals may form.

C Role of the Gallbladder

Cholesterol gallstones occur very rarely in patients who have undergone previous cholecystectomy. Therefore, the gallbladder is believed to play an important role in gallstone formation. The gallbladder has storage, concentrative, absorptive, secretory, and contractile properties that may contribute to development of gallstones.

1 Motor Function

Gallbladder motility is commonly assessed by measuring fasting volume, contracted or residual volume, and fractional emptying. Maximal contraction is seen after meals. Between meals, the gallbladder may undergo partial emptying and filling. During periods of fasting, gallbladder contraction is weak, and bile accumulates in the gallbladder, with sequestration of the circulating bile acid pool. With the resulting fall in bile acid secretion rates, bile becomes progressively more saturated, and cholesterol crystallization or stone formation may occur. Contractile function of the gallbladder is important to empty any saturated bile, sludge, or small stones before larger stones can form (26). Gallbladder contractility is controlled through the endocrine and nervous systems. The most important hormone regulating gallbladder contractility is cholecystokinin (CCK). This hormone is released by the duodenum after meals, and causes gallbladder contraction and sphincter of Oddi relaxation (26). Neural control is mediated through both the vagus nerve and the sympathetic nervous system. Vagal activity enhances gallbladder contraction, while the role of sympathetic innervation is generally inhibitory (26).

Abnormal gallbladder motility, such as increased fasting volume and decreased fractional emptying, has been noted in animals and in a subgroup of patients who form sludge and gallstones (27–34). Some studies also show a slower rate of contraction after a fatty meal in gallstones patients (29). In many conditions that predispose to sludge or gallstone formation, gallbladder emptying is markedly inhibited owing to endocrine or neurologic abnormalities (26). For example, patients who are fasting or receiving total parenteral nutrition will have markedly diminished CCK release and gallbladder hypomotility (35,36). Treatment with the CCK antagonist somatostatin, as in patients with acromegaly, can inhibit gallbladder contractility (37,38), The obese, who are also predisposed to sludge and stone formation, may have diminished responsiveness of the gallbladder wall to CCK (33).

2 Mucosal Function

The gallbladder is generally thought of as a storage organ. However, several recent studies have demonstrated that the gallbladder can concentrate bile and alter its composition. The gallbladder epithelium acidifies bile, actively transports sodium and chloride, and absorbs water by passive osmosis. During this process, initially dilute hepatic bile is concentrated, leading to higher concentrations of biliary lipids, predisposing to cholesterol crystal nucleation. Bile pH and carbonate concentration decrease (39–42). Nucleation times also become more rapid with bile concentration (43).

In addition to its concentrative and absorptive functions, gallbladder epithelium secretes mucin glycoprotein (13). Mucin glycoprotein has extensive hydrophobic domains that can bind biliary lipids. In more concentrated bile, vesicles and micelles are entrapped in these binding sites and come into close and prolonged contact (44–48). Mucin hypersecretion has been shown to precede gallstone formation in prairie dog models, and probably entraps cholesterol within its hydrophobic domains (48–50). The stimulus for mucin hypersecretion is not entirely clear, but may be lithogenic bile, hydrophobic bile salts, prostaglandins, or arachidonic acid (49–51).

3 Nucleation of Cholesterol Crystals

Cholesterol crystal nucleation is the first step in gallstone formation. Nucleation begins with aggregation and fusion of unilamellar vesicles to multilamellar vesicles, with subsequent aggregation of cholesterol molecules to form crystals. This initial aggregation is mediated at least in part by mucin binding of these lipids. Cholesterol that precipitates is derived primarily from biliary vesicles and precipitates using mucin glycoprotein as a nidus (20,44,52,53). Calcium ions are believed to be important in gallstone formation, as they can promote fusion of phospholipid-cholesterol vesicles. Calcium salts can also serve as a nidus for cholesterol precipitation and are usually found in the central core of cholesterol stones (2). Proteins, including albumin and other calcium-binding proteins, are found in the matrix of cholesterol stones, and thus may also serve as sites for nucleation (52,54,55). When cholesterol crystals reach a certain critical size, gallstone formation can occur with further deposition of cholesterol on the surface of the aggregate.

Normal biliary proteins can have pro-nucleating (56–62) and antinucleating (63,64) properties. Proteins with pro-nucleating properties include IgG, haptoglobin, phospholipase C, and aminopeptidase N (56–62). Proteins with antinucleating properties include apolipoprotein A-I and A-II (64), secretory IgA (65), and some small acidic glycoproteins (63). It is felt that these proteins somehow interact with and stabilize biliary lipids and calcium. The existence of proteins with antinucleating properties may explain the prolonged stability of bile that is supersaturated with cholesterol. The presence of proteins with pro-nucleating properties may contribute to nucleation, as high biliary protein concentrations have been found in supersaturated bile with cholesterol crystals (66). Many other, poorly characterized, nonmucin proteins are found in the core of cholesterol gallstones (52,54). The exact nature and role in the gallstone pathogenesis of these proteins is unknown.

4 Growth of Cholesterol Crystals into Stones

Once a crystal of adequate size has formed, cholesterol, calcium bilirubinate, and other biliary lipids can deposit on its surface, leading to formation of visible gallstones. One study has suggested that bile in obese patients promotes more rapid crystal growth than in the nonobese (67). However, this process has not been as extensively studied as crystal nucleation, and little information is available on factors that may influence growth of stones.

III EFFECTS OF OBESITY

Gallstone formation requires three conditions: secretion of supersaturated bile, nucleation of cholesterol crystals from supersaturated bile, and gallbladder stasis. Obesity has direct effects on bile composition and gallbladder motility. This section will review the epidemiology of gallbladder disease and the effects of obesity on bile composition and gallbladder motility that predispose to gallstone formation.

A Epidemiology of Gallbladder Disease

Gallstones occur in populations throughout the world, but the prevalence varies substantially (68–71). In Western countries, the majority of gallstones are composed of cholesterol. Gallstones in the obese are composed primarily of cholesterol. The prevalence of gallstones in females varies from 3.7% in Indians and Pakistanis to 62.2% in Pima Indians (69,70). In males, the prevalence varies from 2.9% in Thailand to 25.9% in Pima Indians (70,71). Both racial and genetic factors likely contribute to the wide variation in prevalence. About two-thirds of patients with known gallstones do not have symptoms of biliary tract disease.

In all populations studied, the prevalence of gallstones increases with age (68–71). The prevalence of gallbladder disease increases markedly in those over 40 years old, such that 10–15% of Caucasian males and 20–40% of Caucasian females over the age of 60 have gallstones ultrasonographically. In the Pima Indians, a group known to have a high prevalence of gallstones, 68% of men and 90% of women over the age of 65 have gallbladder disease by oral cholecystography (70). With aging, biliary cholesterol secretion becomes excessive through mechanisms that are not well understood (72).

At all ages, females have a higher prevalence of gallstones than males, but in older age groups, the female predominance of gallstone incidence is less marked. Other states with higher estrogen stimulation, such as oral contraceptive use, higher parity, and estrogen replacement therapy, also are associated with greater risk of gallstones (73–75). Multiple theories have been put forth to explain this gender difference. Females may have a higher level of the enzyme 12α-hydroxylase, with resulting higher biliary levels of CA and more supersaturated bile. Estrogens increase receptors for lipoproteins B and E, leading to increased hepatic cholesterol uptake (76). High levels of circulating estrogens have been shown to decrease the total bile acid and CDCA pools, with resulting increases in cholesterol saturation (77).

Risk factors other than ethnicity, age, and gender are less well defined and less well understood. Patients with diabetes mellitus or glucose intolerance have a higher incidence of gallstones in some but not all studies, likely secondary to altered gallbladder motility and hepatic lipid metabolism (78–81). A weak negative association between total serum cholesterol or LDL levels and gallstone formation has been seen in some but not all studies (73,74,79,82–84). Gallstone patients have mean triglyceride levels 21–26% higher and HDL cholesterol levels 14–19% lower than matched control patients (73,82–84). There is no clear consensus on the effect of alcohol consumption, smoking, or occupation on the risk of gallbladder disease (76,79,85,86).

Dietary factors have been implicated in gallbladder disease, but there are no clear data on the potential effects or mechanisms. Evidence exists that higher total caloric intake correlates with cholesterol gallstone formation. In the Nurses' Health Study, a significant trend toward higher risk of gallstones was seen with increasing caloric intake (86). However, in a study of Japanese-American men, there was an inverse correlation between total caloric intake and gallstone incidence (85). Studies differ in respect to the roles of total dietary fat, protein, or carbohydrate intake (87–89).

More recently, physical activity has been implicated has been implicated as a risk factor for symptomatic gallstones and cholecystectomy, independently of its effect on overall body mass index and weight loss (89–91). These studies, performed in both men and women, have shown that even moderate levels of recreational physical activity are protective against symptomatic gallstones. The mechanisms behind this phenomenon are unclear, although some have postulated that the effects of exercise on glucose tolerance, insulin levels, and serum lipid levels may be responsible. Recent studies have found no effect of exercise on gallbladder contractility in obese women (92).

B Risk of Gallstones in the Obese

Many studies have shown that obese women are predisposed to gallbladder disease (Table 1). The incidence of gallstones in obese women has been estimated at 2.6 per 100 person-years, with approximately two-thirds of these stones being asymptomatic (95). The relative risk seems to increase as body weight increases (73,74,78,85,86,93,96–99). Thus, the risk of gallstones relative to nonobese women is increased two times in women with a body mass index (BMI) >30 kg/m^2 and seven times in women with a BMI >45 kg/m^2 (86). However, there is not a defined threshhold effect, as the relative risk of gallstones increases with BMI, even in women with a BMI <25 kg/m^2. Obesity seems to confer a greater relative risk in younger populations (98,100,101). In one study of obese adolescents, 55% of adolescent females undergoing cholecystectomy were obese, compared to 23% of adolescent females undergoing nongallbladder surgery, a relative risk of 4.2 (101). This relationship between obesity and gallstones is less striking in men, but several studies have also shown an increased risk of gallstones in men with increasing BMI (79,99,102,103). Up to 43% of men and women undergoing bariatric surgery have gallbladder disease, defined as prior cholecystectomy or gallstones (104,105).

Table 1 Relative Risk of Gallstones with Obesity in Various Populations

Reference	Study population	Diagnostic criteria	Normal population	Obese population	Relative risk
78	Japanese men age 48–56	Screening by US	BMI <22.5	BMI >25	1.9
85	Japanese-American men	Screening by US	BMI <21.65	BMI 21.6–23.8	1.1
				BMI 23.8–25.8	1.4
				BMI >25.8	1.8
86	Nurses' Health Study	Previous cholecystectomy or symptoms	BMI <24	BMI 30–35	3.69
				BMI 35–40	4.72
				BMI 40–45	5.11
				BMI >45	7.36
93	Nurses' Health Study	US if symptomatic	BMI <22	BMI 22–24.9	1.6
				BMI 25–31.9	3.3
				BMI >32	6.3
94	Obese prior to bariatric surgery	Previous cholecystectomy and intraoperative US	BMI <20	BMI 35–40	5
				BMI 40–50	7
				BMI 50–60	8

US, ultrasound.

In addition to the effects of overall obesity, central or truncal adiposity is also correlated with the risk of gallstones in both men and women. In the San Antonio Heart Study of Mexican-American women, the risk for developing gallstone disease was 30% higher for women in the highest quartile of subscapular-triceps skinfold thickness ratio when compared to those in the lowest quartile (106). In a study limited to obese white women, Hartz et al. found the risk of gallbladder disease to be 75% higher in women in the highest quartile of waist-hip circumference ratio compared with those in the lowest quartile (107). Truncal skinfold thickness ratio has been correlated with later symptomatic gallstone formation in men, with men in the highest quartile having risk 2.5 times greater than men in the lowest quartile. This association was not altered after adjusting for initial BMI (108). In support of these findings, the lithogenic index of bile positively correlates with total body fat mass and intra-abdominal fat mass (109).

C Alterations in Serum Lipids

Excessive body weight is associated with increased daily cholesterol synthesis and a larger pool of metabolically active cholesterol in the body. In addition, hepatic conversion of cholesterol into bile acids is impaired in the obese. The obese therefore have dual mechanisms contributing to the higher total cholesterol pool: increased synthesis and decreased degradation (110–112). There are also changes in lipid concetrations in serum, with decreased HDL cholesterol and higher LDL cholesterol levels. In the obese, serum triglycerides are elevated owing to excess hepatic synthesis of VLDL and triglycerides, an effect of peripheral hyperinsulinemia and enhanced peripheral lipolysis. Lower lipoprotein lipase activity leads to decreased triglyceride clearance (113). As discussed previously, gallstone formation has also been correlated with higher serum triglyceride and lower serum HDL levels. However, it is not clear if altered serum lipids are a direct cause of gallstones, or if both disorders are a reflection of an underlying common metabolic derangement.

D Alterations in Bile Composition

Overall, biliary cholesterol secretion is increased in the obese relative to the nonobese with or without gallstones. However, when normalized to subject weight, cholesterol secretion appears normal in obese patients without gallstones. In contrast, in obese patients with gallstones, cholesterol secretion is markedly elevated, even after correction for body weight (114–119). This marked cholesterol hypersecretion, with a resulting higher cholesterol saturation index, is felt to be the primary mechanism predisposing to gallbladder disease in the obese (115–119).

The pathophysiology of cholesterol hypersecretion in the obese is poorly understood. Putative mechanisms of cholesterol hypersecretion include increased cholesterol uptake from lipoproteins (76), increased cholesterol synthesis by HMG CoA reductase (112,120), decreased cholesterol catabolism by cholesterol 7α-hydroxylase (120,121), and decreased esterification of cholesterol within the hepatocyte (112). It seems likely that cholesterol hypersecretion is secondary to a combination of these effects. Recent data suggest that leptin may be a molecular mediator of cholesterol hypersecretion (4) (Fig. 1).

In contrast to the consistent data showing cholesterol hypersecretion, the data on alterations in bile acid secretion are variable. The total pool and biliary secretion of bile acids are felt to be normal to increased in the obese. However, when normalized for body weight, bile acid secretion is lower than in the nonobese, and the relative percentage of bile acids is lower owing to the marked increase in cholesterol secretion (116–118,122–124). The data on phospholipid secre-

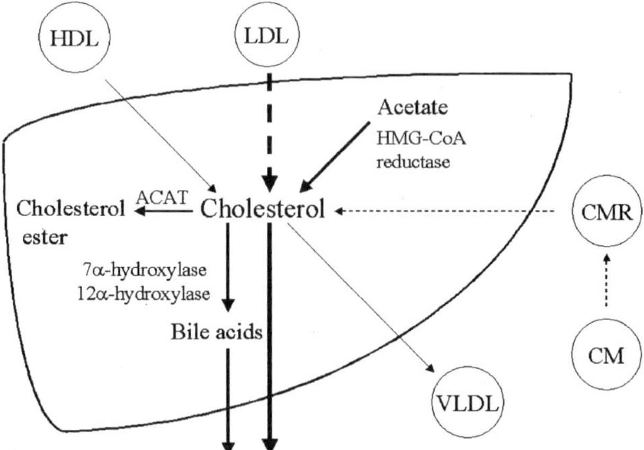

Figure 1 Hepatic cholesterol metabolism. In the liver, cholesterol may be derived from circulating lipid particles or synthesized de novo from acetate via the HMG CoA reductase pathway. Export pathways of cholesterol include incorporation into circulating VLDL particles, esterification via the ACAT enzyme, conversion to bile acids, or secretion into bile. LDL = low-density lipoprotein; HDL = high density lipoprotein; CM = chylomicron; CMR = chylomicron receptor; VLDL = very low density lipoprotein; ACAT = acetyl CoA cholesterol acyl transferase.

tion are also variable, with different studies showing unchanged to elevated total phospholipid secretion (115–118). Evidence also conflicts on the relative percentage of biliary phospholipids. No change in the relative composition of biliary phospholipids is found with obesity (116).

From the previous evidence, it follows that markedly increased cholesterol secretion in the obese, coupled with an unchanged to mildly increased bile acid secretion, leads to an increase in the cholesterol/bile salt ratio (124). Cholesterol saturation index thus increases with BMI, independent of age, gender, or ethnicity (124). As a correlate, bile becomes more lithogenic. In contrast to nonobese individuals, where bile is supersaturated only with fasting, supersaturation of bile is not transient, but persist even after feeding. The obese thus have more supersaturated bile that persists for longer periods of time.

E Alterations in Gallbladder Motility

Gallbladder stasis is an important factor that predisposes to formation of gallstones. Obesity in itself is associated with gallbladder hypomotility and stasis, with many studies showing increased fasting volumes, increased residual volumes, and decreased fractional emptying (30–32,125,126). Multiple mechanisms may predispose to alterations in gallbladder motility in the obese. Alterations in peripheral CCK levels have been postulated, but not yet proven. Diminished gallbladder responsiveness to CCK has also been proposed (126). Another proposed mechanism is related to accelerated gastric emptying. Rapid emptying of a meal would diminish the amount of time that food or chyme is in the duodenum. There would then be a resulting decrease in release of CCK, with lesser stimulation of gallbladder emptying (32).

IV EFFECTS OF WEIGHT LOSS

Obesity itself is associated with a marked increase in the incidence of gallbladder disease. Paradoxically, weight loss, through either dieting or bariatric surgery, is also associated with a further increase in the incidence of gallstone formation (Table 2). This section will review the incidence, pathophysiology, and prevention of gallstone formation during weight loss.

A Incidence of and Risk Factors for Gallstone Formation

1 Incidence

In follow-up of the Nurses' Health study, women losing 4–10 kg had a 44% increase, and those losing >10 kg had a 94% increase in the risk of gallstones (93). Interestingly, the risk of symptomatic gallstones in this population was also influenced by long-term weight

Table 2 Risk of Gallstone Formation with Weight Reduction

Reference	Study population	Method of weight loss	Diagnostic test	Follow-up period	Percent with gallstones
127	Obese undergoing bariatric surgery	Jejunoileal bypass	US if symptomatic	24 months	male 10% female 9%
128	Obese undergoing bariatric surgery	Jejunoileal bypass	Oral cholecystogram	36 months	10.3%
129	Obese undergoing bariatric surgery	Jejunoileal bypass	US if symptomatic	60 months	20%
130	Obese on low-calorie diet	540-kcal diet	US screening	4 weeks 8 weeks	7.8% 25.5%
131	Obese undergoing bariatric surgery	Gastric bypass	US screening	6 months	36%
132	Obese on low-calorie diet	520-kcal diet	US screening	16 weeks	10.9%
133	Obese on low-calorie diet	605-kcal diet	US if symptomatic	6 months	11%
134	Obese undergoing bariatric surgery	Gastric bypass	US screening	6 months 12 months 18 months	37% 37% 37%
135	Obese undergoing bariatric surgery	Gastric bypass	US screening	3 months	43%

US, ultrasound.

patterns (136). Women whose weight fluctuated and women with net weight loss over time had higher prevalence of gallstones than those who maintained a steady weight.

The overall incidence of gallstones ranges up to 25% in the 8–16 weeks after initiating a weight reduction diet (127–130,137). It has been suggested that the risk of gallstone formation increases dramatically if the rate of weight loss exceeds 1.5 kg per week (138). In addition, the composition of the weight loss diet, especially the amount of fat included, may be important. Patients given a diet containing >10 g fat per day are at lower risk of gallstone formation than those who consume <10 g fat per day, perhaps due to maintenance of gallbladder motility (139–142).

Patients losing weight with either low-calorie diets or bariatric surgery seem to be at risk (143). One study has shown a 37% incidence of gallstones 6 months after bariatric surgery. A high percentage of patients will also develop biliary sludge in the first postoperative year (131). The risk for gallstone formation is greatest in the first postoperative year, but may be increased for up to 3 years postoperatively, as weight loss continues. Although these periods are coincident with the periods of greatest weight loss and ongoing weight loss, respectively, the risk for gallstone formation does not necessarily correlate with the degree of weight loss. Twenty-four percent to 40% of those developing gallstones will be symptomatic, and ~28% may need repeat surgery for cholecystectomy (104,105, 131). Asymptomatic gallstones will resolve in about 50% after 1–2 years (144). Gallbladder concentrations of biliary lipids and cholesterol saturation index do not predict who will develop gallstones (94,128,132, 143,145,146).

2 Risk Factors

Both initial BMI and the relative rate of weight loss are predictors of gallstone development (132). Absolute weight loss is more difficult to assess, as it is highly dependent on initial BMI (132). Likewise, the rapidity of weight loss has not been established as a definite risk factor owing to confounding with absolute and relative amounts of weight lost. Higher rates of gallstone formation during weight loss are seen in men. However, this effect is removed when controlling for the higher initial BMI, relative BMI lost, and initial serum triglycerides seen in obese men as compared with obese women (132). Diets in which gallbladder motility is maintained, such as diets with higher caloric or fat contents, do not seem to be associated with as great a risk of gallstone formation (141,147). Repeated cycles of weight loss also seem to predispose to gallstone formation (136). No studies have looked at effects of weight loss due to increases in physical activity in relation to gallstone formation.

B Pathophysiology of Gallstone Formation During Weight Loss

Changes in bile composition that lead to increased lithogenicity are seen with very low calorie diets. CSI in bile increases on average during weight reduction (134,137,139,141,148–151). However, this effect is not seen in all subjects studied; some patients have large increases, and others have large decreases in saturation index. CSI and nucleation time decrease in nearly all patients after a prolonged fast. It is felt that hepatic cholesterol secretion increases during weight loss and decreases again during weight maintenance. Similarly, the molar percentage of cholesterol increases during the weight loss phase and decreases in the weight maintenance phase (131,134,148–151). The excess excreted cholesterol during weight loss is mobilized from peripheral adipose tissue. Counteracting these factors is the fact that low caloric intake lowers cholesterol input and may reduce bile acid secretion and cholesterol synthesis. Biliary cholesterol secretion will reflect a balance of all these variables. In the weight stabilization phase after a low-calorie diet, CSI decreases to below the baseline value. Nucleation time decreases concurrently with these changes (150) (Fig. 2).

Bile acid and phospholipid secretion do not reliably change with weight loss, but generally are lower (122, 134,151,152). The total bile acid pool decreases during weight reduction, but the individual bile acid profile does not change (122). If patients regain weight, the cholesterol saturation index and molar percentage of cholesterol will again increase (153). In weight loss induced after jejunoileal bypass, similar changes in bile composition and lithogenicity are noted. Bile salt pool is initially reduced, and saturation index is increased. However, bile composition reverts to normal by about one year postoperatively (150,151).

Gallbladder motility changes with weight reduction. Decreases in gallbladder motility are seen after major abdominal surgery. With gastric bypass, gallbladder hypomotility may be induced because of intraoperative transection of the vagus nerve (32,141,143,146,154). Many of the changes in bile composition during weight loss could be a reflection of this gallbladder stasis, rather than a direct result of alterations in hepatic secretion or

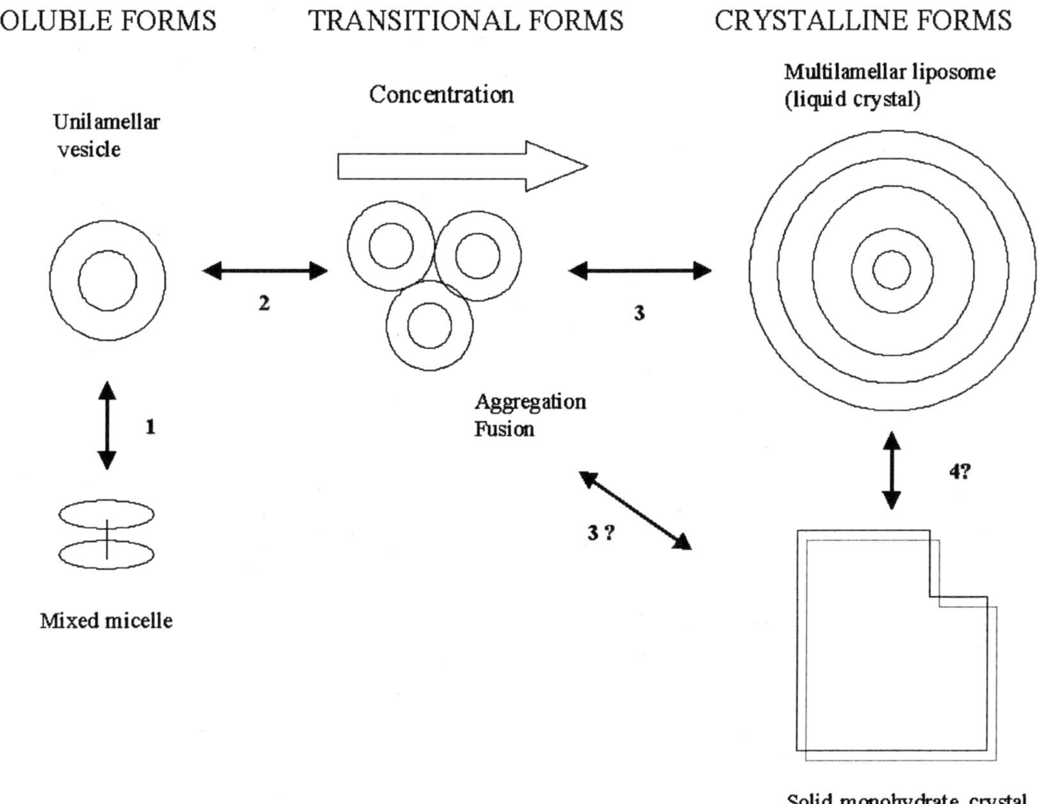

Figure 2 Schematic of cholesterol nucleation. In bile, cholesterol exists in two soluble forms—vesicles and mixed micelles. They are in dynamic equilibrium (1), depending on total bile salt concentration and lipid density. With concentration, the vesicles may be depleted with phospholipid and enriched with cholesterol, resulting in a tendency for the vesicles to aggregate and fuse (2). Pro-nucleators may aid vesicular fusion. The fused vesicles are transitional forms and lead to formation of multilamellar liposomes or liquid crystals (3). Cholesterol separates from the liquid to solid crystalline forms during nucleation (4). It is unclear whether fused vesicles can nucleate into solid cholesterol crystals. (From Ref. 168.)

gallbladder mucosal function. With very low calorie diets, increased fasting and residual gallbladder volumes can be seen (155). This effect may be reversed by inclusion of adequate calories (>800 kcal/d) or dietary fat (>10 g/d) to maximally stimulate gallbladder contractility (139,140,147,155).

C Prevention

1 Screening for Gallstones Prior to Weight Reduction

Patients undergoing bariatric surgery are often screened with preoperative ultrasound to determine the need for concomitant cholecystectomy. However, preoperative ultrasound has a low sensitivity for gallbladder disease in the obese, and may not be the best test to determine need for cholecystectomy. Some have advocated screening for gallbladder disease prior to weight reduction dieting and possibly dietary modification if gallstones are found. However, this approach has not been studied systematically (143). It is not known if patients with preexisting cholelithiasis are at higher risk of complications, such as acute cholecystitis or pancreatitis, with weight reduction.

2 Prophylactic Cholecystectomy

Some authors have advocated prophylactic cholecystectomy at the time of bariatric surgery because of the >30% incidence of gallstones in the initial period of rapid weight loss. From 10% to 25% of patients who have not had a prior cholecystectomy will already have gallstones at the time of surgery, and 95% of patients undergoing cholecystectomy at bariatric surgery will have pathologic evidence of gallbladder disease (104,

105). Cholecystectomy adds only minimally to procedure time (30–45 min), and patients undergoing prophylactic cholecystectomy have not had a higher incidence of perioperative complications or a longer hospital stay. Many centers have moved to routinely performing cholecystectomy at the time of gastric bypass surgery (104, 105). Prophylactic cholecystectomy before initiating weight reduction diets has not been advocated.

3 Bile Acid Supplementation During Weight Loss

Bile acid supplementation has been used as a nonsurgical treatment for gallstones. Certain bile acids, CDCA and ursodeoxycholic acid (UDCA), contribute to cholesterol solubilization and can decrease bile lithogenicity. Bile acid supplementation is generally well tolerated and without significant adverse effects.

In the nonobese, treatment with CDCA desaturates bile and prolongs nucleation times (20,156). However, this effect is not seen consistently in the obese, even with the same doses per kilogram being administered (17,18,157–160). Biliary cholesterol concentrations and saturation indices reliably decrease to unsaturated ranges only with high dose therapy (157–160). HMG CoA reductase activity is reduced during CDCA therapy, with subsequent reduction in hepatic cholesterol synthesis and secretion (122). However, CDCA is a potent inhibitor of cholesterol 7α-hydroxylase, and thus decreases cholesterol catabolism. With oral therapy, this bile acid can increase the total bile acid pool and the rate of bile acid secretion, and in fact, becomes the predominant circulating bile acid. Although it has beneficial effects on bile composition, CDCA may increase gallbladder mucin secretion, and potentially enhance cholesterol crystal nucleation (49–51).

Currently, the use of UDCA has superseded that of CDCA. UDCA is safe and effective. Treatment with UDCA prolongs nucleation times and decreases the concentration of cholesterol and phospholipid present in the vesicular phase (20,135,157–161). Gallbladder bile from patients treated with UDCA contains only a trace of cholesterol in vesicles, the more lithogenic form of transport (162). Similar to CDCA, UDCA decreases biliary cholesterol concentration by decreasing activity of hepatic HMG CoA reductase (122). It has no effect on the activity of cholesterol 7α-hydroxylase. The molar percentage of bile acids is unchanged to slightly increased with UDCA, and UDCA becomes the predominant bile acid during therapy (122,135,161). In addition to its effects on bile composition, UDCA may be able to maintain gallbladder motility in patients losing weight (163). All these factors combined indicate that UDCA may have a role in prophylaxis or treatment of gallstones in the obese. Randomized, controlled studies showed that giving UDCA at 600 mg/d during weight reduction dieting (164) or after gastric bypass surgery (165) can significantly decrease the incidence of biliary sludge and gallstones. In addition, prophylactic use of UDCA has been estimated to be cost saving in patients on weight reduction diets or after gastric bypass surgery (166).

4 Other Pharmacologic Measures

One study looking at high-dose aspirin (1300 mg/d) showed that none of 22 patients receiving aspirin developed gallstones during a weight reduction diet. Three of these patients developed microstones or crystals (167). However, there was no change in the saturation index, cholesterol concentration, bile acid concentration, or biliary glycoprotein concentration. Other studies have shown a possible effect of nonsteroidal anti-inflammatory drugs in inhibiting gallstone recurrence in patients losing weight (163). Although mucin secretion and prostaglandin metabolism may be modified by nonsteroidal anti-inflammatory drugs, the long-term clinical use of these compounds can be associated with substantial complications. The feasibility of using aspirin or nonsteroidal anti-inflammatory drugs for this indication has not been clearly established.

V SUMMARY

Gallstones are a common clinical problem in the obese and the nonobese. Three separate conditions are required for gallstone formation: secretion of supersaturated bile, nucleation of cholesterol crystals, and gallbladder stasis. In obesity, bile is more saturated owing to cholesterol hypersecretion, and gallbladder motor function is impaired, predisposing to gallstone formation. Recent research suggests that leptin may mediate the association between obesity and gallstones. Paradoxically, weight reduction either through dietary modification or through bariatric surgery also predisposes to gallstone formation. The mechanisms of gallstone formation during weight reduction are not entirely clear, but also involve altered bile composition and gallbladder motility. Ursodeoxycholic acid is the only medical therapy that has been studied for gallstones during weight reduction. Further research needs to be done into the risk factors for and treatment of gallstone disease and its prevention in the obese and in those losing weight.

REFERENCES

1. Scharschmidt BF. Bilirubin metabolism, bile formation, and gallbladder and bile duct function. In: Sleisenger MH, Fordtran JS, eds. Gastrointestinal Disease: Pathophysiology, Diagnosis, Management. Philadelphia: W.B. Saunders, 1993:1730–1746.
2. Cooper AD. Epidemiology, pathogenesis, natural history, and medical therapy of gallstones. In: Sleisinger MH, Fordtran JS, eds. Gastrointestinal Disease: Pathophysiology, Diagnosis, Management. Philadelphia: W.B. Saunders, 1993:1788–1804.
3. Somjen GJ, Gilat T. A non-micellar mode of cholesterol transport in human bile. FEBS Lett 1983; 156:265–268.
4. Cohen DE, Ranginani N, Vanpatten S, Rossetti L. Leptin regulates coupling of biliary cholesterol to bile salt secretion in Zucker rats [abstract]. Hepatology 1999; 30:429A.
5. Duggirala R, Mitchell BD, Blangero J, Stern MP. Genetic determinants of variation in gallbladder disease in the Mexican-American population. Genet Epidemiol 1999; 16(2):191–204.
6. Reuben A. Bile formation: sites and mechanisms. Hepatology 1984; 4(suppl 5):15S–24S.
7. Smit JJ, Schinkel AH, Oude Elferink RP, Groen AK, Wagenaar E, Van Deemter L, Mol CA. Homozygous disruption of the murine mdr2 P-glycoprotein gene leads to a complete absence of phospholipid from bile and to liver disease. Cell 1993; 75(3):451–462.
8. Smith AJ, Timmermans-Hereijgers JL, Roelofsen B, Wirtz KW, Van Blitterswijk WJ, Smit JJ, Schinkel AH. The human MDR3 P-glycoprotein promotes translocation of phosphatidylcholine through the plasma membrane of fibroblasts from transgenic mice. FEBS Lett 1994; 354(3):263–266.
9. Reuben A. Biliary proteins. Hepatology 1984; 4(suppl 5):46S–50S.
10. Small DM, Rapo S. Source of abnormal bile in patients with cholesterol gallstones. N Engl J Med 1970; 283:53–57.
11. Admirand WH, Small DM. The physico-chemical basis of cholesterol gallstone formation in man. J Clin Invest 1968; 47:1043–1052.
12. Carey MC, Small DM. The physical-chemistry of cholesterol solubility in bile: relationship to gallstone formation and dissolution in man. J Clin Invest 1978; 61: 998–1026.
13. Lee SP. The mechanism of mucus secretion by the gallbladder epithelium. Br J Exp Pathol 1980; 61:117–119.
14. Lee SP, Park HZ, Madani H, et al. Partial characterization of a non-micellar system of cholesterol solubilization in bile. Am J Physiol 1987; 252:G374–G383.
15. Halpern Z, Dudley MA, Kibe A, Lynn MP, Breuer AC, Holzbach RT. Rapid vesicle formation and aggregation in abnormal human biles. A time-lapse video-enhanced contrast microscopy study. Gastroenterology 1986; 90: 875–885.
16. Kibe A, Dudley MA, Halpern Z, et al. Factors affecting cholesterol monohydrate crystal nucleation time in model systems of supersaturated bile. J Lipid Res 1985; 26: 1102–1111.
17. Halpern Z, Dudley MA, Lynn MP, et al. Vesicle aggregation in model systems of bile: relation to crytal nucleation and lipid composition of the vesicular phase. J Lipid Res 1986; 27:295–306.
18. Somjen GJ, Marikovsky Y, Lelkes P, Gilat T. Cholesterol-phospholipid vesicles in human bile: an ultrastructural study. Biochim Biophys Acta 1986; 879:14–21.
19. Carey MC, Cohen DE. Biliary transport of cholesterol in vesicles, micelles, and liquid crystals. In: Paumgartner G, Stiehl A, Gerok W, eds. Bile Acids and the Liver. Lancaster: MTP Press, 1987:287–300.
20. Hirota I, Chijiiwa K, Noshiro J, Makayama F. Effect of chenodeoxycholate and ursodeoxycholate on nucleation time in human gallbladder bile. Gastroenterology 1992; 102:1668–1674.
21. Zhao XT, Schoenfiel LJ, Bonorris GG, Van de Velde RL, Marks JS. Increased cholesterol in vesicles is associated with rapid nucleation of human gallbladder bile. Hepatology 1994; 20:117A. Abstract.
22. Holzbach RT. Recent progress in understanding cholesterol crystal nucleation as a precursor to human gallstone formation. Hepatology 1986; 6:1403–1406.
23. Holzbach RT, Halpern Z, Dudley MA, et al. Biliary vesicle aggregation and cholesterol crystal nucleation: evidence for a coupled relationship. In: Paumgartner G, Stiehl A, Berok W, eds. Bile Acids and the Liver. Lancaster: MTP, 1987:301–316.
24. Little TE, Lee SP, Madani H, Kaler EW, Chinn K. Interconversions of lipid aggregates in rat and model bile. Am J Physiol 1991; 23:G70–G79.
25. Pattinson NR, Chapman BA. Distribution of biliary cholesterol between mixed micelles and nonmicelles in relation to fasting and feeding in humans. Gastroenterology 1986; 91:697–702.
26. Tierney S, Pitt HA, Lillemoe KD. Physiology and pathophysiology of gallbladder motility. Surg Clin North Am 1993; 73(6):1267–1290.
27. Fridhandler TM, Davison JS, Shaffer EA. Defective gallbladder contractility in the ground squirrel and prairie dog during the early stages of cholesterol gallstone formation. Gastroenterology 1983; 85(4):830–836.
28. Behar J, Lee KY, Thompson WR, Biancani P. Gallbladder contraction in patients with pigment and cho-

lesterol stones. Gastroenterology 1989; 97(6):1479–1484.
29. Pomeranz IS, Shaffer EA. Abnormal gallbladder emptying in a subgroup of patients with gallstones. Gastroenterology 1985; 88(3):787–791.
30. Palasciano G, Serio G, Portincasa P, Palmieri V, Fanelli M, Velardi A, Calo' Gabrieli B. Gallbladder volume in adults, and relationship to age, sex, body mass index, and gallstones: a sonographic population study. Am J Gastroenterol 1992; 87(4):493–497.
31. Kucio C, Besser P, Jonderko K. Gallbladder motor function in obese versus lean females. Eur J Clin Nutr 1988; 42(2):121–124.
32. Marzio L, Capone F, Neri M, Mezzetti A, De Angelis C, Cuccurullo F. Gallbladder kinetics in obese patients. Effect of a regular meal and low-calorie meal. Dig Dis Sci 1988; 33(1):4–9.
33. Vezina WC, Paradis RL, Grace DM, Zimmer RA, Lamont DD, Rycroft KM, King ME. Increased volume and decreased emptying of the gallbladder in large (morbidly obese, tall normal, and muscular normal) people. Gastroenterology 1990; 98(4):1000–1007.
34. Glasbrenner B, Dominguez-Munoz JE, Nelson DK, Pieramico O, Holzwarth C, Riepl RL, Malfertheiner P. Postprandial release of cholecystokinin and pancreatic polypeptide in health and in gallstone disease: relationships with gallbladder contraction [see comments]. Am J Gastroenterol 1994; 89(3):404–410.
35. Cano N, Cicero F, Ranieri F, Martin J, di-Costanzo J. Ultrasonographic study of gallbladder motility during total parental nutrition. Gastroenterology 1986; 91: 313–317.
36. Messing B, Bories C, Kuntslinger F, Benier JJ. Does total parenteral nutrition induce gallbladder sludge formation and lithiasis? Gastroenterology 1983; 84: 1012–1019.
37. Fisher RS, Koch E, Levin G. Effects of somatostatin on gallbladder emptying. Gastroenterology 1987; 92:88–90.
38. Johansson C, Kollberg B, Efendic S, Uvnaswallenstein K. Effects of graded dose of somatostain on gallbladder emptying and pancreatic enzyme output after oral glucose in man. Digestion 1981; 22:24–31.
39. Diamond JM. Transport of salt and water in rabbit and guinea pig gallbladder. J Gen Physiol 1964; 48:1–14.
40. Dietschy JM. Water and electrolyte movement across the wall of the everted rabbit gallbladder. Gastroenterology 1964; 47:395–408.
41. Wood JR, Svanvik J. Gall-bladder water and electrolyte transport and its regulation. Gut 1983; 24(6):579–593.
42. Shiffman ML, Sugerman HJ, Moore EW. Human gallbladder mucosal function: effect of concentration and acidification of bile on cholesterol and calcium solubility. Gastroenterology 1990; 99:1452–1459.
43. Van Erpecum KJ, Van Berge Henegouwen GP, Stoelwinder B, Schmidt YMG, Willekens FLH. Bile concentration is a key factor for nucleation of cholesterol crystals and cholesterol saturation index in gallbladder bile of gallstone patients. Hepatology 1990; 11:1–6.
44. Smith BF. Human gallbladder mucin binds biliary lipids and promotes cholesterol crystal nucleation in model bile. J Lipid Res 1987; 28:1088–1097.
45. Levy PF, Smith BF, LaMont JT. Human gallbladder mucin accelerates nucleation of cholesterol in artificial bile. Gastroenterology 1984; 87:270–275.
46. Gallinger S, Taylor RD, Harvey PRC, Petrunka CN, Strasberg SM. Effect of mucous glycoprotein on nucleation time of human bile. Gastroenterology 1985; 89:648–658.
47. Lee TJ, Smith BF. Bovine gallbladder mucin promotes cholesterol crystal nucleation from cholesterol transporting vesicles in supersaturated model bile. J Lipid Res 1989; 30:491–498.
48. Doty JE, Pitt HA, Kuchenbecker SL, Porter-Fink V, DenBestern LW. Role of gallbladder mucus in the pathogenesis of cholesterol gallstones. Am J Surg 1983; 145:54–61.
49. Lee SP. Hypersecretion of mucus glycoprotein by the gallbladder epithelium in experimental cholelithiasis. Pathology 1981; 134:199–207.
50. Lee SP, LaMont JT, Carey MC. The role of gallbladder mucus hypersecretion in the evolution of cholesterol gallstones: studies in the prairie dog. J Clin Invest 1981; 67:1712–1723.
51. LaMont JT, Turner BS, DiBenedetto D, Handin R, Schafer AI. Arachidonic acid stimulates mucin secretion in prairie dog gallbladder. Am J Physiol 1983; 245(1):G92–G98.
52. Smith BF, LaMont JT. Identification of gallbladder mucin-bilirubin complex in human cholesterol gallstone matrix. Effects of reducing agents on in vitro dissolution of matrix and intact gallstones. J Clin Invest 1985; 76:439–445.
53. Nunes DP, Afdhal NH, Offner GD. A recombinant bovine gallbladder mucin polypeptide binds biliary lipids and accelerates cholesterol crystal appearance time. Gastroenterology 1999; 116(4):936–942.
54. Murray FE, Smith BF. Non-mucin proteins in the matrix of human cholesterol gallstones. Scand J Gastroenterol 1991; 26(7):717–723.
55. Shimizu S, Sabsay B, Veis A, Ostrow JD, Dawes LG, Rege RV. A 12 kDa protein from cholesterol gallstones inhibits precipitation of calcium carbonate and is present in human bile [abstr]. Hepatology 1988; 8: 1257A.
56. Afdhal NH, Gary D, Niu N, Turner B, LaMont JT, Offner GD. Cholesterol cholelithiasis in the prairie dog: role of mucin and nonmucin glycoproteins. Hepatology 1993; 17:693–700.
57. Marks JW, Bonorris GG, Albers G, et al. The sequence

of biliary events preceding the formation of gallstones in humans. Gastroenterology 1992; 103:566.

58. Little TE, Madani H, Lee SP, Kaler EW. Lipid vesicle fusion induced by phospholipase C activity in model bile. J Lipid Res 1993; 34(2):211–217.
59. Luk AS, Kaler EW, Lee SP. Phospholipase C–induced aggregation and fusion of cholesterol-lecithin small unilamellar vesicles. Biochemistry 1993; 32:6965–6973.
60. Groen AK, Stout JPJ, Drapers AG, et al. Cholesterol nucleation influencing activity in T-tube bile. Hepatology 1988; 8:347.
61. Groen AK, Noordam C, Drapers JA, Egbers P, Jansen PL, Tytgat GN. Isolation of a potent cholesterol nucleation-promoting activity from human gallbladder bile: role in the pathogenesis of gallstone disease. Hepatology 1990; 11(4):525–533.
62. Harvey PRC, Upadhya GA, Strasberg SM. Immunoglobulins as nucleating proteins in the gallbladder bile of patients with cholesterol gallstones. J Biol Chem 1991; 266:1–8.
63. Holzbach RT, Kibe A, Thiel E, Howell JH, Marsh M, Hermann RE. Biliary proteins: unique inhibitors of cholesterol crystal nucleation in human gallbladder bile. J Clin Invest 1984; 73:35–45.
64. Kibe A, Holzbach RT, LaRusso NF, et al. Inhibition of cholesterol crystal formation by apolipoproteins in supersaturated model bile. Science 1984; 225:514–516.
65. Busch N, Lammert F, Matern S. Biliary secretory immunoglobulin A is a major constituent of the new group of cholesterol crystal-binding proteins. Gastroenterology 1998; 115(1):129–138.
66. Strasberg SM, Toth JL, Gallinger S, Harvey PRC. High protein and total lipid concentration are associated with reduced metastability of bile in an early stage of cholesterol gallstone formation. Gastroenterology 1990; 98: 739–746.
67. Whiting MJ, Watts J. Supersaturated bile from obese patients without gallstones supports cholesterol crystal growth but not nucleation. Gastroenterology 1984; 86(2):243–248.
68. Rome Group for Epidemiology and Prevention of Cholelithiasis (GREPCO). The epidemiology of gallstone disease in Rome, Italy. Part I. Prevalence data in men. Hepatology 1988; 8(4):904–906.
69. Huang WS. Cholelithiasis in Singapore. Gut 1970; 11: 141.
70. Sampliner RE, Bennett PH, Comers LJ, Rose FA, Burch TA. Gallbladder disease in Pima Indians. Demonstration of high prevalence and early onset by cholecystography. N Engl J Med 1970; 283:1358–1364.
71. Stitnimankarn T. The necropsy incidence of gallstones in Thailand. Am J Med Sci 1960; 240:349.
72. Einarrson K, Nilsell K, Leijd B, et al. Influence of age on secretion of cholesterol and synthesis of bile acids by the liver. N Engl J Med 1985; 313:277.
73. Rome Group for Epidemiology and Prevention of Cholelithiasis (GREPCO). The epidemiology of gallstone disease in Rome, Italy. Part II. Factors associated with the disease. Hepatology 1988; 8(4):907–913.
74. Friedman GD, Kannel WB, Dawber TR. The epidemiology of gallbladder disease: observations in the Framingham study. J Chron Dis 1966; 19:273–292.
75. Sastic JW, Glassman CI. Gallbladder disease in young women. Surg Gynecol Obstet 1982; 155(2):209–211.
76. Everson GT, McKinley C, Kern F. Mechanisms of gallstone formation in women. Effects of exogenous estrogen (Premarin) and dietary cholesterol on hepatic lipid metabolism. J Clin Invest 1991; 87:237–246.
77. Henriksson P, Einarsson K, Eriksson A, Kelter U, Angelin B. Estrogen-induced gallstone formation in males. Relation to changes in serum and biliary lipids during hormonal treatment of prostatic carcinoma. J Clin Invest 1989; 84(3):811–816.
78. Kono S, Shinchi K, Ikeda N, Yanai F, Imanishi K. Prevalence of gallstone disease in relation to smoking, alcohol use, obesity, and glucose tolerance: a study of self-defense officials in Japan. Am J Epidemiol 1992; 136(7):787–794.
79. Kono S, Kochi S, Ohyama S, Wakisaka A. Gallstones, serum lipids, and glucose tolerance among male officials of self-defense forces in Japan. Dig Dis Sci 1988; 33(7):839–844.
80. Lu SN, Chang WY, Wang LY. Risk factors for gallstone among Chinese in Taiwan. J Clin Gastroenterol 1990; 12:542–546.
81. Ruhl CE, Everhart JE. Association of diabetes, serum insulin, and C-peptide with gallbladder disease [see comments]. Hepatology 2000; 31(2):299–303.
82. Thijs C, Knipschild P, Brombacher P. Serum lipids and gallstones: a case-control study. Gastroenterology 1990; 99:843.
83. Laakso M, Suhonen M, Julkunen R, Pyorala K. Plasma insulin, serum lipids and lipoproteins in gall stone disease in non-insulin dependent diabetic subjects: a case control study [see comments]. Gut 1990; 31(3): 344–347.
84. Halpern Z, Rubin M, Harach G, Grotto I, Moser A, Dvir A, Lichtenberg D. Bile and plasma lipid composition in non-obese normolipidemic subjects with and without cholesterol gallstones. Liver 1993; 13(5):246–252.
85. Kato I, Nomura A, Stemmermann GN, Chyou PH. Prospective study of clinical gallbladder disease and its association with obesity, physical activity, and other factors. Dig Dis Sci 1992; 37(5):784–790.
86. Stampfer MJ, Maclure KM, Colditz GA, Manson JE, Willett WC. Risk of symptomatic gallstones in women with severe obesity. Am J Clin Nutr 1992; 55(3):652–658.
87. Moerman CJ, Smeets FW, Kromhout D. Dietary risk factors for clinically diagnosed gallstones in middle-

aged men. A 25-year follow-up study (the Zutphen Study). Ann Epidemiol 1994; 4(3):248–254.
88. Attili AF, Scafato E, Marchioli R, Marfisi RM, Festi D. Diet and gallstones in Italy: the cross-sectional MICOL results. Hepatology 1998; 27(6):1492–1498.
89. Misciagna G, Centonze S, Leoci C, Guerra V, Cisternino AM, Ceo R, Trevisan M. Diet, physical activity, and gallstones—a population-based, case-control study in southern Italy. Am J Clin Nutr 1999; 69(1):120–126.
90. Leitzmann MF, Giovannucci EL, Rimm EB, Stampfer MJ, Spiegelman D, Wing AL, Willett WC. The relation of physical activity to risk for symptomatic gallstone disease in men. Ann Intern Med 1998; 128:417–425.
91. Leitzmann MF, Rimm EB, Willett WC, Spiegelman D, Grodstein F, Stampfer MJ, Colditz GA. Recreational physical activity and the risk of cholecystectomy in women [see comments]. N Engl J Med 1999; 341(11):777–784.
92. Utter AC, Whitcomb DC, Nieman DC, Butterworth DE, Vermillion SS. Effects of exercise training on gallbladder function in an obese female population. Med Sci Sports Exerc 2000; 32(1):41–45.
93. Maclure KM, Hayes KC, Colditz GA, Stampfer MJ, Speizer FE, Willet WC. Weight, diet, and the risk of symptomatic gallstones in middle-aged women. N Engl J Med 1989; 321:563–569.
94. Shiffman ML, Sugerman HJ, Kellum JH, Brewer WH, Moore EW. Gallstones in patients with morbid obesity. Relationship to body weight, weight loss and gallbladder bile cholesterol solubility. Int J Obes Relat Metab Disord 1993; 17(3):153–158.
95. Acalovschi MV, Blendea D, Pascu M, Georoceanu A, Badea RI, Prelipceanu M. Risk of asymptomatic and symptomatic gallstones in moderately obese women: a longitudinal follow-up study. Am J Gastroenterol 1997; 92(1):127–131.
96. Tucker LE, Tangedahl TN, Newmark SR. Prevalence of gallstones in obese Caucasian American women. Int J Obes 1982; 6(3):247–251.
97. Thijs C, Knipschild P, Leffers P. Is gallstone disease caused by obesity or by dieting? Am J Epidemiol 1992; 135(3):274–280.
98. Palasciano G, Portincasa P, Vinciguerra V, Velardi A, Tardi S, Baldassarre G, Albano O. Gallstone prevalence and gallbladder volume in children and adolescents: an epidemiological ultrasonographic survey and relationship to body mass index. Am J Gastroenterol 1989; 84(11):1378–1382.
99. Must A, Spadano J, Coakley EH, Field AE, Colditz G, Dietz WH. The disease burden associated with overweight and obesity. JAMA 1999; 282(16):1523–1529.
100. Petitti DB, Sidney S. Obesity and cholecystectomy among women: implications for prevention. Am J Prev Med 1988; 4(6):327–330.
101. Honore LH. Cholesterol cholelithiasis in adolescent females: its connection with obesity, parity, and oral contraceptive use—a retrospective study of 31 cases. Arch Surg 1980; 115(1):62–64.
102. Weatherall R, Shaper AG. Overweight and obesity in middle-aged British men. Eur J Clin Nutr 1988; 42(3): 221–231.
103. Kodama H, Kono S, Todoroki I, Honjo S, Sakurai Y, Wakabayashi K, Nishiwaki M. Gallstone disease risk in relation to body mass index and waist-to-hip ratio in Japanese men. Int J Obes Relat Metab Disord 1999; 23(2):211–216.
104. Amaral JF, Thompson WR. Gallbladder disease in the morbidly obese. Am J Surg 1985; 149:551.
105. Calhoun R, Willbanks O. Coexistence of gallbladder disease and morbid obesity. Am J Surg 1987; 154(6): 655–658.
106. Haffner SM, Diehl AK, Stern MP, Hazuda HP. Central adiposity and gallbladder disease in Mexican Americans. Am J Epidemiol 1989; 129(3):587–595.
107. Hartz AJ, Rupley DC, Rimm AA. The association of girth measurements with disease in 32,856 women. Am J Epidemiol 1984; 119(1):71–80.
108. Moerman CJ, Berns MP, Smeets FW, Kromhout D. Regional fat distribution as risk factor for clinically diagnosed gallstones in middle-aged men: a 25-year follow-up study (the Zutphen Study). Int J Obes Relat Metab Disord 1994; 18(6):435–439.
109. Hendel HW, Hojgaard L, Andersen T, Pedersen BH, Paloheimo LI, Rehfeld JF, Gotfredsen A. Fasting gall bladder volume and lithogenicity in relation to glucose tolerance, total and intra-abdominal fat masses in obese non-diabetic subjects. Int J Obes Relat Metab Disord 1998; 22(4):294–302.
110. Nestel PJ, Schreibman PH, Ahrens EH Jr. Cholesterol metabolism in human obesity. J Clin Invest 1973; 52(10):2389–2397.
111. Nestel PJ, Whyte HM, Goodman DS. Distribution and turnover of cholesterol in humans. J Clin Invest 1969; 48(6):982–991.
112. Miettinen TA. Cholesterol production in obesity. Circulation 1971; 44(5):842–850.
113. Stamler J. Overweight, hypertension, hypercholesterolemia, and coronary heart disease. In: Mancini M, Lewis B, Contaldo F, eds. Medical Complications of Obesity. London: Academic Press, 1979: 191–216.
114. Bennion LJ, Grundy SM. Effects of obesity and caloric intake on biliary lipid metabolism in man. J Clin Invest 1975; 56:996.
115. Madura JA, Loomis RC, Harris RA, Grosfeld J, Tompkins RK. Relationship of obesity to bile lithogenicity in man. Ann Surg 1979; 189(1):106–111.
116. Angelin B, Einarsson K, Ewerth S, Leijd B. Biliary lipid composition in obesity. Scand J Gastroenterol 1981; 16(8):1015–1019.
117. Mabee TM, Meyer P, DenBesten L, Mason EE. The mechanism of increased gallstone formation in obese human subjects. Surgery 1976; 79(4):460–468.
118. Reuben A, Maton PN, Murphy GM, et al. Biliary lipid

secretion in obese and nonobese individuals with and without gallstones. Clin Sci (Colch) 1985; 69:71.

119. Salen G, Nicolau G, Shefer S, Mosbach EH. Hepatic cholesterol metabolism in patients with gallstones. Gastroenterology 1975; 69(3):676–684.

120. Ahmed HA, Jazrawi RP, Goggin PM, Dormandy J, Northfield TC. Intrahepatic biliary cholesterol and phospholipid transport in humans: effect of obesity and cholesterol cholelithiasis. J Lipid Res 1995; 36(12): 2562–2573.

121. Marcus SN, Heaton KW. Deoxycholic acid and the pathogenesis of gallstones. Gut 1988; 29:522.

122. Mok HY, Von Bergmann K, Croiuse JR, Grundy SM. Bilary lipid metabolism in obesity. Effects of bile acid feeding before and during weight reduction. Gastroenterology 1979; 76(3):556–567.

123. Einarsson K, Hellstrom K, Kallner M. Bile acid kinetics in relation to sex, serum lipids, body weights, and gallbladder disease in patients with various types of hyperlipoproteinemia. J Clin Invest 1974; 54(6):1301–1311.

124. Grundy SM, Duane WC, Adler RD, Aron JM, Metzger AL. Biliary lipid outputs in young women with cholesterol gallstones. Metabolism 1974; 23(1):67–73.

125. Caroli-Bosc FX, Pugliese P, Peten EP, Demarquay JF, Montet JC, Hastier P, Staccini P. Gallbladder volume in adults and its relationship to age, sex, body mass index, body surface area and gallstones. An epidemiologic study in a nonselected population in France. Digestion 1999; 60(4):344–348.

126. Vezina WC, Paradis RL, Grace DM, Zimmer RA, Lamont DD, Rycroft KM, King ME. Increased volume and decreased emptying of the gallbladder in large (morbidly obese, tall normal, and muscular normal) people. Gastroenterology 1990; 98:1000–1007.

127. DeWind LT, Payne JH. Intestinal bypass surgery for morbid obesity. Long-term results. JAMA 1976; 236 (20):2298–2301.

128. Delaney AG, Duerson MC, O'Leary JP. The incidence of cholelithiasis after jejunoileal bypass. Int J Obes 1980; 4(3):243–248.

129. Hocking MP, Duerson MC, O'Leary JP, Woodward ER. Jejunoileal bypass for morbid obesity. Late follow-up in 100 cases. N Engl J Med 1983; 308(17):995–999.

130. Liddle RA, Goldstein RB, Saxton J. Gallstone formation during weight-reduction dieting. Arch Intern Med 1989; 149(8):1750–1753.

131. Shiffman ML, Sugerman HJ, Kellum JM, Brewer WH, Moore EW. Gallstone formation after rapid weight loss: a prospective study in patients undergoing gastric bypass surgery for treatment of morbid obesity. Am J Gastroenterol 1991; 86:1000–1005.

132. Yang H, Petersen GM, Roth MP, Schoenfield LJ, Marks JW. Risk factors for gallstone formation during rapid loss of weight. Dig Dis Sci 1992; 37(6):912–918.

133. Kamrath RO, Plummer LJ, Sadur CN, Adler MA, Strader WJ, Young RL, Weinstein RL. Cholelithiasis in patients treated with a very-low-calorie diet. Am J Clin Nutr 1992; 56(suppl 1):255S–257S.

134. Shiffman ML, Sugerman HJ, Kellum HM, Brewer WH, Engle K, Moore EW. Gallstone formation following rapid weight loss. I Incidence of gallstone formation and relation to gallbladder (GB) bile lipid composition [abstr]. Gastroenterology 1990; 90:A262.

135. Worobetz LJ, Inglis FG, Shaffer EA. The effect of ursodeoxycholic acid therapy on gallstone formation in the morbidly obese during rapid weight loss. Am J Gastroenterol 1993; 88(10):1705–1710.

136. Syngal S, Coakley EH, Willett WC, Byers T, Williamson DF, Colditz GA. Long-term weight patterns and risk for cholecystectomy in women. Ann Intern Med 1999; 130:471–477.

137. Wise L, Stein T. The effect of jejunoileal bypass on bile composition and the formation of biliary calculi. Ann Surg 1978; 187:57–62.

138. Weinsier RL, Wilson LJ, Lee J. Medically safe rate of weight loss for the treatment of obesity: a guideline based on risk of gallstone formation. Am J Med 1995; 98(2):115–117.

139. Gebhard RL, Prigge WF, Ansel HJ. Rapid weight loss, gallbladder function and cholesterol gallstones [abstract]. Hepatology 1994; 20:267A.

140. Stone BG, Ansel HJ, Peterson FJ, Gebhard RL. Gallbladder emptying stimuli in obese and normal-weight subjects. Hepatology 1992; 15:795–798.

141. Festi D, Orsini M, Li Bassi S. Risk of gallstone formation during rapid weight loss: protective role of gallbladder motility [abstract]. Gastroenterology 1993; 102: A311.

142. Gebhard RL, Prigge WF, Ansel HJ, Schlasner L, Ketover SR, Sande D, Holtmeier K. The role of gallbladder emptying in gallstone formation during diet-induced rapid weight loss. Hepatology 1996; 24(3):544–548.

143. Andersen T. Liver and gallbladder disease before and after very-low-calorie diets. Am J Clin Nutr 1992; 56 (suppl 1):235S–239S.

144. Marks JW, Stein T, Schoenfield LJ. Natural history and treatment with ursodiol of gallstones formed during rapid loss of weight in man. Dig Dis Sci 1994; 39(9): 1981–1984.

145. Takahashi T, Yamamura T, Utsonomiya J. Pathogenesis of acute cholecystitis after gastrectomy. Br J Surg 1990; 77:536–539.

146. Bolondi L, Bortolotti M, Santi V, Gaiani S, Testa S. Gallbladder sludge formation during prolonged fasting after gastrointestinal tract surgery. Gut 1985; 26:734–738.

147. Hoy MK, Heshka S, Allison DB, Grasset E, Blank R, Abin M, Heymsfield SF. Reduced risk of liver-function-test abnormalities and new gallstone formation with weight loss on 3350-kJ (800 kcal) formula diets. Am J Clin Nutr 1994; 60:249–254.

148. Reuben A, Qureshi Y, Murphy GM, Dowling RH.

Effect of obesity and weight reduction on biliary cholesterol saturation and the response to chenodeoxycholic acid. Eur J Clin Invest 1985; 16:133–142.

149. Schlierf G, Schellenberg B, Stiehl A, Czygan P, Oster P. Biliary cholesterol saturation and weight reduction—effects of fasting and low calorie diet. Digestion 1981; 21:44–49.
150. Soorensen TIA, Brussgaard A, Pederson LR, Krag E. Lithogenic index of bile after jejunoileal bypass operation for obesity. Scand J Gastroenterol 1977; 12:449–451.
151. Shiffman ML, Sugerman JH, Kellum JM, et al. Changes in gallbladder bile composition following gallstone formation and weight reduction. Gastroenterology 1992; 103:214.
152. Shiffman ML, Shamburek RD, Schwartz CC, Sugerman HJ, Kellum JM, Moore EW. Gallbladder mucin, arachidonic acid, and bile lipids in patients who develop gallstones during weight reduction. Gastroenterology 1993; 105(4):1200–1208.
153. Freeman JB, Meyer PD, Printen KJ, Mason EE, DenBesten L. Analysis of gallbladder bile in morbid obesity. Am J Surg 1975; 129:163–166.
154. Inoue K, Fuchigama A, Higashide S, Sumi S, Kogire M, Suzuki T, Tobe T. Gallbladder sludge and stone formation in relation to contractile function after gastrectomy. Ann Surg 1992; 215:19–26.
155. Festi D, Colecchia A, Orsini M, Sangermano A, Sottili S, Simoni P, Mazzella G. Gallbladder motility and gallstone formation in obese patients following very low calorie diets. Use it (fat) to lose it (well). Int J Obes Relat Metab Disord 1998; 22(6):592–600.
156. Danzinger RG, Hofmann AF, Thistle JL, et al. Effect of oral chenodeoxycholic acid on bile acid kinetics and biliary lipid composition in women with cholelithiasis. J Clin Invest 1972; 52:2809.
157. Mazzella G, Bazzoli F, Festi D, Ronchi M, Aldini R, Roda A, Grigolo B. Comparative evaluation of chenodeoxycholic and ursodeoxycholic acids in obese patients. Effects on biliary lipid metabolism during weight maintenance and weight reduction. Gastroenterology 1991; 101(2):490–496.
158. Iser JH, Maton PN, Murphy GM, Dowling RH. Resistance to chenodeoxycholic acid (CDCA) treatment in obese patients with gall stones. BMJ 1978; 1(6126): 1509–1512.
159. Maton PN, Murphy GM, Dowling RH. Lack of response to chenodeoxycholic acid in obese and nonobese patients. Role of cholesterol synthesis and possible response to ursodeoxycholic acid. Gut 1980; 21 (12):1082–1086.
160. Whiting MJ, Hall JC, Iannos J, Roberts HG, Watts JM. The cholesterol saturation of bile and its reduction by chenodeoxycholic acid in massively obese patients. Int J Obes 1984; 8(6):681–688.
161. Zuin M, Petroni ML, Grandinetti G, Crosignani A, Bertolini E, Battezzati PM, Podda M. Comparison of effects of chenodeoxycholic and ursodeoxycholic acid and their combination on biliary lipids in obese patients with gallstones. Scand J Gastroenterol 1991; 26(3):257–262.
162. Okamoto S, Nakano K, Kosahara K, Kishinaka M, Oda H, Ichimiya H, Chijiiwa K. Effects of pravastatin and ursodeoxycholic acid on cholesterol and bile acid metabolism in patients with cholesterol gallstones. J Gastroenterol 1994; 29(1):47–55.
163. Marks JW, Bonorris GG, Schoenfield LJ. Effects of ursodiol or ibuprofen on contraction of gallbladder and bile among obese patients during weight loss. Dig Dis Sci 1996; 41(2):242–249.
164. Shiffman ML, Kaplan GD, Brinkman-Kaplan V, Vickers FF. Prophylaxis against gallstone formation with ursodeoxycholic acid in patients participating in a very-low-calorie diet program. Ann Intern Med 1995; 122:899–905.
165. Sugerman HJ, Brewer WH, Shiffman ML, Brolin RE, Fobi MA, Linner JH, MacDonald KG. A multicenter, placebo-controlled, randomized, double-blind, prospective trial of prophylactic ursodiol for the prevention of gallstone formation following gastric-bypass-induced rapid weight loss. Am J Surg 1995; 169(1):91–96. Discussion 96–97.
166. Shoheiber O, Biskupiak JE, Nash DB. Estimation of the cost savings resulting from the use of ursodiol for the prevention of gallstones in obese patients undergoing rapid weight reduction. Int J Obes Relat Metab Disord 1997; 21(11):1038–1045.
167. Broomfield PH, Chopra R, Scheinbaum RC, Bonorris GG, Silverman A, Schoenfield LJ, Marks JW. Effects of ursodeoxycholic acid and aspirin on the formation of lithogenic bile and gallstones during loss of weight. N Engl J Med 1988; 319:567–572.
168. Yamada T, ed. Atlas of Gastroenterology. 2d ed. Philadelphia: Lippincott Williams and Wilkins, 1999.

39

Obesity and Pulmonary Function

Shyam Subramanian and Kingman P. Strohl

Case Western Reserve University School of Medicine, Cleveland, Ohio, U.S.A.

I INTRODUCTION

The importance of this chapter lies in the fact that impairment of respiratory function by obesity is potentially reversible and therefore should be a focus for therapeutic intervention (1–12). This review will be composed of three parts. The first will be the description of changes in respiratory mechanics, gas exchange, and control with obesity such as physiological decrements that result in dyspnea, the increased work of breathing, and abnormalities in gas exchange that many obese individuals exhibit. The second part will include a discussion of pathophysiologic staging of respiratory impairment in obesity, using as a basis a classification system proposed by Bates (13). The third part will outline the emerging literature on sleep disordered breathing and obesity, obesity and asthma, and the syndrome of obesity hypoventilation.

II PHYSIOLOGICAL DECREMENTS WITH OBESITY

A Respiratory Compliance and the Work of Breathing

A threshold effect of obesity associated with respiratory compromise has not been defined. While most studies in this literature use a starting point of at least 120% of ideal body weight (IBW), some use different thresholds for entry—150% or 200% IBW, BMI values >30 (males) or >28 (females). The literature is too heterogeneous to combine studies or to examine the relationship of obesity to respiratory function using continuous variables for each condition. Therefore, we will discuss studies that examined categorical effects (obese vs. nonobese subjects).

Respiratory compliance is a measure that relates to the pressure changes that are required to increase lung volume and can be influenced by the mechanical properties of both the lungs and the chest wall (14–16). One major problem in obesity is that increased weight pressing on the thoracic cage and abdomen makes the chest wall stiff and noncompliant (14,15). In addition to increased adiposity around the thoracic cage, chest wall compliance may be decreased because the decreased total thoracic and pulmonary volume may pull the chest wall below its resting level to a flatter portion of its pressure-volume curve. In a study on sedated, paralyzed, postoperative morbidly obese patients, functional residual capacity (FRC) was seen to be markedly low compared to normals, and respiratory compliance was found to be low owing to significant decrease in both lung and chest wall compliance (17).

Total respiratory system resistance was also markedly increased, primarily owing to an increase in lung resistance. Oxygenation was impaired and correlated with total respiratory system compliance. $PaCO_2$ was not different between obese and lean subjects and did not relate to compliance, resistance, or FRC. The same group later compared respiratory mechanics during general anesthesia among groups of normals, overweight subjects, and obese subjects (BMI 25–40) and subjects with morbid obesity (BMI >40) (18). Increasing BMI was correlated to an exponential increase in FRC. Compliance of both the total respiratory system and the lungs decreased; in contrast, the compliance of the chest wall was only minimally affected, and the resistance of the lung and of the total respiratory system increased. Chest wall compliance falls more in obese than lean subjects in moving from the sitting to the supine or even prone position (14,19). In obese patients, prone positioning has been shown to improve pulmonary function, by increasing FRC and lung compliance during general anesthesia (20).

There is a relationship between chest wall compliance and CO_2 retention, independent of body fat. In those obese individuals with an increase in arterial $PaCO_2$ and therefore alveolar hypoventilation, chest wall compliance was one-third of normal, whereas in equally obese but eucapnic subjects, chest wall compliance was in the normal range (16). The mechanism for the differences in chest wall compliance in the two groups was not studied; the interpretation of the results centered on the role of chest wall compliance in CO_2 retention.

The lung itself may be indirectly affected by chest wall mass loading, as lung compliance in addition to chest wall compliance is decreased in some obese individuals (14,21,22). Mechanisms for increased lung stiffness include a large pulmonary blood volume and/or dependent airways, greater collapse of alveolar units and/or intrinsic alterations of the elastic characteristics of lung tissues with surface lining film modifications. Another factor would be the imposition of abdominal fat, producing a cephalad-displaced diaphragm, and restricting lung inflation and promoting recoil in expiration. Experimental mass loading of the chest wall produces dependent bronchioalveolar units with atelectasis which increases further the work of breathing (23). With both an increased lung and chest wall stiffness, in an obese individual there is an increased mechanical work of breathing as well as an oxygen cost of breathing (24,25). Work of breathing can be increased two- to threefold even in obese eucapnic individuals. Another factor contributing to this increased work of breathing is the marked increase in lung and consequently respiratory resistance (18,26).

B Abnormalities in Pulmonary Function Tests

While age and smoking play an important role in determining the rate of decline in the ventilatory capacity, it is clear that body weight is an important risk factor and one that is to be considered both epidemiologically and clinically. Obesity produces a progressively restrictive ventilatory deficit that becomes more evident as BMI is elevated. There occur decreases in the functional residual capacity, the expiratory reserve volume, and total lung capacity (TLC) in those defined as obese (>120% of IBW) (13,15,27–31). Both the forced vital capacity (FVC) and the maximal ventilatory ventilation (MVV) are reduced proportional to the rise in body weight and the decrease in respiratory compliance (13,32–34). Longitudinal analyses have found that weight or BMI gain is associated with accelerated loss of ventilatory function (35,36). In a study on obese snorers with and without sleep apnea, a significant correlation was found between the severity of the apnea-hypopnea index and reductions in expiratory flow rates and specific airway conductance (26). The DLCO is not elevated (34). No differences have been observed in spirometry results in sitting or standing position (37). However, body weight and respiratory compliance appear to account for ~60–70% of the variance in values in obese individuals, indicating that other factors act to reduce FVC and MVV in this population. Body fat deposition may have distinct impacts on ventilatory function measures. A central pattern of adiposity is typically seen in obese men, and a high waist-to-hip ratio, seen in these subjects has been shown to be inversely correlated to spirometry and static lung volumes (38). It seems that the effect of a central pattern of fat distribution is modified by age, since it was seen only in observations from men within the ages of 40 and 59 years (39).

C Gas Exchange and Respiratory Control

Obesity exerts an increased demand to maintain normal arterial PCO_2 and PO_2 levels. The work involved in moving increased body weight results in a larger CO_2 production for height in obese than in nonobese subjects; this effect is present during rest but is more evident with exercise (15,24,25). Obese subjects with increased respiratory system compliance also must work harder to eliminate CO_2 (40). Morbidly obese patients may be dedicating a disproportionately high percentage of total oxygen consumption to conduct respiratory work even during quiet breathing (41).

The majority of obese subjects exhibit an increased ventilatory drive and maintain a eucapnic state (14,27). The subset of patients with obesity-hypoventilation will be discussed in a separate section. In moderately and severely obese individuals (>190% to >200% of IBW), arterial blood gases often show hypoxemia due to a widened alveolar-to-arterial (A-a) gradient (42). The increased A-a gradient arises from a mismatch of ventilation and perfusion, i.e., relating to increased relative perfusion at the lung basis where reduced ventilation occurs due to airway closure and alveolar collapse (42–46). Obese patents who have normal or slightly reduced CO_2 levels have either increased or normal ventilatory drive from hypoxic responses.

Two other factors may contribute to inefficiencies in gas exchange. Obese individuals achieve a minute ventilation with a relatively smaller tidal volume and increased frequency, and while this pattern reduces the work of breathing, it increases the dead space and decreases alveolar ventilation at any given minute ventilation of breathing (47). A second factor is that in severely obese subjects the diaphragm may be overstretched in the supine position (48). Overstretching is a consequence of the mechanical loading by abdominal contents and places the diaphragm at a mechanical disadvantage that contributes to decreased inspiratory strength in the supine posture (48). This factor may be particularly important during sleep when postural muscle tone is decreased (32).

D Dyspnea and Exercise

A common complaint in the obese individual is dyspnea, a sense of shortness of breath on exertion or at rest (49,50). In a recent study, 60% of patients with a BMI > 28 and no comorbid conditions reported some dyspnea at rest (51). Factors that appear to correlate with increased shortness of breath include the decrease in chest wall compliance and the inefficiency of the respiratory control system (see above). The moderately obese individual, though, can sustain a level of ventilation to maintain normal levels of arterial PCO_2 and increase ventilation appropriately with exercise (52). This indicates that the metaboreceptor response to exercise can be intact, at least in moderately obese individuals.

There are three somewhat unique aspects of exercise related to obesity. The first relates to the increased ventilatory demands imposed by the increased weight of the individual. This effect is seen clearly in that ventilation for a given work load on treadmill testing is much greater than that on bicycle testing (15,52–54) and is explained by the weight borne while walking. A second effect relates to the observation that while ventilation is usually increased in relationship to oxygen consumption, in the moderately obese subject studied both at rest and with exercise, arterial oxygen levels increase on exercise with little change in PaO_2. This response is attributed to improved ventilation-perfusion matching (52), indicating that gas exchange abnormalities at rest are functional rather than structural. A third factor is the mechanical constraint on end-expiratory lung volume before and after exercise (55). The lower end-expiratory lung volume during resting breathing in the obese subject is principally due to changes in mechanical properties of the chest wall. Even in simple obesity the pressure-volume curve, while displaced, is linear above end-expiratory lung volume but, unlike normal subjects, very nonlinear below FRC (27). Furthermore, in contrast to lean individuals, obese individuals do not decrease their end-expiratory lung volume during exercise (56). Mechanisms have not been extensively studied. However, it may be that the reduction in chest wall compliance makes the chest wall harder to displace inward or that, below FRC; expiratory muscles operate more inefficiently in expiration in the obese individual. The consequence of a failure to reduce end-expiratory lung volume during exercise is a failure to place the diaphragm at a better mechanical advantage, as well as an inefficient partitioning of the work of breathing between the inspiratory and expiratory muscles (55). An impaired exercise response is seen even in mildly obese individuals and may explain dyspnea on exertion even in those with normal spirometry or gas exchange.

In summary, the metabolic consequences of obesity combined with abnormalities in motor outflow and muscle dysfunction contribute to the respiratory complaints at rest and to exercise intolerance. What is not known is how these develop over time and whether or not certain individuals are predisposed to abnormalities because of factors independent of the level of obesity or factors present as a consequence of the metabolic and cadiovascular syndromes associated with obesity.

III CATEGORIES OF RESPIRATORY COMPROMISE IN OBESITY

Bates (13) proposed that the respiratory effects of obesity be classified into three stages relating to the magnitude of obesity and clinical illness associated with obesity (see Table 1). This staging of dysfunction may have been derived from efforts to classify cardiovascular morbidity from obesity (12). We see a staging scheme as an arbitrary but convenient starting point to discuss the influence that obesity can have on respiratory pathophysiology and illness. What should be emphasized at the onset is that such a classification system serves merely to organize thinking about obesity and its effects on respiratory function and pathophysiology. Individuals will not fall neatly into each category, and the

Table 1 Classification of Obesity-Related[a] Respiratory Compromise

Stage I: Weight-to-height ratio[b] <1, normal FVC and FEV1, reduction in end-expiratory reserve volume, $PaCO_2$ at the lower limit of normal (36–40 mmHg), decrements in exercise capacity related to weight and reserve volumes, independent of conditioning.
Stage II: Weight-to-height ratio >1, impairments in lung volumes, dyspnea at exercise and at rest, increased A-a gradient, decrements in function in the supine posture, normal $PaCO_2$ (40–45 mmHg) or mild hypercapnia at rest may indicate sleep-disordered breathing.
Stage III: Stage II compromise in the presence of illness: pulmonary hypertension and right heart failure, obesity-hypoventilation syndrome, obstructive sleep apnea syndrome, and morbid obesity syndrome.

[a] >120% of ideal body weight.
[b] kg/cm.
Source: Ref. 13.

health outcome effects of an initial classification of individuals are not known with the possible exception of those with morbid obesity. Also, despite its common use in study criteria, we suspect that the distinction among mild, moderate, and severe consequences of obesity may not have, as a defining trait, a numerical value for obesity, expressed as a percent of IBW or BMI. Rather, illness is the result of interaction between sites of fat deposition, time of exposure to obesity, and other inherited or acquired traits of respiratory function or comorbid conditions such as aging or cardiovascular disease.

Patients classified as stage I (Table 1) include those who are mildly obese with a ratio of weight to height (kilograms over centimeters) <1 and body weight of ~120% of IBW. In many of these individuals lung mechanics are usually normal, airway resistance is normal, and the subdivisions of lung volume show only a small reduction in expiratory reserve (17). Arterial blood gases are usually normal at rest. Abnormalities in gas exchange may occur during sleep due to the mechanical effects of chest all loading in interaction with the reduction in postural tone in muscles of the upper airway and chest wall. Exercise tolerance may be reduced by inactivity and/or by a failure to reduce end-expiratory lung volume. Recumbency results in inefficiencies in ventilation, in vascular perfusion, and in diaphragm function.

In stage II, patients are more severely obese with a ratio of weight to height of more than stage I; these individuals are generally >150% of ideal body weight. In these individuals there are decreases in lung as well as chest wall compliance and hypoxemia due to an increasing A-a gradient. These changes are due to ventilation-perfusion mismatching. Gas exchange abnormalities can be reversed, and PaO_2 and oxygen saturation will increase after deep breaths. There is a restrictive defect with FVC and TLC <80% of predicted, and the ratio of FRC to TLC falls to ~25%. In patients with moderate obesity there is a steady decline in ventilation-perfusion ratio from apex to base in the upright posture, and airway closure is further enhanced in the supine posture. Polycythemia may be present, and more severe blood gas changes can be demonstrated during sleep due to ventilation/perfusion mismatch. In this group of patients (stage II), respiratory frequency is increased at rest, tidal volume decreased, and the respiratory drive increased with an increased response to hypoxia but a decreased response to hypercapnia. The ventilatory response to exercise can be normal even in those whose hypercapnic response is depressed. Gas exchange during sleep is impaired by increased closure of lung units and by impairment of muscle function. Apneas during sleep are increased (57), and hypercapnia may occur during sleep secondary to hypoventilation. The presence of hypercapnia during the day may be a consequence of sleep-disordered breathing (58) or coexisting illness (3) or upper-airway obstruction (59). However, sleep-disordered breathing is not accompanied by signs and symptoms of illness during the day; the degree of sleepiness resulting from sleep fragmentation is similar to that in the general population (10). In this group of patients, weight loss achieved either through behavioral modification or through jejunoileal bypass can result in improvement in all these physiological abnormalities (9,11,29,33,60). But it must be noted that many of these good results were reported for younger subjects with moderate obesity. Respiratory complications of surgery for weight loss occur more commonly in older individuals, those who are hypercapnic (perhaps as a result of sleep-disordered breathing), and those who seem to have a reduced expiratory reserve volume prior to surgery (13,32). This impression should be confirmed in longitudinal and prospective studies of outcome assessment.

Stage III or illness-defined obesity impairment includes morbid obesity with edema and cor pulmonale, the obesity-hypoventilation syndrome, and sleep apnea syndrome (both reviewed below). Patients in this category exhibit an inherent predisposition to pulmonary embolism (61,62). Pulmonary hypertension, which can be present in these patients during light exercise, may predispose these patients to inactivity, to dependent edema, and to subsequent risk for venous thrombosis (61). The effects of pulmonary emboli on the lung of an obese individual will be compounded by abnormalities in respiratory function imposed by increased weight alone (62) (see section on OHS). Another confounding factor in this classification is the relationship of respiratory morbidity to the circulatory physiology and pathophysiology of obesity (61,63).

IV SLEEP-DISORDERED BREATHING AND OBESITY

Obstructive sleep apnea (OSA) syndrome is characterized by loud snoring, episodic partial or complete obstruction of the upper airway during sleep, and consequent sleep fragmentation leading to excessive daytime sleepiness. In addition to the morbidity associated with chronic sleepiness, patients with OSA are at increased risk for hypertension, myocardial infarction, and stroke (10). The diagnosis and treatment of OSA have been reviewed elsewhere (10,64–66), although a few key points are mentioned here. When OSA is suspected clinically, the diagnosis is conventionally confirmed via polysomnography, a test in which multiple physiological variables including the electroencephalogram, electrocardiogram, and several measures of respiratory function are recorded during sleep. The most common measure of OSA severity determined in this manner is the total number of apneas (cessation of airflow of 10 sec) and hypopneas (partial obstructions) per hour of sleep (apnea + hypopnea index; AHI). However, other features in the presentation may indicate the need for a therapeutic intervention.

Population studies in the United States and several other countries suggest that the syndrome of obstructive sleep apnea, daytime sleepiness, and cardiovascular disease is present in ~1–4% of working men and women (10,67). There are pockets of higher prevalence, for instance in minority populations and children with tonsillar hypertrophy; however, one of the best-characterized associations is between obesity and OSA. The correlation between body weight and sleep apnea was so strong as to dominate recognition strategies for almost two decades and link sleep apnea almost exclusively with obesity hypoventilation or Pickwickian syndrome (64,66,68); however, in community studies the association of OSA with obesity is not as strong as in clinic-based case collections or reviews from referral centers (10,68). A brief review of this association follows, as does a more thorough account of the literature regarding mechanisms and the effect of weight reduction.

A Association Between Obesity and OSA

In clinical rather than community populations, many are at least 130% of ideal body weight (10), and obesity (expressed as BMI in kg/m^2) is the strongest predictor of AHI in subjects over age 50. Compared to the other factors studied, BMI was twice as strong as gender, and fourfold stronger than age, in predicting AHI, even when subjects with the most severe disease (AHI > 60) were excluded from analysis (69). In a polysomnographic study of 250 obese patients without sleep complaints, only 40% of the men and 3% of the women were found to have sleep apnea severe enough to warrant treatment (70).

The recent population-based study of Wisconsin state employees supports the findings of these clinic-based reports (67). In this cohort of >600 men and women between 30 and 60 years of age, an increase in BMI of 1 SD was associated with a fourfold increase in risk for OSA (defined as an AHI >5/hr). More recently, the same group reported that a weight gain of as little as 10% predicted a sixfold increase in the odds of developing moderate to severe sleep-disordered breathing. Conversely, a loss of 10% of body weight predicted a 26% decrease in the apnea-hypopnea index (71). After examining several measures of body composition and metrics related to fat deposition, neck circumference was the strongest predictor of AHI although all anthropomorphic variables were highly correlated. These and other observations suggest that an upper-body fat deposition profile, rather than a more generalized distribution of body fat, may be important for the development of sleep apnea. Given the strength of the association, defining the causal relationship between excess body weight and OSA remains surprisingly difficult. Studies of mechanisms can be grouped into one or more categories based on hypotheses involving alterations in upper-airway (UA) structure. The major theory is that obesity leads to a change in UA structure or function or alteration in respiratory drive, particularly to muscles regulating nasopharyngeal and oropharyngeal patency. Obesity even in the absence of sleep-disordered breathing can be associated with excessive daytime sleepiness (72). The same study also found that obese patients tend to underestimate their degree of sleepiness. So the recognition profiles designed to detect sleep-disordered breathing that involves sleepiness may not be as specific for OSAHS as it might be in a nonobese individual.

B Obesity and Upper-Airway Function

The major theory is that obesity leads to a change in the UA geometry, either through loading of the pharyngeal wall or by encroachment from periluminal fat deposits, placing it at increased risk of collapse due to physical forces acting on the pharyngeal segment during inspiration. Imaging studies indicate that obese patients with OSA have significant narrowing of the UA compared with nonobese controls while awake using computed tomography (73–75). These studies have demonstrated significant differences in cross-sectional area at naso-, oro-, and hypopharyngeal levels, with obese patients having smaller airways than controls. Although in some of these studies patients and controls were not matched for obesity, the finding of small retropalatal airway in OSA patients compared to weight-matched controls has been shown in additional studies (76,77). Using magnetic resonance imaging to compare obese OSA patients with weight-matched controls, fat deposition was increased at sites removed from the periluminal space, primarily in areas posterior and lateral to the oropharynx at the level of the palate, as well as within the soft palate (78,79). Differences in pharyngeal shape have also been observed between obese OSA patients and normal-weight controls (75,80). Specifically, when the pharynx was viewed in coronal section, awake OSA patients had an elliptically shaped airway channel, the long axes of which were oriented in the anteroposterior plane, while in normals the airway channel was oriented transversely. Obesity by neck fat deposition is associated with a shift in the hyoid bone caudally, possibly altering the pharyngeal patency and/or leading to greater UA collapsibility (81). Patients with OSA have been shown to have necks that are larger in circumference than those of weight-matched controls (82). Some of these features are present in nonobese individuals, and the causality of such associations can be challenged on the basis of the biochemical changes that may result from sleep hypoxemia and fragmentation (10).

Obesity-related decreases in lung volume, as discussed earlier in this chapter, may also result in greater instability of the UA, as lung volume has been directly correlated with UA size (83,84). Moreover, pharyngeal distensibility, or "compliance," has been shown to be greater in both males and females with OSA than in obesity-matched controls using the acoustic reflection technique (85,86). Similar findings were obtained when lung volume was passively altered using continuous positive airway pressure (85). Both increases in lung volume and pharyngeal volume and decreases in this measure of UA distensibility in obese sleep apneics after weight loss have been observed (87,88). Obese patients with a large neck and low FRC tend to have more collapsible velopharynx during wakefulness (89). In one study, a 17% reduction in BMI in moderately obese subjects resulted in both a decline in AHI and a 23% improvement in UA closing pressures during non-REM sleep, which indicates a specific beneficial effect of weight loss on improvement in pharyngeal function and sleep apnea (90). However, another study of weight loss found no correlation between values for UA closing pressure and obesity in patients with OSA. One possible explanation is that weight loss acts indirectly through changes in lung size rather than directly through an effect on UA mechanics. Another is a variability among people in regard to fat distribution and accumulation or susceptibility to OSA. Nevertheless, weight loss in obese individuals is one appropriate and specific therapy for OSA. However, the mechanisms explaining how obesity impairs upper airway structure may be more complex than a simple anatomic enlargement or impairment of structural stability.

V OBESITY HYPOVENTILATION SYNDROME

Most obese patients with OSA are normocapnic when awake; estimates are that 10–15% of morbidly obese patients (BMI > 35) may develop a disorder of the respiratory control system manifested by CO_2 retention during wakefulness (91). This is referred to as the obesity-hypoventilation syndrome (OHS). The term Pickwickian syndrome has also been used to describe this syndrome (92). It has been defined using ABG values of $PCO_2 > 45$ often with a $PO_2 < 55$ (93). Despite a substantial body of literature on the clinical and physiologic factors in obesity, no one mechanism explains the pathogenesis of OHS.

One factor often emphasized is the influence of an impaired ventilatory drive to both hypoxia (94) and hypercapnia (22,95). Although the data are not consistent across all studies, simple obesity may be associated with reduced awake ventilatory chemoresponsiveness, although this is based on data from a limited number of subjects (53,96). Obesity accompanied by OSA may or may not be associated with a reduction in chemoresponsiveness. In an early study, ventilatory and mouth occlusion pressure responses to CO_2 rebreathing were reduced from normals in both eucapnic and hypercapnic OSA patients (97,98), and a relative decrease in the awake ventilatory response to CO_2 in eucapnic obese OSA patients has also been documented more recently (99).

While it is assumed that obesity or body fat explains OHS, there are alternative explanations. These include genetic variations in ventilatory responses, interactions between the metabolic effects of obesity and respiratory control, and/or effects of comorbid cardiovascular or metabolic events also linked to obesity acting on respiratory control (10). Genetically obese (ob/ob) mice exhibit blunted hypercapnic response, independent of the presence of obesity; furthermore, administration of leptin seems to reverse this hypoventilation, irrespective of food intake and weight (100). These studies do make a strong case for the role of central mechanisms in the pathogenesis of obesity-hypoventilation syndrome. Two clinical studies demonstrated that dietary restriction in morbid obesity produces a depression in ventilatory responses and one could speculate that this could relate to lowered leptin levels (101,102). Another factor would be the mechanical impairment to inspiration due to either decreased respiratory system compliance (16,103) or to inspiratory muscle weakness (48). Respiratory drive requires not only activities in the brainstem but also the distribution of neuromuscular drive to the chest wall muscles such as the diaphragm and the intercostal muscles. Muscles can be compromised by fatty infiltration, and their mechanical action on ventilation influenced by abnormalities in chest wall compliance, i.e., the coupling between muscle activity and the generation of pressure for inspiration (13,27,104).

The increase in diaphragmatic electromyogram activity per unit increase in CO_2 in subjects who are morbidly obese is three to four times that found in normal subjects (105). This high value is a reflection of the need to sustain a high level of diaphragm energy expenditure to maintain adequate ventilation, a demand that must increase further with a change to the supine position (48). The reduction in this relationship is indicative of a diminished capacity to increase respiratory muscle activity to meet demands for ventilation. The morbidly obese patient will exhibit static inspiratory pressures 60–70% of normal in both upright and supine positions (14,16,48,104). Therefore, increasing EMG activity acts to move the massive chest wall rather than increase ventilation (95).

The direct effects of obesity on muscle size and function are not resolved. In a Zucker rat model of obesity in which respiratory function changes are similar to those found in human obesity, there are greater size and number of muscle fibers in the diaphragm of obese than of nonobese siblings (106). In contrast, in the obese (ob/ob) mouse model the diaphragm is thinner in obese than lean siblings (E. Schlenker, personal communication). Systematic analysis of respiratory muscle thickness and fiber types in obese individuals are not currently available. The degree of CO_2 retention correlates with decrease in inspiratory strength, decrease in vital capacity, and a decreased ability to sustain a maximal voluntary ventilation (95,105). The latter finding, i.e., an inability to sustain a level of ventilation, may indicate a degree of respiratory muscle fatigue, which contributes to the development of a chronic hypoventilation syndrome (52,107). Disordered breathing during sleep, i.e., OSA, may result in hypoventilation in the awake state (64). Both blunted chemoresponsiveness and load compensation might result from the sleep fragmentation and episodic hypoxemia that occur in OSA. Increases in the ventilatory response to added resistive loads (97) as well as a more brisk CO_2 response curve occur after treatment of OSA with nasal CPAP (108,109). These findings are interpreted to indicate that OSA may play a primary role in the blunting of respiratory responses.

Another factor contributing to hypoventilation is a pattern of breathing (high frequency and lower tidal volume) that leads to an increase in dead space ventilation. The respiratory control system determines ventilation by independent alterations in tidal volume and frequency (47), which must optimize ventilation in the face of challenges like exercise and sleep. Ventilation-perfusion ($\dot{V}/Q$) mismatch results from shallow irregular breathing combined with or without compression by a thick chest wall (110), and is especially pronounced in the lower lung zones (43).

The severity of disease is directly related to the following factors: degree of hypercarbia, degree of coexisting hypoxemia, and presence of complications such as pulmonary hypertension ± cor pulmonale, left ventricular failure, and polycythemia. Table 2 is a useful classification of severity of a hypoventilation syndrome. Patients who are in the mild category may only need periodic follow-up and enrollment in a weight loss program, while those who fall into the moderate to

Table 2 Classification of Obesity-Hypoventilation Syndrome

	Mild	Moderate	Severe
PCO_2	45–50	50–60	> 60
PO_2	> 70	60–70	< 60
Complications	Absent	Absent	Present

severe category need a detailed workup, as outlined in Table 2.

VI MANAGEMENT STRATEGIES FOR OSA AND OHS

A Clinical Studies of Weight Loss

Further evidence for a role of obesity in OSA comes from clinical studies of weight loss in patients with OSA. Some 17 studies have been reported to date, which have included a variety of weight loss methods, patient selection criteria, efficacy and outcome measures, and research designs. Surgical and nonsurgical approaches to weight reduction have been employed in patients with varying degrees of obesity and sleep apnea, and treatment follow-up has ranged from 2 to 24 months. Significant weight loss has been reported in most studies, with varying results. Improvement in sleep-disordered breathing, oxygen hemoglobin saturation sleep fragmentation, and daytime performance; related changes in UA function and to a much more limited extent airway structure have also been evaluated.

Despite this strong support for the role of obesity causal factor in OSA and the potential value of weight loss as a primary treatment intervention for obese patient with OSA, several key issues and concerns remain to be addressed. In particular, it is unclear from these studies whether a critical threshold level for weight loss exists and which patients are most likely to benefit from treatment. Also lacking is information about the relative risks and benefits associated with dietary or surgical weight reduction procedures in patients with OSA and selection of optimal treatment approaches for specific subgroup of patients. The mechanisms of treatment efficacy are also uncertain at this point. Finally, strategies for long-term maintenance of weight loss and associated improvement in OSA need to be developed and tested.

1 Dietary Weight Loss and OSA

Eight small ($n < 30$) uncontrolled studies of dietary weight loss ranging from 25% to 50% of baseline weight yielded mean 30–75% reductions in indices of sleep-disordered breathing (87,111–117). Two controlled dietary weight loss studies found mean weight losses of 9–17% yielded mean AHI decreases of 47% and 61%, respectively (90,118). Two small ($n < 55$) longitudinal studies of SDB change in patients with sleep apnea found no statistically significant correlations between change in AHI and change in BMI (81,119).

Major issues remaining to be addressed in more detail and/or in less selective populations are: (1) the amount of weight needed to achieve significant improvements in both OSA and daytime somnolence; (2) associated structural or functional changes in the upper airway; and (3) maintenance of weight loss beyond the traditional 6 to 12-month observation period. Evidence from other sources suggests that relapse after 1 year is to be expected following weight loss by most methods (120,121).

A brief review of some studies can provide some insight into the level of current understanding. If weight loss treatment consists solely of instructions to reduce caloric intake and no special diets, medications, or behavior modification techniques are provided, there can occur an approximate 10-kg weight loss in the treatment group, associated with a significant decline in mean AHI from 55 to 30 events/hr (90) and improvements can be observed in mean and maximum nocturnal SaO_2 and improvements in sleep quality and daytime alertness. In contrast to the "treatment" group ($n = 15$), no changes were observed in weight, AHI, or nocturnal arterial oxygen saturation in the "control" group ($n = 8$). A significant association was observed between the amount of weight loss achieved and improvement in mean fall in SaO_2 during sleep ($r = 0.69$, $p < 0.01$). In this study, while there was a trend in the direction of a lower AHI with weight loss, in other studies where weight loss is more significant there may occur an improvement in upper airway function and a reduction in OSA in non-REM as well as in REM sleep (118).

The effects of very-low-calorie diets (VLCD) on weight loss and sleep-disordered breathing have been investigated (112,114–116), with similar variability in both the amount of weight loss achieved and the improvement in OSA. In one study (112) it was noted that the effects of weight loss might be attenuated as there was detected a substantial degree of otorhinolaryngeal pathology (e.g., tonsillar hypertrophy, tongue enlargement) (115). Accounting for common upper airway problems, independent of the effect of fat accumulation, would be important in subsequent studies of weight loss using either dietary or surgical interventions. Unfortunately, none of these studies has systematically compared VLCD with more conventional forms of dietary weight loss in patients with OSA.

Finally, a combination of dietary intervention and cognitive behavioral therapy on weight loss, sleep apnea, and hypertension has been reported (113). Following an intensive, 20-week program of dietary intervention, exercise training, and cognitive-behavioral therapy, a mean weight loss of 27 kg was achieved. This was associated with a significant change in AHI (mean decrease = 17 events/hr in seven patients) and improvements in blood pressure, vital capacity, and functional residual capacity. Additionally, a significant decrease in soft palate width has been observed following weight loss. Major weaknesses of the study were the small number of patients, the absence of EEG monitoring of sleep and assessments of daytime alertness, the concomitant use of antihypertensive and other medications, and lack of follow-up evaluation.

2 Anorexiant Drugs

Drug therapy, like other nonsurgical modalities, is accompanied by only a modest (10%) weight reduction and requires continued use to maintain this result. There is a paucity of experience with anorexiants in obese OSA patients. Though it showed initial promise in the long-term treatment of obesity (122), fenfluramine and phenteramine fell out of favor because of the risk for valvular heart disease (123,124) and have subsequently been withdrawn from the market. Newer agents include orlistat, an inhibitor of pancreatic and intestinal lipase, which prevents fat absorption from the gut, and sibutramine, a selective serotonin and norepinephrine reuptake inhibitor, which decreases food intake and increases thermogenesis. Although these agents could help in the medical management of obese patients with sleep-disordered breathing, neither agent has yet been studied in this population in a controlled setting.

3 Surgically Induced Weight Loss and OSA

Surgery directed at reducing obesity appears to have a substantial and consistent trend toward improvements in respiratory symptoms and in some cases respiratory function with weight loss. The Swedish Obese Subjects study randomized >2000 patients to either surgery or conventional treatment arms. The surgically treated group displayed a mean weight loss of 23% compared with the control group in whom the weight remained stable, and this was associated with improvements in dyspnea and reductions in witnessed apnea. In a study on 21 morbidly obese patients undergoing vertical-banded gastroplasty, BMI decreased from a mean of 41.5 preop to 31.7 six months after surgery, and was associated with a significant increase in FVC, TLC, FRC, and a significant improvement in inspiratory muscle endurance assessed by PmPeak/Pimax (125); there was a strong correlation between the degree of weight loss and improvement in respiratory muscle endurance.

Dixon et al. (126) evaluated >300 patients with questionnaires pre- and postsurgery, and found that mean reductions of 48% of baseline weight resulted in a reduction in daytime sleepiness from 39% to 2%, and habitual snoring from 82% to 14%. None of the studies had polysomnographic confirmations of sleep architecture. Several studies have observed marked changes in nocturnal Sao2, and sleep continuing and architecture allowing surgical weight loss interventions. In the first case series (60) jejunoileal bypass surgery in four morbidly obese individuals (mean of 231.0 kg) produced a reduction in mean weight to 123 kg associated with a dramatic decrease in sleep-disordered breathing at 2 years from 78 to 1.4 events per hour. However, one subject died following surgery and was not included in the data analysis, and no long-term follow-up data are provided.

In morbidly obese patients receiving gastric bypass surgery two studies reported similar changes in both the amount of weight loss achieved and associated improvements in OSA and sleep architecture (127,128). Studies were lacking in a detailed description of postsurgical complications or longer-term assessment of treatment outcome.

Sugerman and coworkers (129) emphasized the role of gastric bypass surgery in the management of obesity-hypoventilation, as defined by $PaCO_2 > 45$ mm Hg. Those with significant OSA and apnea-induced arrhythmias also received tracheotomies at the time of gastric surgery. Based on preoperative polysomnography, 10 patients had obesity-hypoventilation syndrome, nine had OSA, and 19 had both. Of these, two died shortly after surgery, and an additional four patients were lost to follow-up. Follow-up studies performed at 3–5 months postsurgery revealed significant weight loss (a 62% reduction in excess body weight) associated with improvements in both OSA and daytime somnolence, as reported subjectively. Percent apnea time (total duration of apneas/total sleep time × 100) declined from a baseline of 44% to 8% following surgery. Unfortunately, no data were provided regarding arterial blood gases, sleep architecture, AHI, or nocturnal SaO_2 before or after surgery. As in the previous studies, these authors also failed to provide long-term assessment of surgical weight loss changes in OSA.

Vertical-banded gastroplasty was reported in morbidly obese patients (BMI >40) with a wide range of symptoms and degrees of OSA (111). Among patients with OSA there was a 30–38% reduction in BMI postsurgery, and a decline in respiratory events during sleep from 85% to 100%. Eight OSA patients were followed and results collected while on dietary management alone, and reductions in BMI were less dramatic; one patient with the greatest amount of weight loss (33% decrease in BMI) was cured of his OSA, and two additional patients showed improvement (i.e., > 50% reduction) in sleep-disordered breathing. Duration of follow-up for either group was not specified.

Overall, impressive results have been observed in terms of weight loss, respiratory function, improvements in sleep quality, and reductions in sleep-disordered breathing. The studies are limited in scope and design and, as a series of case reports, represent a low level of evidence (Sackett level V) for efficacy of a therapeutic intervention (130). Methodological differences have been noted in each of the studies reviewed, including lack of controls for the effects of surgery or other forms of medical intervention, nor have the mechanisms of action been investigated. Insufficient data are provided regarding the risks and benefits associated with surgical weight loss for OSA, although a significant rate of postsurgical complications is to be expected (131). Finally, none of the studies to date has included assessment of waking performance following treatment including such features as arterial blood gases or changes in vigilance as a result of weight loss, nor has adequate long-term assessment of treatment effects been conducted in terms of either weight loss or improvements in sleep and sleep-disordered breathing (132).

B Adjunct Treatments to Weight Loss

1 Noninvasive Ventilation

Initially described by Sullivan et al. in 1981, application of positive airway pressure via a mask (nasal or full face) will restore upper airway patency and probably helps maintain lower airway patency during sleep in obese patients with OSA (133). It has been suggested that in patients with OSA who have OHS nasal CPAP on its own may be insufficient to suppress apneas and correct hypoxemias, particularly during REM sleep. The use of supplemental oxygen or preferably bilevel ventilation has been advocated. For some patients bilevel ventilation may be more comfortable than CPAP because the patient exhales against a lower mask pressure. Also, use of bilevel ventilation has been shown to result in unloading of the diaphragm in grossly obese subjects (134). Successful treatment depends on patient compliance. Studies have shown a reported compliance rate of 65–90% (135–137).

2 Medications

a. Improve Respiratory Drive

Acetazolamide at a dose of 250–500 mg/d will enhance respiratory drive by producing a metabolic acidosis through inhibition of renal tubular H secretion, by producing cerebral vasodilatation, and by direct stimulation of carotid afferents (138,139). Worsening of obstructive apneas was found in another study (140). The most notable side effects are paresthesias and hypokalemia. It may have a role in the treatment of subgroup of patients with periodic breathing or central sleep apnea (141).

Medroxyprogesterone (MPA) acts as a respiratory stimulant. Strohl et al. showed it to be effective in the reduction of apneas in four of nine patients (142). Those who responded had $PaCO_2$ >46 during wakefulness as compared to those who did not respond. MPA does not appear to work in patients with OSA who do not have hypercapnea (143). Side effects include impotence and feminizing effects. Its role is primarily in females with OHS, and it is given at 60–120 mg/d in divided doses.

Theophylline has been shown to be useful for central apnea and periodic breathing, particularly in patients with heart failure. It does not appear to be helpful for OSA, although the number of patients with OSA examined is limited (141,144,145). Its primary drawback is sleep disruption.

b. Management of Daytime Sleepiness

Some studies have examined the role of modafinil in treatment of excess daytime sleepiness in obese patients with OSA. The data, while limited, suggest that modafinil may improve some aspects of alertness in patients with SAHS who remain sleepy during CPAP therapy (146,147).

3 Tracheotomy

Indications include failure of/inability to tolerate medical measures and severe cor pulmonale or serious nocturnal arrhythmias (129). The morbidities, including risks of tracheal stenosis, infection and psychosocial problems, preclude its widespread use. Because these patients have large necks, special tracheotomy techniques are reported, including several skin-flap methods (148) that allow improved and easier stoma care.

4 Treatment of Coexisting Pathology

As re-viewed elsewhere (*Chaps.*), the probability of finding coexisting cardiovascular disease in obese individuals is quite high. Identification and management of congestive heart failure and other causes for edema are likely to improve respiratory function including UA patency. Patients with obesity-hypoventilation tend to retain large volumes of fluid, which further worsens their respiratory mechanics, leading to a vicious cycle. Patients in fluid overload and cor pulmonale should be aggressively diuresed. Care should be taken to avoid excessive metabolic alkalosis by the judicious use of acetazolamide. Identification of upper airway processes like tonsillar enlargement or nasal obstruction are also important (115).

5 Supplemental Oxygen

In severe cases, marked daytime hypoxemia may persist despite of the above measures. These patients need conventional long-term O_2 therapy (> 18 hr/d) in addition to nasal CPAP or BiPAP to halt the progression of PH.

VII OBESITY AND ASTHMA

An association between increase in BMI and asthma has been found in several studies (149). This association seems to be stronger in women. The increasing prevalence of obesity in developed nations may help explain concomitant increases in asthma prevalence. Although individuals with asthma may gain weight as a result of activity limitations, the relationship between BMI and risk of developing asthma is not known.

A Epidemiological Studies

There have been many studies with varied design done in recent years in different age groups, in different parts of the world. These are summarized below.

1 Studies in Adults

In a prospective study looking at factors influencing the rate of decline of ventilatory capacity in a cohort of 181 automobile workers, decrements in the FEV1 in subjects <35 years old were influenced as much by excessive weight gain as by cigarette smoking. Loss of weight in those significantly overweight was frequently associated with improved lung function (150). In another prospective cohort study of female U.S. registered nurses [85,911 participants, aged 26–46 years) between 1991 and 1995, 1596 incident cases of asthma were identified on the basis of self-report of physician-diagnosed asthma. The relative risks of asthma for six increasing categories of BMI in 1991 were 0.9, 1.0, 1.1, 1.6, 1.7, and 2.7 (P for trend <.0001). Women who gained weight after age 18 were at significantly increased risk of developing asthma during the 4-year follow-up period (151). Chen found a 5% prevalence of self-reported asthma in 17,605 subjects aged 12 years or more who participated in the National Population Health Survey in 1994–95. He found that the prevalence of asthma increased with increasing body mass index in females, but not in males (35). Another study looked into the relationship between asthma medication and body weight in an adult Swedish population (n = 17,912). While no significant risk for developing obesity on asthma medication was seen, compared to patients with pharmacologically untreated asthma, they found significantly higher adjusted odds for asthma, in women (OR = 2.74) but not in men (OR = 1.57) with BMI ≥ 30 (152).

In a baseline survey of the Australian Longitudinal Study on Women's Health (n = 14,779), women in the highest BMI category (> or = 30) were found more likely to report asthma (153). Data from the British Cohort Study (BCS70) showed that the prevalence of asthma increased with increasing adult BMI, with a stronger association in women; odds ratios for overweight and obese women were 1.51 and 1.84, respectively. Similar associations with birth weight and adult BMI were present for wheeze but not for hay fever or eczema (154). Another British study, looking at pooled data from 1971 white males, found that severe obesity was a significant risk factor for recent asthma (OR 2.04), wheeze in the previous 12 months (OR 2.6), and asthma medication use in the previous 12 months (OR 2.83), but not for AHR (OR 0.87). FEV1 and FVC were significantly reduced in the group with severe obesity, but FEV1/FVC ratio, peak expiratory flow (PEF) and mid forced expiratory flow were not different from the group with normal BMI. This study suggested that although subjects with severe obesity reported more wheeze and shortness of breath, which may suggest a diagnosis of asthma, their levels of atopy, airway hyperresponsiveness, and airway obstruction did not support the suggestion of a higher prevalence of asthma in this group (155).

2 Studies in the Pediatric Age Group

Multiple population-based studies across different continents have found a strong association between self-reported asthma and obesity in the pediatric population (156–159). This association seems to be stronger among girls (156–158). In a study looking at ED visits in children aged 4–9 years seen with asthma, Belamarich found that in the 9 months after baseline assessment, the obese group had a higher mean number of days of wheeze per 2-week period, and a greater proportion of obese individuals had unscheduled ED visits (160). In a prospective, longitudinal, open-label clinical trial, four groups of children from 8 to 16 years old were studied. Group 1 had 15 asthmatic nonobese children. Group 2 had 15 asthmatic obese children. Group 3 had 15 nonasthmatic obese children. The nonasthmatic obese children had a significant decrease in FEV1; meanwhile, the asthmatic obese children had a deeper decrease in FEV1 than the asthmatic nonobese children. Thus, obesity was seen to be a conditioning factor for bronchial hyperreactivity to the exercise (161). In a review of medical records from a urban community health center there were significantly more children with asthma (30.6%) who were very obese (≥95th BMI percentile) compared with controls (11.6%); the difference was significant for both sexes (162). Gokbel et al. found that pulmonary function changes after the exercise had a significant negative correlation with BMI and subscapular and biceps skinfolds (163). A similar study in children 6–10 years old demonstrated that significantly greater frequency and degree of bronchospasm of the smaller airways occur in obese children was partially related to the amount of subcutaneous fat (164).

B Mechanisms

Possible mechanisms include progressive reductions in airway caliber as a result of chest wall restriction, increased airway resistance, and impairments in small airways function. Obesity predisposes to gastroesophageal reflux disease, an important risk factor for adult-onset asthma. It has also been postulated that the lower tidal volume of obese patients may result in less tidal stretching of airways smooth muscle and could promote airway narrowing and possibly airway hyperreactivity (165).

C Effects of Weight Loss on Asthma

Five studies have all shown a consistent and significant benefit in asthma control in obese asthmatics. Thirty-two patients presenting for LAGB were found to have asthma preoperatively. On follow-up their mean BMI decreased to 32.9 kg/m^2 from 45.7 kg/m^2 prior to operation. All 32 patients recorded a lower asthma score postoperatively. There were significant improvements in all aspects of asthma assessed. These included severity, daily impact, medications needed, hospitalization, sleep, and exercise. The mean preoperative scaled asthma score fell from a mean of 44.5 to 14.3 (126). Hakala measured the effects of weight reduction on peak expiratory flow (PEF) variability and airways obstruction, compared to simultaneous changes in lung volumes and ventilatory mechanics in 14 obese patients with stable asthma (166). The patients were studied before and after a very low calorie diet period of 8 weeks. As patients decreased their BMI from a mean of 37.2 to 32.1, diurnal PEF variation declined from 5.5% to 4.5%, and day-to-day variation declined from 5.3% to 3.1%. The mean morning PEF, FEV1, and FVC increased after weight loss. Functional residual capacity and expiratory reserve volume were significantly higher after weight loss. A significant reduction in R(AW) was found. In another study, 157 severely obese patients underwent silastic ring gastric bypass and were followed for a median 2.5 years. Median preoperative BMI was 45, and decreased significantly to 28 at 2 years post-SRGBP. Before surgery 34 patients were being treated for asthma. Withdrawal of all asthma medication was achieved after surgery in 17 of these patients (167). Similar results were seen in a series of 62 patients undergoing bariatric surgery. Postoperative use of medications for asthma was reduced by 100% (168). In a case-controlled study of 38 obese patients with asthma (BMI kg/m^2 30–42), a supervised weight reduction program including 8-week very low energy diet resulted in a mean loss of 14.5% of their pretreatment weight, and 11.3% after 1 year. Controls had a weight loss of 0.2% at 8 weeks and a gain of 2.2% after 1 year. After the 8-week dieting period the difference in changes in FEV1 percentage from baseline in the treatment and control groups was 7.2%, in FVC was 8.6%, with a 13-mm difference in dyspnea on a visual analog score. These differences were still significant after 1 year. The reduction of rescue medication was 1.2 and 0.1 doses, respectively. The median number of exacerbations in the treatment group was 1 (0–4) and in the controls 4 (0–7) (169).

These data, while supportive, are by no means definitive of a causative basis for obesity in asthma. Management of asthma in obese patients is made difficult by the fact that use of systemic steroids is associated with significant weight gain. Also, smoking cessation frequently causes increased weight gain, which negatively impacts on smoking cessation efforts.

VIII SUMMARY AND CONCLUSIONS

Obesity impairs respiratory structure and function, leading to physiological and pathophysiological impairments. The degree to which increased fat deposition

Table 3 Areas of Needed Research

Epidemiology/Physiology: Sharply defined epidemiological work to capture the intermediate phenotypes for obesity that confer risk for ventilatory impairment and sleep-disordered breathing. Examine interactions between risk factors for sleep apnea (craniofacial anatomy, hormonal status, ventilatory responsiveness, and family history) and obesity. Identify population and clinical subgroups at greatest risk for adverse clinical outcomes from obesity, including those defined by race, gender, or age. The genetic epidemiology of obesity and respiratory lung function, ventilatory control, and gas exchange.
Pathophysiology: Determine if sleep and sleep interruption impact on performance, eating behavior, and growth, particularly in obese school-age children. Describe the various outcomes and independence of interactions between obesity and sleep apnea on daytime performance and cardiovascular risk. Determine the basis for interactions among obesity and age in regard to upper-airway function in sleep apnea.
Treatment: Determine the impact of interventions for obesity on ventilatory function and breathing during sleep, particularly during a preclinical phase (stage I). Compare effectiveness of behavioral interventions for nonapneic and apneic individuals. Estimate the extent of medical care utilization, health care costs, and measures of quality of life.

affects respiratory function may vary according to age, length of the obese condition, comorbidity, and other individual traits, including those related to chemoresponsiveness, load compensation, and sleep-induced alterations in respiratory drive. The influence of obesity on pharyngeal function and the appearance of OSA appears related not only to BMI, but to measures of central obesity and neck size. How neck size is determined and related to other well-studied obese phenotypes remains to be determined by longitudinal studies or by cross-sectional studies in established cohorts being examined for obesity or diabetes. Also needed are outcome-based studies of the impact on obesity on cardiorespiratory morbidity with surgery and with the development of OSA. The classification presented in this chapter is intended to encourage thought and debate in this area. Obesity appears an important variable to examine in regard to respiratory health given that most studies involving weight loss show significant improvement or frank reversal of abnormalities in ventilatory control, respiratory mechanics, and illness like OSA and obesity-hypoventilation syndrome, which suggests that modafinil may improve some aspects of alertness in patients with SAHS who remain sleepy during CPAP therapy. Effective therapy for achieving weight loss would address perhaps half of the current patients diagnosed with OSA syndrome and could play a role in the prevention of OSA. The therapeutic avenues opened by molecular mechanisms for obesity and the obese phenotype will be particularly relevant to understanding sleep-disordered breathing in obesity.

There are gaps in our knowledge; some areas for further research are listed in Table 3. Studies have involved rather small groups of subjects, and the relationship between obesity and respiratory function has been handled by categorical analyses, whereas it is our suspicion that examination of measures of obesity and measures of respiratory function during wakefulness and sleep as continuous variables might disclose new interactions, potentially important not only for therapy but also for public health.

REFERENCES

1. Council on Scientific Affairs. Treatment of obesity in adults. JAMA 1988; 260(17):2547–2551.
2. Allison DB, et al. Annual deaths attributable to obesity in the United States. JAMA 1999; 282(16):1530–1538.
3. Pi-Sunyer FX. Health implications of obesity. Am J Clin Nutr 1991; 53(suppl 6):1595S–1603S.
4. Stunkard AJ. Current views on obesity. Am J Med 1996; 100(2):230–236.
5. Flegal KM, et al. Overweight and obesity in the United States: prevalence and trends 1960–1994. Int J Obes Relat Metab Disord 1998; 22(1):39–47.
6. Redline S, et al. Studies in the genetics of obstructive sleep apnea. Familial aggregation of symptoms associated with sleep-related breathing disturbances. Am Rev Respir Dis 1992; 145(2 pt 1):440–444.
7. Pillar G, Lavie P. Assessment of the role of inheritance in sleep apnea syndrome. Am J Respir Crit Care Med 1995; 151(3 pt 1):688–691.
8. Sims EA. Mechanisms of hypertension in the syndromes of obesity. Int J Obes 1981; 54(suppl 1):9–18.
9. Strohl KP, et al. Biochemical morbidity in sleep apnea. Ear Nose Throat J 1993; 72(1):34, 39–41.
10. Strohl KP, Redline S. Recognition of obstructive sleep apnea. Am J Respir Crit Care Med 1996; 154(2 pt 1): 279–289.
11. Luce JM. Respiratory complications of obesity. Chest 1980; 78(4):626–631.
12. Bjorntorp P. Classification of obese patients and complications related to the distribution of surplus fat. Am J Clin Nutr 1987; 45(suppl 5):1120–1125.
13. Bates D. Respiratory Function in Disease. 3rd ed. Philadelphia: W.B. Saunders, 1989.

14. Sharp JT, Barrocas M, Chokroverty S. The cardiorespiratory effects of obesity. Clin Chest Med 1980; 1(1): 103–118.
15. Ray CS, et al. Effects of obesity on respiratory function. Am Rev Respir Dis 1983; 128(3):501–506.
16. Naimark A, CR. Compliance of the respiratory system in health and obesity. J Appl Physiol 1960; 15:377–382.
17. Pelosi P, et al. Total respiratory system, lung, and chest wall mechanics in sedated-paralyzed postoperative morbidly obese patients. Chest 1996; 109(1):144–151.
18. Pelosi P, et al. The effects of body mass on lung volumes, respiratory mechanics, and gas exchange during general anesthesia. Anesth Analg 1998; 87(3):654–660.
19. Suratt PM, et al. Compliance of chest wall in obese subjects. J Appl Physiol 1984; 57(2):403–407.
20. Pelosi P, et al. Prone positioning improves pulmonary function in obese patients during general anesthesia. Anesth Analg 1996; 83(3):578–583.
21. Douglas FG, Chong PY. Influence of obesity on peripheral airways patency. J Appl Physiol 1972; 33(5): 559–563.
22. Rochester DF, Enson Y. Current concepts in the pathogenesis of the obesity-hypoventilation syndrome. Mechanical and circulatory factors. Am J Med 1974; 57(3):402–420.
23. Sharp JT, HJ, Sweany SK, Meadows WR, Pietras RJ. Effects of mass loading the respiratory system in man. J Appl Physiol 1964; 19:959–966.
24. Dempsey JA, et al. Work capacity determinants and physiologic cost of weight-supported work in obesity. J Appl Physiol 1966; 21(6):1815–1820.
25. Sharp JT, HJ, Sweany SK, Meadows WR, Pietras RJ. The total work of breathing in normal and obese men. J Clin Invest 1964; 43:728–739.
26. Zerah F, et al. Effects of obesity on respiratory resistance. Chest 1993; 103(5):1470–1476.
27. Sharp J. The chest wall and respiratory muscles in obesity, pregnancy and ascites. In: Roussos C, Macklem PT, eds. The Thorax. New York: Marcel Dekker, 1985:999–1021.
28. Barlett HL, Buskirk ER. Body composition and the expiratory reserve volume in lean and obese men and women. Int J Obes 1983; 7(4):339–343.
29. Jacobsen E, Dano P, Skovsted P. Respiratory function before and after weight loss following intestinal shunt operation for obesity. Scand J Respir Dis 1974; 55(6):332–339.
30. Reichel G. Lung volumes, mechanics of breathing and changes in arterial blood gases in obese patients and in Pickwickian syndrome. Bull Physiopathol Respir (Nancy) 1972; 8(5):1011–1020.
31. Stalnecker MC, Suratt PM, Chandler JG. Changes in respiratory function following small bowel bypass for obesity. Surgery 1980; 87(6):645–651.
32. Rocehster DF. Respiratory failure from obesity. In: Mancini M, Contaldo F, eds. Medical Complications of Obesity. New York: Academic Press, 1980:183–190.
33. Farebrother MJ, McHardy GJ, Munro JF. Relation between pulmonary gas exchange and closing volume before and after substantial weight loss in obese subjects. BMJ 1974; 3(927):391–393.
34. Biring MS, et al. Pulmonary physiologic changes of morbid obesity. Am J Med Sci 1999; 318(5):293–297.
35. Chen Y, et al. Increased effects of smoking and obesity on asthma among female Canadians: the National Population Health Survey, 1994–1995. Am J Epidemiol 1999; 150(3):255–262.
36. Dontas AS, et al. Longitudinal versus cross-sectional vital capacity changes and effecting factors. J Gerontol 1984; 39(4):430–438.
37. Gudmundsson G, Cerveny M, Shasby DM. Spirometric values in obese individuals. Effects of body position. Am J Respir Crit Care Med 1997; 156(3 pt 1):998–999.
38. Collins LC, et al. The effect of body fat distribution on pulmonary function tests. Chest 1995; 107(5):1298–1302.
39. Lazarus R, Sparrow D, Weiss ST. Effects of obesity and fat distribution on ventilatory function: the normative aging study. Chest 1997; 111(4):891–898.
40. Sampson MG, Grassino AE. Load compensation in obese patients during quiet tidal breathing. J Appl Physiol 1983; 55(4):1269–1276.
41. Kress JP, et al. The impact of morbid obesity on oxygen cost of breathing (VO(2RESP)) at rest. Am J Respir Crit Care Med 1999; 160(3):883–886.
42. Rorvik S, Bo G. Lung volumes and arterial blood gases in obesity. Scand J Respir Dis Suppl 1976; 95:60–64.
43. Holley HS, et al. Regional distribution of pulmonary ventilation and perfusion in obesity. J Clin Invest 1967; 46(4):475–481.
44. Partridge MR, Ciofetta G, Hughes JM. Topography of ventilation-perfusion ratios in obesity. Bull Eur Physiopathol Respir 1978; 14(6):765–773.
45. Hurewitz AN, Susskind H, Harold WH. Obesity alters regional ventilation in lateral decubitus position. J Appl Physiol 1985; 59(3):774–783.
46. Demedts M. Regional distribution of lung volumes and of gas inspired at residual volume: influence of age, body weight and posture. Bull Eur Physiopathol Respir 1980; 16(3):271–285.
47. Milic-Emili J, Grunstein MM. Drive and timing components of ventilation. Chest 1976; 70(Suppl 1):131–133.
48. Sharp JT, Druz WS, Kondragunta VR. Diaphragmatic responses to body position changes in obese patients with obstructive sleep apnea. Am Rev Respir Dis 1986; 133(1):32–37.
49. American Thoracic Society. Evaluation of impairment/disability secondary to respiratory disorders. Am Rev Respir Dis 1986; 133(6):1205–1209.

50. Sjostrom LV. Mortality of severely obese subjects. Am J Clin Nutr 1992; 55(suppl 2):516S–523S.
51. Sahebjami H. Dyspnea in obese healthy men. Chest 1998; 114(5):1373–1377.
52. Beck KC, BT, Staats BA, Hyatt RE. Dynamics of breathing in exercise. In: Whipp BJ, ed. Exercise: Pulmonary Physiology and Pathophysiology. New York: Marcel Dekker, 1991:67–97.
53. Burki NK, Baker RW. Ventilatory regulation in eucapnic morbid obesity. Am Rev Respir Dis 1984; 129(4): 538–543.
54. Freyschuss U, Melcher A. Exercise energy expenditure in extreme obesity: influence of ergometry type and weight loss. Scand J Clin Lab Invest 1978; 38(8):753–759.
55. Martin JG. The thorax and control of functional residual capacity. In: Roussos C, Macklem PT, eds. The Thorax. New York: Marcel Dekker, 1985:899–921.
56. Babb TG, Buskirk ER, Hodgson JL. Exercise end-expiratory lung volumes in lean and moderately obese women. Int J Obes 1989; 13(1):11–19.
57. Block AJ, et al. Sleep apnea, hypopnea and oxygen desaturation in normal subjects. A strong male predominance. N Engl J Med 1979; 300(10):513–517.
58. Harman E, et al. Sleep-disordered breathing and oxygen desaturation in obese patients. Chest 1981; 79(3): 256–260.
59. Licht JR, Smith WR, Glauser RL. Tonsillar hypertrophy in an adult with obesity-hypoventilation syndrome. The use of the flow-volume loop. Chest 1976; 70(5):672–674.
60. Harman EM, Wynne JW, Block AJ. The effect of weight loss on sleep-disordered breathing and oxygen desaturation in morbidly obese men. Chest 1982; 82(3): 291–294.
61. Pi-Sunyer FX. Medical hazards of obesity. Ann Intern Med 1993; 119(7 pt 2):655–660.
62. Miller A, Granada M. In-hospital mortality in the Pickwickian syndrome. Am J Med 1974; 56(2):144–150.
63. Higgins M, et al. Benefits and adverse effects of weight loss. Observations from the Framingham Study. Ann Intern Med 1993; 119(7 pt 2):758–763.
64. Gastaut H, Tassinari CA, Duron B. Polygraphic study of the episodic diurnal and nocturnal (hypnic and respiratory) manifestations of the Pickwick syndrome. Brain Res 1966; 1(2):167–186.
65. Strohl KP, Cherniack NS, Gothe B. Physiologic basis of therapy for sleep apnea. Am Rev Respir Dis 1986; 134(4):791–802.
66. Strollo PJ, Rogers RM. Obstructive sleep apnea. N Engl J Med 1996; 334(2):99–104.
67. Young T, et al. The occurrence of sleep-disordered breathing among middle-aged adults. N Engl J Med 1993; 328(17):1230–1235.
68. Blondal T, Torebjork E. Hypersomnia and periodic breathing. Report of a case and review of the literature. Scand J Respir Dis 1977; 58(5):273–278.
69. Bliwise DL, et al. Risk factors for sleep disordered breathing in heterogeneous geriatric populations. J Am Geriatr Soc 1987; 35(2):132–141.
70. Vgontzas AN, et al. Sleep apnea and sleep disruption in obese patients. Arch Intern Med 1994; 154(15):1705–1711.
71. Peppard PE, et al. Longitudinal study of moderate weight change and sleep-disordered breathing. JAMA 2000; 284(23):3015–3021.
72. Vgontzas AN, et al. Obesity without sleep apnea is associated with daytime sleepiness. Arch Intern Med 1998; 158(12):1333–1337.
73. Haponik EF, et al. Computerized tomography in obstructive sleep apnea. Correlation of airway size with physiology during sleep and wakefulness. Am Rev Respir Dis 1983; 127(2):221–226.
74. Suratt PM, et al. Fluoroscopic and computed tomographic features of the pharyngeal airway in obstructive sleep apnea. Am Rev Respir Dis 1983; 127(4):487–492.
75. Schwab RJ, et al. Dynamic upper airway imaging during awake respiration in normal subjects and patients with sleep disordered breathing. Am Rev Respir Dis 1993; 148(5):1385–1400.
76. Kuna ST, Bedi DG, Ryckman C. Effect of nasal airway positive pressure on upper airway size and configuration. Am Rev Respir Dis 1988; 138(4):969–975.
77. Rivlin J, et al. Upper airway morphology in patients with idiopathic obstructive sleep apnea. Am Rev Respir Dis 1984; 129(3):355–360.
78. Horner RL, et al. Sites and sizes of fat deposits around the pharynx in obese patients with obstructive sleep apnoea and weight matched controls. Eur Respir J 1989; 2(7):613–622.
79. Mortimore IL, et al. Neck and total body fat deposition in nonobese and obese patients with sleep apnea compared with that in control subjects. Am J Respir Crit Care Med 1998; 157(1):280–283.
80. Rodenstein DO, et al. Pharyngeal shape and dimensions in healthy subjects, snorers, and patients with obstructive sleep apnoea. Thorax 1990; 45(10):722–727.
81. Sforza E, et al. Upper airway collapsibility and cephalometric variables in patients with obstructive sleep apnea. Am J Respir Crit Care Med 2000; 161(2 pt 1): 347–352.
82. Katz I, et al. Do patients with obstructive sleep apnea have thick necks? Am Rev Respir Dis 1990; 141(5 pt 1):1228–1231.
83. Van de Graaff WB. Thoracic influence on upper airway patency. J Appl Physiol 1988; 65(5):2124–2131.
84. Van de Graaff WB. Thoracic traction on the trachea: mechanisms and magnitude. J Appl Physiol 1991; 70(3): 1328–1336.
85. Brown IG, et al. Pharyngeal compliance in snoring

subjects with and without obstructive sleep apnea. Am Rev Respir Dis 1985; 132(2):211–215.

86. Rubinstein I, Hoffstein V, Bradley TD. Lung volume–related changes in the pharyngeal area of obese females with and without obstructive sleep apnoea. Eur Respir J 1989; 2(4):344–351.
87. Rubinstein I, et al. Improvement in upper airway function after weight loss in patients with obstructive sleep apnea. Am Rev Respir Dis 1988; 138(5):1192–1195.
88. Suratt PM, McTier RF, Wilhoit SC. Collapsibility of the nasopharyngeal airway in obstructive sleep apnea. Am Rev Respir Dis 1985; 132(5):967–971.
89. Ryan CF, Love LL. Mechanical properties of the velopharynx in obese patients with obstructive sleep apnea. Am J Respir Crit Care Med 1996; 154(3 pt 1): 806–812.
90. Schwartz AR, et al. Effect of weight loss on upper airway collapsibility in obstructive sleep apnea. Am Rev Respir Dis 1991; 144(3 pt 1):494–498.
91. Vincken WG, Elleker MG, Cosio MG. Flow-volume loop changes reflecting respiratory muscle weakness in chronic neuromuscular disorders. Am J Med 1987; 83(4):673–680.
92. Burwell CS, RE, Whaley RD, et al. Extreme obesity associated with alveolar hypoventilation A Pickwickian syndrome. Am J Med 1956; 21:811–818.
93. Sugerman HJ, et al. Hemodynamic dysfunction in obesity hypoventilation syndrome and the effects of treatment with surgically induced weight loss. Ann Surg 1988; 207(5):604–613.
94. Zwillich CW, et al. Decreased hypoxic ventilatory drive in the obesity-hypoventilation syndrome. Am J Med 1975; 59(3):343–348.
95. Lopata M, et al. Ventilatory control and the obesity hypoventilation syndrome. Am Rev Respir Dis 1979; 119(2 pt 2):165–168.
96. Kunitomo F, et al. Sex differences in awake ventilatory drive and abnormal breathing during sleep in eucapnic obesity. Chest 1988; 93(5):968–976.
97. Greenberg HE, et al. Effect of chronic resistive loading on hypoxic ventilatory responsiveness. J Appl Physiol 1997; 82(2):500–507.
98. Lopata M, Onal E. Mass loading, sleep apnea, and the pathogenesis of obesity hypoventilation. Am Rev Respir Dis 1982; 126(4):640–645.
99. Gold AR, et al. Pulmonary function and respiratory chemosensitivity in moderately obese patients with sleep apnea. Chest 1993; 103(5):1325–1329.
100. O'Donnell CP, et al. Leptin, obesity, and respiratory function. Respir Physiol 2000; 119(2–3):163–170.
101. Emirgil C, Sobol BJ. The effects of weight reduction on pulmonary function and the sensitivity of the respiratory center in obesity. Am Rev Respir Dis 1973; 108(4): 831–842.
102. Chapman KR, Himal HS, Rebuck AS. Ventilatory responses to hypercapnia and hypoxia in patients with eucapnic morbid obesity before and after weight loss. Clin Sci (Colch) 1990; 78(6):541–545.
103. Lopata M, Evanich MJ, Lourenco RV. Quantification of diaphragmatic EMG response to CO2 rebreathing in humans. J Appl Physiol 1977; 43(2):262–270.
104. Rochester DF. Tests of respiratory muscle function. Clin Chest Med 1988; 9(2):249–261.
105. Lourenco RV. Diaphragm activity in obesity. J Clin Invest 1969; 48(9):1609–1614.
106. Farkas GA, et al. Histochemical and mechanical properties of diaphragm muscle in morbidly obese Zucker rats. J Appl Physiol 1994; 77(5):2250–2259.
107. Sampson MG, GA. Diaphragmatic muscle fatigue in the massively obese. Am Rev Respir Dis 1981; 123 (suppl):183.
108. Han F, WH, He Q, Ding D, Strohl KP. Treatment effects of carbon dioxide retention in patients with obstructive sleep apnea syndrome. Chest 2001; 119:1814–1819.
109. Berthon-Jones M, Sullivan CE. Time course of change in ventilatory response to CO_2 with long-term CPAP therapy for obstructive sleep apnea. Am Rev Respir Dis 1987; 135(1):144–147.
110. Bedell GN, Seebohm PM. Pulmonary function in obese persons. Clin Invest 1958; 37:1049–1053.
111. Rajala R, et al. Obstructive sleep apnoea syndrome in morbidly obese patients. J Intern Med 1991; 230(2): 125–129.
112. Suratt PM, et al. Effect of very-low-calorie diets with weight loss on obstructive sleep apnea. Am J Clin Nutr 1992; 56(suppl 1):182S–184S.
113. Kiselak J, et al. The association between hypertension and sleep apnea in obese patients. Chest 1993; 104(3): 775–780.
114. Suratt PM, et al. Changes in breathing and the pharynx after weight loss in obstructive sleep apnea. Chest 1987; 92(4):631–637.
115. Pasquali R, et al. Treatment of obese patients with obstructive sleep apnea syndrome (OSAS): effect of weight loss and interference of otorhinolaryngiatric pathology. Int J Obes 1990; 14(3):207–217.
116. Nahmias J, Kirschner M, Karetzky MS. Weight loss and OSA and pulmonary function in obesity. NJ Med 1993; 90(1):48–53.
117. Noseda A, et al. Sleep apnea after 1 year domiciliary nasal-continuous positive airway pressure and attempted weight reduction. Potential for weaning from continuous positive airway pressure. Chest 1996; 109(1):138–143.
118. Smith PL. Weight loss in mildly to moderately obese patients with obstructive sleep apnea. Ann Intern Med 1985; 103(6 pt 1):850–855.
119. Pendlebury ST, et al. Natural evolution of moderate sleep apnoea syndrome: significant progression over a mean of 17 months. Thorax 1997; 52(10):872–878.
120. Wooley SC, Garner DM. Obesity treatment: the high

cost of false hope. J Am Diet Assoc 1991; 91(10):1248–1251.

121. Jeffery RW, et al. Long-term maintenance of weight loss: current status. Health Psychol 2000; 19(suppl 1):5–16.
122. Weintraub M, Bray GA. Drug treatment of obesity. Med Clin North Am 1989; 73(1):237–249.
123. Connolly HM, et al. Valvular heart disease associated with fenfluramine-phentermine. N Engl J Med 1997; 337(9):581–588.
124. Weissman NJ, et al. An assessment of heart-valve abnormalities in obese patients taking dexfenfluramine, sustained-release dexfenfluramine, or placebo. Sustained-Release Dexfenfluramine Study Group. N Engl J Med 1998; 339(11):725–732.
125. Weiner P, et al. Influence of excessive weight loss after gastroplasty for morbid obesity on respiratory muscle performance. Thorax 1998; 53(1):39–42.
126. Dixon JB, Chapman L, O'Brien P. Marked improvement in asthma after Lap-Band surgery for morbid obesity. Obes Surg 1999; 9(4):385–389.
127. Charuzi I, et al. The effect of surgical weight reduction on sleep quality in obesity-related sleep apnea syndrome. Surgery 1985; 97(5):535–538.
128. Peiser J, et al. Sleep apnea syndrome in the morbidly obese as an indication for weight reduction surgery. Ann Surg 1984; 199(1):112–115.
129. Sugerman HJ, et al. Gastric surgery for respiratory insuffiency of obesity. Chest 1986; 90(1):81–86.
130. Cook DJ, et al. Rules of evidence and clinical recommendations on the use of antithrombotic agents. Chest 1992; 102(suppl 4):305S–311S.
131. Mason EE, Ito C. Gastric bypass. Ann Surg 1969; 170(3):329–339.
132. Garner D, WS. Confronting the failure of behavioral and dietary treatments for obesity. Clin Psychol Rev 1991; 111:779–780.
133. Kessler R, et al. Pulmonary hypertension in the obstructive sleep apnoea syndrome: prevalence, causes and therapeutic consequences. Eur Respir J 1996; 9(4):787–794.
134. Pankow W, et al. Influence of noninvasive positive pressure ventilation on inspiratory muscle activity in obese subjects. Eur Respir J 1997; 10(12):2847–2852.
135. Sanders MH, Gruendl CA, Rogers RM. Patient compliance with nasal CPAP therapy for sleep apnea. Chest 1986; 90(3):330–333.
136. Rolfe I, Olson LG, Saunders NA. Long-term acceptance of continuous positive airway pressure in obstructive sleep apnea. Am Rev Respir Dis 1991; 144(5):1130–1133.
137. Hoffstein V, et al. Treatment of obstructive sleep apnea with nasal continuous positive airway pressure. Patient compliance, perception of benefits, and side effects. Am Rev Respir Dis 1992; 145(4 pt 1):841–845.
138. White DP, et al. Central sleep apnea. Improvement with acetazolamide therapy. Arch Intern Med 1982; 142(10):1816–1819.
139. Tojima H, et al. Effects of acetazolamide in patients with the sleep apnoea syndrome. Thorax 1988; 43(2):113–119.
140. Shore ET, Millman RP. Central sleep apnea and acetazolamide therapy. Arch Intern Med 1983; 143(6):1278, 1280.
141. Hudgel DW, Thanakitcharu S. Pharmacologic treatment of sleep-disordered breathing. Am J Respir Crit Care Med 1998; 158(3):691–699.
142. Strohl KP, et al. Progesterone administration and progressive sleep apneas. JAMA 1981; 245(12):1230–1232.
143. Rajagopal KR, Abbrecht PH, Jabbari B. Effects of medroxyprogesterone acetate in obstructive sleep apnea. Chest 1986; 90(6):815–821.
144. Saletu B, et al. Efficiency of continuous positive airway pressure versus theophylline therapy in sleep apnea: comparative sleep laboratory studies on objective and subjective sleep and awakening quality. Neuropsychobiology 1999; 39(3):151–159.
145. Javaheri S. Treatment of central sleep apnea in heart failure. Sleep 2000; 23(suppl 4):S224–S227.
146. Kingshott RN, et al. Randomized, double-blind, placebo-controlled crossover trial of modafinil in the treatment of residual excessive daytime sleepiness in the sleep apnea/hypopnea syndrome. Am J Respir Crit Care Med 2001; 163(4):918–923.
147. Arnulf I, et al. Modafinil in obstructive sleep apnea-hypopnea syndrome: a pilot study in 6 patients. Respiration 1997; 64(2):159–161.
148. Fee WE, Ward PH. Permanent tracheostomy: a new surgical technique. Ann Otol Rhinol Laryngol 1977; 86(5 pt 1):635–638.
149. Shaheen SO. Obesity and asthma: cause for concern? Clin Exp Allergy 1999; 29(3):291–293.
150. Morgan WK, Reger RB. Rise and fall of the FEV(1). Chest 2000; 118(6):1639–1644.
151. Camargo CA, et al. Prospective study of body mass index, weight change, and risk of adult-onset asthma in women. Arch Intern Med 1999; 159(21):2582–2588.
152. Hedberg A, Rossner S. Body weight characteristics of subjects on asthma medication. Int J Obes Relat Metab Disord 2000; 24(9):1217–1225.
153. Brown WJ, et al. Relationships between body mass index and well-being in young Australian women. Int J Obes Relat Metab Disord 2000; 24(10):1360–1368.
154. Shaheen SO, et al. Birth weight, body mass index and asthma in young adults. Thorax 1999; 54(5):396–402.
155. Schachter LM, et al. Obesity is a risk for asthma and wheeze but not airway hyperresponsiveness. Thorax 2001; 56(1):4–8.
156. Figueroa-Munoz JI, Chinn S, Rona RJ. Association between obesity and asthma in 4–11 year old children in the UK. Thorax 2001; 56(2):133–137.
157. Huang SL, Shiao G, Chou P. Association between body

mass index and allergy in teenage girls in Taiwan. Clin Exp Allergy 1999; 29(3):323–329.
158. Von Kries R, et al. Is obesity a risk factor for childhood asthma? Allergy 2001; 56(4):318–322.
159. Lee SI, et al. Prevalences of symptoms of asthma and other allergic diseases in Korean children: a nationwide questionnaire survey. J Korean Med Sci 2001; 16(2):155–164.
160. Belamarich PF, et al. Do obese inner-city children with asthma have more symptoms than nonobese children with asthma? Pediatrics 2000; 106(6):1436–1441.
161. Del Rio-Navarro B, et al. Exercise induced bronchospasm in asthmatic and non-asthmatic obese children. Allergol Immunopathol (Madr) 2000; 28(1):5–11.
162. Gennuso J, et al. The relationship between asthma and obesity in urban minority children and adolescents. Arch Pediatr Adolesc Med 1998; 152(12):1197–1200.
163. Gokbel H, Atas S. Exercise-induced bronchospasm in nonasthmatic obese and nonobese boys. J Sports Med Phys Fitness 1999; 39(4):361–364.
164. Kaplan TA, Montana E. Exercise-induced bronchospasm in nonasthmatic obese children. Clin Pediatr (Phila) 1993; 32(4):220–225.
165. Fredberg JJ, et al. Airway smooth muscle, tidal stretches, and dynamically determined contractile states. Am J Respir Crit Care Med 1997; 156(6):1752–1759.
166. Hakala K, Stenius-Aarniala B, Sovijarvi A. Effects of weight loss on peak flow variability, airways obstruction, and lung volumes in obese patients with asthma. Chest 2000; 118(5):1315–1321.
167. Dhabuwala A, Cannan RJ, Stubbs RS. Improvement in co-morbidities following weight loss from gastric bypass surgery. Obes Surg 2000; 10(5):428–435.
168. Murr MM, Siadati MR, Sarr MG. Results of bariatric surgery for morbid obesity in patients older than 50 years. Obes Surg 1995; 5(4):399–402.
169. Stenius-Aarniala B, et al. Immediate and long term effects of weight reduction in obese people with asthma: randomised controlled study. BMJ 2000; 320(7238): 827–832.

40

Obesity, Arthritis, and Gout

Anita Wluka and Flavia M. Cicuttini

Monash University, Melbourne, Victoria, Australia

Tim D. Spector

Guy's and St. Thomas' Hospital NHS Trust, London, England

I INTRODUCTION

Musculoskeletal conditions affect 16% of all Americans (1). In 1988 it was estimated that the direct and indirect costs of these to the country were equivalent to 2.5% GNP (2). This was three times as great as the estimated cost in 1980. Musculoskeletal conditions are an important cause of acute and chronic disability, being amongst the most common causes of work disability, because of their prevalence and severity (2). Indeed, in the workplace, the cost of musculoskeletal diseases were the highest and second-highest disease categories in workers with BMI between ~27.5–30 and >30, respectively (3).

The most common musculoskeletal condition is osteoarthritis (OA), which affects 12.1% of Americans between the ages of 25 and 74 years (4). Its prevalence increases with age, so that the socioeconomic burden to society will grow with our aging population. Gout is the most common form of inflammatory arthritis in males over 40 years old.

II OBESITY AND OSTEOARTHRITIS

Osteoarthritis is a disorder of synovial joints characterized by deterioration and abrasion of the joint cartilage and formation of new bone at the joint surfaces. Obesity is likely to be the most important preventable risk factor for knee OA. Overall, results to date suggest that the link between obesity and OA is more consistent in women and is strongest in OA of the knees and less conclusive in other joints. This has important implications since OA is an enormous public health problem in developed countries as it is the commonest single cause of disability (5) and the major reason for hip and knee replacements (6). The combination of its effect on patients and the therapeutic procedures used produces a huge burden on society (7). Recently, efforts have been focused on potential risk factors for OA with a view to identifying possible preventive measures. The management of obesity is likely to be a key factor in the management of OA.

A Association of Obesity and Osteoarthritis of the Knee

Cross-sectional epidemiological studies have consistently shown a relationship between obesity and knee OA, which has generally been stronger in women than in men. The reported increased risks have ranged from two- to seven-fold for women in the top tertile of BMI compared to women in the bottom tertile (8–14) (Table 1). The earliest survey to mention this link

Table 1 Evidence of Association Between Knee OA and Obesity from Some Recent Cross-Sectional and Longitudinal Population-Based Studies

Study	Comparison groups of body weight	Relative risk of knee OA (95% CI)
Cross-sectional		
Felson et al., 1988 (12)	Quintile 5 (MRW ≥129)[a] vs. quintile 1 (MRW <105)	Men 1.51 (1.14, 1.98)
	Quintile 5 (MRW ≥128) vs. quintile 1 (MRW <100)	Women 2.07 (1.67, 2.55)
Davis et al., 1990 (14)	BMI >30 vs. BMI ≤30	3.64 (2.21, 6.02)
Hart et al., 1993 (16)	Tertile 3 (BMI >26.4) vs. tertile 1 (BMI <23.4)	Women 6.17 (3.26–11.71)
Longitudinal		
Anderson, 1988 (13)	Minimum adult weight[b]	
	BMI >27.3 vs. BMI <27.3	Women 2.66 (1.6, 4.42)
	BMI >27.8 vs. BMI <27.8	Men 0.65 (0.10, 4.36)
Felson, 1992 (59)	Weight gain >2 units BMI over the 10 years prior	Per 2 units gain in BMI 1.35 (1.11, 1.64)
Hart, 1999 (24)	Weight at age 20[c] tertile 3 (BMI >26.4) vs. tertile 1 (BMI <23.4)	Osteophytes, 1.76 (0.90, 3.43)
Gelber, 1999 (23)	BMI at 20–29 years old >24.7 vs. BMI <22.8[d]	3.6 (1.5, 8.7)

[a] MRW = Metropolitan Relative Weight, a measure of weight in pounds adjusted for height.
[b] Recalled minimum adult weight.
[c] Recalled weight, adjusted for height, examination, women examined.
[d] Adjusted for year of birth, physical activity, joint injury, men with median follow-up 36 years.

was by Fletcher 1945 (8). In 1958 Kellgren and Lawrence found that knee OA was commoner in obese people and twice as common in females as in males (9). Data from the large National Health and Nutrition Exam Survey (NHANES I), 1971–75, found that the risk of OA increased with degree of obesity and that long-term obesity was significantly associated with knee OA (13,14). Obesity was strongly related to bilateral knee disease (15).

A population-based cross-sectional prevalence study of obesity and OA in middle-aged females confirmed obesity as a strong risk factor for OA knees in women (16). This study showed a nearly 18-fold increased risk for bilateral disease. This same effect was also seen in the subgroup of asymptomatic women. The proportion of OA which was estimated to be attributable to obesity in this group of middle-aged women was 63%.

B Association of Obesity with OA in the Different Knee Compartments

Until recently, little consideration was given to the multicompartmental nature of the knee joint in epidemiological studies of OA. However, recent work has suggested that a significant proportion of symptomatic knee OA may be caused by patellofemoral disease (17–19), which is not visualized by conventional anteroposterior radiography. Consequently, little attention has been focused on whether the risk factors for OA differ among the different knee compartments. A recent population based case control study examined whether risk factors for OA differ between the different knee compartments (20). This study did not show a significant effect of obesity on the patellofemoral joint but showed an effect at the tibiofemoral joint. This case control study, based on small numbers, was the first to consider the possibility that OA in different compartments may have different etiologies and that previously described risk factors such as obesity may have differential effects in the different compartments. In contrast, data from a population-based cross-sectional study of middle-aged women showed it to be an important risk factor for both medial tibiofemoral and patellofemoral joint disease (21). This is an area where further work will be needed to clarify the role of obesity as a risk factor in OA in the different compartments of the knee. This is likely to have important implications for preventive strategies in OA of the knee and for our understanding of the pathogenesis of OA.

C Evidence from Longitudinal Studies of the Association of Obesity with Knee OA

Longitudinal studies have consistently shown an association of obesity with knee OA (Table 1). The Framingham Study examined the association between obesity and knee OA in a longitudinal study. At the time of that study, the group had been followed up for 35 years (22).

Radiographs that were obtained on examination 18 (subjects' mean age 73) were used, together with weights on the same subjects that had been obtained at the beginning of the Framingham Study when the mean age of participants was 37. No radiographs were available at the age of 37, but the assumption when analyzing the data was that the prevalence of OA at age 37 was low. This study was able to look at obesity prior to the development of OA. A strong association between being overweight in 1948–1951 and having knee OA ~36 years later was found. This association was stronger for women than men after controlling for possible confounders such as age, uric acid level, and physical activity. Furthermore, this association was present for both symptomatic and asymptomatic disease. In addition, there was a stronger association with more severe, rather than mild, radiological disease. Similarly, the Johns Hopkins Precursors Study (23) examined the relationship between obesity and subsequent OA in men. In a prospective cohort of 1132, using 84 cases of incident hip and/or knee OA, the investigators were able to demonstrate a dose response relationship for increased body mass index (BMI) at a young age with an increased risk of knee OA. The Chingford population study of incident OA in women (24) found over a 4-year period that the odds ratio of developing incident osteophytes, but not joint space narrowing, was significantly increased in those in the highest tertile for BMI. These results suggest that higher BMI earlier in life may be a more important risk factor for the subsequent development of knee OA than heavier weight later in life.

These data are supported by other studies in which, although data on actual weight preceding the onset of OA were not available, self-reported, recall weights were used. In the NHANES study, the effect of past obesity on the risk of developing OA was examined by using self-reported minimum adult weight as a proxy measure of long-term obesity (13). In this study, past obesity was found to be associated with OA. In the Chingford population study of 1003 middle-aged women, a similar association was observed between self-reported minimum weight at age 20 and OA in middle age (16). In that study it was argued that the recalled weight was probably quite accurate as it coincided with the approximate age at which many of the women got married, thus improving the likelihood of accurate recall of their weight at that time.

Further evidence suggesting that obesity precedes OA, rather than the converse, is that the association between OA and obesity is strong even for individuals with radiological evidence of knee OA who are asymptomatic (13,16,21). This is important as radiological disease has been shown to correlate with later disability (25,26). Furthermore, a strong dose response effect has also been observed between obesity and OA. Those individuals that were obese (BMI > 30) were shown to have a markedly increased risk of knee OA relative to those who were only modestly overweight (BMI > 25 to < =30) (13). This dose response relationship provides additional evidence of a possible etiological effect.

D Evidence from Twin Studies of the Role of Obesity in OA

A further method for examining the association between obesity and osteoarthritis is via twin studies, which have been used to estimate the magnitude of the weight difference associated with the development of OA (21). Twin studies provide a special research methodology that, as well as assessing the relative contributions of genetic and environmental factors to a disease, may also be used to examine environmental risk factors in twin pairs discordant for that disease trait. The twin model used in this study enabled close matching of the diseased and nondiseased twin for genetic similarity and many known or unknown environmental factors, thus providing a useful tool to quantify the magnitude of the difference in obesity between the twin with disease and their cotwin with no disease.

The twin study confirmed that obesity is a strong risk factor for OA of the knee, with twins with OA of the tibiofemoral and patellofemoral joints of the knee tending, on average, to be 3–5 kg heavier than their cotwin (Fig. 1). This weight difference was also observed in asymptomatic women, again suggesting that obesity is a cause of OA rather than the converse. After adjusting for other potential risk factors, the results showed that for every kg increase in weight, a twin had a 14% increased risk of developing tibiofemoral osteophytes and a 32% increased risk of developing patellofemoral osteophytes compared to their cotwin. These results were consistent with a previous population study, in a similar age group of women, that showed that the risk of knee OA increased by 35% for every 5 kg of weight gain (16). This suggests that in middle-aged women even small increases in body weight are associated with significant increases in risk of developing OA. Risks in men, however, cannot be extrapolated from these results, and separate studies are needed.

E Association of Obesity and Osteoarthritis of the Hand

Results regarding the association of obesity with hand OA are conflicting. OA of the distal interphalangeal joints has been associated with obesity in some studies,

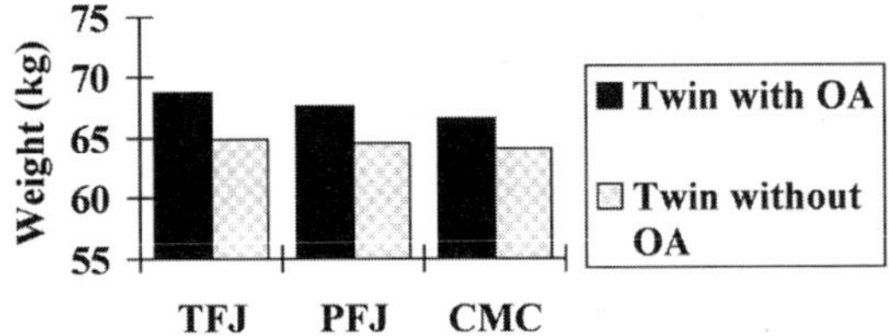

Figure 1 Body weight for twins with osteoarthritis in the tibiofemoral joint (TFJ) of the knee, the patellofemoral joint (PFJ) of the knee, and the carpometacarpal (CMC) joint of the hand. The weight differences between the twins with OA and the twins without OA were significant at all the above joints: TFJ ($P < .001$), PFJ ($P < .001$), CMC ($P < .002$).

although principally in men (9,27). Secondary analysis of data from the National Health Examination Survey showed a significant association of BMI with the presence of hand OA in men after adjustment for age, race, and skinfold thickening but not after adjustment for waist girth and seat breadth (28). An association between radiographic hand OA and BMI in men was also observed in the longitudinal prospective study of 70-year-old people in Goteborg (29). An association between obesity and finger OA was observed in the New Haven Survey, with this association being stronger in females (10). The Fallon Community Health Plan Study of OA (30), a case control study, found that obesity and hand OA were associated.

An association was observed between BMI and the grade of hand OA for women in the Tecumseh Community Health Study (31). Obesity was also modestly associated with distal interphalangeal and carpometacarpal OA, but not but not with the proximal interphalangeal OA in the women in the Chingford Study (16).

Data from a twin study showed a mean weight difference (95% CI) within twin pairs discordant for carpometacarpal osteophytes of 3.06 (0.83, 5.28) kg (21). The results suggested that there was a 9% increase in risk of developing carpometacarpal osteophytes for every kg increase in body weight. However, there was no significant difference in weight within twin pairs discordant for osteophytes at the distal interphalangeal (distal interphalangeal) or proximal interphalangeal (proximal interphalangeal) joints.

However, other studies have found no relationship between obesity and hand OA. No association was observed between indices of obesity and hand OA in men in the Baltimore Longitudinal Study of Aging (32) or for women between BMI and hand OA in the National Health Examination Survey (28). The Ulm Osteoarthritis Study, (33) which examined 809 consecutive patients who underwent hip or knee replacement for OA, also found no association.

F Evidence from Longitudinal Studies of the Association of Obesity with Hand OA

Less information is available on the effect of long-term obesity and hand OA. One of the few studies to examine this was the Tecumseh Community Health Study, a longitudinal study that investigated the role of obesity in the etiology of hand osteoarthritis (34). This study, conducted in Tecumseh, MI, began in 1962 with baseline examinations of clinical, biochemical, and radiologic characteristics. A 1985 reexamination of the cohort characterized osteoarthritis status in 1276 participants (588 males and 688 females) aged 50–74 years at this follow-up. Baseline obesity, as measured by an index of relative weight, was found to be significantly associated with the 23-year incidence of osteoarthritis of the hands among subjects disease free at baseline. Greater baseline relative weight was also associated with greater subsequent severity of osteoarthritis of the hands. However, the difference between baseline and follow-up weight values was not significantly associated with the incidence of osteoarthritis of the hands. Furthermore, there was no evidence that development of osteoarthritis subsequently led to increased incidence of obesity.

G Association of Obesity and Osteoarthritis of the Hip

The available data suggest that there may be a modest association between hip OA and obesity (9,11,27). When data from 4225 persons from the national Health and Nutrition Examination Survey (HANES) were examined by dividing subjects into four groups on the basis of sex and race, relative weight was weakly associated with OA of the hips in white women and nonwhite men (11). A case control study that examined BMI at ages 20, 30, 40, and 50 years in 239 men who had just received a hip prosthesis because of osteoarthritis and in 302 controls randomly selected from the general population (35) showed that men with a BMI > 1 SD above the mean had a greater relative risk of developing severe OA than with men with a BMI < 1 SD below the mean. Those slightly obese at the age of 40 years had a relative risk of 2.5 for later surgery of the hip.

In contrast, data from the First National Health and Nutrition Examination Survey (NHANES-I) did not support this (36). Obesity, and fat distribution were not associated with hip osteoarthritis. The Johns Hopkins Precursors Study (23) found no relationship between BMI in the preceding three decades with subsequent hip OA. Other studies have also found no association between obesity and hip OA (30,33).

H Possible Mechanisms for Obesity in the Pathogenesis of OA

OA is a disease of cartilage in which cartilage breakdown and erosion are accompanied by bony changes such as osteophytes, subchondral sclerosis, and bony cysts. Although the mechanisms by which obesity may lead to OA are unknown, three hypotheses have been proposed (14,15,37): (1) obesity increases the load across the knee joint resulting in increased or abnormal stress and resultant deterioration of the joint structures; (2) obesity acts indirectly by metabolic changes associated with increased fatness such as glucose intolerance, hyperlipidemia, hyperestrogenemia, or changes in bone density; and (3) elements of the diet that result in obesity, such as high fat content and adversely affect bone, cartilage, or other joint structures (Table 2).

Obesity may initiate cartilage breakdown or may promote joint destruction after the initial incipient lesion. Biomechanical characteristics may be accentuated by obesity. In a study of 300 subjects, most of the effect of BMI on the severity of OA in medial tibiofemoral osteoarthritis was explained by varus malalignment of the joint (38). Furthermore, this study showed that obese subjects with valgus malalignment had hardly any increase in OA prevalence. These results suggest that a major mechanical influence of obesity is modified by alignment. Whether obesity influences alignment or the two are independent is unclear. Although obesity possibly leads to disease because it causes increased force on the cartilage, it also may produce disease by increasing subchondral bony stiffness (39) and by making subchondral bone less deformable to impact loads. This stiff bone would then transmit the increased force to underlying cartilage, making it more vulnerable.

Table 2 Possible Mechanisms for Obesity in the Pathogenesis of OA

Mechanical
Increase in load across the joint
Abnormal stresses across a joint
Malalignment
Varus
Valgus
Systemic
Association with raised serum glucose, hypertension, hypercholesterolaemia, hyperuricaemia, and insulin resistance
?Excess endogenous steroids
Genetic association of two common diseases
Dietary
High fat content resulting in abnormal joint structures

A number of factors suggest a metabolic/systemic component to OA. These include the female preponderance, the menopausal onset of generalized OA, the unequal effect of obesity on knee and hip OA, and the inverse relationship with osteoporosis. Furthermore, obesity is also linked to OA of the fingers and the base of the thumb, in which mechanical force is less likely to play an important role.

I Evidence for Obesity Acting Via a Systemic Mechanism

1 Association Between Osteoarthritis and Other Metabolic Conditions

a. Hypertension

On analysis of the data from the 1960s survey in Leigh and Wensleydale, Lawrence found that hypertension was associated with generalize OA in men and with knee OA in hypertensive, nonobese females (40). The relationship was between diastolic blood pressure and knee OA in both obese and nonobese females, and this association remained in each 5-year age group from 45 to 69. The association between hypertension and OA was also observed in the Chingford population study which showed that "ever treated" hypertension was associated with the development of OA and that this association was strongest for those with bilateral knee disease (41).

However, other studies have failed to confirm an association between OA and blood pressure. No association was found in a study of 70-year-old people in Goteborg (29). In univariate analysis of NHANES 1 data, an increase in recorded diastolic and systolic blood pressure was found in females with knee OA, but this association disappeared after adjusting for weight (42). Similarly, in the Baltimore Longitudinal Study of Aging (43), men and women with knee OA had higher unadjusted blood pressure than those with normal radiographs. However, after adjustment for age and weight, the effect was lost in men. Although women with knee OA had higher systolic pressure than those with normal knees, the mean pressure was within the normal range.

b. Cholesterol

A significant association was found with hand OA and above average measured serum cholesterol in women in the 1960s survey in Leigh and Wensleydale (44). However, the association disappeared in those with very high serum cholesterol. Furthermore, Lawrence (40) found that subjects with OA and hypertension in this same population did not have an association with high serum cholesterol or uric acid. In analyses of the data from NHANES 1, the study of 70-year-old people in Goteborg and the Baltimore Longitudinal Study of Aging, serum cholesterol was not significantly associated with either unilateral or bilateral knee OA (15,29,43). In contrast, the data from the Chingford population study suggested an association between bilateral knee disease and hypercholesterolemia (41).

c. Glucose

Few studies have examined the association between blood glucose and OA. Cimmino et al. (45) studied 1026 subjects with OA from clinics and compared them to 220 healthy population controls and found slightly higher levels of plasma glucose in females in the OA group after adjusting for age. A study comparing 25 female diabetic patients with knee OA and 48 non-diabetic females who were matched on age, weight, symptoms, and duration of OA found an increased incidence of osteophytes on the radiographs of the diabetic patients, while the joint space narrowing and sclerosis were equal in the two groups (46). An association between serum glucose and osteoarthritis was also observed in the Chingford population study (41). In this study, raised blood glucose was a significant factor in all forms of knee OA, but the association was strongest for those with bilateral knee disease (41). It has been speculated that the link between diabetes and OA may be through elevated growth hormone levels that alter cartilage metabolism and increase bone density (14,15). Increased bone density associated with obesity has been hypothesised to increased the forces acting on the cartilage, thus predisposing the development of OA (14,15). However, these theories have not been well examined and not all epidemiological studies have shown an association between serum glucose and OA. In the analyses of the NHANES 1 data, self-reported diabetes was not associated with either unilateral or bilateral knee OA (15). Furthermore, no association was observed between blood glucose levels and OA in a study of 70-year-old people in Goteborg (29). Indeed, in the Baltimore Longitudinal Study of Aging, no association was noted between fasting glucose and OA, but men with OA had lower 2-hour glucose in a glucose tolerance test than those without OA(43).

d. Uric Acid

Data from the New Haven population survey showed that a raised serum uric acid level was significantly associated with OA, with the association being stronger in women than in men (6). In univariate analysis of NHANES I data, hyperuricemia was found to be related to knee OA in women, but the association disappeared after adjusting for body weight (13). There was no significant association with either unilateral or bilateral knee OA (15). This is further supported by a study of 70-year-old people in Goteborg (29), where no association was observed between serum uric acid level and OA. In contrast, the data from the Chingford population study suggested a possible association between raised serum uric acid levels and bilateral knee disease (41).

e. Summary

The data suggesting a link between OA and raised serum glucose, cholesterol, uric acid, and hypertension remain inconclusive. However, one possible explanation for an association among hypertension, hyperlipidemia, and OA is insulin resistance or Reavens syndrome (47). This syndrome may be a distinct genetic trait, or it may represent a physiological adaptation to chronic obesity (48).

2 Association Between Osteoarthritis and Body Fat Distribution

Adipose tissue distribution is associated with a number of metabolic complications, with a pattern of central body fat (particularly abdominal fat) indicating increased risk of diabetes, cardiovascular disease, and mortality, independent of degree of obesity (49). Recent interest has focused on the distribution of body fat in OA in an effort to understand whether systemic factors are important in the development of OA. Analysis of the NHANES data showed that BMI correlated best with presence of OA using different anthropomorphic measurements suggesting that body fat may be more important than the absolute weight (37). In this study there was a significant association between hand and foot OA and seat breadth in men, odds ratio 1.45 (1.03–2.06). Although this association was also observed in women, the confidence intervals included one. However, no association was found in this study between a centralized pattern of body fat distribution with hand or knee OA. In fact, this study found some evidence for of an association for a peripheral body fat pattern and combined hand and feet OA (14). Consistent with these observations, the Chingford population study of middle-aged women (41) and the Baltimore Longitudinal Study of Aging (50) of both women and men also failed to show an association between body fat distribution and OA, independent of body weight.

3 Summary

Together these data support a greater contribution of mechanical as opposed to systemic factors to explain the association between obesity and OA. The results would suggest that peripheral distribution of fat may act as a mechanical effect rather than a metabolic cause of OA. However, there is increasing evidence that OA is not a single disorder but a heterogeneous group of disorders. It is postulated that a complex interplay of several factors may result in a common pathway of joint damage. Therefore, it is possible that obesity has a mechanical effect on some joints and a metabolic effect on other joints. Several studies have shown an association of obesity with hand OA (9,10,27,29). Thus, it may be, for example, that obesity causes knee OA because of an increase in mechanical stress across the joint but that the effect of obesity on the small joints of the hand is through metabolic consequences.

J Role of Obesity in Progression of OA

The natural history of knee osteoarthritis is poorly understood, and few studies have any detailed data on prognostic factors such as obesity, although the available data suggest that obesity is important. In a small group of clinical cases followed up for 11 years, there was no clear effect of obesity (51). However, in the EPOZ study, Schouten et al. (52) found that obesity, age, Heberden's nodes and valgus deformity were all associated with cartilage loss over a 12-year period. Factors related to joint space progression in the multicenter French study were obesity and number of affected joints (53). A recent study that examined the rates of incident OA in the contralateral knee in a general population sample showed that in middle-aged women with early unilateral osteoarthritis of the knee, a high percentage (34%) develop OA in the contralateral knee within 2 years, while 22.4% progress radiologically in the index joint. Obesity appeared to have a marked effect on the incidence rates, with nearly a fivefold increase in overweight women compared to thin women. This is supported by a further study that showed that the odds ratio for BMI was 11.1 (3.3 to 37.3) for the fourth versus the first quartile (52). BMI was also found to be related to loss of cartilage in those that had OA (52).

K Association of Obesity with Symptoms and Disability in OA

Most nonfatal chronic conditions are strongly age related (53), their prevalence rising with increasing age of the population. Thus, as the total population continues to age owing to the decrease in birth rate and to recent declines in mortality in the older age groups, the burden of nonfatal diseases and impairments will continue to increase. This has highlighted the need to examine prognostic factors for disability. Using the 1984 Supplement on Aging conducted by the National Center for Health Statistics, the risk factors for disability among U.S. adults aged 55+ who had arthritis were compared to those who did not have arthritis (54). This study showed that obesity was strongly implicated in disability once arthritis was present. Thus, not only obesity is a risk factor for developing OA, but it also contributes to the disability once it occurs. The contribution of obesity to symptom development in individuals who already have the pathological changes of OA is unclear. Studies that have assessed whether obese subjects with concurrent radiographic OA are more likely to have symptoms have yielded conflicting results (11,55).

L Is Weight Loss Effective in Reducing the Symptoms of OA?

An early study examined this question in subjects at least 25% above their ideal weight (56). The study was a placebo-controlled trial of 3 months of therapy with phentermine to achieve weight loss in patients with hip or knee OA. At 6 months, weight loss of 12.6% (6.3 kg) in the phentermine group and 9.2% (4.5 kg) in the control group was achieved. Reduction in pain correlated with weight loss, more strongly for knee than hip pain. A second study examining the effect of weight loss in patients following gastroplasty on musculoskeletal symptoms (57) found a marked reduction in symptoms. However, not all musculoskeletal complaints were related to OA. These data suggest that weight loss reduces the symptoms of OA.

Which component of weight loss contributes most to reduction in symptoms was studied recently (58). Forty new patients with radiographic and symptomatic OA and BMI >26.4 were treated with Ranzsile (NSAID) for at least 4 weeks. Twenty-two were randomized to receive a controlled calorie weight loss diet and Manzidol (an appetite suppressant, Sanorex, Sandoz), and 18 to receive advice only. All were given ongoing NSAID therapy (Rantudil) and advised to walk for up to 30 min continuously per day during the 6-week trial. Three in the control group forgot to wear pedometers for several days and were excluded from the study. The treatment group lost more weight and was more active than the control group. Nineteen of 22 (86.4%) in the treatment group improved symptomatically, compared to 4 of 15 (26.7%) in the advice-only group. In the treatment group, symptomatic relief of knee OA was most strongly associated with reduction in body fat (2.4%, SD 2.6) and physical activity (7.5, SD 1.7 $\times 10^3$ steps per day). Physical activity and reduction in body fat percent were related.

M Is Weight Loss Effective in Reducing the Risk of OA?

Few studies have looked at the effect of weight loss in subjects who have established disease. Felson et al. (59), in the Framingham cohort, observed that weight loss in middle and later adult life substantially reduced the risk of symptomatic OA of the knee. To evaluate the effect of weight loss in preventing symptomatic knee osteoarthritis, women who participated in the Framingham Knee Osteoarthritis Study (1983–85) were examined. Sixty-four out of 796 women studied had recent-onset symptomatic knee osteoarthritis (knee symptoms plus radiographically confirmed osteoarthritis) and were compared with women without disease. Weight change significantly affected the risk for the development of knee osteoarthritis. For example, a decrease in body mass index of 2 units or more (weight loss, ~5 kg) over the 10 years before the current examination decreased the odds for developing osteoarthritis by over 50% (odds ratio, 0.46; 95% Cl, 0.24–0.86). Among those women with a high risk for osteoarthritis due to elevated baseline body mass index (≥25), weight loss also decreased the risk (for 2 units of body mass index, odds ratio, 0.41). Weight gain was associated with a slightly increased risk for osteoarthritis, which was not statistically significant, while weight loss reduced the risk for symptomatic knee osteoarthritis in women. Furthermore, extrapolating from cross-sectional data suggests that risk of knee OA increases by 35% for every 5 kg of weight gain (16).

The available data would suggest that reduction or maintenance of weight may have an important role in the prevention of OA. However, there is little data on whether weight loss affects the long-term progression of OA and this area needs further work.

III OBESITY AND GOUT

There has been an increase in prevalence of gout since World War II (60). Although increased awareness of this disease may in part explain this, and milder cases are being identified, particular interest has focused on the role of changes in diet and weight over this time. The evidence from cross-sectional and prospective studies for an association between obesity and gout is presented in the following sections.

A Evidence from Cross-Sectional Studies for Obesity as a Risk Factor for Gout

A large body of evidence exists to support an association between gout and obesity. The New Haven survey showed that certain metabolic conditions, including hyperuricemia, were associated with obesity (10). In a cross-sectional study of 73,000 women aged 30–49, obesity was shown to be significantly associated with gout ($P < .001$) (61). In 460 apparently healthy Dutch men and women aged 65–79 years, serum uric acid level was found to be positively associated with body weight, body mass index, body fatness, and lean body mass in men but not in women (62). In a study of 7735 middle-aged men in 24 British towns, a positive association was observed between BMI and gout (63).

The association between obesity and hyperuricemia has also been observed in other ethnic groups. A survey of 115 Maori men of working age showed a strong relationship between hyperuricemia and obesity (64). In Melanesian and Asian Indians in Fiji, BMI was shown to have a significant and independent association with plasma uric acid levels in both nondiabetic and diabetic men and women (65). However, the most extreme example of an association between gout and obesity was seen in sumo wrestlers, who do not appear to have any underlying genetic predisposition to gout (66). In a study of 96 sumo wrestlers in Japan, mean serum levels of uric acid were significantly higher than those obtained in 89 age-matched healthy males. Weight correlated significantly with uric acid.

Some recent data have suggested that body fat and the distribution pattern of fat may be more important than total weight as a risk factor for gout (67). The association between fat distribution and gout was examined in 95 overweight adult men and 210 overweight adult women (67). It was found that, adjusted for age and body mas index, a high waist-thigh circumference ratio was a risk factor for gout, particularly in women. The association of waist-hip circumference ratio with gout was less pronounced in men. Visceral fat (estimated from abdominal CT scans) was shown to be independently related to serum uric acid concentration, uric acid clearance, and uric acid/creatinine ratio, while BMI and subcutaneous fat were not (68).

B Evidence from Longitudinal Studies for Obesity as a Risk Factor for Gout

The association of obesity with gout is also supported by longitudinal studies. The Johns Hopkins Precursors study, a cohort study of medical students, was examined with the aim of identifying potentially modifiable risk factors for the development of gout (69). Predominantly young (median age, 22 years), white, male students (n = 1271) received a standardized medical examination and questionnaire during medical school. The outcome measure was the development of gout. Sixty cases of gout (47 primary and 13 secondary) were identified among 1216 men; none occurred among 121 women. In this study, body mass index at age 35 years, excessive weight gain between cohort entry and age 35 years were significant risk factors for gout in univariate analysis. Multivariate analyses confirmed the association of BMI at age 35 years and excessive weight gain as risk factors for gout.

Data from the Harvard Growth Study of 1922–1935 was used to examine the long-term effect of obesity in adolescence on morbidity, including the development of gout (70). A total of 508 lean or overweight adolescents 13–18 years old that participated in the Harvard Growth Study were included in this subanalysis. Overweight adolescents were defined as those with a BMI that on two occasions was greater than the 75th centile in subjects of the same age and sex in a large national survey. Lean adolescents were defined as those with a body mass index between the 25th and 50th centiles. The risk of gout was increased among men who had been overweight in adolescence. Overweight in adolescence was a more powerful predictor of this risk than overweight in adulthood.

In hyperuricemic men, a further increase in BMI has been shown to be a predictor for the development of gout (71).

C Association of Gout and Other Metabolic Disorders

Hyperuricemia has been shown to correlate with a cluster of metabolic and hemodynamic disorders closely associated with insulin resistance syndrome (IRS) in young, apparently healthy individuals (72). After adjustment for sex, serum uric acid concentration showed positive associations with BMI, waist/hip girth, waist/thigh girt, and subscapula/triceps skinfold ratios. Furthermore, serum uric acid was also positively correlated with fasting insulin, serum triglycerides, and LDL cholesterol, and negatively with HDL/total cholesterol ratio. This has been confirmed in other studies (73). Furthermore, urinary uric acid clearance appears to decrease in proportion to increase in insulin resistance in normal volunteers, leading to an increase in serum uric acid concentration. Thus, it appears that modulation of serum uric concentration by insulin resistance is exerted at the level of the kidney (73). Other studies investigating the relationship between gout and hyperuricemia and coronary artery disease have suggested that hyperuricemia, as a component of IRS (but not independently), may act as a risk factor for coronary artery disease (74,75).

Thus, obesity has a number of effects on urate metabolism, which include decreasing urate clearance (73) and increasing urate production (76). It has been suggested that other factors such as muscle mass may also play a role in producing hyperuricemia (77). Weight reduction has been associated with a modest lowering of the serum urate concentration (78).

D Diet

It is thought that the increase in the prevalence of gout the last century may relate to the changing nutritional patterns associated with increasing industrialization (79). Genetic factors and nutrition combine such that the disease may become manifest. Interest has largely focused on the more abundant diet that is also richer in purines. For example, a study in the Ukraine showed that in the period from 1925–28 to 1970–71 there was an increase in the consumption of animal products (milk, meat, fish, eggs), sugar, vegetables, and fruits, and a fall in the consumption of cereals (bakery products, grits, macaroni, beans) and potato (80). In parallel with these dietary changes, the incidence of diseases such as gout increased over the same time period (80).

Population-based studies have confirmed the association between diet and gout. A study of 460 apparently healthy Dutch elderly aged 65–79 years showed that serum uric acid correlated with alcohol intake (men) and consumption of meat and fish (women), and inversely with consumption of bread, margarine, and milk products (women), independently of confounders such as body mass index (62). A community-based survey of 1738 registered residents $\geq$30 years of age in Pu-Li Township, Taiwan, from 1987 to 1988, showed that organ meat consumption significantly correlated with hyperuricemia after simultaneously controlling for weight (81).

Migration studies have also suggested a role for a richer diet in gout. The incidence of hyperuricemia and gout has been well recognized to be higher among Filipinos in Hawaii, Alaska, and mainland United States than in their native country (82). It appears that Filipino hyperuricemia may become manifest because some Filipinos possess a renal defect that may lead to hyperuricemia due to renal inability to compensate for an increased purine intake which may occur in the shift from a low-purine Filipino diet to a high-purine Western diet in the new environment (82).

To examine the effect of ingesting some purine-rich foods (beef liver, haddock filets, and soybeans) on uric acid metabolism, a crossover study was performed where three isoenergetic and isonitrogenous meals were fed to 18 male subjects with no history of gout or kidney disorder during a 3-week period (83). Only the content of uricogenic bases (adenine and hypoxanthine) varied among the test meals. Ingestion of all experimental meals caused an increase in serum uric acid levels at 120 min, and this increase was more marked (about twofold) with haddock and soybean ingestion. In all groups, the postprandial serum uric acid levels at 240 min were lower than those obtained at 120 min, but still remained elevated in comparison to the fasting level. As expected, 24-hr urinary uric acid excretion was similar for the three test meals owing to the isonitrogenous load of proteins and purines. This study suggested that assessment of each purine base content rather than the total purine content of foods may be important in the management of hyperuricemic individuals.

Conversely, Dessein et al. (84) theorized that if hyperuricemia were a component of insulin resistance syndrome, then loss of weight through moderate limitation of caloric and carbohydrate intake, together with an increased proportion of protein and replacement of saturated by unsaturated fat should reduce gout and hyperuricemia—despite this being the converse to the diet recommended to reduce the purine load. In a pilot study of 13 men (one normal BMI, six overweight, six obese) with acute intermittent gout, weight reduction reduced the frequency of episodes of gout and level of hyperuricemia and improved the serum lipid profile. This warrants further investigation.

E Alcohol

Many studies with different study designs and in different populations have now shown a relationship between alcohol consumption and gout (85–91). For example, in a population-based study in Denmark, 5249 males aged between 40 and 59 were interviewed to identify a history of gout (91). A total of 104 men who had experienced gout were compared to 208 computer-selected age-matched controls drawn at random from the entire sample. Alcohol consumption was higher in gout cases than in controls. In a cohort of 2046 initially healthy men in the Normative Aging Study followed for 14.9 years with serial examinations and measurement of urate levels, alcohol intake was a strong predictor of gout when examined in a proportional hazards model (92). In a longitudinal cohort study of hyperuricemic men, persistent alcohol consumption was a predictor of incident gout (71).

Migration studies have also confirmed the association between alcohol and gout. In a study of the prevalence and 14-year incidence of clinical gout in the Polynesian population of Tokelauans living in the Pacific Basin, nonmigrant Tokelauans living in their isolated atoll homeland being compared with migrant Tokelauans living in urban New Zealand (93). Self-reported alcohol consumption at entry to the study was a strong predictor of gout in men. Factors predisposing to acute gout were investigated in a case control study (94) of 70 patients with acute gout and matched for age and sex controls. Gout was significantly associated with obesity (odds ratio 3.7; 95% CI 1.4, 9.1) and high alcohol intake (odds ratio 3.3; 95% CI 1.1, 9.8). In these patients, it was estimated that 23% of gout was attributable to obesity and 16% to high alcohol consumption.

To determine the contribution of alcohol to increased production and decreased excretion of uric acid, a study was performed where oral ethanol (1.8 g/k body weight every 24 hr) for 8 days or intravenous ethanol (0.25–0.35 g/k/hr) for 2 hr was given to six patients with gout (95). The results of this study suggested that ethanol increases urate synthesis by enhancing the turnover of adenine nucleotides (95). A further study showed that chronic oral ethanol administration was associated with increased serum urate, urine uric acid excretion, urine uric acid clearance, and oxypurine excretion (96). The daily rate of uric acid turnover was significantly increased. Intravenous ethanol administration was associated with increased uric acid excretion, increased uric acid clearance, and significantly increased oxypurine excretion. Excretion of radioactivity derived from intravenously administered adenine increased significantly. It concluded that hyperuricemia related to ethanol consumption at lower blood ethanol levels (<150 mg/dL) results from increased production of uric acid probably secondary to accelerated degradation of adenine nucleotides.

Although red wine and not beer drinking has traditionally been linked to gout, beer drinking may have an additional effect on the risk of gout. A recent study of 61 men with gout and 52 control subjects showed that the patients with gout drank significantly more alcohol and that the average daily intake of most other nutrients, including total purine nitrogen, was similar (97). Beer was the most popular beverage, and 25 (41%) of those with gout consumed >60 g alcohol daily (equivalent to 2.5 L beer). The heavy drinkers had a significantly higher intake of purine nitrogen, half of which was derived from beer. Though the effect of ingested purine on the blood uric acid was difficult to estimate in this study, it was probably sufficient to have a clinical effect, augmenting the hyperuricemic effect of alcohol itself. A further study attempted to simulate the beer-drinking habits of gout patients and examine the effect on uric acid levels (98). Beer or squash was drunk over a 4-hr period on two successive days by five gouty and five normouricemic men. Serum lactate increased with beer and squash, but elevation of plasma uric acid was confined to beer drinking. Urate clearane increased with both beverages, but 24-hr uric acid excretion was accentuated only by beer. The purine content of several beers was measured and the principal constituent found to be guanosine, which is probably the most readily absorbed dietary purine. It was concluded that the hyperuricemic effect of beer was mediated by the digestion of purines contained by the beer and by an effect of ethanol on uric acid synthesis. However, there was no evidence that beer taken in usual quantities reduced the renal excretion of uric acid.

IV SUMMARY

Obesity is an important risk factor for osteoarthritis and gout, which are two common, chronic diseases associated with significant morbidity and cost to the community. Preventive efforts to reduce obesity in the population are likely to have a major impact on these two conditions.

ACKNOWLEDGMENTS

We would like to thank Dr. Nisha Manek for her helpful comments.

REFERENCES

1. Yelin EH, Callahan L. The economic cost and social and psychological impact of musculoskeletal conditions. Arthritis Rheum 1995; 38:1351–1362.
2. Yelin EH. The Economic Impact and Functional Impact of Rheumatic Disease in the US. Vol 1. 2d ed. London: Mosby, 1998.
3. Burton WN, Chen C-Y, Schultz AB, Edington DW. The economic costs associated with body mass index in a workplace. J Occup Environ Med 1998; 40(9):786–792.
4. Cunningham LS, Kelsey JL. Epidemiology of musculoskeletal impairments and associated disability. Am J Public Health 1984; 74:574–579.
5. Verbrugge LM. From Sneezes to Adieux: Stages of Health for American Men and Women. New York: Springer, 1987.
6. Bulstrode C. Keeping up with orthopaedic epidemics. BMJ 1987; 295:514.
7. Dieppe P. Osteoarthritis; the Scale and Scope of the Clinical Problem. Osteoarthritis: Current Research and Prospects for Pharmacological Intervention. London: IBC Technical Services Ltd, 1991.
8. Fletcher E, Lewis-Faning E. Chronic rheumatic diseases with special reference to chronic arthritis: a survey based on 1000 cases. Postgrad Med J 1945; 21:51–56.
9. Kellgren JH, Lawrence JS. Osteoarthritis and disk degeneration in an urban population. Ann Rheum Dis 1958; 17:388–396.
10. Acheson RM, Collart AB. New Haven survey of joint diseases. XVII. Relationship between some systemic characteristics and osteoarthrosis in a general population. Ann Rheum Dis 1975; 34(5):379–387.
11. Hartz AJ, Fischer ME, Bril G, Kelber S, Rupley D Jr, Oken B. The association of obesity with joint pain and osteoarthritis in the HANES data. J Chron Dis 1986; 39(4):311–319.
12. Felson DT, Anderson JJ, Naimark A, Walker AM, Meenan RF. Obesity and knee osteoarthritis. The Framingham Study. Ann Intern Med 1988; 109(1):18–24.
13. Anderson JJ, Felson DT. Factors associated with osteoarthritis of the knee in the first national Health and Nutrition Examination Survey (HANES I). Evidence for an association with overweight, race, and physical demands of work. A J Epidemiol 1988; 128(1): 179–189.
14. Davis MA, Ettinger WH, Neuhaus JM. Obesity and osteoarthritis of the knee: evidence from the National Health and Nutrition Examination Survey (NHANES I). Semin Arthritis Rheum 1990; 20(3 suppl 1):34–41.
15. Davis MA, Ettinger WH, Neuhaus JM, Cho SA, Hauck WW. The association of knee injury and obesity with unilateral and bilateral osteoarthritis of the knee. Am J Epidemiol 1989; 130(2):278–288.
16. Hart DJ, Spector TD. The relationship of obesity, fat distribution and osteoarthritis in women in the general population: the Chingford Study. J Rheumatol 1993; 20(2):331–335.
17. Cooper C, Cushnaghan J, Kirwan J, et al. Radiological

asessment of the knee joint in osteoarthritis. Br J Rheum 1992; 51:80–82.
18. McAlindon TE, Snow S, Cooper C, Dieppe PA. Radiographic patterns of knee osteoarhtitis in the community: the importance of the patellofemoral joint. Ann Rheum Dis 1993; 51:844–849.
19. Leadingham J, Regan M, Jones A, Doherty M. Radiographic patterns and associations of osteoarthritis of the knee in patients referred to hospital. Ann Rheum Dis 1993; 52:520–526.
20. Cooper C, McAlindon T, Snow S, Vines K, Young P, Kirwan J. Mechanical and constitutional risk factors for symptomatic knee osteoarthritis: differences between medial tibiofemoral and patellofemoral disease. J Rheumatol 1994; 21(2):307–313.
21. Cicuttini FM, Spector T, Baker J. Risk factors for osteoarthritis in the tibiofemoral and patellofemoral joints of the knee. J Rheumatol 1997; 24(6):1164–1167.
22. Felson DT. Obesity and osteoarthritis of the knee. Bull Rheum Dis 1992; 41(2):6–7.
23. Gelber AC, Hochberg MC, Mead LA, Wang NY, Wigley FM, Klag MJ. Body mass index in young men and the risk of subsequent knee and hip osteoarthritis. Am J Med 1999; 107(6):542–548.
24. Hart DJ, Doyle DV, Spector TD. Incidence and risk factors for radiographic knee osteoarthritis in middle-aged women: the Chingford Study. Arthritis Rheum 1999; 42(1):17–24.
25. Hochberg MC, Lawrence RC, Everett DF, Cornoni-Huntley J. Epidemiologic associations of pain in osteoarthritis of the knee: data from the National Health and Nutrition Examination Survey and the National Health and Nutrion Examination-I Epidemiologic Follow-up Survey. Semin Arthritis Rheum 1989; 18(4 suppl 2):4–9.
26. Acheson RM, Kelsey JL, Ginsburg GN. The New Haven survey of joint diseases. XVI. Impairment, disability and arthritis. Br J Prev Med 1974; 27:168–176.
27. Van Saase JL, Van denbroucke JP, Van Romunde LK, Valkenburg HA. Osteoarthritis and obesity in the general population. A relationship calling for an explanation. J Rheumatol 1988; 15(7):1152–1158.
28. Davis MA, Neuhaus JM, Ettinger WH, Mueller WH. Body fat distribution and osteoarthritis. Am J Epidemiol 1990; 132(4):701–707.
29. Bagge E, Bjelle A, Eden S, Svanborg A. Factors associated with radiographic osteoarthritis: results from the population study 70-year-old people in Goteborg. J Rheumatol 1991; 18:1218–1222.
30. Oliveria SA, Felson DT, Cirillo PA, Reed JI, Walker AM. Body weight, body mass index, and incident symptomatic osteoarthritis of the hand, hip, and knee. Epidemiology 1999; 10(2):161–166.
31. Sowers MF, Zobel D, Weissfeld L, Hawthorne VM, Carman W. Progression of osteoarthritis of the hand and metacarpal bone loss: a twenty-year followup of incident cases. Arthritis Rheum 1991; 34:36–42.
32. Hochberg MC, Lethbridge-Cejku M, Plato CC, Wigley FM, Tobin JD. Factors associated with osteoarthritis of the hand in males: data from the Baltimore Longitudinal Study of Aging. Am J Epidemiol 1991; 134(10):1121–1127.
33. Sturmer T, Gunther KP, Brenner H. Obesity, overweight and patterns of osteoarthritis: the Ulm Osteoarthritis Study. J Clin Epidemiol 2000; 53(3):307–313.
34. Carman WJ, Sowers M, Hawthorne VM, Weissfeld LA. Obesity as a risk factor for osteoarthritis of the hand and wrist: a prospective study. Am J Epidemiol 1994; 139(2): 119–129.
35. Vingard E. Overweight predisposes to coxarthrosis. Body-mass index studied in 239 males with hip arthroplasty. Acta Orthop Scand 1991; 62:106–109.
36. Tepper S, Hochberg MC. Factors associated with hip osteoarthritis: data from the First National Health and Nutrition Examination Survey (NHANES-I). Am J Epidemiol 1993; 137(10):1081–1088.
37. Davis MA, Ettinger WH, Neuhaus JM, Hauck WW. Sex differences in osteoarthritis of the knee. The role of obesity. Am J Epidemiol 1988; 127(5):1019–1030.
38. Sharma L, Lou C, Cahue S, Dunlop DD. The mechanism of the effect of obesity, in knee osteoarthritis: the mediating role of malalignment. Arthritis Rheum 2000; 43(3):568–575.
39. Dequeker J, Goris P, Uytterhoeven R. Osteoporosis and osteoarthritis (osteoarthrosis). Anthropometric distinctions. JAMA 1983; 249(11):1448–1451.
40. Lawrence JS. Hypertension in relation to musculoskeletal disorders. Ann Rheum Dis 1975; 34(5):451–456.
41. Hart DJ, Doyle DV, Spector TD. Association between metabolic factors and knee osteoarthritis in women: the Chingford Study. J Rheumatol 1995; 22(6):111–1123.
42. Davis MA, Ettinger WH, Neuhaus JM. The role of metabolic factors and blood pressure in the association of obesity with osteoarthritis of the knee. J Rheumatol 1988; 15(12):1827–1832.
43. Martin K, Lethbridge-Cejku M, Muller DC, Elahi D, Andres R, Tobin JD. Metabolic correlates of obesity and radiographic features of knee osteoarthritis: data from the Baltimore Longitudinal Study of Aging. J Rheumatol 1997; 24(4):702–707.
44. Kellgren JH. Osteoarthritis in patients and populations. BMJ 1961; 1:1–6.
45. Cimmino MA, Cutolo M. Plasma glucose concentration in symptomatic osteoarthritis: a clinical and epidemiological survey. Clin Exp Rheumatol 1990; 8(3):251–257.
46. Horn CA, Bradley JD, Brandt KD, Kreipke DL, Slowman SD, Kalasinski LA. Impairment of osteophyte formation in hyperglycaemic patients with type II diabetes mellitus and knee osteoarthritis. Arthritis Rheum 1992; 35(3):336–342.
47. Reven GM. Role of insulin resistance in human disease. Diabetes 1988; 37:1595–1607.
48. Eckel RH. Insulin resistance: an adaptation for weight maintenance. Lancet 1992; 340:1452–1453.
49. Joos SK, Mueller WH, Hanis CL, Schull WJ. Diabetes

alert study: weight history and upper body obesity in diabetic and non-diabetic Mexican American adults. Ann Hum Biol 1984; 11(2):167–171.

50. Hochberg MC, Lethbridge-Cejku M, Scott WW Jr, Reichle R, Plato CC, Tobin JD. The association of body weight, body fatness and body fat distribution with osteoarthritis of the knee: data from the Baltimore Longitudinal Study of Aging. J Rheumatol 1995; 22(3):488–493.
51. Spector TD, Dacre JE, Harris PA, Huskisson EC. The radiological progression of osteoarthritis; an eleven year follow-up study of the knee. Ann Rheum Dis 1992; 51:1107–1110.
52. Schouten JS, Van den Ouwel FA, Valkenburg HA. A 12 year follow up study in the general population on prognostic factors of cartilage loss in osteoarthritis of the knee. Ann Rheum Dis 1992; 51(8):932–937.
53. Dougados M, Gueguen A, Nguyen M, Thiesce A, Listrat V, Jacob L. Longitudinal radiologic evaluation of osteoarthritis of the knee. J Rheumatol 1992; 19(3): 378–384.
54. Verbrugge LM, Gates DM, Ike RW. Risk factors for disability among U.S. adults with arthritis. J Clin Epidemiol 1991; 44(2):167–182.
55. Bremmer JM, Bier F. Osteoarthrosis: prevalence in and relationship between symptoms and x-ray changes. Rheum Dis 1966; 25:1–24.
56. Williams RA, Foulsham BM. Weight reduction in osteoarthritis using phentermine. Practitioner 1981; 22S:231–232.
57. McGoey B, Deitel M, Saplys RJ, Kliman ME. Effect of weight loss on musculoskeletal pain in the morbidly obese. J Bone Joint Surg 1990; 72B:322–323.
58. Toda Y, Toda T, Takemura S, Wada T, Morimoto T, Ogawa R. Change in body fat, but not body weight or metabolic correlates of obesity, is related to symptomatic relief of obese patients with knee osteoarthritis after a weight control program. J Rheumatol 1998; 25(11): 2181–2186.
59. Felson DT, Zhang Y, Anthony JM, Naimark A, Anderson JJ. Weight loss reduces the risk for symptomatic knee osteoarthritis in women. The Framingham Study. Ann Intern Med 1992; 116(7):535–539.
60. Mertz DP, Babucke G. Epidemiology and clinical findings in primary gout. Observations between 1948 and 1968. Munch Med Wochensch 1971; 113:617–624.
61. Rimm AA, Werner LH, Yserloo BV, Bernstein R. Relationship of obesity and disease in 73,532 weight-conscious women. Public Health Rep 1975; 90:44–54.
62. Loenen HM, Eshuis H, Lowik MR, Schouten EG, Hulshof KF, Odink I. Serum uric acid correlates in elderly men and women with special reference to body composition and dietary intake (Dutch Nutrition Surveillance System). J Clin Epidemiol 1990; 43:1297–1303.
63. Weatherall R, Shaper AG. Overweight and obesity in middle-aged British men. Eur J Clin Nutr 1988; 42:221–231.
64. Gibson T, Waterworth R, Hatfield P, Robinson G, Bremner K. Hyperuricaemia, gout and kidney function in New Zealand Maori men. Br J Rheum 1984; 23:276–282.
65. Tuomilehto J, Zimmet P, Wolf E, Taylor R, Ram P, King H. Plasma uric acid level and its association with diabetes mellitus and some biologic parameters in a biracial population of Fiji. Am J Epidemiol 1988; 127:321–336.
66. Nishizawa T, Akaoka I, Nishida Y, Kawaguchi Y, Hayashi E. Some factors related to obesity in the Japanese sumo wrestler. Am J Clin Nutr 1976; 29:1167–1174.
67. Seidell JC, Bakx JC, De Boer E, Deurenberg P, Hautvast JG. Fat distribution of overweight persons in relation to morbidity and subjective health. Int J Obes 1985; 9:363–374.
68. Takahashi S, Yamamoto T, Tsutsumi Z, Moriwaki Y, Yamakita J, Higashino K. Close correlation between visceral fat accumulation and uric acid metabolism in healthy men. Metabolism 1997; 46(10):1162–1165.
69. Roubenoff R, Klag MJ, Mead LA, Liang KY, Seidler AJ, Hochberg MCJ. Incidence and risk factors for gout in white men. JAMA 1991; 266:3004–3007
70. Must A, Jacques PF, Dallal GE, Bajema CJ, Dietz WH. Long-term morbidity and mortality of overweight adolescents. A follow-up of the Harvard Growth Study of 1922 to 1935. N Engl J Med 1992; 327:1350–1355.
71. Lin K-C, Lin H-Y, Chou P. The interaction between uric acid level and other risk factors on the development of gout among asymptomatic hyperuricemic men in a prospective study. J Rheumatol 2000; 27:1501–1505.
72. Cigolini M, Targher G, Tonoli M, Manara F, Muggeo M, De Sandre G. Hyperuricaemia: relationships to body fat distribution and other components of the insulin resistance syndrome in 38-year-old healthy men and women. Int J Obes Relat Metab Disord 1995; 19:92–96.
73. Facchini F, Chen YD, Hollenbeck CB, Reaven GM. Relationship between resistance to insulin-mediated glucose uptake, urinary uric acid clearance, and plasma uric acid concentration. JAMA 1995; 66:3008–3011.
74. Wannamethee SG, Shaper AG, Whincup PH. Serum urate and the risk of major coronary heart disease events. Heart 1997; 78:147–153.
75. Culleton BF, Larson MG, Kannel WB, Levy D. Serum uric acid and risk for cardiovascular disease and death: the Framingham Heart Study. Ann Intern Med 1999; 131:7–13.
76. Emmerson BT. Alteration of uric acid metabolism by weight reduction. Aust NZ J Med 1973; 3:410–412.
77. Brauer GW, Prior IAM. A prospective study of gout in New Zealand Maoris. Ann Rheum Dis 1978; 37:466–472.
78. Scott JT. Obesity and uricaemia. Clin Rheum Dis 1977; 3:25–35.
79. Zollner NB. Consequences of malnutrition in prosper-

ous countries. Zentralbl Bakteriol Orig 1976; 163:111–117.
80. Maistruk PN, Priputina LS, Rudenko AK, Smoliar VI. Nutrition and the state of health of the population of the UkrSSR. Vopr Pitan 1976; 1:13–17.
81. Chou P, Soong LN, Lin HY. Community-based epidemiological study on hyperuricemia in Pu-Li, Taiwan. J Formos Med Assoc 1993; 92:597–602.
82. Torralba TP, Bayani Sioson PS. The Filipino and gout. Semin Arthritis Rheum 1975; 4:307–320.
83. Brule D, Sarwar G, Savoie L. Changes in serum and urinary uric acid levels in normal human subjects fed purine-rich foods containing different amounts of adenine and hypoxanthine. J Am Coll Nutr 1992; 11:353–358.
84. Dessein PH, Shipton EA, Stanwix AE, Joffe BI, Ramokgadi I. Beneficial effects of weight loss associated with moderate calorie/carbohydrate restriction, and increased proportional intake of protein and unsaturated fat on serum urate and lipoprotein levels in gout: a pilot study. Ann Rheum Dis 2000; 59(7):539–553.
85. Takahashi S, Yamamoto T, Moriwaki Y, Tsutsumi Z, Higashino K. Impaired lipoprotein metabolism in patients with primary gout—influence of alcohol intake and body weight. Br J Rheumatol 1994; 33:731–734.
86. Lutalo SK, Mabonga N. A clinical assessment of the consequences of alcohol consumption in 'communal' drinkers in the Zimbabwean Midlands. Cent Afr J Med 1992; 38:380–384.
87. al Jarallah KF, Shehab DK, Buchanan WW. Rheumatic complications of alcohol abuse. Semin Arthritis Rheum 1992; 22:162–171.
88. Cook DG, Shaper AG, Thelle DS, Whitehead TP. Serum uric acid, serum glucose and diabetes: relationships in a population study. Postgrad Med J 1986; 62:1001–1006.
89. Tofler OB, Woodings TL. A 13-year follow-up of social drinkers. Med J Aust 1981; 2:479–481.
90. Nishioka K, Mikanagi K. Hereditary and environmental factors influencing on the serum uric acid throughout ten years population study in Japan. Adv Exp Med Biol 1980; 122A:155–159.
91. De Muckadell OB, Gyntelberg F. Occurrence of gout in Copenhagen males aged 40–59. Int J Epidemiol 1976; 5:153–158.
92. Campion EW, Glynn RJ, DeLabry LO. Asymptomatic hyperuricemia. Risks and consequences in the Normative Aging Study. Am J Med 1987; 82:421–426.
93. Prior IA, Welby TJ, Ostbye T, Salmond CE, Stokes YM. Migration and gout: the Tokelau Island migrant study. BMJ 1987; 295:457–461.
94. Waller PC, Ramsay LE. Predicting acute gout in diuretic-treated hypertensive patients. J Hum Hypertens 1989; 3:457–461.
95. Faller J, Fox IH. Ethanol-induced hyperuricemia: evidence for increased urate production by activation of adenine nucleotide turnover. N Engl J Med 1982; 307:1598–1602.
96. Faller J, Fox JH. Ethanol induced alterations of uric acid metabolism. Adv Exp Med Biol 1984; 165(Pt A):457–462.
97. Gibson T, Rodgers AV, Simmonds HA, Court-Brown F, Todd E, Meilton V. A controlled study of diet in patients with gout. Ann Rheum Dis 1983; 42:123–127.
98. Gibson T, Rodgers AV, Simmonds HA, Toseland P. Beer drinking and its effect on uric acid. Br J Rheumatol 1984; 23:203–209.

41

Obesity, Pregnancy, and Infertility

Stephan Rössner

Huddinge University Hospital, Huddinge, Sweden

I GENERAL HORMONAL BACKGROUND

By definition obesity implies an excess of adipose tissue, which is not an inert storage room for triglycerides but actually the largest hormonally active gland of the body (1). Fat cells are known to convert androstenedione to estrone (2,3). Increased concentrations of estrone in obesity may interfere with the feedback system to the hypothalmohypophysial axis, increasing the levels of gonadotropins and androgens (4). As a consequence anovulation may occur. Furthermore, in obesity a reduction in sex hormone–binding globulin (SHBG) concentrations is seen, and the end result is an increased concentration of biologically active free androgens.

Menstrual disturbances are frequent in obesity and may often be normalized after weight reduction (5–7). Several studies have demonstrated that with weight reduction various characteristics of the hormonal profile can be normalized. As early as the 1950s the relationship between obesity and menstrual disorders was reported (8). A particular clinical syndrome associated with obesity and anovulation is the polycystic ovarian syndrome (PCOS), characterized by anovulation, hyperandrogenism, insulin resistance, and altered gonadotropin secretion (9,10). Several investigations have analyzed the relationship between weight loss and menstrual function in PCOS, but often these designs have had clinical and methodological limitations. In some situations, appropriate endocrine characteristics have not been available, and in others no proper control group has been included.

In the study of Guzick (11), on the other hand, a group of obese hyperandrogenic anovulatory women were studied in a prospective randomized controlled fashion before and after a weight loss of 16.2 kg. This weight loss resulted in a significant increase in SHBG, a significant reduction in non-SHBG testosterone levels, and resumed ovulation in two-thirds of these subjects. These changes appeared in spite of nonsignificant reductions in fasting insulin concentrations and LH and FSH concentration characteristics.

The positive effects of weight reduction in obese women with PCOS are underscored by a study of Hamilton-Fairley et al. (12). These authors suggest that all overweight women—whether with PCOS or not—should be advised to lose weight before attempted conception in order to improve their chances of a successful outcome, and furthermore that PCOS women requiring gonadotropin treatment should consider weight loss before treatment to improve their chances of a successful pregnancy.

II OBESITY AFTER PREGNANCY

It is common clinical experience that many overweight women report that each pregnancy has resulted in weight retention after delivery. Since pregnancy can in fact be viewed as an example of weight cycling, increased interest has been focused on the behavioral and metabolic consequences of such repeated body weight cycling (13). Generally, weight cycles have been caused by initial weight loss during dieting programs with subsequent regains after relapse. The weight increase and subsequent fall during pregnancy constitute an interesting biological and "normal" cause of such reversed weight cycling.

Over the years interest has been focused on the possible role of repeated changes in body weight as a risk factor for coronary hearth disease and all-cause mortality (14). When pregnancy-associated weight changes in terms of weight cycling and risk have been discussed, this has mainly been in normal-weight women and in relation to the fat distribution pattern (13).

As part of the Stockholm Pregnancy and Weight Development Study, a retrospective pilot study to obtain an impression of the role of pregnancy on body weight development in severely obese women was carried out (15). Seventy-three percent of these women (83/113) retained >10 kg in association with the pregnancy period and up to 1 year after delivery. Although it has been well documented that the body weight of women increases with parity and that many women have a higher body weight in the beginning of a subsequent pregnancy than in the previous one (16), there is little information concerning the importance of pregnancies in the development of obesity.

Several methodological questions may be raised regarding the validity of the self-reported data and the retrospective design of such studies. For some women, their pregnancies were certainly many years behind them, and it can be argued that memory must have been uncertain. However, most women do indeed remember their pregnancy-associated weight changes quite well. From these data it seems reasonable to assume that for many women, pregnancy has actually resulted in pronounced and sustained weight gain.

III WEIGHT DEVELOPMENT AND PREGNANCY

Maternal weight development can vary to a very great extent and still be compatible with healthy pregnancy outcomes, which makes rigid recommendations meaningless. As reviewed by Johnson (17), weight loss during pregnancy as well as weight increases up to more than 23 kg may result in quite normal birth outcomes. Some factors affecting variation in weight gain are maternal characteristics such as age, prepregnancy weight, parity, multiple pregnancies, ethnic origin, various aspects of socioeconomic status, drug abuse, and physical activity levels.

A Pregnancy, Weight, and Age

Mean body weight and the prevalence of obesity increase with pregnancy. Rookus et al. (18) reviewed the older literature on this issue (16,19–26) and concluded that (1) the cohort sizes varied from 49 to 35,556 deliveries; (2) age correction was seldom carried out; (3) prepregnancy weight was generally not well measured; and (4) the timing of the postpartum weight measurement varied from 4 to 24 months.

In a later extensive review by Harris (27), the general outcome of this literature was summarized as follows: 90% of all studies reviewed found a body weight greater after pregnancy than before (by 0.2-10.6 kg). However, only 3/71 studies in her review (18,28,29) complied with the following quality criteria:

1. Accurate measurements of body weight from conception and onwards must be obtained.
2. Sufficient time for weight lost after delivery must be allowed.
3. The parallel effect of ageing during pregnancy and follow-up must be accounted for.

In this subgroup (18,28,29) the average "cost" of a pregnancy was 0.9-3.3 kg. These differences in weight gain became slightly smaller (0.4-3.0 kg) after control for several sociobehavioral confounders. Thus in the literature it is generally rare that factors such as age, height, education, parity, giving up work, smoking habits, prepregnant weight and activity, alcohol consumption, marital status, morbidity, and dieting behavior obviously of importance in evaluating the role of physical activity, are accounted for (27). This evaluation is further complicated by the fact that changes of these confounders may take place in different ways and during various phases of the entire pregnancy period.

Since body weight also increases with age in the fertile age groups, it has been necessary to analyze weight increase, parity, and age separately. Such studies demonstrate that the weight increase associated with pregnancy is age independent. The relationship between body weight development and parity can be illustrated by Figure 1, derived from a Finnish study (30).

Body weight increases with age, whether women have children or not. Figure 2, based on a representative sample of the entire Swedish adult female population, is a cross-sectional example of the increase in BMI with age, more pronounced in women than in men. It should

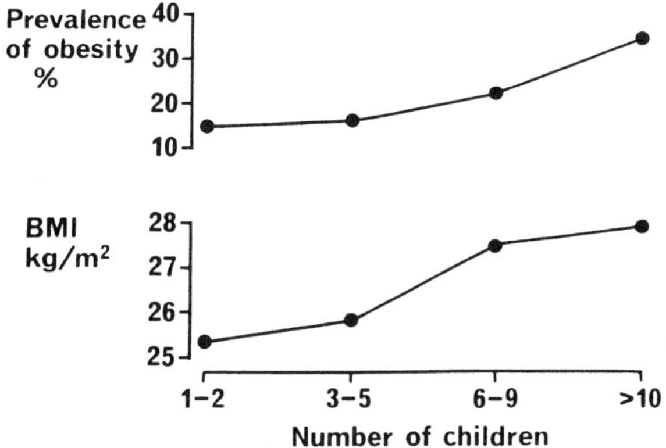

Figure 1 Relationship between body weight and parity. (From Ref. 30.)

be kept in mind that the basal metabolic rate typically decreases by ~1% per year. For an individual who maintains an identical lifestyle with regard to eating habits and exercise, this implies a weight increase of about 3-4 kg per 10 years, which could possibly be regarded as "biological."

The average of reported weight increases with pregnancies thus range from 0.4 to 3.0 kg compared with prepregnancy weights (18). However, as many authors point out, there are several methological complications that have to be taken into account, when these data are evaluated:

1. Women generally do not have recorded weight data at the time of conception. Initial body weight information is hence uncertain.

2. Weight increase during pregnancy consists of several components such as the weight of the fetus, the weight of placenta, amniotic fluid and the enlarged uterus, the whole-body water retention caused by the pregnancy, and finally the adipose tissue increase of the mother (31) (Table 1). For obvious technical and ethical reasons it is not possible to analyze all of these compartments in larger studies.

3. There is the methodological question to consider as when to determine postpregnancy body weight. Many women may change their weight during a considerable period of time after delivery. If the weight measurement is taken soon after delivery, this figure may not be representative of the entire weight development associated with the pregnancy as such. If, on the other hand, the weight after delivery is recorded at a late stage, numerous other life changes may have taken part, not primarily related to the pregnancy and delivery. In women in the active child-producing ages, some will be pregnant again, if the time span measurement is taken to 1 year after delivery.

Generally, a mean weight increase of 12.5 kg is considered normal during an entire pregnancy. In different studies reported by Ash et al. (32), the mean increase has ranged between 10.7 and 15.2 kg. In developing countries the weight increase for obvious reasons is considerably lower. Of the total weight increase a certain proportion consists of maternal adipose tissue, ~ 3-6 kg. This adipose tissue storage occurs mainly during the first two trimesters. From a nutritional point of view it seems reasonable to assume that the adipose tissue storage during pregnancy provides energy for the child during the lactation period.

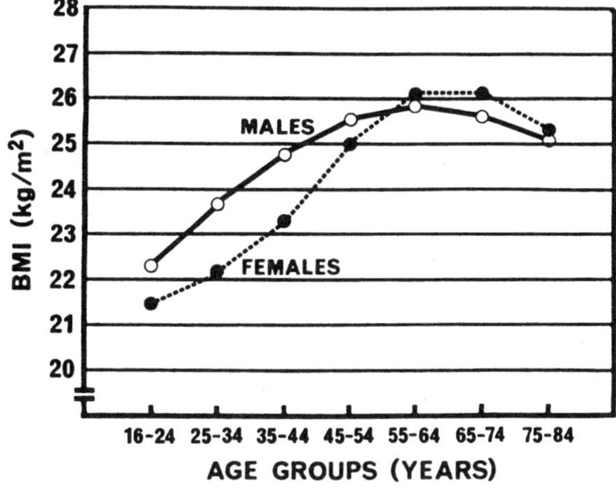

Figure 2 Mean BMI in different Swedish age groups. (From Ref. 95.)

Table 1 Weight Increase (Including Fluid Retention) in Various Tissues at Full Term

	Weight (g)	Fluid weight (g)
Fetus	3300	2340
Placenta	650	540
Amniotic fluid	800	790
Uterus	900	740
Mammary glands	400	300
Blood	1300	1100
Extracellular fluid	1200	1200
Other tissues (mainly fat)	3950	1000
Total	12,500	8010

Source: Ref. 31.

B Menopause and Weight Development

A marked weight increase occurs at the time of menopause. However, it is not clear whether this is related to the loss of the regular menstruations or aging in itself has these effects on body weight development. Weight increase to the degree of overweight and even obesity at the time of menopause may have important health implications, since this is a part of the risk factor pattern associated with atherosclerotic manifestations. It has been demonstrated that with menopause there is an increase in the atherogenic lipoprotein profile (33,34).

In an analysis of the Healthy Women's Study (35), weight changes and the effect of weight change on coronary heart disease risk factors were analyzed prospectively. Four hundred eighty five women were studied when they were premenopausal and aged 42-50 years and then restudied 3 years later. During this time period the average weight gain was 2.3 ± 4.2 kg, but there were no significant differences in weight gain of women who remained premenopausal and those who had a natural menopause. The weight gain observed was significantly associated with increases in conventional risk factors for coronary heart disease. However, it was not possible to predict who would gain weight based on the variables at entry to the study.

During the perimenopausal transition there is not only an increase in body weight but also a redistribution of adipose tissue with an increase in waist circumference and upper-body fat (36). This shift is also related to the change in carbohydrate metabolism (35).

The data from the Healthy Women's Study underscore the fact that much more information is needed concerning the effects of menopause on body weight development. Of particular interest for the future development are studies that are longitudinal and include various populations, since most previous work has almost exclusively been done in whites. It is of interest to note that a prospective study of Pima Indian women at the time of menopause found no changes in body weight with menopause and also no changes in lipoprotein levels (37).

C Energy Metabolism During Pregnancy

It is obvious that nutrient and energy intake should match maternal and fetal requirements in order to ensure an optimal outcome of a pregnancy. Maternal weight gain has been used as an indicator for nutritional status, and several studies have demonstrated that the weight gain is positively related with birth weight up to a certain weight level. Excessive weight gain during pregnancy is a clear risk for future development of obesity, and high weight gain during pregnancy is furthermore a risk factor associated with toxemia although it is likely that the toxemia of pregnancy in this case is rather the cause than the effect.

The body weight increase of the pregnant woman constitutes the sum of several tissues (31). To determine the true energy costs of a pregnancy, longitudinal studies are essential, since interindividual variations are marked. During recent years several such longitudinal studies have been published. In general they describe a similar pattern: in developing countries the energy costs of the pregnancy are low but increases in countries in the Western world. In all studies, however, the observed changes in energy intake over the entire pregnancy seem insufficient to meet the energy costs of the total pregnancy. This has led several researchers to speculate that substantial energy savings must occur during pregnancy.

The weakening of the relationship between gestational weight gain and birth weight with increasing body mass index of the woman suggests that in heavy women the energy supplies are generally sufficient, whereas in undernourished women the development of the fetus is more dependent on the state of the maternal nutrition. Thus different recommendations for suggested weight increase throughout a pregnancy may be appropriate in thin women. Energy balance is less of a problem in overweight women, and recommendations in this group would be adjusted accordingly.

D Energy Metabolism During Lactation

Energy requirements for an entire pregnancy are ~80,000 kcal or ~300 calories per day covering the needs for fetal growth and adipose tissue storage. Lactation has been assumed to facilitate weight loss after delivery, particularly if the period of lactation exceeds 2 months. Lactation has been calculated to increase the energy requirements by 500 kcal/d, which also takes into account that production of milk is an energy requiring process.

After delivery and during lactation, the role of maternal body fat mobilization could theoretically be a matter of conflicting interests. Excessive maternal body fat mobilization during lactation could increase the concentration of fat-soluble contaminants in the breast milk, which theoretically could have adverse health effects for a baby relying entirely on breast feeding. This is a research area that should be addressed in future research. A target group for such research would be older mothers for several reasons. First, body weight increases with age and parity and such mothers could be more inclined to try to use complete breast feeding as help to revert to prepregnancy body weight levels. On the other hand, since environmental contaminants accumulate with time in adipose tissue, the fat stores of these older mothers might contain a higher concentration of such toxins and thus pose a larger risk for the infant. It has recently been reported that PCB trace element concentrations increase in the circulation after weight loss, but the possible clinical significance of that finding is unclear (38).

Studies by Rebuffé-Scrive and others have demonstrated that the characteristics of the adipose tissue change dramatically during pregnancy [39]. Adipose tissue lipolysis in the femoral region is limited during pregnancy, but can be easily stimulated hormonally during lactation. This seems to be a functional adaptation of the adipose tissue to the needs of the mother and the child.

However, the relationships between lactation, energy needs, and energy balance are not fully clarified. In some studies no difference in energy intake was found between lactating and nonlactating women. Other studies suggest that lactation plays a minor roll in weight reduction after delivery (18,40). In the Stockholm Pregnancy and Weight Development Study a minor roll of lactation on body weight regulation was demonstrated (25,41).

From a theoretical point of view weight changes after delivery could also depend on changes in basal metabolic rates. Prentice and Prentice (42) identified three hypothetical mechanisms which could explain the lack of weight loss after delivery: (1) reduced basal metabolism; (2) impaired thermogenesis; and (3) reduced physical activity. These mechanisms could account for reduction in energy requirements of up to 240 calories per day. Thus, it is possible that the energy need during lactation can be provided from different sources such as a combination of an increased energy intake, utilization of adipose tissue in storage, and a metabolic adaption.

These hypotheses, however, were not supported by a Dutch study. Spaiij et al. (43–45) studied prospectively various aspect of energy metabolism in 27 women, who were monitored repeatedly before pregnancy, during each trimester and during lactation. Three different aspects of such energy savings were analyzed: the possibility that the thermic effect of meals is reduced during pregnancy; the possibility that work efficiency improves during pregnancy; and finally the alternative that during lactation the metabolic efficiency is altered.

No changes were observed of any of these three factors, possibly explaining the discrepancy between energy intake and the energy costs of a pregnancy. Therefore the Dutch group reassessed the extra energy needs during pregnancy and concluded that such extra needs may be met by an increase in energy intake but also by substantial behavioral adaptations. As an example, energy savings by reduced physical activity seem to be higher than earlier estimates. The large variations between subjects regarding both energy intake and energy expenditure lead the Dutch group to suggest that energy intake recommendations for well-nourished pregnant women have little value. Since no metabolic adaptations seemed to appear, Spaaij et al. conclude that underestimation of the energy savings by reduced physical activity probably explain the imbalance noted between energy input and output.

In a similar design a Swedish group has monitored energy expenditure of healthy women during pregnancy and lactation (46). In these studies, 23 healthy, normal-weight women were monitored as regards body composition and energy metabolism before a planned pregnancy, and then immediately after delivery and 2 months and 6 months postpartum. Only minor changes were found with a slight increase in resting metabolic rate during lactation and a small energy intake increase during the lactation period of 280 $\pm$ 440 calories per day. In this group the main fat gain during pregnancy was 5.8 $\pm$ 4.2 kg, which was not lost during the first 2 months of lactation but disappeared partly between 2 and 6 months after delivery. These authors underscore the importance of methodological problems in estimating body composition, and suggest that a lack of correlation between changes in body weight and body fat during early pregnancy might be explained by changes in the degree of hydration of the body. Regarding physical activity, the Swedish study suggests that there was a tendency to increased physical activity during early pregnancy (47). The Swedish study supports previous work that lactation does not affect the metabolic efficiency but proposes that with extremely accurate methods it might still be possible to detect minor such differences.

That not only behavioral but also genetic factors at least partly explain weight development after delivery was illustrated in a study by Harris et al. (48). That group monitored women who had given birth and been followed in a project database for up to 2.5 years. They confirmed that body weight dissatisfaction was associated with increased likelihood for weight retention, but that women who selected larger silhouettes in a questionnaire as proxy indicators of the body shapes of their mothers were themselves also more likely to maintain more body weight (48).

IV STOCKHOLM PREGNANCY AND WEIGHT DEVELOPMENT STUDY

To further analyze the relationships between body weight, weight development, pregnancy, lactation, sociodemographic factors, and weight retention, the Stockholm Pregnancy and Weight Development Study was started in the mid-1980s (25,41,49). It is now reopened as "SPAWN" for the study of long-term effects of previous pregnancies on weight history. The study was designed as a combination of retrospective and pro-spective parts. Women who were invited to participate represented a mixture of the southern Stockholm metropolitan area, the Stockholm suburbs, and the countryside. A total of 1423 women completed the entire study. Detailed analyses failed to reveal that the salient results of the study could be explained by a selective dropout mechanism.

From the obstetric records and the questionnaires administered at follow-up, data were computed regarding body weight, age, parity, nationality, occupation, living site, marital status, smoking habits, contraceptive practices, duration of lactation and lactation intensity, weight-losing practices, return to salaried work, eating, and exercise habit. The prepregnancy weight was accepted from the women's own reports.

The validity of the prepregnancy reported weight constitutes an important methological problem. We compared the data with results obtained from a subgroup of 49 women, who were excluded from the 12-month follow-up because of a new pregnancy. This gave us an unforeseen opportunity to compare their reported weight with the weight that was recorded as the starting level for their next pregnancy. The reported mean weight was 0.92 kg lower at the onset of pregnancy than the latest recorded weight obtained under our study conditions. The mean weight loss between 6 and 12 months after delivery was calculated to 0.12 kg from data from the entire study. If we subtract this weight from 0.92 kg, we can estimate that these women have reported an initial body weight at onset of the new pregnancy which was on average 0.8 kg lower than their true body weight.

These results fit reasonably well with studies of a group of Swedish women where true prepregnancy weight data could be obtained since these women were studied and weighed at a time when their intrauterine device was removed before a planned pregnancy (50).

A Weight After Delivery

The mean weight increase 1 year after delivery compared to the reported weight at the time of conception was 1.5 kg (Fig. 3). When we corrected for the estimated underreporting of the weight at conception from our parallel studies (0.8 kg plus the estimated mean weight increase with time 0.2 kg), the net mean weight increase induced by a pregnancy was calculated at 0.5 kg. However, the range was very wide: 1.5% of the women had a mean weight retention of at least 10 kg, and 13% had a weight retention between 5 and 10 kg. The majority (56%) had a weight retention of up to 5 kg. Thirty percent of the women lost weight. The wide weight change distribution one year after delivery is shown in Figure 4.

Table 2 summarizes characteristics of weight development after delivery. The correlations of established behaviors at baseline and changes in behavior with weight change overall exhibited very low r values. Women with > 5 kg weight retention differed from the other women in several respects. Whereas women with a small net increase in weight lost a mean of 2.3 kg between 2.5 and 12 months after delivery, women with larger weight retention increased 0.4 kg during the same time period. Those who retained more weight:

1. Had a larger initial body weight.
2. Had gained more in weight during pregnancy.
3. Were lactating to a lesser extent.
4. Stopped smoking during pregnancy more often.

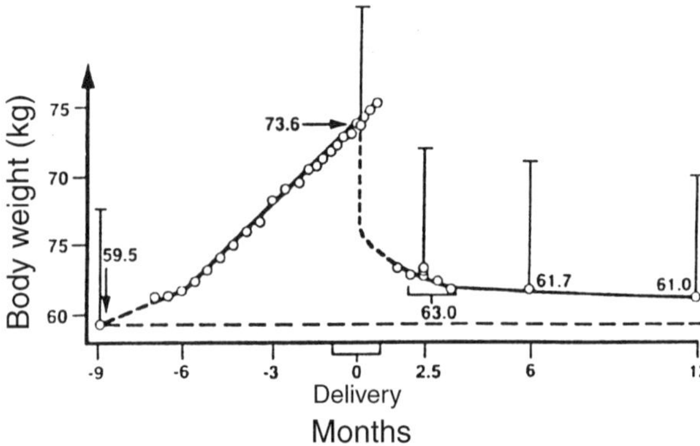

Figure 3 Body weight changes in 1423 Swedish women from conception until 12 months postpartum (kg ± SD). Dashed line shows mean prepregnancy weight. (From Ref. 25.)

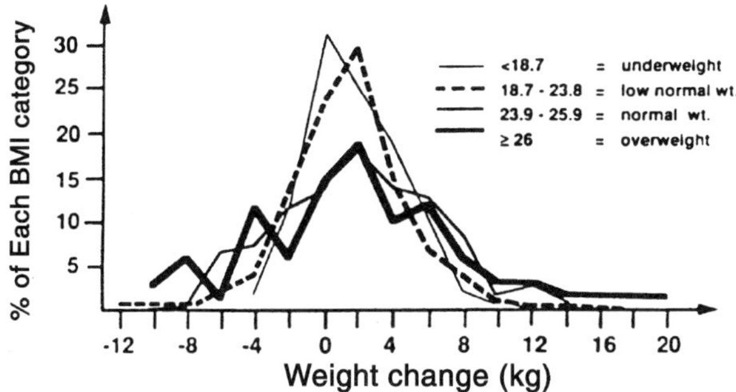

Figure 4 Distribution of weight changes from conception until 12 months postpartum in 1423 Swedish women with different prepregnancy BMI values. (From Ref. 25.)

We also found a less well structured eating pattern of dietary habits before, during, and after pregnancy (Fig. 5) (41). Those women who retained more body weight reported that their energy intake had increased after delivery, since they ate larger portions and snacked more frequently. They had less regular eating habits and did not eat breakfast or lunch as regularly as women who retained less weight. Age and parity did not differ between women who retained >5 kg and those who retained less.

B Lifestyle Trends and Lactation

Figure 6 demonstrates that the weight increase during the first trimester is already predictive of future overall weight increase. This could have preventive implications and suggests that life style recommendations concerning optimal weight increase should start early during pregnancy. In Stockholm, weight retention increased only slightly with age and not with parity. Women who gave up smoking when they became pregnant increased more than others; 45% of these women retained >5 kg.

Interestingly enough, lactation played a small roll for weight control after delivery. Although there was a significant relationship between a lactation score and weight retention, the r value was low ($r = .05$, $P < .01$) (Fig. 7). However, there was a difference with time, in that women with a high lactation score lost more weight during the first half year after delivery. Toward the end of the year, the differences between the groups were limited. Only in a small subset of subjects, those who had been lactating for a whole year, was a significant reduction of body weight compared to prepregnancy weight found.

The lack of importance of lactation for weight loss after delivery may seem surprising, but has been

Table 2 Characteristics of Weight Development After Pregnancy

Risk factors statistically associated with sustained weight retention after delivery	
Weight increase during pregnancy	$r = .36^c$
Lactation	$r = -.09^b$
Age	$r = .06^a$
Irregular eating habits after delivery	$r = -.07^a$
Leisure time physical activity after delivery	$r = -.05^a$
Factors with major effects on weight retention (net weight increase 1 year after delivery compared to prepregnancy weight)	
Smoke cessation	$+3.4$ kg^b
Marked weight changes (±6 kg) previous pregnancy	$+2.5$ kg^a
Factors significantly associated with body weight development 1 year after delivery	
Initial body weight	
Parity	
Previous contraceptive pill	
Social class	
Occupation	
Marital status	
Nationality	
Dietary advice during pregnancy	

[a] $P < .05$,
[b] $P < .01$,
[c] $P < .001$.
Source: Ref. 25.

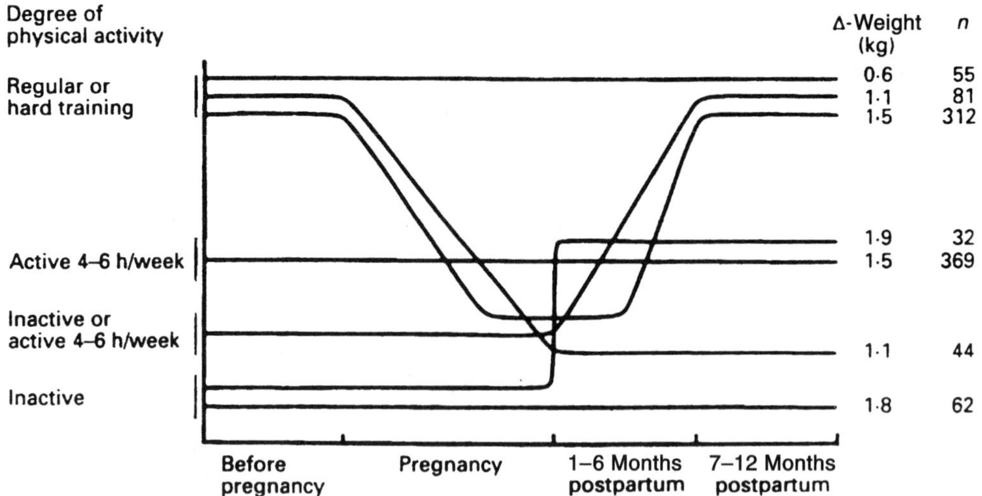

Figure 5 Different trend patterns in physical activity and effects on postpartum body weight development. (From Ref. 41.)

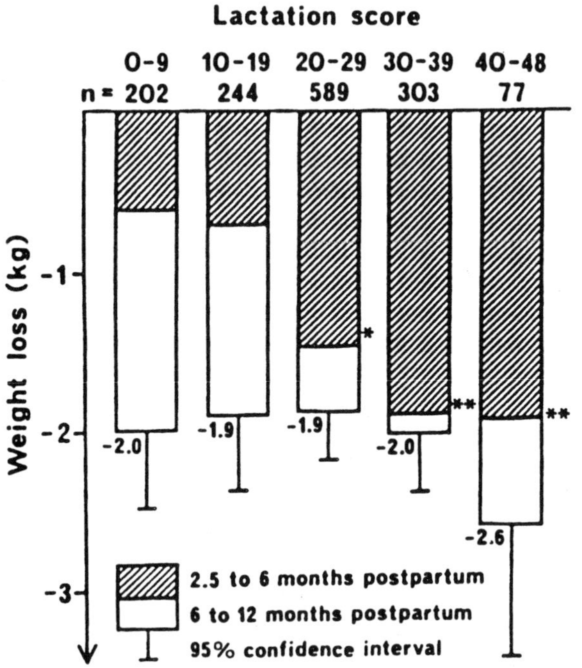

Figure 6 The Stockholm Pregnancy and Weight Development Study. Weight loss in kg from 2.5 to 12 months postpartum in groups with different lactation scores. Statistically significant differences from score 0–9 and 10–19 shown as $*P < .05$ and $**P < .01$. (From Ref. 25.)

reported previously by Rookus (18) and was also described by others, as cited in her review.

In clinical practice, women are often instructed to try to breast-feed as much as possible to revert to normal weight after delivery. This seems logical, since a full lactation requires ~500 calories per day, which may constitute about 20–25% of the daily energy requirement of women in this age group. However, it is possi-

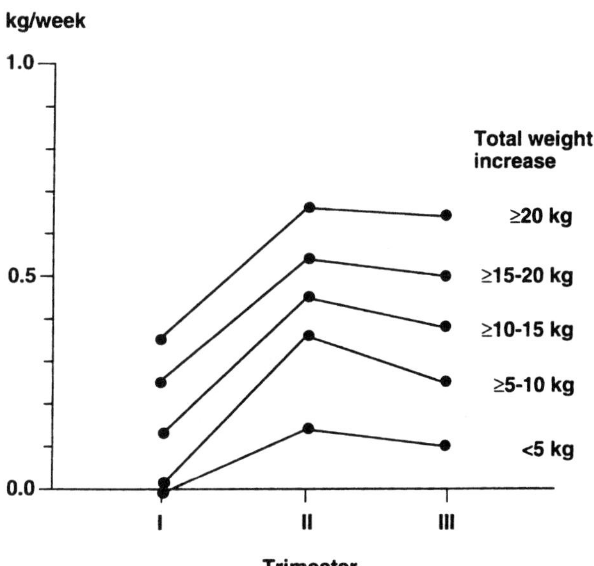

Figure 7 Trimester-related mean weight increase in women with different total weight increase. (From Ref. 96.)

ble that the changes in eating behavior and lifestyle affect women in such a way that they only use their adipose tissue storage when food is not readily available, as has been suggested by Prentice (42).

Questions regarding eating habits, physical activity, and lifestyle revealed that there was a tendency for women who retain more weight to develop a more sedentary and irregular lifestyle. This can, of course, be explained by the new social situation and the lack of opportunities to engage in outdoor physical activities, when the care of the newborn has became a first priority. Women who had received dietary guidance during pregnancy did not have a more favorable weight outcome than those who did not receive such support.

In summary, the metabolic cost of an entire pregnancy seems to be extremely flexible and is influenced by numerous factors, such as maternal prepregnancy nutritional status, energy intake during pregnancy, fetal size, and a combination of these factors. Metabolic adaption may possibly occur to spare some energy for fetal growth, should this be insufficient.

C Maternal Body Weight and Birth Weight

The definition of optimal weight gain during pregnancy remains controversial. The old saying is that a pregnant woman should "eat for two." On the other hand, in affluent societies where overweight is more of a problem than starvation, it is important that the dietary recommendations not expose pregnant vulnerable women to the risk of subsequently developing an excess of fat that they may later have great difficulty in losing. The safety of the newborn is one basic concern, and a low birth weight constitutes a well-known risk, but "eating for two" must be balanced against the adverse effects of overweight and obesity.

A linear relationship has been reported by some authors between birth weight and maternal pregnancy weight gain at all levels of pregnancy weight (23,51,52). Others suggest that as maternal weight increases, the infant's birth weight will increase proportionately less (53–56). As part of the data analyses of the Stockholm Pregnancy and Weight Development Study, the relationships between initial maternal body weight, weight development during pregnancy, and birth weights were studied (57). The birth weight increased with maternal pregnancy weight gain minus birth weight in each group. When divided by quartiles, children of mothers in the two groups with the highest net weight increase were significantly heavier than those of the two groups that increased <10 kg. However, in women who had a net weight gain exceeding 10 kg, no further significant birth weight increase with maternal weight was found. For the total material the correlation between net maternal weight gain and birth weight was $r = .17$ ($P < .001$). Net weight increase (defined as maternal weight increase minus birth weight) explained only 3.0% of the variation in birth weight. When initial body weight was added, these two factors together explained 5.0% of the variation in birth weight.

Numerous factors, such as paternal and maternal heredity, maternal prepregnancy weight, nutrition, and several hormonal factors, ultimately determine the infant's birth weight (58). The Stockholm study is confined to total maternal body weight, and it should be borne in mind that lean body mass rather adipose tissue seems to be the important determinant of birth weight. Our data support the concept that birth weight increases with maternal weight up to a certain level, and then levels off.

V AMERICAN IOM RECOMMENDATIONS

During the past 50 years recommendations for healthy pregnancy weight development have been controversial in many parts of the world. The initial concern was mainly focused on safety for mother and infant. The emerging obesity epidemic, however, has made it more and more important to scrutinize to what extent an extensive and physiologically unnecessary weight gain during pregnancy could be an unfortunate lead into overweight and obesity of the mother.

In countries with low socioeconomic status or with ethnic subgroups containing such individuals, it is clear that a low weight gain during pregnancy is an indicator of poverty, malnourishment, and future risk for high infant mortality, disability, and even mental retardation.

In the United States, the Institute of Medicine (IOM) issued recommendations in 1990, which were more liberal than before and hence caused considerable discussion. Some experts even claimed that these IOM recommendations would not improve perinatal outcome and would have negative consequences for both infant and mother: the liberal weight increase recommended ranges advocated by the IOM would produce overgrown newborns, result in an increased frequency of cesarean sections, and eventually also trigger obesity in the mothers.

Abrams et al. (59) have recently reviewed all studies that examined fetal and maternal outcome. They conclude that there is an impressive body of evidence indicating that weight gains within IOM recommendations are indeed associated with better pregnancy outcome but found no evidence that such pregnancy weight gain is a course of substantive postpartum weight retention. The authors are, however, anxious to point out that the studies on which these conclusions are based are observational and not experimental. They note that maternal weight gain alone may not be a very helpful predictor of poor pregnancy outcome and that a good pregnancy outcome can be associated with a wide variety of weight development patterns throughout pregnancy. Furthermore, these studies are based on data from an American population. Seen the other way around, it is clear that many women, seeking professional help for their overweight and obesity, report their pregnancies as having been major events in their overweight development.

VI PREGNANCY, WEIGHT, AND SMOKING

Smoking affects body weight. Generally, smoking increases the basal metabolic rate by ~10% (60), and smokers are relatively lean (61,62). The weight development pattern in pregnancy is confounded by the fact that many smoking women give up this habit when they learn of their pregnancy.

Smoking mothers seem to gain ~13% less per week than nonsmokers (63). In this study from Australia, "reformed smokers," who decided to quit when they learned of their pregnancy, had the highest weekly weight gain of all groups. Our Stockholm data show similar results, both with a high pregnancy weight gain and also with higher weight retention than in those who never smoked or who continued (25). However, these results are not in agreement with all other studies. In the large Ontario Perinatal Mortality Study of 31,788 women smoking habits were unrelated to maternal weight gain distribution (64).

VII OBESITY, WEIGHT GAIN, AND PREGNANCY COMPLICATIONS

Obesity is considered a risk factor in pregnancy, but knowledge of the relation of the degree of maternal obesity to risk for specific complications and pregnancy outcome remains unclear (65–69). There are several methodological reasons for the lack of precise knowledge about these interrelationships, such as exact definitions of obesity and adequate control groups. In a study from Chile, a group of obese pregnant women were compared with a group matched for age and parity but with normal weight (70). Differences between the two groups were found with regard to gestational hypertension, inadequate pregnancy weight gain, cesarean section frequency, postpartum infections and, large-for-gestational-age infants. No significant increase in the incidence of diabetes, toximia, breech presentation, postpartum hemorrhage, infant morbidity, or lactational failure was noted in the obese women. The authors conclude that although obesity is an important risk factor, methodological aspects of previous studies may have magnified the severity of the problem.

This view is also supported by later studies. In a case control study from California with a similar design, it was shown that massively obese pregnant women were significantly more likely to have a multitude of adverse effects (71). The frequency of cesarean section was doubled, and child malformation or growth retardation were much more prevalent. However, when obese women with diabetes and/or hypertension antedating pregnancy were excluded from the analyses, no statistically significant differences in perinatal outcome persisted. These authors thus conclude that although massively obese pregnant women are at high risk for adverse perinatal outcome, these risks are more related to preexisting morbid conditions than to obesity in itself.

In the Stockholm study the overall frequency of cesarean sections was 12%. There was a tendency, although statistically nonsignificant ($\chi^2 = 2.62$, n.s.), toward a higher frequency of sections in mothers with higher initial BMI values. The mean initial BMI for vaginal deliveries was 21.5 vis-à-vis 21.8 kg/m^2 for cesarean sections.

The frequency of cesarean sections in all women in this study is close to the available Swedish average figure of 12.4%, reported from the corresponding time period. The problem concerning an increased need for cesarean sections in obese mothers is not clear (72).

VIII DIABETES, OBESITY, FAT DISTRIBUTION, AND PREGNANCY

Maternal obesity represents a significant risk factor for the development of gestational diabetes mellitus and subsequent adult-onset diabetes. Obesity in itself is associated with major alterations in carbohydrate metabolism such as insulin resistance and hyperinsulinemia, eventually resulting in hyperglycemia (73). Not only is the degree of overweight important for the likelihood to develop diabetes, but also body fat distribution with upper-body obesity are more important risk factors than generalized increase in body fat (74). In a study of pregnant women with various types of fat distribution, repeated oral glucose tolerance tests were carried out during each trimester and postpartum (75). This study demonstrates that in upper-body obese women, pathological carbohydrate metabolism becames apparent during the second trimester and that a significant relationship between waist/hip ratio and glucose levels, as well as insulin areas were found in late pregnancy in all obese subjects.

IX BODY FAT DISTRIBUTION AND CONCEPTION CAPACITY

Although obesity is common among multiparous women, it is possible that this weight increase is the result of multiple pregnancies rather than a prerequisite for conception. From ancient history the obese female has been considered a symbol of fertility. In some cultures it has been believed that obese women are more likely to bear twins. Although it is well known that underweight women have an impaired capacity to conceive, the effects of overweight and obesity on female fecundity have been less studied. A shift of the hormonal balance toward increased androgenicity in association with an abdominal obesity has been found to lead to menstrual disorders (5,76).

A Weight and Infertility

A moderate degree of overweight may affect the reproductive capacity significantly. In a case control study of body mass index and ovulatory infertility, 597 white infertile women with ovulatory dysfunction were compared with 1695 primiparous control women (77). The study demonstrated an increased risk for primary ovulatory infertility already in women with a body mass index of 27 kg/m^2 or greater. At BMI above 25 kg/m^2, the risk of ovulatory infertility had almost doubled.

Women admitted to an in vitro fertilization unit provide a unique opportunity to study determinants of fecundity while controlling for several other confounders related to conception. In a Dutch study the probability of conception after insemination was studied in 500 women (78). The main reasons for artificial insemination were infertility or subfertility of the partner with azoospermia or oligospermia, respectively. The youngest woman was 20 years old; only a few women were above age 40. Two hundred sixty women reported regular smoking habits. As expected, the women were less likely to conceive with higher ages ($P < .05$). The study demonstrated that a 0.1-unit increase in waist-hip ratio was associated with a 30% decrease in probability of conception per cycle. These data were adjusted for age, overall fatness, clinical indication for insemination, cycle characteristics, smoking habits, and parity. The main finding of this study is that an increase in waist-hip ratio suggesting increased androgenicity was associated with a reduced fecundity. In obese women weight loss often normalizes the regular menstrual cycles and sex hormone concentrations (8,79). This indicates that obesity itself rather than a primary endocrine dysfunction is the cause of the reproductive insufficiency.

B Diabetes, Weight, and Fertility

Type 2 diabetes is associated with obesity as well as with pregnancy. The association between parity and type 2 diabetes has been studied in several populations where either no relationship or a positive association generally has been described. On the other hand, infertility has been associated with a high risk for type 2 diabetes. The complex interrelationship between these factors has recently been studied among Pima Indian women (80). In a longitudinal epidemiological study of diabetes the role of parity and obesity was analyzed after control for age. This study demonstrates that Pima women who had never been pregnant had a higher prevalence of type 2 diabetes but also a higher BMI than women who had been pregnant. To a certain extent this difference could be accounted for by a higher degree of obesity. Possibly high estrogen concentrations could explain the oligomenorrhea or amenorrhea and thus the decreased fertility through a negative feedback mechanism at the hypothalamopituitary level (81).

The fact that there is no consistent relationship between parity and type 2 diabetes may be due to a combination of two effects counteracting each other. On the one hand, pregnancy may be diabetogenic by leading to an accelerated and sustained weight gain that could precipitate a clinically manifest form of type 2 diabetes. On the other hand, it is possible that women of low fertility run a higher risk of developing type 2 diabetes because of a common factor, or several common factors, contributing to both these conditions.

X PREGNANCY, BODY WEIGHT DEVELOPMENT, AND PHYSICAL ACTIVITY

Physical activity is obviously an important determinator of weight development, even in pregnancy (82). A retrospective analysis of the literature, mainly based on an extended Medline search and the Pregnancy and

Childbirth Database (Cochrane), was recently carried out to elucidate the importance of physical activity in determining weight gain characteristics (83).

Several methodological matters complicate the interpretation of the interrelationships: generally body weight and not fat has been measured; sociobehavioral confounders have rarely been accounted for; and the time frame to determine the effect of pregnancy on later weight development has been highly variable. Most studies reviewed concentrate on the role of physical activity, such as recreational activity and sports, on the safety of the pregnant mother and the fetus. Again, less emphasis is put on the potential role of physical activity to prevent or restrict weight retention in obesity-prone women. Advice is general and mostly obvious ("boxing as exercise during pregnancy is discouraged. . .").

One the few studies addressing the question of recreational exercise on pregnancy weight gain and subcutaneous fat deposition is the paper by Clapp (84). This study thus demonstrates that well-educated, nonsmoking, highly motivated women who maintained a balanced diet and were nonobese before pregnancy, accumulated slightly less fat in the last trimester when exercising. Self-selection, nonquatification of the amount exercised, and a very selective group of women limit the possibility of extrapolating these results to the population at isk, for whom pregnancy is major trigger for weight retention and subsequent obesity.

XI SOCIOECONOMIC AND ETHNIC ASPECTS ON PREGNANCY-RELATED WEIGHT GAIN

Women with low education and low income are at increased risk of gaining weight and becoming overweight. Furthermore, there seem to be differences in race. Over a 10-year period the overall mean weight gain for black women was 36% higher than for white women (85). Parker and Abrams (86) have analyzed the 1988 National Maternal and Infant Health Survey to study whether this additional increase in body weight among black women could be explained by factors relating to pregnancy. They found that black mothers were twice as likely to retain at least 20 lb as white mothers (adjusted odds ratio 2.20, 95% CI 1.50-3.22), but that this black-white difference could not be explained by differences in socioeconomic status. There were other differences in the weight increase pattern. Weight attention was more likely to occur in white women who were unmarried, whereas weight retention in black mothers was more associated with high parity. These data suggest that it may be necessary to develop population-specific strategies in helping mothers to return to their prepregnancy body weight.

XII WEIGHT DEVELOPMENT IN PREGNANT ADOLESCENTS

Since maternal weight gain is an important and manageable determinant of infant birth weight among adolescents, some studies have addressed factors related to weight gain in young women. Generally, the women studied have been poor and with numerous psychosocial problems including drug abuse. Stevens-Simon 141 studied pregnant black teenager (87). The group was divided into three different weight gain subgroups. Slow weight gain was associated with a lower quality of food intake. Teenagers who gained more weight during their pregnancies were more compliant with prenatal visits, but also reported more depressive symptoms and more alcohol consumption. An important finding was the substantial variability in the amount of weight gain, ranging from 1.8 to 27.9 kg with a mean weight increase of 14.3 ± 6.0 kg (SD). This study suggests that proper nutritional care in this group of young women may be an effective method to promote optimal gestational weight gain. In the analysis of the 99 pregnant young women (88), most were poor but with an ethnic variability. The authors had anticipated that negative attitudes toward pregnancy weight gain would be more common among these young women and that such attitudes would adversely affect an optimal adolescent maternal weight gain. These teenagers were studies by means of a weight gain attitude scale as well as several other determinants of nutritional status, dietary and health habits, and social history. Surprisingly enough, the authors demonstrated that these young women were not more concerned about staying slim than older pregnant adolescents and adults. Negative weight gain attitudes were more commonly found among heavy and depressed adolescents and those who did not have a family support.

The examples of weight gain–related factors in adolescents given above relate to the problems in the United States. It is reasonable to believe that the situation will be quite different in other cultures, where pregnancy early in the life of a young woman might be considered a normal life event or in societies where the attitude to abortion in pregnant teenagers is different. For this special group of women, appropriate food supplies may be one simple method to ensure optimal weight gain and good pregnancy outcome.

XIII WEIGHT GAIN DURING TWIN PREGNANCIES

Few data are available concerning the optimal weight development during twin gestation. Pederson et al. (89) addressed this question in a retrospective evaluation of the outcome of 217 twin pregnancies. The optimal outcome was associated with a mean weight gain of ~20 kg. These authors were able to construct a weight gain curve for twin gestation, which was compared with the standard weight development curve for singleton pregnancies. During the first half of the pregnancy, curves for singleton and twin pregnancies were similar, after which a more marked increase was seen in twin pregnancies during the second trimester and until term. It is still unknown whether multiple pregnancies require different nutritional needs, but until such data are available it seems practical to use weight gain as a proxy measure of the nutritional status of the mother and her twin fetuses.

XIV GENERAL CLINICAL CONSEQUENCES

Since little weight loss advice is generally offered women after delivery, the results of a prospective, controlled randomized study of the effects of a recent correspondence course are of interest (90). Women taking the 6-month course lost significantly more weight (7.8 vs. 4.9 kg, $P = .03$) than controls. The study indicates that with creativity, weight loss after delivery can be achieved at low cost and with surprising efficiency.

Recent diagnostic and pharmacologic developments have focused renewed attention on polycystic ovary syndrome as an important cause for obesity-associated infertility (91), but subfertility may also occur in obese women who do not suffer from this syndrome. Among choices women can make for themselves to improve their general chances of conceiving, body weight control and proper eating habits are important (92).

For anovulatory women with a weight problem, a general program promoting a better lifestyle with an improved self-esteem has been found to be surprisingly effective in not only improving their quality of life (93) but also their subsequent chances of conceiving. The women were treated with a standard program including diet, exercise, and behavioral modification. In this uncontrolled study the ensuing mean weight loss of 6.3 kg resulted in a marked improvement of the hormonal profile (reductions in testosterone and insulin concentrations) and also conception in 11/13 women, some even without further hormonal stimulation. In what seems an extension of that study, these Australian authors treated 37 obese women and after a mean weight loss of 6.2 kg, only six anxious to become pregnant had not conceived within 36 months. This study is open and uncontrolled, but it may be argued that studies of this kind will probably be difficult to design as proper randomized, prospective controlled trials for several reasons (94).

REFERENCES

1. Arner P, Eckel RH. Adipose tissue as a storage organ. In: Bray GA, Bouchard C, James WPT, eds. Handbook of Obesity New York: Marcel Dekker, 1998:379–396.
2. Siiteri PK, MacDonald PC. Role of extraglandular estrogen in human endocrinology. In: Green PO, Astwood E, eds. Handbook of Physiology. Vol 2. Washington: American Physiological Society, 1973:615–629.
3. MacDonald PC, Edman CD, Hemsell DL, Porter JC, Siiteri PK. Effect of obesity on conversion of plasma androstenedione to estrone in postmenopausal women with and without endometrial cancer. Am J Obstet Gynecol 1978; 130:448–455.
4. Loughlin T, Cunningham SK, Culliton M, Smyth PPA, Meagher DJ, Mckenna TJ. Altered androstenedione and estrone dynamics associated with abnormal hormonal profile in amenhorrheic subjects with weight loss or obesity. Fertil Steril 1985; 43:720–725.
5. Rogers J, Mitchell GWJR. The relation of obesity to menstrual disturbances. N Engl J Med 1952; 257:53–55.
6. Glass AR, Dahms WT, Abraham G, Atkinson RL, Bray GA, Swerdloff RS. Secondary amenorrhea in obesity: etiologic role of weight related androgen excess. Fertil Steril 1978; 30:243–244.
7. Kopelman PG, White N, Pilkington TRE, Jeffcoate SL. The effect of weight loss on sex steroid secretion and binding in massively obese women. Clin Endocrinol 1981; 14:113–116.
8. Mitchell GW, Rogers J. The influence of weight reduction on amenorrhea in obese women. N Engl J Med 1953; 249:835–837.
9. Yen SS, Vela P, Rankin J. Inappropriate secretion of follicle-stimulating hormone and luteninizing hormone in polycystic ovarian disease. J Clin Endocrinol Metab 1970; 30:435–442.
10. Barbieri RL, Smith S, Ryan KJ. The role of hyperinsulinemia in the pathogenesis of ovarian hyperandrogenism. Fertil Steril 1988; 50:197–212.

11. Guzick DS, Wing R, Smith D, Berga SL, Winters SJ. Endocrine consequences of weight loss in obese, hyperandrogenic, anovulatory women. Fertil Steril 1994; 61: 598–604.
12. Hamilton-Fairley D, Kiddy D, Watson H, Paterson C, Franks S. Association of moderate obesity with a poor pregnancy outcome in women with polycystic ovary syndrome treated with low dose gonadotrophin. Br J Obstet Gynaecol 1992; 99:128–131.
13. Rodin J, Radke-Sharpe N, Rebuffé-Scrive M, Greenwood MRC. Weight cycling and fat distribution. Int J Obes 1990; 14:303–310.
14. Lissner L, Odell R, D'Agostino R, et al. Health implications of weight cycling in the Framingham population. Am J Epidemiol 1988; 128:1180–1184.
15. Rössner S. Pregnancy, weight cycling and weight gain. Int J Obes 1992; 16:145–147.
16. Billewicz WZ, Thomson AM. Body weight in parous women. Br J Prev Soc Med 1970; 24:97–104.
17. Johnston EM. Weight changes during pregnancy and the postpartum period. Prog Food Nutr Sci 1991; 15:117–157.
18. Rookus MA, Rokebrand P, Burema J, Deurenberg P. The effect of pregnancy on the body mass index 9 months postpartum in 49 women. Int J Obes 1987; 11:609–618.
19. McKeown T, Record RG. The influence of reproduction on body weight in women. J Endoncrinol 1957; 15:393–409.
20. Abitol MM. Weight gain in pregnancy. Am J Obstet Gynecol 1969; 104:140–157.
21. Garn SM, Shaw HA, McCabe KD. Effect of maternal smoking on weight and weight gain between pregnancies. Am J Clin Nutr 1978; 31:1302–1303.
22. Beazley JM, Swinhoe JR. Body weight in parous women: is there any alteration between successive pregnancies? Acta Obstet Gynecol Scand 1979; 5:45–47.
23. Gormican A, Valentine J, Satter E. Relationships of maternal weight gain, prepregnancy weight, and infant birth weight. J Am Diet Assoc 1980; 77:662–667.
24. Newcombe RG. Development of obesity in parous women. J Epidemiol Community Health 1982; 36:306–309.
25. Öhlin A, Rössner S. Maternal weight development after pregnancy. Int J Obes 1990; 14:159–173.
26. Brown JE, Kaye SA, Folsom AR. Parity-related weight change in women. Int J Obes 1992; 16:627–631.
27. Harris HE, Ellison GTH. Do the changes in energy balance that occur during pregnancy predispose parous women to obesity? Nutr Res Rev 1997; 10:57–81.
28. Smith DE, Lewis CE, Caveny JL, Perkins LL, Burke GL, Bild DE. Longitudinal changes in adiposity associated with pregnancy. JAMA 1994; 271:1747–1751.
29. Williamson DF, Madans J, Pamuk E, Flegal KM, Kendrick JS, Serdula MK. A prospective study of childbearing and 10-year weight gain in US white women 25 to 45 years of age. Int J Obes 1994; 18:561–569.
30. Heliövaara M, Aromaa A. Parity and obesity. J Epidemiol Community Health 1981; 35:197–199.
31. Hytten FE, Leitch I. The Physiology of Human Pregnancy Oxford: Blackwell Scientific, 1971.
32. Ash S, Fischer CC, Truswell AS, Allen JR, Irwing L. Maternal weight gain, smoking, and other factors in pregnancy as predictors of infant birth-weight in Sydney women. Aust NZ J Obstet Gynaecol 1989; 29:212–219.
33. Hjortland MC, McNamara, Kannel WB. Some atherogenic concomitants of menopause: the Framingham Study. Am J Epidemiol 1976; 103:304–311.
34. Lindquist O, Bengtsson C. Serum lipids, arterial blood pressure and body weight in relation to the menopause: results from a population study of women in Goteborg, Sweden. Scand J Clin Lab Invest 1980; 40:629–636.
35. Wing RR, Matthews KA, Kuller LH, Meilahn EN, Plantinga PL. Weight gain at the time of menopause. Arch Intern Med 1991; 151:97–102.
36. Kuller LH, Meilahn EN, Cauley JA, Gutai JP, Matthews KA. Epidemiologic studies of menopause: changes in risk factors and disease. Exp Gerontol 1994; 29:495–509.
37. Hamman RF, Bennett PH, Miller M. The effect of menopause on serum cholesterol in American (Pima) Indian women. Am J Epidemiol 1975; 102:164–169.
38. Chevrier J, Dewailly E, Ayotte P, Mauriege P, Despres JP, Trembley A. Body weight loss increases plasma and adipose tissue concentrations of potentially toxic pollutants in obese individuals. Int J Obes Relat Disord 2000; 24:1272–1278.
39. Rebuffé-Scrive M, Enk L, Crona P, et al. Fat cell metabolism in different regions in women. Effects of menstrual cycle, pregnancy and lactation. J Clin Invest 1985; 75:1973–1976.
40. Illingworth PJ, Jung RT, Howie PW, Isles TE. Reduction in postprandial energy expenditure during lactation. BMJ 1987; 294:1573–1576.
41. Öhlin A, Rössner S. Trends in eating patterns, physical activity and sociodemographic factors in relation to postpartum body weight development. Br J Nutr 1994; 71:457–470.
42. Prentice AM, Prentice A. Energy cost of lactation. Annu Rev Nutr 1988; 8:63–79.
43. Spaaij CJK, Van Raaij JMA, Van der Heijden LJM, et al. No substantial reduction of the thermic effect of a meal in pregnancy in well-nourished Dutch women. Br J Nutr 1994; 71:335–344.
44. Spaaij CJK, Van Raaij JMA, Van der Heijden LJM, de Groot CPGM, Boekholt HA, Hautvast JGAJ. No changes during pregnancy in the net cost of cycling exercise. Eur J Clin Nutr 1994; 48:513–521.
45. Spaaij CJK, Van Raaij JMA, de Groot CPGM, Van der Heijden LJM, Boekholt HA, Hautvast JGAJ. Effect of lactation of resting metabolic rate and on diet- and work-induced thermogenesis. Am J Clin Nutr 1994; 59:42–47.
46. Forsum E, Sadurskis A. Estimation of body fat in

healthy Swedish women during pregnancy and lactation. Am J Clin Nutr 1989; 50:465–473.
47. Forsum E, Kabir N, Sadurskis A, Westerterp K. Total energy expenditure of healthy Swedish women during pregnancy and lactation. Am J Clin Nutr 1992; 56:334–342.
48. Harris HE, Ellison GT, Clement S. Relative importance of heritable characteristics and lifestyle in the development of maternal obesity. J Epidemiol Community Health 1999; 2:66–74.
49. Öhlin A Pregnancy and overweight. (In Swedish.) Thesis, Karolinska Institute, Stockholm, 1991.
50. Sadurskis A, Kabir N, Wager J, Forsum E. Energy metabolism, body composition and milk production in healthy Swedish women during lactation. Am J Clin Nutr 1988; 48:44–49.
51. Harrison GG, Udall JN, Morrow G. Maternal obesity, weight gain in pregnancy, and infant birth weight. Am J Obstet Gynecol 1980; 136:411–412.
52. Luke B, Dickinson C, Petrie RH. Intrauterine growth: correlations of maternal nutritional status and rate of gestational weight gain. Eur J Obstet Gynecol Reprod Biol 1981; 12:113–121.
53. Eastman NJ, Jackson E. Weight relationship in pregnancy. Obstet Gynecol Surv 1968; 23:1003–1024.
54. Niswander KR, Singer J, Westphal M, Weiss W. Weight gain during pregnancy and prepregnancy weight gain. Obstet Gynecol 1969; 33:482–491.
55. Winikoff B, Debrovner CH. Anthropometric determinants of birth weight. Obstet Gynecol 1981; 58:678–684.
56. Abrams BF, Laros RK. Pregnancy weight, weight gain, and birth weight. Am J Obstet Gynecol 1986; 154:503–509.
57. Rössner S, Öhlin A. Maternal body weight and relation to birth weight. Acta Obstet Gynecol Scand 1990; 69:475–478.
58. Langhoff-Roos J Determinants of infant birth weight at term. Thesis, Uppsala University, 1987.
59. Abrams B, Altman SL, Pickett KE. Maternal body weight and relation to birth weight. Am J Clin Nutr 2000; 71(suppl):1233S–1241S.
60. Rössner S. Cessation of cigarette smoking and body weight increase. Acta Med Scand 1986; 219:1–2.
61. Lincoln JE, Morris P. Weight gain after cessation of smoking. JAMA 1969; 210:1765.
62. Dallosso HM, James WPT. The role of smoking in the regulation of energy balance. Int J Obes 1984; 8:365–375.
63. Newnham JP, Patterson L, James I, Reid SE. Effects of maternal cigarette smoking on ultrasonic measurement of fetal growth and on Doppler flow velocity waveforms. Early Hum Dev 1990; 24:23–26.
64. Meyer MB. How does maternal smoking affect birth weight and maternal weight gain? Evidence from the Ontario Perinatal Mortality Study. Am J Obstet Gynecol 1978; 131:888–893.
65. Gross T, Sokol RJ, King K. Obesity in pregnancy: risks and outcome. Obstet Gynecol 1980; 56:446–450.
66. Garbaciak JA Jr, Richter M, Miller S, Barton JJ. Maternal weight and pregnancy complications. Am J Obstet Gynecol 1985; 152:238–245.
67. Johnson SR, Kolberg BH, Warner MW, Railsback LD. Maternal obesity and pregnancy. Surg Gynecol Obstet 1987; 164:431–437.
68. Mitchell MC, Lerner E. A comparison of pregnancy outcome in overweight and normal weight women. J Am Coll Nutr 1989; 8:617–624.
69. Naeye RL. Maternal body weight and pregnancy outcome. Am J Cin Nutr 1990; 52:273–279.
70. Tilton Z, Hodgson MI, Donoso E, Arteaga A, Rosso P. Complications and outcome of pregnancy in obese women. Nutrition 1989; 5:95–99.
71. Perlow JH, Morgan MA, Montgomery D, Towers CV, Porto M. Perinatal outcome in pregnancy complicated by massive obesity. Am J Obstet Gynecol 1992; 167:958–962.
72. Gross TL. Operative considerations in the obese pregnant patient. Clin Perinatol 1983; 10:411–421.
73. Reaven GM. Role of insulin resistance in human disease [Banting Lecture 1988]. Diabetes 1988; 37:593–607.
74. Kissebah AH, Vydelingum N, Murray R. Relation of body fat distribution to metabolic complications of obesity. J Clin Endocrinol Metab 1982; 54:254–260.
75. Landon MB, Osei K, Platt M, O'Dorisio T, Samuels P, Gabbe SG. The differential effects of body fat distribution on insulin and glucose metabolism during pregnancy. Am J Obstet Gynecol 1994; 171:875–884.
76. Hartz AJ, Rupley DC, Rimm AA. The association of girth measurements with disease in 32,856 women. Am J Epidemiol 1984; 119:71–80.
77. Grodstein F, Goldman MB, Cramer DW. Body mass index and ovulatory infertility. Epidemiology 1994; 5:247–250.
78. Zaadstra BM, Seidell JC, Van Noord PAH, et al. Fat and femal fecundity: prospective study of effect of body fat distribution on conception rates. BMJ 1993; 306:484–487.
79. Grenman S, Ronnema T, Irisia K, Kaihola HL, Gross M. Sex steroid, gonadotrophin, cortisol and prolaction levels in healthy, massively obese women: correlation with abdominal fat cell size and effect of weight reduction. J Clin Endocrinol Metab 1986; 63:1257.
80. Charles MA, Pettitt DJ, MCance DR, Hanson RL, Bennett PH, Knowler WC. Gravidity, obesity and non-insulin-dependent diabetes among Pima Indian women. Am J Med 1994; 97:250–255.
81. Edman CD, MacDonald PC. Effect of obesity on conversion of plasma androstenedione to estrone in ovulatory and anovulatory young women. Am J Obstet Gynecol 1978; 130:456–461.
82. Bell R, O'Neill M. Exercise and pregnancy: a review. Birth 1994; 21:85–95.

83. Rössner S. Physical activity and prevention and treatment of weight gain associated with pregnancy: current evidence and research issues. Med Sci Sports Exerc 1999; 31:S560–S563.
84. Clapp JF III, Little KD. Effect of recreational exercise on pregnancy weight gain and subcutaneous fat deposition. Med Sci Sports Exerc 1995; 27:170–177.
85. Kahn HS, Williamson DF, Stevens JA. Race and weight change in US women: the roles of socioeconomic and marital status. Am J Public Health 1991; 81:319–323.
86. Parker JD, Abrams B. Differences in postpartum weight retention between black and white mothers. Obstet Gynecol 1993; 81:768–774.
87. Stevens-Simon C, McAnarney ER. Determinants of weight gain in pregnant adolescents. J Am Diet Assoc 1992; 92:1348–1351.
88. Stevens-Simon C, Nakashima I, Andrews D. Weight gain attitudes among pregnant adolescents. J Adolesc Health 1993; 14:369–372.
89. Pederson AL, Worthington-Roberts B, Hickok DE. Weight gain patterns during twin gestation. J Am Diet Assoc 1989; 89:642–646.
90. Leermakers EA, Anglin K, Wing RR. Reducing postpartum weight retention through a correspondence intervention. Int J Obes Relat Metab Disord 1998; 11: 1103–1109.
91. Hunter MH, Sterrett JJ. Polycystic ovary syndrome: it's not just infertility. Am Fam Physician 2000; 62:1079–1088.
92. Silva PD, Cool JL, Olson KL. Impact of lifestyle choices on female infertility. J Reprod Med 1999; 44:288–296.
93. Clark AM, Ledger W, Galletly C, Tomlinson L, Blaney F, Wang X, Norman RJ. Weight loss results in significant improvement in pregnancy and ovulation rates in anovulatory obese women. Hum Reprod 1995; 10:2705–2710.
94. Galletly C, Clark A, Tomlinson L, Blaney F. Improved pregnancy rates for obese, infertile women following a group treatment program. An open pilot study. Gen Hosp Psychiatry 1996; 18:192–195.
95. Kuskowska-Wolk A, Rössner S. Prevalence of obesity in Sweden: cross-sectional study of a representative adult sample. J Intern Med 1990; 227:241–246.
96. Rössner S. Pregnancy as a risk factor for obesity: lessons from the Stockholm Pregnancy and Weight Development Study. Obes Res 1995; 3(suppl 2):S267–S275.

42

Physical Activity, Obesity, and Health Outcomes

William J. Wilkinson and Steven N. Blair

The Cooper Institute, Dallas, Texas, U.S.A.

I INTRODUCTION

As documented by recent national and international guidelines, obesity is a significant public health problem (1,2). The prevalence of overweight and obesity is increasing in many countries around the world. In the United States it is estimated that at least 55% of adults are overweight or obese (defined as a body mass index [BMI] $\geq$25 kg/m^2), and according to recent surveys, the prevalence of obesity (BMI $\geq$30 kg/m^2) in the United States increased from 12% to 19.8% between 1991 and 2000 (1,3,4). Low levels of energy expenditure from physical activity are likely a major contributing factor to the rapid increase in the prevalence of obesity (5–7). Although there are no direct data, it seems probable that a decline in energy expenditure has taken place due to obvious changes in occupational- and household-related physical activity, as well as urban environments that are increasingly less conducive to leisure-time physical activity.

In the United States, the most recent data indicate that 29.2% of adults are inactive in their leisure time and 43.1% participate in some leisure-time activity but at levels too low to confer significant health benefits. Only 27.7% of U.S. adults are physically active at recommended levels (8,9). Compared with normal-weight and overweight adults, obese individuals are more likely to report being inactive (27.3%, 28%, and 37% respectively) (9). Cross-sectional and cohort studies suggest that differences in amounts of physical activity contribute to differences in body weight and body fatness and play an important role in whether obesity develops (10–13). A recent ecological review of secular trends suggests that the prevalence of obesity is more strongly related to decreases in energy expenditure than to increases in energy intake (14).

A large body of scientific evidence and consensus opinion indicates that physical activity is an essential element, along with dietary and behavioral modification, in the clinical strategy for weight management for patients who are overweight and obese (1,8,15). In recent years, professional and governmental bodies have provided expert consensus recommendations on physical activity for health promotion and disease prevention in all adults (8,16–18). The latest guidelines can be summarized as follows:

All adults should increase their regular physical activity to a level appropriate to their capacities, needs, and interests. The long-term goal is to accumulate 30 min or more of moderate-intensity physical activity (i.e., brisk walking, leisurely cycling, swimming, recreational sports, home repair, and yard work) on most, preferably all, days of the week. People who currently meet these recommended minimal standards may derive additional health and fitness benefits by becoming more physically active or including more vigorous activity.

The recommendation from the National Heart, Lung, and Blood Institute's Clinical Guidelines on the Identification, Evaluation, and Treatment of Overweight and Obesity in Adults for physical activity as part of a comprehensive weight loss program is consistent with the above summary statement and is based on an evidence-based review of the scientific literature (1).

The purpose of this chapter is to review the current scientific evidence on the interrelationships among physical activity, obesity, and health outcomes. We will give particular attention to recent evidence-based consensus statements on physical activity and obesity. We also will review prospective observational studies from the Aerobics Center Longitudinal Study cohort and other investigations that stratify health outcomes based on both markers of body habitus and measures of cardiorespiratory fitness or physical activity. We will review evidence from randomized controlled trials (RCT) on the influence of exercise intervention on obesity-related disease risk factors and conclude the chapter with recommendations in the areas of research, public health, and clinical practice.

II OBESITY AND HEALTH OUTCOMES

Obesity is associated with increased morbidity and mortality (1). The risk of death from all causes, cardiovascular disease (CVD), certain cancers, and other diseases increases throughout the range of moderate and severe overweight for both men and women in all age groups (1,19–21). Although a subject for debate, consensus opinion indicates that mortality rates begin to increase modestly with BMIs >25 kg/m^2 with more significant increases occurring in individuals with a BMI of 30 kg/m^2 or higher (1,2,19,20). There are differences among racial groups in the pattern of the association between BMI and mortality (19). Some experts estimate that obesity is second only to cigarette smoking as a leading cause of death in the United States and is associated with ~300,000 deaths per year among adults (22). Physical inactivity and poor dietary habits may be the main lifestyle factors contributing to the excess deaths associated with obesity (23,24). The contribution of obesity to increased morbidity and mortality appears to be independent of its influence on known risk factors, and this is particularly true for CVD (25,26). Overweight and obesity are directly related to an increased risk of several medical conditions including insulin resistance, glucose intolerance, type 2 diabetes mellitus, hypertension, dyslipidemia, and impaired physical function (1,27). There is strong evidence that weight loss in overweight and obese individuals reduces risk factors for diabetes and CVD (1).

Because of the health consequences of excess body fat, it is likely that the current epidemic of obesity will translate into increased prevalence of adverse health outcomes (28). The total healthcare cost attributable to obesity and its comorbidities represents a substantial economic burden (1,29). Concerns about the rapidly rising rates of obesity and associated negative health outcomes have generated calls to action for significant changes in clinical intervention and public health policy (1,2,30). We believe that regular physical activity, because of its contribution to the regulation of energy balance, and, as we will review in this chapter, favorable effects on several of the comorbidities of obesity, must assume a primary role in both public health and clinical efforts to prevent and manage obesity and its associated comorbidities.

III PHYSICAL ACTIVITY AND HEALTH OUTCOMES

A large body of scientific evidence and consensus opinion confirms that low levels of physical activity and cardiorespiratory fitness are associated with high rates of all-cause and cause-specific mortality across diverse population groups (8,16–18,31,32). Regular physical activity and moderate to high levels of cardiorespiratory fitness are associated with more favorable disease risk profiles and lower all-cause and CVD mortality (8,16, 33–35). The inverse association between physical activity or cardiorespiratory fitness and premature mortality is independent of changes in disease risk factors and other potentially confounding variables (36,37).

Based on a review of 42 prospective cohort studies, Lee and Skerrett concluded that there is clear evidence of an inverse dose-response relation between volume of physical activity (or level of physical fitness) and all-cause mortality rates (34). These studies suggest that physical activity resulting in an energy expenditure of ~1000 kcal/wk is associated with a significant 20–30% reduction in risk of all-cause mortality (33,34). Evidence-based review also supports an inverse dose-response relation between physical activity and incidence and mortality rates from cardiovascular and coronary heart disease (CHD) (33,35). Available data indicate a beneficial effect of physical activity on incidence of colon cancer; however, the evidence is less conclusive for a reduction in risk for other types of cancer, such as cancers of the breast and prostate (33,38).

Physical activity and higher levels of cardiorespiratory fitness are associated with lower risk for type 2 diabetes, hypertension, weight gain, and functional limitations that often occur with aging (33,39–42). Activity and fitness are also associated with improvements in the plasma lipid profile and favorable alterations in coagulation and hemostatic factors (33). Other benefits of physical activity include a reduced incidence of depressive illness and improved symptoms in individuals with mild to moderately severe depressive illness (33,43).

A Aerobics Center Longitudinal Study

In this section, we provide a review of studies from the Aerobics Center Longitudinal Study (ACLS) cohort to describe in more detail evidence supporting a strong and independent effect of moderate to high levels of cardiorespiratory fitness on all-cause and CVD mortality in men and women (31,36,44). These studies also introduce preliminary evidence suggesting a protective effect of cardiorespiratory fitness on mortality independent of body mass.

The ACLS is a prospective observational study of patients between the ages of 30 and 83 examined at least once between 1970 and 1993 at the Cooper Clinic in Dallas, Texas. All participants undergo a thorough evaluation including a medical history, physical examination, anthropometry, blood chemistry, and a determination of cardiorespiratory fitness by a maximal exercise test on a treadmill. Each participant's level of cardiorespiratory fitness is based on age and maximal time on the treadmill. In this cohort, total treadmill time correlates highly ($r = .92$) with measured VO_{2max} (45). The least fit 20% are classified as unfit, the next 40% are classified as moderately fit, and the top 40% as high fit. Anthropometric measures include BMI (kg/m^2) calculated from directly measured height and weight, percent body fat determination by hydrostatic weight and/or sum of seven skinfold measurements, and waist circumference measured at the umbilicus. Mailed follow-up surveys and the National Death Index are used to determine morbidity and mortality endpoints.

In 1989, we published a report in which age-adjusted all-cause death rates were calculated across low, moderate, and high cardiorespiratory fitness categories in 10,224 men and 3120 women who were apparently healthy at baseline (31). The results demonstrated a strong and graded inverse association between cardiorespiratory fitness and mortality due to all causes, CVD, and cancer with the major difference in death rates observed in the moderately fit men and women when compared with those with low fitness. Although not specifically designed to examine the relationship among cardiorespiratory fitness, obesity, and mortality, this study provides preliminary evidence of a protective effect of moderate to high levels of cardiorespiratory fitness in overweight men and women. In this study, we found that the mortality benefits of moderate and high fitness persisted across three different BMI strata (< 20 kg/m^2, 20–25 kg/m^2, ≥25 kg/m^2). Men and women in the moderate and high fitness groups had lower death rates than did the low fit individuals in each BMI strata. High fit men with a BMI ≥25 kg/m^2 had an age-adjusted death rate from all causes of 20 per 10,000 man-years of observation compared to a rate of 48 per 10,000 man-years in unfit men in the same BMI group.

In 1995, we reported on observations from 9777 men from the ACLS who received two preventive medical examinations that included maximal treadmill exercise testing (46). The purpose of the investigation was to evaluate the relationship between changes in cardiorespiratory fitness and risk of mortality in men. The average length of follow-up was 5.1 years, and the main outcomes were all-cause and CVD mortality. The highest all-cause mortality rate was observed in men who were unfit at both examinations and the lowest rate was in men who remained fit at both examinations. Men who moved from unfit at baseline to fit at follow-up had an age-adjusted death rate that was 44% lower than men who were unfit at both examinations. The reduction in all-cause mortality associated with moving from the unfit to the fit category was greater than the reduction associated with a favorable change in any of the other risk factors evaluated, including BMI, and was the only statistically significant reduction in multivariate analyses (Fig. 1). In a similar study examining the influence of changes in physical activity on all-cause mortality, Paffenbarger et al. (47) showed that physically inactive middle-aged men who began to participate in moderately vigorous sports activity during the 11 years of follow-up had a 23% lower risk of dying when compared with men who remained sedentary.

In 1996, we published an investigation on 35,341 men and 7080 women from the ACLS cohort that showed that the relative risks of low cardiorespiratory fitness for all-cause and CVD mortality in both men and women were as strong as or stronger than those associated with cigarette smoking, high blood pressure, elevated cholesterol, elevated fasting glucose, and BMI ≥27 (36). In this study, high-fit persons with multiple risk factors, including cigarette smoking, high blood pressure, and elevated cholesterol, had lower death rates than low-fit persons who had none of these other risk factors.

IV DOES PHYSICAL ACTIVITY INFLUENCE OBESITY-RELATED HEALTH OUTCOMES?

Evidence is accumulating that higher levels of physical activity and cardiorespiratory fitness provide protection against many of the adverse health outcomes

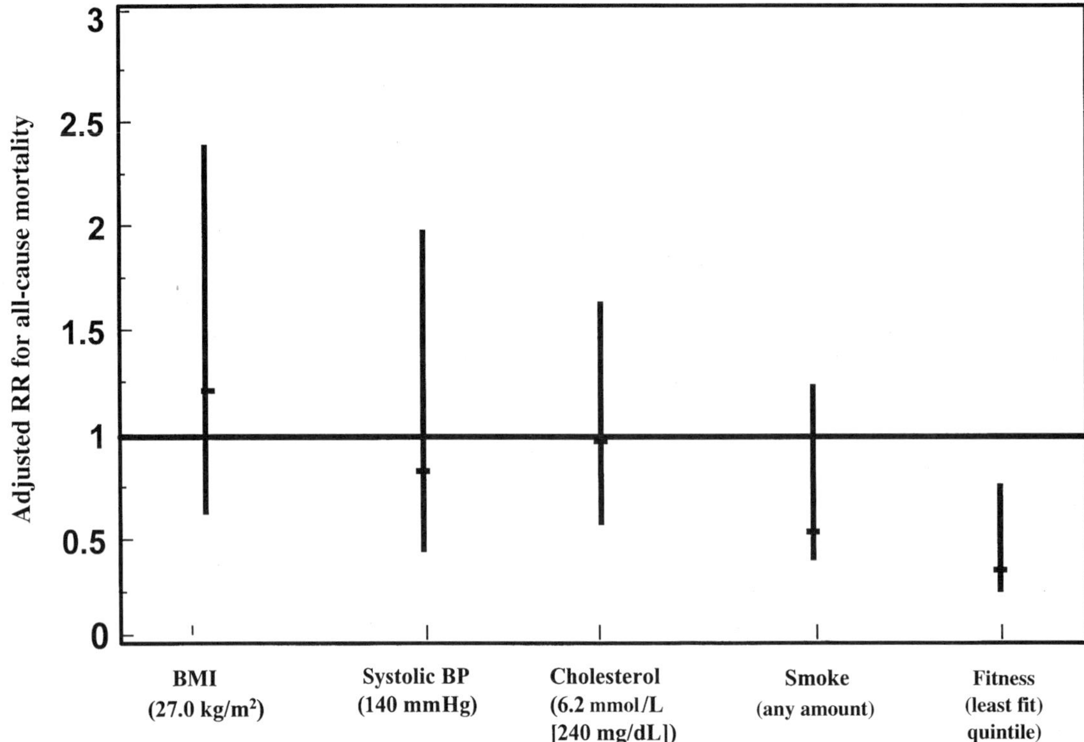

Figure 1 Adjusted relative risk estimates and 95% CI for all-cause mortality for losing weight, lowering blood pressure, reducing cholesterol, stopping smoking, and improving fitness in men at risk for each of these risk factors at the first of two preventive medical examinations. Cutoff points for at-risk categories are in parentheses below each risk factor. Analyses were adjusted for age, family history of coronary heart disease, health status, baseline values, changes for all variables in the figure, and interval in years between examinations. (Adapted from Ref. 46.)

associated with overweight and obesity. Thc National Heart, Lung, and Blood Institute's Obesity Education Initiative convened an expert panel in 1995 to systematically review the scientific literature and determine the most appropriate treatment strategies that would constitute evidence-based clinical guidelines on overweight and obesity. The National Institutes of Health published the evidence report and clinical guidelines (NIH report) from this panel in 1998 (1). The panel followed a categorical system for rating the strength of the evidence using data from RCTs as the strongest level of evidence for evaluating treatment efficacy. The categorical rating system is outlined in Table 1. Of the 39 areas the panel determined required a thorough examination of the relevant scientific literature, six addressed the association of physical activity and cardiorespiratory fitness to health outcomes associated with overweight and obesity. These six evidence statements and corresponding evidence categories are presented in Table 2.

In 1999, the American College of Sports Medicine (ASCM) held a consensus conference to review and report on the scientific evidence on the role of physical activity in the prevention and treatment of obesity and its comorbidities. From this conference, the ACSM released a consensus statement from an independent expert panel and 23 scientific reviews (ACSM report) (48). The consensus statement and reviews provide an indepth review of the role of physical activity in the treatment of overweight and obesity and expand on the evidence presented in the NIH report. Based on the scientific evidence, the ACSM's independent panel issued several consensus statements of which 10 relate to the influence of physical activity on health outcomes associated with overweight and obesity. The consensus statements and evidence categories are presented in Table 2.

A systematic review of the evidence statements from the NIH and ACSM reports reveals that there are seven specific health-related outcomes associated with overweight and obesity where there appears to be sufficient

Table 1 Evidence Categories

Evidence category	Source of evidence	Definition
A	Randomized controlled trials (rich body of data)	Evidence is from endpoints of well-designed RCTs (or trials that depart only minimally from randomization) that provide a consistent pattern of findings in the population for which the recommendation is made. Category A therefore requires substantial numbers of studies involving substantial numbers of participants.
B	Randomized controlled trials (limited body of data)	Evidence is from endpoints of intervention studies that include only a limited number of RCTs, post-hoc, or subgroup analysis of RCTs, or meta-analysis of RCTs. In general, category B pertains when few randomized trials exist, they are small in size, and the trial results are somewhat inconsistent, or the trials were undertaken in a population that differs from the target population of the recommendation.
C	Nonrandomized trials Observational studies	Evidence is from outcomes of uncontrolled or nonrandomized trials or from observational studies.
D	Panel consensus judgment	None of the evidence statements on fitness and health outcomes were placed in this category.

Source: Ref. 1.

evidence for a beneficial and often independent effect of cardiorespiratory fitness and physical activity. As outlined in Table 2, these areas include cardiorespiratory fitness, morbidity and mortality, CVD, insulin resistance and glucose tolerance, hypertension and blood pressure, lipids and dyslipoproteinemias, and cancer. In this section, we will review the scientific evidence on the influence of physical activity and cardiorespiratory fitness on obesity-related health outcomes in each of these seven areas.

A Cardiorespiratory Fitness

The NIH report includes an evidence statement confirming the ability of physical activity to increase cardiorespiratory fitness in overweight and obese individuals independent of weight loss (1). Based on a review of 11 RCTs meeting acceptance criteria, the NIH panel placed the evidence in category A. All 11 studies showed that physical activity increased maximal oxygen uptake in men and women in the exercise groups by an average of 14–18%. Even in studies with modest weight loss (<2%), physical activity increased fitness by an average of 12–16%.

In a more recent RCT, Ross et al. (49) reported on the effects of diet- or exercise-induced weight loss or exercise without weight loss on changes in cardiorespiratory fitness in 52 obese men (mean BMI 31.3 kg/m^2) following a 12-week intervention. The investigators matched treatment groups for total energy deficit of ~700 kcal/d (dietary deficit in the diet-only group and increased energy expenditure in the exercise-only weight loss group). The exercise without weight loss group increased calorie intake by ~700 kcal/d to match the energy expenditure of exercise. Participants in the exercise groups performed daily exercise (brisk walking or light jogging) on a motorized treadmill, at an intensity of 77% of maximal heart rate for ~60 min. Body weight decreased by 7.5 kg (8%) in both weight loss groups and remained stable in the exercise without weight loss group. Maximum oxygen uptake (L/min) increased by 13% and 19% in the exercise weight loss group and exercise weight stable group compared to no change in the control and diet groups. The findings of Ross et al. demonstrate that exercise training significantly increases cardiorespiratory fitness in obese men with or without weight loss. Numerous studies show that exercise training improves VO_{2max} between 5% and 30%, with a minimum expected improvement of 15% when the quantity and quality of training meets recommended levels (50). Therefore, overweight and obese individuals appear to derive expected improvements in cardiores-

Table 2 Evidence Statements for the Influence of Physical Activity and Cardiorespiratory Fitness on Obesity-Related Health Outcomes

NIH evidence statements	Evidence category	ACSM consensus statements	Evidence category
1. Cardiorespiratory fitness			
Physical activity in overweight and obese adults increases cardiorespiratory fitness independent of weight loss.	A	Evidence not reviewed.	
2. Morbidity and mortality			
Evidence statement not given.		Higher levels of physical activity or cardiovascular fitness reduce morbidity and mortality in overweight or obese persons.	C
		Overweight and obese persons who are physically active have a lower risk of morbidity and mortality than normal weight individuals who are sedentary.	C
3. Cardiovascular disease			
Physical activity independently reduces CVD risk factors.	A	Evidence statement not given.	
Physical activity independently reduces risk for cardiovascular disease.	C		
4. Insulin resistance and glucose tolerance			
Increased aerobic activity to increase cardiorespiratory fitness improves glucose tolerance in overweight individuals, but no evidence shows this relationship to be independent of weight loss.	C	Intervention-based RCTs consistently show that increased physical activity improves insulin action, and thus reduces insulin resistance, in obese subjects.	A
		Epidemiological data suggest that exercise alone and exercise combined with weight reduction retard the transition from impaired glucose tolerance to type II diabetes.	C
5. Hypertension and blood pressure			
Increased aerobic activity to increase cardiorespiratory fitness reduces blood pressure independent of weight loss.	A	RCTs provide strong evidence that physical activity can reduce blood pressure in obese subjects and that the reduction is independent of weight loss or changes in body composition. The response does not go beyond the blood pressure reduction obtained by diet alone.	A
		Observational studies support the concept that physical activity reduces the risk for developing hypertension, independent of its effects on body size or body composition.	C
6. Lipids and dyslipoproteinemias			
Increased aerobic activity to increase cardiorespiratory fitness favorably affects blood lipids, particularly if accompanied by weight loss.	A	Physical activity of a volume that results in at least 4.5 kg weight loss will raise HDL-cholesterol and lower triglycerides in men and postmenopausal women.	A
		The addition of physical activity to a low-energy, low-fat diet will reverse the HDL-lowering effect of the low-fat diet in overweight men and women.	A
		In men and postmenopausal women with atherogenic dyslipidemia, the addition of physical activity to a modestly reducing, low-fat diet significantly enhances the LDL-lowering effect of the diet.	A
7. Cancer			
Evidence not reviewed.		Epidemiological studies find a strong inverse relationship between physical activity and colon cancer. The strength and consistency of this association is so strong that a causal connection seems likely.	C

Source: Refs. 1 and 15.

piratory fitness from physical training with or without weight loss.

Data from the ACLS cohort indicate that overweight and obese individuals are more likely than normal-weight persons to be sedentary and unfit (51,52). There is a strong direct association between BMI and low cardiorespiratory fitness in the ACLS cohort (Fig. 2). In this cohort, ~80% of women and >90% of men with a BMI ≥40 kg/m^2 are unfit compared to <10% unfit in individuals with a BMI between 18.5 and 24.9 kg/m^2. However, as can be seen from Figure 2, many obese individuals (BMI ≥30 kg/m^2) are at least moderately fit and, as will be discussed, are likely at a lower risk for many adverse health outcomes than are normal-weight, overweight, and obese individuals who are unfit.

The importance of low cardiorespiratory fitness as a mortality predictor in obese men was demonstrated by a study reported by Wei et al. in 1999 (53). We conducted this study in 25,714 men from the ACLS cohort to compare low cardiorespiratory fitness with established CVD risk factors (type 2 diabetes, high total cholesterol, hypertension, current smoking) as a predictor of mortality in normal-weight, overweight, and obese men. In this study, baseline CVD was the strongest predictor of premature mortality. However, for overweight and obese men, low cardiorespiratory fitness was a strong predictor of mortality, with relative risks comparable with, if not greater than, those for type 2 diabetes, high cholesterol levels, hypertension, and current cigarette smoking (Fig. 3). In the 3293 obese men (BMI ≥30 kg/m^2), low fitness was the most common mortality predictor with a prevalence rate about five times higher than that of type 2 diabetes, which was the least prevalent of the factors evaluated. About 50% of obese men in this study were unfit; 16% had baseline CVD, and 10% had type 2 diabetes. Because of its high prevalence and strength as predictor of premature mortality, low cardiorespiratory fitness had the highest population-attributable risk of the six mortality predictors evaluated in overweight and obese men in this cohort.

B Morbidity and Mortality

The ACSM report issued two evidence statements indicating that (1) higher levels of physical activity or cardiovascular fitness reduce morbidity and mortality in overweight or obese persons, and (2) overweight and obese individuals who are physically active have a lower risk of morbidity and mortality than normal weight individuals who are sedentary (Table 2) (15). The evidence supporting these two statements was judged by the panel to be moderately strong and placed in evidence category C. In this section, we will address the available evidence on the relation of physical activity and cardiorespiratory fitness to all-cause and CVD mortality, CHD risk, and cancer in overweight and obese individuals.

1 All-Cause Mortality

Several prospective observational studies indicate that overweight and obese men who are fit or physically active have lower death rates than unfit or sedentary normal-weight men (54). In some of these studies, overweight and obese men only had elevated mortality if they were unfit or inactive. Unfortunately, only a few studies have included women in their analyses.

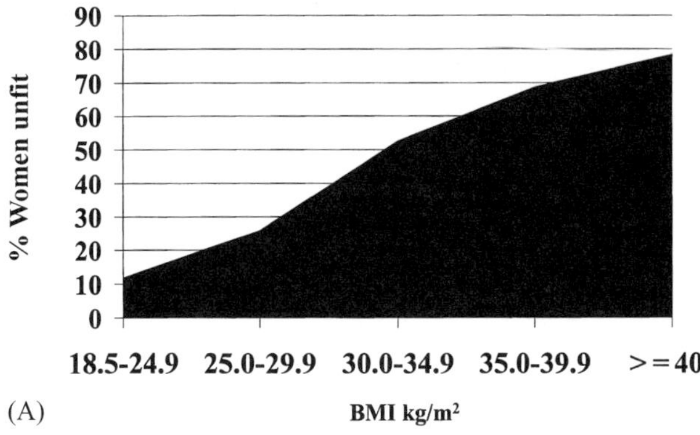

(A)

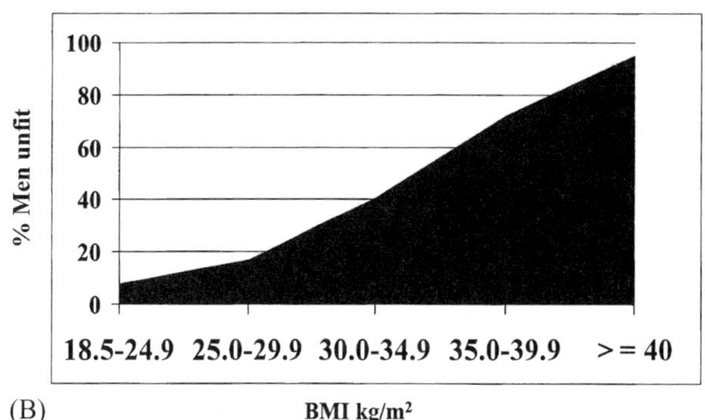

(B)

Figure 2 The association between BMI and the prevalence of low cardiorespiratory fitness (dark area of the figure) in 6840 women (panel A) and 23,190 men (panel B) from the Aerobics Center Longitudinal Study cohort who were free of CHD, cancer, and abnormal ECG. The number of individuals across the BMI strata of 18.5–24.9, 25.0–29.9, 30.0–34.9, 35.0–39.9, and ≥40 were 5499, 959, 262, 83, and 37 for women, and 9838, 10,544, 2308, 361, and 139 for men.

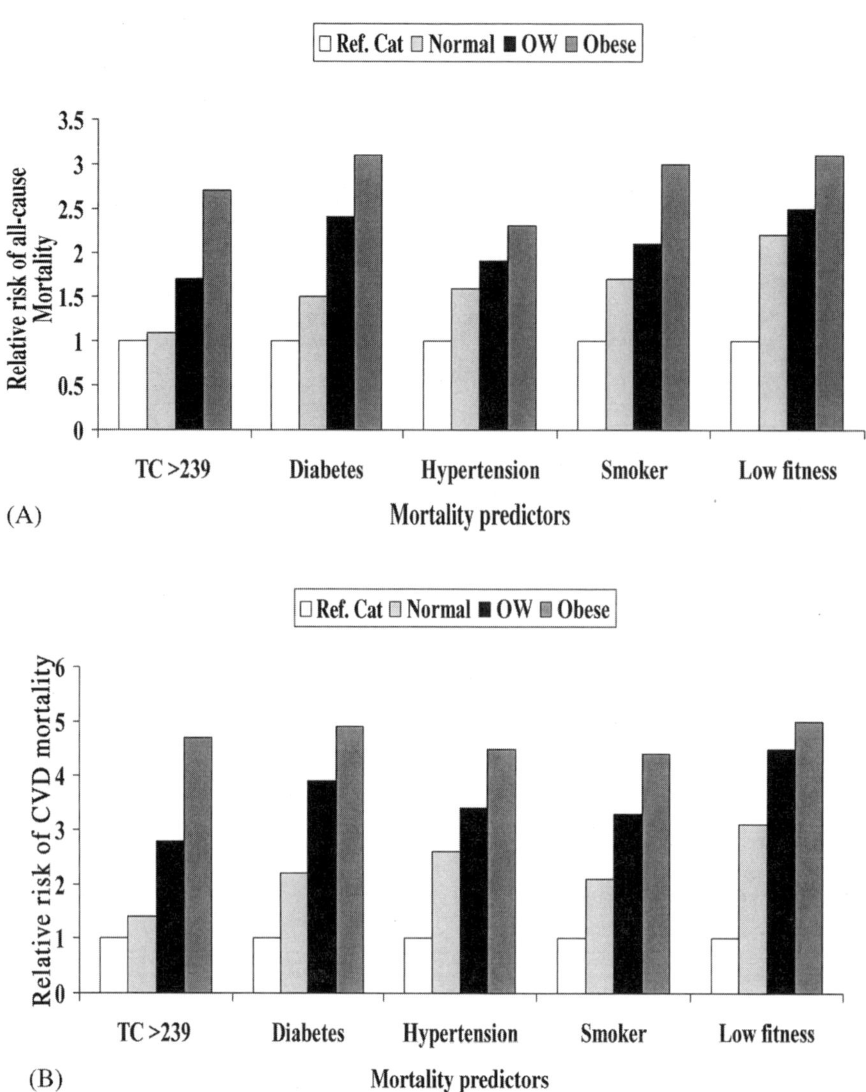

Figure 3 Relative risks for all-cause (panel A) and cardiovascular disease (CVD) (panel B) mortality by BMI and other CVD risk factors in 25,714 men followed for 258,781 man-years of observation (1025 deaths, 439 from CVD). Relative risks were adjusted for age and examination year. The referent group in each of the five analyses was normal-weight men (BMI 18.5–24.9) who did not have the CVD risk factor examined in the specific analysis. Overweight men were those with a BMI of 25.0–29.9, and obese men were those with BMI ≥30.0. (Adapted from Ref. 53.)

In 1995, Barlow et al. (55) investigated the relation of cardiorespiratory fitness to mortality in 25,389 men classified as normal-weight, overweight, or obese (<27 kg/m^2, 27–30 kg/m^2, >30 kg/m^2) from the ACLS cohort (55). In all three BMI categories, moderate and high-fit men had a lower relative risk for all-cause mortality than unfit men. In this report, it was also observed that moderate to high-fit men who were overweight or obese (BMI ≥27 kg/m^2) did not have elevated death rates as compared with high fit men who were normal weight (BMI <27 kg/m^2). The high-fit obese men also had lower death rates than low-fit men who were normal weight. Specifically, obese men (BMI >30 kg/m^2) who were at least moderately fit had an age-adjusted all-cause death rate of 18/10,000 man-years of observation compared with a rate of 52/10,000 man-years in normal-weight men who were unfit. The highest death rate was observed in the unfit obese men (62.1/10,000 man-years of observation).

Extending the observations of Barlow and colleagues, Lee et al. (56) performed a more detailed analysis on the relation of cardiorespiratory fitness to mortality in overweight men in 21,856 men from the ACLS cohort. In this study, men with previous myocardial infarction, stroke, and cancer at baseline were excluded, and the analyses were adjusted for smoking habit and alcohol intake. The men were stratified by BMI and cardiorespiratory fitness. Normal-weight men were classified as a BMI from 19.0 to <25, mild-overweight from 25.0 to <27.8, and overweight ≥27.8 kg/m^2. The investigators used two categories for cardiorespiratory fitness: (1) unfit (bottom 20th centile based on age and treadmill time) and (2) fit (the remaining 80%). Fit normal-weight men were used as the reference group in the analysis. Unfit men had a higher risk of all-cause mortality than their fit counterparts in all three BMI categories. In this study, men who were unfit and overweight had the highest risk for all-cause mortality at follow-up. However, fit and overweight men were not at increased risk when compared with fit normal-weight men and had a lower risk for all-cause mortality at follow-up than the normal-weight but unfit men (Fig. 4A).

Lee et al. (57) extended these observations in 1999 by performing a more detailed investigation of body habitus, cardiorespiratory fitness, and mortality in 21,925 men. The investigators assigned subjects to categories of lean, normal, or obese based on measures of percent body fat (either sum of seven skinfolds or underwater weighing) and waist circumference. The results demonstrated a direct relationship between percent body fat and waist circumference measures and risk of all-cause mortality. Fit men had lower death rates than did their unfit counterparts within each body fatness and waist circumference category. Obese men, classified by either body fatness (≥25%) or waist circumference (≥99 cm), who were fit had a twofold lower risk of all-cause mortality than unfit lean men (body fat <16.7% or waist circumference <87 cm) (Fig. 5A). All-cause mortality rates in the fit obese men were not significantly different from those of fit lean men. In summary, all three of these studies from the ACLS cohort found that overweight

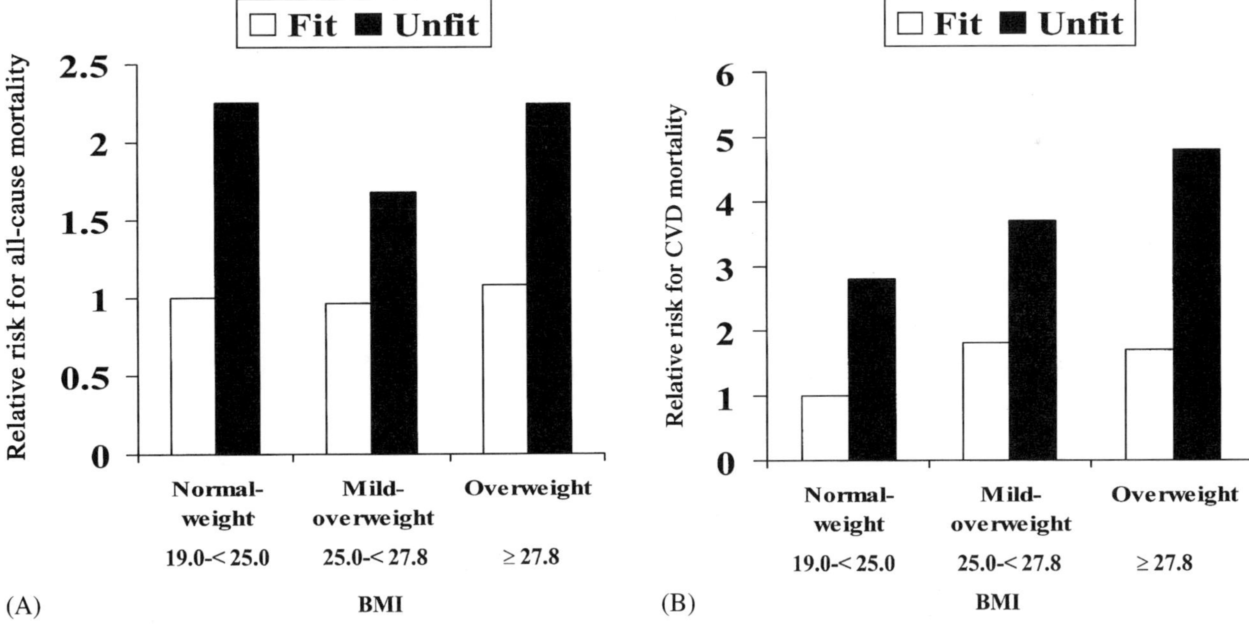

Figure 4 Body mass index and relative risks of all-cause (panel A) and cardiovascular disease (CVD) (panel B) mortality by cardiorespiratory fitness level in 21,856 men from the Aerobics Center Longitudinal Study cohort followed for 176,189 years of observation (427 deaths: 144 CVD, 143 cancer, 140 other). Adjusted for age, examination year, smoking habit, and alcohol intake. Unfit men (black bars) were the least fit 20% in each age group, and all other men were classified as fit. (Adapted from Ref. 56.)

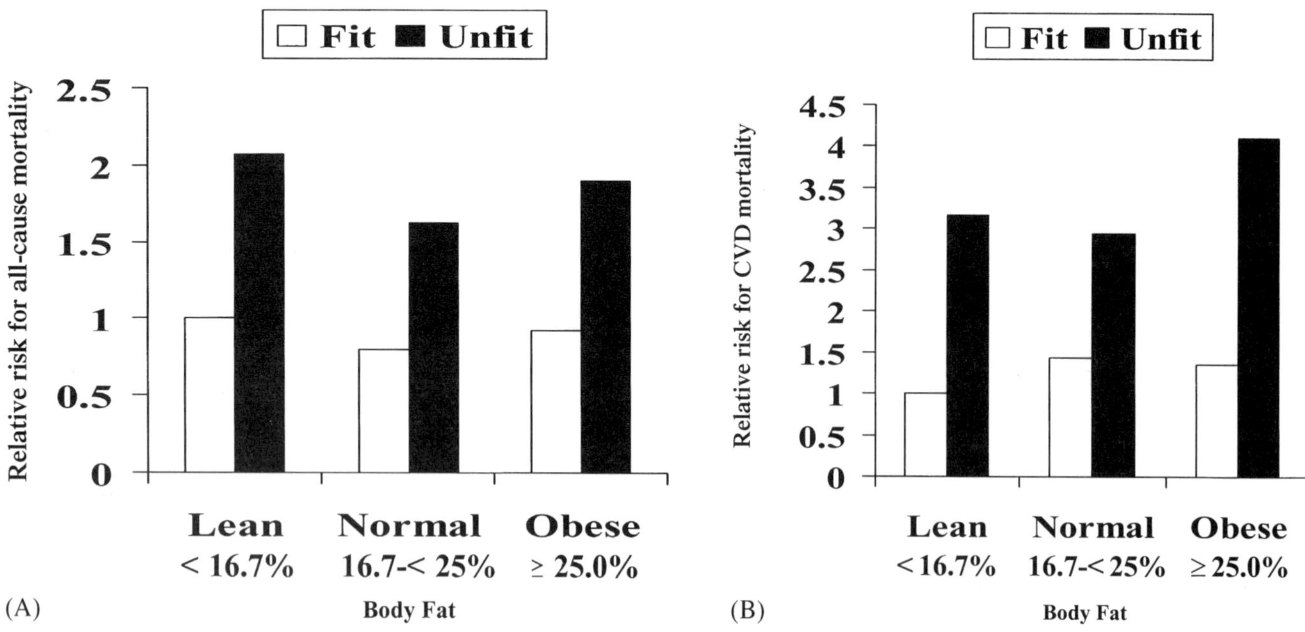

Figure 5 Relative risks for all-cause (panel A) and cardiovascular disease (CVD) (panel B) mortality by percent body fat and cardiorespiratory fitness level in 21,925 men followed for 176,742 man-years of observation (428 deaths: 144 CVD, 143 cancer, 141 other). Relative risks are adjusted for age, examination year, smoking status, alcohol intake, and parental history of coronary heart disease. Unfit men (black bars) were the least fit 20% in each age group, and all other men were classified as fit. (Adapted from Ref. 57.)

and obese men had elevated mortality only if they were also unfit.

A few prospective investigations provide analyses evaluating all-cause mortality as the outcome and physical activity and BMI as the exposure variables. Most of these studies provide evidence indicating that overweight and obese individuals who are physically active have a lower risk of all-cause mortality than normal weight individuals who are sedentary (32,37,54,58,59). In a study investigating the influence of leisure-time physical activity on mortality in 16,936 male Harvard alumni aged 35–74, Paffenbarger et al. (32) performed an analysis to determine the confounding influence of BMI on the inverse association between physical activity and mortality. The investigators reported on the influence of self-reported physical activity (<500, 500–1999, ≥2000 kcal/wk) across categories of BMI (<23.9, 23.9–25.2, ≥25.3 kg/m^2) on all-cause mortality. In this study, BMI was not significantly related to mortality and the relation of BMI to mortality was uneven with men in the lowest and highest BMI groups having the highest death rates. When stratified by both physical activity and BMI, the results indicate lower mortality rates in active men compared to sedentary men in each BMI group. The most active men in the highest BMI group had a lower death rate (60/10,000 man-years) than sedentary men in the two lower BMI categories (81 and 113/10,000 man-years). Rosengren and Wilhelmsen (37) also reported on an analysis investigating whether the reduction in mortality risk by physical activity varied according to baseline BMI. As for the results reported by Paffenbarger et al. (32), death rates were lower with increasing levels of self-report physical activity across all BMI categories. In this study, age-adjusted all-cause mortality rates were lower in active men with a BMI >26.6 kg/m^2 as compared with sedentary men with a BMI <24.1 kg/m^2.

More recently, Dorn et al. (58) reported that physical activity was inversely related to all-cause mortality in nonobese men (27.02 kg/m^2) but not for obese men (BMI ≥27.02 kg/m^2) (58). From their results, the investigators speculated that the benefits of activity on mortality may not override the harmful effects of excess weight in obese men. In this cohort from the Buffalo Health Study, no significant interaction was observed between activity and BMI on mortality in women. Haapaanen-Niemi et al. (59) investigated the interaction of BMI, leisure-time physical activity, and perceived physical fitness with the risk of all-cause mortality (59). The study population was 2212 middle-aged and elderly Finnish men and women followed for 16 years. In this study, low levels of leisure-time physical activity (LTPA) seemed to predict and low perceived physical fitness predicted an increased risk of all-cause mortality among both men and women. However, in contrast to the hypothesis, obesity was not an independent predictor of mortality in this population, and no interaction effect was found between BMI and LTPA or perceived fitness and the relative risk of death. The authors concluded that the beneficial effects of LTPA and fitness are similar among obese and nonobese men and women.

2 Cardiovascular disease

Cardiovascular disease is the leading cause of death in the United States and many industrialized countries. In the United States, CVD is responsible for nearly 950,000 deaths each year (60). Both obesity and a sedentary lifestyle are strong independent predictors of fatal and nonfatal CVD (1,8). While the ACSM report does not make a specific evidence statement on CVD mortality, the review by Blair and Brodney (54) provides a summary of three prospective observational studies from the ACLS cohort that support a reduced risk of CVD mortality in fit overweight and obese men (54). In the two studies by Lee et al. (56,57), described earlier for all-cause mortality, CVD mortality was lower in fit obese men when compared with unfit lean and unfit normal weight men. In these analyses there was a tendency for fit overweight and fit obese men to have higher CVD mortality than fit normal-weight men (Figs. 4B, 5B). This finding is in contrast to the finding of no increased risk between fit normal-weight men and fit obese men for the outcome of all-cause mortality in these two studies. The NIH report contains a specific statement on the independent effect of physical activity in reducing risk for CVD morbidity and mortality, but provides no specific review of scientific literature that examines the evidence supporting reduced CVD mortality in overweight or obese individuals (Table 2).

In a more recent study examining the relation between physical activity and CVD in 1564 female alumnae from the University of Pennsylvania, Sesso et al. (61) found an inverse association for CVD risk only for lean women with a BMI <23 kg/m^2. After multivariate adjustment, lean women who expended ≥1000 kcal/wk had a 37% lower CVD risk than women who expended <500 kcal/wk. In the study from Haapanen-Niemi et al. (59), as discussed for all-cause mortality, BMI did not appear to be an independent risk factor for CVD mortality. More studies are needed to evaluate the protective influence of physical activity on CVD mortality in overweight and obesity.

3 Coronary Heart Disease

Both obesity and physical inactivity are major independent predictors for CHD (1,8,25). In the United States, CHD is responsible for >450,000 deaths each year and is the single leading killer of men and women (60). Neither of the evidence reports makes a specific statement on CHD; however, the review by Blair and Brodney (54) provides a summary of seven prospective observational studies that included the exposure variables of body habitus and physical activity as predictors of fatal and nonfatal CHD. In general, these studies demonstrate a protective effect of physical activity against CHD in men regardless of BMI. In a study from Salonen et al. (62), overweight men (BMI ≥27 kg/m^2) who were active at work and in their leisure time had a CHD death rate of 7.4/1000 men compared with a rate of 25.9/1000 in sedentary men with a BMI <27 kg/m^2. Morris et al. (63) reported a heart attack rate of 7.3/1000 man-years in sedentary overweight (BMI ≥27 kg/m^2) men and only 1.3/1000 man-years in the most active men in the same BMI category. The rate in sedentary normal-weight (BMI <24 kg/m^2) men was 5.5/1000 man-years and 1.9/1000 man-years in regular vigorous exercisers. The lower rate of CHD events in these two studies suggests that physically active overweight men may have lower CHD mortality compared with normal-weight but inactive men.

Unfortunately, none of the studies reviewed by Blair and Brodney (54) were designed to specifically investigate the influence of physical activity on CHD in overweight and obese individuals. Typically, the highest BMI stratum in these studies had a lower bound in the mild-overweight category, so we cannot be certain that the results apply to obese individuals. Only one study included data for women. There are no studies examining CHD as the outcome variable and BMI and cardiorespiratory fitness as exposure variables.

Two more recent studies evaluated the relation of physical activity to CHD mortality in both men and women. In the study by Dorn et al. (58), physical activity was only associated with a decreased risk of CHD mortality in nonobese men. In the study by Haapanen-Niemi and colleagues (59), BMI was not associated with increased risk of CHD mortality in men or women; therefore, no interaction effect was found between physical activity or perceived fitness and BMI for CHD mortality. At this time, some evidence suggests that fatal and nonfatal CHD events are lower in physically active overweight men than in either normal-weight and overweight men who are inactive; however, more evidence is needed to support an evidence-based statement on this question.

4 Cancer

Cancer is the second leading killer of Americans and is responsible for >550,000 deaths each year in the United States (64). Observational studies have found a positive relation between overweight and obesity and the risk for morbidity from several types of cancer, including colon, breast, endometrial, and prostate (1,21, 27,65–67). Cross-sectional and observational studies have also found an inverse relationship between physical activity and total and site-specific cancer; however, the findings are not always consistent (33,38). Etiologic mechanisms for an interaction effect of physical activity and obesity on cancer incidence seem plausible for hormone-dependent cancers; however, the strongest evidence for a protective effect is for colon cancer (38). The most commonly cited mechanism for this effect is reduced bowel transit time, which reduces the period of contact between carcinogens and mucosal cells (38,68, 69). Two recent evidence-based reviews of physical activity and cancer risk concluded that the majority of studies observe a 10% to 70% reduction in the incidence of colon cancer, with the observed relationship being strongest for cancers of the distal colon (38,68).

Several studies also suggest that there is a dose-response association between higher levels of physical activity and decreased risk for colon cancer (33,38). While the NIH report does not make an evidence statement for physical activity and cancer risk in overweight and obese individuals, the ACSM expert panel states that current epidemiological evidence finds a strong inverse relationship between physical activity and colon cancer and that a causal connection seems likely (Table 2) (15). Although the effect of BMI has been taken into account in many studies, few studies have stratified results using both physical activity and body habitus as exposure variables (54). In a case-control study, Slattery et al. (70) stratified the incidence of colon cancer by physical activity patterns and BMI. The results suggest a protective effect of intermediate and high levels of physical activity across BMI categories, particularly in women. Given the significant limitations of current physical activity and colon cancer research, it is difficult to make any statements on the strength of evidence supporting a protective effect of physical activity independent of body habitus.

While evidence is building for a protective effect of physical activity on the risk of developing breast cancer in pre- and postmenopausal women, evidence-based statements cannot be made based on existing data (15, 33,38,68). Because of the complex relationship between body weight and breast cancer risk across the life span and the methodological limitations of current studies, it is not clear to what extent physical activity and body weight might interact to influence risk (68). Also, there are insufficient data to make evidence-based statements on the protective effects of physical activity for other obesity-related cancers such as endometrial and prostate cancers (15,33).

C Comorbidities

Obesity and physical inactivity are directly related to several chronic disease risk factors, such as insulin resistance, hypertension, and dyslipidemia (1,8). In this section, we review the evidence indicating a protective and often independent effect of physical activity on these disease risk factors in overweight and obese individuals.

1 Insulin Resistance and Glucose Tolerance

Type 2 diabetes mellitus is a leading cause of death and disability in many countries (71). In the United States, it is estimated that nearly 15 million individuals have type 2 diabetes, and the prevalence is rising rapidly (4,72,73). Type 2 diabetes is characterized by varying degrees of insulin resistance, relative insulin deficiency, and glucose intolerance. Along with genetic factors, obesity and physical inactivity are strongly implicated in the development of type 2 diabetes (73,74). Both the NIH and ACSM reports make evidence statements about the effects of physical activity and moderate to high cardiorespiratory fitness on insulin action, glucose tolerance, and diabetes risk in overweight and obese individuals (Table 2).

Studies indicate that a single session of acute exercise at an intensity of 55–75% of VO_{2max} and a duration of 45–60 min lowers blood glucose 20–40 $mg{\cdot}dL^{-1}$ (1–2 mmol·dL-1) and reduces insulin resistance for 2–3 days following exercise in subjects with type 2 diabetes mellitus (33,75). Studies show this effect in both obese and nonobese men and women (75). Studies examining the effects of strength training on insulin action have found similar improvements in insulin action as those induced by aerobic exercise (76). Experimental studies indicate that there are several plausible mechanisms for the beneficial effects of acute and chronic physical activity intervention on glucose homeostasis and insulin action. These mechanisms may include reduced hepatic glucose production, increased skeletal muscle insulin sensitivity and glycogen repletion, enhanced glucose uptake, reductions in visceral and abdominal subcutaneous adipose tissue, and depletion of muscle triglycerides (76–79).

For the ACSM consensus conference, Blair and Brodney (54) evaluated prospective observational studies that stratified diabetes risk by both body habitus and cardiorespiratory fitness or physical activity. In these studies the trend was for physically active overweight and obese individuals to have a lower incidence of self-reported type 2 diabetes at follow-up compared with inactive men in the same BMI group; however, the overweight or obese men appeared to remain at higher risk when compared with sedentary normal-weight men. The most convincing evidence of a protective effect comes from a study by Wei et al. (39) in the ACLS cohort. To determine whether cardiorespiratory fitness is associated with risk for developing impaired fasting glucose and diabetes, the investigators followed 8633 nondiabetic men who were examined at least twice and followed for an average of 6 years. The strengths of this study lie in its objective measure of cardiorespiratory fitness and the determination of diabetes incidence by measured fasting plasma glucose at baseline and follow-up. In this study, after adjusting for multiple influencing factors, the investigators reported a 1.9-fold risk (95% CI, 1.5–2.4) for impaired fasting glucose and a 3.7-fold risk (95% CI, 2.4–5.8) for developing type 2 diabetes in men with low cardiorespiratory fitness (the least fit 20% of the cohort) as compared with high-fit men (the most fit 40% of the cohort). The data from this study also demonstrated a steep inverse gradient of risk for developing type 2 diabetes across fitness categories among individuals with BMI of <27 and ≥27 kg/m^2 (Fig. 6). Fit men with a BMI ≥27 kg/m^2 had a slightly lower incidence of type 2 diabetes than unfit men with BMI <27 kg/m^2.

To date, only one RCT has been conducted that examines the influence of increased physical activity on the prevention of type 2 diabetes. The Da Qing study, conducted on 577 Chinese subjects with impaired fasting glucose, found that exercise alone, after adjustment for baseline BMI and fasting glucose, decreased the risk for developing diabetes by 46% (80). This rate of risk reduction was similar to that seen for the diet-only and diet-plus-exercise arms of the study, and the decrease in incidence was similar when individuals were stratified by BMI <25 or ≥25 kg/m^2.

In the ACSM Report, Kelley and Goodpaster (76) reviewed 11 randomized and nonrandomized trials that investigated the effect of aerobic exercise at recommended levels of intensity, duration, and frequency on

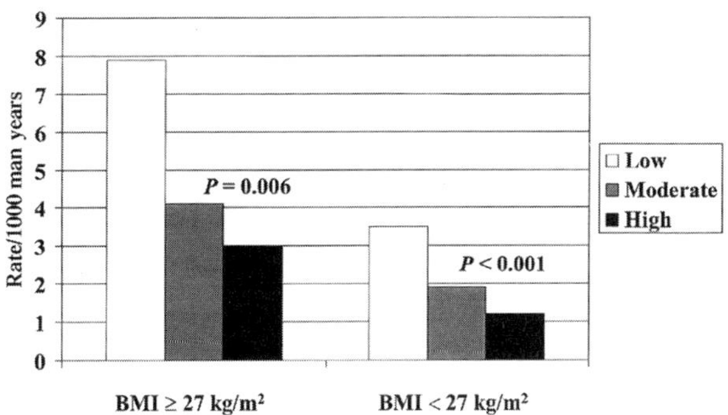

Figure 6 Incidence of type 2 diabetes per 1000 person-years by cardiorespiratory fitness levels according to BMI. Of 8633 nondiabetic men at baseline examination, 149 developed type 2 diabetes during an average follow-up of 6 years. White bars indicate low-fit men (least fit 20%), diagonal lines moderate-fit men (next 40%), and black bars high-fit men (remaining 40%). (Adapted from Ref. 39.)

insulin sensitivity and glucose tolerance in relation to obesity (76). Nine of the trials reviewed indicated that physical activity resulted in improved indices of glucose homeostasis, notably improved insulin resistance, in the absence of weight loss or changes in body composition. Although physical activity appears to have an independent beneficial effect on insulin action and glucose tolerance, data from several studies suggest that greater effects occur in the presence of weight loss or a change in body composition, particularly a reduction in abdominal or visceral fat (76,78,81,82). Dengel et al. (83) reported on a 9-month intervention in 97 men assigned to one of four groups: weight loss, aerobic exercise, exercise plus weight loss, and control. The three intervention groups had significant reductions in glucose and insulin responses to an oral glucose tolerance test (OGTT) compared with the control group; however, the reduction in the insulin response for the exercise plus weight loss group was significantly greater than the other groups. A recent RCT in 52 obese men by Ross and colleagues (49) suggests the importance of weight loss in glucose control. The study found that diet-induced and exercise-induced weight loss groups matched for total energy deficit achieved similar increases in glucose disposal rates compared to the control and exercise without weight loss groups over 12 weeks of intervention. In contrast, Rice et al. (79) reported that obese men randomized to diet plus aerobic exercise or diet plus resistance exercise achieved greater reductions in the insulin area under the curve during an OGTT when compared with men in a diet only group after 16 weeks of intervention. In this study, reductions in weight and visceral and subcutaneous adipose tissue were not different among the three treatments. In summary, while clinical trial data provide evidence that physical activity independently improves insulin action and glucose tolerance independent of weight loss, the combination of exercise plus dietary intervention to induce weight loss appears to produce more favorable changes in glucose homeostasis.

A recent study from the ACLS cohort suggests that physical activity and cardiorespiratory fitness may provide protection against premature mortality in men with type 2 diabetes. In this study, Wei et al. (84) reported on 1263 men with type 2 diabetes followed prospectively for all-cause mortality. During an average follow-up of 12 years there were 180 deaths. After adjusting for multiple influencing factors, men in the low-fitness group (bottom 20th centile based on age and treadmill time) had a risk for all-cause mortality of 2.1 (95% CI, 1.5–2.9) compared with fit men (remaining 80%). Men who reported being physically inactive at baseline had an adjusted risk for mortality of 1.7 (95% CI, 1.2–2.3) compared with physically active men. In this study, fitness had the same protective effect in normal-weight (BMI <25 kg/m^2) and overweight men (BMI ≥ 25 kg/m^2). Hu et al. (85) reported on the influence of physical activity on CVD in 5125 female nurses with type 2 diabetes over 14 years of follow-up. In this study, greater leisure-time physical activity was associated with a reduced risk of CHD and stroke, and the inverse association persisted in a subgroup analysis stratified by BMI. The results of these two studies suggest that physical activity and cardiorespiratory fitness have strong and independent effects on morbidity and mortality in individuals with type 2 diabetes and that the protective effect extends to both normal weight and overweight individuals.

2 Hypertension and Blood Pressure

Hypertension is a leading cause of CVD morbidity and mortality. In the United States it is estimated that >50 million individuals have hypertension, with many cases undiagnosed (60). The long-term complications associated with hypertension include atherosclerotic cardiovascular, cerebrovascular, and peripheral vascular disease. Weight reduction and increased physical activity are widely accepted lifestyle interventions for the management of hypertension (86). Both the NIH and ACSM expert panels conclude that physical activity reduces blood pressure independent of weight loss and place the evidence in category A (Table 2). Observational studies suggest that physical activity reduces the risk for developing hypertension independent of body habitus (15,54,87). Paffenbarger et al. (88,89) followed two cohorts of male college alumni for up to 15 years for the development of incident physician diagnosed hypertension. In general, men participating in vigorous sports play had a lower risk of developing hypertension than sedentary men, with the greatest protection occurring in men in the highest BMI categories. Evidence from cross-sectional surveys and prospective observational studies is supported by RCTs (87). Investigators have identified several plausible mechanisms for this beneficial independent effect of physical activity on blood pressure. Such mechanisms may include reduced peripheral vascular resistance, decrease in plasma catecholamine concentrations, changes in autonomic regulation, and decreased plasma volume (87,90).

There is strong evidence that a single session of exercise at an intensity of 50–100% of VO_{2max} produces a lowering of 18–20 mm Hg in systolic and 7–9 mm Hg in diastolic blood pressure with the maximal changes occurring in individuals with stage I hypertension (33,75). The post exercise hypotension may persist for up to 12–16 hours after exercise, thus offering individuals with hypertension a significant amount of protection on days that activity is performed. A recent meta-analysis of 44 RCTs found that aerobic training from three to five times per week for 30–60 min per session and at an intensity of at least 40–50% of maximal exercise reduces blood pressure, particularly in hypertensives (91). In this review, Fagard determined that aerobic exercise training reduces blood pressure, after controlling for weight loss and dietary change, by an average of 3.4/2.4 mm Hg. The blood pressure reduction in response to exercise training was greater in hypertensive individuals (7.4/5.8 mm Hg). In an earlier meta-analysis and evidence-based review for the ACSM report, Fagard (87) summarized the results from 64 study groups according to whether the average baseline BMI was <25 or ≥ 25 kg/m^2. Reductions in blood pressure associated with exercise training were similar in the two BMI groups, although BMI decreased significantly in the overweight but not in the lean subjects. A metaregression analysis of these data demonstrated that there were no significant relationships between changes in blood pressure associated with exercise training and initial BMI or changes in BMI.

Several recent investigations indicate that exercise training alone, while effective, is less effective for reducing blood pressure than diet-induced weight loss in overweight and obese individuals (82,87). In his review, Fagard also compared exercise training versus dietary intervention in 11 study groups (87). The reduction in blood pressure and BMI with diet alone was significantly greater than that of exercise alone. It is likely that the greater reduction in blood pressure seen with the dietary interventions is due to weight loss. Some studies indicate that exercise-induced and diet-induced weight losses appear to produce similar reductions in blood pressure (92,93). In addition, several studies indicate that there is not a synergistic effect on blood pressure control when exercise is combined with dietary therapy (83,87,92). Fagard compared diet alone with combined diet and exercise in 11 study groups and found that there was not an additive blood pressure lowering effect for the combined intervention, although the combined intervention was more effective in reducing BMI (87). However, a more recent study, by Blumenthal et al. (94), found that the addition of a behavioral weight loss program enhanced the blood pressure lowering effect of exercise alone. It is important to note that in several of these studies exercise training significantly increased fitness compared with no change with diet-induced weight loss (1,8,83,92). Work from our center provides evidence that moderate to high levels of fitness may provide an independent protective effect against premature mortality in normotensive and hypertensive men (95).

3 Lipids and Dyslipoproteinemias

It is widely accepted that blood lipids are a major factor in the process that leads to atherosclerotic CVD (96). Treatment of unfavorable lipid levels reduces the incidence of fatal and nonfatal CHD events (97). A large body of evidence from cross-sectional observational studies, clinical trials, and experimental investigations supports a beneficial effect of physical activity on blood lipids, particularly HDL cholesterol (HDL-C) and triglycerides (15,33,98,99). The most frequently observed change associated with physical activity intervention is an increase in HDL-C. Exercise training also appears to attenuate the reduction in HDL-C accompanying decreased dietary intake of saturated fat and cholesterol. Less frequently observed are decreases in total cholesterol and LDL-C. According to Leon and Sanchez, exercise training in RCTs typically involved moderate to vigorous exercise three to five times per week for 30–60 min and a study duration of 12–52 weeks (98). There is also strong evidence for an acute beneficial effect of endurance exercise on HDL-C and triglycerides (33,75). Experimental investigations have identified several possible mechanisms for the favorable influence of physical activity on lipid levels. The mechanisms include increases in lipoprotein lipase activity, decreases in hepatic triglyceride lipase activity, and depletion of intramuscular triglycerides (75).

Both the NIH and ACSM reports place evidence for a favorable effect of physical activity on blood lipids in overweight and obese individuals in category A, particularly if the physical activity is accompanied by weight loss (Table 2). Although the body of evidence is small, it appears that much, if not most, of the effect of physical activity on lipid levels in overweight and obese individuals is mediated through changes in weight and body composition. The ACSM consensus panel determined that physical activity of a volume that results in at least a 4.5-kg weight loss will raise HDL-C and lower triglycerides in men and postmenopausal women (15). The addition of physical activity to caloric deficit low-fat diet may reverse the HDL-C lowering effect associated with this eating pattern in overweight men and women. Physical activity significantly enhances the LDL-C-lowering effect of a weight-reducing low-fat diet (15,99). However, it is important to note that the number of studies evaluating the effects of physical activity in overweight or obese individuals with adverse lipoprotein profiles is very limited.

In the ACSM report, Stefanick (99) provides an evidence-based review of RCTs on the effects of physical activity on dyslipoproteinemias in overweight and obese men and women (99). Stefanick reviewed six RCTs conducted in men and/or women with a mean BMI of 25 to 29.9 kg/m^2 and five studies in obese men or postmenopausal women (BMI$\geq$30 kg/m^2). In a trial of 132 overweight premenopausal women, diet plus exercise significantly increased HDL-C compared to diet only intervention, but not compared to controls (100). There were no significant differences in total cholesterol, LDL-C, or triglycerides between the intervention groups. The diet only group had a nonsignificant decrease in HDL-C, which indicates that the exercise may have offset the HDL-C-lowering effect of the hypocaloric, low-fat diet. In the five other studies reviewed involving overweight men and women, there were no significant changes in total cholesterol, triglycerides, or HDL-C levels when exercise only groups were compared to controls or when diet plus exercise was compared to diet alone. However, in three trials, the addition of aerobic exercise to diet resulted in significant improvements in lipids compared with controls. In one study, men and women who adopted a National Cholesterol Education Program Step 2 Diet and aerobic exercise significantly reduced LDL-C compared to controls (101). In her review, Stefanick concluded that the addition of exercise to a weight-reducing diet and/or reduced-fat diet in overweight men and women produced only modest benefits in HDL-C, triglycerides, and LDL-C compared to that achieved by diet alone. Of the five studies reviewed in obese men and women, only one demonstrated a favorable effect of diet plus exercise compared to diet alone on HDL-C and triglycerides (100).

V RECOMMENDATIONS

A Research

The current body of evidence evaluating the association of physical activity to obesity-related health outcomes is limited. As reviewed, few studies have specifically evaluated the independent influence of physical activity on obesity-related health outcomes. In addition, most studies evaluating the association of overweight and obesity to morbidity and mortality fail to appropriately account for the potential confounding influence of physical activity and cardiorespiratory fitness on health outcomes. In studies where physical activity is considered, it is often measured so crudely that there is too much misclassification to have high confidence in the data. To determine and account for the independent association of physical activity to morbidity and mortality in overweight and obesity, results from prospective observational studies must be presented by both strata of body habitus and physical activity with better control for potential confounding factors such as changes in diet and health status. Unfortunately, few of the available studies in this area include women, older subjects, or minority groups. In addition, most studies are limited to overweight and class I obesity, with few individuals with higher levels of obesity. The current body of evidence is particularly limited for other obesity-related health outcomes such as cerebrovascular disease, functional disability, osteoarthritis, cancer, prothrombotic states, mood disorders, and health-related quality of life (15,33).

To improve the quality of data, researchers must develop better methods of assessing and quantifying physical activity in overweight and obese individuals. We need improved surveillance methods for monitoring physical activity patterns and trends within populations to better understand and characterize the influence of activity patterns on the increasing prevalence of overweight and obesity. More data are needed to better characterize environmental, psychosocial, and behavioral trends that influence weight, physical activity participation, and health outcomes. The major determinants of physical activity participation by overweight and obese individuals must be assessed and effective public health and clinical interventions developed to promote the adoption and maintenance of beneficial levels of physical activity. Research efforts must be directed at finding effective ways to apply behavioral theories and methods to physical activity counseling and intervention in the clinical setting.

Investigators must employ better design for RCTs to account for the complex interrelationships and synergistic effects between physical activity, body weight, adiposity, dietary change, and health status on health outcomes. More RCTs must be conducted to better characterize the mechanisms by which physical activity influences obesity-related health outcomes and disease risk factors. More research is needed to determine the minimal and optimal levels of physical activity necessary to favorably influence disease risk factors and health outcomes in overweight and obese individuals. Variables of importance include the length of intervention and the frequency, intensity, duration, and total dose of physical activity. The objective of this line of research is to better characterize the quantitative effect or dose-response relationship of physical activity to obesity-related health outcomes.

B Public Health

The public health burdens of physical inactivity and obesity are substantial. Recent reports indicate that obesity and the contributing lifestyle factors of physical inactivity and poor dietary habits are responsible for between 14% and 23% of total mortality in the United States (29). Overall, the total direct healthcare delivery cost associated with obesity and physical inactivity account for some 9.4%, over $94 billion, of national health care expenditures in the United States (29). Given the disease burden and public health impact of obesity and its increasing prevalence, population-based strategies for obesity prevention deserve increasing emphasis and attention. It is likely that the prevalence of low fitness is substantially higher than the prevalence of other obesity-related disease risk factors, such as diabetes. Given the high prevalence of both physical inactivity and obesity and strong association with all-cause and CVD mortality, the population-attributable risk associated with low fitness levels in obese individuals is substantial (53). Ultimately, for obesity control at the population level, public health and environmental policies aimed at increasing opportunities for physical activity are of paramount importance.

Research and clinical experience must be used to help guide public policy decisions. Public health organizations and educational institutions must communicate to governmental agencies and the public the importance of physical activity in improving health and preventing weight gain. Organizations and agencies must help develop and implement effective strategies to promote the adoption of physically active lifestyles among all members of society. We need to take special actions to target population subgroups where physical inactivity and obesity are particularly prevalent. Researchers and clinicians must assume a leadership role in the promotion of physical activity at the public health level. Public health efforts must be directed at strategies to create public environments that are conducive to physical activity, particularly for overweight and obese individuals.

To achieve these public health goals, several things must happen:

1. Communities need resources to develop parks, walking and bicycle paths, playgrounds, recreation centers, and safe neighborhoods.
2. Worksites and public buildings must provide facilities and programs that encourage physical activity and increase access for all individuals.
3. Architectural designs must begin to make stairs more accessible and appealing and include parking areas that encourage walking.
4. School-based programs must capitalize on the opportunity to promote physical activity among a large number of children, adolescents, and their families.
5. Media messages and public awareness campaigns to encourage active lifestyles and healthy weights need to be developed and delivered.
6. More citizens need to develop and apply behavioral skills to avoid the allure of technologies that promote sedentary living.

C Clinical Practice

It is clear that regular physical activity is helpful for weight control and provides important health benefits for overweight and obese individuals. Because of these benefits, professional and governmental bodies have provided expert consensus documents and recommendations on physical activity both for the treatment of overweight and obesity and for health enhancement in the general population (1,8). However, despite general consensus and expert guidelines, the barriers to physical activity counseling and participation present significant challenges for clinicians and patients, respectively. A recent survey of U.S. adults found that, of 44% of women and 29% of men trying to lose weight at any given time, <40% report engaging in the recommended 150 min or more of leisure-time physical activity per week (102). Another survey found that >54% of overweight and obese patients are not receiving exercise counseling from their physicians (103). Health care professionals face several established barriers to physical activity counseling in clinical practice including lack of time, inadequate reimbursement, and little training in physical activity and behavioral counseling. Despite the barriers, available evidence indicates that clinicians must assess physical activity and fitness status in overweight and obese individuals to allow for a more complete risk stratification and enhanced clinical decision making. We feel that it is as important for health care professionals to provide physical activity assessment, prescription, and counseling as it is to assess and treat other obesity-related comorbidities, such as diabetes and hypertension. Given the beneficial effects of physical activity on health outcomes, health care professionals have the responsibility to routinely promote physical activity to increase cardiorespiratory fitness in all patients. Clinical research must guide the development and implementation of policies and programs that will eliminate the barriers to physical activity counseling and participation and promote the application of proven physical activity interventions in clinical practice.

Available evidence favors a combination of dietary, physical activity, and behavioral intervention as the most important strategy for weight loss and maintenance in clinical practice (1). Although questions remain as to the minimal and optimal doses of physical activity needed to favorably influence obesity-related health outcomes, available evidence indicates that current public health recommendations for a minimum of 30 min of moderate-intensity physical activity accumulated on most, preferably all, days of the week will result in significant health benefits for overweight and obese individuals. Some evidence suggests that higher levels of physical activity may be needed to produce significant weight loss or promote long-term weight maintenance (104,105). Applying validated behavior modification techniques in clinical practice and educating patients on alternative approaches to physical activity, such as lifestyle physical activity and the accumulation of short bouts of moderate to vigorous activity, may improve patient participation in and adherence to clinically beneficial levels of physical activity (106–109). It is important to recognize that physical activity is a behavior that requires certain skills to integrate it into one's lifestyle. We believe far more success can be achieved if clinicians and patients focus on developing the behavioral skills (i.e., goal setting, problem solving, and self-monitoring) needed to increase physical activity and improve health rather than the traditional focus on the attributes of weight and body composition. We have published specific guidelines and programs for using physical activity in this way (106,110,111). We also recommend that all healthcare professionals adopt a physically active lifestyle themselves. Clinicians who are active and fit will not only benefit personally, but also be better able to counsel patients on the benefits of adopting and enjoying a physically active lifestyle.

VI CONCLUSIONS

Current evidence indicates that higher levels of physical activity and cardiorespiratory fitness have a beneficial influence on several adverse health outcomes associated with overweight and obesity. For many of these adverse health outcomes, moderate to high levels of physical activity and cardiorespiratory fitness provide benefits independent of changes in weight or body composition. Overweight and obese individuals who are or who become physically active have better risk factor profiles and lower rates of disease and death than overweight and obese individuals who are inactive and unfit. Physical activity appears to work synergistically with dietary intervention and weight loss to produce more favorable risk factor profiles in overweight and obese individuals. Although the current body of research is limited, some evidence suggests that fit overweight and obese men have lower rates of all-cause and CVD mortality when compared with normal-weight men who are unfit. More research is needed to evaluate the extent to which physical activity attenuates mortality risk in overweight and obese individuals. More public health efforts and clinical strategies for promoting physical activity are needed to decrease the incidence of obesity and its associated adverse health outcomes.

ACKNOWLEDGMENTS

We thank Melba Morrow and Ginny Shead for editorial review and assistance with manuscript preparation. We thank Dr. Kenneth H. Cooper and the staff of the Cooper Aerobics Center for making this work possible. The work reported here is supported in part by National Institutes of Health grants AG06945 and HL48597.

REFERENCES

1. National Institutes of Health. Clinical guidelines on the identification, evaluation, and treatment of overweight and obesity in adults-the evidence report. Obes Res 1998; 2:51S–209S.
2. World Health Organization. Obesity: Preventing and Managing the Global Epidemic. Report of a WHO Consultation on Obesity. Geneva: World Health Organization, 1998.
3. Mokdad AH, Bowman BA, Ford ES, et al. The continuing epidemics of obesity and diabetes in the United States, 1991-1998. JAMA 1999; 282:1519–1522.
4. Mokdad AH, Serdula MK, Dietz WH, et al. The continuing epidemic of obesity in the United States. JAMA 2000; 284:1650–1651.
5. Hill JO, Melanson EL. Overview of the determinants of overweight and obesity: current evidence and research issues. Med Sci Sports Exerc 1999; 31:S515–S521.
6. Weinsier RL, Hunter GR, Heini AF, et al. The etiology of obesity: relative contribution of metabolic factors, diet, and physical activity. Am J Med 1998; 105:145–150.
7. Heini AF, Weinsier RL. Divergent trends in obesity and fat intake patterns: the American paradox. Am J Med 1997; 102:259–264.
8. U.S. Department of Health and Human Services. Physical Activity and Health: A Report of the Surgeon General. Atlanta, GA: U.S. Department of Health and Human Services, Centers for Disease Control and Prevention, National Center for Chronic Disease Prevention and Health Promotion, 1996.
9. Pratt M, Macera CA, Blanton C. Levels of physical activity and inactivity in children and adults in the United States: current evidence and research issues. Med Sci Sports Exerc 1999; 31:S526–S533.
10. Williamson DF, Madans J, Anda RF, et al. Recreational physical activity and ten-year weight change in a US national cohort. Int J Obes Relat Metab Disord 1993; 17:279–286.
11. DiPietro L, Kohl HW III, Barlow CE, et al. Improvements in cardiorespiratory fitness attenuate age-related weight gain in healthy men and women: the Aerobics Center Longitudinal Study. Int J Obes Relat Metab Disord 1998; 22:55–62.
12. Ching PL, Willett WC, Rimm EB, et al. Activity level and risk of overweight in male health professionals. Am J Pub Health 1996; 86:25–30.
13. Coakley EH, Rimm EB, Colditz G, et al. Predictors of weight change in men: Results from the Health Professionals Follow-up Study. Int J Obes Relat Metab Disord 1998; 22:89–96.
14. Prentice AM, Jebb SA. Obesity in Britain: gluttony or sloth? BMJ 1995; 311:437–439.
15. Grundy SM, Blackburn G, Higgins M, et al. Physical activity in the prevention and treatment of obesity and its comorbidities. Med Sci Sports Exerc 1999; 31:S502–S508.
16. NIH Consensus Development Panel on Physical Activity and Cardiovascular Health. NIH Consensus Con-

ference: physical activity and cardiovascular health. JAMA 1996; 276:241-246.
17. Fletcher GF, Balady G, Blair SN, et al. Statement on exercise: benefits and recommendations for physical activity programs for all Americans: a statement for health professionals by the Committee on Exercise and Cardiac Rehabilitation of the Council on Clinical Cardiology. American Heart Association. Circulation 1996; 94:857–862.
18. Pate RR, Pratt M, Blair SN, et al. Physical activity and public health: a recommendation from the Centers for Disease Control and Prevention and the American College of Sports Medicine. JAMA 1995; 273:402–407.
19. Calle EE, Thun MJ, Petrelli JM, Rodriguez C, Heath CWJr.. Body-mass index and mortality in a prospective cohort of U.S. adults. N Engl J Med 1999; 341:1097–1105.
20. Manson JE, Willett WC, Stampfer MJ, Colditz GA, Hunter DJ, Hankinson SE, Hennekens CH, Speizer FE. Body weight and mortality among women. N Engl J Med 1995; 333:677–685.
21. Murphy TK, Calle EE, Rodriguez C, Khan HS, Thun MJ. Body mass index and colon cancer mortality in a large prospective study. Am J Epidemiol 2000; 152:847–854.
22. Allison DB, Fontaine KR, Manson JE, et al. Annual deaths attributable to obesity in the United States. JAMA 1999; 282:1530–1538.
23. Hahn RA, Teutsch SM, Rothenberg RB, et al. Excess deaths from nine chronic diseases in the United States, 1986. JAMA 1990; 264:2654–2659.
24. McGinnis JM, Foege WH. Actual causes of death in the United States. JAMA 1993; 270:2207–2212.
25. Eckel RH. Obesity and heart disease: a statement for healthcare professionals from the Nutrition Committee. American Heart Association. Circulation 1997; 96: 3248–3250.
26. Solomon CG, Manson JE. Obesity and mortality: a review of the epidemiologic data. Am J Clin Nutr 1997; 66:1044S–1050S.
27. Pi-Sunyer FX. Comorbidities of overweight and obesity: current evidence and research issues. Med Sci Sports Exerc 1999; 31:S602–S608.
28. Bouchard C, Blair SN. Roundtable introduction: introductory comments for the consensus on physical activity and obesity. Med Sci Sports Exerc 1999; 31:S498–S501.
29. Colditz GA. Economic costs of obesity and inactivity. Med Sci Sports Exerc 1999; 31:S663–S667.
30. Koplan JP, Dietz WH. Caloric imbalance and public health policy. JAMA 1999; 282:1579–1581.
31. Blair SN, Kohl HW III, Paffenbarger RS Jr, et al. Physical fitness and all-cause mortality: a prospective study of healthy men and women. JAMA 1989; 262: 2395–2401.
32. Paffenbarger RS Jr, Hyde RT, Wing AL, Hsieh CC. Physical activity, all-cause mortality, and longevity of college alumni. N Engl J Med 1986; 314:605–613.
33. Kesaniemi YA, Danforth E, Jensen MD, et al. Dose-response issues concerning physical activity and health: an evidence-based symposium. 2001; 33:S351–S358.
34. Lee I-M, Skerrett PJ. Physical activity and all-cause mortality: what is the dose-response relation? Med Sci Sports Exerc 2001; 33:S459–S471.
35. Kohl HW. Physical activity and cardiovascular disease: evidence for a dose response. Med Sci Sports Exerc 2001; 33:S472–S483.
36. Blair SN, Kampert JB, Kohl HW, et al. Influences of cardiorespiratory fitness and other precursors on cardiovascular disease and all-cause mortality in men and women. JAMA 1996; 276:205–210.
37. Rosengren A, Wilhelmsen L. Physical activity protects against coronary death and deaths from all causes in middle-aged men. Ann Epidemiol 1997; 7:69–75.
38. Thune I, Furberg A-S. Physical activity and cancer risk: dose-response and cancer, all sites and site-specific. Med Sci Sports Exerc 2001; 33:S530–S550.
39. Wei M, Gibbons LW, Mitchell TL, et al. The association between cardiorespiratory fitness and impaired fasting glucose and type 2 diabetes mellitus in men. Ann Intern Med 1999; 130:89–96.
40. Blair SN, Goodyear NN, Gibbons LW, Cooper KH. Physical fitness and incidence of hypertension in healthy normotensive men and women. JAMA 1984; 252:487–490.
41. DiPietro L, Kohl HW III, Barlow CE, Blair SN. Improvements in cardiorespiratory fitness attenuate age-related weight gain in healthy men and women: the Aerobics Center Longitudinal Study. Int J Obes Relat Metab Disor 1998; 22:55–62.
42. Huang Y, Macera CA, Blair SN, et al. Physical fitness, physical activity, and functional limitation in adults aged 40 and older. Med Sci Sports Exerc 1998; 30:1430–1435.
43. Dunn AL, Trivedi MH, O'Neal HA. Physical activity dose-response effects on outcomes of depression and anxiety. Med Sci Sports Exerc 2001; 33:S587–S597.
44. Farrell SW, Kampert JB, Kohl HW, et al. Influences of cardiorespiratory fitness levels and other predictors on cardiovascular disease mortality in men. Med Sci Sports Exerc 1997; 30:899–905.
45. Pollock ML, Bohannon RL, Cooper KH. A comparative analysis of four protocols for maximal treadmill stress testing. Am Heart J 1976; 92:39–46.
46. Blair SN, Kohl HW III, Barlow CE, et al. Changes in physical fitness and all-cause mortality: a prospective study of healthy and unhealthy men. JAMA 1995; 273: 1093–1098.
47. Paffenbarger RS Jr, Hyde RT, Wing AL, et al. The association of changes in physical-activity level and other lifestyle characteristics with mortality among men. N Engl J Med 1993; 328:538–545.

48. American College of Sports Medicine. American College of Sports Medicine roundtable: physical activity in the prevention and treatment of obesity and its comorbidities. Med Sci Sports Exerc 1999; 31(11)(suppl): S497–S667.
49. Ross R, Dagnone D, Jones PJH, et al. Reduction in obesity and related comorbid conditions after diet-induced weight loss or exercise-induced weight loss in men: a randomized, controlled trial. Ann Intern Med 2000; 133:92–103.
50. American College of Sports Medicine. The recommended quantity and quality of exercise for developing and maintaining cardiorespiratory and muscular fitness in healthy adults. Med Sci Sports Exerc 1998; 30: 975–991.
51. Cooper KH, Pollock ML, Martin RP, et al. Physical fitness levels vs selected coronary risk factors: a cross-sectional study. JAMA 1976; 236:166–169.
52. Gibbons LW, Blair SN, Cooper KH, et al. Association between CHD risk factors and physical fitness in healthy adult women. Circulation 1983; 67:977–983.
53. Wei M, Kampert JB, Barlow CE, et al. Relationship between low cardiorespiratory fitness and mortality in normal-weight, overweight, and obese men. JAMA 1999; 282:1547–1553.
54. Blair SN, Brodney S. Effects of physical inactivity and obesity on morbidity and mortality: current evidence and research issues. Med Sci Sports Exerc 1999; 31:S646–S662.
55. Barlow CE, Kohl HW III, Gibbons LW, et al. Physical fitness, mortality and obesity. Int J Obes Relat Metab Disord 1995; 19:S41–S44.
56. Lee CD, Jackson AS, Blair SN. US weight guidelines: Is it also important to consider cardiorespiratory fitness? Int J Obes Relat Metab Disord 1998; 22:S2–S7.
57. Lee CD, Blair SN, Jackson AS. Cardiorespiratory fitness, body composition, and all-cause and cardiovascular disease mortality in men. Am J Clin Nutr 1999; 69:373–380.
58. Dorn JP, Cerny FJ, Epstein LH, et al. Work and leisure time physical activity and mortality in men and women form a general population sample. Ann Epidemiol 1999; 9:366–373.
59. Haapanen-Niemi N, Miilunpalo S, Pasanen M, et al. Body mass index, physical inactivity and low level of physical fitness as determinants of all-cause and cardiovascular disease mortality—16y follow-up of middle-aged and elderly men and women. Int J Obes 2000; 24:1465–1474.
60. American Heart Association. 2001 Heart and Stroke Statistical Update. Dallas: American Heart Association, 2000.
61. Sesso HD, Paffenbarger RS, Ha T, et al. Physical activity and cardiovascular disease risk in middle-aged and older women. Am J Epidemiol 1999; 150: 408–416.
62. Salonen JT, Slater JS, Tuomilehto J, et al. Leisure time and occupational physical activity: risk of death from ischemic heart disease. Am J Epidemiol 1988; 127:87–94.
63. Morris JN, Clayton DG, Everitt MG, et al. Exercise in leisure time: coronary attack and death rates. Br Heart J 1990; 63:325–334.
64. American Cancer Society. Cancer Facts and Figures 2001. Atlanta: American Cancer Society, 2001.
65. Huang Z, Hankinson SE, Colditz GA, et al. Dual effects of weight and weight gain on breast cancer risk. JAMA 1997; 278:1407–1411.
66. Goodman MT, Hankin JH, Wilkens LR, et al. Diet, body size, physical activity, and the risk of endometrial cancer. Cancer Res 1997; 57:5077–5085.
67. Lew EA, Garfinkel L. Variations in mortality by weight among 750,000 men and women. J Chron Dis 1979; 32:564–576.
68. Rissanen A, Fogelholm M. Physical activity in the prevention and treatment of other morbid conditions and impairments associated with obesity: current evidence and research issues. Med Sci Sports Exerc 1999; 31:S635–S645.
69. Shephard RJ. Exercise and cancer: linkages with obesity? Int J Obes Relat Metab Disord 1995; 19:S62–S68.
70. Slattery ML, Potter J, Caan B, et al. Energy balance and colon cancer—beyond physical activity. Cancer Res 1997; 57:75–80.
71. Harris MI. Diabetes in America: epidemiology and scope of the problem. Diabetes Care 1998; 21:C11–C14.
72. Centers for Disease Control and Prevention. National Diabetes Fact Sheet: National Estimates and General Information on Diabetes in the United States. Atlanta: U.S. Department of Health and Human Services, Centers for Disease Control and Prevention, 1999.
73. Mokdad AH, Ford ES, Bowman BA, et al. Diabetes trends in the U.S.: 1990–1998. Diabetes Care 2000; 23:1278–1283.
74. Albright A, Franz M, Hornsby G, et al. American College of Sports Medicine position stand. Exercise and type 2 diabetes. Med Sci Sports Exerc 2000; 32:1345–1360.
75. Thompson PD, Crouse SF, Goodpaster B, et al. The acute versus the chronic response to exercise. Med Sci Sports Exerc 2001; 33:S438–S445.
76. Kelley DE, Goodpaster BH. Effects of exercise on glucose homeostasis in type 2 diabetes mellitus. Med Sci Sports Exerc 2001; 33:S495–S501.
77. Thorell A, Hirshman MF, Nygren J, et al. Exercise and insulin cause GLUT-4 translocation in human skeletal muscle. Am J Physiol 1999; 277:E733–E741.
78. Segal KR, Edano A, Abalos A, et al. Effect of exercise training on insulin sensitivity and glucose metabolism in lean, obese, and diabetic men. J Appl Physiol 1991; 71:2402–2411.

79. Rice B, Janssen I, Hudson R, et al. Effects of aerobic or resistance exercise and/or diet on glucose tolerance and plasma insulin levels in obese men. Diabetes Care 1999; 22:684–691.
80. Pan XR, Li GW, Hu YH, et al. Effects of diet and exercise in preventing NIDDM in people with impaired glucose tolerance. the Da Qing IGT and Diabetes Study. Diabetes Care 1997; 20:537–544.
81. Dengel DR, Pratley RE, Hagberg JM, et al. Distinct effects of aerobic exercise training and weight loss on glucose homeostasis in obese sedentary men. J Appl Physiol 1996; 81:318–325.
82. Katzel LI, Bleecker ER, Colman EG, et al. Effects of weight loss vs aerobic exercise training on risk factors for coronary disease in healthy, obese, middle-aged and older men. JAMA 1995; 274:1915–1921.
83. Dengel DR, Galecki AT, Hagberg JM, et al. The independent and combined effects of weight loss and aerobic exercise on blood pressure and oral glucose tolerance in older men. Am J Hypertens 1998; 11:1405–1412.
84. Wei M, Gibbons LW, Kampert JB, et al. Low cardiorespiratory fitness and physical inactivity as predictors of mortality in men with type 2 diabetes. Ann Intern Med 2000; 132:605–611.
85. Hu FB, Stampfer MJ, Solomon CG, et al. The impact of diabetes mellitus on mortality from all causes and coronary heart disease in women: 20 years of follow-up. Arch Intern Med 2001; 61:1717–1723.
86. Sixth report of the Joint National Committee on prevention, detection, evaluation, and treatment of high blood pressure. Arch Intern Med 157 (1997) 2413-2446.
87. Fagard RH. Physical activity in the prevention and treatment of hypertension in the obese. Med Sci Sports Exerc 1999; 31:S624–S630.
88. Paffenbarger RS Jr, Wing AL, Hyde RT, et al. Physical activity and incidence of hypertension in college alumni. Am J Epidemiol 1983; 117:245–257.
89. Paffenbarger RS Jr, Jung DL, Leung RW, et al. Physical activity and hypertension: an epidemiological view. Ann Med 1991; 23:319–327.
90. Duncan JJ, Farr JE, Upton JS, et al. The effects of aerobic exercise on plasma catecholamines and blood pressure in patients with mild essential hypertension. JAMA 1985; 254:2609–2613.
91. Fagard RH. Exercise characteristics and the blood pressure response to dynamic physical training. Med Sci Sports Exerc 2001; 33:S484–S492.
92. Gordon NF, Scott CB, Levine BD. Comparison of single versus multiple lifestyle interventions: are the antihypertensive effects of exercise training and diet-induced weight loss additive? Am J Cardiol 1997; 79:763–767.
93. Fortmann SP, Haskell WL, Wood PD. Effects of weight loss on clinic and ambulatory blood pressure in normotensive men. Am J Cardiol 1988; 62:89–93.
94. Blumenthal JA, Sherwood A, Gullette ECD, et al. Exercise and weight loss reduce blood pressure in men and women with mild hypertension: effects on cardiovascular, metabolic, and hemodynamic functioning. Arch Intern Med 2000; 160:1947–1958.
95. Blair SN, Kohl HW III, Barlow CE, et al. Usefulness of cardiorespiratory fitness as a predictor of all-cause and cardiovascular disease mortality in men with systemic hypertension. Am J Cardiol 2001; 88:651–656.
96. Fuster V, Gotto AM, Libby P. 27th Bethesda Conference: matching the intensity of risk factor management with the hazard for coronary disease events. Task Force 1. Pathogenesis of coronary disease: the biologic role of risk factors. J Am Coll Cardiol 1996; 27:964–976.
97. Expert Panel on Detection, Evaluation, and Treatment of High Blood Cholesterol in Adults. Executive Summary of the Third Report of the National Cholesterol Education Program (NCEP) Expert Panel on Detection, Evaluation, and Treatment of High Blood Cholesterol in Adults (Adult Treatment Panel III). Washington: National Heart, Lung, and Blood Institute; NIH Publication No. 01-3670, 2001.
98. Leon AS, Sanchez OA. Response of blood lipids to exercise training alone or combined with dietary intervention. Med Sci Sports Exerc 2001; 33:S502–S515.
99. Stefanick ML. Physical activity for preventing and treating obesity-related dyslipoproteinemias. Med Sci Sports Exerc 1999; 31:S609–S618.
100. Wood PD, Stefanick ML, Williams PT, et al. The effects on plasma lipoproteins of a prudent weight-reducing diet, with or without exercise, in overweight men and women. N Engl J Med 1991; 325:461–466.
101. Stefanick ML, Mackey S, Sheehan M, Ellsworth N, Haskell WL, Wood PD. Effects of diet and exercise in men and postmenopausal women with low levels of HDL cholesterol and high levels of LDL cholesterol. N Engl J Med 1998; 339:12–20.
102. Serdula MK, Mokdad AH, Williamson DF, et al. Prevalence of attempting weight loss and strategies for controlling weight. JAMA 1999; 282:1353–1358.
103. Wee CC, McCarthy EP, Davis RB, et al. Physician counseling about exercise. JAMA 1999; 282:1583–1588.
104. Klem ML, Wing RR, McGuire MT, et al. A descriptive study of individuals successful at long-term maintenance of substantial weight loss. Am J Clin Nutr 1997; 66:239–246.
105. Schoeller DA, Shay K, Kushner RF. How much physical activity is needed to minimize weight gain in previously obese women? Am J Clin Nutr 1997; 66:551–556.
106. Dunn AL, Marcus BH, Kampert JB, et al. Comparison of lifestyle and structured interventions to increase physical activity and cardiorespiratory fitness: a randomized trial. JAMA 1999; 281:327–334.
107. Jakicic JM, Wing RR, Butler BA, et al. Prescribing exercise in multiple short bouts versus one continuous

bout: effects on adherence, cardiorespiratory fitness, and weight loss in overweight women. Int J Obe Relat Metab Disord 1995; 19:893–901.
108. Andersen RE, Wadden TA, Bartlett SJ, et al. Effects of lifestyle activity vs structured aerobic exercise in obese women: a randomized trial. JAMA 1999; 281:335–340.
109. Calfas KJ, Long BJ, Sallis JF, et al. A controlled trial of physician counseling to promote the adoption of physical activity. Prev Med 1996; 25:225–233.
110. Leermakers EA, Dunn AL, Blair SN. Exercise management of obesity. Med Clin North Am 2000; 84:419–440.
111. Blair SB, Dunn AL, Marcus BH, et al. Active Living Every Day. Champaign, IL: Human Kinetics, 2001.

43

Obesity and Quality of Life

Donald A. Williamson

Pennington Biomedical Research Center, Louisiana State University, Baton Rouge, Louisiana, U.S.A.

Patrick M. O'Neil

Medical University of South Carolina, Charleston, South Carolina, U.S.A.

I OVERVIEW OF RESEARCH EVIDENCE

Quality of life, particularly health-related quality of life, has been defined as the "physical, psychological, and social domains of health, seen as distinct areas that are influenced by a person's experiences, beliefs, expectations, and perceptions" (1). This definition makes it explicit that quality of life includes not only objective indicators but also subjective appraisals of well-being. Further, the growing interest in assessing quality of life reflects the recognition that health is much more than the absence of disease.

Obesity is at once a chronic condition with numerous effects on physical health and functioning, a publicly apparent characteristic with pervasive social implications, and a vexing health problem whose remediation or control requires long-term, often difficult behavioral changes. It is thus expected that obesity may affect quality of life in many ways. A growing body of research has examined the quality of life experienced by obese persons. Quality of life in obesity has been studied with questionnaires explicitly assessing a range of areas of life functioning, with assessment of specific psychiatric disorders or moods, and with examination of other indicators of life quality. We will approach this research from the point of view that different aspects of quality of life may be affected by obesity in different ways, and that various factors influence how obese individuals are affected.

The present section describes measures of overall quality of life, mood and personality, eating behavior and disturbed eating, dietary restraint and overeating/binge eating, and body image. Sections II–IV of this chapter provide a review of research findings pertaining to obesity and quality of life. Section V describes frequently used assessment methods that measure various aspects of quality of life. When reading these sections, the reader may wish to refer to the section on methods if there are questions about the reliability and validity of a particular measure that was used to assess the relationship between obesity and quality of life.

A Obesity and Quality of Life

1 Overall Quality of Life

Two questionnaires that have been frequently used in this research are the Impact of Weight on Quality of Life questionnaire (2) and the Medical Outcomes Study Short-Form Health Survey (SF-36) (3). They are described in more detail later in this chapter. Among a sample of treatment-seeking obese men and women, functioning in most areas of the Impact of Weight on Quality of Life questionnaire was worse with increasing body mass index (BMI). Women reported greater impact on Self-Esteem and Sexual Life than did men (2,4).

Obese persons seeking weight loss treatment have reported worse functioning in all eight domains of the SF-36, especially bodily pain and vitality, compared to population norms. Differences remained after controlling for sociodemographic factors and certain comorbidities including depression. Physical and social functioning was worse among the most severely obese in the sample. Bodily pain scores were comparable to those of migraine sufferers (5).

Again using the SF-36, Fontaine et al. (6) found more impaired functioning among a group of treatment-seeking obese people compared to a group of obese respondents not trying to lose weight. The differences were primarily on measures of physical functioning, consistent with the higher average BMI and higher prevalence of hypertension, chronic pain, and diabetes among the treatment seekers. However, differences on bodily pain, general health and vitality persisted after controlling for sociodemographic and medical variables on which the groups also differed. Further, among an obese treatment-seeking sample, worse physical functioning was related to greater BMI, higher age, report of pain, and male gender, although few such relations were seen with mental functioning scores (7).

With other measures of quality of life, baseline assessment of participants in the Swedish Obese Subjects study (BMIs $\geq$ 34 for males, $\geq$ 38 for females) revealed lower subjective ratings of current health, worse social functioning, and lower rates of employment, compared to population norms and other reference groups. Women reported worse general health than men, while the reverse was true of the measure of social functioning. Indices of somatic morbidity (joint symptoms, angina pectoris, days in hospital) and of previous psychiatric morbidity were associated with worse ratings of current health and social functioning (8).

With a mail survey of nearly 9000 adults in the Oxford region of England, Doll et al. (9) assessed the association of obesity with quality of life as measured by the SF-36. Increasing degrees of obesity were associated with decreasing physical well-being, regardless of the presence or absence of other chronic medical conditions. Emotional well-being was adversely affected only for those obese subjects with chronic medical conditions, and their emotional functioning was not significantly different from that of nonobese subjects with equal degrees of chronic illness. However, the obese subjects were significantly more likely to report having chronic illness.

Brown et al. (10) assessed the effects of obesity among a large population-based sample of Australian women 18–23 years of age, using the SF-36. They found that even among this young group, functioning was lower among overweight and obese groups on the measures of general health, physical functioning, and vitality.

Other objective indicants of quality of life reflect impaired quality of life for many obese people. Obesity in adolescence and/or early adulthood has been found at follow-up 7 years later to predict lower rates of marriage, and for women, lower educational achievement and income and higher rates of poverty in American (11) and British (12) samples. Relative to thinner women, heavier women are more likely to marry men of lower socioeconomic status (13).

Additional evidence regarding the perceived effect of obesity on quality of life may be inferred from the degree of value placed by obese people on achieving a lower weight goal. Rand and MacGregor (14) reported that gastric bypass patients who had lost at least 45 kg (100 lb) indicated that they would prefer to be blind, deaf, dyslexic, diabetic, or an amputee rather than return to their former severely obese status, and stated unanimously that they would forego the opportunity to be a millionaire if it required them to be obese again. In another study, obese treatment seekers and obese and nonobese members of a community sample answered forced-choice items assessing what they would hypothetically sacrifice or endure to reach and maintain their personal weight goal (15). Nearly 90% or more of the treatment-seeking obese, and 40% or more of the non-treatment-seeking obese, said they would be willing to forego a job promotion, retiring with full pay, eliminating the national debt, or winning their dream house or car or an all-expenses-paid vacation. Smaller majorities of the treatment seekers said they would suffer loss of half their income or a job demotion, although relatively few of the community obese sample were willing to incur negative events. Figures 1 and 2 summarize these findings. From the findings of these studies, it is apparent that obesity is a status that is loathed by those who have developed excess adiposity.

2 Psychological Functioning

Although obesity is not a psychiatric diagnosis (16), a lengthy literature has assessed psychological functioning among obese persons. It appears that among nonclinical samples of obese people, rates of diagnosable psychopathology are no greater than among nonobese groups (17–20). However, lifetime prevalence rates of

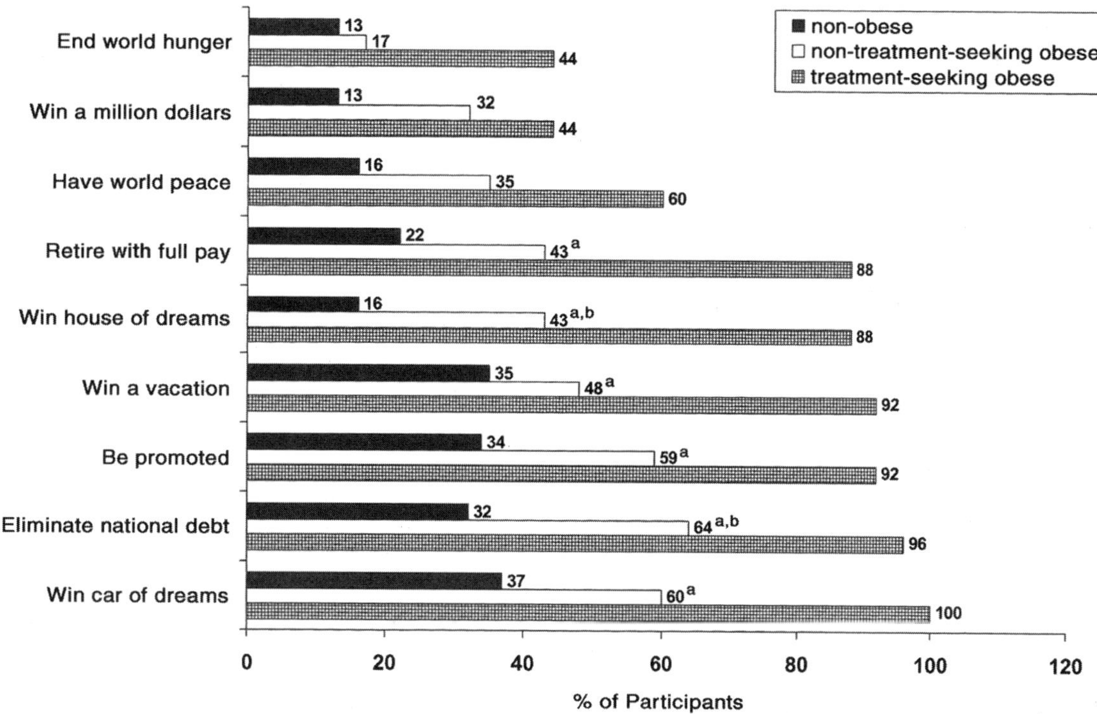

Figure 1 Hypothetical positive events foregone to reach weight goal. [a]Treatment-seeking obese participants differ from non-treatment-seeking obese participants. [b]Non-treatment-seeking obese participants differ from nonobese participants ($P < .01$). (From Ref. 15.)

certain psychiatric disorders in the general population are substantial; thus, any obese group may be expected to include a number of people so afflicted, independent of weight status.

Nonetheless, clinical samples of people seeking treatment for their obesity have been shown to display prevalence rates of psychiatric disorders and other measures of psychopathology higher than those seen among the general population. Among persons seeking professionally directed dietary, pharmacological, or surgical treatment, lifetime prevalence rates of 48–57% have been reported for axis I (e.g., anxiety or depression) psychiatric disorders (21–23). This compares to general population rates of 26–35% (24). One study found the lifetime rate of personality disorder diagnoses was 57% among applicants for outpatient treatment (21).

Moderately to severely obese men and women assessed at entry to the Swedish Obese Subjects study described lower mood states and more symptoms of depression and anxiety compared to a healthy reference group. Further, their overall mood scores were worse than those of samples of rheumatoid arthritis patients, recurrence-free cancer survivors, spinal cord injury victims, and intermittent claudication patients. The obese participants' anxiety and depression scores were also higher than most of these groups (8).

It has been observed that the extent of psychological distress among obese treatment-seeking groups is similar to that observed among other groups of medical or surgical patients (19). This observation suggests that the higher rates of distress among obese subjects observed in clinical studies, compared to population-based studies, reflect a selection bias in which those who are more distressed seek treatment. Indeed, when treatment-seeking obese samples have been compared to nonclinical obese samples, higher rates of psychological disturbance or distress have often been found among the treatment-seeking patients. For example, among obese females, those seeking treatment were more depressed and histrionic than those from a nonclinical sample (25). In another study, obese people applying for weight loss treatment reported more symptoms of borderline personality disorder than groups of nonclinical obese or nonobese controls, and only the treatment-seeking obese subjects showed more psychiatric symp-

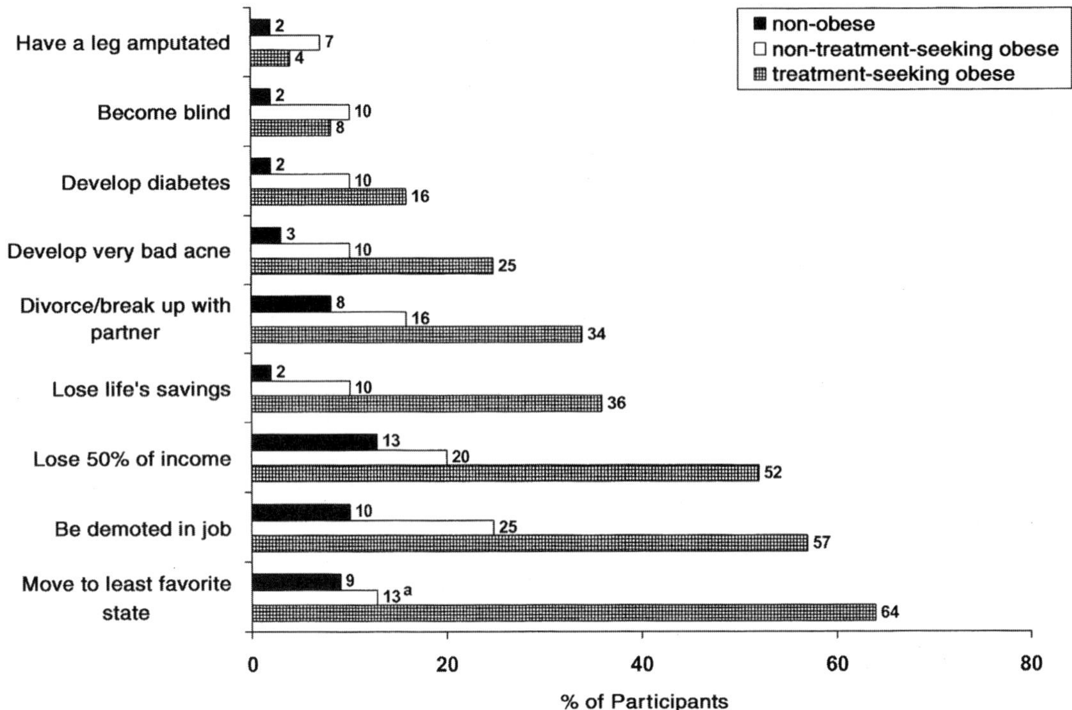

Figure 2 Hypothetical negative events to be incurred to reach weight goal. [a]Treatment-seeking obese participants differ from nontreatment-seeking obese participants ($P < .01$). (From Ref. 14.)

toms than the nonobese controls (17). A sample of treatment-seeking extremely obese adolescents and young adults demonstrated higher prevalence rates of mood, anxiety, somatoform and eating disorders, compared to a less obese population group and a general population group (26).

It has been contended that rather than asking whether obesity per se increases the risk of psychopathology or psychological distress, research should attempt to determine which obese people are more vulnerable to associated psychological disturbance (32). Such studies may reveal not only subgroups that are more susceptible to obesity-related psychological distress, but other subgroups that are more resilient. For example, one study of the relation of BMI to depressive symptoms among an older (50–89 years old) community sample in California found that whereas there was a trend for heavier women to have more depressive symptoms, obese men actually had lower scores on the Beck Depression Inventory than did their nonobese counterparts (27).

Although there are some reports of impaired self-esteem among adult obese patients (2) and, to a lesser degree, nonpatient obese adults (28), much research in this area has focused on children and adolescents. Studies of the effects of obesity on self-esteem among preteenage children have yielded inconsistent results, with some finding lowered self-esteem and others finding no differences. However, the deleterious effects of obesity on self-esteem are more consistent among adolescents and young adults (29–31). While some studies have shown that in some groups (e.g., white and Hispanic females), obesity in the preteen years predicts impaired self-esteem in early adolescence (30), other studies have suggested that causality may be bidirectional. Studies of black middle-school girls and boys and of white adolescent girls found that higher self-esteem scores were associated with lower weight gain over the next 1–3 years (29).

3 Interpersonal Consequences of Obesity

One pervasive, consistent effect of obesity on quality of life is seen in the social realm. It has been widely noted that at least in the United States and other Western societies, obese people inhabit a world that is poised to treat them badly (19,20,32,33). Negative attitudes toward obese people have been demonstrated among adults and children, even preschoolers (19,20,33,34). Unfortunately, they have also been found among health care professionals (35–38). Obese women in weight loss treatment reported less satisfaction with and confidence in their physicians' management of their obesity than of their general health. However, fewer than 10% reported frequent, negative interactions with their physicians concerning their weight (39).

Negative attitudes are frequently reflected in prejudicial behavior against obese people. The extent of discrimination in employment and educational settings has been frequently documented (11,33,40,41). Obese adults frequently report perceived mistreatment due to their weight at the hands of strangers and loved ones alike, with the frequency of such reports related to degree of obesity (42).

One result of repeatedly interacting with a world that is often flinty and at worst hostile may be a reduction in opportunities to develop certain social skills. For example, in a study in which obese and nonobese women conversed on the telephone with anonymous partners who were unaware of their weight status, the obese women were rated by both the partners and reviewers of the taped conversations as being less friendly, less likable, less attractive, and less socially skilled (43). However, the same research team later found no differences between obese and nonobese women in the rated quality of their actual relationships or social behavior, based on ratings by both participants and their friends and coworkers (44). Interestingly, a study of 9-year-old British schoolgirls found that although the overweight and obese girls were less likely than nonoverweight girls to be rated as pretty by peers, they were just as popular as measured by peer nomination questions (45).

B Is There an "Obese Personality"?

Stereotypic views of the personality makeup of obese persons have been long and widely held by the public and by professionals. For example, in 1941 psychoanalyst Hilde Bruch (46) noted: "It is a matter of common knowledge that obese people show certain similarities of character and behavior. According to popular opinion, fat people are cheerful and easygoing. They enjoy life in general, and good, rich food in particular." Bruch (46) took issue with that lay view: "This popular concept has been challenged as incorrect for the obese adult. . . . It certainly is not true for the obese child. On the contrary, obese children are fundamentally unhappy and maladjusted. Timid and retiring, clumsy and slow, they are not capable of holding a secure place among other children."

It is noteworthy that Bruch challenged only the accuracy of the popular stereotypes, not the underlying assumption that there was a common set of personality characteristics that captured the behavioral and psychological functioning of obese adults or children. Personality traits represent psychological and/or behavioral dimensions which vary broadly across members of the normal population, but on which a particular person is generally consistent across time and situations. For example, extraversion/introversion, rigidity/flexibility, masculinity/femininity, dominance/submission, and obsessive-compulsive tendencies may all be considered personality traits. There is little consistent evidence that obese people differ from the nonobese on such general dispositional traits, and little evidence that there are significant personality characteristics that are unique to obese persons (47,48).

In contrast to personality traits, personality type can be thought of as the relative configuration of various individual traits. In order to demonstrate that there is an "obese personality," there should be evidence that the obese population has personality types that are generally homogeneous within that group and generally different from those types seen in the nonobese population. Neither type of evidence has been reported. One cluster analysis of Minnesota Multiphasic Personality Inventory profiles of 170 women applying for obesity surgery found that there were five derived cluster profiles that were similar to those found in other populations. Further, these five nonunique prototypes described barely more than half the subjects (49). It is unlikely that the broader and much more diverse population of obese persons is any more homogeneous or different from nonobese people than was this group of surgery applicants. Given the sheer numbers of the obese population, it is improbable that so many individuals could be described by a very small number of personality types.

C Body Image and Obesity

The term body image has been used to describe many aspects of perceived physical appearance. Generally, body image refers to one's perception or evaluation of body size and shape (50–52). Using this definition, body image is not defined as satisfaction with other aspects of physical appearance, which might include such features as complexion, hair, facial shape, etc. Instead, body image specifically refers to the perception or evaluation of *body shape* or *size*. Body image is often defined as the estimation of body size (including actual and ideal body size) or as body size dissatisfaction. Body size dissatisfaction is often measured using questionnaires about satisfaction with various body parts or with the whole body (53). However, body size dissatisfaction has also been defined as the discrepancy between actual and ideal body size (54), and this actual-ideal discrepancy measure is highly correlated with questionnaire measures of body size dissatisfaction (55,56).

Studies of body size dissatisfaction have found that obese people are more dissatisfied with body size than are nonobese controls, though this relationship is moderated by the *perception* of being overweight, as opposed to actually being overweight (57), as defined by conventional standards such as BMI. Generally, the severity of body size dissatisfaction is positively correlated with actual body size (56), though certain other variables, e.g., ethnicity and gender, moderate this relationship (56–58). One consistent finding is that African-American men and women report lower levels of body size dissatisfaction than white men and women (56). Concerns about body size and shape also differ as a function of gender and sexual orientation. For example, Strong, et al. (59) found that heterosexual women were most highly concerned about body size, followed by gay men and lesbians, who did not differ, and all groups had greater body size concerns than did heterosexual men.

Studies of body size estimation by obese persons have yielded variable results. Some studies have found that obese persons are more likely to overestimate body size (60–62), while other studies have failed to find this phenomenon (32,63,64). In general, as BMI increases, the discrepancy between actual and ideal body size increases dramatically (65). A recent study found that in comparison to black adults, white men and women overestimated actual body size and underestimated ideal body, resulting in greater body size dissatisfaction in overweight/obese white adults (56).

D Dieting and Disturbed Patterns of Eating

Over the past 25 years, there has been a widely held belief that dieting leads to binge eating or overeating (66). This perspective led to the conclusion that dieting may be hazardous to one's health, causing weight cycling, binge eating, and other adverse health consequences (67,68). Other reviews of the literature, e.g., Yanovski (69), found few if any significant short-term or long-term effects of weight cycling. Therefore the validity of the perspective that dieting causes disturbed patterns of eating has been challenged in the past decade. A key concept for this perspective was dietary restraint. According to this view, voluntary intention to restrict energy intake was often disrupted, causing "disinhibited eating," whereby the person overate since the prohibition against eating had been violated (70).

Over the past 25 years, a number of laboratory studies have supported this conclusion (71), but a number of studies have also questioned the validity of this theory (72–75). An important consideration when reviewing this literature is the methodology for measuring dietary restraint. For example, Stunkard and Messick (76) developed a questionnaire that separated dietary restraint and the susceptibility to overeat. Using this questionnaire, a number of studies have found that some people who are attempting to restrict energy intake can successfully do so and, as a consequence, can maintain lower body weight without adverse psychological consequences (72,74). Other studies have suggested that there may be safe (flexible) dieting strategies and unsafe (rigid) dieting strategies (73,77). Flexible dieting strategies are characterized by less rigid rules about weight management and have been found to be associated with less severe binge eating and mood disturbances. However, it should be noted that all of the studies on rigid versus flexible dieting have used cross-sectional research designs, so it is not possible to discern if the relative absence of adverse psychological correlates is a direct consequence of flexible dieting or whether lower levels of psychological disturbance may allow for the presence of less rigid weight control strategies to manage body weight.

Finally, there is some evidence that extreme obesity may be associated with unrestrained overeating (72,74). Lowe (75) has suggested unrestrained overeaters may represent people who have tried unsuccessfully to restrict energy intake in the past, and who gave up in despair, resulting in relatively rapid weight gain until extreme obesity is achieved. A National Task Force on the Prevention and Treatment of Obesity (76) concluded that dieting for weight reduction was relatively safe, with greater potential benefits than costs.

II RISK FACTOR MODELS OF QUALITY OF LIFE ASSOCIATED WITH OBESITY

A Introduction and Basic Concepts

Psychological research over the past 40 years has failed to find that in general, obese people have a higher level of psychological problems than do nonobese people. Instead, this research has found that obese people struggle with specific problems related to being overweight, e.g., body dissatisfaction or strong motivation to restrict energy intake. Within the population of people who are obese, there are some people who experience significant psychological and behavioral disturbances (32) or may live in poverty, and these people may be at risk for chronic obesity and may be less likely to lose weight in structured weight loss trials (58,79). This perspective suggests that there may be certain risk or protective factors for adverse psychological correlates of obesity. The following sections describe some of these factors.

B Gender

Men tend to be less disturbed by obesity than women (32). This phenomenon is generally believed to stem from lower social pressure for thinness, and is reflected in higher self-esteem, quality of life, and marriage prospects among obese males (2,11,13).

C Ethnicity

Minority adults (especially women) tend to be less concerned about overweight status and are less motivated to lose body weight than white adults (79–82). As noted earlier, African-American men and women have lower levels of body size dissatisfaction (56). Therefore, minorities may be at lower risk for developing mood or self-esteem problems associated with obesity, yet may also be less motivated to lose weight.

D Binge Eating

Research has consistently found that obese binge eaters experience more psychological disturbances than obese people who do not frequently engage in binge eating (18,83,84). There has been considerable controversy about the distinction between a psychiatric syndrome called Binge Eating Disorder (BED) and binge eating as a behavioral correlate of obesity (85). Recent research studies that have used very strict definitions and have used structured interview methods for assessing BED have found that the syndrome as defined by the American Psychiatric Association (16) is actually quite rare (1–3%) even in obese people seeking treatment (86). However, binge eating as a symptom of obesity is much more common; significant binge eating is observed in 7–15% of obese adults (85). Men are slightly less likely to report binge eating than women, and most ethnic groups report comparable rates of binge eating. Binge eating and BED are associated with higher rates of depression (85). A recent study reported by Womble et al. (87) found that binge eating was highly correlated with obesity and that the combined influences of negative affect and dietary restraint accounted for binge eating. This study and others (88) have suggested that binge eating is often determined by breaking dietary restraint or reduction of negative emotion. Thus, binge eating appears to be a significant risk factor for lower quality of life and may be viewed as a type of "coping behavior" for body dissatisfaction and negative affect that is commonly associated with obesity (87). Furthermore, binge eating is highly correlated with increased adiposity (89).

E Severity of Obesity

In general, higher levels of obesity are negatively correlated with quality of life. For example, morbidly obese adults who seek obesity surgery report extremely negative reactions to their obesity. Furthermore, a national survey (90) found that obese women with a BMI ≥ 36 were more likely to report histories of rape, sexual molestation, or posttraumatic stress disorder than less overweight women. These data suggest that a history of trauma and/or binge eating may be associated with morbid obesity, significant mood disturbances, and a very low quality of life, but these cross-sectional studies do not inform us about the causes of lower quality of life that is correlated with obesity.

III QUALITY OF LIFE AND WEIGHT LOSS

The process and outcome of weight loss would both be expected to affect quality of life. For most obese and overweight people, losing weight and maintaining the weight loss involves restriction of dietary intake, physiological readjustment, major lifestyle changes, and effort. For patients who undergo surgery, physiological functioning and food consumption are greatly altered beyond their control. Thus, the process of losing weight may have substantial impact on the life of the person engaged in the effort.

When successful, the result of this process would also likely impact one's life. Weight loss may produce improved health, increased work and activity capacity, altered appearance, and evidence of personal ability to change. Additionally, the altered dietary and exercise patterns necessary to maintain a weight loss represent long-term changes in the weight loser's life.

In this section we will review briefly the effects of losing weight on overall quality of life, mood, hunger, and body image. Most of the relevant data come from studies of people participating in weight loss interventions that are under study. Therefore, it is usually difficult to separate the effects of weight loss from the effects of the intervention and process required to achieve that loss. Further, in most cases the process is a structured intervention rather than a self-directed effort. Unless otherwise indicated, the findings reported should be assumed to refer to both the process of losing weight and the resultant weight loss.

A Overall Quality of Life

Weight loss by obese persons is consistently associated with improved quality of life. Kolotkin and colleagues (2) compared scores on the Impact of Weight on Quality of Life scale at days 1 and 28 of a residential weight loss program. They found improvements in self-reported health, social functioning, work, activities of daily living, mobility, sexuality, and self-esteem. In a later study the same group (4) also found improvements in these areas among participants in a 2-week program. Further, the improvements tended to be greater for the 4-week program than for the 2-week program, and improvement in a total score was correlated significantly with amount of weight lost.

Fontaine et al. (91) compared scores on the SF-36 at the beginning and end of 13-week outpatient weight loss programs based on lifestyle modification and either aerobic exercise or lifestyle activity interventions. They found improvements on the physical functioning, role-physical, general health, vitality, and mental health domains, regardless of which physical activity program was encouraged. Other patients losing weight with the assistance of medication have demonstrated improvements in the Health, Mobility, and Activities of Daily Living scales of the Impact of Weight on Quality of Life scale (92). Hypertensive, dyslipidemic, or diabetic patients using prepared meals lost more weight and reported greater improvements on scales assessing physical and mental functioning than did patients in the standard diet condition (93).

Formerly severely obese patients who through gastric bypass surgery lost on average 43 kg showed improvements on all domains of the SF-36, physical and mental, and their postloss scores were equal to or better than population norms (94). The dramatic improvements appear more attributable to the large amount of weight lost than to the surgical procedure. Klem et al. (95) compared two groups of people who had lost on average ~ 66 kg—one group via surgery, and the other with various nonsurgical means; the subjects had maintained those losses for 2–3 years (95). Nearly all persons of both groups reported improvements in mood, self-confidence, quality of life, physical health, mobility, energy level, and activity level. Similar majorities of both groups reported improvements in social interactions and job performance.

There is also evidence for a beneficial effect of weight loss achieved outside of professional programs and clinical trials. For example, Fine et al. (96) administered the SF-36 to a very large cohort of women, aged 46–71 years, at a baseline assessment and 4 years later, comparing changes in scores to changes in weight over the same time. As shown in Figure 3, overweight and obese women who lost weight over the period showed improvements in physical functioning, vitality, and bodily pain. Women who gained weight over the period showed decreased functioning in the same domains. This tended to be true for women over 65 as well as for those in the younger ages.

B Mood

The notion that dieting has negative psychological consequences has had wide currency among the public and some professionals. The idea was first suggested by studies of substantial caloric restriction and weight loss by normal-weight subjects and by descriptions of patients' historical reports of symptoms during prior dieting (66,68,70,71). However, many subsequent, more relevant and highly controlled studies have shown at worst neutral and often beneficial mood changes among obese persons dieting to lose weight (18,97). Obese patients who have lost weight via moderate caloric restriction, very low calorie diets (VLCDs), or surgery frequently demonstrate improvements in depression and trait anxiety. With the dietary approaches, the improvements may be more commonly seen when a behavioral or lifestyle change program accompanies the diet (18, 98). However, anxiety and depression changes during VLCD are not related to diet variables such as whether the diet is food or formula based (99) or whether it is ketogenic (100).

Improvements in mood have also been observed among persons who have lost weight with a variety of means, most outside of professional programs. A group of 784 people who had lost on average 30 kg and maintained it for on average 5.5 years showed levels of distress and of depression lower than psychiatric-patient norms and similar to community norms (101).

The above-noted improvements in mood with weight loss occur in spite of certain physiological changes during dieting that in other circumstances suggest impairment in mood. For example, during VLCD, serum triodothyronine (T3) is reduced substantially, but the degree of reduction is unrelated to changes in depres-

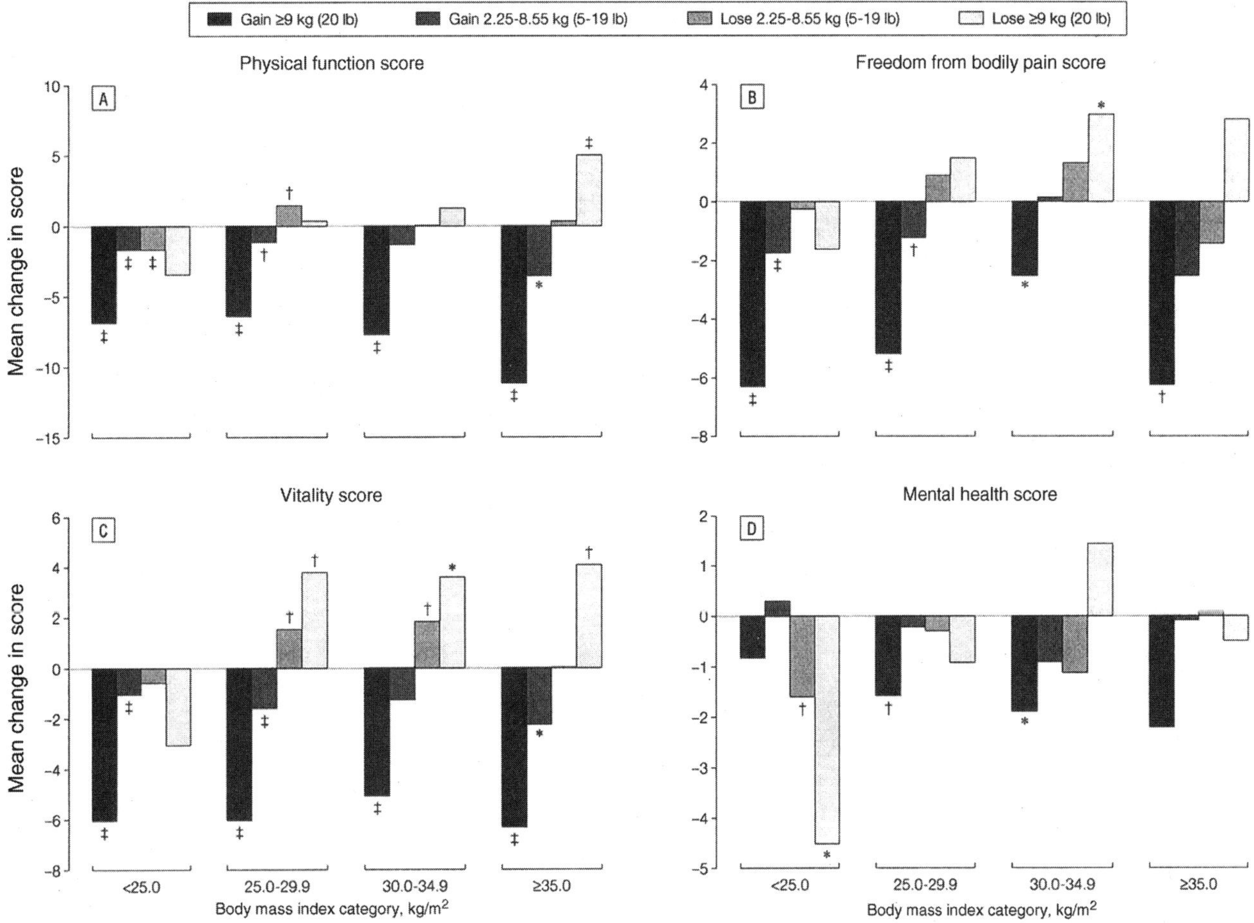

Figure 3 Relationships between weight change and changes in SF-36 subscale scores over a 4-year period in women younger than 65 years. (From Ref. 96.) Asterisk indicates $P < .01$; dagger, $P < .05$; double dagger, $P < .001$; and 5F-36, Medical Outcomes Study Short-Form 36 Health Status Survey. A decrease in the bodily pain score indicates a decrease in functioning due to bodily pain.

sion (102). Nonoverweight volunteers undergoing a 3-week low-calorie diet (103) had indications of reduced availability of tryptophan for serotonin synthesis (lowered total plasma tryptophan, lowered ratiol of tryptophan to competing amino acids). Whether this applies to overweight dieters remains to be seen.

Given the temporary nature of most weight losses, the possible impact of weight regain on mood deserves consideration. It has been asserted (68) that weight cycling may be associated with adverse psychological outcomes. However, there is little evidence in support of this position. Several cross-sectional comparisons of cyclers and noncyclers among clinical samples have failed to reveal consistent differences in psychological functioning (78). Foster et al. (104) used a prospective design to assess mood and eating-related variables among a sample of obese women who had lost on average ~20 kg in dietary and behavioral treatment but after follow-up of more than 4 years were on average above their baseline weight. Despite the regain of more than the original loss, scores on measures of depression, binge eating, hunger, and disinhibition were still lower than at baseline. Changes in these measures were unrelated to amount of weight regain.

Among a community sample balanced on weight status, gender, and age, Foreyt et al. (105) examined the relations of recent and historical weight change patterns to measures of psychological status. Subjects were categorized by changes in measured weight over a 1-year period and by their subjective reports of whether they frequently lost and regained. There were no significant effects of 1-year measured weight change (in either direction) on well-being or depression, but 1-year gainers and losers both reported having experienced more life change events than did 1-year maintainers. Subjects who denied historical patterns of losing and regaining reported greater well-being and control of eating compared to those who described their weight as typically fluctuating.

A related issue is whether weight gain per se, rather than weight gain following a weight loss, may have psychological effects. Analysis of psychological well-being scores for a subset of women in an NHANES I follow-up sample showed that those who had gained weight recently (at least 4.5 kg in the previous 6 months) had lower well-being scores than women who had maintained stable weights (106). This finding was seen in nonoverweight, overweight, and obese women. This study did not distinguish intentional from unintentional weight changes, or gain from regain; however, in this nationally representative sample there is no reason to believe that regain of previously intentionally lost weight accounted for more than a small minority of the cases of weight gain.

C Hunger

It might be assumed that decreasing caloric intake below maintenance needs would inevitably lead to feelings of hunger. Several reports indicate that this is not always so. For example, with VLCDs, after the first week or 2, hunger and preoccupation with food either decrease or remain at prediet levels (99,100,107,108). Method of weight loss may affect level of hunger. Hunger and preoccupation with food have been found lower during a VLCD or following weight loss surgery than during moderate caloric restriction (19,99,107, 108). However, one study comparing VLCD and moderate caloric restriction with type 2 diabetics found no differences in hunger ratings (109).

Another study (110) examined changes on the Perceived Hunger scale of the Eating Inventory (76) of obese women before and after 5–6 months in different treatment programs that included various diets. Across all treatment programs, hunger scored declined by ~18%. At baseline, higher hunger scores were seen among subjects who had higher scores on measures of depression and binge eating. Interestingly, weight loss was unrelated to baseline hunger scores or change in hunger scores (110).

Among the large group of successful weight loss maintainers noted earlier (101), Perceived Hunger scores were as low as those of normal-weight nondieters and lower than those of eating disorder samples. This finding suggests that long-term maintenance of substantially lowered body weight is not accomplished at the cost of chronic hunger.

D Body Image

As noted earlier, dissatisfaction with body size is a common problem associated with obesity, and body size dissatisfaction generally worsens with increased adiposity (56). The association of body size dissatisfaction and BMI has been observed in men and women, but it is less pronounced in African-Americans than in whites (56). Based on these findings, one would hypothesize that weight loss would be associated with improvement of body image. In general, this hypothesis has been supported for persons who lose weight through lifestyle behavior modification and obesity surgery (2,14,19,38, 111). However, many other factors are also associated with improved body image that accompanies weight loss. An important variable is the person's weight loss goals. Foster et al. (112) found that most participants in weight loss trials do not achieve weight losses that meet even minimally acceptable weight goals. These findings suggest that improvement of body image may not be a direct product of weight loss, but instead may be caused by a complex interaction of changes in body weight, ideal body size goals, and personality characteristics related to the importance of thinness and physical appearance for self-esteem.

IV ASSESSMENT OF QUALITY OF LIFE

A Introduction

Quality of life has been measured using a wide variety of assessment procedures, ranging from very general measures of quality of life to very specific behavioral and psychological indicators of quality of life. This section provides a summary of some of the most common methods that have been used in research pertaining to obesity and quality of life.

B Overall Quality of Life

The two questionnaires most widely used to measure overall quality of life in obesity research are the Impact of Weight on Quality of Life questionnaire and the Medical Outcomes Study Short-Form Health Survey (SF-36) (3,113). The Impact of Weight on Quality of Life 74-item questionnaire asks the respondent to indicate the degree to which obesity negatively affects his or her functioning in eight areas: Health, Social/Interpersonal, Work, Mobility, Self-Esteem, Sexual Life, Activities of Daily Living, and Comfort with Food (2,4). Recently, a shorter (31-item) version has been developed (114).

The 36-item Medical Outcomes Study Short Form (SF-36) (113) is a very widely used self-report index of health status and medical outcomes as related to a variety of medical conditions and treatments. It produces scores on eight scales measuring physical and emotional functioning and general health perceptions.

As previously described, both the Impact of Weight on Quality of Life Scale and the SF-36 have shown the ability to detect differences associated with differences in body weight. Further, these measures have been found to be sensitive to changes in body weight and can be used as indices for benefits of weight loss upon health and well-being.

There are a number of brief surveys and questionnaires that have been developed as measures of quality of life (115). Most of these questionnaires assess very general happiness with life (116) and/or family relationships (117). These measures have not received widespread use, in comparison to the SF-36 and Impact of Weight on Quality of Life.

C Mood and Personality

Another common approach for measuring quality of life is to assess global indicators of mood or personality. The Beck Depression Inventory (BDI) (118–120) has been used frequently for this purpose. The BDI has 21 items that measure the symptoms of depression. It has been used in many studies of many different physical and mental health problems over the past 30 years (121), including obesity (122). Studies of mood disturbances associated with obesity (25,123) and clinical trials have found the BDI to be a sensitive and useful tool.

The State-Trait Anxiety Inventory (STAI) (124) is a commonly used measure of situational (state) and generalized (trait) anxiety. The STAI requires rating 40 anxiety symptoms; it has been studied for >30 years and has been found to be a reliable and valid measure of anxiety in a wide variety of physical and mental health disorders, including obesity (54).

The Symptom Checklist-90 (125) measures nine symptom domains ranging from depression and anxiety to obsessive-compulsive disorder and psychotic problems. The SCL-90 also has three global measures of symptom severity that may be more useful as measures of quality of life than the nine scales that measure specific symptom domains. The SCL-90 has been validated in a variety of studies over the past 30 years and has been used extensively in research related to obesity (122).

One of the most frequently used measures of personality is the Minnesota Multiphasic Personality Inventory (126). The MMPI-2 has three validity scales that test for "faking good" and "faking bad." The MMPI-2 also has 10 clinical scales (126) and hundreds of supplemental scales (127,128). In general, obese people do not have high scores on any of the MMPI-2 clinical scales. Furthermore, the MMPI-2 is not sensitive to change during clinical trials. Therefore, the primary purpose of the MMPI-2 is to screen for psychological problems at baseline. However, since it is quite long (567 questions), there are several other less time-consuming methods that can be used for the same purpose.

The PRIME-MD (129) is one alternative to the MMPI-2 for screening of common psychiatric disorders. This method was developed as a cost-efficient procedure to be used by primary care physicians to screen for the presence of depression, anxiety disorders, eating disorders, psychosis, and substance abuse. The original version of the PRIME-MD included a survey of common mental health symptoms that was completed by the patient. The physician then interviewed the patient about specific problem behaviors to establish a psychiatric diagnosis. A more recent version of the PRIME-MD (130) relies exclusively upon the patient's self-report via questionnaire. This method is equally valid as the original PRIME-MD for screening common mental health problems. A much longer interview for psychiatric problems is the Structured Clinical Interview for DSM-IV axis I Disorders (SCID) (131). This semistructured interview format has been found to be a reliable and valid method for establishing psychiatric diagnoses based on the diagnostic criteria established by the American Psychiatric Association (16). The SCID is primarily used in research studies where it is important to screen for a wide variety of mental health problems.

D Eating Behavior/Disturbed Eating

Over the past 20 years, many assessment methods have been developed to measure the symptoms of anorexia nervosa, bulimia nervosa, and binge-eating disorders. Other methods have been established to measure specific behavioral, cognitive, or affective symptoms associated with disturbed patterns of eating.

Two semistructured interviews have been tested as measures of eating disorder symptoms. The Eating Disorder Examination (132–134) was developed to assess the core features of bulimia nervosa. In recent years, the

EDE has been used to define eating disorders, including binge eating disorder. The EDE has undergone 12 revisions and is generally considered to be one of the best methods for assessing core symptoms of eating disorders. The Interview for Diagnosis of Eating Disorders, fourth version (IDED-IV) (135) was developed specifically for the purpose of establishing a diagnosis of anorexia nervosa, bulimia nervosa, binge-eating disorder, or eating disorder not otherwise specified, using the diagnostic criteria established by the American Psychiatric Association (16). The reliability and validity of the IDED-IV has been established in a number of studies, and it has been used to reliably differentiate binge-eating disorder from simple obesity (135). Therefore, the most important use for the IDED-IV in obesity research may be its potential for reliably screening for the presence of eating disorders, including binge-eating disorder.

Several questionnaires have been developed for measuring a wide range of eating behaviors and eating disorder symptoms. The Eating Behavior Inventory (EBI) (136) was developed to assess behaviors prescribed by behavioral weight loss programs, e.g., self-monitoring of food intake and body weight, refusing offers of food, eating at only one place, shopping from a list, and eating in response to emotions. Factor analysis found three scales: control over eating, use of behavioral weight control methods, and use of stimulus control procedures (137). The EBI has been found to be a reliable and valid measure, and it is sensitive to treatment effects. Unfortunately, it has not found widespread use in obesity research.

The most widely used "broad-band" measure of disturbed eating is the Eating Disorder Inventory-2 (EDI-2) (138). The EDI-2 was developed for use with eating disorders, and only two of the EDI-2 scales are applicable to obesity: the bulimia scale, and the body dissatisfaction scale. Thus, despite the established reliability and validity of the EDI, it has only limited potential for use with obesity. Two recently developed questionnaires may be more useful in obesity. One is the Weight Loss Behavior Scale (139). This self-report inventory was developed specifically for use in treatment outcome research related to obesity. The reliability and validity of the WLBS has been supported in a recent study (139), and it measures five symptom domains: (1) concern with dieting and weight; (2) exercise; (3) overeating; (4) avoidance of fattening foods; and (5) emotional eating. Another questionnaire, the Multidimensional Assessment of Eating Disorder Symptoms (140), was developed for assessment of treatment outcome with eating disorders; it has six scales: (1) binge eating; (2) restrictive eating; (3) purgative behavior; (4) fear of fatness; (5) avoidance of forbidden foods; and (6) depression.

E Dietary Restraint and Overeating/Binge Eating

A variety of questionnaires have been developed for measuring intention to restrict caloric intake to manage body weight. As noted earlier, dietary restraint has been hypothesized to result in "disinhibited eating." The first measure of dietary restraint was developed by Herman and Mack (141) and was later revised to a 10-item scale (142). Researchers began to question whether dietary restraint and overeating were necessarily linked. These questions led to the development of two new measures that measured the two constructs, dietary restraint and overeating, as separate variables. Stunkard and Messick (76) developed the Three Factor Eating Questionnaire, and it is now called the Eating Inventory (143). The Eating Inventory has three scales—dietary (cognitive) restraint, disinhibition, and perceived hunger. Later research found that the dietary restraint and disinhibition scales were not correlated, which supports the conclusion that intention to diet and overeating may not be causally linked (74). A series of studies (73,74,77) have reported that flexible approaches to dieting are not associated with overeating, but that rigid approaches to dieting are associated with overeating. This line of research led to the development of a revision of the Dietary Restraint scale that has two dimensions: rigid and flexible dieting (144). At about the time the Three Factor Eating Questionnaire was developed, Van Strien et al. (145) reported a similar self-report inventory called the Dutch Eating Behavior Questionnaire; it measures restrained eating, emotional eating, and external eating. The reliability and validity of these scales have been established in a series of studies (146).

Several questionnaires have been developed as measures of binge eating. The Binge Eating Questionnaire is a nine-item self-report inventory that measures binge eating (147). The Binge Eating Scale is a 16-item questionnaire that has been used more frequently in research studies of binge eating (148). The Questionnaire of Eating and Weight Patterns was developed to screen for the presence of binge-eating disorder (149). Recent studies have found that all of these questionnaires overestimate the prevalence of binge eating and binge-eating disorder (85,86). The Eating Disorder Examination, described earlier, is a semistructured interview method that includes questions for measuring binge eating that provides a more accurate measure of consuming objectively large amounts of food (134). Also as mentioned, the IDED-IV (135) structured interview has been validated as an objective method for defining binge-eating disorder (86).

F Body Image

Until recently, questionnaires have been most frequently used in studies of body image, body dissatisfaction, and obesity. Two of the more frequently used questionnaires are the body dissatisfaction scale of the EDI-2 (138) and the Body Shape Questionnaire (150). Recently, two nonquestionnaire measures of body image associated with obesity have been developed. Williamson et al. (56) validated the Body Image Assessment for Obesity (BIA-O). The BIA-O measures estimates of current, ideal, and reasonable body size, using pictures of body silhouettes that vary in terms of body size and shape (from very thin to very obese). The discrepancy between current and ideal body size estimates was validated as a measure of body size dissatisfaction. The BIA-O has been validated for use with Caucasian men and women and African-American men and women. Stewart et al. (65) validated a computerized body image assessment procedure called the Body Morph Assessment (BMA). The BMA also measures estimates of current, ideal, and reasonable body size and these estimates were validated against the BIA-O. Thus far, the BMA has only been studied with Caucasian women, which limits its use with a diverse population.

V CONCLUSIONS

Research has found that obesity is associated with lower overall quality of life. Obese people experience considerable distress stemming from excess body weight, but only a minority of obese adults develop clinical psychiatric syndromes. In addition to social influences, the impact of obesity on quality of life is also a function of personal characteristics, e.g., severity of obesity, gender, ethnic background, and the presence of behavioral characteristics such as binge eating. Weight loss generally results in improved overall quality of life, mood, hunger, and body image. Conversely, weight gain is associated with worsened quality of life. In recent years, many assessment instruments that measure quality of life have been developed and validated. In conclusion, research on quality of life and obesity has been very active over the past ten years, leading to a much better understanding of how obesity and weight loss (and gain) are related to personal well-being. It is recommended that measures of quality of life routinely be included in obesity treatment outcome studies as additional important indicants of treatment effectiveness.

REFERENCES

1. Testa MA, Simonson DC. Assessment of quality-of-life outcomes. N Engl J Med 1996; 334:835–840.
2. Kolotkin RL, Head S, Hamilton M, Tse C-KJ. Assessing impact of weight on quality of life. Obes Res 1995; 3:49–56.
3. Ware JE Jr, Gandek B. Overview of the SF-36 Health Survey and the International Quality of Life Assessment (IQOLA) Project. J Clin Epidemiol 1998; 51:903–912.
4. Kolotkin RL, Head S, Brookhart A. Construct validity of the Impact of Weight on Quality of Life Questionnaire. Obes Res 1997; 5:434–441.
5. Fontaine KR, Cheskin LJ, Barofsky I. Health-related quality of life in obese persons seeking treatment. J Fam Pract 1996; 43:265–270.
6. Fontaine KR, Barlett SJ, Barofsky I. Health-related quality of life among obese persons seeking and not currently seeking treatment. Int J Eating Disord 2000; 27:101–105.
7. Fontaine KR, Barofsky I, Cheskin LJ. Predictors of quality of life for obese persons. J Nerv Ment Dis 1997; 185:120–122.
8. Sullivan M, Karlsson J, Sjostrom L, Backman L, Bengtsson C, Bouchard C, Dahlgren S, Jonsson E, Larsson B, Lindstedt S, Naslund I, Olbe L, Wedel H. Swedish Obese Subjects (SOS)—an intervention study of obesity. Baseline evaluation of health and psychosocial functioning in the first 1743 subjects examined. Int J Obes 1993; 17:503–512.
9. Doll HA, Petersen SE, Stewart-Brown SL. Obesity and physical and emotional well-being: associations between body mass index, chronic illness, and the physical and mental components of the SF-36 questionnaire. Obes Res 2000; 8(2):160–170.
10. Brown WJ, Mishra G, Kenardy J, Dobson A. Relationships between body mass index and well-being in young Australian women. Int J Obes Relat Metab Disord 2000; 24:1360–1368.
11. Gortmaker SL, Must A, Perrin JM, Sobol AM, Dietz WH. Social and economic consequences of overweight in adolescence and young adulthood. N Engl J Med 1993; 329:1008–1012.
12. Sargent JD, Blanchflower DG. Obesity and stature in adolescence and earnings in young adulthood. Analysis of a British birth cohort. Arch Pediatr Adolesc Med 1994; 148:681–687.
13. Garn SM, Sullivan TV, Hawthorne VM. Educational level, fatness, and fatness differences between husbands and wives. Am J Clin Nutr 1989; 50:740–745.

14. Rand CSW, MacGregor AMC. Successful weight loss following obesity surgery and the perceived liability of morbid obesity. Int J Obes 1991; 15:577–579.
15. O'Neil PM, Smith CF, Foster GD, Anderson DA. The perceived relative worth of reaching and maintaining goal weight. Int J Obes Relat Metab Disord 2000; 24:1069–1076.
16. Diagnostic and Statistical Manual of Mental Disorders. 4th ed. Washington: American Psychiatric Association, 1994.
17. Fitzgibbon ML, Stolley MR, Kirschenbaum DS. Obese people who seek treatment have different characteristics than those who do not seek treatment. Health Psychol 1993; 12:342–345.
18. O'Neil PM, Jarrell MP. Psychological aspects of obesity and dieting. In: Wadden TA, Van Itallie TB, eds. Treatment of the Seriously Obese Patient. New York: Guilford Press, 1992:342.
19. Stunkard AJ, Wadden TA. Psychological aspects of severe obesity. Am J Clin Nutr 1992; 55:524S–532S.
20. Wadden TA, Stunkard JJ. Social and psychological consequences of obesity. Ann Intern Med 1985; 103: 1062–1067.
21. Berman WH, Berman ER, Heymsfeld S, Fauci M, Acherman S. The effect of psychiatric disorders on weight loss in obesity clinic patients. Behav Med 1993; 18:162–167.
22. Goldsmith SJ, Anger-Friedfeld K, Beren S, Rudolph D, Boeck M, Aronne L. Psychiatric illness in patients presenting for obesity treatment. Int J Eating Disord 1992; 12:63–71.
23. Halmi KA, Long M, Stunkard AJ, Mason E. Psychiatric diagnosis of morbidly obese gastric bypass patients. Am J Psychiatry 1980; 137:470–472.
24. Robins LN, Helzer JE, Weissman MM, Orvaschel H, Gurenberg E, Burke JD, Regier DA. Lifetime prevalence of specific psychiatric disorders in three sites. Arch Gen Psychiatry 1984; 41:949–958.
25. Prather RC, Williamson DA. Psychopathology associated with bulimia, binge eating, and obesity. Int J Eating Disord 1988; 7:177–184.
26. Britz B, Siegfried W, Ziegler A, Lamertz C, Herpertz-Dahlmann BM, Remschmidt H, Wittchen HU, Hebebrand J. Rates of psychiatric disorders in a clinical study group of adolescents with extreme obesity and in obese adolescents ascertained via a population based study. Int J Obes Relat Metab Disord 2000; 24:1707–1714.
27. Palinkas LA, Wingard DL, Barrett-Connor E. Depressive symptoms in overweight and obese older adults: a test of the "jolly fat" hypothesis. J Psychosom Res 1996; 40:59–66.
28. Poston WSC, Goodrick GK, Foreyt JP. The Rosenberg Self-Esteem Scale. In: St. Jeor ST, ed. Obesity Assessment: Tools, Methods, Interpretations. New York: Chapman & Hall, 1997:59.
29. French SA, Story M, Perry CL. Self-esteem and obesity in children and adolescents: a literature review. Obes Res 1995; 3:479–490.
30. Strauss RS. Childhood obesity and self-esteem. Pediatrics 2000; 105:e15.
31. Must A, Strauss RS. Risks and consequences of childhood and adolescent obesity. Int J Obes Relat Metab Disord 1999; 23(suppl 2):S2–S11.
32. Friedman MA, Brownell KD. Psychological correlates of obesity: moving to the next research generation. Psychol Bull 1995; 117:3–20.
33. Allon N. The stigma of overweight in everyday life. In: Wolman BB, ed. Psychological Aspects of Obesity: A Handbook. New York: Van Nostrand Reinhold, 1982.
34. Turnbull JD, Heaslip S, McLeod HA. Pre-school children's attitudes to fat and normal male and female stimulus figures. Int J Obes Relat Metab Disord 2000; 24:1705–1706.
35. Blumberg P, Mellis PP. Medical students' attitudes toward the obese and the morbidly obese. Int J Eating Disord 1985; 4:169–175.
36. Oberrieder H, Walker R, Monroe D, Adeyanju M. Attitude of dietetics students and registered dietitians toward obesity. J Am Diet Assoc 1995; 95:914–916.
37. Price JH, Desmond SM, Krol RA, Snyder FF, O'Connell JK. Family practice physician's beliefs, attitudes, and practices regarding obesity. Am J Prev Med 1987; 3:339–345.
38. Rand CSW, MacGregor AMC. Morbidly obese patients' perceptions of social discrimination before and after surgery for obesity. South Med J 1990; 83:1390–1395.
39. Wadden TA, Anderson DA, Foster GD, Bennett A, Steinberg C, Sarwer DB. Obese women's perceptions of their physicians' weight management attitudes and practices. Arch Fam Med 2000; 9:854–860.
40. Klesges RC, Klem ML, Hanson CL, Eck LH, Ernst J, O'Laughlin D, Garrott A, Rife R. The effects of applicant's health status and qualifications on simulated hiring decisions. Int J Obes 1990; 14:527–535.
41. Pringitore R, Dugoni BL, Tindale RS, Spring B. Bias against overweight job applicants in a simulated employment interview. J Appl Psychol 1994; 79:909–917.
42. Falkner NH, French SA, Jeffery RW, Neumark-Sztainer D, Sherwood NE, Morton N. Mistreatment due to weight: prevalence and sources of perceived mistreatment in women and men. Obes Res 1999; 7: 572–576.
43. Miller CT, Rothblum ED, Barbour L, Brand PA, Felicio DM. Do obese women have poorer social relationships than nonobese women? Reports by self, friends, and co-workers. J Person 1990; 58:365–380.
44. Miller CT, Rothblum ED, Brand PA, Felicio DM. Do obese women have poorer social relationships than nonobese women? Reports by self, friends, and co-workers. J Person 1995; 63:65–85.
45. Phillips RG, Hill AJ. Fat, plain, but not friendless: self-

esteem and peer acceptance of obese pre-adolescent girls. Int J Obes Relat Metab Disord 1998; 22:287–293.
46. Bruch H. Obesity in childhood and personality development. Obes Res 1997; 5(2):157–161. (Reprinted from Am J Orthopsychiatry 1941; 11:467–473).
47. Klesges RC. Personality and obesity: global versus specific measures. Behav Ther 1984; 6:347–356.
48. Leon GR, Roth L. Obesity: psychological causes, correlations, and speculations. Psychol Bull 1977; 84:117–139.
49. Blankmeyer BL, Smylie KD, Price DC, Costello RM, McFee AS, Fuller DS. A replicated five cluster MMPI topology of morbidly obese female candidates for gastric bypass. Int J Obes 1990; 14:235–247.
50. Rosen JC. Body image disorder: definition, development and contribution to eating disorders. In: Crowther JH, Tennenbaum DL, Hobfoll SE, Stephens MAP, eds. The Etiology of Bulimia: The Individual and Family Context. Washington: Hemisphere Publishers, 1992: 157–177.
51. Thompson JK. Body image; extent of disturbance, associated features, theoretical models, assessment methodologies, intervention strategies, and a proposal for a new DSM-IV diagnostic category—Body Image Disorder. In: Hersen M, Eisler RM, Miller PM, eds. Progress in Behavior Modification. Sycamore, IL: Sycamore Publishers, 1992:3–54.
52. Wiliamson DA. Body image disturbances in eating disorders: a form of cognitive bias? Eating Disord J Treat Prev 1996; 4:47–58.
53. Thompson JK. Assessment of body image. In: Allison DB, ed. Handbook of Assessment Methods for Eating Behavior and Weight-Related Problems: Measures, Theory, and Research. Thousand Oaks, CA: Sage Publications, 1995:119–148.
54. Williamson DA. Assessment of Eating Disorders: Obesity, Anorexia, and Bulimia Nervosa. New York: Pergamon Press, 1990.
55. Williamson DA, Gleaves DH, Watkins PC, Schlundt DG. Validation of self-ideal body size discrepancy as a measure of body dissatisfaction. J Psychopathol Behav Assess 1993; 15:57–68.
56. Williamson DA, Womble LG, Zucker NL, Reas DL, White MA, Blouin DC, Greenway F. Body Image Assessment for Obesity (BIA-O): development of a new procedure. Int J Obes 2000; 24:1326–1332.
57. Faith MS, Allison DB. Assessment of psychological status among obese persons. In: Thompson JK, ed. Body Image, Eating Disorders, and Obesity. Washington: American Psychological Association, 1996:365–388.
58. Klesges RC, DeBon M, Meyers AW. Obesity in African American women: epidemiology, determinants, and treatment issues. In: Thompson JK, ed. Body Image, Eating Disorders, and Obesity. Washington: American Psychological Association, 1996:461–477.
59. Strong SM, Williamson DA, Netemeyer RG, Geer JH. Eating disorder symptoms and concerns about body differ as a function of gender and sexual orientation. J Social Clin Psychol 2000; 19:240–255.
60. Collins JK. Methodology for the objective measurement of body image. Int J Eating Disord 1987; 6:393–399.
61. Colins JK, Beaumont PJV, Touyz SW, Krass J, Thompson P, Philips T. Variability in body shape perception in anorexic, bulimic, obese, and control subjects. Int J Eating Disord 1987; 6:633–638.
62. Counts CR, Adams HE. Body image in bulimic, dieting, and normal females. J Psychopathol Behav Assess 1985; 7289–7300.
63. Davis CJ, Williamson DA, Goreczny AJ, Bennett SM. Body image disturbances and bulimia nervosa: an empirical analysis of recent revisions of DSM-III. J Psychopathol Behav Assess 1989; 11:61–69.
64. Williamson DA, Prather RC, McKenzie SJ, Blouin DC. Behavioral assessment procedures can differentiate bulimia nervosa, compulsive overeater, obese, and normal subjects. Behav Assess 1990; 12:239–252.
65. Stewart TM, Williamson DA, Smeets MAM, Greenway FL. The Body Morph Assessment: development of a computerized measure of body image. Obes Res 2001; 9:43–50.
66. Polivy J, Herman CP. Dieting and bingeing: a causal analysis. Am Psychol 1985; 40:193–201.
67. Brownell KD, Greenwood MRC, Stellar E, Shrager EE. The effects of repeated cycles of weight loss and regain in rats. Physiol Behav 1986; 38:459–464.
68. Brownell KD, Rodin J. Medical, metabolic and psychological effects on weight cycling. Arch Intern Med 1994; 154:1325–1330.
69. Yanovski SZ, Atkinson RL, Dietz WH, et al. National Task Force on the Prevention and Treatment of Obesity. Weight cycling. JAMA 1994; 272:1196–1202.
70. Herman PC, Polivy J. Anxiety, restraint, and eating behavior. J Abnorm Psychol 1975; 84:666–672.
71. Polivy J, Herman CP. Etiology of binge eating: psychological mechanisms. In: Fairburn CG, Wilson GT, eds. Binge Eating: Nature, Assessment and Treatment. New York: Guilford Press, 1993:173–205.
72. Lawson OJ, Williamson DA, Champagne CM, DeLany JP, Brooks ER, Howat PM, Wozniak PJ, Bray GA, Ryan DH. The association of body weight, dietary intake, and energy expenditure with dietary restraint and disinhibition. Obes Res 1995; 3:433–439.
73. Westenhoefer J. Dietary restraint and disinhibition: is restraint a homogeneous construct? Appetite 1991; 16: 45–55.
74. Williamson DA, Lawson OJ, Brooks ER, Wozniak PJ, Ryan DH, Bray GA, Duchmann EG. Association of body mass with dietary restraint and disinhibition. Appetite 1995; 25:31–41.
75. Lowe MR. The effects of dieting on eating behavior: a three-factor model. Psychol Bull 1993; 114:100–121.

76. Stunkard AJ, Messick S. The Three-Factor Eating Questionnaire to measure dietary restraint, disinhibition, and hunger. J Psychosom Res 1985; 29:71–83.
77. Smith CF, Williamson DA, Bray GA, Ryan DH. Flexible vs. rigid dieting strategies: relationship with adverse behavioral outcomes. Appetite 1999; 32:295–305.
78. National Task Force on the Prevention and Treatment of Obesity. Dieting and the development of eating disorders in overweight and obese adults. Arch Intern Med 2000; 160:2581–2589.
79. Kumanyika S. Obesity in black women. Epidemiol Rev 1987; 9:31–50.
80. Stevens J, Kumanyika SK, Keil JE. Attitudes toward body size and dieting: differences between elderly black and white women. Am J Public Health 1994; 84:1322–1325.
81. Kumanyika S, Wilson JF, Guilford-Davenport M. Weight-related attitudes and behaviors of black women. J Am Diet Assoc 1993; 93:416–422.
82. Powell AD, Kahn AS. Racial differences in women's desires to be thin. Int J Eating Disord 1995; 17:191–195.
83. Kolotkin RL, Revis ES, Kirkley B, Janick L. Binge eating in obesity: associated MMPI characteristics. J Consult Clin Psychol 1987; 55:872–876.
84. Yanovski SZ, Nelson JE, Dubbert BK, Spitzer RL. Association of binge eating disorder and psychiatric comorbidity in obese subjects. Am J Psychiatry 1993; 150:1472–1479.
85. Williamson DA, Martin CK. Binge eating disorder: a review of the literature after publication of DSM-IV. Eating Weight Disord 1999; 4:103–114.
86. Varnado PJ, Williamson DA, Bentz BG, Ryan DH, Rhodes SK, O'Neil PM, Sebastian SB, Barker SE. Prevalence of binge eating disorder in obese adults seeking weight loss treatment. Eating Weight Disord 1998; 2:117–124.
87. Womble LG, Williamson DA, Martin CK, Zucker NL, Thaw JM, Netemeyer R, Lovejoy JC, Greenway FL, Psychosocial variables associated with binge eating in obese males and females. Int J Eating Disord 2001; 30:217–221.
88. Stice E, Akutagawa D, Gaggar A, Agras WS. Negative affect moderates the relation between dieting and binge eating. Int J Eating Disord 2000; 27:218–229.
89. Telch CF, Agras WS, Rossiter EM. Binge eating increases with increasing adiposity. Int J Eating Disord 1988; 7:115–119.
90. Danksy BS, O'Neil PM, Brewerton TD, Kilpatrick DG. The nature of the relationship between obesity and victimization in a national sample of US women [abstr]. Ann Behav Med 1993; 15:S67.
91. Fontaine KR, Barofsky I, Andersen RE, Bartlett SJ, Wiersema L, Cheskin LJ, Franckowiak SC. Impact of weight loss on health-related quality of life. Quality Life Res 1999; 8(3):275–277.
92. McMahon FG, Fujioka K, Singh BN, Mendel CM, Rowe E, Rolston K, Johnson F, Mooradian AD. Efficacy and safety of sibutramine in obese white and African American patients with hypertension: a 1-year, double-blind, placebo-controlled, multicenter trial. Arch Intern Med 2000; 160:2185–2191.
93. Metz JA, Stern JS, Kris-Etherton P, Reusser ME, Morris CD, Hatton DC, Oparil S, Haynes RB, Resnick LM, Pi-Sunyer FX, Clark S, Chester L, McMahon M, Snyder GW, McCarron DA. A randomized trial of improved weight loss with a prepared meal plan in overweight and obese patients: impact on cardiovascular risk reduction. Arch Intern Med 2000; 160:2150–2158.
94. Choban PS, Onyejekwe J, Burge JC, Flancbaum L. A health status assessment of the impact of weight loss following Roux-en-Y gastric bypass for clinically severe obesity. J Am Coll Surg 1999; 188:491–497.
95. Klem ML, Wing RR, Chang CC, Lang W, McGuire MT, Sugerman HI, Hutchison SL, Makovich AL, Hill JO. A case-control study of successful maintenance of a substantial weight loss: individuals who lost weight through surgery versus those who lost weight through non-surgical means. Int J Obes Relat Metab Disord 2000; 24:573–579.
96. Fine JT, Colditz GA, Coakley EH, Moseley G, Manson JE, Willett WC, Kawachi I. A prospective study of weight change and health-related quality of life in women. JAMA 1999; 282:2136–2142.
97. French SA, Jeffry RW. Consequences of dieting to lose weight: effects on physical and mental health. Health Psychol 1994; 13:195–212.
98. Wing RR, Epstein LH, Marcus MD, Kupfer DJ. Mood changes in behavioral weight loss programs. J Psychosom Res 1984; 28:189–196.
99. Wadden TA, Stunkard AJ, Brownell KD, Day SC. A comparison of two very-low-calorie diets: protein-sparing modified fast versus protein-formula-liquid diet. Am J Clin Nutr 1985; 41:533–539.
100. Rosen JC, Hunt DA, Sims EAH, Bogardus C. Comparison of carbohydrate-containing and carbohydrate-restricted hypocaloric diets in the treatment of obesity: effects on appetite and mood. Am J Clin Nutr 1982; 36:463–469.
101. Klem ML, Wing RR, McGuire MT, Seagle HM, Hill JO. Psychological symptoms in individuals successful at long-term maintenance of weight loss. Health Psychol 1998; 17:336–345.
102. Wadden TA, Mason G, Foster GD, Stunkard AJ, Prange AJ. Effects of a very low calorie diet on weight, thyroid hormones, and mood. Int J Obes 1990; 14:249–258.
103. Anderson IM, Parry-Billings M, Newsholme EA, Fairburn CG, Cowen PJ. Dieting reduces plasma tryptophan and alters brain 5-HT function in women. Psychol Med 1990; 20:785–791.
104. Foster GD, Wadden TA, Kendall PC, Stunkard AJ, Vogt RA. Psychological effects of weight loss and re-

gain: a prospective evaluation. J Consult Clin Psychol 1996; 64:752–757.
105. Foreyt JP, Brunner RL, Goodrick GK, Cutter G, Brownell KD, St Jeor ST. Psychological correlates of weight fluctuation. Int J Eating Disord 1995; 17(3):263–275.
106. Rumpel C, Ingram DD, Harris TB, Madans J. The association between weight change and psychological well-being in women. Int J Obes Relat Metab Disord 1994; 18:179–183.
107. Lappalainen R, Sjoden PO, Hursti T, Vesa V. Hunger/craving responses and reactivity to food stimuli during fasting and dieting. Int J Obes 1990; 14:679–688.
108. Wadden TA, Stunkard AJ, Day SC, Gould RA, Rubin CJ. Less food, less hunger: reports of appetite and symptoms in a controlled study of a protein-sparing modified fast. Int J Obes 1987; 11:239–249.
109. Wing RR, Marcus MD, Blair EH, Burton LR. Psychological responses of obese type II diabetic subjects to very-low-calorie diet. Diabetes Care 1991; 14:596–599.
110. Foster GD, Wadden TA, Swain RM, Stunkard AJ, Platte P, Vogt RA. The Eating Inventory in obese women: clinical correlates and relationship to weight loss. Int J Obes Relat Metab Disord 1998; 22:778–785.
111. Kral JG, Sjostrom LV, Sullivan MEE. Assessment of quality of life before and after surgery for severe obesity. Am J Clin Nutr 1992; 55:611S–614S.
112. Foster GD, Wadden TA, Vogt RA, Brewer G. What is a reasonable weight loss? Patients' expectations and evaluations of obesity treatment outcomes. J Consult Clin Psychol 1997; 65:79–85.
113. Ware JE. The MOS 36-item short-form health survey (SF-36). Conceptual framework and item selection. Med Care 1992; 30:473–483.
114. Kolotkin RL, Crosby RD, Kosloski KD, Williams GR. Development of a brief measure to assess quality of life in obesity. Obes Res 2001; 9:102–111.
115. Alfonso VC. Measures of quality of life, subjective well-being, and satisfaction with life. In: Allison DB, ed. Handbook of Assessment Methods for Eating Behavior and Weight-Related Problems: Measures, Theory, and Research. Thousand Oaks, CA: Sage Publications, 1995:23–80.
116. Diener E, Emmons RA, Larsen RJ, Griffin S. The Satisfaction with Life Scale. J Person Assess 1985; 49:71–75.
117. Schumm WR, McCollum EE, Bugaighis MA, Jurich AP, Bollman SR. Characteristics of the Kansas Family Life Satisfaction Scale in a regional sample. Psychol Rep 1986; 58:975–980.
118. Beck AT, Rush AJ, Shaw BR, Emery G. Cognitive Therapy for Depression. New York: Guilford Press, 1979.
119. Beck AT, Steer RA, Garbin MG. Psychometric properties of the Beck Depression Inventory: twenty-five years of evaluation. Clin Psychol Rev 1988; 8:77–100.
120. Beck AT, Brown GK, Steer RA. Beck Depression Inventory-II. San Antonio: Psychological Corporation, 1996.
121. Beck AT, Steer RA, Garbin MG. Psychometric properties of the Beck Depression Inventory: twenty-five years of evaluation. Clin Psychol Rev 1988; 8:77–100.
122. Morey LC, Kurtz JE. Assesment of general personality and psychopathology among persons with eating and weight-related concerns. In: Allison DB, ed. Handbook of Assessment Methods for Eating Behavior and Weight-Related Problems: Measures, Theory, and Research. Thousand Oaks, CA: Sage Publications, 1995:1–22.
123. Marcus MD, Wing RR, Hopkins J. Obese binge eaters: affect, cognition, and response to behavioral weight control. J Consult Clin Psychol 1988; 5:433–439.
124. Spielberger CD, Gorsuch RL, Lushene RE. Manual for the State Trait Anxiety Inventory. Palo Alto, CA: Consulting Psychologists Press, 1970.
125. Derogatis L. Manual for the Symptom Checklist-90, Revised. Baltimore: Johns Hopkins Press, 1977.
126. Butcher JN. MMPI-2 in Psychological Treatment. New York: Oxford University Press, 1990.
127. Wiggins JS. Substantive dimensions of self-report in the MMPI item pool. Psychol Monogr 1966; 80:22 (whole No. 630).
128. Graham JR. The MMPI: A Practical Guide. 2d ed. New York: Oxford University Press, 1987.
129. Spitzer RL, Williams JB, Kroenke K, Linzer M, De Gruy FV, Hahn SR, Brody D, Johnson JG. Utility of a new procedure for diagnosing mental disorders in primary care. The PRIME-MD 1000 study. JAMA 1994; 272:1749–1756.
130. Spitzer RL, Kroenke K, Williams JB. Validation and utility of a self-report version of PRIME-MD: the PHQ primary care study. Primary Care Evaluation of Mental Disorders. Patient Health Questionnairc. JAMA 1999; 282:1737–1744.
131. First MB, Gibbon M, Spitzer RL, Williams JBW. User's Guide for the Structural-Clinical Interview for DSM-IV Axis 1 Disorders (SCID-I, Version 2.0). Washington: American Psychiatric Press, 1995.
132. Fairburn CG, Cooper Z. The eating disorder examination. In: Fairburn CG, Wilson GT, eds. Binge Eating: Nature, Assessment, and Treatment. 12th ed. New York: Guilford Press, 1993:3–14.
133. Williamson DA, Anderson DA, Jackman LP, Jackson SR. Assessment of eating disordered thoughts, feelings, and behaviors. In: Allison DB, ed. Handbook of Assessment Methods for Eating Behavior and Weight-Related Problems: Measures, Theory, and Research. Thousand Oaks, CA: Sage Publications, 1995:327–386.
134. Cooper Z, Fairburn CG. The Eating Disorder Exami-

nation: a semi-structured interview for the assessment of the specific psychopathology of eating disorders. Int J Eating Disord 1987; 6:1–8.
135. Kutlesic V, Williamson DA, Gleaves DH, Barbin JM, Murphy-Eberenz KP. The Interview for the Diagnosis of Eating Disorders IV: application to DSM-IV diagnostic criteria. Psychol Assess 1998; 10:41–48.
136. O'Neil PM, Currey HS, Hirsh AA, Malcom FJ, Sexauer JD, Riddle FE, Tayor CT. Development and validation of the Eating Behavior Inventory. J Behav Assess 1979; 1(suppl 2):123–132.
137. Currey HS, O'Neil PM, Malcolm R, Riddle FE. Factor analysis of the eating behavior inventory. Fourth International Congress on Obesity, New York, October 1983 .
138. Garner DM. Eating Disorder Inventory-2 Manual. Odessa, FL: Psychological Assessment Resources, 1991.
139. Smith CF, Williamson DA, Womble LG, Johnson J, Burke LE. Psychometric development of a multidimensional measure of weight-related attitudes and behaviors. Eating Weight Disord 2000; 5:73–86.
140. Anderson DA, Williamson DA, Duchmann EG, Gleaves DH, Barbin JM. Development and validation of a multifactorial treatment outcome measure for eating disorders. Assessment 1999; 6:7–20.
141. Herman CP, Mack D. Restrained and unrestrained eating. J Personal 1975; 43:647–660.
142. Polivy J, Herman PH, Howard KI. Restraint scale: assessment of dieting. In: Hersen M, Bellack AS, eds. Dictionary of Behavioral Assessment Techniques. New York: Pergamon Press, 1988:377–380.
143. Stunkard AJ, Messick S. The Eating Inventory. San Antonio, TX: Psychological Corporation, 1988.
144. Westenhoefer J, Stunkard AJ, Pudel V. Validation of the flexible and rigid control dimensions of dietary restraint. Int J Eating Disord 1999; 26:53–64.
145. Van Strein T, Frijters JER, Bergers GPA, Defares PB. The Dutch Eating Behavior Questionnaire (DEBQ) for assessment of restrained, emotional, and external eating behavior. Int J Eating Disord 1986; 5:295–315.
146. Gorman BS, Allison DB. Measures of restrained eating. In: Allison DB, ed. Handbook of Assessment Methods for Eating Behavior and Weight-Related Problems: Measures, Theory, and Research. Thousand Oaks, CA: Sage Publications, 1995:149–184.
147. Hawkins RC, Clement PF. Development and construct validation of a self-report measure of binge eating tendencies. Addict Behav 1980; 5:219–226.
148. Gormally J, Black S, Daston S, Rardin D. The assessment of binge eating severity among obese persons. Addict Behav 1982; 7:47–55.
149. Spitzer RL, Devlin M, Walsh BT, Hasin D, Wing RR, Marcus MD, Stunkard A, Wadden T, Yanovski S, Agras S, Mitchell J, Nonas C. Binge Eating Disorder: a multi-site field trial of the diagnostic criteria. Int J Eating Disord 1992; 11:191–203.
150. Cooper PJ, Taylor MJ, Cooper Z, Fairburn CG. Development and validation of the Body Shape Questionnaire. Int J Eating Disord 1987; 6:485–494.

Index

Abdomen
  adipose tissue imaging, 56–58
  circumference and diastolic blood pressure, 877
  computed tomography, 57
  visceral fat, 167–168
Abdominal obesity and diabetes mellitus, 283
Acarbose and diabetes, 908
Acc2, 264
Accelerometers, 633
Accuracy, 65–66
  predictive body composition methods, 83–86
Acetazolamide, 944
Acetylcholine and feeding-related circuits, 336–337
Acetyl CoA carboxylase 2 (Acc2), 264
Acidic fibroblast growth factor (alphaFGF), 331
ACLS, 985
Acomys caharinus, 268
Acromegaly and body fat distribution, 679–680
ACTH, 301
Activity logs, 634
Activity recall, 633
Activity thermogenesis
  quantifying, 634–635
  total daily energy expenditure, 640
Acupuncture, 5
Acylation-stimulation protein (ASP), 266
  visceral adipose tissue (VAT), 595–596
Acyl COA, 264
Adenylyl cyclase regulation, 518
Adipocyte apoptosis
  peroxisome proliferator-activated receptor gamma (PPAR-gamma), 566
Adipocyte binding protein (aP2), 264
Adipocyte differentiation
  peroxisome proliferator-activated receptor gamma (PPAR-gamma), 563–565
Adipocyte differentiation related protein (ADRP), 494
Adipocyte secretory products
  visceral adipose tissue (VAT), 600
Adipocyte-specific genes
  peroxisome proliferator-activated receptor gamma (PPAR-gamma), 566–567
Adipogenesis
  cellular models, 492–494
  molecular mechanisms, 499–504
  peroxisome proliferator-activated receptor gamma (PPAR-gamma), 561–563
    genetic studies, 571–572
  receptor equipment, 494–496
  sequential events, 494–496
  transcriptional activators and repressors, 499–504
Adiponectin, 287
  visceral adipose tissue (VAT), 599
Adipose cell
  differentiation, 495
  plasticity
    cellular models, 492–494
Adipose tissue
  abdomen
    imaging, 56–58

[Adipose tissue]
  anatomic distribution, 38
  development in early life, 483
  differentiation, 482
  distribution, 60–61
  as endocrine organ, 671
  growth, 484–485
  hormonal effects, 485–486
  lipogenesis, 671–672
  lipolysis, 672
  malignancies, 492
  nutrients, 487–488
  ontogeny, 482–483
  peroxisome proliferator-activated receptor gamma (PPAR-gamma), 569–571
  phylogeny, 482–483
  precursor cells, 484
  regional distribution, 658–659
  regional growth, 489
  secretions, 284
  in vitro development, 492–499
  in vivo regulation, 482–490
Adipose tissue cellularity, 490–491
  diet, 490–491
  physiology, 483–489
  weight change, 490–491
Adiposity
  age changes, 123–124
  atomic level, 34–35
  cellular level, 36
  measurement
    body mass index, 773–774
    monkeys, 282–283
  molecular level, 34–36
  tissue organ level, 36–38
  whole-body level, 38
Adolescents
  overweight
    secular trends, 122
ADP, 46–47
ADRB3 gene, 213
Adrenal steroid hormones, 308–309
Adrenal steroids, 225
Aerobics Center Longitudinal Study (ACLS), 985
Afferent receptors
  stomach, 382
Africa, obesity in women, 94
African-Americans
  fat distribution, 137
  hypertension
    prevalence, 877
  major genes, 162
  mortality rate, 775
  quality of life, 1011
  subcutaneous fat, 84
  total body fat
[African-Americans]
    multicomponent measurement, 49
  visceral adipose tissue (VAT), 593
Age
  anthropometry
    Mexican-Americans, 69
    non-Hispanic blacks, 68
    non-Hispanic whites, 67
  exercise, 636
  exercising individual, 643
  food, thermic effect, 622
  mortality rate, 774–775
  pregnancy weight, 968–969
  work efficiency, 639
Age changes
  adiposity, 123–124
Aging
  lipid mobilization, 521
  metabolic syndrome, 792
Aging-associated obesity
  primates, 281–292
Agouti gene, 14, 261
Agouti gene-related peptide (AGRP), 212, 213, 303, 314–315, 543, 662–663
  modifier, 213
  NPY, 213–214
  regulation, 212–213
Agouti locus
  structure, 212
Agouti protein, 543
Agouti-Yellow, 202–215
  identification, 202–203
  modifiers, 203, 212
  normal action, 203
  pigmentation phenocopies, 203
AGRP (*see* Agouti gene-related peptide (AGRP))
AHO, 233–234
AIDS
  visceral adipose tissue (VAT), 600
Air displacement plethysmography (ADP), 46–47
Albright hereditary osteodystrophy (AHO), 233–234
Alcohol
  gout, 962–963
  hypothalamic-pituitary-adrenal axis dysregulation, 791–792
Alcohol intake
  oxidation, 720
All-cause mortality
  physical activity, 989–993
Alpha blockers
  hypertension
    obesity, 889
AlphaFGF, 331
Alpha-glycerol dehydrogenase (alphaGPDH), 265
Alpha-melanocyte stimulating hormone (alpha-MSH), 303, 543

Altered leptin pathway
  experimental obesity models,
    465–466
Alveolar-to-arterial gradient, 937
Amandamide, 318
Amino acids
  feeding-related circuits, 337–338
  substrate oxidation, 717–718
Aminostatic theory, 405
Amitriptyline, 17
Amphetamine, 15
Amylin, 262, 391
Anatomy, historical development of, 6
Androgen receptors
  adipose tissue, 487
Androgens
  body fat distribution, 674–675
Android obesity, 162–163, 851, 901
Androstenedione, 659
Anesthesia, introduction, 15
Angiopoietin-1, 483
Angiotensin-converting enzyme inhibitors
  hypertension
    obesity, 889
Angiotensin II, 499
Aniline, 15
Animal models
  new peptide regulators, 410–412
Anorexia, 322, 393
Anorexiant drugs, 943
ANP, 519–520
Anthropometry, 59–60
  age
    Mexican-Americans, 69
    non-Hispanic blacks, 68
    non-Hispanic whites, 67
  Mexican-Americans, 69
Antiadipogenic factors, 499
Antidiabetic drugs, 17
Anxiety, 1007, 1012
AP2, 264
Apo A-IV, 326–327, 392
ApoE, 600
Apolipoprotein A-IV (apo A-IV), 326–327, 392
Apolipoprotein E (ApoE), 600
Apoptosis, 481
  adipocyte
    peroxisome proliferator-activated receptor gamma
      (PPAR-gamma), 566
  white adipose tissue (WAT), 491–492
Appetite
  anatomy, 432
  food influences, 441
  research, 428–429
Appetite control systems
  compartments, 435–440
Appetite suppressants
  cardiovascular effects, 833–834
Appetite system
  behavior, 431–433
  nature, 431–435
  physiology, 431
Arabic medicine, 6
Arachidonic acid, 498
ARC, 305
Arcuate nucleus (ARC), 305
Arginine vasopressin (AVP), 303
Aromatase, 265
  metabolic syndrome, 800–801
Aromatase-deficient mice, 264
Arrhythmia, 830
Asian-Americans
  visceral adipose tissue (VAT), 593
Asian Indians
  gout, 960
Asians, 103
  body composition, 83
  cardiovascular morbidity, 88
ASIP gene, 204
ASP, 266
  visceral adipose tissue (VAT), 595–596
Aspirin
  weight reduction
    gallstones, 928
Associations, 23
Association studies, 169
Asthma
  obesity, 945–946
  weight loss, 946
Atherogenic dyslipidemias
  waist girth, 862–864
Atherogenic metabolic profile
  visceral adipose tissue (VAT), 857
Atherosclerosis, 283, 907
  peroxisome proliferator-activated receptor gamma
    (PPAR-gamma), 572
  weight loss, 833
Atrial natriuretic peptides
  hypertension, 885
Atrial natriuretic peptides (ANP), 519–520
Australian aborigines
  non-insulin-dependent diabetes mellitus (type 2), 900
Autonomic nervous system
  food, thermic effect, 623
Avicenna medicine, 18
AVP, 303
Ayurveda, 5
A-ZIP/F, 267

7B2, 265
Banting's cure, 19
Bardet Biedl syndrome, 234

Bariatric gastric surgery
  glucose tolerance, 910
Basal lipolysis
  visceral adipose tissue (VAT), 594
Basal metabolic rate (BMR), 341, 618–621, 631–632
  nutrient partitioning, 755
Basophilic adenomas
  pituitary gland, 17
BAT (*see* Brown adipose tissue (BAT))
BDI, 1008, 1015
Beacon, 320
Beaumont, William, 12
Beck Depression Inventory (BDI), 1008, 1015
Behavior
  brain, 338–340
  food intake, 427–428
Behavioral neuroscience, 301–343
Behavior generator system, 338
Behavior inhibition system, 338–339
Behavior modification, 20
Behavior reinforcement system, 338–339
  hypothalamic control, 339
Berardinelli-Seip congenital lipodystrophy syndrome, 237
Beta3-adrenergic receptor gene, 885
Beta3-agonists
  diabetes, 909
Beta3-AR knockout mice, 263
Beta blockers
  hypertension and obesity, 889
Beta-casomorphin, 392
BFLS, 234–235
BIA, 64–65
Biguandines
  hypertension and obesity, 889
Bile, 919
  composition of in gallbladder disease, 924–925
Bile acids, 920
Bile acid supplementation
  weight loss, 928
Biliary lipids
  physical chemistry, 920–921
  synthesis and secretion, 919–920
Binge eaters, 340, 1011, 1016–1017
Binge Eating Questionnaire, 1016
Binge Eating Scale, 1016
Biochemistry, 13
Biogenic amines
  eating, 331–336
Bioimpedance analysis (BIA), 64–65
Biological chemistry, 13–14
Birth body size, 109–110
Birth weight
  maternal body weight, 975
Blacks (*see* African-Americans)
Blood, circulation, 12
Blood flow
  visceral adipose tissue (VAT), 597
Blood pressure
  body fat distribution, 876–877
  body mass index, 876–877
  cuff (*see* Compression cuff)
  measurement, 873–874
    equipment, 874
  physical activity, 996–997
  regulation, 873–890
  weight gain, 875
  weight loss, 875–876
BMI (*see* Body mass index (BMI))
B-mode imaging ultrasound, 59
BMR (*see* Basal metabolic rate (BMR))
BNP, 519–520
BOD POD Body Composition System, 46
Body builders
  body mass index, 85
Body composition, 13, 34
  adiposity-related components, 71
  age-related changes, 135–136
  versus body mass index, 780
  ethnic and geographic influences, 81–90
  exercise, 636
  exercising individual, 643
  fetal nutrition, 110–112
  food
    thermic effect, 622
  monographs, 70–71
  physical activity energy cost, 638
  resting metabolic rate (RMR), 619
  substrate oxidation, 717, 722–723
Body fat, 409
  determination, 82
  distribution, 88–89
    diabetes, 903–904
  genetic epidemiology, 161–162
  physical activity, 644
Body fat distribution
  blood pressure, 876–877
  conception, 977
  dyslipidemia, 850–852
  lipid mobilization, 521
  non-insulin-dependent diabetes mellitus (type 2), 901–902
  osteoarthritis, 958–959
Body fat percent, 83, 86
Body image, 1017
  obesity, 1009–1010
  quality of life, 1014
Body mass
  fetal growth, 113–114
  genetic epidemiology, 161–162
Body mass index (BMI), 39, 85, 120
  adiposity measures, 773–774

[Body mass index (BMI)]
  blood pressure, 876–877
  versus body composition, 780
  cardiorespiratory fitness, 989
  cutoff points, 86–88
  inheritance, 15
  major gene, 162
  mortality, 986
  optimal mortality, 813–815
  predictive value, 158
  versus total body fat, 70
Body size
  birth, 109–110
Body weight
  dopamine, 335
  measurement, 38–40
  physical activity energy cost, 638
Body weight loss, 322
Bombesin, 262–263, 329, 389
Borjeson-Forssman-Lehmann syndrome (BFLS), 234–235
Boyle, Robert, 13
Brain and behavior, 338–340
Brain areas, 305–306
Brain insulin
  energy balance, 469–470
Brain insulin hypothesis, 462
Brain natriuretic peptides (BNP), 519–520
Brain pathways
  peripheral signals, 466
Brain transport
  leptin, 473–475
Brazil, 97
Breast cancer, 796, 818
Breastfeeding and pediatric obesity, 125
Brown adipose tissue (BAT), 258
  apoptosis, 481
  in white fat depots, 541–542
BRS3 gene, 204
Bulimia, 340, 1015–1016
Burnout
  cortisol, 793–794
1-butyrylglycerol, 483

Calcium blockers
  hypertension and obesity, 889
Calipers, 59
Callipyge locus, 204
Caloric partitioning
  leptin deficiency, 216–217
Caloric restriction
  diabetes, 908
Calorie intake in elderly, 138
CAMP-elevating agents, 497
Canada, 95
Canadians
  non-insulin-dependent diabetes mellitus (type 2), 900
Cancer, 818–819
  physical activity, 994
Candidate genes, 15
  linkages, 176
  markers, 170–171
  primates, 284
Carbacyclin, 497
Carbohydrate, 443–445
  satiety, 439
Carbohydrate intake
  glucose oxidation, 718
Carbohydrate metabolism, 264–265
  endocrine control, 758–759
  nutrient partitioning, 756
Carbon, 34
Carboxypeptidase E, 225–226, 258–259
Carboxypeptidase H, 258–259
Cardiac output
  euglycemic hyperinsulinemia, 881–882
Cardiac structure and function, 825–827
  weight loss, 828–829
Cardiorespiratory fitness, 987–989
Cardiovascular disease, 815–817, 984
  physical activity, 993
Cardiovascular risk factors, 88, 887–888
Cardiovascular system, 825–834
CART, 323–324
Casomorphin, 392
Catecholamines, 523–525
  body fat distribution, 673–674
CCAAT enhancer-binding proteins (CEBP), 267
CCK (*see* Cholecystokinin (CCK))
CCKAR gene, 204
CEBP, 267
CEBP gene, 204
Cell surface receptors, 496
CETP, 600
Chaucer, 18
Chemical carcass analyses, 81
Chemistry, 13
Children
  feeding practice in pediatric obesity, 125
  overweight, secular trends, 122
  total body fat, multicomponent measurement, 49
  type 2 diabetes mellitus, 117
Chinese, 102–103
  bioelectrical impedance, 85
  medicine, 4–5
    body composition, 83
  non-insulin-dependent diabetes mellitus (type 2), 900
  pharmacopeia, 5
Cholecystokinin (CCK), 227–228, 262, 303, 310, 328–329, 388, 396, 473
  receptors, 227–228, 436–437
Cholelithiasis
  body mass index, 814

Cholesterol, 919–920
  mortality, 986
  nucleation, 921–922
  osteoarthritis, 958
Cholesterol crystals
  growth into stones, 922
Cholesterol ester transfer protein (CETP), 600
Cholesterol gallstones
  pathogenesis, 919–922
Ciliary neurotropic factor (CNTF), 322, 393
Cinchona bark (quinine), 5
Cinephotography, 633
Circulating factors, 437
Circulating glucocorticoid
  leptin, 471–473
Circulation, blood, 12
Circumference measurement, 59
Circumference ratios, problems, 61
Clinical medicine, 16
Clinical practice
  physical activity, 999–1000
CNTF, 322, 393
Cocaine-and amphetamine-regulated transcript (CART), 323–324
Cognitive behavioral therapy
  OSA, 942–943
Cold exposure and energy expenditure, 712–713
Cold intolerance and leptin deficiency, 216
Colipase, 392
Colon cancer, 818
Component field measurement
  total body fat, 59–65
Component reference methods, 40–59
Compression cuff, 874
  bladder dimensions, 874
  blood pressure measurement, 873–874
Computed tomography, 49–52
Conception, body fat distribution, 977
Confounding deaths, 768
Congenital disorder of glycosylation type 1a, 235
Congenital malformations, 820
Congestive heart failure, 827–828
Congresses, 23
Conicity index, 61
Continuous crossed-circulated rats, 394
Converting enzymes, 265–266
Copernicus, 6
Coronary artery disease, 907
Coronary heart disease, 816–817, 831–833
  body mass index, 814
  deaths, 112
  dyslipidemic phenotypes, 845–850
  growth, 112
  insulin resistance/metabolic syndrome, 850
  physical activity, 993–994
  relative risks, 815
[Coronary heart disease]
  visceral adipose tissue (VAT), 860–864
  weight loss, 833
Corpulency, 22
CORT (*see* Corticosterone (CORT))
Corticoids, 225
Corticosterone (CORT), 301
  hypothalamic peptides, 309
  insulin, 309
  leptin, 309
Corticotropin-releasing factor (CRF), 487
Corticotropin-releasing hormone (CRH), 301, 324–325
Cortisol, 657
  burnout, 793–794
  metabolic syndrome, 789–791
  stress, 799
  visceral adipose tissue (VAT), 597–598
Cortisone-cortisol interconversion
  visceral adipose tissue (VAT), 599–600
CPE
  secretory pathway, 226
CPE^{fat} mutation, 225
CPE gene, 204
Creoles
  non-insulin-dependent diabetes mellitus (type 2), 900
CRF, 487
CRH, 301, 324–325
CRH/urocortin-glucocorticoid system, 262
Crossed-circulated rats
  challenges, 394
  gut nerve sections, 393–397
  interpretation difficulties, 395
  results, 396
Crossed-intestines experiments
  limitation, 386
Cuba, 97
Cuff, blood pressure (*see* Compression cuff)
Culture
  obesity prevalence, 105–106
Cushing's syndrome, 17, 487, 658, 790
  body fat distribution, 679
  visceral adipose tissue (VAT), 597–598
Cyclo(His-Pro), 331
Cyproheptadine, 17
Cytokines, 263, 322–323
  food intake, 393
  metabolic syndrome, 792

DAG, 741
DALY, 149
DBH gene, 205
Deep vein thrombosis, 817
Dehydroepiandrosterone (DHEA), 658
  elderly, 142–143
2-deoxyglucose (2-DG), 407

Depression, 1007–1008, 1012
hypothalamic-pituitary-adrenal axis dysregulation, 791
Dexamethasone suppression, 793
Dexfenfluramine, 833–834
Dextroamphetamine, 15
2-DG, 407
Dgat, 264
DGAT gene, 205
DHEA, 658
elderly, 142–143
DHT, 680
Diabetes
daily food intake in rats, 391
exercise, 906
free fatty acids, 903
gallbladder disease, 922
infertility and weight, 977
insulin resistance, 902
leptin, 909
macrovascular disease risk, 906–907
obesity, 899–910
management, 907–910
Pima Indians, 905–906
pregnancy, 976–977
severity in rodents, 258
visceral adipose tissue (VAT), 903–904
Diabetes allele
identification, 221
Diabetes mellitus
abdominal obesity, 283
sex hormone-binding globulin (SHBG)
women, 795
Diacylglycerol (DAG), 741
Diacylglycerol acyl transferase (Dgat), 264
Diaphragm, stretched, 937
Diastolic blood pressure, abdominal circumference, 877
Diazoxide, 682
Diet, 17–18, 18
adipose tissue cellularity, 490–491
composition
feeding behavior, 440–451
exercise
visceral adipose tissue (VAT), 602–603
gout, 961–962
resting metabolic rate (RMR), 619–620
18th century, 18
Dietary composition
food, thermic effect of, 621–622
Dietary factors in gallbladder disease, 923
Dietary fat
substrate oxidation, 722
thermic effect, 622
Dietary intake, misreporting of, 430
Dietary practice
pediatric obesity, 125
Dietary restraint, 1016–1017
Dietary Restraint Scale, 1016
Dietary weight loss studies in the elderly, 141
Diet composition and food intake, 427–454
Diet-induced obesity, 450
Diet-induced thermogenesis, 714
Dieting, 1010
Digestion, 12
Digit preference, 874
Dihydrotestosterone (DHT), 680
Dilution techniques, 82
Dinitrophenol, 15
Dionysius, 5
Direct calorimetry, 615
Direct costs, 150
cost centers, 154
Disability-adjusted life years (DALY), 149
Disinhibited eating, 1010, 1016
Disturbed eating, 1015–1016
Divine Farmer, 5
Dopamine, 205, 263, 304, 333–336
body weight, 335
hypothalamus, 334
mesolimbic system, 334–335
neurotransmitter release, 335–336
taste reactions, 335
Dorsomedial nucleus (DMN), 305
Doubly labeled water technique, 615–616, 634–635
Douglas bags, 633–634
Dual-energy X-ray absorptiometry (DXA), 47–49
Dutch Eating Behavior Questionnaire, 1016
DXA, 47–49
Dyslipidemia
body fat distribution, 850–852
elderly, 139
spontaneous obesity, 283
visceral adipose tissue (VAT), 852–857, 860–864
cause-effect relationship, 857–860
Dyslipidemic phenotypes
coronary heart disease, 845–850
Dyslipoproteinemias
physical activity, 997–998
Dyspnea, 937

Eastern Mediterranean, 101–102
Eating
biogenic amines, 331–336
disturbed patterns, 1010
hormones, 306–311
peptides, 311–321
Eating behavior, 1015–1016
Eating Behavior Inventory (EBI), 1016
Eating behavior or fuel intake
food intake, 428–429
Eating Disorder Examination, 1015–1016
Eating Inventory, 1016

Eating reduction
  peptides, 321–331
Ebers papyrus, 4
EBI, 1016
Ebstein's diet, 19–20
Economic costs, 149–155
  study requirements, 154–155
  study comparisons, 152–154
  types, 150
Education and exercise, 636
Edwin Smith papyrus, 4
EGF, 499
Egyptian medicine, 4
Elderly, total body fat, multicomponent measurement, 49
Electrocardiogram, 829
Endocrine obesity, 269
Endometrial cancer, 796, 818
Endurance training in the elderly, 142
Energy monitoring, 437
Energy balance, 631
  brain insulin, 469–470
  fuel composition, 720–721
  regulation, 409, 464
  RQ/FQ, 721
  vagotomy, 396
Energy density, 444
  macronutrients, 446
Energy exchange, 34
Energy expenditure, 13, 341
  components, 631–634
  control, 464–465
  daily variability, 715
  elderly, 138
  measurement, 615–618, 616–618, 713–715
  nutrient partitioning, 754–755
  physical activity, 631–646, 714–715
  primates, 287–288
  substrate oxidation, 713–725
  sympathetic nervous systems, 698–700
  uncoupling protein 1 (UCP1), 539–540, 620–621
  weight loss, 625–626
  weight maintenance, 721–722
Energy intake, 34, 447
  food, thermic effect of, 621–622
  tonic control, 440
Energy metabolism
  lactation, 970–973
  pregnancy, 970
Energy turnover
  free-living subjects, 713–714
Enterostatin, 325, 392
Environmental associations
  pediatric obesity, 125–128
Environmental stressors
  hypothalamic-pituitary-adrenal axis dysregulation, 791
Ephedra, 834
Epidemic, explanation of, 103–106
Epidemiology, 768–774
Epidermal growth factor (EGF), 499
Epinephrine and resting metabolic rate (RMR), 620
Esophageal fistula, 378–380
Estimation errors, 65–66
Estradiol, 301
Estradiol alpha-receptor, 264
Estrogen, 264, 680
  body fat distribution, 675
  glucose metabolism, 759
  lipid metabolism, 757
  metabolism, 660
  protein metabolism, 760
Estrogen receptors in adipose tissue, 487
Estrogen replacement therapy and adipose tissue, 487
Ethanol, thermic effect of, 622
Ethnicity
  body composition, 88
  body mass index, 88
  fat distribution, 137
  pediatric obesity, 121
  pregnancy
    weight gain, 978
  quality of life, 1011
  sympathetic nervous systems, 885
Euglycemic clamp studies
  whole-body glucose uptake, 880
Euglycemic hyperinsulinemia
  cardiac output, 881–882
  glucose uptake, 879
Euglycemic insulin infusion
  systolic blood pressure, 884–885
Europe, 98–101, 99
Exercise, 17–18, 413, 632
  age, 636
  amount performed, 635
  body composition, 636
  diabetes, 906
  duration, 641–642
  education, 636
  energy cost, 633–634
  gender, 636
  genetics, 636
  hypertension
    obesity, 889
  intensity, 641
  intraabdominal fat mass, 142
  lipid mobilization, 521
  metabolic cost, 637
  nature and duration quantification, 632–635
  nutrient partitioning, 753–754
  retrospective survey, 632–633
  visceral adipose tissue (VAT), 601–602
Exercise tolerance, 938

Exercise training
  elderly, 141–142
  work efficiency, 639
Exercising individual
  age, 643
  body composition, 643
  characteristics, 642–643
  gender, 642–643
Experimental science, 21–22
Extracellular matrix, 499
Extraordinary obesity, 16–17

Factorial method, 634
Familial partial lipodystrophy dunnigan (FPLD), 237–238
Family history and body mass index, 776–777
Famine, 110
Fascia lata, 736
Fasting and Agouti gene-related peptide, 212–213
Fat, 445–446, 452
  mimetics, 452
  oxidation
    inhibition, 412
  satiety, 439
Fat balance, control of, 465
Fat deposits, 590
  neck, 940
Fat distribution
  classification, 93–94
  endocrine determinants, 671–686
  racial/ethnic characteristics, 137
Fat-free mass (FFM), 81
  age-related changes, 136
  hydration, 35–36
  mortality rate, 774
Fat intake
  fat oxidation, 718–719
Fat mass (FM), 81
  mortality rate, 774
Fat mouse, 258–259
Fat mutation, 225–226
  defective neuropeptide processing, 226
Fat oxidation
  elderly, 138
  fat intake, 718–719
Fat paradox, 446
Fat-sugar seesaw, 445
Fatty acid metabolism in skeletal muscle, 742–745
Fatty acids, 498
  selective mobilization, 517–518
  visceral adipose tissue (VAT), 596
Fatty mutation, 223–224
Fatty oxidation in skeletal muscle, 740–741
Feeding behavior, 432
  diet composition, 440–451
  physiology, 431
  uncoupling protein1 (UCP1), 543–544
Feeding-related circuits
  acetylcholine, 336–337
  amino acids, 337–338
Female hypogonadism and body fat distribution, 679
Fenfluramine, 15, 833–834, 943
Fertility, 682
Fetal growth
  adult body mass, 113–114
  obesity-related disease, 112–113
Fetal nutrition and body composition, 110–112
FFM (*see* Fat-free mass (FFM))
FGF, 331, 499
FGF13 gene, 205
Fibrinolysis and visceral adipose tissue (VAT), 600
Fibroblast growth factor (FGF), 499
Filipinos, diet and gout, 962
Finnish families, 174
Fluoxetene, 834
FM, 81
  mortality rate, 774
Food
  gastrointestinal components, 436–437
  orosensory components, 436
Food addiction models, 339–340
Food consumption, 428–429
Food delivery in the small intestine, 385
Food influences, appetite, 441
Food intake
  behavior, 427–428
  control, 464–465
  cytokines, 393
  diet composition, 427–454
  eating behavior or fuel intake, 428–429
  experimental studies, 373–413
  gastrointestinal tracts, 381
  hibernating rodents, 375
  hormones, 387–390
  inflammatory peptides, 393
  internal signals, 373–376
  liver, 400–404
  obesity, 412–413
  palatability factors, 451
  pancreatic hormones, 390–392
  studies
    demand characteristics, 430
    methodological approaches, 429–431
    po2er, sensitivity, effect, 430
    power, sensitivity and effect size, 430
    precision *vs.* naturalness, 429–430
    regulation, 431
    relevant questions, 430–431
  weight maintenance, 721–722
FPLD, 237–238
FRC, 935–936

Free fatty acids in diabetes, 903
Free-living subjects, energy turnover, 713–714
Fuel composition
  energy balance, 720–721
  substrate oxidation, 717
Functional residual capacity (FRC), 935–936

GABA, 263–264
GAL, 303, 313–314
Galanin (GAL), 303, 313–314
Galaninlike peptide, 313–314
Galectin-12, 290
Galen, 5–6, 18
Gallbladder
  motility alterations, 925
  motor function, 921
  mucosal function, 921
Gallbladder cancer, 818
Gallbladder disease, 819
  epidemiology, 922–925
  obesity, 919–929
  relative risks, 815
  risk factors, 922–923
  weight loss, 925–926
Gallstones, 819
  incidence, 925–926
  obesity, 923–924
  prevention, 927–928
  prophylactic cholecystectomy, 927–928
  risk factors, 926
  during weight loss
    pathophysiology, 926–927
Gamma-aminobutyric acid (GABA), 263–264
Gas exchange, 936–937
Gastric bypass surgery, OSA, 943
Gastric emptying, 380
  rats, 381
Gastric fistula, 378–380
Gastric inhibitory peptide (GIP), 387, 388, 390
Gastric theory, limitation of, 383
Gastroesophageal reflux disease, 946
Gastrointestinal tracts
  food intake, 381
  signals, 377–378
GDF8 gene, 208
Gender
  exercise, 636
  exercising individual, 642–643
  food, thermic effect of, 622
  quality of life, 1011
  visceral adipose tissue (VAT), 592–593, 854
  work efficiency, 639–640
Gene-environment, 176–181
Gene-gene interactions, 176–181
Gene-gene interations, 162
Gene knockout models, 254–256, 260–267
Genes
  location, 183–185
  symbols, 183–185
Genetic epidemiological model-fitting, 181
Genetic epidemiology, 159–168
  findings, 161–168
  methods, 160–170
    combined models, 161
    major gene, 161
    multifactorial, 160–161
Genetics, 14–15, 157–170
  environmental interactions, 724–725
  exercise, 636
  lipolysis, 525–526
  metabolic syndrome, 800–803
  primates, 284–287
  resting metabolic rate (RMR), 620
  visceral adipose tissue (VAT), 598
  work efficiency, 639
Genetic susceptibility, 176
Genome scans
  studies, 172–173
Genomewide explorations, 181–182
Genomewide scans
  linkages, 171–175
Genotype-environment interactions, 176–181
  findings, 179–181
  method, 176–179
  recommendations, 181–183
Geriatric obesity, 135–143
  causes, 137–138
  consequences, 138–140
    functional, 139–140
    metabolic, 138–139
  prevalence, 135–137
  treatment, 140–143
    drug, 142–143
Gestational diabetes, 820
GFAT, 265
Ghrelin, 319–320, 382, 662–663
  body fat distribution, 676
GHRH (*see* Growth hormone-releasing hormone (GHRH)
GHRP, 319
GHS and body fat distribution, 676
GIP, 387, 388, 390
Gi-protein-coupled receptors, 518–519
Glargine and diabetes, 908–909
Glitazones and diabetes, 908
GLP-1 (*see* Glucagonlike peptide 1 (GLP-1))
GLP-2, 398
Glucagon, 327, 390
Glucagonlike peptide 1 (GLP-1), 327–328, 387, 389, 390, 398
  diabetes, 909
Glucocorticoid receptor
  peroxisome proliferator-activated receptor gamma
      (PPAR-gamma), 565–566

Glucocorticoids, 497
adipose tissue, 486–487
body fat distribution, 674
fat distribution, 684–685
glucose metabolism, 759
lipid metabolism, 757–758
nutrient partitioning, 762–763
obesity, 799
protein metabolism, 760–761
Glucose and osteoarthritis, 958
Glucose-induced thermogenesis, 622
Glucose intolerance
gallbladder disease, 922
leptin deficiency, 216
Glucose metabolism
estrogen, 759
glucocorticoids, 759
growth hormone, 758
insulin, 758
testosterone, 758–759
Glucose oxidation and carbohydrate intake, 718
Glucose tolerance and physical activity, 994–995
Glucose transporters, 264–265, 310–311
Glucose uptake
euglycemic hyperinsulinemia, 879
visceral adipose tissue (VAT), 595
Glucostatic theory, 404–405
Glucuronic acid, 682
GLUT4, 488, 657
Glut4, 264–265
Glutamine: fructose-6-phosphate amidotransferase (GFAT), 265
Glycerol, 408
Glycerol dehydrogenase (GPDH), 265
Glycogen, 42
Glycolytic enzyme profiles of skeletal muscle, 739–740
GNAS1 gene, 205
GnRH, 310–311
Go-coupled receptors, tubby mutation, 227
Gonadal steroid hormones, 310
Gonadotrophin-releasing hormone (GnRH), 310–311
Gout and obesity, 960–963
longitudinal studies, 961
GPC3 gene, 205
GPC4 gene, 205
GPDH, 265
G protein alpha subunit, 266
G-protein-coupled receptors, 518
Greco-Roman medicine, 5–6
Growth and coronary heart disease, 112
Growth hormone, 263, 498, 520, 661–662
adipose tissue, 486
body fat distribution, 676
elderly, 142
fat distribution, 683
glucose metabolism, 758
[Growth hormone]
lipid metabolism, 756–757
nutrient partitioning, 761–762
protein metabolism, 760
visceral adipose tissue (VAT), 597
Growth hormone deficiency and body fat distribution, 679
Growth hormone-releasing hormone (GHRH), 310–311, 318–319, 382
gene, 206
Growth hormone-releasing peptides (GHRP), 319
Growth hormone secretagogues (GHS) and body fat distribution, 676
Gs-protein-coupled receptors, 518
Gut nerve sections in crossed-circulated rats, 393–397
Gut-related peptide hormones, 392–393
Gynoid obesity, 168, 851, 901

Hand, osteoarthritis of and obesity, 955–956
Harvey, William, 12
HDL, 283
Health outcomes
obesity, 984
physical activity, 984–985
Heart rate
high-fat diet, 875
24-hour energy expenditure, 713
Hepatic vagotomy, 404
Herbal weight loss aids, 834
HERITAGE family study, 174–175
Hibernating rodents and food intake, 375
High blood pressure (*see* Hypertension)
High-carbohydrate foods, 444
High fat content, 413
overeating, 412
High-fat diet, 875
with sedentary lifestyle
substrate oxidation, 722–723
High sympathetic tone, 341
Hip, osteoarthritis of and obesity, 956–957
Hispanics, fat distribution, 137
Histamine, 263, 304, 336
Histology, 6
Hmgic, 267
HMGIC gene, 206
Holland, diet and gout, 961
Hormones, 260–264, 301–303, 680–685
abbreviations, 302
eating, 306–311
food intake, 387–390
metabolic syndrome, 788–789
substrate oxidation, 723
visceral adipose tissue (VAT), 597–598
Hormone-sensitive lipase (HSL), 264, 515, 517, 672
differences, 522–523
gene expression, 518

24-hour energy expenditure
  heart rate, 713
  metabolic chambers, 713
HPA (*see* Hypothalamic-pituitary-adrenal (HPA) axis)
HSL (*see* Hormone-sensitive lipase (HSL))
5HT, metabolic syndrome, 801–803
Human genetic obesities without mouse homologs, 233–238
Humans, leptin, biological activity of, 467–468
Human single-gene obesities, 228–233
Hunger and quality of life, 1014
Hunger state, 434–435
Hydrodensitometry plethysmography, 45–46
Hydrometry, 43–45
Hydrotherapy, 15
3-hydroxybutyrate, 407
Hyperandrogenicity in women, 794–796
Hypercapnia, 940
Hypercholesterolemia, relative risks of, 815
Hypercortisolemia, 886–887
Hyperglycemia in mice, 224–225
Hyperinsulinemia, 877–878, 906–907
  chronic sodium retention, 879–880
Hyperphagia, 15, 215–216, 444, 656
Hypertension, 826–827
  atrial natriuretic peptides, 885
  body mass index, 814
  elderly, 139
  leptin, 886
  metabolic syndrome, 796–799
  obesity, 874–877
    epidemiological studies, 874–875
    hypothalamic origins, 886–887
    ion transport, 882–883
    management, 888–889
    mechanism, 877–887
    vascular structure and function, 881–882
  osteoarthritis, 957
  physical activity, 996–997
  pregnancy, 820
  prevalence, 877
  relative risks, 815
  skeletal muscle, 882
  sympathetic nervous systems, 884–885
Hyperthyroidism, 620
Hypertriglyceridemic waist, 861–864
Hyperuricemia, 960, 961
Hypothalamic control, reinforcement system, 339
Hypothalamic hypogonadism and leptin deficiency, 217
Hypothalamic obesity, 268–269
Hypothalamic peptides
  corticosterone (CORT), 309
Hypothalamic-pituitary-adrenal (HPA) axis, 487
  fat distribution, 684–685
  metabolic syndrome, 790–792, 802–803
Hypothalamus
  dopamine, 334
  lesions, 374
Hypothyroidism, 485
Hypoxia, 940

ICAM-1, 267
IDED-IV, 1016
IFN-alpha, 393
IGF (*see* Insulinlike growth factor (IGF))
IL-1, 322, 393
IL-6 (*see* Interleukin (IL)-6)
IL-1b, 393
  converting enzyme, 265
Imaging, 49–56
Imhotep, 4
Impact of weight on quality of life, 1005
Inactivity in the elderly, 138
Incas, 5
Indapaminde, hypertension and obesity, 889
India
  non-insulin-dependent diabetes mellitus (type 2), 900
Indian medicine, 5
Indian Ocean islanders
  non-insulin-dependent diabetes mellitus (type 2), 900
Indirect calorimetry, 615, 616–618, 633–634, 713
Indirect costs, 150
Indonesians
  bioelectrical impedance, 85
Infant feeding and obesity, 111–112
Infants, adipose tissue in, 485
Infertility
  leptin deficiency, 217
  weight, 977
Inflammatory peptides and food intake, 393
Innervation and visceral adipose tissue (VAT), 597
Institute of Medicine (IOM) pregnancy recommendations, 975–976
Insulin, 306, 391, 464–465, 473, 497–498
  adipose tissue, 486
  body fat distribution, 521, 672–673
  brain transport, 466
  corticosterone (CORT), 309
  glucose metabolism, 758
  hypertension
    metabolic syndrome, 798
  interaction, 470–471
  lipid metabolism, 756
  lipid oxidation, 744
  Na-K-ATPase, 882–883
  nutrient partitioning, 761
  obesity, 656–657
  peroxisome proliferator-activated receptor gamma (PPAR-gamma), 569–571
  protein metabolism, 759–760
  renin-angiotensin system, 883–884

[Insulin]
  resistance, 283
  substrate oxidation, 717, 723
  visceral adipose tissue (VAT), 594–595
Insulin-dependent diabetes mellitus (type1), 899
Insulinlike growth factor (IGF), 262, 483, 497–498, 661–662
  adipose tissue, 486
  fat distribution, 683
Insulin-mediated glucose transport, 883
Insulinoma, 797
Insulinopenia in mice, 224–225
Insulin receptors, 290, 902
Insulin resistance
  chronic sodium retention, 879–880
  diabetes, 902
  elderly, 138
  hypertension
    obesity, 877–878
  metabolic syndrome, 788
  physical activity, 994–995
  skeletal muscle, 881–882
  tumor necrosis factor-alpha (TNF-alpha), 904–905
Insulin resistance/metabolic syndrome
  coronary heart disease, 850
Insulin resistance syndrome, 848–849
Insulin-resistant glucose metabolism, 745–747
Insulin secretion
  diabetes, 905–906
Insulin-suppressed fatty acids in type 2 diabetes, 747
Intangible costs, 150
Interferon-alpha (IFN-alpha), 393
Interleukin (IL)-1, 322, 393
Interleukin (IL)-6, 322
  body fat distribution, 677
  metabolic syndrome, 792
  visceral adipose tissue (VAT), 599–600
Interleukin (IL)-1b, 393
  converting enzyme, 265
Internal signals
  food intake, 373–376
  types, 376–377
International Diabetes Institute, 103
International Journal of Obesity, 23
Interpersonal consequences
  obesity, 1008–1009
Interview for Diagnosis of Eating Disorders, fourth version (IDED-IV), 1016
Intestines
  meal termination, 386
  signals, 384–387
  stomach emptying, 381
Intra-abdominal fat mass and exercise, 142
Intracellular adhesion molecule 1 (ICAM-1), 267
In vivo lipolysis and visceral adipose tissue (VAT), 595
IOM pregnancy recommendations, 975–976

Japanese-Americans
  fat distribution, 137
  gallbladder disease, 923
  visceral adipose tissue (VAT), 904
Japanese school children, 119
JDCA
  weight loss, 928
Jejunoileal bypass surgery, 397
Journals, 23

Kidney cancer, 818
Kinematic measurements, 633
KK mice, 260
Klinefelter syndrome, 682
Knee, osteoarthritis of and obesity, 953–955
Korotkoff sounds, 874

Lactation
  energy metabolism, 970–973
  lifestyle trends, 973–975
Laxatives, 15
LDL, 283, 907
LDL cholesterol, 845–849
Left ventricular hypertrophy, 827
Leg respiratory quotient, fasting values, 743
Leisure time physical activity (LTPA)
  secular trends, 644–645
LEP Arg105Trp C, 229–230
LEP G398, 228–229
LEP gene, 206
LEP mutations, 229
LEPR (*see* Leptin receptor (LEPR))
Leptin, 14, 215–220, 284–287, 306–308, 383, 410–411, 440, 461–463, 464–465, 473, 657
  Agouti gene-related peptide, 212–213
  biological activity, 466–467
  body fat distribution, 676–677
  brain transport, 466, 473–475
  cardiovascular effects, 886
  cells mediating, 224
  circulating, 218
  circulating glucocorticoid, 471–473
  corticosterone (CORT), 309
  deficiency, 215–216
  diabetes, 909
  expression, 218
  gene, 411–412
  human biological activity, 467–468
  hypertension, 886
    metabolic syndrome, 798
  interaction, 470–471
  melanocortin, 472–473
  metabolic syndrome, 801
  mice, 217
  neuroendocrine system interaction, 473
  NPY, 471

[Leptin]
outside brain, 219–220
reduced brain responsiveness, 469
regulation, 217–218
resistance, 269
resting energy expenditure, 621
rodent biological activity, 466–467
visceral adipose tissue (VAT), 598
Leptin receptor (LEPR), 220–225, 222, 230, 468–469
alleles, 222–223
extinct mutations, 223–224
gene, 207
genomic structure, 221
isoforms, 221–222
Leukemia inhibitory factor (LIF), 497
Level gene, 178
LH, 301
LHRH, 301
LIF, 497
Lifestyle changes, 103–105
Lifestyle physical activity (LSPA)
secular trends, 644–645
Linkage phenotypes, 177
Linkage studies, 171
Lipectomy, 488–489
Lipid, 311
defined, 35
physical activity, 997–998
Lipid metabolism
endocrine control, 756–758
estrogen, 757
genes, 264–267
glucocorticoids, 757–758
growth hormone, 756–757
insulin, 756
nutrient partitioning, 755–756
peroxisome proliferator-activated receptor gamma (PPAR-gamma), 572
skeletal muscle in weight loss, 745
testosterone, 757
Lipid mobilization, 515–527
body fat distribution, 521
Lipid-mobilizing factor (LMF), 520
Lipid oxidation and insulin, 744
Lipid signaling in skeletal muscle, 741–742
Lipin, 266
Lipodystrophies
visceral adipose tissue (VAT), 600
Lipodystrophy syndromes with single-gene basis, 237
Lipogenesis in adipose tissue, 671–672
Lipolysis, 515–527
adipose tissue, 672
basal rate, 522
control, 516
dysregulation, 522–525
genetics, 525–526
[Lipolysis]
hormonal control, 518–520
regulation, 755–756
in vivo regulation, 520–522
Lipolytic agonists
visceral adipose tissue (VAT), 594
Lipoprotein lipase (LPL), 409, 494, 671
visceral adipose tissue (VAT), 596
Lipoprotein metabolism, 845–864
overview, 846
Lipostatic hypothesis, 412
Lipostatic regulation, 438
Lipostatic theory, 408
Liver, 437
food intake, 400–404
signals, 400–404
Liver disease, 819
LMF, 520
Long-chain fatty acids
adipose tissue, 487–488
Longitudinal assessment, 160
Long-term energy balance feedback
nutrient stores, 438–440
Low-birth weight, 110
Low energy expenditure, 697–698
Lower body fat, 168
Lower gut signals, 397–400
Low parasympathetic tone, 341
Low sympathetic tone, 341–342
LPL (*see* Lipoprotein lipase (LPL))
LSPA, secular trends, 644–645
LTPA, secular trends, 644–645
Lung volume, 940
Luteinizing hormone (LH), 301
Luteinizing hormone-releasing hormone (LHRH), 301
Lysophosphatidic acid, 497–498

Macaca, 281
Macaca fascicularis, 283
Macaca mulatta, 284
Macaca nemestrina, 284
Macronutrients, 441–447, 449–541
energy density, 446
Macrophage colony-stimulating factor (MCSF)
adipose tissue, 485
Magas, 5
Magnetic resonance imaging, 52–56
protocol, 55
reliability studies, 54
software, 53
validation studies, 54
Mahoganoid, 203
Mahoganoid gene, 261
Mahogany, 203
Mahogany gene, 261
Major gene, 161

Male hypogonadism and body fat distribution, 679
Males, sex hormones, 682–683
Malignancies and adipose tissue, 492
Malnourished children, 442
M amylin, 329–330
Maori and gout, 960
Massively obesity, 16–17
Maternal body weight and birth weight, 975
Mayans, 5
Mayer's glucostatic theory, 341
MCH, 262, 316–317
MCH gene, 207
MC3R, 215
MC4R, 215, 230–231
MC4R gene, 207, 213
MCSF and adipose tissue, 485
Meal termination in intestines, 386
Mean arterial pressure related to high-fat diet, 875
Medial hypothalamus, 305
Medial preoptic area (MPO), 305
Medical Outcomes Study Short-Form Health Survey (SF-36), 1005–1006
Medroxyprogesterone, 944
Melanesian Indians, gout, 960
Melanin concentrating hormone (MCH), 262, 316–317
Melanocortin, 321–322
  leptin, 472–473
Melanocortin system, 260–261
Melanocyte stimulating hormone (MSH), 303, 543
Menarche, 659
Menopause, 137
  weight development, 970
Menstrual abnormalities, 659
Menstrual cycle and thermic effect of food, 622
Mercaptoacetate, 407
Meso-American medicine, 5
Mesolimbic system and dopamine, 334–335
Mesopotamian medicine, 4
Metabolic chambers and 24-hour energy expenditure, 713
Metabolic disturbances and visceral adipose tissue (VAT), 852–855
Metabolic efficiency
  energy expenditure, 711–712
Metabolic genes, 264–267
Metabolic signals, 404–408
Metabolic syndrome, 605–606, 787–805
  aromatase, 800–801
  cortisol, 789–791
  defined, 787–789
  elderly, 138
  genetics, 800–803
  hypertension, 796–799
  hypothalamic-pituitary-adrenal axis, 790–792
  hypothalamic-pituitary-adrenal (HPA) axis, 802–803
  leptin, 801
  normal LDL cholesterol, 849–850
[Metabolic syndrome]
  obesity, 799–800
  physiological elements, 792–793
  POMC gene, 801
  serotonin (5HT), 801–803
Metabolism, 12
Metabolites, 498
Metallothionein I, 266
Metallothionein II, 266
Metformin
  diabetes, 908
  hypertension and obesity, 889
Metroprolol and hypertension in obesity, 889
Mexican-Americans
  anthropometry, 69
  beta3-adrenergic receptor gene, 885
  diabetes, 901
  hypertension prevalence, 877
  mortality rate, 776
MGL, 516
Mice
  hyperglycemia, 224–225
  insulinopenia, 224–225
  leptin, 217
  leptin receptor (LEPR)
    alleles, 222–223
Micellar cholesterol transport, 921
Michaelis-Menten kinetics, 739
Micronutrients, 447
Microscopic anatomy, 6
Minnesota Multiphasic Personality Inventory, 1015
Minute ventilation, 937
MKKS gene, 207
Molecular biology, 14–15
Molecular genetics, single gene mutations, 201–238
Molecular markers, 168–177
Monkeys
  adiposity measurement, 282–283
  gastric emptying, 381
Monoglyceride lipase (MGL), 516
Monographs
  body composition, 70–71
  obesity, 22
Mood
  assessment, 1015
  weight loss, 1012–1014
Mortality, 813–815, 986
  elderly, 139
  voluntary weight fluctuation in elderly, 140–141
  weight loss, 778–779
Mortality rate, 767–781
  fat-free mass, 774
  fat mass, 774
  potential moderators, 774–779
  recent weight loss, 777
Mother Goddess figurines, 3

Moth1 gene, 227
MPO, 305
MSH, 303, 543
Multicomponent measurement of total body fat, 49
Multiple genes, 162, 267–268
Multiple sensory cues, 432
Multivariate assessment, 160–161
Muscle composition in computed tomography, 51
Muscle sympathetic nerve activity, thermic effect of food, 623
MY09A gene, 207
MYOD1 gene, 208

Na-K-ATPase
  insulin, 882–883
NASH, 152–153, 819
National Health and Nutrition Examinations Surveys (NHANES), 66
National Institutes of Health, 22–23
National Library of Medicine
  Visible Man, 38
Nationwide Nutritional Survey, 102–103
Native Americans
  non-insulin-dependent diabetes mellitus (type 2), 900
Natriuretic peptides, 519–520
N-cells, 397
Neck, fat deposits in, 940
NEFA, 515
Negative energy balance experiments
  genotype-environment interactions, 180–181
Neolithic artifacts, 2
Nerve activity in sympathetic nervous system, 696
Nervous system, 431
Netherlands, 99
Neurochemicals, 303–309
  abbreviations, 302
Neuromedin U, 329
Neuropeptide systems, 260–264
Neuropeptide Y (NPY), 261, 303, 311–313, 662–663
  Agouti gene-related peptide (AGRP), 213–214
  leptin, 471
Neuroscience, 15–16
Neurotensin, 325–326, 389, 397
Neurotransmitter release
  dopamine, 335–336
  sympathetic nervous systems, 696–697
Neurotransmitters, 263–264
Neutron activation analysis in vivo, 41
NHANES, 66
Nhlh2 gene, 208, 267
Nitric oxide, 520
Noise, 429
Nonalcoholic steatohepatitis (NASH), 152–153, 819
Nonesterified fatty acids (NEFA), 515
Nonexercise activities
  amount performed, 635
  energy cost, 633–634
[Nonexercise activities]
  metabolic cost, 637–638
  nature and duration quantification, 633
Non-Hispanic blacks, anthropometry, 68
Non-Hispanic whites, anthropometry, 67
Nonhuman primate obesity
  diet, food intake, activity, energy expenditure, 282
  prevention, 291
Non-insulin-dependent diabetes mellitus (type 2), 100, 899
  body fat distribution, 901–902
  body mass index, 814
  children, 117
  elderly, 138
  global epidemic, 900–901
  insulin-suppressed fatty acids, 747
  physical activity, 994–996
  Pima Indians, 977
  relative risks, 815
  skeletal muscle lipid content, 737–738
Noninvasive ventilation, 944–945
Nonmicellar cholesterol transport, 920
Norepinephrine, 304, 331–332
Normal LDL cholesterol
  metabolic syndrome, 849–850
Novel uncoupling proteins (UCP), 545–557
  biochemical studies, 546–547
  genetic studies, 547–548
  physiological and pathophysiological studies, 548–549
  transgenic mice, 549–550
NPY (*see* Neuropeptide Y (NPY))
NPY/NYPR gene, 208
Nuclear receptors, 496
Nutrient flux, monitoring of, 437
Nutrient partitioning, 753–763
  endocrine control, 756–761
  endocrine influences, 754
  energy expenditure, 754–755
  exercise, 753–754
  fuel processing, 755–756
  glucocorticoids, 762–763
  growth hormone, 761–762
  insulin, 761
  testosterone, 762
Nutrient receptors, 381
Nutrient stores
  long-term energy balance feedback, 438–440
Nutritional status and thermic effect of food, 622

Obese individuals, anatomical dissection of, 6
Obese personality, 1009
Obese rhesus monkeys, 283
Obesity
  adrenocortical function, 657–658
  after pregnancy, 967–968
  asthma, 945–946
  body image, 1009–1010

[Obesity]
classification, 93–94
cutoff points, 86–88
definition, 86–88
diabetes, 899–910
management, 907–910
endocrine determinants, 655–664
fetal origins, 109–114
food and macronutrient intake, 449–541
food intake, 412–413
gallbladder disease, 919–929
gallstones, 923–924
gout, 960–963
cross-sectional studies, 960–961
longitudinal studies, 961
health outcomes, 984
historical development of, 1–23
hypertension, 874–877
epidemiological studies, 874–875
ion transport, 882–883
management, 888–889
mechanism, 877–887
vascular structure and function, 881–882
infant feeding, 111–112
insulin, 656–657
international classification, 103
interpersonal consequences, 1008–1009
late-onset in rodents, 258
metabolic syndrome, 799–800
monographs, 22
osteoarthritis, 953–960
progression, 959
symptoms and disability, 959
overall quality of life, 1005–1006
pathological alterations, 463
physical activity, 983–1000
recommendations, 998–1000
pregnancy complications, 976
prevalence, 93–106, 105–106
pulmonary function, 935–947
quality of life, 1005–1007
severity and quality of life, 1011
WHO region prevalence, 94–103
women
psychosocial outcomes, 118
Obesity and Weight Regulation, 23
Obesity hypoventilation syndrome (OHS), 940–942
classification, 941
management, 942–945
Obesity Research, 23
Obesity Surgery, 23
Obesity syndromes, 233–238
Ob gene, 410–411
Ob/ob mouse, genetic defect in, 14
Obstructive sleep apnea (OSA) syndrome, 939–940
daytime, 944
[Obstructive sleep apnea (OSA) syndrome]
management, 942–945
medications, 944
noninvasive ventilation, 944
obesity, 939–940
supplemental oxygen, 945
tracheotomy, 944
OHS, 940–942
classification, 941
management, 942–945
Old Order Amish population, 175
One-way crossed intestines, 387
rodents, 375, 383–384
Opioid peptides, 317–318
Opioid reward and eating, 317–318
Opioid reward and feeding
inhibition, 318
Opioid subsystems, 317
Orexin, 262, 315–316
Orlistat
diabetes, 909
visceral adipose tissue (VAT), 605
OSA [*see* Obstructive sleep apnea (OSA) syndrome]
Osteoarthritis, 819
body fat distribution, 958–959
cholesterol, 958
glucose, 958
hand obesity, 955–956
hip obesity, 956–957
hypertension, 957
knee obesity, 953–955
obesity, 953–960
pathogenesis, 957
progression, 959
symptoms and disability, 959
twin studies of obesity, 955
uric acid, 958
weight loss, 959–960
Overall quality of life
assessment, 1014–1015
obesity, 1005–1006
weight loss, 1012
Overconsumption, sensorily induced, 428–429
Overeating, 1016–1017
high fat content, 412
reinforcement systems, 338–340
Overfeeding study, 179–180
Overnutrition, 111
Over-the-counter drugs, cardiovascular effects of, 834
Overweight
children, secular trends, 122
cutoff points, 86–88
development, 124–125
international comparisons, 121
Oxidation and alcohol intake, 720
Oxidative enzyme profiles of skeletal muscle, 739–740

Oxidative phosphorylation
  diet composition, 709–710
  efficiency, 713–717
  energy expenditure, 709–710
  energy reserve maintenance, 710
  futile cycles, 710–711
  glucose conversion to fat, 710
  substrate handling and storage costs, 708–709
Oxygen theory, 13
Oxytocin, 303

Pacific Ocean islanders
  non-insulin-dependent diabetes mellitus (type 2), 900
Palatability factors, 451–453
  food intake, 451
Paleolithic artifacts, 2
Paleolithic Venus figurines, 2
Paleomedicine, 2
Pancreatic hormones and food intake, 390–392
Pancreatic peptide YY, 398
Pancreatic polypeptide, 261
Parabrachial nucleus (PBN), 305
Parasympathetic nervous systems, 340–342
Paraventricular nucleus (PVN), 305
Paris-Lille French Study, 173–174
PBN, 305
PC1 gene, 231–232
PCOS, 660–661, 681, 967
PCSK1 gene, 209, 213
Pediatric obesity, 117–129
  behavioral environment, 125–126
  breastfeeding, 125
  child feeding practice, 125
  definition, 119–120
  dietary practice, 125
  environmental associations, 125–128
  identification, 119–120
  physical activity, 125–126
  physical examination, 125
  prevalence, 120–123
  sedentary behavior, 125–126
  social environment, 128
  weight goals, 120
Pedometers, 633
Peptides
  eating, 311–321
  eating reduction, 321–331
Peptide YY (PYY), 389
Perilipin, 264
Peripheral neuroendocrine signals
  brain integration, 464–465
Peripheral signals
  brain pathways, 466
  central integration
    neuroendocrinology, 463–464
Peripheral vascular disease, 833
Peroxisome proliferator-activated receptor gamma (PPAR-gamma), 489–490, 559–576, 681
  activators, 567–569
  adipocyte apoptosis, 566
  adipocyte differentiation, 563–565
  adipocyte-specific genes, 566–567
  adipogenesis, 561–563
    genetic studies, 571–572
  adipose tissue, 569–571
  atherosclerosis, 572
  gene, 559–560
  2 gene, 209, 213, 232–233
  glucocorticoid receptor, 565–566
  insulin, 569–571
  lipid metabolism, 572
  protein, 559–560
  protein-protein interactions, 572–576
  RNA, 559–560
  signal transducers and activators of transcriptions (STAT), 565–566
  structure, 560–561
  thrifty response, 561–566
  transcription factors, 569–571
Peroxisome proliferator-activated receptors (PPAR), 266–267
  primates, 288–291
Peroxisome proliferator-activated receptors (PPAR) alpha
  receptor and agonists, 288–289
Peroxisome proliferator-activated receptors (PPAR) gamma
  receptor and agonists, 289–290
Personal costs, 150
Personality assessment, 1015
PFC, 305
PGE2, 483
Pharmacology, historical development of, 15
Pharmacotherapy, 20–21
Pharynx, distensibility of, 940
Phenothiazines, 17
Phenotypes, 157–159
  linkage, 177
Phlogiston Theory, 13
Phospholipids, 920
Phospholipid transfer protein (PLTP), 600
Physical activity, 341
  all-cause mortality, 989–993
  amount performed, 635–637
  body fatness, 644
  cancer, 994
  cardiovascular disease, 993
  characteristics, 640–641
  clinical practice, 999–1000
  comorbidities, 994–998
  coronary heart disease, 993–994
  energy cost, 637–640, 638–639
  energy expenditure, 631–646, 714–715
  gallbladder disease, 923
  health outcomes, 984–985

[Physical activity]
  increasing, 646
  mortality, 986
  nutrient partitioning, 755
  obesity, 983–1000
    recommendations, 998–1000
  obesity etiology, 643–646
  obesity-related health outcomes, 985–998
  postpartum weight development, 974
  pregnancy
    body weight development, 977–978
  public health, 998–999
  seasonal variations, 636–637
  secular trends, 644–645
  substrate oxidation, 640–643, 722
  weight gain, 645
Physical inactivity, 770–773
  metabolic syndrome, 800
Physiology, 12–13
Pickwickian syndrome, 17, 940–942
  classification, 941
  management, 942–945
Pima Indians
  beta3-adrenergic receptor gene, 885
  diabetes, 901, 905–906
  genomewide scans, 171–173
  non-insulin-dependent diabetes mellitus (type 2), 901, 977
Pioglitazone and hypertension in obesity, 889
Pituitary gland and basophilic adenomas, 17
Pituitary-thyroid axis, 663
PKA, 266, 494
Plasminogen, 499
PLIN gene, 209
PLTP, 600
PMM2 gene, 209
Polycystic ovary syndrome (PCOS), 660–661, 681, 967
Polysarcy, 22
POMC (*see* Proopiomelanocortin (POMC))
Ponderal index, 113
Portal hypothesis
  visceral adipose tissue (VAT), 589–590
Positive airway pressure, 944
Positive energy balance experiments
  genotype-environment interactions, 179–180
Postabsorptive satiety signals, 447
Postexercise energy expenditure, 637
Postpartum weight development and physical activity, 974
Postprandial hyperlipidemia
  visceral adipose tissue (VAT), 855–857
Postreceptor effects, 902–903
PPAR, primates, 288–291
PPAR alpha, receptor and agonists, 288–289
PPAR gamma, receptor and agonists, 289–290
PPAR-gamma (*see* Peroxisome proliferator-activated receptor gamma (PPAR-gamma))
Prader-Willi syndrome (PWS), 210, 235–236
Preadipose cells, 481
Preadolescents and adipose tissue, 485
Precision, 65–66
Predictive body composition methods
  accuracy and validity, 83–86
Pre-eclampsia, 820
Prefrontal cortex (PFC), 305
Pregnancy, 820
  age and weight, 968–969
  body mass index, 85
  body weight development
    physical activity, 977–978
  complications of weight gain, 976
  energy metabolism, 970
  hypertension, 820
  obesity after, 967–968
  physical activity and body weight development, 977–978
  smoking and weight, 976
  weight development, 968–975
    general clinical consequences, 979
  weight development after
    characteristics, 973
  weight gain
    socioeconomic and ethnic aspects, 978
Pregnant adolescents, weight development, 978–979
Prehistoric medicine, 2
Prescientific medicine, 3
Primary endocrine disease, 655–656
Primate models, common features of, 283
Primates
  aging-associated obesity, 281–292
  candidate genes, 284
  energy expenditure, 287–288
  gene-environment interactions, 284
  genetics, 284–287
  in vivo metabolic and endocrine effects, 283–284
  peroxisome proliferator-activated receptors (PPAR), 288–291
PRIME-MD, 1015
Primitive fat organ, 483
Procolipase, 392
Progesterone, 301
  body fat distribution, 675
Prolactin, 320–321, 498
Pro-opiomelanocortin (POMC), 214–215, 231, 260–261, 321–322
  gene, 209, 213
    metabolic syndrome, 801
  mutations, 231
  posttranslational processing, 214
Prophylactic cholecystectomy and gallstones, 927–928
Prostacyclin, 497
Prostaglandin E2 (PGE2), 483
Protein, 441–442, 920
  satiety, 439
  thermic effect, 622

Protein kinase A (PKA), 266, 494
Protein-lipid interactions, 516–518
Protein metabolism
endocrine control, 759–761
insulin, 759–760
nutrient partitioning, 756
Protein-protein interactions
peroxisome proliferator-activated receptor gamma (PPAR-gamma), 572–576
Protein tyrosine phosphate 1B (PTRB), 266
Psammomys obesus, 268
Pseudo-Cushing syndrome, 792
Pseudohypoparathyroidism, 233–234
Psychosocial outcomes, obesity in women, 118
PTRB, 266
Public health and physical activity, 998–999
Pulmonary embolism, 817
Pulmonary function
obesity, 935–947
physiological decrements, 935–937
Pulmonary function tests, abnormalities in, 936
Pulse recorder, 632
PVN, 305
PWS, 210, 235–236
PYY, 389

QTL, 169–170, 268
Quality of life, 149, 820–821
assessment, 1014–1017
body image, 1014
hunger, 1014
obesity, 1005–1007
psychological functioning, 1006–1008
risk factor models
obesity, 1010–1011
weight loss, 1011–1014
Quantitative trait loci (QTL), 169–170, 268
Quebec Family Study, 174
Quetelet Index, 22, 39, 85
Quinine, 5

Race
fat distribution, 137
mortality rate, 775
pediatric obesity, 121
visceral adipose tissue (VAT), 593
Radar tracking, 633
Rats
adipose tissue cellularity, 490
daily food intake in diabetes, 391
gastric emptying, 381
leptin receptor (LEPR)
alleles, 222–223
two-way crossed-intestines, 386
Recent weight loss
mortality rate, 777
Recumbency, 938
Reduced brain responsiveness
leptin, 469
Reference body composition methods, 82–83
Reference values, 66–70
Regional adipose tissue in skeletal muscle, 736
Relative weight, 39
Reliability, 66
Renin-angiotensin system
hypertension, 883–884
insulin, 883–884
visceral adipose tissue (VAT), 600
Repeatability, 66
Reported costs, 150–151
Reproducibility, 66
Reproductive health, 820
Resistance training in elderly, 142
Resistin and body fat distribution, 678–679
Respiratory compliance, 935–936
Respiratory compromise, categories of, 937–939
Respiratory control, 936–937
Resting energy expenditure
leptin, 621
Resting metabolic rate (RMR), 618–621
elderly, 138
genetics, 620
Retinoic acid, 498
Retinoids, 498
Rhesus monkeys
prevention, 291
RMR
elderly, 138
genetics, 620
Rodent models, 253–270
visceral adipose tissue (VAT), 592
Rodents
leptin and biological activity, 466–467
one-way crossed intestines, 375, 383–384
single gene mutations
naturally occurring, 202–214
single gene obesities, 228–233
Rosiglitazone and hypertension in obesity, 889
RQ/FQ, energy balance, 721

Sagittal trunk thickness, 63
Saline emptying, 381
San Antonio Family Heart Study, 173
Sand Rat (*Psammomys obesus*), 268
Santorio, Santorio, 12
Satiation, 433–434, 441–447
Satiety, 428–429, 433–434
signals, 433
postabsorptive satiety, 447
SBPEBP, 267, 741–742
SCID, 1015

Scientific medicine, 6–17
Screening overweight, 128
Seasonal variations in physical activity, 636–637
Second-messenger pathways, 496–499
SEE, 83
Segregation studies, 164–166
Sensory factors, 451–453
Sensory inputs, 338
Serotonin, 304, 332–333, 389
Serotonin (5HT), metabolic syndrome, 801–803
Serum, 466
Serum lipids and gallbladder disease, 924
Sex anthropometry
  Mexican-Americans, 69
  non-Hispanic blacks, 68
  non-Hispanic whites, 67
Sex hormone-binding globulin (SHBG), 660, 680–681, 682, 967
  diabetes mellitus in women, 795
Sex hormones
  males, 682–683
  women, 680–681
Sex steroids
  adipose tissue, 487
  secretion obesity, 659
  visceral adipose tissue (VAT), 597, 599
SHBG (*see* Sex hormone-binding globulin (SHBG))
Short-term satiety signals, 377
Sibutramine, 834, 943
  visceral adipose tissue (VAT), 605
Signaling proteins, 266
Signals
  gastrointestinal tracts, 377–378
  intestines, 384–387
  liver, 400–404
  lower gut, 397–400
  satiety, 433
  stomach, 380–384
Signal transducers and activators of transcriptions (STAT), 266
  peroxisome proliferator-activated receptor gamma (PPAR-gamma), 565–566
SIM1 gene, 210, 233
Simpson-Golabi-Behmel 1 syndrome, 236
Single gene mutations
  molecular genetics, 201–238
  naturally occurring in rodents, 202–214
Single gene obesities in rodents, 228–233
Skeletal muscle, 733–747
  biochemistry, 739–742
  capillary density, 738–739
  CT, 734–735
  distribution, 738
  fatty acid metabolism, 742–745
  fatty oxidation, 740–741
  hypertension, 882
[Skeletal muscle]
  insulin resistance, 881–882
  lipid content, 736–738
  lipid metabolism
    weight loss, 745
  lipid signaling, 741–742
  microscopic studies, 736–739
  molecular biology, 739–742
  MRI, 735
  noninvasive studies, 733–736
  quality, 734–736
  quantity, 733–734
  regional adipose tissue distribution adjacent to, 736
  size, 738
  substrate utilization, 742–745
  type, 738
Skeletal muscle metabolism
  work efficiency, 638–639
Skinfold, 59
  thickness, 84
    age-related changes, 136
  thickness ratios, 61
Sleep apnea, 819
Small-baby syndrome
  metabolic syndrome, 792–793
Small intestine, 436–437
  food delivery, 385
Smell, 377–378
Smoking, 768, 769, 779
  hypothalamic-pituitary-adrenal axis dysregulation, 792
  mortality, 986
  pregnancy and weight, 976
Socioeconomic characteristics of pediatric obesity, 121
Socioeconomic factors in obesity prevalence, 105–106
Sodium retention
  hypertension and obesity, 879–880
Software for magnetic resonance imaging, 53
Soluble leptin receptor, 218
Somatostatin, 391–392
Southeast Asia, 97–98
SOX3 gene, 210
Spermatogenesis, 682
Sphygmomanometer, 874
Spiny Mouse (*Acomys caharinus*), 268
Spontaneous obesity and dyslipidemia, 283
Spontaneous physical activity
  sympathetic nervous system, 699
Stadiometer, 39
STAI, 1015
Standard error of estimate (SEE), 83
STAT, 266
  peroxisome proliferator-activated receptor gamma (PPAR-gamma), 565–566
STAT5A gene, 210
State-Trait Anxiety Inventory (STAI), 1015

Stature
  age-related changes, 136
  measurement, 38–40
Sterol regulatory element binding proteins (SBPEBP), 267, 741–742
Stethoscope, 874
Stomach
  afferent receptors, 382
  distension, 380
  signals, 380–384
  size, 436–437
Stomach emptying, intestines, 381
Stone age, 22
Storage signals, 408–410
Stress
  cortisol, 799
  hypertension, 797–798
  lipid mobilization, 521
Stress eating, 799–800
Stretch receptors, 436–437
Stroke, 817, 833
Structural genes, 267
Structured Clinical Inventory for DSM-IV axis I Disorders (SCID), 1015
Subcutaneous fat
  African-Americans, 84
Subcutaneous skinfold ratio
  trunk-to-extremity (TER), 163
Substrate oxidation
  body composition, 722–723
  daily patterns, 724
  energy expenditure, 713–725
  factors determining, 713–718, 715–720
  glucose turnover, 716
  measurement, 713–715
  obesity predisposition, 724
  physical activity, 640–643
  regulation, 717–720
  starvation ketosis, 716–717
  sympathetic nervous systems, 699
  tissue types, 715–716
Sucrose, 451
Sudden death, 830–831
Sugar intake, 340
Surgery, 21
Sweeteners, 451
Sweetness, 451
Sympathetic nervous systems, 340–342, 693–701
  activity assessment, 696–697
  dietary stimulation, 700–701
  energy expenditure, 698–700
  ethnicity, 885
  factors affecting, 697
  food, thermic effect of, 623
  hypertension, 884–885
  nerve activity, 696
[Sympathetic nervous systems]
  neurotransmitter release, 696–697
  physiological role, 694–696
  stimuli response, 699–700
  structure, 693–694
  weight gain, 700
  weight loss, 700
Sympathomimetics, 834
Symptom Checklist-90, 1015
Syndecan, 261
Syndecan-3, 213
Systolic blood pressure
  euglycemic insulin infusion, 884–885
  mortality, 986

Taiwan, diet and gout, 961
Taste, 377–378
Taste reactions and dopamine, 335
TBX3 gene, 211
TEF [*see* Thermic effect of food (TEF)]
TER and subcutaneous skinfold ratio, 163
Terminology, 22
Testosterone, 659
  adipose tissue, 487
  elderly, 142
  glucose metabolism, 758–759
  lipid metabolism, 757
  nutrient partitioning, 762
  protein metabolism, 760
  visceral adipose tissue (VAT), 597
TGF-beta, 483, 499
Theophylline, 944
Thermic effect of feeding in elderly, 138
Thermic effect of food (TEF), 340–341, 621–624, 622, 631–632
  nutrient partitioning, 755
  sympathetic nervous systems, 699
Thermogenesis, 340–341
Thermogenic pathways, 265–266
Thiazide diuretics and hypertension in obesity, 889
Thiazolidinediones
  diabetes, 908
  hypertension
    obesity, 889
  visceral adipose tissue (VAT), 598
Thigh, computed tomography of, 52
THRB gene, 211
Three Factor Eating Questionnaire, 1016
Thrifty gene, 622
Thrifty phenotype hypothesis, 901
Thymidine kinase, 485
Thyroid extract, 15
Thyroid hormones
  adipose tissue, 485
  body fat distribution, 675–676
  resting metabolic rate (RMR), 620
Thyrotropin-releasing hormone (TRH), 301

Thyroxine, 301
Tibetan medicine, 4–5
Time and motion studies, 633
Timeline, 7–11
TNF alpha [*see* Tumor necrosis factor-alpha (TNF-alpha)]
TOPS family study, 174
Total body bioelectrical impedance, 84
Total body carbon, 41
Total body fat
  versus body mass index, 70
  component field measurement, 59–65
  multicomponent measurement, 49
Total body potassium, 40–41
Total body protein, 42
Total daily energy expenditure
  activity thermogenesis, 640
Total energy expenditures, 624–626
  absolute versus relative values, 624–625
Total fat
  fat tomography, 168
Transcription factors, 266–267, 496
  peroxisome proliferator-activated receptor gamma (PPAR-gamma), 569–571
Transforming growth factor-beta (TGF-beta), 483, 499
Transgenic models, 254–256, 260–267
TRH, 301
Triacylglycerol synthesis
  visceral adipose tissue (VAT), 595–596
Triglycerides, 35
  hydrolysis, 516–518
Tri-idodothyronine, 498
Troglitazone and hypertension in obesity, 889
Truncal fat in youth, 110
Trunk-to-extremity (TER)
  subcutaneous skinfold ratio, 163
Tubby (tub/tub) mouse, 259
Tubby mutation, 226–227
  Go-coupled receptors, 227
TUB gene, 211
Tub/tub mouse, 259
TULP1 gene, 211
Tumor necrosis factor-alpha (TNF-alpha), 322, 492, 499, 520
  body fat distribution, 677–678
  insulin resistance, 904–905
  visceral adipose tissue (VAT), 599
Twin pregnancies, weight gain, 979
Twin studies of osteoarthritis in obesity, 955
Two-way crossed-intestines in rats, 386
Type II steroid receptors, 308–309
Type I steroid receptors, 308–309
Tyrosine-kinase receptors, 519

UCP, 265, 539–551
  gene, 213
UCP1 [*see* Uncoupling protein1 (UCP1)]
UCP2, 550–551
UCP3, 550–551
Ukraine, diet and gout, 961
Ulnar mammary syndrome (UMS), 236–237
  human alleles, 237
Ultrasound, 59
UMS, 236–237
  human alleles, 237
Uncoupling protein1 (UCP1), 539–545
  energy expenditure, 539–540, 620–621
  feeding behavior, 543–544
  knockout mice, 542–544
  regulation, 544–545
  transgenic mice, 540–541, 542–544
Uncoupling protein2 (UCP2), 550–551
Uncoupling protein3 (UCP3), 550–551
Uncoupling proteins (UCP), 265, 539–551
  gene, 213
Undernutrition, 110–111
Underwater weighing, 45–46
United Kingdom, 99
University of Pennsylvania Family Study, 174
Upper-airway function
  obesity, 940
Upper body fat, 162–163
Upper-body obesity, 61
Uric acid and osteoarthritis, 958
Ursodeoxycholic acid (JDCA) and weight loss, 928

Vagotomy and energy balance, 396
Validity of predictive body composition methods, 83–86
Valproate, 17
Valvular heart disease, 943
Variability gene, 178
Vascular endothelial growth factor (VEGF), 483
VAT (*see* Visceral adipose tissue (VAT))
VEGF, 483
Venous thromboembolism, 817
Ventromedial hypothalamus (VMH), 305
Venus figurines, 3, 4
Vertical-banded gastroplasty, OSA, 943–944
Very-low-calorie diets (VLCD), OSA, 942
Vesalius, Andreas, 6
Viscera, defined, 37
Visceral adipose tissue (VAT), 589–605, 657
  anatomical description, 590–592
  anthropometry versus CT, 860–861
  atherogenic metabolic profile, 857
  composition, 593–594
  coronary heart disease, 860–864
  CT, 591, 853
  defined, 591–592
  diabetes, 903–904
  dyslipidemia, 852–857, 860–864
    cause-effect relationship, 857–860
  endocrine and secretory functions, 598–600
  gender, 592–593

[Visceral adipose tissue (VAT)]
genetic determinants, 598
gout, 960–961
historical perspective, 589
Japanese-Americans, 904
measurement, 590–592
metabolic characteristics, 594–596
metabolic disturbances, 852–855
metabolic syndrome, 605–606
MRI, 591
physiological determinants, 596–598
portal hypothesis, 589–590
postprandial hyperlipidemia, 855–857
race, 593
rodent models, 592
therapy, 600–604
triacylglycerol synthesis, 595–596
in vivo lipolysis, 595
Visceral fat
abdomen, 167–168
metabolic syndrome, 788
Visible Man, 38
VLCD, OSA, 942
VLDL, 283, 907
VMH, 305
Voluntary weight fluctuation
mortality in elderly, 140–141
Von Noorden's diet, 19

Waist circumference divided by hip circumference (WHR), 17
Waist girth and atherogenic dyslipidemias, 862–864
Waist/hip ratio (WHR), 61
Waist/thigh ratio (WTR), 61
WAT. *see* White adipose tissue (WAT)
Water in human body, 82
Weight
age-related changes, 135–136
high-fat diet, 875
infertility, 977
Weight change and adipose tissue cellularity, 490–491
Weight development
menopause, 970
pregnant adolescents, 978–979
Weight fluctuation and preexisting disease, 768–769
Weight gain
blood pressure, 875
physical activity, 645
pregnancy complications, 976
prevention, 646
sympathetic nervous systems, 700
twin pregnancies, 979
Weight goals in pediatric obesity, 120
Weight loss
asthma, 946
atherosclerosis, 833
bile acid supplementation, 928

[Weight loss]
blood pressure, 875–876
cardiac structure and function, 828–829
coronary heart disease, 833
diabetes, 908
energy expenditure, 625–626
exercise and visceral adipose tissue (VAT), 601–602
gallbladder disease, 925–926
hypertension in obesity, 888–889
hypothalamus, lesions in, 374
lipid metabolism
skeletal muscle, 745
mood, 1012–1014
mortality, 778–779, 780
OSA, 942–943
osteoarthritis, 959–960
overall quality of life, 1012
repeated cycles and gallstones, 926
surgically induced, OSA, 943
sympathetic nervous systems, 700
ursodeoxycholic acid (JDCA), 928
Weight maintenance
energy expenditure, 721–722
food intake, 721–722
substrate balances, 720–725
Weight-reducing medications, 723–724
Weight regain, prevention of, 645–646
Weight-stature indices, 39
Western Pacific Region, 102–103
White adipose tissue (WAT)
apoptosis, 481, 491–492
dedifferentiation, 491–492
development, 481–504
gain and loss of function, 504–505
genes, 501–503
Whole-body glucose uptake
euglycemic clamp studies, 880
WHR, 17, 61
Women
hyperandrogenicity, 794–796
obesity
Africa, 94
psychosocial outcomes, 118
sex hormones, 680–681
Work efficiency
age, 639
exercise training, 639
gender, 639–640
genetics, 639
skeletal muscle metabolism, 638–639
Work of breathing, 935–936
WTR, 61

Yellow Emperor, 5
Yellow Obese mouse, 14
Yellow (Av/a) obese mouse, 259–260

CONTENTS

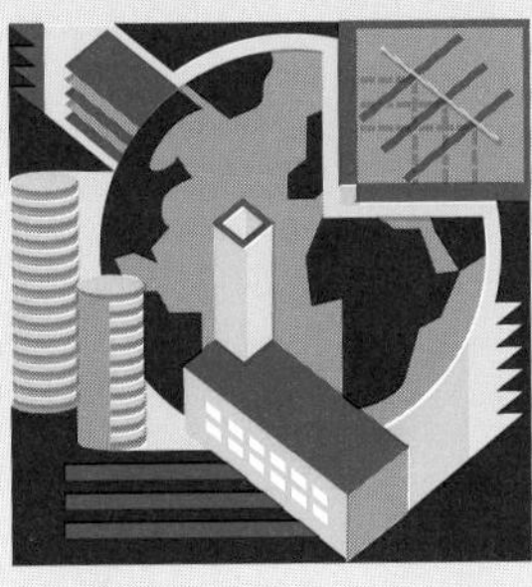

PART 1
INTRODUCTION TO ECONOMICS 1

CHAPTER 1 ECONOMICS, ECONOMIC ISSUES, AND ECONOMIC METHODS 2
Introduction 2
What Is Economics? 2
Economics in Relation to Other Fields 3
Why Study Economics? 3
Scarcity: Limited Resources, Insatiable Wants 4
International Perspective: The Nobel Prize for Economics 7
Society's Choices: The Production Possibilities Curve 8
Theories, Hypotheses, and Models 13
Basic Elements of the Economic Approach 17
Economic Profile: Milton Friedman (1912–) and Paul A. Samuelson (1915–) 18
Three Common Fallacies 20
International Perspective: The United States and the Rest of the World 22
Making Policy Choices 23
Summary 25
New Terms 25
Questions for Discussion 26
Suggestions for Further Reading 27
Appendix: Economic Relationships and Graphs 29

CHAPTER 2 MARKETS, GOVERNMENTS, AND NATIONS: THE ORGANIZATION OF ECONOMIC ACTIVITY 41
Introduction 41
Limited Resources: The Factors of Production 41
The Basic Economic Questions 43
The Circular Flow of Economic Activity 48
The Economic Role of Government 52

International Perspective: Privatization in Britain 54
The Role of the Foreign Sector 59
International Perspective: The Size of the Foreign Sector 60
Economic Profile: Adam Smith (1723–1790) 63
Summary 65
New Terms 65
Questions for Discussion 66
Suggestions for Further Reading 67

CHAPTER 3 SUPPLY AND DEMAND: THE BASICS OF ECONOMIC ANALYSIS 69
Introduction 69
Demand 69
Supply 76
Market Equilibrium 80
International Perspective: Adding Foreign Demand and Supply 81
A Theory of Price Formation 85
Evaluating the Market Process 88
International Perspective: Emerging Markets in Eastern Europe 89
Summary 93
New Terms 94
Questions for Discussion 94
Suggestions for Further Reading 95

PART 2
INTRODUCTION TO MACROECONOMICS 97

CHAPTER 4 MACROECONOMIC GOALS AND FLUCTUATIONS 98
Introduction 98
The Circular Flow Model Revisited 98
Macroeconomic Goals 103
Economic Insight: Constructing an Index 106
Fluctuations in Output, Employment, and Prices 113
International Perspective: The Great Depression in Europe and China 117
Summary 121
New Terms 122
Questions for Discussion 122
Suggestions for Further Reading 123

CHAPTER 5 MEASURING ECONOMIC PERFORMANCE AND NATIONAL INCOME ACCOUNTING 125
Introduction 125
Basic Accounting Concepts 125
Measuring Gross National Product 129
National Income 134
National Income Accounts and the Circular Flow 138
Prices and Price Indices 139
International Perspective: A Price Index for the Dollar 142
Problems in Using GNP Figures 144
Measuring Unemployment 146
International Perspective: Comparing GNP, Inflation, and Unemployment 147
Summary 149
New Terms 149
Questions for Discussion 150
Suggestions for Further Reading 151

CHAPTER 6 AGGREGATE DEMAND AND AGGREGATE SUPPLY 153
Introduction 153
A General Framework for Macroeconomics 153
International Perspective: Foreign Trade and Aggregate Demand 156
Aggregate Supply and Demand and Competing Macroeconomic Ideas 168
Economic Profile: Jean-Baptiste Say (1767–1832) 172
Summary 179
New Terms 179
Questions for Discussion 180
Suggestions for Further Reading 180
Appendix: A Glossary of Symbols 182

PART 3
DETERMINING OUTPUT AND EMPLOYMENT: KEYNESIAN MACROECONOMICS AND FISCAL POLICY 183

CHAPTER 7 CLASSICAL MACROECONOMICS AND THE KEYNESIAN RESPONSE 184
Introduction 184
The Classical View of Macroeconomics 185
International Perspective: Immigration, Employment, and Unemployment 190
The Business Cycle Theorists 199
The Keynesian Revolution 200
Economic Profile: John Maynard Keynes (1883–1946) 202
A Preview of Keynesian Theory and Policy 204
Summary 209
New Terms 209
Questions for Discussion 209
Suggestions for Further Reading 210

CHAPTER 8 THE KEYNESIAN MODEL 211
Introduction 211
The Keynesian Aggregate Expenditure Function 212
Adding Government and the Foreign Sector 223
Changes in Aggregate Expenditure and the Expenditure Multiplier 228
International Perspective: The Keynesian Model in a One-Product Economy 229
The Keynesian Model and Aggregate Demand 233
Summary 235
New Terms 236
Questions for Discussion 236
Suggestions for Further Reading 237
Appendix: The Algebra of the Keynesian Model 238

CHAPTER 9 FISCAL POLICY 241
Introduction 241
Why Fiscal Policy? 241
How Fiscal Policy Works 243
International Perspective: Fiscal Policy in the Open Economy 247
The Tools of Fiscal Policy: Government Spending and Taxes 250
Implementing Fiscal Policy: Automatic Stabilizers 251
Economic Insight: Who Makes Policy? 254
Discretionary Fiscal Policy 255
Fiscal Policy: Pros and Cons 260
International Perspective: Fiscal Policy in Thatcher's Britain 262
Fiscal Policy, Aggregate Demand, and the Price Level 266

Summary 268
New Terms 268
Questions for Discussion 268
Suggestions for Further Reading 269

Chapter 10 Budget Deficits and the National Debt 271
Introduction 271
Debt and Deficits 271
The Growth of the National Debt since 1980 274
International Perspective: The Other Deficit—The Balance of Trade 275
Should the Budget Be Balanced? 278
Do Deficits Matter? 283
Economic Insight: The Third Deficit 284
Summary 288
New Terms 289
Questions for Discussion 289
Suggestions for Further Reading 290

Part 4
Money, Financial Markets, and Monetary Policy 291

Chapter 11 Money: What It Is and Why People Hold It 292
Introduction 292
What Is Money? 293
International Perspective: Yap Island Money 297
Banks and Money 300
International Perspective: Money Around the World 301
Demand for Money 305
Economic Insight: The Underground Economy 306
Money Demand, Money Supply, and Aggregate Demand 309
Summary 313
New Terms 313
Questions for Discussion 313
Suggestions for Further Reading 314

Chapter 12 Money Creation and the Federal Reserve System 315
Introduction 315
What Banks Do 316
Central Banking in the United States 322
Structure and Functions of the Federal Reserve System 325
International Perspective: Central Banking in Europe and the United States 327
International Perspective:
The International Monetary Fund and the World Bank 335
Summary 340
New Terms 340
Questions for Discussion 341
Suggestions for Further Reading 341

Chapter 13 Financial Markets and Interest Rates 343
Introduction 343
Bank Deregulation in the 1980s 343
International Perspective: Financial Markets in Japan 347
The Loanable Funds Market and Interest Rates 350
Stocks, Stockholders, and the Stock Market 357